a LANGE medical book

CURRENT
Pediatric Diagnosis & Treatment

18th Edition

Edited by

William W. Hay, Jr., MD
Professor, Department of Pediatrics
Section of Neonatology and the Division
of Perinatal Medicine
University of Colorado School of Medicine and
The Children's Hospital, Denver

Myron J. Levin, MD
Professor, Departments of Pediatrics and Medicine
Section of Pediatric Infectious Diseases
University of Colorado School of Medicine and
The Children's Hospital, Denver

Judith M. Sondheimer, MD
Professor, Department of Pediatrics,
Section of Pediatric Gastroenterology, Hepatology,
and Nutrition
University of Colorado School of Medicine and
The Children's Hospital, Denver

Robin R. Deterding, MD
Associate Professor, Department of Pediatrics
Section of Pediatric Pulmonary Medicine
University of Colorado School of Medicine and
The Children's Hospital, Denver

and Associate Authors
The Department of Pediatrics at the University of
Colorado School of Medicine is affiliated with
The Children's Hospital of Denver, Colorado.

Lange Medical Books/McGraw-Hill
Medical Publishing Division

New York   Chicago   San Francisco   Lisbon   London   Madrid   Mexico City
Milan   New Delhi   San Juan   Seoul   Singapore   Sydney   Toronto

Current Pediatric Diagnosis & Treatment, Eighteenth Edition

2 3 4 5 6 7 8 9 0 DOC/DOC 0 9 8 7

ISBN-10: 0-07-146300-3; ISBN-13: 978-0-07-146300-3
ISSN: 0093-8556

Notice

This book was set in Adobe Garamond by Silverchair Science + Communications, Inc.
The editors were Anne M. Sydor, Harriet Lebowitz, and Patrick Carr.
The production supervisor was Sherri Souffrance.
The index was prepared by Pam Edwards.
The cover designer was Mary McKeon.
RR Donnelley was printer and binder.

This book is printed on acid-free paper.

INTERNATIONAL EDITION ISBN-10: 0-07-110444-5; ISBN-13: 978-0-07-110444-9

Contents

Authors

Frank J. Accurso, MD
Professor, Department of Pediatrics, Head, Section
of Pediatric Pulmonary Medicine, University of
Colorado School of Medicine; The Children's
Hospital, Denver, Colorado
accurso.frank@tchden.org
Respiratory Tract & Mediastinum
Chemistry & Hematology Reference Intervals

Daniel R. Ambruso, MD
Professor, Department of Pediatrics, Section of
Pediatric Hematology/Oncology/Bone Marrow
Transplant, Associate Medical Director, Belle
Bonfils Blood Center, University of Colorado
School of Medicine; The Children's Hospital,
Denver, Colorado
daniel.ambruso@uchsc.edu
Hematologic Disorders

Marsha S. Anderson, MD
Assistant Professor, Department of Pediatrics,
Section of Pediatric Infectious Diseases,
University of Colorado School of Medicine;
The Children's Hospital, Denver, Colorado
anderson.marsha@tchden.org
Infections: Bacterial & Spirochetal

Vivek Balasubramaniam, MD
Assistant Professor, Department of Pediatrics,
Section of Pediatric Pulmonary Medicine,
University of Colorado School of Medicine; The
Children's Hospital, Denver, Colorado
Vivek.Balasubramaniam@uchsc.edu
Respiratory Tract & Mediastinum

F. Keith Battan, MD, FAAP
Attending Pediatrician, Colorado Permanente
Medical Group, Denver, Colorado
keith@battan.com
Emergencies & Injuries

Timothy A. Benke, MD, PhD
Assistant Professor, Departments of Pediatrics,
Neurology, and Pharmacology, Director, Division
of Child Neurology Residency Training Program,
University of Colorado School of Medicine; The
Children's Hospital, Denver, Colorado
tim.benke@uchsc.edu
Neurologic & Muscular Disorders

Timothy J. Bernard, MD
Departments of Pediatrics and Neurology,
University of Colorado School of Medicine;
The Children's Hospital, Denver, Colorado
tim.bernard@hotmail.com
Neurologic & Muscular Disorders

Mark Boguniewicz, MD
Professor, Divisions of Pediatic Allergy-Immunology,
Department of Pediatrics, National Jewish
Medical and Research Center; University of
Colorado School of Medicine, Denver, Colorado
boguniewiczm@njc.org
Allergic Disorders

Robert M. Brayden, MD
Associate Professor, Department of Pediatrics, Section
of General Academic Pediatrics, University of
Colorado School of Medicine; The Children's
Hospital, Denver, Colorado
brayden.robert@tchden.org
Ambulatory & Community Pediatrics

Jeffrey M. Brown, MD, MPH
Professor, Department of Pediatrics, University of
Colorado School of Medicine; Director, General
Pediatrics Division, Denver Health Medical
Center, Denver, Colorado
jeff.brown@dhha.org
Ambulatory & Community Pediatrics

Joanna M. Burch, MD
Assistant Professor, Departments of Dermatology
and Pediatrics, University of Colorado School of
Medicine, Denver, Colorado
joanna.burch@uchsc.edu
Skin

Todd C. Carpenter, MD
Associate Professor, Department of Pediatrics,
Section of Pediatric Critical Care Medicine,
University of Colorado School of Medicine;
The Children's Hospital, Denver, Colorado
todd.carpenter@uchsc.edu
Critical Care

Keith Cavanaugh, MD
Assistant Professor, Department of Pediatrics,
Section of Pediatric Pulmonary Medicine,

University of Colorado School of Medicine; The
Children's Hospital, Denver, Colorado
cavanaugh.keith@tchden.org
Respiratory Tract & Mediastinum

H. Peter Chase, MD
Professor, Department of Pediatrics, Clinical
Director Emeritus, Barbara Davis Center for
Childhood Diabetes, University of Colorado
School of Medicine, Denver, Colorado
peter.chase@uchsc.edu
Diabetes Mellitus

Matthew F. Daley, MD
Assistant Professor, Department of Pediatrics,
Section of General Academic Pediatrics,
University of Colorado School of Medicine;
The Children's Hospital, Denver, Colorado
daley.matthew@tchden.org
*Ambulatory & Community Pediatrics
Immunization*

Richard C. Dart, MD, PhD
Professor, Department of Surgery, University of
Colorado School of Medicine, Director, Rocky
Mountain Poison and Drug Center, Denver,
Colorado
rdart@rmpdc.org
Poisoning

Bert Dech, MD
Clinical Instructor, Department of Psychiatry, The
Children's Hospital, Denver, Colorado
dech.bert@tchden.org
*Child & Adolescent Psychiatric Disorders &
Psychosocial Aspects of Pediatrics*

Robin R. Deterding, MD
Associate Professor, Department of Pediatrics,
Section of Pediatric Pulmonary Medicine,
University of Colorado School of Medicine;
The Children's Hospital, Denver, Colorado
deterding.robin@tchden.org
Respiratory Tract & Mediastinum

Emily L. Dobyns, MD
Associate Professor, Department of Pediatrics,
Section of Pediatric Critical Care Medicine,
University of Colorado School of Medicine;
The Children's Hospital, Denver, Colorado
dobyns.emily@tchden.org
Critical Care

Arlene Drack, MD
Associate Professor, Departments of Ophthalmology
and Pediatrics, University of Colorado School of
Medicine; Rocky Mountain Lions Eye Institute;
The Children's Hospital, Aurora, Colorado
arlene.drack@uchsc.edu
Eye

Robert E. Eilert, MD
Clinical Professor, Department of Orthopedic
Surgery, University of Colorado School of
Medicine; Chairman, Department of Orthopedic
Surgery, The Children's Hospital, Denver,
Colorado
eilert.robert@tchden.org
Orthopaedics

George S. Eisenbarth, MD, PhD
Professor, Department of Pediatrics, Executive
Director, Barbara Davis Center for Childhood
Diabetes, University of Colorado School of
Medicine, Denver, Colorado
george.eisenbarth@uchsc.edu
Diabetes Mellitus

Ellen R. Elias, MD
Associate Professor, Departments of Pediatrics and
Genetics, Section of Clinical Genetics and
Metabolism, University of Colorado School of
Medicine; Director, Special Care Clinic, The
Children's Hospital, Denver, Colorado
elias.ellen@tchden.org
Genetics & Dysmorphology

Glenn Faries, MD
Assistant Professor, Department of Pediatrics, Co-
Director, Core Clerkship Block in Urgent Care/
Emergency Medicine, University of Colorado
School of Medicine; Medical Director, Continuing
Medical Education, The Children's Hospital,
Denver, Colorado
faries.glenn@tchden.org
Emergencies & Injuries

Margaret A. Ferguson, MD
Clinical Assistant Professor, Department of Pediatrics,
Section of Pediatric Critical Care Medicine,
University of Colorado School of Medicine; The
Children's Hospital, Denver, Colorado
ferguson.margaret@tchden.org
Critical Care

Douglas M. Ford, MD
Professor, Department of Pediatrics, Section of
Pediatric Renal Medicine, University of Colorado
School of Medicine; The Children's Hospital,
Denver, Colorado
ford.douglas@tchden.org
Fluid, Electrolyte, & Acid–Base Disorders & Therapy

Nicholas K. Foreman, MD
Professor, Department of Pediatrics, Section of
Hematology/Oncology/Bone Marrow Transplant,
University of Colorado School of Medicine; The
Children's Hospital, Denver, Colorado
foreman.nicholas@tchden.org
Neoplastic Disease

Norman R. Friedman, MD
Professor Department of Otolaryngology,
University of Colorado School of Medicine; The
Children's Hospital, Denver, Colorado
friedman.norman@tchden.org
Ear, Nose, & Throat

Roger H. Giller, MD
Professor, Department of Pediatrics, Section of
Pediatric Hematology/Oncology/Bone Marrow
Transplant, Director, Pediatric BMT program,
University of Colorado School of Medicine;
The Children's Hospital, Denver, Colorado
giller.roger@tchden.org
Neoplastic Disease

Neil A. Goldenberg, MD
Assistant Professor, Departments of Pediatrics and
Medicine, Center for Cancer and Blood
Disorders; Associate Director, Mountain States
Regional Hemophilia and Thrombosis Center,
Aurora, Colorado; University of Colorado at
Denver and Health Sciences Center; The
Children's Hospital, Denver, Colorado
neil.goldenberg@uchsc.edu
Hematologic Disorders

Edward Goldson, MD
Professor, Department of Pediatrics, Section of
Developmental and Behavioral Pediatrics,
University of Colorado School of Medicine;
The Children's Hospital, Denver, Colorado
goldson.edward@tchden.org
Child Development & Behavior

Doug K. Graham, MD, PhD
Assistant Professor, Department of Pediatrics,
Section of Pediatric Hematology/Oncology/Bone
Marrow Transplant, University of Colorado
School of Medicine; The Children's Hospital,
Denver, Colorado
doug.graham@uchsc.edu
Neoplastic Disease

Eva N. Grayck, MD
Associate Professor, Department of Pediatrics,
Section of Pediatric Critical Care Medicine,
University of Colorado School of Medicine;
The Children's Hospital, Denver, Colorado
Eva.Grayck@uchsc.edu
Critical Care

Brian S. Greffe, MD
Associate Professor, Department of Pediatrics,
Section of Pediatric Hematology/Oncology/Bone
Marrow Transplant, University of Colorado
School of Medicine; The Children's Hospital,
Denver, Colorado
greffe.brian@tchden.org
Neoplastic Disease

Jennifer Hagman, MD
Associate Professor, Department of Psychiatry,
University of Colorado School of Medicine; Co-
Director, Eating Disorders Treatment Program;
The Children's Hospital, Denver, Colorado
hagman.jennifer@tchden.org
*Child & Adolescent Psychiatric Disorders &
Psychosocial Aspects of Pediatrics*

Taru Hays, MD
Professor, Department of Pediatrics, Section of
Pediatric Hematology/Oncology/Bone Marrow
Transplant, University of Colorado School of
Medicine; The Children's Hospital, Denver,
Colorado
hays.taru@tchden.org
Hematologic Disorders

Francis Hoe, MD
Instructor, Department of Pediatrics, Section of
Pediatric Endocrinology, University of Colorado
School of Medicine; The Children's Hospital,
Denver, Colorado
francis.hoe@uchsc.edu
Endocrine Disorders

J. Roger Hollister, MD
Professor, Departments of Pediatrics and Medicine, Head, Section of Pediatric Rheumatology, University of Colorado School of Medicine; The Children's Hospital; Senior Staff Physician, National Jewish Medical and Research Center, Denver, Colorado
Hollister.Roger@tchden.org
Rheumatic Diseases

Candice E. Johnson, MD, PhD
Professor, Department of Pediatrics, Section of General Academic Pediatrics, University of Colorado School of Medicine; The Children's Hospital, Denver, Colorado
johnson.candice@tchden.org
Ear, Nose, & Throat

Richard B. Johnston, Jr., MD
Professor of Pediatrics, Section of Immunology, Associate Dean for Research Development, Executive Vice President for Academic Affairs, National Jewish Medical and Research Center; University of Colorado School of Medicine, Denver, Colorado
richard.johnston@uchsc.edu
Immunodeficiency

Carol S. Kamin, MS, EdD
Associate Professor, Department of Pediatrics, Director, Medical Education Research & Development, Director, Project L.I.V.E (Learning through Interactive Video Education), University of Colorado School of Medicine; The Children's Hospital, Denver, Colorado
kamin.carol@tchden.org
Information Technology in Pediatrics

David W. Kaplan, MD, MPH
Professor, Department of Pediatrics, Head, Section of Adolescent Medicine, University of Colorado School of Medicine; The Children's Hospital, Denver, Colorado
kaplan.david@tchden.org
Adolescence

Michael S. Kappy, MD, PhD
Professor, Department of Pediatrics, Head, Section of Pediatric Endocrinology, University of Colorado School of Medicine; The Children's Hospital, Denver, Colorado
kappy.michael@tchden.org
Endocrine Disorders

Paritosh Kaul, MD
Assistant Professor, Department of Pediatrics, Director, Denver School Based Health Centers, Section of Adolescent Medicine, University of Colorado School of Medicine; The Children's Hospital; Denver Health Medical Center, Denver, Colorado
paritosh.kaul@dhha.org
Substance Abuse

Amy K. Keating, MD
Fellow, Department of Pediatrics, Section of Pediatric Hematology/Oncology/Bone Marrow Transplant, Center for Cancer and Blood Disorders, University of Colorado School of Medicine; The Children's Hospital, Denver, Colorado
keating.amy@tchden.org
Neoplastic Disease

Peggy E. Kelley, MD
Associate Professor, Department of Otolaryngology, University of Colorado School of Medicine; The Children's Hospital, Denver, Colorado
kelley.peggy@tchden.org
Ear, Nose, & Throat

Gwendolyn S. Kerby, MD
Assistant Professor, Department of Pediatrics, Section of Pediatric Pulmonary Medicine, University of Colorado School of Medicine; The Children's Hospital, Denver, Colorado
kerby.gwendolyn@tchden.org
Respiratory Tract & Mediastinum

Nancy F. Krebs, MD, MS
Professor, Department of Pediatrics, Head, Section of Nutrition, University of Colorado School of Medicine; The Children's Hospital, Denver, Colorado
nancy.krebs@uchsc.edu
Normal Childhood Nutrition & Its Disorders

Richard D. Krugman, MD
Professor, Department of Pediatrics, Dean, University of Colorado School of Medicine, Denver, Colorado
richard.krugman@uchsc.edu
Child Abuse & Neglect

Myron J. Levin, MD
Professor, Departments of Pediatrics and
Medicine, Section of Pediatric Infectious
Diseases, University of Colorado School of
Medicine; The Children's Hospital, Denver,
Colorado
myron.levin@uchsc.edu
Infections: Viral & Rickettsial
Infections: Parasitic & Mycotic
Sexually Tansmitted Infections

Andrew H. Liu, MD
Associate Professor, Department of Pediatrics,
Section of Allergy & Clinical Immunology,
National Jewish Medical & Research Center;
University of Colorado School of Medicine,
Denver Colorado
liua@njc.org
Immunodeficiency

Kathryn A. Love-Osborne, MD
Assistant Professor, Department of Pediatrics,
Section of Adolescent Medicine, University of
Colorado School of Medicine; The Children's
Hospital, Denver, Colorado
kathryn.love-osborne@dhha.org
Adolescence

Gary M. Lum, MD
Professor, Departments of Pediatrics and
Medicine, Head, Section of Pediatric Renal
Medicine, University of Colorado School of
Medicine; The Children's Hospital, Denver,
Colorado
lum.gary@tchden.org
Kidney & Urinary Tract

Kelly Maloney, MD
Associate Professor, Department of Pediatrics,
Section of Pediatric Hematology/Oncology/Bone
Marrow Transplant, University of Colorado
School of Medicine; The Children's Hospital,
Denver, Colorado
maloney.kelly@tchden.org
Neoplastic Disease

David K. Manchester, MD
Professor, Department of Pediatrics, Section of
Clinical Genetics and Metabolism, University of
Colorado School of Medicine; Co-Director,
Division of Genetic Services, The Children's
Hospital, Denver, Colorado
manchester.david@tchden.org
Genetics & Dysmorphology

Dennis J. Matthews, MD
Professor and Chairman, Department of
Rehabilitation Medicine, University of
Colorado School of Medicine; Chairman
and Medical Director, The Children's
Hospital Rehabilitation Center, Denver, Colorado
matthews.dennis@tchden.org
Rehabilitation & Sports Medicine

Elizabeth J. McFarland, MD
Associate Professor, Department of Pediatrics,
Section of Pediatric Infectious Diseases,
University of Colorado School of Medicine;
The Children's Hospital, Denver, Colorado
betsy.mcfarland@uchsc.edu
Human Immunodeficiency Virus Infection

Shelley D. Miyamoto, MD
Instructor, Department of Pediatrics, Section of
Pediatric Cardiology, University of Colorado
School of Medicine; The Children's Hospital,
Denver, Colorado
miyamoto.shelley@tchden.org
Cardiovascular Diseases

Paul G. Moe, MD
Professor, Departments of Pediatrics and
Neurology, Division of Child Neurology,
University of Colorado School of Medicine;
The Children's Hospital, Denver, Colorado
moe.paul@tchden.org
Neurologic & Muscular Disorders

Joseph G. Morelli, MD
Professor, Departments of Dermatology and
Pediatrics, University of Colorado School of
Medicine, Denver, Colorado
joseph.morelli@uchsc.edu
Skin

Peter M. Mourani, MD
Assistant Professor, Department of Pediatrics,
Section of Pediatric Critical Care Medicine,
University of Colorado School of Medicine;
The Children's Hospital, Denver, Colorado
peter.mourani@uchsc.edu
Critical Care

William A. Mueller, DMD
Clinical Associate Professor, University of Colorado
  School of Dentistry; The Children's Hospital,
  Denver, Colorado
williammueller@earthlink.net
Oral Medicine & Dentistry

Kristen Nadeau, MD
Assistant Professor, Department of Pediatrics
  Section of Pediatric Endocrinology, University
  of Colorado School of Medicine; The Children's
  Hospital, Denver, Colorado
kristen.nadeau@uchsc.edu
Endocrine Disorders

Michael R. Narkewicz, MD
Professor, Department of Pediatrics, Section of
  Pediatric Gastroenterology, Hepatology and
  Nutrition, The Pediatric Liver Center, University
  of Colorado School of Medicine; The Children's
  Hospital, Denver, Colorado
narkewicz.michael@tchden.org
Liver & Pancreas

Ann-Christine Nyquist, MD, MSPH
Associate Professor, Department of Pediatrics,
  Section of Pediatric Infectious Diseases,
  University of Colorado School of
  Medicine; The Children's Hospital,
  Denver, Colorado
nyquist.ann-christine@tchden.org
Immunization
Sexually Transmitted Infections

John W. Ogle, MD
Professor, Department of Pediatrics, Section of
  Pediatric Infectious Diseases, University of
  Colorado School of Medicine; The Children's
  Hospital; Director, Department of Pediatrics,
  Denver Health Medical Center, Denver
  Colorado
jogle@dhha.org
Antimicrobial Therapy
Infections: Bacterial & Spirochetal

Christopher C. Porter, MD
Fellow, Department of Pediatrics, Section
  of Hematology/Oncology/Bone Marrow
  Transplant, University of Colorado

School of Medicine; The Children's
  Hospital, Denver, Colorado
porter.christopher@tchden.org
Neoplastic Disease

Laura E. Primak, RD, CNSD, CSP
Professional Research Assistant, Nutritionist,
  Section of Nutrition, Department of Pediatrics,
  University of Colorado School of Medicine; The
  Children's Hospital, Denver, Colorado
laura.primak@uchsc.edu
Normal Childhood Nutrition & Its Disorders

Ralph R. Quinones, MD
Associate Professor, Department of Pediatrics,
  Section of Pediatric Hematology/Oncology/Bone
  Marrow Transplant, Director, Pediatric Blood
  and Marrow Processing Laboratory, University of
  Colorado School of Medicine; The Children's
  Hospital, Denver, Colorado
quinones.ralph@tchden.org
Neoplastic Disease

Ann Reynolds, MD
Assistant Professor, Department of Pediatrics,
  Child Development Unit, University of
  Colorado School of Medicine; The Children's
  Hospital, Denver, Colorado
reynolds.ann@tchden.org
Child Development & Behavior

Adam Rosenberg, MD
Professor, Department of Pediatrics, Section of
  Neonatology, Medical Director of the Newborn
  Service, University of Colorado Hospital; Director,
  Pediatric Residency Training Program, University of
  Colorado School of Medicine; The Children's
  Hospital, Denver, Colorado
adam.rosenberg@uchsc.edu
The Newborn Infant

Barry H. Rumack, MD
Clinical Professor, Department of Pediatrics,
  University of Colorado School of Medicine;
  Director Emeritus, Rocky Mountain Poison and
  Drug Center, Denver Health Authority, Denver,
  Colorado
barry@rumack.com
Poisoning

Scott D. Sagel, MD
Assistant Professor, Department of
Pediatrics, Section of Pediatric
Pulmonary Medicine, University of
Colorado School of Medicine; The
Children's Hospital, Denver, Colorado
sagel.scott@tchden.org
Respiratory Tract & Mediastinum

Rebecca Sands, MD
Assistant Professor, Department of Ophthalmology,
University of Colorado School of Medicine;
Rocky Mountain Lions Eye Institute, Denver,
Colorado
rebecca.sands@uchsc.edu
Eye

Kelly D. Sawczyn, MD
Department of Pediatrics, Section of Pediatric
Hematology/Oncology/Bone Marrow Transplant,
University of Colorado School of Medicine; The
Children's Hospital, Denver, Colorado
sawczyn.kelly@tchden.org
Neoplastic Disease

Eric J. Sigel, MD
Assistant Professor, Department of Pediatrics,
Section of Adolescent Medicine, University of
Colorado School of Medicine; The Children's
Hospital, Denver, Colorado
sigel.eric@tchden.org
Eating Disorders
Sexually Transmitted Infections

Eric A. F. Simoes, MD, DCH
Professor, Department of Pediatrics, Section of
Pediatric Infectious Diseases, University of
Colorado School of Medicine; The Children's
Hospital, Denver, Colorado
eric.simoes@uchsc.edu
Immunization

Georgette Siparsky, PhD
Supervisor, Clinical Chemistry Laboratory,
Department of Pathology, The Children's
Hospital, Denver, Colorado
siparsky.georgette@tchden.org
Chemistry and Hematology Reference Intervals

Andrew P. Sirotnak, MD
Associate Professor, Department of
Pediatrics, University of Colorado
School of Medicine; Director, Kempe
Child Protection Team, The Children's
Hospital and Kempe Children's Center for the
Prevention and Treatment of Child Abuse,
Denver, Colorado
sirotnak.andrew@tchden.org
Child Abuse & Neglect

Ronald J. Sokol, MD
Professor and Vice-Chair Head, Department of
Pediatrics, Section of Pediatric
Gastroenterology, Hepatology and Nutrition,
The Pediatric Liver Center; Director, Pediatric
Clinical Translational Research Center,
University of Colorado School of Medicine;
The Children's Hospital, Denver, Colorado
sokol.ronald@tchden.org
Liver & Pancreas

Henry M. Sondheimer, MD
Professor, Department of Pediatrics,
Section of Pediatric Cardiology, Associate
Dean for Admissions, University of Colorado
School of Medicine; The Children's Hospital,
Denver, Colorado
sondheimer.henry@tchden.org
Cardiovascular Diseases

Judith M. Sondheimer, MD
Professor, Department of Pediatrics, Section of
Pediatric Gastroenterology, Hepatology and
Nutrition, University of Colorado School of
Medicine; The Children's Hospital, Denver,
Colorado
sondheimer.judith@tchden.org
Gastrointestinal Tract

Kurt R. Stenmark, MD
Professor, Department of Pediatrics,
Head, Section of Pediatric Critical Care
Medicine, Director, Developmental Lung
Biology Lab, University of Colorado School of
Medicine; The Children's Hospital, Denver,
Colorado
kurt.stenmark@uchsc.edu
Critical Care

Catherine Stevens-Simon, MD
Professor, Department of Pediatrics, Section of
 Adolescent Medicine, University of Colorado
 School of Medicine; The Children's Hospital,
 Denver, Colorado
stevens-simon.catherine@tchden.org
Substance Abuse

Lora J. Stewart, MD
Fellow, Department of Pediatrics, Section of
 Allergy & Clinical Immunology, National
 Jewish Medical & Research Center; University
 of Colorado School of Medicine, Denver,
 Colorado
lstewart@premierallergy.com
Immunodeficiency

Elizabeth H. Thilo, MD
Associate Professor, Department of Pediatrics,
 Section of Neonatology, University of Colorado
 School of Medicine; The Children's Hospital,
 Denver, Colorado
thilo.elizabeth@tchden.org
The Newborn Infant

Janet A. Thomas, MD
Assistant Professor, Department of Pediatrics, Section
 of Clinical Genetics and Metabolism, University of
 Colorado School of Medicine; The Children's
 Hospital, Denver, Colorado
thomas.janet@tchden.org
Inborn Errors of Metabolism

Sharon H. Travers, MD
Associate Professor, Department of Pediatrics,
 Section of Pediatric Endocrinology, University of
 Colorado School of Medicine; The Children's
 Hospital, Denver, Colorado
travers.sharon@tchden.org
Endocrine Disorders

Chun-Hui (Anne) Tsai, MD
Associate Professor, Department of Pediatrics,
 Section of Clinical Genetics and Metabolism,
 University of Colorado School of Medicine;
 The Children's Hospital, Denver, Colorado
tsai.chun-hui@tchden.org
Genetics & Dysmorphology

Johan L. K. Van Hove, MD, PhD, MBA
Associate Professor, Department of Pediatrics,
 Section of Clinical Genetics and Metabolism,
 University of Colorado School of Medicine; The
 Children's Hospital, Denver, Colorado
vanhove.johan@tchden.org
Inborn Errors of Metabolism

Adriana Weinberg, MD
Professor, Departments of Pediatrics and Medicine,
 Director of Clinical Virology Laboratory, Section
 of Pediatric Infectious Diseases, University of
 Colorado School of Medicine; The Children's
 Hospital, Denver, Colorado
adriana.weinberg@uchsc.edu
Infections: Viral & Rickettsial
Infections: Parasitic & Mycotic

Pamela E. Wilson, MD
Assistant Professor, Department of Rehabilitation
 Medicine, University of Colorado School of
 Medicine; The Children's Hospital
 Rehabilitation Center, Denver, Colorado
wilson.pamela@tchden.org
Rehabilitation & Sports Medicine

Angela T. Yetman, MD
Associate Professor, Department of Pediatrics,
 Section of Pediatric Cardiology, University of
 Colorado School of Medicine; The Children's
 Hospital, Denver, Colorado
yetman.angela@tchden.org
Cardiovascular Diseases

Patricia J. Yoon, MD
Assistant Professor, Department of Otolaryngology,
 University of Colorado School of Medicine;
 The Children's Hospital, Denver, Colorado
yoon.patricia@tchden.org
Ear, Nose, & Throat

Philip S. Zeitler, MD, PhD
Associate Professor, Department of Pediatrics,
 Section of Pediatric Endocrinology, University of
 Colorado School of Medicine; The Children's
 Hospital, Denver, Colorado
phil.zeitler@uchsc.edu
Endocrine Disorders

Preface

The 18th edition of *Current Pediatric Diagnosis & Treatment* (CPDT) features practical, up-to-date, well-referenced information on the care of children from birth through infancy and adolescence. CPDT emphasizes the clinical aspects of pediatric care while also covering the important underlying principles. Its goal is to provide a guide to diagnosis, understanding, and treatment of the medical problems of all pediatric patients in an easy-to-use and readable format.

INTENDED AUDIENCE

Like all Lange medical books, CPDT provides a concise yet comprehensive source of current information. Students will find CPDT an authoritative introduction to pediatrics and an excellent source for reference and review. CPDT provides excellent coverage of The Council on Medical Student Education in Pediatrics (COMSEP) curriculum used around the country in pediatric clerkships. Residents in pediatrics (and other specialties) will appreciate the detailed descriptions of diseases as well as diagnostic and therapeutic procedures. Pediatricians, family practitioners, nurses and nurse practitioners, and other health-care providers who work with infants and children also will find CPDT a useful reference on management aspects of pediatric medicine.

COVERAGE

Forty-three chapters cover a wide range of topics, including neonatal medicine, child development and behavior, emergency and critical care medicine, and diagnosis and treatment of specific disorders according to major problems and organ systems. A wealth of tables and figures provides quick access to important information, such as acute and critical care procedures in the delivery room, the office, the emergency room, and the critical care unit; anti-infective agents; drug dosages; immunization schedules; differential diagnosis; and developmental screening tests. The final chapter is a handy guide to normal laboratory values.

NEW TO THIS EDITION

The 18th edition of CPDT has been revised comprehensively by the editors and contributing authors. New references as well as up-to-date and useful Web sites have been added, permitting the reader to consult original material and to go beyond the confines of the textbook. As editors and practicing pediatricians, we have tried to ensure that each chapter reflects the needs and realities of day-to-day practice.

Chapter Revisions: Eight chapters have been extensively revised, with new authors added in several cases, reflecting substantially updated material in each of their areas of pediatric medicine. The information in the previous edition's chapter on drug therapy (which has been deleted) is now incorporated into chapters throughout the book, as appropriate for specific drugs. Especially important are updates to the chapters on infectious diseases, including information on methicillin-resistant staphylococcus and human metapneumovirus, the Respiratory Tract & Mediastium chapter with major revision on bronchiectasis and children's interstitial lung disease, and the chapter on normal hematological and biochemical values. Chapters with major revisions include:

6. Child & Adolescent Psychiatric Disorders & Psychosocial Aspects of Pediatrics
8. Ambulatory & Community Pediatrics
15. Eye
18. Respiratory Tract & Mediastinum
28. Neoplastic Disease
29. Immunodeficiency
37. Human Immunodeficiency Virus Infection
42. Information Technology in Pediatrics
43. Normal Chemistry & Hematology Reference Intervals

All other chapters are substantially revised and references have been updated. Nineteen new authors have contributed to these revisions.

Acknowledgment: The Editors would like to thank Shara Knight for her expert assistance in managing the flow of manuscripts and materials among the chapter authors, editors, and publishers. Her attention to detail was enormously helpful.

William W. Hay, Jr., MD
Myron J. Levin, MD
Judith M. Sondheimer, MD
Robin R. Deterding, MD

Denver, Colorado
August, 2006

The Newborn Infant

Elizabeth H. Thilo, MD, & Adam A. Rosenberg, MD

The first 28 days of life are usually considered the newborn period. In practice, however, neonatal care may extend to many months for sick or very immature infants. Levels of newborn care are classified as level 1 (basic neonatal care including care of well newborns, neonatal resuscitation, and stabilization of ill newborns prior to transport), level 2 (specialty neonatal care including care of prematures > 1500 g) and level 3 (subspecialty care of increasing complexity ranging from 3A to 3D based on the size and gestational age of infants [1000–1500 g or < 1000 g and 28 weeks], availability of general and cardiac surgery, and extracorporeal membrane oxygenation). Level 3 nurseries are often part of a perinatal center offering critical care to the mother and fetus as well as the newborn infant.

■ EVALUATION OF THE NEWBORN INFANT HISTORY

Taking the history in newborn medicine involves three key areas: (1) the medical history of the mother and father, including a relevant genetic history; (2) the history of the mother's previous pregnancies; and (3) the history of the current pregnancy, including antepartum and intrapartum events.

The mother's medical history should include any chronic medical conditions, medications taken during pregnancy, unusual dietary habits, smoking history, occupational exposures to chemicals or infections of potential risk to the fetus, and pertinent aspects of the social history that may suggest increased risks for parenting problems and child abuse. Family illnesses with genetic implications should be sought. The past pregnancy history should include maternal age, gravidity and parity, blood type, and pregnancy outcomes. The current obstetric history should include documentation and results of procedures such as ultrasound, amniocentesis, screening tests (eg, hepatitis B surface antigen [HBsAg], antibody screen, serum quadruple screen for genetic disorders, human immunodeficiency virus [HIV]), and antepartum tests of fetal well-being (eg, biophysical profiles, nonstress tests, or Doppler assessment of fetal blood flow patterns). Information should be sought regarding pregnancy-related illnesses in the mother such as urinary tract infection, pregnancy-induced hypertension or preeclampsia, eclampsia, vaginal bleeding, and preterm labor. Peripartum events of importance include duration of ruptured membranes, maternal fever, fetal distress or meconium-stained amniotic fluid, type of delivery (vaginal or cesarean section), anesthesia and analgesia used, reason for operative or forceps delivery, and condition of the infant at birth, including any resuscitation needed and Apgar scores.

ASSESSMENT OF GROWTH & GESTATIONAL AGE

It is important to know the gestational age because infant behavior and problems can be predicted on this basis. Recall of the date of the last menstrual period is the best indicator of gestational age. Other obstetric observations, such as fundal height and early ultrasound examination, provide supporting information. Postnatal examination can also be used because fetal physical characteristics and neurologic development progress in predictable fashion. Table 1–1 lists the physical and neurologic criteria to be examined. The upper panel is the neuromuscular examination, assessing primarily muscle tone and strength. The lower panel catalogs a variety of physical characteristics. Adding the scores assigned to each characteristic yields a total score corresponding to gestational age.

Disappearance of the anterior vascular capsule of the lens is also helpful in determining gestational age. Until 27–28 weeks' gestation, the lens capsule is covered by vessels; by 34 weeks, this vascular plexus is completely atrophied. Foot length, from the heel to the tip of the longest toe, also correlates with gestational age in appropriately grown infants. The foot measures 4.5 cm at 25 weeks' gestation and increases by 0.25 cm/week until term.

Unless the physical examination indicates a gestational age more than 2 weeks different in either direction from the obstetric dates, the gestational age is as assigned by the dates. Birth weight and gestational

Table 1–1. New Ballard score for assessment of fetal maturation of newly born infants.[a]

Neuromuscular Maturity

Neuromuscular Maturity Sign	Score							Record Score Here
	-1	0	1	2	3	4	5	
Posture								
Square window (wrist)	>90°	90°	60°	45°	30°	0°		
Arm recoil		180°	140° to 180°	110° to 140°	90° to 110°	<90°		
Popliteal angle	180°	160°	140°	120°	100°	90°	<90°	
Scarf sign								
Heel to ear								

Total Neuromuscular Maturity Score

Physical Maturity

Physical Maturity Sign	Score							Record Score Here
	-1	0	1	2	3	4	5	
Skin	Sticky, friable, transparent	Gelatinous, red, translucent	Smooth, pink, visible veins	Superficial peeling &/or rash; few veins	Cracking, pale areas; rare veins	Parchment, deep cracking; no vessels	Leathery, cracked, wrinkled	
Lanugo	None	Sparse	Abundant	Thinning	Bald areas	Mostly bald		
Plantar surface	Heel toe 40–50 mm: -1 <40 mm: -2	> 50 mm: no crease	Faint red marks	Anterior transverse crease only	Creases anterior 2/3	Creases over entire sole		
Breast	Imperceptible	Barely perceptible	Flat areola; no bud	Stippled areola; 1- to 2-mm bud	Raised areola; 3- to 4-mm bud	Full areola; 5- to 10-mm bud		
Eye/Ear	Lids fused loosely: -1 tightly: -2	Lids open; pinna flat; stays folded	Slightly curved pinna; soft; slow recoil	Well-curved pinna; soft but ready recoil	Formed & firm instant recoil	Thick cartilage; ear stiff		
Genitals (male)	Scrotum flat, smooth	Scrotum empty; faint rugae	Testes in upper canal; rare rugae	Testes descending; few rugae	Testes down; good rugae	Testes pendulous; deep rugae		
Genitals (female)	Clitoris prominent & labia flat	Prominent clitoris & small labia minora	Prominent clitoris & enlarging minora	Majora & minora equally prominent	Majora large; minora small	Majora cover clitoris & minora		

Total Physical Maturity Score

Maturity	Score	-10	-5	0	5	10	15	20	25	30	35	40	45	50
Rating	Weeks	20	22	24	26	28	30	32	34	36	38	40	42	44

[a]See text for a description of the clinical gestational age examination.
Reproduced, with permission, from Ballard JL et al: New Ballard Score, expanded to include extremely premature infants. J Pediatr 1991;119:417.

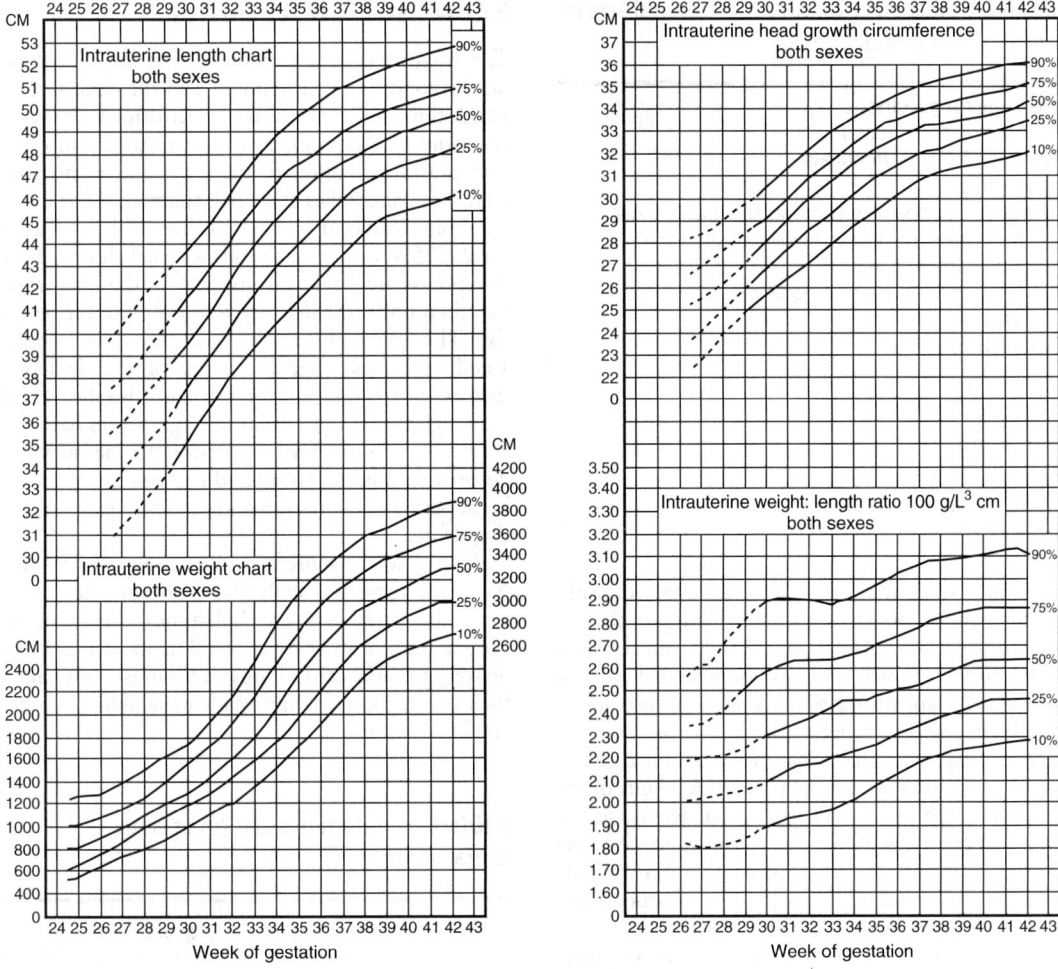

Figure 1–1. Intrauterine growth curves for weight, length, and head circumference for singleton births in Colorado. (Reproduced, with permission, from Lubchenco LO et al: Intrauterine growth in length and head circumference as estimated from live births at gestational ages from 26 to 42 weeks. Pediatrics 1966;37:403.)

age must be plotted on an appropriate standard to determine if the infant's weight is appropriate for gestational age (AGA), small for gestational age (SGA), intrauterine growth restricted (IUGR), or large for gestational age (LGA) (Figure 1–1). Birth weight and gestational age distributions vary in different populations depending on factors such as socioeconomic issues that affect nutrition and access to care; altitude; and environmental factors such as smoking, drug and alcohol use, and race. Whenever possible, standards should be prepared from data derived from the local population. When such information is not available, regional standards may be used. The birth weight–gestational age distribution of an infant is a screening tool that should be supplemented by clinical data

confirming a tentative diagnosis of intrauterine growth restriction or excessive fetal growth. These data include not only the clinical features of the infant determined by physical examination, but also factors such as the size of the parents and the birth weight–gestational age distribution of infants previously born to the parents.

Table 1–2 lists causes of variations in neonatal size in relation to gestational age. An important distinction, particularly in SGA infants, is whether the growth disorder is symmetrical (weight, length, and occipitofrontal circumference [OFC] all ≤ 10%) or asymmetrical (only weight ≤ 10%). Asymmetrical growth restriction implies a problem late in pregnancy, such as pregnancy-induced hypertension or placental insufficiency. Sym-

Table 1–2. Causes of variations in neonatal size in relation to gestational age.

Infants large for gestational age
   Infant of a diabetic mother
Infants small for gestational age
   Asymmetrical
      Placental insufficiency secondary to pregnancy-induced
         hypertension or other maternal vascular disease
      Maternal age > 35 years
      Poor weight gain during pregnancy
      Multiple gestation
   Symmetrical
      Maternal drug use
         Narcotics
         Cocaine
         Alcohol
      Chromosomal abnormalities
      Intrauterine viral infection (eg, cytomegalovirus)

---

metrical growth restriction implies an event of early pregnancy: chromosomal abnormality, drug or alcohol use, or congenital viral infections. In general, the outlook for normal growth and development is better in asymmetrically growth-restricted infants whose intrauterine brain growth has been spared.

The fact that SGA infants have fewer problems (such as respiratory distress syndrome) than AGA infants of the same birth weight but a lower gestational age has led to the misconception that SGA infants have accelerated maturation. SGA infants, when compared with AGA infants of the same gestational age, actually have increased morbidity and mortality rates.

Knowledge of birth weight in relation to gestational age is also helpful in anticipating neonatal problems. LGA babies are at risk for birth trauma, hypoglycemia, polycythemia, congenital anomalies, cardiomyopathy, hyperbilirubinemia, and hypocalcemia. SGA babies are at risk for fetal distress during labor and delivery, polycythemia, hypoglycemia, and hypocalcemia.

American Academy of Pediatrics: *Guidelines for Perinatal Care,* 5th ed. American Academy of Pediatrics, 2002.

American Academy of Pediatrics: Committee on Fetus and Newborn: Levels of neonatal care. Pediatrics 2004;114:1341 [PMID: 15520119].

Cowett RM: Neonatal care of the infant of the diabetic mother. Neoreviews 2002;3:e190.

Leviton A et al: The wealth of information conveyed by gestational age. J Pediatr 2005;146:123 [PMID: 15644836].

Taslimi MM: Doppler ultrasonography in assessment of fetal well-being. Neoreviews 2004;5:e247.

Thureen PJ et al: The small-for-gestational age infant. Neoreviews 2001;2:e139.

EXAMINATION AT BIRTH

The extent of the newborn physical examination depends on the condition of the infant and the environment in which the examination is being performed. In the delivery room, the examination consists largely of observation plus auscultation of the chest and inspection for congenital anomalies and birth trauma. Major congenital anomalies occur in 1.5% of live births and account for 20–25% of perinatal and neonatal deaths. Because the infants are physically stressed by the birth process, examination in the delivery room should not be extensive. The Apgar score (Table 1–3) should be recorded at 1 and 5 minutes of age. In the case of severely depressed infants, a 10-minute score should also be recorded. Although the 1- and 5-minute Apgar scores have almost no predictive value for long-term outcome, serial scores do provide a useful shorthand description of the severity of perinatal depression and the response to resuscitative efforts.

Skin color is a useful indicator of cardiac output. Normally there is a high blood flow to the skin. Any stress that triggers a catecholamine response redirects cardiac output away from the skin to preserve oxygen delivery to more critical organs. Cyanosis and pallor are thus two signs reflecting inadequate skin oxygenation and cardiac output.

Table 1–3. Infant evaluation at birth— Apgar score.[a]

	Score		
	0	**1**	**2**
Heart rate	Absent	Slow (< 100)	> 100
Respiratory effort	Absent	Slow, irregular	Good, crying
Muscle tone	Limp	Some flexion	Active motion
Response to catheter in nostril[b]	No response	Grimace	Cough or sneeze
Color	Blue or pale	Body pink; extremities blue	Completely pink

© 1958 American Medical Association.
[a]One minute and 5 minutes after complete birth of the infant (disregarding the cord and the placenta), the following objective signs should be observed and recorded.
[b]Tested after the oropharynx is clear.
Reproduced, with permission, from Apgar V et al: Evaluation of the newborn infant—Second report. JAMA 1958;168:1985.

Skeletal examination immediately after delivery serves two purposes: (1) to detect any obvious congenital anomalies, and (2) to detect signs of birth trauma, particularly in LGA infants or those born after a protracted second stage of labor—in whom a fractured clavicle or humerus might be found.

The umbilical cord should be examined for the number of vessels. Normally, there are two arteries and one vein. In 1% of deliveries (5–6% of twin deliveries), the cord has only two vessels: an artery and a vein. The latter configuration is considered a minor anomaly, and as with other minor anomalies, carries a slightly increased risk of associated defects. The placenta is usually examined by the physician delivering it. Small placentas are always associated with small infants. The placental examination emphasizes the identification of membranes and vessels—particularly in multiple gestations—as well as the presence and severity of placental infarcts or clots (placental abruption) on the maternal side.

GENERAL EXAMINATION IN THE NURSERY

It is important that the examiner have warm hands and a gentle approach. Start with observation, then auscultation of the chest, and then palpation of the abdomen. Examination of the eyes, ears, throat, and hips should be done last, since these maneuvers are most disturbing to the infant. The heart rate should range from 120–160 beats/min, and the respiratory rate from 30–60 breaths/min; blood pressure is affected by perinatal asphyxia and the need for mechanical ventilation more than by gestational age or birth weight. Systolic blood pressure on day 1 ranges from 50–70 mm Hg and increases steadily during the first week of life. *Note:* An irregularly irregular heart rate, usually caused by premature atrial contractions, is common. This irregularity should resolve in the first days of life and is not of pathologic significance.

Minor anomalies occur in < 4% of the population and should be noted. Approximately 15–20% of healthy newborns have one minor anomaly, with a 3% risk of having an associated major anomaly. Approximately 0.8% of newborns have two minor anomalies, and 0.5% have three or more, with a risk of 10% and 20%, respectively, of a major malformation. Common minor anomalies requiring no diagnostic evaluation if isolated in an otherwise normal infant include preauricular pits (although hearing should be assessed), a sacral dimple without other cutaneous abnormality that occurs within 2.5 cm of the anus, a single transverse palmar crease, and three or fewer café-au-lait spots in a white infant or five or fewer in an African American infant.

Skin

Observe for bruising, petechiae (common over the presenting part), meconium staining, and jaundice. Peripheral cyanosis is commonly present when the extremities are cool or the infant is polycythemic. Generalized cyanosis merits immediate evaluation. Pallor may be caused by acute or chronic blood loss or by acidosis. In dark-skinned infants, pallor and cyanosis should be assessed in the lips, mouth and nail beds. Plethora suggests polycythemia. Note vernix caseosa (a whitish, greasy material covering the body that decreases as term approaches) and lanugo (the fine hair covering the preterm infant's skin). Dry skin with cracking and peeling of the superficial layers is common in postterm infants. Edema may be generalized (hydrops) or localized (eg, on the dorsum of the feet in Turner syndrome). Check for birthmarks such as capillary hemangiomas (lower occiput, eyelids, and forehead) and mongolian spot (bluish black pigmentation over the back and buttocks). Milia, small white keratogenous cysts, can be found scattered over the cheeks, forehead, nose, and nasolabial folds. Miliaria (blocked ducts of sweat glands) occurs in intertriginous areas and on the face or scalp. It can appear as small vesicles (crystallina), small erythematous papules (rubra), or pustules. Erythema toxicum is a benign rash characterized by fleeting erythematous papules and pustules filled with eosinophils. Pustular melanosis leaves pigmented macules when the pustules rupture. The pustules are noninfectious but contain neutrophils. Jaundice in the first 24 hours is considered abnormal and should be evaluated (see section on Neonatal Jaundice).

Head

Check for cephalhematoma (a swelling over one or both parietal bones contained within suture lines) and caput succedaneum (edema over the presenting part that crosses suture lines). Subgaleal hemorrhages (beneath the scalp) are uncommon but can lead to extensive blood loss into this large potential space with resultant hypovolemic shock. Skull fractures may be linear or depressed and may be associated with cephalhematoma. Check for the presence and size of the fontanelles. The anterior fontanelle varies from 1–4 cm in any direction; the posterior fontanelle should be less than 1 cm. A third fontanelle is a bony defect along the sagittal suture in the parietal bones and may be a feature of certain syndromes, such as trisomy 21. Sutures should be freely mobile. Craniosynostosis is a prematurely fused suture.

Face

Odd facies may be associated with a specific syndrome. Bruising from birth trauma (especially with face presentation) and forceps marks should be identified. Face presentation may be associated with soft tissue swelling around the nose and mouth and can cause considerable distortion. Facial nerve palsy is observed when the infant cries; the unaffected side of the mouth moves normally, giving a distorted grimace.

Eyes

Subconjunctival hemorrhages frequently result from birth trauma. Less commonly, a corneal tear may occur and present as a clouded cornea. Ophthalmologic consultation is indicated in such cases. Extraocular movements should be assessed. Occasional uncoordinated eye movements are common, but persistent irregular movements are abnormal. The iris should be inspected for abnormalities such as Brushfield spots (trisomy 21) and colobomas. Look for the retinal red reflex. Red reflexes should be symmetrical. Dark spots, a blunted reflex on one side, lack of a reflex, or a white reflex all require ophthalmologic evaluation. Leukokoria can be caused by glaucoma (cloudy cornea), cataract, or tumor (retinoblastoma). Infants at risk for chorioretinitis (congenital viral infection) should undergo a formal retinal examination with pupils dilated.

Nose

Examine the nose for size and shape. In utero compression can cause deformities. Because babies under age 1 month are obligate nose breathers, any nasal obstruction (eg, bilateral choanal atresia or stenosis) can cause respiratory distress. Unilateral choanal atresia can be diagnosed by occluding each naris. Patency is best checked by holding a cold metal surface (eg, a chilled laryngoscope blade) under the nose, and observing the fog from both nares on the metal. Purulent nasal discharge at birth suggests congenital syphilis.

Ears

Malformed or malpositioned (low-set or posteriorly rotated) ears are often associated with other congenital anomalies. The tympanic membranes should be visualized. Preauricular pits and tags are common minor variants that can be associated with hearing loss.

Mouth

Epithelial (Epstein) pearls are retention cysts along the gum margins and at the junction of the hard and soft palates. Natal teeth may be present and sometimes must be removed to prevent their aspiration. Check the integrity and shape of the palate; rule out cleft lip and cleft palate. A small mandible and tongue with cleft palate is seen with Pierre Robin syndrome and can result in respi-

ratory difficulty, as the tongue occludes the airway. Prone positioning can be very beneficial. A prominent tongue can be seen in trisomy 21 and Beckwith-Wiedemann syndrome. Excessive oral secretions suggests esophageal atresia or a swallowing disorder.

Neck

Redundant skin or webbing is seen in Turner syndrome. Sinus tracts may be seen as remnants of branchial clefts. Check for masses: midline (thyroid), anterior to the sternocleidomastoid (branchial cleft cysts), within the sternocleidomastoid (hematoma and torticollis), and posterior to the sternocleidomastoid (cystic hygroma).

Chest & Lungs

Check for fractured clavicles (crepitus, bruising, and tenderness). Increased anteroposterior diameter (barrel chest) can be seen with aspiration syndromes. Check air entry bilaterally and the position of the mediastinum and heart tones. Decreased breath sounds with respiratory distress and a shift in the mediastinum suggests pneumothorax (tension) or a space-occupying lesion (eg, diaphragmatic hernia). With pneumomediastinum, the heart sounds are muffled. Expiratory grunting and decreased air entry are observed in hyaline membrane disease. Rales are not of clinical significance at this age.

Heart

Examination of the heart is described in detail in Chapter 19. *Note:* Murmurs are commonly present in the first hours and are most often benign. Severe congenital heart disease in the newborn infant may be present with no murmur at all. The two most common presentations of heart disease in the newborn infant are cyanosis and congestive heart failure with abnormalities of pulses. In hypoplastic left heart and critical aortic stenosis, pulses are diminished at all sites. In aortic coarctation and interrupted aortic arch, pulses are diminished in the lower extremities.

Abdomen

Check for softness, distention, and bowel sounds. If polyhydramnios was present or excessive oral secretions are noted, pass a soft catheter into the stomach to rule out esophageal atresia. Palpate the kidneys—most abdominal masses in the newborn infant are associated with kidney disorders (eg, multicystic or dysplastic and hydronephrosis). When the abdomen is relaxed, normal kidneys may be felt but are not prominent. A markedly scaphoid abdomen plus respiratory distress suggests diaphragmatic hernia. Absence of abdominal musculature (prune belly syndrome) may occur in association with renal abnormalities. Check the size of the liver and spleen. These organs are superficial and discernible by light palpation in the newborn infant. The outline of a distended bladder may be seen and palpated above the pubic symphysis.

Genitalia & Anus

Male and female genitals show characteristics according to gestational age (see Table 1–1). In the female during the first few days, a whitish vaginal discharge with or without blood is normal. Check the patency and location of the anus.

Skeleton

Check for obvious anomalies, for example, the absence of a bone, clubfoot, fusion or webbing of digits, and extra digits. Examine for hip dislocation by attempting to dislocate the femur posteriorly and then abducting the legs to relocate the femur. Look for extremity fractures and for palsies (especially brachial plexus injuries). Rule out myelomeningocele and other spinal deformities (eg, scoliosis). Arthrogryposis (multiple joint contractures) results from chronic limitation of movement in utero that may result from lack of amniotic fluid or from congenital neuromuscular disease.

Neurologic Examination

Normal newborns have reflexes that facilitate survival (eg, rooting and sucking reflexes), and have sensory abilities (eg, hearing and smell) that allow them to recognize their mother within a few weeks of birth. Although the retina is well developed at birth, visual acuity is poor (20/400) because of a relatively immobile lens. Acuity improves rapidly over the first 6 months, with fixation and tracking becoming well developed by 2 months.

Observe the newborn's resting tone (normal-term newborns should exhibit flexion of the upper and lower extremities) and spontaneous movements. Look for symmetry of movements. Extension of extremities should result in spontaneous recoil to the flexed position. Assess the character of the cry; a high-pitched cry may indicate disease of the central nervous system (CNS) (eg, hemorrhage). Hypotonia and a weak cry may indicate systemic disease or congenital neuromuscular disorder. Check for newborn reflexes:

1. Sucking reflex in response to a nipple or the examiner's finger in the mouth. This reflex is observed by 14 weeks' gestation.
2. Rooting reflex: Head turns to the side of a facial stimulus. This reflex develops by 28 weeks' gestation.
3. Traction response: The infant is pulled by the arms to a sitting position. Initially, the head lags, then with active flexion comes to the midline briefly before falling forward.
4. Palmar grasp with placement of the examiner's finger in the palm. This reflex develops by 28 weeks' gestation and disappears by age 4 months.
5. Deep tendon reflexes: Several beats of ankle clonus and an upgoing Babinski reflex may be normal.
6. Placing: Rub the dorsum of one foot on the underside of a surface. The infant will flex the knee and bring the foot up.
7. Moro (startle) reflex: Hold the infant and support the head. Allow the head to drop 1–2 cm suddenly. The arms will abduct at the shoulder and extend at the elbow. Adduction with flexion will follow. The hands show a prominent spreading or extension of the fingers. This reflex develops by 28 weeks' gestation (incomplete) and disappears by age 3 months.
8. Tonic neck reflex: Forcibly turn the infant's head to one side, and the arm and leg on that side extend while the opposite arm and leg flex ("fencing position"). This reflex disappears by age 8 months.

Ackerman LL, Menezes AH: Spinal congenital dermal sinuses: A 30-year experience. Pediatrics 2003;112:641 [PMID: 12949296].

Adam M, Hudgins L: The importance of minor anomalies in the evaluation of the newborn. Neoreviews 2003;4:e99.

American Academy of Pediatrics Committee on Quality Improvement, Subcommittee on Developmental Dysplasia of the Hip: Early detection of developmental dysplasia of the hip. Pediatrics 2000;105:896 [PMID: 10742345].

American Academy of Pediatrics Section on Ophthalmology: Red reflex examination in infants. Pediatrics 2002;109:980 [PMID: 11986467].

Eichenfield LF et al (editors): *Textbook of Neonatal Dermatology.* WB Saunders, 2001.

Hernandez JA, Morelli JG: Birthmarks of medical significance. Neoreviews 2003;4:e270.

CARE OF THE WELL NEWBORN INFANT

The primary responsibility of the level 1 nursery is care of the well infant. This includes promoting mother-infant bonding, establishing feeding, and teaching the techniques of newborn care. Surveillance of the infant is a key function of the staff; they must be alert for the signs and symptoms of illness, including temperature instability, change in activity, refusal to feed, pallor, cyanosis, early or excessive jaundice, tachypnea and respiratory distress, delayed (beyond 24 hours) passage of first stool or voiding of urine, and bilious vomiting. Several preventive measures are undertaken routinely in the normal newborn nursery.

Prophylactic treatment with erythromycin ointment to prevent gonococcal ophthalmia is routinely administered within 1 hour of birth.

Vitamin K, 1 mg, is given intramuscularly or subcutaneously within 4 hours of birth to prevent hemorrhagic disease of the newborn.

All infants should be vaccinated against hepatitis B, but the first dose can wait until 1–2 months of age if the mother is HBsAg-negative. Hepatitis B vaccine and hepatitis B immune globulin (HBIG) are administered if the mother is known to be HBsAg-positive. If maternal HBsAg status is unknown, vaccine should be given. Maternal blood should be tested and HBIG given to the neonate before 7 days of age if the test is positive.

Cord blood is collected on all infants at birth and used for blood typing and Coombs testing if the mother is type O or Rh-negative.

Rapid glucose testing should be performed in infants at risk for hypoglycemia (eg, infants of diabetic mothers [IDMs], preterm, SGA, LGA, or stressed infants). Values less than 45 mg/dL should be confirmed by laboratory blood glucose testing and treated. Hematocrit should be measured at age 3–6 hours in infants at risk for or those who have symptoms of polycythemia or anemia.

The state-sponsored newborn genetic screen (for inborn errors of metabolism such as phenylketonuria [PKU], galactosemia, sickle cell disease, hypothyroidism, and cystic fibrosis) is performed just prior to discharge, after 24–48 hours in the hospital if possible. In many states, a repeat test is required at 8–14 days of age because the PKU test is often falsely negative when obtained before 48 hours of age. Not all state-mandated screens include the same panel of diseases; the most recent addition in some states is a screen for congenital adrenal hyperplasia. In infants with prolonged hospital stays, the test should be performed by 1 week of age. In addition to the state-mandated screen, some centers offer expanded newborn screening by tandem mass spectrometry that looks for a variety of other inborn errors such as fatty acid oxidation defects.

Infants should routinely be positioned supine to minimize the risk of sudden infant death syndrome (SIDS). Prone positioning is contraindicated unless there are compelling clinical reasons for another position. Bed sharing with adults and prone positioning are associated with increased risk of SIDS.

FEEDING THE WELL NEWBORN INFANT

Indications that the baby is ready for feeding include (1) alertness and vigor, (2) absence of abdominal distention, (3) good bowel sounds, and (4) normal hunger cry. All of these usually occur within 6 hours after birth, but fetal distress or traumatic delivery may prolong this period.

The healthy full-term infant should be allowed to feed every 2–5 hours on demand. The first breast feeding should occur in the delivery room. For formula-fed babies the first feeding usually occurs by 3 hours of life, and the volume generally increases from 0.5–1 oz per feeding initially to 1.5–2 oz per feeding on day 3. By day 3, the average full-term newborn takes in about 100 mL/kg/d of milk.

Although a wide range of infant formulas can satisfy the nutritional needs of most neonates, breast milk is the standard on which formulas are based. (See also Chapter 10.) Despite the low concentrations of several vitamins and minerals, their bioavailability is high. All of the necessary nutrients, vitamins, minerals, and water are provided by human milk for the first 6 months of life except vitamin K (thus, 1 mg IM is administered at birth), vitamin D (200–300 IU/d if minimal sunlight exposure), and vitamin B_{12} (0.3–0.5 mg/d if the mother is a strict vegetarian and takes no B_{12} supplement). Other advantages of breast milk include (1) the presence of immunologic, antimicrobial, and anti-inflammatory factors, including IgA, cellular, and protein or enzymatic components that decrease the incidence of upper respiratory and gastrointestinal (GI) infections in infancy; (2) the possibility that breast feeding may decrease the frequency and severity of childhood eczema and asthma; (3) promotion of mother-infant bonding; and (4) evidence that breast milk as a nutritional source improves neurodevelopmental outcomes.

Although approximately 70% of mothers in the United States initiate breast feeding, only 33% continue to breastfeed at 6 months. Hospital practices that facilitate successful initiation of breast feeding include rooming-in, nursing on demand, and avoiding supplemental formula (unless medically indicated). The nursery staff must be cognizant of problems associated with breast feeding and be able to provide help and support for mothers in the hospital. It is essential that an experienced professional observe and assist with several feedings to document good latch-on. Good latch-on is important in preventing the common breast-feeding problems of sore nipples, unsatisfied babies, engorgement, poor milk supply, and excessive hyperbilirubinemia ("lack-of-breast-milk jaundice").

Table 1–4 presents guidelines the nursing mother and health care provider can use to assess successful breast feeding.

American Academy of Pediatrics Committee on Fetus and Newborn: Controversies concerning vitamin K and the newborn. Pediatrics 2003;112:191 [PMID: 12837888].

Table 1–4. Guidelines for successful breast feeding.

	First 8 Hours	8–24 Hours	Day 2	Day 3	Day 4	Day 5	Day 6 Onward
Milk supply	You may be able to express a few drops of milk.	Milk should come in between the second and fourth days.				Milk should be in. Breasts may be firm or leak milk.	Breasts should feel softer after feedings.
Baby's activity	Baby is usually wide-awake in the first hour of life. Put baby to breast within 30 min after birth.	Wake up your baby. Babies may not wake up on their own to feed.	Baby should be more cooperative and less sleepy.	Look for early feeding cues such as rooting, lip smacking, and hands to face.			Baby should appear satisfied after feedings.
Feeding routine	Baby may go into a deep sleep 2–4 h after birth.	Feed your baby every 1–4 h or as often as wanted—at least 8–12 times a day.	Use chart to write down time of each feeding.			May go one longer interval (up to 5 h between feeds) in a 24-h period.	
Breast feeding	Baby will wake up and be alert and responsive for several more hours after initial deep sleep.	As long as the mother is comfortable, nurse at both breasts as long as baby is actively sucking.	Try to nurse both sides each feeding, aiming at 10 min per side. Expect some nipple tenderness.	Consider hand expressing or pumping a few drops of milk to soften the nipple if the breast is too firm for the baby to latch on.	Nurse a minimum of 10–30 min per side every feeding for the first few weeks of life. Once milk supply is well established, allow baby to finish the first breast before offering the second.		Mother's nipple tenderness is improving or is gone.
Baby's urine output		Baby must have a minimum of one wet diaper in the first 24 h.	Baby must have at least one wet diaper every 8–11 h.	You should see an increase in wet diapers (up to four to six) in 24 h.	Baby's urine should be light yellow.	Baby should have six to eight wet diapers per day of colorless or light yellow urine.	
Baby's stool	Baby should have a black-green (meconium) stool.	Baby should have a black-green (meconium) stool.	Baby may have a second very dark (meconium) stool.	Baby's stools should be in transition from black-green to yellow.	Baby's stool should be in transition from meconium to yellow.	Baby should have three or four yellow, seedy stools a day.	The number of stools may decrease gradually after 4–6 wk of life.

Modified, with permission, from Gabrielski L: Lactation support services. The Children's Hospital, Denver, 1999.

American Academy of Pediatrics Section on Breastfeeding Policy Statement: Breastfeeding and the use of human milk. Pediatrics 2005;115:496 [PMID: 15687461].

American Academy of Pediatrics Task Force on Infant Sleep Position and Sudden Infant Death Syndrome: Concepts of sudden infant death syndrome: Implications for infant sleeping environment and sleep position. Pediatrics 2000;105:650 [PMID: 10699127].

Dewey KG et al: Risk factors for suboptimal infant breastfeeding behavior, delayed onset of lactation, and excess neonatal weight loss. Pediatrics 2003;112:607 [PMID: 12949292].

Hale TW: Drug therapy and breastfeeding: antidepressants, antipsychotics, antimanics. NeoReviews 2004;5:e45.

Hale TW: Drug therapy and breastfeeding: antibiotics, analgesics and other indications. NeoReviews 2005;6:e233.

Natowicz M: Newborn screening-setting evidence-based policy for protection. N Engl J Med 2005;353:867 [PMID: 16135829].

Ostrea EM et al: Drugs that affect the fetus and newborn via the placenta or breast milk. Pediatr Clin North Am 2004;51:539 [PMID: 15157585].

Schulze A et al: Expanded newborn screening for inborn errors of metabolism by electrospray ionization–tandem mass spectrometry: Results, outcome, and implications. Pediatrics 2003;111:1399 [PMID: 12777559].

EARLY DISCHARGE OF THE NEWBORN INFANT

Discharge at 24–36 hours of age appears safe and appropriate for most newborns if there are no contraindications (Table 1–5) and a follow-up visit 48–72 hours

Table 1–5. Criteria for early newborn discharge.

Contraindications to early newborn discharge
1. Jaundice at ≤ 24 h
2. High risk for infection (eg, maternal chorioamnionitis); discharge allowed at 24 h with a normal transition
3. Known or suspected narcotic addiction or withdrawal
4. Physical defects requiring evaluation
5. Oral defects (clefts, micrognathia)

Relative contraindications to early newborn discharge (infants at high risk for feeding failure, excessive jaundice)
1. Prematurity or borderline prematurity (< 38 weeks' gestation)
2. Birth weight < 2700 g (6 lb)
3. Baby difficult to arouse for feeding; not demanding regularly in nursery
4. Medical or neurologic problems that interfere with feeding (Down syndrome, hypotonia, cardiac problems)
5. Twins or higher multiples
6. ABO blood group incompatibility or severe jaundice in previous child
7. Mother whose previous breast-fed infant gained weight poorly
8. Mother with breast surgery involving periareolar areas (if attempting to nurse)

Table 1–6. Guidelines for early outpatient follow-up evaluation.

History
Rhythmic sucking and audible swallowing for at least 10 minutes total per feeding?
Baby wakes and demands to feed every 2–3 h (at least eight to ten feedings per 24 h)?
Do breasts feel full before feedings, and softer after?
Are there at least six noticeably wet diapers per 24 h?
Are there yellow bowel movements (no longer meconium)—at least four per 24 h?
Is baby still acting hungry after nursing (frequently sucks hands, rooting)?

Physical assessment
Weight, unclothed: should not be more than 8–10% below birth weight
Extent and severity of jaundice
Assessment of hydration, alertness, general well-being
Cardiovascular examination: murmurs, brachial and femoral pulses, respirations

after discharge is ensured. Most infants with severe cardiorespiratory disorders and infections are identified in the first 12 hours of life. The exception may be the infant treated with intrapartum antibiotic prophylaxis for maternal group B streptococcal (GBS) colonization or infection. The Centers for Disease Control and Prevention (CDC) and the American Academy of Pediatrics (AAP) have recommended that these infants be observed in hospital for 48 hours because of the possibility of "partial treatment" with delayed onset of symptoms of infection. Recent data show that exposure to antibiotics in labor does not appear to change the type or timing of symptoms related to GBS infection in full-term infants, and that hospital observation beyond 24 hours may not be necessary for the asymptomatic full-term infant who received intrapartum chemoprophylaxis. Other problems, such as jaundice and difficulties in breast feeding, typically occur after 48 hours and can usually be dealt with on an outpatient basis provided good follow-up has been arranged.

The AAP recommends a follow-up visit within 48–72 hours for newborns discharged before 48 hours of age. Infants who are small or slightly premature—especially if breast feeding—are at particular risk for inadequate intake. Suggested guidelines for the follow-up interview and physical examination are presented in Table 1–6. The optimal timing of discharge must be determined in each case based on medical, social, and financial factors.

CIRCUMCISION

Circumcision is an elective procedure to be performed only in healthy, stable infants. The procedure probably has medical benefits, including prevention of phimosis, paraphimosis, balanoposthitis, and urinary tract infection. Later benefits include decreased incidence of cancer of the penis, cervical cancer (in partners of circumcised men), and sexually transmitted diseases (including HIV). Most parents decide on circumcision for nonmedical reasons. The risks of the procedure include local infection, bleeding, removal of too much skin, and urethral injury. The combined incidence of these complications is less than 1%. Local anesthesia (dorsal penile nerve block or circumferential ring block with 1% lidocaine without epinephrine) or topical application of an anesthetic cream are safe and effective and should always be used. Techniques that allow visualization of the glans throughout the procedure (eg, Plastibell and Gomco clamp) are preferred to a blind technique (eg, Mogen clamp) because occasional amputation of the glans can occur with the latter technique. Circumcision is contraindicated in infants with genital abnormalities (eg, hypospadias). A coagulation screen should be performed prior to the procedure in infants with a confirmed family history of serious bleeding disorders.

HEARING SCREENING

Normal hearing is critical to normal language development. Significant bilateral hearing loss is present in 1–3 infants per 1000 in the well nursery and in 2–4 infants per 100 in the neonatal intensive care unit population. All infants should be screened for hearing loss by auditory brainstem evoked responses or evoked otoacoustic emissions as early as possible. Primary care providers and parents need to be advised of the possibility of hearing loss and offered ready referral in suspect cases.

American Academy of Pediatrics Committee on Fetus and Newborn Policy Statement: Hospital stay for healthy term newborns. Pediatrics 2004;113:1434 [PMID: 15121968].

American Academy of Pediatrics Joint Committee on Infant Hearing: Year 2000 position statement: Principles and guidelines for early hearing detection and intervention programs. Pediatrics 2000;106:798 [PMID: 11015525].

American Academy of Pediatrics Task Force on Circumcision: Circumcision policy statement. Pediatrics 1999;103:686 [PMID: 10049981].

Bromberger P et al: The influence of intrapartum antibiotics on the clinical spectrum of early-onset group B streptococcal infection in term infants. Pediatrics 2000;106:244 [PMID: 10920146].

Farrell PA et al: SIDS, ALTE, apnea and the use of home monitors. Pediatr Rev 2002;23:3 [PMID: 11773587].

Friedman MA, Spitzer AR: Discharge criteria for the term newborn. Pediatr Clin North Am 2004;51:599 [PMID: 15157587].

Kerschner JE: Neonatal hearing screening: to do or not to do. Pediatr Clin North Am 2004;51:725 [PMID: 15157594].

Rhead WJ, Irons M: The call from the newborn screening laboratory: frustration in the afternoon. Pediatr Clin North Am 2004;51:803 [PMID: 15157599].

Sokol J, Hyde M: Hearing screening. Pediatr Rev 2002;23:155 [PMID: 11986491].

Thompson DC et al: Universal newborn hearing screening. Summary of evidence. JAMA 2001;286:2000 [PMID: 11667937].

COMMON PROBLEMS IN THE TERM NEWBORN INFANT

NEONATAL JAUNDICE

General Considerations

Jaundice is a common neonatal problem. Sixty-five percent of newborns develop clinical jaundice with a bilirubin level above 5 mg/dL during the first week of life. Bilirubin is a potent antioxidant and peroxyl scavenger that may help the newborn, who is deficient in most antioxidant substances such as vitamin E, catalase, and superoxide dismutase, to avoid oxygen toxicity in the days after birth. Extremely high levels of bilirubin are not uncommon, with an incidence of approximately 1–2% of infants having a total serum bilirubin (TSB) > 20 mg/dL, 0.16% (1 in 700) having TSB > 25 mg/dL, and 0.03% (1 in 10,000) having TSB > 30 mg/dL. Such high levels can result in an encephalopathy known as kernicterus.

Metabolism of Bilirubin

Heme (iron protoporphyrin) is broken down by heme oxygenase to iron, which is conserved; carbon monoxide, which is exhaled; and biliverdin, which is then further metabolized to bilirubin by the enzyme bilirubin reductase. Each 1 g of hemoglobin breakdown results in the production of 34 mg of bilirubin (1 mg/dL = 17.2 mmol/L of bilirubin). Bilirubin is carried bound to albumin to the liver, where, in the presence of the enzyme uridyldiphosphoglucuronyl transferase (UDPGT; glucuronyl transferase), it is taken up by the hepatocyte and conjugated with two glucuronide molecules. The conjugated bilirubin is then excreted through the bile to the intestine. In the presence of normal gut flora, the conjugated bilirubin is metabolized further to stercobilins and excreted in the stool. In the absence of gut flora—and with slow intestinal motility, as in the first few days of life—the conjugated bilirubin remains in the intestinal lumen, where a mucosal enzyme (β-glucuronidase) can cleave off the glucuronide molecules, leaving unconjugated bilirubin to be reabsorbed (the enterohepatic circulation of bilirubin).

Bilirubin Toxicity

The exact mechanism by which bilirubin is toxic to cells is unknown. It is assumed that if the amount of lipid-soluble unconjugated bilirubin exceeds the available binding sites on albumin, unbound bilirubin will be available to enter neurons and damage them. The blood-brain barrier probably plays an important role in protecting an individual from brain damage, but its integrity is impossible to measure clinically. It is unknown whether a level of bilirubin exists above which brain damage always occurs even in a healthy individual.

The syndrome of bilirubin encephalopathy was well described in the era before exchange transfusion as treatment for Rh isoimmunization. The pathologic correlate is known as kernicterus, named for the yellow staining of the subthalamic nuclei (kerns) seen at autopsy. The symptoms of acute bilirubin encephalopathy consist of lethargy, hypotonia, and poor sucking, progressing to hypertonia, irritability, backward arching of the neck (retrocollis) and the trunk (opisthotonos), and a high-pitched cry. Chronic bilirubin encephalopathy includes athetoid cerebral palsy, sensorineural deafness, limitation of upward gaze, and dental dysplasia. Whether or not bilirubin causes more subtle neurologic abnormalities remains debatable.

Bilirubin encephalopathy is rare with current neonatal management; however, more than 120 cases have been reported to an informal registry since 1990. For decades, the strategy of keeping bilirubin under 20 mg/dL with phototherapy and exchange transfusion if needed eliminated kernicterus in the United States. The reappearance of kernicterus over the past decade has been ascribed to the increased prevalence of breast feeding along with earlier discharge of newborns (before adequate milk supply is established and before jaundice appears or peaks) without timely follow-up, and a failure to recognize, measure, investigate, and treat jaundice aggressively. It is now understood that there are common polymorphisms in the promoter region of the gene coding for UDPGT that significantly decrease this key enzyme activity. Subjects with Gilbert syndrome are homozygous for the variant promoter, with a prevalence of 9% in the population. An additional 40% of the population is heterozygous. The effects of this decreased enzyme activity are additive with other genetic (eg, glucose-6-phosphate dehydrogenase [G6PD] deficiency and hereditary spherocytosis) or nongenetic (eg, ABO incompatibility, increased enterohepatic circulation, and cephalhematoma) causes of increased bilirubin production or decreased excretion. It is possible, and even likely, that such genetic variations explain many cases of extreme hyperbilirubinemia, as well as the ethnic and racial differences seen in the incidence of severe neonatal jaundice.

The risk of bilirubin encephalopathy is probably very small for full-term infants without hemolysis even at bilirubin levels of 25 mg/dL (430 mmol/L). Premature infants are at increased risk because of associated illnesses that may affect the integrity of the blood-brain

barrier as well as reduced albumin levels. For this reason, a lower level of bilirubin is generally assumed to represent the "exchange level" in these infants and is usually determined based on the infant's birth weight, gestational age, and serum albumin level.

Causes of Unconjugated Hyperbilirubinemia

The causes of unconjugated hyperbilirubinemia can be grouped into two main categories: overproduction of bilirubin and decreased conjugation of bilirubin (Table 1–7).

Table 1–7. Causes of jaundice secondary to unconjugated hyperbilirubemia.

Overproduction of bilirubin
1. Increased rate of hemolysis (reticulocyte count elevated)
   a. Patients with a positive Coombs test
      ABO blood group incompatibility
      Rh incompatibility
      Other blood group sensitizations
   b. Patients with a negative Coombs test
      Abnormal red cell shapes
         Spherocytosis
         Elliptocytosis
         Pyknocytosis
         Stomatocytosis
      Red cell enzyme abnormalities
         Glucose-6-phosphate dehydrogenase deficiency
         Pyruvate kinase deficiency
         Hexokinase deficiency
         Other metabolic defects
   c. Patients with bacterial or viral sepsis
2. Nonhemolytic causes of increased bilirubin load (reticulocyte count normal)
   a. Extravascular hemorrhage
      Cephalhematoma
      Extensive bruising
      Central nervous system hemorrhage
   b. Polycythemia
   c. Exaggerated enterohepatic circulation of bilirubin
      Gastrointestinal tract obstruction
      Functional ileus
Decreased rate of conjugation
(Unconjugated bilirubin elevated, reticulocyte count normal)
   Physiologic jaundice
   Crigler-Najjar syndrome
      Type I glucuronyl transferase deficiency, autosomal-recessive
      Type II glucuronyl transferase deficiency, autosomal-dominant
   Gilbert syndrome
   ?Hypothyroidism

A. Increased Bilirubin Production

Increased production of bilirubin results from an increased rate of red blood cell destruction (hemolysis) due to the presence of maternal antibodies against fetal cells (Coombs test–positive), abnormal red cell membrane shape (ie, spherocytosis), or abnormal red cell enzymes (ie, G6PD deficiency). Antibodies can be directed against the major blood group antigens (the type A or type B infant of a type O mother) or the minor antigens (the Rh system: D, E, C, d, e, c, Kell, Duffy, and so on).

1. Antibody-mediated hemolysis (Coombs test-positive)—ABO blood group incompatibility is common, usually not severe, and can accompany any pregnancy in a type O mother. The severity is unpredictable because of variability in the amount of naturally occurring anti-A or anti-B IgG antibodies in the mother. Although 20% of pregnancies are the appropriate "set-ups" for ABO incompatibility (mother O, baby A or B), only about 33% of such infants are Coombs test–positive and only about 20% of these develop excessive jaundice that can be severe enough to require exchange transfusion. In addition to hyperbilirubinemia in the first days of life, these infants may become anemic over the first several weeks and may require transfusion at a few weeks of age.

Rh isoimmunization is much less common and increases in severity with each immunized pregnancy because of increased maternal IgG antibody production each time. Most Rh disease can be prevented by administering high-titer Rho (D) immune globulin to an Rh-negative woman after any invasive procedure during pregnancy as well as after miscarriage, abortion, or delivery of an Rh-positive infant. In severe cases, erythroblastosis fetalis (hydrops or generalized edema with heart failure related to severe anemia in the fetus) occurs and may cause fetal or neonatal death without appropriate antenatal intervention. In less severe cases, hemolysis is the main problem, with resultant hyperbilirubinemia and anemia. The cornerstone of antenatal management is transfusion of the fetus with Rh-negative cells, either directly into the umbilical vein via percutaneous cordocentesis or into the fetal abdominal cavity. Following delivery, phototherapy is usually started immediately, with exchange transfusion (see later discussion) as needed. A 0.5–1 g/kg dose of intravenous immune globulin (IVIG) given to the infant as soon after delivery as the diagnosis is made has been shown to decrease the need for exchange transfusion. Ongoing hemolysis will still occur until all maternal antibody is gone; therefore, these infants need to be followed carefully over the first 2 months of life for development of anemia severe enough to require transfusion.

2. Nonimmune hemolysis (Coombs test–negative)—Hereditary spherocytosis is the most common red cell membrane defect, resulting in hemolysis because of decreased red cell deformability. These infants may have hyperbilirubinemia severe enough to require exchange transfusion. Mild to moderate splenomegaly may be present. Diagnosis is suspected by peripheral blood smear and family history.

G6PD deficiency is the most common red cell enzyme defect resulting in hemolysis and should be suspected in infants of African, Mediterranean, or Asian descent, particularly when the onset of jaundice is later than usual. The importance of this enzyme deficiency in cases of severe neonatal jaundice has likely been underestimated. In most cases, no triggering agent is found, although those infants who develop severe jaundice with G6PD deficiency also are found to have Gilbert syndrome.

3. Nonhemolytic increased bilirubin production—Enclosed hemorrhage, such as cephalhematoma, intracranial hemorrhage, or extensive bruising in the skin, can lead to jaundice as the red blood cells are broken down and removed. Polycythemia leads to jaundice by increased red cell mass, with increased numbers of cells reaching senescence daily. Ileus, either paralytic or mechanical, related to a bowel obstruction, leads to increased enterohepatic circulation.

B. Decreased Rate of Conjugation

1. UDPGT deficiency (Crigler-Najjar syndrome type I [complete deficiency, autosomal recessive] and type II [partial deficiency, autosomal dominant])—These syndromes result from a mutation in the exon or encoding region of the gene for the enzyme UDPGT that causes complete or nearly complete absence of enzyme activity. Both are rare and cause severe unconjugated hyperbilirubinemia, bilirubin encephalopathy, and death without therapy. In type II, the enzyme can be induced with phenobarbital, which may lower bilirubin levels by 30–80%. There is no cure, although phototherapy and liver transplantation prolong survival in type I.

2. Gilbert syndrome—This syndrome is a mild autosomal dominant disorder affecting 9% of the population. It is characterized by decreased hepatic UDPGT levels, resulting from a genetic polymorphism affecting the promoter region of the UDPGT gene. Affected individuals have a greater propensity, in the presence of other icterogenic factors such as G6PD deficiency, hereditary spherocytosis, or other factors that increase bilirubin production, to develop hyperbilirubinemia. They may also be more likely to have prolonged neonatal jaundice.

C. Hyperbilirubinemia Caused by Unknown or Multiple Factors

1. Physiologic jaundice—The contributing factors to physiologic jaundice include UDPGT inactivity at birth, a relatively high red cell mass even in the non-

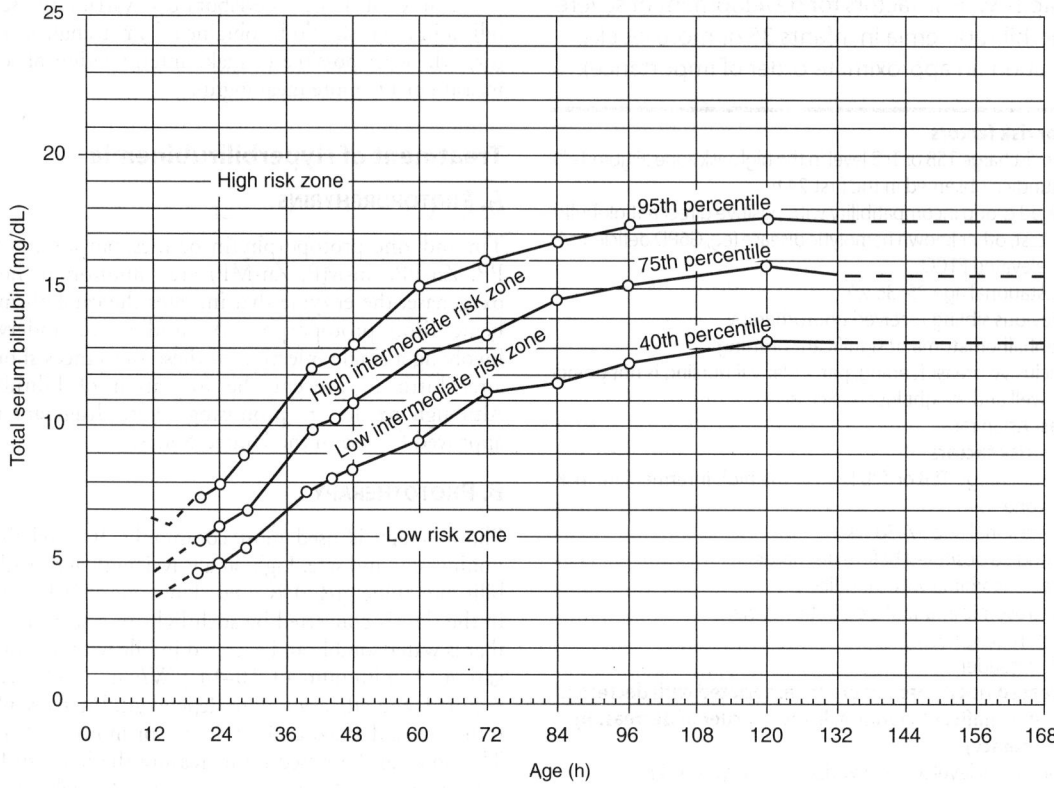

Figure 1–2. Risk designation of full-term and near-term newborns based on their hour-specific bilirubin values. (Reproduced, with permission, from Bhutani VK et al: Predictive ability of a predischarge hour-specific serum bilirubin test for subsequent significant hyperbilirubinemia in healthy term and near-term newborns. Pediatrics 1999;103:6.)

nearly 80% of the sensitized or abnormal red blood cells and offending antibody so that ongoing hemolysis will be decreased. The procedure is invasive and not without risk. The risk of mortality is 1–5% and is greatest in the smallest, most immature, and otherwise unstable infants, but sudden death during the procedure can occur in any infant. Risk of serious complications such as necrotizing enterocolitis (NEC), infection, electrolyte disturbances, or thrombocytopenia is 5–10%. Because of the rarity of the procedure and its inherent risk, it should be performed very cautiously, preferably at a referral center. Albumin 1 g/kg can be given first to aid in binding and removal of bilirubin. IVIG 0.5–1.0 g/kg should be given in cases of severe antibody-mediated hemolysis.

American Academy of Pediatrics Subcommittee on Hyperbilirubinemia: Clinical practice guideline: management of hyperbilirubinemia in the newborn infant 35 or more weeks of gestation. Pediatrics 2004;114:297 [PMID: 15231951].

Bhutani VK et al: Diagnosis and management of hyperbilirubinemia in the term neonate: for a safer first week. Pediatr Clin North Am 2004;51:843 [PMID: 15275978].

Dennery PA et al: Neonatal hyperbilirubinemia. N Engl J Med 2001;344:581 [PMID: 11207355].

Gottstein R, Cooke RWI: Systematic review of intravenous immunoglobulin in hemolytic disease of the newborn. Arch Dis Child Fetal Neonatal Ed 2003;88:F6 [PMID: 12496219].

Johnson LH, Bhutani VK: System-based approach to management of neonatal jaundice and prevention of kernicterus. J Pediatr 2002;140:396 [PMID: 12006952].

Kaplan M et al: Bilirubin genetics for the nongeneticist: Hereditary defects of neonatal bilirubin conjugation. Pediatrics 2003;111:886 [PMID: 12671128].

Shapiro SM: Definition of the clinical spectrum of kernicterus and bilirubin-induced neurologic dysfunction (BIND). J Perinatol 2005;25:54 [PMID: 15578034].

Vreman HJ et al: Phototherapy: current methods and future directions. Semin Perinatol 2004;28:326 [PMID: 15686263]

Watchko JF: Vigintiphobia revisited. Pediatrics 2005;115:1747 [PMID: 15930239].

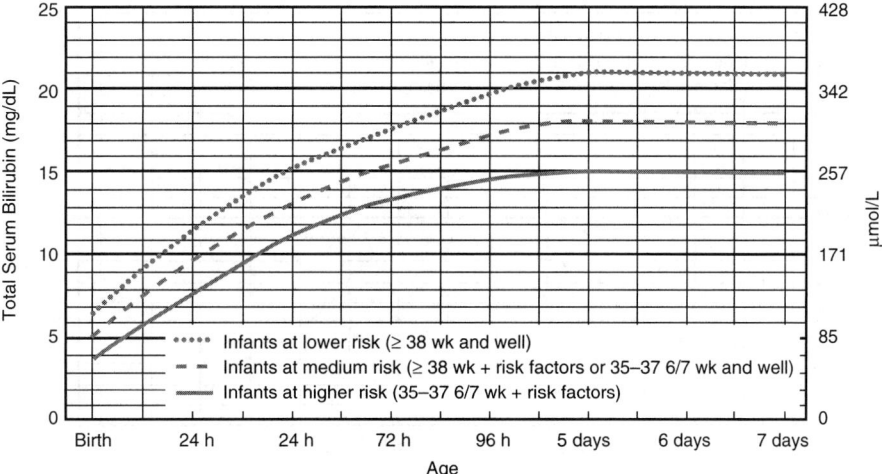

- Use total bilirubin. Do not subtract direct reacting or conjugated bilirubin.
- Risk factors = isoimmune hemolytic disease, G6PD deficiency, asphyxia, significant lethargy, temperature instability, sepsis, acidosis, or albumin < 3.0 g/dL (if measured).
- For well infants 35–37 6/7 wk can adjust TSB levels for intervention around the medium risk line. It is an option to intervene at lower TSB levels for infants closer to 35 wks and at higher TSB levels for those closer to 37 6/7 wk.
- It is an option to provide conventional phototherapy in hospital or at home at TSB levels 2–3 mg/dL (35–50 mmol/L) below those shown but home phototherapy should not be used in any infant with risk factors.

Figure 1–3. Guidelines for phototherapy in hospitalized infants of 35 or more weeks' gestation. These guidelines are based on limited evidence and levels shown are approximations. The guidelines refer to the use of intensive phototherapy (at least 30 μW/cm² in the blue-green spectrum) which should be used when the total serum bilirubin exceeds the line indicated for each category. If total serum bilirubin approaches the exchange level, the sides of the incubator or bassinet should be lined with aluminum foil or white material. (Reproduced, with permission, from the AAP Subcommittee on Hyperbilirubinemia: Management of hyperbilirubinemia in the newborn infant 35 or more weeks of gestation. Pediatrics 2004;114:297.)

HYPOGLYCEMIA

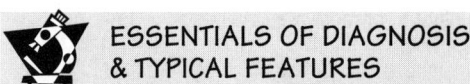

ESSENTIALS OF DIAGNOSIS & TYPICAL FEATURES

- *Defined as blood glucose < 40–45 mg/dL.*
- *LGA, SGA, preterm, and stressed infants at risk.*
- *May be asymptomatic.*
- *Infants can present with lethargy, poor feeding, irritability, or seizures.*

General Considerations

Blood glucose concentration in the fetus is approximately 15 mg/dL less than the maternal glucose con-centration. Glucose concentration normally decreases in the immediate postnatal period, with concentrations below 40–45 mg/dL being considered indicative of hypoglycemia. By 3 hours, the glucose concentration in normal full-term babies stabilizes between 50 and 80 mg/dL. The two most commonly encountered groups of full-term newborn infants at high risk for neonatal hypoglycemia are IDMs and IUGR infants.

Infants of Diabetic Mothers

The IDM has abundant glucose stores in the form of glycogen and fat but develops hypoglycemia because of hyperinsulinemia induced by maternal and fetal hyperglycemia. Other tissues grow abnormally in utero, probably as a consequence of increased flow of nutrients from the maternal circulation. The result is a macrosomic infant at increased risk for trauma during deliv-

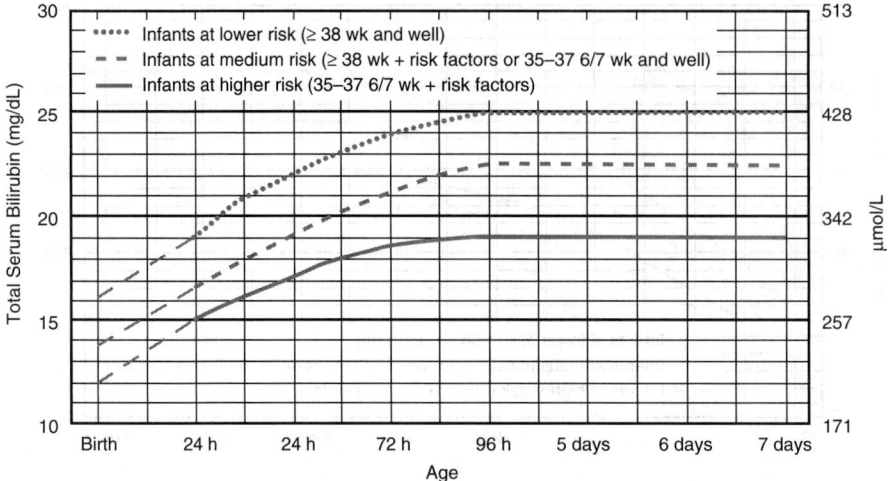

- The dashed lines for the first 24 hours indicate uncertainty due to a wide range of clinical circumstances and a range of responses to phototherapy.
- Immediate exchange transfusion is recommended if infant shows signs of acute bilirubin encephalopathy (hypertonia, arching, retrocolitis, opisthotonos, fever, high pitched cry) or if TSB is ≥ 5 mg/dL (85 µmol/L) above these lines.
- Risk factors—isoimmune hemolytic disease, G6PD deficiency, asphyxia, significant lethargy, temperature instability, sepsis, acidosis.
- Measure serum albumin and calculate B/A ratio (see legend).
- Use total bilirubin. Do not subtract direct reading or conjugated bilirubin.
- If infant is well and 35–37 6/7 wk (median risk) can individualize TSB levels for exchange based on actual gestational age.

Figure 1–4. Guidelines for exchange transfusion in infants 35 or more weeks' gestation. These guidelines represent approximations for which an exchange transfusion is indicated in infants treated with intensive phototherapy. For readmitted infants, if the total serum bilirubin level is above the exchange level, repeat total serum bilirubin measurement every 2–3 hours and consider exchange if the total serum bilirubin remains above the level after 6 hours of intensive phototherapy. The total serum bilirubin/albumin ratio (total serum bilirubin mg/dL/Alb g/dL 8.0 for infants at lower risk, 7.2 for medium risk, and 6.8 for higher risk) can be used together with, but not in lieu of the total serum bilirubin level as an additional factor in determining the need for transfusion. If the total serum bilirubin is at or approaching exchange level, send blood for an immediate type and crossmatch. (Reproduced, with permission, from the AAP Subcommittee on Hyperbilirubinemia: Management of hyperbilirubinemia in the newborn infant 35 or more weeks of gestation. Pediatrics 2004;114:297.)

ery. Other problems related to the in-utero metabolic environment include cardiomyopathy (asymmetrical septal hypertrophy), which can present as a murmur with or without cardiac failure and respiratory distress, and, more rarely, microcolon, which presents as low intestinal obstruction. Infants whose mothers are diabetic at conception are at increased risk for congenital anomalies probably related to first-trimester glucose control. Other neonatal problems include hypercoagulable state and polycythemia, a combination that predisposes the infant to large venous thromboses (eg, renal vein thrombosis). Finally, these infants are some-

what immature for their gestational age and are at increased risk for hyaline membrane disease, hypocalcemia, and hyperbilirubinemia.

Intrauterine Growth Restricted Infants

The IUGR infant has reduced glucose stores in the form of glycogen and body fat and therefore is prone to hypoglycemia despite relatively appropriate endocrine adjustments at birth. In addition to hypoglycemia, marked hyperglycemia and a transient diabetes mellitus–like syndrome may occasionally develop, particularly in the very premature SGA infant. These problems can usually be handled by adjusting glucose intake, though insulin is sometimes needed transiently. Some IUGR infants also have hyperinsulinemia that persists for a week or more.

Other Causes of Hypoglycemia

Hypoglycemia occurs with disorders associated with islet cell hyperplasia (Beckwith-Wiedemann syndrome [macroglossia, omphalocele, and macrosomia], erythroblastosis fetalis, genetic forms of hyperinsulinism, inborn errors of metabolism [glycogen storage disease and galactosemia], and endocrine disorders [panhypopituitarism and other deficiencies of counterregulatory hormones]). It may also occur as a complication of birth asphyxia, hypoxia, or other stresses, including bacterial and viral sepsis. Premature infants are also at risk for hypoglycemia because of decreased glycogen stores.

Clinical Findings

The signs of hypoglycemia in the newborn infant may be nonspecific or subtle: lethargy, poor feeding, irritability, tremulousness, jitteriness, apnea, and seizures. Hypoglycemia is most severe and resistant to treatment if due to hyperinsulinemia. Cardiac failure may occur in severe cases, particularly in IDMs with cardiomyopathy. Hypoglycemia in hyperinsulinemic states can develop very quickly (within the first 30–60 minutes of life).

Blood glucose can be measured by heelstick using a bedside glucometer. All infants at risk should be screened, including IDMs, IUGR infants, premature infants, and any infant with symptoms that could be due to hypoglycemia. All low or borderline values should be confirmed by direct measurement of blood glucose concentration in the clinical laboratory. It is important to continue surveillance of glucose concentration until the baby has been on full enteral feedings without intravenous supplementation for 24 hours. Relapse of hypoglycemia thereafter is unlikely.

Infants with hypoglycemia requiring IV glucose infusions for more than 5 days should be evaluated for less common disorders. This work-up should include evaluation for inborn errors of metabolism, hyperinsulinemic states, and deficiencies of counterregulatory hormones.

Treatment

Therapy is based on provision of glucose either enterally or intravenously. Table 1–10 presents suggested treatment guidelines. In hyperinsulinemic states, boluses of glucose should be avoided and a higher glucose infusion rate used. After initial correction with a bolus of $D_{10}W$, 2 mL/kg, glucose infusion should be increased gradually as needed from a starting rate of 6 mg/kg/min. Finally, in both IDMs and IUGR infants, those with high hematocrits and hypoglycemia are most likely to show clinical signs of hypoglycemia. In such infants,

Table 1–10. Hypoglycemia: suggested therapeutic regimens.

Screening Test[a]	Presence of Symptoms	Action
20–45 mg/dL	No symptoms of hypoglycemia	Draw blood glucose;[b] if the infant is alert and vigorous, feed; follow with frequent glucose monitoring. If the baby continues to have blood glucose < 40–45 mg/dL or is unable to feed, provide intravenous glucose at 6 mg/kg/min ($D_{10}W$ at 3.6 mL/kg/h).
< 45 mg/dL	Symptoms of hypoglycemia present	Draw blood glucose;[b] provide bolus of $D_{10}W$ (2 mL/kg) followed by an infusion of 6 mg/kg/min (3.6 mL/kg/h).
< 20 mg/dL	With or without symptoms of hypoglycemia	Draw blood glucose;[b] provide bolus of $D_{10}W$ followed by an infusion of 6 mg/kg/min. If intravenous access cannot be obtained immediately, an umbilical vein line should be used.

[a]Rapid bedside determination.
[b]Laboratory confirmation.

both the hypoglycemia and the polycythemia should be treated—with IV glucose infusion and partial exchange transfusion, respectively.

Prognosis

The prognosis of hypoglycemia is good if therapy is prompt. CNS sequelae are seen in infants with neonatal seizures resulting from hypoglycemia and are more likely in neonates with persistent hyperinsulinemic hypoglycemia. Hypoglycemia may also potentiate brain injury after perinatal depression and should be avoided.

Cornblath M et al: Controversies regarding definition of neonatal hypoglycemia: Suggested operational thresholds. Pediatrics 2000;105:1141 [PMID: 10790476].

Cowett RM: Neonatal care of the infant of the diabetic mother. Neoreviews 2002;3:e190.

Fourtner SH, Stanley CA: Genetic and nongenetic forms of hyper-insulinism in neonates. NeoReviews 2004;5:e370.

Hussain K, Aynsley-Green A: The effect of prematurity and intra-uterine growth restriction on glucose metabolism in the new-born. NeoReviews 2004;5:e365.

Kahler SG: Metabolic disorders associated with neonatal hypogly-cemia. NeoReviews 2004;5:e377.

Menni F et al: Neurologic outcomes of 90 neonates and infants with persistent hyperinsulinemic hypoglycemia. Pediatrics 2001;107:476 [PMID: 11230585].

Nold JL, Georgieff MK: Infants of diabetic mothers. Pediatr Clin North Am 2004;51:619 [PMID: 15157588].

Salhab WA et al: Initial hypoglycemia and neonatal brain injury in term infants with severe fetal acidemia. Pediatrics 2004;114:361 [PMID: 15286217].

Sperling MA, Menon RK: Differential diagnosis and management of neonatal hypoglycemia. Pediatr Clin North Am 2004;51:703 [PMID: 15157593].

RESPIRATORY DISTRESS IN THE TERM NEWBORN INFANT

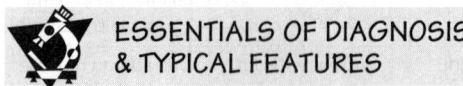

ESSENTIALS OF DIAGNOSIS & TYPICAL FEATURES

- *Tachypnea, respiratory rate > 60 breaths/min.*
- *Retractions (intercostal, sternal).*
- *Expiratory grunting.*
- *Cyanosis on room air.*

General Considerations

Respiratory distress is among the most common symptom complexes seen in the newborn infant. It may result from both noncardiopulmonary and cardiopulmonary causes (Table 1–11). Chest radiography, arterial blood gases, and pulse oximetry are useful in assessing both the cause and the severity of the problem. It is important to consider the noncardiopulmonary causes listed in Table 1–11 because the natural tendency is to focus on the heart and lungs. Most of the noncardiopulmonary causes can be ruled out by the history, physical examination, and a few simple laboratory tests. The evaluation of cardiovascular disorders is discussed in a subsequent section.

The most common pulmonary causes of respiratory distress in the full-term infant are transient tachypnea, aspiration syndromes, congenital pneumonia, and air leaks.

A. TRANSIENT TACHYPNEA (RETAINED FETAL LUNG FLUID)

Respiratory distress is typically present from birth, usually associated with a mild to moderate oxygen require-

Table 1–11. Causes of respiratory distress in the newborn.

Noncardiopulmonary
Hypothermia or hyperthermia
Hypoglycemia
Polycythemia
Metabolic acidosis
Drug intoxications or withdrawal
Insult to the central nervous system
Asphyxia
Hemorrhage
Neuromuscular disease
Phrenic nerve injury
Asphyxiating thoracic dystrophy
Cardiovascular
Left-sided outflow tract obstruction
Hypoplastic left heart
Aortic stenosis
Coarctation of the aorta
Cyanotic lesions
Transposition of the great vessels
Total anomalous pulmonary venous return
Tricuspid atresia
Right-sided outflow obstruction
Pulmonary
Upper airway obstruction
Choanal atresia
Vocal cord paralysis
Lingual thyroid
Meconium aspiration
Clear fluid aspiration
Transient tachypnea
Pneumonia
Pulmonary hypoplasia
Hyaline membrane disease
Pneumothorax
Pleural effusions
Mass lesions
Lobar emphysema
Cystic adenomatoid malformation

Reproduced, with permission, from Rosenberg AA: Neonatal adaptation. In Gabbe SG et al (editors): *Obstetrics: Normal and Problem Pregnancies.* Churchill Livingstone, 1996.

ment (25–50% O_2). The infant may be full-term or near-term, nonasphyxiated, and born following a short labor or cesarean section without labor. Chest radiograph shows perihilar streaking and fluid in interlobar fissures. Resolution usually occurs within 12–24 hours.

B. ASPIRATION SYNDROMES

The infant is typically full-term or near-term, frequently with some fetal distress prior to delivery or depression at delivery. Blood or meconium is usually present in the amniotic fluid, but occasionally the fluid is clear. Respiratory distress is present from birth, in many cases manifested by a barrel chest appearance and coarse breath sounds. An increasing O_2 need from pneumonitis may require intubation and ventilation. Chest radiograph shows coarse irregular infiltrates, hyperexpansion, and in the worst cases, lobar consolidation. In some cases, secondary surfactant deficiency can ensue, with progression to a diffuse homogeneous infiltrate pattern.

When amniotic fluid contains meconium or blood, suctioning the infant's mouth and nose as the head is delivered and before delivery of the chest is no longer recommended to prevent aspiration. If the infant is not vigorous at birth, suctioning of the trachea under direct vision is recommended, especially before commencing resuscitation with positive-pressure ventilation (PPV). Although this procedure is recommended, it will not prevent all cases of meconium or blood aspiration. Aspiration often occurs in utero as the stressed infant gasps. Babies who aspirate are at risk of air leak (pneumothorax) because of uneven aeration with segmental overdistention and are at risk for persistent pulmonary hypertension (see section on Cardiac Problems).

C. CONGENITAL PNEUMONIA

Infants may be of any gestational age, with or without a maternal history of prolonged rupture of membranes, chorioamnionitis, or maternal antibiotic administration. Respiratory distress may begin at birth or may be delayed for several hours. The chest radiograph may resemble that of retained lung fluid or hyaline membrane disease; rarely, there may be a lobar infiltrate.

The lungs are the most common site of infection in the neonate. Infections usually ascend from the genital tract before or during labor, with the vaginal or rectal flora the most likely agents (group B streptococci, *Escherichia coli*, and *Klebsiella*). Shock, poor perfusion, absolute neutropenia (< 2000/mL), and elevated C-reactive protein provide corroborating evidence for pneumonia. Gram stain of tracheal aspirate may be helpful. Because no signs or laboratory findings confirm the presence or absence of pneumonia with certainty, all infants with respiratory distress should have blood cultured and receive broad-spectrum antibiotic therapy (ampicillin 100 mg/kg in two divided doses and gentamicin 4 mg/kg q24h or 2.5 mg/kg q12h) until the diagnosis of bacterial infection can be ruled out.

D. SPONTANEOUS PNEUMOTHORAX

Respiratory distress (primarily tachypnea) is present from birth, typically not severe, and requires mild to moderate supplemental O_2. Breath sounds may be decreased on the affected side; heart tones may be shifted toward the opposite side and may be distant. Chest radiograph will show pneumothorax or pneumomediastinum.

This entity occurs in 1% of all deliveries. Risk is increased by manipulations such as PPV in the delivery room. Treatment usually consists of supplemental O_2 and watchful waiting. Breathing 100% O_2 for a few hours may accelerate reabsorption of extrapulmonary gas by creating a diffusion gradient for nitrogen across the surface of the lung (nitrogen washout technique). This is effective only if the infant was breathing room air or O_2 at low concentration at the time of the pneumothorax. Drainage by needle thoracentesis or tube thoracostomy is occasionally required. A small increased risk of renal abnormalities is associated with spontaneous pneumothorax; therefore, a careful physical examination of the kidneys and observation of urine output are indicated. If pulmonary hypoplasia with pneumothorax is suspected, renal ultrasound would also be indicated.

E. OTHER PULMONARY CAUSES

Other pulmonary causes of respiratory distress are fairly rare. Bilateral choanal atresia should be suspected if there is no air movement when the infant breathes through the nose. These infants at delivery have good color and heart rate while crying but become cyanotic and bradycardiac when they quiet down and resume normal nasal breathing. Other causes of upper airway obstruction are usually characterized by some degree of stridor or poor air movement despite good respiratory effort. Pleural effusions can be suspected in hydropic infants (eg, those with erythroblastosis fetalis or nonimmune hydrops). Space-occupying lesions cause a shift of the mediastinum and asymmetrical breath sounds and would be apparent on chest radiograph.

Treatment

Whatever the cause, the cornerstone of treatment of neonatal respiratory distress is provision of supplemental oxygen to maintain a PaO_2 of 60–70 mm Hg and a saturation by pulse oximetry (SpO_2) of 92–96%. PaO_2 levels less than 50 mm Hg are associated with pulmonary vasoconstriction, which can exacerbate hypoxemia, whereas those greater than 100 mm Hg may increase the risk of oxygen toxicity without additional benefit. Oxygen should be warmed, humidified, and delivered through an air blender. Concentration should be measured with a calibrated oxygen analyzer. An umbilical or peripheral arterial line should be considered in any infant requiring more than 45% FiO_2 by 4–6 hours of life to allow frequent blood gas determinations. Noninvasive monitoring with pulse oximetry should be used.

Other supportive treatment includes IV provision of glucose and water. Unless infection can be unequivocally ruled out, blood cultures should be obtained and broad-spectrum antibiotics started. Volume expansion (normal saline) can be given in infusions of 10 mL/kg over 30 minutes for low blood pressure, poor perfusion, and metabolic acidosis. Sodium bicarbonate (1–2 mEq/kg) is indicated for treatment of documented metabolic acidosis unresponsive to initial oxygen, ventilation, and volume. Specific work-up should be pursued as indicated by the history and physical findings. In most cases, a chest radiographic study, blood gas measurements, CBC, and blood glucose allow a diagnosis.

Intubation and ventilation should be undertaken for signs of respiratory failure (PaO_2 < 60 mm Hg in 60–80% FIO_2, $PaCO_2$ > 60 mm Hg, or repeated apnea). Peak pressures should be adequate to produce chest wall expansion and audible breath sounds (usually 18–24 cm H_2O). Positive end-expiratory pressure (4–6 cm H_2O) should also be used. Ventilation rates of 20–50 breaths/min are usually required. The goal is to maintain a PaO_2 of 60–70 mm Hg and a $PaCO_2$ of 45–55 mm Hg.

Prognosis

Most respiratory conditions affecting the full-term infant are acute and resolve in the first several days. Meconium aspiration and congenital pneumonia are associated with significant long-term pulmonary morbidity (chronic lung disease) and mortality in approximately 10–20%. Mortality rates in these disorders have been reduced by use of high-frequency oscillatory ventilation, inhaled nitric oxide for pulmonary hypertension, and extracorporeal membrane oxygenation (ECMO).

Aly H: Respiratory disorders in the newborn: identification and diagnosis. Pediatr Rev 2004;25:201 [PMID: 15173453].

Flidel-Raman O, Shinwell ES: Respiratory distress in the term and near-term infant. NeoReviews 2005;6:e289.

Ross MG: Meconium aspiration syndrome—more than intrapartum meconium. N Engl J Med 2005;353:946 [PMID: 16135842].

Sasidharan P: An approach to diagnosis and management of cyanosis and tachypnea in term infants. Pediatr Clin North Am 2004;51:999 [PMID: 15275985].

HEART MURMURS (See Also Section on Cardiac Problems)

Heart murmurs are common in the first days of life and do not usually signify structural heart problems. If a murmur is present at birth, however, it should be considered a valvular problem until proved otherwise because the common benign transitional murmurs (eg, patent ductus arteriosus) are not audible until minutes to hours after birth.

If an infant is pink, well-perfused, and in no respiratory distress and has palpable and symmetrical pulses (right brachial pulse no stronger than the femoral pulse), the murmur is most likely transitional. Transitional murmurs are soft (grade 1–3/6), heard at the left upper to midsternal border, and generally loudest during the first 24 hours. If the murmur persists beyond 24 hours, blood pressure in the right arm and a leg should be determined. If there is a difference of more than 15 mm Hg (arm > leg) or if the pulses in the lower extremities are difficult to appreciate, cardiology consultation should be arranged to evaluate for coarctation of the aorta. If there is no difference, the infant can be discharged home with follow-up in 2–3 days for auscultation and evaluation for signs of congestive failure. If signs of failure or cyanosis are present, the infant should be referred for evaluation without delay. If the murmur persists without these signs, the infant can be referred for elective evaluation at age 2–4 weeks. Some centers now recommend routine pulse oximetry screening in the nursery to identify infants with congenital heart disease, with a saturation < 95% at sea level triggering an echocardiogram. Further studies will need to be performed to document the accuracy, specificity, and cost-effectiveness of this technique.

Frommelt MA: Differential diagnosis and approach to a heart murmur in term infants. Pediatr Clin North Am 2004;51:1023 [PMID: 15331284].

Koppel RI et al: Effectiveness of pulse oximetry screening for congenital heart disease in asymptomatic newborns. Pediatrics 2003;111:451 [PMID: 12612220].

Reich JD et al: The use of pulse oximetry to detect congenital heart disease. J Pediatr 2003;142:268 [PMID: 12640374].

BIRTH TRAUMA

Most birth trauma is associated with difficult delivery, particularly with a large infant, abnormal position, or fetal distress requiring rapid extraction. The most common injuries are soft tissue bruising, fractures (clavicle, humerus, or femur), and cervical plexus palsies, although skull fractures, intracranial hemorrhage (primarily subdural and subarachnoid), and cervical spinal cord injuries can also occur.

Fractures are often diagnosed by the obstetrician, who may feel and hear a snap during delivery. Clavicular fractures may cause decreased spontaneous movement of the arm, with tenderness and crepitus over the area. Humeral or femoral fractures may cause tenderness and swelling over the shaft with a diaphyseal fracture, with limited spontaneous extremity motion in all cases. Epiphyseal fractures are harder to diagnose radiographically owing to the cartilaginous nature of the epiphysis. After 8–10 days, callus appears and is visible on radiographs. Treatment in all cases is gentle handling, with immobilization for 8–10 days: the humerus against the chest with elbow flexed; the femur with a posterior splint from below the knee to the buttock.

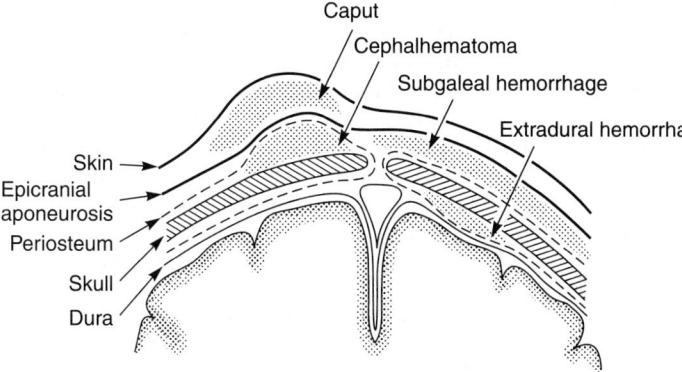

Figure 1–5. Sites of extracranial bleeding in the newborn. (Adapted and reproduced, with permission, from Pape KE, Wigglesworth JS: *Haemorrhage Ischemia and the Perinatal Brain.* JB Lippincott, 1979.)

Brachial plexus injuries may result from traction as the head is pulled away from the shoulder during delivery. Injury to the C5–C6 roots is most common and results in Erb-Duchenne paralysis. The arm is limp, adducted, and internally rotated, extended and pronated at the elbow, and flexed at the wrist (so-called waiter's tip posture). Grasp is present. If the lower nerve roots (C8–T1) are involved, the hand is flaccid (Klumpke palsy). Isolated involvement of these roots is rare. If the entire plexus is injured, the arm and hand are flaccid, with an associated sensory deficit.

Early treatment for brachial plexus injury is conservative, because function usually returns over several weeks. Referral should be made to a physical therapist so that parents can be instructed on range-of-motion exercises, splinting, and further evaluation if needed. Return of function begins in the deltoid and biceps, with recovery by 3 months in most cases.

Spinal cord injury can occur at birth, especially in difficult breech extractions with hyperextension of the neck, or in midforceps rotations when the body fails to turn with the head. Infants are flaccid, quadriplegic, and without respiratory efforts at birth, although facial movements are preserved. The long-term outlook for such infants is grim.

Facial nerve palsy is sometimes associated with forceps use but more often results from in-utero pressure of the baby's head against the mother's sacrum. The infant has asymmetrical mouth movements and eye closure with poor movement on the affected side. Most cases resolve spontaneously within a few days to weeks.

Subgaleal hemorrhage into the large potential space under the scalp (Figure 1–5) is associated with difficult vaginal deliveries and repeated attempts at vacuum extraction. It can lead to hypovolemic shock and death from ongoing blood loss and severe coagulopathy triggered by both consumption of clotting factors and release of thromboplastin from accompanying brain injury. This is an emergency requiring rapid replacement of blood and clotting factors.

Gardella C et al: The effect of sequential use of vacuum and forceps for assisted vaginal delivery on neonatal and maternal outcomes. Am J Obstet Gynecol 2001;185:896 [PMID: 11641674].

Rosenberg AA: Traumatic birth injuries. Neoreviews 2003;4:e270.

Towner D et al: Effect of mode of delivery in nulliparous women on neonatal intracranial injury. N Engl J Med 1999;341:1709 [PMID: 10580069].

Uhring MR: Management of birth injuries. Clin Perinatol 2005; 32:19 [PMID: 15777819].

INFANTS OF MOTHERS WHO ABUSE DRUGS

The problem of newborn infants born to mothers who abuse drugs is increasing in all communities. The drugs most commonly abused are tobacco, alcohol, marijuana, and cocaine. Because these mothers may abuse many drugs and give an unreliable history of drug usage, it may be difficult to pinpoint which drug is causing the morbidity seen in a newborn infant. Early hospital discharge makes discovery of these infants based on physical findings and abnormal behavior much more difficult.

1. Cocaine

Cocaine is currently the most commonly abused hard drug, identified in up to 20–40% of infants on urban delivery services by anonymous screening of urine or meconium; moreover, cocaine is often used in association with other drugs. The obstetric effects include maternal hypertension, decreased uterine blood flow, fetal hypoxemia, and uterine contractions. The rates of stillbirth, placental abruption, and preterm delivery are increased two- to fourfold over rates for nonusers, and IUGR is increased two- to fourfold over that for nonusers. Methamphetamines cause similar problems. In high-risk populations (no prenatal care, placental abruptions, and preterm labor), urine toxicology screens should be performed in mothers and infants. Analysis of meconium enhances diagnosis by indicating cumulative drug use prior to delivery.

As with other illegal drugs, cocaine may have long-term neurobehavioral effects, but multiple drug use and environmental factors preclude assigning specific effects to cocaine with certainty. The risk of SIDS is increased three to seven times over the risk in nonusers (0.5–1% of exposed infants), but may be lessened by supine infant positioning.

2. Opioids

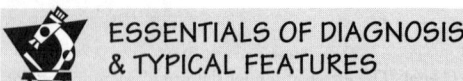

ESSENTIALS OF DIAGNOSIS & TYPICAL FEATURES

- Irritability, hyperactivity, incessant hunger, and salivation.
- Vomiting, diarrhea, excessive weight loss.
- Tremors, seizures.
- Nasal stuffiness, sneezing.
- Often IUGR.

Clinical Findings

The withdrawal signs in infants born to mothers who are addicted to heroin or who have been in methadone maintenance programs are similar. The clinical findings in infants born to methadone-maintained mothers may actually be more severe and prolonged than those seen with heroin. Clinical manifestations begin usually within 1–2 days. The clinical picture is typical enough to suggest a diagnosis even if a maternal history of drug abuse has not been obtained. Confirmation should be attempted with urine toxicology, but results will be negative unless the last drug dose was taken within a few days before delivery. Meconium can also be tested for illicit drugs and is more likely to be positive because the substances accumulate throughout pregnancy.

Treatment

Careful observation of the infant is a requirement. If opioid abuse or withdrawal is suspected, the baby is not a candidate for early discharge. Supportive treatment includes swaddling the infant and providing a quiet, dimly-lit environment. In general, specific treatment should be avoided unless the infant has severe symptoms or excessive weight loss. No single drug has been uniformly effective, and the first choice varies among nurseries. The drugs that have been used include phe-

nobarbital at an initial loading dose of 10–20 mg/kg IM, followed by a maintenance dose of 5 mg/kg/d in two divided doses, usually given orally. Opioids, diazepam, and clonidine have also been used, although the present authors prefer phenobarbital for irritability alone because of its safety and predictability. If diarrhea and weight loss are prominent findings, or if adequate control of symptoms has not been achieved, tincture of opium (25-fold dilution to 0.4 mg/mL morphine equivalent; 0.1 mL/kg q4h to start) titrated to improve symptoms, or methadone 0.05–0.1 mg/kg q6h will be more beneficial than phenobarbital alone. Treatment can be tapered over several days to a week. Both handling and procedures in the nursery should be kept to a minimum. It is also important to review maternal tests for syphilis, HIV, hepatitis B, and gonorrhea, as all are common in women who use cocaine or opiates.

Prognosis

These infants demonstrate long-term neurobehavioral handicaps. However, it is difficult to distinguish the effects of in-utero drug exposure from those of environmental influences during upbringing. Infants of opioid abusers have a four- to fivefold increased risk of SIDS.

3. Alcohol

The legal substances alcohol and tobacco have much greater effects on perinatal outcome than any illicit substances. Alcohol is the only recreational drug of abuse that is clearly teratogenic and is the most common preventable cause of mental retardation. The effects of alcohol on the fetus and the newborn are roughly proportionate to the degree of ethanol abuse, but there is no established safe dose. Fetal growth and development are adversely affected, and infants can experience withdrawal similar to that associated with maternal opioid abuse. Features observed are listed in Table 1–12. Clinical features of fetal alcohol syndrome (FAS) are often not obvious in the newborn period.

Children with full-blown FAS demonstrate postnatal growth deficiency and mild to moderate mental retardation. Those with lesser effects are at increased risk for attention-deficit/hyperactivity disorder and subtle developmental delays.

4. Tobacco Smoking

Smoking has been shown to have a negative effect on the growth rate of the fetus. The more the mother smokes, the greater the degree of IUGR. There is a twofold increase in low birth weight even in light smokers (< 10 cigarettes/day). Smoking during pregnancy has been associated with mild neurodevelopmental handicaps. The possible effects of multiple drug abuse apply

Table 1–12. Features observed in fetal alcohol syndrome in the newborn.

Craniofacial
Short palpebral fissures
Short, upturned nose
Flat midface
Thin vermillion of upper lip
Flattened philtrum
Growth
Prenatal and postnatal growth deficiency (small for gestational age, failure to thrive)
Central nervous system
Microcephaly
Partial or complete agenesis of the corpus callosum
Optic nerve hypoplasia
Hypotonia, poor feeding

to this category as well, and the potential interaction of multiple factors on fetal growth and development must be considered.

5. Toluene Embryopathy

Solvent abuse (paint, lacquer, or glue sniffing) is relatively common. The active organic solvent in these agents is toluene. Features attributable to in-utero toluene exposure include prematurity, IUGR, microcephaly, craniofacial abnormalities similar to those associated with in-utero alcohol exposure (Table 1–12), nail hypoplasia, and renal anomalies. Long-term effects include postnatal growth deficiency and developmental delay.

6. Marijuana

Marijuana is the most frequently used illegal drug. It does not appear to be teratogenic, and although a mild abstinence-type syndrome has been described, infants exposed to marijuana in utero rarely require treatment. Some long-term neurodevelopmental problems, particularly disordered sleep patterns, have been noted.

7. Other Drugs

Drugs and their effects on the newborn should be considered in two categories. In the first are drugs to which the fetus is exposed because of the mother's exposure. In many cases these are drugs prescribed for therapy of maternal conditions. The human placenta is relatively permeable, particularly to lipophilic solutes. Whenever possible, maternal drug therapy should be postponed until after the first trimester. Drugs with potential fetal toxicity include antineoplastics, antithyroid agents, benzodiazepines, warfarin, lithium, angiotensin-converting enzyme inhibitors (eg, captopril and enalapril), and immunosuppressants.

In the second category are drugs the infant acquires from the mother during breast feeding. Most drugs taken by the mother at this time achieve some concentrations in breast milk, although they usually do not present a problem to the infant. If the drug is one that could have adverse effects on the baby, timing breast feeding to coincide with trough concentrations in the mother may be useful. The AAP (see second reference in the following list) has reviewed drugs contraindicated in the breast-feeding mother.

American Academy of Pediatrics Committee on Drugs: Neonatal drug withdrawal. Pediatrics 1998;101:1079 [PMID: 9614425].

American Academy of Pediatrics Committee on Drugs: The transfer of drugs and other chemicals into human milk. Pediatrics 2001;108:776 [PMID: 11533352].

American Academy of Pediatrics Committee on Substance Abuse and Committee on Children with Disabilities: Fetal alcohol syndrome and alcohol-related neurodevelopmental disorders. Pediatrics 2000;106:358 [PMID: 10920168].

Boyle RJ: Effects of certain prenatal drugs on the fetus and newborn. Pediatr Rev 2002;23:17 [PMID: 11773589].

Chan O et al: New methods for neonatal drug screening. NeoReviews 2003;4:e236.

Chasnoff IJ: Prenatal substance exposure: maternal screening and neonatal identification and management. NeoReviews 2003; 4:e228.

Coyle MG et al: Diluted tincture of opium (DTO) and phenobarbital versus DTO alone for neonatal opiate withdrawal in term infants. J Pediatr 2002;140:561 [PMID: 12032522].

Frank DA et al: Growth, development, and behavior in early childhood following prenatal cocaine exposure. A systematic review. JAMA 2001;285:1613 [PMID: 11268270].

Gleason CA: Fetal alcohol exposure: Effects on the developing brain. Neoreviews 2001;2:e231.

Holmes LB et al: The teratogenicity of anticonvulsant drugs. N Engl J Med 2001;344:1132 [PMID: 11297704].

Hoyme HE et al: A practical clinical approach to diagnosis of fetal alcohol spectrum disorders: clarification of the 1996 Institute of Medicine criteria. Pediatrics 2005;115:39 [PMID: 15629980].

Johnson K et al: Treatment of neonatal abstinence syndrome. Arch Dis Child Fetal Neonatal Ed 2003;88:F2 [PMID: 12496218].

Singer LT et al: Cognitive outcomes of preschool children with prenatal cocaine exposure. JAMA 2004;291:2448 [PMID: 15161895].

Sokol RH et al: Fetal alcohol spectrum disorder. JAMA 2003; 290:2996 [PMID: 14665662].

Ventura SJ et al: Trends and variations in smoking in pregnancy and low birth weight: Evidence from the birth certificate, 1999–2000. Pediatrics 2003;111:1176 [PMID: 12728134].

MULTIPLE BIRTHS

Twinning has historically occurred as a demographic variation in one of 80 pregnancies (1.25%). The incidence of twinning and higher-order multiple births in the United States has been increasing as a consequence of the increased use of in-vitro fertilization and other assisted reproductive technologies. In 2002, twins occurred in 1/32 live births in the United States, with multiple births accounting for 3.3% of all births.

A distinction should be made between dizygotic (fraternal) and monozygotic (identical) twins. Race, maternal parity, and maternal age affect the incidence only of dizygotic twinning. Drugs that induce ovulation, such as clomiphene citrate and gonadotropins, increase the incidence of dizygotic or polyzygotic twinning. Monozygotic twinning can be viewed as a birth defect; the incidence of malformations is also increased in identical twins and may affect only one of the twins. If a defect is found in one, the other should be examined carefully for lesser degrees of the same defect.

Examination of the placenta can help establish the type of twinning: Two amnionic membranes and two chorionic membranes are found in all dizygotic twins and in one-third of monozygotic twins; a single chorionic membrane always indicates monozygotic twins.

Complications of Multiple Births

A. INTRAUTERINE GROWTH RESTRICTION

There is some degree of IUGR in most multiple pregnancies after 34 weeks. If prenatal care is good, however, the growth restriction is rarely significant. There are two exceptions: The first is the monochorial twin pregnancy in which an arteriovenous shunt occurs from one twin's circulation to that of the other (twin-twin transfusion syndrome). The infant on the venous side becomes plethoric and considerably larger than the smaller anemic twin. Morbidity and mortality rates are considerable in twin-twin transfusion syndrome. Discordance in size—birth weights that are significantly different—can also occur when separate placentas are present. One placenta develops poorly, presumably because of a poor implantation site. In this instance, no fetal exchange of blood takes place but the growth rates of the two infants are significantly different.

B. PRETERM DELIVERY

Gestation length tends to be inversely related to the number of fetuses. The prematurity rate is 5–10 times that of singletons, with 50% of twins and 90% of triplets born before 37 weeks. The prematurity rate tends to increase the mortality or morbidity rates occurring in twin pregnancies.

C. OBSTETRIC COMPLICATIONS

Polyhydramnios, pregnancy-induced hypertension, premature rupture of membranes, abnormal fetal presentations, and prolapsed umbilical cord occur more frequently in women with multiple fetuses. In general, most of the complications can be avoided or minimized by good obstetric management. Multiple pregnancy

should always be identified prenatally with ultrasound examinations; doing so allows the obstetrician and pediatrician or neonatologist to plan management jointly. The neonatal complications are usually related to prematurity. Prolongation of pregnancy, therefore, leads to a significant reduction in neonatal morbidity.

Follow-up studies of twin pregnancies have yielded conflicting results. In general, the studies do not suggest that twinning has a significant effect on later development, especially if prematurity is excluded as a separate risk factor.

Banek CS et al: Long-term neurodevelopmental outcome after intrauterine treatment for severe twin-twin transfusion syndrome. Am J Obstet Gynecol 2003;188:876 [PMID: 1272079].

Mari G et al: Perinatal morbidity and mortality rates in severe twin-twin transfusion syndrome: Results of the International Amnioreduction Registry. Am J Obstet Gynecol 2001;185:708 [PMID: 11568802].

Martin JA et al: Annual summary of vital statistics 2003. Pediatrics 2005;115:619 [PMID: 15741364].

Reynolds MA et al: Trends in multiple births conceived using assisted reproductive technology, United States, 1997–2000. Pediatrics 2003;111:1159 [PMID: 12728130].

NEONATAL INTENSIVE CARE

PERINATAL RESUSCITATION

Perinatal resuscitation refers to the steps taken by the obstetrician to support the infant during labor and delivery, as well as the traditional resuscitative steps taken by the pediatrician after delivery. Intrapartum support includes maintaining maternal blood pressure with volume expanders if needed, maternal oxygen therapy, positioning the mother to improve placental perfusion, readjusting oxytocin infusions or administering a tocolytic if appropriate, minimizing trauma to the infant (particularly important in infants of very low birth weight), suctioning the nasopharynx upon delivery of the head if meconium is present in the amniotic fluid, obtaining all necessary cord blood samples, and completing an examination of the placenta.

Steps taken by the pediatrician or neonatologist focus on temperature support, initiation and maintenance of effective ventilation, maintenance of perfusion and hydration, and glucose regulation.

A number of conditions associated with pregnancy, labor, and delivery place the infant at risk for birth asphyxia: (1) maternal diseases such as diabetes, pregnancy-induced hypertension, heart and renal disease, and collagen-vascular disease; (2) fetal conditions such as prematurity, multiple births, growth restriction, and fetal anomalies; and (3) labor and delivery conditions, including fetal distress with or without meconium in the amniotic fluid, and administration of anesthetics and opioid analgesics.

Physiology of Birth Asphyxia

Birth asphyxia can be the result of several mechanisms: (1) acute interruption of umbilical blood flow (eg, prolapsed cord with cord compression), (2) premature placental separation, (3) maternal hypotension or hypoxia, (4) chronic placental insufficiency, and (5) failure to execute newborn resuscitation properly.

The neonatal response to asphyxia follows a predictable pattern that has been demonstrated in many species (Figure 1–6). The initial response to hypoxia is an increase in frequency of respiration and a rise in heart rate and blood pressure. Respirations then cease (primary apnea) as heart rate and blood pressure begin to fall. This initial period of apnea lasts 30–60 seconds. Gasping respirations (3–6/min)

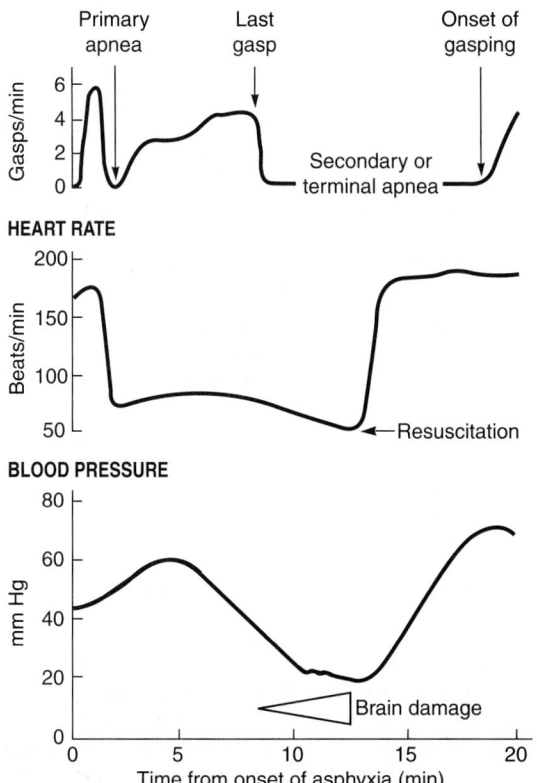

Figure 1–6. Schematic depiction of changes in rhesus monkeys during asphyxia and on resuscitation by positive-pressure ventilation. (Adapted and reproduced, with permission, from Dawes GS: *Fetal and Neonatal Physiology.* Year Book, 1968.)

then begin, while heart rate and blood pressure gradually decline. Secondary or terminal apnea then ensues, with further decline in heart rate and blood pressure. The longer the duration of secondary apnea, the greater the risk for hypoxic organ injury. A cardinal feature of the defense against hypoxia is the underperfusion of certain tissue beds (eg, skin, muscle, kidneys, and GI tract), which allows the perfusion of core organs (ie, heart, brain, and adrenals) to be maintained.

Response to resuscitation also follows a predictable pattern. During the period of primary apnea, almost any physical stimulus causes the baby to initiate respirations. Infants in secondary apnea require PPV. The first sign of recovery is an increase in heart rate, followed by an increase in blood pressure with improved perfusion. The time required for rhythmic, spontaneous respirations to occur is related to the duration of the secondary apnea. As a rough rule, for each minute past the last gasp, 2 minutes of PPV is required before gasping begins, and 4 minutes is required to reach rhythmic breathing. These times can vary depending on the degree and duration of intrauterine asphyxia. Not until some time later do spinal and corneal reflexes return. Muscle tone gradually improves over the course of several hours.

Delivery Room Management

When asphyxia is anticipated, a resuscitation team of at least two persons should be present: one to manage the airway and one to monitor the heartbeat and provide assistance. The necessary equipment and drugs are listed in Table 1–13.

A. STEPS IN THE RESUSCITATION (SEE FIGURE 1–7)

1. Dry the infant well, and place him or her under the radiant heat source. Do not allow the infant to become hyperthermic.

2. Gently suction the mouth, then the nose.

3. Quickly assess the infant's condition. The best criteria are the infant's respiratory effort (apneic, gasping or, regular) and heart rate (> 100 or < 100 beats/min). A depressed heart rate—indicative of hypoxic myocardial depression—is the single most reliable indicator of the need for resuscitation.

4. Infants who are breathing and have heart rates over 100 beats/min usually require no further intervention. Infants with heart rates less than 100 beats/min and apnea or irregular respiratory efforts should be stimulated vigorously. The baby's back should be rubbed with a towel while oxygen is provided near the baby's face.

5. If the baby fails to respond to tactile stimulation within a few seconds, begin bag and mask ventilation, using a soft mask that seals well around the mouth and nose. For the initial inflations, pressures of 30–40 cm H_2O may be necessary to overcome surface-active forces in

Table 1–13. Equipment for neonatal resuscitation.

Clinical Needs	Equipment
Thermoregulation	Radiant heat source with platform, mattress covered with warm sterile blankets, servocontrol heating, temperature probe
Airway management	**Suction:** Bulb suction, mechanical suction with sterile catheters (6F, 8F, 10F), meconium aspirator
	Ventilation: Manual infant resuscitation bag connected to manometer or with a pressure-release valve capable of delivering 100% oxygen, appropriate masks for term and preterm infants, oral airways, stethoscope
	Intubation: Neonatal laryngoscope with No. 0 and No. 1 blades; endotracheal tubes (2.5, 3.0, 3.5 mm outer diameter with stylet): extra bulbs and batteries for laryngoscope; scissors, adhesive tape, gloves, end tidal CO_2 detection device
Gastric decompression	Nasogastric tube: 8F with 20-mL syringe
Administration of drugs and volume replacement	Sterile umbilical catheterization tray, umbilical catheters (3.5F and 5F), volume expanders, normal saline, drug box[a] with appropriate neonatal vials and dilutions, sterile syringes, needles, and alcohol sponges
Transport	Warmed transport isolette with oxygen source

[a]Epinephrine 1:10,000; naloxone hydrochloride 1 mg/mL; sodium bicarbonate 4.2% (5 mEq/10 mL); 10% dextrose.
Modified, with permission, from Rosenberg AA: Neonatal adaptation. In: Gabbe SG et al (editors). *Obstetrics: Normal and Problem Pregnancies.* Churchill Livingstone, 1996.

the lungs. Adequacy of ventilation is assessed by observing expansion of the infant's chest accompanied by an improvement in heart rate, perfusion, and color. After the first few breaths, lower the peak pressure to 15–20 cm H_2O. The baby's chest movement should resemble that of an easy breath rather than a deep sigh. The rate of bagging should be 40–60 breaths/min.

6. Most neonates can be resuscitated effectively with a bag and mask. If the infant does not respond to bag and mask ventilation, try to reposition the head (slight extension), reapply the mask to achieve a good seal, consider suctioning the mouth and the oropharynx, and try

ventilating with the mouth open. If the infant does not respond within 30 seconds, intubation is appropriate.

Failure to respond to intubation and ventilation can result from (1) mechanical difficulties (Table 1–14), (2) profound asphyxia with myocardial depression, and (3) inadequate circulating blood volume.

Quickly rule out the mechanical causes listed in Table 1–14. Check to ensure that the endotracheal tube passes through the vocal cords. A CO_2 detector placed between the endotracheal tube and the bag can be very helpful as a rapid confirmation of proper tube position in the airway. Occlusion of the tube should be suspected when there is resistance to bagging and no chest wall movement. Very few neonates (approximately 0.1%) require either cardiac massage or drugs during resuscitation. Almost all newborns respond to ventilation if done effectively. Although current AAP Neonatal Resuscitation Program (NRP) guidelines recommend 100% oxygen for neonatal resuscitation, there is some evidence that this may increase the risk of post-resuscitative oxidative injury. Resuscitation with room air may be equally effective unless lung pathology is present. At a minimum when possible, blended oxygen should be available in the delivery room.

7. If mechanical causes are ruled out and the heart rate remains below 60 beats/min after intubation and PPV for 30 seconds, cardiac compression should be initiated. Simultaneous delivery of chest compressions and PPV is likely to decrease the efficiency of ventilation. Therefore, chest compressions should be interspersed with ventilation at a 3:1 ratio (90 compressions and 30 breaths/min).

8. If drugs are needed, the drug and dose of choice is epinephrine 1:10,000 solution, 0.1–0.3 mL/kg given via the endotracheal tube or preferably through an umbilical venous line. Sodium bicarbonate, 1–2 mEq/kg of the neonatal dilution (0.5 mEq/mL), can be used in prolonged resuscitation efforts in which the response to other measures is poor. If volume loss is suspected, 10 mL/kg of a volume expander (normal saline) should be administered through an umbilical vein line.

B. CONTINUED RESUSCITATIVE MEASURES

The appropriateness of continued resuscitative efforts should be reevaluated in an infant who fails to respond to the previously described efforts. In current practice, resuscitative efforts are made even in apparent stillbirths (ie, infants whose Apgar score at 1 minute is 0–1). Modern resuscitative techniques have led to an increasing survival rate for these infants, with 60% of survivors showing normal development. It is clear from a number of studies that initial resuscitation of these infants should proceed; however, subsequent continued support must depend on response to resuscitation. All studies emphasize that if the Apgar score is not improving markedly over the first 10

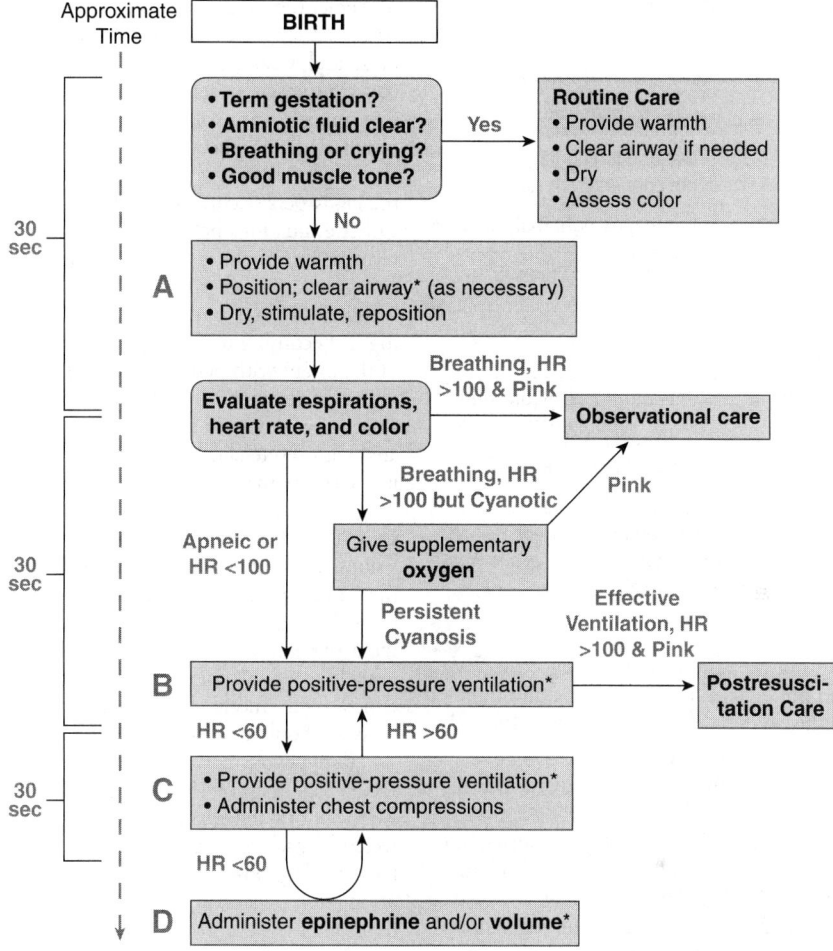

Approximate
Time

BIRTH

• **Term gestation?**
• **Amniotic fluid clear?**   Yes →   **Routine Care**
• **Breathing or crying?**   • Provide warmth
• **Good muscle tone?**   • Clear airway if needed
                                          • Dry
                                          • Assess color

No ↓

30
sec

A   • Provide warmth
      • Position; clear airway* (as necessary)
      • Dry, stimulate, reposition

Evaluate respirations,   Breathing, HR
heart rate, and color   >100 & Pink →   **Observational care**

                    Breathing, HR
                    >100 but Cyanotic   Pink
Apneic or
HR <100   Give supplementary
30   **oxygen**
sec
                    Persistent   Effective
                    Cyanosis   Ventilation, HR
                                        >100 & Pink

B   Provide positive-pressure ventilation*   →   **Postresusci-
                                                    tation Care**

      HR <60   HR >60

30   C   • Provide positive-pressure ventilation*
sec   • Administer chest compressions

      HR <60

↓ D   Administer **epinephrine** and/or **volume***

*Endotracheal intubation may be considered at several steps

Figure 1–7. Delivery room management. (Reproduced, with permission, from American Heart Association, American Academy of Pediatrics: Neonatal Resuscitation Guidelines. Circulation 2005;112:14.)

minutes of life, the mortality rate and the incidence of severe developmental handicaps among survivors are high.

C. SPECIAL CONSIDERATIONS

1. Preterm Infants—
a. Minimizing heat loss improves survival, so pre-warmed towels should be available. The environmental temperature of the delivery suite should be raised to > 25°C (especially for infants weighing < 1500 g). Providing a polyethylene occlusive skin cover can also aid in minimizing heat loss in the extremely low birth weight (< 1000 g) infant.
b. The lungs of preterm infants may be especially prone to injury from PPV due to volutrauma. For this reason, if possible, ventilation efforts should be sup-

ported with nasal continuous positive airway pressure (CPAP) rather than PPV. Whether this will result in improved outcomes and less chronic lung disease is still under study.
c. In the extremely low birth weight infant (< 1000 g), proceed more quickly to intubation.
d. Volume expanders and sodium bicarbonate (if needed) should be infused more slowly to minimize rapid swings in blood pressure and serum osmolality.
2. Narcotic depression—In the case of opioid administration to the mother within 4 hours of delivery, perform the resuscitation as described earlier. When the baby is stable with good heart rate, color, and perfusion, but still has poor respiratory effort, a trial of naloxone (0.1 mg/kg IM, SC, IV, or IT) is indicated.

Table 1–14. Mechanical causes of failed resuscitation.

Cause	Examples
Equipment failure	Malfunctioning bag, oxygen not connected or running
Endotracheal tube malposition	Esophagus, right main stem bronchus
Occluded endotracheal tube	
Insufficient inflation pressure to expand lungs	
Space-occupying lesions in the thorax	Pneumothorax, pleural effusions, diaphragmatic hernia
Pulmonary hypoplasia	Extreme prematurity, oligohydramnios

Reproduced, with permission, from Rosenberg AA: Neonatal adaptation. In: Gabbe SG et al (editors): *Obstetrics: Normal and Problem Pregnancies.* Churchill Livingstone, 1996.

Naloxone should not be administered in place of PPV. Naloxone should not be used in the infant of an opioid-addicted mother because it will precipitate withdrawal.

3. Meconium-stained amniotic fluid—
a. The obstetrician carefully suctions the oropharynx and the nasopharynx after birth.
b. If the baby is active and breathing, requiring no resuscitation, the airway need not be inspected—only further suctioning of the mouth and nasopharynx is required.
c. The airway of any depressed infant requiring ventilation must be checked and cleared (by passage of a tube below the vocal cords) before PPV is instituted. Special adapters are available for use with regulated wall suction to allow suction to be applied directly to the endotracheal tube.
d. Since most severe cases of meconium aspiration syndrome with pulmonary hypertension likely have their origins in utero, resuscitative efforts should not be excessively delayed with attempts to clear the airway of meconium.

4. Universal precautions—In the delivery room, universal precautions should always be observed.

Treatment of the Asphyxiated Infant

Asphyxia is manifested by multiorgan dysfunction, seizures, hypoxic-ischemic encephalopathy, and metabolic acidemia. The infant who has experienced a significant episode of perinatal hypoxia and ischemia is at risk for dysfunction of multiple end organs (Table 1–15). The organ of greatest concern is the brain.

The clinical features of hypoxic-ischemic encephalopathy progress over time: birth to 12 hours, decreased level of consciousness, poor tone, decreased spontaneous movement, periodic breathing or apnea, and possible seizures; 12–24 hours, more seizures, apneic spells, jitteriness, and weakness; after 24 hours, decreased level of consciousness, further respiratory abnormalities (progressive apnea), onset of brainstem signs (oculomotor and pupillary disturbances), poor feeding, and hypotonia.

The severity of clinical signs and the length of time the signs persist correlate with the severity of the insult. Other evaluations helpful in assessing severity in the full-term infant include electroencephalogram (EEG) and computed tomography (CT) scan. Magnetic resonance imaging (MRI), particularly diffusion-weighted imaging, is becoming useful, especially in the early evaluation of the infant with perinatal asphyxia.

Markedly abnormal EEGs with voltage suppression and slowing evolving into a burst-suppression pattern are associated with severe clinical symptomatology. A CT scan early in the course may demonstrate diffuse hypodensity and loss of gray/white matter tissue differentiation, whereas later scans may demonstrate brain atrophy and focal ischemic lesions. In most instances, it is not necessary to use all of these tests, but some are obtained to confirm a poor prognosis. Management is directed at supportive care and treatment of specific abnormalities. Fluids should be restricted initially to 60–80 mL/kg/d; oxygenation should be maintained (with mechanical ventilation if necessary); blood pressure should be supported with judicious volume expansion (if hypovolemic) and pressors; and glucose should be in the normal range of 45–100 mg/dL. Hypocalcemia, coagulation abnormalities, and metabolic acidemia should be corrected and seizures treated with IV phenobarbital (20 mg/kg as loading dose, with total initial 24-hour dosing up to 40 mg/kg). Phenobarbital in large doses (40 mg/kg IV 1–6 hours after the event) given as a neuroprotective therapy is associated with improvement in neurologic outcome with minimal adverse effects on blood pressure, respirations, or

Table 1–15. Signs and symptoms caused by asphyxia.

Hypoxic-ischemic encephalopathy, seizures
Respiratory distress due to aspiration or secondary surfactant deficiency, pulmonary hemorrhage
Persistent pulmonary hypertension
Hypotension due to myocardial dysfunction
Transient tricuspid valve insufficiency
Anuria or oliguria due to acute tubular necrosis
Feeding intolerance; necrotizing enterocolitis
Elevated aminotransferases due to liver injury
Adrenal insufficiency due to hemorrhage
Disseminated intravascular coagulation
Hypocalcemia
Hypoglycemia
Persistent metabolic acidemia
Hyperkalemia

blood gases. Other anticonvulsants should be reserved for refractory seizures. Hypothermia, in particular using selective head cooling with mild systemic hypothermia initiated within 6 hours of birth, has been shown to improve outcome at an 18-month follow-up in infants with moderate neurologic symptoms as defined clinically and with a 1-lead amplitude-integrated EEG. Efficacy has not been proven in the most severe cases of neonatal encephalopathy.

Birth Asphyxia: Long-Term Outcome

Fetal heart rate tracings, cord pH, and 1-minute Apgar scores are imprecise predictors of long-term outcome. Apgar scores of 0–3 at 5 minutes in full-term infants result in an 18–35% risk of death in the first year of life and an 8% risk of cerebral palsy among survivors. The risks of mortality and morbidity increase with more prolonged depression of the Apgar score. The single best predictor of outcome is the severity of clinical hypoxic-ischemic encephalopathy (severe symptomatology including coma carries a 75% chance of death and a 100% rate of neurologic sequelae among survivors). The major sequela of hypoxic-ischemic encephalopathy is cerebral palsy with or without associated mental retardation and epilepsy. Other prognostic features include elevated nucleated red blood cell counts, prolonged seizures refractory to therapy, markedly abnormal EEGs, and CT or MRI scans with evidence of major ischemic injury. Other clinical features required to support perinatal hypoxia as the cause of cerebral palsy include the presence of fetal distress prior to birth, a low cord pH of < 7.00, evidence of other end-organ dysfunction, and absence of a congenital brain malformation.

Allan WC: The clinical spectrum and prediction of outcome in hypoxic-ischemic encephalopathy. Neoreviews 2002;3:e108.

Aly H et al: Is it safer to intubate premature infants in the delivery room? Pediatrics 2005;115:1660 [PMID: 15930230].

American Heart Association and American Academy of Pediatrics: *Textbook of Neonatal Resuscitation,* 5th ed. American Heart Association/American Academy of Pediatrics, 2006.

Davis PG et al: Resuscitation of newborn infants with 100% oxygen or air: a systematic review and meta-analysis. Lancet 2004;364:1329 [PMID: 15474135].

Ferriero DM: Neonatal brain injury. N Engl J Med 2004;351:1985 [PMID: 15525724].

Fraser WD et al: Amnioinfusion for the prevention of the meconium aspiration syndrome. N Engl J Med 2005;353:909 [PMID: 16135835].

Gluckman PD et al: Selective head cooling with mild systemic hypothermia after neonatal encephalopathy: multicentre randomized trial. Lancet 2005;365:663 [PMID: 15721471].

Grow J, Barks JDE: Pathogenesis of hypoxic-ischemic cerebral injury in the term infant: Current concepts. Clin Perinatol 2002;29:585 [PMID: 12516737].

Hamkins GDV, Spear M: Defining the pathogenesis and pathophysiology of neonatal encephalopathy and cerebral palsy. Obstet Gynecol 2003;102:628 [PMID: 12962954].

Huppi PS: Advances in postnatal neuroimaging: Relevance to pathogenesis and treatment of brain injury. Clin Perinatol 2002;29:827 [PMID: 12516748].

Morley C, Davis P: Continuous positive airway pressure: current controversies. Curr Opin Pediatr 2004;16:141 [PMID: 15021191].

Mosler D et al: The association of Apgar score with subsequent death and cerebral palsy: A population-based study in term infants. J Pediatr 2001;138:798 [PMID: 11391319].

Phelan JP et al: Birth asphyxia and cerebral palsy. Clin Perinatol 2005;32:61 [PMID: 15777821].

Ramji S, Saugstad OD: Use of 100% oxygen or room air in neonatal resuscitation. NeoReviews 2005;6:e172.

Shankaran S: The postnatal management of the asphyxiated term infant. Clin Perinatol 2002;29:675 [PMID: 12516741].

Thomson MA: Early nasal continuous positive airway pressure to minimize the need for endotracheal intubation and ventilation. NeoReviews 2005;6:e184.

Vain NE et al: Oropharyngeal and nasopharyngeal suctioning of meconium-stained neonates before delivery of their shoulders: multicentre, randomized, controlled trial. Lancet 2004; 364:597 [PMID: 15313360]

Vento M et al: Oxidative stress in asphyxiated term infants resuscitated with 100% oxygen. J Pediatr 2003;142:240 [PMID:12640369].

Vobra S et al: Heat loss prevention (HELP) in the delivery room: a randomized controlled trial of polyethylene occlusive skin wrapping in very preterm infants. J Pediatr 2004;145:750 [PMID: 15580195]

Willoughby RE Jr, Nelson KB: Chorioamnionitis and brain injury. Clin Perinatol 2002;29:603 [PMID: 12516738].

Wiswell TE et al: Delivery room management of the apparently vigorous meconium-stained neonate: Results of the multicenter, international collaborative trial. Pediatrics 2000;105:1 [PMID: 10617696].

THE PRETERM INFANT

Premature infants account for the majority of high-risk newborns. The preterm infant faces a variety of physiologic handicaps:

1. The ability to suck, swallow, and breathe in a coordinated fashion is not achieved until 34–36 weeks' gestation. Therefore, enteral feedings must be provided by gavage. Furthermore, preterm infants frequently have gastroesophageal reflux and an immature gag reflex, which increases the risk of aspiration of feedings.

2. Decreased ability to maintain body temperature.

3. Pulmonary immaturity-surfactant deficiency, often with structural immaturity in infants of less than 26 weeks' gestation. Their condition is complicated by the combination of noncompliant lungs and an extremely compliant chest wall.

4. Immature control of respiration, leading to apnea and bradycardia.

5. Persistent patency of the ductus arteriosus, leading to further compromise of pulmonary gas exchange because of overperfusion of the lungs.

6. Immature cerebral vasculature, predisposing the infant to subependymal or intraventricular hemorrhage and periventricular leukomalacia.

7. Impaired substrate absorption by the GI tract, compromising nutritional management.

Table 1–16. Use of parenteral alimentation solutions.

	Volume (mL/kg/d)	Carbohydrate (g/dL)	Protein (g/kg)	Lipid (g/kg)	Calories (kcal/kg)
Peripheral: Short-term (7–10 days)					
Starting solution	100–150	$D_{10}W$	2	1	46–64
Target solution	150	$D_{12.5}W$	3–3.5	3	102
Central: Long-term (> 10 days)					
Starting solution	100–150	$D_{10}W$	2	1	46–64
Target solution	130	$D_{20}W$	3–3.5	3	123

Notes:
1. Advance dextrose in central hyperalimentation as tolerated by 2.5% per day as long as blood glucose remains normal.
2. Advance lipids by 1.0 g/kg/d as long as triglycerides are normal. Use 20% concentration.
3. Total water should be 100–150 mL/kg/d, depending on the child's fluid tolerance.

Monitoring:
1. Blood glucose two or three times a day when changing dextrose concentration, then daily.
2. Electrolytes daily, then twice a week when the child is receiving a stable solution.
3. Every other week blood urea nitrogen and serum creatinine; total protein and serum albumin; serum calcium, phosphate, magnesium, direct bilirubin, and CBC with platelet counts.
4. Triglyceride level after 24 h at 2 g/kg/d and 24 h at 3 g/kg/d; then every other week.

treated with erythropoietin (epoetin alfa) for prevention or treatment of anemia of prematurity require a higher dosage of 4–8 mg/kg/d.

Berseth CL et al: Prolonging small feeding volumes early in life decreases the incidence of necrotizing enterocolitis in very low birth weight infants. Pediatrics 2003;111:529 [PMID: 12612232].

Carver JD et al: Growth of preterm infants fed nutrient-enriched or term formula after hospital discharge. Pediatrics 2001;107:683 [PMID: 11335744].

Clandinin MT et al: Growth and development of preterm infants fed infant formulas containing docosahexaenoic acid and arachidonic acid. J Pediatr 2005;146:461 [PMID: 15812447].

Embleton NE et al: Postnatal malnutrition and growth retardation: An inevitable consequence of current recommendations in preterm infants. Pediatrics 2001;107:270 [PMID: 11158457].

Thureen PJ, Hay WW: Early aggressive nutrition in preterm infants. Semin Neonatol 2001;6:403 [PMID: 11988030].

Zeigler EE et al: Aggressive nutrition of the very low birth weight infant. Clin Perinatol 2002;29:225 [PMID: 12168239].

1. Apnea in the Preterm Infant

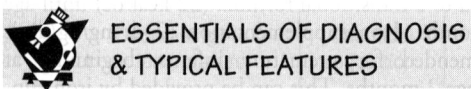

ESSENTIALS OF DIAGNOSIS & TYPICAL FEATURES

- *Respiratory pause of sufficient duration to result in cyanosis or bradycardia.*

- *Most common in infants born at < 34 weeks' gestation with onset at < 2 weeks of age.*
- *Methylxanthines (eg, caffeine) provide effective treatment for apnea of prematurity.*

General Considerations

In preterm infants, recurrent apneic episodes are a common problem. Apnea is defined as a respiratory pause lasting more than 20 seconds—or any pause accompanied by cyanosis and bradycardia. Shorter respiratory pauses associated with cyanosis or bradycardia also qualify as significant apnea but must be differentiated from periodic breathing, which is common in full-term as well as preterm infants. Periodic breathing is defined as regularly recurring ventilatory cycles interrupted by short pauses not associated with bradycardia or color change. Although apnea in premature infants is often not associated with a predisposing factor, a variety of processes may precipitate apnea (Table 1–17). These processes should at least be considered before a diagnosis of apnea of prematurity can be established.

Apnea of prematurity is the most frequent cause of apnea. Most apnea of prematurity is mixed apnea characterized by a centrally (brainstem) mediated respiratory pause preceded or followed by airway obstruction. Less common is pure central or pure obstructive apnea. Apnea of prematurity is the result of immaturity of both the cen-

Table 1–17. Causes of apnea in the preterm infant.

Temperature instability—both cold and heat stress
Response to passage of a feeding tube
Gastroesophageal reflux
Hypoxemia
    Pulmonary parenchymal disease
    Patent ductus arteriosus
    ?Anemia
Infection
    Sepsis (viral or bacterial)
    Necrotizing enterocolitis
Metabolic causes
    Hypoglycemia
    Hyponatremia
Intracranial hemorrhage
Posthemorrhagic hydrocephalus
Seizures
Drugs (eg, morphine)
Apnea of prematurity

---

tral respiratory regulatory centers and protective mechanisms that aid in maintaining airway patency.

Clinical Findings

Onset, typically during the first 2 weeks of life, is gradual, with the frequency of spells increasing over time. Pathologic apnea can be suspected in an infant with a sudden onset of frequent or very severe apneic spells. Apnea presenting from birth or on the first day of life is unusual but can occur in the preterm infant who does not require mechanical ventilation for respiratory distress syndrome. In the full-term or near-term infant, this presentation can suggest neuromuscular abnormalities of an acute (asphyxia, birth trauma, or infection) or chronic (eg, congenital hypotonia or structural CNS lesion) nature.

The work-up depends on the clinical presentation. All infants—regardless of the severity and frequency of apnea—require a minimum screening evaluation, including a general assessment of well-being (eg, tolerance of feedings, stable temperature, normal physical examination), a check of the association of spells with feeding, measurement of PaO_2 or SaO_2, blood glucose, hematocrit, and a review of the drug history. Infants with severe apnea of sudden onset may require a more extensive evaluation, including evaluation for infection. Other specific tests are dictated by relevant signs, for example, evaluation for necrotizing enterocolitis in an infant with apnea and abdominal distention or feeding intolerance.

Treatment

The physician should first address any underlying cause. If the apnea is due simply to prematurity, treat-

ment is dictated by the frequency and severity of apneic spells. Apneic spells frequent enough to interfere with other aspects of care (eg, feeding), or severe enough to necessitate bag and mask ventilation to relieve cyanosis and bradycardia, require treatment. First-line therapy is with methylxanthines. Caffeine citrate (20 mg/kg as loading dose and then 5–10 mg/kg/d) is the drug of choice because of once-daily dosing, wider therapeutic index, and fewer side effects than theophylline. Side effects of methylxanthines include tachycardia, feeding intolerance, and (with overdosing) seizures. The dose used should be the smallest dose necessary to decrease the frequency of apnea and eliminate severe spells. Desired drug levels are usually in the range of 10–20 μg/mL for caffeine. Nasal CPAP (continuous positive airway pressure), by treating the obstructive component of apnea, can be effective treatment for some infants. Intubation and ventilation can eliminate symptomatic apneic spells but carry the risks associated with long-term endotracheal intubation.

Prognosis

In the majority of premature infants, apneic and bradycardiac spells cease by 34–37 weeks postconception. Spells that require intervention cease prior to self-resolved episodes. In infants born at less than 28 weeks' gestation, episodes may continue past term. Whether to provide home monitoring or outpatient methylxanthine therapy for such infants is controversial. Apneic and bradycardiac episodes in the nursery are not predictors of later SIDS, although the incidence of SIDS is slightly increased in preterm infants. Therefore, home monitoring in infants still experiencing self-resolving apnea and bradycardia at the time of hospital discharge may be indicated in some cases.

2. Hyaline Membrane Disease

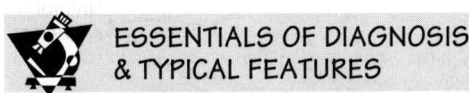

ESSENTIALS OF DIAGNOSIS & TYPICAL FEATURES

- *Tachypnea, cyanosis, and expiratory grunting.*
- *Poor air movement despite increased work of breathing.*
- *Chest radiograph showing hypoexpansion and air bronchograms.*

General Considerations

The most common cause of respiratory distress in the preterm infant is hyaline membrane disease. The incidence increases from 5% of infants born at 35–36 weeks' gestation to more than 50% of infants born at 26–28 weeks' gestation. This condition is caused by a deficiency of surfactant. Surfactant decreases surface tension in the alveolus during expiration, allowing the alveolus to remain partly expanded and in that way maintaining a functional residual capacity. The absence of surfactant results in poor lung compliance and atelectasis. The infant must expend a great deal of effort to expand the lungs with each breath, and respiratory failure ensues (Figure 1–9).

Clinical Findings

Infants with hyaline membrane disease demonstrate all the clinical signs of respiratory distress. On auscultation, air movement is diminished despite vigorous respiratory effort. Chest radiograph demonstrates diffuse bilateral atelectasis, causing a ground-glass appearance. Major airways are highlighted by the atelectatic air sacs, creating air bronchograms. In the unintubated child, doming of the diaphragm and underexpansion occur.

Treatment

Supplemental oxygen, use of nasal CPAP, early intubation for surfactant administration and ventilation, and placement of umbilical artery and vein lines are the initial interventions required. A ventilator that can deliver breaths synchronized with the infant's respiratory efforts (synchronized intermittent mandatory ventilation) should be used. High-frequency ventilators are also available for rescue of infants doing poorly on conventional ventilation or who have air leak problems.

Surfactant replacement therapy, used both in the delivery room as prophylaxis and with established hyaline membrane disease as rescue, decreases both the mortality rate in preterm infants and air leak complications of the disease. During the acute course, ventilator settings and oxygen requirements are significantly lower in surfactant-treated infants than in control subjects. The dose of the bovine-derived beractant (Survanta) is 4 mL/kg, the calf lung surfactant extract (Infasurf) is 3 mL/kg, and the porcine-derived poractant (Curosurf) is 1.25–2.5 mL/kg, given intratracheally. When the first dose is given in the delivery room to prevent hyaline membrane disease, the usual dosing schedule is a total of two or three doses given 6–12 hours apart as long as the infant remains ventilated on over 30–40% inspired oxygen concentration. Rescue surfactant is given as two to four doses 6–12 hours apart. The first dose is administered as soon as possible after birth, preferably before 2–4 hours of age. As the disease process evolves, proteins that inhibit surfactant function leak into the air spaces, making surfactant replacement less effective. The second dose should be administered to infants who continue to require mechanical ventilation and more than 30–40% inspired oxygen concentration. A prophylactic strategy offers some advantage in those infants born at 26 weeks' gestation or less. For infants over 26 weeks' gestation, early rescue therapy (as soon as a diagnosis of surfactant deficiency can be made) is the strategy of choice. In stable infants, a trial of nasal CPAP at 5–6 cm H_2O pressure can be attempted prior to intubation and surfactant administration. For those who do require mechanical ventilation, extubation to nasal CPAP should be done as early as possible to minimize lung injury and evolution of chronic lung disease. Antenatal administration of corticosteroids to the mother is an important strategy used by obstetricians to accelerate lung maturation. Infants whose mothers were given corticosteroids more than 24 hours prior to preterm birth have less respiratory distress syndrome and a lower mortality rate.

3. Chronic Lung Disease in the Premature Infant

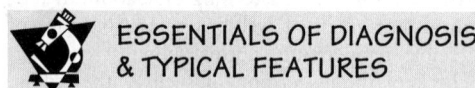

ESSENTIALS OF DIAGNOSIS & TYPICAL FEATURES

- *Oxygen requirement, respiratory symptoms, and abnormal chest radiograph at 36 weeks post conceptual age.*
- *Incidence greatest in infants of the lowest gestational ages.*

General Considerations

Chronic lung disease in the premature infant, defined as respiratory symptoms, oxygen requirement, and chest

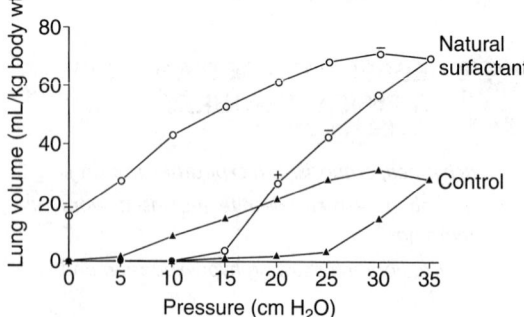

Figure 1–9. Pressure-volume relationships for the inflation and deflation of surfactant-deficient and surfactant-treated preterm rabbit lungs. (Reproduced, with permission, from Jobe AH: The developmental biology of the lung. In: Fanaroff AA, Martin RJ [editors]: *Neonatal-Perinatal Medicine: Diseases of the Fetus and Infant,* 6th ed. Mosby, 1997.)

radiograph abnormalities at 36 weeks postconception, occurs in about 20% of infants ventilated for surfactant deficiency. The incidence is higher at lower gestational ages and in infants exposed to chorioamnionitis prior to birth. The development of chronic lung disease is a function of lung immaturity at birth, inflammation, and exposure to high oxygen concentrations and ventilator volutrauma. The use of surfactant replacement therapy or early nasal CPAP has, in general, diminished the severity of the chronic lung disease. The mortality rate from this complication is now very low, but significant morbidity still exists secondary to reactive airway symptoms, and hospital readmissions during the first 2 years of life for intercurrent respiratory infection.

Treatment

Continued use of supplemental oxygen, mechanical ventilation, and nasal CPAP are the primary therapies for chronic lung disease of the premature. Diuretics (Lasix 1–2 mg/kg/d or Aldactazide 1–2 mg/kg/d), inhaled β_2 adrenergics, inhaled corticosteroids (fluticasone or budesonide), and systemic corticosteroids (dexamethasone 0.2–0.5 mg/kg/d or hydrocortisone 1–3 mg/kg/d) have been used as adjunctive therapy. Use of systemic corticosteroids remains controversial. Although a decrease in lung inflammation can aid infants in weaning off of ventilator support, there are data associating dexamethasone use in the first several weeks of life with an increased incidence of cerebral palsy. This risk must be balanced against the higher risk of neurodevelopmental handicap in infants with severe chronic lung disease. There is likely a point in the course of these infants at which the benefit of using systemic corticosteroids for the shortest amount of time at the lowest dose possible outweighs the risk of continued mechanical ventilation with its associated volutrauma and persistent lung inflammation. After hospital discharge, some of these infants will continue to require oxygen at home. This can be monitored by pulse oximetry with a target SaO_2 of 94–96%.

American Academy of Pediatrics Committee on Fetus and Newborn: Apnea, sudden infant death syndrome, and home monitoring. Pediatrics 2003;111:914 [PMID: 12671135].

American Academy of Pediatrics Committee on Fetus and Newborn, Canadian Paediatric Society: Postnatal corticosteroids to treat or prevent chronic lung disease in preterm infants. Pediatrics 2002;109;330 [PMID: 11826218].

Baird TM et al: Clinical association, treatment, and outcome of apnea of prematurity. Neoreviews 2002;3:e66.

Doyle LW et al: Impact of postnatal systemic corticosteroids on mortality and cerebral palsy in preterm infants: effect modification by risk for chronic lung disease. Pediatrics 2005;115:655 [PMID: 15741368].

Eichenwald EC et al: Apnea frequently persists beyond term gestation in infants delivered at 24–28 weeks. Pediatrics 1997; 100:354 [PMID: 9282705].

Jobe AH, Bancalari E: Bronchopulmonary dysplasia. Am J Respir Crit Care Med 2001;163:1723 [PMID: 11401896].

Jobe AH: Postnatal corticosteroids for preterm infants—do what we say, not what we do. N Engl J Med 2004;350:1349 [PMID: 15044647].

Kattwinkel J et al: High- versus low-threshold surfactant replacement for neonatal respiratory distress syndrome. Pediatrics 2000;106:282 [PMID: 10920152].

Lodygensky GA et al: Structural and functional brain development after hydrocortisone treatment for neonatal chronic lung disease. Pediatrics 2005;116:1 [PMID: 15995023].

Martin RJ et al: Pathophysiologic mechanisms underlying apnea of prematurity. Neoreviews 2002;3:e59.

Murphy BP et al: Impaired cerebral cortical gray matter growth after treatment with dexamethasone for neonatal chronic lung disease. Pediatrics 2001;107:217 [PMID: 11158449].

Ramanathan R et al: Cardiorespiratory events recorded on home monitors: Comparison of healthy infants with those at increased risk for SIDS. JAMA 2001;285:2199 [PMID: 11325321].

Stark AR: Risks and benefits of postnatal corticosteroids. NeoReviews 2005;6:e99.

Suresh GK, Soll RF: Current surfactant use in premature infants. Clin Perinatol 2001;28:671 [PMID: 11570160].

Vaucher Y: Bronchopulmonary dysplasia: An enduring challenge. Pediatr Rev 2002;23:349 [PMID: 12359869].

Yeh TF et al: Outcomes at school age after postnatal dexamethasone therapy for lung disease of prematurity. N Engl J Med 2004;350:1304 [PMID: 15044641].

4. Patent Ductus Arteriosus

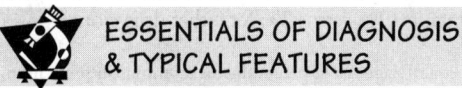

ESSENTIALS OF DIAGNOSIS & TYPICAL FEATURES

- *Hyperdynamic precordium.*
- *Widened pulse pressure.*
- *Hypotension.*
- *Presence of a systolic heart murmur in many cases.*

General Considerations

Clinically significant patent ductus arteriosus usually presents on days 3–7 as the respiratory distress from hyaline membrane disease is improving. Presentation can be on days 1 or 2, especially in infants born at less than 28 weeks' gestation and in those who have received surfactant replacement therapy. The signs include a hyperdynamic precordium, increased peripheral pulses, and a widened pulse pressure with or without a systolic heart murmur. Early presentations are sometimes manifested by systemic hypotension without a murmur or hyperdynamic circulation. These signs are often accompanied by an increase in respiratory support and a metabolic acidemia. The presence of significant patent ductus arteriosus can be confirmed by echocardiography.

Treatment

The ductus arteriosus is managed by medical or surgical ligation. A clinically significant ductus causing compromise in the infant can be closed (in about two-thirds of cases) with indomethacin, 0.1–0.2 mg/kg IV q12–24h for three doses. If the ductus reopens or fails to close completely, a second course of drug may be used. If indomethacin fails to close the ductus or if a ductus reopens a second time, surgical ligation is appropriate. In some cases, a more prolonged course of indomethacin is being used to prevent recurrences. In addition, in the extremely low birth weight infant (< 1000 g) who is at very high risk of developing a symptomatic ductus, a prophylactic strategy starting indomethacin (0.1 mg/kg q24h for 3–5 days) on the first day of life can be used. The major side effect of indomethacin is transient oliguria, which can be managed by fluid restriction until urine output improves. There may also be an increased incidence of necrotizing enterocolitis with more prolonged therapy. Transient decreases in intestinal and cerebral blood flow caused by indomethacin can be ameliorated by giving the drug as a slow infusion over 1–2 hours. The drug should not be used if the infant is hyperkalemic, if the creatinine is > 2 mg/dL, or if the platelet count is < 50,000/mL. There is an increased incidence of intestinal perforation if used concomitantly with hydrocortisone in extremely low birth weight infants (9% versus 2% for either drug alone).

Evans N et al: Diagnosis of patent ductus arteriosus in preterm infants. NeoReviews 2004;5:e86.

Lee J et al: Randomized trial of prolonged low dose versus conventional dose indomethacin for treating patent ductus arteriosus in very low birth weight infants. Pediatrics 2003;112:345 [PMID: 12897285].

Narayan-Sankar M, Clyman RI: Pharmacologic closure of patent ductus arteriosus in the neonate. Neoreviews 2003;4:e215.

Schmidt B et al: Long-term effects of indomethacin prophylaxis in extremely-low-birth-weight infants. N Engl J Med 2001;344:1966 [PMID: 11430325].

Watterberg KL et al: Prophylaxis of early adrenal insufficiency to prevent bronchopulmonary dysplasia: a multicenter trial. Pediatrics 2004;114:1649 [PMID: 15574629].

5. Necrotizing Enterocolitis

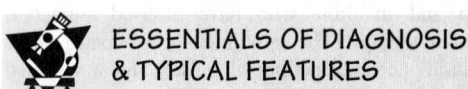

ESSENTIALS OF DIAGNOSIS & TYPICAL FEATURES

- *Feeding intolerance with gastric aspirates or vomiting.*
- *Bloody stools.*
- *Abdominal distention and tenderness.*
- *Pneumatosis intestinalis on abdominal radiograph.*

General Considerations

Necrotizing enterocolitis is the most common acquired GI emergency in the newborn infant; it most often affects preterm infants, with an incidence of 10% in infants of birth weight < 1500 g. In full-term infants, it occurs in association with polycythemia, congenital heart disease, and birth asphyxia. The pathogenesis of the disease is multifactorial. Previous intestinal ischemia, bacterial or viral infection, and immunologic immaturity of the gut are all thought to play a role in the genesis of the disorder. In up to 20% of affected infants, the only risk factor is prematurity.

Clinical Findings

The most common presenting sign is abdominal distention. Other signs include vomiting or increased gastric residuals, heme-positive stools, abdominal tenderness, temperature instability, increased apnea and bradycardia, decreased urine output, and poor perfusion. The CBC may show an increased white blood cell count with an increased band count or, as the disease progresses, absolute neutropenia. Thrombocytopenia is often observed along with stress-induced hyperglycemia and metabolic acidosis. Diagnosis is confirmed by the presence of pneumatosis intestinalis (air in the bowel wall) on radiograph. There is a spectrum of disease, and milder cases may exhibit only distention of bowel loops with bowel wall edema (thickened-appearing walls on radiograph).

Treatment

A. MEDICAL TREATMENT

Necrotizing enterocolitis is managed by decompression of the gut by nasogastric tube, maintenance of oxygenation, mechanical ventilation if necessary, and IV fluids (normal saline) to replace third-space GI losses. Enough fluid should be given to restore a good urine output. Other measures consist of broad-spectrum antibiotics (usually ampicillin, a third-generation cephalosporin or an aminoglycoside, and possibly additional anaerobic coverage), close monitoring of vital signs, serial physical examinations, and laboratory studies (blood gases, white blood cell count, platelet count, and radiographs). Although there are no proven strategies to prevent NEC, cautious advancement of feeds and use of probiotics in sick tiny infants may prove to provide some protection against NEC.

B. Surgical Treatment

Indications for surgery are evidence of perforation (free air present on a left lateral decubitus or cross-table lateral film), a fixed dilated loop of bowel on serial radiographs, abdominal wall cellulitis, or progressive deterioration despite maximal medical support. All of these signs are indicative of necrotic bowel. In the operating room, necrotic bowel is removed and ostomies are created. In extremely low birth weight infants, the initial surgical management may simply be the placement of peritoneal drains. Reanastomosis in infants with ostomies is performed after the disease is resolved and the infant is bigger (usually > 2 kg and after 4–6 weeks).

C. Course & Prognosis

Infants treated either medically or surgically should not be refed until the disease is resolved (normal abdominal examination and resolution of pneumatosis on radiograph), usually in 10–14 days. Nutritional support during this time should be provided by total parenteral nutrition.

Death occurs in 10% of cases. Surgery is needed in less than 25% of cases. Long-term prognosis is determined by the amount of intestine lost. Infants with short bowel require long-term support with IV nutrition and therefore have very long hospitalizations. Even for those infants, however, the outcome is favorable because of improved parenteral nutrition formulations. Late strictures—about 3–6 weeks after initial diagnosis—occur in 8% of patients whether treated medically or surgically, and generally require operative management. Infants with surgically managed NEC have an increased risk of poor neurodevelopmental outcome.

Berseth CL et al: Prolonged small feeding volumes early in life decreases the incidence of necrotizing enterocolitis in very low birth weight infants. Pediatrics 2003;111:529 [PMID: 12612232].

Caplan MS, Jilling T: The pathophysiology of necrotizing enterocolitis. Neoreviews 2001;2:e103.

Dimmit RA, Moss LR: Clinical management of necrotizing enterocolitis. Neoreviews 2001;2:e110.

Hintz SR et al: Neurodevelopmental and growth outcomes of extremely low birthweight infants after necrotizing enterocolitis. Pediatrics 2005;115:696 [PMID: 15741374].

Lin H-C et al: Oral probiotics reduce the incidence and severity of necrotizing enterocolitis in very low birth weight infants. Pediatrics 2005;115:1 [PMID: 15629973].

6. Anemia in the Premature Infant

General Considerations

In the premature infant, the hemoglobin reaches its nadir at approximately 8–12 weeks and is 2–3 g/dL lower than that in the full-term infant. The lower nadir in premature infants appears to be the result of a decreased erythropoietin response to the low red cell mass. Symptoms of anemia include poor feeding, lethargy, increased heart rate, poor weight gain, and perhaps apnea.

Treatment

The decision to transfuse is based on the presence of clinical symptoms. Transfusion is not indicated in an asymptomatic infant simply because of an arbitrary hematocrit. Most infants become symptomatic if the hematocrit drops below 20%. With risks of transfusion, alternative therapies have been explored. Epoetin alfa, 250 U/kg, given subcutaneously three times per week or added daily with iron dextran to parenteral nutrition, has been shown to increase hematocrit and reticulocyte count and to decrease the frequency and volume of transfused blood. This treatment should be reserved for the highest-risk infants (those born at less than 28–30 weeks' gestation and below 1000–1200 g). For optimal effect, supplemental iron at a dosage of 4–8 mg/kg/d should be given. Other options include rescue epoetin alfa at 300 U/kg/d for 7–10 days for hematocrits < 28% or a late transfusion from the same blood unit used for an infant's early transfusions.

Murray NA, Roberts IAG: Neonatal transfusion practice. Arch Dis Child Fetal Neonatal Ed 2004;89:F101 [PMID: 14977890].

Ohls RK: Human recombinant erythropoietin in the preterm and treatment of anemia of prematurity. Paediatr Drugs 2002; 4:111 [PMID: 11888358].

7. Intraventricular Hemorrhage

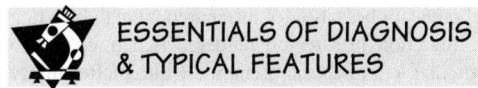

ESSENTIALS OF DIAGNOSIS & TYPICAL FEATURES

- *Large bleeds are accompanied by hypotension, metabolic acidosis, and altered neurologic status. Smaller bleeds can be asymptomatic.*
- *Routine cranial ultrasound scanning is essential for diagnosis in infants born at less than 32 weeks' gestation.*

General Considerations

Periventricular-intraventricular hemorrhage occurs almost exclusively in premature infants. The incidence is 20–30% in infants born at less than 31 weeks' gestation and weighing less than 1500 g at birth. The highest incidence is observed in babies of the lowest gestational age (< 26 weeks). Bleeding most commonly occurs in the sub-

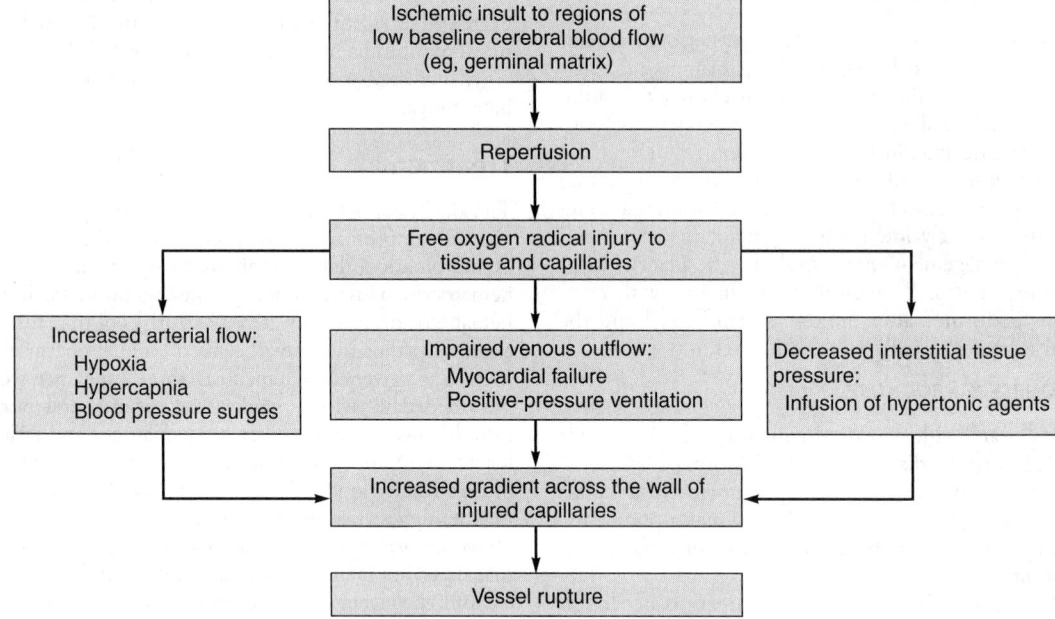

Figure 1–10. Pathogenesis of periventricular and intraventricular hemorrhage.

ependymal germinal matrix (a region of undifferentiated cells adjacent to or lining the lateral ventricles). Bleeding can extend into the ventricular cavity. The proposed pathogenesis of bleeding is presented in Figure 1–10. The critical event is ischemia with reperfusion injury to the capillaries in the germinal matrix that occurs in the immediate perinatal period. The actual amount of bleeding is also influenced by a variety of factors that affect the pressure gradient across the injured capillary wall. This pathogenetic scheme applies also to intraparenchymal bleeding (venous infarction in a region rendered ischemic) and to periventricular leukomalacia (ischemic white matter injury in a watershed region of arterial supply). Central nervous system complications in preterm infants are more frequent in infants exposed antenatally to intrauterine infection.

Clinical Findings

Up to 50% of hemorrhages occur at less than 24 hours of age, and virtually all occur by the fourth day. The clinical syndrome ranges from rapid deterioration (coma, hypoventilation, decerebrate posturing, fixed pupils, bulging anterior fontanelle, hypotension, acidosis, or acute drop in hematocrit), to a more gradual deterioration with more subtle neurologic changes, to absence of any specific physiologic or neurologic signs.

The diagnosis can be confirmed by real-time ultrasound scan. This can be performed whenever bleeding is clinically suspected. If symptoms are absent, routine scanning should be done at 10–14 days in all infants born at

< 29 weeks' gestation. Hemorrhages are graded as follows: grade I, germinal matrix hemorrhage only; grade II, intraventricular bleeding without ventricular enlargement; grade III, intraventricular bleeding with ventricular enlargement; and grade IV, any infant with intraparenchymal bleeding. The amount of bleeding is minor (grade I or II) in 75% of infants and major in the remainder.

Follow-up ultrasound examinations are based on the results of the initial scan. Infants with no bleeding or germinal matrix hemorrhage require only a single late scan at age 4–6 weeks to look for periventricular leukomalacia. Any infant with blood in the ventricular system is at risk for posthemorrhagic ventriculomegaly. This is usually the result of impaired absorption of cerebrospinal fluid (CSF), but it can also occur secondary to obstructive phenomena. An initial follow-up scan should be done 1–2 weeks after the initial scan. Infants with intraventricular bleeding and ventricular enlargement should be followed every 7–10 days until ventricular enlargement stabilizes or decreases. Infants without ventriculomegaly should have one additional scan at age 4–6 weeks. In addition, all infants born at 29–32 weeks' gestation should have at least a late scan (4–6 weeks) to look for ventriculomegaly and periventricular leukomalacia.

Treatment

During acute hemorrhage, supportive treatment (including restoration of volume and hematocrit, oxygenation, and ventilation) should be provided to avoid further cerebral ischemia. Progressive posthemorrhagic hydro-cephalus (if it develops) is treated initially with a sub-galeal shunt. When the infant is large enough, this can be converted to a ventriculoperitoneal shunt.

Although the incidence and severity of intracranial bleeding have decreased in premature infants, strategies to prevent this complication are still needed. Use of antenatal corticosteroids appears to be important in decreasing this complication, and phenobarbital may have a role in the mother who has not been prepared with steroids and is delivering at less than 28 weeks' gestation. The route of delivery may also play a role, with babies delivered by cesarean section showing a decreased rate of intracranial bleeds, but this issue remains controversial. Postnatal strat-egies appear less promising. Early indomethacin adminis-tration may have some benefit in minimizing bleeding, especially in males, with unclear influence on long-term outcome.

Prognosis

No deaths occur as a result of grade I and grade II hemor-rhages, whereas grade III and grade IV hemorrhages carry a mortality rate of 10–20%. Posthemorrhagic ventricular enlargement is rarely seen with grade I hemorrhages but is seen in 54–87% of grade II–IV hemorrhages. Very few of these infants will require a ventriculoperitoneal shunt. Long-term neurologic sequelae are seen no more fre-quently in infants with grade I and grade II hemorrhages than in preterm infants without bleeding. In infants with grade III and grade IV hemorrhages, severe sequelae occur in 20–25% of cases, mild sequelae in 35% of cases, and no sequelae in 40% of cases. The presence of severe periven-tricular leukomalacia, large parenchymal bleeds, and pro-gressive ventriculomegaly greatly increases the risk of neu-rologic sequelae. It is important to note that extremely low birth weight infants without major ultrasound findings remain at increased risk for both cerebral palsy and cogni-tive delays. Recent reports using quantitative MRI scans demonstrate that subtle gray and white matter findings not seen with ultrasound are prevalent in preterm survivors and are predictive of neurodevelopmental handicap. Again, this is especially true in those infants born at less than 1000 g and 28 weeks' gestation.

Inder TE et al: Abnormal cerebral structure is present at term in pre-mature infants. Pediatrics 2005;115:286 [PMID: 15687434].

Laptook AR et al: Adverse neurodevelopmental outcome among extremely low birth weight infants with normal head ultra-sound: prevalence and antecedents. Pediatrics 2005;115:673 [PMID: 15741371].

Ramsey PS, Rouse DJ: Therapies administered to mothers at risk for preterm birth and neurodevelopmental outcome in their infants. Clin Perinatol 2002;29:725 [PMID: 12616743].

Schmidt B et al: Long-term effects of indomethacin prophylaxis in ex-tremely-low-birth-weight infants. N Engl J Med 2001;344:1966 [PMID: 11430325].

Volpe JJ: Cerebral white matter injury of the premature infant—More common than you think. Pediatrics 2003;112:176 [PMID: 12737883].

Volpe JJ: Encephalopathy of prematurity includes neuronal abnor-malities. Pediatrics 2005;116:221 [PMID: 15995055].

Whitelaw et al: Post haemorrhagic ventricular dilation. Arch Dis Child Fetal Neonatal Ed 2002;86:72 [PMID: 11882544].

8. Retinopathy of Prematurity

Retinopathy of prematurity occurs only in the incom-pletely vascularized retina of the premature infant. The incidence of any acute retinopathy in infants weighing < 1250 g is 66%, whereas only 6% have reti-nopathy severe enough to warrant intervention. The incidence is highest in babies of the lowest gestational age. The condition appears to be triggered by an ini-tial injury to the developing retinal vessels. Hypoxia, shock, asphyxia, vitamin E deficiency, and light expo-sure have been associated with this initial injury. After the initial injury, normal vessel development may fol-low or abnormal vascularization may occur with ridge formation on the retina. The process can still regress at this point or may continue, with growth of fibrovas-cular tissue into the vitreous associated with inflam-mation, scarring, and retinal folds or detachment. The disease is graded by stages of abnormal vascular devel-opment and retinal detachment (I–V), by the zone of the eye involved (1–3, with zone 1 being the posterior region around the macula), and by the amount of the retina involved, in "clock hours" (eg, a detachment in the upper, outer quadrant of the left eye would be defined as affecting the left retina from 12 to 3 o'clock).

Initial eye examination should be performed at 4–6 weeks of age in infants with a birth weight < 1500 g or in those born at < 28 weeks' gestation, as well as in infants weighing > 1500 g with an unstable clinical course. Follow-up is done at 1- to 2-week intervals until the retina is fully vascularized. Infants with threshold disease are candidates for laser therapy. Although this treatment does not always prevent retinal detachment, it reduces the incidence of poor outcomes based on visual acuity and retinal anatomy.

American Academy of Pediatrics Section on Ophthalmology, American Academy of Ophthalmology and Association for Pediatric Ophthalmology and Strabismus: Screening ex-amination of premature infants for retinopathy of prema-turity. Pediatrics 2006;117:572 [PMID: 16452383].

Early treatment for retinopathy of prematurity cooperative group: Re-vised indications for the treatment of retinopathy of prematurity. Arch Ophthalmol 2003;121:1684 [PMID: 14662586].

Early treatment for retinopathy of prematurity cooperative group: The incidence and course of retinopathy of prematurity: find-ings from the early treatment for retinopathy of prematurity study. Pediatrics 2005;116:15 [PMID: 15995025].

Maden A: Angiogenesis and antiangiogenesis in the neonate: relevance to retinopathy of prematurity. NeoReviews 2003; 4:e356.

Phelps DL: Retinopathy of prematurity: history, classification, and pathophysiology. Neoreviews 2001;2:e153.

Phelps DL: The early treatment for retinopathy of prematurity study: better outcomes changing strategy. Pediatrics 2004; 114:490 [PMID: 15286325].

9. Discharge & Follow-Up of the Premature Infant

Hospital Discharge

Medical criteria for discharge of the premature infant include the ability to maintain temperature in an open crib, nippling all feeds and gaining weight, and the absence of apneic and bradycardiac spells requiring intervention. Infants going home on supplemental oxygen should not desaturate too badly (< 80%) in room air or should demonstrate the ability to arouse in response to hypoxia. Factors such as support for the mother at home and the stability of the family situation play a role in the timing of discharge. Home nursing visits and early physician follow-up can be used to hasten discharge.

Follow-Up

With advances in obstetric and maternal care, survival for infants born at > 28 weeks' gestation or with birth weights as low as 1000 g is now better than 90%. Seventy to 80% survive at 26–27 weeks' gestation and birth weights of 800–1000 g. Survival at gestational age 25 weeks and birth weight 700–800 g is 50–70%, with a considerable drop-off below this level (Figure 1–11).

These high rates of survival do come with a price in terms of morbidity. Major neurologic sequelae, including cerebral palsy, cognitive delay, and hydrocephalus, is reported in 10–25% of survivors with birth weights < 1500 g. The rate of these sequelae tends to be higher in infants with lower birth weights. In addition to a higher incidence of severe neurologic sequelae, infants with birth weights < 1000 g have an increased rate of lesser disabilities, including learning, behavioral and psychiatric problems. Risk factors for neurologic sequelae include seizures, grade III or IV intracranial hemorrhage, periventricular leukomalacia, ventricular dilatation, severe IUGR, poor early head growth, need for mechanical ventilation, chronic lung disease, NEC, and low socioeconomic class. Maternal fever and chorioam-

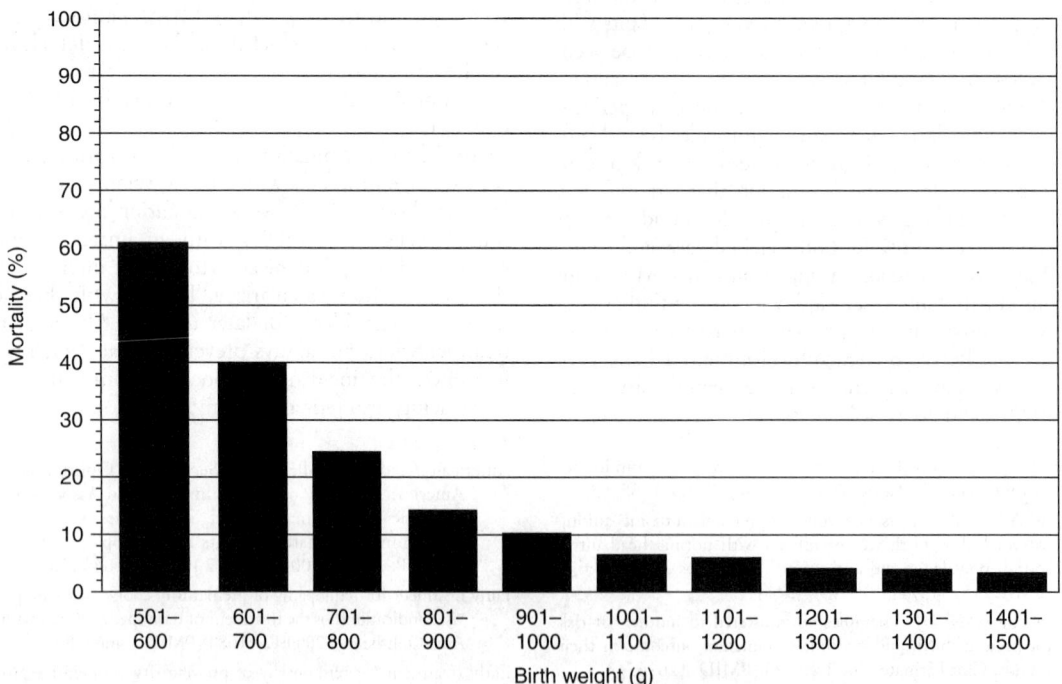

Figure 1–11. Mortality rates before discharge by 100-g birth weight subgroups in 2004. (Reproduced, with permission, from the Vermont Oxford Network, 2005.)

nionitis have also been associated with an increased risk of cerebral palsy. Other morbidities in these infants include chronic lung disease and reactive airway disease, resulting in an increased risk from respiratory infections and hospital readmissions in the first 2 years; retinopathy of prematurity with associated loss of visual acuity and strabismus; hearing loss; and growth failure. All of these issues require close multidisciplinary outpatient follow-up. Infants with residual lung disease are candidates for monthly palivizumab (Synagis) injections during their first winter after hospital discharge to prevent severe infection with respiratory syncytial virus. Routine immunizations should be done by chronologic age and not age-corrected for prematurity.

American Academy of Pediatrics. Committee on Infectious Diseases and Committee on Fetus and Newborn: Revised indications for the use of palivizumab and respiratory syncytial virus immune globulin intravenous for the prevention of respiratory syncytial virus infection. Pediatrics 2003;112:1442 [PMID: 14654628].

Bhutta AT et al: Cognitive and behavioral outcomes of school-aged children who were born preterm. A meta-analysis. JAMA 2002;288:728 [PMID: 12169077].

Doyle LW and the Victorian Infant Collaborative Study Group: Outcome at 5 years of age of children 23–27 weeks gestation: Refining the prognosis. Pediatrics 2001;108:134 [PMID: 11433066].

Hack M et al: Behavioral outcomes and evidence of psychopathology among very low birth weight infants at age 20 years. Pediatrics 2004;114:932 [PMID: 15466087].

Hack M et al: Chronic conditions, functional limitations, and special healthcare needs of school-aged children born with extremely low-birth-weight in the 1990's. JAMA 2005;294:318 [PMID: 16030276].

Hack M et al: Outcomes in young adulthood for very-low-birth-weight infants. N Engl J Med 2002;346:149 [PMID: 11796848].

Horbar JD et al: Trends in mortality and morbidity for very low birth weight infants 1991–1999. Pediatrics 2002;110:143 [PMID: 12093960].

Latal-Hajnal B et al: Postnatal growth in VLBW infants: significant association with neurodevelopmental outcome. J Pediatr 2003;143:163 [PMID: 12970627].

Marlow N et al: Neurologic and developmental disability at six years of age after extremely preterm birth. N Engl J Med 2005;352:9 [PMID: 15635108].

Ment LR et al: Change in cognitive function over time in very-low-birth-weight infants. JAMA 2003;289:705 [PMID: 12585948].

O'Connor AR et al: Long-term ophthalmic outcome of low birth weight children with and without retinopathy of prematurity. Pediatrics 2002;109:12 [PMID: 11773536].

Saari TN and the Committee on Infectious Diseases: Immunization of preterm and low birth weight infants. Pediatrics 2003;112:193 [PMID: 12837889].

Schmidt B et al: Impact of bronchopulmonary dysplasia, brain injury, and severe retinopathy on the outcome of extremely low-birth-weight infants at 18 months: Results from the trial of indomethacin prophylaxis in preterms. JAMA 2003; 289: 1124 [PMID: 12622582].

Wilson-Costello D et al: Improved survival rates with increased neurodevelopmental disability for extremely low birth weight infants in the 1990's. Pediatrics 2005;115:997 [PMID: 15805376].

Wood NS et al: Neurologic and developmental disability after extremely preterm birth. N Engl J Med 2000;343:378 [PMID: 10933736].

■ CARDIAC PROBLEMS IN THE NEWBORN INFANT

STRUCTURAL HEART DISEASE

1. Cyanotic Presentations

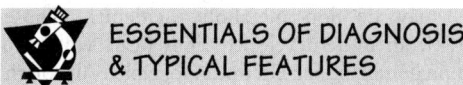

ESSENTIALS OF DIAGNOSIS & TYPICAL FEATURES

- *Cyanosis, initially without associated respiratory distress.*
- *Failure to increase PaO_2 with supplemental oxygen.*
- *Chest radiograph with decreased lung markings suggests right heart obstruction, while increased lung markings suggest transposition or venous obstruction.*

General Considerations

The causes of cyanotic heart disease that occurs in the newborn period are transposition of the great vessels, total anomalous pulmonary venous return, truncus arteriosus (some types), tricuspid atresia, and pulmonary atresia or critical pulmonary stenosis.

Clinical Findings

Infants with these disorders present with early cyanosis. The hallmark of many of these lesions is cyanosis in an infant without associated respiratory distress. In most of these infants, tachypnea develops over time either because of increased pulmonary blood flow or secondary to metabolic acidemia from progressive hypoxemia. Diagnostic aids include comparing the blood gas or oxygen saturation in room air to that in 100% FIO_2. Failure of PaO_2 or SaO_2 to increase suggests cyanotic heart disease. Note: A PaO_2, if feasible, is the preferred measure. Saturation in the newborn may be misleadingly high despite pathologically low PaO_2 due to the left-shifted oxyhemoglobin dissociation curve seen with fetal hemoglobin. Other useful aids are chest radiograph, electrocardiography, and echocardiography.

Transposition of the great vessels is the most common form of cyanotic heart disease presenting in the newborn period. Examination generally reveals a systolic murmur and single S2. Chest radiograph shows a generous heart size and a narrow mediastinum with normal or increased lung markings. There is little change in PaO_2 or SaO_2 with supplemental oxygen. Total anomalous pulmonary venous return, in which venous return is obstructed, presents early with severe cyanosis and tachypnea because the pulmonary venous return is obstructed, resulting in pulmonary edema. The chest radiograph typically shows a small to normal heart size with marked pulmonary edema. Infants with right heart obstruction (pulmonary and tricuspid atresia, critical pulmonary stenosis, and some forms of truncus arteriosus) have decreased lung markings on chest radiograph and, depending on the severity of hypoxia, may develop metabolic acidemia. Those lesions with an underdeveloped right heart will have left-sided predominance on electrocardiography. Although tetralogy of Fallot is the most common form of cyanotic heart disease, the obstruction at the pulmonary valve is often not severe enough to result in cyanosis in the newborn. In all cases, diagnosis can be confirmed by echocardiography.

2. Acyanotic Presentations

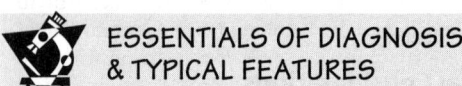

ESSENTIALS OF DIAGNOSIS & TYPICAL FEATURES

- *Most newborns who present with acyanotic heart disease have left-sided outflow obstruction.*
- *Differentially diminished pulses (coarctation) or decreased pulses throughout (aortic atresia).*
- *Metabolic acidemia.*
- *Chest radiograph showing large heart and pulmonary edema.*

General Considerations

Newborn infants who present with serious acyanotic heart disease usually have congestive heart failure secondary to left-sided outflow tract obstruction. Infants with left-to-right shunt lesions (eg, ventricular septal defect) may have murmurs in the newborn period, but clinical symptoms do not occur until pulmonary vascular resistance drops enough to cause significant shunt-

ing and subsequent congestive heart failure (usually at 3–4 weeks of age).

Clinical Findings

Infants with left-sided outflow obstruction generally do well the first day or so until the ductus arteriosus—the source of all or some of the systemic flow—narrows. Tachypnea, tachycardia, congestive heart failure, and metabolic acidosis develop. On examination, all of these infants have abnormalities of the pulses. In aortic atresia (hypoplastic left heart syndrome) and stenosis, pulses are all diminished, whereas in coarctation syndromes, differential pulses (diminished or absent in the lower extremities) are evident. Chest radiographic films in these infants show a large heart and pulmonary edema. Diagnosis is confirmed with echocardiography.

3. Treatment of Cyanotic & Acyanotic Lesions

Early stabilization includes supportive therapy as needed (eg, IV glucose, oxygen, ventilation for respiratory failure, and pressor support). Specific therapy includes infusions of prostaglandin E_1, 0.025–0.1 µg/kg/min, to maintain ductal patency. In some cyanotic lesions (eg, pulmonary atresia, tricuspid atresia, and critical pulmonary stenosis) in which lung blood flow is ductus-dependent, this improves pulmonary blood flow and PaO_2 by allowing shunting through the ductus to the pulmonary artery. In left-sided outflow tract obstruction, systemic blood flow is ductus-dependent; prostaglandins improve systemic perfusion and resolve the acidosis. Further specific management—including palliative surgical and cardiac catheterization procedures—is discussed in Chapter 19.

PERSISTENT PULMONARY HYPERTENSION IN THE NEWBORN INFANT

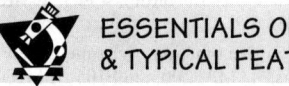

ESSENTIALS OF DIAGNOSIS & TYPICAL FEATURES

- *Onset of symptoms on day 1 of life.*
- *Hypoxia with poor response to high concentrations of inspired oxygen.*
- *Right-to-left shunts through the foramen ovale, ductus arteriosus, or both.*
- *Most often associated with parenchymal lung disease.*

General Considerations

Persistent pulmonary hypertension of the newborn (PPHN) results when the normal decrease in pulmonary vascular resistance after birth does not occur. Most infants so affected are full term or postterm, and many have experienced perinatal asphyxia. Other clinical associations include hypothermia, meconium aspiration syndrome, hyaline membrane disease, polycythemia, neonatal sepsis, chronic intrauterine hypoxia, and pulmonary hypoplasia.

There are three underlying pathophysiologic mechanisms of PPHN: (1) acute vasoconstriction due to perinatal hypoxia related to an acute event such as sepsis or asphyxia, (2) a prenatal increase in pulmonary vascular smooth muscle development often associated with meconium aspiration syndrome, and (3) decreased cross-sectional area of the pulmonary vascular bed associated with lung hypoplasia (eg, diaphragmatic hernia).

Clinical Findings

Clinically, the syndrome is characterized by onset on the first day of life, usually from birth. Respiratory distress is prominent, and PaO_2 is usually poorly responsive to high concentrations of inspired oxygen. Many of the infants have associated myocardial depression with resulting systemic hypotension. Echocardiography reveals right-to-left shunting at the level of the ductus arteriosus or foramen ovale (or both). Chest radiograph usually shows lung infiltrates related to associated pulmonary pathology (eg, meconium aspiration and hyaline membrane disease). If the majority of right-to-left shunt is at the ductal level, pre- and postductal differences in PaO_2 and SaO_2 will be observed.

Treatment

Therapy for PPHN involves supportive therapy for other postasphyxia problems (eg, anticonvulsants for seizures, careful fluid and electrolyte management for renal failure). IV glucose should be provided to maintain normal blood sugar, and antibiotics should be administered for possible infection. Specific therapy is aimed at both increasing systemic arterial pressure and decreasing pulmonary arterial pressure to reverse the right-to-left shunting through fetal pathways. First-line therapy includes oxygen and ventilation (to reduce pulmonary vascular resistance) and crystalloid infusions (10 mL/kg, up to 30 mL/kg) to improve systemic pressure. Ideally, systolic pressure should be greater than 60 mm Hg. With compromised cardiac function, systemic pressors can be used as second-line therapy (eg, dopamine, 5–20 μg/kg/min; dobutamine, 5–20 μg/kg/min; or both). Metabolic acidemia should be corrected with sodium bicarbonate because acidemia exacerbates pulmonary vasoconstriction. In some cases, a mild respiratory alkalosis may improve oxygenation. Pulmonary vasodilation can be enhanced using the inhaled gas nitric oxide, which is identical or very similar to endogenous endothelium-derived relaxing factor, at doses of 5–20 ppm. In addition, use of high-frequency oscillatory ventilation has proved effective in many of these infants, particularly those with severe associated lung disease.

Infants for whom conventional therapy is failing (poor oxygenation despite maximum support) may require extracorporeal membrane oxygenation (ECMO). The infants are placed on bypass, with blood exiting the baby from the right atrium and returning to the aortic arch after passing through a membrane oxygenator. The lungs are essentially at rest during the procedure, and with resolution of the pulmonary hypertension the infants are weaned from ECMO back to ventilator therapy. This therapy can save infants who might otherwise die, but has major side effects that must be considered prior to its institution. Neurodevelopmental outcome among survivors of ECMO is similar to that of infants with PPHN managed without the procedure. Approximately 10–15% of survivors have significant neurologic sequelae, with cerebral palsy or cognitive delays. Other sequelae such as chronic lung disease, sensorineural hearing loss, and feeding problems have also been described in this population.

ARRHYTHMIAS

Irregularly irregular heart rates, commonly associated with premature atrial contractions and less commonly with premature ventricular contractions, are noted often in the first days of life in well newborns. These arrhythmias are benign and of no consequence. Clinically significant bradyarrhythmias are seen in association with congenital heart block. Heart block can be seen in an otherwise structurally normal heart (associated with maternal lupus) or with structural cardiac abnormalities. If fetal hydrops is absent, the bradyarrhythmia has been well tolerated. Indications for cardiac pacing include symptoms of inadequate cardiac output.

On electrocardiography, tachyarrhythmias can be either wide complex (eg, ventricular tachycardia) or narrow complex (eg, supraventricular tachycardia). Supraventricular tachycardia is the most common tachyarrhythmia in the neonate and may be a sign of structural heart disease, myocarditis, left atrial enlargement, and aberrant conduction pathways. Acute treatment is ice to the face, and if unsuccessful, IV adenosine at a dose of 50–200 μg/kg. If there is no response, the dose can be increased to 300 μg/kg. Long-term therapy is with digoxin or propranolol. Digoxin should not be used in Wolff-Parkinson-White syndrome. Cardioversion is rarely needed for supraventricular tachycardia but is needed acutely for hemodynamically unstable ventricular tachycardia.

Beck AE, Hudgins L: Congenital cardiac malformations in the neonate: Isolated or syndromic? Neoreviews 2003;4:e105.

Carriedo H, Deming D: Therapeutic techniques: neonatal ECMO. NeoReviews 2003;4:e212.

Frommelt MA: Differential diagnosis and approach for a heart murmur in term infants. Pediatr Clin North Am 2004;51:1023 [PMID:15331284].

Kinsella JP, Abman SH: Inhaled nitric oxide: Current and future uses in neonates. Semin Perinatol 2000;24:387 [PMID: 11153900].

Larmay HJ, Strasburger JF: Differential diagnosis and management of the fetus and newborn with an irregular or abnormal heart rate. Pediatr Clin North Am 2004;51:1033 [PMID: 15275987].

Walsh MC, Stork EK: Persistent pulmonary hypertension of the newborn: Rationale therapy based on pathophysiology. Clin Perinatol 2001;28:609 [PMID: 11570157].

GASTROINTESTINAL & ABDOMINAL SURGICAL CONDITIONS IN THE NEWBORN INFANT (See Also Chapter 20.)

ESOPHAGEAL ATRESIA & TRACHEOESOPHAGEAL FISTULA

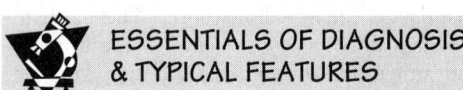

ESSENTIALS OF DIAGNOSIS & TYPICAL FEATURES

- *Polyhydramnios.*
- *Baby with excessive drooling and secretions, choking with attempted feeding.*
- *Unable to pass an orogastric tube to the stomach.*

General Considerations

This group of anomalies are characterized by a blind esophageal pouch and a fistulous connection between the proximal and/or distal esophagus and the airway. In 85% of infants, the fistula is between the distal esophagus and the airway. Polyhydramnios is common because of high GI obstruction.

Clinical Findings

Infants present in the first hours of life with copious secretions, choking, cyanosis, and respiratory distress.

Diagnosis is confirmed with chest radiograph after careful placement of a nasogastric (NG) tube to the point at which resistance is met. The tube will be seen radiographically in the blind pouch. If a tracheoesophageal fistula is present to the distal esophagus, gas will be present in the bowel. In esophageal atresia without tracheoesophageal fistula, there is no gas in the bowel.

Treatment

The NG tube in the proximal pouch should be placed on low intermittent continuous suction to drain secretions and prevent aspiration. The head of the bed should be elevated to prevent reflux of gastric contents through the distal fistula into the lungs. IV glucose and fluids should be provided and oxygen administered as needed. Definitive treatment is surgical and the technique used depends on the distance between the segments of esophagus. If the distance is not too great, the fistula can be ligated and the ends of the esophagus anastomosed. If the ends of the esophagus cannot be brought together, the initial surgery is fistula ligation and a feeding gastrostomy. Echocardiography should be performed prior to surgery to rule out a right-sided aortic arch. In those cases, a left-sided thoracotomy would be preferred.

Prognosis

Prognosis is determined primarily by the presence or absence of associated anomalies. Vertebral, anal, cardiac, renal, and limb anomalies are the most likely to be observed (VACTERL association). Evaluation for associated anomalies should be initiated early.

INTESTINAL OBSTRUCTION

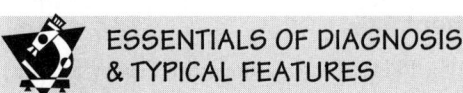

ESSENTIALS OF DIAGNOSIS & TYPICAL FEATURES

- *Infants with high intestinal obstruction present soon after birth with emesis.*
- *Bilious emesis suggests intestinal malrotation with midgut volvulus until proved otherwise.*
- *Low intestinal obstruction is characterized by abdominal distention and late onset of emesis.*

General Considerations

A history of polyhydramnios is common, and the fluid, if bile-stained, can easily be confused with thin meconium staining. The higher the obstruction in the intestine, the earlier the infant will develop vomiting and the less prominent the distention will be. The opposite is true for lower intestinal obstructions. Most obstructions are bowel atresias, believed to be caused by an ischemic event during development. Approximately 30% of cases of duodenal atresia are associated with Down syndrome. Meconium ileus is a distal small bowel obstruction caused by the viscous meconium produced in utero by infants with pancreatic insufficiency secondary to cystic fibrosis. Hirschsprung disease is caused by a failure of neuronal migration to the myenteric plexus of the distal bowel. The distal bowel lacks ganglion cells, causing a lack of peristalsis in that region with a functional obstruction.

Malrotation with midgut volvulus is a surgical emergency that appears in the first days to weeks as bilious vomiting without distention or tenderness. If malrotation is not treated promptly, torsion of the intestine around the superior mesenteric artery will lead to necrosis of the small bowel. For this reason, bilious vomiting in the neonate always demands immediate attention and evaluation.

Clinical Findings

Diagnosis of intestinal obstructions depends on plain abdominal radiographs with either upper GI series (high obstruction suspected) or contrast enema (lower obstruction apparent) to define the area of obstruction. Table 1–18 summarizes the findings expected.

Infants with meconium ileus are presumed to have cystic fibrosis. Infants with pancolonic Hirschsprung disease,

colon pseudo-obstruction syndrome, or colonic dysgenesis or atresia may also present with meconium impacted in the distal ileum. Definitive diagnosis of cystic fibrosis is by the sweat chloride test (Na^+ and Cl^- concentration > 60 mEq/L) or by genetic testing. Approximately 10–20% of infants with cystic fibrosis have meconium ileus. Infants with cystic fibrosis and meconium ileus generally have a normal immunoreactive trypsinogen test result on their newborn screen because of the associated severe exocrine pancreatic insufficiency in utero.

Intestinal perforation in utero results in meconium peritonitis with residual intra-abdominal calcifications. Many perforations are completely healed at birth. If the infant has no signs of obstruction, no immediate evaluation is needed. A sweat test to rule out cystic fibrosis should be done at a later date.

Low intestinal obstruction may present with delayed stooling (> 24 hours in term infants is abnormal) with mild distention. Radiographic findings of gaseous distention should prompt contrast enema to diagnose (and treat) meconium plug syndrome. If no plug is found, the diagnosis may be small left colon syndrome (occurring in IDMs) or Hirschsprung disease. Rectal biopsy will be required to clarify these two diagnoses. Imperforate anus is generally apparent on physical examination, although a rectovaginal fistula with a mildly abnormal-appearing anus can occasionally be confused with normal. High imperforate anus in males may be associated with recto-urethral or recto-vesical fistula.

Table 1–18. Intestinal obstruction.

Site of Obstruction	Clinical Findings	Plain Radiographs	Contrast Study
Duodenal atresia	Down syndrome (30%); early vomiting, sometimes bilious	"Double bubble" (dilated stomach and proximal duodenum, no air distal)	Not needed
Malrotation and volvulus	Bilious vomiting with onset anytime in the first few weeks	Dilated stomach and proximal duodenum; paucity of air distally (may be normal gas pattern)	UGI shows displaced duodenojejunal junction with "corkscrew" deformity of twisted bowel
Jejunoileal atresia, meconium ileus	Bilious gastric contents > 25 mL at birth; progressive distention and bilious vomiting	Multiple dilated loops of bowel; intra-abdominal calcifications if in-utero perforation occurred (meconium peritonitis)	Barium or osmotic contrast enema shows microcolon; contrast refluxed into distal ileum may demonstrate and relieve meconium obstruction (successful in about 50%)
Meconium plug syndrome; Hirschsprung disease	Distention, delayed stooling (> 24 h)	Diffuse bowel distention	Barium or osmotic contrast enema outlines and relieves plug; may show transition zone in Hirschsprung disease; delayed emptying (> 24 h) suggests Hirschsprung disease

UGI, upper gastrointesinal tract.

Treatment

Nasogastric suction to decompress the bowel, IV glucose, fluid and electrolyte replacement, and respiratory support as necessary should be instituted. Antibiotics are usually indicated. The definitive treatment for these conditions (with the exception of meconium plug syndrome, small left colon syndrome, and some cases of meconium ileus) is surgery.

Prognosis

Up to 10% of infants with meconium plug syndrome are subsequently found to have cystic fibrosis or Hirschsprung disease. For this reason, some surgeons advocate performance of a sweat chloride test and rectal biopsy in all of these infants before discharge. The infant with meconium plug syndrome who is still symptomatic after contrast enema should have a rectal biopsy.

In duodenal atresia associated with Down syndrome, the prognosis depends on associated anomalies (eg, heart defects) and the severity of prestenotic duodenal dilation and subsequent duodenal dysmotility. Otherwise, these conditions usually carry an excellent prognosis after surgical repair.

ABDOMINAL WALL DEFECTS

1. Omphalocele

Omphalocele is a membrane-covered herniation of abdominal contents into the base of the umbilical cord. There is a high incidence of associated anomalies (cardiac, GI, and chromosomal—eg, trisomy 13). The sac may contain liver and spleen as well as intestine.

Acute management of omphalocele involves covering the defect with a sterile dressing soaked with warm saline to prevent fluid loss, nasogastric decompression, IV fluids and glucose, and antibiotics. If the contents of the omphalocele will fit into the abdomen, a primary surgical closure is done. If not, a staged closure is performed, with gradual reduction of the omphalocele contents into the abdominal cavity and a secondary closure. Postoperatively, third-space fluid losses may be extensive; fluid and electrolyte therapy, therefore, must be monitored carefully.

2. Gastroschisis

In gastroschisis, the intestine extrudes through an abdominal wall defect lateral to the umbilical cord. There is no membrane or sac and no liver or spleen outside the abdomen. Gastroschisis is associated with no other anomalies except intestinal atresia in approximately 10%. The herniation is thought to be related to

abnormal involution of the right umbilical vein, although the exact cause is unknown.

Therapy is as described for omphalocele.

DIAPHRAGMATIC HERNIA

This congenital malformation consists of herniation of abdominal organs into the hemithorax (usually left) through a posterolateral defect in the diaphragm. It presents in the delivery room as severe respiratory distress in an infant with poor breath sounds and scaphoid abdomen. The rapidity and severity of presentation—as well as ultimate survival—depend on the degree of pulmonary hypoplasia, which is a result of compression by the intrathoracic abdominal contents in utero. Affected infants are prone to development of pneumothorax.

Treatment includes intubation and ventilation as well as decompression of the GI tract with a nasogastric tube to intermittent suction. An IV infusion of glucose and fluid should be started. Chest radiograph confirms the diagnosis. Surgery to reduce the abdominal contents from the thorax and to close the diaphragmatic defect is performed after the infant is stabilized. The postoperative course is often complicated by severe pulmonary hypertension, requiring therapy with high-frequency oscillatory ventilation, inhaled nitric oxide, or ECMO. The mortality rate for this condition is 25–40%, with survival dependent on the degree of pulmonary hypoplasia and presence of congenital heart disease.

GASTROINTESTINAL BLEEDING

Upper Gastrointestinal Bleeding

Upper GI bleeding is not uncommon in the newborn nursery. Old blood ("coffee-grounds" material) may be either swallowed maternal blood or infant blood from a bleeding gastric irritation such as gastritis or stress ulcer. Bright red blood from the stomach is most likely acute bleeding, again due to gastritis. Treatment generally consists of gastric lavage (a sample can be sent for Apt testing to determine if it is mother's or baby's blood) and antacid medication. If the volume of bleeding is large, intensive monitoring, fluid and blood replacement, and endoscopy are indicated. (See Chapter 20.)

Lower Gastrointestinal Bleeding

Rectal bleeding is less common than upper GI bleeding in the newborn and is associated with infections (eg, *Salmonella* acquired from the mother perinatally), milk intolerance (blood streaks with diarrhea), or in stressed infants, necrotizing enterocolitis. An abdominal radiograph should be obtained to rule out pneumatosis intestinalis (air in the wall of the bowel) or other abnormalities in gas pattern (eg, obstruction). If the radiograph is negative and the examination is benign, a protein hydrolysate or predigested formula (eg, Nutramigen or Pregestimil) should be tried or the mother instructed to avoid all dairy products in her diet if nursing. If the amount of rectal bleeding is large or persistent, endoscopy will be needed.

GASTROESOPHAGEAL REFLUX
(See Also Chapter 20.)

All normal people reflux occasionally, and physiologic regurgitation is common in infants. Reflux is pathologic and should be treated when it results in failure to thrive owing to excessive regurgitation, poor intake due to dysphagia and irritability, apnea or cyanotic episodes (acute life-threatening events), or chronic respiratory symptoms of wheezing and recurrent pneumonias. Diagnosis is clinical, with confirmation by pH probe or impedance study. Barium radiograph is helpful to rule out anatomic abnormalities but is not diagnostic of pathologic reflux.

Initial steps in treatment include thickened feeds (rice cereal, 1 tbsp/oz of formula) for those with frequent regurgitation and poor weight gain. Gastric acid suppressants such as ranitidine (2 mg/kg bid) or lansoprazole (1.5 mg/kg/d) can also be used, especially if there is associated irritability. Because most infants improve by 12–15 months of age, surgery is reserved for the most severe cases, especially those with chronic neurologic or respiratory conditions that exacerbate reflux and those who have life-threatening events caused by reflux.

Bohn D: Congenital diaphragmatic hernia. Am J Respir Crit Care Med 2002;166:911 [PMID: 12359645].

Cass DL, Wesson DE: Advances in fetal and neonatal surgery for gastrointestinal anomalies and disease. Clin Perinatol 2003; 29:1 [PMID: 11917733].

Cohen MS et al: Influence of congenital heart disease on survival in children with congenital diaphragmatic hernia. J Pediatr 2002;141:25 [PMID: 12091847].

Jadcherla SR: Gastroesophageal reflux in the neonate. Clin Perinatol 2002;29:135 [PMID: 11917735].

Rodgers BM: Upper gastrointestinal hemorrhage. Pediatr Rev 1999;20:171 [PMID: 10233176].

Squires RH: Gastrointestinal bleeding. Pediatr Rev 1999;20:95 [PMID: 10073071].

■ INFECTIONS IN THE NEWBORN INFANT

The fetus and the newborn infant are susceptible to infections. There are three major routes of perinatal infection: (1) blood-borne transplacental infection of the fetus (eg, cytomegalovirus [CMV], rubella, and syphilis); (2) ascending infection with disruption of the barrier provided by the amniotic membranes (eg, bacterial infections after 12–18 hours of ruptured membranes); and (3) infection on passage through an infected birth canal or exposure to infected blood at delivery (eg, herpes simplex, hepatitis B, HIV, and bacterial infections).

Susceptibility of the newborn infant to infection is related to immaturity of both the cellular and humoral immune systems at birth. This feature is particularly evident in the preterm neonate. Passive protection against some organisms is provided by transfer of IgG across the placenta during the third trimester of pregnancy. Preterm infants, especially those born at less than 30 weeks' gestation, do not have the full amount of this passively acquired antibody.

BACTERIAL INFECTIONS
1. Bacterial Sepsis

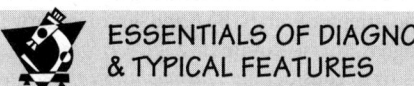

ESSENTIALS OF DIAGNOSIS & TYPICAL FEATURES

- *Most infants with early-onset sepsis present at <24 hours of age.*
- *Respiratory distress is the most common presenting symptom.*
- *Hypotension, acidemia, and neutropenia are associated clinical findings.*
- *The presentation of late-onset sepsis is more subtle.*

General Considerations

The incidence of early-onset (< 5 days) neonatal bacterial infection is 4–5 per 1000 live births. If rupture of the membranes occurs more than 24 hours prior to delivery, the infection rate increases to 1 per 100 live births. If early rupture of membranes with chorioamnionitis occurs, the infection rate increases further to 1 per 10 live births. Regardless of membrane rupture, infection rates are five times higher in preterm than in full-term infants.

Clinical Findings

Early-onset bacterial infections appear most commonly on day 1 of life, and the majority of cases appear at < 12 hours. Respiratory distress due to pneumonia is the most common presenting sign. Other features include unexplained low Apgar scores without fetal distress, poor perfusion, and hypotension. Late-onset bacterial infection (at > 5 days of age) presents in a more subtle manner, with poor feeding, lethargy, hypotonia, temperature instability, altered perfusion, new or increased oxygen requirement, and apnea. Late-onset bacterial sepsis is more often associated with meningitis or other localized infections.

Low total white counts, absolute neutropenia (< 1000/mL), and elevated ratios of immature to mature neutrophils are suggestive of neonatal bacterial infection. Thrombocytopenia is also a common feature. Other laboratory signs are hypoglycemia or hyperglycemia with no change in glucose administration, unexplained metabolic acidosis, and elevated C-reactive protein. In early-onset bacterial infection, pneumonia is invariably present; chest radiography shows infiltrates, but these infiltrates cannot be distinguished from those resulting from other causes of neonatal lung disease. Presence of a pleural effusion makes a diagnosis of pneumonia more likely. Definitive diagnosis is made by positive cultures from blood, CSF, and the like.

Early-onset infection is most often caused by group B β-hemolytic streptococci (GBS) and gram-negative enteric pathogens (most commonly *Escherichia coli*). Other organisms to consider are *Haemophilus influenzae* and *Listeria monocytogenes*. Late-onset sepsis is caused by coagulase-negative staphylococci (most common in infants with indwelling central venous lines), *Staphylococcus aureus*, GBS, *Enterococcus* and gram-negative organisms.

Treatment

A high index of suspicion is important in diagnosis and treatment of neonatal infection. Table 1–19 presents guidelines for the evaluation and treatment of full-term infants with risk factors or clinical signs of infection. Because the risk of infection is greater in the preterm infant and because respiratory disease is a common sign of infection, any preterm infant with respiratory disease requires blood cultures and broad-spectrum antibiotic therapy for 48–72 hours pending the results of cultures. Early-onset sepsis is usually caused by GBS or gram-negative enteric organisms; broad-spectrum coverage, therefore, should include ampicillin plus an aminoglycoside or third-generation cephalosporin—for example, ampicillin, 100–150 mg/kg/d divided q12h, and gentamicin, 2.5 mg/kg/dose q12–24h (depending on gestational age), or cefotaxime, 100 mg/kg/d divided q12h. In infants > 34 weeks' gestation, gentamicin can also be given at a dose of 4 mg/kg q24h. Late-onset infections can also be caused by the same organisms, but coverage may need to be expanded to include staphylococci. In particular, the preterm infant with an indwelling line is at risk for infection with coagulase-negative staphylococci, for which vancomycin is the drug of choice in a dosage of 10–15

Table 1–19. Guidelines for evaluation of neonatal bacterial infection in the full-term infant.

Risk Factor	Clinical Signs of Infection	Evaluation and Treatment
Delivery 12–18 h after rupture of membranes	None	Observation
Delivery > 12–18 h after rupture of membranes, chorioamnionitis	None	Complete blood cell count (CBC), blood culture, broad-spectrum antibiotics for 48–72 h[c]
Delivery > 12–18 h after rupture of membranes, chorioamnionitis, maternal antibiotics[a]	None	CBC, blood culture, broad-spectrum antibiotics for 48–72 h[c]
With or without risk factors	Present	CBC, blood and CSF cultures, perhaps urine culture (see below); broad-spectrum antibiotics[b]

[a]Minimum of 24 h of observation is indicated if no treatment is given.
[b]Irrespective of age at presentation, any infant who appears infected by clinical criteria should undergo cerebrospinal fluid (CSF) examination. Urine culture is indicated in the evaluation of infants who were initially well but have developed symptoms after 2–3 d of age.
[c]If clinical signs are absent, close observation without treatment may be sufficient.

mg/kg q8–24h depending on gestational and postnatal ages. Initial broad-spectrum coverage should also include a third-generation cephalosporin (cefotaxime or ceftazidime 100 mg/kg/d divided q12h when *Pseudomonas aeruginosa* is strongly suspected). To prevent the development of vancomycin-resistant organisms, vancomycin should be stopped as soon as cultures and sensitivities indicate that it is not needed for ongoing therapy. Other supportive therapy includes the administration of IVIG (500–750 mg/kg) to infants with known overwhelming infection. The duration of treatment for proved sepsis is 10–14 days of IV antibiotics. In sick infants, the essentials of good supportive therapy should be provided: IV glucose and nutritional support, volume expansion, use of pressors as needed, and oxygen and ventilator support.

Prevention of neonatal GBS infection has been achieved with intrapartum administration of penicillin given > 4 hours prior to delivery. The current clinical guideline (Figure 1–12) is to perform a vaginal and rectal GBS culture at 35–37 weeks' gestation for all pregnant

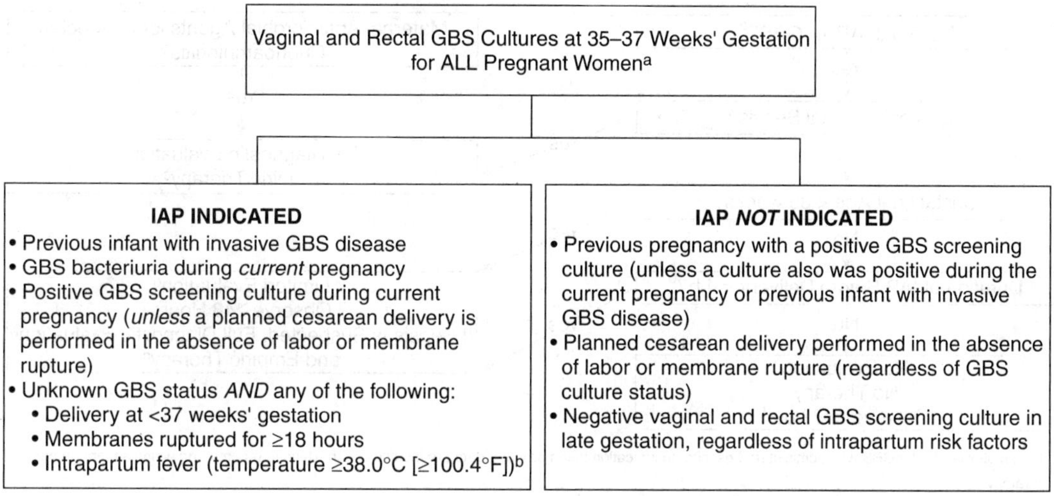

```
┌─────────────────────────────────────────────────┐
│  Vaginal and Rectal GBS Cultures at 35–37 Weeks' Gestation  │
│              for ALL Pregnant Womenᵃ              │
└─────────────────────────────────────────────────┘
```

IAP INDICATED
- Previous infant with invasive GBS disease
- GBS bacteriuria during *current* pregnancy
- Positive GBS screening culture during current pregnancy (*unless* a planned cesarean delivery is performed in the absence of labor or membrane rupture)
- Unknown GBS status *AND* any of the following:
  - Delivery at <37 weeks' gestation
  - Membranes ruptured for ≥18 hours
  - Intrapartum fever (temperature ≥38.0°C [≥100.4°F])ᵇ

IAP *NOT* INDICATED
- Previous pregnancy with a positive GBS screening culture (unless a culture also was positive during the current pregnancy or previous infant with invasive GBS disease)
- Planned cesarean delivery performed in the absence of labor or membrane rupture (regardless of GBS culture status)
- Negative vaginal and rectal GBS screening culture in late gestation, regardless of intrapartum risk factors

ᵃ Exceptions: women with GBS bacteriuria during the current pregnancy or women with a previous infant with invasive GBS disease.

ᵇ If chorioamnionitis is suspected, broad-spectrum antimicrobial therapy that includes an agent known to be active against GBS should replace GBS IAP.
  GBS = group B streptococcus, IAP = intrapartum antimicrobial prophylaxis.

Figure 1–12. Indications for intrapartum antimicrobial prophylaxis to prevent early-onset GBS (group B streptococcal) disease using a universal prenatal culture screening strategy at 35–37 weeks' gestation for all pregnant women. (Reproduced, with permission, from the American Academy of Pediatrics: Red Book 2003 Report of the Committee on Infectious Disease, 2003.)

women. Prophylaxis with penicillin is given to GBS-positive women as well as those who have unknown GBS status at delivery with risk factors for infection. Figure 1–13 presents a suggested strategy for the infant born to a mother who received intrapartum prophylaxis for prevention of early-onset GBS or for suspected chorioamnionitis. Some authors also recommend selective neonatal prophylaxis with 50,000 U/kg of penicillin G given IM if adequate intrapartum treatment has not been given.

2. Meningitis

Any newborn with bacterial sepsis is also at risk for meningitis. The incidence is low in infants with early-onset sepsis but much higher in infants with late-onset infection. The work-up for any newborn with possible signs of CNS infection should include a spinal tap since blood cultures can be negative in neonates with meningitis. Diagnosis is suggested by a CSF protein > 150 mg/dL, glucose < 30 mg/dL, > 25 leukocytes/mL, and a positive Gram stain. The diagnosis is confirmed by culture. The most common organisms are GBS and gram-negative enteric bacteria. Although sepsis can be treated with antibiotics for 10–14 days, meningitis often requires 21 days. The mortality rate of neonatal meningitis is approximately 10%, with significant neurologic morbidity present in one-third of the survivors.

3. Pneumonia

The respiratory system can be infected in utero or on passage through the birth canal. Early-onset neonatal infection is usually associated with pneumonia. Pneumonia should also be suspected in older neonates with a recent onset of tachypnea, retractions, and cyanosis. In infants already receiving respiratory support, an increase in the requirement for oxygen or ventilator support may indicate pneumonia. Not only common bacteria but also viruses (CMV, respiratory syncytial virus, adenovirus, influenza, herpes simplex, and parainfluenza) and *Chlamydia* can cause the disease. In infants with preexisting respiratory disease, intercurrent pulmonary infections may contribute to the ultimate severity of chronic lung disease.

4. Urinary Tract Infection

Infection of the urine is uncommon in the first days of life. Urinary tract infection in the newborn can occur in association with genitourinary anomalies and is caused by gram-negative enteric pathogens, *Enterococcus,* or other organisms. Urine should always be evaluated as part of the work-up for late-onset infection. Culture should be obtained either by suprapubic aspiration or bladder catheterization. Antibiotic IV therapy is continued for 7–10 days if the blood culture is negative and

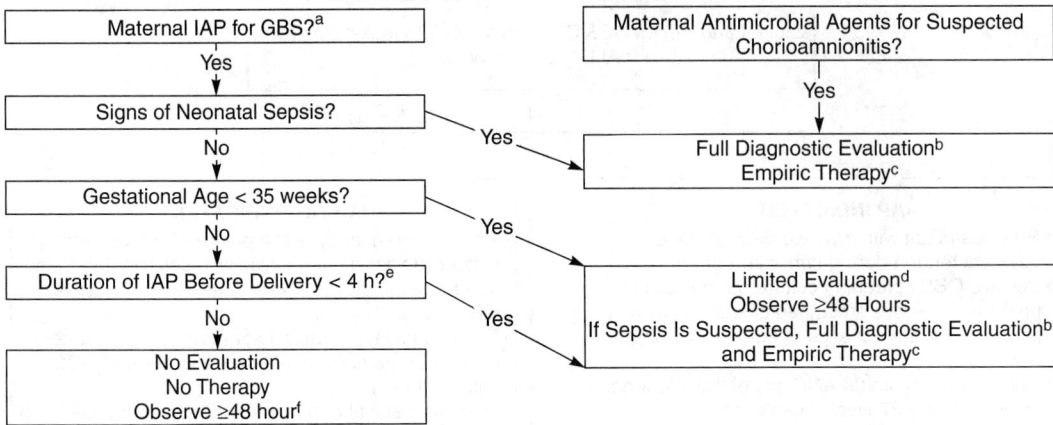

a If no maternal IAP for GBS was administered despite an indication being present, data are insufficient on which to recommend a single management strategy.

b Includes complete blood cell (CBC) count with differential, blood culture, and chest radiograph if respiratory abnormalities are present. When signs of sepsis are present, a lumber puncture, if feasible, should be performed.

c Duration of therapy varies depending on results of blood culture, cerebrospinal fluid findings (if obtained), and the clinical course of the infant. If laboratory results and clinical course do not indicate bacterial infection, duration may be as short as 48 hours.

d CBC including (WBC) count with differential and blood culture.

e Applies only to penicillin, ampicillin, or cefazolin and assumes recommended dosing regimens.

f A healthy-appearing infant who was ≥38 weeks' gestation at delivery and whose mother received ≥4 hours of IAP before delivery may be discharged home after 24 hours if other discharge criteria have been met and a person able to comply fully with instructions for home observation will be present. If any one of these conditions is not met, the infant should be observed in the hospital for at least 48 hours and until criteria for discharge are achieved.

Figure 1–13. Empiric management of a neonate born to a mother who received intrapartum antimicrobial prophylaxis (IAP) for prevention of early-onset GBS (group B streptococcal) disease or chorioamnionitis. (Reproduced, with permission, from the American Academy of Pediatrics: Red Book 2003 Report of the Committee on Infectious Disease, 2003.)

clinical signs resolve quickly. Evaluation for genitourinary anomalies, starting with an ultrasound examination and a voiding cystourethrogram, should be done subsequently.

5. Omphalitis

A normal umbilical cord stump will atrophy and separate at the skin level. A small amount of purulent material at the base of the cord is common but can be minimized by keeping the cord open to air and cleaning the base with alcohol several times a day. The cord can become colonized with streptococci, staphylococci, or gram-negative organisms that can cause local infection. Infections are more common in cords manipulated for venous or arterial lines. Omphalitis is diagnosed when redness and edema develop in the soft tissues around the stump. Local and systemic cultures should be obtained. Treatment is with broad-spectrum IV antibiotics (usually nafcillin 50–75 mg/kg/d divided q8–12h or vancomycin and a third-generation cephalosporin). Complications are determined by the degree of infection of the cord vessels and include septic thrombophlebitis, hepatic abscess,

necrotizing fasciitis, and portal vein thrombosis. Surgical consultation should be obtained because of the potential for necrotizing fasciitis.

Gerdes JS: Diagnosis and management of bacterial infections in the neonate. Pediatr Clin North Am 2004;51:939 [PMID: 15275982].

Philip AGS: Neonatal meningitis in the new millennium. Neoreviews 2003;4:e73.

Pomeranz A: Anomalies, abnormalities, and care of the umbilicus. Pediatr Clin North Am 2004;51:819 [PMID: 15157600].

Puopolo KM et al: Early-onset group B streptococcal disease in the era of maternal screening. Pediatrics 2005;115:1240 [PMID: 15867030].

Schrag SJ et al: A population based comparison of strategies to prevent early-onset group B streptococcal disease in neonates. N Engl J Med 2002;347:233 [PMID: 12140298].

Schrag S et al: Prevention of perinatal group B streptococcal disease: Revised guidelines from CDC. MMWR Morb Mortal Wkly Rep 2002;51(RR11):1 [PMID: 12211284].

Schrag SJ et al: Group B streptococcal disease in the era of intrapartum antibiotic prophylaxis. N Engl J Med 2000;342:15 [PMID: 10620644].

Schrag S, Schuchat A: Prevention of neonatal sepsis. Clin Perinatol 2005;32:601 [PMID: 16085022].

Sinha A et al: Intrapartum antibiotics and neonatal invasive infections caused by organisms other than group B streptococcus. J Pediatr 2003;142:492 [PMID: 12756379].

Stoll BJ et al: Changes in pathogens causing early onset sepsis in very-low-birth-weight infants. N Engl J Med 2002;347:240 [PMID: 12140299].

Velaphi S et al: Early-onset group B streptococcal infection after a combined maternal and neonatal group B streptococcal chemoprophylaxis strategy. Pediatrics 2003;111:541 [PMID: 12612234].

FUNGAL SEPSIS

With the survival of smaller, sicker infants, infection with *Candida* species has become more common. Infants of low birth weight with central lines who have had repeated exposures to broad-spectrum antibiotics are at highest risk. For infants of birth weight < 1500 g, colonization rates of 27–64% have been demonstrated, with many of these infants developing cutaneous lesions, although the GI tract appears to be the initial site of colonization. A much smaller percentage (2–5%) develop systemic disease.

Clinical features of fungal sepsis can be indistinguishable from those of late-onset bacterial sepsis but may be more subtle. Thrombocytopenia may be the earliest and only sign. Deep organ involvement (renal, eye, or endocarditis) is commonly associated with systemic candidiasis. Treatment is with amphotericin B (0.5–1.5 mg/kg/d). In severe infections, flucytosine (50–150 mg/kg/d) can be added for synergistic coverage. (See Chapter 39.) Prophylaxis with oral mycostatin at 0.5–1 mL PO qid or fluconazole at 3–6 mg/kg/d as a single dose diminishes intestinal colonization with yeast and decreases the frequency of systemic disease.

Malassezia furfur is also seen in infants with central lines receiving IV fat emulsion. To eradicate this organism, as well as *Candida* species, it is necessary to remove the indwelling line.

Benjamin DK et al: When to suspect fungal infection in neonates: A clinical comparison of *Candida albicans* and *Candida parapsilosis* fungemia with coagulase-negative staphylococcal bacteremia. Pediatrics 2000;106:712 [PMID: 11015513].

Kicklighter SD: Antifungal agents and fungal prophylaxis in the neonate. Neoreviews 2002;3:e249.

CONGENITAL VIRAL & PARASITIC INFECTIONS (See Also Chapters 36 & 39.)

1. Cytomegalovirus Infection

CMV is the most common virus transmitted in utero. The incidence of congenital infection ranges from 0.2–2.2% of live births. Transmission of CMV can occur during either primary or reactivated infection in the mother. An important source of infection is children (especially those in a day care setting), who transmit the virus to parents and workers. The incidence of primary infection in pregnancy is 1–4%, with a 40% transplacental transmission rate to the fetus. Of these infants, 85–90% are asymptomatic at birth, whereas 10–15% have clinically apparent disease—hepatosplenomegaly, petechiae, small size for gestational age, microcephaly, direct hyperbilirubinemia, thrombocytopenia, intracranial calcifications, and chorioretinitis. The risk of neonatal disease is higher when the mother acquires the infection in the first half of pregnancy. The incidence of reactivated infection in pregnancy is less than 1%, with an incidence of clinically apparent disease of 0–1%. Diagnosis in the neonate should be confirmed by culture of the virus from urine. Rapid diagnosis is possible with antigen detection techniques and polymerase chain reaction (PCR) testing. Diagnosis can also be confirmed in utero from an amniocentesis specimen. Although not routinely recommended, ganciclovir therapy has been used in some severely ill neonates.

The mortality rate in patients with symptomatic congenital CMV may be as high as 20%. Sequelae such as hearing loss, mental retardation, delayed motor development, chorioretinitis and optic atrophy, seizures, language delays, and learning disability occur in 90% of symptomatic survivors. The incidence of complications is 5–15% in asymptomatic infants; the most frequent complication is hearing loss, which can be progressive.

Perinatal infection can also occur with acquisition of virus around the time of delivery. These infections are generally asymptomatic and without sequelae. Postnatal infection is usually asymptomatic but can cause hepatitis, pneumonitis, and neurologic illness in compromised seronegative premature infants. The virus can be acquired postnatally through transfusions or ingestion of CMV-infected breast milk. Transfusion risk can be minimized by using frozen, washed red blood cells or CMV antibody–negative donors.

2. Rubella

Congenital rubella infection occurs as a result of rubella infection in the mother during pregnancy. The frequency of infection and damage to the fetus is as high as 80% in mothers infected during the first trimester. Fetal infection rates decline in the second trimester before increasing again in the third trimester. Fetal damage generally does not occur in infections acquired after 18 weeks' gestation. Clinical features of congenital rubella include adenopathy, bone radiolucencies, encephalitis, cardiac defects (pulmonary arterial hypoplasia and patent ductus arteriosus), cataracts, retinopathy, growth retardation, hepatosplenomegaly, thrombocytopenia, and purpura. Affected infants can be asymptomatic at birth but develop clinical sequelae during the first year of life. The diagnosis should be suspected in cases of a characteristic clinical illness in the mother (rash, adenopathy, and arthritis) confirmed by serologic testing. Diagnosis can be confirmed by an increase in serum rubella-specific IgM or culture of pharyngeal secretions in the baby. Congenital rubella is now rare because of widespread immunization.

3. Varicella

Congenital varicella infection is rare (< 5% after infection acquired during the first or second trimester) but may cause a constellation of findings, including limb hypoplasia, cutaneous scars, microcephaly, cortical atrophy, chorioretinitis, and cataracts. Perinatal exposure (5 days before to 2 days after delivery) can cause severe to fatal disseminated varicella in the infant. If maternal varicella infection develops within this perinatal risk period, 1 vial of varicella immune globulin should be given to the newborn. If this has not been done, the illness can be treated with IV acyclovir (30 mg/kg/d divided q8h).

Hospitalized premature infants of at least 28 weeks' gestation whose mothers have no history of chickenpox—and all infants of less than 28 weeks' gestational age—should receive varicella immune globulin following any postnatal exposure. Susceptible women of childbearing age should be immunized with varicella vaccine.

4. Toxoplasmosis

Toxoplasmosis is caused by the protozoan *Toxoplasma gondii*. Maternal infection occurs in 0.1–0.5% of pregnancies and is usually asymptomatic. When primary infection occurs during pregnancy, up to 40% of the fetuses become infected, of whom 15% have severe damage. The sources of transmission include exposure to cat feces and ingestion of raw or undercooked meat. Although the risk of transmission increases to 90% near term, fetal damage is most likely to occur when maternal infection occurs in the second to sixth month of gestation.

Clinical findings include growth retardation, chorioretinitis, seizures, jaundice, hydrocephalus, microcephaly, cerebral calcifications, hepatosplenomegaly, adenopathy, cataracts, maculopapular rash, thrombocytopenia, and pneumonia. The majority of affected infants are asymptomatic at birth but show evidence of damage (chorioretinitis, blindness, low IQ, and hearing loss) at a later time. The serologic diagnosis is based on a positive IgA or IgM in the first 6 months of life or a persistent IgG beyond 12 months. Infants with suspected infection should have eye and auditory examinations and a CT scan of the brain. Organism isolation from placenta or cord blood and PCR tests are also available for diagnosis in the neonate and from amniocentesis specimens.

Spiramycin treatment of primary maternal infection is used to try to reduce transmission to the fetus. Neonatal treatment using pyrimethamine and sulfadiazine with folinic acid can improve long-term outcome. (See Chapter 39.)

PERINATALLY ACQUIRED VIRAL INFECTIONS

1. Herpes Simplex (See Also Chapter 36.)

Herpes simplex virus infection is most commonly acquired at the time of birth during transit through an infected birth canal. The mother may have either primary or reactivated secondary infection. Primary maternal infection, because of the high titer of organism and the absence of maternal antibodies, poses the greatest risk to the infant. The risk of neonatal infection with vaginal delivery in this setting is 33–50%. Seventy percent of mothers with primary herpes at the time of delivery are asymptomatic. The risk to an infant born to a mother with recurrent herpes simplex is much lower (< 0–5%). Time of presentation of localized (skin, eye, or mouth) or disseminated disease (pneumonia, shock, or hepatitis) in the infant is usually 5–14 days of age. CNS disease usually presents at 14–28 days with lethargy and seizures. In about 10% of cases, presentation can be as early as day 1 of life. Disease appearing this early suggests in-utero infection. In about one-third of patients, localized skin, eye, and mouth disease is the first indication of infection. In another third, disseminated or CNS disease precedes skin, eye, and mouth findings, whereas the remaining third have disseminated or CNS disease in the absence of skin, eye, and mouth disease. Preliminary diagnosis can be made by scraping the base of a vesicle and finding multinucleated giant cells. Viral culture from vesicles, usually positive in 24–72 hours, makes the definitive diagnosis. PCR technology can assist in diagnosis, but may be falsely negative in the CSF early in the course. If a lumbar puncture performed shortly after the onset of symptoms is negative, a repeat should be performed if herpes simplex virus disease is considered a strong possibility.

Acyclovir (60 mg/kg/d given q8h) is the drug of choice for neonatal herpes infection. Localized disease is treated for 14 days, and a 21-day course is used for disseminated or CNS disease. Treatment improves survival of neonates with CNS and disseminated disease and prevents the spread of localized disease. Prevention is possible by not allowing delivery through an infected birth canal (eg, by cesarean section within 6 hours after rupture of the membranes). However, antepartum cervical cultures are poor predictors of the presence of virus at the time of delivery. Furthermore, given the low incidence of infection in the newborn from secondary maternal infection, cesarean section is not indicated for asymptomatic mothers with a history of herpes. Cesarean sections are performed in mothers with active lesions (either primary or secondary) at the time of delivery. Infants born to mothers with a history of herpes simplex virus infection but no active lesions can be observed closely after birth. Cultures should be obtained and acyclovir treatment initiated only for clinical signs consistent with herpes virus infection. Infants born to mothers with active lesions—regardless of the route of delivery—should be cultured (eye, oropharynx, umbilicus, and rectum) 24 hours after delivery. If the infant is colonized (positive cultures) or if symptoms consistent with herpes infection develop, treatment with acyclovir should be started. In cases of maternal primary infection at the time of vaginal delivery, the infant should be cultured and started on acyclovir pending the results of cultures. The major problem facing perinatologists is the high percentage of asymptomatic primary maternal infection. In these cases, infection in the neonate is currently not preventable. Therefore, any infant who presents at the right age with symptoms consistent with neonatal herpes should be cultured and started on acyclovir pending the results of those cultures.

The prognosis is good for truly localized skin and mucosal disease that does not progress. The mortality rate for both disseminated and CNS herpes is high, with significant rates of morbidity among survivors despite treatment. Recurrences are common, and examination of the CSF should occur each time.

2. Hepatitis B & C
(See Also Chapter 21.)

Infants can be infected with hepatitis B at the time of birth. Clinical illness is rare in the neonatal period, but infants exposed in utero are at high risk of becoming chronic HBsAg carriers and developing chronic active hepatitis, and later hepatocellular carcinoma. The presence of HBsAg should be determined in all pregnant women. If the result is positive, the infant should receive HBIG and hepatitis B vaccine as soon as possible after birth, followed by two subsequent vaccine doses at 1 and 6 months of age. If HBsAg has not been tested prior to birth in a mother at risk, the test should be run after delivery and hepatitis B vaccine given within 12 hours after birth. If the mother is subsequently found to be positive, HBIG should be given as soon as possible (preferably within 48 hours, but not later than 1 week after birth). Subsequent vaccine doses should be given at 1 and 6 months of age. In premature infants born to HBsAg-positive mothers, vaccine and HBIG should be given at birth, but a three-vaccine hepatitis B series should be given after a weight of 2000 g is attained.

Hepatitis C perinatal transmissions occur in about 5% of infants born to mothers who carry the virus. At the present time, no prevention strategies exist. Up to 12 months of age, the only reliable screen for hepatitis C infection is PCR. After that time, the presence of hepatitis C antibodies in the infant strongly suggests that infection has occurred.

3. Enteroviral Infection

Enteroviral infections occur with greatest frequency in the late summer and early fall. Infection is usually acquired in the perinatal period. There is often a history of maternal illness (fever, diarrhea, and rash) in the week prior to delivery. The illness appears in the infant in the first 2 weeks of life and is most commonly characterized by fever, lethargy, irritability, diarrhea, and rash, but is not severe. More severe forms occasionally occur, especially if infection occurs before 1 week of age, including meningoencephalitis and myocarditis, as well as a disseminated illness with hepatitis, pneumonia, shock, and disseminated intravascular coagulation. Diagnosis can be confirmed by culture (rectum, CSF, or blood) or by the more rapid PCR techniques.

No therapy has proved efficacy. The prognosis is good for all symptom complexes except severe disseminated disease, which carries a high mortality rate.

4. HIV Infection
(See Also Chapter 37.)

Human immunodeficiency virus (HIV) can be acquired in utero or at the time of delivery, or can be transmitted postpartum via breast milk. The majority of transmission occurs during the 2 weeks prior to delivery and during delivery. Transmission of virus occurs in 13–30% of births. Administration of zidovudine during pregnancy starting at 14–34 weeks' gestation, intrapartum, and for the first 6 weeks of life in the newborn at a dosage of 2 mg/kg PO qid decreases vertical transmission to 7%. Shorter courses of zidovudine are also associated with decreased disease transmission, as is cesarean delivery. The combination of zidovudine treatment and cesarean delivery can lower transmission to 2%. The addition of other anti-HIV therapy may further reduce the risk of ante- and intrapartum viral transmission. Current guidelines for use of antiretroviral drugs in pregnant HIV-infected women are similar to those for nonpregnant patients (eg, highly active antiretroviral combination therapy). In cases of unknown HIV status at presentation in labor, rapid HIV testing and intrapartum treatment should be offered. The risk of transmission is increased in mothers with advanced disease, high viral loads, low CD4 counts, and p24 antigenemia. Prematurity, vaginal delivery, ruptured membranes for over 4 hours, and chorioamnionitis also increase the transmission rate. Diagnosis is based on clinical, immunologic, and serologic findings. Newborns with congenitally acquired HIV are often free of symptoms. Jaundice, neonatal giant-cell hepatitis, and thrombocytopenia have been reported at birth. Failure to thrive, lymphadenopathy, hepatosplenomegaly, oral thrush, chronic diarrhea, bacterial infections with common organisms, and an increased incidence of upper and lower respiratory diseases, including lymphoid interstitial pneumonitis, may appear early in life or may be delayed for months to years.

Infants born to HIV-infected women should be tested by HIV DNA PCR at < 48 hours, at 1–2 months of age, and at 2–4 months old. In an infant who is age 4 months with no positive PCR, infection can be reasonably excluded. HIV-positive mothers should be counseled not to breastfeed their infants.

Protection of health care workers is an important issue. Testing should be performed in all pregnant women. Because such testing will fail to identify some infected patients, however, universal precautions should be used. Gloves should be worn during all procedures involving blood and blood-contaminated fluids, intubation, and any invasive procedures using needles. When a splash exposure is possible (eg, in the delivery room), a mask and eye covers should be used.

OTHER INFECTIONS

1. Congenital Syphilis

The infant is usually infected in utero by transplacental passage of *Treponema pallidum*. Active primary and secondary maternal syphilis leads to fetal infection in nearly 100% of infants; latent disease in 40%; and late disease in 10%. Fetal infection is rare at under 18 weeks' gestation. Fetal infection can result in stillbirth or prematurity. Findings consistent with early congenital syphilis (presentation at under 2 years) include mucocutaneous lesions, lymphadenopathy, hepatosplenomegaly, bony changes, and hydrops. However, in the newborn period, infants are often asymptomatic, so diagnosis is based on maternal and infant serologic testing and is only presumptive. Later manifestations (at over age 2 years) include Hutchinson teeth and mulberry molars, keratitis, chorioretinitis, glaucoma, hearing loss, saddle nose, saber shins, and mental retardation. An infant should be evaluated for congenital syphilis if it is born to a mother with positive nontreponemal tests confirmed by a positive treponemal test but without documented adequate treatment (parenteral penicillin G), including the expected fourfold decrease in nontreponemal antibody titer. Infants of mothers treated less than 1 month before delivery also require evaluation. Evaluation should include physical examination, a quantitative nontreponemal serologic test for syphilis, CSF examination for cell count, protein and Venereal Disease Research Laboratory testing, long bone radiographs, and antitreponemal IgM. A definitive diagnosis can be made on rare occasions when the organism is identified by dark-field microscopy or pathologic examination of the placenta. Guidelines for therapy are presented in Table 1–20. Infants should be treated for congenital syphilis if they have proven or probable disease, as evidenced by (1) physical or radiographic evidence, (2) quantitative nontreponemal antibody titers four times higher than the mother, (3) elevated CSF protein or cell count or positive Venereal Disease Research Laboratory test, or (4) a positive antitreponemal IgM test. Asymptomatic infants should be treated if the mother did not receive adequate treatment for syphilis.

2. Tuberculosis (See Also Chapter 38.)

Congenital tuberculosis (TB) is rare but may occur in the infant of a mother with hematogenously spread TB or by aspiration of infected amniotic fluid in cases of tuberculous endometritis. Women with pulmonary TB are not likely to infect the fetus until after delivery. Postnatal acquisition is the most common mechanism of neonatal infection. Management in these cases is based on the mother's evaluation.

1. Mother or other household contact with a positive skin test and negative chest radiograph, or mother with an abnormal chest radiograph but no evidence of tuberculous disease after clinical evaluation: Investigate family contacts. Treat the mother with isoniazid.

2. Mother has an abnormal chest radiograph consistent with tuberculous disease: Mother and infant should be separated until the mother is evaluated for active TB. If active TB is found, maintain separation until the mother has received antituberculosis therapy for 2 weeks. Investigate family contacts.

3. Mother with clinical or radiographic evidence of acute and possibly contagious TB: Evaluate the infant for congenital TB (skin test, chest radiograph, lumbar puncture, and cultures) and HIV. Treat the mother and infant. If the infant is receiving isoniazid and the mother has no risks for multidrug-resistant TB, separation is not necessary.

If congenital TB is suspected, multidrug therapy should be initiated.

3. Conjunctivitis

Neisseria gonorrhoeae may colonize an infant during passage through an infected birth canal. Gonococcal ophthalmitis presents at 3–7 days with copious purulent conjunctivitis. The diagnosis can be suspected when gram-negative intracellular diplococci are seen on a Gram-stained smear and confirmed by culture. Treatment is with IV or IM ceftriaxone, 25–50 mg/kg (not to exceed 125 mg) given once. Prophylaxis at birth is with 0.5% erythromycin ointment. Infants born to mothers with known gonococcal disease should also receive a single dose of ceftriaxone.

Chlamydia trachomatis is another important cause of conjunctivitis, appearing at 5 days to several weeks of age with congestion, edema, and minimal discharge. The organism is acquired at birth after passage through an infected birth canal. Acquisition occurs in 50% of infants born to infected women, with a 25–50% risk of conjunctivitis. Prevalence in pregnancy is over 10% in some populations. Diagnosis is by isolation of the organism or by

Table 1–20. Recommended treatment of neonates (≤ 4 wk of age) with proven or possible congenital syphilis.

Clinical Status	Antimicrobial Therapy[a]
Proven or highly probable disease[b]	Aqueous crystalline penicillin G, 100,000–150,000 U/kg/d, administered as 50,000 U/kg per dose, IV, every 12 h during the first 7 d of life and every 8 h thereafter for a total of 10 d **OR** Penicillin G procaine,[c] 50,000 U/kg/d, IM, in a single dose for 10 d
Asymptomatic: normal CSF examination results, CBC and platelet count, and radiographic examination; and follow-up is certain with the following maternal treatment history:	
• (a) No penicillin treatment or inadequate or no documentation of penicillin treatment[d]; (b) mother was treated with erythromycin or other nonpenicillin regimen; (c) mother received treatment ≤ 4 wk before delivery; (d) sequential serologic tests on the mother do not demonstrate a fourfold or greater decrease in a nontreponemal antibody titer	Aqueous crystalline penicillin G, IV, for 10–14 d[b] **OR** Penicillin G procaine,[c] 50,000 U/kg/d, IM, in a single dose for 10 d **OR** Clinical, serologic follow-up, and penicillin G benzathine,[c] 50,000 U/kg, IM in a single dose
• (a) Adequate therapy given >1 mo before delivery; (b) mother's nontreponemal titers decreased fourfold after appropriate therapy for early syphilis and remained stable and low for late syphilis; (c) mother has no evidence of reinfection or relapse	Clinical, serologic follow-up, and penicillin G benzathine, 50,000 U/kg, IM in a single dose[e]

[a]See text for details.
[b]If more than 1 day of therapy is missed, the entire course should be restarted.
[c]Penicillin G benzathine and penicillin G procaine are approved for IM administration *only*.
[d]See text for definition (includes infants in whom a serum quantitative nontreponemal serologic titer is the same or less than fourfold the maternal titer). If any part of the infant's evaluation is abnormal or not performed or if the CSF analysis is uninterpretable, the 10-day course of penicillin is required.
[e]Some experts would not treat the infant but would provide close serologic follow-up.
CBC, complete blood cell; CSF, cerebrospinal fluid; IM, intramuscularly; IV, intravenously.
Reprinted, with permission, from the American Academy of Pediatrics: Red Book 2003 Report on Infectious Diseases, 2003.

rapid antigen detection tests. Treatment is with oral erythromycin (30 mg/kg/d in divided doses q8–12h) for 14 days. Topical treatment alone will not eradicate nasopharyngeal carriage, leaving the infant at risk for the development of pneumonitis.

4. Parvovirus B19 Infection

Parvovirus B19 is a small, nonenveloped, single-stranded DNA virus that causes erythema infectiosum (fifth disease) in children, with a peak incidence at ages 6–7 years. Transmission to the mother is primarily by respiratory secretions. The virus replicates initially in erythroid progenitor cells, and induces cell-cycle arrest resulting in severe anemia, myocarditis, and nonimmune hydrops in approximately 3%, and fetal death in up to 10% of fetuses infected in the second trimester. Resolution of the hydrops may occur in utero, either spontaneously or after fetal transfusion. Mothers who have been exposed may have specific serologic testing for antibody response, and

serial ultrasound, Doppler exams, and percutaneous umbilical cord blood sampling of the fetus for anemia. If the fetus survives, the long-term outcome is good with no late effects from the infection.

American Academy of Pediatrics and Canadian Paediatric Society Clinical Report: Evaluation and treatment of the human immunodeficiency virus-1-exposed infant. Pediatrics 2004;114: 497 [PMID: 15286240].

American Academy of Pediatrics Committee on Infectious Diseases: Report of the committee on infectious diseases, 26th ed. Red Book 2003. American Academy of Pediatrics, 2003.

Boppana SB et al: Intrauterine transmission of cytomegalovirus to infants of women with preconceptional immunity. N Engl J Med 2001;344:1366 [PMID: 12359792].

Brown ZA et al: Effect of serologic status and cesarean delivery on transmission rates of herpes simplex virus from mother to infant. JAMA 2003;289:203 [PMID: 12517231].

Bulterys M et al: Rapid HIV-1 testing during labor: a multicenter study. JAMA 2004;292:219 [PMID: 15249571].

Centers for Disease Control and Prevention: US Public Health Service Task Force recommendations for use of antiretroviral drugs in pregnant HIV-1 infected women for maternal health and interventions to reduce perinatal HIV-1 transmission in the US. MMWR Morb Mortal Wkly Rep 2002;51(RR-18):1 [PMID: 12489844].

Fowler KB et al: Maternal immunity and prevention of congenital cytomegalovirus infection. JAMA 2003;289:1008 [PMID: 12597753].

Frenkel LM: Challenges in the diagnosis and management of neonatal herpes simplex virus encephalitis. Pediatrics 2005;115:795 [PMID: 15741389].

Havens PL, Waters D: Management of the infant born to a mother with HIV infection. Pediatr Clin North Am 2004;51:909 [PMID: 15275981].

Hill J, Roberts S: Herpes simplex virus in pregnancy: new concepts in prevention and management. Clin Perinatol 2005;32:657 [PMID: 16085025]

Hollier LM, Grissom H: Human herpes viruses in pregnancy: cytomegalovirus, Epstein-Barr virus, and varicella zoster virus. Clin Perinatol 2005;32:671 [PMID: 16085026].

Kimberlin DW et al: Natural history of neonatal herpes simplex virus infections in the acyclovir era. Pediatrics 2001;108:223 [PMID: 11483781].

Kimberlin DW et al: Effect of ganciclovir therapy on hearing in symptomatic cytomegalovirus disease involving the central nervous system: A randomized, controlled trial. J Pediatr 2003;143:16 [PMID: 12915819].

Kumar ML, Abughali NF: Perinatal parvovirus B19 infection. NeoReviews 2005;6:e32.

Michelow IC et al: Central nervous system infection in congenital syphilis. N Engl J Med 2002;346:1792 [PMID: 12050339].

Peters V et al: Missed opportunities for perinatal HIV prevention among HIV-exposed infants born 1996–2000, pediatric spectrum of HIV disease cohort. Pediatrics 2003;111:1186 [PMID: 12728136].

Shetty AK, Maldonado Y: Advances in the prevention of perinatal HIV-1 transmission. NeoReviews 2005;6:e12.

Stehel EK, Sanchez PJ: Cytomegalovirus infection in the fetus and neonate. NeoReviews 2005;6:e38.

Tuomala RE et al: Antiretroviral therapy during pregnancy and the risk of an adverse outcome. N Engl J Med 2002;346:1863 [PMID: 12063370].

Watts H: Management of human immunodeficiency virus infection in pregnancy. N Engl J Med 2002;346:1879 [PMID: 12063373].

HEMATOLOGIC DISORDERS IN THE NEWBORN INFANT

BLEEDING DISORDERS

Neonatal coagulation is discussed in Chapter 27. Bleeding in the newborn infant may result from inherited clotting deficiencies (eg, factor VIII deficiency) or acquired disorders—hemorrhagic disease of the newborn, disseminated intravascular coagulation, liver failure, and thrombocytopenia.

1. Vitamin K Deficiency Bleeding of the Newborn

Vitamin K deficiency bleeding is caused by the deficiency of the vitamin K–dependent clotting factors (II, VII, IX, and X). Bleeding occurs in 0.25–1.7% of newborns who do not receive vitamin K prophylaxis after birth, generally in the first 5 days to 2 weeks, but as late as 12 weeks in an otherwise well infant. Early vitamin K deficiency bleeding (0–2 weeks) can be prevented by either parenteral or oral vitamin K administration, whereas late disease is most effectively prevented by administering parenteral vitamin K. Sites of ecchymoses and surface bleeding include the GI tract, umbilical cord, circumcision site, and nose, although devastating intracranial hemorrhage can occur. Bleeding from vitamin K deficiency is more likely to occur in exclusively breast-fed infants because of very low amounts of vitamin K in breast milk, with slower and more restricted intestinal colonization. Differential diagnosis includes disseminated intravascular coagulation and hepatic failure, both occurring in ill infants (Table 1–21).

Treatment consists of 1 mg of vitamin K SC or IV. IM injections should be avoided in infants who are actively bleeding.

2. Thrombocytopenia

Infants with thrombocytopenia have generalized petechiae (not just on the presenting part) and platelet counts < 150,000/mL (usually < 50,000/mL, may be < 10,000/mL). Neonatal thrombocytopenia can be isolated or may occur in association with a deficiency of clotting factors. The differential diagnosis for thrombocytopenia with distinguishing clinical features is presented in Table 1–22. Treatment of neonatal thrombocytopenia is transfusion of platelets (10 mL/kg of platelets increases the platelet count by approximately 70,000/mL). Indications for transfusion in the full-term infant are clinical bleeding or a total platelet count < 10,000–20,000/mL. In the preterm infant at risk for intraventricular hemorrhage, transfusion is indicated for counts < 40,000–50,000/mL.

Isoimmune thrombocytopenia (analogous to Rh isoimmunization, with a human platelet antigen [HPA]-1a–negative mother and HPA-1a–positive fetus) requires transfusion of maternal platelets, because 98% of the random population will also be HPA-1a–positive. The mother would be the most readily available known HPA-1a–negative donor. Treatment with steroids has been disappointing. Treatment with IVIG infusion, 1 g/kg/d for 2–3 days or until the platelet count has doubled or is

Table 1–21. Features of infants bleeding from vitamin K deficiency (VKDB), disseminated intravascular coagulation (DIC), or liver failure.

	VKDB	DIC	Liver Failure
Clinical	Well infant; no prophy-lactic vita-min K	Sick infant; hypoxia, sepsis, etc	Sick infant; hepatitis, in-born errors of metabolism, shock liver
Bleeding	GI tract, um-bilical cord, circumci-sion, nose	Generalized	Generalized
Onset	2–3 d	Any time	Any time
Platelet count	Normal	Decreased	Normal or de-creased
Prothrom-bin time	Prolonged	Prolonged	Prolonged
Partial throm-boplastin time	Prolonged	Prolonged	Prolonged
Fibrinogen	Normal	Decreased	Decreased
Factor V	Normal	Decreased	Decreased

GI, gastrointestinal.

over 50,000/mL, is recommended. Antenatal therapy of the mother with IVIG with or without steroids is also beneficial, since 20–30% of infants with isoimmune thrombocytopenia will experience intracranial hemorrhage, half of them before birth.

Infants born to mothers with idiopathic thrombocytopenic purpura are at low risk for serious hemorrhage despite the thrombocytopenia, and treatment is usually unnecessary. If bleeding does occur, IVIG can be used.

ANEMIA

The newborn infant with anemia from acute blood loss presents with signs of hypovolemia (tachycardia, poor perfusion, and hypotension), with an initially normal hematocrit that falls after volume replacement. Anemia from chronic blood loss is evidenced by pallor without signs of hypovolemia, with an initially low hematocrit and reticulocytosis.

Anemia can be caused by hemorrhage, hemolysis, or failure to produce red blood cells. Anemia occurring in the first 24–48 hours of life is the result of hemorrhage or hemolysis. Hemorrhage can occur in utero (fetopla-cental, fetomaternal, or twin-to-twin), perinatally (cord rupture, placenta previa, or incision through the placenta at cesarean section), or internally (intracranial hemorrhage, cephalhematoma, or ruptured liver or spleen). Hemolysis is caused by blood group incompatibilities, enzyme or membrane abnormalities, infection, and disseminated intravascular coagulation, and is accompanied by significant hyperbilirubinemia.

Initial evaluation should include a review of the perinatal history, assessment of the infant's volume status, and a complete physical examination. A Kleihauer-Betke test for fetal cells in the mother's circulation should be done. A CBC, blood smear, reticulocyte count, and direct and indirect Coombs tests should be performed. This simple evaluation should suggest a

Table 1–22. Differential diagnosis of neonatal thrombocytopenia.

Disorder	Clinical Tips
Immune Passively acquired anti-body; idiopathic throm-bocytopenic purpura, systemic lupus erythe-matosus, drug-induced	Proper history, maternal thrombocytopenia
Isoimmune sensitization to HPA-1a antigen	No rise in platelet count from random donor platelet trans-fusion. Positive antiplatelet antibodies in baby's serum, sustained rise in platelets by transfusion of mother's platelets
Infections Bacterial infections Congenital viral infec-tions	Sick infants with other signs consistent with infection
Syndromes Absent radii Fanconi anemia	Congenital anomalies, associ-ated pancytopenia
Disseminated intravascular coagulation (DIC)	Sick infants, abnormalities of clotting factors
Giant hemangioma	
Thrombosis	Hyperviscous infants, vascu-lar catheters
High-risk with respiratory distress syndrome, pul-monary hypertension, etc	Isolated decrease in platelets is not uncommon in sick in-fants even in the absence of DIC (? localized trapping)

HPA, human platelet antigen.

diagnosis in most infants. It is important to remember that hemolysis related to blood group incompatibility can continue for weeks after birth. Serial hematocrits should be followed.

POLYCYTHEMIA

Polycythemia in the newborn is manifested by plethora, cyanosis, mild respiratory distress with tachypnea and oxygen need, hypoglycemia, poor feeding, emesis, and lethargy. The capillary hematocrit is > 68%, the venous hematocrit > 65%.

Elevated hematocrits occur in 2–5% of live births. Although 50% of polycythemic infants are AGA, the prevalence of polycythemia is greater in the SGA and LGA populations. Causes of increased hematocrit include (1) twin-twin transfusion, (2) maternal-fetal transfusion, (3) intrapartum transfusion from the placenta, and (4) chronic intrauterine hypoxia (SGA infants and LGA infants of diabetic mothers).

The consequence of polycythemia is hyperviscosity with decreased perfusion of the capillary beds. Clinical symptomatology can affect several organ systems (Table 1–23). Screening can be done by measuring a capillary (heelstick) hematocrit. If the value is greater than 68%, a peripheral venous hematocrit should be measured. Values greater than 65% should be considered consistent with hyperviscosity.

Treatment is recommended for symptomatic infants. Treatment for asymptomatic infants based strictly on hematocrit is controversial. Definitive treatment is accomplished by an isovolemic partial exchange transfusion with normal saline, effectively decreasing the hematocrit. The amount to exchange (in milliliters) is calculated using the following formula:

$$\frac{PVH - DH}{PVH} \times \frac{BV}{kg} \times Wt$$

where PVH = peripheral venous hematocrit, DH = desired hematocrit, BV = blood volume, kg = kilogram, and Wt = weight.

Blood is withdrawn at a steady rate from an umbilical venous line while the replacement solution is infused at the same rate through a peripheral IV line over 15–30 minutes. The desired hematocrit value is 50–55%; the assumed blood volume is 80 mL/kg.

American Academy of Pediatrics Committee on the Fetus and Newborn: Controversies concerning vitamin K and the newborn. Pediatrics 2003;122:191 [PMID: 12837888].

Bizzarro MJ et al: Differential diagnosis and management of anemia in the newborn. Pediatr Clin North Am 2004;51:1087 [PMID: 15275990].

Chalmers EA: Neonatal coagulation problems. Arch Dis Child Fetal Neonatal Ed 2004;89:F475 [PMID: 15499133].

Table 1–23. Organ-related symptoms of hyperviscosity.

Central nervous system	Irritability, jitteriness, seizures, lethargy
Cardiopulmonary	Respiratory distress, secondary to congestive heart failure, or persistent pulmonary hypertension
Gastrointestinal	Vomiting, heme-positive stools, distention, necrotizing enterocolitis
Renal	Decreased urinary output, renal vein thrombosis
Metabolic	Hypoglycemia
Hematologic	Hyperbilirubinemia, thrombocytopenia

Pappas A, Delaney-Black V: Differential diagnosis and management of polycythemia. Pediatr Clin North Am 2004;51:1063 [PMID: 15275989].

Wong W, Glader B: Approach to the newborn who has thrombocytopenia. NeoReviews 2004;5:444.

RENAL DISORDERS IN THE NEWBORN INFANT

Renal function depends on postconceptional age. The glomerular filtration rate is 20 mL/min/1.73 m² in full-term neonates and 10–13 mL/min/1.73 m² in infants born at 28–30 weeks' gestation. The speed of maturation after birth also depends on postconceptional age. Creatinine can be used as a clinical marker of glomerular filtration rate. Values in the first month of life are shown in Table 1–24. Creatinine at birth reflects the maternal level and should decrease slowly over the first 3–4 weeks. An increasing serum creatinine is never nor-

Table 1–24. Normal values of serum creatinine (mg/dL).

Gestational Age at Birth (weeks)	Postnatal Age (days)	
	0–2	28
< 28	1.2	0.7
29–32	1.1	0.6
33–36	1.1	0.45
36–42	0.8	0.3

mal. The ability to concentrate urine and retain sodium also depends on gestational age. Infants born at less than 28–30 weeks' gestation are compromised in this respect and if not observed carefully can become dehydrated and hyponatremic. Preterm infants also have an increased bicarbonate excretion and a low tubular maximum for glucose (approximately 120 mg/dL).

RENAL FAILURE

Renal failure is most commonly seen in the setting of birth asphyxia, hypovolemia, or shock from any cause. The normal rate of urine flow is 1–3 mL/kg/h. After a hypoxic or ischemic insult, acute tubular necrosis may ensue. Typically, 2–3 days of anuria or oliguria is associated with hematuria, proteinuria, and a rise in serum creatinine. The period of anuria or oliguria is followed by a period of polyuria and then gradual recovery. During the polyuric phase, excessive urine sodium and bicarbonate losses may be seen.

The initial step in management is restoration of the infant's volume status as needed. Thereafter, restriction of fluids to insensible water loss (40–60 mL/kg/d) without added electrolytes, plus milliliter-for-milliliter urine replacement, should be instituted. Serum and urine electrolytes and body weights should be followed frequently. These measures should be continued through the polyuric phase. After urine output has been reestablished, urine replacement should be decreased to between 0.5 and 0.75 mL for each milliliter of urine output to see if the infant has regained normal function. If that is the case, the infant can be returned to maintenance fluids.

Finally, many of these infants experience fluid overload and should be allowed to lose enough water through urination to return to birth weight. Hyperkalemia, which may become life-threatening, may occur in this situation despite the lack of added IV potassium. If the serum potassium reaches 7–7.5 mEq/L, therapy should be started with glucose and insulin infusion, giving 1 unit of insulin for every 3 g of glucose administered, in addition to binding resins. Calcium chloride (20 mg/kg bolus) and correction of metabolic acidosis with bicarbonate are also helpful for arrhythmia resulting from hyperkalemia.

Peritoneal dialysis is occasionally needed for the management of neonatal acute renal failure.

URINARY TRACT ANOMALIES

Abdominal masses in the newborn are most frequently caused by renal enlargement. Most common is a multicystic or dysplastic kidney; congenital hydronephrosis is second in frequency. Chromosomal abnormalities and syndromes with multiple anomalies frequently include renal abnormalities. An ultrasound examination is the first step in diagnosis. In pregnancies associated with oligohydramnios, renal agenesis or obstruction secondary to posterior urethral valves should be considered.

Only bilateral disease or disease in a solitary kidney is associated with oligohydramnios, significant morbidity, and death. Such infants will generally also have pulmonary hypoplasia and die from pulmonary rather than renal insufficiency.

Prenatal ultrasonography identifies infants with renal anomalies (most often hydronephrosis) prior to birth. Postnatal evaluation of these infants should include renal ultrasound and a voiding cystourethrogram at about 1–6 weeks of age, depending on the severity of the antenatal findings. Until genitourinary reflux is ruled out, these infants should receive antibiotic prophylaxis with low-dose penicillin or amoxicillin.

RENAL VEIN THROMBOSIS

Renal vein thrombosis occurs most often in IDMs and in the context of dehydration and polycythemia. Of particular concern is the IDM who is also polycythemic. If fetal distress is superimposed on these problems, prompt reduction in blood viscosity is indicated. Thrombosis usually begins in intrarenal venules and can extend into larger veins. Clinically, the kidney may be enlarged, and blood and protein may be found in the urine. With bilateral renal vein thrombosis, anuria ensues. Diagnosis can be confirmed with an ultrasound examination that includes Doppler flow studies of the kidneys. Treatment involves correcting the predisposing condition and systemic heparinization for the thrombosis. Use of thrombolytics for this condition is controversial. Prognosis for a full recovery is uncertain. Some infants will go on to develop significant atrophy of the affected kidney and systemic hypertension.

Andreoli SP: Acute renal failure in the newborn. Semin Perinatol 2004;28:112 [PMID: 15200250].

Kennedy WA: Assessment and management of fetal hydronephrosis. Neoreviews 2002;3:e214.

Mesrobian HG et al: Urologic problems of the neonate. Pediatr Clin North Am 2004;51:1051 [PMID: 15275988].

NEUROLOGIC PROBLEMS IN THE NEWBORN INFANT

SEIZURES

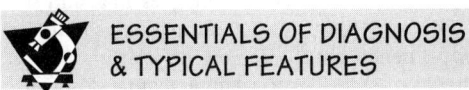

ESSENTIALS OF DIAGNOSIS & TYPICAL FEATURES

• *Usual onset at 12–48 hours.*

- *Most common seizure type is characterized by a constellation of findings.*
- *Most common causes include hypoxic-ischemic encephalopathy, intracranial bleeds, and infection.*

Newborns rarely have well-organized tonic-clonic seizures because of their incomplete cortical organization and a preponderance of inhibitory synapses. The most common type of seizure is characterized by a constellation of findings, including horizontal deviation of the eyes with or without jerking; eyelid blinking or fluttering; sucking, smacking, drooling, and other oral-buccal movements; swimming, rowing, or paddling movements; and apneic spells. Strictly tonic or multifocal clonic episodes are also seen.

Clinical Findings

The differential diagnosis of neonatal seizures is presented in Table 1–25. Most neonatal seizures occur between 12 and 48 hours of age. Later-onset seizures suggest meningitis, benign familial seizures, or hypocalcemia. Information regarding antenatal drug use, the presence of birth asphyxia or trauma, and family history (regarding inherited disorders) should be obtained. Physical examination focuses on neurologic features, other signs of drug withdrawal, concurrent signs of infection, dysmorphic features, and intrauterine growth. Screening work-up should include blood glucose, ionized calcium, and electrolytes in all cases. Further work-up depends on diagnoses suggested by the history and physical examination. If there is any suspicion of infection, a spinal tap should be done. Hemorrhages and structural disease of the CNS can be addressed with real-time ultrasound and CT scan. Infarctions are most easily seen on diffusion-weighted MRI scan. Metabolic work-up should be pursued when appropriate. EEG should be done; the presence of spike discharges must be noted and the background wave pattern evaluated. At times correlation between EEG changes and clinical seizure activity is absent.

Treatment

Adequate ventilation and perfusion should be ensured. Hypoglycemia should be treated immediately with a 2-mL/kg infusion of $D_{10}W$ followed by 6 mg/kg/min of $D_{10}W$ (100 mL/kg/d). Other treatments such as calcium or magnesium infusion and antibiotics are indicated to treat hypocalcemia, hypomagnesemia, and suspected infection. Electrolyte abnormalities should be corrected. Phenobarbital, 20 mg/kg IV, should be administered to stop seizures. Supplemental doses of 5 mg/kg can be used if seizures persist, up to a total of 40 mg/kg. In most cases, phenobarbital controls seizures.

Table 1–25. Differential diagnosis of neonatal seizures.

Diagnosis	Comment
Hypoxic-ischemic encephalopathy	Most common cause (60%), onset in first 24 hours
Intracranial hemorrhage	Up to 15% of cases, periventricular-intraventricular hemorrhage, subdural or subarachnoid bleeding, stroke
Infection	12% of cases
Hypoglycemia	Small for gestational age, infant of a diabetic mother (IDM)
Hypocalcemia, hypomagnesemia	Infant of low birth weight, IDM
Hyponatremia	Rare, seen with syndrome of inappropriate secretion of antidiuretic hormone (SIADH)
Disorders of amino and organic acid metabolism, hyperammonemia	Associated acidosis, altered level of consciousness
Pyridoxine dependency	Seizures refractory to routine therapy; cessation of seizures after administration of pyridoxine
Developmental defects	Other anomalies, chromosomal syndromes
Drug withdrawal	
No cause found	10% of cases
Benign familial neonatal seizures	

If seizures continue, therapy with fosphenytoin, sodium valproate, or lorazepam may be indicated. For refractory seizures, a trial of pyridoxine is indicated.

Prognosis

Outcome is related to the underlying cause of the seizure. The outcomes for hypoxic-ischemic encephalopathy and intraventricular hemorrhage have been discussed earlier in this chapter. In these settings, seizures that are difficult to control carry a poor prognosis for normal development. Seizures resulting from hypoglycemia, infection of the CNS, some inborn errors of metabolism, and developmental defects also have a high rate of poor outcome. Seizures caused by hypocalcemia or isolated subarachnoid hemorrhage generally resolve without sequelae.

HYPOTONIA

One should be alert to the diagnosis of congenital hypotonia when a mother has polyhydramnios and a history of poor fetal movement. The newborn may present with poor respiratory effort and birth asphyxia. For a discussion of causes and evaluation, see Chapter 23.

INTRACRANIAL HEMORRHAGE[1]

1. Subdural Hemorrhage

Subdural hemorrhage is related to birth trauma; the bleeding is caused by tears in the veins that bridge the subdural space. Prospective studies relating incidence to specific obstetric complications are not available.

The most common site of subdural bleeding is in ruptured superficial cerebral veins with blood over the cerebral convexities. These hemorrhages can be asymptomatic or may cause seizures, with onset on days 2–3 of life, vomiting, irritability, and lethargy. Associated findings include retinal hemorrhages and a full fontanelle. The diagnosis is confirmed by CT scan.

Specific treatment entailing needle drainage of the subdural space is rarely necessary. Most infants survive; 75% are normal on follow-up.

2. Primary Subarachnoid Hemorrhage

Primary subarachnoid hemorrhage is the most common type of neonatal intracranial hemorrhage. In the full-term infant, it can be related to trauma of delivery, whereas subarachnoid hemorrhage in the preterm infant is seen in association with germinal matrix hemorrhage. Clinically, these hemorrhages can be asymptomatic or can present with seizures and irritability on day 2, or rarely, a massive hemorrhage with a rapid downhill course. The seizures associated with subarachnoid hemorrhage are very characteristic—usually brief, with a normal examination interictally. Diagnosis can be suspected on lumbar puncture and confirmed with CT scan. Long-term follow-up is uniformly good.

3. Neonatal Stroke

Focal cerebral ischemic injury can occur in the context of intraventricular hemorrhage in the premature infant and hypoxic-ischemic encephalopathy. Neonatal stroke has also been described in the context of underlying disorders of thrombolysis, maternal drug use (cocaine), a history of infertility, preeclampsia, prolonged membrane rupture and chorioamnionitis. In some cases, the origin is unclear. The injury often occurs antenatally. The most common clinical presentation of an isolated cerebral infarct is with seizures, and diagnosis can be confirmed acutely with diffusion-weighted MRI scan. The most frequently described distribution is that of the middle cerebral artery.

Treatment is directed at controlling seizures. Long-term outcome is variable, ranging from near-normal to hemiplegias and cognitive deficits.

Brunquell PJ et al: Prediction of outcome based on clinical seizure type in newborn infants. J Pediatr 2002;140:707 [PMID: 12072874].

Chalmers EA: Perinatal stroke—risk factors and management. Br J Haematol 2005;130:333 [PMID: 16042683].

Hahn JS, Olson DM: Etiology of neonatal seizures. NeoReviews 2004;5:e327.

Lee J et al: Maternal and infant characteristics associated with perinatal arterial stroke in the infant. JAMA 2005;293:723 [PMID: 15701914].

Mercuri E et al: Neonatal cerebral infarction and neuromotor outcome at school age. Pediatrics 2004;113:95 [PMID: 14702455].

Zupanc ML: Neonatal seizures. Pediatr Clin North Am 2004;51:961 [PMID: 15275983].

◼ METABOLIC DISORDERS IN THE NEWBORN INFANT[2]

HYPERGLYCEMIA

Hyperglycemia may develop in preterm infants, particularly those of extremely low birth weight who are also SGA. Glucose concentrations may exceed 200–250 mg/dL, particularly in the first few days of life. This transient diabeteslike syndrome usually lasts approximately 1 week.

Management may include simply reducing glucose intake while continuing to supply IV amino acids to prevent protein catabolism with resultant gluconeogenesis. Intravenous insulin infusions will be needed in infants who remain hyperglycemic despite glucose infusion rates of only 5–6 mg/kg/min or less.

HYPOCALCEMIA

Calcium concentration in the immediate newborn period decreases in all newborn infants. The concentration in fetal plasma is higher than that of the neonate or adult. Hypocalcemia is usually defined as a total serum concentration less than 7 mg/dL (equivalent to a calcium activ-

---

[1]Intraventricular hemorrhage is discussed in the section on Care of the Premature Infant.

[2]Hypoglycemia is discussed in the section on Common Problems in the Term Newborn Infant.

ity of 3.5 mEq/L), although the physiologically active fraction, ionized calcium, should be measured whenever possible. Ionized calcium is usually normal even when total calcium is as low as 6–7 mg/dL. An ionized calcium level of greater than 0.9 mmol/L (1.8 mEq/L; 3.6 mg/dL) is not likely to be detrimental.

Clinical Findings

The clinical signs of hypocalcemia and hypocalcemic tetany include a high-pitched cry, jitteriness, tremulousness, and seizures.

Hypocalcemia tends to occur at two different times in the neonatal period. Early-onset hypocalcemia occurs in the first 2 days of life and has been associated with prematurity, maternal diabetes, asphyxia, and rarely, maternal hypoparathyroidism. Late-onset hypocalcemia occurs at approximately 7–10 days and is observed in infants receiving modified cow's milk rather than infant formula (high phosphorus intake) or in infants with hypoparathyroidism (DiGeorge syndrome, 22q11 deletion). Mothers in underdeveloped countries may have vitamin D deficiency, which can also contribute to late-onset hypocalcemia.

Treatment

A. Oral Calcium Therapy

The oral administration of calcium salts, often along with vitamin D, is the preferred method of treatment for chronic forms of hypocalcemia resulting from hypoparathyroidism. (See Chapter 30.)

B. Intravenous Calcium Therapy

Intravenous calcium therapy is usually needed for infants with symptomatic hypocalcemia or an ionized calcium less than 0.9 mmol/L. A number of precautions must be observed when calcium is given intravenously. The infusion must be given slowly so that there is no sudden increase in calcium concentration of blood entering the right atrium, which could cause severe bradycardia and even cardiac arrest. Furthermore, the infusion must be observed carefully, because an IV infiltrate containing calcium can cause full-thickness skin necrosis requiring grafting. For these reasons, IV calcium therapy should be given judiciously and through a central venous line if possible. Intravenous administration of 10% calcium gluconate is usually given as a bolus of 100–200 mg/kg (1–2 mL/kg) over approximately 10–20 minutes, followed by a continuous infusion (0.5–1 g/kg/d) over 1–2 days. Ten percent calcium chloride (20 mg/kg or 0.2 mL/kg per dose) may result in a larger increment in ionized calcium and greater improvement in mean arterial blood pressure in sick hypocalcemic infants and thus may have a role in the newborn. *Note:* Calcium salts cannot

be added to IV solutions that contain sodium bicarbonate because they precipitate as calcium carbonate.

Prognosis

The prognosis is good for neonatal seizures entirely caused by hypocalcemia that is promptly treated.

INBORN ERRORS OF METABOLISM

The individual inborn errors of metabolism are rare, but collectively have an incidence of 1/1000 live births. Expanded newborn genetic screening will undoubtedly aid in the diagnosis of these disorders. Nevertheless, many infants will present prior to these results being available. The diseases are considered in detail in Chapter 32. These diagnoses should be entertained when infants who were initially well present with sepsislike syndromes, recurrent hypoglycemia, neurologic syndromes (seizures or altered levels of consciousness), or unexplained acidosis (suggestive of organic acidemias).

In the immediate neonatal period, urea cycle disorders present as an altered level of consciousness secondary to hyperammonemia. A clinical clue that supports this diagnosis is hyperventilation with primary respiratory alkalosis, along with a lower-than-expected blood urea nitrogen. The other major diagnostic category to consider consists of infants with severe acidemia secondary to organic acidemias.

Burton BK: Inborn errors of metabolism in infancy: A guide to diagnosis. Pediatrics 1998;102:e69 [PMID: 9832597].

Enns GM, Packman S: Diagnosing inborn errors of metabolism in the newborn: clinical features. Neoreviews 2001;2:e183.

Hemachandra AH, Cowett RM: Neonatal hyperglycemia. Pediatric Rev 1999;20:e16.

REFERENCES

Printed Resources

Fanaroff AA, Martin RJ (editors): *Neonatal-Perinatal Medicine. Diseases of the Fetus and Infant,* 8th ed. Elsevier Mosby, 2005.

Jones KL (editor): *Smith's Recognizable Patterns of Human Malformation,* 6th ed. Elsevier Saunders, 2005.

Thureen PJ et al (editors): *Assessment and Care of the Well Newborn,* 2nd ed. Elsevier Saunders, 2005.

Young TE, Mangum B (editors): *Neofax 2004,* 17th ed. Acorn Publishing, 2000.

Web Resources

[Cochrane neonatal database]

www.nichd.nih.gov/cochraneneonatal/

[Neoreviews]

http://neoreviews.aapjournals.org/

[Neonatal resuscitation program]

www.aap.org/profed/nrp/nrpmain.html

Child Development & Behavior

Edward Goldson, MD, & Ann Reynolds, MD

The field of developmental and behavioral pediatrics has emerged as a subspecialty that addresses not only typical development but also the diagnosis and evaluation of atypical behavior and development. This chapter will provide an overview of typical development, identify developmental variations, and discuss several developmental disabilities. First, it discusses normal development, but does not cover the newborn period or adolescence (see Chapters 1 and 3, respectively). Second, it addresses behavioral variations, emphasizing that these variations reflect the spectrum of normal development and not pathology. Third, it deals with developmental and behavioral disorders and their treatment. The developmental principle, that is, the concept of ongoing change and maturation, is integral to the daily practice of pediatrics. For example, we recognize that a 3-month-old infant is very different from a 3-year-old and from a 13-year-old adolescent, not only with respect to what the child can do, but also in terms of the kind of illness he or she might have. From the perspective of the general pediatrician all of these areas should be viewed in the context of a Medical Home. The Medical Home is defined as the setting that provides consistent, continuous, culturally competent, comprehensive and sensitive care to children and their families. It is a setting that advocates for all children, whether they are typical or if they have developmental challenges or disabilities. By incorporating the principles of child development—the concept that children are constantly changing—the Medical Home is the optimum setting to understand and enhance typical development and to address variations, delays and deviations, as they may occur in the life-trajectory of the child and family.

▩ NORMAL DEVELOPMENT

Typical children follow a trajectory of increasing physical size (Figures 2–1 through 2–10) and increasing complexity of function (Figures 2–7 and 2–8 and Tables 2–1 and 2–2). Table 2–3 provides the theoretical perspectives of human behavior, taking into consideration the work of Freud, Erikson, and Piaget.

The first 5 years of life are a period of extraordinary physical growth and increasing complexity of function. The child triples his or her birth weight within the first year and achieves two-thirds of his or her brain size by age 2¹/₂–3 years. The child progresses from a totally dependent infant at birth to a mobile, verbal person who is able to express his or her needs and desires by age 2–3 years. In the ensuing 3 years the child further develops the capacity to interact with peers and adults, achieves considerable verbal and physical prowess, and becomes ready to enter the academic world of learning and socialization.

It is critical for the clinician to identify disturbances in development during these early years because there may be windows of time or sensitive periods when appropriate interventions may be instituted to effectively address developmental issues.

THE FIRST TWO YEARS

From a motor perspective, children develop in a cephalocaudal direction. They can lift their heads with good control at 3 months, sit independently at 6 months, crawl at 9 months, walk at 1 year, and run by 18 months. The child learning to walk has a wide-based gait at first. Next, he or she walks with legs closer together, the arms move medially, a heel-toe gait develops, and the arms swing symmetrically by 18–24 months.

Clinicians often focus on gross motor development, but an appreciation of fine motor development and dexterity, particularly the grasp, can be instructive not only in monitoring normal development but also in identifying deviations in development. The grasp begins as a raking motion involving the ulnar aspect of the hand at age 3–4 months. The thumb is added to this motion at about age 5 months as the focus of the movement shifts to the radial side of the hand. The thumb opposes the fingers for picking up objects just before age 7 months, and the neat pincer grasp emerges at about age 9 months. Most young children have symmetrical movements. Children should not have a significant hand preference before 1 year of age and typically develop handedness between 18 and 30 months.

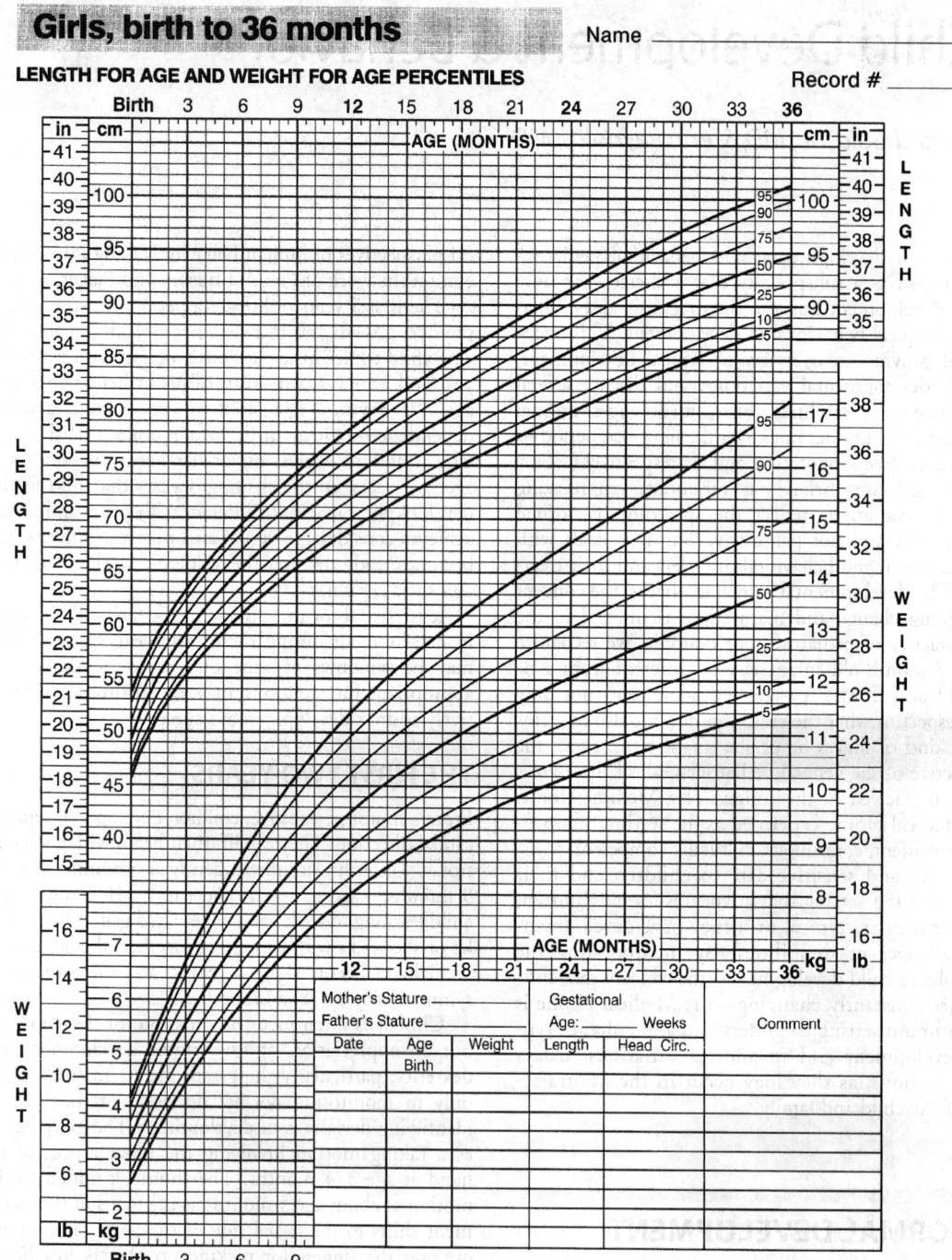

Figure 2–1. Percentile standards for length for age and weight for age in girls, birth to age 36 months. (Centers for Disease Control and Prevention.)

Girls, birth to 36 months

Name _____

HEAD CIRCUMFERENCE FOR AGE AND WEIGHT FOR LENGTH PERCENTILES

Record # _____

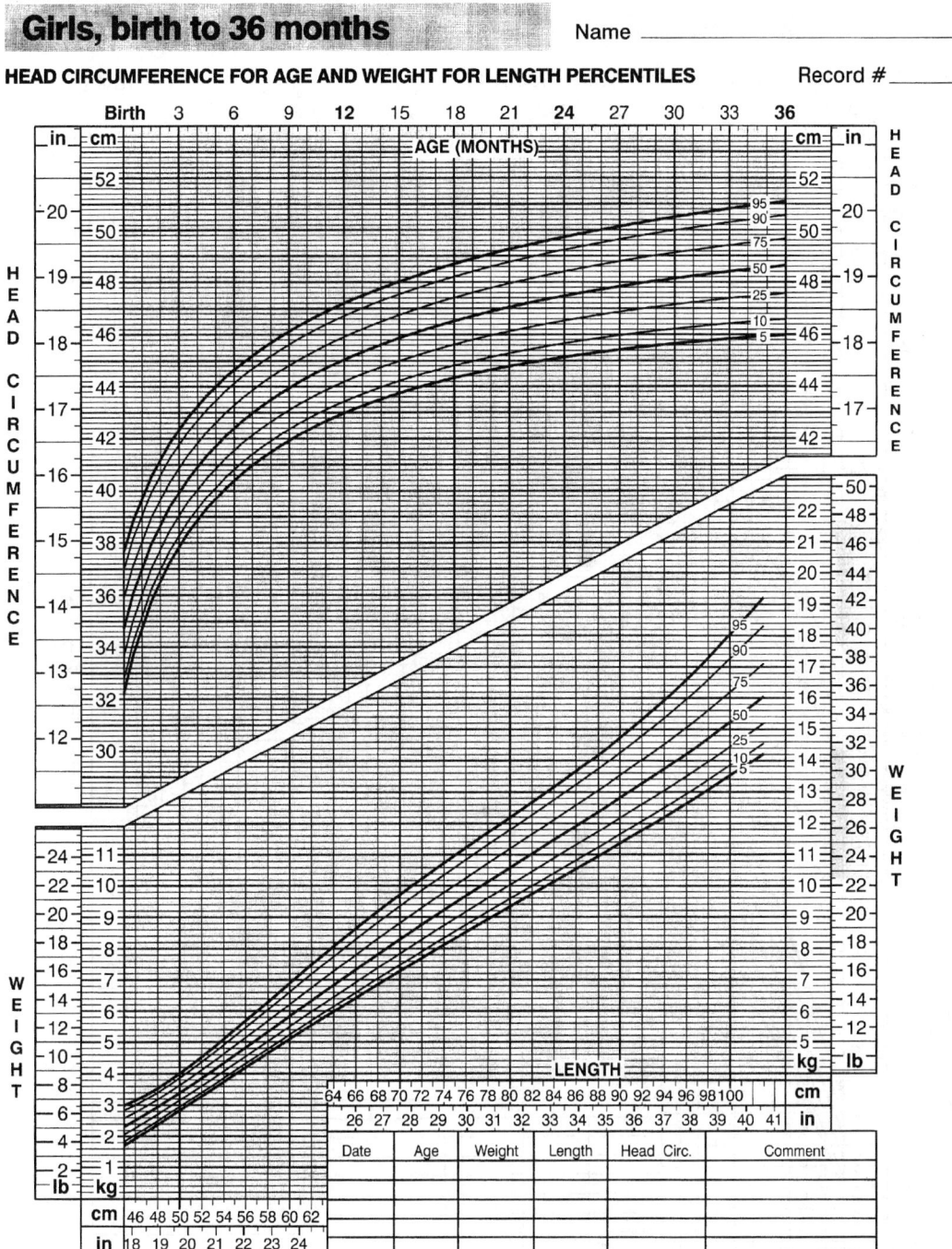

Figure 2–2. Percentile standards for head circumference for age and weight for length in girls, birth to age 36 months. (Centers for Disease Control and Prevention.)

Boys, birth to 36 months

Name _____

LENGTH FOR AGE AND WEIGHT FOR AGE PERCENTILES

Record #_____

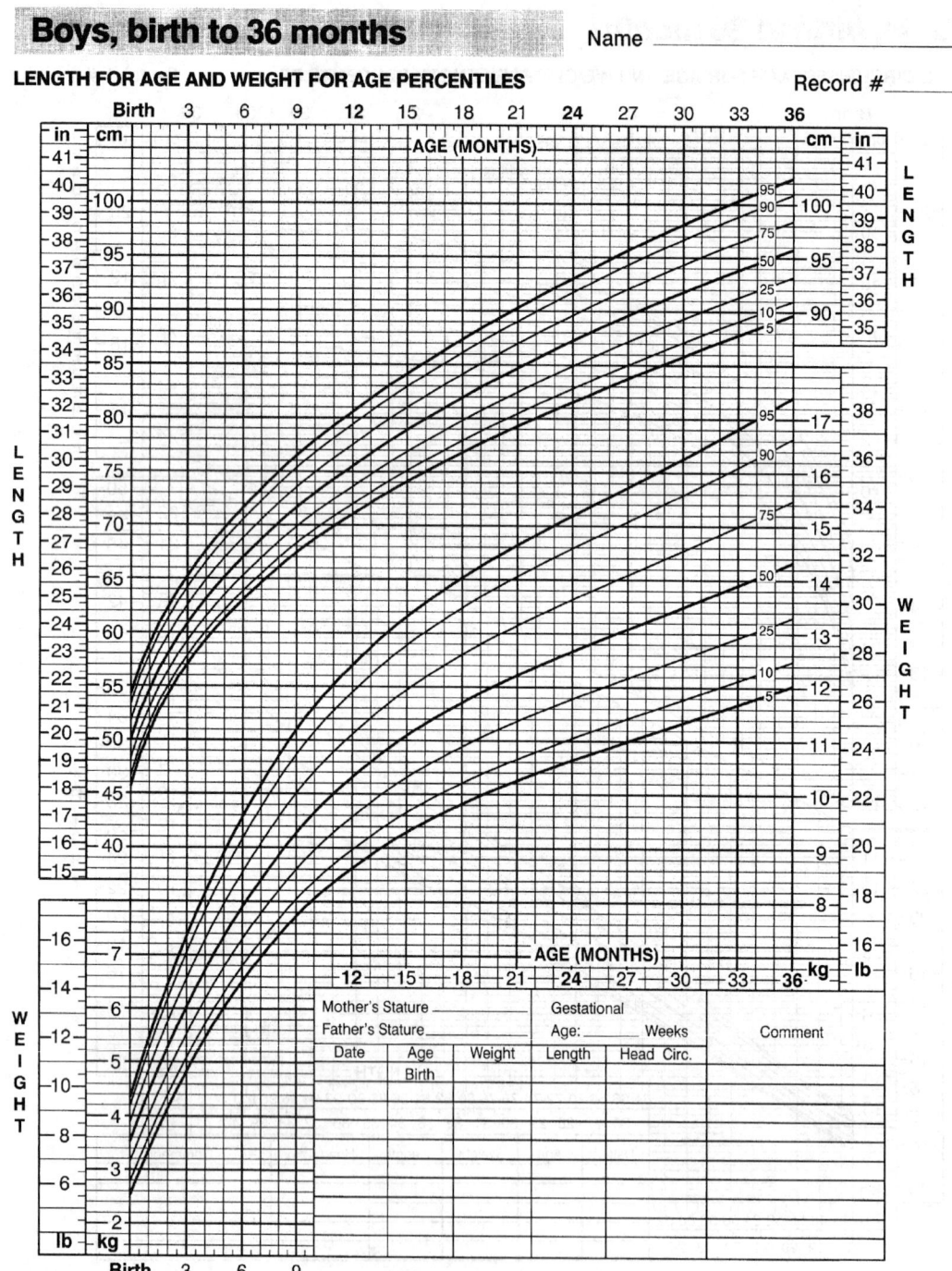

Figure 2–3. Percentile standards for length for age and weight for age in boys, birth to age 36 months. (Centers for Disease Control and Prevention.)

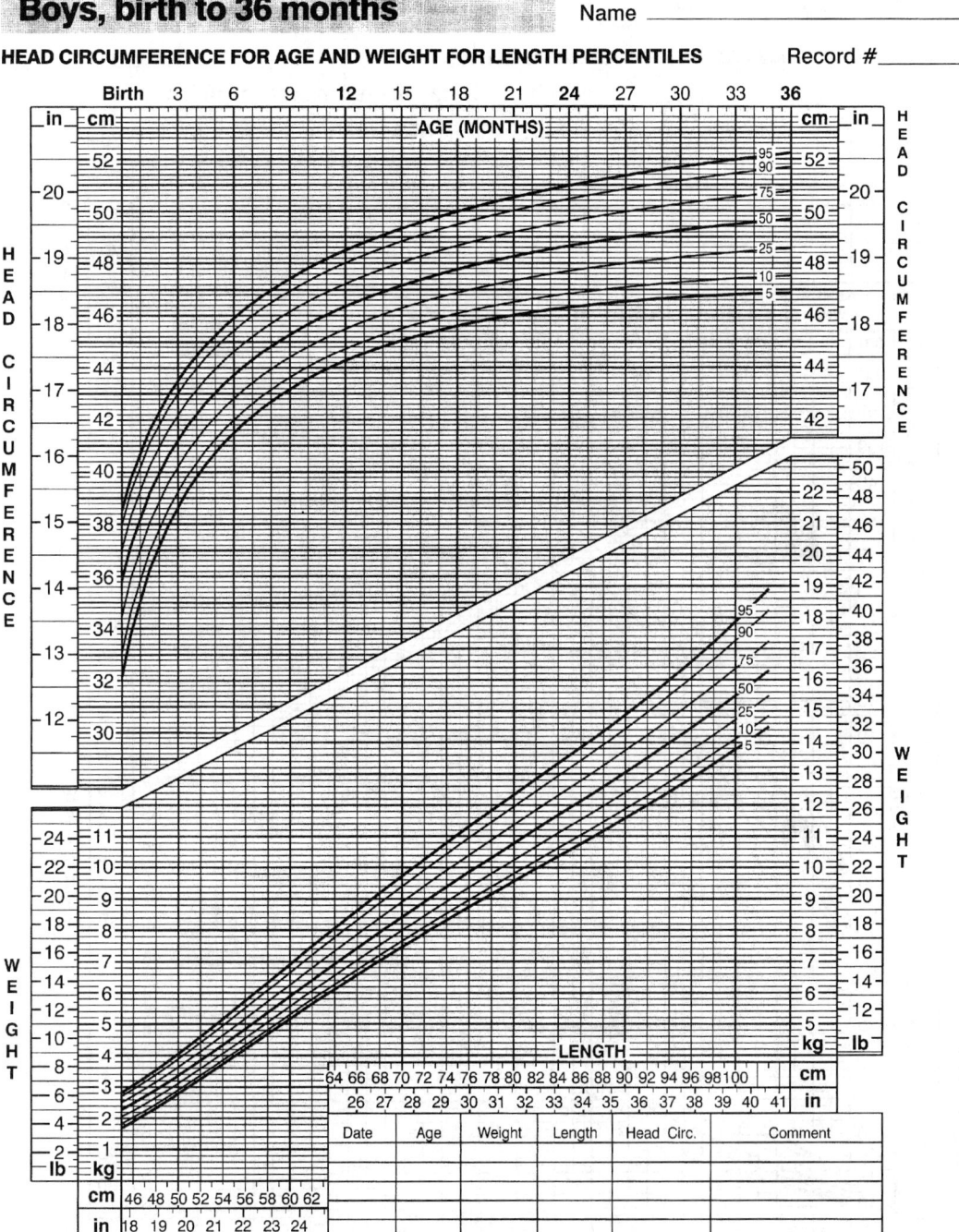

Figure 2–4. Percentile standards for head circumference for age and weight for length in boys, birth to age 36 months. (Centers for Disease Control and Prevention.)

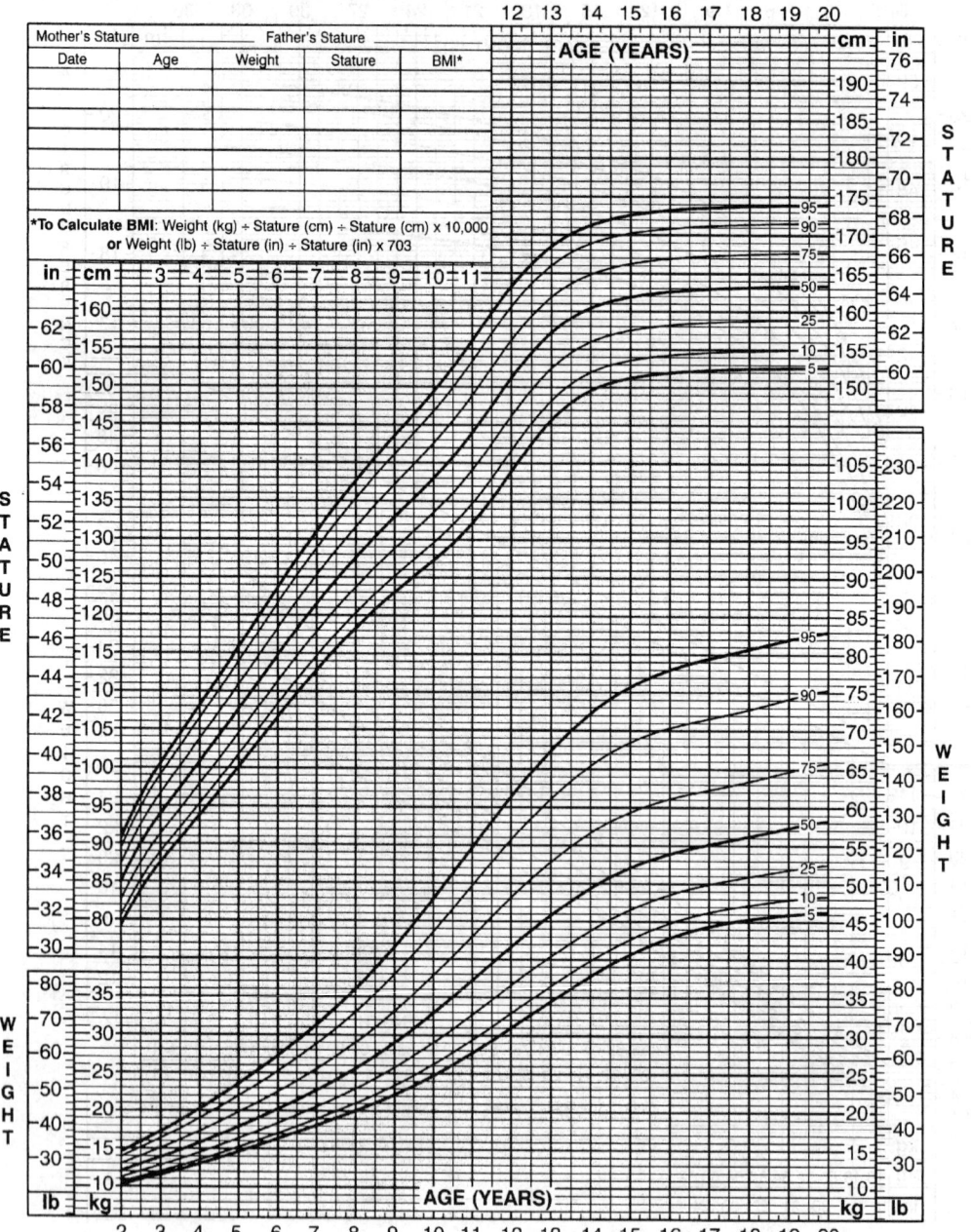

Figure 2–5. Percentile standards for stature for age and weight for age in girls, 2–20 years. (Centers for Disease Control and Prevention.)

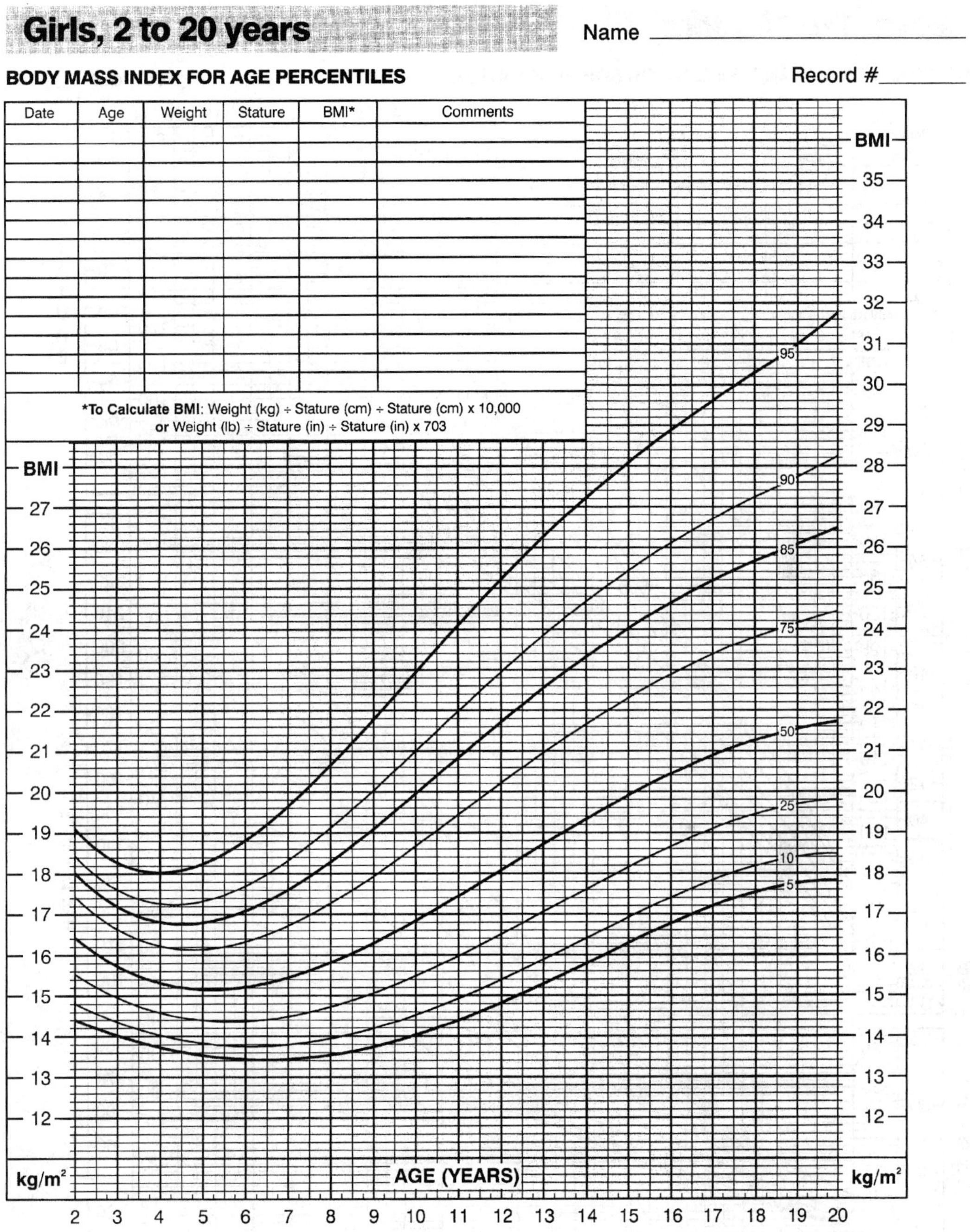
Girls, 2 to 20 years
Name
BODY MASS INDEX FOR AGE PERCENTILES
Record #
Date
Age
Weight
Stature
BMI*
Comments
*To Calculate BMI: Weight (kg) ÷ Stature (cm) ÷ Stature (cm) x 10,000
or Weight (lb) ÷ Stature (in) ÷ Stature (in) x 703
BMI
35
34
33
32
31
30
29
28
27
26
25
24
23
22
21
20
19
18
17
16
15
14
13
12
kg/m²
AGE (YEARS)
95
90
85
75
50
25
10
5
2
3
4
5
6
7
8
9
10
11
12
13
14
15
16
17
18
19
20

Figure 2–6. Percentile standards for body mass index for age in girls, 2–20 years. (Centers for Disease Control and Prevention.)

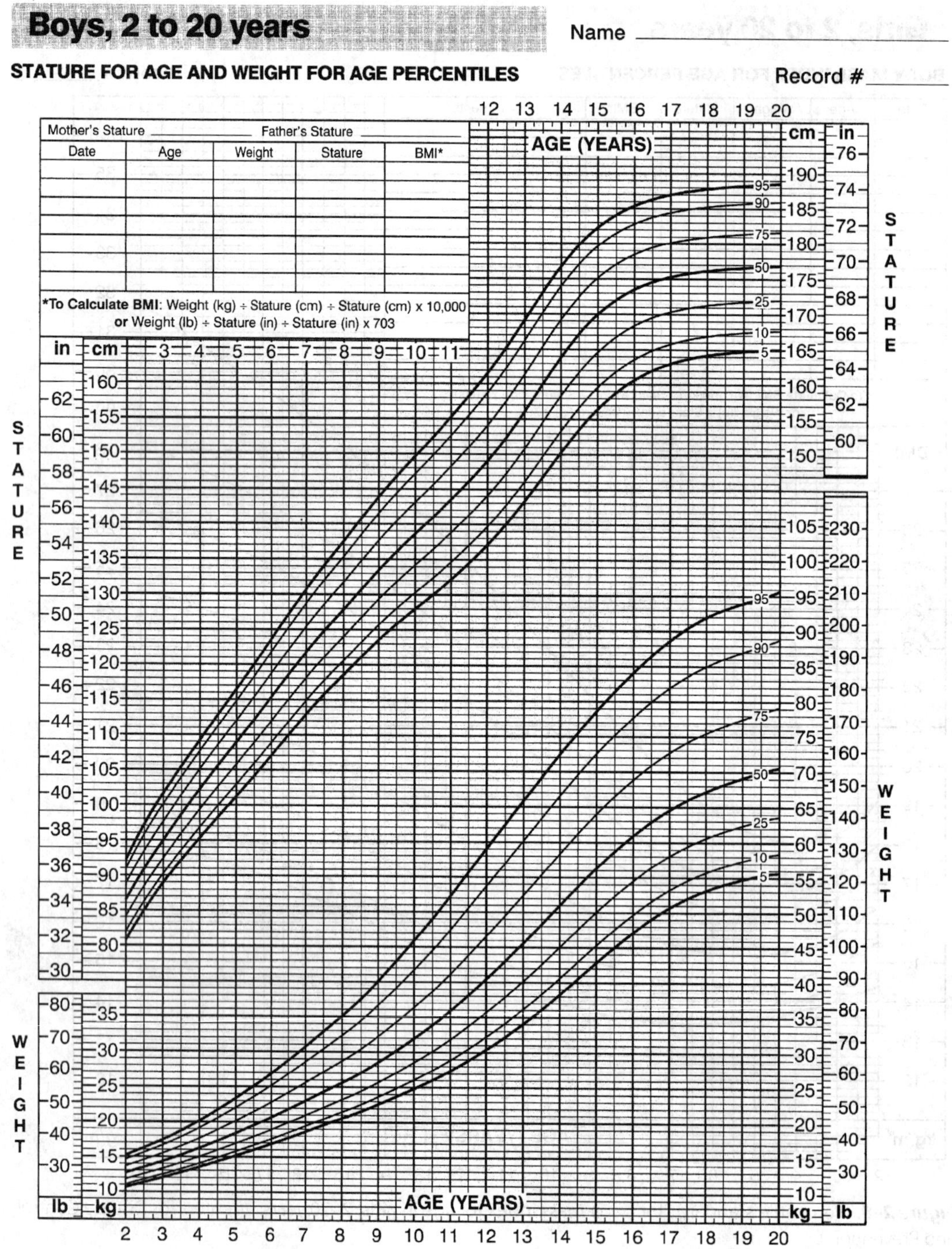

Boys, 2 to 20 years

Name _____

STATURE FOR AGE AND WEIGHT FOR AGE PERCENTILES

Record # _____

Figure 2–7. Percentile standards for stature for age and weight for age in boys, 2–20 years. (Centers for Disease Control and Prevention.)

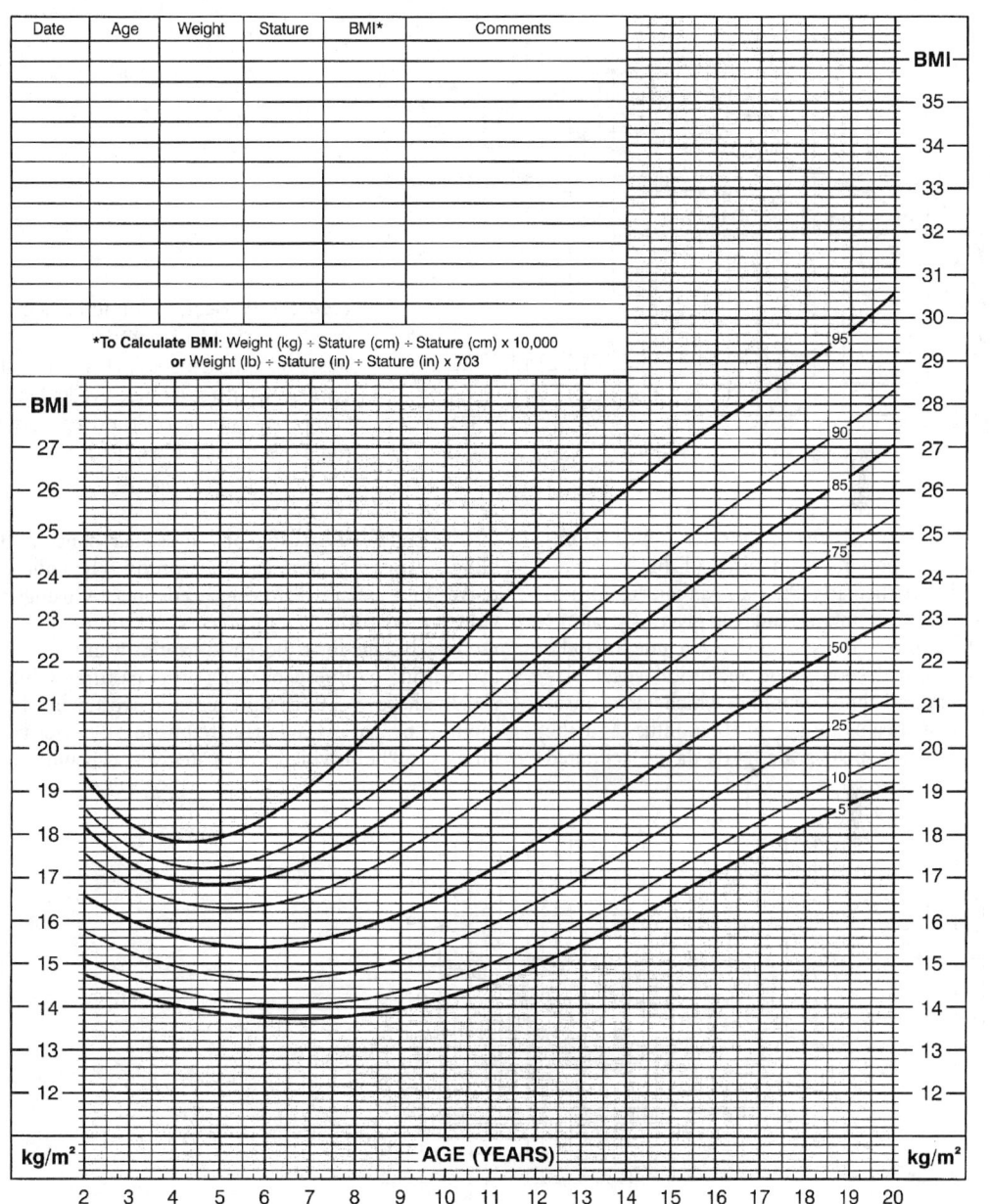

Figure 2–8. Percentile standards for body mass index for age in boys, 2–20 years. (Centers for Disease Control and Prevention.)

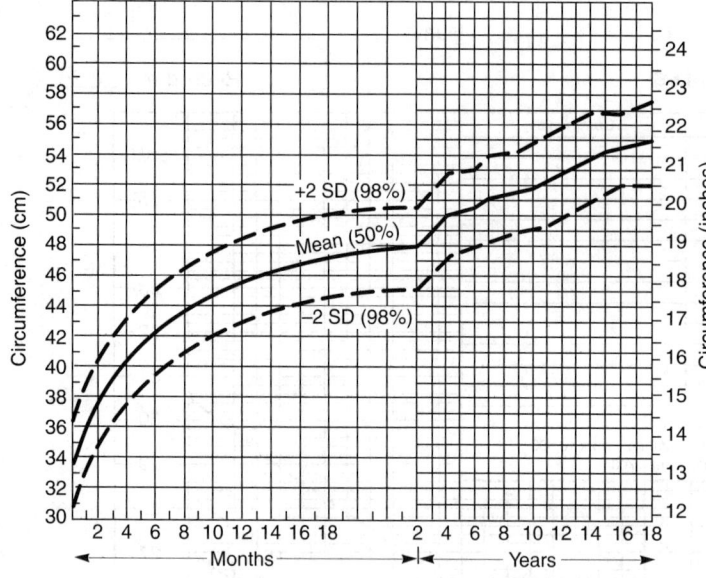

Figure 2–9. Head circumference of girls. (Modified and reproduced, with permission, from Nelhaus G: Head circumference from birth to eighteen years. Practical composite international and interracial graphs. Pediatrics 1968;41:106.)

Language is a critical area to consider as well. Communication is important from birth (Table 2–2 and Figure 2–11), particularly the nonverbal, reciprocal interactions between infant and caregiver. By age 2 months, these interactions begin to include melodic vowel sounds called cooing and reciprocal vocal play between parent and child. Babbling, which adds consonants to vowels, begins by age 6–10 months, and the repetition of sounds such as "da-da-da-da" is facilitated by the child's increasing oral muscular control. Babbling reaches a peak at age 12 months. The child then moves into a stage of having needs met by using individual words to represent objects or actions. It is common at this age for children to express wants and needs by pointing to objects or using other gestures. Children usually have 5–10 comprehensible words by 12–18 months; by age 2 years they are putting 2–3 words into phrases, 50% of which their caregivers can understand

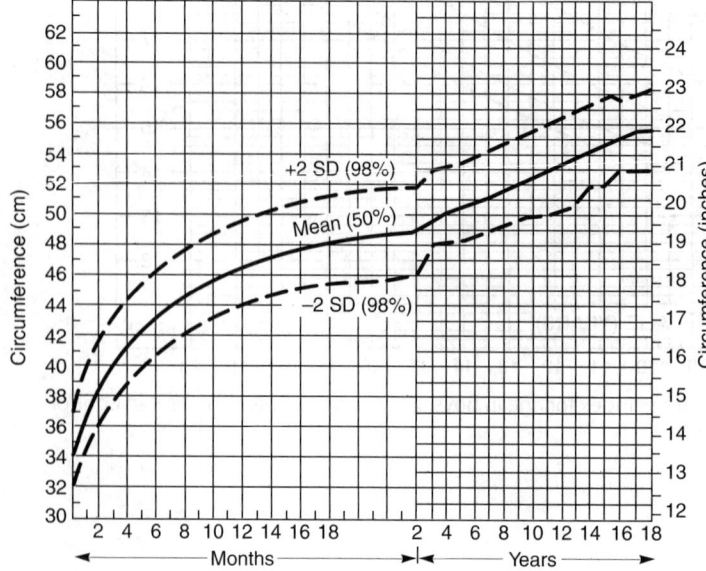

Figure 2–10. Head circumference of boys. (Modified and reproduced, with permission, from Nelhaus G: Head circumference from birth to eighteen years. Practical composite international and interracial graphs. Pediatrics 1968;41:106.)

Table 2–1. Developmental charts.

1–2 months

Activities to be observed:
Holds head erect and lifts head.
Turns from side to back.
Regards faces and follows objects through visual field.
Drops toys.
Becomes alert in response to voice.
Activities related by parent:
Recognizes parents.
Engages in vocalizations.
Smiles spontaneously.

3–5 months

Activities to be observed:
Grasps cube—first ulnar then later thumb opposition.
Reaches for and brings objects to mouth.
Makes "raspberry" sound.
Sits with support.
Activities related by parent:
Laughs.
Anticipates food on sight.
Turns from back to side.

6–8 months

Activities to be observed:
Sits alone for a short period.
Reaches with one hand.
First scoops up a pellet then grasps it using thumb opposition.
Imitates "bye-bye."
Passes object from hand to hand in midline.
Babbles.
Activities related by parent:
Rolls from back to stomach.
Is inhibited by the word *no*.

9–11 months

Activities to be observed:
Stands alone.
Imitates pat-a-cake and peek-a-boo.
Uses thumb and index finger to pick up pellet.
Activities related by parent:
Walks by supporting self on furniture.
Follows one-step verbal commands, eg, "Come here," "Give it to me."

1 year

Activities to be observed:
Walks independently.
Says "mama" and "dada" with meaning.
Can use a neat pincer grasp to pick up a pellet.
Releases cube into cup after demonstration.

Gives toys on request.
Tries to build a tower of 2 cubes.
Activities related by parent:
Points to desired objects.
Says 1 or 2 other words.

18 months

Activities to be observed:
Builds tower of 3–4 cubes.
Throws ball.
Seats self in chair.
Dumps pellet from bottle.
Activities related by parent:
Walks up and down stairs with help.
Says 4–20 words.
Understands a 2-step command.
Carries and hugs doll.
Feeds self.

24 months

Activities to be observed:
Speaks short phrases, 2 words or more.
Kicks ball on request.
Builds tower of 6–7 cubes.
Points to named objects or pictures.
Jumps off floor with both feet.
Stands on either foot alone.
Uses pronouns.
Activities related by parent:
Verbalizes toilet needs.
Pulls on simple garment.
Turns pages of book singly.
Plays with domestic mimicry.

30 months

Activities to be observed:
Walks backward.
Begins to hop on one foot.
Uses prepositions.
Copies a crude circle.
Points to objects described by use.
Refers to self as I.
Holds crayon in fist.
Activities related by parent:
Helps put things away.
Carries on a conversation.

3 years

Activities to be observed:
Holds crayon with fingers.
Builds tower of 9–10 cubes.

(continued)

Table 2–1. Developmental charts. (continued)

Imitates 3-cube bridge.
Copies circle.
Gives first and last name.
Activities related by parent:
Rides tricycle using pedals.
Dresses with supervision.

3–4 years

Activities to be observed:
Climbs stairs with alternating feet.
Begins to button and unbutton.
"What do you like to do that's fun?" (Answers using plurals, personal pronouns, and verbs.)
Responds to command to place toy *in, on,* or *under* table.
Draws a circle when asked to draw a person.
Knows own sex. ("Are you a boy or a girl?")
Gives full name.
Copies a circle already drawn. ("Can you make one like this?")
Activities related by parent:
Feeds self at mealtime.
Takes off shoes and jacket.

4–5 years

Activities to be observed:
Runs and turns without losing balance.
May stand on one leg for at least 10 seconds.
Buttons clothes and laces shoes. (Does not tie.)
Counts to 4 by rote.
"Give me 2 sticks." (Able to do so from pile of 4 tongue depressors.)
Draws a person. (Head, 2 appendages, and possibly 2 eyes. No torso yet.)
Knows the days of the week. ("What day comes after Tuesday?")
Gives appropriate answers to: "What must you do if you are sleepy? Hungry? Cold?"
Copies + in imitation.
Activities related by parent:
Self-care at toilet. (May need help with wiping.)
Plays outside for at least 30 minutes.
Dresses self except for tying.

5–6 years

Activities to be observed:
Can catch ball.
Skips smoothly.
Copies a + already drawn.
Tells age.
Concept of 10 (eg, counts 10 tongue depressors). May recite to higher number by rote.

Knows right and left hand.
Draws recognizable person with at least 8 details.
Can describe favorite television program in some detail.
Activities related by parent:
Does simple chores at home (eg, taking out garbage, drying silverware).
Goes to school unattended or meets school bus.
Good motor ability but little awareness of dangers.

6–7 years

Activities to be observed:
Copies a $\triangle$.
Defines words by use. ("What is an orange?" "To eat.")
Knows if morning or afternoon.
Draws a person with 12 details.
Reads several one-syllable printed words. (My, dog, see, boy.)

7–8 years

Activities to be observed:
Counts by 2s and 5s.
Ties shoes.
Copies a $\Diamond$
Knows what day of the week it is. (Not date or year.)
No evidence of sound substitution in speech (eg, *fr* for *thr*).
Draws a man with 16 details.
Reads paragraph #1 Durrell:
Reading:
Muff is a little yellow kitten. She drinks milk. She sleeps on a chair. She does not like to get wet.
Corresponding arithmetic:

7	6	6	8
$+4$	$+7$	-4	-3

Adds and subtracts one-digit numbers.

8–9 years

Activities to be observed:
Defines words better than by use. ("What is an orange?" "A fruit.")
Can give an appropriate answer to the following:
"What is the thing for you to do if . . .
—you've broken something that belongs to someone else?"
—a playmate hits you without meaning to do so?"
Reads paragraph #2 Durrell:
Reading:
A little black dog ran away from home. He played with two big dogs. They ran away from him. It began to rain. He

(continued)

Table 2–1. Developmental charts. (continued)

went under a tree. He wanted to go home, but he did not know the way. He saw a boy he knew. The boy took him home.

Corresponding arithmetic:

$$67 \quad \begin{array}{r} 45 \\ 16 \\ +27 \end{array} \quad \begin{array}{r} 14 \\ -8 \end{array} \quad \begin{array}{r} 84 \\ -36 \end{array}$$

$$\begin{array}{r} 67 \\ +4 \end{array}$$

Is learning borrowing and carrying processes in addition and subtraction.

9–10 years

Activities to be observed:
Knows the month, day, and year.
Names the months in order. (15 seconds, 1 error.)
Makes a sentence with these 3 words in it: (1 or 2. Can use words orally in proper context.)
  1. work . . . money . . . men
  2. boy . . . river . . . ball
Reads paragraph #3 Durrell:
Reading:
  Six boys put up a tent by the side of a river. They took things to eat with them. When the sun went down, they went into the tent to sleep. In the night, a cow came and began to eat grass around the tent. The boys were afraid. They thought it was a bear.
  Should comprehend and answer the question: "What was the cow doing?"
Corresponding arithmetic:

$$\begin{array}{r} 5204 \\ -530 \end{array} \quad \begin{array}{r} 23 \\ \times 3 \end{array} \quad \begin{array}{r} 837 \\ \times 7 \end{array}$$

Learning simple multiplication.

10–12 years

Activities to be observed:
Should read and comprehend paragraph #5 Durrell:
Reading:
  In 1807, Robert Fulton took the first long trip in a steamboat. He went one hundred and fifty miles up the Hudson River. The boat went five miles an hour. This was faster than a steamboat had ever gone before. Crowds gathered on both banks of the river to see this new kind of boat. They were afraid that its noise and splashing would drive away all the fish.
  Answer: "What river was the trip made on?"
  Ask to write the sentence: "The fishermen did not like the boat."
Corresponding arithmetic:

$$\begin{array}{r} 420 \\ \times 29 \end{array} \quad 9\overline{)72} \quad 31\overline{)62}$$

Should do multiplication and simple division.

12–15 years

Activities to be observed:
Reads paragraph #7 Durrell:
Reading:
  Golf originated in Holland as a game played on ice. The game in its present form first appeared in Scotland. It became unusually popular and kings found it so enjoyable that it was known as "the royal game." James IV, however, thought that people neglected their work to indulge in this fascinating sport so that it was forbidden in 1457. James relented when he found how attractive the game was, and it immediately regained its former popularity. Golf spread gradually to other countries, being introduced in America in 1890. It has grown in favor until there is hardly a town that does not boast of a private or public course.
  Ask to write a sentence: "Golf originated in Holland as a game played on ice."
  Answers questions:
    "Why was golf forbidden by James IV?"
    "Why did he change his mind?"
Corresponding arithmetic:

$$536\overline{)4762} \qquad \begin{array}{r} \frac{1}{3} \\ +\frac{1}{3} \end{array} \qquad \begin{array}{r} 7\frac{1}{6} \\ -\frac{3}{4} \end{array}$$

Reduce fractions to lowest forms.
Does long division, adds and subtracts fractions.

Modified from Leavitt SR, Goodman H, Harvin D: Use of developmental charts in teaching well child care. Pediatrics 1963;31:499.

(see Tables 2–1 and 2–2 and Figure 2–11). The acquisition of expressive vocabulary varies greatly between 12 and 24 months of age. As a group, males and children who are bilingual tend to develop expressive language more slowly during that time. It is important to note, however, that for each individual, milestones should still fall within the expected range. Gender and exposure to two languages should never be used as an excuse for failing to refer a child who has significant delay in the acquisition of speech and language for further evaluation. It is also important to note that most children are not truly bilingual. Most children have one primary language, and any other languages are secondary.

Receptive language usually develops more rapidly than expressive language. Word comprehension begins to increase at age 9 months, and by age 13 months the child's receptive vocabulary may be as large as 20–100 words. After age 18 months, expressive and receptive vocabularies increase dramatically, and by the end of the second year there is typically a quan-

Table 2–2. Normal speech and language development.

Age	Speech	Language	Articulation
1 month	Throaty sounds		Vowels: \ah\, \uh\, \ee\
2 months	Vowel sounds ("eh"), coos		
2 ½ months	Squeals		
3 months	Babbles, initial vowels		
4 months	Guttural sounds ("ah," "go")		Consonants: m, p, b
5 months			Vowels: \o\, \u\
7 months	Imitates speech sounds		
8 months			Syllables: da, ba, ka
10 months		"Dada" or "mama" nonspecifically	Approximates names: baba/bottle
12 months	Jargon begins (own language)	One word other than "mama" or "dada"	Understandable: 2–3 words
13 months		Three words	
16 months		Six words	Consonants: t, d, w, n, h
18–24 months		Two-word phrases	Understandable 2-word phrases
24–30 months		Three-word phrases	Understandable 3-word phrases
2 years	Vowels uttered correctly	Approximately 270 words; uses pronouns	Approximately 270 words; uses phrases
3 years	Some degree of hesitancy and uncertainty common	Approximately 900 words; intelligible 4-word phrases	Approximately 900 words; intelligible 4-word phrases
4 years		Approximately 1540 words; intelligible 5-word phrases or sentences	Approximately 1540 words; intelligible 5-word phrases
6 years		Approximately 2560 words; intelligible 6- or 7-word sentences	Approximately 2560 words; intelligible 6- or 7-word sentences
7–8 years	Adult proficiency		

Data on articulation from Berry MF: *Language Disorders of Children.* Appleton-Century-Crofts, 1969; and from Bzoch K, League R: *Receptive-Expressive Emergent Language Scale.* University Park Press, 1970.

tum leap in language development. The child begins to put together words and phrases and begins to use language to represent a new world, the symbolic world. Children begin to put verbs into phrases and focus much of their language on describing their new abilities, for example, "I go out." They begin to incorporate prepositions, such as "I" and "you" into speech and ask "why?" and "what?" questions more frequently. They also begin to appreciate time factors and to understand and use this concept in their speech (see Table 2–1).

The Early Language Milestone Scale (see Figure 2–11) is a simple tool for assessing early language development in the pediatric office setting. It is scored in the same way as the Denver II (Figure 2–12) but tests receptive and expressive language areas in greater depth.

One may easily memorize the developmental milestones that characterize the trajectory of the typical child; however, these milestones become more meaningful and clinically useful if placed in empirical and theoretical contexts. The work of Piaget and others is quite instructive and provides some insight into behavioral and affective development (see Table 2–3). Piaget described the first 2 years of life as the sensorimotor period, during which infants learn with increasing sophistication how to link sensory input from the environment with a motor response. Infants build on primitive reflex patterns of behavior (termed sche-

Table 2–3. Perspectives of human behavior.

Age	Theories of Development			Skill Areas		Psychopathology
	Freud	Erikson	Piaget	Language	Motor	
Birth to 18 months	Oral	Basic trust versus mistrust	Sensorimotor	Body actions; crying; naming; pointing	Reflex sitting, reaching, grasping, walking	Autism; anaclitic depression, colic; disorders of attachment; feeding, sleeping problems
18 months–3 years	Anal	Autonomy versus shame, doubt	Symbolic (preoperational)	Sentences; telegraph jargon	Climbing, running	Separation issues; negativism; fearfulness; constipation; shyness, withdrawal
3–6 years	Oedipal	Initiative versus guilt	Intuition (preoperational)	Connective words; can be readily understood	Increased coordination; tricycle; jumping	Enuresis; encopresis; anxiety; aggressive acting out; phobias; nightmares
6–11 years	Latency	Industry versus inferiority	Concrete operational	Subordinate sentences; reading and writing; language reasoning	Increased skills; sports, recreational cooperative games	School phobias; obsessive reactions; conversion reactions; depressive equivalents
12–17 years	Adolescence (genital)	Identity versus role confusion	Formal operational	Reason abstract; using language; abstract manipulation	Refinement of skills	Delinquency; promiscuity; schizophrenia; anorexia nervosa; suicide

Adapted and reproduced, with permission, from Dixon S: Setting the stage: Theories and concepts of child development. In Dixon S, Stein M (editors): *Encounters with Children,* 2nd ed. Year Book, 1992.

mata; sucking is an example) and constantly incorporate or assimilate new experiences. The schemata evolve over time as infants accommodate new experiences and as new levels of cognitive ability unfold in an orderly sequence. Enhancement of neural networks through dendritic branching and pruning (apoptosis) occurs.

In the first year of life, the infant's perception of reality revolves around itself and what it can see or touch. The infant follows the trajectory of an object through the field of vision, but before age 6 months the object ceases to exist once it leaves the infant's field of vision. At age 9–12 months, the infant gradually develops the concept of object permanence, or the realization that objects exist even when not seen. The development of object permanence correlates with enhanced frontal activity on the electroencephalogram. The concept attaches first to the image of the mother or primary caregiver because of his or her emotional importance and is a critical part of attachment behavior (discussed

later). In the second year, children extend their ability to manipulate objects by using instruments, first by imitation and later by trial and error.

Freud described the first year of life as the oral stage because so many of the infant's needs are fulfilled by oral means. Nutrition is obtained through sucking on the breast or bottle, and self-soothing occurs through sucking on fingers or a pacifier. During this stage of symbiosis with the mother, the boundaries between mother and infant are blurred. The baby's needs are totally met by the mother, and the mother has been described as manifesting "narcissistic possessiveness" of the infant. This is a very positive interaction in the bidirectional attachment process called bonding. The parents learn to be aware of and to interpret the infant's cues, which reflect its needs. A more sensitive emotional interaction process develops that can be seen in the mirroring of facial expressions by the primary caregiver and infant and in their mutual engagement in cycles of attention and

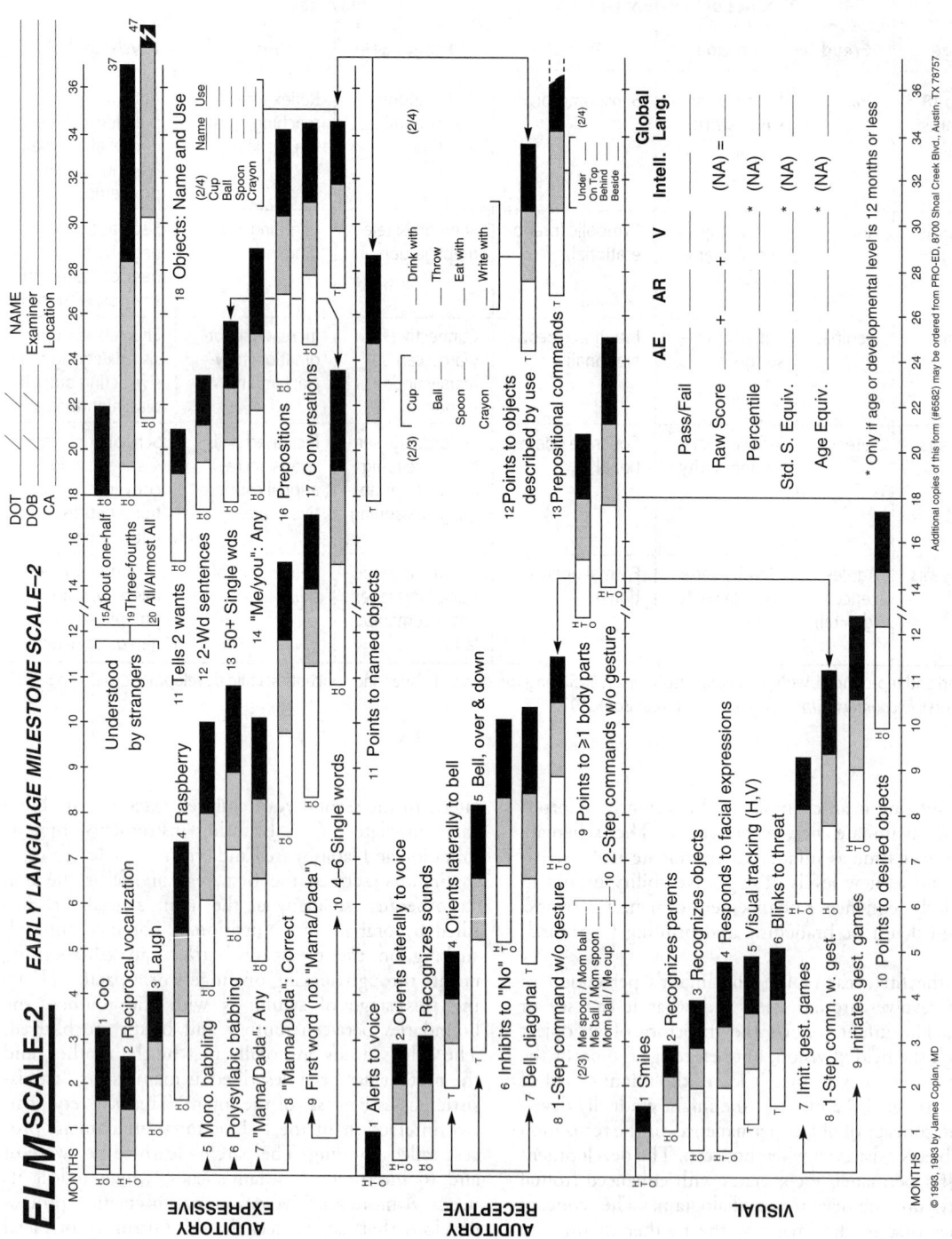

Figure 2–11. Early Language Milestone Scale-2. (Reproduced, with permission, from Coplan J: *Early Language Milestone Scale*. Pro Ed, 1993.)

80

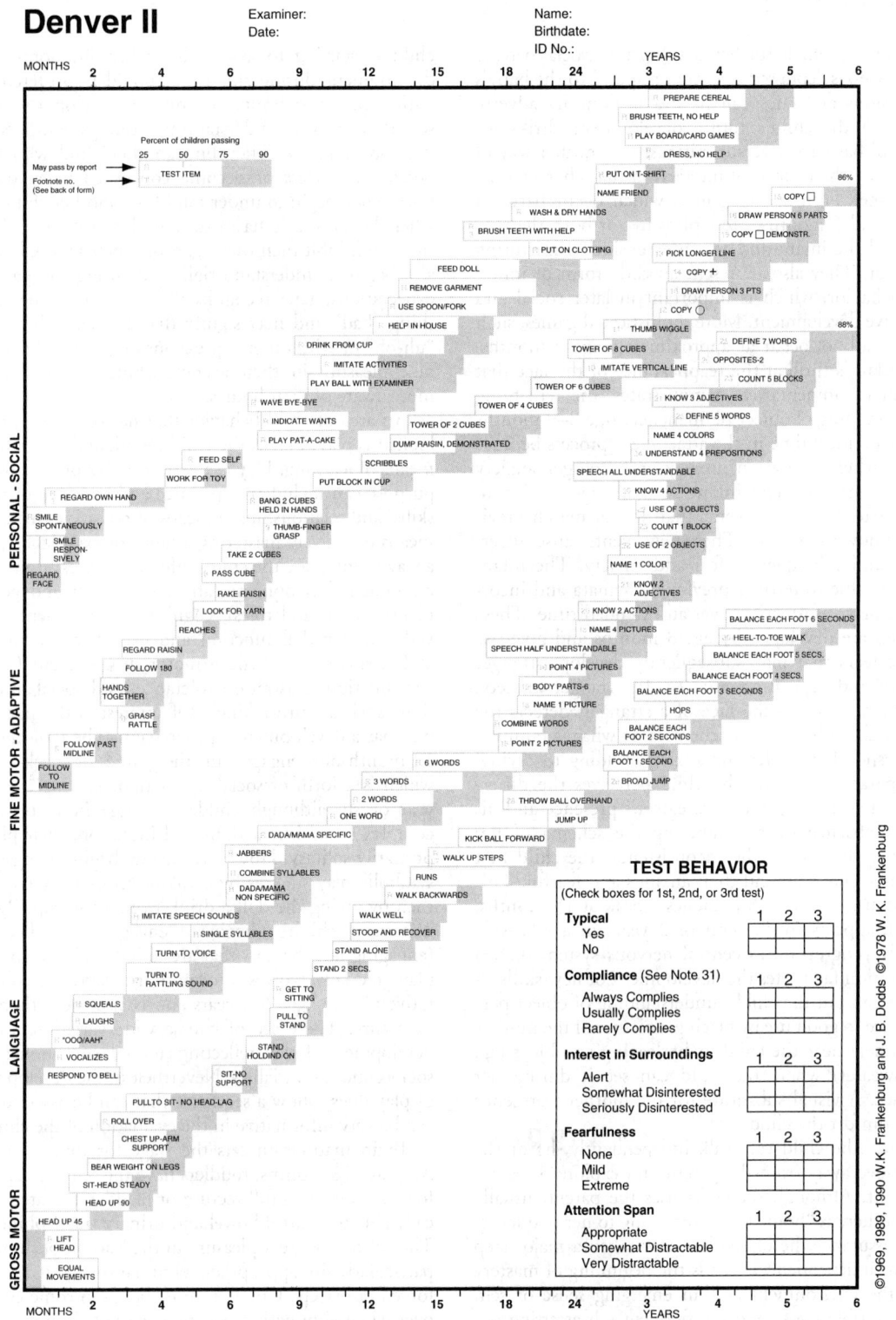

Figure 2–12. Denver II. (Copyright © 1969, 1989, 1990 WK Frankenburg and JB Dodds. © 1978 WK Frankenberg.)

inattention, which further develop into social play. A parent who is depressed or cannot respond to the baby's expressions and cues can have a profoundly adverse effect on the child's future development. Erikson's terms of basic trust versus mistrust are another way of describing the reciprocal interaction that characterizes this stage. Turn-taking games, which occur between ages 3 and 6 months, are a pleasure for both the parents and the infant and are an extension of mirroring behavior. They also represent an early form of imitative behavior, which is important in later social and cognitive development. More sophisticated games, such as peek-a-boo, occur at approximately age 9 months. The infant's thrill at the reappearance of the face that vanished momentarily demonstrates the emerging understanding of object permanence. Age 8–9 months is also a critical time in the attachment process because this is when separation anxiety and stranger anxiety become marked. The infant at this stage is able to appreciate discrepant events that do not match previously known schemata. These new events cause uncertainty and subsequently fear and anxiety. The infant must be able to retrieve previous schemata and incorporate new information over an extended time. These abilities are developed by age 8 months and give rise to the fears that may subsequently develop: stranger anxiety and separation anxiety. In stranger anxiety, the infant analyzes the face of a stranger, detects the mismatch with previous schemata or what is familiar, and responds with fear or anxiety, leading to crying. In separation anxiety, the child perceives the difference between the primary caregiver's presence and his or her absence by remembering the schema of her presence. Perceiving the inconsistency, the child first becomes uncertain and then anxious and fearful. This begins at age 8 months, reaches a peak at 15 months, and disappears by the end of 2 years in a relatively orderly progression as central nervous system (CNS) maturation facilitates the development of new skills. A parent can put the child's understanding of object permanence to good use by placing a picture of the mother (or father) near the child or by leaving an object (eg, her sweater) where the child can see it during her absence. A visual substitute for the mother's presence may comfort the child.

Once the child can walk independently, he or she can move away from the parent and explore the environment. Although the child uses the parent, usually the mother, as "home base," returning to her frequently for reassurance, he or she has now taken a major step toward independence. This is the beginning of mastery over the environment and an emerging sense of self. The "terrible twos" and the frequent self-asserting use of "no" are the child's attempt to develop a better idea of what is or might be under his or her control. The

child is starting to assert his or her autonomy. Ego development during this time should be fostered but with appropriate limits. As children develop a sense of self, they begin to understand the feelings of others and develop empathy. They hug another child who is in perceived distress or become concerned when one is hurt. They begin to understand how another child feels when he or she is harmed, and this realization helps them to inhibit their own aggressive behavior. Children also begin to understand right and wrong and parental expectations. They recognize that they have done something "bad" and may signify that awareness by saying "uh-oh" or with other expressions of distress. They also take pleasure in their accomplishments and become more aware of their bodies.

An area of child behavior that has often been overlooked is play. Play is the child's work and a significant means of learning. Play is a very complex process whose purpose can include the practice and rehearsal of roles, skills, and relationships; a means of revisiting the past; a means of actively mastering a range of experiences; and a way to integrate the child's life experiences. It involves emotional development (affect regulation and gender identification and roles), cognitive development (nonverbal and verbal function and executive functioning and creativity), and social/motor development (motor coordination, frustration tolerance, and social interactions such as turn-taking). Of interest is the fact that play has a developmental progression. The typical 6- to 12-month-old engages in the game of peek-a-boo, which is a form of social interaction. During the next year or so, although children engage in increasingly complex social interactions and imitation, their play is primarily solitary. However, they do begin to engage in symbolic play such as by drinking from a toy cup and then by giving the doll a drink from a toy cup. By age 2–3 years children begin to engage in parallel play (engaging in behaviors that are imitative). This form of play gradually evolves into more interactive or collaborative play by age 3–4 years and is also more thematic in nature. There are of course wide variations in the development of play, reflecting cultural, educational, and socioeconomic variables. Nevertheless, the development of play does follow a sequence that can be assessed and can be very informative in the evaluation of the child.

Brain maturation sets the stage for toilet training. After age 18 months, toddlers have the sensory capacity for awareness of a full rectum or bladder and are physically able to control bowel and urinary tract sphincters. They also take great pleasure in their accomplishments, particularly in appropriate elimination, if it is reinforced positively. Children must be given some control over when elimination occurs. If parents impose severe restrictions, the achievement of this developmental milestone can become a battle between parent and child. Freud termed this period the anal stage because the developmental issue of bowel control is the major task requiring mastery. It encompasses a more generalized theme of socialized behavior and overall body cleanliness, which is usually taught or imposed on the child at this age.

TWO TO FOUR YEARS

Piaget characterized the 2- to 6-year-old stage as preoperational. This stage begins when language has facilitated the creation of mental images in the symbolic sense. The child begins to manipulate the symbolic world; sorts out reality from fantasy imperfectly; and may be terrified of dreams, wishes, and foolish threats. Most of the child's perception of the world is egocentric or interpreted in reference to his or her needs or influence. Cause-effect relationships are confused with temporal ones or interpreted egocentrically. For example, children may focus their understanding of divorce on themselves ("My father left because I was bad" or "My mother left because she didn't love me"). Illness and the need for medical care are also commonly misinterpreted at this age. The child may make a mental connection between a sibling's illness and a recent argument, a negative comment, or a wish for the sibling to be ill. The child may experience significant guilt unless the parents are aware of these misperceptions and take time to deal with them.

At this age, children also endow inanimate objects with human feelings. They also assume that humans cause or create all natural events. For instance, when asked why the sun sets, they may say, "The sun goes to his house" or "It is pushed down by someone else." Magical thinking blossoms between ages 3 and 5 years as symbolic thinking incorporates more elaborate fantasy. Fantasy facilitates development of role playing, sexual identity, and emotional growth. Children test new experiences in fantasy, both in their imagination and in play. In their play, children often create magical stories and novel situations that reflect issues with which they are dealing, such as aggression, relationships, fears, and control. Children often invent imaginary friends at this time, and nightmares or fears of monsters are common. At this stage, other children become important in facilitating play, such as in a preschool group. Play gradually becomes more cooperative; shared fantasy leads to game playing. Freud described the oedipal phase between ages 3 and 6 years, when there is strong attachment to the parent of the opposite sex. The child's fantasies may focus on play-acting the adult role with that parent, although by age 6 years oedipal issues are usually resolved and attachment is redirected to the parent of the same sex.

EARLY SCHOOL YEARS: AGES 5–7 YEARS

Attendance at kindergarten at age 5 years marks an acceleration in the separation-individuation theme initiated in the preschool years. The child is ready to relate to peers in a more interactive manner. The brain has reached 90% of its adult weight. Sensorimotor coordination abilities are maturing and facilitating pencil-and-paper tasks and sports, both part of the school experience. Cognitive abilities are still at the preoperational stage, and children focus on one variable in a problem at a time. However, most children have mastered conservation of length by age $5^1/_2$ years, conservation of mass and weight by $6^1/_2$ years, and conservation of volume by age 8 years.

By first grade, there is more pressure on the child to master academic tasks—recognizing numbers, letters, and words and learning to write. Piaget described the stage of concrete operations beginning after age 6 years, when the child is able to perform mental operations concerning concrete objects that involve manipulation of more than one variable. The child is able to order, number, and classify because these activities are related to concrete objects in the environment and because these activities are stressed in early schooling. Magical thinking diminishes greatly at this time, and the reality of cause-effect relationships is better understood. Fantasy and imagination are still strong and are reflected in themes of play.

MIDDLE CHILDHOOD: AGES 7–11 YEARS

Freud characterized ages 7–11 years as the latency years, during which children are not bothered by significant aggressive or sexual drives but instead devote most of their energies to school and peer group interactions. In reality, throughout this period there is a gradual increase in sex drive, manifested by increasingly aggressive play and interactions with the opposite sex. Fantasy still has an active role in dealing with sexuality before adolescence, and fantasies often focus on movie and music stars. Organized sports, clubs, and other activities are other modalities that permit preadolescent children to display socially acceptable forms of aggression and sexual interest.

For the 7-year-old child, the major developmental tasks are achievement in school and acceptance by peers. Academic expectations intensify and require the child to concentrate on, attend to, and process increasingly complex auditory and visual information. Children with significant learning disabilities or problems with attention, organization, and impulsivity may have difficulty with academic tasks and subsequently may receive negative reinforcement from teachers, peers, and even parents. Such children may develop a poor self-image manifested as behavioral difficulties. The pediatrician must evaluate potential learning disabilities in any child who is not developing adequately at this stage or who presents with emotional or behavioral problems. The developmental status of school-age children is not documented as easily as that of younger children because of the complexity of the milestones. In the school-age child, the quality of the response, the attentional abilities, and the child's emotional approach to the task can make a dramatic difference in success at school. The clinician must consider all of these aspects in the differential diagnosis of learning disabilities and behavioral disorders.

Bjorklund FP: *Children's Thinking.* Brooks/Cole, 1995.

Dixon SD, Stein MT: *Encounters with Children: Pediatric Behavior and Development,* 4th ed. Mosby-Year Book, 2006.

Feldman HM: Evaluation and management of language and speech disorders in preschool children. Pediatr Rev 2005;26:131.

Frankenberg WK et al: The Denver II: A major revision and restandardization of the Denver Developmental Screening Test. Pediatrics 1991;89:91.

Glascoe FP, Dworkin PH: The role of parents in the detection of developmental and behavioral problems. Pediatrics 1995; 95:829 [PMID: 7539122].

Green M, Palfrey JS (editors): *Bright Futures: Guidelines for Health Supervision of Infants, Children, and Adolescents,* 2nd ed revised. National Center for Education in Maternal and Child Health Georgetown University, 2002.

Levine MD, Carey WB, Crocker AC (editors): *Developmental-Behavioral Pediatrics,* 3rd ed. WB Saunders, 1999.

Parker S, Zuckerman B (editors): *Behavioral and Developmental Pediatrics: A Handbook for Primary Care.* Lippincott, Williams & Wilkins, 2005.

behavioral complaints are by and large normal variations in behavior, a reflection of each child's individual biologic and temperament traits and the parents' responses. There are no cures for these behaviors, but management strategies are available that can enhance the parents' understanding of the child and the child's relationship to the environment. These strategies also facilitate the parents' care of the growing infant and child.

The last section of this chapter discusses developmental disorders of cognitive and social competence. Diagnosis and management of these conditions requires a comprehensive and often multidisciplinary approach. The health care provider can play a major role in diagnosis, in coordinating the child's evaluation, in interpreting the results to the family, and in providing reassurance and support.

American Academy of Pediatrics, Medical Home Initiatives for Children with Special Health Care Needs Project Advisory Committee, 2002: The Medical Home. Pediatrics 2002; 110:184.

Capute AJ, Accardo PJ (editors): *Developmental Disabilities in Infancy and Childhood,* 2nd ed. Vol. 1, *Neurodevelopmental Diagnosis and Treatment.* Vol. 2, *The Spectrum of Developmental Disabilities.* Brookes/Cole, 1996.

Greydanus DE, Wolraich ML (editors): *Behavioral Pediatrics.* Springer, 1992.

Levine MD, Carey WB, Crocker AC (editors): *Developmental-Behavioral Pediatrics,* 3rd ed. WB Saunders, 1999.

Parker S, Zuckerman B (editors): *Behavioral and Developmental Pediatrics: A Handbook for Primary Care.* Lippincott, Williams & Wilkins, 2005.

Wolraich ML (editor): *Disorders of Development and Learning: A Practical Guide to Assessment and Management,* 3rd ed. BC Decker, 2003.

Wolraich ML, Felice ME, Drotar D: *The Classification of Child and Adolescent Mental Diagnoses in Primary Care: Diagnostic and Statistical Manual for Primary Care (DSM-PC) Child and Adolescent Version.* American Academy of Pediatrics, 1996.

■ BEHAVIORAL & DEVELOPMENTAL VARIATIONS

Behavioral and developmental variations and disorders encompass a wide range of issues of importance to pediatricians. Practitioners will be familiar with most of the problems discussed in this chapter; however, with increasing knowledge of the factors controlling normal neurologic and behavioral development in childhood, new perspectives on these disorders and novel approaches to their diagnosis and management are emerging.

Variations in children's behavior reflect a blend of intrinsic biologic characteristics and the environments with which the children interact. The next section focuses on some of the more common complaints about behavior encountered by those who care for children. These

■ NORMALITY & TEMPERAMENT

The physician confronted by a disturbance in physiologic function rarely has doubts about what is abnormal. Variations in temperament and behavior are not as straightforward. Labeling such variations as disorders implies that a disease entity exists.

The behaviors described in this section are viewed as part of a continuum of responses by the child to a variety of internal and external experiences. Variations in temperament have been of interest to philosophers and writers since ancient times. The Greeks believed there were four temperament types: choleric, sanguine, melancholic, and phlegmatic. In more recent times, folk wisdom has defined temperament as a genetically influenced behavioral disposition that is stable over time. Although a number of models of temperament have been proposed, the one usually used by pediatricians in clinical practice is that of Thomas and Chess, who describe temperament as being the "how" of behavior as distinguished from the "why" (motivation) and the "what" (ability). Temperament is an independent psychological attribute that is expressed as a response to an external stimulus. The influence of temperament is bidirectional: The effect of a particular experience will be influenced by the child's temperament, and the child's temperament will influence the responses of others in the child's environment. Temperament is the style with which the child interacts with the environment.

The perceptions and expectations of parents must be considered when a child's behavior is evaluated. A child that one parent might describe as hyperactive might not be characterized as such by the other parent. This truism can be expanded to include all the dimensions of temperament. Thus, the concept of "goodness of fit" comes into play. For example, if the parents want and expect their child to be predictable but that is not the child's behavioral style, the parents may perceive the child as being bad or having a behavioral disorder rather than as having a developmental variation. An appreciation of this phenomenon is important because the physician may be able to enhance the parents' understanding of the child and influence their responses to the child's behavior. When there is goodness of fit, there will be more harmony and a greater potential for healthy development not only of the child but also of the family. When goodness of fit is not present, tension and stress can result in parental anger, disappointment, frustration, and conflict with the child.

Other models of temperament include those of Rothbart, Buss and Plomin, and Goldsmith and Campos (Table 2–4). All models seek to identify intrinsic behavioral characteristics that lead the child to respond to the world in particular ways. One child may be highly emotional and another less so (ie, calmer) in response to a variety of experiences, stressful or pleasant. The clinician must recognize that each child brings some intrinsic, biologically based traits to its environment and that such characteristics are neither good nor bad, right nor wrong, normal nor abnormal; they are simply part of the child. Thus, as one looks at variations in development, one should abandon the illness model and consider this construct as an aid to understanding the nature of the child's behavior and its influence on the parent-child relationship.

Barr RG: Normality: A clinically useless concept: The case of infant crying and colic. J Dev Behav Pediatr 1993;14:264 [PMID: 8408670].

Table 2–4. Theories of temperament.

Thomas and Chess	Temperament is an independent psychologic attribute, biologically determined, which is expressed as a response to an external stimulus. It is the child's behavioral style: an interactive model.
Rothbart	Temperament is a function of biologically based individual differences in reactivity and self-regulation. It is subsumed under the concept of "personality" and goes beyond mere "behavioral style."
Buss and Plomin	Temperament is a set of genetically determined personality traits that appear early in life and are different from other inherited and acquired personality traits.
Goldsmith and Campos	Temperament is the individual's differences in the probability of experiencing emotions and arousal.

Goldsmith HH et al: Roundtable: What is temperament? Four approaches. Child Dev 1987;58:505 [PMID: 3829791].

Prior M: Childhood temperament. J Child Psychol Psychiatr 1992;33:249 [PMID: 1737829].

Thomas A, Chess S: *Temperament and Development.* Brunner/Mazel, 1977.

■ COMMON DEVELOPMENTAL CONCERNS

COLIC

Infant colic is characterized by severe and paroxysmal crying that occurs mainly in the late afternoon. The infant's knees are drawn up and its fists are clenched, flatus is expelled, the facies is pained, and there is minimal response to attempts at soothing. Studies in the United States have shown that among middle-class infants, crying occupies about 2 hours per day at 2 weeks of age, about 3 hours per day by 6 weeks, and gradually decreases to about 1 hour per day by 3 months. The word "colic" is derived from Greek *kolikos* ("pertaining to the colon"). Although colic has traditionally been attributed to gastrointestinal disturbances, this has never been proved. Colic is a behavioral sign or symptom that begins in the first few weeks of life and peaks at age 2–3 months. In about 30–40% of cases, colic continues into the fourth and fifth months.

A colicky infant, as defined by Wessel, is one who is healthy and well fed but cries for more than 3 hours a day, for more than 3 days a week, and for more than 3 weeks—commonly referred to as the rule of threes. The important word in this definition is "healthy." Thus, before the diagnosis of colic can be made, the pediatrician must rule out diseases that might cause crying. With the exception of the few infants who respond to elimination of cow's milk from its own or the mother's diet, there has been little firm evidence of an association of colic with allergic disorders. Gastroesophageal reflux is often suspected as a cause of colicky crying in young infants. Undetected corneal abrasion, urinary tract infection, and unrecognized traumatic injuries including child abuse must be among the physical causes of crying considered in evaluating these infants. Some attempts have been made to eliminate gas with simethicone and to slow gut motility with dicyclomine. Simethicone has not been shown to ameliorate colic. Dicyclomine has been associated with apnea in infants and is contraindicated.

This then leaves characteristics intrinsic to the child (ie, temperament) and parental caretaking patterns as contributing to colic. Behavioral states have three features: (1) they are self-organizing—that is, they are maintained until it is necessary to shift to another one; (2) they are stable over several minutes; and (3) the same stimulus elicits a state-specific response that is different from other states. The behavioral states are (among others) a crying state, a quiet alert state, an active alert state, a transitional state, and a state of deep sleep. The states of importance with respect to colic are the crying state and the transitional state. During transition from one state to another, infant behavior may be more easily influenced. Once an infant is in a stable state (eg, crying), it becomes more difficult to bring about a change (eg, to soothe). How these transitions are accomplished is probably influenced by the infant's temperament and neurologic maturity. Some infants move from one state to another easily and can be diverted easily; other infants sustain a particular state and are resistant to change.

The other component to be considered in evaluating the colicky infant is the feeding and handling behavior of the caregiver. Colic is a behavioral phenomenon that involves interaction between the infant and the caregiver. Different caregivers perceive and respond to crying behavior differently. If the caregiver perceives the crying infant as being spoiled and demanding and is not sensitive to or knowledgeable about the infant's cues and rhythms—or is hurried and "rough" with the baby—the infant's ability to organize and soothe itself or respond to the caregiver's attempts at soothing may be compromised. Alternatively, if the temperament of an infant with colic is understood and the rhythms and cues deciphered, crying can be anticipated and the caregiver can intervene before the behavior becomes "organized" in the crying state and more difficult to extinguish.

Management of Colic

A number of approaches can be taken to the management of colic.

1. Parents may need to be educated about the developmental characteristics of crying behavior and made aware that crying increases normally into the second month and abates by the third to fourth month.

2. Parents may need reassurance, based on a complete history and physical examination, that the infant is not sick. Although these behaviors are stressful, they are a normal variant and are usually self-limited. This discussion can be facilitated by having the parent keep a diary of crying and weight gain. If there is a diurnal pattern and adequate weight gain, an underlying disease process is less likely to be present. Parental anxiety must be relieved, because it may be contributing to the problem.

3. For parents to effectively soothe and comfort the infant, they need to understand the baby's cues. The pediatrician can help by observing the infant's behavior and devising interventions aimed at calming both the infant and the parents. One can encourage a quiet environment without excessive handling. Rhythmic stimulation such as gentle swinging or rocking, soft music, drives in the car, or walks in the stroller may be helpful, especially if the parents are able to anticipate the onset of crying. Another approach is to change the feeding habits so that the infant is not rushed, has ample opportunity to burp, and if necessary can be fed more frequently so as to decrease gastric distention if that seems to be contributing to the problem.

4. Medications such as phenobarbital elixir and dicyclomine have been found to be somewhat helpful, but their use is to be discouraged because of the risk of adverse reactions and overdosage. A trial of ranitidine hydrochloride might be of help if gastroesophageal reflux is contributing to the child's discomfort.

5. For colic that is refractory to behavioral management, a trial of changing the feedings, and eliminating cow's milk from the formula or from the mother's diet if she is nursing, may be indicated.

Barr RG: Colic and crying syndromes in infants. Pediatrics 1998;102:1282 [PMID: 9794970].

Barr RG et al (editors): *Crying as a Sign, a Symptom, and a Signal: Clinical, Emotional, and Developmental Aspects of Infant and Toddler Crying.* MacKeith Press, 2000.

Barr RG, Geertsma MA: Colic: The pain perplex. In: Schechter NL et al (editors): *Pain in Infants, Children and Adolescents.* Williams & Wilkins, 1993.

Dhigo SK: New strategies for the treatment of colic: Modifying the parent-infant interaction. J Pediatr Health Care 1998;12: 256.

Lucassen PL et al: Effectiveness of treatments for infantile colic: A systematic review. Br Med J 1998;316:1563 [PMID: 1945549].

Miller AR, Barr RG: Infantile colic: Is it a gut issue? Pediatr Clin North Am 1991;38:1407.

Treem WR: Infant colic: A pediatric gastroenterologist's perspective. Pediatr Clin North Am 1994;41:1121 [PMID: 7936776].

Turner JL, Palamountain S: Clinical features and etiology of colic. In: Rose BD (editor): UpToDate. UpToDate, 2005.

Turner JL, Palamountain S: Evaluation and management of colic. In: Rose BD (editor): UpToDate. UpToDate, 2005.

FEEDING DISORDERS IN INFANTS & YOUNG CHILDREN

Children have feeding problems for various reasons including oral motor dysfunction, cardiopulmonary disorders leading to fatigue, gastrointestinal disturbances causing pain, social/emotional issues and problems with regulation. The common denominator, however, is usually food refusal. Infants and young children may refuse to eat if they find eating painful or frightening. They may have had unpleasant experiences (emotional or physiologic) associated with eating, they may be depressed, or they may be engaged in a developmental conflict with the caregiver that is being played out in the arena of feeding. The infant may refuse to eat if the rhythm of the feeding experience with the caregiver is not harmonious. The child who has had an esophageal atresia repair and has a stricture may find eating uncomfortable. The very young infant with severe oral candidiasis may refuse to eat because of pain. The child who has had a choking experience associated with feeding may be terrified to eat (oral motor dysfunction or aspiration). The child who is forced to eat by a maltreating parent or an overzealous caregiver may refuse feeds. Children who have required nasogastric feedings or who have required periods of fasting and intravenous nutrition in the first 1–2 months of life are more likely to display food refusal behavior upon introduction of oral feedings.

Depression in children may be expressed through food refusal. Food refusal may develop when the infant's cues around feeding are not interpreted correctly by the parent. The baby who needs to burp more frequently or who needs time between bites but instead is rushed will often passively refuse to eat. Some will be more active refusers, turning their heads away to avoid the feeder, spitting out food, or pushing away food.

Chatoor and coworkers have proposed a developmental and interactive construct of the feeding experience. The stages through which the child normally progresses are establishment of homeostasis (0–2 months), attachment (2–6 months), and separation and individuation (6 months to 3 years). During the first stage, feeding can be accomplished most easily when the parent allows the infant to determine the timing, amount, pacing, and preference of food intake. During the attachment phase, allowing the infant to control the feeding permits the parent to engage the infant in a positive manner. This paves the way for the separation and individuation phase. When a disturbance occurs in the parent-child relationship at any of these developmental levels, difficulty in feeding may ensue, with both the parent and the child contributing to the dysfunctional interaction. One of the most striking manifestations of food refusal occurs during the stage of separation and individuation. Conflict may arise if the parent seeks to dominate the child by intrusive and controlling feeding behavior at the same time the child is striving to achieve autonomy. The scenario then observed is of the parent forcing food on the child while the child refuses to eat. This often leads to extreme parental frustration and anger, and the child may be inadequately nourished and developmentally and emotionally thwarted.

When the pediatrician is attempting to sort out the factors contributing to food refusal, it is essential first to obtain a complete history, including a social history. This should include information concerning the parents' perception of the child's behavior and their expectations of the child. Second, a complete physical examination should be performed, with emphasis on oral-motor behavior and other clues suggesting neurologic, anatomic, or physiologic abnormalities that could make feeding difficult. The child's emotional state and developmental level must be determined. This is particularly important if there is concern about depression or a history of developmental delays. If evidence of oral-motor difficulty is suspected, evaluation by an occupational therapist is warranted. Third, the feeding interaction needs to be observed live, if possible. Finally, the physician needs to help the parents understand that infants and children may have different styles of eating and different food preferences and may refuse foods they do not like. This is not necessarily abnormal but reflects temperamental differences and variations in the child's way of processing olfactory, gustatory, and tactile stimuli.

Management of Feeding Disorders

The goal of intervention is to identify factors contributing to the disturbance and to work to overcome them. The parents may be encouraged to view the child's behavior differently and try not to impose their expectations and desires. Alternatively, the child's behavior may need to be modified so that the parents can provide adequate nurturing.

When the chief complaint is failure to gain weight, a different approach is required. The differential diagnosis should include not only food refusal but also medical disorders and maltreatment. The most common reason for failure to gain weight is inadequate caloric intake. Excessive weight loss may be due to vomiting or diarrhea, to malabsorption, or to a combination of these factors. In this situation more extensive diagnostic evaluation may be needed. Laboratory studies may include a complete blood count; erythrocyte sedimentation rate; urinalysis and urine culture; blood urea nitrogen; serum electrolytes and creatinine; and stool examination for fat, occult blood, and ova and parasites. Some practitioners also include liver and thyroid profiles. Occasionally an assessment of swallowing function or evaluation for the presence of gastroesophageal reflux may be indicated. Because of the complexity of the problem, a team approach to the diagnosis and treatment of failure to thrive, or poor weight gain, may be most appropriate. The team should include a physician, nurse, social worker, and dietitian. Occupational and physical therapists, developmentalists, and psychologists may be required.

The goals of treatment of the child with poor weight gain are to establish a normal pattern of weight gain and to establish better family functioning. Guidelines to accomplishing these goals include the following: (1) establish a comprehensive diagnosis that considers all factors contributing to poor weight gain; (2) monitor the feeding interaction and ensure appropriate weight gain; (3) monitor the developmental progress of the child and the changes in the family dynamics that facilitate optimal weight gain and psychosocial development; and (4) provide support to the family as they seek to help the child.

Benoit D: Phenomenology and treatment of failure to thrive. Child Adolesc Psychiatr Clin North Am 1993;2:61.

Chatoor I et al: Failure to thrive and cognitive development in toddlers with infantile anorexia. Pediatrics 2004;113:e440.

Krugman SD, Dubowitz H: Failure to thrive. Am Fam Physician 2003;68:879.

Macht J: *Poor Eaters.* Plenum, 1990.

Reilly SM et al: Oral-motor dysfunction in children who fail to thrive: Organic or non-organic. Dev Med Child Neurol 1999;41:115.

Skuse D: Epidemiologic and definitional issues in failure to thrive. Child Adolesc Psychiatr Clin North Am 1993;2:37.

SLEEP DISORDERS

Sleep is a complex physiologic process influenced by intrinsic biologic properties, temperament, cultural norms and expectations, and environmental conditions. Between 20% and 30% of children experience sleep disturbances at some point in the first 4 years of life. The percentage decreases to 10–12% in school-age children. Sleep disorders fall into two categories. Dyssomnias refer to problems with initiating and maintaining sleep or to excessive sleepiness. Parasomnias refer to abnormalities of arousal, partial arousal, and transitions between stages of sleep.

Sleep is controlled by two different biologic clocks. The first is a circadian rhythm–daily sleep/wake cycle. The second is an ultradian rhythm that occurs several times per night—the stages of sleep. Sleep stages cycle every 50–60 minutes in infants to every 90 minutes in adolescents. The circadian clock has a 25-hour cycle. Environmental cues entrain the sleep-wake cycle into a 24-hour cycle. The cues are light-dark, ambient temperature, core body temperature, noise, social interaction, hunger, pain, and hormone production. Without the ability to perceive these cues (ie, blindness or autism) a child might have difficulty entraining a 24-hour sleep-wake cycle.

Two major sleep stages have been identified clinically and with the use of polysomnography (electroencephalography, electro-oculography, and electromyelography): rapid eye movement (REM) and nonrapid eye movement (NREM) sleep. In REM sleep, muscle tone is relaxed, the sleeper may twitch and grimace, and the eyes move erratically beneath closed lids. In adults and children, REM sleep occurs throughout the night but is increased during the latter half of the night. NREM sleep is divided into four stages. In the process of falling asleep, the individual enters stage 1, light sleep, characterized by reduced bodily movements, slow eye rolling, and sometimes opening and closing of the eyelids. Stage 2 sleep is characterized by slowing of eye movements, slowing of respirations and heart rate, and relaxation of the muscles but with repositioning of the body. Most mature individuals spend about half of their sleep time in this stage. Stages 3 and 4 (also called delta or slow-wave sleep) are the deepest NREM sleep stages, during which the body is relaxed, breathing is slow and shallow, and the heart rate is slow. The deepest NREM sleep occurs during the first 1–3 hours after going to sleep. Most parasomnias occur early in the night during deep NREM sleep. Dreams and nightmares that occur later in the night occur during REM sleep.

Sleep is clearly a developmental phenomenon. Infants are not born with a sleep-wake cycle. REM sleep is more common than NREM sleep in newborns and decreases by 3–6 months of age. Sleep spindles and vertex waves are usually not seen until 9 weeks of age. By 3–6 months, stage 1 through 4 NREM sleep can be seen. By 6–12 months an infant's electroencephalogram (EEG) can be read using adult criteria. Infants also do not make melatonin until 9–12 weeks of age. Melatonin is a hormone that decreases core body temperature which appears to play a role in sleep onset and sleep maintenance. This hormone is sensitive to light. It crosses the placenta and is present in breast milk.

Like the sleep EEG, sleep patterns slowly mature throughout infancy, childhood, and adolescence until they become adultlike. Newborns sleep 16–20 hours per day in 2- to 5-hour blocks. Over the first year of life the infant slowly consolidates sleep at night into a 9- to 12-hour block and naps gradually decrease to one per day by about 12 months. Most children stop napping between 3 and 5 years of age. School-age children typically sleep 10–11 hours per night without a nap. Adolescents need 9–9$^1/_2$ hours per night but often only get 7–7$^1/_4$ hours per night. This is complicated by an approximate 2-hour sleep phase delay in adolescence which is due to physiologic changes in hormonal regulation of the circadian system. Often the adolescent is not tired until 2 hours later than their typical bedtime but still has to get up at the same time in the morning. Some school districts have implemented later start times for high school students because of this phenomenon.

1. Parasomnias

Parasomnias, consisting of arousal from deep NREM sleep, are probably the most frightening for parents. They include night terrors, sleeptalking, and sleepwalking (somnambulism).

Night Terrors & Sleepwalking

Night terrors commonly occur within 2 hours after falling asleep, during the deepest stage of NREM sleep, and are often associated with sleepwalking. They occur in about 3% of children. During a night terror, the child may sit up in bed screaming, thrashing about, and exhibiting rapid breathing, tachycardia, and sweating. The child is often incoherent and unresponsive to comforting. The episode may last up to half an hour, after which the child goes back to sleep and has no memory of the event the next day. The parents must be reassured that the child is not in pain and that they should let the episode run its course.

Management of night terrors is by reassurance of the parents plus measures to avoid stress, irregular sleep schedule, or sleep deprivation which prolongs deep sleep when night terrors occur. Scheduled awakening (awakening the child 30–45 minutes before the time the night terrors usually occur) can be used in children with nightly or frequent night terrors.

Sleepwalking also occurs during slow-wave sleep and is common between 4 and 8 years of age. It is typically benign except that injuries can occur while the child is walking around. Steps should be taken to ensure that the environment is free of obstacles and that doors to the outside are locked. Parents may also wish to put a bell on their child's door to alert them that the child is out of bed. As with night terrors, steps should be taken to avoid stress and sleep deprivation. Scheduled awakenings may also be used if the child sleep walks frequently and at a predictable time.

Nightmares

Nightmares are frightening dreams that occur during REM sleep, typically followed by awakening, which usually occurs in the latter part of the night. The peak occurrence is between ages 3 and 5 years, with an incidence between 25% and 50%. A child who awakens during these episodes is usually alert. He or she can often describe the frightening images, recall the dream, and talk about it during the day. The child seeks and will respond positively to parental reassurance. The child will often have difficulty going back to sleep and will want to stay with the parents. Nightmares are usually self-limited and need little treatment. They can be associated with stress, trauma, anxiety, sleep deprivation that can cause a rebound in REM sleep, and medications that increase REM sleep.

2. Dyssomnias

The dyssomnias include problems going to sleep and maintaining sleep/nighttime awakenings. Although parasomnias are frightening, dyssomnias are frustrating. They can result in daytime fatigue for both the parents and the child, parental discord about management, and family disruption. A number of factors contribute to these disturbances. The quantity and timing of feeds in the first years of life will influence nighttime awakening. Most infants beyond age 6 months can go through the night without being fed. Thus, under normal circumstances, night waking for feeds is probably a learned behavior and is a function of the child's arousal and the parents' response to that arousal. Bedtime habits can influence settling in for the night as well as nighttime awakening. If the child learns that going to sleep is associated with pleasant parental behavior such as rocking, singing, reading, or nursing, going back to sleep after nighttime arousal without these pleasant parental attentions may be difficult. This is called a sleep onset association disorder and usually is the reason for night waking. Every time that the child gets to the light sleep portion of the sleep-wake cycle they may wake up. This is usually brief and not remembered the next morning, but for the child who does not have strategies for getting to sleep, getting back to sleep may require the same interventions needed to get to sleep initially such as rocking, patting, and drinking or sucking. Most of these interventions require a parent. Night waking occurs in 40–60% of infants and young children. Parents need to set limits for the child while acknowledging the child's individual biologic rhythms. They should resist the child's attempts to put off bedtime or to engage them during nighttime awakenings. The goal is to establish clear bedtime rituals, to put the child to bed while still awake, and to create a quiet, secure bedtime environment. The child's temperament is another factor contributing to sleep. It has been reported that children with low sensory thresholds and less rhythmicity (regulatory disorder) are more prone to night waking. Night waking often starts at about 9 months as separation anxiety is beginning. Parents should receive anticipatory guidance prior to that time so that they know to reassure their child without making the interaction prolonged or pleasurable. Finally, psychosocial stressors and changes in routine can play a role in night waking.

3. Sleep Disordered Breathing

Sleep disordered breathing or obstructive sleep apnea is characterized by obstructed breathing during sleep accompanied by loud snoring, chest retractions, morning headaches and dry mouth, and daytime sleepiness. Obstructive sleep apnea occurs in 1–3% of preschoolers. It has its highest peak in childhood between the ages of 2 and 6 which corresponds with the peak in adenotonsillar hypertrophy. It has been associated with daytime behavioral disorders including attention-deficit/hyperactivity disorder. A good physical examination is important to look for adenotonsillar hypertrophy, hypotonia, and facial anomalies which may predispose the child to obstruction during sleep. Lateral neck films may be helpful. The gold standard for diagnosis is polysomnography.

4. Restless Leg Syndrome & Periodic Limb Movement Disorder

Restless leg syndrome and periodic limb movement disorder are common disorders in adults and frequently occur together. The frequency of these disorders in children is unknown. Restless leg syndrome is associated with an uncomfortable sensation in the lower extremities that is relieved by movement and occurs at night when trying to fall asleep, and is sometimes described by children as "creepy/crawly" or "itchy bones." Periodic limb movement disorder is stereotyped, repetitive limb movements often associated with a partial arousal or awakening. The etiology of these disorders is unknown but there has been some association with iron deficiency. A diagnosis of restless leg syndrome is generally made by history and a diagnosis of periodic limb movement disorder can be made with a sleep study.

Management of Sleep Disorders

A complete medical and psychosocial history should be obtained and a physical examination performed. A detailed sleep history and diary should be maintained to which both parents contribute. Lateral neck films and polysomnography may be indicated to complete the evaluation, especially if sleep disordered breathing is suspected. It is important to consider disorders such as gastroesophageal reflux, which may cause discomfort or pain when recumbent.

The key to treatment of children who have difficulty going to sleep or who awaken during the night and disturb others is to recognize that both the child and the parents play significant roles in initiating and sustaining what may be an undesirable behavior. Thus, it becomes important for the physician and parents to understand normal sleep patterns, the parents' responses that inadvertently reinforce undesirable sleep behavior, and the child's individual temperament traits. It is also important to remember that individual circadian rhythms do not change immediately; they require consistency and regularity over a period of time before change will occur. Keeping sleep logs or diaries and patience are essential.

Chervin RD et al: Inattention, hyperactivity, and symptoms of sleep-disordered breathing. Pediatrics 2002;109:449 [PMID: 11875140].

Ferber R: Clinical assessment of child and adolescent sleep disorder. Child Adolesc Psychiatr Clin North Am 1996;5:569.

France KG et al: Fact, act, and tact: A three-stage approach to treating the sleep problems of infants and young children. Child Adolesc Psychiatr Clin North Am 1996;5:581.

Grigg-Damberger M: Neurologic disorders masquerading as pediatric sleep problems. Pediatr Clin North Am 2004;51:89.

Mindel JA, Owens JA: *A Clinical Guide to Pediatric Sleep: Diagnosis and Management of Sleep Problems.* Lippincott Williams & Wilkins, 2003.

www.kidzzzsleep.org

TEMPER TANTRUMS & BREATH-HOLDING SPELLS

1. Temper Tantrums

Temper tantrums are common between ages 12 months and 4 years, occurring about once a week in 50–80% of children in this age group. The child may throw him- or herself down, kick and scream, strike out at people or objects in the room, and hold his or her breath. These behaviors may be considered normal as the young child seeks to achieve autonomy and mastery over the environment. They are often a reflection of immaturity as the child strives to accomplish age-appropriate developmental tasks and meets with difficulty because of inadequate motor and language skills, impulsiveness, or parental restrictions. In the home, these behaviors may be annoying. In public, they are embarrassing.

Some children tolerate frustration well, are able to persevere at tasks, and cope easily with difficulties; others have a much greater problem dealing with experiences beyond their developmental level. Parents can minimize tantrums by understanding the child's temperament and what he or she is trying to communicate.

Parents must also be committed to supporting the child's drive to master his or her feelings.

Management of Temper Tantrums

Appropriate intervention can provide an opportunity for enhancing the child's growth. The tantrum is a loss of control on the child's part that may be a frightening event and a blow to the child's self-image. The parents and the physician need to view these behaviors within the child's developmental context rather than from a negative, adversarial, angry perspective.

Several suggestions can be offered to parents and physicians to help manage tantrums:

1. Minimize the need to say "no" by "child-proofing" the environment so that fewer restrictions need to be enforced.
2. Use distraction when frustration increases; direct the child to other, less frustrating activities; and reward the positive response.
3. Present options within the child's capabilities so that he or she can achieve mastery and autonomy.
4. Fight only those battles that need to be won, and avoid those that arouse unnecessary conflict.
5. Do not abandon the preschool child when a tantrum occurs. Stay nearby during the episode without intruding. A small child may need to be restrained. An older child can be asked to go to his or her room. Threats serve no purpose and should not be used.
6. Do not use negative terms when the tantrum is occurring. Instead, point out that the child is out of control and give praise when he or she regains control.
7. Never let a child hurt him- or herself or others.
8. Do not "hold a grudge" after the tantrum is over, but do not grant the child's demands that led to the tantrum.
9. Seek to maintain an environment that provides positive reinforcement for desired behavior. Do not overreact to undesired behavior, but set reasonable limits and provide responsible direction for the child.
10. Approximately 5–20% of young children have severe temper tantrums that are frequent and disruptive. Such tantrums may result from a disturbance in the parent-child interaction, poor parenting skills, lack of limit-setting, and permissiveness. They may be part of a larger behavioral or developmental disorder or may emerge under adverse socioeconomic conditions, in circumstances of maternal depression and family dysfunction, or when the child is in poor health. Referral to a psychologist or psychiatrist is appropriate while the pediatrician continues to support and work with the family.

2. Breath-Holding Spells

Whereas temper tantrums can be frustrating to parents, breath-holding spells can be terrifying. The name for this behavior may be a misnomer in that it connotes prolonged inspiration. In fact, breath-holding occurs during expiration and is reflexive—not volitional—in nature. It is a paroxysmal event occurring in 0.1–5% of healthy children from age 6 months to 6 years. The spells usually start during the first year of life, often in response to anger or a mild injury. The child is provoked or surprised, starts to cry—briefly or for a considerable time—and then falls silent in the expiratory phase of respiration. This is followed by a color change. Spells have been described as either pallid (acyanotic) or cyanotic, with the latter usually associated with anger and the former with an injury such as a fall. The spell may resolve spontaneously, or the child may lose consciousness. In severe cases, the child may become limp and progress to opisthotonos, body jerks, and urinary incontinence. Only rarely does a spell proceed to asystole or a seizure.

Management of Breath-Holding Spells

For the child with frequent spells, underlying disorders such as seizures, orthostatic hypotension, obstructive sleep apnea, abnormalities of the CNS, tumors, familial dysautonomia, and Rett syndrome need to be considered. An association exists among breath-holding spells, pica, and iron-deficiency anemia. These conditions can be ruled out on the basis of the history, physical examination, and laboratory studies. Once it has been determined that the child is healthy, the focus of treatment is behavioral. Parents should be taught to handle the spells in a matter-of-fact manner and monitor the child for any untoward events. The reality is that parents cannot completely protect the child from upsetting and frustrating experiences and probably should not try to do so. Just as in temper tantrums, parents need to help the child control his or her responses to frustration. Parents need to be careful not to be too permissive and submit to the child's every whim for fear the child might have a spell. If loss of consciousness occurs, the child should be placed on his or her side to protect against head injury and aspiration. Maintaining a patent oral airway is essential, but cardiopulmonary resuscitation should be avoided. There are no prophylactic medications. Atropine, 0.01 mg/kg given subcutaneously, has been used with some benefit in spells accompanied by bradycardia or asystole.

Breningstall GN: Breath holding spells. Pediatr Neurol 1996;14:91 [PMID: 8703234].

DiMario FJ Jr: Breath-holding spells in childhood. Am J Dis Child 1992;146:125 [PMID: 1736640].

Greene RW: *The Explosive Child.* Quill, 2001.

Needleman R et al: Psychosocial correlates of severe temper tantrums. J Dev Behav Pediatr 1991;12:77.

Needleman R et al: Temper tantrums: When to worry. Contemp Pediatr 1989;6:12.

DEVELOPMENTAL DISORDERS

Developmental disorders include abnormalities in one or more aspects of development, such as verbal, motor, visual-spatial, attentional, and social abilities. These problems are diagnosed by comparing the child's performance level with norms accumulated from observation and testing of children of the same age. Problems with development are often noted by parents when a child does not meet typical motor and language milestones. Developmental disorders may also include difficulties with behavior or attention. Attention-deficit/hyperactivity disorder (ADHD) is the most common neurodevelopmental disorder. ADHD occurs in 2–10% of school-age children and may occur in combination with a variety of other learning or developmental issues. Mild developmental disorders are often not noted until the child is of school age.

Many biologic and psychosocial factors may influence a child's performance on developmental tests. In the assessment of the child, it is important to document adverse psychosocial factors, such as neglect or poverty, which can negatively influence developmental progress. Many of the biologic factors that influence development are genetic and are discussed throughout this section.

Evaluation

The neurodevelopmental evaluation must focus on (1) defining the child's level of developmental abilities in a variety of domains, including language, motor, visual-spatial, attentional, and social abilities; (2) attempting to determine the etiology for the child's developmental delays; and (3) planning a treatment program. These objectives are best achieved by a multidisciplinary team that includes the physician, a psychologist, a speech or language therapist, an occupational therapist, and an educational specialist. The psychologist will usually carry out standardized testing of intellectual ability appropriate to the child's age. The motor and language specialists will also carry out clinical testing to document the deficits in their areas and to organize a treatment program. The educational specialist will usually carry out academic testing for the school-age child and plan a course of special education support through the school. The physician is usually the integrator of the information from the team and must also obtain a detailed medical and developmental history and conduct the physical and neurologic examinations.

Medical and Neurodevelopmental Examination

The medical history should begin with pregnancy, labor, and delivery to identify conditions that might compromise the child's central nervous system. The physician must ask the child's parents about prenatal exposures to toxins, medications, alcohol, drugs, smoking, and infections; maternal chronic illness; complications of pregnancy or delivery and neonatal course. Problems such as failure to thrive, chronic illnesses, hospitalizations, and abuse can interfere significantly with normal development. Major illnesses or hospitalizations should be discussed. Any CNS problems, such as trauma, infection, or encephalitis should be documented. The presence of metabolic diseases, such as diabetes or phenylketonuria, and exposure to environmental toxins such as lead should be determined. Chronic diseases such as chronic otitis media, hyper- or hypothyroidism, and chronic renal failure can interfere with normal development. The presence of motor or vocal tics, seizures, or sleep disturbances should be documented. In addition, parents should be questioned about any motor, cognitive, or behavioral regression.

The physician should review and document the child's temperament, difficulties with feeding, and subsequent developmental milestones. The child's difficulties with tantrums, poor attention, impulsivity, hyperactivity, or aggression should be documented.

A detailed history of school-related events should be recorded, including previous special education support, evaluations through the school, history of repeating grades, difficulties with specific academic areas, problems with peers, and the teacher's impressions of the child's difficulties, particularly related to attentional problems, impulsivity, or hyperactivity. Input from teachers can be invaluable and should be sought prior to the evaluation.

Perhaps the most important aspect of the medical history is a detailed family history of learning strengths and weaknesses, emotional or behavioral problems, learning disabilities, mental retardation, or psychiatric disorders. Parental learning strengths and weaknesses, temperament difficulties, or attentional problems may be passed on to the child. For instance, dyslexia (deficits in decoding skills resulting in reading difficulties) is often inherited.

The neurodevelopmental examination should include a careful assessment of dysmorphic features such as epicanthal folds, palpebral fissure size, shape of the philtrum, low-set or posteriorally-rotated ears, prominent ear pinnae, unusual dermatoglyphics (eg, a single palmar crease), hyperextensibility of the joints, syndactyly, clino-dactyly, or other unusual features. A detailed physical and neurologic examination needs to be carried out with an emphasis on both soft and hard neurologic findings. Soft signs can include motor incoordination, which can relate to handwriting problems and academic delays in written language or drawing. Visual motor coordination abilities can be assessed by having the child write, copy designs, or draw a person.

The child's growth parameters, including height, weight, and head circumference, need to be assessed, along with hearing and visual acuity. Cranial nerve abnormalities and oral motor coordination problems need to be noted. The examiner should watch closely for motor or vocal tics. Both fine and gross motor abilities should be assessed. Dyspraxia (motor planning difficulties or imitating complex motor movements) and disorders of fine motor coordination are fairly common. Tandem walking, one-foot balancing, and coordinating a skip may often show surprising abnormalities. Tremors can be noted when watching a child stack blocks or draw.

The developmental aspects of the examination can include an assessment of auditory processing and perceptual ability with simple tasks, such as twofold to fivefold directions, assessing right and left directionality, memory for a series of spoken words or digit span, and comprehension of a graded paragraph. In assessing expressive language abilities, the examiner should look for difficulties with word retrieval, formulation and articulation, and adequacy of vocabulary. Visual-perceptual abilities can be assessed by simple visual memory tasks, puzzles, or object assembly, and evaluating the child's ability to decode words or organize math problems. Visual motor integration and coordination can be assessed again with handwriting, design copying, and drawing a person. Throughout the assessment the clinician should pay special attention to the child's ability to focus attention and concentrate, and to other aspects of behavior such as evidence of depression or anxiety.

Additional questionnaires and checklists—such as the Child Behavior Checklist by Achenbach; ADHD scales such as the Conners' Parent/Teacher Rating Scale; and the Swanson, Nolan and Pelham Questionnaire-IV, which includes the *Diagnostic and Statistical Manual of Mental Disorders, Fourth Edition, Text Revision* (DSM-IV-TR) criteria for ADHD—can be used to help with this assessment.

Referral of family to community resources is critical as is a Medical Home. A Medical Home provides accessible, continuous, comprehensive, family-centered, compassionate, culturally-effective care that is well coordinated with subspecialists.

American Academy of Pediatrics, Medical Home Initiatives for Children with Special Health Care Needs Project Advisory Committee. 2002. The Medical Home. Pediatrics 2002; 110:184.

http://www.nichcy.org

Levine MD et al (editors): *Developmental-Behavioral Pediatrics,* 3rd ed. WB Saunders, 1999.

Reynolds CR, Mayfield JW: Neuropsychological assessment in genetically linked neurodevelopmental disorders. In Goldstein S, Reynolds CR (editors): *Handbook of Developmental and Genetic Disorders in Children.* Guilford, 1999.

Wolraich ML (editor): *Disorders of Development and Learning,* 3rd ed. BC Decker, 2003.

ATTENTION-DEFICIT/HYPERACTIVITY DISORDER

Attention-deficit/hyperactivity disorder (ADHD) is a common neurodevelopmental disorder that may affect 2–10% of school-age children and may persist into adolescence and adulthood. It is associated with a triad of symptoms: impulsivity, inattention, and hyperactivity. DSM-IV-TR has described three ADHD subtypes: hyperactive impulsive, inattentive, and combined. To be classified according to either subtype, the child must exhibit six or more of the symptoms listed in Table 2–5.

Table 2–5. Attention-deficit/hyperactivity disorder subtypes.

Subtype	Symptoms[a]
Hyperactive-impulsive	Fidgetiness Difficulty remaining seated in the class Excessive running or climbing Difficulty in engaging in quiet activities Excessive talking and blurting out answers before questions have been completed Difficulty awaiting turns Interrupting and intruding on others
Inattentive	Failure to give close attention to detail Difficulty sustaining intention in task Failure to listen when spoken to directly Failure to follow instructions Difficulty organizing tasks and activities Reluctance to engage in tasks Losing utensils necessary for tasks or activities Easy distractibility Forgetfulness in daily activities

[a]The child must exhibit six or more of these symptoms.
Adapted, with permission, from American Psychiatric Association: Diagnostic and Statistical Manual of Mental Disorders, 4th ed. American Psychiatric Association, 1994.

The majority of children with ADHD have a combined type with symptoms of inattention as well as hyperactivity and impulsivity. Although symptoms begin in early childhood, they can diminish between ages 10 and 25 years. Hyperactivity declines more quickly, and impulsivity and inattentiveness often persist into adolescence and adulthood. ADHD may be combined with other psychiatric conditions, such as mood disorder in approximately 20% of patients, conduct disorders in 20%, and oppositional defiant disorder in up to 40%. Up to 25% of children with ADHD seen in a referral clinic have tics or Tourette syndrome. Conversely, well over 50% of individuals with Tourette syndrome also have ADHD.

ADHD has a substantial genetic component. Several candidate genes have been identified, although there is strong evidence that ADHD is a disorder involving multiple genes. ADHD is also associated with a variety of genetic disorders related to developmental disorders, including fragile X syndrome, Williams syndrome, Angelman syndrome, XXY syndrome (Klinefelter syndrome), and Turner syndrome. Fetal alcohol syndrome (FAS) is also strongly associated with ADHD. CNS trauma, CNS infections, prematurity, and a difficult neonatal course with brain injury can also be associated with later ADHD. Metabolic problems such as hyperthyroidism can sometimes cause ADHD. These organic causes of ADHD should be considered in the evaluation of any child presenting with attentional problems, hyperactivity, or impulsivity. However, in the majority of children who have ADHD the cause remains unknown.

Treatment

The treatment of ADHD varies depending on the complexity of the individual case. It is important to educate the family regarding the symptoms of ADHD and to clarify that it is a neurologic disorder that at times is difficult for the child to control. Behavior modification techniques usually help these children and should include structure with consistency in daily routine, positive reinforcement whenever possible, and time out for negative behaviors. It is important to try to boost the child's self-esteem because psychological complications are common in ADHD.

A variety of educational interventions can be helpful, including preferential seating in the classroom, a system of consistent positive behavior reinforcement, consistent structure, the repetition of information when needed, and the use of instruction that incorporates both visual and auditory modalities. Many children with ADHD have significant social difficulties, and social skills training can be helpful. Individual counseling is beneficial in alleviating poor self-esteem, oppositional behavior, and conduct problems.

The use of medication, specifically stimulant medication such as methylphenidate (Ritalin) and dextroamphet-amine, is helpful. Medications combined with behavioral intervention is felt to be most helpful. This is particularly so when there are comorbid conditions. A newer medication, atomoxetine has been found to be effective in some children with ADHD as a second-line drug. Pemoline is no longer recommended because of its association with liver injury.

It is most important that, no matter what medication is used, the diagnosis is correct and the correct dosage is prescribed. A recent study has demonstrated that one of the major factors contributing to treatment failure is inadequate dosing or the failure to recognize the presence of comorbid conditions such as learning disability, anxiety disorders, and depression.

In children with normal intellectual abilities, 70–90% respond well to stimulant medications. Stimulants enhance both dopamine and norepinephrine neurotransmission, which seems to improve impulse control, attention, and hyperactivity. Metabolic studies of the CNS (eg, using positron emission tomography scanning) have demonstrated enhanced metabolism in several areas of the brain, including the caudate and the frontal regions.

The side effects of methylphenidate and dextroamphetamine include appetite suppression and resulting weight loss as well as sleep disturbances. Atomoxetine has a similar side-effect profile. Some individuals experience increased anxiety, particularly with higher doses of stimulant medications. Stimulants may exacerbate psychotic symptoms. They may also exacerbate motor tics in 30% of patients, but in 10% motor tics may be improved. Long-acting and short-acting forms of stimulant medication are available. The initial dose of methylphenidate can be 5, 10, 15, or 20 mg daily divided two or three times a day. Adderall is another stimulant that combines four dextro and levo amphetamine salts. This is a more long-acting medication, and often a single morning dose suffices for the day. Starting doses can be 5, 7.5, 10, 12.5, or 15 mg, although the medication comes in higher doses also.

Alternative medications for the treatment of ADHD include clonidine or guanfacine, which are α_2-adrenergic presynaptic agonists that decrease norepinephrine levels. They are particularly helpful for individuals who are hyperreactive to stimuli and may be helpful in decreasing motor tics in patients who have Tourette syndrome. Tricyclic antidepressant medications such as imipramine may also be effective treatment for ADHD, but the cardiovascular side effects at high dosages can include severe arrhythmias. Bupropion is an antidepressant medication that can also be effective for treatment of ADHD symptoms. Its use is contraindicated in patients with a history of seizures, because it will lower the seizure threshold. It has also been known to cause seizures in individuals who have anorexia or bulimia. It is used more commonly in adolescents and adults with ADHD than in children with the disorder.

American Academy of Pediatrics: Clinical practice guideline: Treatment of the school-aged child with attention-deficit/hyperactivity disorder. Pediatrics 2001;108:1033.

Elia J et al: Treatment of attention deficit hyperactivity disorder. N Engl J Med 1999;340:780 [PMID: 1007214].

Goldman LS et al: Diagnosis and treatment of attention deficit hyperactivity disorder in children and adults. JAMA 1998;79:1100 [PMID: 9546570].

http://www.add.org

http://www.chadd.org

Jensen PS et al: Findings from the NIMS Multimodal Treatment Study of ADHD (MTA): Implications and applications for primary care providers. J Develop Behav Pediatr 2001;22:60 [PMID: 11265923].

Krull KA: Evaluation and diagnosis of attention deficit hyperactivity disorders in children. In Rose BD (editor): UpToDate. UpToDate, 2005.

Krull KA: Treatment and prognosis of attention deficit hyperactivity disorders in children. In Rose BD (editor): UpToDate. UpToDate, 2005.

Reiff MI: *ADHD: A Compete Authoritative Guide.* American Academy of Pediatrics, 2004.

AUTISM SPECTRUM DISORDERS

Autism is a neurologic disorder characterized by (1) qualitative impairments in social interaction; (2) qualitative impairments in communication; and (3) restricted repetitive and stereotyped patterns of behavior, interests, and activities. Autism is currently grouped under the Pervasive Developmental Disorders in the DSM-IV with Asperger Disorder, Pervasive Developmental Disorder Not Otherwise Specified, Childhood Disintegrative Disorder, and Rett Syndrome. Asperger disorder is characterized by impairment in social interaction and restricted interest/repetitive behaviors. Individuals with Asperger disorder should not have significant delays in cognitive, language, or self-help skills. Pervasive developmental disorder not otherwise specified is characterized by an impairment in reciprocal social interaction along with an impairment in communication skills, or restricted interest or repetitive behaviors. Children with pervasive developmental disorder not otherwise specified do not meet full criteria for autism due to mild or atypical symptoms. Childhood disintegrative disorder is characterized by typical development for at least 2 years followed by a regression in at least two of the following three areas: social interaction, communication, and behavior (characterized by restricted interests or repetitive behaviors.) Rett syndrome is a genetic syndrome caused by a mutation on the X chromosome that is characterized by regression in skills in the first year of life.

Autism spectrum disorders are relatively common, occurring in approximately 1 in 166 to 1 in 500 children. No known etiology can be found in 80–90% of cases. A genetic syndrome such as fragile X syndrome or chromosome 15q duplication is found in 10–20% of cases. There is a strong familial component. Parents of one child with autism of unknown etiology have a 2–9% chance of having a second child with autism. The concordance rate among monozygotic twins is high, and there is an increased incidence of speech, language, reading, attention, and affective disorders in family members of children with autism.

Evaluation & Treatment

Children with autism are often not diagnosed until age 3–4 years, when their disturbances in reciprocal social interaction and communication become more apparent. However, impairments in communication and behavior can often be recognized in the first 12–18 months of life. The three most striking characteristics during the first year are a consistent failure to orient to one's name, failure to regard people directly, and failure to develop speech. By 18 months a child should have "joint attention," which occurs when two people attend to the same thing at the same time. This is usually accomplished by shifting eye gaze, pointing or saying "look." Toddlers should point to get needs met ("I want that") and to show ("look at that") by 1 year of age and they should do it regularly. By 18 months a toddler should be able to follow a point and engage in functional play (using toys in the way that they are intended to be used, such as rolling a car, throwing a ball, or holding a baby).

Because there is evidence that early intervention is particularly important for children with autism, great interest has arisen in developing a screening instrument that can be used in very young children. The Modified Checklist for Autism in Toddlers is designed for children 16–30 months of age. It is a parent report measure with 23 yes/no questions. This test is still undergoing study to determine sensitivity and specificity but preliminary outcomes show good sensitivity and specificity. Much work is still needed to determine the best tools and the best way to screen for autism.

When behaviors consistent with autism are noted, the child should be referred to a team of specialists experienced in the assessment of autism spectrum disorders. The child should also be referred to their local early intervention program and to a speech and language pathologist to get therapy started as soon as possible. All children with autism should have a formal audiology evaluation because of their language disorder. Laboratory tests for high-resolution chromosomes, DNA for fragile X syndrome, and fluorescence in situ hybridization (FISH) for 15q duplication should be considered. Metabolic screening, lead level, thyroid studies, and a Wood lamp test for tuberous sclerosis may also be done if indicated by findings in the history and physical examination. Neuroimaging is not routinely indicated even in the presence of macrocephaly since children with autism often have relatively large heads. Neuroimaging should be done if there is microcephaly or focal neurologic signs. Approximately 15–30% of children with autism demonstrate plateauing or loss of skills (usually language and social skills only) between 12 and 24 months of age. This usually occurs before attaining 10 words. If a child presents with regression they should be referred to a child neurologist. A sleep-deprived EEG or an overnight EEG should be considered when there is a history of regression. The EEG must have adequate sampling of slow-wave sleep to rule out epileptiform discharges during slow-wave sleep. It should be noted that the recommendations for treatment of that type of EEG abnormality are still being debated.

Much controversy surrounds the appropriate treatment and educational approaches for children with autistic spectrum disorders. As with any child, treatment should be based on the individual needs of the child. It is clear, however, that intervention must begin early and must be comprehensive and intensive. Many advocate 20–25 hours or more per week of structured behavioral treatments such as applied behavioral analysis, that target development of social attention, peer interactions, functional language, and appropriate play. There are many models for this type of intervention and much variability in what is available in different areas of the country. Families should be encouraged to find a model that best suits the needs of their child.

There are many complementary and alternative treatments for autism. Research is currently underway to evaluate some of these treatments.

Baird G et al: A screening instrument for autism at 18 months of age: A 6-year follow-up study. J Am Acad Child Adolesc Psychiatr 2000;39:694 [PMID: 108946303].

Baird G et al: Current topic: Screening and surveillance for autism and pervasive developmental disorders. Arch Dis Child 2001;84:468 [PMID: 11369559].

Cohen DJ, Volkman FR (editors): Handbook of Autism and Pervasive Developmental Disorders, 2nd ed. John Wiley & Sons, 1997.

Dumont-Mathieu T, Fein D: Screening for autism in young children: The Modified Checklist for Autism in Toddlers (M-CHAT) and other measures. Ment Retard Dev Disabil Res Rev 2005;11:253.

Filipek PA et al: Practice parameter: Screening and diagnosis of autism: Report of the Quality Standards Subcommittee of the American Academy of Neurology and Child Neurology Society. Neurology 2000;55:468 [PMID: 10953176].

Gabriels RL, Hill DE (editors): Autism: From Research to Individualized Practice. Jessica Kingsley Publishers, 2002.

Gilberg C, Coleman M (editors): The Biology of the Autistic Syndromes. MacKeith Press, 2000.

http://firstsigns.org

http://teacch.com

http://www.autism-society.org

http://www.cdc.gov/ncbddd/autism/actearly/

Lord C, McGee JP (editors): Educating Children with Autism. National Academy of Sciences Press, 2001.

Ozonoff S et al (editors): Autism Spectrum Disorders: A Research Review for Practitioners. American Psychiatric Publishing, 2003.

Rogers SJ: Empirically supported comprehensive treatments for young children with autism. J Clin Child Psychol 1998; 27:168 [PMID: 9648034].

MENTAL RETARDATION

Severe deficits in the development of language, motor skills, attention, abstract reasoning, visual-spatial skills, and academic or vocational achievement are associated with mental retardation. Deficits on standardized testing in cognitive and adaptive functioning greater than two standard deviations below the mean for the population are considered to fall in the range of mental retardation (Table 2–6). The most common way of reporting the results of these tests is by using an intelligence quotient. The intelligence quotient is a statistically derived number reflecting the ratio of age-appropriate cognitive function and the child's actual level of cognitive function. A number of accepted standardized measurement tools, such as the Wechsler Intelligence Scale for Children, 3rd edition, can be used to assess these capacities. To receive a diagnosis of mental retardation a child must not only have an intelligence quotient of less than 70, but also must demonstrate adaptive skills more than two standard deviations below the mean. Adaptive function refers to the child's ability to function in his or her environment and can be measured by a parent or teacher interview recorded using an instrument such as the Vineland Adaptive Behavior Scales.

The prevalence of mental retardation is approximately 3% in the general population, although some states have reported a prevalence of less than 2%. Mild levels of mental retardation are more common and more likely to have a sociocultural cause than are more severe levels. Poverty, deprivation, or a lack of exposure to a stimulating environment can contribute to developmental delays and poor performance on standardized

Table 2–6. Categories of mental retardation.

Mental Retardation Range	Intelligence Quotient (IQ)
Mild mental retardation	50–69
Moderate mental retardation	35–49
Severe mental retardation	20–34
Profound mental retardation	< 20

Table 2-7. Causes of mental retardation.

Cause	Percentage of Cases
Chromosomal abnormalities	4–28
Fragile X syndrome	2–5
Monogenetic conditions	4–14
Structural CNS abnormalities	7–17
Complications of prematurity	2–10
Environmental or teratogenic causes	5–13
"Cultural-familial" mental retardation	3–12
Metabolic or endocrine causes	1–5
Unknown	30–50

Adapted from Curry CJ et al: Evaluation of mental retardation: Recommendations of a consensus conference. Am J Med Genet 1997;72:468.

tests. In addition, physical problems such as hearing loss, blindness, and brain trauma can lead to developmental delays and low intelligence quotient test scores. Great strides in our identification of genetic causes of mental retardation have been made since the 1990s because of the Human Genome Project. Over 750 genetic disorders have been associated with mental retardation, and over 200 of those disorders are carried on the X chromosome alone. In approximately 60% of cases, the cause of the mental retardation can be identified. Table 2–7 summarizes the findings of several studies on the causes of mental retardation.

Evaluation

Children who present with developmental delays should be evaluated by a team of professionals as described at the beginning of this section. For children 0–3$\frac{1}{2}$ years of age, the Bayley Scales of Infant Development, 2nd edition, is a well-standardized developmental test. For children older than 3 years of age standardized cognitive testing, such as the Wechsler Preschool and Primary Scale of Intelligence-Revised; the Wechsler Intelligence Scale for Children, 3rd edition; the Stanford-Binet IV; or the Kaufman Assessment Battery for Children should be administered to assess cognitive function over a broad range of abilities, including verbal and nonverbal scales. For the nonverbal patient, a scale such as the Leiter-R will assess skills that do not involve language.

A full psychological evaluation in school-age children should include an emotional assessment if psychiatric or emotional problems are suspected. Such problems are common in children with developmental delays or mental retardation. A hearing test and a vision screening or ophthalmologic evaluation are important to determine whether hearing and vision are normal.

Diagnostic testing should be carried out in an effort to find the cause of mental retardation. Because chromosomal abnormalities occur in 4–28% of patients with mental retardation, cytogenetic testing is important in cases without a known cause. A consensus panel has recommended a high-resolution karyotype so that small deletions or duplications can be visualized. In addition, FISH studies are available. These studies use a fluorescent DNA probe that hybridizes to a region of DNA where a deletion or duplication is suspected. Microdeletion syndromes such as Prader-Willi syndrome or Angelman syndrome, caused by a deletion at 15q; velocardiofacial syndrome, caused by a deletion at 22q; Smith-Magenis syndrome, caused by a deletion at 17p; and Williams syndrome, caused by a 7p deletion—can be assessed with FISH studies. Sometimes the deletion is so small that it may not be visualized through the microscope even with high-resolution cytogenetic studies. If clinical features consistent with any of the microdeletion syndromes are present, then FISH studies should be ordered to look for a small deletion in a specific region. In addition, duplications may be present. For example, a duplication at 15q has been associated with pervasive developmental disorder or autistic spectrum disorders and with general mental retardation. This duplication can be identified by FISH testing.

Structural abnormalities of the brain can occur in many individuals with mental retardation. Magnetic resonance imaging is superior to computed tomography in identifying structural and myelination abnormalities. Computed tomography is the study of choice in evaluation of intracranial calcifications, such as those seen in congenital infections or tuberous sclerosis. The value of computed tomography and magnetic resonance imaging studies in a child with a normal-sized head and no focal neurologic signs is unclear, and they are not routinely carried out. Neuroimaging is important in patients with microcephaly, macrocephaly, seizures, loss of psychomotor skills, or specific neurologic signs such as spasticity, dystonia, ataxia, or abnormal reflexes. Neuroimaging is not routinely carried out in known genetic disorders such as Down syndrome, fragile X syndrome, or microdeletion syndromes because the CNS abnormalities have been well described and documentation of the abnormalities usually does not affect management.

Metabolic screening has a relatively low yield (0–5%) in children who present with developmental delay or mental retardation. Many patients with metabolic disorders such as hypothyroidism, phenylketonuria, and galactosemia are identified through newborn screening. Most patients with metabolic problems will present with specific indications for more focused testing, such as failure to thrive, recurrent unexplained illnesses, plateauing or loss of developmental skills, coarse facial features, cataracts, recurrent coma, abnormal sexual differentiation, arachnodactyly, hepatosplenomegaly, deafness, structural hair abnormalities, muscle tone changes, and skin abnormalities. Thyroid function studies should be carried out in any patient who has a palpably abnormal thyroid or exhibits clinical features associated with hypothyroidism. Serum amino acids, urine organic acid, and mucopolysaccharide screens should be considered in children with developmental delays and a suggestive history. Preliminary laboratory findings such as lactic acidosis, hyperuricemia, hyperammonemia, or a low or high cholesterol level require additional metabolic work-up.

Serial follow-up of patients is important because the physical and behavioral phenotype changes over time and diagnostic testing improves with time. Although cytogenetic testing may have been negative 10 years earlier, advances in high-resolution techniques, FISH testing, and fragile X DNA testing may now reveal an abnormality that was not identified previously. A stepwise approach to diagnostic testing may also be more cost-effective, so that the test most likely to be positive is done first.

Treatment

Once a diagnosis of mental retardation is made, treatment should include a combination of individual therapies, such as speech and language therapy, occupational therapy or physical therapy, special education support, behavioral therapy or counseling, and medical intervention, which may include psychopharmacology. To illustrate how these interventions work together, three disorders are described in detail in the next section.

Burack JA et al (editors): *Handbook of Mental Retardation and Development.* Cambridge University Press, 1999.

Curry CJ et al: Evaluation of mental retardation: Recommendations of a consensus conference. Am J Med Genet 1997;72:468 [PMID: 9375733].

Hagerman RJ: *Neurodevelopmental Disorders: Diagnosis and Treatment.* Oxford University Press, 1999.

http://www.TheArc.org

SPECIFIC FORMS OF MENTAL RETARDATION & ASSOCIATED TREATMENT ISSUES

1. Fragile X Syndrome

The most common inherited cause of mental retardation is fragile X syndrome, which is caused by a trinucleotide expansion (CGG repeated sequence) within the fragile X mental retardation I (*FMR1*) gene. Individuals with mental retardation of unknown origin

should receive *FMR1* DNA testing to see if they have an expansion of the CGG repeat causing dysfunction of this gene. The CGG sequence at *FMR1* in the normal population includes 5–50 repeats. Carriers of the premutation have 54–200 repeats, and have been considered unaffected. However, there is mounting evidence for a specific phenotype in these individuals. Women with the premutation have a higher incidence of premature ovarian failure, anxiety, and mild facial dysmorphisms. Individuals with the premutation have normal levels of FMR1 protein but increased levels of mRNA. It should be noted that seemingly unaffected females can pass an expansion of the CGG repeat to the next generation. Approximately 1 in 250 women and 1 in 700 men in the general population are premutation carriers. When a premutation of more than 90 repeats is passed on by a female to her offspring, it will expand to a full mutation (more than 200 repeats) 100% of the time, which usually causes mental retardation or learning disabilities. The full mutation is associated with methylation of the gene, which turns off transcription, resulting in a deficiency in the FMR1 protein product. These deficiencies result in mental retardation or significant learning and emotional problems.

Fragile X syndrome includes a broad range of symptoms. Patients can present with shyness, social anxiety, and learning problems, or they can present with mental retardation. Girls are usually less affected by the syndrome because they have a second X chromosome that is producing FMR1 protein. Approximately 70% of girls with the full mutation have cognitive deficits in addition to emotional problems, such as mood lability, ADHD, anxiety, and shyness. Approximately 85% of males with the syndrome have mental retardation and autisticlike features, such as poor eye contact, hand flapping, hand biting, and tactile defensiveness. About 20% of fragile X males meet the criteria for autism.

Children with fragile X syndrome usually present with language delays, hyperactivity, and tantrum behavior in early childhood. Although prominent ears and hyperextensible finger joints are common, approximately 30% of children with the syndrome may not have these features, and the diagnosis must be suspected because of behavioral problems and developmental delays alone. As the boys move into puberty, macroorchidism develops with an average adult volume of 50 mL, or twice the normal volume. The child's face may become longer during puberty, and the majority of these children continue to have prominent ears.

Treatment

All young children with fragile X syndrome benefit from language and motor therapy because delays in these areas are universal. Because approximately 10% of boys with the syndrome will be nonverbal at age 5 years, the use of augmentative communication techniques—such as signing; the use of pictures to represent food, toys, or activities; or the use of computers that can be programmed for communication—are helpful. Tantrums and hyperarousal to stimuli, along with hyperactivity, are common. Sensory integrative occupational therapy can be helpful in calming hyperarousal to stimuli and in improving the child's fine and gross motor coordination and motor planning. Speech and language therapy can decrease oral hypersensitivity, improve articulation, enhance verbal output and comprehension, and stimulate abstract reasoning skills.

If the behavioral problems are severe, it can be helpful to involve a behavioral psychologist who emphasizes positive reinforcement, time outs, consistency in routine, and the use of both auditory and visual modalities, such as a picture sequence, to help with difficult transition times and new situations.

Psychopharmacology can also be useful to treat ADHD, aggression, anxiety, or severe mood instability. Clonidine or guanfacine may be helpful in low doses, beginning in the preschool period to treat hyperarousal, tantrums, or severe hyperactivity. Stimulant medications such as methylphenidate, dextroamphetamine, and Adderall are usually beneficial by age 5 years and occasionally earlier. Relatively low doses are used (eg, 0.2–0.3 mg/kg/dose of methylphenidate) because irritability is often a problem with higher doses.

Shyness and social anxiety combined with mild ADHD are commonly seen in girls who have fragile X syndrome. The social anxiety is sometimes so severe that selective mutism (refusal to speak in some environments, especially school) is seen in girls who have the full mutation. The treatment for selective mutism includes fluoxetine, language therapy, and counseling.

Anxiety may also be a significant problem for boys with fragile X syndrome, and the use of a selective serotonin reuptake inhibitor (SSRI) such as fluoxetine, sertraline, fluvoxamine, or paroxetine is often helpful. SSRIs may also decrease aggression or moodiness, although in approximately 25% of cases, an increase in agitation or even hypomania may occur. The use of a more limited serotonin agent, buspirone, may also be helpful for anxiety, particularly if the patient cannot tolerate SSRIs.

Anticonvulsants such as carbamazepine, valproic acid, and gabapentin can be used to treat seizures, which occur in 20% of children with fragile X syndrome. They can also be helpful in treating more severe mood instability that does not improve with an SSRI, clonidine, or a stimulant medication. The use of carbamazepine and valproic acid requires careful monitoring of blood levels, liver function studies, electrolytes, blood count, and platelet level.

Aggression may become a significant problem in childhood or adolescence for boys with fragile X syndrome. Counseling can often be helpful, although medication may be needed. Stimulants, clonidine, and an SSRI may decrease aggression, although sometimes an atypical antipsychotic may be needed. If psychotic features are present, such as paranoia, delusions, or hallucinations, or if thinking is severely disorganized, then an atypical antipsychotic is usually helpful. Risperidone has been used most frequently in pediatrics and has a low risk for extrapyramidal symptoms. Side effects include sedation, excessive appetite and subsequent weight gain, and an increase in prolactin, which can cause breast tenderness and gynecomastia in boys. Usually a low dose of risperidone is well tolerated, and 0.5–2 mg at bedtime usually improves aggression, decreases hyperactivity, and stabilizes mood.

An important component of treatment is genetic counseling. Parents should meet with a genetic counselor after the diagnosis of fragile X syndrome is made because there is a high risk that other family members are carriers or may be affected by the syndrome. A detailed family history is essential, and all siblings of the proband should have *FMR1* DNA testing. If the mother received the gene from her father, then all of her sisters are obligate carriers, and their children are at 50% risk of having the fragile X mutation.

It is also helpful to link up a newly diagnosed family to a parent support group. Educational materials and parent support information may be obtained by calling The National Fragile X Foundation at 1-800-688-8765.

Hagerman RJ: *Fragile X Syndrome in Neurodevelopmental Disorders: Diagnosis and Treatment.* Oxford University Press, 1999.

Hagerman RJ, Cronister AC (editors): *Fragile X Syndrome: Diagnosis, Treatment, and Research,* 3rd ed. Johns Hopkins University Press, 2001.

http://www.FragileX.org

http://www.fraxa.org

2. Fetal Alcohol Spectrum Disorders

Alcohol exposure in utero is associated with a broad spectrum of developmental problems, ranging from learning disabilities to severe mental retardation. Fetal alcohol spectrum disorders (FASD) is an umbrella term describing the range of effects that can occur in an individual exposed to alcohol prenatally. The Institute of Medicine in 1996 defined the diagnostic categories in individuals with documented prenatal maternal alcohol exposure as follows.

A. FETAL ALCOHOL SYNDROME

Fetal alcohol syndrome (FAS) refers to the full syndrome associated with prenatal alcohol exposure. The diagnosis of FAS requires the presence of a characteristic pattern of facial abnormalities (short palpebral fissures, thin upper lip, and indistinct or smooth philtrum, for which there are standard measurements), growth deficiency, and evidence of CNS damage and neurodevelopmental abnormalities.

B. Partial Fetal Alcohol Syndrome

The diagnosis of partial fetal alcohol syndrome requires the presence of some but not all components of the facial anomalies as well as growth retardation, CNS neurodevelopmental abnormalities, or behavioral or cognitive abnormalities that are inconsistent with the child's developmental level and cannot be explained by familial background or environment.

Partial fetal alcohol syndrome is a category that has been controversial and some feel that the criteria are too vague and imprecise to be of clinical help. What is most important, if the child does not have all of the criteria for FAS, is the documentation of prenatal alcohol exposure and the presence of neurodevelopmental dysfunction (encephalopathy).

C. Alcohol-Related Neurodevelopmental Disorder

Alcohol-related neurodevelopmental disorder does not require the presence of dysmorphic facial features, but it does require the presence of neurodevelopmental abnormalities or evidence of a pattern of behavioral or cognitive abnormalities. These abnormalities may include learning disabilities; poor impulse control; and problems in memory, attention, and judgment.

D. Alcohol-Related Birth Defects

The diagnosis of alcohol-related birth defects requires the presence of congenital anomalies including malformations and dysplasias in cardiac, skeletal, renal, ocular, or auditory areas (ie, sensorineural hearing loss).

Animal and human data support these diagnostic categories, including the controversial alcohol-related neurodevelopmental disorder diagnosis, which does not include dysmorphic features. The prevalence of FAS, partial fetal alcohol syndrome, and alcohol-related neurodevelopmental disorder combined is approximately 1 per 100 in the general population. These are common problems. Thus, the physician should always ask about alcohol (and other drug) intake during pregnancy. This is particularly true when evaluating a child presenting with developmental disturbances. The exact amount of alcohol consumption that leads to teratogenesis remains unclear. However, there is strong evidence that binge drinking during the first trimester, the critical period of embryogenesis, leads to FASD.

Evaluation & Treatment

Essential to the evaluation of a child with FASD, or one suspected of having FASD, is an assessment by a multidis-

ciplinary team. Growth deficiency, facial features, brain dysfunction, and the documentation of prenatal alcohol exposure are the most significant areas to be assessed.

The majority of children with alcohol-related syndromes present with ADHD symptoms, with or without significant developmental delays. To adequately assess involvement in other organs the following tests are recommended: an ophthalmologic examination, a hearing test, and a careful cardiac examination, with ultrasonography if abnormalities are detected. A careful examination for dysmorphic features and bony abnormalities is necessary. Renal function studies (ie, creatinine) should be conducted and a renal ultrasound obtained. Mental health problems are observed in over 90% of children and adolescents affected by alcohol in utero. Depression, panic attacks, anxiety, and mood instability are common. Because psychotic ideation is present in 20–40% of individuals with alcohol-related syndromes, a thorough emotional or psychiatric evaluation is essential. Long-term therapy and special education services are usually needed, and psychopharmacologic intervention may be helpful.

For treatment of ADHD symptoms, a dextroamphetamine preparation should be tried initially, although methylphenidate may also be helpful. SSRIs can help relieve anxiety, panic attacks, and depression, although mania or hypomanias, a side effect, may occur in 25–50% of patients. Mood instability may be severe, although it usually responds to a mood stabilizer such as valproate or carbamazepine. One should be cautious with lithium because kidney dysfunction, secondary to malformations or hypoplasia, occasionally occurs. Psychotic features can be treated with an atypical or typical antipsychotic agent. However, consultation with a psychiatrist is advised under these circumstances. A speech and language evaluation and an occupational therapy evaluation in childhood usually lead to documentation of problems, and ongoing therapy is usually helpful. The most significant problem in FASD is the high rate of legal problems, incarceration, and alcohol or drug abuse in adolescence and adulthood. A coordinated intensive treatment program must be put in place early on if the outcome for these children is to be improved. Long-term counseling and advocacy, along with intensive job training can be of help in preventing social and legal problems for children with FASD.

Claren SK: Fetal alcohol syndrome. In Wolraich ML (editor). *Disorders of Development and Learning,* 3rd ed. BC Decker, 2003.

Hagerman RJ, Cronister AC (editors): *Fragile X Syndrome: Diagnosis, Treatment, and Research,* 2nd ed. Johns Hopkins University Press, 1996.

Hagerman RJ: *Fetal Alcohol Syndrome in Neurodevelopmental Disorders: Diagnosis and Treatment.* Oxford University Press, 1999.

http://www.nofas.org

Stratton KR et al: *Fetal Alcohol Syndrome: Diagnosis, Epidemiology, Prevention, and Treatment.* National Academy Press, 1996.

Streissguth AP: *Fetal Alcohol Syndrome: A Guide for Families and Communities.* Brookes/Cole, 1997.

REFERENCES

Web resources

[Title V Program Information: Institute for Child Health Policy]
www.ichp.edu

[Parent Training and Information Centers: Alliance Coordinating Office]
www.taalliance.org

[Advocacy: The Arc of the United States]
www.TheArc.org

[American with Disabilities Act Information: National Access for Public Schools Project]
www.adaptenv.org

[General: NADDC-National Association of Developmental Disabilities Councils]
www.naddc.org

Adolescence

3

David W. Kaplan, MD, MPH, & Kathryn Love-Osborne, MD

Adolescence is a period of rapid physical, emotional, cognitive, and social growth and development. Generally, adolescence begins at age 11–12 years and ends between ages 18 and 21. Most teenagers complete puberty by age 16–18 years; in western society, however, for educational and cultural reasons, the adolescent period is prolonged to allow for further psychosocial development before the individual assumes adult responsibilities.

The developmental passage from childhood to adulthood encompasses the following steps: (1) completing puberty and somatic growth; (2) developing socially, emotionally, and cognitively, moving from concrete to abstract thinking; (3) establishing an independent identity and separating from the family; and (4) preparing for a career or vocation.

DEMOGRAPHY

In the United States in 2005, there were 20.6 million adolescents between ages 15 and 19 years and 21.0 million between ages 20 and 24 years. Adolescents and young adults (ages 15–24 years) constitute 14% of the U.S. population. Over the next several decades, the proportion of racial and ethnic minority adolescents is expected to increase. It is projected that by 2040 the percentage of non-Hispanic whites will drop below 50%. Hispanics are becoming the second most populous racial/ethnic group.

MORTALITY DATA

For the adolescent population, cultural and environmental rather than organic factors pose the greatest threats to life. The three leading causes of death in the adolescent population (ages 15–19 years) in 2002 were unintentional injury (51.6%), homicides (13.7%), and suicides (11.0%). These three causes of violent death accounted for 76.3% of all adolescent deaths. Although deaths from automobile crashes have decreased over the last decade, alcohol use remains the underlying cause of most teenage motor vehicle deaths. Almost two-thirds of motor vehicle deaths involving young drinking drivers occur on

Friday, Saturday, or Sunday, and 70% occur between 8:00 pm and 4:00 am.

There is continued concern in the United States with the problem of youth violence. This concern is rooted in the high rate of homicides involving handguns among young males, the number of firearm-related suicides, and school shootings. Youths ages 12–17 are twice as likely as adults to be victims of serious violent crimes, which include aggravated assault, rape, robbery, and homicide. Violent crimes committed by juveniles constitute about one in four of all violent crimes. Nationally, 17.1% of high-school students reported carrying a weapon at least once in the preceding 30 days. Violent crime victimization among adolescents has declined substantially since the early 1990s. In 2003, adolescents ages 12–15 were victimized at a rate of 51.6 per 1000 and youth ages 16–19 were victimized at an all-time low rate of 53.0 per 1,000. These rates are less than half of what they were as recently as 1994. Adolescents who have been violently victimized are more likely to have physical and mental health problems, substance abuse problems, and problems at school.

MORBIDITY DATA

Demographic and economic changes in the American family since the mid 1970s have had a profound effect on children and adolescents. Between 1955 and 1990, the divorce rate rose from about 400,000 to nearly 1.2 million a year. Between 1960 and 1990, the number of children involved in divorce each year increased from 460,000 to 1.1 million. The percentage of children and adolescents living in two-parent households has decreased significantly, from 79% in 1980 to 68% in 2004. After peaking at 22% in 1992, the percentage of children living in families whose income was below the official poverty threshold fell during the late 1990s to about 16% in 1999. However, the rate of poverty differs significantly by race and family structure. In 2004, 33% of black children and 29% of Hispanic children lived in families with incomes below the official poverty threshold. In 2004, 42% of children living in single-mother families were poor, compared with 9% of children living in married-couple families.

The major causes of morbidity during adolescence are psychosocial and often correlated with poverty: unintended pregnancy, sexually transmitted infections (STIs), substance abuse, smoking, dropping out of school, depression, running away from home, physical violence, and juvenile delinquency. High-risk behavior in one area is frequently associated with problems in another (Figure 3–1). For example, teenagers who live in a dysfunctional family (eg, problems related to drinking or physical or sexual abuse) are much more likely than other teenagers to be depressed. A depressed teenager is at greater risk for drug and alcohol abuse, academic failure, inappropriate sexual activity, STIs, pregnancy, and suicide.

Early identification of the teenager at risk for these problems is important in preventing immediate complications and future associated problems. Early indicators for problems related to depression include the following:

1. Decline in school performance.
2. Excessive school absences or cutting class.
3. Frequent or persistent psychosomatic complaints.
4. Changes in sleeping or eating habits.
5. Difficulty in concentrating or persistent boredom.
6. Signs or symptoms of depression, extreme stress, or anxiety.

7. Withdrawal from friends or family, or change to a new group of friends.
8. Unusually severe violent or rebellious behavior, or radical personality change.
9. Conflict with parents.
10. Sexual acting-out.
11. Conflicts with the law.
12. Suicidal thoughts or preoccupation with themes of death.
13. Drug and alcohol abuse.
14. Running away from home.

American Academy of Pediatrics Committee on Injury and Poison Prevention: Firearm-related injuries affecting the pediatric population. Pediatrics 2000;105:888 [PMID: 10742344].

Anderson RN, Smith BL: Deaths: leading causes for 2002. Natl Vital Stat Rep 2005;53:1 [PMID: 1578662].

Committee on Adolescents. American Academy of Pediatrics: Suicide and suicide attempts in adolescents. Pediatrics 2000; 105(4 Pt 1):871 [PMID: 10742340].

Emery RE, Laumann-Billings L: Practical and emotional consequences of parental divorce. Adolesc Med State Art Rev 1998;9:271 [PMID: 10961235].

Grunbaum JA et al: Youth risk behavior surveillance—United States, 2003. MMWR Surveill Summ 2004;53:1. Erratum in: MMWR Morb Mortal Wkly Rep 2004;53:536; MMWR Morb Mortal Wkly Rep 2005;54:608 [PMID: 15152182].

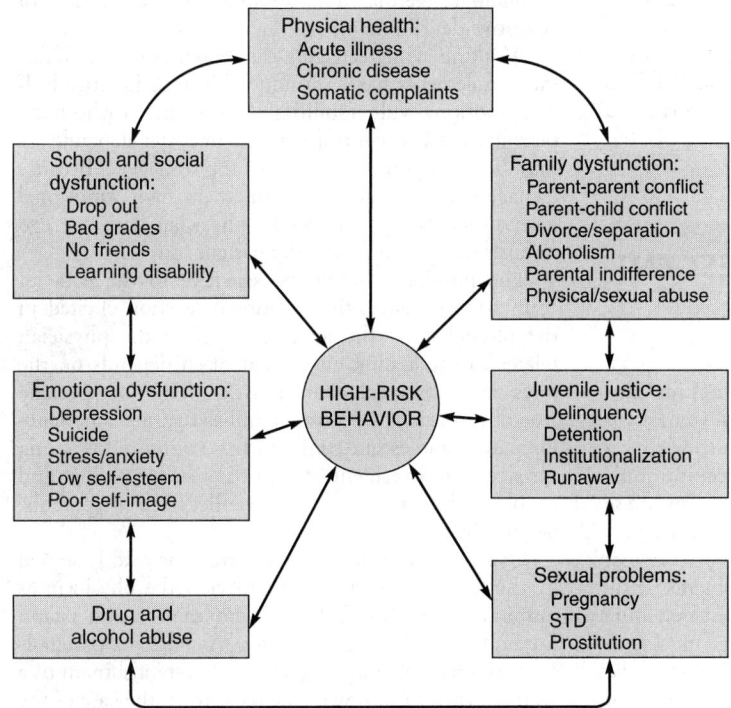

Figure 3–1. Interrelation of high-risk adolescent behavior.

Healthy People 2010: National Health Promotion and Disease Prevention Objectives. U.S. Government Printing Office, Washington, 2000.

O'Malley PM, Johnston LD: Unsafe driving by high school seniors: national trends from 1976 to 2001 in tickets and accidents after use of alcohol, marijuana and other illegal drugs. J Stud Alcohol 2003;64:305 [PMID: 12817818].

Resnick MD et al: Protecting adolescents from harm: Findings from the national longitudinal study on adolescent health. JAMA 1997;278:823 [PMID: 9293990].

Steinberg L: Gallagher lecture. The family at adolescence: Transition and transformation. J Adolesc Health 2000;27:170 [PMID: 10960215].

DELIVERY OF HEALTH SERVICES

How, where, why, and when adolescents seek health care depends on ability to pay, distance to health care facilities, availability of transportation, accessibility of services, time away from school, and privacy. Many common teenage health problems, such as unintended pregnancy and the need for contraception; STIs; and substance abuse, depression, and other emotional problems, have moral, ethical, and legal implications. Teenagers are often reluctant to confide in their parents for fear of punishment or disapproval. Recognizing this reality, health care providers have established many specialized programs such as teenage family planning clinics, drop-in centers, STI clinics, hotlines, and adolescent clinics. For the physician, establishing a trusting and confidential relationship is basic to meeting an adolescent patient's health care needs. A patient who senses that the physician will inform the parents about a confidential problem may lie or fail to disclose information essential for proper diagnosis and treatment.

■ GUIDELINES FOR ADOLESCENT PREVENTIVE SERVICES

The American Medical Association guidelines for adolescent preventive services and the National Center for Education in Maternal and Child Health's *Bright Futures* cover health screening and guidance, immunization, and health care delivery. The goals of these guidelines are (1) to deter adolescents from participating in behaviors that jeopardize health; (2) to detect physical, emotional, and behavioral problems early and intervene promptly; (3) to reinforce and encourage behaviors that promote healthful living; and (4) to provide immunization against infectious diseases. The guidelines recommend that adolescents between ages 11 and 21 years have annual routine health visits.

Health services should be developmentally appropriate and culturally sensitive, and confidentiality between patient and physician should be ensured.

RELATING TO THE ADOLESCENT PATIENT

Adolescence is one of the physically healthiest periods in life. The challenge of caring for adolescents lies not in managing complex organic disease, but in accommodating the cognitive, emotional, and psychosocial growth that influences health behavior.

How the physician initially approaches the adolescent may determine the success or failure of the visit. The physician should behave simply and honestly, without an authoritarian or excessively professional manner. Because the self-esteem of many young adolescents is fragile, the physician must be careful not to overpower and intimidate the patient. To establish a comfortable and trusting relationship, the physician should strive to present the image of an ordinary person who has special training and skills.

Because individuals vary greatly in the onset and termination of puberty, chronologic age may be a poor indicator of physical, physiologic, and emotional development. In communicating with an adolescent, the physician must be sensitive to the patient's developmental level, recognizing that outward appearance and chronologic age may not give an accurate assessment of cognitive development.

Working with teenagers can be emotionally draining. Adolescents have a unique ability to identify hidden emotional vulnerabilities. The physician who has a personal need to control patients or foster dependency may be disappointed in caring for teenagers. Because teenagers are consumed with their own emotional needs, they rarely provide the physician with the ego rewards that younger or older patients do.

The physician should be sensitive to the issue of countertransference, the emotional reaction elicited in the physician by the adolescent. How the physician relates to the adolescent patient often depends on the physician's personal characteristics. This is especially true of physicians who treat families that are experiencing parent-adolescent conflicts. It is common for young physicians to overidentify with the teenage patient and for older physicians to see the conflict from the parents' perspective.

Overidentification with the parents is readily sensed by the teenager, who is likely to view the physician as just another authority figure who cannot understand the problems of being a teenager. Assuming a parental-authoritarian role may jeopardize the establishment of a working relationship with the patient. In the case of the young physician, overidentification with the teenager may cause the parents to become defensive about their parenting role and discount the physician's experience and ability.

THE SETTING

Adolescents respond positively to a setting and to services that communicate a sensitivity to their age. A pediatrician's waiting room with toddlers' toys and examination tables too short for a young adult make adolescent patients feel they have outgrown the practice. Similarly, a waiting room filled with geriatric or pregnant patients can make a teenager feel out of place.

It is not uncommon to see a teenage patient who has been brought to the office against his or her wishes, especially for evaluations of drug and alcohol use, parent-child conflict, school failure, depression, or a suspected eating disorder. Even in cases of acute physical illness, the adolescent may feel anxiety about having a physical examination. If future visits are to be successful, the physician must spend time on the first visit to foster a sense of trust and an opportunity to feel comfortable.

CONFIDENTIALITY

It is helpful at the beginning of the visit to talk with the adolescent and the parents about what to expect. The physician should address the issue of confidentiality, telling the parents that two meetings, one with the teenager alone and one with only the parents, will take place. Adequate time must be spent with both the patient and the parents, or important information may be missed. At the beginning of the interview with the patient, it is useful to say, "I am likely to ask you some personal questions. This is not because I am trying to pry into your personal affairs, but because these questions may be important to your health. I want to assure you that what we talk about is confidential, just between the two of us. If there is something I feel we should discuss with your parents, I will ask your permission first unless I feel it is life-threatening."

THE STRUCTURE OF THE VISIT

Caring for adolescents is a time-intensive process. In many adolescent practices, a 40–50% no-show rate is not unusual. The stated chief complaint may conceal the patient's real concern. For example, a 15-year-old girl may say she has a sore throat but actually may be worried about being pregnant.

By age 11 or 12 years, patients should be seen alone. This gives them an opportunity to ask questions they may be embarrassed to ask in front of a parent. Because of the physical changes that take place in early puberty, some adolescents are too self-conscious to undress in front of a parent. If an adolescent comes in willingly, either for an acute illness or for a routine physical examination, it may be helpful to meet with the adolescent and parent together to obtain the history. In the case of angry adolescents brought in against their will, it is useful to meet with the parents and patient just long enough to have the parents describe the conflict and voice their concerns. This meeting should last no longer than 3–5 minutes, and the adolescent should then be seen alone. This approach conveys that the physician is primarily interested in the adolescent patient, yet gives the physician an opportunity to acknowledge the parents' concerns.

The Interview

The first few minutes may dictate the success of the visit, whether or not a trusting relationship can be established. A few minutes just getting to know the patient is time well spent. For example, immediately asking, "Do you smoke marijuana?" when a teenager is brought in for suspected marijuana use confirms the adolescent's negative preconceptions about the physician and the purpose of the visit.

It is preferable to spend a few minutes asking nonthreatening questions, such as "Tell me a little bit about yourself so I can get to know you," "What do you like to do most?" "Least?" and "What are your friends like?" Neutral questions help defuse some of the patient's anger and anxiety. Toward the end of the interview, the physician can ask more directed questions about psychosocial concerns.

Medical history questionnaires for the patient and the parents are useful in collecting historical data (Figure 3–2).

The history should include an assessment of progress with psychodevelopmental tasks and of behaviors potentially detrimental to health. The review of systems should include questions about the following:

1. Nutrition: Number and balance of meals; calcium, iron, and cholesterol intake; body image.
2. Sleep: Number of hours, problems with insomnia or frequent waking.
3. Seat belt or helmet: Regularity of use.
4. Self-care: Knowledge of testicular or breast self-examination, dental hygiene, and exercise.
5. Family relationships: Parents, siblings, relatives.
6. Peers: Best friend, involvement in group activities, gangs, boyfriends, girlfriends.
7. School: Attendance, grades, activities.
8. Educational and vocational interests: College, career, short-term and long-term vocational plans.
9. Tobacco: Use of cigarettes, snuff, chewing tobacco.

TEEN HEALTH HISTORY

This information is *strictly confidential*. Its purpose is to help your caregiver give you better care. We request that you fill out the form completely, but you may skip any question that you do not wish to answer.

NAME _____ DATE _____
       FIRST   MIDDLE INITIAL   LAST

BIRTHDATE _____ AGE _____ GRADE _____ Name that you like to be called _____

1. Why did you come to the clinic today? _____
_____
_____

STRICTLY CONFIDENTIAL

Medical History
2. Are you allergic to any medicines? .... YES NO
   Name of medicines _____
3. Are you taking any medicines now? .... YES NO
   Name of medicines _____
4. Do you have any long-term health conditions? .... YES NO
   Conditions _____
5. Date or age at your last tetanus (or dT) shot_____

School Information
6. What grade do you usually make in English? _____
   (Example: A, B, C, D, E, F)
7. What grade do you usually make in Math? _____
8. How many days were you absent from school last semester? _____
9. How many days were you absent last semester because of illness? _____
10. How do you get along at school? _____
_____

1	2	3	4	5	6	7
TERRIBLE						GREAT

11. Have you ever been suspended? .... YES NO
12. Have you ever dropped out of school? .... YES NO
13. Do you plan to graduate from high school? .... YES NO

Job/Career Information
14. Are you working? .... YES NO
   If YES, What is your job? _____
   How many hours do you work per week?_____
15. What are your future plans or career goals? _____

Family Information
16. Who do you live with? (Check all that apply.)

_____ Both natural parents	_____ Stepmother	_____ Brother(s)-ages: _____
_____ Mother	_____ Stepfather	_____ Sister(s)-ages: _____
_____ Father	_____ Guardian	_____ Other:Explain _____
_____ Adoptive parents	_____ Alone	

17. Have there been any changes in your family? Check all that apply.

_____ a. Marriage	_____ d. Serious illness	_____ g. Births
_____ b. Separation	_____ e. Loss of job	_____ h. Deaths
_____ c. Divorce	_____ f. Move to new home	_____ i. Other

18. Father's/stepfather's occupation or job: _____
   Mother's/stepmother's occupation or job: _____

Figure 3–2. Adolescent medical history questionnaire. (Reproduced, with permission, from *AMA Guidelines for Adolescent Preventive Services: Recommendations and Rationale.* American Medical Association, 1995.) (continued)

19. How do you get along at home?

1	2	3	4	5	6	7
TERRIBLE						GREAT

20. Have you ever run away from home? . . . .   YES NO
21. Have you ever lived in foster care or an institution? . . . .   YES NO

Self Information

22. On the whole, how do you like yourself?

1	2	3	4	5	6	7
NOT VERY MUCH						A LOT

23. What do you do best?_____

24. If you could, what would you like to change about yourself? _____
_____

25. List any habits you would like to break. _____
_____

26. Do you feel people expect too much from you? . . . .   YES NO
27. How do you get along with your friends/peers?

1	2	3	4	5	6	7
TERRIBLE						GREAT

28. Do you feel you have friends you can count on? . . . .   YES NO
29. Have you ever felt really sad or depressed for more than 3 days in a row? . .   YES NO
30. Have you ever thought of suicide as a solution to your problems? . . . .   YES NO
31. Have you gotten into any trouble because of your anger/temper? . . . .   YES NO

Health Concern

32. On a scale of 1–7, how would you rate your general health?

1	2	3	4	5	6	7
TERRIBLE						GREAT

33. Do you have any questions or concerns about any of the following? (Check those that apply.)

____ Height/weight
____ Blood pressure
____ Head/headaches
____ Dizziness/passing out
____ Eyes/vision
____ Ears/hearing/earaches
____ Nose/frequent colds
____ Mouth/teeth
____ Neck/back
____ Chest/breathing/coughing
____ Breasts
____ Heart
____ Stomach/pain/vomiting
____ Diarrhea/constipation

____ Skin rash
____ Arms, legs/muscle or joint pain
____ Frequent or painful urination
____ Wetting the bed
____ Sexual organs/genitals
____ Trouble sleeping
____ Tiredness
____ Diet food/appetite
____ Eating disorder
____ Smoking/drugs/alcohol
____ Future plans/jobs
____ Worried about parents

____ Family violence/physical abuse
____ Feeling down or depressed
____ Dating
____ Sex
____ Worried about VD/STD
____ Masturbation
____ Sexual abuse/rape
____ Having children/parenting/adoption
____ Cancer/or dying
____ Other (explain) _____

Health Behavior Information

34. Have you lost or gained any weight in the last year? . . . .   YES NO
    Gained ( ) How much? _____
    Lost ( ) How much? _____
35. In the past year, have you tried to lose weight or control your weight by vomiting, taking diet pills or laxatives, or starving yourself? . . . .   YES NO
36. Do you ever drive after drinking or when high? . . . .   YES NO
37. Do you ever smoke cigarettes or use snuff or chewing tobacco? . . . .   YES NO
38. Do you ever smoke marijuana? . . . .   YES NO
39. Do you ever drink alcoholic beverages? . . . .   YES NO
40. Do you ever use street drugs (speed, cocaine, acid, crack, etc.)? . . . .   YES NO
41. Does anyone in your household smoke? . . . .   YES NO
42. Does anyone in your family have a problem with drugs or alcohol? . . . .   YES NO

Figure 3–2. Continued

43. Have you ever been in trouble with the police or the law? . . . .   YES NO
44. Have you begun dating? . . . .   YES NO
45. Do you currently have a boyfriend or girlfriend? . . . .   YES NO
    If YES, how old is he/she? _____
46. Do you think you might be gay/lesbian/homosexual? . . . .   YES NO
47. Have you ever had sex (sexual intercourse)? . . . .   YES NO
48. Are you interested in receiving information on preventing pregnancy? . . . . . .   YES NO
49. If you have had sex, are you (or your partner) using any kind of birth control?   YES NO
50. If you have had sex, have you ever been treated for gonorrhea or chlamydia
    or any other sexually transmitted disease? . . . .   YES NO

For males only
51. Have you been taught how to use a condom correctly? . . . .   YES NO
52. If you have had sex, do you use a condom every time or almost every time?   YES NO
53. Have you ever fathered a child? . . . .   YES NO

For females only
54. How old were you when your periods began? . . . .   _____
55. What date did your last period start? . . . .   _____
56. Are your periods regular (once a month)?. . . . .   YES NO
57. Do you have painful or excessively heavy periods? . . . .   YES NO
58. Have you ever had a vaginal infection or been treated for a female disorder?   YES NO
59. Do you think you might be pregnant? . . . .   YES NO
60. Have you ever been pregnant? . . . .   YES NO

Everyone
61. Do you have any other problems you would like to discuss with the caregiver?   YES NO

Past Medical History
62. Were you born prematurely or did you have any serious problems as an infant?   YES NO
63. Are you allergic to any medicines? . . . .   YES NO
    If YES, what? _____
    _____

64. List any medications that you are taking and the problems for which the
    medication was given:
    MEDICATION   REASON   HOW LONG
    _____   _____   _____
    _____   _____   _____

65. Have you ever been hospitalized? . . . .   YES NO
    If YES, describe your problem and your age at the time.
    AGE   PROBLEM
    _____   _____
    _____   _____

66. Have you had any injuries? . . . .   YES NO
    If YES, describe the injury and your age when it occurred.
    AGE   KIND OF INJURY
    _____   _____
    _____   _____

67. Have you had any serious illnesses? . . . .   YES NO
    If YES, state the kind of illness and your age when it started.
    AGE   ILLNESS
    _____   _____
    _____   _____

Figure 3–2. Continued

STRICTLY CONFIDENTIAL

Family History

Have any members of your family, alive or dead (parents, grandparents, uncles, aunts, brothers or sisters), had any of the following problems? If YES, please state the age of the person when the condition occurred and the person's relationship to you.

PROBLEM	YES	NO	DON'T KNOW	AGE	RELATIONSHIP
A. Seizure disorder Epilepsy					
B. Mental retardation Birth defects					
C. Migraine headaches					
D. High blood pressure High cholesterol					
E. Heart attack or stroke at less than age 60					
F. Lung disease Tuberculosis					
G. Liver or intestinal disease					
H. Kidney disease					
I. Allergies Asthma Eczema					
J. Arthritis					
K. Diabetes					
L. Endocrine problems Other glandular problems					
M. Obesity Eating disorder					
N. Cancer					
O. Blood disorders Sickle cell anemia					
P. Emotional problems Suicide					
Q. Alcoholism Drug problems					

Figure 3–2. Continued

10. Substance abuse: Frequency, extent, and history of alcohol and drug use.

11. Sexuality: Sexual activity, contraceptive use, pregnancies, history of sexually transmitted infection, number of sexual partners, risk for human immunodeficiency virus infection.

12. Emotional health: Signs of depression and excessive stress.

The physician's personal attention and interest is likely to be a new experience for the teenager, who has probably received medical care only through a parent. The teenager should leave the visit with a sense of having a personal physician.

Physical Examination

During early adolescence, many teenagers may be shy and modest, especially with a physician of the opposite sex. The examiner should address this concern directly, because it can be allayed by acknowledging the uneasiness verbally and by explaining the purpose of the examination, for example, "Many boys that I see who are your age are embarrassed to have their penis and testes examined. This is an important part of the examination for a couple of reasons. First, I want to make sure that there aren't any physical problems, and second, it helps me determine if your development is proceeding normally." This also introduces the subject of sexual development for discussion.

A pictorial chart of sexual development is useful for showing the patient how development is proceeding and what changes to expect. Figure 3–3 shows the relationship between height, penis and testes development, and pubic hair growth in the male, and Figure 3–4 shows the relationship between height, breast development, menstruation, and pubic hair growth in the female. Many teenagers do not openly admit that they are interested in this subject, but they are usually attentive when it is raised. This discussion is particularly useful in counseling teenagers who lag behind their peers in physical development.

Because teenagers are sensitive about their changing bodies, it is useful to comment during the examination: "Your heart sounds fine. I feel a small lump under your right breast. This is very common during puberty in boys. It is called gynecomastia and should disappear in

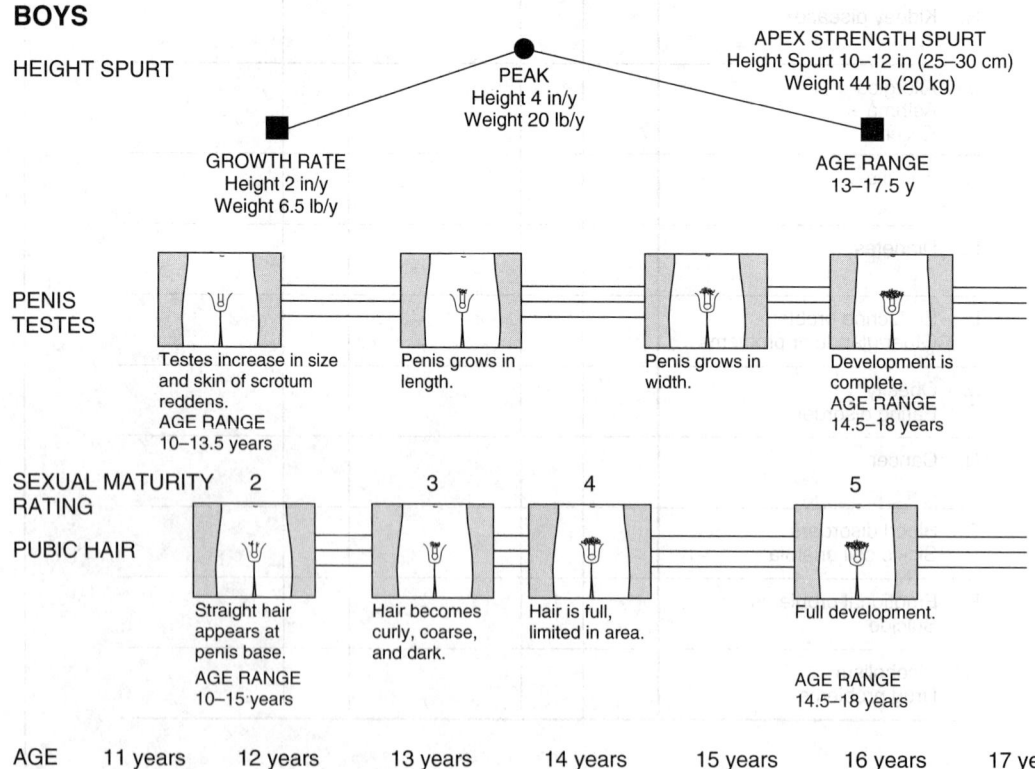

Figure 3–3. Adolescent male sexual maturation and growth. (Adapted, with permission, from Tanner JM: *Growth at Adolescence.* Blackwell Scientific, 1962.)

GIRLS

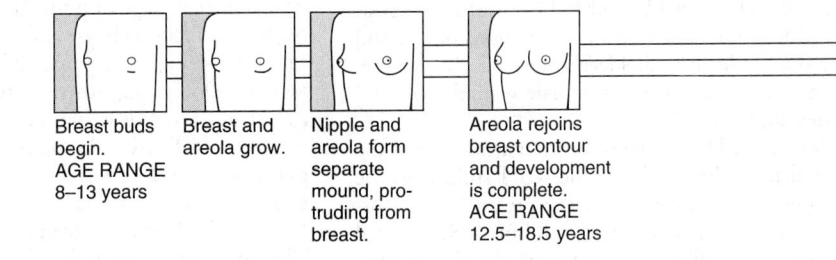

HEIGHT SPURT

PEAK
Height 3 in/y
Weight 17.5 lb/y

GROWTH RATE
Height 2 in/y
Weight 6 lb/y

AGE RANGE
11.5–16.5 y

MENARCHE

Age Range 10–16.5 y
Average Height 62.5 in (158.5 cm)
Average Weight 106 lb (48 kg)

BREAST

Breast buds begin.
AGE RANGE
8–13 years

Breast and areola grow.

Nipple and areola form separate mound, protruding from breast.

Areola rejoins breast contour and development is complete.
AGE RANGE
12.5–18.5 years

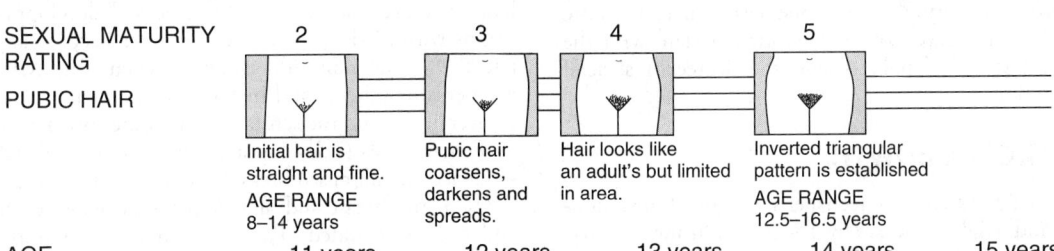

SEXUAL MATURITY RATING

2   3   4   5

PUBIC HAIR

Initial hair is straight and fine.
AGE RANGE
8–14 years

Pubic hair coarsens, darkens and spreads.

Hair looks like an adult's but limited in area.

Inverted triangular pattern is established
AGE RANGE
12.5–16.5 years

AGE   11 years   12 years   13 years   14 years   15 years

Figure 3–4. Adolescent female sexual maturation and growth. (Adapted, with permission, from Tanner JM: *Growth at Adolescence.* Blackwell Scientific, 1962.)

6 months to a year. Don't worry, you are not turning into a girl."

If a teenage girl has not been sexually active and has no gynecologic complaints or abnormalities, a pelvic examination is usually not necessary until about age 18 years. The following are indications for a pelvic examination in a younger teenage girl:

1. A history of sexual intercourse. (The pelvic examination should be done for purposes of contraceptive counseling and to rule out sexually transmitted infection.)
2. Abnormal vaginal discharge.
3. Menstrual irregularities.
4. Suspicion of anatomic abnormalities, such as imperforate hymen.
5. Pelvic pain.
6. Patient request for an examination.

Ford C, English A, Sigman G: Confidential Health Care for Adolescents: position paper for the Society for Adolescent Medicine. J Adolesc Health 2004;35:160.

Metzl JD: Preparticipation examination of the adolescent athlete: Part 1. Pediatr Rev 2001;22:199 [PMID: 11389307].

Metzl JD: Preparticipation examination of the adolescent athlete: Part 2. Pediatr Rev 2001;22:227 [PMID: 11435624].

■ GROWTH & DEVELOPMENT

PUBERTY

Pubertal growth and physical development are a result of activation of the hypothalamic-pituitary-gonadal axis in late childhood. Before the onset of puberty, pituitary and gonadal hormone levels are low. With the onset of puberty, the inhibition of gonadotropin-releasing hormone in the hypothalamus is removed, allowing pulsatile production and release of the gonadotropins: luteinizing hormone (LH) and follicle-stimulating hormone (FSH). In early to middle adolescence, pulse frequency and amplitude of LH and FSH secretion increase, which stimulates the gonads to produce sex steroids (estrogen or testosterone). In the female, FSH stimulates ovarian maturation, granulosa cell function, and estradiol secretion. LH is important in ovulation and is involved also in corpus luteum formation and progesterone secretion. Initially, estradiol has an inhibitory effect on the release of LH and FSH. Eventually, estradiol becomes stimulatory, and the secretions of LH and FSH become cyclic. Estradiol levels progressively increase, resulting in maturation of the female genital tract and breast development.

In the male, LH stimulates the interstitial cells of the testes, which produce testosterone. FSH stimulates the production of spermatocytes in the presence of testosterone. The testes also produce inhibin, a Sertoli cell protein that also inhibits the secretion of FSH. During puberty, circulating testosterone levels increase more than 20-fold. Levels of testosterone correlate with the physical stages of puberty and the degree of skeletal maturation.

PHYSICAL GROWTH

During adolescence, a teenager's weight almost doubles, and height increases by 15–20%. During puberty, major organs double in size, with the exception of lymphoid tissue, which decreases in mass. Before puberty, there is little difference in the muscular strength of boys and girls. The body's musculature increases both in size and in strength during puberty, with maximal strength lagging behind the increase in size by many months. Boys attain greater strength and mass, and strength continues to increase into late puberty. Although motor coordination lags behind growth in stature and musculature, it continues to improve as strength increases.

The pubertal growth spurt begins nearly 2 years earlier in girls than in boys. Girls reach their peak height velocity between ages $11^1/2$ and 12 years; boys, between ages $13^1/2$ and 14 years. Linear growth at peak velocity is 9.5 cm/y ± 1.5 cm for boys and 8.3 cm/y ± 1.2 cm for girls. Pubertal growth usually takes 2–4 years and continues longer in boys than in girls. By age 11 years in girls and age 12 years in boys, 83–89% of ultimate height has been attained. An additional 18–23 cm in females and 25–30 cm in males will be achieved during further pubertal growth. Following menarche, growth is rarely more than 5–7.5 cm.

In boys, the quantity of body fat increases before onset of the height spurt. They then lose fat until the growth spurt has finished and gradually again increase in fat. Muscle mass doubles between ages 10 and 17 years. Girls, by contrast, gradually store fat from about age 6 years and do not decrease the quantity of fat, although its location changes, with an increase of subcutaneous fat in the region of the pelvis, breasts, and upper back.

SEXUAL MATURATION

Sexual maturity rating (SMR) is useful clinically for categorizing genital development. SMR staging includes age ranges of normal development and specific descriptions for each stage of pubic hair growth, penis and testis development in boys, and breast maturation in girls. Figures 3–3 and 3–4 graphically represent this chronologic development with reference to each sexual maturity stage. SMR 1 is prepuberty and SMR 5 is adult maturity. In SMR 2 the pubic hair is sparse, fine, nonpigmented, and downy; in SMR 3, the hair becomes pigmented and curly and increases in amount; and in SMR 4, the hair is adult in texture but limited in area. The appearance of pubic hair precedes that of axillary hair by more than 1 year. Male genital development begins with SMR 2, in which the testes become larger and the scrotal skin reddens and coarsens. In SMR 3, the penis lengthens; and in SMR 4, the penis enlarges in overall size and the scrotal skin becomes pigmented.

Female breast development follows a predictable sequence. Small, raised breast buds appear in SMR 2. In SMR 3, the breast and areolar tissue generally enlarge and become elevated. The areola and papilla (nipple) form a separate mound from the breast in SMR 4, and in SMR 5 the areola assumes the same contour as the breast.

Great variability exists in the timing and onset of puberty and growth, and psychosocial development does not necessarily parallel physical changes. Because of this variability, chronologic age may be a poor indication of physiologic and psychosocial development. Skeletal maturation correlates well with growth and pubertal development.

Teenagers have been entering puberty at increasingly earlier ages during the last century because of better nutrition and improved socioeconomic conditions. In the United States, the average age at menarche is 12.16 years in African-American girls and 12.88 in white girls. Among girls reaching menarche, the average weight is 48 kg, and the average height is 158.5 cm. However, menarche may be delayed until age 16 years or may begin as early as age 10. Although the first measurable sign of puberty in girls is the beginning of the height spurt, the first conspicuous sign usually is development of breast buds between ages 8 and 11 years. Although breast development usually precedes the growth of pubic hair, in some girls the sequence may be reversed. A common concern for girls at this time is whether the breasts will be of the right size and shape, especially because it is not unusual for one breast to grow faster than the other. Among girls, the growth spurt starts at about age 9 years and reaches a peak at age $11^1/_2$, usually at SMR 3–4 breast development and stage 3 pubic hair development. The spurt usually ends by age 14 years. Girls who mature early will reach their peak height velocity sooner and attain their final height earlier. Girls who mature late will attain a greater ultimate height because of the longer period of growth before the growth spurt. Final height is related to skeletal age at onset of puberty as well as genetic factors. The height spurt correlates more closely with breast developmental stages than with pubic hair stages.

The first sign of puberty in the male, usually between ages 10 and 12 years, is scrotal and testicular growth. Pubic hair usually appears early in puberty but may do so any time between ages 10 and 15 years. The penis begins to grow significantly a year or so after the onset of testicular and pubic hair development, usually between ages 10 and $13^1/_2$. The first ejaculation usually occurs about 1 year after initiation of testicular growth, but its timing is highly variable. About 90% of boys have this experience between ages 11 and 15 years. Gynecomastia, a hard nodule under the nipple, occurs in a majority of boys, with a peak incidence between ages 14 and 15 years. Gynecomastia usually disappears within 6 months to 2 years. The height spurt begins at age 11 years but increases rapidly between ages 12 and 13, with the peak height velocity reached at age $13^1/_2$ years. The period of pubertal development lasts much longer in boys and may not be completed until age 18 years. The height velocity is higher in males (8–11 cm/y) than in females (6.5–9.5 cm/y). The development of axillary hair, deepening of the voice, and the development of chest hair in boys usually occur in midpuberty, about 2 years after onset of growth of pubic hair. Facial and body hair begin to increase at age 16–17 years.

Biro FM et al: Pubertal maturation in girls and the relationship to anthropometric changes: pathways through puberty. J Pediatr 2003;142:643 [PMID: 12838192].

Molgaard C et al: Influence of weight, age and puberty on bone size and bone mineral content in healthy children and adolescents. Acta Paediatr 1998;87:494 [PMID: 9641728].

Rogol AD, Roemmich JN, Clark PA: Growth at puberty. J Adolesc Health 2002;31(6 Suppl):192.

Rosen DS: Physiologic growth and development during adolescence. Pediatr Rev 2004;25:194.

Tanner JM, Davies PW: Clinical longitudinal standards for height and height velocity for North American children. J Pediatr 1985;107:317 [PMID: 3875704].

PSYCHOSOCIAL DEVELOPMENT

Adolescents are struggling to find out who they are, what they want to do in the future, and, in relation to that goal, what their personal strengths and weaknesses are. These questions arise primarily because teenagers are in the process of establishing their own identity. Adolescence is a period of progressive individuation and separation from the family. Because of the rapid physical, emotional, cognitive, and social growth occurring during adolescence, it is useful to divide the period into three sequential phases of development. Early adolescence occurs roughly between ages 10 and 13 years; middle adolescence, between ages 14 and 16 years; and late adolescence, at age 17 years and later.

Early Adolescence

Early adolescence (ages 10–13 years) is characterized by rapid growth and development of secondary sex characteristics. Because of the rapid physical changes during this period, body image, self-concept, and self-esteem fluctuate dramatically. Concerns about how personal growth and development deviate from that of peers may be a great worry, especially short stature in boys and delayed breast development or delayed menarche in girls. Although there is a certain curiosity about sexuality, young adolescents tend to feel more comfortable with members of the same sex. Peer relationships become increasingly important. Young teenagers still think concretely and cannot easily conceptualize about the future. They may have vague and unrealistic professional goals, such as becoming a movie star or a lead singer in a rock group.

Middle Adolescence

During middle adolescence (ages 14–16 years), as the rapid pubertal growth rate subsides, teenagers become more comfortable with their new bodies. Intense emotions and wide swings in mood are typical. Although some teenagers go through this experience relatively peacefully, others struggle desperately. Cognitively, teenagers move from concrete thinking to formal operations and develop the ability to think abstractly. With this new mental power comes a sense of omnipotence and a belief that the world can be changed by merely thinking about it. Sexually active teenagers may believe they do not need to worry about using contraception because they can't get pregnant, "it won't happen to me." Sixteen-year-old drivers believe they are the best drivers in the world and think the insurance industry is conspiring against them by charging such high rates for automobile insurance. With the onset of the ability to think abstractly, teenagers begin to see themselves as others see them and may become extremely self-centered. Because they are establishing their own identities, relationships with other people, including peers, are primarily narcissistic, and experimenting with different images is quite common. Peers determine the standards for identification, behavior, activities, and fashion and provide emotional support, intimacy, empathy, and the sharing of guilt and anxiety during the struggle for autonomy. The struggle for independence and autonomy is often a difficult and stressful period for both the teenager and the parents.

As sexuality increases in importance during this time, adolescents may begin dating and experimenting with sex. Relationships usually tend to be one-sided and narcissistic.

Late Adolescence

During late adolescence (age 17 years and older), the young person generally becomes less self-centered and begins caring more about others. Social relationships shift from the peer group to the individual. Dating becomes much more intimate. By 10th grade, 41% of adolescents have had sexual intercourse, and by 12th grade, 61%. The ability to think abstractly allows older adolescents to think more realistically in terms of future plans, actions, and careers. Older adolescents have rigid concepts of what is right or wrong. This is a period of idealism.

Sexual Orientation

Sexual orientation develops during early childhood. One's gender identity is established by age 2 years, and a sense of masculinity or femininity usually solidifies by age 5 or 6 years. Homosexual adults describe homosexual feelings during late childhood and early adolescence, years before engaging in overt homosexual acts.

Although only 5–10% of American young people acknowledge having had homosexual experiences and only 5% feel that they are or could be gay, homosexual experimentation is common, especially during early and middle adolescence. Experimentation may include mutual masturbation and fondling the genitals and does not by itself cause or lead to adult homosexuality. Theories about the causes of homosexuality include genetic, hormonal, environmental, and psychological models.

The development of homosexual identity in adolescence commonly progresses through two stages. The adolescent feels different, develops a crush on a person of the same sex without clear self-awareness of a gay identity, and then goes through a coming-out phase in which the homosexual identity is defined for the individual and revealed to others. The coming-out phase may be a very difficult period for the young person and the family. The young adolescent is afraid of society's bias and seeks to reject homosexual feelings. This struggle with identity may include episodes of both homosexual and heterosexual promiscuity, STIs, depression, substance abuse, attempted suicide, school avoidance and failure, running away from home, and other crises.

In a clinical setting, the issue of homosexual identity most often surfaces as a result of a teenager being seen for an STI, family conflict, school problem, attempted suicide, or substance abuse rather than as a result of a consultation about sexual orientation. Pediatricians should be aware of the psychosocial and medical implications of homosexual identity and be sensitive to the possibility of these problems in gay adolescents. Successful management depends on the physician's ability to gain the trust of the gay adolescent and on the physician's knowledge of the wide range of medical and psychological problems for which gay adolescents may be at risk. Pediatricians must be nonjudgmental in posing sexual questions if they are to be effective in encouraging the teenager to share concerns. Physicians who for religious or other personal reasons cannot be objective must refer the homosexual patient to another professional for treatment and counseling.

Frankowski BL: American Academy of Pediatrics Committee on Adolescence. Sexual orientation and adolescents. Pediatrics 2004;113:1827 [PMID: 15173519].

Garofalo R et al: Sexual orientation and risk of suicide attempts among a representative sample of youth. Arch Pediatr Adolesc Med 1999;153:487 [PMID: 10323629].

Gutgesell ME, Payne N: Issues of adolescent psychological development in the 21st century. Pediatr Rev 2004;25:79.

Russell ST, Joyner K: Adolescent sexual orientation and suicide risk: Evidence from a national study. Am J Public Health 2001;91:1276 [PMID: 11499118].

Ryan C, Futterman D: Caring for gay and lesbian teens. Contemp Pediatr 1998;15:107.

■ BEHAVIOR & PSYCHOLOGICAL HEALTH

It is not unusual for adolescents to seek medical attention for seemingly minor complaints. During early adolescence, teenagers may worry about normal developmental changes such as gynecomastia. They may present with vague symptoms, whereas the hidden agenda may be concerns about pregnancy or an STI. Adolescents with emotional disorders often present with somatic symptoms, for example, abdominal pain, headaches, dizziness or syncope, fatigue, sleep problems, and chest pain, that appear to have no biologic cause. The emotional basis of such complaints may be varied: somatoform disorder, depression, or stress and anxiety.

PSYCHOPHYSIOLOGIC SYMPTOMS & CONVERSION REACTIONS

The most common somatoform disorders during adolescence are conversion disorders or conversion reactions.

(A conversion reaction is a psychophysiologic process in which unpleasant feelings, especially anxiety, depression, and guilt, are communicated through a physical symptom.) Psychophysiologic symptoms result when anxiety activates the autonomic nervous system, resulting in tachycardia, hyperventilation, and vasoconstriction. The emotional feeling may be threatening or unacceptable to the individual, who expresses it as a physical symptom rather than verbally. This process is unconscious, and the anxiety or unpleasant feeling is dissipated by the somatic symptom. The degree to which the conversion symptom lessens anxiety, depression, or the unpleasant feeling is referred to as primary gain. Conversion symptoms not only diminish unpleasant feelings but also release the adolescent from conflict or an uncomfortable situation. This is referred to as secondary gain. Secondary gain may intensify the symptoms, especially with increased attention from concerned parents and friends. Adolescents with conversion symptoms tend to have overprotective parents and become increasingly dependent on their parents as the symptom becomes the major focus of concern in the family.

Clinical Findings

The symptom may appear at times of stress. Nervous, gastrointestinal, and cardiovascular symptoms are common and include paresthesias, anesthesia, paralysis, dizziness, syncope, hyperventilation, abdominal pain, nausea, and vomiting. Specific symptoms may reflect existing or previous illness (eg, pseudoseizures in adolescents with epilepsy) or modeling of a close relative's symptom (eg, chest pain in a boy whose grandfather died of a heart attack).

Conversion symptoms are more common in girls than boys. They occur in patients from all socioeconomic levels; however, the complexity of the symptom may vary with the sophistication and cognitive level of the patient.

Differential Diagnosis

The history and physical findings are usually inconsistent with anatomic and physiologic concepts. Conversion symptoms are exhibited most frequently at times of stress and in the presence of individuals meaningful to the patient. The patient often exhibits a characteristic personality pattern, including egocentricity, emotional lability, and dramatic and attention-seeking behaviors.

Conversion reactions must be differentiated from hypochondriasis, which is a preoccupation with developing or having a serious illness despite medical reassurance that there is no evidence of disease. Over time, the fear of one disease may give way to concern about another. In contrast to patients with conversion symp-

toms, who seem relieved if an organic cause is considered, patients with hypochondriasis become more anxious when such a cause is considered.

Malingering is uncommon during adolescence. The malingering patient consciously and intentionally produces false or exaggerated physical or psychological symptoms. Such patients are motivated by external incentives such as avoiding work, evading criminal prosecution, obtaining drugs, or obtaining financial compensation. These patients may be hostile and aloof. Parents of patients with conversion disorders and malingering have a similar reaction to illness. They have an unconscious psychological need to have sick children and reinforce their child's behavior.

Somatic delusions are physical symptoms, often bizarre, that accompany other signs of mental illness. Examples are visual or auditory hallucinations, delusions, incoherence or loosening of associations, rapid shifts of affect, and confusion.

Treatment

The physician must emphasize from the onset that both physical and emotional causes of the symptom need to be considered. The relationship between physical causes of emotional pain and emotional causes of physical pain should be described to the family, using examples such as stress causing an ulcer or making a severe headache worse. The patient should be encouraged to understand that the symptom may persist and that at least a short-term goal is to continue normal daily activities. Medication is rarely helpful. If the family will accept it, psychological referral is often the best initial step toward psychotherapy. If the family resists psychiatric or psychological referral, the pediatrician may need to begin to deal with some of the emotional factors responsible for the symptom while building rapport with the patient and family. Regular appointments should be scheduled. During the sessions, the teenager should be seen first and encouraged to talk about school, friends, the relationship with the parents, and the stresses of life. Discussion of the symptom itself should be minimized; however, the physician should be supportive and must never suggest that the pain is not real. As the parents gain further insight into the cause of the symptom, they will become less indulgent of the complaints, facilitating the resumption of normal activities. If management is successful, the adolescent will increase coping skills and become more independent, while decreasing secondary gain.

If the symptom continues to interfere with daily activities and if the patient and parents feel that no progress is being made, psychological referral is indicated. A psychotherapist experienced in treating adolescents with conversion reactions is in the best position to establish a strong therapeutic relationship with the patient and family. After referral is made, the pediatrician should continue to follow the patient to ensure compliance with psychotherapy.

American Psychiatric Association: *Diagnostic and Statistical Manual of Mental Disorders,* 4th ed. American Psychiatric Press, 1994.

Gold MA, Friedman SB: Conversion reactions in adolescents. Pediatr Ann 1995;24:296 [PMID: 7659461].

Silber TJ, Pao M: Somatization disorders in children and adolescents. Pediatr Rev 2003;24:255 [PMID: 12897265].

Wood BL: Physically manifested illness in children and adolescents: A biobehavioral family approach. Child Adolesc Psychiatr Clin North Am 2001;10:543 [PMID: 11449811].

DEPRESSION (See Also Chapter 6.)

Symptoms of clinical depression (lethargy, loss of interest, sleep disturbances, decreased energy, feelings of worthlessness, and difficulty concentrating) are common during adolescence. The intensity of feelings, often in response to seemingly trivial events such as a poor grade on an examination or not being invited to a party, makes it difficult to differentiate severe depression from normal sadness or dejection. In less severe depression, sadness or unhappiness associated with problems of everyday life is generally short-lived. The symptoms usually result in only minor impairment in school performance, social activities, and relationships with others. Symptoms respond to support and reassurance.

Clinical Findings

The presentation of serious depression in adolescence may be similar to that in adults, with vegetative signs such as depressed mood, crying spells or inability to cry, discouragement, irritability, a sense of emptiness and meaninglessness, negative expectations of oneself and the environment, low self-esteem, isolation, a feeling of helplessness, diminished interest or pleasure in activities, weight loss or weight gain, insomnia or hypersomnia, fatigue or loss of energy, feelings of worthlessness, and diminished ability to think or concentrate. However, it is not unusual for a serious depression to be masked because the teenager cannot tolerate the severe feelings of sadness. Such a teenager may present with recurrent or persistent psychosomatic complaints, such as abdominal pain, chest pain, headache, lethargy, weight loss, dizziness and syncope, or other nonspecific symptoms. Other behavioral manifestations of masked depression include truancy, running away from home, defiance of authorities, self-destructive behavior, vandalism, drug and alcohol abuse, sexual acting out, and delinquency.

Differential Diagnosis

A complete history and physical examination, including a careful review of the patient's medical and psychoso-

cial history, should be performed. The family history should be explored for psychiatric problems.

The teenager should be questioned about the previously listed symptoms of depression, and specifically about suicidal ideation or preoccupation with thoughts of death. The history should include an assessment of school performance, looking for signs of academic deterioration, excessive absence or cutting class, changes in work or other outside activities, and changes in the family (eg, separation, divorce, serious illness, loss of employment by a parent, a recent move to a new school, increasing quarrels or fights with parents, or the death of a close relative). The teenager may have withdrawn from friends or family or switched allegiance to a new group of friends. The physician should seek to develop a history of drug and alcohol abuse, conflicts with the police, sexual acting out, running away from home, unusually violent or rebellious behavior, or radical personality changes. Patients with vague somatic complaints or concerns about having a fatal illness may have an underlying affective disorder.

Adolescents presenting with symptoms of depression require a thorough medical evaluation to rule out any contributing or underlying medical illness. Among the medical conditions associated with affective disorders are eating disorders, organic central nervous system disorders (tumors, vascular lesions, closed head trauma, and subdural hematomas), metabolic and endocrinologic disorders (systemic lupus erythematosus, hypothyroidism, hyperthyroidism, Wilson disease, hyperparathyroidism, Cushing syndrome, Addison disease, or premenstrual syndrome), infections (infectious mononucleosis or syphilis), and mitral valve prolapse. Marijuana use, phencyclidine abuse, amphetamine withdrawal, and excessive caffeine intake can cause symptoms of depression. Common prescription and over-the-counter medications, including birth control pills, anticonvulsants, and β-blockers, may cause depressive symptoms.

Some routine laboratory studies are indicated in the depressed patient to rule out organic disease: a complete blood count and erythrocyte sedimentation rate, urinalysis, serum electrolytes, blood urea nitrogen, serum calcium, thyroxine and thyroid-stimulating hormone (TSH), Venereal Disease Research Laboratory or rapid plasma reagin, and liver enzymes. Although metabolic markers such as abnormal secretion of cortisol, growth hormone, and thyrotropin-releasing hormone have been useful in confirming major depression in adults, these neurobiologic markers are less reliable in adolescents.

The risk of depression appears to be greatest in families with a history of early-onset and chronic depression. Depression of early onset and bipolar illness are more likely to occur in families with a strong multigenerational history of depression. The lifetime risk of depressive illness in first-degree relatives of adult depressed patients has been estimated to be between 18% and 30%.

Treatment

The primary care physician may be able to counsel adolescents and parents if depression is mild or is the result of an acute personal loss or frustration and if the patient is not contemplating suicide or other life-threatening behaviors. If, however, there is evidence of a long-standing depressive disorder, suicidal thoughts, or psychotic thinking, or if the physician does not feel competent or has no interest in counseling the patient, psychological referral should be made.

Counseling involves establishing and maintaining a positive supportive relationship; following the patient at least weekly; remaining accessible to the patient at all times; encouraging the patient to express emotions openly, defining the problem and clarifying negative feelings, thoughts, and expectations; setting realistic goals; helping to negotiate interpersonal crises; teaching assertiveness and social skills; reassessing the depression as it is expressed; and staying alert to the possibility of suicide.

Patients with a clinical course consistent with bipolar disease or those who have a significant depression that is unresponsive to supportive counseling should be referred to a psychiatrist for evaluation for antidepressant medication. Tricyclic antidepressant medication may be extremely useful in treating serious adolescent depression, especially if there is a family history of depression that was responsive to medication. The Food and Drug Administration has issued a "black box warning" alerting providers that using antidepressants in children and adolescents my increase the risk of suicidal thoughts and behavior (suicidality). Adolescents taking these medications should be monitored closely.

Belmaker RH: Bipolar disorder. N Engl J Med 2004;351:476 (Review) [PMID: 15282355].

Brent DA, Birmaher B: Clinical practice. Adolescent depression. N Engl J Med 2002;347:667 [PMID: 12200555].

Jellinek MS, Snyder JB: Depression and suicide in children and adolescents. Pediatr Rev 1998;19:255 [PMID: 9707715].

March J et al: Fluoxetine, cognitive-behavioral therapy, and their combination for adolescents with depression: Treatment for Adolescents with Depression Study (TADS) randomized controlled trial. JAMA 2004;292:807 [PMID: 15315995].

Whooley MA, Simon GE: Managing depression in medical outpatients. N Engl J Med 2000;343:1942 [PMID: 11136266].

ADOLESCENT SUICIDE (See Also Chapter 6.)

In 2000, 3994 people age 15–24 years committed suicide, there were 1621 suicides among those age 15–19 years, and 2378 among those age 20–24 years. In the younger group, males had a suicide rate five times higher than females, and white males had the highest rate, 15.5 per 100,000. The incidence of unsuccessful suicide attempts is three times higher in females than in males. The estimated ratio of attempted suicides to actual suicides is estimated to be 100:1–50:1. Firearms account for 67% of suicide deaths in both males and females.

With the normal mood swings of adolescence, short periods of depression are common, and a teenager may have thoughts of suicide. Normal mood swings during this period rarely interfere with sleeping, eating, or participating in normal activities. Acute depressive reactions (transient grief responses) to the loss of a family member or friend may result in depression lasting for weeks or even months. An adolescent who is unable to work through this grief can become increasingly depressed. A teenager who is unable to keep up with schoolwork, does not participate in normal social activities, withdraws socially, has sleep and appetite disturbances, and has feelings of hopelessness and helplessness should be considered to be at increased risk for suicide.

Another group of suicidal adolescents is composed of angry teenagers attempting to influence others by their actions. They may be only mildly depressed and may not have a long-standing wish to die. Teenagers in this group, usually females, may attempt suicide or make a suicidal gesture as a way of getting back at someone or gaining attention by frightening another person.

The last group at risk for suicide are adolescents with a serious psychiatric problem such as acute schizophrenia or a true psychotic depressive disorder.

Risk Assessment

The physician must determine the extent of the teenager's depression and assess the risk of inflicting self-harm. The evaluation should include interviews with both the teenager and the family. The history should include the medical, social, emotional, and academic background. The physician should inquire about:

1. Common signs of depression
2. Recent events that could be the cause of an underlying depression
3. Evidence of long-standing problems in the home, at school, or with peers
4. Drug or substance use and abuse
5. Signs of psychotic thinking, such as delusions or hallucinations
6. Evidence of masked depression, such as rebellious behavior, running away from home, reckless driving, or other acting-out behavior

When seeing depressed patients, the physician should always inquire about thoughts of suicide, for example by asking, "Are things ever so bad that life doesn't seem worth living?" If the response is affirmative, a more specific question should be asked, for example, "Have you thought of taking your life?" If the patient has thoughts of suicide, the immediacy of risk can be assessed by determining if the patient has a concrete, feasible plan. Although patients who are at greatest risk have a concrete plan that can be carried out in the near future, especially if they have rehearsed the plan, the physician should not dismiss the potential risk of suicide in the adolescent who does not describe a specific plan. The physician should pay attention to his or her gut feelings. Subtle nonverbal signs may indicate that the patient is at greater risk than may be apparent.

Treatment

The primary care physician is often in a unique position to identify an adolescent at risk for suicide, because many teenagers who attempt suicide seek medical attention in the weeks preceding the attempt. These visits are often for vague somatic complaints. If the patient shows evidence of depression, the physician must assess the severity of the depression and suicidal risk. The pediatrician should always seek emergency psychological consultation for any teenager who is severely depressed, psychotic, or acutely suicidal. It is the psychologist's or psychiatrist's responsibility to assess the seriousness of suicidal ideation and decide whether hospitalization or outpatient treatment is most appropriate. Adolescents with mild depression and at low risk for suicide should be followed closely, and the extent of the depression should be assessed on an ongoing basis. If at any point it appears that the patient is worsening or the teenager is not responding to supportive counseling, referral should be made.

American Academy of Child and Adolescent Psychiatry: Summary of the practice parameters for the assessment and treatment of children and adolescents with suicidal behavior. J Am Acad Child Adolesc Psychiatry 2001;40:495 [PMID: 11314578].

American Academy of Pediatrics Committee on Adolescence: Suicide and suicide attempts in adolescents. Pediatrics 2000; 105:871 [PMID: 10742349].

Grossman DC et al: Self-inflicted and unintentional firearm injuries among children and adolescents: The source of the firearm. Arch Pediatr Adolesc Med 1999;153:875 [PMID: 10437764].

Hatcher-Kay C, King CA: Depression and suicide. Pediatr Rev 2003;24:363.

Zametkin AJ et al: Suicide in teenagers: Assessment, management, and prevention. JAMA 2001;286:3120 [PMID: 11754678].

SUBSTANCE ABUSE

Substance abuse is a complex problem for adolescents and the broader society. See Chapter 4 for an in-depth look at this issue.

EATING DISORDERS (See Chapter 5.)

OVERWEIGHT (See Chapter 10.)

Overweight is defined as body mass index (BMI) greater than the 95th percentile for age (Figures 3–5 and 3–6). At risk for overweight is defined as BMI greater than the 85th percentile for age. It is important to note that mean BMI changes dramatically with age. For a 13-year-old, a BMI > 25 constitutes overweight, whereas in adolescents older than 18, the adult standard of BMI > 30 defines obesity (Figure 3–7). The term obesity is generally not used in the pediatric patient.

Background

Data from the National Health and Nutrition Examination Survey showed an increase in overweight in adolescents ages 12–19 from 5% in 1966–1970 to 16% in 1999–2002. The changes in BMI during and after adolescence have been shown to be important predictors of adult adiposity. In general, the longer a child remains overweight, the more likely obesity will persist into adulthood. The medical risks associated with obesity are discussed in Chapter 10. The psychosocial hazards of overweight tend to be great for adolescents, who may experience alienation, distorted peer relations, poor self-esteem, guilt, depression, or altered body image.

Diagnosis

Patients can be identified as at risk for overweight based on current weight relative to height, growth, and weight trends, and weights of family members. In addition, the provider needs to assess a patient's readiness to make lifestyle changes. When overweight is diagnosed, the following data can be collected: height; weight; BMI; blood pressure; condition of the skin, thyroid, heart, and abdomen; hematocrit; and urinalysis. Acanthosis nigricans is a cutaneous finding characterized by velvety hyperpigmentation, most prominent behind the neck, in the axilla, and in the groin. Acanthosis nigricans is more commonly seen in dark-skinned persons and is a marker for insulin resistance. Endocrine causes of obesity, such as hypothyroidism and Cushing disease, can generally be excluded on the basis of the history and physical examination. If an adolescent is healthy and has no delay of growth or sexual maturation, an underlying endocrinologic, neurologic, or genetic cause is unlikely.

Treatment

Poorly motivated adolescents may be alienated by an aggressive discussion of weight loss. Instead, providers may give basic information about healthy diet and regular exercise and be available for future visits if patients become interested in weight loss. For the highly moti-

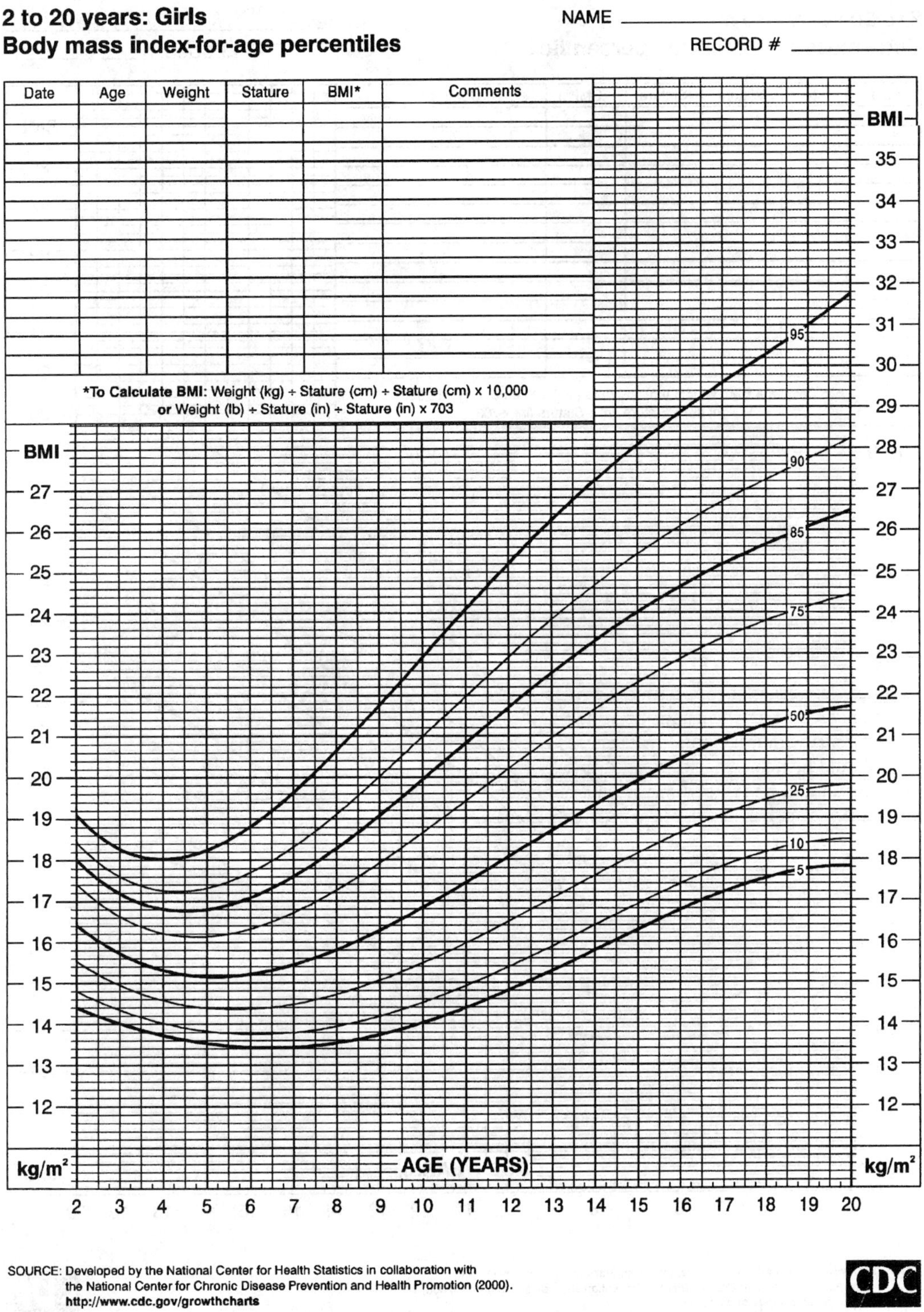

2 to 20 years: Girls
Body mass index-for-age percentiles

NAME _____

RECORD # _____

Date	Age	Weight	Stature	BMI*	Comments

*To Calculate BMI: Weight (kg) ÷ Stature (cm) ÷ Stature (cm) x 10,000
or Weight (lb) ÷ Stature (in) ÷ Stature (in) x 703

Figure 3–5. Percentile values for BMI (kg/m²) in girls. (Centers for Disease Control and Prevention.)

2 to 20 years: Boys
Body mass index-for-age percentiles

NAME _____

RECORD # _____

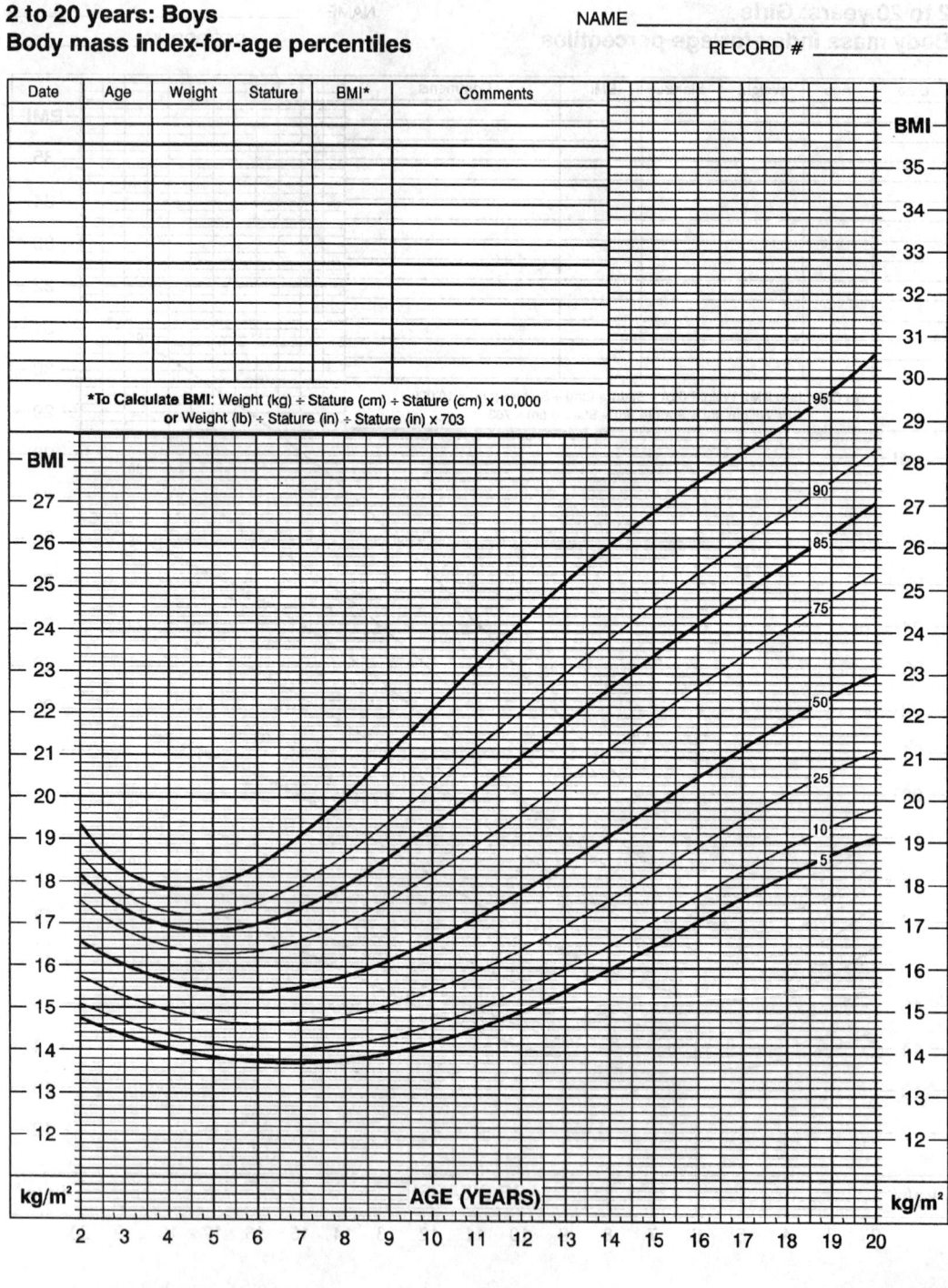

*To Calculate BMI: Weight (kg) ÷ Stature (cm) ÷ Stature (cm) x 10,000
or Weight (lb) ÷ Stature (in) ÷ Stature (in) x 703

SOURCE: Developed by the National Center for Health Statistics in collaboration with
the National Center for Chronic Disease Prevention and Health Promotion (2000).
http://www.cdc.gov/growthcharts

Figure 3–6. Percentile values for BMI (kg/m²) in boys. (Centers for Disease Control and Prevention.)

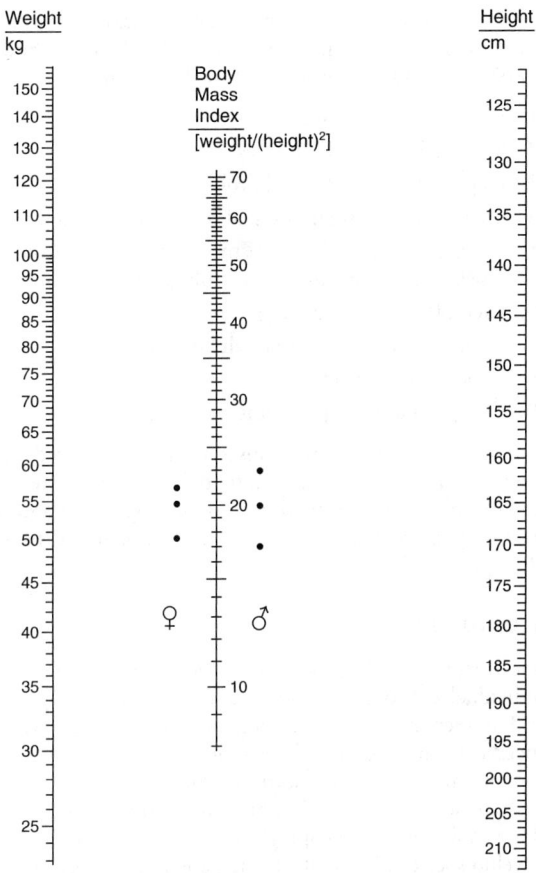

Weight
kg

Body
Mass
Index
[weight/(height)²]

Height
cm

Figure 3–7. Nomogram for determining body mass index (BMI) from height and weight. A straight-edge connecting weight and height allows one to read BMI (weight in kg ÷ [height in m²]). The three dots on the left side of the BMI line represent 50th percentile values for females age 20 years (**top**), 15 years (**middle**), and 10 years (**bottom**). The dots on the right side are for similar-aged males. (Reproduced, with permission, from Forbes GR: Nutrition and Growth. In Mcanarney ER et al [editors]: *Textbook of Adolescent Medicine.* WB Saunders, 1992.)

vated patient, treatment should be appropriate to age and developmental level. The adolescent should be taught appropriate eating and exercise habits to maintain weight reduction yet meet nutritional needs for growth and development. Providers may be more likely to engage the average adolescent by helping him or her to choose concrete, obtainable goals (decreasing soda or other sugared drinks from three to two per day, or walking with a friend 3 days a week instead of watching television). Appetite-suppressing drugs, fasting, and bypass surgery have no role in the management of over-weight adolescents unless severe comorbidities of over-weight are present. An age-appropriate behavior modification program incorporating good dietary counseling and exercise is optimal, although a report from the U.S. Preventive Services Task Force did not find sufficient evidence that behavioral counseling is effective. Studies indicate that increased activity may be more important than dietary changes in long-term weight management. Lifestyle activity recommendations, such as walking and taking the stairs, may be more effective in the long run than regimented exercise programs. Avoiding labeling any food as "forbidden" may improve long-term success with healthful eating behaviors. Behavioral treatment involving parents has been shown to improve long-term maintenance of weight loss in children; parental involvement in adolescent weight loss programs has shown mixed results. In general, the most important factor in successful weight loss and weight maintenance is motivation of the adolescent. Monthly follow-up visits may help to maintain motivation, especially initially. Unfortunately, no program has been proven effective for long-term weight reduction.

National Center for Health Statistics: Prevalence of overweight among children and adolescence: United States, 1999–2002. http://www.cdc.gov/nchs/products/pubs/pubd/hestats/overwght99.htm

U.S. Preventive Services Task Force: Screening and Interventions for overweight in children and adolescents: recommendation statement. Pediatrics 2005;116:205.

SCHOOL AVOIDANCE

Any teenager who has missed more than 1 week of school for a physical illness or symptom, and whose clinical picture is inconsistent with a serious illness, should be suspected of harboring primary or secondary emotional factors that contribute to the absence. Investigation of absences may show a pattern, such as missing morning classes or missing the same days at the beginning or end of the week. Emotional factors for school absenteeism are usually attributed to physical symptoms in this age group.

School avoidance should be suspected in children who are consistently absent in spite of parents' and professionals' attempts to encourage school attendance. Adolescents with school avoidance problems often have a history of excessive absences or separation difficulties as a younger child. They may also have a record of recurrent somatic complaints. Parents of a school avoider often feel helpless to compel their adolescent to attend school, may lack the sophistication to distinguish malingering from illness, or may have an underlying need to keep the teenager at home.

A complete history and physical examination should be performed, reviewing the patient's medical, educational, and psychiatric history. Signs of emotional problems should be explored. After obtaining permission from the patient and parents, the physician may find it helpful to speak directly with school officials and some key teachers. The adolescent may be having problems with particular teachers or subjects or experiencing adversity at school (eg, schoolyard bullying or an intimidating instructor). Some students get so far behind academically that they see no way of catching up and feel overwhelmed. Separation anxiety, sometimes of long duration, may be manifested in subconscious worries that something may happen to the mother while the teenager is at school.

The school nurse may give useful information, including the number of visits to the nurse during the last school year. An important part of the history is how the parents respond to the absences and somatic complaints. The parent(s) may be making a subconscious attempt to keep the adolescent at home, which may be coupled with secondary gains for the patient, such as increased parental attention.

Treatment

The importance of returning to school quickly after a period of school avoidance needs to be emphasized. The pediatrician should facilitate this process by offering to speak with school officials to excuse missed examinations, homework, and papers. The pediatrician should speak directly with teachers who are punitive. The objective is to make the transition back to school as easy as possible. The longer adolescents stay out of school, the more anxious they may become about returning and the more difficult the return becomes. If an illness or symptom becomes so severe that an adolescent cannot go to school, the patient and the parents must be informed that a visit to a medical office is necessary. The physician focuses visits on the parents as much as on the adolescent to alleviate any parental guilt about sending the child to school. If the adolescent cannot stay in school, hospitalization should be recommended for an in-depth medical and psychiatric evaluation. Parents should be cautioned about the possibility of relapse after school holidays, summer vacation, or an acute illness.

Klerman LV: School absence: A health perspective. Pediatr Clin North Am 1988;35:1253 [PMID: 3059298].

SCHOOL FAILURE

When children graduate from grade school to middle school or junior high school, the amount and complexity of course work increase significantly. This occurs at about the same time as the rapid physical, social, and emotional changes of puberty. To perform well academically, young adolescents must have the necessary cognitive capacity, study habits, concentration, motivation, interest, and emotional focus. Academic failure presenting at adolescence has a broad differential:

1. Limited intellectual abilities
2. Specific learning disabilities
3. Depression or emotional problems
4. Physical causes such as visual or hearing problems
5. Excessive school absenteeism secondary to chronic disease such as asthma or neurologic dysfunction
6. Lack of ability to concentrate
7. Attention-deficit/hyperactivity disorder
8. Lack of motivation
9. Drug and alcohol problems

Each of these possible causes must be explored in depth. Evaluation of this differential requires a careful history, physical examination, and appropriate laboratory tests, as well as standardized educational and psychological testing.

Treatment

Treatment depends on the cause. Management must be individualized to address specific needs, foster strengths, and implement a feasible program. For children with specific learning disabilities, an individual prescription for regular and special education courses, teachers, and extracurricular activities is important. Counseling helps these adolescents gain coping skills, raise self-esteem, and develop socialization skills. If the patient has a history of hyperactivity or attention-deficit disorder along with poor ability to concentrate, a trial of stimulant medication (eg, methylphenidate or dextroamphetamine) may be useful. If the teenager appears to be depressed or if other serious emotional problems are uncovered, further psychological evaluation should be recommended.

Reiff MI: Adolescent school failure. Failure to thrive in adolescence. Pediatr Rev 1998;19:199 [PMID: 9613171].

Shaywitz SE: Dyslexia. N Engl J Med 1998;338:307 [PMID: 9445412].

Wilens TE, Faraone SV, Biederman J: Attention-deficit/hyperactivity disorder in adults. JAMA 2004;292:619.

Wolraich ML et al: Attention-deficit/hyperactivity disorder among adolescents: A review of the diagnosis, treatment, and clinical implications. Pediatrics 2005;115:1734.

■ BREAST DISORDERS

The breast examination should become part of the routine physical examination in girls as soon as breast budding occurs. The preadolescent thus comes to accept breast examination as a routine part of health care, and the procedure serves as an opportunity to offer reassurance about any concerns she may have. The breast examination begins with inspection of the breasts for symmetry and Tanner or sexual maturity rating (SMR) stage. Asymmetrical breast development is common, especially in young adolescents, and is generally transient, although 25% of women may continue to have some degree of asymmetry into adulthood. Unusual causes of breast asymmetry include unilateral breast hypoplasia, amastia, absence of the pectoralis major muscle, and unilateral virginal hypertrophy (massive enlargement of the breast during puberty).

Palpation of the breasts can be performed with the patient in the supine position and the patient's ipsilateral arm placed behind her head. The examiner palpates the breast tissue with the flat of the fingers in concentric circles from the sternum, clavicle, and axilla in to the areola. The areola should be compressed gently to check for discharge.

Instructions for breast self-examination and its purpose can be given to older adolescents approaching age 18 years during this portion of the physical examination, and the patient should be encouraged to begin monthly self-examination after each menstrual flow after age 18 years. Because the vast majority of breast lesions in teens are benign, teaching young adolescents breast self-examination may lead to unnecessary anxiety and overconcern with normal variants.

BREAST MASSES

Most breast masses in adolescents are benign (Table 3–1); however, cancer does occasionally occur in adolescents. Malignancies include hemangiosarcoma, rhabdomyosarcoma, ductal carcinoma, cystosarcoma phyllodes, and metastatic tumor.

Fibroadenoma

Fibroadenoma (which accounts for approximately two-thirds of all breast masses in adolescents) presents as a rubbery, well-demarcated, slowly growing, nontender mass that may occur in any quadrant, but is most commonly found in the upper outer quadrant. The average size is 2–3 cm in diameter. In 10–25% of cases, multiple or recurrent lesions occur. Quiescence can be expected after the teenage years.

Cysts

Breast cysts are generally tender and spongy, with exacerbation of symptoms premenstrually and improvement after menses. Often they are multiple. Spontaneous regression occurs over two or three menstrual cycles in about 50% of cases.

Table 3–1. Breast masses in adolescent females.

Common
Fibroadenoma
Fibrocystic changes
Breast cysts
Breast abscess/mastitis
Less common or rare (benign)
Lymphangioma
Hemangioma
Giant fibroadenoma
Neurofibromatosis
Nipple adenoma/keratoma
Mammary duct ectasia
Lipoma
Hematoma
Rare (malignant potential)
Adenocarcinoma
Cystosarcoma phyllodes
Intraductal papilloma
Rhabdomyosarcoma
Lymphosarcoma
Hemangiosarcoma
Metastatic cancer

It is reasonable to follow breast masses that are consistent with fibroadenoma or cyst in adolescents for two or three menstrual cycles. Approximately 25% of fibroadenomas become smaller, and approximately 50% of cysts resolve. If a presumed fibroadenoma does not change after this time, ultrasound will differentiate a solid tumor from a cyst. Patients with solid tumors larger than 2.5 cm in diameter should be referred for fine-needle aspiration or excisional biopsy. Those with tumors less than 2.5 cm in diameter may be followed every 3–6 months, because many of these tumors will shrink or remain the same. Persistent cystic lesions may be drained by needle aspiration. Patients with suspicious lesions should be referred immediately to a breast surgeon (Table 3–2).

Fibrocystic Breasts

Fibrocystic breast disease sometimes occurs in older adolescents and becomes more common with age. It is characterized by cyclic tenderness and nodularity bilaterally and is believed to be influenced by the estrogen-progesterone balance.

Reassuring the young woman about the benign nature of the process and emphasizing the importance of breast self-examination as she becomes an adult may be all that is needed. Support bras may provide symptomatic relief. Oral contraceptive pills (OCPs) often improve symptoms. Studies have shown no association between methylxanthines and fibrocystic breasts; how-

Table 3–2. Breast lesions.

Fibroadenoma	Rubbery, well demarcated, nontender, slowly growing; most commonly found in the upper outer quadrant of the breast. Usually < 5 cm.
Adenocarcinoma	Hard, nonmobile, well-circumscribed, painless mass; generally indolent clinical course; occurs also in males but less frequently.
Cystosarcoma phyllodes	Firm, rubbery mass that may suddenly enlarge; associated with skin necrosis; most often benign.
Giant juvenile fibroadenoma	Remarkable large fibroadenoma with overlying dilated superficial veins; accounts for 5–10% of fibroadenomas in adolescents; benign but requires excision to prevent breast atrophy and for cosmetic reasons.
Intraductal papilloma	A cylindric tumor arising from the ductal epithelium; often subareolar but may be in the periphery of the breast in adolescents, with associated nipple discharge. Most are benign but require excision for cytologic diagnosis.
Fat necrosis	Localized inflammatory process in one breast; follows trauma in about half of cases. Subsequent scarring may be confused with cancer.
Virginal or juvenile hypertrophy	Massive enlargement of both breasts or, less often, one breast; attributed to end-organ hypersensitivity to normal hormonal levels just before or within a few years after menarche.
Miscellaneous	Fibroma, galactocele, hemangioma, intraductal granuloma, interstitial fibrosis, keratoma, lipoma, granular cell myoblastoma, papilloma, sclerosing adenosis.

ever, some women report reduced symptoms when they discontinue caffeine intake. The efficacy of vitamins E, B_1, and A is unknown. Evening primrose oil was beneficial in 44% of patients in one study. A trial of 1000 mg three times a day for 3 months may be helpful.

Breast Abscess

The female with a breast abscess usually complains of unilateral breast pain, and examination reveals overlying inflammatory changes. Often the examination is misleading in that the infection may extend much deeper than suspected. A palpable mass is found only late in the course. Although breast feeding is the most common cause of mastitis, trauma and eczema involving the areola are frequent factors in teenagers. *Staphylococcus aureus* is the most common pathogen, but other aerobic and anaerobic organisms have also been implicated.

Cyclic mastodynia, fibrocystic disease, or chest wall pain may also be causes of breast pain, but no associated inflammatory signs should be present.

Fluctuant abscesses should be surgically incised and drained. Fluid should be sent for culture. Oral antibiotics with appropriate coverage for methicillin-resistant *S aureus* (dicloxacillin or trimethoprim-sulfamethoxazole) should be given for 2–4 weeks. Ice packs for the first 24 hours and heat thereafter may relieve symptoms.

GALACTORRHEA

In teenagers, galactorrhea is most often benign; however, a careful history and work-up are necessary. Prolactinomas are the most common pathologic cause of galactorrhea in adolescents of both sexes and generally present as amenorrhea or failure of sexual maturation. Hypothyroidism is the second most common cause in the adolescent years but has been reported only in girls, usually prepubertally.

Galactorrhea may be present after spontaneous or induced abortions as well as postpartum. Numerous prescribed and illicit drugs are associated with galactorrhea (Table 3–3). In addition, stimulation of the intercostal nerves (following surgery or due to herpes zoster infection), stimulation of the nipples, central nervous system disorders (hypothalamic injury), or significant emotional distress may produce galactorrhea.

Clinical Findings

If the teenager has no history of pregnancy or drug use, TSH and serum prolactin levels should be determined. An elevated TSH confirms the diagnosis of hypothyroidism. An elevated prolactin and normal TSH, often accompanied by amenorrhea, suggest a hypothalamic or pituitary tumor, and a magnetic resonance imaging scan is indicated. When the prolactin level is normal, uncommon causes such as adrenal, renal, or ovarian tumors should be considered. Males with a negative work-up and normal puberty need to be followed intensively. Males with elevated prolactin levels require a magnetic resonance imaging scan every 12–18 months even if the galactorrhea resolves, because of the significant risk of a small pituitary adenoma that may become apparent with serial examinations.

Treatment

Treatment depends on the underlying cause. Prolactinomas may be removed surgically or suppressed with dopamine agonists such as bromocriptine. Bromocriptine may also be beneficial to some amenorrheic females with nor-

Table 3–3. Medications and herbs associated with galactorrhea.

Antidepressants and anxiolytics	Other drugs
Alprazolam (Xanax)	Amphetamines
Buspirone (BuSpar)	Anesthetics
Monoamine oxidase inhibitors	Arginine
Moclobemide (Manerix;	Cannabis
available in Canada)	Cisapride (Propulsid)
Selective serotonin reuptake	Cyclobenzaprine (Flexeril)
inhibitors	Danazol (Danocrine)
Citalopram (Celexa)	Dihydroergotamine
Fluoxetine (Prozac)	(DHE 45)
Paroxetine (Paxil)	Domperidone (Motilium;
Sertraline (Zoloft)	available in Canada
Tricyclic antidepressants	and Mexico)
Antihypertensives	Isoniazid (INH)
Atenolol (Tenormin)	Metoclopramide
Methyldopa (Aldomet)	(Reglan)
Reserpine (Serpasil)	Octreotide (Sandostatin)
Verapamil (Calan)	Opiates
Antipsychotics	Rimantadine (Flumadine)
Histamine H$_2$-receptor blockers	Sumatriptan (Imitrex)
Cimetidine (Tagamet)	Valproic acid (Depak-
Famotidine (Pepcid)	ene)
Ranitidine (Zantac)	Herbs
Hormones	Anise
Conjugated estrogen and	Blessed thistle
medroxyprogesterone	Fennel
(Premphase, Prempro)	Fenugreek seed
Medroxyprogesterone contra-	Marshmallow
ceptive injections (Depo-	Nettle
Provera)	Red clover
Oral contraceptive formula-	Red raspberry
tions	
Phenothiazines	
Chlorpromazine (Thorazine)	
Prochlorperazine (Compazine)	
Others	

Reprinted, with permission, from American Family Physician.

mal serum prolactin levels. The female with a negative work-up and persistent galactorrhea may be followed with menstrual history and serum prolactin level every 6–12 months. In many cases, symptoms resolve spontaneously and no diagnosis is made. The female with an elevated serum prolactin concentration but negative prolactinoma work-up may be treated with bromocriptine if her symptoms are bothersome or may be observed with a magnetic resonance imaging scan every 1–2 years for several years.

GYNECOMASTIA

Gynecomastia is a common concern of male adolescents, most of whom (60–70%) develop transient sub-

areolar breast tissue during SMR stages 2 and 3. Proposed causes include testosterone-estrogen imbalance, increased serum prolactin level, and abnormal serum protein binding levels.

Clinical Findings

In type I idiopathic gynecomastia, the adolescent presents with a unilateral (20% bilateral) tender, firm mass beneath the areola. More generalized breast enlargement is classified as type II. Pseudogynecomastia is the term for excessive fat tissue or prominent pectoralis muscles.

Differential Diagnosis

Gynecomastia may be drug-induced (Table 3–4). Testicular, adrenal, or pituitary tumors, Klinefelter syndrome, primary hypogonadism, thyroid or hepatic dysfunction, or malnutrition may also be associated with gynecomastia (Table 3–5). Onset of gynecomastia in late (rather than early or middle) adolescence is more likely indicative of pathology.

Treatment

If gynecomastia is idiopathic, reassurance about the common and benign nature of the process can be given. Resolution may take up to 2 years. Medical reduction has been achieved with pharmacotherapeutic agents, such as dihydrotestosterone, danazol, clomiphene, and tamoxifen, but these agents should be reserved for patients in whom no decrease in breast size occurs after 2 years. Surgery is reserved for those with significant psychological trauma or severe breast enlargement.

Table 3–4. Drugs associated with gynecomastia.

Antibiotics	**Drugs and substances of abuse**
Isoniazid	Alcohol
Ketoconazole	Amphetamines
Metronidazole	Marijuana
Anti-ulcer drugs	Opiates
Cimetidine	**Hormones or related agents**
Omeprazole	Anabolic steroids
Ranitidine	Estrogens
Cardiovascular drugs	Chorionic gonadotropin
Captopril	**Psychoactive medications**
Digoxin	Tricyclic antidepressants, eg,
Enalapril	amitriptyline
Methyldopa	Antipsychotics, eg, chlorproma-
Reserpine	zine, fluphenazine, haloperidol
Verapamil	Anxiolytics, eg, chlordiaze-
Chemotherapeutic drugs	poxide, diazepam
Busulfan	
Vincristine	

Table 3–5. Disorders associated with gynecomastia.

Klinefelter syndrome
Traumatic paraplegia
Male pseudohermaphroditism
Testicular feminization syndrome
Reifenstein syndrome
17-Ketosteroid reductase deficiency
Endocrine tumors (seminoma, Leydig cell tumor, teratoma,
  feminizing adrenal tumor, hepatoma, leukemia, hemophilia,
  bronchogenic carcinoma, leprosy, etc)
Hypothyroidism
Hyperthyroidism
Cirrhosis
Herpes zoster
Friedreich ataxia

Arca MJ, Caniano DA: Breast disorders in the adolescent patient. Adolesc Med Clin 2004;15:473 [PMID: 15625988].

Lazala C, Saenger P: Pubertal gynecomastia. J Pediatr Endocrinol Metab 2002;15:553 [PMID: 12014513].

■ GYNECOLOGIC DISORDERS IN ADOLESCENCE

PHYSIOLOGY OF MENSTRUATION

The ovulatory menstrual cycle is divided into three consecutive phases: follicular (the first 14 days), ovulatory (midcycle), and luteal (days 16–28). During the follicular phase, pulsatile gonadotropin-releasing hormone from the hypothalamus stimulates anterior pituitary secretion of FSH and LH. Under the influence of FSH and LH, a dominant ovarian follicle emerges by days 5–7 of the menstrual cycle, and the other follicles become atretic. Rising estradiol levels produced by the maturing follicle cause proliferation of the endometrium. By the midfollicular phase, FSH is beginning to decline secondary to estradiol-mediated negative feedback, whereas LH continues to rise as a result of estradiol-mediated positive feedback.

The rising LH initiates progesterone secretion and luteinization of the granulosa cells of the follicle. Progesterone in turn further stimulates LH and FSH. This leads to the LH surge, which causes the follicle to rupture and expel the oocyte.

During the luteal phase, LH and FSH gradually decline. The corpus luteum secretes progesterones. The endometrium enters the secretory phase in response to rising levels of estrogen and progesterone, with maturation 8–9 days after ovulation. If no pregnancy occurs or placental human chorionic gonadotropin is released, luteolysis begins; estrogen and progesterone levels decline; and the endometrial lining is shed as menstrual flow approximately 14 days after ovulation (Figure 3–8).

During the first 2 years after menarche, the majority of cycles are anovulatory (50–80%). Between 10% and 20% of cycles remain anovulatory for up to 5 years after menarche.

PELVIC EXAMINATION

A pelvic examination may be indicated to evaluate abdominal pain or menstrual disorders or to detect a suspected STI in the adolescent. It has previously been recommended that a routine pelvic examination be done at age 18 years to obtain the first Papanicolaou (Pap) smear and to evaluate reproductive anatomy. Recommendations have changed to delay the first Pap smear until age 21 years in the absence of menstrual problems in patients who have never had intercourse. The first Pap smear should be performed within 3 years of the initiation of sexual activity. Pap smears should be performed earlier in adolescents with a history of sexual abuse with penile penetration. The adolescent may be apprehensive about the first examination. It should not be rushed, and an explanation of the procedure and its purpose should precede it. The patient can be encouraged to relax by slow, deep breathing and by relaxation of her lower abdominal and inner thigh muscles. A young adolescent may wish to have her mother present during the examination, but the history should be taken privately. A female chaperone should be present with male examiners.

The pelvic examination begins by placing the patient in the dorsal lithotomy position after equipment and supplies are ready (Table 3–6). The examiner inspects the external genitalia, noting the pubic hair maturity rating, the size of the clitoris (2–5 mm is normal), Skene glands just inside the urethral meatus, and Bartholin glands at 4 o'clock and 8 o'clock outside the hymenal ring. In cases of alleged sexual abuse or assault, the horizontal measurement of the relaxed prepubertal hymenal opening should be recorded and the presence of any lacerations, bruises, scarring, or synechiae about the hymen, vulva, or anus should be noted.

A vaginal speculum is then inserted at a 45-degree twist and angled 45 degrees downward. (A medium Pedersen speculum is most often used in sexually experienced patients; a narrow Huffman is used for virginal patients.) The vaginal walls are inspected for estrogen effects, inflammation, or lesions. The cervix should be dull pink. Cervical ectropion is commonly observed in adolescents; the columnar epithelium extends outside

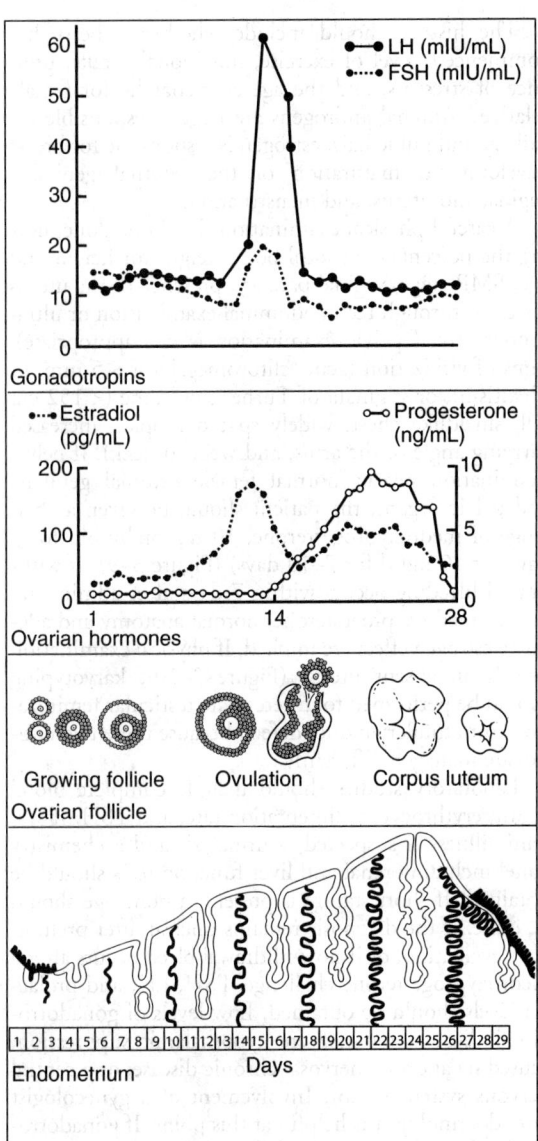

Figure 3–8. Physiology of the normal ovulatory menstrual cycle; gonadotropin secretion, ovarian hormone production, follicular maturation, and endometrial changes during one cycle. FSH, follicle-stimulating hormone, LH, luteinizing hormone. (Reproduced, with permission, from Emans SJH et al: *Pediatric and Adolescent Gynecology,* 4th ed. Little, Brown, 1998.)

the cervical os onto the face of the cervix until later adolescence, when it recedes.

Specimens are obtained, including a wet preparation for leukocytes, trichomonads, and clue cells (vaginal epi-

Table 3–6. Items for pelvic exam tray.

Medium and virginal speculums (warm)
Gloves
Applicator sticks, sterile
Large swabs to remove excess discharge
Cervical spatulas, cervical brushes
Microscope slides and cover slips (frosted and labeled)
Centrifuge tube or test tube (if swab is to be placed in drop of saline and slide prepared later)
NaCl dropper bottle
KOH dropper bottle
Slide container to send to lab
Gonorrhea test media
Chlamydia test media
Lubricant
Facial tissue

thelial cells stippled with adherent bacteria); potassium hydroxide preparation for yeast and whiff test; cervical swab for gonorrhea and *Chlamydia;* and endocervical and cervical samples for Pap smear testing if indicated. A cervical brush provides a higher yield of cells for the endocervical Pap slide. Pap smears should be interpreted by a cytopathologist at a laboratory using the Bethesda system of classification. Liquid-based Pap testing is often used with reflex human papillomavirus testing if the Pap result is atypical squamous cells of uncertain etiology.

The speculum is then removed, and bimanual examination is performed to assess uterine size and position, adnexal enlargement or tenderness, or cervical motion tenderness. Bimanual examination may reveal beading in the adnexa secondary to endometriosis.

MENSTRUAL DISORDERS

1. Amenorrhea

Amenorrhea is the lack of onset of menses when normally anticipated. Primary amenorrhea is no menstrual periods or secondary sex characteristics by age 14 years or no menses in the presence of secondary sex characteristics by age 15 years. Constitutional delay is normal pubertal progression at a delayed onset or rate. Secondary amenorrhea is defined as the absence of menses for at least three cycles after regular cycles have been present. In some instances, evaluation should begin immediately, without waiting for the specified age or duration of lapsed periods, such as in patients with suspected pregnancy, short stature with the stigmata of Turner syndrome, or an anatomic defect.

Evaluation for Primary Amenorrhea

Primary amenorrhea may be the result of anatomic abnormalities, chromosomal deviations, or physiologic delay (Table 3–7).

Table 3–7. Causes of amenorrhea.

Hypothalamic-pituitary axis
Hypothalamic repression
  Emotional stress
  Depression
  Chronic disease
  Weight loss
  Obesity
  Severe dieting
  Strenuous athletics
  Drugs (post–birth control pills, phenothiazines)
Central nervous system lesion
  Pituitary lesion: adenoma, prolactinoma
  Craniopharyngioma, brainstem, or parasellar tumors
  Head injury with hypothalamic contusion
  Infiltrative process (sarcoidosis)
  Vascular disease (hypothalamic vasculitis)
Congenital conditions[a]
  Kallmann syndrome
Ovaries
Gonadal dysgenesis[a]
  Turner syndrome (XO)
  Mosaic (XX/XO)
Injury to ovary
  Autoimmune disease
  Infection (mumps, oophoritis)
  Toxins (alkylating chemotherapeutic agents)
  Irradiation
  Trauma, torsion (rare)
Polycystic ovary syndrome
Ovarian failure
  Premature menopause
  Resistant ovary
Uterovaginal outflow tract
Müllerian dysgenesis[a]
  Congenital deformity or absence of uterus, uterine tubes, or vagina
  Imperforate hymen, transverse vaginal septum, vaginal agenesis, agenesis of the cervix[a]
Testicular feminization (absent uterus)[a]
Uterine lining defect
  Asherman syndrome (intrauterine synechiae post-curettage or endometritis)
  Tuberculosis, brucellosis
Defect in hormone synthesis or action (virilization may be present)
Adrenal hyperplasia[a]
Cushing disease
Adrenal tumor
Ovarian tumor (rare)
Drugs (steroids, ACTH)

[a]Indicates condition that usually presents as primary amenorrhea.
ACTH, adrenocorticotropic hormone.

The history should include whether puberty has commenced, level of exercise, nutritional intake, presence of stressors, and the age at menarche for female relatives. Adrenal androgens are largely responsible for axillary and pubic hair; estrogen is responsible for breast development, maturation of the external genitalia, vagina, and uterus, and menstruation.

A careful physical examination should be done, noting the percentage of ideal body weight for height and age, SMR stage, vaginal patency, presence of the uterus (assessed through rectoabdominal examination or ultrasonography if pelvic examination is not appropriate), signs of virilization (acne, clitoromegaly of > 5 mm, or hirsutism), or stigmata of Turner syndrome (< 152 cm tall, shieldlike chest, widely spaced nipples, increased carrying angle of the arms, and webbed neck). If pelvic examination reveals normal female external genitalia and pelvic organs, the patient should be given a challenge of medroxyprogesterone, 10 mg orally bid for 5 days (or 10 mg/d for 7–10 days) (Figure 3–9). If withdrawal bleeding occurs within 7 days after administration of medroxyprogesterone, normal anatomy and adequate estrogen effect are implied. If physical examination reveals an absent uterus (Figure 3–10), karyotyping should be performed to differentiate testicular feminization from müllerian duct defect, because these two entities are managed differently.

Laboratory studies should include complete blood count, erythrocyte sedimentation rate, and TSH. If systemic illness is suspected, a urinalysis and a chemistry panel including renal and liver function tests should be obtained. If short stature is present, a bone age should be done. If the diagnosis remains unclear after preliminary evaluation, or if no withdrawal bleed occurs after a medroxyprogesterone challenge, FSH, LH, and prolactin levels should be obtained. Low levels of gonadotropins indicate a more severe hypothalamic suppression, caused by anorexia nervosa, chronic disease, or a central nervous system tumor. Involvement of a gynecologist or endocrinologist is helpful at this point. If gonadotropin levels are high, ovarian failure or gonadal dysgenesis is implied, and a karyotype should be obtained.

Evaluation & Treatment of Secondary Amenorrhea

Secondary amenorrhea results when estrogen stimulation is unopposed, maintaining the endometrium in the proliferative phase. The most common causes are pregnancy, stress, and polycystic ovary syndrome (PCOS). Ovarian failure can also present as secondary amenorrhea, caused by mosaic Turner syndrome or autoimmune oophoritis.

The history should focus on issues of stress, chronic illness, drugs, weight change, strenuous exercise, sex-

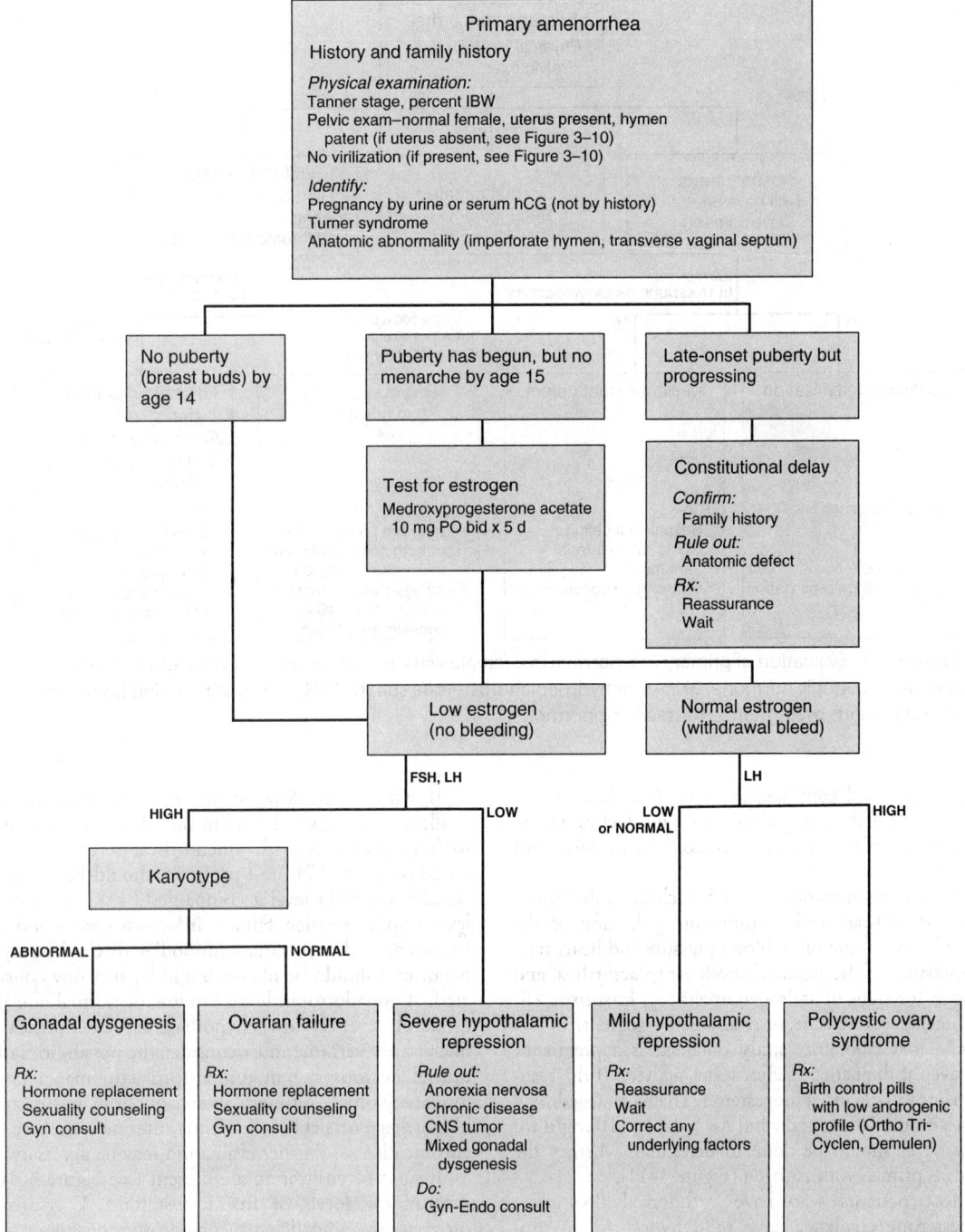

Figure 3–9. Evaluation of primary amenorrhea in a normal female. CNS, central nervous system; FSH, follicle-stimulating hormone; IBW, ideal body weight; LH, luteinizing hormone.

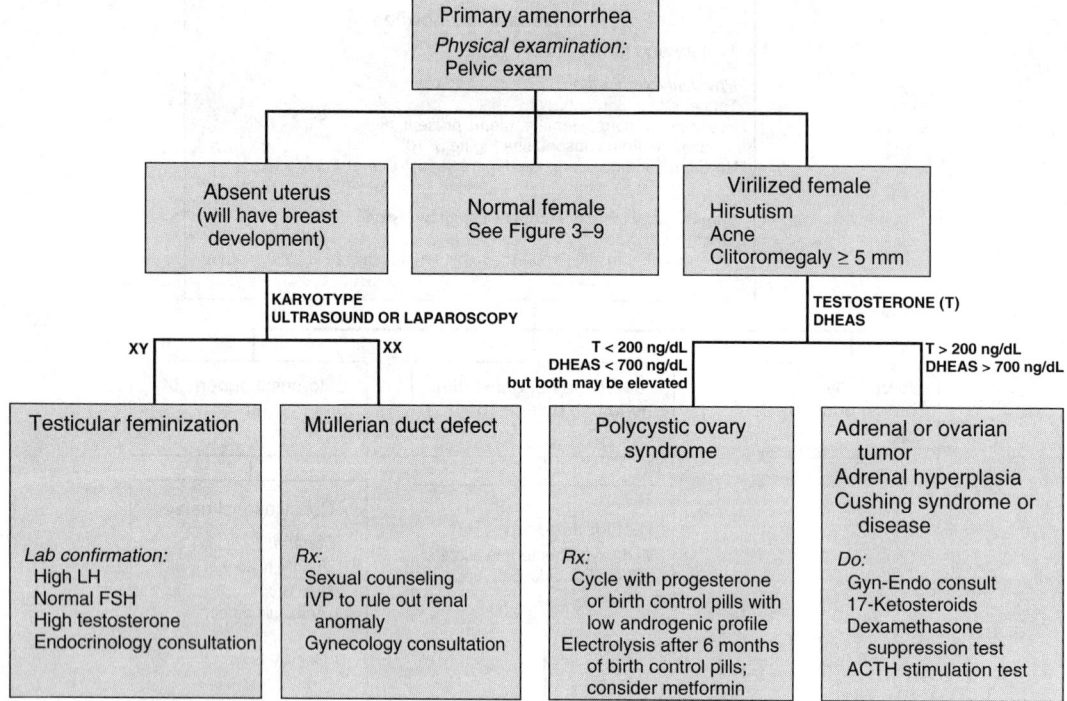

Figure 3–10. Evaluation of primary amenorrhea in a female without a uterus or with virilization. ACTH, adrenocorticotropic hormone; DHEAS, dehydroepiandrosterone sulfate; FSH, follicle-stimulating hormone; IVP, intravenous pyelogram; LH, luteinizing hormone.

ual activity, and contraceptive use. A review of systems should include questions about headaches, visual changes, hirsutism, constipation, cold intolerance, and galactorrhea.

Physical examination should include ophthalmoscopic and visual field examination, palpation of the thyroid, determination of blood pressure and heart rate, compression of the areola to check for galactorrhea, and a search for signs of androgen excess (eg, hirsutism, clitoromegaly, severe acne, or ovarian enlargement).

The first laboratory study obtained is a pregnancy test, even if the patient denies sexual activity. If the teenager is not pregnant, a progesterone challenge (medroxyprogesterone, 10 mg orally bid for 5 days or 10 mg/d for 7–10 days) should be done to determine whether the uterus is primed with estrogen (Figure 3–11).

Most patients who have withdrawal flow after progesterone challenge have mild hypothalamic suppression due to weight change, athletics, stress, or illness; however, disorders such as PCOS, adrenal disorders, ovarian tumors, thyroid disease, and diabetes mellitus should be excluded by history and physical examination and appropriate laboratory studies. (See section on Primary Amenorrhea and Figure 3–10.)

If withdrawal flow occurs after the progesterone challenge (see Figure 3–9), but the adolescent continues to have problems with amenorrhea, serum levels of estradiol, FSH, LH, and prolactin should be checked. An elevated FSH level accompanied by a low estrogen level implies ovarian failure, in which case blood for karyotype and antiovarian antibodies (if the karyotype is normal) should be obtained and laparoscopy considered. If gonadotropin levels are low or normal and the estradiol level is low, hypothalamic amenorrhea is likely; however, one must consider the possibilities of a central nervous system tumor (prolactinoma or craniopharyngioma), pituitary infarction from postpartum hemorrhage or sickle cell anemia, uterine synechiae, or chronic disease. Further evaluation may be necessary.

If signs of virilization are present (see Figure 3–10), determining levels of free testosterone, 17-hydroxyprogesterone, and dehydroepiandrosterone sulfate will help to distinguish PCOS from adrenal causes of virilization and amenorrhea. Although elevation of testosterone and dehydroepiandrosterone sulfate may occur in patients with PCOS, the elevation is not as dramatic as with androgen-producing adrenal or ovarian tumors, adrenal hyperplasia, or Cushing syndrome. Endocrino-

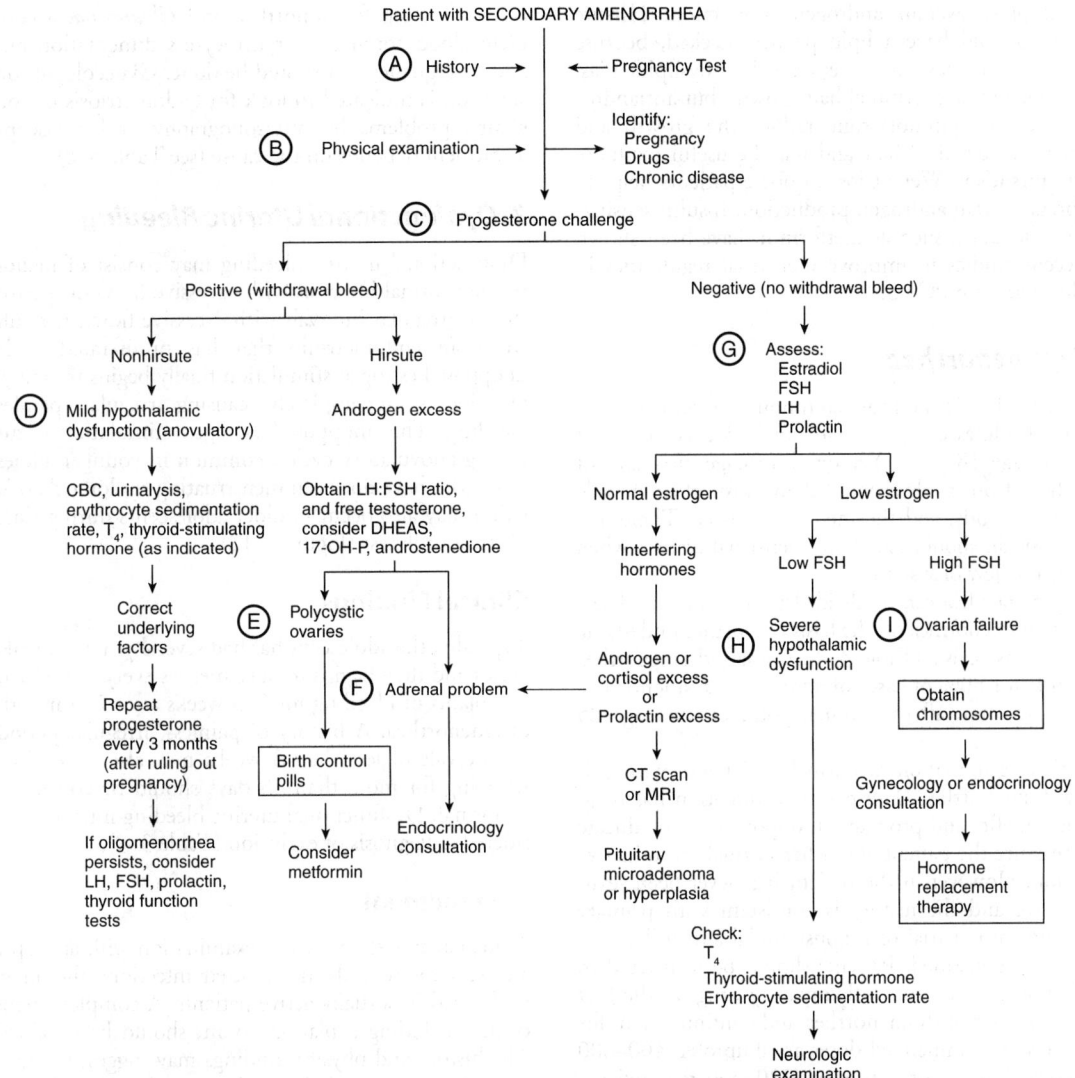

Figure 3–11. Evaluation of secondary amenorrhea. CBC, complete blood count; DHEAS, dehydroepiandrosterone sulfate; FSH, follicle-stimulating hormone; LH, luteinizing hormone; MRI, magnetic resonance imaging scan; T$_4$, thyroxine.

logic consultation will assist in differentiating the cause of significantly elevated androgens.

PCOS is a spectrum of disorders accompanied by symptoms of obesity, insulin resistance, hirsutism, acne, oligomenorrhea, and infertility. PCOS is very common, with a prevalence estimated at 5–10%. Although a classic LH:FSH ratio of greater than 2.5:1 is described in PCOS, up to 40% of patients do not have elevated LH levels. Because of insufficient FSH, androstenedione cannot be converted to estradiol in the ovarian follicle,

and anovulation and production of excess androgens result. Thus another term for PCOS is functional hyperandrogenic anovulation.

Oral contraceptive pills containing a low androgenic progestin (desogestrel or norgestimate) such as Desogen or Ortho Tri-Cyclen help to regulate menses and improve acne and hirsutism. Patients who do not wish to take an oral contraceptive pill can be given progesterone, 10 mg daily, for the first 10 days of each month to allow withdrawal flow; however, this treatment does not suppress ovarian androgen production. Hirsute patients should have a lipid profile checked, because PCOS patients have an increased risk of dyslipidemias. OCPs may reduce terminal hair growth, but antiandrogens such as spironolactone reduce the growth and diameter of terminal hair and may be useful for more severe hirsutism. Weight loss in obese patients helps to suppress ovarian androgen production. Insulin sensitizing medications, such as metformin, have been shown in recent studies to improve menstrual regularities in adolescents with PCOS.

2. Dysmenorrhea

Dysmenorrhea is the most common gynecologic complaint of adolescent girls, with an incidence of about 80% by age 18 years. Yet many teenage girls do not seek help from a physician, relying instead on female relatives, friends, and the media for advice. Therefore, the physician should ask about menstrual cramps when taking a review of systems.

Dysmenorrhea can be divided into primary and secondary dysmenorrhea on the basis of whether underlying pelvic disease exists (Table 3–8). Primary dysmenorrhea accounts for 80% of cases of adolescent dysmenorrhea and most often affects women younger than age 25 years.

Pelvic examination is normal in females with primary dysmenorrhea. The pelvic examination has diagnostic benefits and provides an opportunity to educate and reassure the patient about her normal reproductive function. However, if the patient has never been sexually active and the history is consistent with primary dysmenorrhea, a trial of a nonsteroidal anti-inflammatory drug is justified. Patients should be instructed to begin nonsteroidal anti-inflammatory drugs at the first sign of menses or dysmenorrhea and continue them for 2–3 days. Recommended doses are ibuprofen 400–800 mg every 6 hours or naproxen (220–550 mg) twice a day. If the patient does not respond to nonsteroidal anti-inflammatory drugs, oral contraceptive pills are an effective treatment for primary dysmenorrhea. If patients do not respond to either of these treatments, secondary dysmenorrhea is more likely and a pelvic examination is indicated.

Secondary dysmenorrhea is menstrual pain due to an underlying pelvic lesion (see Table 3–8). Although uncommon in adolescents, when present it is most often due to infection or endometriosis. In one study of adolescent females with chronic pelvic pain, more than 40% who had not received a definitive diagnosis by the third visit were found to have endometriosis.

The clinician evaluating a patient with secondary dysmenorrhea should take a sexual history and conduct a pelvic examination even if the patient is not sexually active. Testing for gonorrhea and *Chlamydia,* a complete blood count and erythrocyte sedimentation rate, and a pregnancy test should be done. Gynecologic consultation is indicated to look for endometriosis or congenital problems by ultrasonography or laparoscopy. Treatment depends on the cause (see Table 3–8).

3. Dysfunctional Uterine Bleeding

Dysfunctional uterine bleeding may consist of menorrhagia (normal intervals with excessive flow) or metrorrhagia (irregular intervals with excessive flow). It results when an endometrium that has proliferated under unopposed estrogen stimulation finally begins to slough, but does so incompletely, causing irregular, painless bleeding. The unopposed estrogen stimulation occurs during anovulatory cycles, common in younger adolescents who have not been menstruating for long. Anovulation may also occur in older adolescents during times of stress or illness (Figure 3–12).

Clinical Findings

Typically, the adolescent has had several years of regular cycles and then begins to have menses every 2 weeks, or complains of bleeding for 2–3 weeks after 2–3 months of amenorrhea. A history of painless, irregular periods at intervals of less than 3 weeks may also be elicited. Bleeding for more than 10 days should be considered abnormal. Dysfunctional uterine bleeding must be considered a diagnosis of exclusion (Table 3–9).

Management

A pregnancy test and pelvic examination with appropriate tests for sexually transmitted infections should be performed in sexually active patients. A complete blood count, including a platelet count, should be obtained. The history and physical findings may suggest the need for additional coagulation or hormonal studies. Coagulation studies should be done if the patient presents with severe anemia, especially within 1 year after menarche. Management depends on the severity of the problem (Table 3–10). It is important to treat for a minimum of 3–4 months to progressively reduce the endometrium to baseline thickness.

4. Mittelschmerz

Mittelschmerz is midcycle pain caused by irritation of the peritoneum due to spillage of fluid from the ruptured follicular cyst at the time of ovulation. The patient presents with a history of midcycle, unilateral dull or aching abdominal pain lasting a few minutes to as long as 8 hours. This pain rarely mimics the abdominal findings of acute appendicitis, torsion or rupture of

Table 3–8. Dysmenorrhea in the adolescent.

Primary Dysmenorrhea—no pelvic pathology

	Etiology	Onset and Duration	Symptoms	Pelvic Exam	Treatment
Primary	Excessive amount of prostaglandin $F_2\alpha$, which attaches to myometrium, causing uterine contractions, hypoxia, and ischemia. Also, directly sensitizes pain receptors.	Begins with onset of flow or just prior and lasts 1–2 d. Does not start until 6–18 mos after menarche, when cycles become ovulatory.	Lower abdominal cramps radiating to lower back and thighs. Associated nausea, vomiting, diarrhea, and urinary frequency also due to excess prostaglandins.	Normal. May wait to examine if never sexually active and history is consistent with primary dysmenorrhea.	Mild—heating pad, warm baths, non-prescription analgesics. Moderate to severe—prostaglandin inhibitors at onset of flow or pain. Consider oral contraceptives.

Secondary Dysmenorrhea—underlying pathology present. (Always perform pelvic exam if secondary dysmenorrhea suspected or patient is sexually active. Tests for *Chlamydia* and gonorrhea, CBC, and ESR should be obtained.)

Infection	Most often due to an STI such as chlamydia or gonorrhea.	Recent onset of pelvic cramps.	Pelvic cramps, excessive bleeding, intermenstrual spotting or vaginal discharge.	Mucopurulent or purulent discharge from cervical os, cervical friability, cervical motion tenderness, adnexal tenderness, positive test for STI.	Appropriate antibiotics.
Endometriosis	Aberrant implants of endometrial tissue in pelvis or abdomen; may result from reflux.	Generally starts more than 2 y after menarche.	Pelvic pain, may occur intermenstrually.	Two thirds are tender on exam, especially during late luteal phase.	Hormonal suppression by oral contraceptives or danazol. Surgery may be necessary for extensive disease.
Complication of pregnancy	Spontaneous abortion, ectopic pregnancy.	Acute onset.	Pelvic cramps associated with a delay in menses.	Positive hCG, enlarged uterus or adnexal mass.	Immediate gynecologic consult.
Congenital anomalies	Transverse vaginal septum, septate uterus, or cervical stenosis.	Onset at menarche.	Pelvic cramps.	Underlying congenital anomaly may be apparent. May require exam under anesthesia.	Gynecologic consult for ultrasound, hysteroscopy, or laparoscopy.
IUD	Increased uterine contractions, or increased risk for pelvic infection.	Onset after placement of IUD or acutely if due to infection.	Pelvic cramps, heavy menstrual bleeding, may have vaginal discharge.	Normal, or see infection above.	Prostaglandin inhibitors of mefenamic acid may be drug of choice because they also reduce flow. Appropriate antibiotics and consider removal of IUD if infection is present.
Pelvic adhesions	Previous abdominal surgery or pelvic inflammatory disease.	Delayed onset after surgery or PID.	Abdominal pain, may or may not be associated with menstrual cycles; possible alteration in bowel pattern.	Variable.	Surgery. Consider a trial of tricyclic antidepressants.

CBC, complete blood count; ESR, erythrocyte sedimentation rate; hCG, human chorionic gonadotropin; STI, sexually transmitted infection; IUD, intrauterine device; PID, pelvic inflammatory disease.

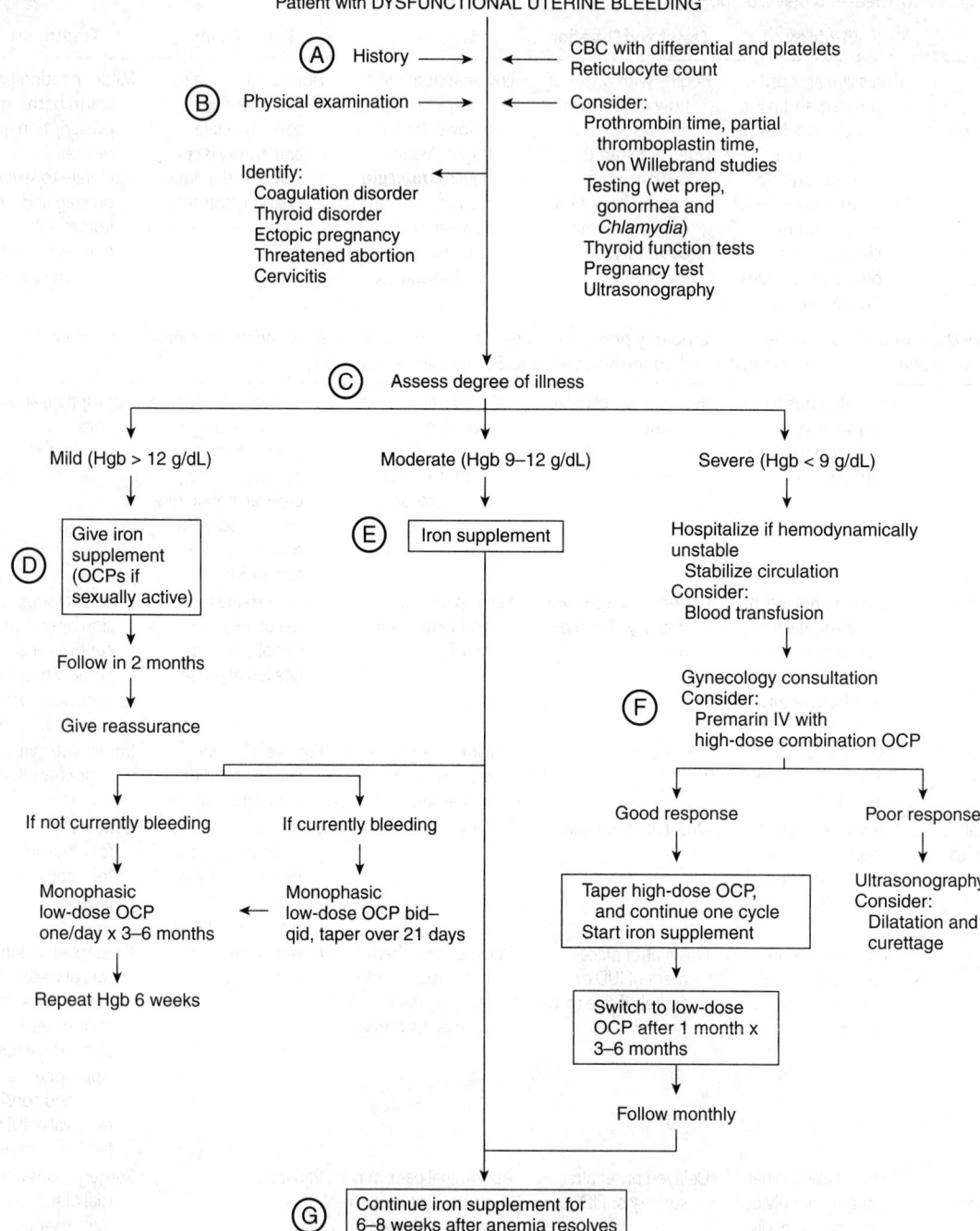

Figure 3–12. Evaluation of dysfunctional uterine bleeding. CBC, complete blood count; Hgb, hemoglobin, OCP, oral contraceptive pills.

Table 3–9. Differential diagnosis of dysfunctional uterine bleeding in adolescents.

Anovulation
Sexually transmitted infections
   Cervicitis
   Pelvic inflammatory disease
Pregnancy complications
   Ectopic pregnancy
   Spontaneous abortion
Bleeding disorders
   von Willebrand disease
   Thrombocytopenia
   Coagulopathy
Endocrine disorders
   Hypothyroidism
   Hyperprolactinemia
   Adrenal hyperplasia
   Polycystic ovary syndrome
Anatomic abnormalities
Uterine fibroids
Trauma
Foreign body
Chronic illness
Malignancy
   Leukemia
   Carcinoma
Drugs
   Birth control pills
   Depo-Provera

---

an ovarian cyst, or ectopic pregnancy. The patient should be reassured and treated symptomatically. If the findings are severe enough to warrant consideration of the previously mentioned diagnoses, laparoscopy may be done.

5. Premenstrual Syndrome

Premenstrual syndrome (PMS) refers to a cluster of physical and psychological symptoms that are temporally related to the luteal phase of the menstrual cycle and are alleviated by the onset of menses. PMS should be distinguished from major depression, idiopathic cyclic edema, fibromyalgia, chronic fatigue syndrome, and psychosomatic disorders. This may be difficult because of the diversity of symptoms ascribed to PMS and the variability from month to month in the same patient. Premenstrual behavioral symptoms most commonly cited include emotional lability, anxiety, depression, irritability, impulsivity, hostility, and impaired social function. Physical symptoms include bloating, breast tenderness, fatigue, and appetite changes. Previously thought to be a disorder limited to adult women, studies indicate that adolescents also experience premenstrual symptoms. Although a number of causes have been proposed (progesterone deficiency, hyperprolactinemia, estrogen excess or imbalance of the estrogen-progesterone ratio, vitamin B_{12} deficiency, fluid retention, low levels of endorphins and prostaglandins, hypoglycemia, and psychosomatic factors), none has been proven. Hormones may play a role; women who have undergone hysterectomy but not oophorectomy may have cyclic symptoms resembling PMS, whereas postmenopausal women have no such symptoms.

Several treatments have been advocated but are without consistent benefits. OCPs or nonsteroidal antiinflammatory drugs may be beneficial for some women. Sertraline (50–100 mg) has been shown to be significantly better than placebo for treatment of premenstrual dysphoria.

6. Ovarian Cysts

Functional cysts account for 20–50% of ovarian tumors in adolescents and are a result of the normal physiologic process of ovulation. They may be asymptomatic or may cause menstrual irregularity, constipation, or urinary frequency. Functional cysts, unless large, rarely cause abdominal pain; however, torsion or hemorrhage of an ovarian cyst may present as an acute abdomen. Follicular cysts account for the majority of ovarian cysts. They are produced every cycle but occasionally are not resorbed. Follicular cysts are unilateral, usually not larger than 4 cm in diameter, and resolve spontaneously. If the patient is asymptomatic, she can be reexamined monthly. The patient should be referred to a gynecologist for laparoscopy if she is premenarcheal, if the cyst has a solid component or is larger than 5 cm by ultrasonography, if she has symptoms or signs suggestive of hemorrhage or torsion, or if the cyst fails to regress within 2 months. Luteal cysts occur less commonly and may be 5–10 cm in diameter. The patient may have associated amenorrhea, or as the cyst becomes atretic, heavy vaginal bleeding. The patient may be monitored for 3 months but should have a laparoscopy if the cyst is larger than 5 cm, does not resolve within 2 months, or if there is pain or bleeding from the cyst.

Dickerson LM et al: Premenstrual syndrome. Am Fam Physician 2003;67:1743 [PMID: 12725453].

Slap GB: Menstrual disorders in adolescence. Best Pract Res Clin Obstet Gynaecol 2003;17:75 [PMID: 12758227].

CONTRACEPTION

Among high school students, 45% of females and 48% of males have had sexual intercourse. According to the 2002 National Survey of Family Growth, teens were more likely to use contraception when they began having intercourse; 79% in 1999–2002, up from 61% in the

Table 3–10. Management of dysfunctional uterine bleeding.[a]

	Mild	**Moderate**	**Severe**
	Hgb > 12 g/dL	Hgb 9–12 g/dL	Hgb < 9 g/dL (or dropping); orthostatic symptoms and signs
Acute treatment	Menstrual calendar Iron supplementation NSAID with menses may help reduce flow Consider oral contraceptive pills if patient is sexually active and desires contraception	Monophasic oral contraceptive pills up to four pills per day and taper over 2–3 wk; may need antiemetic. Bleeding should stop in a few days. Begin tapering dose 2–3 d after bleeding stops. Expect withdrawal flow a few days after last dose.	Fluids, blood transfusion as needed, admit to hospital if Hgb < 7 g/dL or patient is hemodynamically unstable For hemostasis, consider: conjugated estrogens (Premarin), 25 mg IV every 4–6 h for 24 h or until bleeding stops. Provide antiemetic medication. Then: oral contraceptive pills (1/50) cycle: 4 pills/d for 4 d 3 pills/d for 4 d 2 pills/d for 17 d withdrawal bleeding for 7 d[b]
Long-term management	Monitor menstrual calendar and Hgb Follow-up in 2–3 mo	Cycle with either: (1) Medroxyprogesterone acetate, 10 mg PO daily for 10 d starting on day 14 of each cycle for 3–6 mo, or (2) Oral contraceptive pills for 3–6 mo beginning the Sunday after withdrawal bleeding starts. Provide iron supplementation. Monitor Hgb Follow-up within 2–3 wk and every 3 mo	Next: Oral contraceptive pills cycle (using 28-d packs) for 3 mo Begin the Sunday after withdrawal bleeding begins. Length of use dependent on resolution of anemia. Monitor hemoglobin Follow-up within 2–3 wk and every 3 mo

[a]Diagnosis: Prolonged (> 8 d) painless menses; heavy flow (> 6 tampons/pads per day); short cycles (< 21 d); no cause found.
[b]This schedule will use three 21-d packages.
Hgb, hemoglobin; PO, by mouth; NSAID, nonsteroidal anti-inflammatory drug.
Modified from Blythe M: Common menstrual problems. Part 3. Abnormal uterine bleeding. Adolesc Health Update 1992;4:1.

1980s. Teens were also more likely to have used contraception at their most recent intercourse in 2002 (83% in 2002 compared with 71% in 1995). Still, an estimated 50% of adolescent pregnancies occur within the first 6 months of initiation of sexual activity. Adolescents often delay seeing a clinician for prescription contraceptives for a year or more after initiating sexual activity.

Abstinence & Decision Making

Many adolescents have given little thought to how they feel about their developing sexuality or how they will handle sexual situations. By talking with teenagers about sexual intercourse and its implications, and alternatives to intercourse, providers can help teens make informed decisions before they find themselves with an unplanned pregnancy or a sexually transmitted infection.

If an adolescent chooses to remain abstinent, the clinician should reinforce that decision. Encouraging adolescents to use contraception when they do engage in sexual intercourse does not lead to higher rates of sexual activity. Another approach to decreasing teen pregnancy is to educate adolescent males on the importance of hormonal contraception and emergency contraception for their partners, in addition to condom use. The teen pregnancy, birth, and abortion rates are higher in the United States than in any other developed country, despite similar rates of sexual experience.

Emergency Contraception

A discussion of emergency contraception (EC), which could potentially prevent 50–90% of unintended pregnancies and elective abortions, should be part of antici-

Table 3–11. Emergency postcoital contraception regimens.

Pill	Dosage	Each Dose Achieves:
Plan B[a]	Two tablets orally	Levonorgestrel 1.5 mg
Nordette[b]	Four tablets orally and repeat in 12 h	Levonorgestrel 0.6 mg
Lo-Ovral[b]	Four tablets orally and repeat in 12 h	Norgestrel 1.2 mg
Alesse[b]	Five pink pills orally and repeat in 12 h	Levonorgestrel 0.5 mg
Triphasil[b]	Four yellow pills orally and repeat in 12 h	Levonorgestrel 0.5 mg

[a]Both doses can be given at the same time.
[b]An antiemetic drug taken 30 minutes before the dose may help reduce nausea.

patory guidance given to both female and male teenagers. Indications for EC include unprotected intercourse within the past 120 hours (5 days), condom breakage, more than two missed oral contraceptive pills, and more than 14 weeks since the last Depo-Provera injection. The pregnancy rate after EC is 1.8%, compared with 6.8% without such intervention. (See Table 3–11 for dosages.) EC works best within 24 hours of intercourse but can be taken up to 120 hours afterward. It should be verified that other instances of unprotected intercourse beyond 120 hours have not occurred. The only contraindication to the use of EC is pregnancy. Plan B is a progestin-only method that causes significantly less nausea and vomiting than combined estrogen/progesterone methods. A recent study showed that the two pills can be given at the same time if there is a single episode of unprotected intercourse; patients with multiple episodes of unprotected intercourse should receive the doses 12 hours apart. If this method is not available, certain combined OCPs can be used for EC. It is important to note that the newer progestin-containing contraceptives are **not** approved for EC. A follow-up appointment should be held in 2–3 weeks, to test for pregnancy if menses have not occurred, to screen for STIs if indicated, and to counsel regarding contraceptive use.

Condoms & Spermicides

The use of condoms has gained popularity as a result of the educational and marketing efforts driven by the acquired immunodeficiency syndrome epidemic. Condom use has increased over the past several decades.

Regardless of whether another method is used, all sexually active adolescents should be counseled to use condoms. Condoms offer protection against STIs by decreasing (but not eliminating) the transmission of gonorrhea, *Chlamydia,* syphilis, herpes simplex, hepatitis, and the human immunodeficiency virus. Spermicides containing nonoxynol-9 are no longer recommended, as evidence has suggested that repeated use of spermicide may increase transmission of human immunodeficiency virus. Aside from the diaphragm and cervical cap, barrier methods do not require a medical visit or prescription and are widely available. The polyurethane vaginal pouch, or female condom, is also available. Although it has pregnancy and STI prevention properties similar to those of the male condom, its higher cost and greater difficulty of insertion make it less appealing to adolescents.

Oral Contraceptives

OCPs have a three-pronged mechanism of action: (1) suppression of ovulation; (2) thickening of the cervical mucus, thereby making sperm penetration more difficult; and (3) atrophy of the endometrium, which diminishes the chance of implantation. The latter two actions are progestin effects.

A. COMBINATION ORAL AND CUTANEOUS CONTRACEPTIVES

Combination OCPs contain both estrogen and progestin. Ethinyl estradiol is the estrogen currently used in nearly all OCPs in the United States. A number of progestins are used in OCPs and differ in their estrogenic, antiestrogenic, and androgenic effects. As estrogen doses decreased in OCPs, the androgenic side effects of progestins became more apparent, leading to the development of two progestins (desogestrel and norgestimate) with lower androgenic potential. Ortho Tri-Cyclen has been advertised as a treatment for acne. All of the lower androgenic pills improve acne and may especially benefit patients with polycystic ovary syndrome. Reports of increased risk of thromboembolism associated with the newer progestins are likely related to an excess of first-time users among desogestrel patients. Factor V Leiden has been identified as a risk factor for venous thrombosis; 5% of patients of European ancestry are carriers of factor V Leiden. Carriers have a 30- to 50-fold increased risk for thrombosis. Testing family members with a history of venous thrombosis for factor V Leiden and other conditions such as the prothrombin gene mutation, proteins C and S, and antithrombin III before prescribing estrogen-containing OCPs to the adolescent may prevent these complications. OCPs have many noncontraceptive benefits, including improvement of dysmenorrhea, menorrhagia, acne, and PMS; suppression of ovarian and breast cysts; and lower risk of anemia, pelvic inflammatory disease, and ectopic pregnancy. A pill containing 30–35 mg of ethinyl estradiol with norgestimate, desogestrel, or 0.5 mg norethindrone is recommended for adolescents beginning OCPs.

Ortho Evra is a combined estrogen/progesterone patch, which is worn 3 weeks out of every 4. It releases 150 μg of norelgestromin and 20 μg of ethinyl estradiol per day. Side effects are similar to those of combined OCPs. Recent reports of increased thrombotic events reinforce the importance of screening patients for risk factors for thrombosis (personal or family history of thrombosis) prior to prescription of the patch. Five percent of patients report having a patch come off. Two percent report skin irritation. Efficacy may be reduced in patients weighing more than 200 pounds. The patch is an attractive alternative to OCPs for adolescents who have difficulty remembering to take a pill every day, as compliance is increased. The failure rate for the patch is reported to be 1%.

B. PROGESTIN-ONLY PILLS

Progestin-only pills contain no estrogen. Their chief use is in women who experience unacceptable estrogen-related side effects with combination OCPs or who have a contraindication to estrogen-containing pills. Their lack of estrogen, however, is also responsible for the main side effect, less predictable menstrual patterns. For this reason, progestin-only pills are not often desirable for adolescents. Their mechanism of action relies on the progestin-mediated actions, and ovulation is suppressed in only 15–40% of cycles.

C. INDICATIONS AND CONTRAINDICATIONS

Combined OCPs may be the method of choice for sexually active adolescents who frequently have unplanned intercourse; however, the patient must be able to comply with a daily dosing regimen. Most states allow OCPs to be prescribed to minors confidentially. Ideally, it is best to wait until 6–12 regular menstrual cycles have occurred before beginning hormonal contraception; however, if the teenager is already sexually active, the medical and social risks of pregnancy outweigh the risks of hormonal contraception.

OCPs or the contraceptive patch may also be used to treat dysmenorrhea, menorrhagia, dysfunctional uterine bleeding, and acne (see previous discussion).

Contraindications to combined OCPs or the contraceptive patch can be categorized as absolute and relative (Table 3–12). When use of estrogenic agents is contraindicated, progestin-only pills and Depo-Provera are alternatives.

D. BEGINNING BIRTH CONTROL PILLS OR THE CONTRACEPTIVE PATCH AND FOLLOW-UP

Before a patient begins taking OCPs or the patch, a careful menstrual history, medical history, and family

Table 3–12. Contraindications to combined birth control pills.

Absolute contraindications
Pregnancy
Lactation (first 6 wk postpartum to allow milk supply to become established)
History of thrombophlebitis, thromboembolic disorder, cerebrovascular disease, or ischemic heart disease
Structural heart disease with endocarditis, atrial fibrillation, or pulmonary hypertension
Breast cancer
Migraine headaches with neurologic changes (numbness or unilateral weakness)
History of active liver disease or tumor
Hypertension SBP > 160 mm Hg or DBP > 100 mm Hg
Prolonged immobilization after surgery on legs or pelvis

Relative contraindications
First 3 wk postpartum due to decreased milk supply
Lactation (6 wk–6 mo)
Active gallbladder disease
Use of drugs that affect liver enzymes (rifampin, griseofulvin, phenytoin, carbamazepine, barbiturates)

SBP, systolic blood pressure; DBP, diastolic blood pressure; OCPs, oral contraceptives.

medical history should be taken. In addition, baseline weight and blood pressure should be established; breast and pelvic examinations should be performed; and specimens for urinalysis, Pap smear, and gonorrhea and *Chlamydia* testing should be obtained if indicated. If patients have not yet initiated intercourse, pelvic examination can be deferred until after intercourse is initiated. If time constraints are present and a patient has no symptoms suggesting an STI, OCPs or the patch may be started and a pelvic examination scheduled as soon as possible.

If the teen has no contraindications (see Table 3–12), she may begin her first pack of pills or the patch with her next menstrual period (either the first Sunday after flow begins or the first day of flow, depending on the brand). A low-dose monophasic combined oral contraceptive or a triphasic pill of low androgenic profile is used for those without contraindications to use of estrogen. With adolescents, it is wise to use 28-day packs rather than 21-day packs to reduce the chance of confusion. The patient should be instructed on the use of her pills and on the possible risks and side effects and their warning signs. To ensure protection, she should use a back-up method, such as condoms, for the first 2 weeks. In addition, the patient should be advised to use condoms at every intercourse to prevent STIs. A follow-up visit every 3 months for the first year may improve compliance, because teenagers often discontinue birth control pills because of nonmedical reasons or minor side effects. Teenagers may need reassurance about the safety of birth control pills and their added benefits (Table 3–13).

E. MANAGEMENT OF SIDE EFFECTS

A different type of combined oral contraceptive should be tried if a patient has a persistent minor side effect for more than the first 2–3 months. Adjustments should be made on the basis of hormonal effects desired (Table 3–14). Changes are most often made for persistent breakthrough bleeding not related to missed pills.

Injectable Hormonal Contraceptives

The depot form of medroxyprogesterone acetate (DMPA), or Depo-Provera, is a long-acting injectable progestational contraceptive. It is given as a deep intramuscular injection of 150 mg into the gluteal or deltoid muscle every 13 weeks. The first injection should be given within the first 5 days of the menstrual cycle to ensure immediate contraceptive protection. Patients more than 1 week late for their injection should have two pregnancy tests 2 weeks apart before restarting DMPA, unless they have not been sexually active since missing the DMPA injection. If an adolescent is not able to reliably remain abstinent for 2 weeks, DMPA may be given, but the patient should be informed of the chance of pregnancy and should return in 2 weeks for a repeat pregnancy test. DMPA works chiefly by blocking the LH surge, thereby suppressing ovulation, but it also thickens cervical mucus and alters the endometrium to inhibit implantation. With a failure rate of less than 0.3%, minimal compliance issues, long-acting nature, reversibility, lack of interference with intercourse, and lack of estrogen-related side effects, it may be an attractive contraceptive for many adolescents. Patients should be warned about unpredictable menstrual patterns, the possibility of weight gain or mood changes, and the potential for decreased bone density. The FDA has issued a black box warning about decreased bone density with Depo-Provera. Whether this decrease in bone density is reversible remains under investigation. Current recommendations are for adolescents to consider another method of contraception after 2 years of DMPA. Providers must take into consideration the risk of pregnancy, including deleterious effects on bone density with pregnancy. DMPA may reduce intravascular sickling and increase hemoglobin and red cell survival in patients with sickle cell disease. Moreover, DMPA may be the preferred method for patients with seizure disorders, because it has been found to reduce the number of seizures in some patients. DMPA may also be helpful for adolescents with von Willebrand disease, since amenorrhea (which decreases blood loss) is a common effect of DMPA. Studies have shown no increased risk of liver cancer, breast cancer, or invasive squamous cell cervical cancer among users of DMPA, and the risk of endometrial and ovarian cancers is also reduced.

Implantable Contraceptive Methods Available Outside of the United States

No implantable contraceptive methods are currently marketed in the United States.

Implanon is a single implant, effective for 3 years. It contains etonogestrel. It has been used in Europe and has a failure rate approaching 0%. Side effects include irregular bleeding, headache, nausea, breast pain, and depression. Return to fertility is rapid following removal. Insertion and removal are reportedly significantly easier than with Norplant. Other implantable progesterones used in other countries include Norplant II (Jadelle) which contains 2 rods of 75 mg levonorgestrel with a .3% cumulative pregnancy rate over 3 years and a 1.1% pregnancy rate over 5 years. The implantable contraceptives do not lead to decreased bone density, likely due to lower levels of progestins.

Contraceptive Vaginal Ring

The NuvaRing is a vaginal ring that releases 15 μg of ethinyl estradiol and 120 μg of etonogestrel per day. The ring is placed inside the vagina for 3 weeks, followed by 1 week without the ring to allow for withdrawal bleeding. A new ring is inserted each month. The failure rate is 1%. Side effects include vaginitis in 5%, headache in 6%, and foreign body sensation in

Table 3–13. Noncontraceptive health benefits of oral contraceptive pills.

Protection against life-threatening conditions
Ovarian cancer
Endometrial cancer
Pelvic inflammatory disease
Ectopic pregnancy
Morbidity and mortality due to unintended pregnancies

Alleviate conditions affecting quality of life
Iron deficiency anemia
Benign breast disease
Dysmenorrhea
Irregular cycles
Functional ovarian cysts
Premenstrual syndrome
Acne

Mounting evidence
Improved bone density

Table 3–14. Estrogenic, progestogenic, and androgenic effects of oral contraceptive pills.

Estrogenic Effects	Progestogenic Effects	Androgenic Effects
Nausea	Breast tenderness	Decreased production of testosterone, improved acne, less oily skin, and improved hirsutism. The progestin component may have androgenic as well as progestational effects:
Increased breast size (ductal and fatty tissue)	Headaches	
Cyclic weight gain due to fluid retention	Hypertension	
Leukorrhea	Myocardial infarction (rare)	
Cervical eversion or ectopy		Increased appetite and weight gain
Hypertension		Depression, fatigue
Telangiectasia		Decreased libido
Thromboembolic complications including pulmonary emboli (rare), deep venous thrombosis, cerebrovascular accident, or myocardial infarction (rare)		Increased breast tenderness or breast size
		Increased LDL cholesterol levels
		Decreased HDL cholesterol levels
		Decreased carbohydrate tolerance; increased insulin resistance
		Pruritus

LDL, low-density lipoprotein; HDL, high density lipoprotein.
Adapted, with permission, from Hatcher RA et al: *Contraceptive Technology,* 17th ed. Ardent Media, 1998.

2.5%. The vaginal ring is easier to insert correctly than the diaphragm. However, like the diaphragm, adolescents are often reluctant to use contraception requiring insertion into the vagina.

Contraceptive Methods Not Usually Recommended for Teenagers

Adolescents should understand the menstrual cycle and be taught that ovulation typically occurs 2 weeks before the next menstrual period and may be difficult to predict. Because teenagers frequently have irregular cycles, the rhythm, or calendar, method is not effective. Adolescents also need to be taught that withdrawal is not a reliable method of contraception. Diaphragms and cervical caps require professional fitting and skill with insertion and are not popular among teenagers. Adolescents who have never been pregnant or who engage in behaviors that carry a risk of STIs should not use an intrauterine device.

Centers for Disease Control and Prevention: Youth Risk Behavior Surveillance—United States, 2003. MMWR Morb Moral Wkly Rep 2004:53(SS-2):1. Available at: www.cdc.gov/healthyyouth/yrbs/index.html

Gallo MF et al: Skin patch and vaginal ring versus combined oral contraceptives for contraception. Cochrane Database Syst Rev 2003;(1):CD003552 [PMID: 12535478].

Meirik O et al: Implantable contraceptives for women. Hum Reprod Update 2003;9:49 [PMID: 12638781].

Petitti DB: Clinical practice: Combination estrogen-progestin oral contraceptives. N Engl J Med 2003;349:1443 [PMID: 14534338].

PREGNANCY

Approximately 900,000 adolescents younger than age 19 become pregnant every year. The birth rate fell to 43 births per 1000 females 15–19 years of age in 2002, a 5% decline from 2001 and a 28% decline from 1990. The decline in the birth rate for younger teens, 15–17 years of age, is even more substantial, dropping 38% from 1990 to 2002 compared with a drop of 18% for teens 18–19 years of age.

Abortions in adolescents have also decreased over the past decade, down 39% from 1990 to 1999. Despite decreasing rates, the United States still has the highest adolescent pregnancy rate of any developed country. Young maternal age and associated maternal risk factors have been linked to adverse neonatal outcome, including higher rates of low birth weight babies (< 2500 g) and neonatal mortality. The psychosocial consequences for the teenage mother and her infant are listed in Table 3–15. Teenagers who are pregnant require additional support from their caregivers. Clinics for young mothers may be the best providers.

Presentation

Adolescents may present with delayed or missed menses or may even request a pregnancy test, but often they present with an unrelated concern or have a hidden agenda. Because of the high level of denial, they may come in with complaints of abdominal pain, urinary frequency, dizziness, or other nonspecific symptoms

Table 3–15. Psychosocial consequences of pregnancy for the adolescent mother and her infant.

Mother	Infant
Increased morbidity related to pregnancy	**Greater health risks**
Greater risk of eclampsia, anemia, prolonged labor, premature labor	Increased chance of low birth weight or prematurity
Increased chance of miscarriages, stillbirths	Increased risk of infant death
Increased chance of maternal mortality	Increased risk of injury and hospitalization by age 5
Decreased educational attainment	**Decreased academic achievement**
Less likely to get high school diploma, go to college, or graduate	Lower cognitive scores
Lower occupational attainment and prestige	Decreased development
	Greater chance of being behind grade or needing remedial help
Less chance of stable employment (some resolution over time)	Lower chance of advanced academics
Lower job satisfaction	Lower academic aptitude as a teenager and perhaps a higher probability of dropping out of school
Lower income/wages	
Greater dependence on public assistance	**Psychosocial consequences**
Less stable marital relationships	Greater risk of behavior problems
Higher rates of single parenthood	Poverty
Earlier marriage (though less common than in the past)	Higher probability of living in a nonintact home while in high school
Accelerated pace of marriage, separation, divorce, and remarriage	Greater risk of adolescent pregnancy
Faster pace of subsequent childbearing	
High rate of repeat unintended pregnancy	
More births out of marriage	
Closer spacing of births	
Larger families	

and have no concern about pregnancy. A history of symptoms such as weight gain, nausea, engorged breasts, an unusually light or mistimed period, or urinary frequency may be present. Denial contributes to the delay in seeking prenatal care. Clinicians need to have a low threshold of suspicion of pregnancy. If any suspicion exists, a urine pregnancy test should be obtained.

Diagnosis

The history and physical examination may assist in making the diagnosis. Bluish coloring and softening of the cervix may be noted on speculum examination. The uterine fundus may be palpable on abdominal examination if sufficient time has elapsed. If uterine size on bimanual examination does not correspond to dates, one must consider ectopic pregnancy, incomplete or missed abortion, twin gestation, or inaccurate dates.

Enzyme-linked immunosorbent assay test kits specific for the β-human chorionic gonadotropin subunit and sensitive to less than 50 mIU/mL of human chorionic gonadotropin can be performed on urine (preferably the first morning-voided specimen, because it is more concentrated) in less than 5 minutes and are accurate by the expected date of the missed period in almost 100% of patients. Serum radioimmunoassay is also specific for the β subunit, is accurate within 7 days after conception, and is helpful in ruling out ectopic pregnancy or threatened abortion.

The timing of pregnancy tests is important, because human chorionic gonadotropin levels rise initially after conception, peak at about 60–70 days, then drop to levels not detected by routine office slide tests after 16–20 weeks.

Special Issues in Management

When an adolescent presents for pregnancy testing, it is helpful, before performing the test, to find out what she hopes the result will be and what she thinks she will do if the test is positive. If she wants to be pregnant and the test is negative, further counseling about the implications of teen pregnancy should be offered. Prenatal vitamins should be prescribed. For those who do not wish to be pregnant, contraception should be discussed, because teens with a negative pregnancy test have a high risk of pregnancy within the next 2 years.

If the adolescent is pregnant, the physician must discuss her support systems and her options with her (abortion, adoption, or raising the baby). Many teenagers need help in telling and involving their parents. It is important to remain available for further assistance with decision making. Patients should be informed of the gestational age and time frames required for the different options. If the patient knows what she wants to do, she should be referred to the appropriate resources. Because teenagers are often ambivalent about their plans and may have a high level of denial, it is prudent to follow-up in 1 week to be certain that a decision has been made. Avoiding a decision reduces the adolescent's options and may result in poor pregnancy outcomes. Providers can help ensure that the patient obtains prenatal care if she has chosen to continue the pregnancy. In addition, brief counseling about healthful diet; folic acid supplementation (400 µg/d); and avoiding alcohol, tobacco, and other drugs is helpful.

Young maternal age, low maternal prepregnancy weight, poor weight gain, delay in prenatal care, and low socioeconomic status contribute to low birth weight and poor fetal outcome. The poor nutritional status of some teenagers; their erratic diets, smoking, drinking, or substance abuse; and their high incidence of STIs also play a role. Teenagers are also at greater risk than adult women for preeclampsia, eclampsia, iron deficiency anemia, cephalopelvic disproportion, prolonged labor, premature labor, and maternal death. Early prenatal care and good nutrition can make a difference with a number of these problems.

Because of the high risk of a second unintended pregnancy within the next 2 years, postpartum contraceptive counseling and follow-up are imperative. Combined OCPs or the contraceptive patch can be started 3 weeks after delivery in adolescents who are not breast feeding; progestin-only methods can be started immediately postpartum, even in breast feeding adolescents. Pregnancy prevention is the most cost-effective means of reducing the consequences of teenage pregnancy. Sexual decision making, contraceptive counseling, and close follow-up of sexually active adolescents of both sexes can make a difference. Adolescents who receive sexuality and contraceptive education are not more likely to have intercourse, but are less likely to become pregnant than their counterparts who do not receive such instruction.

Ectopic Pregnancy

In the United States, 100,000 ectopic pregnancies occur each year, accounting for 2% of pregnancies. Adolescents have the highest mortality rate from ectopic pregnancy, most likely related to delayed entry into health care. Risk factors include history of pelvic inflammatory disease or chlamydial infection. Conception while on progestin-only methods of contraception also increases the risk of ectopic pregnancy, because of the progestin-mediated decrease in tubal motility. Providers should have a high level of suspicion with any adolescent presenting with vaginal bleeding and abdominal pain.

Abma JC et al: Teenagers in the United States: sexual activity, contraceptive use, and childbearing, 2002 Vital Health Stat 2004;24:1 [PMID: 15648540].

Elfenbein DS et al: Adolescent pregnancy. Pediatr Clin North Am 2003;50:781, viii [PMID: 12964694].

Klein DJ: Adolescent pregnancy: current trends and issues. Pediatrics 2005;116:281 [PMID: 15995071].

National Center for Health Statistics: Teen Birth Rate Continues to Decline; African-American Teens Show Sharpest Drop; Final 2002 United States Birth Data Now Available. http://www.cdc.gov/nchs/pressroom/03facts/teenbirth.htm

VULVOVAGINITIS

Vaginitis may be due to pathogens or to indigenous flora after a change in milieu of the vagina. Candidal vulvovaginitis and bacterial vaginosis (formerly called *Gardnerella, Haemophilus,* or nonspecific vaginitis) may occur in patients who are not sexually active. These are examples of indigenous flora that may cause symptoms. Bacterial vaginosis, however, is more prevalent in those who are sexually active. In sexually active patients, *Trichomonas* infection or cervicitis due to sexually transmitted pathogens must be considered (see Chapter 40). For this reason, appropriate specimens should be taken from sexually active patients or suspected victims of sexual abuse in order to detect STIs, even if yeast forms are present or bacterial vaginosis is identified.

1. Physiologic Leukorrhea

Leukorrhea is the normal vaginal discharge that begins around the time of menarche. The discharge is typically clear or white, and its consistency may vary according to cyclic hormonal influences. There should be no odor. Girls in early adolescence may have concerns about such a discharge and need reassurance that it is normal. This may be a good time to tell girls that there is no need for douching. If a vaginal wet preparation is examined, a few squamous epithelial cells may be revealed, but there should be fewer than five polymorphonuclear cells per high-power field.

2. Candidal Vulvovaginitis

Candidal vulvovaginitis is caused by yeast (*Candida albicans*). It typically occurs after a course of antibiotics, after which the normal perineal flora are altered and yeast is allowed to proliferate. Diabetic patients, those with compromised immune systems, and those who are pregnant or receiving OCPs are more prone to develop candidal infections.

Clinical Findings

The patient usually complains of vulvar pruritus or dyspareunia and a thick vaginal discharge, frequently beginning the week before menses. Examination of the vulva reveals erythematous mucosa, sometimes with excoriation, and a thick, white, cheesy discharge. The discharge may be adherent to the walls of the vagina. Leukocytes may be seen on a wet preparation, and a potassium hydroxide preparation may reveal budding yeast or mycelia. The vaginal preparations are often not helpful, and the patient should be treated on the basis of the clinical examination. Vaginal culture for yeast is usually unnecessary.

Treatment

Butoconazole, clotrimazole, miconazole, terconazole, or tioconazole vaginal creams or suppositories designed for seven nightly doses are effective in most patients. Fluconazole (150 mg once orally) is also effective and may be beneficial in virginal adolescents. Patients with recurrent episodes should be given prophylactic treatment whenever they take antibiotics. It may be helpful to simultaneously treat the partners of sexually active patients with recurrent candidal infections.

3. Bacterial Vaginosis

Bacterial vaginosis may be caused by any of the indigenous vaginal flora, such as *Gardnerella, Bacteroides, Peptococcus, Mycoplasma hominis,* lactobacilli, or other anaerobes.

Clinical Findings

The patient generally complains of a malodorous discharge or wetness. On examination, a thin, homogeneous, grayish white discharge is found adhering to the vaginal wall. A whiff test, in which a drop of potassium hydroxide is added to a smear of the discharge on a slide, results in the release of amines, causing a fishy odor. Wet preparation reveals an abundance of clue cells and small pleomorphic rods.

Treatment

Treatment for bacterial vaginosis is with metronidazole (500 mg orally bid for 7 days) or clindamycin (300 mg orally bid for 7 days). Topical metronidazole or clinda-mycin may also be effective. Ampicillin (500 mg orally four times a day for 7 days) is the alternative for pregnant patients.

4. Other Causes of Vulvovaginitis

Sexually Transmitted Infections

STIs are a common cause of vaginal discharge in adolescents (see Chapter 40). *Chlamydia* and gonorrhea testing should be done whenever a sexually active adolescent complains of vaginal discharge even when the cervix appears normal.

Foreign Body Vaginitis

Foreign bodies (most commonly retained tampons or condoms) cause extremely malodorous vaginal discharges. Treatment consists of removal, for which ring forceps may be useful. Further treatment is generally not necessary.

Allergic or Contact Vaginitis

Bubble baths, feminine hygiene sprays, or vaginal contraceptive foams or suppositories may cause chemical irritation of the vaginal mucosa. Discontinuing use of the offending agent is indicated.

REFERENCES

Brook I: Microbiology and management of polymicrobial female genital tract infections in adolescents. J Pediatr Adolesc Gynecol 2002;15:217 [PMID: 12459228].

Substance Abuse

4

Paritosh Kaul, MD, & Catherine Stevens-Simon, MD

The use and abuse of mood-altering substances—alcohol, marijuana, opioids, cocaine, amphetamines, sedative-hypnotics, hallucinogens, inhalants, nicotine, anabolic steroids, γ-hydroxybutyrate (GHB), and methylene-dioxymethamphetamine (ecstasy)—continues to be a serious public health problem. The short- and long-term health, social, emotional, legal, and behavioral consequences of substance abuse are particularly damaging during childhood and adolescence. Not only does early substance use portend chronic, severe polysubstance abuse later in life, but substance use may also compromise physical, cognitive, and psychosocial aspects of adolescent development if this maladaptive behavior becomes the preferred response to environmental stressors.

Substance abuse tends to be a chronic, progressive disease. The first or initiation stage—from nonuser to user—is such a common feature of becoming an American adult that many authorities call it normative behavior. At this stage, substance use is typically limited to experimentation with tobacco or alcohol (so-called gateway substances). During adolescence, young people are expected to establish an independent, autonomous identity. They try out a variety of behaviors within the safety of their family circles and peer groups. This process often involves experimentation with psychoactive substances, usually in culturally acceptable circumstances. Progression to the second or continuation stage of substance abuse is a nonnormative risk behavior with the potential to compromise adolescent development. The American Psychiatric Association criteria listed in Table 4–1 can be used to judge the severity of substance use that progresses beyond the experimentation stage to substance abuse or substance dependency. Maintenance and progression within a class of substances (eg, from beer to liquor) and progression across classes of substances (eg, from alcohol to marijuana) represent the third and fourth stages of substance abuse. Individuals at these stages are polysubstance abusers, and most manifest one or more of the symptoms of dependency listed in Table 4–1. The transition from one stage to the next is typically a cyclic process of regression, cessation, and relapse. Common symptoms and physiologic effects of intoxication (which can occur at any stage) and withdrawal (a symptom of dependency) for the major classes of substances are presented in Tables 4–2 and 4–3.

American Psychiatric Association: *Diagnostic and Statistical Manual of Mental Disorders,* 4th ed. Text Revision. American Psychiatric Association, 2000.

Barkin SL, Smith KS, DuRant RH: Social skills and attitudes associated with substance use behaviors among young adolescents. J Adolesc Health 2002;30:448 [PMID: 12039515].

Comerci GD, Schwebel R: Substance abuse: An overview. Adolesc Med State Art Rev 2000;11:79 [PMID: 10640340].

Greydanus DE, Patel DR: Substance abuse in adolescents: a complex conundrum for the clinician. Pediatr Clin North Am 2003;50:1179 [PMID: 14558685].

U.S. Department of Health and Human Services: *Healthy People 2010,* 2nd ed, with *Understanding and Improving Health and Objectives for Improving Health* (2 vols.). U.S. Government Printing Office, 2000.

SCOPE OF THE PROBLEM

The best source of information about the prevalence of substance abuse among American children and adolescents is the annual Monitoring the Future Study, which tracks health-related behaviors in a sample of 50,000 8th, 10th, and 12th graders in about 400 public and private schools across the United States. This study probably understates the magnitude of the problem of substance abuse because it excludes two of the most abuse-prone groups of young people—school dropouts and runaways. Although the exclusion of these youngsters may minimize prevalence estimates only moderately for the entire population, errors in estimating drug use among subgroups with high rates of school dropout (eg, urban minority youths) are thought to be substantial. Data from this survey and others show that alcohol is the most frequently abused substance in our society. Experimentation with alcohol typically begins in or before middle school; is more common among boys than girls; and is most common among whites, less common among Hispanics and Native Americans, and least common among blacks and Asians. Over 50% of children consume alcohol before high school, and over 90% do so before graduation. Over 25% of eighth graders and over 50% of high-school students seen in an average American pediatric practice have used alcohol within the last 30 days, and half have consumed five or more drinks on at least one occasion. Use of tobacco, marijuana, and other mood-altering substances is less

Table 4–1. Substance abuse and substance dependency.

Diagnostic criteria for substance abuse

A. A maladaptive pattern of substance use leading to clinically significant impairment or distress, as manifested by one or more of the following occurring within a 12-month period:

  1. Recurrent substance use resulting in a failure to fulfill major role obligations at work, school, or home (eg, repeated absences or poor work performance related to substance use; substance-related absences, suspensions, or expulsions from school; neglect of children or household).

  2. Recurrent substance use in situations in which it is physically hazardous (eg, driving an automobile or operating a machine when impaired by substance use).

  3. Recurrent substance-related legal problems (arrests for substance-related disorderly conduct).

  4. Continued substance use despite having persistent or recurrent social or interpersonal problems caused or exacerbated by the effects of the substance (eg, arguments with spouse about consequences of intoxication, physical fights).

B. The symptoms have never met criteria for substance dependence for this class of substance.

Diagnostic criteria for substance dependency

A maladaptive pattern of substance use, leading to clinically significant impairment or distress, as manifested by three or more of the following, occurring at any time in the same 12-month period:

  1. Tolerance, as defined by either of the following:

    a. Need for markedly increased amounts of the substance to achieve intoxication or desired effect.

    b. Markedly diminished effect with continued use of the same amount of the substance.

  2. Withdrawal, as manifested by either of the following:

    a. The characteristic withdrawal syndrome for the substance (criteria A and B of the criteria for withdrawal from the specific substance).

    b. The same (or closely related) substance taken to relieve or avoid withdrawal symptoms.

  3. The substance often taken in larger amounts or over a longer period than was intended.

  4. There is a persistent desire or unsuccessful efforts to cut down or control substance use.

  5. A great deal of time spent in activities necessary to obtain the substance (eg, visiting multiple doctors, driving long distances), use the substance (chain-smoking), or recover from its effects.

  6. Important social, occupational, or recreational activities given up or reduced because of substance use.

  7. The substance use is continued despite knowledge of having a persistent or recurrent physical or psychological problem that is likely to have been caused or exacerbated by the substance (eg, current cocaine use despite recognition of cocaine-induced depression, or continued drinking despite recognition that an ulcer was made worse by alcohol consumption).

Reprinted, with permission, from the *Diagnostic and Statistical Manual of Mental Disorders*, 4th ed. Text Revision. Copyright 2000. American Psychiatric Association.

common (Table 4–4). Marijuana is the most commonly used illicit drug in the United States. First experiences with marijuana and the substances listed in Table 4–4 typically occur during middle school and early high school. Initiation of substance abuse is rare after age 20 years.

The level of substance abuse among American youth rose in the 1960s and 1970s, declined in the 1980s, reached a nadir in 1990, and rose again in the early and mid-1990s, peaking among eighth graders in 1996 (see Table 4–4). Use declined slightly in the late 1990s and was stable in 2000. Marijuana accounted for most of the increased drug use during the 1990s. Table 4–4 shows that marijuana use is still widespread among American youth. Use of most other drugs, including crack cocaine, declined during the 1990s. The major exception to this encouraging trend has been the increased use of ecstasy and anabolic steroids in 1999 and 2000. However, use of both drugs showed a decline in 2002. Overall drug and alcohol use also decreased in 2002. Studies indicate that the rise and fall in use of a substance is heralded by changes in the perceived risks and benefits of using the substance. Increased availability has been a major factor in the rising use of anabolic steroids and ecstasy. The age at initiation of alcohol and other substance abuse dropped significantly in the early 1990s. Currently, most first-time users are between 12 and 14 years of age. Inhalants such as glue and gasoline are predominantly a choice of younger adolescents. This statistic is particularly worrisome because early-onset substance use is one of the best predictors of persistent abuse later in life.

Dyer JE, Roth B, Hyman BA: Gamma-hydroxybutyrate withdrawal syndrome. Ann Emerg Med 2001;37:147 [PMID: 11174231].

Gilpin EA, Choi WS, Berry C, et al: How many adolescents start smoking each day in the United States? J Adolesc Health 1999;25:248 [PMID: 10505842].

Table 4–2. Physiologic effects of commonly abused mood-altering substances.[a]

EYES/PUPILS	
Mydriasis	Amphetamines, MDMA, or other stimulants, cocaine, glutethimide, jimson weed, LSD Withdrawal from alcohol and opioids
Miosis	Alcohol, barbiturates, benzodiazepines, opioids, PCP
Nystagmus	Alcohol, barbiturates, benzodiazepines, inhalants, PCP
Conjunctival injection	LSD, marijuana
Lacrimation	Inhalants, LSD. Withdrawal from opioids
CARDIOVASCULAR	
Tachycardia	Amphetamines, MDMA, or other stimulants, cocaine, LSD, marijuana, PCP. Withdrawal from alcohol, barbiturates, benzodiazepines
Hypertension	Amphetamines, MDMA, or other stimulants, cocaine, LSD, marijuana, PCP. Withdrawal from alcohol, barbiturates, benzodiazepines
Hypotension	Barbiturates, opioids. Orthostatic: marijuana. Withdrawal from depressants
Arrhythmia	Amphetamines, MDMA, or other stimulants, cocaine, inhalants, opioids, PCP
RESPIRATORY	
Depression	Opioids, depressants, GHB
Pulmonary edema	Opioids, stimulants
CORE BODY TEMPERATURE	
Elevated	Amphetamines, MDMA, or other stimulants, cocaine, PCP. Withdrawal from alcohol, barbiturates, benzodiazepines, opioids
Decreased	Alcohol, barbiturates, benzodiazepines, opioids, GHB
PERIPHERAL NERVOUS SYSTEM RESPONSE	
Hyperreflexia	Amphetamines, MDMA, or other stimulants, cocaine, LSD, marijuana, methaqualone, PCP Withdrawal from alcohol, barbiturates, benzodiazepines
Hyporeflexia	Alcohol, barbiturates, benzodiazepines, inhalants, opioids
Tremor	Amphetamines or other stimulants, cocaine, LSD Withdrawal from alcohol, barbiturates, benzodiazepines, cocaine
Ataxia	Alcohol, amphetamines, MDMA, or other stimulants, barbiturates, benzodiazepines, inhalants, LSD, PCP, GHB
CENTRAL NERVOUS SYSTEM RESPONSE	
Hyperalertness	Amphetamines, MDMA, or other stimulants, cocaine
Sedation, somnolence	Alcohol, barbiturates, benzodiazepines, inhalants, marijuana, opioids, GHB
Seizures	Alcohol, amphetamines, MDMA, or other stimulants, cocaine, inhalants, methaqualone, opioids (particularly meperidine, propoxyphene) Withdrawal from alcohol, barbiturates, benzodiazepines
Hallucinations	Amphetamines, MDMA, or other stimulants, cocaine, inhalants, LSD, marijuana, PCP Withdrawal from alcohol, barbiturates, benzodiazepines
GASTROINTESTINAL	
Nausea, vomiting	Alcohol, amphetamines or other stimulants, cocaine, inhalants, LSD, opioids, peyote, GHB Withdrawal from alcohol, barbiturates, benzodiazepines, cocaine, opioids

[a]GHB, gamma hydroxybutyrate, LSD, lysergic acid diethylamide, MDMA, methylenedioxymethamphetamine (ecstasy), PCP, phencyclidine hydrochloride.
Adapted, with permission, from Schwartz B, Alderman EM: Substance abuse. Pediatr Rev 1997;18:215.

Gruber AJ, Pope HG Jr: Marijuana use among adolescents. Pediatr Clin North Am 2002;49:389 [PMID: 11993290].

Halpern-Felsher BL, Cornell JL: Preventing underage alcohol use: where do we go from here? J Adolesc Health 2005;37:1 [PMID: 15963895].

Johnston LD, O'Malley PM, Bachman JG: *The Monitoring the Future National Survey Results on Adolescent Drug Use: Overview of Key Findings.* National Institute on Drug Abuse, US Department of Health and Human Services, 2006 (NIH Publication No. 06–5882). National Institute on Drug Abuse. www.monitoringthefuture.org

Koesters SC, Rogers PD, Rajasingham CR: MDMA ('ecstasy') and other 'club drugs.' The new epidemic. Pediatr Clin North Am 2002;49:415 [PMID: 11993291].

Kurtzman TL, Otsuka KN, Wahl RA: Inhalant abuse by adolescents. J Adolesc Health 2001;28:1616 [PMID: 11226839].

O'Malley PM, Johnston LD: Drinking and driving among US high school seniors, 1984–1997. Am J Public Health 1999;89:678 [PMID: 10224978].

Sung HE, Richter L, Vaughan R, et al: Nonmedical use of prescription opioids among teenagers in the United States: trends and correlates. J Adolesc Health. 2005;37:44 [PMID: 15963906].

Table 4–3. Effects of commonly abused mood-altering substances.

Substance	Pharmacology	Intoxication	Withdrawal	Chronic Use
Alcohol (ethanol)	Depressant; 10 g/drink Drink: 12 oz beer, 4 oz wine, 1 $\frac{1}{2}$ oz liquor; one drink increases blood level by approximately 0.025 g/dL (varies by weight)	Legal: 0.05–0.1 g/dL (varies by state) Mild: < 0.1 g/dL; disinhibition, euphoria, mild sedation and impaired coordination Moderate: 0.1–0.2 g/dL; impaired mentation and judgment, slurred speech, ataxia Severe: > 0.3 g/dL; confusion, stupor; > 0.4 g/dL; coma, depressed respiration	Mild: headache, tremors, nausea and vomiting ("hangover") Severe: fever, sweaty, seizure, agitation, hallucination, hypertension, tachycardia Delirium tremens (chronic use)	Hepatitis, cirrhosis, cardiac disease, Wernicke encephalopathy, Korsakoff syndrome
Marijuana (cannabis)	Delta-9-tetrahydrocannabinol (THC); 4–6% in marijuana; 20–30% in hashish	Low: euphoria, relaxation, impaired thinking High: mood changes, depersonalization, hallucinations Toxic: panic, delusions, paranoia, psychosis	Irritability, disturbed sleep, tremor, nystagmus, anorexia, diarrhea, vomiting	Cough, gynecomastia, low sperm count, infertility, amotivational syndrome, apathy
Cocaine	Stimulant; releases biogenic amines; concentration varies with preparation and route of administration	Hyperalert, increased energy, confident, insomnia, anxiety, paranoia, dilated pupils, tremors, seizures, hypertension, arrhythmia, tachycardia, fever, dry mouth Toxic: coma, psychosis, seizure, myocardial infarction, stroke, hyperthermia, rhabdomyolysis	Drug craving, depression, dysphoria, irritability, lethargy, tremors, nausea, hunger	Nasal septum ulceration, epistaxis, lung damage, intravenous drug use
Opioids (heroin, morphine, codeine, methadone, opium, fentanyl, meperidine, propoxyphene)	Depressant; binds central opioid receptor; variable concentrations with substance	Euphoria, sedation, impaired thinking, low blood pressure, pinpoint pupil, urinary retention Toxic: hypotension, arrhythmia, depressed respiration, stupor, coma, seizure, death	Only after > 3 weeks of regular use: drug craving, rhinorrhea, lacrimation, muscle aches, diarrhea, anxiety, tremors, hypertension, tachycardia	Intravenous drug use: cellulitis, endocarditis, embolisms, HIV
Amphetamines	Stimulant; sympathomimetic	Euphoria, hyperalert state, hyperactive, hypertension, arrhythmia, fever, flushing, dilated pupils, tremor, ataxia, dry mouth	Lethargy, fatigue, depression, anxiety, nightmares, muscle cramps, abdominal pain, hunger	Paranoia, psychosis

(continued)

Table 4–3. Effects of commonly abused mood-altering substances. (continued)

Substance	Pharmacology	Intoxication	Withdrawal	Chronic Use
		Toxic: coma, circulatory collapse, hypertensive crisis, cerebral hemorrhage		
MDMA (ecstasy)	Stimulant, psychedelic; releases serotonin, dopamine, and norepinephrine; inhibits reuptake of neurotransmitters; increases dopamine synthesis; inhibits MAO	Enhanced empathy, euphoria, increased energy and self-esteem, tachycardia, hypertension, increased pyschomotor drive, sensory enhancement, illusions, difficulty concentrating and retaining information, headaches, palpitations, flushing, hyperthermia Toxic: frank psychosis, coma, seizures, intracranial hemorrhage, cerebral infarction, asystole, pulmonary edema, multisystem organ failure, acute renal or heptic failure, ARDS, DIC, SIADH, death	None	Paranoid pyschosis
GHB (liquid ecstasy)	Depressant, endogenous CNS transmitter; influences dopaminergic activity, higher levels of GABA-B activity	10 mg/kg: sleep 30 mg/kg: memory loss 50 mg/kg: general anesthesia Toxic: CNS and respiratory depression, aggressiveness, seizures, bradycardia, apnea	Only after chronic use with dosing every 3 h Early: mild tremor, tachycardia, hypertension, diaphoresis, moderate anxiety, insomnia, nausea, vomiting Progressive: confusion, delirium, hallucinations, autonomic instability, death	Wernicke-Korsakoff syndrome
Sedative-hypnotics (barbiturates, benzodiazepines, methaqualone)	Depressant	Sedation, lethargy, slurred speech, pinpoint pupils, hypotension, psychosis, seizures Toxic: stupor, coma, cardiac arrest, seizure, pulmonary edema, death	Only after weeks of use: agitation, delirium, psychosis, hallucinations, fever, flushing, hyper- or hypotension, death	Paranoia

(continued)

Table 4–3. Effects of commonly abused mood-altering substances. (continued)

Substance	Pharmacology	Intoxication	Withdrawal	Chronic Use
Hallucinogens (LSD, peyote, mescaline, mushrooms, nutmeg, jimson weed)	Inhibition of serotonin release	Illusions, depersonalization, hallucination, anxiety, paranoia, ataxia, dilated pupils, hypertension, dry mouth Toxic: coma, terror, panic, "crazy feeling"	None	Flashbacks
Phencyclidine	Dissociative anesthetic	Low dose (< 5 mg): illusions, hallucinations, ataxia, hypertension, flushing Moderate dose (5–10 mg): hyperthermia, salivation, myoclonus High dose: (> 10 mg): rigidity, seizure, arrhythmia, coma, death	None	Flashbacks
Inhalants (toluene, benzene, hydrocarbons and fluorocarbons)	Stimulation progressing to depression	Euphoria, giddiness, impaired judgment, ataxia, rhinorrhea, salivation, hallucination Toxic: respiratory depression, arrhythmia, coma, stupor, delirium, sudden death	None	Permanent damage to nerves, liver, heart, kidney, brain
Nicotine	Releases dopamine, 1 mg nicotine per cigarette	Relaxation, tachycardia, vertigo, anorexia	Drug craving, irritability, anxiety, hunger, impaired concentration	Permanent damage to lung, heart, cardiovascular system
Anabolic steroids[a]	Bind steroid receptor Stacking: use many types simultaneously; pyramiding: increase dosage	Increased muscle bulk, strength, endurance, increased drive, hypogonadism, low sperm count, gynecomastia, decreased libido, virilization, irregular menses, hepatitis, early epiphysial closure, aggressiveness	Drug craving, dysphoria, irritability, depression	Tendon rupture, cardiomyopathy, atherosclerosis, peliosis hepatis (orally active C17 derivatives of testosterone are especially hepatotoxic)

[a]Despite conventional assumptions, scientific studies show that anabolic steroids do not improve aerobic athletic performance and improve strength only in athletes trained in weight lifting before they begin using steroids who continue to train and take a high-protein diet.
ARDS, acute respiratory distress syndrome; CNS, central nervous system; DIC, disseminated intravascular coagulation; GABA, γ-aminobutyric acid; GHB, γ-hydroxybutyrate; HIV, human immunodeficiency virus; LSD, lysergic acid diethylamide; MAO, monoamine oxidase; MDMA, methylenedioxymethamphetamine; SIADH, syndrome of inappropriate secretion of antidiuretic hormone.

Swaim R et al: The effect of school dropout rates on estimates of adolescent substance use among three racial/ethnic groups. Am J Public Health 1997;87:51 [PMID: 9065226].

Tomar SL, Giovino GA: Incidence and predictors of smokeless tobacco use among US youth. Am J Public Health 1998;88:20 [PMID: 9584028].

Wakefield M, Kloska DD, O'Malley PM, et al: The role of smoking intentions in predicting future smoking among youth: findings from Monitoring the Future data. Addiction 2004; 99:914 [PMID: 15200587].

Zamboanga BL, Bean JL, Pietras AC, et al: Subjective evaluations of alcohol expectancies and their relevance to drinking game

Table 4–4. Prevalence of pediatric substance use and abusers by year.

	Lifetime					Annual					30-day				
	1991	1996	2002	2003	2004	1991	1996	2002	2003	2004	1991	1996	2002	2003	2004
Any illicit drug															
8th grade	18.7	31.2	24.5	22.8	21.5	11.3	23.6	17.7	16.1	15.2	5.7	14.6	10.4	9.7	8.4
10th grade	30.6	45.4	44.6	41.4	39.8	21.4	37.5	34.8	32.0	31.1	11.6	23.2	20.8	19.5	18.3
12th grade	44.1	50.8	53.0	51.1	51.1	29.4	40.2	41.0	39.3	38.8	16.4	24.6	25.4	24.1	23.4
Marijuana/hashish															
8th grade	10.2	23.1	19.2	17.5	16.3	6.2	18.3	14.6	12.8	11.8	3.2	11.3	8.3	7.5	6.4
10th grade	23.4	39.8	38.7	36.4	35.1	16.5	33.6	30.3	28.2	27.5	8.7	20.4	17.8	17.0	15.9
12th grade	36.7	44.9	47.8	46.1	45.7	23.9	35.8	36.2	34.9	34.3	13.8	21.9	21.5	21.2	19.9
Inhalants															
8th grade	17.6	21.2	15.2	15.8	17.3	9.0	12.2	7.7	8.7	9.6	4.4	5.8	3.8	4.1	4.5
10th grade	15.7	19.3	13.5	12.7	12.4	7.1	9.5	5.8	5.4	5.9	2.7	3.3	2.4	2.2	2.4
12th grade	17.6	16.6	11.7	11.2	10.9	6.6	7.6	4.5	3.9	4.2	2.4	2.5	1.5	1.5	1.5
MDMA (ecstasy)															
8th grade	—	3.4	4.3	3.2	2.8	—	2.3	2.9	2.1	1.7	—	1.0	1.4	0.7	0.8
10th grade	—	5.6	6.6	5.4	4.3	—	4.6	4.9	3.0	2.4	—	1.8	1.8	1.1	0.8
12th grade	—	6.1	10.5	8.3	7.5	—	4.6	7.4	4.5	4.0	—	2.0	2.4	1.3	1.2

MDMA, methylenedioxymethamphetamine.
Reproduced, with permission, from Monitoring the Future Study, 2006. Available at www.monitoringthefuture.org.

involvement in female college students. J Adolesc Health 2005;37:77 [PMID: 15963914].

MORBIDITY ASSOCIATED WITH SUBSTANCE ABUSE

Use and abuse of alcohol or other mood-altering substances is associated with the leading causes of adolescent and young adult deaths and injuries in the United States (ie, motor vehicle crashes, other unintentional injuries, homicide, and suicide), which are typically outcomes of high-risk or violent behaviors combined with impaired judgment. Substance abuse is also associated with physical and sexual abuse. Up to two-thirds of sexual assaults and acquaintance or date rapes are linked to alcohol or other drug use. Drug use and abuse also contribute to other high-risk behaviors, such as unsafe and increased sexual activity, leading to unintended pregnancy and sexually transmitted diseases. The use of drugs during periods of low self-esteem and depression increases the risk of suicide.

The well-known long- and short-term risks associated with tobacco, alcohol, and cocaine are listed in Table 4–3. Less well known are the long- and short-term morbidities connected with the currently most popular illicit drugs among adolescents (eg, marijuana and ecstasy). The active ingredient in marijuana, δ-9-tetrahydrocannabinol (THC), transiently causes tachycardia, mild hypertension, and bronchodilation. Regular use can cause lung changes similar to those seen in tobacco smokers. Heavy use decreases fertility in both sexes, leads to immunosuppression, and can cause the destruction of hippocampal and basal ganglia nuclei, resulting in disruption in cognition, learning, coordination, and memory. This may explain the development of so-called amotivational syndrome in heavy users, characterized by decreased attention to environmental stimuli and impaired goal-directed thinking and behavior. Also of concern is the increasing potency of available marijuana. Recent analysis of confiscated marijuana has shown a three- to fivefold increase in the concentration of THC since the 1970s and 1980s.

Ecstasy, which is gaining in popularity with teens and becoming more accessible, can cause permanent brain damage. Chronic use destroys the serotonin system of the brain and has been associated with progressive decline of immediate and delayed memory and with alterations in mood, sleep, and appetite. Even first-time users may develop frank psychosis indistinguishable from schizophrenia. Irreversible cardiomyopathy, noncardiogenic pulmonary edema, and pulmonary hypertension may occur with long-term use. Overdose can cause hyperthermia and multiorgan system failure.

Environmental and prenatal exposure to abused substances carry significant health risks. Parental tobacco smoking has been associated with low birth weight in newborns, sudden infant death syndrome, bronchiolitis, asthma, otitis media, and fire-related injuries. Paternal use of marijuana during pregnancy is associated with an increased risk of sudden infant death syndrome. In utero exposure to cocaine and alcohol can result in fetal malformations, intrauterine growth restriction, and brain injury.

American Academy of Pediatrics Committee on Substance Abuse: Tobacco's Toll: Implications for the pediatrician. Pediatrics 2001;107:794 [PMID: 11335763].

Burd L, Wilson H: Fetal, infant, and child mortality in a context of alcohol use. Am J Med Genet C Semin Med Genet 2004; 15;127:51 [PMID: 15095472].

Gouzoulis-Mayfrank E et al: Impaired cognitive performance in drug free users of recreational ecstasy (MDMA). J Neurol Neurosurg Psychiatr 2000;68:719 [PMID: 10811694].

Graeme K: New drugs of abuse. Emerg Med Clin North Am 2000;18:625 [PMID: 11130930].

Klonoff-Cohen H, Lam-Kruglick P: Maternal and paternal recreational drug use and sudden infant death syndrome. Arch Pediatr Adolesc Med 2001;155:765 [PMID: 11434841].

Knishkowy B, Amitai Y: Water-pipe (narghile) smoking: an emerging health risk behavior. Pediatrics 2005;116:e113 [PMID: 15995011].

Ownby DR, Johnson CC, Peterson EL: Passive cigarette smoke exposure in infants. Arch Pediatr Adolesc Med 2000;154:1237 [PMID: 11115309].

Tapert SF et al: Adolescent substance use and sexual risk-taking behavior. J Adolesc Health 2001;28:181 [PMID: 11226840].

Tschann JM, Flores F, Pasch LA, et al: Emotional distress, alcohol use, and peer violence among Mexican-American and European-American adolescents. J Adolesc Health 2005;37:11 [PMID: 15963902].

Van Beurden E, Zask A, Brooks L, et al: Heavy episodic drinking and sensation seeking in adolescents as predictors of harmful driving and celebrating behaviors: implications for prevention. J Adolesc Health 2005;37:37 [PMID: 15963905].

Wu LT, Schlenger WE, Ringwalt CL: Use of nitrite inhalants ("poppers") among American youth. J Adolesc Health 2005; 37:52 [PMID: 15963907].

SUPPLEMENT USE AND ABUSE

Use of supplements or special diets to enhance athletic performance dates back to antiquity, when warriors and athletes ate certain animals to acquire their characteristics. Today, many elite and casual athletes use ergogenic supplements in an attempt to improve performance. The most popular products among the pediatric population are protein supplements, creatine, and the prohormones. Strength athletes (ie, weight lifters) use protein powders and shakes to enhance muscle repair and mass. The typical amount of protein consumed by athletes far exceeds the recommended daily allowance for resistance-training athletes such as weight lifters (1.6–1.7 g/kg/d).

Excess consumption of protein provides no added strength or muscle mass and can provoke renal failure in teens with underlying renal dysfunction.

Creatine is the most popular nutritional supplement, with annual sales of $400 million. It is a combination of glycine, arginine, and methionine. Creatine is produced naturally in the liver, kidneys, and pancreas. It facilitates the production of adenosine triphosphate and increases free energy for muscle contraction. It maximizes power during short-duration, intense exercise, and improves baseline strength in adults. In contrast, creatine does not improve performance in longer-duration, aerobic exercise, nor has its effectiveness been analyzed in children. Although the American College of Sports Medicine discourages use of the synthetic product by people under 18 years of age, recent studies show that creatine is extensively used by athletes in grades 6–12. Use by high-school juniors and seniors mirrors that of college athletes. Side effects include weight gain, headache, abdominal pain, diarrhea, and increased muscle strain. There are conflicting reports about the risk of renal damage.

Most disturbing for health care providers is the growing availability and use of prohormones, specifically dehydroepiandrosterone (DHEA) and androstenedione. Sold as dietary supplements, these precursors to testosterone and other sex hormones are sold without federal regulation. Endogenous DHEA is produced in the adrenal cortex as a precursor of gonadal hormones. Putative benefits of DHEA include increased fat catabolism; increased muscle mass; increased libido; "improved" immune function; and decreased memory loss, heart disease, cancer, type 2 diabetes mellitus, and Alzheimer and Parkinson disease. Although its effects on strength and performance in athletes remain unstudied and unproven, the advertised benefits are attractive to many athletes. Its effect on young, healthy individuals (ie, those with higher baseline DHEA levels) has not been studied. In adults, two studies have shown that its use at 50 mg/d and 100 mg/d increases androgenic steroid plasma levels and improves subjective perception of physical and psychological well-being. Users of DHEA report few adverse effects.

Androstenedione, which is banned by the International Olympic Committee, National Collegiate Athletic Association, and National Football League, is converted to testosterone by the liver. A recent study of young athletes concluded that oral androstenedione does not increase plasma testosterone concentrations, and in young eugonadal men has no anabolic effect on muscle protein metabolism. Other studies have shown increased biologically active estrogen levels. No long-term studies of androstenedione have been conducted. Its side effects are believed to be similar to those of other anabolic and androgenic agents. Most side effects are secondary to androgen excess—hyperlipidemia, hypertension, insulin resistance, hyperinsulinism, depression, aggression, paranoia, acne, male pattern baldness, alopecia, priapism, and others. Most effects are reversible with cessation of the product's use. Irreversible side effects include virilization in females (hair loss, clitoromegaly, hirsutism, and voice-deepening) and gynecomastia in males.

As the use of supplements and herbs increases, it will be increasingly important for pediatric care providers to be familiar with their common side effects. The Internet has become a source of information and sales of these products, which could lead to their increased use. The easy accessibility, perceived low risk, and low cost of these products significantly increase the likelihood that they will become significant substances of abuse by the pediatric population.

Ahrendt DM: Ergogenic aids: Counseling the athlete. Am Fam Physician 2001;63:913 [PMID: 11261867].

Bahrke MS, Yesalis CE, Kopstein AN, et al: Risk factors associated with anabolic-androgenic steroid use among adolescents. Sports Med 2000;29:397 [PMID: 10870866].

Congeni J, Miller S: Supplements and drugs used to enhance athletic performance. Pediatr Clin North Am. 2002;49:435 [PMID: 11993292].

Metzl JD et al: Creatine use among young athletes. Pediatrics 2001;108:421 [PMID: 11483809].

Morris CA, Avorn J: Internet marketing of herbal products. JAMA 2003;290:1505 [PMID: 13129992].

Rasmussen BB: Androstenedione does not stimulate muscle protein anabolism in young healthy men. J Clin Endocrinol Metab 2000;85:55 [PMID: 10634363].

Terjung RL, Clarkson P, Eichner ER et al: American College of Sports Medicine roundtable. The physiological and health effects of oral creatine supplementation. Med Sci Sports Exerc 2000;32:706 [PMID: 10731017].

RESPONSE TO THE PROBLEM

Federal, state, and local governments attempt to control the damage caused by substance abuse by prohibiting use and by legislating against associated high-risk behaviors (eg, enacting drunk-driving laws and nighttime curfews). However, neither these legal actions nor the large sums of money spent on school- and community-based drug abuse prevention and treatment programs have curbed the problem. Hence, the American Academy of Pediatrics (AAP) recommends that pediatricians become knowledgeable about the extent and nature of drugs used in their community, provide anticipatory guidance to parents starting with the first prenatal visit, and be aware of community referral and treatment resources for adolescents. The Internet makes this task more difficult. For example, poor methods for age verification make it easy for minors to purchase tobacco products online.

Hogan MJ: Diagnosis and treatment of teen drug use. Med Clin North Am 2000;84:927 [PMID: 10928196].

Kodjo CM, Klein JD: Prevention and risk of adolescent substance abuse. The role of adolescents, families, and communities. Pediatr Clin North Am 2002;49:257 [PMID: 11993282].

Kulig JW: American Academy of Pediatrics Committee on Substance Abuse. Tobacco, alcohol, and other drugs: the role of the pediatrician in prevention, identification, and management of substance abuse. Pediatrics 2005;115:816 [PMID: 15741395].

Ribisl KM et al: Internet sales of cigarettes to minors. JAMA 2003;290:1356 [PMID: 12966128].

PREDICTING THE PROGRESSION FROM USE TO ABUSE

Most adolescents who use mood-altering substances do so only intermittently or experimentally. The challenge to pediatric health care providers is to recognize the warning signs, identify potential abusers early, and intervene in an effective and timely fashion before acute or chronic use results in morbidity. The best predictors of ethanol and drug abuse are male sex, young age at first use, and associating with drug-using peers. It is still unclear why only a minority of the young people exhibiting the high-risk characteristics listed in Table 4–5 go on to abuse substances. Substance abuse is a symptom of personal and social maladjustment as often as it is a cause. Because a direct relationship exists between the number of risk factors listed in Table 4–5 and the frequency of substance abuse, a combination of risk factors is the best indicator of risk. Even so, most teenagers who exhibit multiple risk characteristics never develop a substance abuse problem, presumably because the protective factors listed in Table 4–5 give them enough resiliency to cope with stress in more socially adaptive ways.

Being aware of the risk domains listed in Table 4–5 will help physicians identify youngsters most apt to need counseling about substance abuse. Theories concerning the mechanisms responsible for the association between the risk factors listed in Table 4–5 and substance abuse are listed in Table 4–6. These theories provide a framework for understanding why individual patients may be at risk for progressing from occasional to established or compulsive substance abuse. Most theories emphasize social influences as the most reliable predictors of both the onset and the progression of substance abuse. For example, most teenage smokers report smoking at home and cite smoking parents or relatives as a reason to continue smoking.

Problem behavior theory is one of the most frequently cited concepts in the substance abuse literature. Its main argument is that socially disapproved behaviors tend to cluster and to resist intervention because they have both negative and positive consequences for the individual. Expectancy theory, which takes up where problem behavior theory leaves off, proposes a potentially modifiable mechanism by which learning experiences influence substance abuse. Measuring alcohol- and drug-related expectations has been found to provide a more accurate assess-

Table 4–5. Factors that influence the progression from substance use to substance abuse.

Enabling Risk Factors	Potentially Protective Factors
SOCIETAL AND COMMUNITY	
Experimentation encouraged by media	Regular involvement in church activities
Illicit substances available	Support for norms and values of society
Extreme economic deprivation	Strict enforcement of laws prohibiting substance
Neighborhood disorganization, crowding	use among minors and abuse among adults
Tolerance of licit and illicit substance use	Neighborhood resources, supportive adults
SCHOOL	
Lack of commitment to school or education	Strong commitment to school or education
Truancy	Future-oriented goals
Academic failure	Achievement oriented
Early, persistent behavior problems	
FAMILY	
Models of substance abuse and other unconventional behavior	Models of conventional behavior
Dysfunctional parenting styles; excessive authority or permissiveness	Attachment to parents
High family conflict; low bonding	Cohesive family
	Nurturing parenting styles
PEERS	
Peer rejection in elementary grades	Popular with peers
Substance use prevalent among peers	Abstinent friends
Peer attitudes favorable to substance abuse and unconventional behavior	Peer attitudes favor conventional behavior
INDIVIDUAL	
Genetic predisposition	Positive self-concept, good self-esteem
Psychological diagnoses (attention-deficit/hyperactivity disorder; antisocial personality)	Intolerance of deviance
Depression and low self-esteem	Internally motivated, takes charge of problems
Alienation and rebelliousness	
Sexual or physical abuse	
Early onset of deviant behavior or delinquency	
Early onset of sexual behavior	
Aggressive	

ment of risk than any of the factors listed in Table 4–5. Expectations about the effects of substances are important determinants of social and psychological reactions to them. Furthermore, these expectations are longitudinally related to different patterns of substance abuse. For example, within homogeneous groups of nondrinkers, low-risk drinkers, and high-risk drinkers, expectations about outcomes differ significantly both at entry into college and 3 years later. At each level alcohol abusers who progress to the next level of drinking expect more positive outcomes from the drinking. Conversely, evidence that negative experiences with alcohol transform some high-risk freshmen drinkers into nondrinking seniors suggests that it may be possible to influence indulgence patterns by altering expectancies. Here intervention is critical. Without guidance, most youngsters do not draw sobering conclusions from their negative experiences with drugs and alcohol. Despite serious accidents and socially unrewarding experiences, positive expectancies about the effects of alcohol tend to increase rather than decrease during the first 3 years of college. Similarly the expectation of weight loss and improved mood leads to initiation of smoking or reluctance to quit.

Brown RT: Risk factors for substance abuse in adolescents. Pediatr Clin North Am 2002;49:247 [PMID: 11993281].

Comerci GD, Schwebel R: Substance abuse: An overview. Adolesc Med 2000;11:79 [PMID: 10640340].

Table 4–6. Theories accounting for the progression from substance use to substance abuse.[a]

Theory	Key Constructs and Assumptions	Major Protagonist
Problem Behavior	Socially problematic behaviors[b] occur together and reflect a common underlying cause. The common antecedent is the reflection of the interaction among individual personality traits (eg, unconventionality), the perceived environment (eg, models of deviance), and a nondominant pattern of socialization (eg, low value on education).	Jessor R, Jessor R: *Problem Behavior and Psychosocial Development.* Academic Press, 1977.
Social Learning	Problem behavior theory plus a scheme to explain reinforcement of these behaviors. The risk of problem behavior increases when youngsters have the opportunity to become skillful in unconventional settings and are rewarded for doing so.	Bandura A: *Social Learning Theory.* Prentice-Hall, 1977.
Reasoned Action	Behavior is determined by the interaction between perceived consequences and attitudes toward those consequences. The risk of problem behavior increases when the perceived costs are low or the perceived benefits high.	Ajzen I, Fishbein M: *Understanding Attitudes and Predicting Behavior.* Prentice-Hall, 1980.
Health Belief	Health behaviors reflect assessments of perceived risk or harm, potential to avoid that harm through alternative behaviors, and ability to access requisite resources. The risk of unhealthy behavior increases when the perceived health risk is low or the ability to avoid that risk is perceived to be low or unrelated to the behavior.	Becker MH: The health belief model and personal health behavior. Health Educ Monogr 1974;2:324.
Social Control	Behavior is determined by the bonds an individual establishes with society. The risk of problem behavior increases when attachment to those who express conventional values is weak, commitment to participation in conventional activities is low, little time is spent in these activities, and the central value system of society is not fully accepted.	Hirschi T: *Causes of Delinquency.* University of California Press; 1969.
Peer Cluster	The socialization process that accompanies adolescent development results in the formation of peer clusters. Family sanctions, religious identifications, and school adjustment affect behavior indirectly through their effects on peer clusters.	Oetting ER, Beauvais F: Peer cluster theory. Counseling Psychol 1987;34:205.
Expectancy	Problem behavior and reasoned action theories plus a mechanism by which learning experiences exert an influence on future behavior. The risk of problem behavior increases when experiences reinforce preexisting positive expectancies about the effects of deviant behavior.	Werner MJ: Relation of alcohol expectancies to change in problem drinking among college students. Arch Pediatr Adolesc Med 1995;149:733.
Self-Medication	Individuals are predisposed to addiction when they experience painful affective states or psychiatric disorders; symptom relief perpetuates the use of specific substances.	Khantzian EJ: The self-medication hypothesis. Am J Psychiatry 1985;142:1259.

[a]Ordered by frequency of citation in the literature.
[b]A problem behavior is defined as any behavior compromising the accomplishment of normal developmental tasks of adolescence; most are hard to change because they also serve functions central to the psychosocial development of adolescents who lack conventional alternatives.

Hill KG, Hawkins JD, Catalano RF, et al: Family influences on the risk of daily smoking initiation. J Adolesc Health 2005;37:202 [PMID: 16109339].

Nash SG, McQueen A, Bray JH: Pathways to adolescent alcohol use: family environment, peer influence, and parental expectations. J Adolesc Health 2005;37:19 [PMID: 15963903].

MANAGEMENT OF SUBSTANCE ABUSE

It is critical that pediatric care providers have the knowledge and skill to diagnose, treat, and advocate for their substance-using and abusing patients. The AAP Committee on Substance Abuse recommends that pediatricians include discussions of substance abuse as part of their anticipatory care, starting with parents at the first prenatal visit.

Office Screening

Given the high incidence of substance abuse and the subtlety of its early signs and symptoms, a general psychosocial assessment is the best way to screen for substance abuse. Interviewing and counseling techniques and methods for taking a psychosocial history are discussed in Chapter 3. In an atmosphere of trust and confidentiality, physicians must ask routine screening questions of all patients and be alert for addictive diseases, especially in light of the high level of denial often present in addicted patients. The universal screening approach outlined in the American Medical Association (AMA) Guidelines for Adolescent Preventive Services (GAPS) is a good guide for routine screening and diagnosis. Clues to possible substance abuse include truancy, failing grades, problems with interpersonal relationships, delinquency, depressive affect, chronic fatigue, recurrent abdominal pains, chest pains or palpitations, headache, chronic cough, persistent nasal discharge, and recurrent complaints of sore throat. Substance abuse should be included in the differential diagnosis of all behavioral, family, psychosocial, and medical problems. Pediatricians seeing patients in emergency departments, trauma units, or prison must have an especially high index of suspicion. A family history of drug addiction or abuse should raise the level of concern about drug abuse in the pediatric patient. Possession of promotional products such as T-shirts and caps with cigarette or alcohol logos should also be a red flag because teenagers who own these items are more likely to use the products they advertise.

Albers AB, Biener L: Adolescent participation in tobacco promotions: Role of psychosocial factors. Pediatrics 2003;111:402 [PMID: 12563070].

Collins RL, Ellickson PL, McCaffrey DF et al: Saturated in beer: awareness of beer advertising in late childhood and adolescence. J Adolesc Health 2005;37:29 [PMID: 15963904].

Dias PJ: Adolescent substance abuse. Assessment in the office. Pediatr Clin North Am 2002;49:269 [PMID: 11993283].

Gruber EL, Thau HM, Hill DL et al: Alcohol, tobacco and illicit substances in music videos: a content analysis of prevalence and genre. J Adolesc Health 2005;37:81 [PMID: 15963915].

Levy S, Vaughan BL, Knight JR: Office-based intervention for adolescent substance abuse. Pediatr Clin North Am 2002;49:329 [PMID: 11993286].

Schydlower M (editor): Substance Abuse: A Guide for Health Professionals. American Academy of Pediatrics, 2000.

Weddle M, Kokotailo P: Adolescent substance abuse. Confidentiality and consent. Pediatr Clin North Am 2002;49:301 [PMID: 11993284].

Diagnosis

Although few children and adolescents will have been abusing substances long enough to have developed overt

Table 4–7. Diagnostic interview for substance abuse.

I. Define the extent of the problem by determining:
Age at onset of substance use
Which substances are being used
Circumstances of use
Where?
When?
With whom?
To what extent substances are being used
How frequently?
How much (quantity)?
With what associated symptoms (eg, tolerance, withdrawal)?
With what result?
What does the patient gain from becoming high?
Does the patient get into risky situations while high?
Does the patient engage in behaviors while high that are later regretted?
II. Define the cause of the problem by developing a differential diagnosis

signs and symptoms, it is important to look for them on physical examination. Positive physical findings can be a tool to penetrate a patient's denial and convince him or her of the significance of the alcohol or drug use.

When the psychosocial history suggests the possibility of substance use, the primary tasks of the diagnostic interview are the same as for the evaluation of other medical problems (Table 4–7).

First, specific information about the extent of the problem must be gathered. Eliciting multiple-choice answers is a useful technique. For example, "Has anything really good ever happened to you when you are high?" or "Some of my patients like to get high because they feel good; others find it helps them relax and be sociable with friends; and some find it helps them forget their problems. Are any of these things true for you?"

Second, the provider needs to determine why the patient has progressed from initiation to the continuation or maintenance phase of substance abuse. The cause may be different at different periods of development. Although peer group characteristics are one of the best predictors of substance use among early and middle adolescents, this is not so among older adolescents and young adults.

Brief questionnaires can be used if time does not allow for more detailed investigation. Two instruments evaluated rigorously in primary care settings are the CAGE questionnaire and the Perceived Benefits of Drinking Scale. CAGE is a mnemonic derived from the first four questions listed in Table 4–8. A score of 2 or more is highly suggestive of substance abuse. The Per-

Table 4–8. Substance abuse screening questionnaires.

CAGE Questionnaire
CUT DOWN: Have you ever felt you ought to cut down on your drinking (drug use)?
ANNOYED: Have people annoyed you by criticizing your drinking (drug use)?
GUILTY: Have you ever felt bad about your drinking (drug use)?
EYE OPENER: Have you ever had a drink (used drugs) to steady your nerves in the morning?
(Score 1 point for each positive answer; refer if total points ≥ 2)
Used, with permission, from Ewing JE: Detecting alcoholism: The CAGE questionnaire. JAMA 1984;252:1905.
Perceived Benefits Scales
1. Drinking (drug use) helps me forget my problems.
2. Drinking (drug use) helps me be friendly.
3. Drinking (drug use) helps me feel good about myself.
4. Drinking (drug use) helps me relax.
5. Drinking (drug use) helps me be friends with others who drink (use drugs).
(Score 1 point for each positive answer; refer if total points ≥ 3)
Used, with permission, from Petchers MK, Singer MI: Perceived-Benefit-of-Drinking Scale. J Pediatr 1987;110:977.

ceived-Benefit-of-Drinking Scale consists of the next five statements listed in Table 4–8. Patients who endorse more than three statements deserve further evaluation. Because CAGE is more predictive of substance use problems among males and the Perceived-Benefit-of-Drinking Scale is more predictive among females, many clinicians combine the two scales. Including an additional question about use of tobacco and a question about the patient's best friend's use of mood-altering substances further enhances the diagnostic accuracy of these screening tools.

Although constructed as screening tools for alcohol abuse in adults, the questions in Table 4–8 can be adapted to elicit similar information about use of other mood-altering substances by pediatric patients and by their close contacts (eg, parents and older siblings). Finally, clinicians may find it helpful to use these questionnaires to stimulate discussion of the patient's self-perception of his or her substance use. For example, if an adolescent admits to a previous attempt to cut down on drinking, this provides an opportunity to inquire about events that may have led to the attempt.

Additional screening instruments include the following:

1. The Simple Screening Instrument for Alcohol and Other Drug Abuse (SSI-AOD), from the Center for Treatment of Substance Abuse, is a quick, 16-item screen that has proven reliable among adolescent medical patients.
2. The Personal Experience Inventory is a comprehensive, standardized 260-item self-report measure of chemical involvement and the psychosocial aspect of substance use.
3. The Personal Experience Screening Questionnaire is a quick, 38-item screen that evaluates the severity of the problem and associated psychosocial risks.
4. The Adolescent Diagnostic Interview is a structured interview based on the American Psychiatric Association's diagnostic criteria for substance abuse (see Table 4–1).

Although these instruments may be too time-consuming for routine office use, they may prove helpful in the evaluation of patients who pose diagnostic or therapeutic dilemmas.

Knight JR, Sherritt L, Harris SK et al: Validity of brief alcohol screening tests among adolescents: a comparison of the AUDIT, POSIT, CAGE, and CRAFFT. Alcohol Clin Exp Res 2003;27:67 [PMID: 12544008].

Knight JR, Sherritt L, Shrier LA et al: Validity of the CRAFFT substance abuse screening test among adolescent clinic patients. Arch Pediatr Adolesc Med 2002;156:607 [PMID: 12038895].

Knight JR, Sherritt L, Van Hook S et al: Motivational interviewing for adolescent substance use: a pilot study. J Adolesc Health 2005;37:167 [PMID: 16026730].

Wilson CR, Sherritt L, Gates E et al: Are clinical impressions of adolescent substance use accurate? Pediatrics 2004;114:e536 [PMID: 15520086].

Comorbidity

It is important for pediatric care providers to recognize the possibility of multiple diagnoses in patients who are abusing substances. Alcohol and substance abusers are more likely than are their nonabusing counterparts to have another psychiatric disorder. Affective disorders, anxiety disorders, and mania rank among the disorders most strongly associated with alcohol and drug dependence. Adolescents with depression are likely to use drugs in an attempt to feel pleasure, but this type of self-medication may exacerbate their condition. In addition to identifying psychiatric comorbidities, it is imperative that providers look for medical conditions that can mimic symptoms of drug withdrawal or intoxication. Patients with significant primary medical conditions may use illicit substances to relieve symptoms (severe pain or chemotherapeutic side effects). Although it is often difficult to determine which diagnosis is primary, it is important for pediatric health care providers to recognize the possibility of a comorbid condition and provide appropriate treatment.

Comerci GD, Schwebel R: Substance abuse: An overview. Adolesc Med 2000;11:79 [PMID: 10640340].

Jellinek MS: Depression and suicide in children and adolescents. Pediatr Rev 1998;19:255 [PMID: 9797715].

Substance use problems and associated psychiatric symptoms among adolescents in primary care. Pediatrics 2003;111:e699 [PMID: 12777588].

Pharmacologic Screening

The use of urine and blood testing for detecting substance abuse is controversial. The consensus is that pharmacologic screening should be reserved for situations in which behavioral dysfunction is of sufficient concern to outweigh the practical and ethical drawbacks of testing. The AAP recommends screening under certain circumstances (eg, an inexplicably obtunded patient in the emergency department) but discourages routine screening for the following reasons: (1) Voluntary screening programs are rarely truly voluntary owing to the negative consequences for those who decline to participate; (2) infrequent users or individuals who have not used substances recently may be missed; (3) confronting substance-abusing individuals with objective evidence of their use has little or no effect on their behavior; (4) the AAP reminds providers that their role is counseling and treatment, not law enforcement, so drug testing should not be done for the purpose of detecting illegal use. If testing is to be performed, the provider should discuss the plan for screening with the patient, explain the reasons for it, and obtain informed consent. The AAP does not consider parental request and permission sufficient justification for involuntary screening of mentally competent minors.

Beyond the ethical concerns, there are also practical concerns. If testing is to be performed, it is imperative that it be done accurately and that the limitations of testing be understood by all parties. Tests range from simple, inexpensive, chromatographic spot tests, which can be performed in the office, to gas chromatography and mass spectrometry, which require specialized laboratory equipment and are usually reserved for forensic investigations. Most commercial medical laboratories use the enzyme multiplication immunoassay technique, in which a sample of the fluid to be tested is added to a test reagent consisting of a known quantity of the radiolabeled index drug (ie, the drug being tested for). If the index drug is also present in the patient's urine or serum, it competes with the radiolabeled drug for binding sites on the test kit antibody. The unbound or excess drug can then be quantified with a spectropho-

Table 4–9. Causes of false-positive drug screens.

Opioids
Poppy seeds
Dextromethorphan
Chlorpromazine
Diphenoxylate
Amphetamines
Ephedrine
Phenylephrine
Pseudoephedrine
N-acetylprocainamide
Chloroquine
Procainamide
Phencyclidines
Dextromethorphan
Diphenhydramine
Chlorpromazine
Doxylamine
Thioridazine

tometer. Most of the commonly abused mood-altering substances, with the exception of solvents and inhalants, can be detected by this method.

Caution is necessary in interpreting results because false-positives may be obtained as a result of antibody cross-reactions with the medications and substances listed in Table 4–9 or from passive exposure to illicit substances. The most common cause of false-negative tests is infrequent use. Table 4–10 shows the duration of detectability in the urine after last use by class of substance and duration of use. Detectability ranges from a few hours for alcohol to several weeks for regular marijuana use. False-negative results can occur if the patient alters or adulterates the specimen, either by drinking a large volume of fluid or adding such substances as bleach, vinegar, or goldenseal powder to the specimen. (Teenagers should be advised that despite street lore, ingesting these compounds is an ineffective and potentially dangerous way to prevent drug detection in the urine.) Close observation during collection and pretesting the temperature, specific gravity, and pH of urine samples may detect attempts at deception.

American Academy of Pediatrics Committee on Substance Abuse: Testing for drugs of abuse in children and adolescents. Pediatrics 1996;98:305 [PMID: 8692638].

Casavant MJ: Urine drug screening in adolescents. Pediatr Clin North Am 2002;49:317 [PMID: 11993285].

Perrone J: Drug screening versus history in detection of substance use in ED psychiatric patients. Am J Emerg Med 2001;19:49 [PMID: 11146019].

Schwartz RH, Silber TJ, Heyman RB et al: Urine testing for drugs of abuse: a survey of suburban parent-adolescent dyads. Arch Pediatr Adolesc Med 2003;157:158 [PMID: 12580685].

Table 4–10. Duration of urine positivity for selected drugs.

Drug Class	Detection Time
Amphetamines	< 48 hours
Barbiturates	Short-acting: 1 d Long-acting: 2–3 wk
Benzodiazepines	Single dose: 3 d Habitual use: 4–6 wk
Cocaine metabolites	Acute use: 2–4 d Habitual use: 2 wk
Ethanol	2–14 h
Methadone	Up to 3 d
Opioids	Up to 2 d
Propoxyphene	6–48 h
Cannabinoids	Moderate use: 5 d Habitual use: 10–20 d
Methaqualone	2 wk
Phencyclidine	Acute use: 1 wk Habitual use: 3 wk
Anabolic steroids	Days to weeks

Reprinted, with permission, from Woolf A, Shannon M: Clinical toxicology for the pediatrician. Pediatr Clin North Am 1995;42:317.

TREATMENT & REFERRAL

Office-Based Treatment

The AMA and the AAP recommend that all children and adolescents receive counseling about the dangers of substance use and abuse from their primary health care providers. By offering confidential health care services and routinely counseling about the risks associated with drug abuse, pediatricians can help most of their patients avoid the adverse consequences of experimentation with mood-altering substances. However, more intervention is required for youngsters in environments where substance abuse is regarded as acceptable recreational behavior. Because substance use is often deeply embedded in the fabric of these young peoples' lives, most have little interest in prevention or treatment. Counseling strategies appropriate for patients who wish to change their behavior may be ineffective for a patient who does not consider use of mood-altering substances to be a problem. It may therefore be preferable to begin discussions about treatment by helping youngsters consider alternative ways of meeting the needs that substance use is currently providing. The clinician may in this way help the patient devise alternatives that are more attractive than substance use. Realistically, few substance-abusing teenagers will choose to quit because of a single conversation with even a highly respected health care provider. The message is most effective when offered repeatedly from a variety of sources—family, peers, guidance counselors, and teachers.

Because an assessment of the patient's readiness to change is the critical first step in office-based intervention, clinicians should consider the construct presented in Table 4–11. In theory, individuals pass through this series of stages in the course of changing problem behaviors. Thus, to be maximally effective, providers should tailor their counseling messages to the patient's stage of readiness to change.

Once it has been established that a patient is prepared to act on information about treatment, the next step is to select the program that best fits his or her individual needs. Most drug treatment programs are not designed to recognize and act on the individual vulnerabilities that have predisposed the patient to substance abuse. When programs are individualized, even brief (5- to 10-minute) counseling sessions may promote reductions in cigarette smoking and drinking. This strategy appears to be most effective when the

Table 4–11. Stages of change and intervention tasks.

Patient Stage	Motivation Tasks
Precontemplation	Create doubt, increase the patient's awareness of risks and problems with current patterns of substance use
Contemplation	Help the patient weigh the relative risks and benefits of changing substance use; evoke reasons to change and risks of not changing; strengthen the patient's self-efficacy for changing current use
Determination	Help the patient determine the best course of action to change substance use from among available alternatives
Action	Help the patient establish a clear plan of action toward changing substance use
Maintenance	Help the patient identify and use strategies to prevent relapse
Relapse	Help the patient renew the process of change starting at contemplation

Reprinted, with permission, from Werner MJ: Principles of brief intervention for adolescent alcohol, tobacco, and other drug use. Pediatr Clin North Am 1995;42:341.

health care provider's message is part of an office-wide program so that the entire staff reinforces the cessation message with every patient. Specific steps to help youngsters quit smoking are discussed in the next section and summarized in Table 4–12. These same strategies and principles can be applied to the treatment of drug and alcohol use.

Smoking Cessation in Pediatrics

Although more than half of adolescents who smoke regularly say they want to quit and have tried to quit, only a minority report that they have been advised or helped to do so by a health care provider. Practitioners unfamiliar with approaches to smoking cessation may feel that smoking cessation interventions are time-consuming, nonreimbursable, and impractical in a busy office. In reality, studies conducted by the National Cancer Institute indicate that health care providers can help their patients stop smoking with short office interventions. Some of the most effective smoking cessation interventions are self-help programs consisting of a series of short (typically under 5 minutes) physician interventions reinforced by the entire office staff using the simple protocol outlined in Table 4–12.

The first step is motivational. Provide patients with a list of reasons for quitting. Suggest that they call 1-800-4CANCER to obtain the National Cancer Institute's "Quit for Good" or "Why Do You Smoke?" pamphlets and materials.

However, motivation alone is not enough. Learning to use coping skills to prevent relapse and to avoid discouragement at the time of relapse appear to be important to ultimate success. Smoking cessation is a process that takes time. Relapse must be regarded as a normal part of quitting rather than evidence of personal failure or a reason to forgo further attempts. Patients can actually benefit from relapses if they are helped to identify the circumstances that led to the relapse and to devise strategies to prevent subsequent relapses or respond to them in a different manner. Because nicotine is a physically and psychologically addictive substance, replacement therapy may relieve withdrawal symptoms. Three types of nicotine replacement therapies are available. Nicotine gum and transdermal nicotine patches are recommended for teens. Nicotine replacement therapy improves smoking cessation rates and provides relief from withdrawal symptoms. Providers should be aware that adolescents may not exhibit the same symptoms of nicotine dependence as adults, that symptoms may occur rapidly, with autonomy lost within only 4 weeks. Those who are not comfortable prescribing and monitoring nicotine replacement therapies should limit their involvement with patients who smoke to those who do not exhibit signs of nicotine dependency (eg, patients who smoke less than a pack of cigarettes a day or do not

Table 4–12. How to help your patients stop smoking.

Ask about smoking at every opportunity.
1. Do you smoke? How old were you when you started?
2. How much?
3. How soon after waking do you have your first cigarette?
4. Do you have friends who smoke? family members? relatives? role models?
5. Are you interested in stopping smoking?
6. Have you ever tried to stop before? If so, what happened?

Advise all smokers to stop.
1. State your advice clearly, for example: "As your physician, I must advise you to stop smoking now."
2. Personalize the message to quit. Refer to the patient's clinical condition, smoking history, family history, personal interests, or social roles (see Table 4–13).

Assist the patient in stopping.
1. Set a quit date. Help the patient pick a date within the next 4 weeks, acknowledging that no time is ideal.
2. Provide self-help materials. The smoking cessation coordinator or support staff member can review the materials with the patient.
3. Discuss the importance of a smoke-free environment.
4. Rehearse through role-playing how to respond to social situations where others are smoking.
5. Elicit support of parents and relatives; encourage them to stop smoking with their teen.
6. Encourage participation in activities that are incompatible with smoking.
7. Consider prescribing replacement therapy (patch or gum) for highly addicted patients (those who smoke a pack or more daily or who smoke their first cigarette within 30 minutes after waking).
8. Consider signing a stop-smoking contract with the patient.
9. If the patient is not willing to quit now, provide motivating literature and flag the chart and do remember to ask again at the next visit.

Arrange follow-up visits.
1. Set a follow-up visit within 1–2 weeks after the quit date.
2. Have a member of the office staff call or write the patient within 7 days after the initial visit, reinforcing the decision to stop and reminding the patient of the quit date.
3. At the first follow-up visit, ask about the patient's smoking status to provide support and help prevent relapse.
4. Set a second follow-up visit in 1 month.
5. Remind the teen that relapse is common—indeed the norm. When it happens, discuss the circumstances and encourage the patient to think of alternative responses and to try again.

Adapted, with permission, from Glynn T, Manley M: *How to Help Your Patients Stop Smoking: A National Cancer Institute Manual for Physicians.* National Institutes of Health, 1989.

feel a craving to smoke their first cigarette within 30 minutes after waking). In addition to nicotine replacement therapies, sustained-release forms of the antidepressants bupropion, clonidine, and nortriptyline have been shown in randomized trials to help smokers quit and to decrease relapse rates fivefold.

Two tobacco-use prevention curricula have been selected by The Division of Adolescent and School Health of the Centers for Disease Control and Prevention for adoption by schools—Botvin's Life Skills Training Program and Project Toward No Tobacco. The first is the more comprehensive of the two curricula. It is designed to target the primary causes of substance use, including tobacco, alcohol, and other drugs, by teaching a combination of health information, general life skills, and skills in resisting tobacco and other drugs. Program effectiveness has been demonstrated among white, African American, and Hispanic youth.

Project Toward No Tobacco, the second curriculum and the more effective of the two, was designed to target the primary causes of cigarette smoking, smokeless tobacco use, and cigar and pipe smoking among teens. Compared with the subjects who received the standard school health education, subjects in Project Toward No Tobacco were less likely to start using smokeless tobacco or cigarettes, and less likely to use them regularly. The program was equally effective in boys and girls, and was effective during the transitional period from junior to senior high school.

American Academy of Pediatrics Committee on Substance Abuse: Tobacco's toll: Implications for the pediatrician. Pediatrics 2001;107:794 [PMID: 11335763].

DiFranza JR et al: Initial symptoms of nicotine dependence in adolescents. Tobacco Control 2000;9:313 [PMID: 10982576].

DiFranza JR et al: Measuring the loss of autonomy over nicotine use in adolescents: The DANDY (development and assessment of nicotine dependence in youth) Study. Arch Pediatr Adolesc Med 2002;156:397 [PMID: 11929376].

Heyman RB: Reducing tobacco use among youth. Pediatr Clin North Am 2002;49:377 [PMID: 11993289].

Irwin CE Jr: Tobacco use during adolescence and young adulthood: The battle is not over. J Adolesc Health 2004;35:169 [PMID: 15313497].

Moolchan ET: A review of tobacco smoking in adolescents: Treatment implications. J Am Acad Child Adolesc Psychiatry 2000;39:682 [PMID: 10846302].

Wheeler KC, Fletcher KE, Wellman RJ, et al: Screening adolescents for nicotine dependence: the Hooked On Nicotine Checklist. J Adolesc Health 2004;35:225 [PMID: 15313504].

Referral

There is no consensus about which substance-abusing patients can be adequately treated in the office, which require referral, and which require hospitalization. Factors to be considered are summarized in Table 4–13.

Table 4–13. Factors to consider prior to referral for substance abuse.

Duration and frequency of substance use
The type of substances being used
Presence of other psychological disorders
Attention-deficit/hyperactivity disorder
Depression
Antisocial personality disorder
Presence of other social morbidities
School failure
Delinquency
Homelessness
Ongoing or past physical or sexual abuse
Program evaluation
View on substance abuse as primary disorder vs symptom
Offers comprehensive evaluation of patient and can manage associated problems identified in initial assessment (eg, co-morbid conditions)
Adherence to abstinence philosophy
Patient:staff ratios
Separate adolescent and adult treatment programs
Follow-up and continuing care

When doubt exists about the seriousness of the problem or the advisability of office management, consultation with a specialist should be sought.

Although most primary pediatric providers will not assume responsibility for the treatment of substance-abusing youngsters, clinicians can be instrumental in motivating their patients to seek treatment and in guiding them to appropriate treatment resources. Substance-abusing teenagers must be treated in teen-oriented treatment facilities. Despite the similarities between adult and adolescent substance abuse, adult programs are usually developmentally inappropriate and ineffective for adolescents. As discussed in Chapter 3, many adolescents are concrete thinkers. Their inability to reason deductively, especially about emotionally charged issues, makes it difficult for them to understand the abstract concepts (such as denial) that are an integral component of most adult-oriented programs. This invariably frustrates counselors who misinterpret lack of comprehension as resistance to therapy, and concrete responses as evidence of deceit.

Treatment programs range from low-intensity, outpatient, school-based student assistance programs, which rely heavily on peers and nonprofessionals, to residential, hospital-based programs staffed by psychiatrists and other professionals. Outpatient counseling programs are most appropriate for motivated patients who do not have significant mental health or behavioral problems and are not at risk for withdrawal. Some investigators have raised the concern that in pediatric settings, low-problem users may actually experience a strengthening of the drug subculture by associating with high-problem users in group therapy. More intensive day treatment programs are available for those who require a structured environment. Inpatient treatment should be considered for patients who need medical care and detoxification in addition to counseling, education, and family therapy.

Finally, special dual-diagnosis facilities are available for substance-abusing patients who also have other psychological conditions. These patients are difficult to diagnose and treat because it is often unclear whether their symptoms are a consequence of substance use or a symptom of a comorbid psychological disorder. Recognition of such disorders is critical because they must be treated in programs that include psychiatric expertise.

Approaches to the treatment of substance abuse in children and adolescents are typically modeled after adult treatment programs. Most notable are the 12-step programs modeled after Alcoholics Anonymous. These programs are attractive because they demand total abstinence and acknowledge that substance abuse is a chronic disease requiring a lifelong commitment to abstinence and long-term support from family, peers, and community. Although treatment is usually effective, relapse is common. Because efficacy research has lagged behind practice and implementation (especially among low-intensity programs), there is little empirical evidence on which to base recommendations for one program or another. Various forms of treatment appear to have the potential to be effective. Thus, in practice, referral recommendations should be based on the significance of the problem for the individual and the availability of affordable programs in the community.

Anton RF, Swift RM: Current pharmacotherapies of alcoholism: a U.S. perspective. Am J Addict 2003;12:S53 [PMID: 14972780].

Bertholet N, Daeppen JB, Wietlisbach V et al: Reduction of alcohol consumption by brief alcohol intervention in primary care: systematic review and meta-analysis. Arch Intern Med 2005;165:986 [PMID: 15883236].

Cox LS, Patten CA, Niaura RS et al: Efficacy of bupropion for relapse prevention in smokers with and without a past history of major depression. J Gen Intern Med 2004;19:828 [PMID: 15242467].

Heyman RB: Turning the tide: Tobacco and the 21st century. Adolesc Med 2000;11:69 [PMID: 10640339].

PREVENTION OF SUBSTANCE ABUSE

Prevention of substance abuse has been a public health priority since the 1980s. Pediatric health care providers are important as advocates and educators of the community and government on developmentally appropriate programs. *Primary level* programs focus on preventing the initiation of substance use. The Drug Awareness and Resistance Education program is a familiar example of a primary prevention program that attempts to educate elementary and middle school students about the adverse consequences of substance abuse and enable them to resist peer pressures.

Secondary level programs target populations at increased risk for substance use. The aim is to prevent progression from initiation to continuance and maintenance, relying on individualized intervention to reduce the risk and enhance the protective factors listed in Table 4–5. This approach enables the provider to focus scarce resources on those who are most likely to benefit from them. Alateen, which supports the children of alcoholic parents, typifies secondary level prevention.

Tertiary level prevention programs target young people who have been identified as substance abusers. The aim is to prevent the morbid consequences of substance use. One example is identifying adolescents who misuse alcohol and drugs at parties and providing them with a safe ride home. Because prevention is more effective when targeted at reducing the initiation of substance use than at decreasing use, tertiary prevention is the least effective approach.

Very few population-based programs undergo rigorous scientific evaluation. It is the consensus among drug educators that primary prevention programs, such as Drug Awareness and Resistance Education, have minimal effect in decreasing the use of illicit substances. During the 1990s, when these programs were most popular, a smaller proportion of middle- and high-school students perceived illicit drug and alcohol use as dangerous, and substance use actually increased. Even when knowledge- and resistance-based programs do increase student understanding of adverse consequences, there is no evidence that they change attitudes or abuse rates.

The failure of resistance education programs has fostered interest in a potentially more effective type of program, exemplified by the Adolescents Training and Learning to Avoid Steroids program. This program, a same-sex, peer-educator program designed to simultaneously reduce the use of steroids and improve dietary and exercise habits of teen athletes has proven effective in randomized controlled trials. Pediatric health care providers should promote developmentally appropriate prevention programs like this one that address the social and psychological problems predisposing youngsters to substance abuse and which provide realistic alternative solutions.

Parents and others should understand that most adolescents who abuse alcohol and drugs do not do so just for the high. Rather, these behaviors are often purposeful, developmentally appropriate coping strategies. To the extent that these behaviors meet young peoples' developmental needs, they are not apt to be abandoned unless equally attractive alternatives are available. For example, even though many teenagers cite stress and anxiety as reasons for smoking, teen-oriented smoking cessation programs rarely address the young smoker's need for alternative coping strategies by offering stress management training. Similarly, for the youngster growing up in an impoverished urban environment, the real costs of substance abuse may be too low and the rewards too high to be influenced by talk and knowledge alone. It is unreasonable to expect a talk-based intervention to change attitudes and behaviors in a direction that is opposite to that of the child's own social milieu. The efficacy of the most promising prevention models and interventions is apt to decay over time unless changes in the social environment provide substance-abusing children and adolescents with realistic alternative ways to meet their developmental needs.

Goldberg L, Elliot DL, MacKinnon DP et al: Drug testing athletes to prevent substance abuse: background and pilot study results of the SATURN (Student Athlete Testing Using Random Notification) study. J Adolesc Health 2003;32:16 [PMID: 12507797].

Goldberg L et al: The adolescents' training and learning to avoid steroids program: Preventing drug use and promoting health behaviors. Arch Adolesc Med 2000;154:332 [PMID: 10768668].

Perry CL, Komro KA, Veblen-Mortenson S et al: A randomized controlled trial of the middle and junior high school D.A.R.E. and D.A.R.E. Plus programs. Arch Pediatr Adolesc Med 2003;157:178 [PMID: 12580689].

REFERENCES

Web Resources

[Monitoring the Future Study detailed information and longitudinal data]
www.monitoringthefuture.org

[Information on Trends from National Institute on Drug Abuse]
www.nida.nih.gov

[National Clearinghouse Drug and Alcohol Abuse Gives information and resources including free publications for providers, parents, and adolescents]
www.health.org

[Substance use and mental health services administration resources for both substance use and mental health services]
www.samhsa.org

Eating Disorders

5

Eric J. Sigel, MD

Teenagers and younger children continue to develop eating disorders at a significant rate. The spectrum of eating disorders includes anorexia nervosa, bulimia nervosa, eating disorders not otherwise specified, and binge-eating disorder. The relationship between biology and environment in the development of eating disorders is complex: these disorders are best defined in a biopsychosocial context.

ETIOLOGY

In general, it is thought that patients have a genetic susceptibility to developing eating disorders. Factors from the environment—stressors such as psychological changes in the home, social pressure to lose weight, and the presence of a drive for thinness—influence the biologic milieu, setting into motion a chain reaction that ultimately leads to the development of eating disorders.

Increasing evidence supports a genetic predisposition for eating disorders. There is a 7% incidence of anorexia nervosa in first-degree relatives of anorexic patients compared with a 1–2% incidence in the general population. Twin studies have shown a 55% concordance rate in monozygotic twins, compared with 7% in dizygotic twins. Twin studies have estimated the heritability of anorexia nervosa (AN) to be between 33% and 84%, and bulimia nervosa (BN) to be between 28% and 83%. A study of males with AN showed a relative risk of 20 for first-degree female relatives. Most studies have found a higher incidence of eating disorders among first-degree relatives of bulimic patients as well. Genomic regions on chromosome 1 for AN and chromosome 10 for BN are likely to harbor susceptibility genes. Genetics and eating disorders continue to be an active area of investigation.

Leptin, a hormone secreted by adipocytes that regulates energy homeostasis and satiety signaling, does not appear to contribute to the etiology of AN primarily, but may mediate energy changes that impact the hypothalamic-pituitary axis and play a role in the perpetuation of AN. Leptin physiology is deranged in patients with AN. Leptin levels are decreased in people with low body weight, and increase to excessive levels as they regain weight. The idiosyncratic higher levels of leptin may contribute to the difficulty patients have when try-

ing to regain weight, as higher leptin signals the body to decrease energy intake. Leptin also plays a significant role in some of the sequelae of AN, with low levels signaling the hypothalamus to inhibit reproductive hormone production. In a systematic review, Bosanac et al concluded that there is evidence of persistently altered serotonergic and dopaminergic function in AN. Other alterations in neuropeptides and gut peptides are found both in AN and BN. Adiponectin appears elevated in AN, though it is unclear as to whether it is due to the malnourished state, or elevated independently of malnourishment. Cholecystokinin is decreased in BN, perhaps contributing to the lack of post-ingestion satiety that perpetuates a binge. An alteration in dopamine has also been recognized, though its significance has not been elucidated. Ghrelin, a gut peptide, is elevated in patients with AN. Ghrelin does not decrease in the normal fashion after a meal in patients with AN. Though significant research has been done on the neurobiology of eating disorders, it remains unclear as to whether alterations contribute to the development of eating disorders, or are present as a consequence of the physiologic changes that occur. Patients with BN or binge-eating disorder appear to have a blunted serotonin response to eating and satiety. With a decreased satiety response, patients continue to eat, leading to a binge. Treatment with selective serotonin reuptake inhibitors (SSRIs) tends to equilibrate satiety regulation. More research is needed to determine which factors are causative and which are results of the eating disorder.

Traditional psychological theory has suggested many factors that might lead to the development of eating disorders. Enmeshment of mother with daughter to the point that the teenager cannot develop her own identity (a key developmental marker of adolescence) may be a predisposing factor. The teenager may cope by asserting control over food, as she senses her lack of control in the developmental realm. A second theory involves father-daughter distancing. As puberty progresses and a girl's sexuality blossoms, a father may experience difficulty in dealing with his daughter as a sexual being and may respond by withdrawing both emotionally and physically. The teenage girl may intuitively recognize this and subconsciously decrease her food intake in order to become prepubertal again. A third theory is

163

related to puberty itself. Some teenagers may fear or dislike their changing bodies. By restricting food intake they lose weight, stop menstruating, and effectively reverse pubertal development.

In addition, society has provided the message that being thin or muscular is necessary for attractiveness and success. The ease of access to diet products—foods and diet pills—as well as Internet instructions (pro-anorexia sites) makes it simple for adolescents to embark on a quest for thinness or muscularity.

Genetic predisposition, psychological factors, and environmental factors combine to create a milieu that promotes adolescent eating disorders.

Bailer UF, Kaye WH: A review of neuropeptide and neuroendocrine dysregulation in anorexia and bulimia nervosa. Curr Drug Target CNS Neurol Disord 2003;2:53 [PMID: 12769812].

Bosanac P et al: Serotonergic and dopaminergic systems in anorexia nervosa: a role for atypical antipsychotics? Aust N Z J Psychiatry 2005;39:146 [PMID: 15701063].

Bulik CM, Tozzi F: Genetics in eating disorders: state of the science. CNS Spectrums 2005;9:511 [PMID: 15208510].

Chan JL, Manzoros CS: Role of leptin in energy deprived states: normal human physiology and clinical implications for hypothalamic amenorrhea and anorexia nervosa. Lancet 2005;366:74 [PMID: 15993236].

Strober M et al: Males with anorexia nervosa: A controlled study of eating disorders in first-degree relatives. Int J Eat Disord 2001;29:263 [PMID: 11262504].

Tolle V et al: Balance in ghrelin and leptin plasma levels in anorexia nervosa patients and constitutionally thin women. J Clin Endocrinol Metab 2003;88:109 [PMID: 12519838].

INCIDENCE

Among teenage girls in the United States, anorexia nervosa is the third most common chronic illness. The incidence in the United States has been increasing steadily since the 1930s. Ascertaining exact incidence is difficult. Most studies show that 1–2% of teenagers develop anorexia nervosa and 2–4% develop bulimia nervosa. Adolescents outnumber adults 5 to 1, although the number of adults with eating disorders is rising. The incidence is also increasing among younger children. Often prepubertal patients have significant associated psychiatric diagnoses. Males represent approximately 10% of the total eating disorder population, though recent studies show increasing prevalence in males. Prevalence of full or partial syndrome BN is 1.1% of males and 3.2% of females, representing a 2.9:1 female:male ratio. For full or partial syndrome AN, prevalence in males is .9% and 1.8% in females, a 2:1 female:male ratio. The increasing number of males diagnosed with eating disorders correlates with the increased media emphasis on muscular, chiseled appearance as the male ideal. In the recent Youth Risk Behavior Survey (2003) of U.S. teenagers, 59% of females

and 29% of males were attempting to lose weight during the preceding 30 days of the survey. Thirteen percent of youth fasted for more than 24 hours to lose weight. Overall, 9.2% of youth had used diet pills, powders, or liquids as a weight loss method in the previous 30 days—11.3% of girls and 6.1% of boys. Self-induced vomiting or laxative use (or both) was also common: 8.4% of females and 3.7% of males were using one or the other to lose weight. For males, this represented a 27% increase compared to 2001 data. Binge-eating disorder has a 1.1% incidence in the teenage population. Forty-six percent of females and 30% of males report at least one bingeing episode during their lifetime.

Centers for Disease Control and Prevention: Youth Risk Behavior Surveillance System 2003. http://www.cdc.gov/mmwr/preview/mmwrhtml/ss5302a1.htm

Woodside DB, Garfinkel PE et al: Comparisons of men with full or partial eating disorders, men without eating disorders, and women with eating disorders in the community. Am J Psychol 2001;158:570.

PREDISPOSING FACTORS

In the past, the typical anorexic patient was described as a high-achieving, athletic, straight-A student from a middle class socioeconomic background. Demographics have changed, and eating disorders now occur across all racial and ethnic groups. In fact, Shaw et al found that blacks, Asians, Hispanics, and whites experienced no difference in eating disorder symptoms or eating disorder risk factors. Children involved in gymnastics, figure skating, and ballet—activities that emphasize (and in which coaches often require) thin bodies—are at higher risk for anorexia than are children in sports that do not emphasize body image. Sudden changes in dietary habits, such as becoming vegetarian, may be a first sign of anorexia, especially if the change is abrupt and without good reason.

The typical bulimic patient is more impulsive, tending to engage in risk-taking behavior such as alcohol use, drug use, and sexual experimentation. Bulimic patients are often an appropriate weight for height or slightly overweight, and they get average grades. Some studies have found that 50% of bulimic patients have been sexually abused. Patients with diabetes also have an increased risk of BN. In males, wrestling and homosexual orientation predispose to BN. A recent prospective study revealed that attempting a diet to lose weight and social pressure to be thin were sensitive predictors of future-onset eating disorders.

Shaw H, Ramirez L et al: Body image and eating disturbances across ethnic groups: more similarities than differences. Psychol Addict Behav 2004;18:8 [PMID: 15008651].

DIAGNOSIS

1. Anorexia Nervosa

Table 5–1 lists the diagnostic criteria for anorexia nervosa, according to the *Diagnostic and Statistical Manual of Mental Disorders,* 4th edition (DSM-IV). There are two forms of anorexia nervosa. In the restricting type, patients do not regularly engage in binge eating or purging. In the purging type, classic anorexia nervosa is combined with binge eating or purging behavior (or both). Differentiating between the two is important because of differing implications for prognosis and treatment. Additionally, there is debate regarding criteria for AN, as some experts have argued to eliminate amenorrhea as a specific criterion. Though patients may not demonstrate all features of AN, they may still exhibit the deleterious symptoms associated with AN.

Clinical Findings

A. SYMPTOMS AND SIGNS

Clinicians should recognize the early symptoms and signs of anorexia nervosa because intervention may prevent the full-blown syndrome from developing. Patients may show some of the behaviors and psychology of anorexia nervosa, such as reduction in dietary fat and intense concern with body image, even before weight loss or amenorrhea occurs.

Making the diagnosis of anorexia nervosa can be challenging because adolescents may try to conceal their illness. Assessing the patient's body image is essential to

Table 5–1. Diagnostic criteria for anorexia nervosa.

A. Refusal to maintain body weight at or above a minimally normal weight for age and height (eg, weight loss leading to maintenance of body weight less than 85% of that expected; or failure to make expected weight gain during a period of growth, leading to body weight less than 85% of that expected).

B. Intense fear of gaining weight or becoming fat, even though underweight.

C. Disturbance in the way in which one's body weight or shape is experienced, undue influence of body weight or shape on self-evaluation, or denial of the seriousness of the current low body weight.

D. In postmenarchal females, amenorrhea, ie, the absence of at least three menstrual cycles. (A woman is considered to have amenorrhea if her periods occur only following hormone, eg, estrogen, administration.)

Reprinted, with permission, from the *Diagnostic and Statistical Manual of Mental Disorders,* 4th ed. Text Revision. Copyright 2000. American Psychiatric Association.

Table 5–2. Screening questions to help diagnose anorexia and bulimia nervosa.

How do you feel about your body?
Are there parts of your body you might change?
When you look at yourself in the mirror, do you see yourself as overweight, underweight, or satisfactory?
If overweight, how much do you want to weigh?
If your weight is satisfactory, has there been a time that you were worried about being overweight?
If overweight/underweight, what would you change?
Have you ever been on a diet?
What have you done to help yourself lose weight?
Do you count calories or fat grams?
Do you keep your intake to a certain number of calories?
Have you ever used nutritional supplements, diet pills, or laxatives to help you lose weight?
Have you ever made yourself vomit to get rid of food or lose weight?

determining the diagnosis. Table 5–2 lists screening questions that help to tease out a teenager's perceptions of body image. Additional diagnostic screening tools include the Eating Attitudes Test or other questionnaires that assess a range of eating and dieting behaviors. Parental observations are critical in determining whether a patient has expressed dissatisfaction over body habitus as well as revealing what weight loss techniques the child has attempted. In the teenager who is not ready to share his or her concerns about body image, the clinician may find clues to the diagnosis by carefully considering other presenting symptoms. Weight loss from a baseline of normal body weight is an obvious red flag and should raise the clinical suspicion of an eating disorder. Additionally, anorexia nervosa should be considered in any girl with secondary amenorrhea who has lost weight.

Physical symptoms are usually secondary to weight loss and proportional to the degree of malnutrition. The body effectively goes into hibernation, becoming functionally hypothyroid (euthyroid sick) to save as much energy as possible. Body temperature decreases, and patients report being colder than normal. Patients become bradycardic, especially in the supine position. Dizziness, lightheadedness, and occasional syncope may ensue, as orthostasis and hypotension secondary to impaired cardiac function occur. Left ventricular mass is decreased (as all striated muscle throughout the body loses mass), stroke volume is compromised, and peripheral resistance is increased, contributing to left ventricular systolic dysfunction. Patients can develop prolonged QT syndrome and increased QT dispersion, putting them at risk for cardiac arrhythmias. Peripheral circulation is reduced. Hands and feet may be blue and cool.

Hair thins, nails become brittle, and the skin is dry. Lanugo develops as a primitive response to starvation. The gastrointestinal tract may be affected. Inability to take in normal quantities of food, early satiety, and gastroesophageal reflux can develop as the body adapts to reduced intake. The normal gastrocolic reflex may be temporarily lost due to lack of stimuli, leading to delayed gastric emptying and constipation. A recent study showed that delayed gastric emptying is present in both AN restricting type and AN purging type. Long-term physical rehabilitation improves symptoms of gastric emptying and dyspeptic symptoms in AN restricting type, but not in purgers.

Neurologically, patients may experience decreased cognition, inability to concentrate, increased irritability, and depression, which may be related to structural brain changes and decreased cerebral blood flow.

A combination of malnutrition and stress causes hypothalamic hypogonadism. The hypothalamic-pituitary-gonadal axis shuts down as the body struggles to survive, directing finite energy resources to support more vital functions. This may be mediated by the effect of low levels of leptin on the hypothalamic-pituitary axis. Both males and females experience decreased libido and interruption of pubertal development, depending on the timing of the illness. Skeletal growth may be interrupted as well.

Nutritional assessment is vital. Often patients eliminate fat from their diets and may eat as few as 100–200 kcal/d. A gown-only weight after urination is the most accurate way to assess weight. Patients tend to wear bulky clothes and may hide weights in their pockets or drink excessive amounts of fluid (water-loading) to trick the practitioner. Calculating body mass index (BMI)—weight in kilograms divided by height in meters squared—is an efficient way to interpret degree of malnutrition. A BMI less than the 25th percentile (using BMI growth curves) indicates risk for malnutrition, and less than the fifth percentile significant malnutrition. Additionally, ideal body weight (IBW) for height should be calculated, using the 50th percentile of BMI for age. A weight less than 85% IBW is one of the diagnostic criteria for anorexia nervosa.

A hallmark physical feature of anorexia nervosa in girls is amenorrhea, which occurs for two reasons. The hypothalamic-pituitary-ovarian axis shuts down under stress, causing hypothalamic amenorrhea. Additionally, adipose tissue is needed to convert estrogen to its activated form. When weight loss is significant, adipose tissue is lost and there is not enough substrate to activate estrogen. Resuming normal menses depends on increasing both body weight and body fat. Approximately 73% of postmenarcheal girls will resume menstruating if they reach 90% of their IBW. An adolescent female needs, on average, 17% body fat to restart menses and 22% body fat if she has primary amenorrhea. A recent study demonstrated that target weights for return of menses are approximately 1 kg greater than the weight at which menses was lost.

B. LABORATORY FINDINGS

Most organ systems can potentially suffer some degree of damage in the anorexic patient, related both to severity and duration of illness (Table 5–3). Initial screening should include complete blood count with differential, and serum levels of electrolytes, blood urea nitrogen/creatinine, phosphorus, calcium, magnesium, and thyroid-stimulating hormone, as well as liver function tests and urinalysis. An electrocardiogram should be performed, because significant electrocardiographic abnormalities may be present, most importantly prolonged QT syndrome. Bone densitometry should be done if amenorrhea has persisted for 6 months, as patients begin to accumulate risk for osteoporosis.

Differential Diagnosis

If the diagnosis is unclear (ie, the patient has lost a significant amount of weight but does not have typical body image distortion or fat phobia), then the clinician must consider the differential diagnosis for weight loss in adolescents. This includes inflammatory bowel disease, diabetes, hyperthyroidism, malignancy, and depression. Less common diagnoses include adrenal insufficiency and malabsorption syndromes such as celiac disease. The history and physical examination should direct laboratory and radiologic evaluation.

Table 5–3. Laboratory findings: anorexia nervosa.

Increased blood urea nitrogen/creatinine secondary to renal insufficiency

Decreased white blood cells, platelets, and less commonly red blood cells/hematocrit secondary to bone marrow suppression or fat atrophy of the bone marrow

Increased AST and ALT secondary to malnutrition

Increased cholesterol, thought to be related to fatty acid metabolism

Decreased alkaline phosphatase secondary to zinc deficiency

Low to low-normal thyroid-stimulating hormone and thyroxine

Decreased follicle-stimulating hormone, luteinizing hormone, estradiol, and testosterone secondary to shutdown of hypothalamic-pituitary-gonadal axis

Abnormal electrolytes related to hydrational status

Decreased phosphorus

Decreased insulin-like growth factor

Increased cortisol

Decreased urine specific gravity in cases of intentional water intoxication

ALT, alanine aminotransferase; AST, aspartate aminotransferase.

Table 5–4. Diagnostic criteria for bulimia nervosa.

A. Recurrent episodes of binge eating. An episode of binge eating is characterized by both of the following:
  (1) eating, in a discrete period of time (eg, within any 2-hour period), an amount of food that is definitely larger than most people would eat during a similar period of time and under similar circumstances.
  (2) a sense of lack of control over eating during the episodes (eg, a feeling that one cannot stop eating or control what or how much one is eating).
B. Recurrent inappropriate compensatory behavior in order to prevent weight gain, such as self-induced vomiting; misuse of laxatives, diuretics, enemas, or other medications; fasting; or excessive exercise.
C. The binge eating and inappropriate compensatory behaviors both occur, on average, at least twice a week for 3 months.
D. Self-evaluation is unduly influenced by body shape and weight.
E. The disturbance does not occur exclusively during episodes of anorexia nervosa.

Reprinted, with permission, from the *Diagnostic and Statistical Manual of Mental Disorders,* 4th ed. Text Revision. Copyright 2000. American Psychiatric Association.

2. Bulimia Nervosa

Table 5–4 lists the diagnostic criteria for bulimia nervosa. Binge eating is either eating excessive amounts of food during a normal mealtime or having a meal (or other eating episode) last longer than usual, consuming food throughout. Bulimic individuals feel out of control while eating, unable or unwilling to recognize satiety signals. Any type of food may be included in a binge, though typically it is either carbohydrates or junk food. Extreme guilt is often associated with the episode. At some point, either prior to or during a binge, bulimic individuals often decide to purge. The amount of food consumed feels overwhelming, and they do not want to gain weight. The most common ways to purge are self-induced vomiting, exercise, and laxative use. Some individuals will vomit multiple times during a purge episode, after using large amounts of water to cleanse their system. This can induce significant electrolyte abnormalities such as hyponatremia and hypokalemia, which may put the patient at acute risk for arrhythmia or seizure. Other methods of purging include diuretics, diet pills, cathartics, and nutritional supplements, including Metabolife.

Diagnosing bulimia nervosa can be difficult unless the teenager is forthcoming or parents or caregivers can supply direct observations. Often bulimic patients are average or slightly above average in body weight, without any physical abnormalities. Screening all teenagers for body image concerns is crucial. If the teenager expresses concern about being overweight, then the clinician needs to screen the patient about dieting methods. Asking whether patients have binged, feel out of control while eating, or whether they cannot stop eating can clarify the diagnosis. Parents may report that significant amounts of food are missing or disappearing more quickly than normal. If the physician is suspicious, direct questioning about all the ways to purge should follow. Indicating first that the behavior in question is not unusual can make the questioning less threatening and more likely to elicit a truthful response. For example, the clinician might say, "Some teenagers who try to lose weight make themselves vomit after eating. Have you ever considered or done that yourself?"

Clinical Findings

A. SYMPTOMS AND SIGNS

Symptoms are related to the mechanism of purging. Gastrointestinal problems are most prominent. Abdominal pain is a frequent complaint. This can be due to gastroesophageal reflux, as the lower esophageal sphincter is compromised due to repetitive vomiting. Frequent vomiting may result in esophagitis or gastritis, as the mucosa is irritated from increased exposure to acid. Early satiety, involuntary vomiting, and complaints of food "coming up" on its own are frequent. Less common but more serious is hematemesis or esophageal rupture. Patients may report bowel problems—diarrhea or constipation—if laxatives have been used. Sialadenitis—parotid pain and enlargement—may occur secondary to frequent vomiting. Erosion of dental enamel may result from increased exposure to acidity during vomiting. Because comorbid depression is common in bulimia nervosa, patients may report difficulty sleeping, decreased energy, decreased motivation, and headaches. Lightheadness or syncope may develop secondary to dehydration.

It is important to note that most purging methods are ineffective. When patients binge, they may consume thousands of calories. Digestion begins rapidly. Although the patient may be able to vomit some of the food, much is actually digested and absorbed. Laxatives work in the large intestine, leading to fluid and electrolyte loss. Consumed calories are still absorbed from the small intestine. Use of diuretics may result in decreased fluid weight and electrolyte imbalance.

On physical examination, bulimic patients may be dehydrated and have orthostatic hypotension. Sialadenitis, tooth enamel loss, dental caries, and abdominal tenderness are the most common findings. Abrasion of the proximal interphalangeal joints may occur secondary to scraping the fingers against teeth while inducing vomiting. Rarely a heart murmur is heard. An irreversible cardiomyopathy can develop secondary to ipecac use. Tachycardia and hypertension may occur secondary to caffeine and diet pill use.

B. Laboratory Findings

Electrolyte disturbances are characteristic of bulimic patients. The method of purging results in specific abnormalities. Vomiting causes metabolic alkalosis, hypokalemia, and hypochloremia. If laxatives are used, then a metabolic acidosis develops with hypokalemia and hypochloremia. Amylase may be increased secondary to chronic parotid stimulation.

American Psychiatric Association: *Diagnostic and Statistical Manual of Mental Disorders*, 4th ed. Text Revision. American Psychiatric Association, 2000.

Benini L, Todesco T et al: Gastric emptying in patients with restricting and binge/purging subtypes of anorexia nervosa. Am J Gastroenterol 2004;99:1448 [PMID: 15307858].

Kreipe RE, Birndorf SA: Eating disorders in adolescents and young adults. Med Clin North Am 2000;84:1027 [PMID: 10928200].

Miller KK et al: Medical findings in outpatients with anorexia nervosa. Arch Intern Med 2005;165:561 [PMID: 15767533].

Panagiotopoulos C et al: Electrocardiographic findings in adolescents with eating disorders. Pediatrics 2000;105:1100 [PMID: 10790469].

Swenne I: Weight requirements for return of menstruations in teenage girls with eating disorders, weight loss, and secondary amenorrhea. Acta Paediatrica 2004;93:1449 [PMID: 08035253].

3. Binge-Eating Disorder

The diagnostic category of binge-eating disorder was created in DSM-IV. Officially, it is still considered a research diagnosis. Studies show that most adults who have binge-eating disorder (a prevalence of 2–4%) develop symptoms during adolescence. Table 5–5 lists the diagnostic criteria.

Clinical Findings

A. Symptoms and Signs

Binge-eating disorder most often occurs in patients who are overweight or obese. Eighteen percent of such patients report bingeing at least once in the past year. Patients with binge-eating disorder have an increased incidence of depression and substance abuse. Using the DSM-IV diagnostic criteria as a guide for evaluation, the suspicion of binge-eating disorder should be raised for any significantly overweight patient. Specific questionnaires are available for evaluating patients suspected of having binge-eating disorder.

B. Laboratory Findings

The clinician should assess causes and complications of obesity, and laboratory evaluation should include thy-

Table 5–5. Diagnostic criteria for binge-eating disorder.

A. Recurrent episodes of binge eating. An episode of binge eating is characterized by both of the following:
  (1) eating, in a discrete period of time (eg, within any 2-hour period), an amount of food that is definitely larger than most people would eat in a similar period of time under similar circumstances.
  (2) a sense of lack of control over eating during the episode (eg, a feeling that one cannot stop eating or control what or how much one is eating).
B. The binge-eating episodes are associated with three (or more) of the following:
  (1) eating much more rapidly than normal
  (2) eating until feeling uncomfortably full
  (3) eating large amounts of food when not feeling physically hungry
  (4) eating alone because of being embarrassed by how much one is eating
  (5) feeling disgusted with oneself, depressed, or very guilty after overeating
C. Marked distress regarding binge eating at present.
D. The binge eating occurs, on average, at least 2 days a week for 6 months.
E. The binge eating is not associated with regular use of inappropriate compensatory behaviors (eg, purging, fasting, excessive exercise) and does not occur exclusively during the course of anorexia nervosa or bulimia nervosa.

Reprinted, with permission, from the *Diagnostic and Statistical Manual of Mental Disorders*, 4th ed. Text Revision. Copyright 2000. American Psychiatric Association.

roid function tests and measurement of cholesterol and triglyceride levels.

Fairburn CG et al: The natural course of bulimia nervosa and binge eating disorder in young women. Arch Gen Psychiatry 2000;57:659 [PMID: 10891036].

Johnson WG et al: Measuring binge eating in adolescents: Adolescent and parent versions of the questionnaire of eating and weight patterns. Int J Eat Disord 1999;26:301 [PMID: 10441246].

Schneider M: Bulimia nervosa and binge eating disorder in adolescents. Adolesc Med State Art Rev 2003;14:119 [PMID: 12529196].

4. Eating Disorder Not Otherwise Specified

An additional diagnostic category found in DSM-IV is eating disorder not otherwise specified. Patients do not meet all the criteria for either anorexia nervosa or bulimia nervosa, but have features of either or both. Table 5–6 lists the diagnostic criteria. This has become a "catch-all" category; some researchers describe this as

Table 5–6. Diagnostic criteria for eating disorder not otherwise specified.

The eating disorder not otherwise specified category is for disorders of eating that do not meet the criteria for any specific eating disorder. Examples include

1. For females, all of the criteria for anorexia nervosa are met except that the individual has regular menses.
2. All of the criteria for anorexia nervosa are met except that, despite significant weight loss, the individual's current weight is in the normal range.
3. All of the criteria for bulimia nervosa are met except that the binge eating and inappropriate compensatory mechanisms occur at a frequency of less than twice a week or for a duration of less than 3 months.
4. The regular use of inappropriate compensatory behavior by an individual of normal body weight after eating small amounts of food (eg, self-induced vomiting after the consumption of two cookies).
5. Repeatedly chewing and spitting out, but not swallowing, large amounts of food.

Reprinted, with permission, from the *Diagnostic and Statistical Manual of Mental Disorders*, 4th ed. Text Revision. Copyright 2000. American Psychiatric Association.

an atypical eating disorder, or partial syndrome eating disorder. Incidence of eating disorder not otherwise specified appears significant, as studies show a range of .5–14% in the general adolescent population. Careful attention by clinicians to patient concerns about body weight and dieting behavior can provide clues to the diagnosis. Symptoms and sequelae depend on patient behaviors. Some patients with eating disorder not otherwise specified will go on to develop full blown AN or BN, and early recognition and treatment may decrease further complications.

Chamay-Weber C, Narring F, Michaud PA: Partial eating disorders among adolescents: a review. J Adolesc Health 2005; 37:417.

COMPLICATIONS (Table 5–7)

1. Anorexia Nervosa

Short-Term Complications

A. EARLY SATIETY

Patients may have significant difficulty digesting modest quantities as their bodies adapt to increased caloric intake. Patients may benefit from a gastric-emptying agent such as metoclopramide. This complication usually resolves after a patient has become used to larger meals.

B. SUPERIOR MESENTERIC ARTERY SYNDROME

As patients become malnourished, the fat pad between the superior mesenteric artery and the duodenum may shrink, compressing the transverse duodenum and causing vomiting and intolerance of oral intake, especially solids. Diagnosis is made by an upper GI series, which shows to and fro movement of barium in the descending and transverse duodenum proximal to the obstruction. Treatment involves a liquid diet or nasoduodenal

Table 5–7. Complications of anorexia and bulimia nervosa.

Cardiovascular	**Hematologic**
Bradycardia	Leukopenia
Postural hypotension	Anemia
Arrhythmia, sudden death	Thrombocytopenia
Congestive heart failure (during refeeding)	↓ESR
Pericardial effusion	Impaired cell-mediated immunity
Mitral valve prolapse	**Metabolic**
ECG abnormalities (prolonged QT, low voltage, T-wave abnormalities, conduction defects)	Dehydration
	Acidosis
	Hypokalemia
Endocrine	Hyponatremia
↓LH, FSH	Hypochloremia
↓T_3, ↑rT_3; ↓T_4, TSH	Hypochloremic alkalosis
Irregular menses	Hypocalcemia
Amenorrhea	Hypophosphatemia
Hypercortisolism	Hypomagnesemia
Growth retardation	Hypercarotenemia
Delayed puberty	**Neurologic**
Gastrointestinal	Cortical atrophy
Dental erosion	Peripheral neuropathy
Parotid swelling	Seizures
Esophagitis, esophageal tears	Thermoregulatory abnormalities
Delayed gastric emptying	↓REM and slow-wave sleep
Gastric dilatation (rarely rupture)	**Renal**
Pancreatitis	Hematuria
Constipation	Proteinuria
Diarrhea (laxative abuse)	↓Renal concentrating ability
Superior mesenteric artery syndrome	**Skeletal**
Hypercholesterolemia	Osteopenia
↑Liver function tests (fatty infiltration of the liver)	Fractures

LH, luteinizing hormone; ECG, electrocardiogram; FSH, follicle-stimulating hormone; T_3, triiodothyronine; rT_3, resin triiodothyronine uptake; T_4, thyroxine; TSH, thyroid-stimulating hormone; ESR, erythrocyte sedimentation rate; REM, rapid eye movement.

feedings until restoration of the fat pad has occurred, coincident with weight gain.

C. CONSTIPATION

Patients may have prolonged constipation, often not having a bowel movement for a week or longer. Two mechanisms contribute to this symptom: loss of the gastrocolic reflex and loss of colonic muscle tone. Typically stool softeners do not help because the colon has decreased peristaltic amplitude. Agents that induce peristalsis, such as bisacodyl and polyethylene glycol-electrolyte solution (MiraLax), are helpful. Constipation can persist for up to 6–8 weeks after refeeding. Occasionally patients need enemas.

D. REFEEDING SYNDROME

This is described in the Treatment section.

Long-Term Complications

A. OSTEOPOROSIS

Approximately 90% of females with anorexia nervosa have reduced bone mass at one or more sites. The development of osteopenia and osteoporosis is multifactorial. Estrogen and testosterone are essential to potentiate bone development. Higher ghrelin levels is an independent predicator of bone density in healthy adolescents; however, it does not appear to contribute to bone loss in patients with anorexia nervosa. Teenagers are particularly at risk as they accrue 40% of their bone mineral during adolescence. Low body weight is most predictive of bone loss. Amenorrhea, an indicator of estrogen deficiency and hypothalamic amenorrhea, is also highly correlated with osteoporosis. Bone minerals begin to resorb without estrogen. Elevated cortisol levels and decreased insulin-like growth factor-1 also contribute to bone resorption. Studies show that as few as 6 months of amenorrhea can lead to osteopenia or osteoporosis. In one study, 44% of adolescents with anorexia had osteopenia of the lumbar spine. Males also can develop osteoporosis due to decreased testosterone and elevated cortisol.

A recent finding has shown that the presence of depression in adolescent females with AN contributes to a higher risk of osteoporosis, compared to AN alone. Depression as a risk factor for osteoporosis needs to be further studied.

The only proven treatment for osteoporosis in anorexia nervosa in girls is regaining sufficient weight and body fat to restart the menstrual cycle. Controversy exists regarding the use of hormone replacement therapy. Most studies do not support use of hormone replacement therapy to improve bone recovery; however, some evidence indicates that use of hormone replacement therapy may stop further bone loss and may be of particular benefit for patients with extremely low body weight (less than 70% IBW). Some practitioners use hormone replacement therapy if amenorrhea is prolonged (> 1 year) and the patient is not able to achieve normal body weight. The bisphosphonates used to treat postmenopausal osteoporosis are currently being studied in adolescents. Two small randomized controlled trials have shown small but positive effects on bone density with two of the bisphosphonates—alendronate and risedronate—though clinical effectiveness has not yet been determined. Newer treatments in research trials have shown some promise, including recombinant insulin-like growth factor-1 injection and use of dehydroepiandrosterone, though they are both still under investigation.

B. BRAIN CHANGES

As malnutrition becomes more pronounced, brain tissue—both white and gray matter—is lost and a concomitant increase in cerebrospinal fluid occurs in the sulci and ventricles. Follow-up studies of weight-recovered anorexic patients show a persistent loss of gray matter, although white matter returns to normal. Functionally there does not seem to be a specific relationship between cognition and brain tissue loss, though studies have shown a decrease in cognitive ability, as well as decreased cerebral blood flow in more severe malnourished states. Communicating to the patient and the family that brain tissue can be lost can have a significant effect on the perception of the seriousness of this disorder.

Castro J et al: Bone mineral density in male adolescents with anorexia nervosa. J Am Acad Child Adolesc Psychiatry 2002; 41:613 [PMID: 12014794].

Golden NH et al: Alendronate for the treatment of osteopenia in anorexia nervosa: A randomized, double-blind, placebo-controlled trial. J Clin Endocrinol Metab 2005;90:3179 [PMID: 15784715].

Golden NH: Osteopenia and osteoporosis in anorexia nervosa. Adolesc Med State Art Rev 2003;14:97 [PMID: 12529194].

Karlsson MK: Bone size and volumetric density in women with anorexia nervosa receiving estrogen replacement therapy and in women recovered from anorexia nervosa. J Clin Endocrinol Metab 2000;85:3177 [PMID: 10999805].

Kerem NC, Katzman DK: Brain structure and function in adolescents with anorexia nervosa. Adolesc Med State Art Rev 2003;14:109 [PMID: 12529195].

Konstantynowicz J et al: Depression in anorexia nervosa: a risk factor for osteoporosis. J Clin Endocrinol Metab 2005;90:5382 [PMID: 15941868].

Mortality

Patients with eating disorders are at a higher risk of dying than the general population. Meta-analysis has shown the risk of dying to be 5.9% in such patients. Mortality estimates vary between 0% and 18%, depending on the patient population studied and the length of the study. One study showed the risk of dying to be 0.56% per year. Death in anorexic patients is due to suicide, abnormal electrolytes, and resultant cardiac arrhythmias.

Herzog DB et al: Mortality in eating disorders: A descriptive study. Int J Eat Disord 2000;28:20 [PMID: 10800010].

2. Bulimia Nervosa

Short-Term & Long-Term Complications

Complications for normal-weight bulimic patients are related to their mechanisms of purging, and many of these complications were listed earlier in the Symptoms and Signs section. If the bulimic patient is significantly malnourished, the complications may be the same as those encountered in the anorexic patient. Other complications of bulimia include esophageal rupture, acute or chronic esophagitis, and rarely, Barrett syndrome. Chronic vomiting can lead to metabolic alkalosis, and laxative abuse may cause metabolic acidosis. Patients may develop aspiration pneumonia from vomiting. Diet pill use can cause insomnia, hypertension, tachycardia, palpitations, seizures, and sudden death.

Patients who stop taking laxatives can have trouble with bowel function, most often constipation. Treating constipation can be difficult psychologically, because the practitioner may need to prescribe agents similar to the drugs of abuse used during the eating disorder.

Mortality

The mortality rate in bulimic patients is similar to that in anorexic patients. Death usually results from suicide or electrolyte derangements.

TREATMENT

Many treatment modalities are available. Factors that determine treatment interventions are severity of illness, length of illness, specific manifestations of disease, previous treatment approaches and outcomes, program availability, financial resources, and insurance coverage. Treatment options include outpatient management, day treatment hospitalization, and inpatient hospitalization of either a medical or psychiatric nature. Residential treatment is most often used when outpatient management or short-term hospitalization fails and the eating disorder becomes chronic. Residential treatment usually lasts 2–6 months. Day treatment programs are a good intervention for patients who do not yet need inpatient care but who are not improving with outpatient management. Treatment is costly. Many patients do not have insurance benefits that adequately cover the cost of

treatment, leaving parents and practitioners with profound dilemmas as to how to best provide treatment in the face of financial constraints.

Regardless of type of treatment program, a multidisciplinary approach is most effective. Treatment should include medical monitoring, nutrition therapy, and individual and family psychotherapy by practitioners experienced with eating disorder patients. Family therapy is especially helpful with younger teenagers, whereas older teenagers tend to benefit more from individual therapy, although both should be encouraged. Family therapy is an important means by which to help families understand the development of the disease and address the issues that may be barriers to recovery. Both types of therapy are encouraged in most treatment programs, and recovery without psychotherapy is unusual. The average length of therapy is roughly 6–9 months, although some individuals continue therapy for extended periods. Adjunctive modalities include art and horticulture therapy, therapeutic recreation, and massage therapy.

A newer family therapy approach, manualized family therapy, developed in Britain by Maudsley and adapted by Lock and LeGrange, has shifted the therapeutic approach to adolescents with AN. Traditional therapy allowed the adolescent to control their eating, and for the parents to back off the food portion of recovery. This manualized approach gives power and control back to parents. Treatment is prescribed for 20 weekly sessions. The first 10 are devoted to empowering parents, putting them in control of their child's nutrition and exercise. Parents are educated about the dangers of malnutrition, and supervise each meal. The next phase—sessions 11–16—returns control over eating back to the adolescent once the adolescent accepts the demands of the parents. The last phase of treatment, sessions 17–20, occurs when the patient is maintaining a healthy weight, and shifts the focus away from the eating disorder and examines the impact that the eating disorder has had on establishing a healthy adolescent identity. This approach has led to 90% of adolescents achieving good or intermediate outcomes.

Careful instruction in nutrition is important in helping the teenager and family dispel misconceptions about nutrition, identify realistic nutritional goals, and normalize eating. Initially, nutrition education may be the most important intervention as the teenager slowly works through his or her fears of fat-containing foods and weight gain. The teenager begins to trust the nutrition therapist and begins to restore body weight, by eventually eating in a well-balanced, healthy manner.

1. Anorexia Nervosa

The key to determining level of intervention depends on the degree of malnutrition, the rapidity of weight loss, the degree of medical compromise, and the presence of life-threatening electrolyte abnormalities. No absolute criteria determine level of intervention. The practitioner must examine the degree of medical compromise and consider immediate risks and the potential for an individual to reverse the situation on his or her own.

A. INPATIENT TREATMENT

Table 5–8 lists the criteria for hospital admission generally used in the medical community. It is usually quite difficult for a patient who is losing weight rapidly (> 2 lb/wk) to reverse the weight loss because the body is in a catabolic state.

If a patient is hospitalized the initial goal is to stop weight loss. The clinician can begin with a meal plan containing approximately 250 kcal more than the patient has been routinely eating. Depending on the sophistication of the program and support staff, this can usually be accomplished orally. Ideally, with the help of a nutritionist, patients should start with a well-balanced meal plan, with appropriately divided carbohydrates, proteins, and fats. Usually patients tolerate oral meals. If the patient resists, a nasogastric tube or intravenous alimentation can be used for a short time. Aside from caloric needs, the clinician needs to pay attention to the patient's hydration status, including the appropriate amount of fluid with the meal plan. Dehydration should be corrected slowly. The oral route is usually adequate. Aggressive intravenous fluid administration should be avoided because left ventricular mass is compromised and a rapid increase in volume may not be tolerated. Regulating fluid intake is important, because water intoxication can contribute to abnormal electrolytes and falsified weights.

During the initial introduction of food, the clinician needs to monitor the patient for refeeding syndrome, a phenomenon that occurs if caloric intake is increased too rapidly. Signs of refeeding syndrome are decreased serum phosphate (as the body finally starts making adenosine triphosphate), decreased serum potassium (as increased insulin causes shifting of K^+ from extracellular fluid into K^+-depleted cells), and edema related to fluid shifts as well as from congestive heart failure.

Table 5–8. Criteria for inpatient treatment of anorexia nervosa.

Body weight < 75% of ideal body weight
Supine heart rate < 45/min
Symptomatic hypotension or syncope
Hypokalemia: K^+ < 2.5 mEq/L
Rapid weight loss that cannot be interrupted as outpatient
Failure of outpatient management
Acute food refusal

Caloric intake can be increased 250 kcal/d as long as refeeding syndrome does not occur. Weight goals vary depending on programmatic approach. Typically intake is adjusted to reach a goal of 0.1–0.25 kg/d weight gain.

Overnight monitoring for bradycardia is helpful in assessing degree of metabolic compromise. Usually the more rapid and severe the weight loss, the worse the bradycardia. Improving bradycardia correlates with weight recovery. Orthostatic hypotension is most severe around hospital day 4, improving steadily and correcting by the third week of nutritional rehabilitation. An electrocardiogram should be obtained because the patient is at risk for prolonged QT syndrome and junctional arrhythmias related to the severity of bradycardia.

It usually takes 2–3 weeks to reach the initial goals of hospitalization—steady weight gain, toleration of oral diet without signs of refeeding syndrome, corrected bradycardia (heart rate > 45/min for three consecutive nights), and orthostasis. Specific weight criteria are used by many programs when considering discharge. This depends partly on admission weight. Ideally a patient gains at least 5% of his or her ideal weight. Some programs set discharge at 80%, 85%, or 90% IBW. Patient outcomes are improved with discharge at a higher body weight. One study has shown that patients do better if discharged at 95% IBW. Frequently, insurance companies do not cooperate and will not pay beyond strict medical stabilization (normal vital signs and normal electrolytes). In many practitioners' experience, relapse rate is high if patients are discharged at less than 75% IBW.

Extremely malnourished patients may not benefit from individual psychotherapy or nutritional instruction initially because they may be cognitively impaired. Beginning family psychotherapy at first, with the addition of individual psychotherapy after the first week of refeeding, may prove more effective.

Use of psychotropic medications has been commonplace in attempting to treat anorexia nervosa, despite lack of solid evidence. The most promising class of medication has been the atypical antipsychotics. Several open label trials support the use of atypical antipsychotics (risperidone and olanzapine), which target specifically the body image distortion that these patients experience. A recent pilot study, the first randomized controlled trial of olanzapine in patients with AN, showed a decrease in rumination in those who received olanzapine. Further studies need to be done before there is enough scientific evidence to support the use of atypical antipsychotics.

Though vigorously studied, SSRIs repeatedly have been shown to not be helpful in treating anorexia nervosa initially. However, once the patient has achieved approximately 85% IBW, then SSRIs (fluoxetine, citalopram, or sertraline) help prevent relapse.

To help address the malnourished state, a multivitamin with iron and zinc supplementation may be beneficial. Zinc has been found to be depleted in anorexia nervosa. Supplementation helps restore appetite as well as improve depressive moods. Symptomatic treatment for disturbances in the gastrointestinal system should be used appropriately until symptoms resolve.

B. OUTPATIENT TREATMENT

Not all patients diagnosed with anorexia nervosa need inpatient treatment, especially if parents and clinicians recognize the warning signs early. These patients can receive treatment in the outpatient setting, employing the same multidisciplinary team approach. Appropriate nutrition counseling is vital in guiding a patient and family through the initial stages of recovery. As the nutrition therapist is working at increasing the patient's caloric intake, a practitioner needs to monitor the patient's weight and vital signs. Often activity level needs to be decreased to help reverse the catabolic state. A reasonable weight gain goal may be 0.2–0.5 kg/wk. If weight loss persists, careful monitoring of vital signs, including supine heart rate, is important in determining whether an increased level of care is needed. Concomitantly, the patient should be referred to a psychotherapist, and if indicated, assessed by a psychiatrist.

2. Bulimia Nervosa

Treatment of bulimia nervosa depends on the frequency of bingeing and purging and the severity of biochemical and psychiatric derangement. If K^+ is less than 3.0 mEq/L, then inpatient medical admission is warranted. Typically extracellular K^+ is spared at the expense of intracellular K^+, so that a patient may become hypokalemic several days after the serum K^+ concentration appears to be corrected. Usually cessation of purging is sufficient to correct K^+ concentration and is the recommended intervention for K^+ greater than 3.0 mEq/L; if K^+ is 2.5–2.9 mEq/L, oral supplementation is suggested; if K^+ is less than 2.5 mEq/L, then intravenous therapy is recommended. Supplements can be stopped once K^+ levels are greater than 3.5 mEq/L. Once serum K^+ corrects and remains normal 2 days after supplements are stopped, the clinician can be confident that total body K^+ has returned to normal. Continued hospitalization depends on the patient's psychological status.

Many of these patients abuse laxatives and may be chronically dehydrated. The renin-angiotensin-aldosterone axis, as well as the antidiuretic hormone level, may be elevated to compensate. These systems do not shut down automatically when laxatives are stopped, and fluid retention of up to 10 kg/wk may result. This puts patients at risk for congestive heart failure and can

scare them as their weight increases dramatically. A diuresis often occurs after approximately 7–10 days. Parents and patients should be advised of this possible complication of initial therapy to help maintain their confidence in the care plan.

Another reason to hospitalize bulimic patients is failure of outpatient management. The binge-purge cycle is addictive and can be difficult for patients to interrupt on their own. Hospitalization can offer a forced break from the cycle, allowing patients to normalize their eating, interrupt the addictive behavior, and regain ability to recognize satiety signals.

Outpatient management can be pursued if patients are medically stable. Cognitive-behavioral therapy is crucial to help bulimic patients understand their disease and to offer suggestions for decreasing bingeing and purging. Nutrition therapy offers patients ways to regulate eating patterns so that they can avoid the need to binge. Medical monitoring should be done to check electrolytes periodically, depending on the purging method used.

SSRIs are generally quite helpful in treating the binge-purge cycle. Fluoxetine has been studied most extensively; a dose of 60 mg/d is most efficacious in teenagers. Other SSRIs are thought to work similarly and are worth trying if the patient experiences side effects while taking fluoxetine. Treatment for gastroesophageal reflux and gastritis should be used when appropriate. The pain and swelling of enlarged parotid glands can be helped by sucking on tart candy and by the application of heat.

Bacaltchuk J et al: Antidepressant versus placebo for the treatment of bulimia nervosa: A systematic review. Aust N Z J Psychiatry 2000;34:310 [PMID: 10789536].

Kaye W et al: Double blind placebo-controlled administration of fluoxetine in restricting- and restricting–purging-type anorexia nervosa. Biol Psychiatry 2001;49:644 [PMID: 11297722].

LeGrange D, Binford R, Loeb KL: Manualized family-based treatment for anorexia nervosa: a case series. J Am Acad Child Adolesc Psychiatry 2005;44:41 [PMID: 15608542].

Mehler P: Bulimia nervosa. N Engl J Med 2003;349:875 [PMID: 12944574].

Mondraty N et al: Randomized controlled trial of olanzapine in the treatment of cognitions in anorexia nervosa. Australas Psychiatry 2005;13:72 [PMID: 15777417].

Newman-Toker J: Risperidone in anorexia nervosa. J Am Acad Child Adolesc Psychiatry 2000;39:941 [PMID: 10939220].

3. Binge-Eating Disorder

A combination of cognitive-behavioral therapy and antidepressant medication has been helpful in treating binge-eating disorder in adults. Use of SSRIs for binge-eating disorder in adolescents has not been studied, but in adults, fluoxetine and citalopram help decrease binge episodes, improve depression, and the decreased appetite that contributes to weight loss. This evidence suggests that SSRIs in adolescents with binge eating disorder may be helpful as well.

McElroy SL et al: Citalopram in the treatment of binge-eating disorder: A placebo-controlled trial. J Clin Psychiatry 2003; 64:807 [PMID: 12934982].

PROGNOSIS

Outcome in eating disorders, especially anorexia nervosa, has been studied extensively. Unfortunately, most studies have focused on specific inpatient treatment programs, and few have evaluated the less ill patients who do not need hospitalization. About 40–50% of patients receiving treatment recover; 20–30% have intermittent relapses; and 20% have chronic, unremitting illness. As time from initial onset lengthens, the recovery rate decreases and mortality associated with anorexia nervosa and bulimia nervosa increase.

The course of anorexia nervosa often includes significant weight fluctuations over time, and it may be a matter of years until recovery is certain. The course of bulimia nervosa often includes relapse episodes of bingeing and purging, although bulimic patients initially recover faster than do anorexic patients. Up to 50% of anorexic patients may develop bulimia, as well as major psychological sequelae, including depression, anxiety, and substance abuse disorders. Bulimic patients also develop similar psychological illness but rarely develop anorexia. Long-term medical sequelae, aside from low body weight and amenorrhea, have not been studied in an outcome format, although anorexia nervosa is known to have multiple medical consequences including osteoporosis and structural brain changes.

It is unclear whether age at onset affects disease course. Shorter length of time between symptom onset and therapy tends to improve outcome. Various treatment modalities can be equally effective. Favorable outcomes have been found with brief medical hospitalization and long psychiatric or residential hospitalization. Higher discharge weight seems to improve the initial outcome. It is difficult to compare treatment regimens, because the numbers are small and the type of patient and illness varies between studies. No existing studies compare outpatient to inpatient treatment or the effects of day treatment on recovery.

Binge-eating disorder has been recognized only recently, and outcomes have not been studied. Intervention with an SSRI appears to help the bingeing, but little is known regarding long-term prognosis.

Fisher M: The course and outcome of eating disorders in adults and in adolescents: A review. Adolesc Med State Art Rev 2003;14:149 [PMID: 12529198].

Herzog D et al: Recovery and relapse in anorexia and bulimia nervosa: A 7.5 year follow-up study. J Am Acad Child Adolesc Psychiatry 1999;38:829 [PMID: 10405500].

REFERENCES

Kreipe RE, Birndorf SA: Eating disorders in adolescents and young adults. [Review] [32 refs] Med Clin North Am 2000;84:1027 [PMID: 10928200].

Rome E et al: Children and adolescents with eating disorders: State of the art. Pediatrics 2003;111:e98 [PMID: 12509603].

Strober M, Freeman R, Morrell W: The long-term course of severe anorexia nervosa in adolescents: Survival analysis of recovery, relapse, and outcome predictors of 10–15 years in a prospective study. Int J Eat Disord 1997;22:339 [PMID: 9356884].

Yager J, Anderson AA. Anorexia nervosa. N Engl J Med 2005; 353:1481 [PMID:16207850].

Child & Adolescent Psychiatric Disorders & Psychosocial Aspects of Pediatrics

Jennifer Hagman, MD, & Bert Dech, MD

Mental illness affects between 14% and 20% of children and adolescents. Unfortunately, the shortage of mental health providers, stigma attached to receiving mental health services, chronic underfunding of the public mental health system, decreased reimbursement to mental health providers, and disparate insurance benefits have contributed to the fact that only 2% of these children are actually seen by mental health specialists. In contrast, about 75% of children with psychiatric disturbances are seen in primary care settings, and half of all pediatric office visits involve behavioral, psychosocial, or educational concerns.

As a result, primary care physicians are compelled to play an important role in the assessment and treatment of mental health issues in children and adolescents. This role has become more important over the past decade as advances in mental health awareness and treatment have improved early identification and interventions. However, child psychiatry remains a critically underserved medical specialty, with only 7000 board certified child and adolescent psychiatrists in the United States. With more than 50,000 board certified pediatricians in the U.S., pediatricians are in a unique position to identify issues impacting the emotional health of children and initiate treatment and/or referrals to other providers.

Emotional problems that develop during childhood and adolescence can significantly impact development and may continue into adulthood. Early interventions can significantly improve outcomes in most situations. If pediatricians and schools do not appropriately identify these health concerns and encourage interventions, childhood-onset disorders may persist and lead to a downward spiral of school and social difficulties, poor employment opportunities, and poverty in adulthood.

Pediatricians and other primary care providers may be the first or sometimes only medical professional in a position to identify a mental health problem. This chapter will review screening for mental illness, situations that may arise in the context of such assessments, illnesses that are often diagnosed during childhood or adolescence, current recommendations for interventions and use of psychotropic medications, and indications for referral to mental health professionals.

DeAngelis C et al: Final report of the POPE II pediatric workforce workgroup. Pediatrics 2000;106:1245 [PMID: 11073554].

SCREENING FOR PSYCHOSOCIAL PROBLEMS & PSYCHIATRIC DISORDERS IN THE CONTEXT OF HEALTH MAINTENANCE VISITS

Most families seek help from their primary care providers when they are concerned about a child's health, growth, or development. The most efficient indicator in screening for psychosocial problems is the history provided by parents or guardians, and interview and observation of the child. Information can also be obtained from checklists and symptom-specific questionnaires (such as depression or eating disorder self-report inventories). Questions can be incorporated into the general pediatric office screening forms, or specific questionnaires can be used.

Like vital signs, which represent an essential component of the physical evaluation, the essential components of the screening for mental health concerns should generally include a review of the youth's general functioning in different aspects of their life. Five questions forming the mnemonic **PSYCH** can be addressed to parents and youth as a means of uncovering areas of concern.

1. **P**arent-child interaction: How are things going with you and your parents?
2. **S**chool: How are things going in school? (academically and behaviorally)

3. **Y**outh: How are things going with peer relationships?
4. **C**asa: How are things going at home? (including siblings, family stresses, and relationship with parents)
5. **H**appiness: How would you describe your mood?

ASSESSMENT OF BEHAVIORAL & EMOTIONAL SIGNS & SYMPTOMS

When an emotional problem or mental illness is suspected, a thorough evaluation is indicated. At least 30 minutes should be scheduled, and additional appointments may be necessary to gather information or perform tests to clarify a diagnosis. Examples for more thorough questions and observation are given in Table 6–1.

It is useful to see both parents and the child first together, then the parents alone, and then the child alone. This sequence enables the physician to observe interactions among family members and gives the parents and the child an opportunity to talk confidentially about their concerns. Parents and children often feel shame and guilt about some personal inadequacy they perceive to be causing the problem. The physician can facilitate the assessment by acknowledging that the family is trying to cope and that the ultimate task of assessment is to seek solutions and not to assign blame. An attitude of nonjudgmental inquiry can be communicated with supportive statements such as, "Let's see if we can figure out what might be happening here and find some ways to make things better."

History of the Presenting Problem

First, obtain a detailed description of the problem.

- When did it start?
- Were there unusual stresses at that time?
- How are the child's life and the family's functioning affected?
- What does the child say about the problem?
- What attempts have been made to alleviate the problem?
- Do the parents have any opinions about the cause of the problem?

Techniques for Interviewing Children and Adolescents

A. INTERVIEWING THE PRESCHOOL CHILD

Preschool children should be interviewed with their parents. As the parents discuss their concerns, the physician can observe the child's behavior, including their activity level and any unusual behaviors or symptoms. It is helpful to have toy human figures, animals, or puppets, and crayons and paper available that the child can use to express him- or herself. After hearing the history from the parents and observing and talking with the child, the physician can begin to develop an impression about the problem and formulate a treatment plan to discuss with the family.

B. INTERVIEWING THE SCHOOL-AGE CHILD

Most school-age children have mastered separation anxiety sufficiently to tolerate at least a brief interview alone with the physician. In addition, they may have important information to share about their own worries. The child should be told beforehand by the parents or physician (or both) that the doctor will want to talk to the child about his or her feelings. School-age children understand and even appreciate parental concern about unhappiness, worries, and difficulty in getting along with people. At the outset, it is useful to explore the child's thoughts about certain issues raised by the parents and ask whether the child thinks that a problem exists (eg, unhappiness, anxiety, or sleep disturbance) and any other concerns the child may have. The physician should ask the child to describe the problem in his or her own words and ask what he or she thinks is causing the problem. It is important to ask the child how the problem affects the child and the family. At the end of the interview with the child, it is important to share or reiterate the central points derived from the interview and to state that the next step is to talk with the parents about ways to make things better for the child. At that time, it is good to discuss any concerns or misgivings the child might have about sharing information with parents so that the child's right to privacy is not arbitrarily violated. Most children want to make things better and thus will allow the physician to share appropriate concerns with the parents.

C. INTERVIEWING THE ADOLESCENT

The physician usually begins by meeting briefly with the parents and adolescent together to define the concerns. Because the central developmental task of adolescence is to create an identity separate from that of the parents, the physician must show respect for the teen's point of view. The physician should then meet alone with the adolescent. After the physician has interviewed the adolescent and talked further with the parents, he or she should formulate thoughts and recommendations. Whenever possible, it is helpful to discuss these with the adolescent before presenting them to the parents and teen together. The issue of confidentiality must be discussed early in the interview: "What we talk about today is between you and me unless we decide together that someone should know or unless it appears to me that you might be in a potentially dangerous situation."

The interview with the adolescent alone might start with a restatement of the parents' concerns. The patient should be encouraged to describe the situation in his or her own words and say what the adolescent would like to be different. The physician should ask questions about the adolescent's primary concerns, predominant

Table 6–1. Screening for psychosocial problems.

Developmental history

1. Review the landmarks of psychosocial development
2. Summarize the child's temperamental traits
3. Review stressful life events and the child's reactions to them
   a. Separations
   b. Losses
   c. Marital conflict
   d. Illnesses, injuries, and hospitalizations
4. Obtain details of past mental health problems and their treatment

Family history

1. Marital history
   a. Overall satisfaction with the marriage
   b. Conflicts or disagreements within the relationship
   c. Quantity and quality of time together away from children
   d. Whether the child comes between or is a source of conflict between the parents
   e. Marital history prior to having children
2. Parenting history
   a. Feelings about parenthood
   b. Whether parents feel united in dealing with the child
   c. "Division of labor" in parenting
   d. Parental energy or stress level
   e. Sleeping arrangements
   f. Privacy
   g. Attitudes about discipline
   h. Interference with discipline from outside the family (eg, ex-spouses, grandparents)
3. Stresses on the family
   a. Problems with employment
   b. Financial problems
   c. Changes of residence
   d. Illness, injuries, and deaths
4. Family history of mental health problems
   a. Depression? Who?
   b. Suicide attempts? Who?
   c. Psychiatric hospitalizations? Who?
   d. "Nervous breakdowns"? Who?
   e. Substance abuse or problems? Who?
   f. Nervousness or anxiety? Who?

Observation of the parents

1. Do they agree on the existence of the problem or concern?
2. Are they uncooperative or antagonistic about the evaluation?
3. Do the parents appear depressed or overwhelmed?
4. Can the parents present a coherent picture of the problem and their family life?
5. Do the parents accept some responsibility for the child's problems, or do they blame forces outside the family and beyond their control?
6. Do they appear burdened with guilt about the child's problem?

Observation of the child

1. Does the child acknowledge the existence of a problem or concern?
2. Does the child want help?
3. Is the child uncooperative or antagonistic about the assessment?
4. What is the child's predominant mood or attitude?
5. What does the child wish could be different (eg, "three wishes")?
6. Does the child display unusual behavior (activity level, mannerisms, fearfulness)?
7. What is the child's apparent cognitive level?

Observation of parent-child interaction

1. Do the parents show concern about the child's feelings?
2. Does the child control or disrupt the joint interview?
3. Does the child respond to parental limits and control?
4. Do the parents inappropriately answer questions addressed to the child?
5. Is there obvious tension between family members?

Data from other sources

1. Waiting room observations by office staff
2. School (teacher, nurse, social worker, counselor)
3. Department of social services

mood state, relationships with family members, level of satisfaction with school and peer relationships, plans for the future, drug and alcohol use, and sexual activity.

In concluding the interview, the physician should summarize his or her thoughts and develop a plan with the teenager to present to the parents. If teenagers participate in the solution, they are more likely to work with the family to improve the situation. This should include a plan either for further investigation or for ways of dealing with the problem and arranging subsequent appointments with the physician or an appropriate referral to a mental health care provider.

DIAGNOSTIC FORMULATION & INTERPRETATION OF FINDINGS

Diagnosis starts with a description of the presenting problem, which is then evaluated within the context of the child's age, developmental needs, the stresses and strains on the child and the family, and the functioning of the family system.

The physician's first task is to decide whether a problem exists. For example, how hyperactive must a 5-year-old child be before he or she is too hyperactive? When a child's functioning is impaired in major domains of life, such as learning, peer relationships, family relationships, authority relationships, and recreation, or when a substantial deviation from the trajectory of normal developmental tasks occurs, a differential diagnosis should be sought based on the symptom profile. The physician then develops an etiologic hypothesis based on the information gathered:

1. The behavior falls within the range of normal given the child's developmental level.

2. The behavior is a temperamental variation.

3. The behavior is related to central nervous system impairment (eg, prematurity, exposure to toxins in utero, seizure disorder, or genetic disorders).

4. The behavior is a normal reaction to stressful circumstances (eg, medical illness, change in family structure, or loss of a loved one).

5. The problem is primarily a reflection of family dysfunction (eg, the child is the symptom bearer, scapegoat, or the identified patient for the family).

6. The problem indicates a possible psychiatric disorder.

7. The problem is complicated by an underlying medical condition.

8. Some combination of the above.

The physician's interpretation is then presented to the family. The interpretive process includes the following components:

1. An explanation of how the presenting problem or symptom is a reflection of a suspected cause

2. A suggested plan of intervention based on the presumed cause

3. A discussion of any further evaluation necessary to confirm or refine a diagnosis

A joint plan involving the physician, parents, and child is then negotiated to address the child's symptoms and developmental needs in light of the family structure and stresses. If an appropriate plan cannot be developed, or if the physician feels that further diagnostic assessment is required, referral to a mental health practitioner should be recommended.

Cassidy SJ, Jellinek M: Approaches to recognition and management of childhood psychiatric disorders in pediatric primary care. Pediatr Clin North Am 1998;45:1037 [PMID: 9884674].

Fritz G: Promoting effective collaboration between pediatricians and child and adolescent psychiatrists. Pediatr Ann 2003;32:387 [PMID: 12846016].

Gardner W et al: Primary care clinicians' use of standardized tools to assess child psychosocial problems. Ambul Pediatr 2003; 3:191 [PMID: 12882596].

Glazebrook C et al: Detecting emotional and behavioural problems in paediatric clinics. Child Care Health Dev 2003;29:141 [PMID: 12603359].

Hack S, Jellenik M: Early identification of emotional and behavioral problems in a primary care setting. Adolesc Med State Art Rev 1998;9:335 [PMID: 10961240].

Luby JL et al: The preschool feelings checklist: a brief and sensitive screening measure for depression in young children. J Am Acad Child Adolesc Psychiatry 2004;43:708 [PMID: 15167087].

Mayes LC: Child mental health consultation with families of medically compromised infants. Child Adolesc Psychiatr Clin N Am 2003;12:401 [PMID: 12910815].

Nicholson J, Clayfield JC: Responding to depression in patients. Pediatr Nurs 2004;30:136 [PMID: 15185736].

Richardson LP, Katzenellenbogen R: Childhood and adolescent depression: the role of primary care providers in diagnosis and treatment. Curr Probl Pediatr Adolesc Health Care 2005;35:6 [PMID: 15611721].

Williams J et al: Diagnosis and treatment of behavioral health disorders in pediatric practice. Pediatrics 2004;114:601 [PMID: 15342827].

Screening Tools for Mental Illness Available for Use in the Primary Physician's Office Setting

A. STRENGTHS AND DIFFICULTIES QUESTIONNAIRES

The Strengths and Difficulties Questionnaires are brief behavioral screening questionnaires targeting patients 3–16 years old. They exist in several versions to meet the needs of researchers, clinicians, and educators. They have been well validated and are available on the Internet without cost.

Many child and adolescent mental health clinics now use the Strengths and Difficulties Questionnaires as part of the initial assessment, asking parents, teachers, and young people over the age of 11 years old to complete questionnaires prior to the first clinical assessment. The findings can then influence how the assessment is carried out and which professionals are involved in that assessment.

Strengths and Difficulties Questionnaire: A pilot study of a new computer version of the self report scale. Eur Child Adolesc Psychiatry 2003;12:9 (www.sdqinfo.com) [PMID: 12601559].

B. VANDERBILT ASSESSMENT SCALES FOR ATTENTION-DEFICIT/HYPERACTIVITY DISORDER

American Academy of Pediatrics/National Initiative for Children's Health Quality (AAP/NICHQ) Attention-Deficit/Hyperactivity Disorder Practitioner's Toolkit.

www.nichq.org/resources/toolkit/

C. Depression Collaborative Tool Kit

This manual outlines all of the key elements of a system of care for people with depression. It contains a Depression Care Model, an Improvement Model, and a Plan-Do-Study-Act cycle to test and implement changes in real work or school settings.

www.healthdisparities.net.

D. The MacArthur Foundation Initiative on Depression and Primary Care: Dartmouth & Duke Depression Tool Kit

This tool kit is intended to help primary care clinicians recognize and manage depression. It includes instruments and information sources to assist with: recognizing and diagnosing depression; educating patients about depression, assessing treatment preferences, engaging their participation and explaining the process of care; and using evidence-based guidelines and management tools for treating depression and monitoring patient response to treatment.

www.depression-primarycare.org/

E. Mental Health in Primary Care Review in the National Electronic Library for Health

This resource provides support of primary care professionals, primary care organizations, and local user groups in their delivery of primary care mental health services.

www.library.nhs.uk/mentalhealth

Situations That May Require Hospitalization or Referral for More Extensive Psychiatric Assessment

If there is any concern about the child's safety the provider must also evaluate the risk of danger to self (suicidal attempts or ideation), danger to others (assault, aggression, or homicidal ideation), and screen for other factors that could heighten the risk of danger to self or others, such as physical or sexual abuse or illicit substance use or abuse. The presence of drug or alcohol abuse in adolescent patients may require referral to community resources specialized for the treatment of these addictive disorders.

The following questions should be asked of the youth. The parents should be asked similar questions about what they have observed. Specific details about the circumstances should be asked if any question below is answered with "yes."

1. Have you ever been sad for more than a few days at a time such that it affected your sleep or appetite?
2. Have you ever been so sad that you wished you weren't alive?

3. Have you ever thought of ways of killing yourself or made a suicide attempt?
4. Have you ever thought about killing someone else, or tried to kill someone?
5. Has anyone ever hit you and left marks? (If yes, ask who, when, and under what circumstances, and if it was reported.)
6. Has anyone ever touched your privates when they weren't supposed to? (If yes, ask who, when, and under what circumstances, and if it was reported.)
7. Do you use alcohol, tobacco, or illicit drugs? (If yes, ask what, when, with whom, and how much.)

Civil Commitment and Involuntary Mental Health "Holds"

If further assessment indicates a need for inpatient hospitalization, it is optimal if the patient and guardian give consent for this care. In a situation in which the guardian is unwilling or unable to give consent for emergency department–based assessment or inpatient hospitalization of a child or adolescent, an involuntary mental health "hold" may become necessary.

The term **involuntary mental health "hold"** refers to a legal process that can be initiated by physicians, police officers, and certified mental health professionals, that allows the individual to be prevented from leaving the emergency department or hospital for up to 72 hours. This allows the physician to establish a safe environment and prevent the individual from harming themselves or others, and allows sufficient time to determine if the individual is a risk to him- or herself or others due to mental illness. Each state has specific laws that specify rules and regulations which must be followed as part of this process. A specific form must be completed and the patient and family informed of their rights. As this involves revoking the civil rights of a patient or their guardian, it is critical to implement the procedure correctly. All physicians should be familiar with their state laws regulating this process.

Although the precise wording and conditions of involuntary mental health holds may vary slightly from state to state, they are generally quite similar. A 72-hour involuntary mental health hold is for the purpose of acute evaluation and determination of the patient's safety when the evaluator elicits sufficient information to confirm a significant risk exists of danger to self or others. Additional criteria for involuntary psychiatric admission include a determination that the patient is "gravely disabled" by virtue of impaired judgment, which renders him or her unable to provide food, clothing, or shelter for themselves, or in the case of a child or adolescent, he or she is unable to eat and perform normal activities of daily living.

Circumstances under which a mental health hold may be discontinued:

At any time after their acute admission but within 72 hours, one of three possibilities must be chosen by the physician or psychiatric treatment team.

1. The clinician may determine that the patient is safe for further treatment in a less restrictive setting and may decide to end the 72-hour mental health hold and discharge the patient from the emergency department or the inpatient psychiatric setting. This requires assessment and documentation that the patient is now safe and a physician signature on an order form to discontinue the hold.

2. The patient or their guardian may agree to inpatient psychiatric treatment and offer to remain in the hospital as a voluntary psychiatric inpatient. In this case, the mental health hold is discontinued and the patient and guardian signs a request for voluntary mental health treatment.

3. Finally, the clinician and patient or guardian may continue to disagree about the need for inpatient psychiatric treatment. In this case, when the psychiatrist believes the patient continues to be a risk to him- or herself or others or is gravely disabled, the psychiatrist may petition the mental health court to place the patient on a "short term certification" (this is the term in use in Colorado, but other states have different terms and processes) for continued involuntary mental health treatment on an inpatient psychiatric unit by completing the appropriate evaluation and paperwork. In Colorado a short term certification can remain in effect for up to 90 days, or can be discontinued any time prior to that time at the clinician's discretion or by a judge. Short term certification also mandates that a patient has access to legal representation in the form of their own lawyer, or if they are unable to afford legal council, a court-appointed attorney. They have the right to contest their involuntary commitment in front of a mental health judge. If the case goes to court, the health care providers must also be present at the hearing. It is always preferable to work with the guardian and the patient to obtain informed consent for treatment and to minimize the need for legal proceedings.

Mandatory Reporting of Mental Health or Abuse

Mandatory reporting by a physician of suspicion of physical or sexual abuse or neglect to the local human services agency is discussed in greater detail in Chapter 7. The "Tarasoff Rule" refers to a California legal case which led to a "duty to warn": Physicians are mandated to warn potential victims of harm when plans are disclosed to them about serious threats to harm specific individuals. Documentation of a phone call and registered letter to the individual being threatened are mandated. Under such circumstances, arrangement for the involuntary civil commitment of the potential perpetrator of harm is likely to be in order as well.

Referral of Patients to Mental Health Care Professionals

Primary care physicians often refer patients to a child and adolescent psychiatrist when the diagnosis or treatment plan is uncertain, or when medication is indicated and the pediatrician prefers that a specialist initiate or manage treatment of the mental illness (Table 6–2). For academic difficulties not associated with behavioral difficulties, a child psychologist may be most helpful in assessing patients for learning disorders and potential remediation. For cognitive difficulties associated with head trauma or brain tumors, a referral to a child neuropsychologist may be indicated.

Patients with private mental health insurance need to contact their insurance company for a list of local mental health professionals trained in the assessment and treatment of children and adolescents who are on their insurance panel. Patients with Medicaid or without mental health insurance coverage can usually be assessed and treated at their local mental health care center. As the referring pediatrician, you or your staff should assist the family by providing information to put them in touch with the appropriate services.

Pediatricians who feel comfortable implementing the recommendations of a mental health professional with whom they have a collaborative relationship should consider remaining involved in the treatment of mental illness in their patients. The local branches of the American Academy of Child and Adolescent Psychiatry and the American Psychological Association should be able to provide you a list of mental health professionals who are trained in the evaluation and treatment of children and adolescents.

Consultation-Liaison Psychiatry

The field of consultation-liaison psychiatry was developed to address the need for mental health assessment and inter-

Table 6–2. When to consider consultation or referral to a child and adolescent psychiatrist.

The diagnosis is not clear
The pediatrician feels that further assessment is needed
The pediatrician believes medication may be needed, but will not be prescribing it
The pediatrician has started medications and needs further psychopharmacologic consultation
Individual, family, and/or group psychotherapy is needed
Psychotic symptoms (hallucinations, paranoia) are present
Bipolar affective disorder is suspected

vention of medically hospitalized pediatric patients. Psychiatric consultation on the medical floor can be complex and often requires assessment and intervention beyond the individual patient. The psychiatric consultation, in addition to evaluating the patient's symptom presentation, should also include assessment of family dynamics as related to the patient, and may include evaluation of how the medical team is addressing care of the patient and family. The psychiatric consultation focuses on the various hierarchies related to the interaction of the patient and staff, or staff and staff, in addition to the patient per se, and can be quite enlightening and may lead to more productive interventions.

When requesting a psychiatric consultation, as with any medical specialty it is critical that the concern and focus of the consultation request be as specific as possible. Psychiatric consultation on the medical floor is often requested when the patient's emotional state is impacting their response to medical care, or when an underlying mental illness may be contributing to the presenting symptoms. Patients admitted to the intensive care unit or a medical floor after a suicide attempt or overdose should be evaluated by a psychiatric consultant before discharge.

Another common reason for requesting a psychiatric consultation on the medical floor is change in mental status. Be alert to the likelihood that acute mental status changes in the medical setting can represent delirium, as this has significant assessment and treatment implications. Delirium is defined as an acute and fluctuating disturbance of the sensorium (ie, alertness and orientation). Delirium can be manifested by a variety of psychiatric symptoms including paranoia, hallucinations, anxiety, and mood disturbances. However, aside from dementia and possibly dissociation and malingering, primary psychiatric presentations do not typically involve disturbances of alertness and orientation that are always present in delirium.

THE CHRONICALLY ILL CHILD

Advances in the treatment of pediatric and adolescent illness have transformed a number of previously fatal conditions into life-threatening but potentially survivable conditions. This includes advances in the fields of neonatal medicine as well as hematology-oncology including bone marrow transplantation. Additionally, solid organ transplantation including heart, liver, kidney, and lung, among others has revolutionized the potential treatment options for a whole host of once-fatal illnesses.

However, the intensity of treatment can in itself be highly stressful, and even traumatic physically, financially, and psychologically, for children as well as their parents and siblings. Survivors are at risk of long-term medical and psychological sequelae. Those who are fortunate enough to survive the initial treatment of a potentially life-threatening condition often exchange a life-threatening illness for a chronic condition.

Phase Oriented Intervention

Psychosocial interventions should vary depending on the developmental level of the patient, siblings, and family, and the phase of the illness. A first crisis is dealt with differently than interventions made during a long course of illness or interventions made during a period of stabilization or remission.

With this in mind, the Organ Procurement and Transplantation Network/United Network for Organ Sharing established new by-laws in August 2004 which set minimum requirements for the psychosocial services available as part of an accredited solid organ transplant program. Included in these guidelines is the establishment of a transplantation psychiatrist, psychologist, nurse practitioner, and psychiatric social worker.

Additional guidelines include psychiatric evaluation including substance abuse screening of prospective transplantation candidates as well as any potential renal or hepatic living donors. These guidelines include the availability of individual supportive counseling, crisis intervention, support groups, and death, dying, and bereavement counseling to transplantation patients and their families.

Reactions to Chronic Physical or Mental Illness and Disability

Between 5% and 10% of individuals experience a prolonged period of medical illness or disability during childhood, and another 5–10% experience the onset of mental illness in childhood. The psychosocial effects for the child and the family are often profound. Although the specific effect of illness on children and their families depends on the characteristics of the illness, the age of the child, and premorbid functioning, it can be expected that both the child and the parents will go through stages toward eventual acceptance of the disease state. It may take months for a family to accept the diagnosis, to cope with the stresses, and to resume normal life to the extent possible. These stages resemble those that follow the loss of a loved one. If anxiety and guilt remain prominent within the family, a pattern of overprotection can evolve. Likewise, when the illness is not accepted as a reality to be dealt with, a pattern of denial may become prominent. The clinical manifestations of these patterns of behavior are presented in Table 6–3.

Children are very observant and intuitive when it comes to understanding their illness and its general prognosis. At the same time, their primary concerns usually are the effects of the illness on everyday life, feeling sick, and limitations on normal activities. Children are also keenly aware of the family's reactions and may be reluc-

Table 6–3. Patterns of coping with chronic illness.

Overprotection
  Persistent anxiety or guilt
  Few friends and peer activities
  Poor school attendance
  Overconcern with somatic symptoms
  Secondary gain from the illness
Effective coping
  Realistic acceptance of limits imposed by illness
  Normalization of daily activities with peers, play, and school
Denial
  Lack of acceptance of the illness
  Poor medical compliance
  Risk-taking behaviors
  Lack of parental follow-through with medical instructions
  General pattern of acting-out behavior

---

tant to bring up issues they know are upsetting to their parents. Whenever possible, parents should be encouraged to discuss the child's illness and to answer questions openly and honestly, including exploration of the child's fears and fantasies. Such interactions promote closeness and relieve the child's sense of isolation. Even with these active attempts to promote effective sharing between the child and the family, ill children frequently experience fear, anxiety, irritability, and anger over their illness, and guilt over causing family distress. Sleep disturbances, tears, and clinging, dependent behavior are not infrequent or abnormal.

The Vicious Cycle of Disease Empowerment

Submission to illness' power, resulting, for example, in staying in bed longer than strictly necessary or withdrawing from friends and family reduces a variety of opportunities to experience normal life. When reinforced by further relapses, increased helplessness and apprehension due to symptoms raise the idea that symptoms and relapse strike unpredictably and cannot be influenced by the patient. Consequently, the patient experiences an increase in fear of illness and a reduction of activity because it can be interrupted at any time by unpredictable relapse. This submission to fear of illness by waiting for relapse reinforces the status of the chronically ill with increased helplessness. Both cycles result in lowering self-esteem and disempowerment.

Families of chronically ill patients sometimes continue to use the same behavior and strategies, favoring rigidity and predictable long-standing habits. Although such rigidity is constraining, families often consider change as being unsafe. Past, present, and future collapse into a timeless dimension under the tyranny of illness. To address this, one can highlight and amplify differences in the past-future timeline. Stressing how hypothetical differences could occur may open up alternative scenarios for the future. Rituals and metaphors serve the purpose of introducing distinctions in time. Rituals have always been used to demarcate different phases in life and to celebrate significant moments. Introducing different rituals that are consistent with family growth and helping the family to seek out their developmental priorities can represent an important intervention.

Treatments designed to interrupt the vicious cycle of disease empowerment can be quite powerful. Discussions and interventions which take into account both emotional and medical symptoms will help the child and family better understand their experiences and attitude toward illness and life. The family and child will benefit from discussions about such questions as "What is the real nature of this illness? Why has it affected us? What will be our future? What does the treatment do to me?" Such discussions can be quite enlightening and empowering, as they encourage open discussion for the child and parents and an active role in treatment.

THE TERMINALLY ILL CHILD

The diagnosis of fatal illness in a child is a severe blow even to families who have reason to suspect that outcome. The discussion with parents (and the child) about terminal illness is one of the most difficult tasks for a physician working with children and adolescents. Although parents want and need to know the truth, they are best told in stepwise fashion beginning with temporizing phrases such as "The news is not good" and "This is a life-threatening illness." The parents' reactions and questions can then be observed for clues about how much they want to be told at any one time. The physician must also attempt to gauge how much of the information the parents are able to comprehend during the initial discussion and consider involvement of appropriate support services. Parents' reactions may proceed in a grief sequence including initial shock and disbelief lasting days to weeks, followed by anger, despair, and guilt over weeks to months, and ending in acceptance of the reality of the situation. These responses vary in their expression, intensity, and duration for each member of the family.

Developmental and phase–oriented perspectives of patients, siblings, parents, and caretakers are reviewed in Table 6–4. Although most children do not fully understand the permanency of death until about age 8, most ill children experience a sense of danger and doom that is associated with death before that age. Even so, the question of whether to tell a child about the fatal nature of a disease should in most cases be answered in the affirmative

Table 6–4. Death and childhood.

Age (y)	Before	During (Sudden)	During (Acute)	During (Chronic)	After (Sudden)	After (Acute)	After (Chronic)
0–5	Ideas on death; Abandonment; punishment		Avoidance of pain; need for love	Withdrawal; separation anxiety			
5–10	Concepts of inevitability; confusion; Castration anxiety		Guilt (bad), regression, denial	Guilt (religious), regression, denial			
10–15	Control of body and other developmental tasks; Reality		Depression; despair for future	Depression; despair, anxiety, anger			
Parents	(Acute) Anxiety; concern; hopefulness — (Chronic) Premature mourning, guilt, anticipatory grief, reaction formation and displacements, need for information	Disbelief; displaced rage; accelerated grief; prolonged numbness	Desperate concern; denial; guilt	Denial; remorse; resurgence of love	Guilt; mourning	Anger at doctors; need for follow-up, over-idealizing, fantasy loss	Remorse; relief and guilt

Siblings

Age (y)		After
0–5	Reactions to changes in parents (sense of loss of love and withdrawal)	1. Respond to reaction of parents 2. Survivor guilt
5–10	Concern about their implications; fearful for themselves	
10–15	Generally supportive	

Staff

Before	During	After
Anxiety; conspiracy of silence	Reaction: Withdraw Tasks: 1. Correct distortions (e.g., "Am I safe?", "Will someone be with me?", "Will be helped to feel better?") 2. Comfort parents 3. Allow hope and promote feeling of actively coping 4. Protect dignity of patient	Need for aftercare of survivors; autopsy request tactful; accurate information regarding disposal of body; delay billing

Reproduced, with permission, from Lewis M: *Clinical Aspects of Child Development*, 2nd ed. Lea & Febiger, 1982.

183

unless the parents object. When the parents object, this should alert the physician to involve the unit social worker, who can work with the family to ensure their decision is in the best interest of the child. Refusal of the adults to tell the child, especially when the adults themselves are very sad, leads to a conspiracy of silence that increases fear of the unknown in the child and leads to feelings of loneliness and isolation at the time of greatest need. In fact, children who are able to discuss their illness with family members are less depressed, have fewer behavior problems, have higher self-esteem, feel closer to their families, and adapt better to the challenges of their disease and its treatment.

The siblings of dying children are also significantly affected. They may feel neglected and deprived because of the time their parents must spend with the sick child. Anger and jealousy may then give rise to feelings of guilt over having such feelings about their sick sibling. Awareness of the emotional responses, coping abilities, and available resources for support of other family members can diminish these feelings and make a significant difference in the family's overall ability to cope with the illness.

After the child dies, the period of bereavement may last for years. Family members may need outside help in dealing with their grief through supportive counseling services or peer-support groups. Bereavement usually does not substantially interfere with overall life functioning for more than 2–3 months. Most parents and siblings are able to return to work and school within a month, although their emotional state and thoughts may continue to be dominated by the loss for some time. When the individual is unable to function in his or her societal and family role beyond this time frame, a diagnosis of complicated bereavement, major depression, posttraumatic stress disorder (PTSD), or adjustment disorder should be considered and appropriate interventions recommended, such as referral for counseling or psychotherapy and possibly antidepressant medication.

Long-Term Coping

The process of coping with a chronic or terminal illness is complex and varies with the dynamics of each individual child and family. Each change in the course of the illness and each new developmental stage present different challenges for the child. It is important for health care providers to continually assess the family and child's needs and coping abilities over time and to provide appropriate support, information, and access to interventions.

Assistance from Health Care Providers

A. EDUCATE THE PATIENT AND FAMILY

Children and their families should be given information about the illness, including its course and treatment, at frequent intervals. Factual, open discussions minimize anxieties. The explanation should be compre-

hensible to all, and time should be set aside for questions and answers. The setting can be created with an invitation such as "Let's take some time together to review the situation again."

B. PREPARE THE CHILD FOR CHANGES AND PROCEDURES

The physician should explain, in an age-appropriate manner, what is expected with a new turn in the illness or with upcoming medical procedures. This explanation enables the child to anticipate and in turn to master the new development and promotes trust between the patient and the health care providers.

C. ENCOURAGE NORMAL ACTIVITIES

The child should attend school and play with peers as much as the illness allows. Individual education plans should be requested from the school if accommodation beyond the regular classroom is necessary. At the same time, parents should be encouraged to apply the same rules of discipline and behavior to the ill child as to the siblings.

D. ENCOURAGE COMPENSATORY ACTIVITIES, INTERESTS, AND SKILL DEVELOPMENT

Children who experience disability or interruption of their usual activities and interests should be encouraged to explore new interests, and the family should be supported in adapting the child's interests for their situation, and in presenting new opportunities.

E. PROMOTE SELF-RELIANCE

Children often feel helpless when others must do things for them, or assist with their daily needs. The health care provider should guide and encourage parents in helping ill children assume responsibility for some aspects of their medical care and continue to experience age-appropriate independence and skills whenever possible.

F. PERIODICALLY REVIEW FAMILY COPING

Families are often so immersed in the crisis of their child's illness that they neglect their own needs or the needs of other family members. From time to time, the physician should ask "How is everyone doing?" The feelings of the patient, the parents, and other children in the family are explored. Parents should be encouraged to stay in touch with people in their support system, and to encourage their children in such efforts as well. Feelings of fear, guilt, anger, and grief should be monitored and discussed as normal reactions to difficult circumstances. If these experiences are interfering with the family's functioning, involvement of the pediatric social worker or a therapist can be helpful.

Appropriate lay support groups for the patient and family should be recommended. Many hospitals have such groups, and hospital social workers can facilitate participation for the patient and family.

Browning D: To show our humanness—Relational and communicative competence in pediatric palliative care. Bioethics Forum 2002;18:23 [PMID: 12744267].

Christian B: Growing up with chronic illness: Psychosocial adjustment of children and adolescents with cystic fibrosis. Annu Rev Nurs Res 2003;21:151 [PMID: 12858696].

Feudtner C, Haney J, Dimmers MA: Spiritual care needs of hospitalized children and their families: a national survey of pastoral care providers' perceptions. Pediatrics 2003;111:e67 [PMID: 12509597].

Freeman K, O'Dell C, Meola C: Childhood brain tumors: children's and siblings' concerns regarding the diagnosis and phase of illness. J Pediatr Oncol Nurs 2003;20:133 [PMID: 12776261].

Freeman K, O'Dell C, Meola C: Childhood brain tumors: parental concerns and stressors by phase of illness. J Pediatr Oncol Nurs 2004;21:87 [PMID: 15125552].

Geist R, Grdisa V, Otley A: Psychosocial issues in the child with chronic conditions. Best Pract Res Clin Gastroenterol 2003; 17:141 [PMID: 12676111].

Haase JE: The adolescent resilience model as a guide to interventions. J Pediatr Oncol Nurse 2004;21:289 [PMID: 15381798].

Kübler-Ross E: *On Children and Death.* Collier Books, Macmillan Publishing, 1983.

Laws T: Fathers struggling for relevance in the care of their terminally ill child. Contemp Nurse 2004;18:34 [PMID: 15729796].

Lewis M, Vitulano LA: Biopsychosocial issues and risk factors in the family when the child has a chronic illness. Child Adolesc Psychiatr Clin N Am 2003;12:389 [PMID: 12910814].

Meyer EC et al: Parental perspective on end-of-life care in the pediatric intensive care unit. Crit Care Med 2002;30:226 [PMID: 11902266].

Oliver RC et al: Beneficial effects of a hospital bereavement intervention program after traumatic childhood death. J Trauma 2001;50:440 [PMID: 11265051].

Stewart JL: Children living with chronic illness; An examination of their stressors, coping responses and health outcomes. Annu Rev Nurs Res 2003;21:203 [PMID: 12858698].

Suris JC: Chronic conditions and adolescence. J Pediatr Endocrinol Metab 2003;16(Suppl)2:247 [PMID: 12729399].

Van Riper M: The sibling experience of living with childhood chronic illness and disability. Annu Rev Nurs Res 2003;21:279 [PMID: 12858700].

Waugh S: Parental views on disclosure of diagnosis to their HIV-positive children. AIDS Care 2003;15:169 [PMID: 12856338].

■ PSYCHIATRIC DISORDERS OF CHILDHOOD & ADOLESCENCE

A psychiatric disorder is defined as a characteristic cluster of signs and symptoms (eg, emotions, behaviors, thought patterns, and mood states) that are associated with subjective distress or maladaptive behavior. This definition presumes that the individual's symptoms are of such intensity, persistence, and duration that the ability to adapt to life's challenges is compromised.

Psychiatric disorders have their origins in neurobiologic, genetic, psychological (life experience), or environmental sources. The neurobiology of childhood disorders is one of the most active areas of investigation in child and adolescent psychiatry. Although much remains to be clarified, data from genetic studies point to heritable transmission of ADHD, schizophrenia, mood and anxiety disorders, eating disorders, pervasive developmental disorders, learning disorders, and tic disorders, among others. About 3–5% of children and 10–15% of adolescents are personally affected by psychiatric disorders and will benefit from psychiatric treatment.

The *Diagnostic and Statistical Manual of Mental Disorders, Fourth Edition, Text Revision* (DSM-IV-TR) is the formal reference text for psychiatric disorders and includes the criteria for each of the mental illnesses, including those that begin in childhood and adolescence. Psychiatric diagnoses are given on five axes to allow the physician to address the developmental, medical, psychosocial, and overall adaptive issues that contribute to the primary diagnosis on axis I or II.

Axis I: Clinical disorders and other conditions that may be a focus of clinical attention

Axis II: Personality disorders, mental retardation, learning disabilities

Axis III: General medical conditions

Axis IV: Psychosocial and environmental problems

Axis V: Global assessment of functioning (on a scale of 0–100, with 100% being the highest level of functioning)

American Psychiatric Association: *Diagnostic and Statistical Manual of Mental Disorders, Fourth Edition, Text Revision.* American Academy of Pediatrics, 2000.

PERVASIVE DEVELOPMENTAL DISORDERS & AUTISM

Pervasive developmental disorders (PDDs) and childhood autism are early-onset, severe neuropsychiatric disorders that were once referred to as childhood psychoses. PDDs (including autistic disorder) are now distinguished from childhood schizophrenia on the basis of clinical differences and family histories. The term PDD denotes a group of disorders with the common findings of impairment of socialization skills and characteristic behavioral abnormalities. Speech and language deficits are common as well.

1. Autistic Disorder

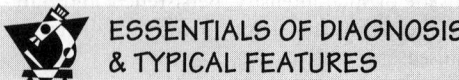

ESSENTIALS OF DIAGNOSIS & TYPICAL FEATURES

- *Severe deficits in social responsiveness and interpersonal relationships.*
- *Abnormal speech and language development.*
- *Behavioral peculiarities such as ritualized, repetitive, or stereotyped behaviors; rigidity; and poverty of age-typical interests and activities.*
- *Onset in infancy or early childhood (before age 3 years).*

General Considerations

Improved identification of autistic disorder has led to earlier interventions. Autism is more common than was once thought, with an incidence of approximately 16–40 cases per 10,000 school-age children. More boys than girls are affected (3:1). Although the cause of autism is unknown, central nervous system dysfunction is suggested by its higher incidence in populations affected by perinatal disorders: rubella, phenylketonuria, tuberous sclerosis, infantile spasms, encephalitis, and fragile X syndrome. Studies of twins reveal over 90% concordance for autistic disorder in monozygotic twins compared with 24% in dizygotic twins. Twenty-five percent of families with an autistic child have other family members with language-related disorders. (See also Chapter 2.) Although there has been much debate over the past decade about a possible link between vaccines or dietary factors and the onset of autism spectrum disorders, research studies have not supported these as causal factors.

Rutter M: Incidence of autism spectrum disorders: changes over time and their meaning. Acta Paediatrica 2005;94:2 [PMID: 15858952].

Clinical Findings

Severe deficits in reciprocal social interaction (eg, delayed or absent social smile, failure to anticipate interaction with caregivers, and a lack of attention to a primary caregiver's face) are often evident even in the first year of life. In toddlers, findings include deficiencies in imitative play and a relative lack of interest in interactions with others. Language development is often quite delayed. In fact, children are often first referred for audiologic evaluation because of failure to respond as expected to sounds. When speech does begin to develop, it may be echolalic or nonsensical. Children with autism often display peculiar interests; bizarre responses to sensory stimuli; repetitive, stereotypical motor behaviors (eg, twirling and hand-flapping); odd posturing; self-injurious behavior; abnormal patterns of eating and sleeping; and unpredictable mood changes. Thematic pretend play is often impaired. An intense preoccupation with an age-unusual interest (eg, power poles) may replace the usual broad range of interests of the child's age-mates. About 40–60% of children with autism have intelligence quotients under 70.

Differential Diagnosis

A hearing or visual impairment must be ruled out with appropriate screening. Children with developmental speech and language disorders typically show better interpersonal interactions than children with autism. Evaluation should include investigations for metabolic disorders and fragile X syndrome.

Complications

Approximately 30% of individuals with autism develop a seizure disorder, with the onset often occurring during puberty. The onset of puberty can also be associated with worsening of aggression, hyperactivity and self-destructive behaviors. These symptoms, along with the development of a seizure disorder, are more common in the individuals with low IQ associated with their autism diagnosis. Comorbid psychiatric disorders should be screened for if significant changes in mood and behavior occur. Some adolescents with autism who have higher cognitive skills become depressed as their awareness of their differences from their peers increases.

Treatment

Parents and families need strong support as well as education in caring for a child with autism. Early interventions to facilitate the development of reciprocal interactions, language, and social skills are critical. Occupational therapy for sensory integration is also an integral component of the comprehensive assessment. Sensory integration interventions help the family better support the child and adapt the environment to their specific needs.

Behaviorally oriented special education classes or day treatment programs are vital in supporting the development of more appropriate social, linguistic, self-care, and cognitive skills.

No specific medications are available to treat autistic disorder. Pharmacotherapy is aimed at reducing specific target symptoms and must be continually assessed and reevaluated for efficacy and side effects. Coexisting diagnoses must be carefully considered. Neuroleptic medications (eg, risperidone, olanzapine, and haloperidol) may modify a variety of disruptive symptoms, including hyperactivity and aggressiveness. Psychostimulants may improve inattentive or hyperactive symptoms but can sometimes worsen behavior or mood. Antidepressants—especially the selective serotonin reuptake inhibitors (SSRIs)—may benefit both mood symptoms and symptoms of excessive rigidity or obsessive behavior. Mood stabilizers may diminish irritability, mood swings, or episodic dyscontrol. Naltrexone may help control severe self-injurious behavior or stereotypes. Controlled studies do not support the use of secretin for autism.

Prognosis

Autism is a lifelong disorder. The best prognosis is for children who have normal intelligence and have developed symbolic language skills by age 5 years. Individuals with autism may not be able to live independently and may require significant support and supervision throughout their lives. Approximately one-sixth of children with autism become gainfully employed as adults, and another one-sixth are able to function in sheltered workshops or special work and school environments. Placement in specialized residential homes or programs may be necessary for some individuals whose guardians are unable to meet their special needs or provide a secure and safe home environment.

Chakrabarti S, Fombonne E: Pervasive developmental disorders in preschool children. JAMA 2002;285:3093 [PMID: 11427137].

Dunn-Geier J, Ho H, Auersperg E et al: Effect of secretin on children with autism: A randomized controlled trial. Dev Med Child Neurol 2000;42:796 [PMID: 11132252].

McDougle CJ et al: Research Units on Pediatric Psychopharmacology (RUPP) Autism Network: Background and rationale for an initial controlled study of risperidone. Child Adolesc Psychiatr Clin North Am 2000;9:201 [PMID: 10674197].

Prater CD, Zylstra RG: Autism: A medical primer. Am Fam Physician 2002;66:1667 [PMID: 12449265].

Santosh PJ, Baird G: Pharmacotherapy of target symptoms in autistic spectrum disorders. Indian J Pediatr 2002;68:427 [PMID: 11407159].

Volkmar F, Cook EH Jr, Pomeroy J, et al: Practice parameters for the assessment and treatment of children, adolescents and adults with autism and other pervasive developmental disorders. J Am Acad Child Adolesc Psychiatry 1999;38(12 Suppl):32S [PMID: 10624084].

2. Nonautistic Pervasive Developmental Disorders

Asperger syndrome, childhood disintegrative disorder, pervasive developmental disorder not otherwise specified (PDD-NOS), and Rett syndrome (Table 6–5).

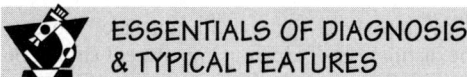

ESSENTIALS OF DIAGNOSIS & TYPICAL FEATURES

- *Substantial social impairment, either primary or representing a loss of previously acquired social skills.*
- *Abnormalities in speech and language development or behavior resembling autistic disorder.*
- *Onset by early childhood (may be as late as age 9 years in childhood disintegrative disorder).*

General Considerations

Children with nonautistic PDDs display a wide range of deficits in social, language, and behavioral skills that are similar to those in children with autistic disorder. However, these children deviate from the clinical profile for autistic disorder by failing to meet all the

Table 6–5. Characteristics of pervasive developmental disorders.

Disorder	Age at Onset	Clinical Features
Asperger syndrome	Early childhood	"Odd" individuals (probably more common in males) with normal intelligence, motor clumsiness, eccentric interests, and a limited ability to appreciate social nuances
Childhood disintegrative disorder	3–4 years	Profound deterioration to severe autistic disorder
Pervasive developmental disorder	Early childhood	Two to three times more common than autistic disorder, with similar but less severe symptoms
Rett syndrome	5 months to 4 years old	Females with reduced head circumference and loss of social relatedness who develop stereotyped hand movements and have impaired language and mental functioning
Autistic disorder	Before age 1	Severe deficit in social interaction, poor language development, abnormal eating and sleeping patterns.

necessary diagnostic criteria, by failing to fulfill the severity threshold (ie, milder functional impairment), by manifesting atypical symptomatology (eg, the characteristic hand-wringing or gender distribution [female] in Rett syndrome), or by experiencing onset at a later age. In the past, many of these children would have been classified in the group manifesting so-called atypical development. Children with nonautistic PDDs probably outnumber autistic children by as much as 2–3:1. The majority of Rett syndrome cases are now known to be due to a mutation in the *MECP2* gene.

Differential Diagnosis

Specific developmental speech and language disorders should be distinguished. Hearing impairment should be ruled out with appropriate screening.

Treatment

The backbone of treatment for Asperger syndrome and PDD-NOS is a cognitive behavioral approach aimed at teaching and reinforcing more appropriate social and language skills and behaviors. Rett syndrome and childhood disintegrative disorder have much worse prognoses and call for multidisciplinary, often milieu-based interventions (as for autistic disorder). Occupational therapy for sensory integration interventions may be helpful. In all cases, family education and support are important.

Children should be screened for the presence of other psychiatric conditions, including mood disorders, obsessive-compulsive disorder (OCD), ADHD, and anxiety disorders, and appropriate interventions should be initiated. Medications may be helpful for treating specific target symptoms as described for autistic disorder.

Prognosis

These are lifelong disorders. The prognosis is variable depending on the severity of social and language deficits and response to treatment interventions.

Starr E et al: Stability and change among high-functioning children with pervasive developmental disorders: A 2-year outcome study. J Autism Dev Disord 2003;33:15 [PMID: 12708576].

Tanguay P: Pervasive developmental disorders: A 10 year review. J Am Acad Child Adolesc Psychiatry 2000;39:1079 [PMID: 10986804].

Tidmarsh L, Volkmar FR: Diagnosis and epidemiology of autism spectrum disorders. Can J Psychiatry 2003;48:517 [PMID: 14574827].

Volkmar FR et al: Nonautistic pervasive developmental disorders. In Coffey CE, Brombach RA (editors): *Textbook of Pediatric Neuropsychiatry*. American Psychiatric Press, 1998.

MOOD DISORDERS

1. Depression in Children & Adolescents

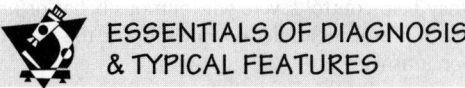

ESSENTIALS OF DIAGNOSIS & TYPICAL FEATURES

- Dysphoric mood, mood lability, irritability or depressed appearance, persisting for days to months at a time.
- Characteristic neurovegetative signs and symptoms (changes in sleep, appetite, concentration, and activity levels).
- Suicidal ideation, feeling of hopelessness.

General Considerations

The incidence of depression in children increases with age, from 1–3% before puberty to around 8% for adolescents. The rate of depression in females approaches adult levels by age 15. The lifetime risk of depression ranges from 10–25% for women and 5–12% for men. The incidence of depression in children is higher when other family members have been affected by depressive disorders. The sex incidence is equal in childhood, but with the onset of puberty the rates of depression for females begin to exceed those for males by 5:1.

Clinical Findings

Clinical depression can be defined as a persistent state of unhappiness or misery that interferes with pleasure or productivity. The symptom of depression in children and adolescents is as likely to be an irritable mood state accompanied by tantrums or verbal outbursts as it is to be a sad mood. Typically, a child or adolescent with depression begins to look unhappy and may make comments such as "I have no friends," "Life is boring," "There is nothing I can do to make things better," or "I wish I were dead." A change in behavior patterns usually takes place that includes social isolation, deterioration in schoolwork, loss of interest in usual activities, anger, and irritability. Sleep and appetite patterns commonly change, and the child may complain of tiredness and nonspecific pain such as headaches or stomach aches (Table 6–6).

Differential Diagnosis

Clinical depression can be usually be identified simply by asking about the symptoms. Children are often more accurate than their caregivers in describing their own mood

Table 6–6. Clinical manifestations of depression in children and adolescents.

Depressive Symptom	Clinical Manifestations
Anhedonia	Loss of interest and enthusiasm in play, socializing, school, and usual activities; boredom; loss of pleasure
Dysphoric mood	Tearfulness; sad, downturned expression; unhappiness; slumped posture; quick temper; irritability; anger
Fatigability	Lethargy and tiredness; no play after school
Morbid ideation	Self-deprecating thoughts, statements; thoughts of disaster, abandonment, death, suicide, or hopelessness
Somatic symptoms	Changes in sleep or appetite patterns; difficulty in concentrating; bodily complaints, particularly headache and stomach ache

state. When several depressive symptoms cluster together over time and are persistent (2 weeks or more) and severe, a major depressive disorder may be present. When depressive symptoms are of lesser severity but have persisted for 1 year or more, a diagnosis of dysthymic disorder should be considered. Milder symptoms of short duration in response to some stressful life event may be consistent with a diagnosis of adjustment disorder with depressed mood.

The Child Depression Inventory, the Beck Depression Rating Scale, and the Reynolds Adolescent Depression Scale are self-report rating scales that are easily used in primary care.

Depression often coexists with other mental illnesses such as ADHD, conduct disorders, anxiety disorders, eating disorders, and substance abuse disorders. Medically ill patients also have an increased incidence of depression. Every child and adolescent with a depressed mood state should be asked directly about suicidal ideation and physical and sexual abuse. Depressed adolescents should also be screened for hypothyroidism and substance abuse.

Complications

The risk of suicide is the most significant risk associated with depressive episodes. In addition, adolescents are likely to self-medicate their feelings through substance abuse, or indulge in self-injurious behaviors such as cutting or burning themselves (without suicidal intent). School performance usually suffers during a depressive episode, as children are unable to concentrate or moti-

vate themselves to complete homework or projects. The irritability, isolation, and withdrawal that often result from the depressive episode can lead to loss of peer relationships and tense dynamics within the family.

Treatment

Treatment includes developing a comprehensive plan to treat the depressive episode and help the family to respond more effectively to the patient's emotional needs. Referrals should always be made for individual and family therapy. Cognitive behavioral therapy (CBT) has been shown to effectively improve depressive symptoms in children and adolescents. CBT includes a focus on building coping skills to change negative thought patterns that predominate in depressive conditions. CBT also helps the young person to identify, label, and verbalize feelings and misperceptions. In therapy, efforts are also made to resolve conflicts between family members and improve communication skills within the family.

When the symptoms of depression are moderate to severe and persistent and have begun to interfere with relationships and school performance, antidepressant medications may be indicated (Table 6–7). Mild depressive symptoms often do not require antidepressant medications and may improve with psychotherapy alone. A positive family history of depression increases the risk of early-onset depression in children and adolescents and the chances of a positive response to antidepressant medication.

Controversy continues regarding the efficacy and safety of antidepressants in children and adolescents. (See Psychopharmacology section.) Medication for depression should be monitored carefully, especially in the first 4 weeks and subsequent 3 months, watching carefully for any increase in suicidal ideation or self-injurious urges.

Prognosis

A comprehensive treatment intervention, including psychoeducation for the family, individual and family psychotherapy, medication assessment, and evaluation of school and home environments, often leads to complete remis-

Table 6–7. Interventions for the treatment of depression.

Adjustment disorder	Refer for psychotherapy	Medications usually not needed
Mild depression	Refer for psychotherapy	Medications may not be needed
Moderate depression	Refer for psychotherapy	Consider antidepressant medication
Severe depression	Refer for psychotherapy	Strongly encourage antidepressant medication

sion of depressive symptoms over a 1- to 2-month period. If medications are started and prove effective, they must be continued for 6–9 months after remission of symptoms to prevent relapse. Early-onset depression (before age 15) is associated with increased risk of recurrent episodes and the potential need for longer-term treatment with antidepressants. Education of the family and child (or adolescent) will help them identify depressive symptoms sooner and limit the severity of future episodes with earlier interventions. Some studies suggest that up to 30% of preadolescents with major depression manifest bipolar disorder at 2-year follow-up. It is important to reassess the child or adolescent with depressive symptoms regularly for at least 6 months and to maintain awareness of the depressive episode in the course of well-child care.

American Academy of Child and Adolescent Psychiatry: Practice parameters for the assessment and treatment of children and adolescents with depressive disorders. J Am Acad Child Adolesc Psychiatry 1998;37(10 Suppl):63S [PMID: 9785729].

Birmaher B, Arbalaez C, Brent D: Course and outcome of child and adolescent major depressive disorder. Child Adolesc Psychiatr Clin North Am 2002;11:619 [PMID: 12222086].

Compton SN et al: Cognitive-behavioral psychotherapy for anxiety and depressive disorders in children and adolescents; an evidence-based medicine review. J Am Acad Child Adolesc Psychiatry 2004;43:930 [PMID: 15266189].

Emslie GJ et al: Fluoxetine for acute treatment of depression in children and adolescents: A placebo-controlled randomized clinical trial. J Am Acad Child Adolesc Psychiatry 2002;41:1205 [PMID: 12364842].

Emslie GJ, Mayes TL, Laptook RS, Batt M: Predictors of response to treatment in children and adolescents with mood disorders. Psychiatr Clin North Am 2003;26:435 [PMID: 12778842].

Louters LL: Don't overlook childhood depression. JAAPA 2004;17:18 [PMID: 15500189].

Olsen AL et al: Primary care pediatrician's roles and perceived responsibility in the identification and management of depression in children and adolescents. Ambulatory Pediatr 2001;1:91 [PMID: 11888379].

Ryan ND: Medication treatment for depression in children and adolescents. CNS Spectr 2003;8:283 [PMID: 1267943].

The Treatment for Adolescents with Depression Study (TADS): Demographic and clinical characteristics. J Am Acad Child Adolesc Psychiatry 2005;44:28 [PMID: 1560841].

Wond IB, Besag FM, Santosh PJ, Murray ML: Use of selective serotonin reuptake inhibitors in children and adolescents. Drug Saf 2004;27:991 [PMID: 15471506].

2. Bipolar Affective Disorder

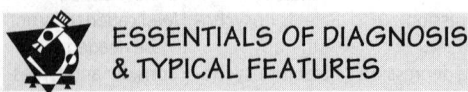

ESSENTIALS OF DIAGNOSIS & TYPICAL FEATURES

- *Periods of abnormally and persistently elevated, expansive, or irritable mood, and heightened levels of energy and activity.*

- *Associated symptoms: grandiosity, diminished need for sleep, pressured speech, racing thoughts, impaired judgment.*

- *Not caused by prescribed or illicit drugs.*

General Considerations

Bipolar affective disorder (previously referred to as manic-depressive disorder) is an episodic mood disorder manifested by alternating periods of mania and major depressive episodes or, less commonly, manic episodes alone. Children and adolescents often exhibit a variable course of mood instability combined with aggressive behavior and impulsivity. At least 20% of bipolar adults experience onset of symptoms before age 20 years. Onset of bipolar disorder before puberty is uncommon; however, symptoms often begin to develop and may be initially diagnosed as ADHD or other disruptive behavior disorders. The lifetime prevalence of bipolar disorder in middle to late adolescence approaches 1%.

Clinical Findings

In about 70% of patients, the first symptoms are primarily those of depression; in the remainder, manic, hypomanic, or mixed states dominate the presentation. Patients with mania display a variable pattern of elevated, expansive, or irritable mood along with rapid speech, high energy levels, difficulty in sustaining concentration, and a decreased need for sleep. The child or adolescent may also have hypersexual behavior, usually in the absence of a history or sexual abuse. (It is critical to rule out abuse, or be aware of abuse factors contributing to the clinical presentation.) Patients often do not acknowledge any problem with their mood or behavior. The clinical picture can be quite dramatic, with florid psychotic symptoms of delusions and hallucinations accompanying extreme hyperactivity and impulsivity. Other illnesses on the bipolar spectrum are Bipolar Type II, which is characterized by recurrent major depressive episodes alternating with hypomanic episodes (lower-intensity manic episodes that do not cause social impairment and do not typically last as long as manic episodes) and Cyclothymic Disorder, which is diagnosed when the child or adolescent has had 1 year of hypomanic symptoms alternating with depressive symptoms that do not meet criteria for major depression.

It is also common for individuals diagnosed with bipolar spectrum disorders to have a history of attentional and hyperactivity problems in childhood and some will have a diagnosis of ADHD as well. ADHD and bipolar disorder are highly comorbid; however, it is also felt that attentional and hyperactivity problems accompanied by mood swings can be an early sign of bipolar disorder before full criteria for the disorder have emerged and clustered together in a specific pattern.

Differential Diagnosis

Differentiating ADHD, Bipolar Disorder, and agitated atypical Major Depressive Disorder can be a challenge even for the seasoned clinician. The situation is further complicated by the potential for the coexistence of ADHD and mood disorders in the same patient.

A history of the temporal course of symptoms can be most helpful. ADHD is typically a chronic disorder of lifelong duration. However, it may not be a problem until the patient enters the classroom setting. Mood disorders are typically characterized by a normal baseline followed by an acute onset of symptoms usually associated with acute sleep, appetite, and behavior changes. If it was not a problem a year ago, it's unlikely to be ADHD. Typically, all of these disorders are quite heritable, so a good family history for other affected individuals can be enlightening. Successful treatment of relatives can offer guidance for appropriate treatment.

In prepubescent children, mania may be difficult to differentiate from ADHD and other disruptive behavior disorders. In both children and adolescents, preoccupation with violence, decreased need for sleep, impulsivity, poor judgement, intense and prolonged rages or dysphoria, hypersexuality, and some cycling of symptoms suggest bipolar disorder. Table 6–8 further defines points of differentiation between ADHD, conduct disorder, and bipolar disorder.

Physical or sexual abuse and exposure to domestic violence can also cause children to appear mood labile, hyperactive, and aggressive, and PTSD should be considered by reviewing the history for traumatic life events in children with these symptoms. Diagnostic considerations should also include substance abuse disorders, and an acute organic process, especially if the change in personality has been relatively sudden, or is accompanied by other neurologic changes. Individuals with manic psychosis may resemble those with schizophrenia. Psychotic symptoms associated with bipolar disorder should clear with resolution of the mood symptoms, which should also be prominent. Hyperthyroidism should be ruled out.

Complications

Children and adolescents with bipolar disorder are more likely to be inappropriate and/or aggressive toward peers and family members. Their symptoms almost always create significant interference with academic learning and peer relationships. The poor judgment associated with manic episodes predisposes to dangerous, impulsive, and sometimes criminal activity. Legal difficulties can arise from impulsive acts, such as excessive spending, and acts of vandalism, theft, or

Table 6–8. Differentiating behavior disorders.

	ADHD	Conduct Disorder	Bipolar Disorder
School problems	Yes	Yes	Yes
Behavior problems	Yes	Yes	Yes
Defiant attitude	Occasional	Constant	Episodic
Motor restlessness	Constant	May be present	May wax and wane
Impulsivity	Constant	May be present	May wax and wane
Distractibility	Constant	May be present	May wax and wane
Anger expression	Short-lived (minutes)	Plans revenge	Intense rages (minutes to hours)
Thought content	May be immature	Blames others	Morbid or grandiose ideas
Sleep disturbance	May be present	No	May wax and wane
Self-deprecation	Briefly, with criticism	No	Prolonged, with or without suicidal ideation
Obsessed with ideas	No	No	Yes
Hallucinations	No	No	Diagnostic, if present
Family history	May be a history of school problems	May be a history of antisocial behavior	May be a history of mood disorders

ADHD, attention-deficit/hyperactivity disorder.

aggression, that are associated with grandiose thoughts. Affective disorders are associated with a 30-fold greater incidence of successful suicide. Substance abuse may be a further complication, often representing an attempt at self-medication for the mood problem.

Treatment & Prognosis

Most patients with bipolar disorder respond to pharmacotherapy with mood stabilizers such as lithium, carbamazepine, or valproate, either alone or in combination. The atypical neuroleptics are increasingly being used as primary mood stabilizers to treat bipolar disorder as primary agents, and olanzapine and risperidone have been approved by the Food and Drug Administration (FDA) for the treatment of bipolar affective disorder. Quetiapine and aripiprazole are also being studied as primary medications for this illness. If the individual is being treated primarily for manic episodes with a non-neuroleptic mood stabilizer (such as lithium) the addition of a neuroleptic medication may be necessary if psychotic symptoms (hallucinations, paranoia, or delusions) or significant aggression is also present. In cases of severe impairment, hospitalization is required to maintain safety and initiate treatment. Although it is often possible to discontinue the neuroleptic medication after remission of psychotic symptoms, it is usually necessary to continue the mood stabilizer for at least a year, and longer if the individual has had recurrent episodes. It is not uncommon for the patient to need lifelong medication. Supportive psychotherapy for the patient and family and education about the recurrent nature of the illness are critical. Family therapy should also include improving skills for conflict management and appropriate expression of emotion.

In its adult form, bipolar disorder is an illness with a remitting course of alternating depressive and manic episodes. The time span between episodes can be years or months depending on the severity of illness and ability to comply with medication interventions. In childhood, the symptoms may be more pervasive and not fall into the intermittent episodic pattern until after puberty.

Blumberg HP et al: Significance of adolescent neurodevelopment for the neural circuitry of bipolar disorder. Ann NY Acad Sci 2004;1021:376 [PMID: 1521913].

Carlson GA: Early onset bipolar disorder: clinical and research consideration. J Clin Child Adolesc Psychol 2005;34:333 [PMID: 15901234].

Emslie GJ et al: Predictors of response to treatment in children and adolescents with mood disorders. Psychiatr Clin North Am 2003;26:435 [PMID: 12778842].

Findling RL: Update on the treatment of bipolar disorder in children and adolescents. Eur Psychiatry 2005;20:87 [PMID: 15797690].

Kent L, Craddock N: Is there a relationship between attention deficit hyperactivity disorder and bipolar disorder? J Affect Disord 2003;73:211 [PMID: 12547289].

Kowatch RA, Delbello MP: The use of mood stabilizers and atypical antipsychotics in children and adolescents with bipolar disorders. CNS Spectr 2003;8:273 [PMID: 12679742].

Kowatch RA et al: Treatment guidelines for children and adolescents with bipolar disorder. J Am Acad Child Adolesc Psychiatry 2005;44:213.

Lofthouse N, Fristad MA: Psychosocial interventions for children with early-onset bipolar spectrum disorder. Clin Child Fam Psychol Rev 2004;7:71 [PMID: 15255173].

McElroy SL: Diagnosing and treating comorbid (complicated) bipolar disorder. J Clin Psychiatry 2004;65(Suppl 15):35 [PMID: 15554795].

Pavuluri MN, Birmaher B, Naylor MW: Pediatric bipolar disorder: A review of the past 10 years. J Am Acad Child Adolesc Psychiatr 2005;44:846 [PMID: 16113615].

Quinn CA, Fristad MA: Defining and identifying early onset bipolar spectrum disorder. Curr Psychiatry Rep 2004;6:101 [PMID: 15038912].

Shapiro NA: Bipolar disorders in children and adolescents. J Pediatr Health Care 2005;19:131 [PMID: 15867828].

Wagner KD: Diagnosis and treatment of bipolar disorder in children and adolescents. J Clin Psychaitry 2004;65(Suppl 15): 30 [PMID: 15554794].

Wozniak J: Recognizing and managing bipolar disorder in children. J Clin Psychiatry 2005;66(Suppl 1):18 [PMID: 15693748].

Youngstrom EA, Youngstrom JK: Clinician's guide to evidence based practice: Assessment of pediatric bipolar disorder. J Am Acad Child Adolesc Psychiatr 2005;44:823 [PMID: 16034285].

SUICIDE IN CHILDREN & ADOLESCENTS

The suicide rate in young people has remained high for several decades. In 1997, suicide was the third leading cause of death among children and adolescents age 10–24 years in the United States. The suicide rate among adolescents age 15–19 years quadrupled from approximately 2.7 to 11.3 per 100,000 since the 1960s. It is estimated that each year, approximately 2 million U.S. adolescents attempt suicide, yet only 700,000 receive medical attention for their attempt. Suicide and homicide rates for children in the United States are two to five times higher than those for the other 25 industrialized countries combined, primarily due to the prevalence of firearms in the United States. For children younger than 10 years old, the rate of completed suicide is low, but from 1980 to 1992 it increased by 120%, from 0.8 to 1.7 per 100,000.

Adolescent girls make three to four times as many suicide attempts as boys of the same age, but the number of completed suicides is three to four times greater in boys. Firearms are the most commonly used method in successful suicides, accounting for 40–60% of cases; hanging, carbon monoxide poisoning, and drug overdoses each account for approximately 10–15% of cases.

Suicide is almost always associated with a psychiatric disorder and should not be viewed as a philosophic choice about life or death or as a predictable response to overwhelming stress. Most commonly it is associated with a mood disorder and the hopelessness that accompanies a severe depressive episode. Although suicide attempts are more common in individuals with a history of behavior problems and academic difficulties, other suicide victims are high achievers who are temperamentally anxious and perfectionistic and who commit suicide impulsively after a failure or rejection, either real or perceived. Mood disorders (in both sexes, but especially in females), substance abuse disorders (especially in males), and conduct disorders are commonly diagnosed at psychological autopsy in adolescent suicide victims. Some adolescent suicides reflect an underlying psychotic disorder, with the young person usually committing suicide in response to auditory hallucinations or psychotic delusions.

The vast majority of young people who attempt suicide give some clue to their distress or their tentative plans to commit suicide. Most show signs of dysphoric mood (anger, irritability, anxiety, or depression). Over 60% make comments such as "I wish I were dead" or "I just can't deal with this any longer" within the 24 hours prior to death. In one study, nearly 70% of subjects experienced a crisis event such as a loss (eg, rejection by a girlfriend or boyfriend), a failure, or an arrest prior to completed suicide.

Assessment of Suicide Risk

Any clinical assessment for depression must include direct questions about suicidal ideation. If a child or adolescent expresses suicidal thinking, the physician must ask if he or she has an active plan. Suicidal ideation accompanied by any plan warrants immediate referral for a psychiatric crisis assessment. This can usually be accomplished at the nearest emergency department.

Assessment of suicide risk calls for a high index of suspicion and a direct interview with the patient and their parents or guardians. The highest risk of suicide is among white adolescent boys. High-risk factors include previous suicide attempts, a suicide note, and a viable plan for suicide with the availability of lethal means, close personal exposure to suicide, conduct disorder, and substance abuse. Other risk factors are signs and symptoms of major depression or dysthymia, a family history of suicide, a recent death in the family, and a view of death as a relief from the pain in their lives.

Principles of Intervention

Suicidal ideation and any suicide attempt must be considered a serious matter. The patient should not be left alone, and one should express concern and convey a desire to help. The physician should meet with the patient and the family, both alone and together, and listen carefully to their problems and perceptions. It should be made clear that with the assistance of mental health professionals, solutions can be found.

The majority of patients who express suicidal ideation and all who have made a suicide attempt should be referred for psychiatric evaluation and possible hospitalization. If the patient has suicidal ideation without a plan, has a therapist they can see the next day, is able to "contract for safety," and the family is able to provide supervision and support, then the physician can consider sending the patient and family home that day from the office without referral for further assessment in an emergency department. If there appears to be potential for suicide as determined by suicidal ideation with a plan, there are no available resources for therapy, and the patient is not able to cooperate with a plan to ensure safety, if they are severely depressed or intoxicated, if the family does not appear to be appropriately concerned, or if there are practical limitations on providing supervision and support to ensure safety, the individual should be hospitalized on an inpatient psychiatric unit. The physician should err on the side of caution and referral for further assessment is always appropriate when there is concern about suicidal thinking and behavior. Any decision to send the patient home from the emergency department without hospitalization should be made only after consultation with a mental health expert. The decision should be based on lessening of the risk of suicide and assurance of the family's ability to follow through with outpatient therapy and provide appropriate support and supervision. Guns, knives, and razor blades should be removed from the home, and as much as possible, access to them outside the home must be denied. Medications and over-the-counter drugs should be kept locked in a safe place with all efforts made to minimize the risk of the patient having access (eg, key kept with a parent, or use of combination lock on the medicine chest). The patient should be restricted from driving for at least the first 24 hours to lessen the chance of impulsive motor vehicle crashes. Instructions and phone numbers for crisis services should be given, and the family must be committed to a plan for mental health treatment.

Suicide prevention efforts include heightened awareness in the community and schools to promote identification of at-risk individuals and increasing access to services, including hotlines and counseling services. Restricting young people's access to firearms is also a critical factor, as firearms are responsible for 85% of deaths due to suicide or homicide in youth in the United States.

Finally, the physician should be aware of his or her own emotional reactions to dealing with suicidal adolescents and their families. Because the assessment can require considerable time and energy, the physician should be on guard against becoming tired, irritable, or angry. The physician should not be afraid of precipitating suicide by direct and frank discussions of suicidal risk.

Borowsky IW, Ireland M, Resnick MD: Adolescent suicide attempts: Risks and protectors. Pediatrics 2001;107:485 [PMID: 11230587].

Borowsky IW: The role of the pediatrician in preventing suicidal behavior. Minerva Pediatr 2002;54:41 [PMID: 11862165].

Gould MS et al: Youth suicide risk and prevention interventions: A review of the past 10 years. J Am Acad Child Adolesc Psychiatry 2003;42:386 [PMID: 12649626].

Kennedy SP et al: Emergency department management of suicidal adolescents. Ann Emerg Med 2004;43:452 [PMID: 15039687].

Pelkonen M, Marttunen M: Child and adolescent suicide: epidemiology, risk factors and approaches to prevention. Paediatr Drugs 2003;5:243 [PMID: 12662120].

Practice Parameters for the assessment and treatment of children and adolescents with suicidal behavior. J Am Acad Child Adolesc Psychiatry 2001;40(7 Suppl):24S [PMID: 11314578].

Schmidt P et al: Suicide in children, adolescents, and young adults. Forensic Sci Int 2002;127:161 [PMID: 12175945].

Spirito A, Overholser J: The suicidal child: assessment and management of adolescents after a suicide attempt. Child Adolesc Psychiatr Clin N Am 2003;12:649 [PMID: 14579644].

Weller EB et al: Overview and assessment of the suicidal child. Depress Anxiety 2001;14:157 [PMID: 11747125].

ADJUSTMENT DISORDERS

The most frequent and most disturbing stresses for children and adolescents are marital discord, separation and divorce, family illness, the loss of a loved one, a change of residence, and for adolescents, peer relationship problems. When faced with stress, children can experience many different symptoms, including changes in mood, changes in behavior, anxiety symptoms, and physical complaints. Key findings include the following:

- The precipitating event or circumstance is identifiable.
- The symptoms have appeared within 3 months after the occurrence of the stressful event.
- Although the child experiences distress or some functional impairment, the reaction is not severe or disabling.
- The reaction does not persist more than 6 months after the stressor has terminated.

Differential Diagnosis

When symptoms are a reaction to an identifiable stressor but are severe, persistent, or disabling, depressive disorder, anxiety disorder, and conduct disorders must be considered.

Treatment

The mainstay of treatment is the doctor's assurance that the emotional or behavioral change is a predictable consequence of the stressful event. This validates the child's reaction and encourages the child to talk about the stressful occurrence and its aftermath. Parents are asked to understand the child's reaction and encourage appropriate verbal expression of feelings, while defining boundaries for behavior that prevent the child from feeling out of control.

Prognosis

The duration of symptoms in adjustment reactions depends on the severity of the stress; the child's personal sensitivity to stress and vulnerability to anxiety, depression, and other psychiatric disorders; and the available support system.

SCHIZOPHRENIA

The incidence of schizophrenia is about 1 per 10,000 per year. The onset of schizophrenia is typically between the middle to late teens and early 30s, with onset before puberty being relatively rare. Symptoms usually begin after puberty, although a full "psychotic break" may not occur until the young adult years. Childhood onset (before puberty) of psychotic symptoms due to schizophrenia is uncommon and usually indicates a more severe form of the spectrum of schizophrenic disorders. Childhood-onset schizophrenia is more likely to be found in boys.

Schizophrenia is a biologically based disease with a strong genetic component. Other psychotic disorders that may be encountered in childhood or adolescence include schizoaffective disorder and psychosis not otherwise specified. Psychosis not otherwise specified may be used as a differential diagnosis when psychotic symptoms are present, but the cluster of symptoms is not consistent with a schizophrenia diagnosis.

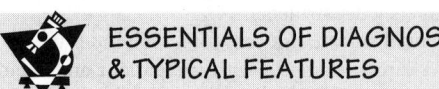

ESSENTIALS OF DIAGNOSIS & TYPICAL FEATURES

- *Delusional thoughts.*
- *Disorganized speech (rambling or illogical speech patterns).*
- *Disorganized or bizarre behavior.*
- *Hallucinations (auditory, visual, tactile, olfactory).*
- *Paranoia, ideas of reference.*
- *Negative symptoms (ie, flat affect, avolition, alogia).*

Clinical Findings

Children and adolescents display many of the symptoms of adult schizophrenia. Hallucinations or delusions, bizarre and morbid thought content, and rambling and illogical speech are typical. Affected individuals tend to withdraw into an internal world of fantasy and may then equate fantasy with external reality. They generally have difficulty with schoolwork and with peer relationships. Adolescents may have a prodromal period of depression prior to the onset of psychotic symptoms. The majority of patients with childhood-onset schizophrenia have had nonspecific psychiatric symptoms or symptoms of delayed development for months or years prior to the onset of their overtly psychotic symptoms.

Differential Diagnosis

Obtaining the family history of mental illness is critical when assessing children and adolescents with psychotic symptoms. Psychological testing is often helpful in identifying or ruling out psychotic thought processes. Psychotic symptoms in children younger than age 8 years must be differentiated from manifestations of normal vivid fantasy life or abuse-related symptoms. Children with psychotic disorders often have learning disabilities and attention difficulties in addition to disorganized thoughts, delusions, and hallucinations. In psychotic adolescents, mania is differentiated by high levels of energy, excitement, and irritability. Any child or adolescent exhibiting new psychotic symptoms requires a medical evaluation that includes physical and neurologic examinations (including consideration of magnetic resonance imaging and electroencephalogram), drug screening, and metabolic screening for endocrinopathies, Wilson disease, and delirium.

Treatment

The treatment of childhood and adolescent schizophrenia focuses on four main areas: (1) decreasing active psychotic symptoms, (2) supporting development of social and cognitive skills, (3) reducing the risk of relapse of psychotic symptoms, and (4) providing support and education to parents and family members. Antipsychotic medications (neuroleptics) are the primary psychopharmacological intervention. In addition, a supportive, reality-oriented focus in relationships can help to reduce hallucinations, delusions, and frightening thoughts. A special school or day treatment environment may be necessary depending on the child's or adolescent's ability to tolerate the school day and classroom activities. Support for the family emphasizes the importance of clear, focused communication and an emotionally calm climate in preventing recurrences of overtly psychotic symptoms.

Prognosis

Schizophrenia is a chronic disorder with exacerbations and remissions of psychotic symptoms. It is generally believed that earlier onset (prior to age 13 years), poor premorbid functioning (oddness or eccentricity), and predominance of negative symptoms (withdrawal, apathy, or flat affect) over positive symptoms (hallucinations or paranoia) predict more severe disability, while later age of onset, normal social and school functioning prior to onset, and predominance of positive symptoms are generally associated with better outcomes and life adjustment to the illness.

Arango C, Parellada M, Moreno DM: Clinical effectiveness of new generation antipsychotics in adolescent patients. Eur Neuropsychopharmacol 2004;14(Suppl 4):S471 [PMID: 15572266].

Calderoni D et al: Differentiating childhood-onset schizophrenia from psychotic mood disorders. J Am Acad Child Adolesc Psychiatry 2001;40:1190 [PMID: 11589532].

American Academy of Child and Adolescent Psychiatry: Practice parameters for the assessment and treatment of children and adolescents with schizophrenia. J Am Acad Child Adolesc Psychiatry 2001;40(7 Suppl):4S [PMID: 11434484].

Shaeffer JL, Ross RG: Childhood onset schizophrenia: Premorbid and prodromal diagnostic and treatment histories. J Am Acad Child Adolesc Psychiatry 2002;41:538 [PMID: 12014786].

Toren P et al: Benefit-risk assessment of atypical antipsychotics in the treatment of schizophrenia and comorbid disorders in children and adolescents. Drug Saf 2004;27:1135 [PMID: 15554747].

CONDUCT DISORDERS

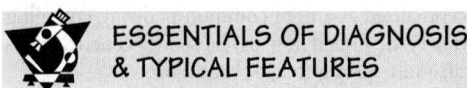

ESSENTIALS OF DIAGNOSIS & TYPICAL FEATURES

A Persistent Pattern of Behavior That Includes the Following:

- *Defiance of authority.*
- *Violating the rights of others' or society's norms.*
- *Aggressive behavior toward persons, animals, or property.*

General Considerations

Disorders of conduct affect approximately 9% of males and 2% of females younger than 18 years. This is a very heterogeneous population, and overlap occurs with ADHD, substance abuse, learning disabilities, neuropsychiatric disorders, mood disorders, and family dysfunction. Many of these individuals come from homes where domestic violence, child abuse, drug abuse, shifting parental figures, and poverty are environmental risk factors. Although social learning partly explains this correlation, the genetic heritability of aggressive conduct and antisocial behaviors is currently under investigation.

Clinical Findings

The typical child with conduct disorder is a boy with a turbulent home life and academic difficulties. Defiance of authority, fighting, tantrums, running away, school failure, and destruction of property are common symptoms. With increasing age, fire-setting and theft may occur, followed in adolescence by truancy, vandalism, and substance abuse. Sexual promiscuity, sexual perpetration, and other criminal behaviors may develop. Hyperactive, aggressive, and uncooperative behavior patterns in the preschool and early school years tend to predict conduct disorder in adolescence with a high degree of accuracy, especially when ADHD goes untreated. A history of reactive attachment disorder is an additional childhood risk factor. The risk for conduct disorder increases with inconsistent and severe parental disciplinary techniques, parental alcoholism, and parental antisocial behavior.

Differential Diagnosis

Young people with conduct disorders, especially those with more violent histories, have an increased incidence of neurologic signs and symptoms, psychomotor seizures, psychotic symptoms, mood disorders, ADHD, and learning disabilities. Efforts should be made to identify these associated disorders (see Table 6–8) because they may suggest specific therapeutic interventions. Conduct disorder is best conceptualized as a final common pathway emerging from a variety of underlying psychosocial, genetic, environmental, and neuropsychiatric conditions.

Treatment

Effective treatment can be complicated by the psychosocial problems often found in the lives of children and adolescents with conduct disorders and related difficulty achieving compliance with treatment recommendations. Efforts should be made to stabilize the environment and improve functioning within the home, particularly as it relates to parental functioning and disciplinary techniques. Identification of learning disabilities and placement in an optimal school environment is also critical. Any associated neurologic and psychiatric disorders should be addressed.

Residential treatment may be needed for some individuals whose symptoms do not respond to lower level interventions, or whose environment is not able to meet their needs for supervision and structure. It is not unusual for the juvenile justice system to be involved when conduct disorder behaviors lead to illegal activities, theft, or assault.

Medications such as mood stabilizers, neuroleptics, stimulants, and antidepressants have all been studied in youth with conduct disorders, yet none has been found to be consistently effective in this population. Early involvement in programs such as Big Brothers, Big Sisters, scouts, and team sports in which consistent adult mentors and role models interact with youth decreases the chances that the youth with conduct disorders will develop antisocial personality disorder. Multisystemic therapy is being used increasingly as an intervention for youth with conduct disorders and involvement with the

legal system. Multisystemic therapy is an intensive home-based model of care that seeks to stabilize and improve the home environment and to strengthen the support system and coping skills of the individual and family.

Prognosis

The prognosis is based on the ability of the child's support system to mount an effective treatment intervention consistently over time. The prognosis is generally worse for children in whom the disorder presents before age 10 years; those who display a diversity of antisocial behaviors across multiple settings; and those who are raised in an environment characterized by parental antisocial behavior, alcoholism or other substance abuse, and conflict. Nearly half of individuals with a childhood diagnosis of conduct disorder develop antisocial personality disorder as adults.

1. Oppositional Defiant Disorder

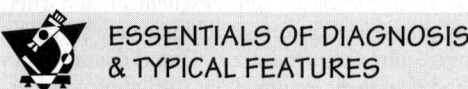

ESSENTIALS OF DIAGNOSIS & TYPICAL FEATURES

- A pattern of negativistic, hostile, and defiant behavior lasting at least 6 months.
- Loses temper, argues with adults, defies rules.
- Blames others for own mistakes and misbehavior.
- Angry, easily annoyed, vindictive.
- Does not meet criteria for conduct disorder.

Oppositional defiant disorder usually is evident before 8 years of age and may be an antecedent to the development of conduct disorder. The symptoms usually first emerge at home, but then extend to school and peer relationships. The disruptive behaviors of oppositional defiant disorder are generally less severe than those associated with conduct disorder and do not include hurting other individuals or animals, destruction of property, or theft.

Oppositional defiant disorder is more common in families in whom caregiver dysfunction is present, and in children with a history of multiple changes in caregivers; inconsistent, harsh, or neglectful parenting; or serious marital discord.

Interventions include careful assessment of the psychosocial situation and recommendations to support parenting skills and optimal caregiver functioning. Assessment for comorbid psychiatric diagnoses such as learning disabilities, depression, and ADHD should be pursued and appropriate interventions recommended.

American Academy of Child and Adolescent Psychiatry: Practice parameters for the assessment and treatment of children and adolescents with conduct disorder. J Am Acad Child Adolesc Psychiatry 1997;36(Suppl):122S [PMID: 9334568].

Burke JH, Loeber R, Birmaher B: Oppositional defiant disorder and conduct disorder: Review of the past 10 years, part II. J Am Acad Child Adolesc Psychiatry 2002;41:1275 [PMID: 12410070].

Cunningham CE, Boyle MH: Preschoolers at risk for ADHD and ODD: Family, parenting and behavioral correlates. J Abnorm Child Psychol 2002;30:555 [PMID: 12481971].

Farmer EM et al: Review of the evidence base for treatment of childhood psychopathology: Externalizing disorders. J Consult Clin Psychol 2002;70:1267 [PMID: 12472301].

Flory K et al: Relation between childhood disruptive behavior disorders and substance use and dependence in young adulthood. Psychol Addictive Behav 2003;17:151 [PMID: 12814279].

Greene RW et al: Psychiatric comorbidity, family dysfunction and social impairment in referred youth with oppositional defiant disorder. Am J Psychiatry 2002;159:1214 [PMID: 12091202].

Kutcher S et al: International consensus statement on attention-deficit/hyperactivity disorder (ADHD) and disruptive behavior disorders (DBDs): clinical implications and treatment practice suggestions. Eur Neuropsychopharmacol 2004;14:11 [PMID: 14659983].

Loeber R et al: Oppositional defiant and conduct disorder: A review of the past 10 years. Part 1. J Am Acad Child Adolesc Psychiatry 2000;39:1468 [PMID: 11128323].

Waschbusch DA et al: Reactive aggression in boys with disruptive behavior disorders; behavior, physiology and affect. J Abnorm Child Psychol 2002;30:641 [PMID: 12481977].

Violent Behavior in Youth

Of particular concern to physicians today, as well as to society at large, is the tragic increase in teen violence, including school shootings. There is strong evidence that screening and initiation of interventions by primary care providers can make a significant difference in violent behavior in youth. Although the prediction of violent behavior remains a difficult and imprecise endeavor, physicians can support and encourage several important prevention efforts.

• The vast majority of the increase in youth violence including suicides and homicides involves the use of firearms. Thus the presence of firearms in the home, the method of storage and safety measures taken when present, and access to firearms outside the home should be explored regularly with all adolescents as part of their routine medical care.

• Violent behavior is often associated with suicidal impulses. In the process of screening for violent behavior, suicidal ideation should not be overlooked. In general, the suicidal youth is somewhat easier to identify than the homicidal youth, and in many cases may be one and the same (see the section on Suicide in Children and Adolescents). Any comment about wishes to be dead or hopelessness should be taken seriously and help sought.

• Parents and guardians should be aware of their child's school attendance and performance and peer groups. They should know their children's friends and be aware of who they are going out with, where they will be, what they will be doing, and when they will be home. Any concerns should be discussed with the teen and interventions sought if necessary.

• Most students involved in school violence could have benefited from earlier interventions to address problems in social and educational functioning in the school environment. Many communities and school districts have increased their efforts to identify and intervene with students whom teachers, peers, or parents recognize as having difficulty.

Birnbaum AS et al: School functioning and violent behavior among young adolescents: A contextual analysis. Health Educ Res 2003;18:389 [PMID: 12828239].

Borowsky IW, Mozayeny S, Steunkel K, Ireland M: Effects of a primary care based intervention on behavior and injury in children. Pediatrics 2004;4:e392 [PMID: 15466063].

Denninghoff KR et al: Emergency medicine: Competencies for youth violence prevention and control. Acad Emerg Med 2002;9:947 [PMID: 12208685].

Fergus S, Zimmerman MA: Adolescent resilience: a framework for understanding healthy development in the face of risk. Annual Rev Public Health 2005;26:399 [PMID: 15760295].

Grant KE et al: Stressors and child and adolescent psychopathology: Moving from markers to mechanisms of risk. Psychol Bull 2003;129:447 [PMID: 12784938].

Group for the Advancement of Psychiatry, Committee on Preventive Psychiatry: Violent behavior in children and youth: Preventive intervention from a psychiatric perspective. J Am Acad Child Adolesc Psychiatry 1999;38:235 [PMID: 10087683].

Johnson SB et al: Urban youths' perspective on violence and the necessity of fighting. Inj Prev 2004;10:287 [PMID: 15470008].

Kruesi MJP et al: Suicide and violence prevention: Parent education in the emergency department. J Am Acad Child Adolesc Psychiatry 1999;38:250 [PMID: 10087685].

Pontin LE: *The Romance of Risk, Why Teenagers Do the Things They Do.* Basic Books, 1997.

Rappaport N, Thomas C: Recent research findings on aggressive and violent behavior in youth: implications for clinical assessment and intervention. J Adolesc Health 2004;35:260 [PMID: 15450540].

Tremblay RE et al: Physical aggression during early childhood: trajectories and predictors. Pediatrics 2004;114:e43 [PMID: 15231972].

ANXIETY DISORDERS

1. Anxiety-Based School Refusal (School Avoidance)

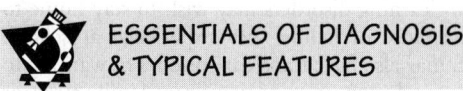

ESSENTIALS OF DIAGNOSIS & TYPICAL FEATURES

• *A persistent pattern of school avoidance related to symptoms of anxiety.*

- *Somatic symptoms on school mornings, with symptoms resolving if the child is allowed to remain at home.*
- *No organic medical disorder that accounts for the symptoms.*
- *High levels of parental anxiety are commonly observed.*

General Considerations

Anxiety-based school refusal should be considered if a child presents with a medically unexplained absence from school for more than 2 weeks. Anxiety-based school refusal is a persistent behavioral symptom rather than a diagnostic entity. It refers to a pattern of school nonattendance resulting from anxiety, which may be related to a dread of leaving home (separation anxiety), a fear of some aspect of school, or a fear of feeling exposed or embarrassed at school (social phobia). In all cases, a realistic cause of the fear (eg, an intimidating teacher or a playground bully) should be ruled out. In most cases, anxiety-based school refusal is related to developmentally inappropriate separation anxiety. The incidence between males and females is about equal, and there are peaks of incidence at ages 6–7 years, again at ages 10–11 years, and in early adolescence.

Clinical Findings

In the preadolescent years, school refusal often begins after some precipitating stress in the family. The child's anxiety is then manifested either as somatic symptoms or in displacement of anxiety onto some aspect of the school environment. The somatic manifestations of anxiety include dizziness, nausea, and stomach distress. Characteristically, the symptoms become more severe as the time to leave for school approaches and then remit if the child is allowed to remain at home for the day. In older children, the onset is more insidious and often associated with social withdrawal and depression. The incidence of anxiety and mood disorders is increased in these families.

Differential Diagnosis

The differential diagnosis of school nonattendance is presented in Table 6–9. Medical disorders that may be causing the somatic symptoms must be ruled out. Children with learning disorders may wish to stay home to avoid the sense of failure they experience at school. Children may also have transient episodes of wanting to stay at home during times of significant family stress or loss. The onset of school avoidance in middle or late adolescence may be related to the onset of schizophrenia. Children who are avoiding school for reasons related

Table 6–9. Differential diagnosis of school nonattendance.[a]

I. Emotional or anxiety-based refusal[b]
A. Separation anxiety disorder (50–80% of anxious refusers)
B. Generalized anxiety disorder
C. Mood/depressive disorder (with or without combined anxiety)
D. Social phobia
E. Specific phobia
F. Panic disorder
G. Psychosis
II. Truancy[c] behavior disorders
A. Oppositional defiant disorder, conduct disorder
B. Substance abuse disorders
III. Situation-specific school refusal
A. Learning disability, unaddressed or undetected
B. Bullying or gang threat
C. Psychologically abusive teacher
D. Family-sanctioned nonattendance
1. For companionship
2. For child care
3. To care for the parent (role-reversal)
4. To supplement family income
E. Socioculturally sanctioned nonattendance (school is not valued)
F. Gender concerns
IV. Undiagnosed medical condition (including pregnancy)

[a]Medically unexplained absence of more than 2 weeks.
[b]Subjectively distressed child who generally stays at home.
[c]Nonsubjectively distressed and not at home.

to oppositional defiant disorder or conduct disorder can be differentiated on the basis of their chronic noncompliance with adult authority and their preference for being with peers rather than at home.

Complications

The longer a child remains out of school, the more difficult it is to return and the more strained the relationship between child and parent becomes. Many parents of nonattending children feel tyrannized by their defiant, clinging child. Children often feel accused of making up their symptoms, leading to further antagonism between the child, parents, and medical caregivers.

Treatment

Once the comorbid diagnoses and situations related to school avoidance/refusal have been identified and interventions begun (ie, educational assessment if learning disabilities are suspected, medication if necessary for depression or anxiety, or addressing problems in the home), the goal of treatment is to help the child confront anxiety and overcome it by returning to school. This requires a strong alliance between the parents and the health care provider. The parent must understand that no underlying medical disorder exists, that the child's symptoms are a manifestation of anxiety, and that the basic problem is anxiety that must be faced to be overcome. Parents must be reminded that being good parents in this case means helping a child cope with a distressing experience. Children must be reassured that their symptoms are caused by worry and that they will be overcome on return to school.

A plan for returning the child to school is then developed with parents and school personnel. Firm insistence on full compliance with this plan is essential. The child is brought to school by someone not likely to give in, such as the father or an older sibling. If symptoms develop at school, the child should be checked by the school nurse and then returned to class after a brief rest. The parents must be reassured that school staff will handle the situation at school and that school personnel can reach the primary health care provider if any questions arise.

If these interventions are ineffective, increased involvement of a therapist and consideration of a day treatment program may be necessary. For children with persistent symptoms of separation that do not improve with behavioral interventions, medications such as SSRIs should be considered. Comorbid diagnoses of panic disorder, generalized anxiety disorder, or major depression should be carefully screened for, and if identified, treated appropriately.

Prognosis

The vast majority of preadolescent children improve significantly with behavioral interventions and return to school. The prognosis is worsened by the length of time the child remains out of school. Long-term outcomes are influenced by comorbid diagnoses and responsiveness to behavioral or medication interventions. A history of school refusal is more common in adults with panic and anxiety disorders and agoraphobia than in the general population.

DelBello M, Greevich S: Phenomenology and epidemiology of childhood psychiatric disorders that may necessitate treatment with atypical antipsychotics. J Clin Psychiatry 2004; 65(Suppl 6):12-9 [PMID: 15104522].

Egger HL, Coatello EJ, Angold A: School refusal and psychiatric disorders: A community study. J Am Acad Child Adolesc Psychiatry 2003;42:797 [PMID: 12819439].

King NJ, Bernstein GA: School refusal in children and adolescents: A review of the past 10 years. J Am Acad Child Adolesc Psychiatry 2001;40:197 [PMID: 11211368].

Masi G, Mucci M, Millepiedi S: Separation anxiety disorder in children and adolescents: Epidemiology, diagnosis, and management. CNS Drugs 2001;15:93 [PMID: 11460893].

Murray RM et al: A developmental model for similarities and dissimilarities between schizophrenia and bipolar disorder. Schizophr Res 2004;71:405 [PMID: 15474912].

Tyrell M: School phobia. J Sch Nurs 2005;21:147.

2. Generalized Anxiety Disorder & Panic Disorder

Anxiety can be manifested either directly or indirectly, as shown in Table 6–10. The characteristics of anxiety disorders in childhood are listed in Table 6–11. Community-based studies of school-age children and adolescents suggest that nearly 10% of children have some type of anxiety disorder. The differential diagnosis of symptoms of anxiety is presented in Table 6–12.

The evaluation of anxiety symptoms in children must consider the age of the child, the developmental fears that can normally be expected at that age, the form of the symptoms and their duration, and the degree to which the symptoms disrupt the child's life. The family and school environment should be evaluated for potential stressors, marital discord, family violence, harsh or inappropriate disciplinary methods, sexual abuse, neglect, and emotional overstimulation. The child's experience of anxiety and its relationship to life events should be explored, and therapy to incorporate specific cognitive and behavioral techniques to diminish the anxiety should be recommended. Finally, when panic attacks or anxiety symptoms do not remit with cognitive, behavioral, and environmental interventions,

Table 6–10. Signs and symptoms of anxiety in children.

Psychological
 Fears and worries
 Increased dependence on home and parents
 Avoidance of anxiety-producing stimuli
 Decreased school performance
 Increased self-doubt and irritability
 Frightening themes in play and fantasy
Psychomotor
 Motoric restlessness and hyperactivity
 Sleep disturbances
 Decreased concentration
 Ritualistic behaviors (eg, washing, counting)
Psychophysiologic
 Autonomic hyperarousal
 Dizziness and lightheadedness
 Palpitations
 Shortness of breath
 Flushing, sweating, dry mouth
 Nausea and vomiting
 Panic
 Headaches and stomach aches

Table 6–11. Anxiety disorders in children and adolescents.

Disorder	Major Clinical Manifestations
Generalized anxiety disorder	Intense, disproportionate or irrational worry, often about future events
Panic disorder	Unprovoked, intense fear with sympathetic hyperarousal, and often palpitations or hyperventilation
Posttraumatic stress disorder	Fear of a recurrence of an intense, anxiety-provoking traumatic experience, causing sympathetic hyperarousal, avoidance of reminders, and the reexperiencing of aspects of the traumatic event
Separation anxiety disorder	Developmentally inappropriate wish to maintain proximity with caregivers; morbid worry of threats to family integrity or integrity of self upon separation; intense homesickness
Social phobia	Painful shyness or self-consciousness; fear of humiliation with public scrutiny
Specific phobia	Avoidance of specific feared stimuli

and they significantly affect life functioning, psychopharmacologic agents may be helpful. SSRIs may be effective across a broad spectrum of anxiety symptoms.

Prognosis

There is continuity between high levels of childhood anxiety and anxiety disorders in adulthood. Anxiety disorders are thus likely to be lifelong conditions, yet with effective interventions, individuals can minimize their influence on overall life functioning.

American Academy of Child and Adolescent Psychiatry: Practice parameters for the assessment and treatment of children and adolescents with anxiety disorders. J Am Acad Child Adolesc Psychiatry 1997;36(Suppl):69S [PMID: 9334566].

Arnold P et al: Childhood anxiety disorders and developmental issues in anxiety. Curr Psychiatry Rep 2003;5:252 [PMID: 12857528].

Arnold PD, Zai G, Richter MA: Genetics of anxiety disorders. Curr Psychiatry Rep 2004;6:243 [PMID: 15260939].

Blanco C, Antia SX, Lebowitz MR: Pharmacotherapy of social anxiety disorder. Biol Psychiatry 2002;51:1098 [PMID: 11801236].

Chavira DA et al: Comorbidity of generalized social anxiety disorder and depression in a pediatric primary care sample. J Affect Disord 2004;80:163 [PMID: 15207929].

Compton SN et al: Cognitive-behavioral psychotherapy for anxiety and depressive disorders in children and adolescents: an evidence based medicine review. J Am Acad Child Adolesc Psychiatr 2004;43:930 [PMID: 15266189].

Hudson JL, Deveney C, Taylor L: Nature, assessment and treatment of generalized anxiety disorder in children. Pediatr Ann 2005;34:97 [PMID: 15768686].

Kelly MN: Recognizing and treating anxiety disorder in children. Pediat Ann 2005;34:147 [PMID: 15768691].

Ginsburg GS, Grover RL: Assessing and treating social phobia in children and adolescents. Pediatr Ann 2005;34:119 [PMID: 15768688].

Jursbergs N, Ledley DR: Separation anxiety disorder. Pediatr Ann 2005;34:108 [PMID: 15768687].

Rynn MA, Siqueland L, Rickels K: Placebo-controlled trial of sertraline in the treatment of children with generalized anxiety disorder. Am J Psychiatry 2001;158:2008 [PMID: 11729017].

Scott RW, Mughelli K, Deas D: An overview of controlled studies of anxiety disorders treatment in children and adolescents. J Natl Med Assoc 2005;97:13 [PMID: 15710867].

Velosa JF, Riddle MA: Pharmacologic treatment of anxiety disorders in children and adolescents. Child Adolesc Psychiatr Clin N Am 2000;9:119 [PMID: 10674193].

Wren FJ, Bridge JA, Birmaher B: Screening for childhood anxiety symptoms in primary care: integrating child and parent reports. J Am Acad Child Adolesc Psychiatry 2004;43:1364 [PMID: 15502595].

Table 6–12. Differential diagnosis of symptoms of anxiety.

I. **Normal developmental anxiety**
  A. Stranger anxiety (5 months to 2 $^1/_2$ years, with a peak at 6–12 months)
  B. Separation anxiety (7 months to 4 years, with a peak at 18–36 months)
  C. The child is fearful or even phobic of the dark and monsters (3–6 years)
II. **"Appropriate" anxiety**
  A. Anticipating a painful or frightening experience
  B. Avoidance of a reminder of a painful or frightening experience
  C. Child abuse
III. **Anxiety disorder (see Table 6–11), with or without other comorbid psychiatric disorders**
IV. **Substance abuse**
V. **Medications and recreational drugs**
  A. Caffeinism (including colas and chocolate)
  B. Sympathomimetic agents
  C. Idiosyncratic drug reactions
VI. **Hypermetabolic or hyperarousal states**
  A. Hyperthyroidism
  B. Pheochromocytoma
  C. Anemia
  D. Hypoglycemia
  E. Hypoxemia
VII. **Cardiac abnormality**
  A. Dysrhythmia
  B. High-output state
  C. Mitral valve prolapse

OBSESSIVE-COMPULSIVE DISORDER

ESSENTIALS OF DIAGNOSIS & TYPICAL FEATURES

- *Recurrent obsessive thoughts, impulses, or images that cause marked anxiety or distress and are not simply excessive worries about real-life problems.*
- *The individual attempts to ignore or suppress the thoughts or impulses.*
- *Repetitive compulsive behaviors or mental acts that the person feels driven to perform in response to the obsessive thought aimed at preventing or reducing distress.*
- *The obsessions and compulsions cause marked distress, are time-consuming, and interfere with normal routines.*

Obsessive-compulsive disorder (OCD) is an anxiety disorder that often begins in early childhood, but may not be diagnosed until the teen or even young adult years. The essential features of OCD are recurrent obsessions or compulsions that are severe enough to be time-consuming or cause marked distress and functional impairment. Obsessions are persistent ideas, thoughts, or impulses that are intrusive and often inappropriate. Children may have obsessions about contamination or cleanliness; ordering and compulsive behaviors will follow, such as frequent handwashing, counting, or ordering objects. The goal of the compulsive behavior for the individual with OCD is to reduce anxiety and distress. There may be significant avoidance of situations due to obsessive thoughts or fears of contamination. OCD is often associated with major depressive disorder. OCD is a biologically based disease and has a strong genetic/familial component. Pediatric autoimmune disorders associated with group B *Streptococcus* have also been implicated in the development of OCD for some children. The prevalence of OCD is estimated to be around 2%, and the rates are equal between males and females.

Trichotillomania, while technically classified as an impulse disorder, is also thought to be related to OCD. It involves the recurrent pulling out of hair, often to the point of bald patches, and can also involve pulling out eyelashes, eyebrows, and hair from any part of the body. Trichotillomania should be considered in the differential diagnosis for any patient with alopecia. Treatment often includes the same medications used to treat OCD, and behavior therapy to decrease hair-pulling and restore normal social functioning.

Treatment

OCD is best treated with a combination of cognitive behavioral therapy (CBT) specific to OCD and medications in more severe cases. SSRIs are effective in diminishing OCD symptoms. Fluvoxamine and sertraline have FDA approval for the treatment of pediatric OCD. The tricyclic antidepressant (TCA) clomipramine has FDA approval for the treatment of OCD in adults.

Prognosis

Although OCD is usually a lifelong condition, most individuals can achieve significant remission of symptoms with the combination of CBT and medications. A minority of individuals with OCD are completely disabled by their symptoms.

American Academy of Child and Adolescent Psychiatry: Practice parameters for the assessment and treatment of children and adolescents with OCD. J Am Acad Child Adolesc Psychiatry 1998;37(10 Supp):27S [PMID: 9785727].

Comer JS et al: Obsessing/worrying about the overlap between obsessive-compulsive disorder and generalized anxiety disorder in youth. Clin Psychol Rev 2004;24:663 [PMID: 15385093].

Cook EH et al: Long-term sertraline treatment of children and adolescents with obsessive–compulsive disorder. J Am Acad Child Adolesc Psychiatry 2001;40:1175 [PMID: 11589530].

Freeman JB et al: Family based treatment of early onset obsessive-compulsive disorder. J Child Adolesc Psychopharmacol 3004;13(Suppl 1):S71 [PMID: 12880502].

Geller DA et al: Fluoxetine treatment for OCD in children and adolescents: A placebo controlled trial. J Am Acad Child Adolesc Psychiatry 2001;40:773 [PMID: 11437015].

Kaplan A, Hollander D: A review of pharmacologic treatment for obsessive-compulsive disorder. Psychiatr Serv 2003;54:1111 [PMID: 12883138].

March JS: Cognitive-behavioral psychotherapy for children and adolescents with OCD: A review and recommendations for treatment. J Am Acad Child Adolesc Psychiatry 1995;34:7.

March JS et al: Cognitive-behavioral psychotherapy for pediatric obsessive–compulsive disorder. J Clin Child Psychol 2001;30:8 [PMID: 11294080].

Riddle MA et al: Fluvoxamine for children and adolescents with OCD: A randomized, controlled, multicenter trial. J Am Acad Child Adolesc Psychiatry 2001;40:222 [PMID: 11211371].

Snider LA, Swedo SE: PANDAS: current status and directions for research. Mol Psychiatry 2004;9:900 [PMID: 1521433].

Stewart SE et al: Long-term outcome of pediatric obsessive-compulsive disorder: a meta-analysis and qualitative review of the literature. Acad Psychiatr Scand 2004;110:4 [PMID: 15180774].

Tay YK, Levy ML, Metry DW: Trichotillomania in childhood: case series and review. Pediatrics 2004;113:e494 [PMID: 15121993].

The Pediatric obsessive–compulsive disorder treatment study: rationale, design and methods. J Child Adolesc Psychopharmacol 2003;13(Suppl 1):S39 [PMID: 12880499].

Waters TL et al: Cognitive-behavioral family treatment of child-hood obsessive–compulsive disorder: Preliminary findings. Am J Psychother 2001;55:372 [PMID: 11641879].

POSTTRAUMATIC STRESS DISORDER

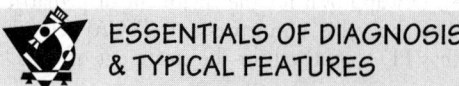

ESSENTIALS OF DIAGNOSIS & TYPICAL FEATURES

- *Signs and symptoms of autonomic hyperarousal such as easy startle, increased heart rate, and hypervigilance.*
- *Avoidant behaviors and numbing of responsiveness.*
- *Flashbacks to a traumatic event, such as nightmares and intrusive thoughts.*
- *All of the preceding following the experience of traumatic events such as exposure to violence, physical or sexual abuse, natural disasters, car accidents, dog bites, and unexpected personal tragedies.*

General Considerations

Factors that predispose individuals to the development of posttraumatic stress disorder (PTSD) include proximity to the traumatic event or loss, a history of exposure to trauma, preexisting depression or anxiety disorder, and lack of an adequate support system. PTSD can develop in response to natural disasters, terrorism, motor vehicle crashes, and significant personal injury, in addition to physical, sexual, and emotional abuse. Natural disasters such as hurricanes, fires, flooding, and earthquakes, for example, can create situations in which large numbers of affected individuals are at heightened risk for PTSD. Individuals who have a previous history of trauma, or an unstable social situation are at greatest risk of PTSD.

Long-overdue attention is now being paid to the substantial effects of family and community violence on the psychological development of children and adolescents. Abused children are most likely to develop PTSD and to suffer wide-ranging symptoms and impaired functioning. As many as 25% of young people exposed to violence develop symptoms of PTSD.

Heightened concern about terrorism in the United States has created increased awareness of PTSD and community-based interventions to decrease the risk of PTSD. Studies after the terrorist attacks of September 11, 2001, and the Oklahoma City bombing reported up to 40% of children and adolescents experienced PTSD symptoms. Studies after the Space Shuttle Challenger explosion and the Oklahoma City bombing strongly suggested that over-

exposure to media coverage of these tragic events also led to symptoms of PTSD for some children and adults.

Clinical Findings

Children and adolescents with PTSD show persistent evidence of fear and anxiety and are hypervigilant to the possibility of repetition. They may regress developmentally and experience fears of strangers, of the dark, and of being alone, and avoid reminders of the traumatic event. Children also frequently reexperience elements of the events in nightmares and flashbacks. In their symbolic play, one can often notice a monotonous repetition of some aspect of the traumatic event. Children with a history of traumatic experiences or neglect in infancy and early childhood are likely to show signs of reactive attachment disorder and have difficulty forming relationships with caregivers.

Treatment

The cornerstone of treatment for PTSD is education of the child and family regarding the nature of the disorder so that the child's emotional reactions and regressive behavior are not mistakenly viewed as crazy or manipulative. Support, reassurance, and repeated explanations and understanding are needed. It is critical that the child be living in a safe environment, and if caregivers have been abusive, concerns must be reported to social services. Efforts should be made to establish or maintain daily routines as much as possible, especially after a trauma or disaster that interrupts the family's environment. In the case of media coverage of a disaster or event, children's viewing should be avoided or limited. Interventions to maintain safety of the child are imperative. Individual and family psychotherapy are central features of treatment interventions. Specific fears usually wane with time, and behavioral desensitization may help. A supportive relationship with a caregiving adult is essential.

For children with more severe and persistent symptoms, assessment for treatment with medication is indicated. Sertraline has approval for the treatment of PTSD in adults. Target symptoms (eg, anxiety, depression, nightmares, and aggression) should be clearly identified and appropriate medication trials initiated with close monitoring. Some of the medications used to treat children with PTSD include clonidine or guanfacine (Tenex), mood stabilizers, antidepressants, and neuroleptics. Children who have lived for an extended time in abusive environments or who have been exposed to multiple traumas are more likely to require treatment with medications. Occupational therapy for sensory integration can also be effective in decreasing reactivity to stimuli and helping the child and caregivers develop and implement self-soothing skills. Individuals who have suffered single-episode traumas usually benefit significantly from psychotherapy and may require limited treatment with medication to address symptoms of anxiety, nightmares, and sleep disturbance.

Psychotherapy that includes eye movement desensitization and reprocessing may also be useful.

Prognosis

At 4- to 5-year follow-up investigations, many children who have been through a traumatic life experience continue to have vivid and frightening memories and dreams and a pessimistic view of the future. The effects of traumatic experiences can be far-reaching. The ability of caregivers to provide a safe, supportive, stable, empathic environment enhances the prognosis for individuals with PTSD. Timely access to therapy and use of therapy over time to work through symptoms also enhance prognosis. Evidence is growing to support a connection between victimization in childhood and unstable personality and mood disorders in later life.

American Academy of Child and Adolescent Psychiatry: Practice parameters for the assessment and treatment of children and adolescents with posttraumatic stress disorder. J Am Acad Child Adolesc Psychiatry 1998;37(Suppl):4S [PMID: 9785726].

Brown DJ: Clinical characteristics and efficacious treatment of posttraumatic stress disorder in children and adolescents. Pediatr Ann 2005;34:138 [PMID: 15768690].

Carr A: Interventions for post-traumatic stress disorder in children and adolescents. Pediatr Rehabil 2004;7:231 [PMID: 15513767].

Fremont WP, Ptaki C, Beresin EV: The impact of terrorism on children and adolescents: terror in the skies, terror on television. Child Adolesc Psychiatr Clin N Am 2005;14:429 [PMID: 15936667].

Fremont WP: Childhood reactions to terrorism-induced trauma: a review of the past 10 years. J Am Acad Child Adolesc Psychiatry 2004;43:381 [PMID: 15187798].

Gurwitch RH et al: When disaster strikes: responding to the needs of children. Prehospital Disaster Med 2004;19:21 [PMID: 15453156].

Margolin G: Children's exposure to violence: exploring developmental pathways to diverse outcomes. J Interpers Violence 2005;20:72 [PMID: 15618563].

Pine DS: Developmental psychobiology and response to threats: Relevance to trauma in children and adolescents. Biol Psychiatry 2003;53:796 [PMID: 12725972].

Scheeringa MS et al: New findings on alternative criteria for PTSD in preschool children. J Am Acad Child Adolesc Psychiatry 2003;42:561 [PMID: 12707560].

Strand VC, Sarmiento TL, Pasquale LE: Assessment and screening tools for trauma in children and adolescents. Trauma Violence Abuse 2005;6:55 [PMID: 15574673].

SOMATOFORM DISORDERS

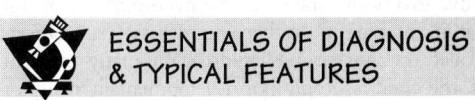

ESSENTIALS OF DIAGNOSIS & TYPICAL FEATURES

• *A symptom suggesting physical dysfunction.*

• *No physical disorder accounting for the symptom.*

• *Symptoms causing distress, dysfunction, or both.*

• *Symptoms not voluntarily created or maintained, as in malingering.*

Clinical Findings

Hypochondriasis, somatization, and conversion disorders involve an unhealthy overemphasis and preoccupation with somatic experiences and symptoms. Somatoform disorders are defined by the presence of physical illness or disability for which no organic cause can be identified, although neither the patient nor the caregiver is consciously fabricating the symptoms. The category includes body dysmorphic disorder, conversion disorder, hypochondriasis, somatization disorder, and somatoform pain disorder (Table 6–13).

Conversion symptoms most often occur in school-age children and adolescents. The exact incidence is unclear, but in pediatric practice they are probably seen more often as transient symptoms than as chronic disorders requiring help from mental health practitioners. A conversion symptom is thought to be an expression of underlying psychological conflict. The specific symptom may be symbolically determined by the underlying conflict; the symptom may resolve the dilemma created by the underlying wish or fear (eg, a seemingly paralyzed child need not fear expressing his underlying rage or aggressive retaliatory impulses). Although children can present with

Table 6–13. Somatoform disorders in children and adolescents.

Disorder	Major Clinical Manifestations
Body dysmorphic disorder	Preoccupation with an imagined defect in personal appearance
Conversion disorder	Symptom onset follows psychologically stressful event; symptoms express unconscious feelings and result in secondary gain
Hypochondriasis	Preoccupation with worry that physical symptoms manifest unrecognized and threatening condition; medical assurance does not provide relief from worry
Somatization disorder	Long-standing preoccupation with multiple somatic symptoms
Somatoform pain disorder	Preoccupation with pain that results in distress or impairment beyond what would be expected from physical findings

a variety of symptoms, the most common include neurologic and gastrointestinal complaints. Children with conversion disorder may be surprisingly unconcerned about the substantial disability deriving from their symptoms. Symptoms include unusual sensory phenomena, paralysis, vomiting, abdominal pain, intractable headaches, and movement or seizurelike disorders.

In the classic case of conversion disorder, the child's symptoms and examination findings are not consistent with the clinical manifestations of any organic disease process. The physical symptoms often begin within the context of a family experiencing stress, such as serious illness, a death, or family discord. On closer examination, the child's symptoms are often found to resemble symptoms present in other family members. Children with conversion disorder may have some secondary gain associated with their symptoms. A number of reports have pointed to the increased association of conversion disorder with sexual overstimulation or sexual abuse. As with other emotional and behavioral problems, health care providers should always screen for physical and sexual abuse.

Differential Diagnosis

It is sometimes not possible to rule out medical disease as a source of the symptoms. Medical follow-up is required to monitor for changes in symptoms and response to recommended interventions.

Somatic symptoms are often associated with anxiety and depressive disorders (see Table 6–10). Occasionally, psychotic children have somatic preoccupations and even somatic delusions.

Treatment & Prognosis

In most cases, conversion symptoms resolve quickly when the child and family are reassured that the symptom is a way of reacting to stress. The child is encouraged to continue with normal daily activities, knowing that the symptom will abate when the stress is resolved. Treatment of conversion disorders includes acknowledging the symptom rather than telling the child that the symptom is not medically justified and responding with noninvasive interventions such as physical therapy while continuing to encourage normalization of the symptoms. If the symptom does not resolve with reassurance, further investigation by a mental health professional is indicated. Comorbid diagnoses such as depression and anxiety disorders should be addressed, and treatment with psychopharmacologic agents may be helpful.

Patients presenting with somatoform disorders are often resistant to mental health treatment, in part fearing that any distraction from their vigilance will put them at greater risk of succumbing to a medical illness. Psychiatric consultation is often helpful and for severely incapacitated patients, referral psychiatric consultation is always indicated.

Somatoform disorder is not associated with the increased morbidity and mortality associated with other psychiatric disorders such as mood disorders or psychotic illness. Somatoform patients are best treated with regular, short scheduled medical appointments to address the complaints at hand. In this way they don't need to precipitate emergencies to elicit medical attention. Avoid invasive procedures unless clearly indicated and offer sincere concern and reassurance. Avoid telling the patient "it's all in your head" and don't abandon or avoid the patient, as somatoform patients are at great risk of seeking multiple alternative treatment providers and potentially unnecessary treatments.

Campo JV et al: Recurrent abdominal pain, anxiety and depression in primary care. Pediatrics 2004;113:817 [PMID: 15060233].

Campo JV et al: Somatization in pediatric primary care: Association with psychopathology, functional impairment, and use of services. J Am Acad Child Adolesc Psychiatry 1999;38:1093 [PMID: 10504807].

Campo JV, Fritz G: A management model for pediatric somatization. Psychosomatics 2001;42:467 [PMID: 11815681].

Dhossche D et al: Somatoform disorders in children and adolescents: A comparison with other internalizing disorders. Ann Clin Psychiatry 2002;14:23 [PMID: 12046637].

Fritz GK et al: Somatoform disorders in children and adolescents: A review of the past 10 years. J Am Acad Child Adolesc Psychiatry 1997;36:1329 [PMID: 9334545].

ELIMINATION DISORDERS

Elimination disorders are defined as problems with age-appropriate bowel and bladder control. These disorders are often identified and addressed by primary care providers. Enuresis and encopresis are not always associated with mental health problems and can simply be due to delayed development of consistent bowel and bladder control, or parental difficulty in managing this developmental stage. Elimination disorders may also treated by child psychiatrists when they are found to be comorbid with other mental health problems, such as posttraumatic stress disorder, anxiety disorders, and developmental disabilities.

1. Enuresis

It is important for the primary care provider to carefully assess the developmental age of the child, the situation in which enuresis is occurring, and to screen for medical concerns before deciding that the enuresis or encopresis is attributable to a behavioral or emotional disorder. It is not uncommon for parents to have unrealistic expectations about toilet training young children. In many cases of enuresis, the child is simply not developmentally ready or sometimes is unable to remain dry at night. Most children with enuresis are able to remain dry by age 9.

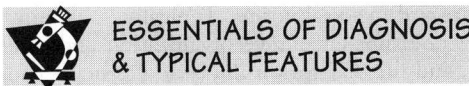

ESSENTIALS OF DIAGNOSIS & TYPICAL FEATURES

- *Urinary incontinence in a child age 5 years (or developmental equivalent) or older.*
- *No medication or general medical condition is causing the urinary incontinence.*

General Considerations

Enuresis is the passage of urine into bedclothes or undergarments, whether involuntary or intentional. At least 90% of enuretic children have primary nocturnal enuresis—that is, they wet only at night during sleep and have never had a sustained period of dryness. Diurnal enuresis (daytime wetting) is much less common, as is secondary enuresis, which develops after a child has had a sustained period of bladder control. The latter two varieties are much more commonly associated with emotional stress, anxiety, and psychiatric disorders. Primary nocturnal enuresis is most often a parasomnia, a deep-sleep (stage 3 or stage 4) event. Etiologically, it is generally viewed as a developmental disorder or maturational lag that children will outgrow. Only infrequently is it associated with a serious psychopathologic disorder.

Clinical Findings

Primary nocturnal enuresis is common (Table 6–14). The incidence is three times higher in boys than in girls. Most children with enuresis become continent by adolescence or earlier. The family history in such cases frequently reveals other members, especially fathers, who have had prolonged nighttime bed-wetting problems. Although the cause of primary nocturnal enuresis is not established, it appears to

Table 6–14. Incidence of enuresis in children.

Age (years)	Primary Nocturnal Enuresis (%)	Occasional Daytime Enuresis (%)[a]
5	15	8
7–8	7	—
10	3–5	—
12	2–3	1
14	1	—

[a]Diurnal (daytime) enuresis tends to resolve by developmental age 6 years, with a slight recurrence around age 12 years in early adolescence.

be related to maturational delay of sleep and arousal mechanisms or to delay in development of increased bladder capacity.

Daytime wetting most often occurs in timid and shy children or in children with ADHD. It occurs with about equal frequency in boys and girls, and 60–80% of daytime wetters also wet at night. Secondary enuresis typically follows a stressful event, such as the birth of a sibling, a loss, or discord within the family. The symptom can be seen as the result of regression in response to stress or as a more symbolic expression of the child's feelings.

Differential Diagnosis

The differential diagnosis includes urinary tract infections, neurologic diseases, seizure disorders, diabetes mellitus, and structural abnormalities of the urinary tract. Urinalysis and urine culture and observing the child's urinary stream can rule out the majority of organic causes of enuresis.

Complications

The most common complication of enuresis is low self-esteem in response to criticism from caregivers and embarrassment if peers are aware of the problem. Older children with enuresis may be reluctant to attend sleepovers and be self-conscious with peers.

Treatment

Treatment should emphasize that the symptom of nocturnal enuresis is a developmental lag and often will be outgrown even without treatment. Even with these interventions, many children will have difficulty remaining dry. If the child chooses to pursue treatment, a program of bladder exercises can be prescribed: fluids should be limited after dinner; the child should attempt to hold urine as long as possible during the day and then start and stop the stream at the toilet bowl; the child is instructed to practice getting up from bed and going to the bathroom at bedtime before sleep. These procedures are helpful in perhaps 30–40% of children with nighttime wetting. Another option is a "potty pager." This is a beeper-like object that attaches to the child's underwear and vibrates when the child is wet in an attempt to rouse the child into a wakeful state and increase awareness of the need to urinate.

Desmopressin acetate (DDAVP), administered intranasally at bedtime, can result in complete remission of nocturnal enuresis in 50% of children as long as they continue the treatment. DDAVP is expensive, but can be useful until the child develops the ability to hold urine through the night or awaken to use the bathroom. For others, a trial of the TCA imipramine is worthwhile, at dosages of 25–50 mg at bedtime for children under age 12 years and 50–75 mg for older children. Because many patients relapse once the drug is stopped, its primary use is for camp attendance or overnight visits. Mental health treatment is more often needed for children with daytime wetting or secondary enuresis. The focus is on the verbal expression of feelings that may be associated with perpetuation of the symptom and behavioral interventions to work toward dryness and cope with episodes of wetting.

2. Encopresis

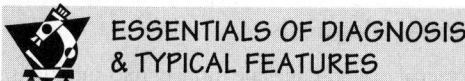

ESSENTIALS OF DIAGNOSIS & TYPICAL FEATURES

- Fecal incontinence in a child age 4 years (or developmental equivalent) or older.
- Not due to medication or a medical disorder.

General Considerations

Functional encopresis is defined as the repeated passage of feces in inappropriate places by a child of at least the developmental equivalent of age 4 years. It may be either involuntary or intentional, although most often it is involuntary. It affects approximately 1–1.5% of school-age children, boys four times more often than girls. Functional fecal incontinence is rare in adolescence.

Clinical Findings

Functional encopresis can be divided into four types: retentive, continuous, discontinuous, and toilet phobia.

A. RETENTIVE ENCOPRESIS

In retentive encopresis, also called psychogenic megacolon, the child withholds bowel movements, leading to the development of constipation, fecal impaction, and the seepage of soft or liquid feces around the margins of the impaction into the underclothing. Marked constipation and painful defecation often contribute to a vicious cycle of withholding, thus creating larger impaction and further seepage. These children often have a history of crossing their legs to resist the urge to defecate and of infrequent bowel movements large enough to stop up the toilet, and they are found on examination to have large fecal masses in their rectal vaults. The soiling that occurs distresses most of these children.

B. CONTINUOUS ENCOPRESIS

Children with continuous encopresis have never gained primary control of bowel function. The bowel movement is usually randomly deposited in underclothing without regard to social norms. Typically, the family structure does not encourage organization and skill training, and for that reason the child has never had adequate bowel training. These children and their parents are more apt to be socially or intellectually disadvantaged.

C. DISCONTINUOUS ENCOPRESIS

Children with discontinuous encopresis have a history of normal bowel control for an extended period. Loss of control often occurs in response to a stressful event, such as the birth of a sibling, a separation, family illness, or marital disharmony. These children may soil their pants or on occasion defecate on the floor or smear feces as an expression of anger or of a wish to be perceived as younger. They typically display relative indifference to the symptom.

D. TOILET PHOBIA

In the infrequent case of toilet phobia, a young child views the toilet as a frightening structure to be avoided. These children may view the bowel movement as an extension of themselves, which is then swept away in a frightening manner. They may think that they, too, may be swept away down the toilet.

Differential Diagnosis

Differential diagnosis includes the medical causes of constipation and retentive encopresis. Hirschsprung disease can be ruled out with reasonable certainty by the history of passing large-caliber bowel movements in the past and by the presence of palpable stool in the rectal vault. Neurologic disorders, hypothyroidism, hypercalcemia, and diseases of smooth muscle must be considered as well. The child should be examined for anal fissures, which tend to encourage the withholding of bowel movements. In addition, fecal soiling can be a presenting symptom in childhood depression and is sometimes a concomitant finding in children with ADHD. If the child engages in fecal smearing, an underlying psychotic disorder should be considered.

Treatment

Identifying the type of encopresis is important in treatment planning. Another important variable is the child's own concern about the symptom. Encopresis in children who display denial or indifference is much harder to treat. Children with coexisting depression or ADHD need to receive treatment for those conditions before focusing treatment on soiling.

With the most common type of encopresis, the retentive type, efforts are made to soften stool so that constipation and painful defecation do not perpetuate the behavior. These children are then taught to adopt a regular schedule of sitting on the toilet after meals. A system of positive reinforcement can be added in which the child is rewarded for each day with no soiled underclothes. The responsibility for rinsing soiled clothing and depositing it in the appropriate receptacle rests with the child. In the case of continuous encopresis, the family is taught to train the child. For toilet phobia, a progressive series of rewarded desensitization steps is necessary. Children with discontinuous encopresis that persists over a number of weeks often need psychotherapy to help them recognize and verbally express their anger and wish to be dependent, rather than express themselves through fecal soiling.

Prognosis

Although the ultimate prognosis is excellent, parental distress and parent-child conflict may be substantial prior to the cessation of symptoms. The natural history of soiling is that it resolves by adolescence in all but the most severely disturbed teenagers.

Bonner L, Dobson P: Children who soil: Guidelines for good practice. J Fam Health Care 2003;13:32 [PMID: 12793299].

Borowitz SM et al: Treatment of childhood encopresis: A randomized trial comparing three treatment protocols. J Pediatr Gastroenterol Nutr 2002;34:378 [PMID: 11930093].

Cedron M: Removing the stigma: Helping reduce the psychosocial impact of bedwetting. Urol Nurs 2002;22:286 [PMID: 12242905].

Cox DF et al: Psychological differences between children with and without chronic encopresis. J Pediatr Psychol 2002;27:585 [PMID: 12228330].

Fishman L et al: Trends in referral to a single encopresis clinic over 20 years. Pediatrics 2003;111(5 pt 1):e604 [PMID: 12728118].

Fritz G, Rockney R: Summary of the practice parameter for the assessment and treatment of children and adolescents with enuresis. J Am Acad Child Adolesc Psychiatry 2004;43:23 [PMID: 14691370].

Gottsegen DN: Curing bedwetting on the spot: A review of one-session cures. Clin Pediatr 2003;42:273 [PMID: 12739927].

Loening-Baucke V: Encopresis. Curr Opin Pediatr 2002;14:570 [PMID: 12352250].

Mercer R: Dry at night. Treating nocturnal enuresis. Adv Nurs Pract 2003;11:26 [PMID: 12640815].

Mikkelson EJ: Enuresis and encopresis: Ten years of progress. Am J Child Adolesc Psychiatr 2001;40:1146 [PMID: 11589527].

Thiedke CC: Nocturnal enuresis. Am Fam Physician 2003;67:1499 [PMID: 12722850].

Van Ginkel R et al: Childhood constipation: Longitudinal follow-up beyond puberty. Gastroenterology 2003;125:357 [PMID: 12891536].

Other psychiatric conditions not covered in this chapter:

Attention-Deficit/Hyperactivity Disorder (ADHD), See Chapter 2

Eating Disorders, See Chapter 5

Mental Retardation, See Chapter 2

Substance Abuse, See Chapter 4

Tourette Syndrome, See Chapter 23

OVERVIEW OF PEDIATRIC PSYCHOPHARMACOLOGY

Pediatric psychopharmacology has improved significantly over the past decade with increasing study of the effect of psychoactive medications on mental illness in childhood and adolescence. Although relatively few medications are approved for use in children, many of the same psychopharmacologic agents used in adults are used in children and adolescents.

As with any medication, the risks as well as the benefits of administering psychoactive medications must be discussed with the child's parent or guardian and with the child and adolescent, as is age-appropriate. A recommendation for medication is warranted if the symptoms observed and reported by the child and family are associated with a psychiatric diagnosis known to respond to a particular medication or class of medications. Medication is more likely to be recommended if the disorder is interfering with psychosocial development, interpersonal relationships, daily functioning, or the patient's sense of personal well-being, and if there is significant potential for benefit with the medication and relatively low risk of harm. Informed consent should be given by the parent or guardian and noted in the record. The recommendation and target symptoms for medication should be discussed with both children and adolescents, and adolescents should also provide informed consent for treatment. In some states adolescents age 15 and older must give informed consent. Informed consent includes a discussion of the diagnosis, target symptoms, possible common side effects, any side effects that should be closely monitored, potential benefits associated with the medication, and documentation of informed consent in the medical record. Psychopharmacologic agents are seldom the only treatment for a psychiatric disorder. They are best used in combination with other interventions such as individual and family psychotherapy and psychosocial interventions, including assessment of school functioning and special needs.

When considering the use of psychoactive medications, specific target symptoms of the medication should be identified and followed to evaluate the efficacy of treatment. These symptoms should be also measured either by self-report rating scales (child and/or family) and clinician-rated scales. When initiating treatment, start with low doses and increase slowly (in divided doses, if indicated) while monitoring for side effects along with therapeutic effects. When a medication is discontinued, it should usually be tapered over 2–4 weeks to minimize withdrawal effects. When multiple choices exist, one should select the medication that has a pediatric FDA approval, or has been studied for the specific indication for which is it being prescribed, ideally in the age range of the patient. The side-effect profile of each option should be carefully considered, and the medication selected with the fewest and least serious risks and side effects. Polypharmacy should be avoided by choosing one drug that might diminish most or all of the target symptoms before considering the simultaneous administration of two or more agents.

Only the stimulants for ADHD, fluvoxamine and sertraline for OCD, and fluoxetine for pediatric depression have FDA approval for specific use in children and adolescents.

In the text that follows, the major classes of psychopharmacologic agents with clinical indications in child and adolescent psychiatry are represented. The more commonly prescribed drugs from each class are reviewed with reference to indications, relative contraindications, initial medical screening procedures (in addition to a general pediatric examination), dosage, adverse effects, drug interactions, and medical follow-up recommendations. This is meant to be a brief reference guide, and the physician should consult a child and adolescent psychopharmacology textbook for additional information on specific medications.

MEDICATIONS FOR ATTENTION-DEFICIT/HYPERACTIVITY DISORDER

Adderall

Atomoxetine (Strattera)

Dextroamphetamine (Dexedrine)

Dexmethylphenidate (Focalin)

Methylphenidate (Concerta, Metadate, Methylin, Ritalin)

A. INDICATIONS

Approximately 75% of children with ADHD experience improved attention span, decreased hyperactivity, and decreased impulsivity when given stimulant medications. Children with ADHD who do not respond favorably to one stimulant may respond well to another. Children and adolescents with ADHD without prominent hyperactivity (ADHD, predominantly inattentive type) are also likely to be responsive to stimulant medications. Atomoxetine (Strattera) and bupropion (Wellbutrin) are nonstimulant medications used to treat ADHD. Atomoxetine has FDA approval for the treatment of ADHD and is a selec-

tive noradrenergic reuptake inhibitor. Bupropion is primarily used as an antidepressant, and blocks serotonin, dopamine, and norepinephrine reuptake.

B. CONTRAINDICATIONS

Stimulants should be used cautiously in individuals with a personal or family history of motor tics or Tourette syndrome, as stimulants can cause or worsen motor tics. Caution should also be taken if there is a personal or family history of substance abuse or addictive disorders, as these medications can be abused or sold as drugs of abuse. Stimulants are also contraindicated for individuals with psychotic disorders, as they can significantly worsen psychotic symptoms. Stimulants should be used with caution in individuals with comorbid bipolar affective disorder and ADHD and consideration of concurrent mood stabilization is critical.

C. INITIAL MEDICAL SCREENING

The child should be observed for involuntary movements. Height, weight, pulse, and blood pressure should be recorded. (See also Chapter 2.)

D. ADVERSE EFFECTS

These are often dose-related and time-limited.

1. Common adverse effects—Anorexia, weight loss, abdominal distress, headache, insomnia, dysphoria and tearfulness, irritability, lethargy, mild tachycardia, and mild elevation in blood pressure.

2. Less common effects—Interdose rebound of ADHD symptoms, emergence of motor tics or Tourette syndrome, behavioral stereotypy, tachycardia or hypertension, depression, mania, and psychotic symptoms. Reduced growth velocity occurs only during active administration. Growth rebound occurs during periods of discontinuation. Ultimate height is not usually noticeably compromised. Treatment with stimulant medications does not predispose to future substance abuse.

E. DRUG INTERACTIONS

Additive stimulant effects are seen with sympathomimetic amines (ephedrine and pseudoephedrine).

F. MEDICAL FOLLOW-UP

Pulse, blood pressure, height, and weight should be recorded every 3–4 months and at times of dosage increases. Assess for abnormal movements such as motor tics at each visit.

G. DOSAGE

1. Methylphenidate—The usual starting dose is 5 mg once or twice a day (before school and at noon), gradually increasing as clinically indicated. The maximum daily dose should not exceed 60 mg, and a single dose should not exceed 0.7 mg/kg. Administration on weekends and during vacations is determined by the need at those times. The duration of action is approximately 3–4 hours. Extended-release forms can prevent the need for taking medication at school. Dexmethylphenidate (Focalin) is typically administered 2.5 mg twice a day (8 am and noon, for example), to a maximum dose of 20 mg.

2. Dextroamphetamine sulfate—The dosage is 2.5–10 mg twice daily, before school and at noon, with or without another dose at 4 pm. A sustained-release preparation may have clinical effects for up to 8 hours. There is also an extended-release form.

3. Pemoline—Pemoline is generally not recommended for the treatment of ADHD due to a significant risk of liver failure.

4. Atomoxetine Hydrochloride—The starting dose for children and adolescents up to 70 kg is 0.5 mg/kg, with titration to a maximum dose of 1.2 mg/kg, in single or divided dosing.

ANTIDEPRESSANTS

The "black box warning" that was issued in October 2005 for all antidepressants has had a significant impact on prescription of these medications for children. The black box warning reads "Pooled analysis of short term (4–16 weeks) placebo-controlled trials of antidepressant drugs (SSRIs and others) in children and adolescents with Major Depressive Disorder (MDD), Obsessive-Compulsive Disorder (OCD) and other psychiatric disorders (a total of 24 trials involving more than 4400 patients) has revealed a greater risk of adverse events representing suicidal thinking or behavior (suicidality) during the first few months of treatment in those receiving antidepressants. The average risk of such events was 4%, twice the placebo risk of 2%. No suicides occurred in these trials."

The "medication guide" created for consumers along with the black box warning which now appears in all antidepressant packaging, recommends the following monitoring schedule for health care providers when starting an antidepressant:

* Once every week for the first 4 weeks
* Every 2 weeks for the next 4 weeks
* After taking the antidepressant for 12 weeks
* After 12 weeks, follow your health care provider's advice on how often to come back.

The Treatment of Adolescent Depression Study found that cognitive behavioral therapy combined with fluoxetine led to the best outcomes in the treatment of pediatric depression.

It is important to be cognizant of evidence-based medical practice when prescribing for any indication. Target symptoms should be carefully monitored for

improvement or worsening, and it is important to ask and document the responses about any suicidal thinking and self-injurious behaviors. When recommending an antidepressant, the physician should also firmly recommend cognitive behavioral therapy and discuss the options for medication treatment, including which medications have FDA approval for pediatric indications.

1. Selective Serotonin Reuptake Inhibitors

> Citalopram, escitalopram (Celexa, Lexapro)
> Fluoxetine (Prozac, Sarafem)
> Fluvoxamine (Luvox)
> Paroxetine (Paxil)
> Sertraline (Zoloft)

A. INDICATIONS

The SSRIs have become the agents of first choice for the treatment of depression and anxiety. Fluvoxamine and sertraline both have approval from the FDA for treatment of pediatric OCD and fluoxetine has approval for pediatric depression. Although no other SSRIs have FDA approval for pediatric indications, some published studies support the efficacy of SSRIs for the treatment of depression, anxiety, and OCD in pediatric populations. Each SSRI has different FDA indications. However, once an indication is obtained for one SSRI, it is widely believed that other SSRIs are likely to be effective as well for the same indication. The FDA-approved indications are the following:

> Major depression (> 18 years of age): fluoxetine (and age 6–17), paroxetine, citalopram, sertraline
> Panic disorder (> 18 years): paroxetine, sertraline
> OCD (> 6 years): sertraline, fluvoxamine
> Bulimia (> 18 years): fluoxetine
> PTSD (> 18 years): sertraline
> Premenstrual dysphoric disorder (> 18 years): fluoxetine

B. CONTRAINDICATIONS

Caution should be used in cases of known liver disease, because all SSRIs are metabolized in the liver. Caution should be used when prescribing for an individual with a family history of bipolar disorder, or when the differential diagnosis includes bipolar disorder, because antidepressants can induce manic or hypomanic symptoms.

C. INITIAL MEDICAL SCREENING

General medical examination.

D. ADVERSE EFFECTS

Often dose-related and time-limited: GI distress and nausea (can be minimized by taking medication with food), headache, tremulousness, decreased appetite, weight loss, insomnia, sedation (10%), sexual dysfunction (25%). Irritability, social disinhibition, restlessness, and emotional excitability can occur in approximately 20% of children taking SSRIs. Monitor for improvement and onset or worsening of suicidal or self-injurious thinking, in addition to other target symptoms.

E. Drug Interactions

All SSRIs inhibit the efficiency of the hepatic microsomal enzyme system. The order of inhibition is: fluoxetine > fluvoxamine > paroxetine > sertraline > citalopram. This can lead to higher-than-expected blood levels of other drugs, including antidepressants, antiarrhythmics, antipsychotics, β-blockers, opioids, and antihistamines. Taking tryptophan while on an SSRI may result in a serotonergic syndrome of psychomotor agitation and GI distress. A potentially fatal interaction that clinically resembles neuroleptic malignant syndrome may occur when the SSRIs are administered concomitantly with the monoamine oxidase inhibitors. Fluoxetine has the longest half-life of the SSRIs and should not be initiated within 14 days of the discontinuation of a monoamine oxidase inhibitor, or a monoamine oxidase inhibitor initiated within at least 5 weeks of the discontinuation of fluoxetine.

F. Dosage (Table 6–15)

The SSRIs are usually given once a day, in the morning with breakfast. One in ten individuals may experience sedation and prefer to take the medication at bedtime. The alternative antidepressants and fluvoxamine are usually given in twice-daily dosing. Paroxetine, bupro-

pion, and venlafaxine are now available in a sustained- and extended-release form. Therapeutic response should be expected 4–6 weeks after a therapeutic dose has been reached. The starting dose for a child younger than 12 years old is generally half the starting dose for an adolescent.

2. Other Antidepressants

Bupropion (Wellbutrin), bupropion SR (sustained-release)

Venlafaxine (Effexor), venlafaxine XR (extended-release)

Mirtazapine (Remeron)

Nefazodone (Serzone)

Bupropion

A. Indications

Bupropion is an antidepressant that inhibits reuptake of primarily serotonin, but also norepinephrine and dopamine. It is approved for treatment of major depression in adults, but is receiving favorable attention for its therapeutic effects with major depressive disorder in adolescents and with ADHD in children and adolescents. Like the SSRIs, bupropion has very few anticholinergic or cardiotoxic effects.

B. Contraindications

History of seizure disorder or bulimia nervosa.

C. Initial Medical Screening and Follow-Up

General medical examination.

Table 6–15. Medications used to treat depression in adolescents.

Generic	Trade Name	Adolescent Starting Dose	Target Dose (Average Effective Dose)	Maximum Dose
Selective serotonin reuptake inhibitors				
Citalopram	Celexa	20 mg q AM	20 mg q AM	40–60 mg q AM
Escitalopram	Lexapro	10 mg	10 mg	30 mg
Fluoxetine	Prozac	10 mg q AM	20 mg q AM	60 mg q AM
Fluvoxamine	Luvox	50 mg qhs	100–150 mg qd	100 mg bid
Paroxetine	Paxil	10 mg q AM	20 mg q AM	60 mg q AM
Paroxetine CR	Paxil CR	25 mg	25 mg	50 mg
Sertraline	Zoloft	25 mg q AM	50 mg q AM	150 mg q AM
Alternative antidepressants				
Bupropion	Wellbutrin	75 mg q AM	150 mg bid	200 mg bid
Bupropion SR	Wellbutrin SR	100 mg q AM	100 mg bid	150 mg bid
Mirtazapine	Remeron	7.5 mg qhs	15 mg qhs	30 mg qhs
Venlafaxine	Effexor	37.5 mg q AM	75 mg bid	150 mg bid
Venlafaxine XR	Effexor XR	37.5 mg q AM	150 mg qd	225 mg qd

q AM, every morning; qhs, every night at bedtime; qd, every day; bid, twice a day.

D. Adverse Effects

Psychomotor activation (agitation or restlessness), headache, GI distress, nausea, anorexia with weight loss, insomnia, tremulousness, precipitation of mania, and induction of seizures with doses above 450 mg/d.

Venlafaxine

Venlafaxine is an antidepressant that primarily inhibits reuptake of serotonin and norepinephrine.

A. Indications

It is approved for the treatment of major depression in adults.

B. Contraindications

Hypertension.

C. Initial Medical Screening and Follow-Up

General medical examination.

D. Adverse Effects

The most common adverse effects are nausea, nervousness, and sweating. Hypertension is likely with doses over 300 mg or over 225 mg of the extended-release version. Venlafaxine must be discontinued slowly to minimize withdrawal symptoms: severe headaches, dizziness, and significant flulike symptoms. It is also available in an extended-release form.

Mirtazapine

Mirtazapine is an α_2-antagonist that enhances central noradrenergic and serotonergic activity.

A. Indications

It is approved for the treatment of major depression in adults.

B. Contraindications

Mirtazapine should not be given in combination with monoamine oxidase inhibitors. Very rare side effects are acute liver failure (1 case per 250,000–300,000), neutropenia, and agranulocytosis.

C. Initial Medical Screening and Follow-Up

General medical examination.

D. Adverse Effects

Dry mouth, increased appetite, constipation, weight gain.

3. Tricyclic Antidepressants

Imipramine
Desipramine (Norpramin)
Clomipramine (Anafranil)
Nortriptyline
Amitriptyline (Elavil)

With the introduction of the SSRIs and alternative antidepressants, use of the TCAs has become uncommon for the treatment of depression and anxiety disorders. The TCAs have more significant side-effect profiles, require more substantial medical monitoring, and are quite cardiotoxic in overdose. For these reasons, in general, SSRIs or alternative antidepressants should be considered before recommending a TCA.

A. Indications

TCAs have been prescribed for chronic pain syndromes, migraines, headache, depression, anxiety, enuresis, bulimia nervosa, OCD, and PTSD in children and adolescents. Imipramine and desipramine have FDA approval for the treatment of major depression in adults and enuresis for children older than 6 years of age. Some published studies have demonstrated clinical efficacy in the treatment of ADHD, panic disorder, anxiety-based school refusal, separation anxiety disorder, bulimia, night terrors, and sleepwalking. But as yet, the FDA has not approved their use for these indications. Studies have not supported efficacy in major depression in children and adolescents. Nortriptyline has FDA approval for the treatment of major depression in adults. Clomipramine has FDA approval for the treatment of depression and OCD in adults and may be helpful for obsessive symptoms in autism.

B. Contraindications

Known cardiac disease or arrhythmia, undiagnosed syncope, known seizure disorder, family history of sudden cardiac death or cardiomyopathy, known electrolyte abnormality (with bingeing and purging).

C. Initial Medical Screening

The family history should be examined for sudden cardiac death; the patient's history for cardiac disease, arrhythmias, syncope, seizure disorder, or congenital hearing loss (associated with prolonged QT interval). Other screening procedures include serum electrolytes and blood urea nitrogen in patients who have eating disorders, cardiac examination, and a baseline electrocardiogram (ECG).

D. Medical Follow-Up

Measure pulse and blood pressure (monitor for tachycardia and orthostatic hypotension) with each dosage increase, and obtain an ECG to monitor for arteriovenous block with each dosage increase; after reaching steady state, record pulse, blood pressure, and ECG every 3–4 months.

E. Adverse Effects

1. Cardiotoxic effects—The cardiotoxic effects of TCAs appear to be more common in children and adolescents than in adults. In addition to anticholinergic effects, TCAs have quinidinelike effects that result in slowing of cardiac conduction. Increased plasma levels appear to be weakly associated with an increased risk of cardiac conduction abnormalities. Steady-state plasma levels of desipramine or of desipramine plus imipramine should therefore not exceed 300 ng/mL. In addition, each dosage increase above 3 mg/kg/d must be carefully monitored with pulse, blood pressure, and repeated ECGs to monitor for arteriovenous block. Upper limits for cardiovascular parameters when administering TCAs to children and adolescents are listed in Table 6–16.

2. Anticholinergic effects—Tachycardia, dry mouth, stuffy nose, blurred vision, constipation, sweating, vasomotor instability, withdrawal syndrome (GI distress and psychomotor activation).

3. Other effects—Orthostatic hypotension and dizziness, lowered seizure threshold, increased appetite and weight gain, sedation, irritability and psychomotor agitation, rash (often associated with yellow dye No. 5), headache, abdominal complaints, sleep disturbance and nightmares, mania.

F. Drug Interactions

TCAs may potentiate the effects of CNS depressants and stimulants; barbiturates and cigarette smoking may decrease plasma levels; phenothiazines, methylphenidate, and oral contraceptives may increase plasma levels; SSRIs given in combination with TCAs will result in higher TCA blood levels due to inhibition of TCA metabolism by liver enzymes (eg, cytochrome P-450 isoenzymes).

G. Dosage

Refer to a pediatric psychopharmacology text for dosages. Daily dosage requirements vary considerably with different clinical disorders.

Table 6–16. Upper limits of cardiovascular parameters with tricyclic antidepressants.

Heart rate	130/min
Systolic blood pressure	130 mm Hg
Diastolic blood pressure	85 mm Hg
PR interval	0.2 s
QRS interval	0.12 s, or no more than 30% over baseline
QT corrected	0.45 s

MOOD STABILIZERS

Carbamazepine (Tegretol)
Gabapentin (Neurontin)
Lamotrigine (Lamictal)
Lithium carbonate (Eskalith, Eskalith CR, Lithobid, Lithotabs)
Valproic acid (Depakote, Depakote ER)
Olanzapine (Zyprexa, atypical neuroleptic)
Risperidone (Risperdal, atypical neuroleptic)

Lithium, valproic acid, and olanzapine (neuroleptic) are FDA approved for the treatment of bipolar disorder. Carbamazepine and oxcarbazepine, although not FDA approved for treatment of bipolar disorder, may also be effective and carry less risk of weight gain. Lamotrigine (Lamictal) was recently approved for the treatment of bipolar depression in adults. Other antiepileptic medications, such as gabapentin and topiramate, have also been used with varying efficacy. Medications that are effective as mood stabilizers may be helpful also in the treatment of severe aggressive symptoms.

Lithium

A. Indications

Lithium remains a front-line drug in the treatment of bipolar disorder and has been shown to have an augmenting effect when combined with SSRIs for treatment-resistant depression and OCD.

B. Contraindications

Lithium is contraindicated in patients with known renal, thyroid, or cardiac disease; those at high risk for dehydration and electrolyte imbalance (eg, vomiting and purging); and those who may become pregnant (teratogenic effects).

C. Initial Medical Screening

General medical screening with pulse, blood pressure, height, and weight; complete blood cell count (CBC); serum electrolytes, blood urea nitrogen, and creatinine; and thyroid function tests including thyroid-stimulating hormone levels.

D. Dosage

For children the starting dose is usually 150 mg once or twice a day, with titration in 150- to 300-mg increments. (Dose may vary with the brand of lithium used; consult a psychopharmacology textbook for medication-specific information.) Oral doses of lithium should be titrated to maintain therapeutic blood levels of 0.8–1.2 mEq/L. The drug is generally given in two doses. Blood samples should be drawn 12 hours after the last dose.

E. ADVERSE EFFECTS

1. Lithium toxicity—Lithium has a narrow therapeutic index. Blood levels required for therapeutic effects are close to those associated with toxic symptoms. Mild toxicity may be indicated by increased tremor, GI distress, neuromuscular irritability, and altered mental status (confusion), and can occur when blood levels exceed 1.5 mEq/L. Moderate to severe symptoms of lithium toxicity are associated with blood levels above 2 mEq/L. Acute renal failure can occur at levels over 2.5–3 mEq/L.

2. Side effects—Lithium side effects include intention tremor, GI distress (including nausea and vomiting and sometimes diarrhea), hypothyroidism, polyuria and polydipsia, drowsiness, malaise, weight gain, acne, and granulocytosis.

F. DRUG INTERACTIONS

Excessive salt intake and salt restriction should be avoided. Thiazide diuretics and nonsteroidal anti-inflammatory agents (except aspirin and acetaminophen) can lead to increased lithium levels. Ibuprofen should be avoided by individuals on lithium due to combined renal toxicity. Precautions against dehydration are required in hot weather and during vigorous exercise.

G. MEDICAL FOLLOW-UP

Serum lithium levels should be measured 5–7 days following a change in dosage and then quarterly at steady state; serum creatinine and thyroid-stimulating hormone concentrations should be determined every 3–4 months.

Valproic Acid

A. INDICATIONS

Valproate has FDA approval for the treatment of bipolar disorder in adults. Its efficacy in acute mania equals that of lithium, but it is generally better tolerated. Valproate is more effective than lithium in patients with rapid-cycling bipolar disorder (more than four cycles per year) and in patients with mixed states (coexisting symptoms of depression and mania). Valproate may be more effective than lithium in adolescents with bipolar disorder because they often have rapid cycling and mixed states.

B. CONTRAINDICATIONS

Liver dysfunction.

C. INITIAL MEDICAL SCREENING

CBC and liver function tests (LFTs).

D. DOSAGE

Usually starts at 15 mg/kg/d and is increased in increments of 5–10 mg/kg/d every 1–2 weeks to a range of 500–1500 mg/d in two or three divided doses. Trough levels in the range of 80–120 mg/mL are thought to be therapeutic.

E. ADVERSE EFFECTS

Between 10% and 20% of patients experience sedation or anorexia, especially early in treatment or if the dose is increased too rapidly. GI upset occurs in 25% of patients, and when severe, can usually be treated with cimetidine. Increased appetite and weight gain can be troublesome for children and adolescents. Blurred vision, headache, hair loss, and tremor occur occasionally. Slight elevations in aminotransferases are frequent. Severe idiosyncratic hepatitis, pancreatitis, thrombocytopenia, and agranulocytosis occur only rarely.

F. MEDICAL FOLLOW-UP

LFTs should be checked monthly for 3–4 months; subsequently, LFTs, a CBC, and trough valproate levels should be obtained every 3–4 months.

Carbamazepine

A. INDICATIONS

Similarly to lithium and valproate, carbamazepine may be effective for treating bipolar disorder or for the target symptoms of mood instability, irritability, or behavioral dyscontrol. Some data suggest that it is more effective than valproate for the depressive phases of bipolar disorder. A new form of carbamazepine—oxcarbazepine (Trileptal)—is also being used for pediatric mood disorders; however, its efficacy has not been established. Reportedly, it does not have the worrisome side effects of bone marrow suppression and liver enzyme induction. Blood levels cannot be monitored, and the dose range is similar to that of carbamazepine.

B. CONTRAINDICATIONS

History of previous bone marrow depression or adverse hematologic reaction to another drug; history of sensitivity to a TCA.

C. INITIAL MEDICAL SCREENING

Obtain a CBC with platelets, reticulocytes, serum iron, and blood urea nitrogen; LFTs; urinalysis.

D. DOSAGE

Usually start at 10–20 mg/kg/d, in two divided doses, in children younger than age 6 years; 100 mg twice daily in children ages 6–12 years; and 200 mg twice daily in children over age 12 years. Doses may be increased weekly until there is effective symptom control. Total daily doses should not exceed 35 mg/kg/d in children younger than age 6 years; 1000 mg/d in children ages 6–15 years; and 1200 mg/d in adolescents older than age 15 years. Plasma levels in the range of 4–12 mg/mL are thought to be therapeutic.

E. ADVERSE EFFECTS

Nausea, dizziness, sedation, headache, dry mouth, diplopia, and constipation reflect the drug's mild anticholinergic properties. Rashes are more common with carbamazepine than with other mood stabilizers. Aplastic anemia and agranulocytosis are rare. Leukopenia and thrombocytopenia are more common, and if present, should be monitored closely for evidence of bone marrow depression. These effects usually occur early and transiently and then spontaneously revert toward normal. Liver enzyme induction may significantly change the efficacy of medications given concurrently.

F. MEDICAL FOLLOW-UP

Hematologic, hepatic, and renal parameters should be followed at least every 3 months for the first year. White blood cell counts below 3000/mL and absolute neutrophil counts below 1000/mL call for discontinuation of the drug and referral for hematology consultation.

Lamotrigine

Lamotrigine is approved for the treatment of bipolar depression in adults. Lamotrigine has a serious side effect of serious rashes that can require hospitalization and can include Stevens-Johnson syndrome (0.8% incidence). This medication should be used very carefully. The starting dose is 25 mg, with a slow titration of increasing the dose by 25 mg per week to a target dose (as clinically indicated) of 300 mg/d.

Gabapentin

Like valproate and carbamazepine, gabapentin is an anticonvulsant that has been used as a mood stabilizer in some adult populations. It may be used along with either valproate or carbamazepine in individuals with treatment-resistant disorders. The usual adult dose range for seizure disorders is 900–1800 mg/d in three divided doses and may need to be adjusted downward in individuals with renal impairment. Although its use among adolescents and even children is increasing, it is not approved for this indication, and reports of its efficacy remain largely anecdotal. Some reports suggest it may worsen behavioral parameters in children with underlying ADHD.

NEUROLEPTICS

1. Atypical (Newer) Neuroleptics

Aripiprazole (Abilify)
Clozapine (Clozaril)

Olanzapine (Zyprexa)
Risperidone (Risperdal)
Quetiapine (Seroquel)
Ziprasidone (Geodon)

2. Conventional Neuroleptics

Chlorpromazine
Thioridazine
Haloperidol
Thiothixene
Molindone
Trifluoperazine
Perphenazine

The neuroleptics, also known as antipsychotics, are indicated for psychotic symptoms in patients with schizophrenia. Some now have an FDA-approved indication for Bipolar Affective Disorder in adults (risperidone and olanzapine). They are also used for acute mania and as adjuncts to antidepressants in the treatment of psychotic depression (with delusions or hallucinations). The neuroleptics may be used cautiously in refractory PTSD, in refractory OCD, and in individuals with markedly aggressive behavioral problems unresponsive to other interventions. They may also be useful for the body image distortion and irrational fears about food and weight gain associated with anorexia nervosa.

The "atypical neuroleptics" differ from conventional neuroleptics in their receptor specificity and effect on serotonin receptors. Conventional neuroleptics are associated with a higher incidence of movement disorders and extrapyramidal symptoms (EPS) due to their wider effect on dopamine receptors. The introduction of the atypical neuroleptics has significantly changed neuroleptic prescribing patterns. The atypical neuroleptics have a better side-effect profile for most individuals and comparable efficacy for the treatment of psychotic symptoms and aggression. Atypical neuroleptics have a decreased incidence of EPS and tardive dyskinesia (TD). Significant side effects can include substantial weight gain and sedation. Because of their increased use over conventional neuroleptics, this section will focus primarily on the atypical neuroleptics.

Aripiprazole

Aripiprazole (Abilify) is the newest atypical neuroleptic and is indicated for the treatment of schizophrenia. It is a partial dopamine blocker and a serotonin agonist. Side effects include nausea and vomiting and fatigue. It is not associated with weight gain. Doses over 30 mg are more likely to be associated with EPS. The dose range is 10–30 mg, and pills can be split.

Olanzapine

The FDA has approved this agent for the treatment of schizophrenia and bipolar disorder in adults. Olanzapine (Zyprexa) has greater affinity for type 2 serotonin receptors than dopamine-2 receptors and also has an effect on muscarinic, histaminic, and α-adrenergic receptors. As with the other atypical neuroleptics, it may be more helpful for treating the negative symptoms of schizophrenia (flat affect, isolation and withdrawal, and apathy) than conventional neuroleptics. Anecdotal and case report data support its utility in child and adolescent psychotic disorders. The adult dose range of 5–15 mg/d administered in a single bedtime dose is probably applicable to adolescents as well. Weight gain can be a significant side effect. The starting dose for children is usually 1.25 mg.

Quetiapine

Quetiapine (Seroquel) is an antagonist at multiple receptor sites, including serotonin ($5\text{-}HT_{1A}$ and $5\text{-}HT_2$), dopamine (D_1 and D_2), histamine, and adrenergic receptors. Quetiapine is given in 25- to 50-mg increments up to 800 mg for the treatment of psychotic symptoms. It is thought to be a weight-neutral medication, and the primary side effect is sedation.

Risperidone

Risperidone (Risperdal) blocks type 2 dopamine receptors (similarly to haloperidol) and type 2 serotonin receptors. It is approved for the treatment of schizophrenia and bipolar affective disorder in adults. Risperidone has also demonstrated clinical efficacy in the treatment of Tourette syndrome. The initial dose is 1–2 mg/d. It is typically titrated up in 0.5–1 mg increments to a maximum dose of 4–10 mg for psychotic disorders. Side effects include weight gain and sedation.

Ziprasidone

Ziprasidone (Geodon) has affinity for multiple serotonin receptors ($5\text{-}HT_2$, $5\text{-}HT_{1A}$, $5\text{-}HT_{1D}$, and $5\text{-}HT_{2C}$) and dopamine-2 receptors, and it moderately inhibits norepinephrine and serotonin reuptake. It also has moderate affinity for H_1 and α_1 receptors. Ziprasidone has a greater effect on cardiac QT intervals and requires a baseline ECG and ECG monitoring when a dose of 80 mg is reached and with each dose change above 80 mg to monitor for QT prolongation. Ziprasidone is reported to cause minimal weight gain. The initial dose of ziprasidone is 20 mg, with dose changes in 20-mg increments to a total daily dose of 140 mg for the treatment of psychotic symptoms in adults. There are no studies of ziprasidone in children and adolescents at this time.

Clozapine

Clozapine (Clozaril) is usually reserved for individuals who have not responded to multiple other neuroleptics due to its side effect of agranulocytosis. Clozapine blocks type 2 dopamine receptors weakly and is virtually free of EPS, apparently including TD. It was very effective in about 40% of adult patients with chronic schizophrenia who did not respond to conventional neuroleptics.

Non–dose-related agranulocytosis occurs in 0.5–2% of subjects. Some case reports note benefit from clozapine in child and adolescent schizophrenic patients who were resistant to other treatment. Contraindications are concurrent treatment with carbamazepine and any history of leukopenia. Initial medical screening should include CBC and LFTs. The daily dose is 200–600 mg in two divided doses. Because of the risk of neutropenia, patients taking clozapine must be registered with the Clozapine Registry and a white blood cell count must be obtained biweekly before a 2-week supply of the drug is dispensed. If the white count falls below 3000/mL, clozapine is usually discontinued. Other side effects include sedation, weight gain, and increased salivation. The incidence of seizures increases with doses above 600 mg/d.

3. General Neuroleptic Information

The following adverse effects of neuroleptics apply to both typical and atypical neuroleptics, but are thought to have a significantly lower incidence with the atypical neuroleptics.

A. INITIAL MEDICAL SCREENING

One should observe and examine for tremors and other abnormal involuntary movements and establish baseline values for CBC and LFTs. An ECG should be taken if there is a history of cardiac disease or arrhythmia, and to establish a baseline QT interval (cardiac repolarization) prior to initiation of the neuroleptics that have a greater effect on the QT interval (eg, ziprasidone and thioridazine). Neuroleptics can cause QT prolongation leading to ventricular arrhythmias, such as torsades de pointes. Medications that affect the cytochrome P-450 isoenzyme pathway (including SSRIs) may increase the neuroleptic plasma concentration and increase risk of QTc prolongation.

B. ADVERSE EFFECTS

The most troublesome adverse effects of the atypical neuroleptics are cognitive slowing, sedation, orthostasis, and weight gain. The conventional neuroleptics have an increased incidence of EPS and TD. Sedation, cognitive slowing, and EPS all tend to be dose-related. Because of the risk of side effects, neuroleptic medications should be used with caution and monitored regularly. The risk:benefit ratio of the medication for the identified target symptom should be carefully considered and reviewed with the parent or guardian.

1. Extrapyramidal side effects—EPS and acute dystonic reactions are tonic muscle spasms, often of the tongue, jaw, or neck. EPS symptoms can be mildly uncomfortable or may result in such dramatically distressing symptoms as oculogyric crisis, torticollis, and even opisthotonos. The onset usually occurs within days after a dosage change and may occur in up to 25% of children treated with conventional neuroleptics. Acute neuroleptic-induced dystonias are quickly relieved by anticholinergics such as benztropine (Cogentin) and diphenhydramine.

2. Tardive dyskinesias—TDs are involuntary movement disorders that are often irreversible and may appear after long-term use of neuroleptic medications. Choreoathetoid movements of the tongue and mouth are most common, but the extremities and trunk may also be involved. The risk of TD is small in patients on atypical neuroleptics, and those on conventional neuroleptics for less than 6 months. There is no universally effective treatment.

3. Pseudoparkinsonism—Pseudoparkinsonism is usually manifested 1–4 weeks after the start of treatment. It presents as muscle stiffness, cogwheel rigidity, masklike facial expression, bradykinesia, drooling, and occasionally pill-rolling tremor. Anticholinergic medications or dosage reductions are helpful.

4. Akathisia—Akathisia is usually manifested after 1–6 weeks of treatment. It presents as a unpleasant feeling of driven motor restlessness that ranges from vague muscular discomfort to a markedly dysphoric agitation with frantic pacing. Anticholinergic agents or β-blockers are sometimes helpful.

5. Neuroleptic malignant syndrome—Neuroleptic malignant syndrome is a very rare medical emergency associated primarily with the conventional neuroleptics, although it has been reported also with atypical neuroleptics. It is manifested by severe muscular rigidity, mental status changes, fever, autonomic lability, and myoglobinemia. Neuroleptic malignant syndrome can present without muscle rigidity with atypical neuroleptics and should be considered in the differential diagnosis of any patient on neuroleptics who presents with high fever and altered mental status. Mortality as high as 30% has been reported. Treatment includes immediate medical assessment, withdrawal of the neuroleptic, and may require transfer to an ICU.

6. Withdrawal dyskinesias—Withdrawal dyskinesias are reversible movement disorders that appear following withdrawal of neuroleptic medications. Dyskinetic movements develop within 1–4 weeks after withdrawal of the drug and may persist for months.

7. Other adverse effects—These include cardiac arrhythmias, irregular menses, gynecomastia and galactorrhea due to increased prolactin, sexual dysfunction, photosensitivity, rashes, lowered seizure threshold, hepatic dysfunction, and blood dyscrasias.

C. DRUG INTERACTIONS

Potentiation of CNS depressant effects or the anticholinergic effects of other drugs may occur, as well as increased plasma levels of antidepressants.

D. MEDICAL FOLLOW-UP

One should examine the patient at least every 3 months for signs of the side effects listed. An Abnormal Involuntary Movement Scale can be used to monitor for TD for patients taking neuroleptics.

ADRENERGIC AGONISTS

Clonidine and Guanfacine (Tenex)

A. INDICATIONS

Clonidine is a nonselective α-adrenergic agonist that is clinically useful in decreasing states of hyperarousal seen in children and adolescents with PTSD and ADHD. Guanfacine is a selective agonist for α_2-adrenergic receptors with advantages over the nonselective agonist clonidine. Guanfacine is less sedating and less hypotensive and has a longer half-life, allowing for twice-daily dosing. Case reports find guanfacine effective in ADHD and Tourette syndrome with comorbid ADHD. Bedtime doses of adrenergic agonists can be helpful for the delayed onset of sleep and nightmares that can occur with PTSD, for the difficulty settling for sleep seen in ADHD, or for ameliorating the side effects of stimulant medications. They are also effective in the treatment of tics in Tourette syndrome

B. CONTRAINDICATIONS

Adrenergic agonists are contraindicated for patients with known renal or cardiovascular disease and for those with a family or personal history of depression.

C. INITIAL MEDICAL SCREENING

The pulse and blood pressure should be recorded prior to starting an adrenergic agonist.

D. DOSAGE

The initial dosage of clonidine is usually 0.025–0.05 mg at bedtime. The dosage can be increased after 3–5 days by giving 0.05 mg in the morning. Further dosage increases are made by adding 0.05 mg first in the morning, then at noon, and then in the evening every 3–5 days to a maximum total daily dose of 0.3 mg in three or four divided doses per day. The half-life of clonidine is in the range of 3–4 hours. Although a clinical response generally becomes apparent by about 4 weeks, treatment effects may increase over 2–3 months. Therapeutic doses of methylphenidate can frequently be decreased by 30–50% when used in conjunction with clonidine. Transdermal administration of clonidine using a skin patch can be quite effective but may result in skin irritation in 40% of patients. Patches are generally changed every 5 days.

The starting dosage of guanfacine is usually 0.5–1 mg once a day, increasing as clinically indicated after 3–5 days to 2–4 mg/d in two or three divided doses per day. Adverse effects include transient headaches and stomach aches in 25% of patients. Sedation and hypertension are mild. For medical follow-up, pulse and blood pressure should be checked every 1–2 weeks for 2 months and then at 3-month intervals.

E. ADVERSE EFFECTS

Sedation can be prominent. Side effects include fatigability, dizziness associated with hypotension, increased appetite and weight gain, headache, sleep disturbance, GI distress, skin irritation with transdermal clonidine administration, and rebound hypertension with abrupt withdrawal. Bradycardia can occasionally be marked.

F. DRUG INTERACTIONS

Increased sedation with CNS depressants; possible increased anticholinergic toxicity. Several case reports have mentioned cardiac toxicity with clonidine when combined with methylphenidate, although other medications and clinical factors were present in each case.

G. MEDICAL FOLLOW-UP

Pulse and blood pressure should be recorded every 2 weeks for 2 months and then every 3 months. The discontinuation of clonidine or guanfacine should occur gradually, with stepwise dosage decreases every 3–5 days to avoid rebound hypertension. Blood pressure should be monitored during withdrawal.

REFERENCES

Ambrosini PJ et al: Multicenter open-label sertraline study in adolescent outpatients with major depression. J Am Acad Child Adolesc Psychiatry 1999;38:566 [PMID: 10230188].

Baumgartner JL, Emslie GJ, Crismon ML: Citalopram in children and adolescents with depression or anxiety. Ann Pharmacother 2002;36:1692 [PMID: 12398561].

Biederman J: Attention-deficit/hyperactivity disorder: a selective overview. Biol Psychiatry 2005;57:1215 [PMID: 15949990].

Birmaher B et al: Fluoxetine for the treatment of childhood anxiety disorders. J Am Acad Child Adolesc Psychiatry 2003;42:415 [PMID: 12649628].

Campbell M et al: Antipsychotics in children and adolescents. J Am Acad Child Adolesc Psychiatry 1999;38:537 [PMID: 10230185].

Compton SN et al: Sertraline in children and adolescents with social anxiety disorder: An open trial. J Am Acad Child Adolesc Psychiatry 2001;40:564 [PMID: 11349701].

Courtney DB: Selective serotonin reuptake inhibitor and venlafaxine use in children and adolescents with major depressive disorder: a systematic review of published randomized controlled trials. Can J Psychiatry 2004;49:557 [PMID: 1543105].

DelBello M, Greevich S: Phenomenology and epidemiology of childhood psychiatric disorders that may necessitate treatment with atypical antipsychotics. J Clin Psychiatry 2004;65(Suppl 6):12 [PMID: 15104522].

Emslie GJ et al: Fluoxetine for acute treatment of depression in children and adolescents; a placebo-controlled randomized clinical trial. J Am Acad Child Adolesc Psychiatry 2002;41:1205 [PMID: 12364842].

Emslie GJ et al: Predictors of response to treatment in children and adolescents with mood disorders. Psychiatr Clin North Am 2003;26:435 [PMID: 12778842].

Galanter CA et al: Response to methylphenidate in children with ADHD and manic symptoms in the multimodal treatment study of children with ADHD titration trial. J Child Adolesc Psychopharmacol 2003;13:123 [PMID: 12880507].

Geller B et al: Critical review of tricyclic antidepressant use in children and adolescents. J Am Acad Child Adolesc Psychiatry 1999;38:513 [PMID: 10230182].

Greenhill LL et al: Developing methodologies for monitoring long-term safety of psychotropic medications: Report on the NIMH conference, Sept. 25, 2000. J Am Acad Child Adolesc Psychiatry 2003;42:651 [PMID: 12921472].

Green WH: *Child and Adolescent Psychopharmacology,* 3rd ed. Lippincott Williams & Wilkins, 2001.

Hellings JA et al: Weight gain in a controlled study of risperidone in children, adolescents and adults with mental retardation and autism. J Child Adolesc Psychopharmacol 2001;11:229 [PMID: 11642473].

Hughes CW et al: The Texas Children's Medication Algorithm Project: Report of the Texas Consensus Conference Panel on Medication Treatment of Childhood Major Depressive Disorder. J Am Acad Child Adolesc Psychiatry 1999;38:1442 [PMID: 10560232].

Kaftantaris V et al: Lithium treatment of acute mania in adolescents: A large open trial. J Am Acad Child Adolesc Psychiatry 2003;42:1038 [PMID: 12960703].

Keller MB et al: Efficacy of paroxetine in the treatment of adolescent major depression: A randomized controlled trial. J Am Acad Child Adolesc Psychiatry 2001;40:762 [PMID: 11437014].

Kowatch RA, Delbello MP: The use of mood stabilizers and atypical antipsychotics in children and adolescents with bipolar disorders. CNS Spectr 2003;8:273 [PMID: 12679742].

Kowatch RA et al: Combination pharmacotherapy in children and adolescents with bipolar disorder. Biol Psychiatry 2003;53:978 [PMID: 12788243].

Kowatch RA et al: Effect size of lithium, divalproex sodium and carbamazepine in children and adolescents with bipolar disorder. J Am Acad Child Adolesc Psychiatry 2000;39:713 [PMID: 10846305].

Kratochvil CJ et al: Pharmacotherapy of childhood anxiety disorders. Curr Psychiatry Rep 2002;4:264 [PMID: 12126594].

Labellarte MJ et al: The relevance of prolonged QTc measurement to pediatric psychopharmacology. J Am Acad Child Adolesc Psychiatry 2003;42:642 [PMID: 12921471].

March JS, Vitiello B: Advances in paediatric neuropsychopharmacology: An overview. Int J Neuropsychopharmacol 2001; 4:141 [PMID: 11466164].

McClellan JM, Werry JS: Evidence-based treatments in child and adolescent psychiatry. J Am Acad Child Adolesc Psychiatry 2003;42:1388 [PMID: 14627873].

Pliszka SR et al: A feasibility study of the children's medication algorithm project (CMAP) for the treatment of ADHD. J Am Acad Child Adolesc Psychiatry 2003;42:279 [PMID: 12595780].

Plizka SR: Non-stimulant treatment of attention-deficit/hyperactivity disorder. CNS Spectr 2003;8:253 [PMID: 12679740].

Rosenberg DR et al: *Pocket Guide for the Textbook of Child and Adolescent Psychiatric Disorders.* Taylor & Francis, 1998.

Ryan ND: Child and adolescent depression: Short-term treatment effectiveness and long-term opportunities. Int J Methods Psychiatr Res 2003;12:44 [PMID: 12830309].

Ryan ND et al: Mood stabilizers in children and adolescents. J Am Acad Child Adolesc Psychiatry 1999;38:529 [PMID: 10230184].

Ryan ND: Medication treatment for depression in children and adolescents. CNS Spectr 2003;8:283 [PMID: 12679743].

Scahill L et al: Lithium in children and adolescents. J Child Adolesc Psychiatr Nurs 2001;14:89 [PMID: 11883628].

Simeon J, Milin R, Walker S: A retrospective chart review of risperidone use in treatment-resistant children and adolescents with psychiatric disorders. Prog Neuropsychopharmacol Biol Psychiatry 2002;26:267 [PMID: 11817503].

Steiner H et al: Psychopharmacologic strategies for the treatment of aggression in juveniles. CNS Spectr 2003;8:298 [PMID: 12679744].

Wagner KD: Pharmacotherapy for major depression in children and adolescents. Prog Neuropsychopharmacol Biol Psychiatry 2005;29:819 [PMID: 15908090].

Walkup J et al: Treatment of pediatric anxiety disorders: An open-label extension of the research units pediatric psychopharmacology anxiety study. J Child Adolesc Psychopharmacol 2002;12:175 [PMID: 12427292].

Whittington CJ et al: Selective serotonin reuptake inhibitors in childhood depression: systematic review of published vs. unpublished data. Lancet 2004;363:1341 [PMID: 15110490].

Child Abuse & Neglect

7

Andrew P. Sirotnak, MD, & Richard D. Krugman, MD

The problem of child abuse and neglect, barely recognized as a significant problem in the early editions of this textbook, has grown to a problem of such serious proportions that in 1990 the U.S. Advisory Board on Child Abuse and Neglect called the present state of the nation's ability to protect children a "national emergency." Over a decade later and into the 21st century, the emergency is still with us. What Dr. Henry Kempe and his colleagues first called battered child syndrome was thought to affect 749 children in the United States in 1960. The best data now available suggest that 1–1.5% of American children are abused or neglected annually. In 2004 an estimated 3 million children were reported to child protective service agencies as alleged victims of child abuse and neglect, which translates to an approximate national referral rate of 43 referrals per 1000 children. Just under one million of these cases were substantiated by child protective services in 2004, yielding an abuse victimization rate of 11.9 per 1000 American children. At least 2000 children are victims of fatal child abuse each year and in 2004 the rate of child abuse death was 2.03 per 100,000 children. This dramatic increase in cases has resulted from increased recognition of the problem by professionals, partly in response to statutory reporting mandates, a broadening of the definitions of abuse and neglect from the original battered child concept, and changes in the demography and social structure of families and neighborhoods over the past several decades. Substance abuse, poverty and economic strains, parental capacity and skills, and domestic violence are cited as the most common presenting problems in abusive families.

Abuse and neglect of children are best considered in an ecological perspective, which recognizes the individual, family, social, and psychological influences that come together to contribute to the problem. For most pediatric health care professionals, however, their involvement will be limited to individual cases. This chapter focuses on the knowledge necessary for the recognition, intervention, and follow-up of the more common forms of child maltreatment and highlights the role of pediatric professionals in prevention.

FORMS OF CHILD MALTREATMENT

Child maltreatment may occur either within or outside the family. The proportion of intrafamilial to extrafa-milial cases varies with the type of abuse as well as the gender and age of child. Each of the following conditions may exist as separate or concurrent diagnoses. Neglect is the most commonly reported and substantiated form of child maltreatment annually.

Physical Abuse

Physical abuse of children is most often inflicted by a caregiver or family member but occasionally by a stranger. The most common manifestations include bruises, burns, fractures, head trauma, and abdominal injuries. A small but significant number of unexpected pediatric deaths, particularly in infants and very young children (eg, sudden infant death syndrome or sudden unexpected infant death), are related to physical abuse.

Sexual Abuse

Sexual abuse is defined as the engaging of dependent, developmentally immature children in sexual activities that they do not fully comprehend and to which they cannot give consent, or activities that violate the laws and taboos of a society. It includes all forms of incest, sexual assault or rape, and pedophilia. This includes fondling, oral-genital-anal contact, all forms of intercourse or penetration, exhibitionism, voyeurism, exploitation or prostitution, and the involvement of children in the production of pornography.

Emotional Abuse

Emotional or psychological abuse has been defined as the rejection, ignoring, criticizing, isolation, or terrorizing of children, all of which have the effect of eroding their self-esteem. The most common form is verbal abuse or denigration. Children who witness domestic violence should be considered emotionally abused.

Physical Neglect

Physical neglect is the failure to provide the necessary food, clothing, and shelter and a safe environment in which children can grow and develop. Although often associated with poverty or ignorance, physical neglect involves a more serious problem than just lack of resources. There is often a component of emotional neglect and either a failure or an inability, intentionally or otherwise, to recognize and respond to the needs of the child.

Emotional Neglect

The most common feature of emotional neglect is the absence of normal parent-child attachment and a subsequent inability to recognize and respond to an infant's or child's needs. A common manifestation of emotional neglect in infancy is nutritional (nonorganic) failure to thrive.

Medical Care Neglect

Medical care neglect is failure to provide the needed treatment to infants or children with life-threatening illness or other serious or chronic medical conditions.

Münchhausen Syndrome By Proxy

Münchhausen syndrome by proxy is a relatively unusual disorder in which a caregiver, usually the mother, either simulates or creates the symptoms or signs of illness in a child. The child can present with a long list of medical problems or often bizarre recurrent complaints. Persistent doctor shopping and enforced invalidism (eg, not accepting that the child is healthy and reinforcing that the child is somehow ill) are also described in the original definition of Münchhausen syndrome by proxy. Fatal cases have been reported.

RECOGNITION OF ABUSE & NEGLECT

The most common features suggesting a diagnosis of child abuse are summarized in Tables 7–1 and 7–2. Obvious signs of injury, sexual abuse, or neglect may be present. Classic radiographic and laboratory findings are discussed later in this chapter. Psychosocial factors may indicate risk for or confirm child maltreatment.

Table 7–1. Common historical features in child abuse cases.

Discrepant, evolving, or absent history
Delay in seeking care
Event or behavior by child that triggers a loss of control of caregiver
History of abuse in the caregiver's childhood
Inappropriate affect of the caregiver
Pattern of increasing severity or number of injuries if no intervention
Social or physical isolation of the child or the caregiver
Stress or crisis in the family or the caregiver
Unrealistic expectations of caregiver for the child

Table 7–2. Presentations of sexual abuse.

General or direct statements about sexual abuse
Sexualized knowledge, play, or behavior in developmentally immature children
Sexual abuse of other children by the victim
Behavioral changes
Sleep disturbances (eg, nightmares and night terrors)
Appetite disturbances (eg, anorexia, bulimia)
Depression, social withdrawal, anxiety
Aggression, temper tantrums, impulsiveness
Neurotic or conduct disorders, phobias or avoidant behaviors
Guilt, low self-esteem, mistrust, feelings of helplessness
Hysterical or conversion reactions
Suicidal, runaway threats or behavior
Excessive masturbation
Medical conditions
Recurrent abdominal pain or frequent somatic complaints
Genital, anal, or urethral trauma
Recurrent complaints of genital or anal pain, discharge, bleeding
Enuresis or encopresis
Sexually transmitted infections
Pregnancy
Promiscuity or prostitution, sexual dysfunction, fear of intimacy
School problems or truancy
Substance abuse

Recognition of any form of abuse and neglect of children can occur only if child abuse is entertained in the differential diagnosis of the child's presenting medical condition. The approach to the family should be supportive, nonaccusatory, and empathetic. The individual who brings the child in for care may not have any involvement in the abuse. Approximately one-third of child abuse incidents occur in extrafamilial settings. Nevertheless, the assumption that the caregiver is "nice," combined with the failure to consider the possibility of abuse, can be costly and even fatal. Raising the possibility that a child has been abused is not the same as accusing the caregiver of being the abuser. The health professional who is examining the child can explain to the family that several possibilities might explain the child's injuries or abuse-related symptoms. If the family or presenting caregiver is not involved in the child's maltreatment, they may actually welcome the necessary report and investigation.

History

A. Physical Abuse

The medical diagnosis of physical abuse is based on the presence of a discrepant history, in which the history offered by the caregiver is not consistent with the clinical findings. The discrepancy may exist because the history is absent, partial, changing over time, or simply illogical or improbable. The presence of a discrepant history should prompt a request for consultation with a multidisciplinary child protection team or a report to the child protective services agency. This agency is mandated by state law to investigate reports of suspected child abuse and neglect. Investigation by social services and possibly law enforcement officers, as well as a home visit, may be required to sort out the circumstances of the child's injuries. Other common historical features in child abuse cases are listed in Table 7–1.

B. Sexual Abuse

Sexual abuse may come to the clinician's attention in different ways: (1) The child may be brought in for routine care or for an acute problem, and sexual abuse may be suspected by the medical professional as a result of the history or the physical examination. (2) The parent or caregiver, suspecting that the child may have been sexually abused, may bring the child to the health care provider and request an examination to rule in or rule out abuse. (3) The child may be referred by child protective services or the police for an evidentiary examination following either disclosure of sexual abuse by the child or an allegation of abuse by a parent or third party. Table 7–2 lists the presentations of child sexual abuse. It should be emphasized that with the exception of acute trauma, certain sexually transmitted infections (STIs), or forensic laboratory evidence, none of these presentations is specific. The presentations listed should arouse suspicion of the possibility of sexual abuse and lead the practitioner to ask the appropriate questions—again, in a compassionate and nonaccusatory manner. The American Academy of Pediatrics has published guidelines for the evaluation of child sexual abuse as well as other guidelines relating to child maltreatment.

C. Emotional Abuse

Emotional abuse may cause nonspecific symptoms in children. Loss of self-esteem or self-confidence, sleep disturbances, somatic symptoms (eg, headaches and stomach aches), hypervigilance, or avoidant or phobic behaviors (eg, school refusal or running away) may be presenting complaints. These complaints may also be seen in children who experience domestic violence. Emotional abuse can occur in the home or day care, school, sports team, or other settings.

D. Neglect

Even though in 2004 there were three times as many reports of neglect of children as of physical abuse, neglect is not easily documented on history. Physical neglect—which must be differentiated from the deprivations of poverty—will be present even after adequate social services have been provided to families in need. Emotionally neglectful parents appear to have an inability to recognize the physical or emotional states of their children. For example, an emotionally neglectful parent may ignore an infant's cry if the cry is perceived incorrectly as an expression of anger. This misinterpretation leads to inadequate nutrition and failure to thrive. The clinician must evaluate the psychosocial history and family dynamics when neglect is a consideration, and a careful social services investigation of the home and entire family may be required.

E. Failure to Thrive

The history offered in cases of failure to thrive is often at odds with the physical findings. Infants who have experienced a significant deceleration in growth are probably not receiving adequate amounts or appropriate types of food despite the dietary history provided. Medical conditions causing poor growth in infancy and early childhood can be ruled out with a detailed history and minimal laboratory tests. A psychosocial history may reveal maternal depression, family chaos or dysfunction, or other previously unknown social risk factors (eg, substance abuse, violence, poverty, or psychiatric illness). Placement of the child with another caregiver or hospitalization of the severely malnourished patient is usually followed by a dramatic weight gain.

Physical Findings

A. Physical Abuse

The findings on examination of physically abused children may include abrasions, alopecia, bites, bruises, burns, dental trauma, fractures, lacerations, ligature marks, or scars. Injuries may be in multiple stages of healing. Bruises in physically abused children are sometimes patterned (eg, belt marks, looped cord marks, or grab or pinch marks) and are typically found over the soft tissue areas of the body. Toddlers or older children typically sustain accidental bruises over bony prominences such as shins and elbows. Any bruise in an infant not developmentally mobile should be viewed with concern. (Other child abuse emergencies are listed in Table 7–3.) Lacerations of the frenulum or tongue and bruising of the lips may be associated with force feeding. Pathognomonic burn patterns include stocking or glove distribution; immersion burns of the buttocks, sometimes with a "doughnut hole" area of sparing; and branding burns such as with cigarettes or hot objects (eg, grill, curling iron, or lighter). The absence of splash marks or a pattern consistent with spillage may be helpful in differentiating accidental from nonaccidental scald burns.

Head and abdominal trauma may present with signs and symptoms consistent with those injuries. Inflicted head trauma (eg, shaken baby syndrome) and abdominal injuries may have no visible findings on

Table 7–3. Potential child abuse medical emergencies.

Any infant with bruises (especially head, facial, or abdominal), burns, or fractures

Any infant or child under age 2 years with a history of suspected "shaken baby" head trauma or other inflicted head injury

Any child who has sustained suspicious or known inflicted abdominal trauma

Any child with burns in stocking or glove distribution or in other unusual patterns, burns to the genitalia, and any unexplained burn injury

Any child with disclosure or sign of sexual assault within 48–72 hours after the alleged event if the possibility of acute injury is present or if forensic evidence exists

---

examination. The finding of retinal hemorrhages in an infant without an appropriate medical condition (eg, leukemia, congenital infection, or clotting disorder) should arouse concern about possible inflicted head trauma. Retinal hemorrhages are not commonly seen after cardiopulmonary resuscitation in either infants or children.

B. SEXUAL ABUSE

The genital and anal findings of sexually abused children, as well as the normal developmental changes and variations in prepubertal female hymens, have been described in journal articles and visual diagnosis guides. The majority of victims of sexual abuse exhibit no physical findings. The reasons for this include delay in disclosure by the child, abuse that may cause no physical trauma (eg, fondling, oral-genital contact, or exploitation by pornographic photography), or rapid healing of minor injuries such as labial, hymenal, or anal abrasions, contusions, or lacerations. Nonspecific abnormalities of the genital and rectal regions such as erythema, rashes, and irritation may not suggest sexual abuse in the absence of a corroborating history, disclosure, or behavioral changes. Finally, some medical conditions may be misdiagnosed as sexual abuse (eg, vulvovaginitis, lichen sclerosus, dermatitis, labial adhesions, congenital urethral or vulvar disorders, Crohn's disease, and accidental straddle injuries to the labia) and can be ruled out by careful history and examination.

Certain STIs should strongly suggest sexual abuse. *Neisseria gonorrhoeae* infection or syphilis beyond the perinatal period are diagnostic of sexual abuse. *Chlamydia trachomatis,* herpes simplex virus, trichomoniasis, and human papillomavirus are all sexually transmitted, although the course of these perinatally acquired infections may be protracted. In the case of human papillomavirus, an initial appearance of venereal warts beyond the toddler age should raise concerns about sexual abuse. Finally, sexual abuse must be considered with the diagnosis of human immunodeficiency virus infection when other modes of transmission (eg, transfusion or perinatal acquisition) have been ruled out. The Centers for Disease Control and Prevention and many sexual abuse atlases list guidelines for the screening and treatment of STIs in sexually abused children and adolescents. Finally, non-culture tests such as nucleic acid amplification tests have not yet been approved for the screening of STIs in sexual abuse victims or for children under 12 years of age due to specificity and sensitivity concerns. Symptomatic patients should be cultured.

C. NEGLECT AND NONORGANIC FAILURE TO THRIVE

Infants and children with nonorganic failure to thrive have a relative absence of subcutaneous fat in the cheeks, buttocks, and extremities. Other conditions associated with poor nutrient and vitamin intake may be present. If the condition has persisted for some time, these patients may also appear and act depressed. Older children who have been chronically emotionally neglected may also have short stature (ie, deprivation dwarfism). The head circumference is usually normal in cases of nonorganic failure to thrive. Microcephaly may signify a prenatal condition, congenital disease, or chronic nutritional deprivation and increases the likelihood of more serious and possibly permanent developmental delay.

D. MÜNCHHAUSEN SYNDROME BY PROXY

Children with Münchhausen syndrome by proxy may present with the signs and symptoms of whatever illness is factitiously produced or simulated. They may be actually ill or, more often, are reported to be ill and have a normal clinical appearance. Among the most common reported presentations are recurrent apnea, dehydration from induced vomiting or diarrhea, sepsis when contaminants are injected into a child, change in mental status, fever, gastrointestinal bleeding, and seizures.

Radiologic & Laboratory Findings

A. PHYSICAL ABUSE

Certain radiologic findings are strong indicators of physical abuse. Examples are metaphyseal "corner" or "bucket handle" fractures of the long bones in infants, spiral fracture of the extremities in nonambulatory infants, rib fractures, spinous process fractures, and fractures in multiple stages of healing. Skeletal surveys in children age 3 years or younger should be performed when a suspicious fracture is diagnosed. Computed tomography or magnetic resonance imaging findings of subdural hemorrhage in infants—in the absence of a clear accidental history—are highly correlated with abusive head trauma, especially after the advent of infant seat restraint laws that have reduced the incidence of head trauma in infants. Abdominal computed tomography is the preferred test in suspected abdominal trauma. Any infant or very young child with suspected abuse-related head or abdominal trauma should be evaluated immediately by an emergency physician or trauma surgeon.

Coagulation studies and a complete blood cell count with platelets are useful in children who present with multiple or severe bruising in different stages of healing. Coagulopathy conditions may confuse the diagnostic picture but can be excluded with a careful history, examination, laboratory screens, and hematologic consultation if necessary.

The differential diagnosis of all forms of physical abuse can be considered in the context of a detailed trauma history, family medical history, radiographic findings, and laboratory testing. The diagnosis of osteogenesis imperfecta or other collagen disorders, for example, may be considered in the child with skin and joint findings or multiple fractures with or without the classic radiographic presentation and is best made in consultation with a geneticist, an orthopedic surgeon, and a radiologist. Trauma—accidental or inflicted—leads the differential diagnosis list for subdural hematomas. Coagulopathy; disorders of copper, amino acid, or organic acid metabolism (eg, Menkes syndrome and glutaric acidemia type 1); chronic or previous central nervous system infection; birth trauma; or congenital central nervous system malformation (eg, arteriovenous malformations or cerebrospinal fluid collections) may need to be ruled out in some cases. It should be recognized, however, that children with these rare disorders can also be abuse victims.

B. Sexual Abuse

The forensic evaluation of sexually abused children should be performed in a setting that prevents further emotional distress. If the history indicates that the child may have had contact with the ejaculate of a perpetrator within 72 hours, an examination looking for semen or its markers (eg, acid phosphatase) should be performed according to established protocols. This should occur in an emergency department or clinic where chain of custody for specimens can be assured. More important, if there is a history of possible sexual abuse within the past 48–72 hours, and the child reports a physical complaint or a sign is observed (eg, genital or anal bleeding or discharge), the child should be examined for signs of trauma. The most experienced examiner (pediatrician, nurse examiner, or child advocacy center) is preferable. The laboratory and serologic evaluation of STIs should be guided by the type of contact reported and the epidemiology of these infections in the community.

C. Neglect and Growth Failure

Children with failure to thrive or malnutrition may not require an extensive work-up. Complete blood cell count, urinalysis, electrolyte panel, and liver function tests are sufficient screening. Newborn screening should be documented as usual. Other tests should be guided by any clinical history that points to a previously undiagnosed condition (eg, thyroid or metabolic studies). A skeletal survey and head computed tomography scan may be helpful if concurrent physical abuse is suspected. The best screening method, however, is placement in a setting in which the child can be fed and monitored. Hospital or foster care placement may be required. Weight gain may not occur for several days to a week in severe cases.

Any child with recurrent polymicrobial sepsis (especially in children with indwelling catheters), recurrent apnea, chronic dehydration of unknown cause, or other highly unusual unexplained laboratory findings should raise the suspicion of Münchhausen syndrome by proxy.

MANAGEMENT & REPORTING OF CHILD ABUSE & NEGLECT

Physical abuse injuries, STIs, and medical sequelae of neglect should be treated immediately. Children with failure to thrive related to emotional and physical neglect need to be placed in a setting in which they can be fed and cared for. Likewise, the child in danger of recurrent abuse or neglect needs to be placed in a safe environment.

In the United States, clinicians and many other professionals who come in contact with or care for children are mandated reporters. If abuse or neglect is suspected, a report must be made to the local or state agency designated to investigate such matters. In most cases, this will be the child protective services agency. Law enforcement agencies may also receive such reports. The purpose of the report is to permit professionals to gather the information needed to determine whether the child's environment (eg, home, school, day care setting, or foster home) is safe. Many hospitals and communities make child protection teams or consultants available when there are questions about the diagnosis and management in a child abuse case. A listing of pediatric consultants in child abuse is available from the American Academy of Pediatrics.

Except in extreme cases, the reporting of emotional abuse is not likely to generate a response from child protection agencies. This should not deter reporting, especially if the concern is in the context of domestic violence or other forms of abuse or neglect. Practitioners can encourage parents to get involved with parent effectiveness training programs (eg, Healthy Families America or Parents Anonymous) or to seek mental health consultation. Support for the child may also include mental health counseling or age-appropriate peer and mentoring activities in school or the community.

PREVENTION OF CHILD ABUSE & NEGLECT

Physical abuse is preventable in many cases. Extensive experience with and evaluation of high-risk families have shown that the provision of home visitor services to families at risk can prevent abuse and neglect of children. These services can be provided by public health nurses or trained paraprofessionals, although more data are available describing public health nurse intervention. This makes it as easy for the family to pick up the telephone and ask for help before they abuse a child as it is for a neighbor or physician to report an episode of abuse after it has occurred. Parent education and anticipatory guidance may also be helpful, particularly with respect to handling situations that stress parents (eg, colic, crying behavior, and toilet training), age-appropriate discipline, and general developmental issues. Prevention of abusive injuries perpetrated by nonparent caregivers (eg, babysitters, nannies, and unrelated adults in the home) may be addressed by education and counseling of mothers about safe child care arrangements and advocating for affordable day care for all families.

The prevention of sexual abuse is more difficult. Most efforts in this area involve teaching children to protect themselves and their "private parts" from harm or interference. These programs are useful but are in general not as efficacious as they are necessary. The age of toilet training is a good anticipatory guidance time to encourage parents to consider this discussion. The most rational approach is to place the burden of responsibility of prevention on the adults who supervise the child and the medical providers rather than on the children themselves.

Efforts to prevent emotional abuse of children have been undertaken through extensive media campaigns. No data are available to assess the effectiveness of this approach. The primary care physician can promote positive, nurturing, and nonviolent behavior in parents. Screening for domestic violence during anticipatory guidance discussions on discipline and home and safety can be effective in identifying parents and children at risk.

REFERENCES

2002 Guidelines for the treatment of sexually transmitted diseases. MMWR Morb Mortal Wkly Rep 2002;(RR-6):51. Available at: www.cdc.gov/std/treatment/rr5106.pdf

American Academy of Pediatrics: Clinical Report: The Evaluation of Sexual Abuse of Children. Pediatrics 2005;116:506 [PMID: 16061610].

American Academy of Pediatrics: Diagnostic imaging of child abuse. Pediatrics 2000;105:1345 [PMID:10835079]

American Academy of Pediatrics: Rotational cranial injury—technical report. Pediatrics 2001;108:206 [PMID:11433079].

American Academy of Pediatrics: *Visual Diagnosis of Child Abuse.* [CD ROM], 2nd ed, 2002.

American Academy of Pediatrics: *Visual Diagnosis of Child Sexual Abuse.* [Slide Set Atlas] American Academy of Pediatrics, 2002.

Augustyn M, McAlister B: If we don't ask, they aren't going to tell: screening for domestic violence. Contemp Pediatr 2005;22:43.

Berkowitz CD: Recognizing and responding to domestic violence. Pediatr Ann 2005;34:395.

DeBellis MD: The psychobiology of neglect [Review]. Child Maltreat 2005;10:150 [PMID: 15798010].

Giardino AP, Finkel MA: Evaluating child sexual abuse [Review]. Pediatr Ann 2005;34:382 [PMID: 15948349].

Horner G: Domestic violence and children. J Pediatr Health Care 2005;19:206 [PMID: 16010259].

Johnson CF: Child sexual abuse [Review]. Lancet 2004;364:462 [PMID: 15288746].

Krous HF et al: Sudden infant death syndrome and unclassified sudden infant deaths: a definitional and diagnostic approach. Pediatrics 2004;114:234 [PMID: 15231934].

Malloy MH, MacDorman M: Changes in the classification of sudden infant deaths: United States 1992–2001. Pediatrics 2005;115:1247 [PMID: 15867031].

Mears DP, Visher CA: Trends in understanding and addressing domestic violence. J Interpers Violence 2005;20:204 [PMID: 15601793].

Olds DL et al: Effects of home visits by paraprofessionals and by nurses: age 4 follow-up results of a randomized trial. Pediatrics 2004;114:1560 [PMID: 15574615].

Olds DL: Prenatal and infancy home visitation by nurses: From randomized trials to community replication. Prev Sci 2002;3:153 [PMID: 12387552].

Schreier H: Münchhausen Syndrome by Proxy [Review]. Current Probl Pediatr Adolesc Health Care 2004;34:126 [PMID 15039661].

Sirotnak AP, Grigsby T, Krugman RD: Physical abuse of children. Pediatr Rev 2004;25:264 [PMID: 15286272].

Thompson S: Accidental or inflicted? [Review] Pediatr Ann 2005;34:372.

U.S. Department of Health and Human Services: Administration for Children, Youth, and Families. Child Maltreatment 2003. Available at: http//www.acf.hhs.gov/programs/cb/stats_research/index.htm

Ambulatory & Community Pediatrics

8

Robert M. Brayden, MD, Matthew F. Daley, MD, & Jeffrey M. Brown, MD, MPH

Pediatric ambulatory outpatient services provide children and adolescents with comprehensive longitudinal care comprised of preventive health care and acute and chronic care management services and consultations. In this chapter, special attention is given to the pediatric history and physical examination, normal developmental stages, office telephone management, and community pediatrics.

The development of a physician-patient-parent relationship is crucially important if the patient and parent are to effectively confide their concerns. This relationship develops over time with increasing numbers of visits and is facilitated by the continuity of clinicians and other staff members. This clinical relationship is based on trust that comes as a result of several experiences in the context of the office visit. Perhaps the greatest factor to facilitate the relationship is for patients or parents to experience advice as valid and effective. Skills such as choosing vocabulary that communicates understanding and competence, commitment of time and attention to the concern, and respect for areas that the patient or parent does not wish to address (assuming the lack of physical/sexual abuse or neglect concerns) are important. Parents and patients expect that their concerns will be managed confidentially and that the clinician understands and sympathizes with those concerns. The effective physician-patient-parent relationship is one of the most satisfying aspects of ambulatory pediatrics.

■ PEDIATRIC HISTORY

A unique feature of pediatrics is that the history represents an amalgam of parents' objective reporting of facts (eg, fever for 4 days), parents' subjective interpretation of their child's symptoms (eg, an infant crying that is interpreted by parents as abdominal pain), and for older children their own history of events. Parents and patients may provide a specific and detailed history, or a vague history that necessitates more focused probing. Parents may or may not be able to distinguish whether symptoms are caused by organic illness or a psychological concern. It is often helpful to ask specifically what problems the parents wish to address in order to determine what really prompted the office visit. Some visits are occasioned by problems at school, such as low grades or troublesome peer relationships. Understanding the family and its hopes for and concerns about the child can help in the process of distinguishing organic illness from emotional or behavioral conditions, thus minimizing unnecessary testing and intervention.

Although the parents' concerns need to be understood, it is essential also to obtain as much of the history as possible directly from the patient. Direct histories not only provide first-hand information, but also give the child a degree of control over a potentially threatening situation and may reveal important information about the family.

Obtaining a comprehensive pediatric history is time-consuming. Many offices provide questionnaires for parents to complete before the clinician sees the child. Data from questionnaires can make an outpatient visit more productive, allowing the physician to address problems in detail while more quickly reviewing areas that are not of concern. Questionnaires may be more productive than face-to-face interviews in revealing sensitive parts of the history. However, failure to review and assimilate this information prior to the interview may cause a parent or patient to feel that the time and effort have been wasted.

Elements of the history that will be useful over time should be readily accessible in the medical record. Such information can be accumulated on a summary sheet, as illustrated in Figure 8–1. Demographic data; a problem list; information about chronic medications, allergies, and previous hospitalizations; and the names of other physicians providing care for the patient are commonly included. Documentation of immunizations, including all data required by the National Childhood Vaccine Injury Act, should be kept on a second page.

25

Name _____ Nickname _____ D.O.B. _____

Mother _____ Father _____ Sibs _____

S.S. # _____ Insurance _____

Problems			Chronic Medications		
Date of onset	Description	Date resolved	Start date		Stop date
			Allergies (Center)		
			Date		
Date	**Hospitalizations/Injuries/Procedures**		Date	**Consultants**	

Figure 8–1. Use of a summary sheet such as this at the front of the record facilitates reorienting the caregiver and his or her partners to the patient. Some practices keep track of health supervision visits on this sheet to tell the physician whether the child is likely to have received the appropriate preventive services. A second page documenting immunizations should record data required by the National Childhood Vaccine Injury Act. When an allergy with potential for anaphylaxis is identified, the patient should wear a medical alert bracelet and obtain an epinephrine kit, if appropriate.

The components of a comprehensive pediatric history are listed in Table 8–1. Ideally, this information should be obtained at the first office visit. The first seven items may be included on a summary sheet at the front of the medical record. Items 8 and 9, and a focused review of systems, are dealt with at each acute or chronic care visit. The entire list should be reviewed and augmented with relevant updates at each health supervision visit.

■ PEDIATRIC PHYSICAL EXAMINATION

In approaching the child, time must be taken to allow the patient to become familiar with the examiner. Interactions and instructions help the child understand what

Table 8–1. Components of the pediatric historical database.[a]

1. Demographic data	Patient's name and nickname, date of birth, social security number, sex, race, parents' names (first and last), siblings' names, and payment mechanism.
2. Problem list	Major or significant problems, including dates of onset and resolution.
3. Allergies	Triggering allergen, nature of the reaction, treatment needed, and date allergy diagnosed.
4. Chronic medications	Name, concentration, dose, and frequency of chronically used medications.
5. Birth history	Maternal health during pregnancy, medications, street drugs used, complications of pregnancy; duration and ease of labor; form of delivery; analgesics and anesthetics used; need for monitoring; and labor complications. Infant's birth weight, gestational age, Apgar scores, and problems in the neonatal period.
6. Screening procedures	Results of newborn screening, vision and hearing screening, any health screen, or screening laboratory tests. (Developmental screening results are maintained in the development section; see item 14, below.)
7. Immunizations	Date of each immunization administered, vaccine manufacturer and lot number, and name and title of the person administering the vaccine; previous reaction and contraindication to immunization (eg, immunodeficiency or an evolving neurologic problem).
8. Reasons for visit	The patient's or parents' concerns, stated in their own words, serve as the focus for the visit.
9. Present illness	A concise chronologic summary of the problems necessitating a visit, including the duration, progression, exacerbating factors, ameliorating interventions, and associations.
10. Medical history	A statement regarding the child's functionality and general well-being, including a summary record of significant illnesses, injuries, hospitalizations, and procedures.
11. Diet	Eating patterns, likes and dislikes, use of vitamins, and relative amounts of carbohydrates, fat, and protein in the diet.
12. Family history	Information about the illnesses of relatives, preferably in the form of a family tree.
13. Social history	Family constellation, relationships, parents' educational background, religious preference, and the role of the child in the family; socioeconomic profile of the family to identify resources available to the child, access to services that may be needed, and anticipated stressors.
14. Development	(1) Attainment of developmental milestones (including developmental testing results); (2) social habits and milestones (toilet habits, play, major activities, sleep patterns, discipline, peer relationships); (3) school progress and documentation of specific achievements and grades.
15. Sexual history	Family's sexual attitudes, sex education, sexual development and activity, sexually transmitted diseases, and birth control measures.
16. Review of systems (ROS)	This area tends to be overlooked because of the work required to obtain a complete ROS and integrate data into the patient's problems list and care plan. A focused ROS is essential if any problem is to be addressed adequately.

[a]The components of this table should be included in a child's medical record and structured to allow easy review and modification. The practice name and address should appear on all pages.

is occurring and what is expected. A gentle, friendly manner and a quiet voice help establish a setting that yields a nonthreatening physical examination. The order in which the child's organ systems are examined should take into consideration the need for a quiet child, the extent of trust established, and the possibility of an emotional response. Painful or unpleasant procedures should be deferred until the end of the examination. Whether or not the physician can establish rapport with the child, the process should proceed efficiently and systematically.

Because young children may fear the examination and become fussy, simple inspection is very important. For example, during an acute care visit for fever, the examiner should observe the child's work of breathing prior to beginning the examination. During a health supervision visit, observation will provide the examiner with an opportunity to assess parent-child interactions.

Clothing should be removed slowly and gently to avoid threatening the child. A parent or the child himself or herself is usually the best person to do this. Modesty should always be respected, and gown or drapes should be provided. Examinations of adolescents should be chaperoned whenever a pelvic examination or a stressful or painful procedure is performed.

Examination tables are convenient, but a parent's lap is a safe haven for a young child. For most purposes, an adequate examination can be conducted on a "table" formed by the parent's and examiner's legs as they sit facing each other.

Although a thorough physical examination is important at every age, at some ages the examination tends to focus on specific issues and concerns. At any age, an astute clinician can detect signs of important clinical conditions in an asymptomatic child. In infancy, for example, physical examination can reveal the presence of craniosynostosis, congenital heart disease, or developmental dysplasia of the hip. Similarly, examination of a toddler may reveal pallor (from iron deficiency anemia) or strabismus. The routine examination of an adolescent may reveal scoliosis or acanthosis nigricans (a finding associated with insulin resistance).

■ HEALTH SUPERVISION VISITS

One of several timetables for recommended health supervision visits is illustrated in Figure 8–2. (**Note:** A PDF printable format of this figure is available at aap.org.) The federal Maternal and Child Health Bureau has developed comprehensive health supervision guidelines through their Bright Futures program (www.brightfutures.org). In areas where evidence-based information is lacking, expert opinion has been used as the basis for these plans. For example, immunizations are proven to be effective and necessary (Centers for Disease Control and Prevention, www.cdc.gov/nip), whereas there is disagreement about whether screening for certain metabolic diseases is universally warranted. Practitioners should remember that guidelines are not meant to be rigid; services should be individualized according to the child's needs.

During health supervision visits, the practitioner should review child development and acute and chronic problems, conduct a complete physical examination, order appropriate screening tests, and anticipate future developments. New historical information should be elicited through an interval history. Development should be assessed by parental report and clinician observation at each visit. Developmental surveillance is augmented with systematic use of parent-directed questionnaires or

screening tests. Growth is carefully recorded, and the growth chart is brought up to date. (See Chapter 2.) Vision and hearing should be assessed subjectively at each visit, with objective assessments at intervals beginning after the child is old enough to cooperate with the screening test, usually at 3 or 4 years of age. A variety of laboratory screening tests may also be part of the visit.

A major portion of the health supervision visit is anticipatory guidance. This portion of the visit enables the health care provider to address behavioral, developmental, injury prevention, nutritional issues, school problems, and other age-appropriate issues that will arise before the next well-child care visit.

American Academy of Pediatrics Committee on Practice and Ambulatory Medicine: Recommendations for Preventive Pediatric Health Care. Pediatrics 2000;105:645.

DEVELOPMENTAL & BEHAVIORAL ASSESSMENT

Addressing developmental and behavioral problems is one of the central features of pediatric primary care. The term *developmental delay* refers to the circumstance in which a child has not demonstrated a developmental skill (such as walking independently) by an age at which the majority of normally developing children have accomplished this task. Developmental delays are in fact quite common: approximately 18% of children under 18 years of age either have developmental delays, or have conditions that place them at risk for developmental delays.

Pediatric practitioners are in a unique position to assess the development of their patients. This developmental assessment should ideally take the form of *developmental surveillance,* in which a skilled individual monitors development over time as part of providing routine care. Developmental surveillance includes several key elements: listening to parent concerns; obtaining a developmental history; making careful observations during office visits; periodically screening all infants and children for delays using validated screening tools; recognizing conditions and circumstances that place children at increased risk of delays; and referring children who fail screening tests for further evaluation and intervention.

The prompt recognition of children with developmental delays is important for a number of reasons. The presence of delays may lead practitioners to diagnose unsuspected but important conditions, such as genetic syndromes or metabolic disorders. Children with delays can be referred for a wide range of developmental therapies, such as those provided by physical therapists and speech/language therapists. Importantly, children with delays, regardless of the cause, make bet-

Recommendations for Preventive Pediatric Health Care (RE9939)

Committee on Practice and Ambulatory Medicine

Each child and family is unique; therefore, these **Recommendations for Preventive Pediatric Health Care** are designed for the care of children who are receiving competent parenting, have no manifestations of any important health problems, and are growing and developing in satisfactory fashion. **Additional visits may become necessary** if circumstances suggest variations from normal.

These guidelines represent a consensus by the Committee on Practice and Ambulatory Medicine in consultation with national committees and sections of the American Academy of Pediatrics. The Committee emphasizes the great importance of **continuity of care** in comprehensive health supervision and the need to avoid **fragmentation of care.**

AGE[1]	PRENATAL[1]	NEWBORN[2]	2-4d[2,3]	By 1mo	2mo	4mo	6mo	9mo	12mo	15mo	18mo	24mo	3y	4y	5y	6y	8y	10y	11y	12y	13y	14y	15y	16y	17y	18y	19y	20y	21y
HISTORY Initial/Interval	●	●	●	●	●	●	●	●	●	●	●	●	●	●	●	●	●	●	●	●	●	●	●	●	●	●	●	●	●
MEASUREMENTS Height and Weight		●	●	●	●	●	●	●	●	●	●	●	●	●	●	●	●	●	●	●	●	●	●	●	●	●	●	●	●
Head Circumference		●	●	●	●	●	●	●	●	●	●	●																	
Blood Pressure													●	●	●	●	●	●	●	●	●	●	●	●	●	●	●	●	●
SENSORY SCREENING Vision		S	S	S	S	S	S	S	S	S	S	S	O	O	O	O	O	O	S	O	S	S	O	S	S	O	S	O	S
Hearing		O	S	S	S	S	S	S	S	S	S	S	O	O	O	O	O	O	S	O	S	S	O	S	S	O	S	O	S
DEVELOPMENTAL/ BEHAVIORAL ASSESSMENT[8]		●	●	●	●	●	●	●	●	●	●	●	●	●	●	●	●	●	●	●	●	●	●	●	●	●	●	●	●
PHYSICAL EXAMINATION[9]		●	●	●	●	●	●	●	●	●	●	●	●	●	●	●	●	●	●	●	●	●	●	●	●	●	●	●	●
PROCEDURES–GENERAL[10] Hereditary/Metabolic Screening[11]		←—→																											
Immunization[12]		●	●	●	●	●	●	●	●	●	●	●	●	●	●	●	●	●	●	●	●	●	●	●	●	●	●	●	●
Hematocrit or Hemoglobin[13]			←—————————→						●							●								●					
Urinalysis		●																											●
PROCEDURES–PATIENTS AT RISK Lead Screening[16]								←—————————————————————→																					
Tuberculin Test[17]										★					★			★											
Cholesterol Screening[18]																		★											
STD Screening[19]																			★	★	★	★	★	★	★	★	★	★	★
Pelvic Exam[20]																			★	★	★	★	★	★	★	★	★	★	★
ANTICIPATORY GUIDANCE[21] Injury Prevention[22]	●	●	●	●	●	●	●	●	●	●	●	●	●	●	●	●	●	●	●	●	●	●	●	●	●	●	●	●	●
Violence Prevention[23]	●	●	●	●	●	●	●	●	●	●	●	●	●	●	●	●	●	●	●	●	●	●	●	●	●	●	●	●	●
Sleep Positioning Counseling[24]	●	●	●	●	●	●	●																						
Nutrition Counseling[25]	●	●	●	●	●	●	●	●	●	●	●	●	●	●	●	●	●	●	●	●	●	●	●	●	●	●	●	●	●
DENTAL REFERRAL[26]													←——————————————————————————————→																

1. A prenatal visit is recommended for parents who are at high risk, for first-time parents, and for those who request a conference. The prenatal visit should include anticipatory guidance, pertinent medical history, and a discussion of benefits of breastfeeding and planned method of feeding per AAP statement "The Prenatal Visit"(1996).
2. Every infant should have a newborn evaluation after birth. Breastfeeding should be encouraged and instruction and support offered. Every breastfeeding infant should have an evaluation 48-72 hours after discharge from the hospital to include weight, formal breastfeeding evaluation, encouragement, and instruction as recommended in the AAP statement "Breastfeeding and the Use of Human Milk" (1997).
3. For newborns discharged in less than 48 hours after delivery per AAP statement "Hospital Stay for Healthy Term Newborns" (1995).
4. Developmental, psychosocial, and chronic disease issues for children and adolescents may require frequent counseling and treatment visits separate from preventive care visits.
5. If a child comes under care for the first time at any point on the schedule, or if any items are not accomplished at the suggested age, the schedule should be brought up to date at the earliest possible time.
6. If the patient is uncooperative, rescreen within 6 months.
7. All newborns should be screened per the AAP Task Force on Newborn and Infant Hearing statement, "Newborn and Infant Hearing Loss: Detection and Intervention" (1999).
8. By history and appropriate physical examination; if suspicious, by specific objective developmental testing. Parenting skills should be fostered at every visit.
9. At each visit, a complete physical examination is essential, with infant totally unclothed, older child undressed and suitably draped.
10. These may be modified, depending upon entry point into schedule and individual need.
11. Metabolic screening (eg, thyroid, hemoglobinopathies, PKU, galactosemia) should be done according to state law.
12. Schedule(s) per the Committee on Infectious Diseases, published annually in the January edition of Pediatrics. Every visit should be an opportunity to update and complete a child's immunizations.
13. See AAP Pediatric Nutrition Handbook (1998) for a discussion of universal and selective screening options. Consider earlier screening for high-risk infants (eg, premature infants and low birth weight infants). See also "Recommendations to Prevent and Control Iron Deficiency in the United States" MMWR. 1998;47 (RR-3);1-29.
14. All menstruating adolescents should be screened annually.
15. Conduct dipstick urinalysis for leukocytes annually for sexually active male and female adolescents.
16. For children at risk of lead exposure consult the AAP statement "Screening for Elevated Blood Levels"(1998). Additionally, screening should be done in accordance with state law where applicable.
17. TB testing per recommendations of the Committee on Infectious Diseases, published in the current edition of Red Book: Report of the Committee on Infectious Diseases. Testing should be done upon recognition of high-risk factors.
18. Cholesterol screening for high-risk patients per AAP statement "Cholesterol in Childhood"(1998). If family history cannot be ascertained and other risk factors are present, screening should be at the discretion of the physician.
19. All sexually active patients should be screened for sexually transmitted diseases (STDs).
20. All sexually active females should have a pelvic examination. A pelvic examination and routine pap smear should be offered as a part of preventive health maintenance between the ages of 18 and 21 years.
21. Age-appropriate discussion and counseling should be an integral part of each visit for care per the AAP Guidelines for Health Supervision III (1998).
22. From birth to age 12, refer to the AAP Injury prevention program (TIPP®) as described in A Guide to Safety Counseling in Office Practice (1994).
23. Violence prevention and management for all patients per AAP Statement "The Role of the Pediatrician in Youth Violence Prevention in Clinical Practice and at the Community Level" (1999).
24. Parents and caregivers should be advised to place healthy infants on their backs when putting them to sleep. Side positioning is a reasonable alternative but carries a slightly higher risk of SIDS. Consult the AAP statement "Changing Concepts of Sudden Infant Death Syndrome: Implications for Infant Sleeping Environment and Sleep Position"(2000).
25. Age-appropriate nutrition counseling should be an integral part of each visit per the AAP Handbook of Nutrition (1998).
26. Earlier initial dental examinations may be appropriate for some children. Subsequent examinations as prescribed by dentist.

Key:
● = to be performed
S = subjective, by history
★ = to be performed for patients at risk
O = objective, by a standard testing method
↕ = the range during which a service may be provided, with the dot indicating the preferred age.

American Academy of Pediatrics

Figure 8–2. Recommendations for preventive health care.

ter developmental progress if they receive appropriate developmental therapies than if they do not. Finally, many infants and toddlers under 3 years of age with developmental delays are eligible to receive a range of therapies and other services, often provided in the home, at no cost to families. Children 3 years and older with delays are also eligible for developmental services at no cost through the local school system.

While the benefits of early detection of developmental delays are clear, it is often difficult to incorporate developmental surveillance into busy outpatient practice. Only 30% of pediatricians routinely use formal screening tests, most relying on clinical judgment alone. However, when screening tests are not used, delays are often not detected until school age, particularly when the delays are not severe. There are several practical barriers to performing routine surveillance using standardized screening tools: perceived lack of time to screen all children at every well-child visit; lack of familiarity with the various screening tools; not wanting to concern parents by identifying a possible delay; and not knowing where in the community to refer patients with suspected delays. There are some solutions to these barriers, such as using parent developmental questionnaires rather than provider-administered tests to save time, getting to know one or two screening tests well, and making use of Internet-based resources. For example, the National Dissemination Center for Children and Youth with Disabilities maintains a website with links to a wide variety of resources in each state (www.nichcy.org).

There are a number of parent-administered and physician-administered developmental screening tools available. The Parents' Evaluation of Developmental Status, the Ages and Stages Questionnaires, and the Child Development Inventories are screening tests that rely on parent reports. The Denver II screening test (reproduced in Chapter 2, Figure 2–12), the Early Language Milestone Scale-2 (see Chapter 2, Figure 2–11), and the Bayley Infant Neurodevelopmental Screener all involve the direct observation of a child's skills by a care provider. All developmental screening tests have their strengths and weaknesses. The Denver II is familiar to many pediatric providers and is widely used. However, while the Denver II has relatively high sensitivity for detecting possible developmental delays, the specificity is poorer, and this may lead to the overreferral of normal children for further developmental testing.

Regardless of the approach taken to developmental screening, there are number of important considerations: (1) the range of normal childhood development is broad, and therefore a child with a single missing skill in a single developmental area is less likely to have a significant developmental problem than a child showing multiple delays in several developmental areas (eg, gross motor *and* language delays); (2) continuity of care is important,

because development is best assessed over time; (3) it is beneficial to routinely use formal screening tests to assess development; (4) if developmental delays are detected in primary care, these patients need referral for further testing, and likely will benefit from receiving developmentally-focused therapies; and (5) parents appreciate when attention is paid to their child's development, and generally react positively to referrals for appropriate developmental therapies.

Several developmental charts with age-based expectations for normal development are presented in Chapter 2 (Table 2–1, Table 2–2, and Table 2–3), as well as a discussion of the recommended medical and neurodevelopmental evaluation of a child with a suspected developmental disorder.

In addition to developmental issues, pediatric providers are an important source of information and counseling for parents regarding a broad range of behavioral issues. The nature of the behavioral problems, of course, varies with the child's age. Some common issues raised by parents, discussed in detail in Chapter 2, include colic, feeding disorders, sleep problems, temper tantrums, breath-holding spells, and noncompliance. Behavioral issues in adolescents are discussed in Chapter 3.

Albrecht SJ et al: Common behavioral dilemmas of the school-aged child. Pediatr Clin North Am 2003;50:841 [PMID: 12964697].

King TM, Glascoe FP: Developmental surveillance of infants and young children in pediatric primary care. Curr Opin Pediatr 2003;15:624 [PMID: 14631210].

Rydz D et al: Developmental screening. J Child Neurol 2005;20:4 [PMID: 15791916].

GROWTH PARAMETERS

Pediatric growth charts are based on a broad sampling of the U.S. population, with representation of young infants, breast-fed infants, and certain ethnic minorities. The 2- to 18-year growth charts include a chart of body mass index (BMI) for age. The BMI is calculated as the weight (in kilograms) divided by the squared height (in meters). The BMI is useful for determining overweight (BMI ≥ 95th percentile for age) and underweight status (BMI ≤ 5th percentile for age). The BMI is highly correlated with secondary complications of overweight.

Height, weight, and head circumference are carefully measured and plotted at each visit during the first 3 years. (See growth charts in Chapter 2.) For children older than 3 years, height and weight should be measured at each well-child examination. To ensure accurate weight measurements for longitudinal comparisons, infants should be undressed completely, and young children should be wearing underpants only. Recumbent length is plotted on the chart from birth to 3 years (see Figures 2–1 and 2–3). When the child is old enough to be measured upright, height should be plotted on the charts for ages 2–18 years (see Figures 2–5 and 2–7). If circumferential head growth has been steady for the first 2 years, routine measurements may be suspended. However, if a central nervous system problem exists or develops, or if the child has growth deficiency, this measurement continues to be useful. Tracking the growth velocity for each of these parameters allows early recognition of deviations from normal.

Kuczmarski RJ et al: *CDC Growth Charts: United States. Advance Data from Vital and Health Statistics,* no. 314. National Center for Health Statistics, 2000.

www.cdc.gov/growthcharts/default.htm

BLOOD PRESSURE

Blood pressure screening at well-child visits starts at age 3 years. If the child has a renal or cardiovascular abnormality, a blood pressure reading should be obtained at each visit regardless of age. Accurate determination of blood pressure requires proper equipment (stethoscope, manometer and inflation cuff, or an automated system) and a cooperative, seated subject. Although automated blood pressure instruments are widely available and easy to use, blood pressure readings from these devices are typically 5 mm Hg higher for diastolic and 10 mm Hg higher for systolic blood pressure compared with auscultatory techniques. Therefore, the diagnosis of hypertension should not be made on the basis of automated readings alone. Additionally, blood pressure varies somewhat by the height and weight of the individual. Consequently, hypertension is diagnosed as a systolic or diastolic blood pressure greater than the 95th percentile based on the age and height (or weight) percentile of the patient.

The width of the inflatable portion of the cuff should be 40–50% of the circumference of the limb. Obese children need a larger cuff size to avoid a falsely elevated blood pressure reading. Cuffs that are too narrow will overestimate and those that are too wide will underestimate the true blood pressure. Blood pressure norms are provided in Chapter 19.

Norwood VF: Hypertension. Pediatr Rev 2002;23:197 [PMID: 12042594].

Park MK, Menard SW, Yuan C: Comparison of auscultatory and oscillometric blood pressures. Arch Pediatr Adolesc Med 2001;155:50 [PMID: 11177062].

VISION & HEARING SCREENING

Examination of the eyes and an assessment of vision should be performed at every health supervision visit.

Parents should be queried about any concerns regarding vision, eye alignment, or any other eye problems. For example, parental observation of photophobia or excessive tearing may be suggestive of glaucoma.

For children from birth to 3 years of age, the eyes and eyelids should be inspected, the movement and alignment of the eyes assessed, and the pupils and red reflexes examined. The red reflex, performed on each pupil individually and then on both eyes simultaneously, is used to detect eye opacities (eg, cataracts or corneal clouding) and retinal abnormalities (eg, retinal detachment or retinoblastoma). In children younger than 3 years of age or in nonverbal children of any age, vision can be assessed by testing a child's ability to fixate on and follow an object.

For children 3 years and older, in addition to the eye evaluations, formal testing of visual acuity should be done. This can be performed in the office with a variety of tests, including the tumbling E chart or picture tests such as Allen cards. Each eye is tested separately, with the nontested eye completely covered. Credit is given for any line on which the child gets more than 50% correct. Children 4 years and older who are unable to cooperate should be retested, ideally within 1 month, and those who cannot cooperate with repeated attempts should be referred to an ophthalmologist. Because visual acuity improves with age, results of the test are interpreted using the cutoff values in Table 8–2. However, any two-line discrepancy between the two eyes, even within the passing range (for example, 20/20 in one eye, 20/30 in the other in a child ≥ 6 years of age) should be referred to an ophthalmologist. Throughout childhood and adolescence, clinicians should screen for undetected strabismus (ocular misalignment) and decreased visual acuity. The random dot E test is recommended for detecting strabismus. The corneal light reflex test, the cover test, and visual acuity tests are described further in Chapter 15.

Hearing loss, if undetected, can lead to substantial impairments in speech, language, and cognitive development. Because significant bilateral hearing loss is one of the more common major anomalies found at birth, and early detection and intervention of hearing loss

Table 8–2. Age-appropriate visual acuity.[a]

Age (years)	Minimal Acceptable Acuity
3–5	20/40
6 and older	20/30

[a]Refer to an ophthalmologist if minimal acuity is not met at a given age or if there is a difference in scores of two or more lines between the eyes.

leads to better outcomes for children, universal hearing screening of all infants is required in many parts of the United States. Hearing in infants is assessed using either auditory brainstem responses or evoked otoacoustic emissions. Because universal newborn hearing screening will inevitably be associated with some false-positive test results, confirmatory audiology testing is required for all abnormal tests.

Informal behavioral testing of hearing, such as observing an infant's response to a shaken rattle, may be unreliable. In fact, parental concerns about hearing are of greater predictive value than the results of informal tests, and such concerns should be taken seriously. Pure tone audiometry in the office is feasible beginning at age 3 years. Any evidence of hearing loss should be substantiated by repeated testing, and if still abnormal, a referral for a formal hearing evaluation should be made. A number of inherited or acquired conditions increase the risk of hearing loss. Children with any risk factors for hearing loss should be closely followed and periodically screened. Additional details regarding hearing assessment are provided in Chapter 17.

American Academy of Pediatrics et al: Eye examination in infants, children, and young adults by pediatricians. Pediatrics 2003; 111:902 [PMID: 12671132].

Cunningham M et al: Hearing assessment in infants and children: Recommendations beyond neonatal screening. Pediatrics 2003;111:436 [PMID: 12563074].

Elden LM et al: Screening and prevention of hearing loss in children. Curr Opin Pediatr 2002;14:723 [PMID: 12436045].

LABORATORY SCREENING

Newborn Screening

Newborn screening involves population-wide testing for metabolic and genetic diseases. Blood samples are collected by heelstick from newborns before hospital discharge, and results are usually available within 1 week. Some states routinely repeat blood testing between 7 and 14 days of life, while others recommend it if the child is discharged in less than 24 hours. Repeat testing may be necessary to detect diseases of protein (eg, phenylketonuria) or sugar metabolism (eg, galactosemia) which may not be discovered if the first newborn blood screen is performed before the child has had substantial milk intake.

All state newborn screening programs include tests for phenylketonuria and congenital hypothyroidism. If undiagnosed, both diseases result in severe mental retardation. Early treatment maintains cognitive function in the normal range. All states also test for classic galactosemia and sickle cell disease. Additional diseases screened for in the majority of states include congenital adrenal hyperplasia, homocystinuria, maple syrup urine disease, and biotinidase deficiency. Tyrosinemia, cystic fibrosis, and tests for the infectious diseases toxoplasmosis and human immunodeficiency virus are conducted in some states.

Infants with a positive screen result should receive close follow-up, with additional confirmatory studies performed. Screening tests are usually accurate, but the sensitivity and specificity of a particular screening test must be carefully considered. If the screening test result is reported as positive, a confirmatory test must be performed. If symptoms of a disease are present despite a negative screening test, the infant should be tested further. Once a diagnosis is confirmed, the infant will need further evaluation and treatment.

Advances in science and technology, such as tandem mass spectroscopy and the Human Genome Project (http://www.nhgri.nih.gov), have created the potential to test for numerous additional inherited diseases. Treatments for these additional diseases varies from highly effective to ineffective. The risks and benefits of early detection of these conditions have been little studied but widely speculated upon. Preliminary results suggest that the early identification of rare metabolic diseases by screening leads to improved child health outcomes and reduced parent stress. The long-term effect of false-positive screens on parents is unknown.

Lead Screening

The developing infant and child are at risk of lead poisoning because of their propensity to place objects in the mouth and their efficient absorption of the metal. High blood levels (> 70 μg/dL) can cause severe health problems such as seizures and coma. Numerous neuropsychological deficits have been associated with increased lead levels. Blood lead levels below 10 μg/dL have been correlated with lower intelligence quotients. The primary source of lead exposure in this country remains lead-based paint, even though most of its uses have been banned since 1977. Lead levels have declined nationally from a mean of 16 μg/dL in 1976 to 2 μg/dL in 2001. However, considerable variation in lead levels exists in different regions of the United States, and a majority of children at risk of lead toxicity are not currently screened. To eliminate childhood lead poisoning by 2010 (a national health objective—http://www.healthypeople.gov), health care providers need to be vigilant about this environmental health threat.

The Centers for Disease Control and Prevention (www.cdc.gov/lead/) recommends universal lead screening for children at ages 1 and 2 and targeted screening for older children living in communities with a high percentage of old housing (> 27% of houses built before 1950) or a high percentage of children with elevated blood lead levels (> 12% of children with levels above 10 μg/dL).

Communities with inadequate data regarding local blood lead levels should also undergo universal screening. Medicaid requires that all children (ages 1–5 years) be screened twice. Caregivers of children between ages 6 months and 6 years may be interviewed by questionnaire about environmental risk factors for lead exposure (Table 8–3), although the data to support the use of this screening are inconclusive. If risk factors are present, a blood lead level should be obtained.

A venous blood sample is preferred over a capillary specimen. An elevated capillary (fingerstick) blood sample should always be confirmed by a venous sample. No action is required for blood lead levels below 10 µg/dL. The cognitive development of children with confirmed blood levels over 14 µg/dL should be evaluated and attempts made to identify the environmental source. Iron deficiency should be treated if present. Chelation of lead is indicated for levels of 45 µg/dL or more, and is urgently required for levels over 70 µg/dL. All families should receive education to decrease the risk of lead exposure. With any elevated lead level (> 10 µg/dL) rescreening should be performed at recommended intervals.

Iron Deficiency

Iron deficiency is the most common nutritional deficiency in the United States. Severe iron deficiency causes anemia, behavioral problems, and cognitive effects, but recent evidence suggests that even iron deficiency without anemia may cause behavioral and cognitive difficul-

Table 8–3. Elements of a lead risk questionnnaire.

Recommended questions
1. Does your child live in or regularly visit a house built before 1950? This could include a day care center, preschool, the home of a baby-sitter or relative, and so on.
2. Does your child live in or regularly visit a house built before 1978 with recent, ongoing, or planned renovation or remodeling?
3. Does your child have a sister or brother, housemate, or playmate being followed for lead poisoning?

Questions that may be considered by region or locality
1. Does your child live with an adult whose job (eg, at a brass/copper foundry, firing range, automotive or boat repair shop, or furniture refinishing shop) or hobby (eg, electronics, fishing, stained-glass-making, pottery-making) involves exposure to lead?
2. Does your child live near a work or industrial site (eg, smelter, battery recycling plant) that involves the use of lead?
3. Does your child use pottery or ingest medications that are suspected of having a high lead content?
4. Does your child have exposure to burning lead-painted wood?

ties. Furthermore, the developmental effects of iron deficiency may be present after 10 years, even if iron deficiency is corrected in infancy. Risk factors for iron deficiency include preterm or low-birth-weight births, multiple pregnancy, iron deficiency in the mother, use of nonfortified formula or cow's milk before age 12 months, and an infant diet that is low in iron-containing foods. Infants and toddlers consuming more than 24 oz of cow's milk per day are at risk, as are children with chronic illness, restricted diet, or extensive blood loss.

Primary prevention of iron deficiency should be achieved through dietary means, including feeding infants iron-containing cereals by age 6 months, avoiding low-iron formula during infancy, and limiting cow's milk to 24 oz/d in children age 1–5 years. Selective early screening for iron deficiency should be considered with the presence of any of the preceding risk factors. A screening hemoglobin or hematocrit should be obtained for high-risk children between ages 9–12 months and again at 15–18 months, and it should be considered annually through age 5 years. Premature and low-birth-weight infants may need testing before 6 months of age. Universal anemia screening at 9 and 15 months of age is appropriate for children in communities or patient populations in which anemia is found in 5% or more of those tested. Biochemical tests of iron deficiency such as ferritin (low in the absence of inflammation), transferrin saturation (low), and erythrocyte protoporphyrin (elevated) are sensitive measures. Lead poisoning can cause iron deficiency anemia and should be explored as a cause for at-risk infants and children. A screening hematocrit is recommended for pregnant teenagers.

Hypercholesterolemia & Hyperlipidemia

The benefits of screening and treatment for hypercholesterolemia and hyperlipidemia in children are not fully known. However, the American Academy of Pediatrics (www.aap.org) and the American Heart Association (www.americanheart.org) recommend obtaining a total cholesterol measurement in children older than 2 years who have a parent with elevated cholesterol (above 240 mg/dL). If there is a family history of cardiovascular disease before age 55 years, a complete lipoprotein analysis (fasting cholesterol, high-density lipoproteins, low-density lipoproteins, and triglycerides) is recommended. For all children, a prudent diet is advised (see Nutrition Counseling section).

Tuberculosis

In 2003, 14,871 cases of tuberculosis were reported in the United States, with 922 of these cases occurring in children younger than age 15 years. Well-child care should include assessment of the risk of tuberculosis, and tuberculosis screening should be based on high-risk status. High risk is defined as contact with a person with known or suspected tuberculosis; having symptoms or radiographic findings suggesting tuberculosis; birth, residence, or travel to a region with high tuberculosis prevalence (Asia, the Middle East, Africa, or Latin America); contact with a person with the acquired immunodeficiency syndrome or human immunodeficiency virus; or contact with a prisoner, migrant farm worker, illicit drug user, or a person who is or has been recently homeless. The Mantoux test (5 tuberculin units of purified protein derivative) is the only recommended screening test. It can be done as early as 3 months of age and should be repeated annually if the risk persists. The tine test should not be used. Previous vaccination with bacille Calmette-Guérin is not a contraindication to tuberculosis skin testing.

Screening of Adolescent Patients

Screening adolescents for blood cholesterol, tuberculosis, and human immunodeficiency virus should be offered based on high-risk criteria outlined in this chapter and in Chapter 37. Females with heavy menses, weight loss, poor nutrition, or athletic activity should have a screening hematocrit. During routine visits, adolescents should be questioned sensitively about sexually transmitted infection risk factors (eg, multiple partners or early onset of sexual activity, including child sexual abuse) and their symptoms (eg, genital discharge, infectious lesions, or pelvic pain). A dipstick urinalysis for leukocytes is generally recommended for sexually active adolescents. Teenage girls who are sexually active and all girls regardless of sexual experience age 18 years and older should have a pelvic examination with Papanicolaou (Pap) smear. A Pap smear should be performed at least every 3 years thereafter and more frequently in patients with risk factors for sexually transmitted infections. Because females with sexually transmitted infections are often not symptomatic, gonococcal and chlamydial cultures and screening tests for syphilis and trichomoniasis are appropriate at the time of each pelvic examination.

American Academy of Pediatrics, Committee on Environmental Health: Lead Exposure in Children: Prevention, Detection, and Management. Pediatrics 2005;116:1036 [PMID: 16199720].

American Academy of Pediatrics Committee on Nutrition: Cholesterol in children. Pediatrics 1998;101:141 [PMID: 11345978].

American Academy of Pediatrics: Tuberculosis. In Pickering LK (editor): *2003 Red Book: Report of the Committee on Infectious Diseases,* 26th ed., p. 642. American Academy of Pediatrics, 2000.

Centers for Disease Control and Prevention, National Center for HIV, STD and TB Prevention: http://www.cdc.gov/nchstp/tb/surv/surv2003/default.htm

Centers for Disease Control and Prevention: www.cdc.gov/lead/factsheets.htm

National Newborn Screening Status Report, updated September 2005. http://genes-r-us.uthscsa.edu

ANTICIPATORY GUIDANCE

An essential part of the health supervision visit is anticipatory guidance. During this counseling, the clinician directs the parent's or the older child's attention to issues that may arise in the future. Guidance must be appropriate to age, focus on concerns expressed by the parent and patient, and address issues in depth rather than run through a number of issues superficially. A combination of oral and printed materials is used. Handouts are an important supplement to anticipatory guidance. A routine schedule for preventive handouts is shown in Table 8–4. Areas of concern include diet, injury prevention, developmental and behavioral issues, and health promotion. Injury prevention is discussed in the next section; other topics are found in other chapters of this book.

Injury Prevention

Injuries are the leading cause of death in children and adolescents after the first year of life (Figure 8–3). For young people age 15–24 years, injuries are responsible for more than 50% of all deaths. Each year, 16 million visits to emergency departments are occasioned by injuries to children and adolescents, and more than 500,000 of these patients are hospitalized. In the case of physical injury to a young child, the physician must recognize that some injuries may be intentional or the result of parental neglect. (See Chapter 7.)

Table 8–4. Preventive handouts for health supervision visits.

Age	Suggested Topics
2 weeks	Breast feeding
2 months	Attachment
4 months	Language and motor development
6 months	Nutrition
12 months	Safe and constructive family relationships
18 months	Toilet training basics
2 years	Time-out technique
3 years	Chores and social competence
4 years	Sexuality education across the ages
5 years	Media and child health
6 years	School work: Encouraging success
8 years	Sibling rivalry
10 years	Social competence
12 years	Adolescents: Promoting responsibility

Children 1–4 years

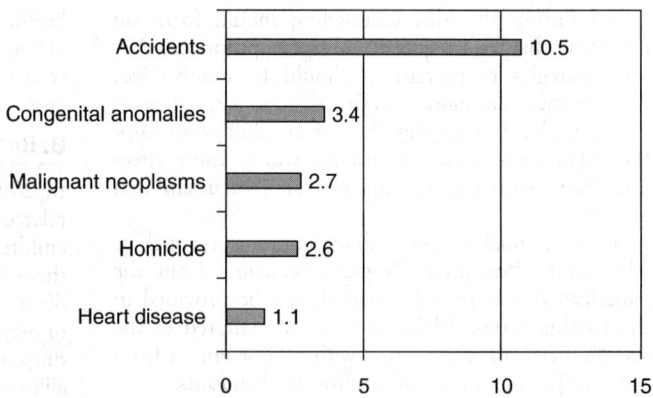

Children 5–14 years

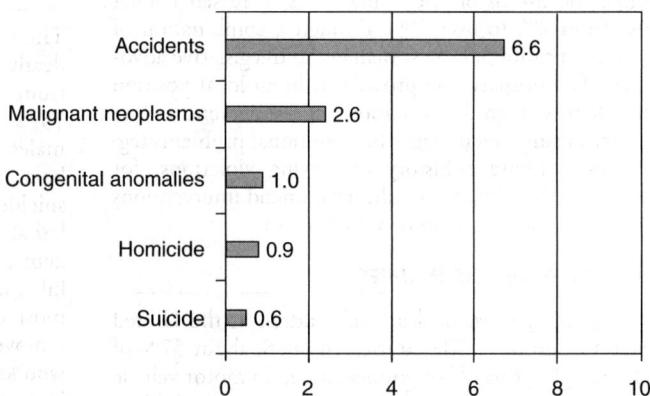

Young adults 15–24 years

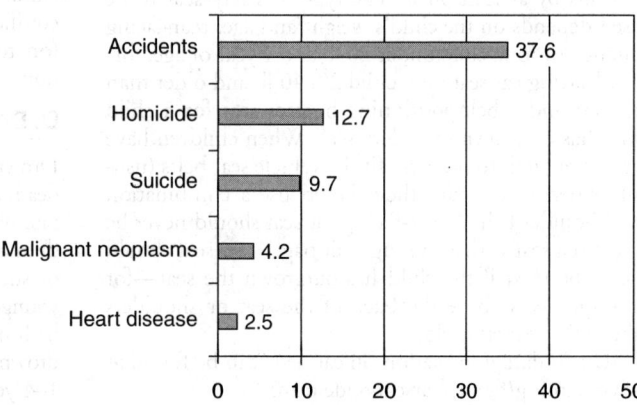

Figure 8–3. Leading causes of death in children at 1–4 years, at 5–14 years, and at 15–24 years (the 2002 rate per 100,000 population). (National Center for Health Statistics, 2002.)

Injury prevention counseling is an important component of each health supervision visit and can be reinforced during all visits. Counseling should focus on problems that are frequent and age-appropriate. Passive strategies of prevention should be emphasized, because these are more effective than active strategies; for example, encouraging the use of childproof cupboard latches to prevent poisoning will be more effective than instructing parents to watch their children closely.

Informational handouts about home safety, such as The Injury Prevention Program (available from the American Academy of Pediatrics), can be provided in the waiting room. Advice can then be tailored to the specific needs of each family, with reinforcement from age-specific Injury Prevention Program handouts.

The pediatrician's influence can extend beyond the office to advocate for safer communities. For example, a community program in Seattle, Washington, to promote the use of bicycle helmets has increased helmet use from 2% to over 60% through a combination of office education, low-cost helmets, and legislative advocacy. The primary care provider is in an ideal position to identify high-risk situations and intervene before injury occurs. If a teenager has emotional problems (eg, depression) and a history of driving violations, for example, the clinician should recommend interventions that could prevent a motor vehicle crash.

A. Motor Vehicle Injuries

The primary cause of death of children in the United States is motor vehicle injuries. In 1998, about 57% of children 15 years old or younger killed in motor vehicle crashes were unrestrained. Car safety seats for children are required in all U.S. states, and their proper use could reduce vehicle-associated fatalities and hospitalizations by at least 50%. The type of safety seat to be used depends on the child's weight and age: rear-facing infant seat for a child under 20 lb and 1 year of age; forward-facing car seat for a child 20–40 lb and older than 1 year; and a belt-positioning booster seat for a child who has outgrown the safety seat. When children have grown enough to properly fit the vehicle seat belts (usually when 4 feet tall), they should use a combination lap/shoulder belt. A rear-facing car seat should never be used in a seat with a passenger air bag. A car seat should never be used if the child has outgrown the seat—for example, ears above the back of the seat or shoulders above the seat strap slots.

Up-to-date information on car seats can be found at www.aap.org/family/carseatguide.htm.

When a child is a passenger in a car crash, the case fatality rate is 1%; for children hit by cars, the risk of fatality increases threefold. Pedestrian safety skills should be taught to children early in childhood; however, paren-

tal supervision of children near roadways continues to be required for many years. A final motor vehicle risk for health involves the use of portable electronic devices. Using a cellular telephone while driving is associated with a fourfold increase in motor vehicle crashes. Parents and teenage drivers should avoid this risk.

B. Bicycle Injuries

In 2001, over 400,000 Americans sustained a bicycle-related injury, and two-thirds of these injuries involved children or adolescents. Head trauma accounts for three-fourths of all bicycle-related fatalities. More than 85% of brain injuries can be prevented through the use of bicycle helmets, and the rate of fatality to bicyclists is dropping. Therefore, bike riders—parents and children alike—should wear a helmet every time they ride. Unfortunately, low bicycle helmet use rates are still common in many communities.

C. Firearm Injuries and Violence Prevention

The United States has a higher rate of firearm-related death than any other industrialized country. Injuries from firearms are more frequent for young people age 15–24 years than for any other age group, and black males are especially vulnerable. Some gun deaths may be accidental, but most are the result of homicide or suicide. A gun in the home doubles the likelihood of a lethal suicide attempt. Although handguns are often kept in homes for protection, a gun is more likely to kill a family member or a friend than an intruder. The most effective way to prevent firearm injuries is to remove guns from the home and community. Families who keep firearms at home should lock them in a cabinet or drawer and store ammunition in a separate locked location.

A nonviolent environment should be provided to all children. Secure parent-infant attachments, social and conflict-resolution skills, and the avoidance of violence (on television or actual) all have a role in promoting nonviolence.

D. Drowning and Near Drowning

Drowning is the second leading cause of injury-related death in children, and those age 1–3 years have the highest rate of drowning. For every death by drowning, six children are hospitalized for near drowning, and up to 10% of survivors experience severe brain damage. Children younger than age 1 year are most likely to drown in the bathtub. Buckets filled with water also present a risk of drowning to the older infant or toddler. For children age 1–4 years, drowning or near drowning occurs most often in home swimming pools; and for school-age children and teens, drowning occurs most often in large bodies of water (eg, swimming pools or open water). After the age of 5 years, the risk of drowning in a swimming pool is much greater for black males than white males. School-age children should be taught to swim, and recreational swimming should always be supervised. Home pools must be fenced securely, and parents should know how to perform cardiopulmonary resuscitation.

E. FIRE AND BURN INJURIES

Fires and burns are the leading cause of injury-related deaths in the home. Categories of burn injury include smoke inhalation; flame contact; scalding; and electrical, chemical, and ultraviolet burns. Scalding is the most common type of burn in children. Most scalds involve foods and beverages, but nearly one-fourth of scalds are with tap water, and for that reason it is recommended that hot water heaters be set to less than 54 °C (130 °F). The greatest number of fire-related deaths result from smoke inhalation. Smoke detectors can prevent 85% of the injuries and deaths caused by fires in the home. Families should practice emergency evacuation from the home.

Sunburn is a common thermal injury, perhaps because symptoms of excessive sun exposure do not begin until after the skin has been damaged. Sunburn and excessive sun exposure are associated with skin cancers. Prevention of sunburn is best achieved by sun avoidance, particularly during the midday hours of 10 AM to 3 PM. Sunscreen using a sun protection factor of 15 or greater extends the period of time that a child can spend in the sun without sunburn. Hats, sunglasses, and special precautions for fair-skinned individuals and infants are also important aspects of safe sun exposure. The safety of sunscreen is not established for infants younger than 6 months; thus sun avoidance, appropriate clothing, and hats are recommended for this age group.

American Academy of Pediatrics, Committee on Injury and Poison Prevention: Bicycle helmets. Pediatrics 2001;108:1030 [PMID: 11581464].

American Academy of Pediatrics, Committee on Injury and Poison Prevention: Firearm-related injuries affecting the pediatric population. Pediatrics 2000;105:888 [PMID: 10742344].

American Academy of Pediatrics, Committee on Injury and Poison Prevention: Reducing the number of deaths and injuries from residential fires. Pediatrics 2000;105:1355 [PMID: 10835082].

Brenner RA et al: Where children drown, United States, 1995. Pediatrics 2001;108:85 [PMID: 11433058].

NUTRITION COUNSELING

Screening for nutritional problems and guidance for age-appropriate dietary choices should be part of every health supervision visit. Undernutrition, overnutrition, and eating disorders can be detected early by a careful analysis of dietary and activity patterns interpreted in the context of a child's growth pattern. When obtaining a dietary history, it is helpful to assess the following: who purchases and prepares food; who feeds the child; whether meals and snacks occur at consistent times and in a consistent setting; whether children are allowed to snack or "graze" between meals; the types and portion sizes of food and drinks provided; the frequency of eating meals in restaurants or eating take-out food; and whether the child eats while watching television.

Iron-fortified formula or breast milk should be used for the first year of life, after which whole cow's milk can be given. Because of continued rapid growth and high energy needs, children should continue to drink whole milk until age 2 years. Baby foods are generally introduced around ages 4–6 months.

For children 2 years old and older, a prudent diet consists of diverse food sources, encourages eating high-fiber foods (eg, fruits, vegetables, and grain products), and limits sodium and fat intake. Foods to be avoided or limited include processed foods, soft drinks, and candy. Parents should be gently reminded that they are modeling for a lifetime of eating behaviors in their children, both in terms of the types of foods they provide, and the structure of meals (eg, the importance of the family eating together). For additional information on nutritional guidelines, undernutrition, and obesity, see Chapter 10; for eating disorders, see Chapter 5; for adolescent obesity, see Chapter 3.

American Academy of Pediatrics, Committee on Nutrition: Prevention of pediatric overweight and obesity. Pediatrics 2003; 112:424 [PMID: 12897303].

COUNSELING ABOUT TELEVISION & OTHER MEDIA

The average child in the U.S. watches approximately 3 hours of television per day, and this does not include time spent watching videotapes/DVDs, playing video games, or playing on computers. Having a television set in the bedroom is associated with watching more television, and 32% of 2- to 7-year-olds and 65% of 8- to 18-year-olds have a bedroom television set.

The excessive watching of television has a negative and potentially long-lasting impact on the health and well-being of children. Television viewing has been shown to have negative effects with respect to violence, sexuality, substance abuse, nutrition, and body self-image. More recent data suggest that excessive television viewing in childhood may have a long-lasting negative effect on cognitive development and academic achievement.

There are educational television programs that would not be expected to adversely affect children, and may in fact have some benefit. Regardless, it is important that clinicians assess media exposure in their patients, and offer parents concrete advice. The American Academy of Pediatrics recommends that children < 2 years old should not be allowed to watch any television, and that children 2 years of age and older be limited to 2 hours total of all media time. Additionally, parents should monitor what their children watch, remove television sets from their children's bedrooms, and encourage alternative activities.

Borzekowski DLG, Robinson TN: The remote, the mouse, and the No. 2 pencil—the household media environment and academic achievement among third grade students. Arch Pediatr Adolesc Med 2005;159:607 [PMID: 15996991].

Hancox RJ et al: Association of television viewing during childhood with poor educational achievement. Arch Pediatr Adolesc Med 2005;159:614 [PMID: 15996992].

Jordan A: The role of media in children's development: an ecological perspective. J Dev Behav Pediatr 2004;25:196 [PMID: 15194905].

IMMUNIZATIONS

A child's immunization status should be assessed at every clinic visit and every opportunity should be taken to vaccinate. Even though parents may keep an immunization record, it is critical that providers also keep an accurate record of a child's immunizations. This information may be written in a prominent location in the chart or kept in a electronic immunization registry.

Despite high overall national immunization coverage levels, areas of underimmunization continue to exist in the United States. Therefore it is important that clinicians screen records and administer required immunizations at all types of visits, and administer all needed vaccinations simultaneously. Additionally, clinicians should operate reminder/recall systems, in which parents of underimmunized children are prompted by mail or telephone to visit the clinic for immunization. The assessment of clinic-wide immunization levels and feedback of these data to providers has also been shown to increase immunization rates.

Immunization schedules and other details of specific vaccines are presented in Chapter 9. A wealth of information for parents and providers about immunizations is also available at the National Immunization Program's website (http://www.cdc.gov/nip).

Santoli JM et al: Immunization pockets of need: Science and practice. Am J Prev Med 2000;19(1S):89 [PMID: 11024333].

Task Force on Community Preventive Services: Recommendations regarding interventions to improve vaccination coverage in children, adolescents, and adults. Am J Prev Med 2000;18(1S):92 [PMID: 10806981].

■ OTHER TYPES OF GENERAL PEDIATRIC SERVICES

ACUTE-CARE VISITS

Acute-care visits account for 30% or more of the general pediatrician's office visits. These visits are conducted in an efficient, structured way. Office personnel should determine the reason for the visit; if there is an emergent situation, obtain a brief synopsis of the child's symptoms; carefully document vital signs; and list known drug allergies. The pediatric clinician should document the events related to the presenting problem and carefully describe them in the medical record. The record should include supporting laboratory data and a diagnosis. Treatments and follow-up instructions must be recorded, including when to return to the office if the problem is not ameliorated. Immunization status should be screened and appropriate vaccinations given. As time allows, age-appropriate health maintenance screenings and anticipatory guidance should be provided. Careful documentation of these visits is important for medicolegal reasons.

PRENATAL VISITS

Ideally, a couple's first trip to a physician's office should take place before the birth of their baby. A prenatal visit goes a long way toward establishing trust and enables a pediatric provider to learn about a family's expectations, concerns, and fears regarding the anticipated birth. If the infant develops a problem during the newborn period, a provider who has already met the family is in a better position to maintain rapport and communication with the new parents.

In addition to helping establish a relationship between parents and pediatric providers, the prenatal visit can be used to gather information about the parents and the pregnancy, provide information and advice, and identify high-risk situations. A range of information can be provided to parents, such as that regarding feeding choices and the benefits of breast feeding; injury prevention including sleeping position and the appropriate use of car seats; and techniques for managing colic. Potential high-risk situations that may be identified include mental health issues in the parents, a history of domestic violence, or maternal medical problems that may affect the infant.

Serwint JR: The prenatal pediatric visit. Pediatr Rev 2003;24:31 [PMID: 12509543].

SPORTS PHYSICALS

The purpose of the preparticipation health evaluation is to determine whether a child can safely participate in organized sports activity. Attention should be directed toward those parts of the body that are most vulnerable to the stresses of sports. The history and physical examination should focus on the following systems: cardiovascular (stenotic lesions, hypertension, and surgery), respiratory (asthma), vision, genitourinary (absence or loss of function of one testicle), gastrointestinal (hepatosplenomegaly and hernia), skin (infection), musculoskeletal (inflammation and dysfunction), and neurologic (concussions and uncontrolled seizures). The sports physical should include counseling about medication usage (eg, diuretic, steroid, and β-blocker abuse, and changes in insulin requirements), protective equipment, proper supervision and instruction, injury management, and the emotional aspects of competition and teamwork. The physician should suggest sports that will be compatible with the child's size, strength, endurance, agility, and chronic illness history. The potential for mild menstrual irregularities should be explained to the adolescent female athlete. The athlete with moderate to severe menstrual irregularities should be referred for endocrinologic evaluation. Anticipatory guidance should address nutritional needs to maintain growth, cessation of activity when pain occurs, and fluid and electrolyte availability to avoid dehydration. (See Chapter 25 for a more detailed discussion of sports medicine.)

CHRONIC DISEASE MANAGEMENT

Chronic disease in pediatrics is defined as illness that has been present for more than 3 months. Twenty-five percent of children and 35% of adolescents have illnesses that meet the definition of a chronic illness. The most common chronic illnesses in pediatric practice include asthma, otitis media with effusion, skin disorders, and allergic diseases.

The goal of chronic disease management is to optimize quality of life while minimizing the side effects of treatment interventions. The child and family's emotional responses to chronic illness should be addressed, and referrals to counselors should be offered if needed. Pediatric subspecialty referrals need to be arranged and monitored and results recorded in the chart in an organized manner. Chronic problems often mean chronic use of medications and the need to monitor their use. Documentation should be made in the medical record whenever a prescription is refilled. A medication summary page in the chart allows easy access to the drug history and is a convenient place to make notes such as when the anticonvulsant level was last checked and what it was at that time (Figure 8–4). Children with medical appliances such as gastrostomy tubes and indwelling intravenous and bladder catheters need advice on their management. Nutritional intake is often complicated and must be closely and carefully monitored.

Ludder-Jackson P, Vessey JA: *Primary Care of the Child with a Chronic Condition,* 3rd ed. Mosby-Year Book, 2000.

COUNSELING

Topics amenable to office counseling include behavioral issues such as negativism and noncompliance, temper tantrums, oppositional behavior, and biting; childhood fears and feeding disorders; school problems;

family upheavals such as separation, divorce, or remarriage; attention-deficit/hyperactivity disorder; and deaths of family members or close friends. Forty-five minutes is usually enough time for the therapeutic process to evolve, and this time should be protected from interruption. The young child is usually interviewed with the parent; school-age children and adolescents benefit from time alone with the physician. After assessing the situation in one or two sessions, the primary care physician must decide whether the child's and family's needs are within his or her area of expertise or whether referral to another professional such as a psychologist or an education specialist would be appropriate. The pediatrician should know the warning signs for childhood depression and bipolar disorder and have a low threshold for referral of these concerns to the appropriate mental health professional.

CONSULTATIONS

Physicians, other professionals, and parents may initiate consultations with a general pediatrician. The general pediatrician may be called on to evaluate many different types of problems both in the hospital and in the ambulatory setting. Parents sometimes desire a second opinion regarding a specific concern while maintaining a relationship with another clinician for their child's primary care. Subspecialists, family physicians, or professionals such as school officials, psychologists, or social workers may also seek medical consultation. Finally, an insurance company representative may want a second opinion before authorizing a set of services.

Consultations usually require one or two 45- to 60-minute appointments. When the patient is referred to a pediatric consultant, the number of visits and the extent of service should be specified. A screening questionnaire, completed in advance by a parent, should delineate the patient's physical, behavioral, and developmental (or school) problems and serve as an initial database.

The types of consultations the general pediatrician may be asked to do include an evaluation only, an evaluation and interpretation, or an evaluation and treatment of an isolated problem. The type of consultation being requested should be clearly determined at the time of referral of the patient. This understanding should be clarified with the patient's insurance company so that appropriate authorization and reimbursement for the visit can occur.

Communication with the Referring Source

Communication is the key to a satisfactory referral process. The pediatric consultant frequently sends the referral source a brief note acknowledging the referral and requesting additional information. The final consultation report should be sent promptly, with content

Medication: _____

Date: Visit (V) or Phone Call (PC)	Tablet Size or Liquid Concentration	Sig.	Disp.	Number of Refills	Approved by	Called by	Pharmacy and Phone No.

Notes (eg, levels): _____

Figure 8–4. Medication summary sheet.

appropriate for the referring source. School officials usually want to know only whether the patient is physically healthy, or if not, what their responsibility is. A referring physician expects a full report. Recommendations should be specific (eg, drugs, dosages, other forms of therapy, duration of therapy, and specific laboratory tests). A copy of or reference to a recent review article on the subject will also be appreciated.

A medical evaluation should contain a factual summary of the history, physical examination, and laboratory and radiologic findings. Families are grateful if a copy is sent to them for their information and records. At the end of the consultation, the parents should be told when the patient should see the primary physician—usually in 1–2 weeks. Positive comments about the referring physician's competence and judgment serve to support the primary physician-patient relationship. The parents must feel confident that the primary physician can provide the necessary follow-up care. If the referring physician had tentatively made the correct diagnosis prior to referral, the consultant's corroboration should be made clear to the parents and included in the consultation report.

TELEPHONE TRIAGE & ADVICE & WEB-BASED INFORMATION

Providing appropriate, efficient, and timely clinical advice over the telephone is a critical element of pediatric primary care in the office setting. An estimated 20–30% of all clinical care delivered by general pediatric offices is provided by telephone. Telephone calls to and from patients occur both during regular office hours and after the office has closed (termed after-hours), and the personnel and systems in place to handle office-hours versus before- and after-hours calls may differ. In either circumstance, several principles are important: (1) advice is given only by clinicians or other staff with formal medical education (eg, nurse or medical assistant), (2) staff is given additional training in providing telephone care, (3) documentation is made of all pertinent information from calls, (4) standardized protocols covering the most common pediatric symptoms are used, and (5) a physician is always available to handle urgent or difficult calls.

During routine office hours, approximately 20–25% of all telephone calls made to pediatric offices are regarding clinical matters. Many of these calls, however, are routine in nature, and an experienced nurse within the office can screen calls and provide appropriate advice by telephone. Calls from inexperienced or anxious parents about simple concerns should be answered with understanding and respect. Certain types of calls received during office hours should be promptly transferred to a physician: (1) true emergencies, (2) calls regarding hospitalized patients, (3) calls from other medical professionals, and (4) calls from parents who demand to speak with a physician. Nurses should also seek help from a clinician whenever they are uncertain about how to handle a particular call. When in doubt about the diagnosis or necessary treatment, nurses giving telephone advice should err on the side of having the patient seen in the office.

Several different options are available for handling after-hours pediatric telephone care. Clinicians may choose to take all calls from their patients, may rely on "advice" nurses without specific pediatric protocols or training, or may use a system specifically designed for pediatric telephone care, called a pediatric after-hours call center. Pediatric call centers, although not available in all communities and potentially more expensive than other options for after-hours care, have certain benefits. Calls are managed using standardized protocols, the call centers are typically staffed by nurses with abundant pediatric experience, the calls are well-documented, and call centers often perform ongoing quality assurance. Extensive research on pediatric call centers has revealed a high degree of appropriate referrals to emergency departments, and a high level of parent satisfaction with the process.

In general, after-hours pediatric telephone calls tend to be more serious than calls made during regular office hours. Deciding which patients need to be seen, and how urgently, are the most important aspects of these after-hours telephone "encounters." Several factors influence this final patient disposition: (1) the age of the patient, (2) the duration and type of symptom, (3) the presence of any underlying chronic condition, (4) whether the child appears "very sick" to the caller, and (5) the anxiety level of the caller. Once all the pertinent medical information is gathered, a decision is made about whether the child should be seen immediately (by ambulance versus car), seen in the office later (today versus tomorrow), or whether the illness can be safely cared for at home. At the end of the call, it should be confirmed that parents understand and feel comfortable with the plan for their child.

The use of the World Wide Web (Internet) has become common in the pediatric office setting. Many practices routinely use the Internet to give information about the practice, care for common minor problems, when to make an appointment, and insurance issues, among other items. With time, the Internet is sure to become a larger part of the ambulatory pediatric practice.

Kempe A et al: Delivery of pediatric after-hours care by call centers: A multicenter study of parental perceptions and compliance. Pediatrics 2001;108:e111 [PMID: 11731638].

Luberti AA: After-hours telephone care: Options for the pediatrician. Pediatr Ann 2001;30:249 [PMID: 11383464].

Poole SR: Creating an after-hours telephone triage system for office practice. Pediatr Ann 2001;30:268 [PMID: 11383466].

Liederman EM, Morefield CS: Web messaging: a new tool for patient-physician communication. J Am Med Inform Assoc 2003;10:260. [PMID: 12626378].

COMMUNITY PEDIATRICS

According to the American Academy of Pediatrics, community pediatrics is "a perspective that enlarges the pediatrician's focus from one child to all children in the community." Pediatricians have historically been very involved in supporting and developing services for vulnerable children in their communities. As a group, pediatricians recognize that communities are integral determinants of a child's health and that the synthesis of public health and personal health principles and practices is important in the practice of community pediatrics. As well, pediatricians have a long commitment to work with other professionals in the community and advocate for the needs of all children. For example, pediatricians have been instrumental in the passage of laws requiring protective fencing around swimming pools.

Pediatricians in practice are frequently instrumental in referring children and families to valuable services and resources. For example, uninsured children can be enrolled in either their state Medicaid program or State Children's Health Insurance Program. Children with special health care needs may be eligible for services typically funded through state health departments and through programs such as those provided based on the Individuals with Disabilities Education Act (IDEA). A variety of community-based immunization programs can provide access to needed immunizations for eligible children. Food and nutrition programs such as the federally funded Women, Infants, and Children program provide sources of food at no cost to eligible families. Finally, subsidized preschool and child care services such as the federally funded Head Start program provide needed preschool programs. Pediatricians are in a unique position to make referrals to these important services from the ambulatory and hospital-based practice settings.

American Academy of Pediatrics: The pediatrician's role in community pediatrics. Pediatrics 2005;115:1092 [PMID: 15805396].

Duggan A et al: The essential role of research in community pediatrics. Pediatrics 2005;115(Supp):1195 [PMID: 15821310].

Satcher D et al: The expanding role of the pediatrician in improving child health in the 21st century. Pediatrics 2005; 115 (Supp):1124 [PMID: 15821293].

COMMON GENERAL PEDIATRIC ISSUES

FEVER

Definition & Measurement

Fever is one of the most common reasons for pediatric office visits, emergency department encounters, and after-hours telephone calls. Several different definitions of fever exist, but most experts define fever as a rectal temperature of 38 °C or above. Temperature in pediatric patients can be measured in a variety of manners: rectal (using a mercury or digital thermometer), oral (mercury or digital), axillary (mercury, digital, or liquid crystal strip), forehead (liquid crystal strip), or tympanic (using a device that measures thermal infrared energy from the tympanic membrane). Tympanic measurement of temperature is quick and requires little patient cooperation. Several cautions apply to the use of this technique: tympanic temperatures have been shown to be less accurate in infants younger than 3 months old and are subject to false readings if the instrument is not positioned properly or the external ear canal is occluded by wax.

Causes of Fever

Fever occurs when there is a rise in the hypothalamic set-point in response to endogenously produced pyrogens. A tremendously broad range of conditions cause fever, including infections, malignancies, autoimmune diseases, metabolic diseases, chronic inflammatory conditions, medications (including immunizations), central nervous system abnormalities, and exposure to excessive environ-

mental heat. In most settings, the majority of fevers in pediatric patients are caused by self-limiting viral infections. Teething does not cause fever over 38.4 °C.

Evaluation

A. GENERAL CONSIDERATIONS

When evaluating a child with fever, one should elicit from the parents information about the duration of fever, the maximum temperature of fever documented at home, all associated symptoms, any chronic medical conditions, any medications taken, medication allergies, fluid intake, urine output, exposures and travel, and any additional features of the illness that concern the parents (Table 8–5). In the office, a temperature, heart rate, respiratory rate, and blood pressure should be documented, as well as an oxygen saturation if the child has any increased work of breathing. A complete physical examination, including a neurologic examination, should then be performed, with particular attention paid to the child's degree of toxicity and hydration status. A well-appearing, well-hydrated child with evidence of a routine viral infection can be safely sent home with symptomatic treatment and careful return precautions.

Table 8–5. Guidelines for evaluating children with fever.

A. See immediately if:
  (1) The child is less than 3 months old.
  (2) The fever is over 40.6 °C.
  (3) The child is crying inconsolably or whimpering.
  (4) The child is crying when moved or even touched.
  (5) The child is difficult to awaken.
  (6) The child's neck is stiff.
  (7) Purple spots or dots are present on the skin.
  (8) The child's breathing is difficult, and not better after the nasal passages are cleared.
  (9) The child is drooling saliva and is unable to swallow anything.
  (10) A convulsion has occurred.
  (11) The child acts or looks "very sick."

B. See within 24 hours if:
  (1) The child is 3–6 months old (unless fever occurs within 48 hours after a diphtheria-tetanus-pertussis vaccination and the infant has no other serious symptoms).
  (2) The fever exceeds 40 °C (especially if the child is under age 3 years).
  (3) Burning or pain occurs with urination.
  (4) The fever has been present for more than 24 hours without an obvious cause or identified site of infection.
  (5) The fever has subsided for more than 24 hours and then returned.
  (6) The fever has been present for more than 72 hours.

Depending on the age of the patient, presence of underlying conditions, type of infection, and the provider's assessment of toxicity and hydration, many focal bacterial infections can also be treated on an outpatient basis, with appropriate oral antibiotics as discussed in Chapter 38.

B. FEVER WITHOUT A FOCUS OF INFECTION

Children who present with fever but without any symptoms or signs of a focal infection are often a diagnostic and management challenge. When assessing a child with fever but no apparent source of infection on examination, the provider needs to carefully consider the likelihood of a serious but hidden or occult bacterial infection. With the widespread use of effective vaccines against *Haemophilus influenzae* type b and *Streptococcus pneumoniae,* two of the most common causes of invasive bacterial infections in unimmunized children, the incidence of occult bacterial infections has declined. However, vaccines are not 100% effective, and other organisms cause serious occult infections in children; therefore febrile children will always demand careful evaluation and observation. Appropriate choices for empiric antibiotic therapy of children with fever without focus are discussed in Chapter 35.

Febrile infants 28 days old or younger, because of their susceptibility to serious disease including sepsis, should always be treated conservatively. Hospitalization and parenteral antibiotics should be strongly considered in all circumstances. An initial diagnostic evaluation should include complete blood cell count; blood culture; urinalysis; urine culture; Gram stain, protein, and glucose tests of cerebrospinal fluid; and cerebrospinal fluid culture. Consideration should also be given to the possibility of a perinatal herpes simplex virus infection (neonatal herpes is described in more detail in Chapter 36). A chest radiograph should be obtained for any infant with increased work of breathing.

Infants age 29–90 days are at risk of a variety of invasive bacterial infections, including perinatally acquired organisms (eg, group B streptococci) or infections acquired in the household (eg, pneumococci or meningococci). Febrile infants without a focus of infection can be divided into those who appear toxic versus nontoxic, and those at low risk versus higher risk of invasive bacterial disease. As with febrile neonates, toxic children in this age group should be admitted to the hospital for parenteral antibiotics and close observation. In nontoxic infants, low risk has been defined as previously healthy; no focal infection on examination; white blood cell count between 5000 and 15,000/mm^3; band cells < 1500/ mm^3; normal urinalysis; and, when diarrhea is present, < 5 white blood cells/high-power field. Nontoxic low-risk infants in this age group are typically treated as outpatients with close follow-up. Clinicians should be confident that lumbar puncture is unnecessary if they decide not to perform this procedure.

In an era of increasing immunization coverage against the most commonly invasive pneumococcal serotypes, it is difficult to estimate the risk of occult bacteremia in febrile 3- to 36-month-old children with no focus of infection. Nevertheless, for children 3–36 months old with temperatures ≥ 39 °C, urine cultures should be considered in all male children younger than 6 months of age and in all females younger than 2 years of age. Chest radiographs should be performed in any child with increased work of breathing and should also be considered in children with high (≥ 20,000/ mm^3) white blood cell counts but no respiratory symptoms. Depending on the child's appearance, underlying medical condition, and the severity of fever, blood cultures should also be obtained. Empiric antibiotic therapy may be considered, particularly for children with temperature of ≥ 39 °C and white blood cell count ≥ 15,000/mm^3. However, in previously healthy, well-appearing, fully immunized children with reassuring laboratory studies, observation without antibiotics is appropriate.

Treatment of Fever

Fever phobia is a term that describes parents' anxious response to the fevers that all children experience. In a recent study, 91% of caregivers thought that a fever could cause harmful effects. Seven percent of parents thought that if they did not treat the fever, it would keep going higher. Parents need to be reassured that fevers < 41.7 °C cause no brain damage. Parents need to be counseled that, although fevers can occasionally (≈ 4%) cause seizures, in which case their child needs to be seen, febrile seizures are generally harmless and also cause no brain damage.

Several safe and effective medications are available for the treatment of fever. Acetaminophen is indicated for children older than 2 months of age for fevers of 39 °C or if the child is uncomfortable. Acetaminophen is given in a dosage of 15 mg/kg of body weight per dose and can be given every 4–6 hours. The other widely used antipyretic is ibuprofen. Ibuprofen is given in a dosage of 10 mg/kg of body weight per dose and can be given every 6–8 hours. Ibuprofen and acetaminophen are similar in safety and their ability to reduce fever; however, ibuprofen is longer lasting. Aspirin should not be used for treating fever in any child or adolescent, because of its association with the development of Reye syndrome (particularly during infections with varicella and influenza).

Crocetti M, Moghbeli N, Serwint J: Fever phobia revisited: Have parental misconceptions about fever changed in 20 years? Pediatrics 2001;107:1241 [PMID: 11389237].

Klein JO: Management of the febrile child without a focus of infection in the era of universal pneumococcal immunization. Pediatr Infect Dis J 2002;21:584 [PMID: 12182394].

McCarthy PL: Fever without apparent source on clinical examination. Curr Opin Pediatr 2002;14:103 [PMID: 11880744].

Rehm KP: Fever in infants and children. Curr Opin Pediatr 2001; 13:83 [PMID: 11216593].

GROWTH DEFICIENCY

Growth deficiency—formerly termed failure to thrive—is deceleration of growth velocity resulting in crossing two major percentile lines on the growth chart. The diagnosis is warranted also if a child younger than age 6 months has not grown for 2 consecutive months or if a child older than age 6 months has not grown for 3 consecutive months. Growth deficiency occurs in about 8% of children.

Patterns of growth deficiency suggest, but are not specific for, different causes. In type I growth deficiency, the head circumference is preserved and the weight is depressed more than the height. This most common type results from inadequate caloric intake, excessive loss of calories, excessive intake of calories, or inability to use calories peripherally. Most such cases result from inadequate delivery of calories. This may be the result of poverty, lack of caregiver understanding, poor caregiver-child interaction, abnormal feeding patterns, or a combination of factors. Type II growth deficiency, which is associated with genetically determined short stature, endocrinopathies, constitutional growth delay, heart or renal disease, or various forms of skeletal dysplasias, is characterized by normal head circumference and proportionate diminution of height and weight. In type III growth deficiency, all three parameters of growth—head circumference, weight, and height—are lower than normal. This pattern is associated with central nervous system abnormalities, chromosomal defects, and in utero or perinatal insults.

Clinical Findings

A. INITIAL EVALUATION

The history and physical examination will identify the cause of growth reduction in the vast majority of cases (Table 8–6). The physical examination should focus on signs of organic disease or evidence of abuse or neglect: dysmorphic features, skin lesions, neck masses, adventitial breath sounds, heart murmurs, abdominal masses, and neuromuscular tone and strength. Throughout the evaluation, the physician should observe the caregiver-child interaction and the level of family functioning. Developmental screening and laboratory screening tests (complete blood count, blood urea nitrogen, creatinine, electrolytes, urinalysis, and urine culture) complete the initial office evaluation.

Table 8–6. Components of initial evaluation for growth deficiency.

Birth history: Newborn screening result. Rule out intrauterine growth retardation, anoxia, congenital infections.
Feeding and nutrition: Difficulty sucking, chewing, swallowing. Feeding patterns. Intake of formula, milk, juice, solids.
Stooling and voiding of urine: Diarrhea, constipation, vomiting, poor urine stream.
Growth pattern: Several points on the growth chart are crucial.
Recurrent infections.
Hospitalizations.
Human immunodeficiency virus risk factors.
Developmental history.
Social and family factors: Family composition, financial status, supports, stresses. Heritable diseases, heights and weights of relatives.
Review of systems.

B. FURTHER EVALUATION

A prospective 3-day diet record should be a standard part of the evaluation. This is useful in assessing undernutrition even when organic disease is present. The diet history is evaluated by a pediatric dietitian for calories, protein, and micronutrients as well as for the pattern of eating. Additional laboratory tests should be ordered based on the history and physical examination. For example, stool collection for fat determination is indicated if a history of diarrhea suggests malabsorption. Moderate or high amounts of proteinuria should prompt work-up for nephrotic syndrome. Vomiting should suggest a gastrointestinal, metabolic, neurologic, infectious, or renal cause. The tempo of evaluation should be based on the severity of symptoms and the magnitude of growth failure.

Treatment

A successful treatment plan addresses the child's diet and eating patterns, the child's development, caregiver skills, and any organic disease. High-calorie diets and frequent monitoring (every 1 or 2 weeks initially) are essential. Acceptable weight gain varies by age (Table 8–7).

The child with growth deficiency may also be developmentally delayed because of living in an environment that fails to promote development or from the effect on the brain of nutrient deprivation. Restoring nutrition does not fully reverse the deficit but does reduce the long-term consequences.

Education in nutrition, child development, and behavioral management as well as psychosocial support of the primary caregiver is essential. If family dysfunction is mild, behavior modification and counseling will be useful. Day care may benefit the child by providing a structured environment for all activities, including eating. If family dysfunction is severe, the local department of social services

Table 8–7. Acceptable weight gain by age.

Age (months)	Weight Gain (g/d)
Birth to 3	20–30
3–6	15–20
6–9	10–15
9–12	6–11
12–18	5–8
18–24	3–7

can help provide structure and assistance to the family. Rarely, the child may need to be temporarily or permanently removed from the home. Hospitalization is reserved for management of dehydration, for cases in which home therapy has failed to result in expected growth, for children who show evidence of abuse or willful neglect, for management of an illness that compromises a child's ability to eat, or for care pending foster home placement.

Weston JA: Growth deficiency. In Berman S (editor): *Pediatric Decision Making,* 4th ed. Mosby-Year Book, 2003.

Immunization

Matthew F. Daley, MD, Ann-Christine Nyquist, MD, MSPH, & Eric A.F. Simoes, MB, BS, DCH, MD

Immunization is used either to prevent primary infection or to prevent the secondary consequences of an infection. Any assessment of the benefits of a proposed immunization program must take into account the likelihood of occurrence of infection in a defined population or specific individual, the consequence of infection, and the likelihood that the vaccination will prevent that infection. The anticipated benefit of immunization must be weighed against the risk to the individual of adverse consequences. The physician must present this information to the parents so they can give informed consent to immunization. The immunization recommendations outlined in this chapter are current but will change as technology evolves and our understanding of the epidemiology of vaccine-preventable diseases changes. The most useful sources for regularly updated information about immunization are the following:

1. *Morbidity and Mortality Weekly Report.* Published weekly by the Centers for Disease Control and Prevention (CDC), Atlanta, GA 30333. Available at http://www.cdc.gov/mmwr.
2. *The Red Book: Report of the Committee on Infectious Diseases.* Published at 2- to 3-year intervals by the American Academy of Pediatrics (AAP). The 2003 *Red Book* is available from the AAP. Updates are published in the journal *Pediatrics* and can be accessed at http://www.aap.org/.
3. Centers for Disease Control and Prevention: National Immunization Program Information Hotline. Provides services to consumers and health care professionals regarding new vaccines, new schedules, and safety issues. 1-800-232-2522 (Spanish 1-800-232-0233). Operates from 8:00 AM to 11:00 PM Monday through Friday. Printed information can be obtained at http://cdc.gov/nip/.
4. Centers for Disease Control and Prevention: Advisory Committee on Immunization Practice (ACIP). Available at http://www.cdc.gov/nip/ACIP.

STANDARDS FOR PEDIATRIC IMMUNIZATION PRACTICES

In the United States, every infant requires between 15 and 19 doses of vaccine by age 18 months to be pro-

tected against 12 childhood diseases. For the first time, in the U.S. in 2004 vaccination rates in children 18–35 months old exceeded 80% coverage for the recommended vaccination series, exceeding the *Healthy People 2010* goal. However, data from the Vaccine Safety Datalink Project shows that only 36% of children < 2 years old were completely compliant with vaccination recommendations, 30% had a missed opportunity for immunization, 20% had an invalid immunization, and 12% received an extra immunization (costing an estimated $26.5 million. The AAP recommends the following specific proven practices to improve these defects: (1) sending caretakers reminder and recall notices, (2) using prompts during all visits, (3) periodic measurement of immunization rates, and (4) having standing orders for vaccines.

The National Childhood Vaccine Injury Act of 1986 requires that for each vaccine covered under the Vaccine Injury Compensation Program, caretakers should be advised about the risks and benefits of vaccination in a standard manner, using the Vaccine Information Statements. In addition the CDC and AAP have the requirements and recommendations summarized later on. Each time a Vaccine Injury Compensation Program–covered vaccine is administered, the current version of Vaccine Information Statements must be provided to the non-minor patient or legal caretaker. Documentation is required in the medical record, including the vaccine manufacturer, lot number, and its date of administration and expiration. The name and address of the person administering the vaccine, Vaccine Information Statement version and date, and site and route of administration should also be recorded.

The use of disposable syringes and needles or some other form of single-dose delivery of vaccine is preferred to minimize the opportunity for contamination. A 70% solution of alcohol is appropriate for disinfection of the stopper of the vaccine container and of the skin at the injection site. A 5% topical emulsion of lidocaine-prilocaine cream applied to the site of vaccination for 30–60 minutes prior to the injection minimizes the pain, especially when multiple vaccines are administered.

The manufacturer's recommendations for route and site of administration of injectable vaccines are critical for safety and efficacy. All vaccines containing an adjuvant must be administered intramuscularly to avoid granuloma formation or necrosis. Such injections should be given at a 90 degree angle into the anterolateral thigh (not intragluteally) in infants (< age 18 months) and may be given in the deltoid or triceps in older children. A 22-gauge needle $^7/8$–$1^1/4$ inches long is recommended for children, but a 25-gauge $^7/8$–1 inch needle may be sufficient for young infants. Aspiration prior to intramuscular injection is suggested by many experts. Vaccines may be administered intramuscularly, subcutaneously, or intradermally. Subcutaneous injections should be administered at a 45-degree angle into the anterolateral aspect of the thigh or the upper outer triceps area using a 25-gauge $^5/8$-inch needle. Intradermal injections should be administered on the volar surface of the forearm with the bevel facing upward using a $^3/8$–$^3/4$ inch 25- to 27-gauge needle. A 25-gauge $^3/4$–$^5/8$ inch needle is recommended. A separate syringe and needle should be used for each vaccine.

It is safe to administer many combinations of vaccines simultaneously without increasing the risk of adverse effects or compromising response. Up to seven injections may be necessary at the 12- to 15-month visit. (See the following individual preparations for further discussion.) Inactivated vaccines (with the exception of cholera and yellow fever) can be given simultaneously or at any time after a different vaccine. Parenteral live-virus vaccines, if not administered on the same day, should be given at least 30 days apart (eg, measles-mumps-rubella [MMR] and varicella [VAR]). Lapses in the immunization schedule do not call for reinstitution of the series. Extra doses of hepatitis B (HepB), *Haemophilus influenzae* type B (Hib), MMR, or VAR are not harmful, but repetitive exposure to tetanus vaccine beyond the recommended intervals can result in hypersensitivity reactions and should be avoided. If an immunoglobulin (Ig) or blood product has been administered, live-virus vaccination should be delayed 3–11 months, depending on the product, to avoid interference with the immune response (eg, 3 months for tetanus Ig, hepatitis A Ig, and hepatitis B Ig, 5–6 months for measles Ig or cytomegalovirus Ig (CMVIg), and 11 months for intravenous Ig for Kawasaki disease).

With the large number of vaccine preparations available, interchangeability of vaccines is an issue. All brands of Hib conjugate, hepatitis B, and hepatitis A vaccines are interchangeable. For vaccines containing acellular pertussis antigens, it is recommended that the same brand be used, but when the brand is unknown or the same brand is unavailable, any DTaP (diphtheria, tetanus toxoids, and acellular pertussis vaccine) should be used to continue vaccination. Longer than a recommended interval between vaccinations does not reduce final antibody titers and thus lapsed schedules do not require restarting the series.

Atkinson WL et al: Centers for Disease Control and Prevention: General recommendations on immunization: Recommendations of the Advisory Committee on Immunization Practices (ACIP) and the American Academy of Family Physicians (AAFP). MMWR Recomm Rep 2002;51(RR-2):1 [PMID: 11848294].

Berman S et al: Impact of a decline in Colorado Medicaid managed care enrollment on access and quality of preventive primary care services. Pediatrics 2005;116:1474 [PMID: 16322173].

Centers for Disease Control and Prevention: National, state and urban area vaccination coverage among children aged 19–35 months—United States 2005. MMWR Morb Mortal Wkly Rep 2005;54:717 [PMID: 16049420].

Mell LK et al: Compliance with national immunization guidelines for children younger than 2 years, 1996–1999. Pediatrics 2005;115:461 [PMID: 15687456].

■ THE COMPOSITION OF IMMUNIZING AGENTS

ACTIVE IMMUNIZATION

The immune response to immunization varies. A small proportion of children receiving certain antigens simply do not mount a response capable of conferring protection. For this reason, every vaccine has a definable failure rate.

The immunogen is suspended or dissolved in sterile water or saline, or in more complex media such as tissue culture medium, which may contain constituents from the biologic system used to produce the immunogen. Most vaccines contain preservatives and trace amounts of antibiotics such as neomycin to prevent bacterial overgrowth. Some vaccines contain adjuvants such as aluminum hydroxide or phosphate that retain the immunogen at the site of inoculation for a prolonged time, thus increasing antigenic stimulation. The theoretical cumulative toxicity of mercury in thimerosal-containing vaccines has led to the development of thimerosal-free vaccines. All vaccines routinely administered to children are now available as free of thimerosal.

Rarely vaccine administration has unforeseen adverse consequences. Thus vaccines should be administered where there is ready access to emergency resuscitative equipment and drugs (eg, epinephrine and antihistamines).

PASSIVE IMMUNIZATION

Immune globulin (Ig) is derived from pooled donations of large numbers of individuals (more than 1000 per lot). Ig is prepared by alcohol fractionation, is sterile, and will not transmit any infectious agents (including hepatitis B and C viruses and human immunodeficiency virus

[HIV]). Ig is a 16.5% solution consisting primarily of IgG with very small amounts of IgA and IgM.

ROUTINE CHILDHOOD & ADOLESCENT IMMUNIZATIONS

Table 9–1 sets forth a schedule of routine immunizations for normal infants and children. The routine immunization schedule is updated annually. Table 9–2 presents recommended schedules for children who did not start vaccination at the recommended time during the first year of life. Variations from these schedules may be necessitated by epidemiologic or individual clinical circumstances. Recommendations for minimum ages and intervals between doses are shown in Table 9–2.

Combination vaccines represent a solution to the problem of large numbers of injections during any single clinic visit. Currently available combination vaccines include MMR, measles-mumps-rubella-varicella [MMRV], and various combinations of Hib, HepB, and diphtheria, tetanus, and pertussis vaccines, and more recently a diphtheria, tetanus, acellular pertussis, hepatitis B, inactivated polio virus (DTaP-HepB-IPV) combination vaccine.

Additional combination vaccines and vaccines specifically for older children and adolescents are in development. Separate vaccines should not be combined into one syringe by the provider unless approved by the Food and Drug Administration (FDA), because this could decrease the efficacy of each component vaccine.

Safe Handling of Vaccines

The numerous vaccines and other immunologic substances, such as antibody preparations and immunoglobulins for routine use by the practitioner, vary in the storage temperatures required. Vaccines that require routine freezing are VAR, oral poliovirus (OPV) and live attenuated intranasal influenza vaccine (LAIV). Yellow fever vaccine may also be stored frozen. Product package inserts should be consulted for detailed information on vaccine storage conditions and shelf life.

Centers for Disease Control and Prevention: Recommended childhood and adolescent immunization schedule—United States, January–June 2006. MMWR Morb Mortal Wkly Rep 2006; 55:1.

■ SAFETY OF IMMUNIZATION

VACCINE FACTORS

The safety standards for all vaccines licensed for use in the United States are established by the FDA and involve reg-

ular examination of manufacturing techniques as well as production lots of vaccine. No incidents of bacterial or viral contamination of vaccines at the factory level have been reported in the United States for decades.

HOST FACTORS

The contraindications and precautions relating to immunization presented in Table 9–3 reflect the current recommendations of the ACIP and the Committee of Infectious Diseases of the AAP (*Red Book*). For more recently licensed vaccines (eg, MMRV and DTaP), information on contraindications and precautions presented in Table 9–3 are based on provisional ACIP recommendations or package insert information.

Healthy Children

Minor acute illnesses, with or without low-grade fever, are not contraindications (see Table 9–3) to vaccination, because there is no evidence that vaccination under these conditions increases the rate of adverse effects or decreases efficacy. A moderate to severe febrile illness may be a reason to postpone vaccination. Routine physical examination and temperature assessment are not necessary before vaccinating healthy infants and children.

Children with Chronic Illnesses

Most chronic diseases are not contraindications to vaccination; in fact, children with chronic diseases may be at greater risk of complications from vaccine-preventable diseases such as influenza and pneumococcal infections. Premature infants are a good example. They should be immunized according to their chronologic, not gestational, age. Vaccine doses should not be reduced for preterm or low-birth-weight infants. The one exception to this rule may be children with progressive central nervous system (CNS) disorders. Vaccination may be deferred or avoided entirely for such children, whereas children with static CNS diseases are candidates for vaccination.

Immunodeficient Children

Congenitally immunodeficient children should not be immunized with live-virus (OPV, MMR, VAR, yellow fever, or LAIV) or live-bacteria vaccines (bacille Calmette-Guérin [BCG] or Ty21a). Depending on the nature of the immunodeficiency, other vaccines are safe, but may fail to evoke an immune response. Children with cancer and children receiving high-dose corticosteroids or other immunosuppressive agents should not be vaccinated with live-virus or live-bacteria vaccines. This contraindication does not apply if the malignancy is in remission and chemotherapy has not been administered for at least 90 days. Live-virus vaccines may also be administered to previously healthy children receiving low to moderate doses of corticosteroids

Table 9–1. Recommended childhood and adolescent immunization schedule: United States, 2006.

Vaccine ▼ Age ▶	Birth	1 month	2 months	4 months	6 months	12 months	15 months	18 months	24 months	4–6 years	11–12 years	13–14 years	15 years	16–18 years
Hepatitis B¹	HepB	HepB		HepB¹	HepB						HepB Series			
Diphtheria, Tetanus, Pertussis²			DTaP	DTaP	DTaP		DTaP			DTaP	Tdap	Tdap		
Haemophilus influenzae type b³			Hib	Hib	Hib³	Hib								
Inactivated Poliovirus			IPV	IPV	IPV					IPV				
Measles, Mumps, Rubella⁴						MMR				MMR	MMR			
Varicella⁵						Varicella					Varicella			
Meningococcal⁶							Vaccines within broken line are for selected populations		MPSV4		MCV4	MCV4		MCV4
Pneumococcal⁷			PCV	PCV	PCV	PCV			PCV		PPV			
Influenza⁸					Influenza (Yearly)						Influenza (Yearly)			
Hepatitis A⁹						HepA Series								

Range of recommended ages   Catch-up immunization   11–12 year old assessment

This schedule indicates the recommended ages for routine administration of currently licensed childhood vaccines, as of December 1, 2005, for children through age 18 years. Any dose not administered at the recommended age should be administered at any subsequent visit when indicated and feasible. ▇ Indicates age groups that warrant special effort to administer those vaccines not previously administered. Additional vaccines may be licensed and recommended during the year. Licensed combination vaccines may be used whenever any components of the combination are indicated and other components of the vaccine are not contraindicated and if approved by the Food and Drug Administration for that dose of the series. Providers should consult the respective ACIP statement for detailed recommendations. Clinically significant adverse events that follow immunization should be reported to the Vaccine Adverse Event Reporting System (VAERS). Guidance about how to obtain and complete a VAERS form is available at **www.vaers.hhs.gov** or by telephone, **800-822-7967.**

1. Hepatitis B vaccine (HepB). *AT BIRTH:* All newborns should receive monovalent HepB soon after birth and before hospital discharge. **Infants born to mothers who are HBsAg-positive** should receive HepB and 0.5 mL of hepatitis B immune globulin (HBIG) within 12 hours of birth. **Infants born to mothers whose HBsAg status is unknown** should receive HepB within 12 hours of birth. The mother should have blood drawn as soon as possible to determine her HBsAg status; if HBsAg-positive, the infant should receive HBIG as soon as possible (no later than age 1 week). **For infants born to HBsAg-negative mothers,** the birth dose can be delayed in rare circumstances but only if a physician's order to withhold the vaccine and a copy of the mother's original HBsAg-negative laboratory report are documented in the infant's medical record. *FOLLOWING THE BIRTHDOSE:* The HepB series should be completed with either monovalent HepB or a combination vaccine containing HepB. The second dose should be administered at age 1–2 months. The final dose should be administered at age ≥24 weeks. It is permissible to administer 4 doses of HepB (e.g., when combination vaccines are given after the birth dose); however, if monovalent HepB is used, a dose at age 4 months is not needed. **Infants born to HBsAg-positive mothers** should be tested for HBsAg and antibody to HBsAg after completion of the HepB series, at age 9–18 months (generally at the next well-child visit after completion of the vaccine series).

2. Diphtheria and tetanus toxoids and acellular pertussis vaccine (DTaP). The fourth dose of DTaP may be administered as early as age 12 months, provided 6 months have elapsed since the third dose and the child is unlikely to return at age 15–18 months. The final dose in the series should be given at age ≥4 years. **Tetanus and diphtheria toxoids and acellular pertussis vaccine (Tdap – adolescent preparation)** is recommended at age 11–12 years for those who have completed the recommended childhood DTP/DTaP vaccination series and have not received a Td booster dose. Adolescents 13–18 years who missed the 11–12-year Td/Tdap booster dose should also receive a single dose of Tdap if they have completed the recommended childhood DTP/DTaP vaccination series. Subsequent **tetanus and diphtheria toxoids (Td)** are recommended every 10 years.

3. *Haemophilus influenzae* **type b conjugate vaccine (Hib).** Three Hib conjugate vaccines are licensed for infant use. If PRP-OMP (PedvaxHIB® or ComVax® [Merck]) is administered at ages 2 and 4 months, a dose at age 6 months is not required. DTaP/Hib combination products should not be used for primary immunization in infants at ages 2, 4 or 6 months but can be used as boosters after any Hib vaccine. The final dose in the series should be administered at age ≥12 months.

4. Measles, mumps, and rubella vaccine (MMR). The second dose of MMR is recommended routinely at age 4–6 years but may be administered during any visit, provided at least 4 weeks have elapsed since the first dose and both doses are administered beginning at or after age 12 months. Those who have not previously received the second dose should complete the schedule by age 11–12 years.

5. Varicella vaccine. Varicella vaccine is recommended at any visit at or after age 12 months for susceptible children (i.e., those who lack a reliable history of chickenpox). Susceptible persons aged ≥13 years should receive 2 doses administered at least 4 weeks apart.

6. Meningococcal vaccine (MCV4). Meningococcal conjugate vaccine (MCV4) should be given to all children at the 11–12 year old visit as well as to unvaccinated adolescents at high school entry (15 years of age). Other adolescents who wish to decrease their risk for meningococcal disease may also be vaccinated. All college freshmen living in dormitories should also be vaccinated, preferably with MCV4, although **meningococcal polysaccharide vaccine (MPSV4)** is an acceptable alternative. Vaccination against invasive meningococcal disease is recommended for children and adolescents aged ≥2 years with terminal complement deficiencies or anatomic or functional asplenia and certain other high risk groups (see *MMWR* 2005;54 [RR-7]:1-21); use MPSV4 for children aged 2–10 years and MCV4 for older children, although MPSV4 is an acceptable alternative.

7. Pneumococcal vaccine. The heptavalent **pneumococcal conjugate vaccine (PCV)** is recommended for all children aged 2–23 months and for certain children aged 24–59 months. The final dose in the series should be given at age ≥12 months. **Pneumococcal polysaccharide vaccine (PPV)** is recommended in addition to PCV for certain high-risk groups. See *MMWR* 2000; 49(RR-9):1-35.

8. Influenza vaccine. Influenza vaccine is recommended annually for children aged ≥6 months with certain risk factors (including, but not limited to, asthma, cardiac disease, sickle cell disease, human immunodeficiency virus [HIV], diabetes, and conditions that can compromise respiratory function or handling of respiratory secretions or that can increase the risk for aspiration), healthcare workers, and other persons (including household members) in close contact with persons in groups at high risk (see *MMWR* 2005;54[RR-8]:1-55). In addition, healthy children aged 6–23 months and close contacts of healthy children aged 0–5 months are recommended to receive influenza vaccine because children in this age group are at substantially increased risk for influenza-related hospitalizations. For healthy persons aged 5–49 years, the intranasally administered, live, attenuated influenza vaccine (LAIV) is an acceptable alternative to the intramuscular trivalent inactivated influenza vaccine (TIV). See *MMWR* 2005;54(RR-8):1-55. Children receiving TIV should be administered a dosage appropriate for their age (0.25 mL if aged 6–35 months or 0.5 mL if aged ≥3 years). Children aged ≤8 years who are receiving influenza vaccine for the first time should receive 2 doses (separated by at least 4 weeks for TIV and at least 6 weeks for LAIV).

9. Hepatitis A vaccine (HepA). HepA is recommended for all children at 1 year of age (i.e., 12–23 months). The 2 doses in the series should be administered at least 6 months apart. States, counties, and communities with existing HepA vaccination programs for children 2–18 years of age are encouraged to maintain these programs. In these areas, new efforts focused on routine vaccination of 1-year-old children should enhance, not replace, ongoing programs directed at a broader population of children. HepA is also recommended for certain high risk groups (see *MMWR* 1999; 48[RR-12]1-37).

The Childhood and Adolescent Immunization Schedule is approved by:
Advisory Committee on Immunization Practices www.cdc.gov/nip/acip • American Academy of Pediatrics www.aap.org • American Academy of Family Physicians www.aafp.org

Reproduced, with permission, from CDC: Recommended childhood and adolescent immunization schedule—U.S., 2006. MMWR Morb Mortal Wkly Rep 2006;54:Q1–Q4.

Table 9–2. Recommended immunization schedule for children and adolescents who start late or who are more than 1 month behind: United States, 2006.

Catch-Up Schedule for Children Aged 4 Months–6 Years				
Dose 1 (Minimum Age)	Minimum Interval between Doses			
	Dose 1 to Dose 2	Dose 2 to Dose 3	Dose 3 to Dose 4	Dose 4 to Dose 5
DTaP (6 wk)	4 wk	4 wk	6 mo	6 mo[a]
IPV (6 wk)	4 wk	4 wk	4 wk[b]	
HepB[c] (birth)	4 wk	8 wk (and 16 wk after 1st dose)		
MMR (12 mo)	4 wk[d]			
VAR (12 mo)				
Hib[e] (6 wk)	4 wk: if 1st dose given at age < 12 mo 8 wk (as final dose): if 1st dose given at age 12–14 mo No further doses needed: if 1st dose given at age ≥ 15 mo	4 wk[f]: if current age < 12 mo 8 wk (as final dose)[f]: if current age ≥ 12 mo and 2nd dose given at age < 15 mo No further doses needed: if previous dose given at age ≥ 15 mo	8 wk (as final dose): this dose only necessary for children aged 12 mo–5 y who received 3 doses before age 12 mo	
PCV[g] (6 wk)	4 wk: if 1st dose given at age < 12 mo and current age < 24 mo 8 wk (as final dose): if 1st dose given at age ≥ 12 mo or current age 24–59 mo No further doses needed: for healthy children if 1st dose given at age ≥ 24 mo	4 wk: if current age < 12 mo 8 wk (as final dose): if current age ≥ 12 mo No further doses needed: for healthy children if previous dose given at age ≥ 24 mo	8 wk (as final dose): this dose only necessary for children aged 12 mo–5 y who received 3 doses before age 12 mo	

Catch-Up Schedule for Children Aged 7–18 Years		
Minimal Interval between Doses		
Dose 1 to Dose 2	Dose 2 to Dose 3	Dose 3 to Booster Dose
Td[h]: 4 wk	Td[h]: 6 mo	Td[h]: 6 mo: if 1st dose given at age <12 mo and current age <11 y; otherwise, 5 y
IPV[i]: 4 wk	IPV[i]: 4 wk	IPV[b,i]
HepB: 4 wk	HepB: 8 wk (and 16 wk after 1st dose)	
MMR: 4 wk		
VAR[i]: 4 wk		

Note: The tables give catch-up schedules and minimum intervals between doses for children who have delayed immunizations. There is no need to restart a vaccine series regardless of the time that has elapsed between doses. Use the chart appropriate for the child's age.

[a]**Diphtheria and tetanus toxoids and acellular pertussis vaccine (DTaP):** The fifth dose is not necessary if the fourth dose was given after the fourth birthday.

[b]**Inactivated polio vaccine (IPV):** For children who received an all-IPV or all-oral poliovirus (OPV) series, a fourth dose is not necessary if third dose was given at age ≥ 4 years. If both OPV and IPV were given as part of a series, a total of 4 doses should be given, regardless of the child's current age.

(defined as up to 2 mg/kg/d of prednisone or prednisone equivalent, with a 20 mg/d maximum) for less than 14 days; children receiving low to moderate doses of alternate-day corticosteroids; children being maintained on physiologic corticosteroid therapy without other immunodeficiency; and children using only topical, inhaled, or intra-articular corticosteroids.

Contraindication of live-pathogen vaccine also applies to children with HIV infection who are severely immunosuppressed. In general those who receive MMR should have at least 15% CD4 cells and a CD4 lymphocyte count equivalent to CDC immunologic class 2. MMR for these children is recommended at 12 months of age (after 6 months during an epidemic). The booster dose may be given as early as 1 month later, but doses given before 1 year of age should not be considered part of a complete series. VAR vaccination is also recommended for HIV-infected children with CD4 cells preserved as listed above. OPV is contraindicated and is no longer recommended in the United States. The ACIP recommends routine vaccination for all children with an all inactivated poliovirus vaccine (IPV) vaccination schedule. Thus immunodeficient children should no longer be exposed to oral polio vaccine through household contacts. MMR and VAR are not contraindicated in household contacts of immunocompromised children.

Allergic or Hypersensitive Children

Hypersensitivity reactions are rare following vaccination, occurring in 1.53 cases/million doses. They are generally attributable to a trace component of the vaccine rather than to the antigen itself. MMR, IPV, and VAR contain microgram quantities of neomycin, and IPV also contains trace amounts of streptomycin and polymyxin B. Children with known anaphylactic responses to these antibiotics should not be given these vaccines. Trace quantities of egg antigens may be present in both inactivated and live influenza and yellow fever vaccines and MMR. Children who have had anaphylactic reactions to eggs should not be given these vaccines; children with less serious reactions to eggs may generally be safely immunized. If doubt exists about the nature of a child's egg sensitivity, a skin testing procedure is outlined in the *Red Book*. Some vaccines (MMR, VAR, and yellow fever) contain gelatin, a substance to which persons with known food allergy may develop an anaphylactic reaction. Skin testing before vaccination may be an option in such cases.

Special Circumstances

Detailed recommendations for preterm low-birth-weight babies; pediatric transplant recipients; Alaskan Natives/ American Indians; children in residential institutions or military communities; or refugees, new immigrants, or travelers are available in the AAP *Red Book*.

American Academy of Pediatrics: *2003 Red Book: Report of the Committee on Infectious Diseases,* 26th ed. American Academy of Pediatrics, 2003.

Bohlke K et al: Vaccine Safety Datalink Team: Risk of anaphylaxis after vaccination of children and adolescents. Pediatrics 2003;112:815 [PMID: 14523172].

DIPHTHERIA

The risk for exposure to toxigenic strains of *Corynebacterium diphtheriae* in the United States is low (53 prob-

---

[c]**Hepatitis B vaccine (HepB):** Administer the 3-dose series to all children and adolescents < 19 years of age if they were not previously vaccinated.

[d]**Measles, mumps, and rubella vaccine (MMR):** The second dose of MMR is recommended routinely at age 4–6 years, but may be given earlier if desired.

[e]*Haemophilus influenzae* **type B (Hib) conjugate vaccine:** Vaccine is not generally recommended for children aged ≥ 5 years.

[f]**Hib:** If current age is < 12 months and the first 2 doses were PRP-OMP (PedvaxHIB® or ComVax® [Merck]), the third (and final) dose should be given at age 12–15 months and at least 8 weeks after the second dose.

[g]**Pneumococcal conjugate vaccine (PCV):** Vaccine is not generally recommended for children aged ≥ 5 years.

[h]**Tetanus and diphtheria toxoids (Td):** Adolescent tetanus, diphtheria, and pertussis vaccine (Tdap) may be substituted for any dose in a primary catch-up series or as a booster if age appropriate for Tdap. A 5-year interval from the last Td dose is encouraged when Tdap is used as a booster dose. See Advisory Committee on Immunization Practices recommendations for further information.

[i]**IPV:** Vaccine is not generally recommended for persons aged ≥ 18 years.

[j]**Varicella vaccine (VAR):** Administer the 2-dose series to all susceptible adolescents aged ≥ 13 years.

Report adverse reactions to vaccines through the federal Vaccine Adverse Event Reporting System. For information on reporting reactions following immunization, please visit www.vaers.hhs.gov or call the 24-hour national toll-free information line 800-822-7967. Report suspected cases of vaccine-preventable diseases to your state or local health department. For additional information about vaccines, including precautions and contraindications for vaccination and vaccine shortages, please visit the National Immunization Program Website at www.cdc.gov/nip or contact 800-CDC-INFO (800-232-4636). (In English, En Espanol: 24/7)

Reproduced, with permission, from CDC: Recommended childhood and adolescent immunization schedule—United States, 2006. MMWR Morb Mortal Wkly Rep 2006:54;Q1–Q4.

Table 9–3. Guide to contraindications and precautions[a] to commonly used vaccines.

Vaccine	True Contraindications and Precautions[a]	Untrue (Vaccines Can Be Administered)
General for all vaccines, including diphtheria and tetanus toxoids and acellular pertussis vaccine (DTaP); pediatric diphtheria-tetanus toxoid (DT); adult tetanus-diphtheria toxoid (Td); inactivated poliovirus vaccine (IPV); measles-mumps-rubella vaccine (MMR); *Haemophilus influenzae* type b vaccine (Hib); hepatitis A vaccine; hepatitis B vaccine; varicella vaccine; pneumococcal conjugate vaccine (PCV); influenza vaccine; and pneumococcal polysaccharide vaccine (PPV)	**Contraindications** Serious allergic reaction (eg, anaphylaxis) after a previous vaccine dose Serious allergic reaction (eg, anaphylaxis) to a vaccine component **Precautions** Moderate or severe acute illness with or without fever	Mild acute illness with or without fever Mild to moderate local reaction (ie, swelling, redness, soreness); low-grade or moderate fever after previous dose Lack of previous physical examination in well-appearing person Current antimicrobial therapy Convalescent phase of illness Premature birth (hepatitis B vaccine is an exception in certain circumstances)[b] Recent exposure to an infectious disease History of penicillin allergy, other nonvaccine allergies, relatives with allergies, receiving allergen extract immunotherapy
DTaP	**Contraindications** Severe allergic reaction after a previous dose or to a vaccine component Encephalopathy (eg, coma, decreased level of consciousness; prolonged seizures) within 7 days of administration of previous dose of DTP or DTaP Progressive neurologic disorder, including infantile spasms, uncontrolled epilepsy, progressive encephalopathy: defer DTaP until neurologic status clarified and stabilized. **Precautions** Fever of > 40.5 °C ≤ 48 h after vaccination with a previous dose of DTP or DTaP Collapse or shock-like state (ie, hypotonic hyporesponsive episode) ≤ 48 h after receiving a previous dose of DTP/DTaP Seizure ≤ 3 d of receiving a previous dose of DTP/DTaP[c] Persistent, inconsolable crying lasting ≥ 3 h ≤ 48 hours after receiving a previous dose of DTP/DTaP Moderate or severe acute illness with or without fever	Temperature of < 40.5 °C, fussiness or mild drowsiness after a previous dose of diphtheria toxoid-tetanus toxoid-pertussis vaccine (DTP)/DTaP Family history of seizures[c] Family history of sudden infant death syndrome Family history of an adverse event after DTP or DTaP administration Stable neurologic conditions (eg, cerebral palsy, well-controlled convulsions, developmental delay)
DT, Td	**Contraindications** Severe allergic reaction after a previous dose or to a vaccine component **Precautions** Guillain-Barré syndrome ≤ 6 wk after previous dose of tetanus toxoid-containing vaccine Moderate or severe acute illness with or without fever	—

(continued)

Table 9–3. Guide to contraindications and precautions[a] to commonly used vaccines. (continued)

Vaccine	True Contraindications and Precautions[a]	Untrue (Vaccines Can Be Administered)
Tdap	**Contraindications** Severe allergic reaction to a vaccine component Encephalopathy (eg, coma, prolonged seizures) not attributable to an identifiable cause within 7 days of administration of a vaccine with pertussis components **Precautions** Guillain-Barré syndrome ≤ 6 wk after a previous dose of a tetanus toxoid–containing vaccine Progressive neurologic disorder, uncontrolled epilepsy, or progressive encephalopathy until the condition has stabilized Moderate or severe acute illness with or without fever History of an Arthus reaction after a tetanus toxoid–containing and/or diphtheria toxoid–containing vaccine administered < 10 y previously	—
IPV	**Contraindications** Severe allergic reaction to previous dose or vaccine component **Precautions** Pregnancy Moderate or severe acute illness with or without fever	—
MMR[d]	**Contraindications** Severe allergic reaction after a previous dose or to a vaccine component Pregnancy Known severe immunodeficiency (eg, hematologic and solid tumors; congenital immunodeficiency; long-term immunosuppressive therapy,[e] or severely symptomatic human immunodeficiency virus [HIV] infection) **Precautions** Recent (≤ 11 mo) receipt of antibody-containing blood product (specific interval depends on product)[g] History of thrombocytopenia or thrombocytopenic purpura Moderate or severe acute illness with or without fever	Positive tuberculin skin test Simultaneous TB skin testing[f] Breast feeding Pregnancy of recipient's mother or other close or household contact Recipient is child-bearing–age female Immunodeficient family member or household contact Asymptomatic or mildly symptomatic HIV infection Allergy to eggs
MMRV	**Contraindications** Severe allergic reaction after a previous dose or to a vaccine component Known severe immunodeficiency (eg, hematologic malignancies, congenital immunodeficiency, long-term immunosuppressive therapy,[e] or symptomatic HIV infection)	—

(continued)

Table 9–3. Guide to contraindications and precautions[a] to commonly used vaccines. (continued)

Vaccine	True Contraindications and Precautions[a]	Untrue (Vaccines Can Be Administered)
MMRV (*continued*)	Active febrile illness with fever > 101.3 °F Active untreated tuberculosis Pregnancy **Precautions** History of thrombocytopenia Recent (≤ 11 mo) receipt of antibody-containing blood product (specific interval depends on product)[g]	
Hib	**Contraindications** Severe allergic reaction after a previous dose or to a vaccine component Age < 6 wk **Precaution** Moderate or severe acute illness with or without fever	—
Hepatitis B	**Contraindication** Severe allergic reaction to yeast, to any vaccine component, or after a previous dose **Precautions** Infant weighing < 2000 g[b] Moderate or severe acute illness with or without fever	Pregnancy Autoimmune disease (eg, systemic lupus erythematosus or rheumatoid arthritis)
Hepatitis A	**Contraindications** Severe allergic reaction after a previous dose or to a vaccine component **Precautions** Pregnancy Moderate or severe acute illness with or without fever	—
Varicella[d]	**Contraindications** Severe allergic reaction after a previous dose or to a vaccine component Substantial suppression of cellular immunity Pregnancy **Precautions** Recent (≤ 11 mo) receipt of antibody-containing blood product (specific interval depends on product)[g] Moderate or severe acute illness with or without fever	Pregnancy of recipient's mother or other close or household contact Immunodeficient family member or household contact[h] Asymptomatic or mildly symptomatic HIV infection Humoral immunodeficiency (eg, agammaglobulinemia)
PCV	**Contraindication** Severe allergic reaction after a previous dose or to a vaccine component **Precautions** Moderate or severe acute illness with or without fever	—

Table 9–3. Guide to contraindications and precautions[a] to commonly used vaccines. (continued)

Vaccine	True Contraindications and Precautions[a]	Untrue (Vaccines Can Be Administered)
Meningococcal (MCV4)	**Contraindications** Severe allergic reaction to any vaccine component, including diphtheria toxoid, or to dry natural rubber latex Pregnancy (no data available regarding safety) **Precautions** Prior history of Guillain-Barré syndrome Moderate or severe acute illness with or without fever	—
Influenza	**Contraindication** Severe allergic reaction to previous dose or vaccine component, including egg protein **Precautions** Moderate or severe acute illness with or without fever	Nonsevere (eg, contact) allergy to latex or thimerosal Concurrent administration of coumadin or aminophylline
PPV	**Contraindication** Severe allergic reaction after a previous dose or to a vaccine component **Precaution** Moderate or severe acute illness with or without fever	—

[a]Events or conditions listed as precautions should be reviewed carefully. Benefits and risks of administering a specific vaccine to a person under these circumstances should be considered. If the risk from the vaccine is believed to outweigh the benefit, the vaccine should not be administered. If the benefit of vaccination is believed to outweigh the risk, the vaccine should be administered. Whether and when to administer DTaP to children with proven or suspected underlying neurologic disorders should be decided on a case-by-case basis.

[b]Hepatitis B vaccination should be deferred for infants weighing < 2000 g if the mother is documented to be hepatitis B surface antigen (HbsAg)-negative at the time of the infant's birth. Vaccine should be given 1 month after birth or at hospital discharge. For infants born to HbsAg-positive women, hepatitis B immunoglobulin and hepatitis B vaccine should be administered at or soon after birth regardless of weight. See text for details.

[c]Acetaminophen or other appropriate antipyretic can be administered to children with a personal or family history of seizures at the time of DTaP vaccination and every 4–6 h for 24 h thereafter to reduce the possibility of postvaccination fever (**Source:** American Academy of Pediatrics. Active immunization. In Pickering LK, [editor]: 2000 Red Book: Report of the Committee on Infectious Diseases. 25th ed. Elk Grove Village, IL: American Academy of Pediatrics, 2000).

[d]MMR and varicella vaccines can be administered on the same day. If not administered on the same day, these vaccines should be separated by ≥ 28 d.

[e]Substantially immunosuppressive steroid dose is considered to be ≥ 2 wk of daily receipt of 20 mg or 2 mg/kg body weight of prednisone or equivalent.

[f]Measles vaccination can suppress tuberculin reactivity temporarily. Measles-containing vaccine can be administered on the same day as tuberculin skin testing. If testing cannot be performed until after the day of MMR vaccination, the test should be postponed for ≥ 4 weeks after the vaccination. If an urgent need exists to do skin test, do so with the understanding that reactivity might be reduced by the vaccine.

[g]See text for details.

[h]If a vaccinee experiences a presumed vaccine-related rash 7–25 d after vaccination, avoid direct contact with immunocompromised persons for the duration of the rash.

DT, diphtheria-tetanus vaccine; DTaP, diphtheria-tetanus–accelular pertussis vaccine; Hib, *Haemophilus influenzae* vaccine; IPV, inactivated poliovirus vaccine; MCV4, meningococcal conjugate vaccine; MMR, measles-mumps-rubella vaccine; MMRV, measles-mumps-rubella-varicella vaccine; PCV, pneumococcal conjugate vaccine; PPV, pneumococcal polysaccharide vaccine; Td, tetanus-diphtheria vaccine; Tdap, diphtheria-tetanus–acellular pertussis vaccine.

Adapted, with permission, from MMWR Recomm Rep 2002:51(RR-2)1–35 [PMID: 11848294].

able cases reported to the CDC between 1980 and 2001 and 1 fatal case in an unimmunized traveler to Haiti in 2003); however, diphtheria remains endemic in many countries. Diphtheria toxoid is prepared by the formaldehyde inactivation of diphtheria toxin. The protective efficacy of diphtheria toxoid has never been measured on a mass scale, but is estimated to be greater than 85%.

Preparations Available

1. Diphtheria toxoid is used only when tetanus toxoid and pertussis vaccine are both contraindicated.
2. Diphtheria-tetanus vaccine (DT) (pediatric) is used when pertussis vaccine is contraindicated. DT contains more diphtheria toxoid per dose than preparations used for adults and should not be used in persons older than 5 years of age because of a high frequency of severe local adverse reactions.
3. Tetanus-diphtheria vaccine (Td) (adult) is for use in persons age 7 years or older. It is less likely to produce local reactions while still eliciting a good immunogenic response in this population.
4. Diphtheria-tetanus-pertussis vaccine (DTP) was the standard immunizing agent for healthy children prior to availability of DTaP. DTP is no longer manufactured in the United States.
5. Diphtheria-tetanus–acellular pertussis vaccine (DTaP) contains an amount of diphtheria toxins similar to DTP and is recommended as the standard immunizing agent for healthy children.
6. Diphtheria-tetanus–acellular pertussis and *H influenzae* type b conjugate vaccine (DTaP-Hib) is licensed only for the fourth dose in the DTP-Hib series (age 15–18 months). Earlier use may result in suboptimal response to the Hib component.
7. Diphtheria-tetanus–acellular pertussis–hepatitis B–inactivated poliovirus (DTaP-HepB-IPV) is licensed for use in infants ages 2, 4, and 6 months.
8. Diphtheria-tetanus–acellular pertussis (Tdap) is licensed for use in persons 11–64 years of age (ADACEL, Sanofi Pasteur) and 10–18 years of age (BOOSTRIX, GlaxoSmithKline).

Dosage & Schedule of Administration

The preceding preparations are given intramuscularly in a dose of 0.5 mL. The use of jet injection may be associated with more local reactions. See Table 9–1 for the routine schedule and Table 9–2 for immunization of children not appropriately immunized during the first year of life. A booster dose of Tdap should be administered at ages 11–12 and every 10 years thereafter.

Adverse Effects

No significant adverse reactions have been associated with diphtheria toxoid alone.

Antibody Preparations

Equine diphtheria antitoxin is available for the treatment of diphtheria. Dosage depends on the size and location of the diphtheritic membrane and an estimate of the patient's level of intoxication. Before using this preparation, the presence or absence of equine serum sensitivity must be determined using a scratch test of a 1:1000 dilution. If the test is positive, desensitization must be undertaken. If negative, the doses shown in Table 9–4 are suggested.

Diphtheria antitoxin is no longer commercially available in the United States but may be obtained from the National Immunization Program at the CDC.

Centers for Disease Control and Prevention: Fatal diphtheria in a US traveler to Haiti—Pennsylvania, 2003. MMWR Morb Mortal Wkly Rep 2004;52:1285 [PMID: 14712177].

Thierry-Carstensen B et al: Spontaneously reported adverse reactions after diphtheria-tetanus revaccination at 4–6 years of age—a comparison of two vaccines with different amounts of diphtheria toxoid. Vaccine 2004;23:668 [PMID: 15542188].

TETANUS

When anaerobic *Clostridium tetani* colonizes devitalized tissue, the exotoxin tetanospasmin is disseminated to inhibitory motor neurons, resulting in tetanus. Tetanus primarily occurs in unvaccinated or inadequately vaccinated persons. Tetanus-prone wounds include (1) puncture wounds, including those acquired due to body piercing, tattooing, and intravenous drug abuse; (2) animal bites; (3) lacerations or abrasions; and (4) wounds resulting

Table 9–4. Suggested dosing for equine diphtheria antitoxin.

Site	Duration of Lesion	Toxic (?)	Dose (units)
Pharyngeal or laryngeal	≤ 48 h	NA	20,000–40,000
Nasopharyngeal	NA	NA	40,000–60,000
Extensive or brawny swelling of the neck	≥ 72 h	Yes	80,000–120,000
Cutaneous[a]	NA	NA	20,000–40,000

[a]Recommended by some but not all expert sources.
NA, not applicable.

from nonsterile delivery and umbilical cord care (neonatal tetanus). Intravenous drug abusers are an increasing proportion of tetanus patients in the United States, accounting for up to 20–40% of cases in some states.

Tetanus toxoid is prepared by inactivating the toxin with formaldehyde. Its protective efficacy is high.

Preparations Available

1. Tetanus toxoid (fluid) is used rarely—only when rapid immunization is desirable.
2. Tetanus toxoid adsorbed on aluminum phosphate is the standard single-antigen booster toxoid.
3. Tetanus-diphtheria vaccines (pediatric DT and adult Td) are the standard dual-antigen booster toxoids and are more often used for prophylaxis in routine wound management over the single-antigen preparation.
4. DTaP with or without Hib (discussed in the section on Hib).
5. DTaP-HepB-IPV.
6. Tdap.

Dosage & Schedule of Administration

The preceding preparations are administered intramuscularly in a dose of 0.5 mL. See Table 9–1 for the routine schedule and Table 9–2 for vaccination of children not appropriately immunized during the first year of life. A booster dose of Tdap should be scheduled at age 11–12 years (or ages 13–18 years for catch-up) with Td

every 10 years thereafter to protect against tetanus and diphtheria. More frequent administration may lead to sensitization and is not recommended.

Table 9–5 summarizes recommendations for the use of tetanus prophylaxis in routine wound management. Patients with non–tetanus-prone wounds should be boosted if more than 10 years have elapsed since their last immunization; those with tetanus-prone wounds should receive a booster if more than 5 years have elapsed.

Adverse Effects

Significant reactions to tetanus toxoid, historically an extremely safe preparation, are very unusual. Anaphylaxis, Guillain-Barré syndrome, and brachial neuritis related to tetanus toxoid are extremely rare.

Antibody Preparations

Tetanus immune globulin (TIg) (human) is indicated in the management of tetanus-prone wounds in individuals who have had an uncertain number or fewer than three tetanus immunizations with tetanus toxoid, as described earlier. Persons fully immunized with at least three doses do not require TIg, regardless of the nature of their wounds (see Table 9–5). The dose is 300–600 units (one or two vials) intramuscularly. Part of the dose may be infiltrated locally.

Centers for Disease Control and Prevention: Tetanus Surveillance—United States, 1998–2000. MMWR Morb Mortal Wkly Rep 2003;52(SS-3):1 [PMID: 12825541].

Table 9–5. Summarized recommendations for the use of tetanus prophylaxis in routine wound management.

History of Adsorbed Tetanus Toxoid	Clean, Minor Wounds		All Other Wounds[a]	
	Tdap, Td, or DT[b]	TIg[c]	Tdap, Td, or DT[b]	TIg[c]
Unknown or < 3 doses	Yes	No	Yes	Yes
≥ 3 doses[d]	No[e]	No	No[f]	No

[a]Such as, but not limited to, wounds contaminated with dirt, feces, soil, or saliva; puncture wounds; avulsions; and wounds resulting from missiles, crushing, burns, or frostbite.
[b]For children less than 7 years old, DTaP is given (or DT, if pertussis vaccine is contraindicated). For persons 7–9 years of age, Td is used. For persons 10–11 years or older (depending on whether BOOSTRIX or ADACEL is used), Tdap is preferred instead of Td if the person has not previously received Tdap. If Tdap is not available or was previously administered, Td should be given to this age group.
[c]TIg, tetanus immune globulin.
[d]If only three doses of fluid toxoid have been received, a fourth dose of toxoid—preferably an adsorbed toxoid—should be administered.
[e]Yes, if more than 10 years have elapsed since the last dose.
[f]Yes, if more than 5 years have elapsed since the last dose. More frequent boosters are not needed and can accentuate side effects.
Reproduced, with permission, from CDC: Diphtheria, tetanus, and pertussis: recommendations for vaccine use and other preventive measures. MMWR Morb Mortal Wkly Rep 1991;40:1 [PMID: 1865873].

PERTUSSIS

Pertussis is increasingly recognized as a disease affecting older children and adults, including fully vaccinated persons with waning immunity. Maintaining vaccination in young infants will protect against severe disease in this age group, but a reservoir of disease among those with waning immunity is a continuing problem. In the U.S., the most dramatic increases in pertussis incidence are among adolescents and young adults, prompting development of booster pertussis vaccines for this population. Recent FDA approval in 2005 of Tdap was based on comparable seroresponse to pertussis antigens and a safety profile similar to control Td. Adolescent and young adult immunization has the capacity to limit spread of pertussis to infants and decrease overall pertussis endemicity.

Pertussis vaccines currently used in the United States for initial immunization contain purified components of pertussis antigens. The DTaP preparations have a protective efficacy of about 70–90% after three doses, depending on the source. Further evidence of the efficacy of pertussis vaccine is provided by the observation of a large increase in pertussis cases in Great Britain and Japan after those countries reduced or abandoned use of the vaccine.

Preparations Available

1. DTaP
2. DTaP-Hib
3. DTaP-HepB-IPV
4. Tdap

Dosage & Schedule of Administration

Each of the available preparations is administered in a dose of 0.5 mL intramuscularly. See Table 9–1 for the routine schedule and Table 9–2 for vaccination of those children not appropriately immunized during the first year of life.

Adverse Effects

A large number of adverse reactions have been attributed to pertussis vaccine. These can be divided into three categories: local reactions, mild to moderate systemic reactions (that occur in up to half of children), and severe systemic reactions. The estimated rates of these reactions within the first 48 hours after vaccination are shown in the following discussion. The only absolute contraindications to the further use of pertussis vaccine are an anaphylactic reaction to the vaccine or a severe acute neurologic illness within 7 days after vaccination (see Table 9–3). Precaution is urged for the following associations: a convulsion within 3 days (1:1750); persistent, severe,

inconsolable screaming or crying for over 3 hours (1:100); a hypotonic-hyporesponsive episode within 48 hours (1:1750); and an unexplained temperature rise to 40.5 °C within 48 hours (1:330).

Controversy continues regarding the causation of serious neurologic illness by pertussis vaccine. The only large-scale case-controlled study with enough statistical power to examine this issue—the British National Childhood Encephalopathy Study—has minimized any potential relationship.

It was calculated that although the attributable risk for serious acute neurologic injury ranges from less than 1:1,000,000 to 1:140,000, the risk for permanent brain damage is even lower, if indeed there is any risk. This reassessment, along with new studies, has led the AAP, the Canadian National Advisory Committee, and the British Pediatric Association to conclude that pertussis vaccine has not been proven to cause brain damage and to reaffirm the safety and effectiveness of routine pertussis vaccine in immunization programs for infants and children.

The 1991 National Academy of Sciences Institute of Medicine report concluded that the vaccine was causally related to only four adverse effects: acute encephalopathy, the range of excess risk being nil to 10.5 per million immunizations; shock (and an unusual shock-like state), 3.5–291 cases per 100,000 immunizations; anaphylaxis, 2 cases per 100,000 injections of DTP; and protracted, inconsolable crying, 0.1–6% of recipients. Thus, although epidemiologic evidence may be consistent with a causal relationship, pertussis toxin has no proven role in severe neurologic reactions to DTP.

DIPHTHERIA-TETANUS-PERTUSSIS VACCINE

DTP has been used for the vaccination of healthy infants against diphtheria, tetanus, and pertussis for more than 40 years. It has the combined clinical efficacy of the three single-dose preparations, and the efficacy of pertussis vaccine may even be enhanced by the adjuvant effect of the diphtheria and tetanus toxoids. DTP is no longer manufactured in the United States.

As of 1999, DTaP is the recommended vaccination against diphtheria, tetanus, and pertussis for all doses in the routine vaccination series (the DTaP-Hib combination vaccine can only be used as the fourth dose).

Two basic types of acellular (DTaP) vaccines have been studied. The T-type vaccines are produced by extraction and purification of *Bordetella pertussis* cultures. In contrast, the B-type vaccines contain combinations of pertussis toxin (PT), filamentous hemagglutinin (FHA), pertactin, and fimbriae. It has been hypothesized that immunity against PT alone may be sufficient to protect against pertussis, but this view has been challenged, and it has been claimed that antibodies against FHA, pertactin, and fimbriae may be required for optimal protection.

Efficacy trials of various acellular pertussis vaccines in Sweden, Germany, Italy, and Senegal have established a 2- to 10-fold lower frequency of minor adverse events and reduced rates of more serious events (hypotonic-hyporesponsive episodes, persistent crying, temperatures higher than 40 °C, and seizures) compared with the whole-cell vaccine, good immunogenicity, and a protective efficacy ranging from 59–89%. Tripedia (Sanofi Pasteur) is licensed for use as the complete five-dose series. Infanrix (GlaxoSmithKline) and DAPTACEL (Sanofi Pasteur) are approved for use for the first four doses of the five-dose series. Licensure of other DTaP vaccines as a five-dose series is anticipated. For children with adverse reactions in the precaution category to DTP, DTaP may be substituted. In those with a true contraindication, neither vaccine should be used. Studies are underway to evaluate the efficacy and safety of acellular vaccines containing reduced quantities of pertussis antigens for use as boosters in adolescents.

Preparations Available

1. DTaP (Tripedia [Sanofi Pasteur]) contains diphtheria toxoid, tetanus toxoid, PT, and FHA.
2. DTaP (Infanrix [GlaxoSmithKline]) contains diphtheria toxoid, tetanus toxoid, PT, FHA, and pertactin.
3. DTaP (DAPTACEL [Sanofi Pasteur]) contains PT, FHA, pertactin, and fimbriae types 2 and 3.
4. DTaP-Hib (TriHIBit [Sanofi Pasteur]) has been licensed for use as the fourth dose (booster) in the DPT immunization series.
5. DTaP-HepB-IPV (PEDIARIX [GlaxoSmithKline]) contains PT, FHA, and pertactin and is licensed for the first three doses beginning at 2 months of age.
6. Tdap (BOOSTRIX [GlaxoSmithKline] and ADACEL [Sanofi Pasteur]).

Dosage & Schedule of Administration

DTaP is administered in a dose of 0.5 mL intramuscularly. See Table 9–1 for the routine schedule and Table 9–2 for the procedure in children not immunized during the first year. The ACIP/AAP and American Academy of Family Physicians (AAFP) recommend a series of five vaccinations before age 7 years (at 2, 4, 6, and 15–18 months and at 4–6 years). Whenever feasible, the same brand of DTaP should be used for all doses. See Table 9–1 for Tdap schedule.

Adverse Effects

Local reactions, fever, and other mild systemic effects occur with one-fourth to two-thirds the frequency noted following whole-cell DTP vaccination. Moderate to severe systemic effects, including fever of 40.5 °C, persistent inconsolable crying lasting 3 hours or more, and hypotonic-hyporesponsive episodes, are less frequent than with whole-cell DTP. These are without sequelae. Severe neurologic effects have not been temporally associated with DTaP vaccinations in use in the United States. A recent study from Canada showed no evidence of encephalopathy related to pertussis vaccine (< 1:3 million doses of DTP and < 1:3.5 million doses of DTaP). Data are limited regarding differences in reactogenicity among currently licensed acellular pertussis vaccines. With all currently licensed DTaP vaccines, reports of the frequency and magnitude of substantial local reactions at injection sites have increased with increasing dose number (including swelling of the thigh or entire upper arm after receipt of the fourth and fifth doses).

Halperin SA: Canadian experience with implementation of an acellular pertussis vaccine booster-dose program in adolescents: implications for the United States. Pediatr Infect Dis J 2005;24(6 Suppl):S141 [PMID: 15931142].

Moore DL et al: Lack of evidence of encephalopathy related to pertussis vaccine: active surveillance by IMPACT, Canada, 1993–2002. Pediatr Infect Dis J 2004;23:568 [PMID: 15194842].

Pichichero ME et al: Combined tetanus, diphtheria, and 5-component pertussis vaccine for use in adolescents and adults. JAMA 2005;293:3003 [PMID: 15933223].

Ward JI et al: Efficacy of an acellular pertussis vaccine among adolescents and adults. N Engl J Med 2005;353:1555 [PMID: 16221778].

POLIOMYELITIS

Vaccines directed against poliovirus infections have eliminated the naturally occurring disease in developed countries. In the United States, the number of reported cases of paralytic poliomyelitis has fallen from more than 18,000 in 1954 to 0–10 per year currently. In September 2005, four infections with a type 1 vaccine-derived poliovirus were recorded in unvaccinated Amish children in Minnesota, the first report in the U.S. since 2000, when OPV use was discontinued. Vaccine-derived polioviruses emerge from OPV because of continuous replication in immunodeficient persons such as the index case in this outbreak, or by circulation in populations with low vaccine coverage (cVDPVs). As of December 8, 2005, 1598 confirmed wild-virus polio cases and 35 vaccine-associated cases were reported worldwide since the beginning of the year. This is three times the number in 2003. It is now endemic in India, Pakistan, Afghanistan, Egypt, and Nigeria; transmission has been reestablished in Africa, in Niger, Chad, Mali, Cameroon, and Sudan, with imported outbreaks in Ethiopia, Eritrea, Somalia,

Madagascar, Angola, Yemen, and Indonesia. cVDPV outbreaks have occurred in Hispaniola, Philippines, and Madagascar in 2001, while retrospective studies detected endemic cVDPV circulation in Egypt from 1988–1993. The risk appears to be highest with the type 2 strain, however wild-type 2 poliovirus has not circulated globally since 1999. The main risk factor for cVDPV circulation appears to be low levels of vaccine coverage, be it in Hispaniola or Egypt or unimmunized children in the U.S. It has also been estimated that the global burden of vaccine-associated paralytic poliomyelitis varies from 250–500 annually, now becoming more common than wild-type poliovirus. The rate of this in the U.S. was 1 case of paralytic disease per 760,000 first doses of OPV distributed. Ninety-three percent of recipient cases and 76% of vaccine-associated paralytic poliomyelitis occurred after administration of the first or second dose of OPV. The risk of paralysis in the immunodeficient recipient may be as much as 6800 times that in normal subjects.

The World Health Organization has reset the target of 2008 for global eradication of poliomyelitis and the endgame strategy for polio eradication has changed. Global synchronous cessation of OPV may need to be coordinated by the World Health Organization after coordinated mass campaigns. Transition to IPV in developed countries with high rates of immunization coverage is encouraged.

The injectable poliovirus vaccine of enhanced potency (IPV-E), which has a higher content of antigens than the old IPV, is the only vaccine against poliomyelitis available in the United States since 2000. IPV is incapable of causing poliomyelitis by virtue of being inactivated, whereas OPV can do so rarely.

Completely immunized adult visitors to areas of continuing wild-type poliovirus circulation should receive a booster dose of IPV-E. Unimmunized or incompletely immunized adults and children should have received two (preferably three) doses of the vaccine prior to travel to these and other areas with circulation of wild-type or vaccine-type virus.

Preparations Available

1. IPV-E (IPOL [Sanofi Pasteur]) contains antigens of types 1, 2, and 3 poliovirus.
2. DTaP-HepB-IPV (PEDIARIX [GlaxoSmithKline Biologicals]) contains diphtheria and tetanus toxoids and acellular pertussis adsorbed, hepatitis B, and inactivated poliovirus vaccine.

Dosage & Schedule of Administration

IPV-E is administered in a dose of 0.5 mL subcutaneously. The DTaP-HepB-IPV combination vaccine can be used in the primary series at 2, 4, and 6 months, and

can be used to complete the primary series. It can be administered with Hib and pneumococcal conjugate (PCV) vaccines at separate sites, but is not approved for the fourth dose of IPV or fourth and fifth doses of DTaP.

Adverse Effects

IPV has essentially no adverse effects associated with it other than possible rare hypersensitivity reactions to trace quantities of antibiotics. The DTaP-HepB-IPV combination has similar rates of local and systemic adverse responses to three doses administered separately except for fever, which is higher in the combination-vaccinated children.

Aristegui J et al: Comparison of the reactogenicity and immunogenicity of a combined diphtheria, tetanus, acellular pertussis, hepatitis B, inactivated polio (DTPa-HBV-IPV) vaccine, mixed with the *Haemophilus influenzae* type b (Hib) conjugate vaccine and administered as a single injection, with the DTPa-IPV/Hib and hepatitis B vaccines administered in two simultaneous injections to infants at 2, 4, and 6 months of age. Vaccine 2003;21:3593 [PMID: 12922087].

Centers for Disease Control and Prevention: FDA licensure of diphtheria and tetanus toxoids and acellular pertussis adsorbed, hepatitis B (recombinant), and poliovirus vaccine combined, (PEDIARIX) for use in infants. MMWR Morb Mortal Wkly Rep 2003;52:203 [PMID: 12653460].

Hennessey KA et al: Poliovirus vaccine shedding among persons with HIV in Abidjan, Cote d'Ivoire. J Infect Dis 2005; 192:2124 [PMID: 16288377].

Kew OM et al: Circulating vaccine-derived polioviruses: Current state of knowledge. Bull World Health Organ 2004;82:16 [PMID: 15106296].

MEASLES

In the 20 years after the 1963 introduction of measles vaccination in the United States, the annual number of reported cases decreased from 500,000 to fewer than 1500. However, between 1989 and 1991 there was a resurgence of measles, with 55,622 cases reported. The major reasons for the increase in cases and the resulting deaths were failure to provide vaccine to preschool children aged 15 months or older, the presence in the community of susceptible children younger than age 15 months, and the growing number of appropriately vaccinated but nonimmune individuals (primary vaccine failures: 2–10%) in schools and colleges. These reasons have led to recommendations for a two-dose vaccination schedule at 12–15 months and at 4–6 years of age. By 2001 almost all states had implemented a two-dose requirement for school entry, and now measles cases in school-age children are at an all time low (from 10,000/year in 1989–90 to < 50/year in 1997–2001). This is the cornerstone of the measles eradication policy in the U.S. In Mexico, a regional pandemic in 1989–1990 resulted in 5899 deaths, leading to intense efforts to administer two doses of vaccine to children 1–6 years old. With coverage of 97.6% of children age 6–10 years having received two doses by 1997, Mexico has succeeded in interrupting endemic transmission of measles. Globally, in 2003, 164 (85%) of all countries offered two doses of vaccine. Following the polio eradication initiative of supplementary immunization activities in 30 of 45 "priority countries," almost 200 million children have received measles vaccine, which may be partly responsible for the overall global decrease in measles mortality by 40%. This raises the possibility that the elimination of endemic transmission of measles using two doses of vaccine is an attainable public health goal.

Recently, reports in the medical and lay press have suggested a possible association between MMR vaccination, autism, and gastrointestinal inflammation. This association has been refuted because of the limited number of patients studied, methods of case and control selection, and means of determining developmental regression. Several large epidemiologic studies subsequently found no association between MMR vaccination and either autism or bowel inflammation. Also, no evidence has been found to support the separate administration of measles, mumps, and rubella vaccines (as opposed to the MMR combination). However, the influence of the lay press is most profound in the United Kingdom, where low vaccination rates with measles vaccine have led to a resurgence of measles, with a distinct possibility that it will become an endemic disease in the United Kingdom.

Preparations Available

1. Measles vaccine, MR, and MMR: The Moraten strain is a live attenuated vaccine derived from the Edmonston B strain after multiple passages in chick embryo tissue culture. The Moraten strain is available as a monovalent vaccine or in combination with rubella vaccine (MR) or in the MMR combination.

2. MMRV: Recently (September 2005) the FDA licensed a combined live attenuated measles, mumps, rubella, and varicella vaccine (MMRV, Proquad, Merck) for use in children 1–12 years of age. It is identical in composition to MMR with the exception that the varicella component is $2\frac{1}{2}$–3 times more than in the VAR vaccine. The MMRV is as immunogenic as the MMR and VAR components administered simultaneously; however, MMRV recipients had a slight increase in fever and a measles-like rash compared to MMR and VAR administered separately. The ACIP recommends that MMRV can be administered on or after the first birthday, with a second dose of MMR at least 1 month later. Concomitant administration of MMRV, DTaP, Hib, and HepB vaccines showed that the immune

responses to all the antigens when administered simultaneously were comparable to sequential administration of MMRV and the other antigens.

Dosage & Schedule of Administration

A. Routine Vaccination

Measles vaccine should be given as MMR at 12–15 months and again at 4–6 years of age. A dose of 0.5 mL, whether alone or in combination, should at least be given subcutaneously. The second dose of MMR is recommended at school entry to help prevent school-based measles outbreaks. Children not reimmunized at school entry should receive their second MMR by 11–12 years of age. If an infant receives the vaccine before 12 months of age, two doses are required to complete the series, the first after at least 12 months of age and the second at least 1 month later. Ig interferes with the immune response to the attenuated vaccine strains of MMR. Therefore, MMR immunization after Ig administration should be deferred by 3–11 months, depending on the type of Ig product received. Consult the AAP's *2003 Red Book* for specific recommendations.

MMRV is preferred over separate vaccine administration. At least 1 month should elapse between a dose of MMR and MMRV, and should the need arise for a second dose of varicella vaccine (eg, in an epidemic) it should be at least 3 months later.

B. Vaccination of Travelers

People traveling abroad should be immune to measles. In high-risk areas, age at primary vaccination should be as soon as possible after the first birthday (ie, at 12 months). However, younger infants 6–11 months of age traveling to high-risk areas should receive the monovalent vaccine followed by two doses at 12–15 months given at least 4 weeks apart, and should complete the series at 4–6 years.

C. Revaccination Under Other Circumstances

Persons entering college and other institutions for education beyond high school, medical personnel beginning employment, and persons traveling abroad should have documentation of immunity to measles, defined as receipt of two doses of measles vaccine after their first birthday, birth before 1957, or a documented measles history or immunity.

D. Outbreak Control

A community outbreak is defined as a single documented case of measles. Control depends on immediate protection of all susceptible persons (defined as persons who have no documented immunity to measles in the affected community). In the case of unvaccinated individuals, the following recommendations hold: (1) age 6–11 months, monovalent measles vaccine (or MMR) if cases are occurring in children younger than age 1 year, followed by two doses of MMR at age 12–15 months and again at age 4–6 years; and (2) age 12 months or older, MMR followed by revaccination at 4–6 years. A child with an unclear or unknown vaccination history should be reimmunized with MMR. Anyone with a known exposure who is not certain of receiving two doses of MMR should receive an additional dose. Unimmunized persons who are not immunized within 72 hours of exposure should be excluded from contact with potentially infected persons until at least 2 weeks after the onset of rash of the last case of measles.

Measles vaccination is contraindicated in pregnant women, women intending to become pregnant within the next 28 days, immunocompromised persons (except those with asymptomatic HIV or those with HIV infection who are not severely immunocompromised), and persons with anaphylactic egg or neomycin allergy. It is also contraindicated in children receiving high-dose steroid therapy (greater than or equal to 2 mg/kg/day, or 20 mg/day total, for longer than 14 days) with the exception of those receiving physiologic replacement doses. In these patients, an interval of 1 month between cessation of steroid therapy and vaccination is sufficient. Leukemic patients who have been in remission and off chemotherapy for at least 3 months can receive MMR safely. Children with minor acute illnesses (including febrile illnesses), nonanaphylactic egg allergy, or a history of tuberculosis should be immunized. Monovalent measles or MMR may be safely administered simultaneously with other routine pediatric immunizations.

Adverse Effects

Between 5% and 15% of vaccinees become febrile to 39.5 °C or higher about 6–12 days following vaccination, lasting approximately 1–2 days, and 5% may develop a transient morbilliform rash. Transient thrombocytopenia occurs in 1:25,000 to 1:100,000 persons. Encephalitis and other CNS conditions such as aseptic meningitis and Guillain-Barré syndrome are reported to occur at a frequency of 1 case per 3 million doses in the United States. This rate is lower than the rate of these conditions in the general unvaccinated population, implying that the relationship between them and measles vaccination may not be causal. MMR vaccination is associated with an increased risk of febrile seizures 8–14 days after vaccination, but no subsequent long-term complications have been seen. A recent study found an increase in female mortality in Guinea Bissau after receiving the high-titered measles vaccine at less than 6 months of age.

Antibody Preparations

If a child is seen within 72 hours after exposure, vaccination is the preferred method of protection. If vaccine is

contraindicated, Ig, given intramuscularly at a dose of 0.25 mL/kg (0.5 mL/kg in immunocompromised patients; maximum dose in either circumstance is 15 mL), is effective in preventing or modifying measles if it is given within 6 days after exposure. Measles vaccine should be given 5 months later to children receiving the 0.25 mL/kg dose and 6 months later for the higher dose. For children receiving regular intravenous immune globulin, a dose of 100–400 mg/kg should be adequate for measles prophylaxis for exposures occurring within 3 weeks of the last dose.

Aaby P et al: Differences in female–male mortality after high-titer measles vaccine and association with subsequent vaccination with diphtheria–tetanus–pertussis and inactivated poliovirus: Reanalysis of West African studies. Lancet 2003;361:2183 [PMID: 14643138].

Centers for Disease Control and Prevention: Progress in reducing measles mortality—worldwide, 1999–2003. MMWR Morb Mortal Wkly Rep 2005;54:2005 [PMID: 15744229].

Centers for Disease Control and Prevention: Licensure of a combined live attenuated measles, mumps, rubella and varicella vaccine. MMWR Morb Mortal Wkly Rep 2005;54:1212.

Jansen VA et al: Measles outbreaks in a population with declining vaccine uptake. Science 2003;301:804 [PMID: 12907792].

Kolasa MS et al: Progress toward implementation of a second dose measles immunization requirement for all school children in the United States. J Infect Dis 2004;189:(Suppl 1)S98 [PMID: 15106097].

Santos JI et al: Measles in Mexico, 1941–2001: Interruption of endemic transmission and lessons learned. J Infect Dis 2004; 189:(Suppl 1)S243 [PMID: 15106118].

Wilson K et al: Association of autistic spectrum disorder and the measles, mumps, and rubella vaccine: A systematic review of current epidemiological evidence. Arch Pediatr Adolesc Med 2003;157:628 [PMID: 12860782].

MUMPS

Mumps vaccine has dramatically reduced this infection and its complications in the United States, from 185,691 cases in 1967 to 226 cases in 2001. Most reported cases of mumps are in children age 5–14 years, despite high vaccine coverage (> 95%) and may be due to primary or secondary vaccine failure (waning immunity).

Preparations Available

The Jeryl Lynn Strain is the only mumps vaccine available in the U.S. It is prepared from virus isolated from a child and passaged in embryonated eggs and in chick embryo tissue culture. The vaccine is available as a monovalent vaccine, and in its preferred form in the MMR or MMRV combination.

Dosage & Schedule of Administration

Mumps vaccine is given to children in the combination vaccine MMR at age 12–15 months and again at age 4–

6 years. Despite the greater than 95% efficacy of the mumps vaccine, outbreaks have been reported in highly vaccinated populations. Most cases were attributed to primary vaccine failure. It is hoped that the two-dose schedule (with the second dose given before school entry) will prevent school-based outbreaks. As monovalent vaccine, it is safe and effective if given after the first birthday. The dose of either monovalent or MMR vaccine is 0.5 mL subcutaneously. Use of the monovalent vaccine is limited to susceptible individuals with proven immunity to the other constituents of MMR. Revaccination with mumps vaccine or any of the vaccines in MMR is not harmful; therefore, anyone with an unclear vaccination history should be immunized with MMR. The same recommendations and contraindications apply to mumps vaccine as to measles vaccine, except as relates to travel. Because maternal antibody to mumps is present in most infants, and the disease is not severe in infancy, infants younger than 12 months of age traveling to endemic countries need not routinely be given mumps vaccine (see previous discussion).

Adverse Effects

Reactions after mumps vaccination are rare and include parotitis, low-grade fever, and orchitis. In 1989, a nationwide surveillance of neurologic complications after a mumps vaccine was conducted in Japan. At least 311 cases of mild aseptic meningitis (96 had vaccine-type mumps virus in the cerebrospinal fluid) occurred among 630,157 recipients. However, this was not the strain used in the U.S. vaccine. There were no sequelae. A high rate of aseptic meningitis was also found in Brazil but not in Germany, where different vaccine strains were used.

Schlipkoter U et al: Surveillance of measles–mumps–rubella vaccine–associated aseptic meningitis in Germany. Infection 2002;30:351 [PMID: 12478324].

Vandermeulen C et al: Outbreak of mumps in a vaccinated child population: a question of vaccine failure. Vaccine 2004;22:2713 [PMID: 15246601].

RUBELLA

The use of rubella vaccine represents an important deviation from the public health philosophy underlying the other vaccines discussed in this chapter. It is not intended to protect individuals from rubella infection, but rather to prevent the serious consequences of rubella infection during pregnancy: miscarriage, fetal demise, and congenital rubella syndrome. Congenital rubella syndrome is a group of birth defects including deafness, cataracts, heart defects, and mental retardation. In the United States and the United Kingdom, the approach has been to vaccinate young children. The intent is to reduce transmission to susceptible women

of childbearing age via a herd immunity effect. Immunity lasts for at least 15 years. With the use of rubella vaccines since 1970, rubella incidence rates have declined more than 99%. However, approximately 10% of young adults are now susceptible to rubella. Rubella is rare in the United States. Currently most cases of rubella are seen in foreign-born adults, and outbreaks have occurred in poultry and meat processing plants that employ many foreign-born workers. Similarly, most infants with congenital rubella syndrome are born to foreign-born mothers.

Preparations Available

The RA 27/3 strain is the only vaccine available in the United States. It is grown in human diploid cells. The RA 27/3 strain is available as a monovalent vaccine, in combined preparations with measles vaccine, or in measles and mumps vaccines. In most circumstances, MMR or MMRV vaccination is the recommended means of immunizing against rubella.

Dosage & Schedule of Administration

Either the monovalent or combined form should be administered subcutaneously in a dose of 0.5 mL. Current practice is to administer MMR or MMRV vaccine at age 12–15 months and MMR again at 4–6 years. A person can be considered immune only with documentation of either serologic immunity to rubella or vaccination with at least one dose of rubella vaccine after age 1 year, or if born before 1957. A clinical diagnosis of rubella is unacceptable. Susceptible pubertal girls and postpubertal women identified by premarital or prenatal screening should also be immunized. Whenever rubella vaccination is offered to a woman of childbearing age, pregnancy should be ruled out and the woman advised to prevent conception for 3 months following vaccination. If a pregnant woman is vaccinated or becomes pregnant within 3 weeks of vaccination, she should be counseled regarding the risk to her fetus. It has been estimated that the risk of serious malformations attributable to giving the RA 27/3 vaccine to pregnant women is from 0 to 1.6%. This is much less than the 20–85% risk of congenital rubella syndrome after maternal infection in the first trimester of pregnancy. All susceptible adults in institutional settings (including colleges), day care center personnel, military personnel, and hospital and health care personnel should be immunized.

Adverse Effects

In children, adverse effects from rubella vaccination are very unusual. Between 5% and 15% of children develop rash, fever, or lymphadenopathy 5–12 days after vaccination. Rash also occurs alone or as a mild rubella illness in 2–4% of adults. Arthralgia and arthritis occur in 10–25% of adult vaccinees, as opposed to only 0–2% of 6- to 16-year-old vaccinees. Chronic arthritis may be causally related to RA 27/3 vaccinations and occurs more often in women age 45 or older, starting 10–11 days after the vaccination and lasting for up to a year. Rare complications include peripheral neuritis and neuropathy, transverse myelitis, and diffuse myelitis.

Castillo-Solorzano C et al: New horizons in the control of rubella and prevention of congenital rubella syndrome in the Americas. J Infect Dis 2003;187(Suppl)1:S146 [PMID: 12721906].

Danovaro-Holliday MC et al: Identifying risk factors for rubella susceptibility in a population at risk in the United States. Am J Public Health 2003;93:289 [PMID: 12554568].

Geier DA, Geier MR: A one-year follow-up of chronic arthritis following rubella and hepatitis B vaccination based upon analysis of the Vaccine Adverse Events Reporting System (VAERS) database. Clin Exp Rheumatol 2002;20:767 [PMID: 12508767].

HAEMOPHILUS INFLUENZAE TYPE B INFECTION

The first vaccine licensed against *Haemophilus influenzae* type b in the United States, composed of the capsular polysaccharide of *H influenzae* type b polyribosyl ribitol phosphate (PRP), was moderately effective in preventing *H influenzae* type b disease in children older than 18 months of age. Conjugation of the PRP with protein carriers confers T-cell–dependent characteristics on the vaccine and enhances the immunologic response to PRP in infancy. Since 1993, the incidence of *H influenzae* type b invasive disease in children younger than age 5 years has declined by > 99% in the United States.

Three conjugate vaccines are currently available in the United States (Table 9–6). Studies in infants ages 2–6 months demonstrated the immunogenicity of each of these vaccines except DTaP-Hib, which is approved only

for the fourth (booster) dose. A geometric mean titer of 1 µg/mL of antipolysaccharide antibody 3 weeks postvaccination has correlated with long-term protection from invasive disease. After three doses at ages 2, 4, and 6 months, each of the three vaccines produces protective levels of antibody. Regardless of the vaccine used in the primary series, booster vaccination of children older than age 12 months with any licensed vaccine elicits an adequate response. Furthermore, each vaccine is immunogenic as a single dose given after age 15 months. Limited information on interchangeability of different *H influenzae* type b vaccines suggests that any combination of the *H influenzae* type b conjugate vaccines will provide adequate protection.

If PRP-OMP is administered as only part of a primary series, the recommended number of doses to complete the series is determined by the other Hib conjugate vaccine.

Because of the differences in the immunogenic response and the different regimens used for these vaccines, the recommendations for use of HbOC, PRP-T, and PRP-OMP differ and are summarized in Table 9–7. Regardless of the regimen implemented, it is crucial to complete the series, because cases of invasive *H influenzae* type b disease have been described in partially vaccinated children. Because high antibody responses occur after the first dose of PRP-OMP, this vaccine is recommended for the first dose in the series for Native American and Alaskan Native children who are at increased risk of disease in early infancy. PRP-OMP-HepB (Comvax) is licensed for use in infants as young as 6 weeks of age. Antibody responses are comparable to those for HbOC and DTP or PRP-OMP and HepB administered separately. In addition, PRP-T-DTaP (TriHIBit) has been licensed for use only as a booster because use in the primary series may result in insufficient titers to Hib. If the exact conjugate vaccine previously administered is unknown, it is recommended that at least three doses of conjugate vaccine be adminis-

Table 9–6. *Haemophilus influenzae* type b conjugate vaccines for children.

Vaccine	Trade Name and Manufacturer	Polysaccharide	Linkage	Protein Carrier
HbOC	HibTITER (Wyeth)	Small	None	CRM[197] mutant *Corynebacterium diphtheriae* toxin protein
PRP-OMP	PedvaxHIB (Merck)	Medium	Thioether	*Neisseria meningitidis* outer membrane protein complex
PRP-T	ACTHIB (Sanofi Pasteur)	Large	Six-carbon	Tetanus toxoid
PRP-T -DTaP	TriHIBit (Sanofi Pasteur)	Large	Six-carbon	See above for PRP-T
PRP-OMP-Hepatitis B	Comvax (Merck)	Medium	Thioether	See above for PRP-OMP

Table 9–7. Schedule for *Haemophilus influenzae* type b conjugate vaccine administration.

Vaccine	Age at First Vaccination	Primary Series (Same Vaccine If Possible)	Booster (Any Conjugate Vaccine)
HbOC or PRP-T[a]	2–6 mo	Three doses 2 mo apart	12–15 mo
	7–11 mo	Two doses 2 mo apart	12–19 mo
	12–14 mo	One dose	2 mo later
	15–59 mo	One dose	...
PRP-OMP[b]	2–10 mo	Two doses 2 mo apart	12–15 mo
	11–14 mo	Two doses 2 mo apart	...
	15–71 mo	One dose	...

[a]A booster dose of DTP or DTaP should be administered at 4–6 y of age, before kindergarten or elementary school. This booster is not necessary if the fourth vaccinating dose was administered after the fourth birthday. DTaP-Hib (TriHIBit) is only approved for the fourth (booster) dose.

[b]Comvax may be administered by the same schedule for primary immunization as PRP-OMP. It should only be used in infants of hepatitis B–negative mothers. Three doses should be given if started in infants (≤ 10 mo), two doses if started at 11–14 mo, and one dose if started at age 15–71 mo. However, three doses of hepatitis B vaccine are required regardless of age of starting immunization.

tered to children between ages 2 and 6 months. Unvaccinated or partially vaccinated children younger than age 2 years who experience invasive *H influenzae* type b disease should receive a complete series of vaccinations as if they had received no previous Hib vaccine doses. Children older than age 2 years mount an adequate immune response to invasive *H influenzae* type b disease and do not require further vaccinations. Unimmunized children age 5 years or older with a chronic illness known to be associated with invasive *H influenzae* type b disease, such as sickle cell anemia and asplenia, should be given a single dose of any of the licensed conjugate vaccines.

Preparations Available

See Table 9–6.

Dosage & Schedule of Administration

The dose for all preparations is 0.5 mL, given intramuscularly (schedule outlined in Table 9–7).

Adverse Effects

Fewer than 5% of those immunized develop systemic reactions (including fever) to the vaccine. About 25% of recipients develop mild transient local reactions. Adverse effects following the second dose of PRP-OMP are more frequent than those following the first dose and more frequent following the third dose of HbOC than following the first two doses.

Kelly DF et al: *Haemophilus influenzae* type b conjugate vaccines. Immunology 2004;113:163 [PMID: 15379976].

Centers for Disease Control and Prevention: Progress toward elimination of *Haemophilus influenzae* type b invasive disease among infants and children—United States, 1998–2000. MMWR Morb Mortal Wkly Rep 2002;51:234 [PMID: 11925021].

PNEUMOCOCCAL INFECTIONS

Streptococcus pneumoniae is the most common cause of invasive bacterial infection in children, with most invasive disease occurring in children younger than age 2 years. Two kinds of vaccines are currently available against pneumococci: a 23-valent polysaccharide vaccine (23-PS) and a 7-valent protein-conjugated polysaccharide vaccine (pneumococcal conjugate vaccine, 7-PCV). Valency indicates the number of serotypes included in the vaccine. A nine-valent (9-PCV) vaccine has undergone clinical trials (in South Africa and The Gambia) while an 11-PCV is undergoing clinical trials in the Philippines. The serotypes represented in these vaccines were chosen for their frequency in disease among adults (23-PS) or children in industrialized countries (7-PCV). Additional serotypes needed in developing countries have been included in 9-PCV and 11-PCV. As in Hib vaccine, the carrier protein may be CRM 197 (Pnc-CRM), protein D of *H influenzae* (PD), tetanus and diphtheria toxoids (TT/DT) or OMP (Pnc-OMP). Prior to the year 2000, the available pneumococcal polysaccharide vaccine had an overall efficacy of 57%, was not effective in children younger than 2 years, and therefore was only indicated for certain high-risk children age 2 years or older. The 7- and 9-valent PCVs have been evaluated for efficacy against invasive pneumococcal disease in four trials (in the

U.S., South Africa, Gambia, and the Navajo Indian Nation). The pooled efficacy estimate from the first three trials of the vaccine was 93% (95% CI 81 and 98.2) against invasive disease caused by serotypes in the vaccine. The effect of the vaccine on pneumococcal pneumonia per se is difficult to define given the problems of establishing bacterial etiology of pneumonia. Three studies (in the U.S., South Africa, and Gambia) have evaluated the impact of the vaccine on radiographic pneumonia. These studies showed 20–37% reduction in radiographically confirmed pneumonia. One additional study evaluating the effect of 11-PCV on radiologic pneumonia is ongoing in the Philippines; results from this study are expected by the end of 2005. Three field trials have evaluated the efficacy of PCV against otitis media. Though two trials in Finland using 7-valent Pnc-CRM or Pnc-OMP showed significant reduction in culture-confirmed pneumococcal otitis caused by vaccine serotypes, there was no net reduction of otitis media in the vaccinated children. This was due to an increase in the rates of otitis media due to non-vaccine types of pneumococci, *H influenzae* and *Moraxella catarrhalis*. However, a trial in Northern California showed that Pnc-CRM had a protective effect against frequent otitis media. There was a 10% reduction in the risk of 3 visits to a 26% reduction in the risk of 10 visits within a 6-month period. Furthermore, otitis requiring tympanostomy tube placement was reduced by 24%. However, a trial in 383 Dutch children with recurrent acute otitis media showed no efficacy in this population. Finally in the Gambian trial, which was conducted in a rural area where access to round-the-clock curative care is difficult, there was a 16% (95% CI 3 to 38) reduction in mortality.

Postlicensure, its routine implementation in infancy has led not only to a remarkable 97% reduction in invasive disease in children younger than 2 years, but also a 46% reduction against vaccine serotypes in adults and 47% effectiveness against disease in the elderly caused by the serotypes in the vaccine.

In the second half of 2000, the 7-PCV was included in routine vaccination of infants and children under 2 years in the United States. By 2001 the incidence of all invasive pneumococcal disease had declined in this age group by 69%; disease due to vaccine and related serotypes declined by 78%. Similar reductions were confirmed in a study in northern California. A slight increase in rates of invasive disease caused by non-vaccine serotypes of pneumococcus was observed, but not large enough to offset the substantial reduction in disease due to vaccine and related serotypes. The vaccine has also significantly reduced the racial disparities in the incidence of invasive pneumococcal disease in the United States. Prior to vaccine introduction the incidences were 440 and 133 per 100,000, respectively, in black and white children under 2 years of age, (black:white ratio = 3.30). In 2002 they fell to 48 and 30 per 100,000, respectively (black:white ratio = 1.58). Interestingly, there was also significant reduction in invasive pneumococcal disease in unvaccinated adults, especially in those 20–39 years and 65+ years of age, suggesting that vaccination of young children exerted considerable herd effect in the community.

Universal immunization of all infants with PCV-7 is now recommended, with four doses given at 2, 4, 6, and 12–15 months of age. Children age 24–59 months at high risk of invasive pneumococcal disease should receive both the conjugate vaccine (PCV-7) and the 23-valent polysaccharide vaccine (23-PS). Although definitive data about using PCV-7 and 23-PS in combination are not available for invasive disease, it did reduce acute otitis media in one study. It is also known that immunization with PCV-7 induces immunologic memory that is boosted by some of the serotypes in 23-PS. Additionally, 23-PS provides coverage against a broader range of serotypes than does PCV-7. Recommendations for using PCV-7 and 23-PS in high-risk children age 24–59 months are found in Table 9–8. Children at high risk of invasive pneumococcal disease include those with chronic cardiovascular, pulmonary (cystic fibrosis but not asthma), or liver diseases, and those with anatomic and functional asplenia (including sickle cell disease), nephrotic syndrome, chronic renal failure, diabetes mellitus, cerebrospinal fluid leak, or immunosuppression (including those with HIV infection, complement deficiencies, malignancies, prolonged use of steroids, and organ transplants). Penicillin prophylaxis of patients with sickle cell disease should be continued regardless of vaccination with PCV-7 or 23-PS. Insufficient data are available to provide definitive recommendations for pneumococcal vaccination for immunocompromised children 5 years and older. Providers can consider giving one dose each of PCV-7 and 23-PS, separated by 6–8 weeks, to older children at risk of invasive pneumococcal disease. An additional 23-PS booster should be given 3–5 years later. Additionally, because otherwise healthy Alaskan Natives and American Indians are at moderately increased risk of invasive pneumococcal disease, they also may benefit from receiving both PCV-7 and 23-PS.

Preparations Available

Pneumococcal conjugate vaccine (Prevnar) is composed of seven purified capsular polysaccharides, each coupled to a nontoxic modified diphtheria toxin. Serotypes included in the vaccine and potentially cross-reacting serotypes accounted for 86% of bacteremia, 83% of meningitis, and 65% of acute otitis media cases caused by pneumococcus during the period 1978–1994. The

Table 9–8. Recommended pneumococcal (PCV-7 and 23-PS) immunization of children at high risk of invasive pneumococcal disease.

Age	Previous Doses	PCV-7	23-PS
2–6 mo	None	3 doses, 6–8 wk apart 1 booster dose at 12–15 mo	1 dose at 24 mo[a] 2nd dose 3–5 y after the first dose of 23-PS
7–11 mo	None	2 doses, 6–8 wk apart 1 booster dose at 12–15 mo	1 dose at 24 mo[a] 2nd dose 3–5 y after the first dose of 23-PS
12–23 mo	None	2 doses, 6–8 wk apart	1 dose at 24 mo[a] 2nd dose 3–5 y after the first dose of 23-PS
24–59 mo	4 doses of PCV-7	None	1 dose, 6–8 wk after last dose of PCV-7 2nd dose 3–5 y after the first dose of 23-PS
24–59 mo	1–3 doses of PCV-7	1 dose, 6–8 wk after the last dose of PCV-7	1 dose, 6–8 wk after last dose of PCV-7 2nd dose 3–5 y after the first dose of 23-PS
24–59 mo	1 dose of 23-PS	2 doses, 6–8 wk apart, starting 6–8 wk after 23-PS dose	1 dose 3–5 y after the first dose of 23-PS
24–59 mo	None	2 doses, 6–8 wk apart	1 dose, 6–8 wk after last dose of PCV-7 2nd dose 3–5 y after the first dose of 23-PS

[a]The dose of 23-PS should be given at least 8 weeks after the last dose of PCV-7.
Modified, with permission, from American Academy of Pediatrics. Pneumococcal infections. In Pickering LK (editor): *Red Book 2003 Report of the Committee on Infectious Diseases,* 20th ed. American Academy of Pediatrics, 2003.

vaccine is licensed for use in children age 6 weeks to 9 years.

The 23-valent polysaccharide vaccine (Pneumovax) is only for use in persons 2 years and older. It contains 25 μg of each purified capsular polysaccharide antigen of 23 serotypes of *S pneumoniae.* These 23 types cause 88% of cases of pneumococcal bacteremia and meningitis in adults and nearly 100% of those in children in the U.S. Cross-reactive antibody responses may protect against an additional 8% of bacteremic serotypes in adults.

Dosage & Schedule of Administration

PCV-7 is given as a 0.5-mL intramuscular dose. The first dose can be given as early as 6 weeks of life, with a recommended vaccination schedule of 2, 4, 6, and 12–15 months. Children who receive their first dose of PCV-7 at 7–11 months of age should receive two doses separated by 6–8 weeks, followed by a booster dose at 12–15 months. Children who receive their first dose of PCV-7 at 12–23 months require two doses total, separated by 6–8 weeks. PCV-7 may be given concurrently with the other routinely recommended childhood immunizations.

Children older than 23 months at high risk of invasive pneumococcal disease should receive both PCV-7 and 23-PS, as outlined in Table 9–8. PCV-7 and 23-PS should not be given simultaneously, and when both are indicated, they should be given 6–8 weeks apart. The dose of 23-PS is 0.5 mL, given intramuscularly. If splenectomy or immunosuppression can be anticipated, vaccination should be done at least 2 weeks beforehand. Revaccination with 23-PS may be considered after 3–5 years in children at high risk of fatal pneumococcal infection.

Adverse Effects

The most common adverse effects associated with PCV-7 administration are fever, induration, and tenderness at the site of the injection. When it is given simultaneously with DTaP, no increase in febrile seizures has been seen when compared with administration of DTaP alone. Vaccination with PCV-7 is contraindicated for individuals with a known hypersensitivity to any component of the vaccine.

With 23-PS, 50% of all vaccine recipients develop pain and redness at the injection site. Fewer than 1% develop systemic side effects such as fever and myalgia. Anaphylaxis is rare. Vaccine safety has not been evaluated during pregnancy.

Fireman B et al: Impact of the pneumococcal conjugate vaccine on otitis media. Pediatr Infect Dis J 2003;22:10 [PMID: 12544402].

Kilpi T et al: Finnish Otitis Media Study Group: Protective efficacy of a second pneumococcal conjugate vaccine against pneumococcal acute otitis media in infants and children: Randomized, controlled trial of a 7-valent pneumococcal polysaccharide-meningococcal outer membrane protein complex conjugate vaccine in 1666 children. Clin Infect Dis 2003;37:1155 [PMID: 14557958].

O'Brien KL et al: Efficacy and safety of seven-valent conjugate pneumococcal vaccine in American Indian children: Group randomised trial. Lancet 2003;362:355 [PMID: 12907008].

Simoes EAF et al: Respiratory diseases in children. In Jamison DT et al (editors): *Disease Control Priorities in Developing Countries,* 2nd ed. The World Bank, 2006.

Veenhoven R et al: Effect of conjugate pneumococcal vaccine followed by polysaccharide pneumococcal vaccine on recurrent acute otitis media: A randomised study. Lancet 2003;361:2189 [PMID: 12842372].

Whitney CG et al: Active bacterial core surveillance of the emerging infections program network. Decline in invasive pneumococcal disease after the introduction of protein-polysaccharide conjugate vaccine. N Engl J Med 2003;348:1737 [PMID: 12724479].

MENINGOCOCCAL DISEASE

For the first time ever in the United States, a vaccine against meningococcal disease has been recommended for universal use in certain age groups. Building upon the technology used to develop conjugate *Haemophilus influenzae* type b (Hib) and *Streptococcus pneumoniae* vaccines, a tetravalent meningococcal polysaccharide-protein conjugate vaccine (MCV4) was licensed in 2005 for use in persons 11–55 years of age. This vaccine, protecting against meningococcal serogroups A, C, Y, and W-135, is currently recommended for routine use in young adolescents (age 11–12 years), those entering high school (at approximately 15 years of age), and college freshmen living in dormitories, as well as other groups at increased risk of meningococcal disease.

Infections with *Neisseria meningitidis* cause significant morbidity and mortality, with an estimated 1400 to 2800 cases of meningococcal disease occurring in the U.S. annually. Even with appropriate treatment, meningococcal disease has an estimated case-fatality rate of 10–14%, and up to 19% of survivors are left with serious disabilities, such as neurologic deficits, loss of limbs or limb function, or hearing loss. Five serogroups of meningococcus (A, B, C, W-135, and Y) cause the vast majority of disease worldwide. Serogroups B, C, and Y are the predominant causes of invasive meningococcal disease in the U.S., while serogroups A and C cause most disease in developing countries. Intensive research efforts have been made to develop an effective vaccine against serogroup B, which causes > 50% of cases among children under 1 year of age. However, the bacterial capsule proteins of serogroup B are poorly immunogenic in humans, presenting a significant obstacle to vaccine development.

It is important to highlight the characteristics of the new MCV4 vaccine compared with the only other meningococcal vaccine available in the U.S., a tetravalent meningococcal polysaccharide vaccine (MPSV4), which was licensed in 1981. Both MCV4 and MPSV4 protect against the same four strains of meningococcus, and both are safe and immunogenic. MCV4 is licensed for use in persons 11–55 years old, while MPSV4 is licensed for persons 2 years and older. The bacterial polysaccharides used in MPSV4 produce B-cell immune stimulation but no T-cell response. Therefore, MPSV4 does not produce long-lasting immunity, nor does it produce an anamnestic response after a subsequent exposure to the same bacterial antigens. In the case of MCV4, bacterial polysaccharides are conjugated (linked) to a modified diphtheria toxoid, which leads to the stimulation of a T-cell–dependent immune response. MCV4 immunogenicity data, as well as the experience with Hib and pneumococcal conjugate vaccines, supports the premise that MCV4 will produce longer-lasting immunity than MPSV4 and will produce a memory immune response that does not occur with MPSV4.

In October 2005, the CDC reported five cases of Guillain-Barré syndrome (GBS) among recipients of MCV4. The five cases of GBS occurred in individuals 17–18 years of age, and followed MCV4 vaccination by 14–31 days. Approximately 2.5 million doses of MCV4 have been distributed in the U.S. Therefore, while GBS is an uncommon disorder (approximately 1–2 cases per 100,000 person-years), the number of cases of GBS reported might have been expected in the population by chance alone. However, the timing of GBS cases in the weeks following vaccination raises the possibility that there is an uncommon but real association between MCV4 vaccination and GBS. The CDC has recommended that the routine use of MCV4 continue, given the known morbidity and mortality caused by meningococcus and the insufficient evidence to date to conclude that MCV4 causes GBS.

A single dose of MCV4 is recommended for young adolescents (age 11–12 years) and for adolescents entering high school (approximately 15 years of age). It is hoped that by 2008 there will be adequate vaccine supplies and financing mechanisms to routinely provide MCV4 to adolescents of all ages. Meningococcal vaccination is also recommended for certain groups at increased risk of invasive meningococcal disease, including: (1) college freshmen living in dormitories; (2) persons living in or traveling to countries with endemic or hyperendemic meningococcal disease; (3) persons with complement deficiencies; (4) persons with functional or anatomic asplenia; (5) military recruits; and (6) microbiologists who work with *N meningitidis.* Whenever meningococcal vaccination is indicated, MCV4 is preferred for persons 11–55 years old while MPSV4 should be used for persons 2–10 years or > 55 years old. If MCV4 is not available, MPSV4 is an appropriate alternative for persons 11–55 years old.

Preparations Available

1. Meningococcal tetravalent conjugate vaccine, MCV4 (Menactra, Sanofi Pasteur). A single 0.5-mL dose contains 4 μg each of capsular polysaccharide from serogroups A, C, Y, and W-135 conjugated to 48 μg of diphtheria toxoid. Available in single-dose vials only.
2. Meningococcal tetravalent polysaccharide vaccine, MPSV4 (Menomune-A/C/Y/W-135, Sanofi Pasteur). Each dose consists of 50 μg each of the four bacterial capsular polysaccharides. Available in single-dose and 10-dose vials.

Dosage & Schedule of Administration

1. MCV4 is given as a single intramuscular dose of 0.5 mL.
2. MPSV4 is administered as a single subcutaneous dose of 0.5 mL.

MCV4 and MPSV4 can be given at the same time as other vaccines, at a different anatomic site. Protective antibody levels are typically achieved within 10 days of vaccination. Persons 11–55 years old who received MPSV4 more than 3–5 years previously, and who remain at increased risk of meningococcal disease, should be considered for an additional dose of MCV4 vaccination, although data are limited about the need and effectiveness of revaccination.

Precautions & Contraindications

MCV4 and MPSV4 are contraindicated in anyone with a known severe allergic reaction to any component of the vaccine, including diphtheria toxoid (for MCV4) and rubber latex. In most circumstances, MCV4 vaccination should be avoided in someone with a prior history of Guillain-Barré syndrome. Both MCV4 and MPSV4 can be given to individuals who are immunosuppressed. MPSV4 is thought to be safe during pregnancy; no information is available regarding the safety of MCV4 during pregnancy.

Adverse Effects

Both MCV4 and MPSV4 are generally well tolerated in adolescent patients. Local vaccination reactions (redness, swelling, or induration) occurred in 11–16% of persons 11–18 years old receiving MCV4 and 4–6% of persons the same age receiving MPSV4. More severe systemic reactions (presence of any of the following:

fever ≥ 39.5 °C; headache, fatigue, malaise, chills, or arthralgias requiring bed rest; anorexia; multiple episodes of vomiting or diarrhea; rash; or seizures) occurred in 4.3% of MCV4 recipients and 2.6% of MPSV4 recipients. As noted above, there have been five cases of Guillain-Barré syndrome among recipients of MCV4, but there is insufficient evidence to support any causal relationship between MCV4 vaccination and the disorder.

Postexposure Prophylaxis

Close contacts of a patient with invasive meningococcal disease should receive antimicrobial prophylaxis to prevent the spread of disease. Because the rate of disease among close contacts is highest immediately after exposure, postexposure prophylaxis should be started as soon as possible, ideally within 24 hours of exposure. Close contacts are defined as: (1) household members; (2) day care center contacts; and (3) anyone encountering an infected patient's secretions, such as through kissing, mouth-to-mouth resuscitation, or endotracheal intubation. Rifampin or ceftriaxone are used for chemoprophylaxis in children; rifampin, ceftriaxone, or ciprofloxacin may be used for adults.

American Academy of Pediatrics, Committee on Infectious Diseases: Prevention and control of meningococcal disease: recommendations for use of meningococcal vaccines in pediatric patients. Pediatrics 2005;116:496 [PMID: 15995007].

Centers for Disease Control and Prevention: Guillain-Barré syndrome among recipients of Menactra meningococcal conjugate vaccine—United States, June–July 2005. MMWR Morb Mortal Wkly Rep 2005;54:1023 [PMID: 16224452].

Centers for Disease Control and Prevention: Prevention and control of meningococcal disease—recommendations of the Advisory Committee on Immunization Practices (ACIP). MMWR Recomm Rep 2005;54(RR-7):1 [PMID: 15917737].

Keyserling H et al: Safety, immunogenicity, and immune memory of a novel meningococcal (groups A, C, Y, and W-135) polysaccharide diphtheria toxoid conjugate vaccine (MCV-4) in healthy adolescents. Arch Pediatr Adolesc Med 2005;159:907 [PMID: 16203934].

Pichichero M et al: Comparative trial of the safety and immunogenicity of quadrivalent (A, C, Y, W-135) meningococcal polysaccharide-diphtheria conjugate vaccine versus quadrivalent polysaccharide vaccine in two- to ten-year-old children. Pediatr Infect Dis J 2005;24:57 [PMID: 15665711].

Shepard CW et al: Cost-effectiveness of conjugate meningococcal vaccination strategies in the United States. Pediatrics 2005; 115:1220 [PMID: 15867028].

HEPATITIS A

The incidence of hepatitis A in the United States has decreased dramatically in recent years. In 2003, annual reported hepatitis A cases had declined by 76% compared to the time period 1990–1997, and the 2003 rate was the lowest recorded in the 40 years since surveillance began. While hepatitis A rates naturally fluctuate in multi-year cycles, a novel vaccination strategy appears to be significantly contributing to declining hepatitis A rates.

Hepatitis A vaccines first became available in the U.S. in 1995. The following year, the ACIP recommended hepatitis A vaccination of certain high-risk groups, such as travelers, users of illegal drugs, and homosexual or bisexual men. However, most hepatitis A infections occur in individuals without known risk factors for exposure to the disease. More than 50% of all infections are thought to occur in children, children are more likely than adults to be asymptomatic while infected, and children are often the mechanism by which hepatitis A is spread through households and communities.

In recognition of these epidemiologic features of hepatitis A, the ACIP in 1999 greatly expanded the population targeted for vaccination. Routine hepatitis A vaccination since then has been recommended for all children 24 months and older living in 11 states with more than twice the national average of hepatitis A cases, and vaccination was encouraged in an additional six states with disease rates exceeding (but less than twice) the national average. Following the implementation of this vaccination strategy, hepatitis A incidence rates in targeted states decreased to levels seen in other low-incidence parts of the country. Despite only modest immunization coverage levels among children in targeted states, hepatitis A incidence rates have declined in both children and adults, suggesting that herd immunity is occurring.

As the next step in reducing hepatitis A incidence in the U.S., the recommendation for 2006 will be that all children nationwide ages 12–23 months routinely receive hepatitis A vaccine.

In addition hepatitis A vaccination is indicated for the following groups: (1) travelers to countries with high hepatitis A rates; (2) children with chronic hepatitis B or hepatitis C infections or other chronic liver disease; (3) children with clotting factor disorders; (4) homosexual or bisexual males; (5) persons with an occupational exposure to hepatitis A; and (6) illegal drug users.

Hepatitis A vaccines are considered very safe; tens of millions of doses have been administered, and no serious adverse events have definitively been caused by the vaccine. Vaccine efficacy is 94–100% at protecting against clinical hepatitis A.

Preparations Available

Two inactivated hepatitis A vaccines are currently available for children: Havrix (GlaxoSmithKline) and Vaqta (Merck). Havrix contains a preservative (2-phenoxyethanol), but Vaqta does not. Both vaccines are approved for children 12 months and older. A combination vaccine against hepatitis A and hepatitis B is also available, but is only licensed in the U.S. for persons 18 years and older.

Dosage & Schedule of Administration

Havrix is available in two formulations. For individuals between the ages of 1 and 18 years, 720 ELU (enzyme-linked immunosorbent assay [ELISA] units) is administered in two doses of 0.5 mL, separated by 6–12 months. For persons older than 18 years, a higher dose (1440 ELU) is recommended, also in two doses.

Vaqta also has two formulations. For persons 1–17 years of age, two doses of 25 ELU (0.5 mL) are given, separated by 6–18 months. Individuals older than 17 years old are given 50 ELU (1.0 mL) in a two-dose schedule.

Both vaccines should be shipped and stored at 2–8 °C and should not be frozen. Hepatitis A vaccines are given intramuscularly, and may be given simultaneously with other vaccines, including hepatitis B vaccine.

Adverse Effects

Adverse reactions are mild and consist of pain and induration at the injection site, feeding problems, and headache. The vaccine should not be administered to children with hypersensitivity to 2-phenoxyethanol (in the case of Havrix) or alum (for both preparations).

Antibody Preparations

For children younger than age 12 months at increased risk of hepatitis A infection (eg, those traveling to endemic areas or those with clotting factor disorders), immunoglobulin (Ig) should be used as preexposure prophylaxis. The recommended dosages are 0.02 mL/kg in a single intramuscular dose if the duration of exposure is likely to be less than 3 months and 0.06 mL/kg if exposure is likely to be more than 3 months. For long-term prophylaxis of persons not eligible for vaccination, prophylactic doses can be repeated every 5 months.

Postexposure prophylaxis with Ig should be given to previously unvaccinated persons exposed within the prior 2 weeks to hepatitis A. Postexposure Ig is recommended for household or sexual contacts of persons with serologically confirmed hepatitis A, and for day care staff and attendees in outbreak situations. Individuals given one dose of hepatitis A vaccine at least 1 month before exposure do not need Ig. When indicated, a single intramuscular dose of Ig (0.02 mL/kg) should be given as soon as possible, but not more than 2 weeks after the last exposure. If vaccination is also indicated, it may be given simultaneously with Ig, but at a different anatomic injection site.

Centers for Disease Control and Prevention: Hepatitis A vaccination coverage among children aged 24–35 months—United States, 2003. MMWR Morb Mortal Wkly Rep 2005;54:141 [PMID: 15716804].

Craig AS, Schaffner W: Prevention of hepatitis A with the hepatitis A vaccine. N Engl J Med 2004;350:476 [PMID: 14749456].

Wasley A et al: Incidence of hepatitis A in the United States in the era of vaccination. JAMA 2005;294:194 [PMID: 16014593].

HEPATITIS B

Hepatitis B virus infection rates among children have declined steadily since 1991, the year the United States adopted a comprehensive strategy for hepatitis B elimination. Infection rates have declined 89% among persons 0–18 years old during the time interval 1990–2002, with decreasing rates seen in all childhood age groups and all races. Racial disparities in hepatitis B incidence among children have also narrowed significantly. Of the 19 verified cases of acute hepatitis B among children reported in 2001 and 2002, eight were born outside the U.S., including six orphans adopted from abroad.

Hepatitis B vaccine (HepB), when given with hepatitis B immune globulin (HBIg), is 95% effective in preventing vertical (perinatal) transmission of hepatitis B virus. HepB alone is 90–95% effective in preventing horizontal hepatitis B transmission in susceptible children and adults. Between 1982 and 2002 an estimated 40 million children and 30 million adults in the United States received hepatitis B vaccine. The use of HepB is also increasing internationally, with approximately two-thirds of all World Health Organization member countries reporting childhood HepB vaccination programs.

All pregnant women should be routinely screened for hepatitis B surface antigen (HBsAg). Women with positive reactions are highly likely to transmit the infection to their offspring. Infants born to HBsAg-positive mothers should receive both HepB and HBIg immediately after birth. Infants for whom the maternal HBsAg status is unknown should receive HepB (but not HBIg) within 12 hours of birth, and the mother's HBsAg status (and thus the newborn's need for HBIg) should be determined as soon as possible. For all infants, the hepatitis B immunization series should be started at birth, with the first dose given prior to when the infant is discharged from the hospital. This approach reduces the risk of perinatal transmission of hepatitis B, and also increases the likelihood that the vaccination series will be completed. In order to facilitate the birth dose the ACIP has recommended that the decision to avoid the birth dose should require an explanation about this in the chart and this should be accompanied by a copy of the mother's negative HBsAg test which is placed in the chart.

Routine immunization with HepB is recommended for all infants and all previously unvaccinated children 0–18 years of age. A two-dose schedule (as opposed to the standard pediatric three doses) is available for adolescents (see following discussion). Since initiating universal recommendations, the percentage of children age 19–35 months receiving three doses of HepB increased from less than 10% in 1991 to 92% in 2004.

In addition to the universal immunization of children, older persons in several risk categories have been identified as target populations for preexposure vaccination. Those that are relevant to physicians caring for children include residents and staff in institutions for the developmentally delayed, residents and staff of hemodialysis units, recipients of clotting factor concentrates, homosexually active males, users of illicit injectable drugs, household contacts of chronic hepatitis B carriers, incarcerated juveniles, long-term international travelers to endemic areas, and all health care personnel. Screening for markers of past infection before HepB immunization is generally not indicated for children and adolescents, but may be considered for high-risk individuals. Because vaccines consist of a purified inactive subunit of the virus and are not infectious, they are not contraindicated in immunosuppressed individuals or in pregnant women.

HepB is immunogenic in infants, children, and young adults. The protective efficacy of HepB correlates well with antibody levels, and virtually all persons with levels of 10 mIU/mL or more are protected in clinical trials.

Preparations Available

1. HepB (Recombivax HB, Merck) contains recombinant hepatitis B vaccine only.

2. HepB (Engerix-B, GlaxoSmithKline) contains recombinant hepatitis B vaccine only.

3. HepB-Hib (Comvax, Merck) contains Recombivax HB and *Haemophilus influenzae* type b (PRP-OMP) vaccine.

4. DTaP-HepB-IPV (PEDIARIX, GlaxoSmithKline) contains diphtheria and tetanus toxoids and acellular pertussis (DTaP), Engerix-B, and inactivated poliovirus (IPV) vaccines.

A combination vaccine against hepatitis A and hepatitis B (Twinrix, GlaxoSmithKline) is also available, but is only licensed in the U.S. for persons 18 years and older.

Only the single-antigen vaccines (Recombivax HB and Engerix-B) can be given between birth and 6 weeks of age. Any single or combination vaccine (except Twinrix) may be used to complete the hepatitis B vaccination series. All pediatric formulations contain trace to no thimerosal.

Dosage & Schedule of Administration

HepB is administered as part of the primary childhood immunization schedule for infants. Table 9–9 presents the vaccination schedules for newborn infants, by maternal HBsAg status. Infants born to mothers with positive or unknown HBsAg status should receive hepatitis B vaccine within 12 hours of birth; infants born to HbsAg-negative mothers should receive HepB prior to hospital discharge.

For children younger than 11 years of age not previously immunized, three intramuscular doses of HepB are needed. Adolescents age 11–15 years have two options: the standard pediatric three-dose schedule or two doses of adult Recombivax HB (1.0-mL dose), with the second dose administered 4–6 months after the first dose. Simultaneous administration with other vaccines at different sites is safe and effective. HepB should be given intramuscularly in either the anterolateral thigh or deltoid, depending on the age and size of the patient.

A. NEONATAL

Infants of HBsAg-positive mothers should be cleansed of blood in the delivery room. Both HepB (see Table 9–9) and HBIg (0.5 mL intramuscularly) should be administered simultaneously at different sites within 12 hours of birth. The vaccine should be repeated at 1–2 months and 6 months. After completion of the HepB series, at 9–15 months of age, immunized infants should be tested for HepB antibodies. If the antibody assay is positive, vaccination has been effective. If the result is negative, HBsAg should be tested for; if that

Table 9–9. Hepatitis B vaccine schedules for newborn infants, by maternal hepatitis B surface antigen (HBsAg) status.[a]

Maternal HBsAg Status	Single-Antigen Vaccine		Single Antigen + Combination Vaccine	
	Dose	Age	Dose	Age
Positive	1[b]	Birth (≤ 12 h)	1[b]	Birth (≤ 12 h)
	HBIg[c]	Birth (≤ 12 h)	HBIg	Birth (≤ 12 h)
	2	1–2 mo	2	2 mo
			3	4 mo
	3[d]	6 mo	4[d]	6 mo (PEDIARIX) or 12–15 mo (Comvax)
Unknown[e]	1[b]	Birth (≤ 12 h)	1[b]	Birth (≤ 12 h)
	2	1–2 mo	2	2 mo
			3	4 mo
	3[d]	6 mo	4[d]	6 mo (PEDIARIX) or 12–15 mo (Comvax)
Negative	1[b,f]	Birth (before discharge)	1[b,f]	Birth (before discharge)
	2	1–2 mo	2	2 mo
			3	4 mo
	3[d]	6–18 mo	4[d]	6 mo (PEDIARIX) or 12–15 mo (Comvax)

[a]See text for vaccination of preterm infants weighing < 2000 g.

[b]Recombivax HB or Engerix-B should be used for the birth dose. Comvax and PEDIARIX cannot be administered at birth or before age 6 weeks.

[c]Hepatitis B immune globulin (HBIg) (0.5 mL) administered intramuscularly in a separate site from vaccine.

[d]The final dose in the vaccine series should not be administered before age 24 wk (164 days).

[e]Mothers should have blood drawn and tested for HBsAg as soon as possible after admission for delivery; if the mother is found to be HBsAg-positive, the infant should receive HBIg as soon as possible but no later than age 7 days.

[f]On a case-by-case basis and only in rare circumstances, the first dose may be delayed until after hospital discharge for an infant who weighs ≥ 2000 g and whose mother is HGsAg-negative, but only if a physician's order to withhold the birth dose and a copy of the mother's original HBsAg-negative laboratory report are documented in the infant's medical record.

Reproduced, with permission, from Centers for Disease Control and Prevention: A comprehensive immunization strategy to eliminate transmission of hepatitis B virus infection in the U.S. MMWR Morb Mortal Wkly Rep 2005;54:1.

test result is positive, immunization has failed and the infant is a chronic carrier. If both HBsAg and HepB antibodies are negative, the series should be repeated at 0, 1, and 6 months, followed by repeat antibody testing 1 month after the third dose.

For infants born to mothers of unknown HBsAg status, the same schedule should be followed, except that HBIg should be withheld until the HBsAg status of the mother is known. If the mother is HBsAg-positive, HBIg should be initiated as soon as possible but no later than 7 days after birth.

For infants born to HBsAg-negative mothers, the first dose should be administered prior to hospital discharge. The recent recommendation of the ACIP (see above) provides a strong mandate to give the birth dose to all newborns. The doses and the schedule for routine vaccination of these infants are set forth in Table 9–9. For preterm infants with birth weights of less than 2 kg born to HBsAg-negative mothers, initiation of HepB should be delayed until 30 days of chronologic age if the infant is medically stable or prior to hospital discharge if discharged before 30 days of age.

If maternal screening is not possible, the infant should receive the first dose of HepB within 12 hours after birth, the second at age 1–2 months, and the third at 6 months. There should be at least 1 month between the first and second doses. The third dose should be administered at least 4 months after the first dose and at least 2 months after the second dose, but not before the child is 6 months old.

B. OLDER CHILDREN AND ADOLESCENTS

All children should receive HepB as part of the routine schedule. The universal immunization of all adolescents is recommended, on either a two- or three-dose schedule.

C. IMMUNOSUPPRESSED PERSONS AND DIALYSIS PATIENTS

Hemodialysis patients and other immunocompromised persons should be vaccinated with larger doses or an increased number of doses (doses are listed in CDC HepB recommendations listed in references).

D. LAPSED HEPATITIS B IMMUNIZATION

The HepB series can be completed regardless of the interval from the last vaccine dose. There is no need to start the series over or to test routinely for anti-HBs in healthy children unless the child's mother is HBsAg-positive.

E. POSTEXPOSURE PROPHYLAXIS

Postexposure prophylaxis is indicated for unvaccinated persons with perinatal, sexual, household, percutaneous, or permucosal exposure to hepatitis B. When prophylaxis is indicated, unvaccinated individuals should receive HBIg

(0.06 mL/kg) and the first dose of HepB at a separate anatomic site. For sexual contact or household blood exposure with an acute case of hepatitis B, HBIg and HepB should be given. Sexual and household contacts of someone with chronic infection should receive immunization (but not HBIg). For individuals with percutaneous or permucosal exposure to blood, HepB should be given, and HBIg considered depending on the HBsAg status of the person who was the source of the blood and on the vaccination response status of the exposed person. All previously vaccinated persons exposed to hepatitis B should be retested for anti-HBs. If antibody levels are adequate (≥ 10 mIU/mL), no treatment is necessary. If levels are inadequate and the exposure was to HBsAg-positive blood, HBIg and vaccination are required.

Adverse Effects

The overall rate of adverse effects is low and minor, and effects include fever (1–6%) and pain at the injection site (3–29%). There is no evidence of an association between vaccination and sudden infant death syndrome, multiple sclerosis, autoimmune disease, or chronic fatigue syndrome.

Antibody Preparations

HBIg is prepared from HIV-negative and hepatitis C virus–negative donors with high titers of hepatitis B surface antibody. The process used to prepare this product inactivates or eliminates HIV and hepatitis C virus. The use of HBIg is described earlier in this section.

Centers for Disease Control and Prevention: A comprehensive immunization strategy to eliminate transmission of hepatitis B virus infection in the United States: recommendations of the Advisory Committee on Immunization Practices (ACIP). MMWR Morb Mortal Wkly Rep 2005;54(RR-16):1 [PMID: 16371945].

Centers for Disease Control and Prevention: Acute hepatitis B among children and adolescents—United States, 1990–2002. MMWR Morb Mortal Wkly Rep 2004;53:1015 [PMID: 15525899].

Centers for Disease Control and Prevention: Global progress toward universal childhood hepatitis B vaccination, 2003. MMWR Morb Mortal Wkly Rep 2003;52:868 [PMID: 12970620].

Centers for Disease Control and Prevention: Hepatitis B vaccination—United States, 1982–2002. MMWR Morb Mortal Wkly Rep 2002;51:549 [PMID: 12118536].

VARICELLA

Prior to the availability of vaccine, about 4 million cases of varicella-zoster virus (VZV) infection occurred annually in the United States, mostly in children younger than 10 years old. This resulted in 11,000 hospitalizations and 100 deaths per year due to severe complications such as secondary bacterial infections, pneumonia, encephalitis, hepatitis, and Reye syndrome.

A live, attenuated varicella vaccine (VAR) has been licensed in the U.S. since 1995, and routine immunization of children 12 month of age and older has been recommended since that time. The vaccine has been shown to be > 95% effective at preventing severe disease. As of 2004, approximately 87% of children age 19–35 months in the United States had received at least one dose of VAR. However, VAR immunization rates vary widely by state: in 2003, state coverage ranged from 67–93%, and 28 states reported vaccination levels < 85%. States with school and day care requirements for varicella vaccination have higher immunization rates than states without such mandates.

The morbidity, mortality, and medical costs associated with varicella infection have significantly declined since VAR was first licensed in the U.S. While there is no national system of surveillance for varicella disease in place, a variety of data sources have all shown a consistent pattern of > 85% reduction in varicella-associated disease. In an investigation using national mortality data, varicella-related deaths were shown to have decreased 75% in recent years, with decreases in mortality seen in all ages, races, and ethnic groups. In a separate study, hospitalizations due to varicella decreased by 88% in 2002 compared to a pre-vaccination period, and outpatient visits for varicella decreased by 59%. Additionally, varicella-related hospital charges have declined by nearly $100 million per year since the onset of routine VAR use.

In the decade since the routine use of VAR has been recommended, there have been reports of breakthrough varicella occurring in immunized patients. However, most cases of chickenpox among previously immunized children are mild. There are limited data about the potential effectiveness, costs, and benefits of giving a booster dose of VAR. This is currently under consideration as a means of decreasing the remaining endemic disease and the mild breakthrough cases. Currently, only a single dose of VAR is recommended for children < 13 years old.

Data from U.S. and Japanese studies suggest that vaccine is also effective in preventing or modifying VZV severity in susceptible individuals exposed to VZV if used within 3–5 days of exposure. A study in the United States suggests that the efficacy of postexposure vaccination is 95% for prevention of any disease and 100% for prevention of moderate or severe disease. There is no evidence that postexposure prophylaxis will increase the risk for vaccine-related adverse events or interfere with development of immunity.

In addition to routine childhood immunization, it is now recommended that all susceptible adults or adolescents older than 13 years receive the varicella vaccine. Special attention is suggested for susceptible pregnant women after the birth of their child. A second dose of vaccine is recommended for outbreak control for relevant children who have had a single dose of vaccine.

Preparations Available

1. A cell-free preparation of OKA strain VZV is produced and marketed in the United States (Merck). Each dose of VAR contains not less than 1350 plaque-forming units of VZV and trace amounts of neomycin and gelatin. Storage in a freezer at a temperature of –15 °C or colder provides a shelf life of 15 months. VAR may be stored for 72 hours at refrigerator temperature in its lyophilized state, and it must be administered within 30 minutes after thawing and reconstitution.

2. The availability of MMRV (measles-mumps-rubella-varicella, Proquad, Merck) for use in children 1–12 years of age simplifies the administration of these antigens. MMRV is well tolerated and provides adequate immune response to all of the antigens it contains. Concomitant administration of MMRV with DTaP, Hib, and HepB vaccines is acceptable.

Dosage & Schedule of Administration

One dose (0.5 mL) of VAR is recommended for immunization for all healthy children age 12 months to 12 years who lack a history of VZV infection. Children 13 years or older require two doses of VAR 1 month apart. Asymptomatic or mildly symptomatic HIV-infected children (> 15% CD4 cells and CD4 number at CDC class 2 or better) should receive two doses of vaccine (with a 3-month interval between doses). VAR may be given simultaneously with MMR at separate sites. If not given simultaneously, the interval between administration of VAR and MMR must be greater than 28 days. Simultaneous VAR administration does not appear to affect the immune response to other childhood vaccines. VAR should be delayed 5 months after intravenous immune globulin infusion. MMRV can be administered on or after the first birthday, with a second dose of MMR at least 1 month later.

Adverse Events

Since the approval of VAR in 1995, more than 50,000,000 doses have been distributed in the United States. The most commonly recognized adverse reactions, occurring in approximately 20% of vaccinees, are minor injection site reactions. Additionally, 3–5% of patients will develop a localized rash, and an additional 3–5% will develop a sparse generalized varicelliform rash. These rashes typically consist of two to five lesions and may appear 5–26 days after immunization. Transmission of vaccine virus from healthy patients to healthy recipients is very rare; has never occurred in the absence of a rash in the index case; and has only resulted in mild disease. One case involved transmission from a vaccinee to a susceptible pregnant female. The pregnancy was terminated, but polymerase chain reaction analysis of the fetus showed no evidence of VZV infection. Based on data from the Vaccine Adverse Event Reporting System (VAERS), rates of serious adverse events following VAR are not increased compared with rates expected after natural infection or the background rates of similar events in the community. Herpes zoster infection has occurred following VAR administration in immunocompetent and immunocompromised persons within 25–722 days after immunization. Many of these cases were due to presumably unappreciated latent wild-type virus. Furthermore, based on preliminary data, the age-specific risk of herpes zoster infection seems to be lower in immunocompetent children following VAR immunization than after natural infection.

Contraindications

Table 9–3 lists contraindications to VZV immunization, such as known hypersensitivity or allergy to any VAR component, including neomycin. Because VAR and MMRV are live-virus vaccines, they are also contraindicated in children who have cellular immunodeficiencies, including those with leukemia, lymphoma, other malignancies affecting the bone marrow or lymphatic systems, and congenital T-cell abnormalities (although VAR vaccine administration to children with acute lymphocytic leukemia is under investigation). The exception to this rule is the recommendation that VAR be administered to HIV-infected children who are not severely immunosuppressed. Children receiving immunosuppressive therapy, including high-dose steroids, should not receive VAR or MMRV. Household contacts of immunodeficient patients should be immunized. VAR should not be given to pregnant women; however, the presence of a pregnant mother in the household is not a contraindication to immunization of a child within that household.

Antibody Preparations

Varicella-zoster immune globulin (VZIg) is prepared from plasma harvested from persons known to have high titers of anti-VZV antibody. It has been reliably used in high-risk susceptible persons who are exposed to VZV, for example, immunocompromised individuals without a history of chickenpox, susceptible pregnant women, newborns whose mothers develop varicella 5 days prior to delivery or within 48 hours after delivery, hospitalized premature infants of 28 weeks or more gestation (whose mother lacks a history of chickenpox or is seronegative), and hospitalized premature

infants less than 28 weeks gestation (regardless of maternal history or serostatus). Exposure is defined as a household contact or playmate contact (over 1 h/d), hospital contact (in the same or contiguous room or ward), intimate contact with a person with zoster deemed contagious, or a newborn contact. Susceptibility is defined as the absence of a reliable history of varicella in persons born after 1966. Uncertainty in this diagnosis can be resolved with an appropriate test for anti-VZV antibody. VZIg should be given as soon as possible after exposure, but should be administered within 96 hours. Newborns should be given one vial (125 U) intramuscularly. The dose for all others is 125 U/10 kg body weight intramuscularly (maximum dose, 625 U). VZIg should be readministered following reexposure of susceptible persons if more than 3 weeks has elapsed since a prior dose of VZIg.

The availability of VZIg may become limited as the sole U.S. manufacturer has stopped production. If VZIg is not available, it is recommended that intravenous Ig (IGIV) be utilized in its place. The dose is 400 mg/kg administered once. A subsequent exposure does not require additional prophylaxis if this occurs within 3 weeks of IGIV administration.

Centers for Disease Control and Prevention: Varicella-related deaths—United States, January 2003–June 2004. MMWR Morb Mortal Wkly Rep 2005;54:272 [PMID: 15788992].

Davis MM et al: Decline in varicella-related hospitalizations and expenditures for children and adults after introduction of varicella vaccine in the United States. Pediatrics 2004;114:786 [PMID: 15342855].

Davis MM, Gaglia MA: Associations of daycare and school entry vaccination requirements with varicella immunization rates. Vaccine 2005;23:3053 [PMID: 15811652].

Nguyen HQ et al: Decline in mortality due to varicella after implementation of varicella vaccination in the United States. N Engl J Med 2005;352:450 [PMID: 15689583].

Vazquez M et al: Effectiveness over time of varicella vaccine. JAMA 2004;291:851 [PMID: 14970064].

Zhou F et al: Impact of varicella vaccination on health care utilization. JAMA 2005;294:797 [PMID: 16106004].

INFLUENZA

Influenza occurs each winter and early spring, often associated with significant morbidity and mortality rates in certain high-risk persons. Up to 36,000 deaths per year in the United States are attributable to influenza, and global epidemics (pandemics) can occur. The current threat of a global pandemic with the avian influenza virus (H5N1 strain) is very real. Globally 135 cases of avian influenza with 65 deaths have been reported as of December 7, 2005, from Vietnam (93), Thailand (21), Indonesia (13), China, and Cambodia (4 each). Currently there are no vaccines available for the H5N1 virus, but several candidates are in preclinical trials, and it has been estimated that vaccines may be available by 2007. Children at high risk of influenza-related complications include those with hemoglobinopathies and those with chronic cardiac, pulmonary (including asthma), metabolic, renal, and immunosuppressive diseases. Children and adolescents receiving long-term aspirin therapy are also at risk of substantial morbidity from influenza-related Reye syndrome. Additionally, healthy children younger than 2 years of age are at increased risk of hospitalization during influenza season.

Annual influenza vaccination is indicated for all children older than 6 months of age who have a chronic health condition that places them at higher risk of complications from influenza infection. Members (including other children) of households with persons in high-risk groups should also be immunized. The vaccine may be administered to healthy children older than age 6 months, and the inactivated vaccine is now routinely recommended for all children ages 6–23 months. Physicians should identify high-risk children in their practices and encourage parents to seek influenza vaccination for them each fall. In pandemic years, it may be important to advocate vaccination in all children regardless of their usual state of health. In high-risk groups, it may be even more effective in preventing lower respiratory disease or other secondary complications, thereby decreasing hospitalizations and deaths. Each year, recommendations are formulated in the spring and summer regarding the constituents of influenza vaccine for the coming season. These recommendations are based on the results of surveillance in Asia and the southern hemisphere during the spring and summer. The vaccine each year is a trivalent inactivated vaccine containing antigens from two strains of influenza A and one strain of influenza B, chosen as those likely to circulate in the United States during the upcoming winter.

To eliminate the need for injections, and potentially to enhance mucosal and systemic immune response to vaccination, a live attenuated intranasal vaccine has been developed. This vaccine is trivalent (containing two type A strains and one type B strain), cold-adapted, and temperature-sensitive. These viruses replicate poorly in the lower respiratory tract but well in the nasal mucosa (thereby producing immunity). The vaccine is effective in preventing influenza in healthy children. However, because of questions regarding its possible association with asthma in vaccinees aged 12–60 months, it is currently licensed only for otherwise healthy children and adults age 5–49 years of age. It should not be used in children < 5 years of age; those with asthma, chronic respiratory, cardiovascular, endocrine, or renal dysfunction; or those with hemoglobinopathies or immune deficiency. It is also contraindicated in children on aspi-

rin therapy, and those with a history of Guillain-Barré syndrome or anaphylaxis to any LAIV components or eggs. During shortages of the inactivated vaccines, the LAIV should be used for healthy subjects while the inactivated one should be prioritized for use in high-risk patients.

Preparations Available

The inactivated influenza vaccine virus is grown in eggs, formalin-inactivated, and may contain trace quantities of thimerosal as a preservative. Only split-virus or purified surface antigen preparations are available in the U.S. Several manufacturers produce similar vaccines each year. Fluzone split-virus (Sanofi Pasteur) is approved for children 6 months and older; Fluvirin (Chiron) is approved only for children 4 years and older.

The intranasal trivalent live attenuated influenza virus vaccine (LAIV) (FluMist, MedImmune) is also produced in a trivalent formulation using identical virus strains to the killed vaccine. It is also made in eggs and comes in a single-use prefilled sprayer. It should be stored at −15 °C in a frost-free freezer. It may be thawed and stored in a 4–8 °C refrigerator for less than 60 hours prior to use. It should not be refrozen after thawing.

Dosage & Schedule of Administration

A. INACTIVATED INFLUENZA VIRUS VACCINE

Because influenza can circulate yearly from November through early March in the U.S., the key time to initiate vaccination is between October and early November of each year. However, providers should continue vaccinating individuals as long as vaccine is available and there is still influenza activity in the community. Children younger than age 6 months should not be immunized. Two doses are recommended for children younger than age 9 years who are receiving influenza vaccine for the first time; subsequent seasons require single doses. Older children receiving vaccine for the first time require only a single dose. The dose for children ages 6–35 months is 0.25 mL given intramuscularly; for older children, 0.5 mL given intramuscularly. The recommended site of vaccination is the antero-lateral aspect of the thigh for younger children and the deltoid for older children. Because this vaccine is inactivated, pregnancy is not a contraindication to its use. The vaccine is recommended for all pregnant women and those contemplating pregnancy during the influenza season. Influenza vaccine has been shown in some but not all studies to transiently increase HIV replication. Nevertheless, the CDC currently recommends influenza vaccination for all HIV-infected persons.

Simultaneous administration with other routine vaccinations is acceptable.

B. LIVE ATTENUATED INFLUENZA VIRUS VACCINE

This vaccine is supplied in a prefilled single-use sprayer containing 0.5 mL of the vaccine, approximately half of which is sprayed into each nostril. A dose divider clip is provided to assist in dividing the dose. If the patient sneezes during administration, the dose should not be repeated. It can be administered to children with minor illnesses, but should not be given if significant nasal congestion is present. Because it is a live vaccine it should be administered 48 hours after cessation of therapy in children receiving anti-influenza antivirals, and antivirals should not be given for 2 weeks after vaccination. Unvaccinated children aged 5–8 years should receive two doses of vaccine 6–10 weeks apart, and one dose is required for previously vaccinated children aged 5–8, or any older individuals 9–49 years of age.

Adverse Effects

A. INACTIVATED VACCINE

The killed vaccine is safe. A small proportion of children will experience some systemic toxicity, consisting of fever, malaise, and myalgias. These symptoms generally begin 6–12 hours after vaccination and may last 24–48 hours. Cases of Guillain-Barré syndrome followed the swine influenza vaccination program in 1976–1977, but careful study by the Institute of Medicine showed no association with that vaccine in children and young adults—nor in any age with vaccines given in subsequent years. For patients with anaphylactic egg allergies in whom influenza vaccination is indicated, a protocol for influenza vaccination is referenced in later discussion.

B. LIVE VACCINE

In 20 studies of the vaccine in which 28,000 doses were administered to more than 20,000 children, signs and symptoms reported more in vaccinees than placebo recipients were runny nose and nasal congestion (20–75%), headache (2–46%), fevers (0–26%), myalgias (0–21.5%), vomiting (3–13%), and abdominal pain (2%). These were reported more frequently with the first dose and were all self-limited. However, in a study of the vaccine in children age 1–17 years of age, significant increases in asthma or reactive airway disease occurred in the subset aged 11–59 months. Hence, it is not recommended in high-risk patients or in children younger than 5 years of age. Early studies from a day care in Finland demonstrated one young child with virus excretion at 21 days. However, studies in adults showed very limited excretion at very low titer for 3–4 days.

Chemoprophylaxis & Treatment

In the United States four influenza antiviral agents are available: amantadine, rimantadine, zanamivir, and oseltamivir. The prophylactic and therapeutic uses of these drugs are discussed in Chapter 36. Chemoprophylaxis is not a substitute for vaccination, and chemoprophylaxis does not interfere with vaccine immunogenicity.

Beigel JH, et al: Avian influenza A (H5N1) infection in humans. N Engl J Med 2005;353:1374 [PMID: 16192482].

Centers for Disease Control and Prevention: Estimated influenza vaccination coverage among adults and children—United States, September 1, 2004–January 31, 2005. MMWR Morb Mortal Wkly Rep 2005;54:304 [PMID: 15800475].

Centers for Disease Control and Prevention: Tiered use of inactivated influenza vaccine in the event of a vaccine shortage. MMWR Morb Mortal Wkly Rep 2005;54:749 [PMID: 16079741].

Centers for Disease Control and Prevention: Update: influenza vaccine supply and recommendations for prioritization during the 2005–06 influenza season. MMWR Morb Mortal Wkly Rep 2005;54:850 [PMID: 16138422].

Harper SA et al: Prevention and control of influenza. Recommendations of the Advisory Committee on Immunization Practices (ACIP). MMWR Recomm Rep 2005;54(RR-8): 1 [PMID: 16086456].

Jefferson T et al: Assessment of the efficacy and effectiveness of influenza vaccines in healthy children: systematic review. Lancet 2005;365:773 [PMID: 15733718].

Talbot TR et al: Duration of virus shedding after trivalent intranasal live attenuated influenza vaccination in adults. Infect Control Hosp Epidemiol 2005;26:494 [PMID: 15954490].

VACCINATIONS FOR SPECIAL SITUATIONS

RABIES

After symptoms of infection develop, rabies is almost invariably fatal in humans. Only six persons are known to have recovered from rabies infection, five of whom had either been vaccinated prior to infection or received some form of postexposure prophylaxis. In 2004, a 15-year-old girl in Wisconsin survived rabies infection; her treatment included induction of a coma while her natural immune response developed, and she did not receive rabies vaccine or rabies immune globulin. Despite this patient's survival, rabies should not be regarded as curable once symptoms develop. However, rabies in humans can be prevented by proper wound care and administration of postexposure prophylaxis when indicated.

The incidence of human rabies in the United States is very low, with fewer than three cases per year nationwide. Of the 36 human cases of rabies reported in the U.S. from

1980–1996, bat exposure was suspected in 21 cases. However, there was a definite history of bite in only one or two of these cases. Although dogs represent the most important vector for human rabies worldwide, in the U.S., because of widespread vaccination of dogs and cats, bats are the most important cause of human rabies. Rabies is also common in skunks, raccoons, and foxes; it is uncommon in rodents.

Human rabies is preventable with appropriate and timely postexposure prophylaxis. Postexposure care consists of local wound care, passive immunization, and active immunization. Immediately after an animal bite, all wounds should be flushed and aggressively cleaned with soap and water. If possible, the wound should not be sutured. Passive immunization after high-risk exposure consists of the injection of rabies immune globulin near the wound, as described later. Active immunization is accomplished by completing a schedule of immunization with one of the three rabies vaccines licensed in the U.S. It is important to keep in mind that bites from bats are often unrecognized; prophylaxis should be given if a bat is found indoors even if there is no history of contact, especially if found in the same room with a sleeping or unattended child or with an intoxicated or otherwise incapacitated individual.

Local public health officials should be consulted before postexposure rabies prophylaxis is started to avoid unnecessary vaccination and to assist in the proper handling of the animal (if confinement or testing of the animal is appropriate). To facilitate consultation, the physician should know the species of animal, its availability for testing or confinement, the nature of the attack (provoked or unprovoked), and the nature of the exposure (bite, scratch, lick, or aerosol of saliva). Preexposure prophylaxis is indicated for veterinarians, animal handlers, and any persons whose work or home environment potentially places them in close contact with animal species in which rabies is endemic. Rabies immunization should also be considered for children traveling to countries where rabies is endemic; this is particularly important for travelers who will not have prompt access to medical care should an exposure occur.

Preparations Available

Rabies vaccines stimulate immunity after 7–10 days, and the immunity persists for 2 years or more postvaccination. Three preparations are licensed in the U.S.:

1. Imovax Rabies (Sanofi Pasteur)
2. RabAvert (Chiron)
3. Rabies vaccine absorbed (BioPort). This vaccine is not currently available in the U.S.

Dosage & Schedule of Administration

The three rabies vaccines licensed in the U.S. are equally safe and efficacious for both preexposure and postexposure prophylaxis. For all three vaccines, 1.0 mL is given intramuscularly in the deltoid (for adults and older children) or anterolateral thigh (for infants and young children). The volume of the dose is not reduced for children. Vaccine should not be given in the gluteal region.

A. PRIMARY PREEXPOSURE VACCINATION

Preexposure rabies immunization should be considered for individuals at high risk for exposure to rabies, for example, veterinarians, animal handlers, spelunkers, and people moving to or extensively traveling in areas with endemic rabies. Three intramuscular injections in the deltoid area of 1 mL of any vaccine are given on days 0, 7, and 21 or 28.

B. POSTEXPOSURE PROPHYLAXIS

After an individual has possibly been exposed to rabies, decisions about whether to initiate postexposure prophylaxis need to be made urgently, in consultation with local public health officials.

1. In previously unvaccinated individuals—After proper wound care has been provided, an individual exposed to rabies should receive rabies vaccination and human rabies immune globulin (RIg). Vaccination is given on the day of exposure and on days 3, 7, 14, and 28 following exposure. RIg should also be given as soon as possible after exposure, ideally on the day of exposure, in a recommended dose of 20 IU/kg. If anatomically possible, the entire dose of RIg should be infiltrated into and around the wound. Any remaining RIg should be administered intramuscularly at an anatomic site other than the location used for rabies vaccination. Postexposure failures occurred only when some deviation from the approved protocol occurred (eg, less than usual amount of RIg, no RIg at the wound site, no cleansing of the wound, or vaccination in the gluteal area).

2. In previously vaccinated individuals—RIg is not necessary, and only two doses of vaccine on days 0 and 3 after exposure are needed.

C. BOOSTER VACCINATION

Previously vaccinated individuals with potential continued exposure to rabies should have a serum sample tested for rabies antibody every 2 years. If the titer is less than 1:5 for virus neutralization, a booster dose of rabies vaccine should be administered.

Adverse Effects

The rabies vaccines are relatively free of serious reactions. Approximately 15–74% of adults experience pain, swelling, induration, or erythema at the injection site; 10–25% may have mild systemic reactions such as headache, nausea, muscle aches, and dizziness. An immune complex–like reaction occurs in about 6% of persons 2–21 days after receiving booster doses of the Imovax Rabies vaccine.

Travelers to countries where rabies is endemic may need immediate postexposure prophylaxis and may have to use locally available vaccines and RIg. In many developing countries, the only vaccines readily available may be nerve tissue vaccines derived from the brains of adult animals or suckling mice, and the RIg may be of equine origin. Although adverse reactions to RIg are uncommon and typically mild, the nervous tissue vaccines may induce neuroparalytic reactions in 1:200 to 1:8000 vaccinees; this is a significant risk and may justify preexposure vaccination prior to travel in circumstances in which exposure to potentially rabid animals is likely.

Antibody Preparations

In the U.S., RIg is prepared from the plasma of human volunteers hyperimmunized with rabies vaccine. The recommended dose is 20 IU/kg body weight. The rabies-neutralizing antibody content is 150 IU/mL, supplied in 2-mL or 10-mL vials. It is very safe.

Rupprecht CE et al: Clinical practice: prophylaxis against rabies. N Engl J Med 2004;351:2626 [PMID: 15602023].

Wilde H et al: Rabies update for travel medicine advisors. Clin Infect Dis 2003;37:96 [PMID: 12830414].

Willoughby RE Jr et al: Survival after treatment of rabies with induction of coma. N Engl J Med 2005;352:2508 [PMID: 15958806].

TYPHOID FEVER

Globally, the burden of typhoid fever is substantial, causing an estimated 22 million illnesses and 220,000 deaths each year. In the United States, typhoid fever is relatively uncommon, with approximately 150–300 laboratory-confirmed cases each year, the majority acquired abroad. In a review of typhoid fever cases reported to the CDC, 74% of patients reported recent travel outside the U.S., only 4% of whom had received typhoid vaccination in the preceding 5 years. Approximately 40% of cases were seen in patients < 18 years old, and both short-term and long-term travel was associated with infection.

Two vaccines against *Salmonella enterica typhi,* the bacterium which causes typhoid fever, are currently available in the U.S.: a live attenuated vaccine given orally (Ty21a), and an inactivated vaccine composed of purified capsular polysaccharide (ViCPS) given parenterally. Both vaccines have been shown to protect 50–80% of vaccine recipients. The oral vaccine is most commonly used because of its ease of administration. However, noncompliance with the oral vaccine dosing sched-

ule occurs frequently, and correct usage should be stressed or the parenteral ViCPS vaccine used.

Routine typhoid vaccination is recommended only for children who are traveling to typhoid-endemic areas or who reside in households with a documented typhoid carrier. While current CDC recommendations emphasize typhoid vaccination for travelers expected to have long-term exposure to potentially contaminated food and drink, vaccination should also be considered for short-term travel to high-risk countries. While typhoid fever occurs throughout the world, areas of highest incidence include southern Asia and southern Africa. Travelers should be advised that because the typhoid vaccines are not fully protective, and because of the potential for other food- and water-borne illnesses, careful selection of food and drink and appropriate hygiene remain necessary when traveling internationally.

Preparations Available

1. Parenteral ViCPS (Typhim Vi, Sanofi Pasteur) is for intramuscular use.
2. Oral live attenuated Ty21a vaccine (Vivotif Berna Vaccine, Swiss Serum and Vaccine Institute) is supplied as enteric-coated capsules.

Dosage & Schedule of Administration

ViCPS is administered as a single intramuscular dose (0.5 mL), with boosters needed every 2 years if exposure continues. It is approved for children 2 years and older.

The dose of the oral preparation is one capsule every 2 days for a total of four capsules, taken 1 hour before meals. The capsules should be taken with cool liquids, and should be kept refrigerated. A full course of four capsules is recommended every 5 years if exposure continues. This vaccine is not approved for children younger than age 6 years. As with all live attenuated vaccines, Ty21a should not be given to immunocompromised patients.

Adverse Reactions

Both the oral and parenteral vaccines are well tolerated, and adverse reactions are uncommon and usually self-limited. The oral vaccine may cause gastroenteritis-like illness, fatigue, and myalgia, while the parenteral vaccine may cause abdominal pain, dizziness, and pruritus.

Begier EM et al: Postmarketing safety surveillance for typhoid fever vaccines from the Vaccine Adverse Event Reporting System, July 1990 through June 2002. Clin Infect Dis 2004;38:771 [PMID: 14999618].

Steinberg EB et al: Typhoid fever in travelers: who should be targeted for prevention? Clin Infect Dis 2004;39:186 [PMID: 15307027].

CHOLERA

Cholera causes significant morbidity and mortality world-wide. It may present only as traveler's diarrhea. For travelers, the risk of developing cholera per month of stay in a developing country is low, ranging from 0.001% to approximately 0.01%. No cholera vaccines are available in the United States. Because the causative bacterium *Vibrio cholerae* is not invasive, and because secretory IgA is crucial, newer vaccines available in other countries are administered orally. Two oral vaccines (one consisting solely of live attenuated bacteria and the other in combination with the B subunit of cholera toxin) are safe and immunogenic. Cholera vaccination is no longer required for international travel or for entry into any countries.

Centers for Disease Control and Prevention: http://www.cdc.gov/ncidod/dbmd/diseaseinfo/cholera_g.htm

TUBERCULOSIS

During 1993–2003 the incidence of tuberculosis (TB) in the U.S. decreased by 44%, setting the stage for possible elimination of the disease. However, nearly 40% of new cases of TB occur in persons born in other countries. Bacille Calmette-Guérin vaccine (BCG) consists of live attenuated *Mycobacterium bovis*. BCG is not currently indicated for mass use in the U.S., chiefly because of doubts about its efficacy. BCG is the most widely used vaccine in the world and has been administered to over 3 billion people (71% of infants worldwide are vaccinated) with a low incidence of serious complications. It is inexpensive, can be given any time after birth, sensitizes the vaccinated individual for 5–50 years, and stimulates both B-cell and T-cell immune responses. BCG is useful in two circumstances in the U.S.: (1) in tuberculin-negative infants or older children residing in households with untreated or poorly treated individuals with active infection with isoniazid- and rifampin-resistant *Mycobacterium tuberculosis,* and (2) in infants or children found to live under constant exposure without the possibility of removal from continuous exposure or access to prophylaxis and treatment. BCG reduces the risk of tuberculous meningitis and disseminated TB in pediatric populations by 50–100% when administered in the first month of life. BCG appears to have had little epidemiologic effect on TB, despite a reported efficacy of 50% in a meta-analysis of 26 vaccine trials, with the greatest protection against pulmonary disease. The two currently licensed BCG vaccines in the U.S. are produced by Connaught Laboratories and Organon Teknika Corporation. They are given intradermally in a dose of 0.05 mL for newborns and 0.1 mL for all other children. Mantoux testing is advised 2–3 months later, and revaccination is advised if the Mantoux test is negative. Adverse effects occur in 1–10% of healthy individuals, including local ulceration, regional lymph node enlargement, and lupus vulgaris. The vaccine is contraindicated in pregnant women and in immunocompromised individuals, including those with HIV infection, because it has caused disseminated or fatal infection.

Factors associated with increased probability that a positive TB skin test is due to *M tuberculosis* infection include (1) larger reactions, (2) contact with an individual known to be infected, (3) family history of TB, (4) longer interval between BCG administration and skin testing, and (5) country of origin with increased incidence of endemic TB. The details and cutoff observations for TB skin testing are described in Chapter 38. To ensure that those infected with TB are evaluated, a 5-mm or greater cutoff for a positive Mantoux test is used in immunocompromised children. In immunocompetent persons, the cutoff is 10 mm or above, whereas it is 15 mm or above when no risk factors are present in the absence of clinical disease (eg, screening). Recently, a case-control study from New York identified that contact with an adult with active TB, foreign birth, foreign travel, or a relative with a positive TB skin test predicted latent TB (with use of the TB skin test). This may justify routinely testing children with these risk factors as well. In 2001 a new test (Quanti-Feron-TB) that measures the release of interferon-γ in whole blood in response to stimulation with purified protein derivative was approved by the FDA. This test is not recommended for persons with symptoms of active TB who are at increased risk for progression to active TB, but may be used instead of a TB skin test in those at increased or low risk for latent TB infection, including as screening for recent immigrants. The whole blood interferon-γ assay is a better indicator of the risk of TB infection than the Mantoux test.

BCG almost invariably causes its recipients to be tuberculin-positive (5–7 mm), but the reaction often becomes negative after 3–5 years. However, a positive Mantoux test in a child with a history of BCG vaccination who is being investigated for TB as a case contact should be interpreted as indicating infection with *M tuberculosis*.

Centers for Disease Control and Prevention: Controlling tuberculosis in the United States of America. Recommendations from the American Thoracic Society, CDC and the Infectious Diseases Society of America. MMWR Morb Mortal Wkly Rep 2005;54:RR-12 [PMID: 16267499].

Kamath AT et al: New live mycobacterial vaccines: The Geneva consensus on essential steps towards clinical development. Vaccine 2005;23:3753 [PMID: 15893612].

Kang YA et al: Discrepancy between the tuberculin skin test and the whole blood interferon-γ assay for the diagnosis of latent tuberculosis in an intermediate tuberculosis burden country. JAMA 2005;293:2756 [PMID: 15941805].

Mazurek GH, Villarino ME: Centers for Disease Control and Prevention. Guidelines for using the QuantiFeron-TB test for diagnosing latent *Mycobacterium tuberculosis* infection. MMWR Morb Mortal Wkly Rep 2003;52(RR-2):15 [PMID: 12583541].

YELLOW FEVER

Immunization against yellow fever is indicated for children as young as age 4 months traveling to endemic areas or to countries that require it for entry, but otherwise immunization should be delayed until age 9 months or older. Public health authorities maintain updated information on these requirements and must be consulted. Yellow fever vaccine is a live vaccine made from the 17D yellow fever attenuated virus strain grown in chick embryos. It is contraindicated in infants younger than age 4 months due to an increased susceptibility to vaccine-associated encephalitis; in pregnant women; in persons with anaphylactic egg allergy; and in immunocompromised individuals. It can only be administered at licensed yellow fever vaccination locations (usually public health departments). A single subcutaneous injection of 0.5 mL of reconstituted vaccine is administered. The International Health Regulations require revaccination at 10-year intervals, but immunity may be lifelong. Adverse reactions are generally mild—consisting of fever, mild headache, and myalgia 5–10 days after vaccination occurring in less than 25% of vaccinees. The risk for vaccine-associated encephalitis within 30 days following vaccination has been estimated to be less than 1/8,000,000 persons. Recently, a new serious adverse reaction syndrome was described. This complication, vaccine-associated viscerotropic disease, consists of severe multiple organ system failure and death within 1–2 weeks postvaccination, especially in older adults. The estimated incidence of this complication among vaccine recipients in the U.S. is 2.5 per million doses distributed. Health care providers should be careful to administer yellow fever vaccine only to persons truly at risk for exposure to yellow fever. There is no contraindication to giving other live-virus vaccines simultaneously with yellow fever vaccine or at intervals of a day to a month.

Centers for Disease Control and Prevention: Yellow fever vaccine: Recommendations of the Advisory Committee on Immunization Practices (ACIP), 2002. MMWR Morb Mortal Wkly Rep 2002;51(RR-17):1 [PMID: 22324159].

Marfin AA et al: Yellow fever and Japanese encephalitis vaccines: indications and complications. Infect Dis Clin North Am 2005;19:151 [PMID: 15701552].

PASSIVE PROPHYLAXIS

Intramuscular Immune Globulin

Ig may prevent or modify infection with hepatitis A virus if administered in a dose of 0.02 mL/kg within 14 days after exposure. Measles infection may be prevented or modified in a susceptible person if Ig is given in a dose of 0.25 mL/kg within 6 days after exposure. Special forms of Ig include tetanus Ig, hepatitis B Ig, rabies Ig, smallpox Ig, and varicella-zoster Ig. These are obtained from donors known to have high titers of antibody against the organism in question. Their use has been described earlier in this chapter. Palivizumab is a humanized monoclonal antibody against respiratory syncytial virus (RSV) and is used to prevent RSV infection in high-risk populations with monthly doses during RSV season.

Ig must be given intramuscularly. The dose varies depending on the clinical indication. Adverse reactions include pain at the injection site, headache, chills, dyspnea, nausea, and anaphylaxis, although all but the first are rare.

Intravenous Immune Globulin

The primary indications for IVIg are for replacement therapy in antibody-deficient individuals; for the treatment of Kawasaki disease, idiopathic thrombocytopenic purpura, Guillain-Barré syndrome, and other autoimmune diseases; and chronic B-cell lymphocytic leukemia. IVIg may be beneficial in some children with HIV infection, toxic shock syndrome, and for anemia caused by parvovirus B19. Specific antibody-enriched IVIg preparations have also been developed for the prevention and treatment of the following viral infections: cytomegalovirus immune globulin for prevention and treatment of CMV disease, and respiratory syncytial virus immune globulin for prevention of RSV illness in high-risk children (no longer commercially available). Prophylaxis to prevent RSV in infants and children at increased risk for severe disease is available in an intramuscular (palivizumab) preparation. Palivizumab should be considered for (1) infants and children younger than age 2 years with chronic lung disease who have required medical therapy (supplemental oxygen, bronchodilator, diuretic, or corticosteroid therapy) for their disease within 6 months before the anticipated RSV season; (2) infants born between 33 and 35 weeks' (32 weeks 1 day and 35 weeks 0 days) gestation or earlier without chronic lung disease with two or more risk factors (child care attendance, school-age siblings, exposure to environmental air pollution, congenital airway abnormalities, or severe neuromuscular disease) up to age 6 months; (3) infants born at 29–32 weeks' gestation up to 6 months of age; (4) up to age 12 months for infants born at 28 weeks' gestation or earlier; and (5) infants and children who are 24 months old or younger with hemodynamically significant cyanotic or acyanotic congenital heart disease. Those most likely to benefit from prophylaxis are infants (< 1 year of age) who are receiving medication to control congestive heart disease, with moderate to severe pulmonary hypertension and cyanotic heart disease. RSV prophylaxis should be initiated at the onset of the RSV season and continued until the end of the season, regardless of breakthrough RSV illness during that RSV season.

RSV intramuscular monoclonal antibody, palivizumab (Synagis [MedImmune]), is a humanized monoclonal antibody directed against the F glycoprotein of RSV, a surface protein that is highly conserved among RSV isolates. It is administered in a dose of 15 mg/kg once a month and is packaged in 50- and 100-mg vials.

Palivizumab does not interfere with response to routine childhood vaccinations.

Feltes TF et al: Palivizumab prophylaxis reduces hospitalization due to respiratory syncytial virus in young children with hemodynamically significant congenital heart disease. J Pediatr 2003; 143:532 [PMID: 14571236].

Meissner HC, Long SS, American Academy of Pediatrics Committee on Infectious Diseases and Committee on Fetus and Newborn: Revised indications for the use of palivizumab and respiratory syncytial virus immune globulin intravenous for the prevention of respiratory syncytial virus infections. Pediatrics 2003;112(6 Pt 1):1447 [PMID: 14654628].

Simoes EA: Immunoprophylaxis of respiratory syncytial virus: Global experience. Respir Res 2002;3(Suppl 1):S26 [PMID: 12119055].

Antitoxins & Antivenins

Igs of animal origin are available for use in certain situations. These include botulinum antitoxin, tetanus antitoxin, diphtheria antitoxin, and snake and spider antivenins. A variety of adverse reactions, including acute febrile responses, anaphylaxis, and serum sickness, may develop after use of these products. A schedule for hypersensitivity testing and desensitization for antisera of equine origin can be found in the *Red Book*.

VACCINE SAFETY AND LEGAL ISSUES

The National Vaccine Injury Compensation Program was established in 1988 with the purpose of providing no-fault compensation for persons thought to be injured by certain vaccines. Under the terms of the act, liability claims against those who administer or manufacture vaccines must go before a federal compensation board before a civil suit may be filed. Compensation may be sought for certain events following certain immunizations within specified time intervals. The compensation system is funded by a continuing surcharge levied against the manufacturers for each dose sold of the specified vaccines. The Vaccine Injury Compensation Program can be reached on the Internet at http://www.hrsa.gov/osp/vicp, or by telephone at 1-800-338-2382.

Physicians administering vaccines are obliged to report serious adverse events following immunization to the Vaccine Adverse Events Reporting System (VAERS). This is a nationwide passive surveillance program for vaccine safety managed cooperatively by the CDC and the FDA. VAERS can be reached on the Internet at http://vaers.hhs.gov, or by telephone at 1-800-822-7967. Reports of possible adverse events related to vaccination may be made via the Internet or by mail.

Recognizing the need to improve its capability to study vaccine safety, the CDC has also participated in numerous studies using large linked databases of computerized vaccination and medical records. The Vaccine Safety Datalink Project (which is a network of several health maintenance organizations' computerized information on immunizations, medical outcomes, and potential confounders) was initiated in 1989 and serves as a useful tool to accumulate and analyze data as new vaccine issues arise.

Vaccine information statements (VIS) are educational sheets designed by the CDC to discuss the indications, benefits, and risks of routinely administered vaccines. Federal law requires that vaccine recipients (or their legal guardians) be given VIS forms prior to the administration of most vaccines. There are different VIS forms for each routinely administered vaccine, that explain in short, easy-to-understand language, important features of the vaccine. VIS forms may be obtained from the CDC at: http://www.cdc.gov/nip/publications/VIS/default.htm.

Centers for Disease Control and Prevention: General recommendations on immunization: Recommendations of the Advisory Committee on Immunization Practices (ACIP) and the American Academy of Family Physicians (AAFP). MMWR Recomm Rep 2002;51(RR-2):1 [PMID: 11848294].

Davis RL et al: Active surveillance of vaccine safety: a system to detect early signs of adverse events. Epidemiology 2005;16:336 [PMID: 15824549].

Iskander JK et al: The role of the Vaccine Adverse Event Reporting system (VAERS) in monitoring vaccine safety. Pediatr Ann 2004;33:599 [PMID: 15462575].

Zhou W et al: Surveillance for safety after immunization: Vaccine Adverse Event Reporting System (VAERS)–United States, 1991–2001. MMWR Surveill Summ 2003;52:113 [PMID: 12825543].

Normal Childhood Nutrition & Its Disorders

Nancy F. Krebs, MD, MS, Laura E. Primak, RD, CNSD, CSP

■ NUTRITIONAL REQUIREMENTS

NUTRITION & GROWTH

The nutrient requirements of children are influenced by (1) growth rate, (2) body composition, and (3) composition of new growth. These factors vary with age and are especially important during early postnatal life. Growth rates are higher in early infancy than at any other time, including the adolescent growth spurt (Table 10–1). Growth rates decline rapidly starting in the second month of postnatal life (proportionately later in the premature infant). Because of their more rapid growth rate in early infancy, nutrient requirements are slightly higher in males than in females.

Nutrient requirements also depend on body composition. In the adult, the brain, which accounts for only 2% of body weight, contributes 19% to the total basal energy expenditure. In contrast, in a full-term neonate, the brain accounts for 10% of body weight and for 44% of total energy needs under basal conditions. Thus, in the young infant, total basal energy expenditure and the energy requirement of the brain are relatively high.

Composition of new tissue is a third factor influencing nutrient requirements. For example, fat accounts for about 40% of weight gain between birth and 4 months but for only 3% between 24 and 36 months. The corresponding figures for protein are 11% and 21%; for water, 45% and 68%. The high rate of fat deposition in early infancy has implications not only for energy requirements but also for the optimal composition of infant feedings.

Because of the high nutrient requirements for growth and the body composition, the young infant is especially vulnerable to undernutrition. Slowed physical growth rate is an early and prominent sign of undernutrition in the young infant. The limited fat stores of the very young infant mean that energy reserves are unusu-ally modest. The relatively large size and continued growth of the brain render the central nervous system (CNS) especially vulnerable to the effects of malnutrition in early postnatal life.

ENERGY

The major determinants of energy expenditure are basal metabolism, metabolic response to food, physical activity, and growth. The efficiency of energy use may be a significant factor, and thermoregulation may contribute in extremes of ambient temperature if the body is inadequately clothed. Because adequate data on requirements for physical activity in infants and children are unavailable and because individual growth requirements vary, recommendations have been based on calculations of actual intakes by healthy subjects. The recent trend toward lower figures for infants reflects a move away from hypercaloric and possibly inappropriate feeding practices that were in vogue in past decades. Suggested guidelines for energy intake of infants and young children are given in Table 10–2. Also included in this table are calculated energy intakes of infants who are exclusively breast-fed, which have been verified recently in a number of centers. Growth velocity of breast-fed infants during the first 3 months equals and often exceeds the 50th percentile for the Centers for Disease Control and Prevention 2000 growth charts. At 6–12 months infants who are breast-fed typically weigh less than formula-fed babies and may show a decrease in growth velocity. The recommended dietary allowances (RDAs) of the Food and Nutrition Board, National Academy of Sciences, and National Research Council (10th edition) are not synonymous with requirements. The RDAs do not take into account the rapid changes in requirements that occur during infancy, especially the first 6 months, therefore RDAs should be used cautiously for calculating energy requirements of infants.

After the first 4 years, energy requirements expressed on a body weight basis decline progressively. The estimated daily energy requirement is about 40 kcal/kg/d

Table 10–1. Changes in growth rate, energy required for growth, and body composition in infants and young children.

Age (months)	Growth Rate (g/d)			Energy Requirements for Growth (kcal/kg/d)	Body Composition		
	Male	Both	Female		Water	Protein	Fat
0–0.25		0[a]			75	11.5	11
0.25–1	40		35	50			
1–2	35		30	25			
2–3	28		25	16			
3–6		20		10	60	11.5	26
6–9		15					
9–12		12					
12–18		8					
18–36		6		2	61	16	21

[a]Birth weight is regained by 10 d. Weight loss of more than 10% of birth weight indicates dehydration or malnutrition; this applies to both formula-fed and breast-fed infants.
Data reprinted with permission, from Fomon SJ (editor): *Infant Nutrition,* 2nd ed. WB Saunders, 1974.

at the end of adolescence. Approximate daily energy requirements can be calculated by adding 100 kcal per year to the base of 1000 kcal per day at age 1 year. Appetite and growth are reliable indices of caloric needs in most healthy children, but intake also depends to some extent on the energy density of the food offered. Individual energy requirements of healthy infants and children vary considerably, and malnutrition and dis-

Table 10–2. Recommendations for energy and protein intake.

Age	Energy (kcal/kg/d)			Protein (g/kg/d)	
	Based on Measurements of Energy Expenditure	Intake from Human Milk	Guidelines for Average Requirements	Intake from Human Milk	Guidelines for Average Requirements
10 days to 1 month	—	105	120	2.05	2.5
1–2 months	110	110	115	1.75	2.25
2–3 months	95	105	105	1.36	2.25
3–4 months	95	75–85	95	1.20	2.0
4–6 months	95	75–85	95	1.05	1.7
6–12 months	85	70	90	—	1.5
1–2 years	85	—	90	—	1.2
2–3 years	85	—	90	—	1.1
3–5 years	—	—	90	—	1.1

Data reprinted with permission, from Krebs NF et al: Growth and intakes of energy and zinc in infants fed human milk. J Pediatr 1994;124:32; Garza C, Butte NF: Energy intakes of human milk-fed infants during the first year. J Pediatr 1990;117:(S)124.

ease increase the variability. Premature infant energy requirements can exceed 120 kcal/kg/d, especially during illness or when catch-up growth is desired.

One method of calculating requirements for malnourished patients is to base the calculations on the ideal body weight (ie, 50th percentile weight for the patient's length-age, 50th percentile weight-for-height, or weight determined from current height and the 50th percentile body mass index (BMI) for age) rather than actual weight. Alternatively, the extra daily energy requirement for catch-up growth can be calculated as:

$$\frac{5 \times \text{Weight (g) deficit below IBW}}{\text{Interval (days) for correction of deficit}}$$

where 5 kcal is the energy cost of each gram of new tissue deposited. These calculations should be adjusted according to the growth response.

World Health Organization: Report of a Joint FAO/WHO/UNO Expert Consultation: Energy and Protein Requirements. WHO Tech Rep Ser No. 724, 1985;724.

De Onis M, Oyango AW: The Centers for Disease Control and Prevention 2000 growth charts and the growth of breastfed infants. Acta Paediatr 2003;92(4):413 [PMID: 12801105].

PROTEIN

Only amino acids and ammonium compounds are usable as sources of nitrogen in humans. Amino acids are provided through the digestion of dietary protein. Nitrogen is absorbed from the intestine as amino acids and short peptides. Absorption of nitrogen is more efficient from synthetic diets that contain peptides in addition to amino acids. Some intact proteins are absorbed in early postnatal life, a process that may be important in the development of protein tolerance or allergy.

The liver plays a central role in amino acid metabolism, including regulation of the absorbed amino acids. Excess amino acids, including essential amino acids, are degraded in the liver, except for the branched-chain amino acids, which pass into the systemic circulation and are taken up primarily by muscle. Insulin stimulates this uptake and suppresses muscle protein catabolism. Protein turnover rates far exceed intake, indicating a reuse of amino acids. However, some of these amino acids released from protein turnover are degraded. After removal of the amino group, the keto acids are either used directly for energy or converted to carbohydrate and fat. Nitrogen is excreted primarily via the kidney as urea.

Because there are no major stores of body protein, a regular dietary supply of protein is essential. In infants and children, optimal growth depends on an adequate dietary protein supply. Relatively subtle effects of protein deficiency are now recognized, especially those affecting tissues with rapid protein turnover rates, such as the immune system and the gastrointestinal (GI) mucosa.

Relative to body weight, rates of protein synthesis and turnover and accretion of body protein are exceptionally high in the infant, especially the premature infant. Eighty percent of the dietary protein requirement of a premature infant is used for growth, compared with only 20% in a 1-year-old child. Protein requirements per unit of body weight decline rapidly during infancy as growth velocity decreases. The recommendations in Table 10–2 are derived chiefly from the Joint FAO/WHO/UNO Expert Committee and are similar to the RDAs. They deliver a protein intake above the quantity provided in breast milk. The protein intake required to achieve protein deposition equivalent to the in utero rate in very low birth weight infants is 3.7–4.0 g/kg/day simultaneous with adequate energy intake. Protein requirements increase in the presence of skin or gut losses, burns, trauma, and infection. Requirements also increase during times of catch-up growth accompanying recovery from malnutrition (approximately 0.2 g of protein per gram of new tissue deposited). Young infants experiencing rapid recovery may need as much as 1–2 g/kg/d of extra protein. By age 1 year, the extra protein requirement is unlikely to be more than 0.5 g/kg/d. Inadequate protein intake may occur in breastfed infants fed low-protein supplements (eg, fruit juices), in infants with malabsorption (cystic fibrosis), or in infants fed low-protein weaning food (eg, cassava or dilute cereal gruels) as the dietary staple.

The quality of protein depends on its amino acid composition. Infants require 43% of protein as essential amino acids, and children require 36%. Adults cannot synthesize eight essential amino acids: isoleucine, leucine, lysine, methionine, phenylalanine, threonine, tryptophan, and valine. Histidine may be added to this list. Cysteine and tyrosine are considered partially essential because their rates of synthesis are limited and may be inadequate in certain circumstances. In young infants, synthetic rates for cysteine, tyrosine, and perhaps taurine are insufficient for needs. Taurine, an amino acid used to conjugate bile acids, may also be conditionally essential in infancy. Lack of an essential amino acid leads to weight loss within 1–2 weeks. Wheat and rice are deficient in lysine, and legumes are deficient in methionine. Appropriate mixtures of vegetable protein are therefore necessary to achieve high protein quality.

Because the mechanisms for removal of excess nitrogen are efficient, moderate excesses of protein are not harmful and may help to ensure an adequate supply of certain micronutrients. Adverse effects of excessive protein intake may include increased calcium losses in urine and, over a life span, increased loss of renal mass. Excessive protein intake may also cause elevated blood urea nitrogen, acidosis, hyperammonemia, and, in the premature infant, failure to thrive, lethargy, and fever.

Thureen P, Heird WC: Protein and energy requirements of the pre-term/low birth weight (LBW) infant. Pediatr Res 2005; 57(5 Pt 2):95R [PMID: 15817496].

LIPIDS

Fats are the main dietary energy source for infants and account for up to 50% of the energy in human milk. Over 98% of breast milk fat is triglyceride, which has an energy density of 9 kcal/g. Fats can be stored efficiently in adipose tissue with a minimal energy cost of storage. This is especially important in the young infant. Fats are required for the absorption of fat-soluble vitamins and for myelination of the central nervous system. Fat also provides essential fatty acids (EFAs) necessary for brain development, for phospholipids in cell membranes, and for the synthesis of prostaglandins and leukotrienes. The EFAs are polyunsaturated fatty acids, linoleic acid ($18:2\omega6$) and linolenic acid ($18:3\omega3$). Arachidonic acid ($20:4\omega6$) is derived from dietary linoleic acid and is present primarily in membrane phospholipids. Oxygenation of arachidonic acid (ARA) through the lipoxygenase pathway yields leukotrienes, and oxygenation through the cyclooxygenase pathway yields prostaglandins. Important derivatives of linolenic acid are eicosapentaenoic acid ($20:6\omega3$) and docosahexaenoic acid (DHA, $22:6\omega3$) found in human milk and brain lipids. Visual acuity and possibly psychomotor development of formula-fed premature infants is improved in formulae supplemented with DHA ($22:6\omega3$) and ARA ($20:4\omega6$). Neurologic developmental outcomes at 18 months in healthy term infants fed formula supplemented with DHA and ARA do not appear to be different from controls, thus the role of supplementing long-chain fatty acids in healthy formula-fed term infant remains unclear (though safety has been established).

Clinical features of EFA $\omega6$ deficiency include growth failure, erythematous and scaly dermatitis, capillary fragility, increased fragility of erythrocytes, thrombocytopenia, poor wound healing, and susceptibility to infection. The clinical features of deficiency of $\omega3$ fatty acids are less well defined, but dermatitis and neurologic abnormalities including blurred vision, peripheral neuropathy, and weakness have been reported. Fatty fish are the best dietary source of $\omega3$ fatty acids. A high intake of fatty fish is associated with decreased platelet adhesiveness and decreased inflammatory response.

Up to 5–10% of fatty acids in human milk are polyunsaturated. Most of these are $\omega6$ series with smaller amounts of long-chain $\omega3$ fatty acids. About 40% of breast milk fatty acids are monounsaturates, primarily oleic acid (18:1), and up to 10% of total fatty acids are medium-chain triglycerides (MCTs) (C_8 and C_{10}) with a calorie density of 7.6 kcal/g. In general, the percentage of calories derived from fat is a little lower in infant formulas than in human milk. Infant formulas have traditionally contained a relatively high percentage of linoleic acid but minimal long-chain $\omega3$ fatty acid.

The American Academy of Pediatrics recommends that infants receive at least 30% of calories from fat, with at least 2.7% of total fat as linoleic acid, and 1.75% of total fatty acids as linolenic. Since 2002, formulas in the United States contain long-chain polyunsaturated fatty acids (LC-PUFA), specifically ARA and DHA. There is controversy regarding long-term neurologic benefits to the term infant, but the potential benefits on development and visual acuity in premature infants are more convincing.

It is appropriate that 40–50% of energy requirements be provided as fat during at least the first year of life. Children older than 2 years should be switched gradually to a diet containing approximately 30% of total calories from fat, with no more than 10% of calories either from saturated fats or polyunsaturated fats.

During digestion, triglycerides are hydrolyzed to monoglycerides, free fatty acids, and glycerol in the lumen of the gut. Substantial hydrolysis of triglycerides in milk formulas occurs in the stomach by the action of lingual and gastric lipases. Pancreatic lipases and bile salt levels are relatively low in early postnatal life, but breast milk contains a bile salt-stimulated lipase that is effective in the lumen of the duodenum. Bile salts promote the formation of the colipase–lipase complex, which adheres to the triglycerides prior to hydrolysis. Bile salts also have a major role in the emulsification of fatty acids, allowing their passage through the unstirred water layer to the surface of the mucosal cell. After passage into the enterocyte, long-chain ($\geq C_{12}$) fatty acids and monoglycerides are reesterified to triglycerides and are packaged with phospholipids, cholesterol, and protein into chylomicrons, which are transported in the lymphatics to the liver and thence the circulation. At the capillary endothelial surface of adipose and muscle tissue, lipoprotein lipase (LPL) hydrolyzes triglycerides from chylomicrons, releasing free fatty acids and glycerol, which are taken up by the adjacent cells. LPL also hydrolyzes triglycerides synthesized in the liver and transported to peripheral tissues as very low density lipoproteins.

Beta-oxidation of fatty acids occurs in the mitochondria of muscle and liver. Carnitine is necessary for oxidation of the fatty acids, which must cross the mitochondrial membranes as acylcarnitine. Carnitine is synthesized in the human liver and kidney from lysine and methionine. Carnitine needs of infants are met by breast milk or formulas, and carnitine is now added routinely to soy-based formulas. In the liver, substantial quantities of fatty acids are converted to ketone bodies, which are then released into the circulation as an important fuel for the brain of the young infant.

MCTs are sufficiently soluble that micelle formation is not required for transport across the intestinal mucosa. They are transported directly to the liver via the portal circulation. MCTs are rapidly metabolized in the liver, undergoing β-oxidation or ketogenesis. They do not require carnitine to enter the mitochondria. Ketones are formed from MCTs even when provided orally. MCTs are useful for patients with luminal phase defects, absorptive defects, and chronic inflammatory bowel disease. The potential side effects of MCT administration include diarrhea when given in large quantities; high octanoic acid levels in patients with cirrhosis; and, if they are the only source of lipids, deficiency of EFA.

Bouwstra H et al: Long-chain polyunsaturated fatty acids and neurological developmental outcome at 18 months in healthy term infants. Acta Paediatr 2005;94(1):26 [PMID: 15858956].

McCann JC, Ames BN: Is docosahexaenoic acid, an n-3 long chain polyunsaturated fatty acid, required for development of normal brain function? An overview of evidence from cognitive and behavioral tests in humans and animals. Am J Clin Nutr 2005;82:281 [PMID: 16087970].

CARBOHYDRATES

The energy density of carbohydrate is 4 kcal/g. Approximately 40% of caloric intake in human milk is in the form of lactose, or milk sugar. Lactose supplies 20% of the total energy in cow's milk. The percent of total energy in infant formulas from carbohydrate is similar to that of human milk.

After the first 2 years of life, 50–60% of energy requirements should be derived from carbohydrates, with no more than 10% from simple sugars. These dietary guidelines are, unfortunately, not reflected in the diets of North American children, who typically derive 25% of their energy intake from sucrose and less than 20% from complex carbohydrates.

The rate at which lactase hydrolyzes lactose to glucose and galactose in the intestinal brush border determines how quickly milk carbohydrates are absorbed. Lactase levels are highest in young infants, and decline with age depending on genetic factors. About 20% of non-white Hispanic and black children less than 5 years of age have lactase deficiency. White children typically do not develop symptoms of lactose intolerance until they are at least 4 or 5 years of age, while non-white Hispanic, Asian-American, and black children may develop these symptoms by 2 or 3 years of age. Lactose-intolerant children have varying symptoms depending on the specific activity of their intestinal lactase and the amount of lactose consumed. Galactose is preferentially converted to glycogen in the liver prior to conversion to glucose for subsequent oxidation. Infants with galactosemia, an inborn metabolic disease caused by deficient galactose-1-phosphate uridyltransferase, require a lactose-free diet starting in the neonatal period.

Starch is broken down in the gut lumen into disaccharides and oligosaccharides, which are hydrolyzed into glucose by maltase, isomaltase, and glucoamylase in the brush border. Glucoamylase, which hydrolyzes oligosaccharides of 4–9 glucose units, is located predominantly at the base of the villi, where it may be protected during periods of mucosal injury. Glucose polymers of this length are used extensively in infant formulas and as caloric supplements. Advantages include a relatively low osmolality and better hydrolysis by damaged mucosa. Glucose and galactose are absorbed actively with sodium. This provides the theoretic basis for the composition of oral rehydration solutions in the management of diarrhea. Glucose enhances absorption of sodium and water and also supplies some energy.

During and immediately following a meal, plasma glucose levels are maintained by glucose absorption. If less than 10% of dietary energy is regularly provided by carbohydrate, ketosis may result. Between 2–4 hours after a meal, maintenance of plasma glucose concentration depends increasingly on hepatic glycogen stores. These provide only 100–150 g glucose in the adult and only 6 g in the neonate. After liver glycogen is depleted, the body progressively depends on gluconeogenesis. Glucose is the principal fuel for the brain and is the main energy source for other tissues, including red and white blood cells.

Children and adolescents in North America consume large quantities of sucrose and high-fructose corn syrup in soft drinks and other sweetened beverages, candy, syrups, and sweetened breakfast cereals. Added sugar intake has been reported to average approximately 15% of total energy intake in adolescents, far exceeding recommended intakes. A high intake of these sugars, especially in the form of sweetened beverages, may predispose to obesity and is a major risk factor for dental caries. Sucrase hydrolyzes sucrose to glucose and fructose in the brush border of the small intestine. Fructose is absorbed more slowly than and independent of glucose by facilitated diffusion. Fructose does not stimulate insulin secretion or enhance leptin production. Since both insulin and leptin play a role in regulation of food intake, consumption of fructose (eg, as high-fructose corn syrup) may contribute to increased energy intake and weight gain. Fructose is also easily converted to hepatic triglycerides, which may be undesirable in malnourished patients or in patients with insulin resistance/metabolic syndrome and cardiovascular disease risk.

Dietary fiber can be classified in two major types: nondigested carbohydrate (β1-4 linkages) and noncarbohydrate (lignin). Insoluble fibers (cellulose, hemicellulose, and lignin) increase stool bulk and water content and decrease gut transit time. They may impair mineral absorption. Soluble fibers (pectins, mucilages, oat bran) bind bile acids and reduce lipid and cholesterol absorption. Pectins also slow gastric emptying and the rate of nutrient absorption. Few data regarding the fiber needs of children are available. The Dietary Reference Intakes recommend 14 grams fiber/1000 kcals consumed. The American Academy of Pediatrics recommends that children over 2 years consume in grams per day an amount of fiber equal to 5 plus the age in years. Fiber intakes are often low in North America. Children who have higher dietary fiber intakes have been found to consume more nutrient-dense diets than children with low fiber intakes. In general, higher fiber diets are associated with lower risk of chronic diseases such as obesity, cardiovascular disease, and diabetes.

Bray GA et al: Consumption of high-fructose corn syrup in beverages may play a role in the epidemic of obesity. Am J Clin Nutr 2004;80(4):537 [PMID 15051594].

Heyman M and the Committee on Nutrition, American Academy of Pediatrics: Clinical features of lactose intolerance in infants, children and adolescents. Pediatrics 2005, in press.

Kranz S et al: Dietary fiber intake by American preschoolers is associated with more nutrient-dense diets. J Am Diet Assoc 2005;105(2):221 [PMID: 15668678].

MAJOR MINERALS

(See Table 10–3 for recommended intakes.)

Calcium

A. DIETARY SOURCES

The major dietary sources of calcium are milk and dairy products. Although some calcium is available from legumes, broccoli, some green leafy vegetables, and fortified cereals, it is difficult to achieve an adequate calcium intake without dairy products or calcium supplementation.

B. ABSORPTION/METABOLISM

Average calcium absorption, is 20–30%, but calcium absorption from human milk is 60%. Absorption is enhanced by lactose, glucose, and protein and is impaired by phytate, fiber, oxalate, and unabsorbed fat. Control of calcium absorption is exerted primarily by variations in serum 1,25-dihydroxycholecalciferol (calcitriol), which increases in response to increases in circulating parathyroid hormone (PTH). PTH is secreted in response to a fall in plasma-ionized calcium. It also promotes the release of calcium from bone. Calcium is excreted primarily via the kidney. It is the most abundant mineral in the body, and more than 99% is in the skeleton. Many vital cellular processes depend on calcium, especially free cytosolic calcium.

C. DEFICIENCY

Dietary calcium deficiency can occur in premature infants and lactating adolescents as a result of restricted milk intake and also in patients with steatorrhea. Deficient calcium intake results in decreased bone density.

Table 10–3. Summary of dietary reference intakes for selected minerals and trace elements.

	0–6 mo	7–12 mo	1–3 yr	4–8 yr	9–13 yr	14–18 yr male	14–18 yr female
Calcium (mg/d)	210[a]	270[a]	500[a]	800[a]	1300[a]	1300[a]	1300[a]
Phosphorus (mg/d)	100[a]	275[a]	460[a]	500	1250	1250	1250
Magnesium (mg/d)	30[a]	75[a]	80	130	240	410	360
Iron (mg/d)	0.27[a]	11	7	10	8	11	15
Zinc (mg/d)	2[a]	3	3	5	8	11	9
Copper (µg/d)	200[a]	220[a]	340	440	700	890	890
Selenium (µg/d)	15[a]	20[a]	20	30	40	55	55

[a]Adequate Intakes (AI). All other values represent the recommended Dietary Allowances (RDA). Both the RDA and AI may be used as goals for individual intakes.
Reproduced, with permission, from National Academy of Sciences, Food and Nutritional Board, Institute of Medicine: *Dietary Reference Intakes, Applications in Dietary Assessment*. National Academy Press, 2000:287–289. Available online at: http://www.nap.edu

Bone density increases with increasing calcium intake up to a daily intake of more than 1000 mg in adolescents. Maximizing bone density in adolescence has important implications for achieving peak bone density and minimizing postmenopausal osteoporosis.

Phosphorus

A. DIETARY SOURCES

Phosphorus is abundant in meats, eggs, dairy products, grains, legumes, and nuts. Phosphorus levels are high in processed foods and very high in colas and other soft drinks.

B. ABSORPTION/METABOLISM

Approximately 80% of dietary phosphorus is absorbed; the kidney is responsible for homeostatic control. PTH decreases tubular reabsorption of phosphorus. More than 85% of body phosphorus is in bone. Phosphorus is also a component of many organic compounds with vital metabolic roles, including adenosine triphosphate and 2,3-diphosphoglycerate. Many of the clinical effects of phosphorus depletion are attributable to cellular energy depletion from lack of adenosine triphosphate or to cellular anoxia secondary to impaired release of oxygen from hemoglobin. Other key compounds containing phosphorus include cell membrane phospholipids and nucleotides.

C. DEFICIENCY

Nutritional phosphorus deficiency is rare but has occurred in very premature infants fed human milk, in whom deficiency can produce osteoporosis and rickets. Deficiency may also occur in patients with severe protein-energy malnutrition. Nonnutritional phosphorus depletion may result from chronic diarrhea, Fanconi tubulopathy, and the ingestion of phosphorus-binding antacids. Severe hypophosphatemia results from a deficiency together with an acute extracellular-to-intracellular shift in phosphorus. This shift can be triggered by glucose, by insulin, or during nutritional rehabilitation of the malnourished patient (eg, refeeding syndrome). Phosphorus deficiency affects most organ systems, including muscle (weakness progressing to rhabdomyolysis), cellular components of blood (both physiologic and functional changes), the GI system, the central nervous system, and bone (bone pain, osteomalacia). Respiratory insufficiency may result from weakness of the diaphragm. Phosphate depletion in the premature infant can cause hypercalcemia. Phosphorus depletion can be treated with phosphorus salts or skim milk. Phosphorus excess may cause neonatal tetany due to decreased serum calcium. Phosphorus retention in chronic renal disease leads to metabolic bone disease.

Magnesium

A. DIETARY SOURCES

Two-thirds of dietary magnesium is derived from vegetables, cereals, and nuts.

B. ABSORPTION/METABOLISM

The kidney controls magnesium homeostasis by minimizing excretion when intake is low. Magnesium is the second most abundant intracellular cation; 50% is in bone. Levels in the cytosol are 10 times that in the extracellular fluids and are especially high in mitochondria. Magnesium activates many enzymes, especially phosphorus-hydrolyzing and phosphorus-transferring enzymes involved in energy metabolism. Magnesium also plays major roles in nucleic acid metabolism.

C. DEFICIENCY

Dietary magnesium deficiency is not recognized except as a component of protein-energy malnutrition (eg, refeeding syndrome), but magnesium depletion may occur secondary to renal disease, intestinal malabsorption, or medications inducing magnesium loss from the gut or kidney. Hypomagnesemia produces neuromuscular excitability, muscle fasciculation, neurologic abnormalities, and electrocardiographic changes (depression of ST segment and T waves). Magnesium modulates PTH secretion and action, albeit to a lesser extent than calcium. Thus, magnesium depletion can cause secondary hypocalcemia. Acute magnesium depletion can be treated with a 50% solution of $MgSO_4$, providing 0.3–1.0 mEq of magnesium per kilogram given intravenously over a 24-hour period. Magnesium excess can cause respiratory depression, lethargy, and coma.

Sodium

A. DIETARY SOURCES

In the United States and western Europe, only 10% of sodium intake is derived from unprocessed foods; 15% is derived from salt added while cooking and 75% from salt added to processed foods during manufacturing. The 10% derived from unprocessed foods is sufficient to meet normal requirements. Current dietary recommendations suggest that North Americans should reduce sodium intake so as to restore a normal ratio of dietary sodium to potassium. The present ratio is approximately 2:1, but in other cultures and in other mammalian species the ratio is 0.25:1. A high sodium-to-potassium ratio has been implicated in the pathogenesis of hypertension, especially if the intake of dietary calcium is low.

Excessive sweating or high sweat sodium (as in cystic fibrosis) may increase the requirement for dietary sodium.

Sodium deficiency occurs most commonly as a result of diarrhea and vomiting. Anorexia, vomiting, and mental apathy may result from chronic depletion of sodium chloride. Hyponatremic and hypernatremic dehydration are discussed in Chapter 42.

B. DEFICIENCY

Severe malnutrition and severe stress or hypermetabolism can disturb the ionic gradient across cell membranes and lead to excess intracellular sodium, which can adversely affect cellular metabolism. Sodium should be administered with great caution in these circumstances. Suggested dietary intake of sodium for infants is 50 mg/kg/d; for children older than 1 year, it is 250–500 mg/d.

Chloride

A. DIETARY SOURCES

Chloride is mainly obtained from table salt or sea salt, which is primarily sodium chloride. It is also found in many vegetables. Foods with higher amounts of chloride are seaweed, rye, tomatoes, lettuce, celery, and olives. Potassium chloride is found in most foods and is the usual ingredient of salt substitutes.

B. ABSORPTION/METABOLISM

The intake and homeostasis of dietary chloride are closely linked with those of sodium. However, chloride is itself important in the physiologic mechanisms of the kidney and the gut. Active chloride transport in the ascending loop of Henle is necessary for the passive reabsorption of sodium. Deficiency of chloride leads to a decrease in the absorption of sodium in the ascending loop of Henle and an increase in the amount of sodium presented to the distal tubule. This sodium is exchanged for H^+ and K^+, which can result in hypokalemic alkalosis.

C. DEFICIENCY

Infants fed formulas low in chloride have experienced a nutritional deficiency of chloride. Other causes of chloride deficiency include cystic fibrosis, pyloric stenosis and other causes of vomiting, familial chloride diarrhea, chronic diuretic (furosemide) therapy, and Bartter syndrome. Chloride deficiency has been associated with failure to thrive and may especially affect head growth. Other features include anorexia, lethargy, muscle weakness, vomiting, dehydration, and hypovolemia. Laboratory features include hypochloremia, hypokalemia, metabolic alkalosis, and hyperreninemia. Suggested chloride content of infant formulas is 50–150 mg/100 kcal; for children older than 1 year, suggested daily intake is 700 mg/d.

Potassium

A. DIETARY SOURCES

Potassium is readily available in unprocessed foods, including nuts, whole grains, meats and fish, beans, bananas, and orange juice. Relatively high potassium intakes are encouraged except in the presence of renal failure.

B. ABSORPTION/METABOLISM

The kidneys control potassium homeostasis via the aldosterone–renin–angiotensin endocrine system. Potassium is the principal intracellular cation. The amount of total body potassium, therefore, depends on lean body mass.

C. DEFICIENCY

Potassium deficiency occurs in protein-energy malnutrition (eg, in refeeding syndrome) and can be a cause of sudden death from cardiac failure if not treated aggressively during the initial phase of rehabilitation. Because of loss of lean body mass, excessive potassium is excreted in the urine in any catabolic state. This too requires aggressive replenishment during recovery. During acidosis, intracellular potassium is exchanged for H^+. Potassium is shifted into the extracellular fluid, and large amounts may be lost in the urine (eg, in diabetic ketoacidosis) despite normal or elevated plasma potassium. Other causes of potassium deficiency are diarrhea and diuretics. Potassium deficiency may produce muscle weakness, mental confusion, and sudden death from arrhythmias. Electrocardiographic findings include depression of the ST segment and low T waves. Hyperkalemia may result from renal insufficiency. Suggested dietary intake of potassium for infants is 80 mg/kg/d; for children older than 1 year, it is 800 mg/d.

Afzal NA et al: Refeeding syndrome with enteral nutrition in children: A case report, literature review, and clinical guidelines. Clin Nutr 2002;21(6):515 [PMID: 12468372].

TRACE ELEMENTS

Trace elements with a recognized role in human nutrition are iron, iodine, zinc, copper, selenium, manganese, molybdenum, chromium, cobalt (as a component of vitamin B_{12}), and fluoride. Dietary requirements of trace elements are summarized in Table 10–3. Iron deficiency is discussed in Chapter 27.

A. DIETARY SOURCES

Human milk, meats, shellfish, legumes, nuts, and whole-grain cereals are good sources of trace elements. Fish are a good source of selenium.

B. ABSORPTION

Absorption of iron, zinc, copper, and other trace elements from human milk is efficient. Healthy full-term breast-fed infants generally do not require exogenous trace elements, including iron, until approximately 6 months. Factors affecting trace element absorption include the quantity in the diet, the simultaneous ingestion of foods promoting the formation of insoluble complexes (phytate, fiber, phosphate, oxalate), the oxidation state of the element (ascorbic acid increases iron absorption and decreases copper absorption), its chemical form in the diet (heme versus nonheme iron), competitive inhibition of mucosal absorption (interactions of iron, zinc, and copper), and host factors such as nutritional status, diarrhea, and intestinal function. The GI tract is the major site of homeostatic control for iron and zinc; the liver for copper; the intestinal tract and liver for manganese; and the kidneys for selenium, chromium, and iodine.

C. DEFICIENCIES

Iron, zinc, and possibly copper deficiencies occur in the free-living population. In certain geographic regions iodine and selenium deficiencies are common because of low content of the minerals in soil and water. Infants exclusively fed cow's milk are at risk for iron and copper deficiency. Excessive loss and impaired absorption can cause iron, zinc, or copper deficiency. Trace element deficiencies have been associated with the use of synthetic diets and especially intravenous (IV) nutrition. Protein-energy malnutrition may be complicated by deficiencies in iron, zinc, copper, selenium, or chromium. Deficiencies in zinc, copper, iron, and molybdenum occur as a result of specific genetic diseases affecting the absorption or metabolism of these elements. (See Chapter 33.)

Zinc

A. FUNCTION

Zinc is a component of many enzymes and plays important roles in gene transcription and nucleic acid metabolism, protein synthesis, and membrane structure and function.

B. DEFICIENCY

Zinc deficiency is the result of diets low in available zinc (high phytate) and synthetic diets (oral or IV) lacking adequate zinc supplements. Diseases associated with impaired absorption (regional enteritis, celiac disease, cystic fibrosis) or excessive loss (chronic diarrhea), and inborn diseases of zinc metabolism may produce a state of zinc deficiency. Although the zinc in human milk is very efficiently absorbed, the zinc concentration in breast milk steadily declines over time. After 6 months, the exclusively breast-fed infant is likely to need additional zinc from complementary foods.

Several recent large trials have shown that zinc supplementation in infants and young children is associated with a significant reduction in the incidence of pneumonia and of acute and chronic diarrhea. Improved zinc status has also been associated with improved immunocompetence. Low birth weight infants appear to be particularly vulnerable to zinc deficiency, and randomized trials of zinc supplementation in developing countries have shown significant improvements in growth as well as reduction in the mortality and morbidity associated with infection. Mild deficiency is associated with impaired growth and poor appetite. Severe deficiency is characterized by mood changes, irritability, and lethargy. Impairment of the immune system, especially T-cell function, has been linked to increased susceptibility to infection. The most severe deficiency state is characterized by an acroorificial skin rash, usually accompanied by diarrhea and alopecia. These features occur in patients with acrodermatitis enteropathica, an inborn error of zinc metabolism, in subjects receiving IV feeding without adequate zinc supplements, and in some breast-fed infants whose mothers have a defect in the secretion of zinc by the mammary gland. Plasma zinc collected before breakfast is below 6 µmol/L (40 µg/dL) in patients with severe zinc deficiency and 6–9 µmol/L (40–60 µg/dL) in patients with moderate zinc deficiency. In patients with mild zinc deficiency, plasma zinc concentration may be within the normal range (60–100 µg/dL).

C. TREATMENT

Dietary zinc deficiency can be treated with 1 mg/kg/d of elemental zinc for 3 months (eg, 4.5 mg of $ZnSO_4$ + 7 H_2O/kg/d), preferably administered separately from meals and iron supplements. Sustained clinical remission in acrodermatitis enteropathica is usually achieved with 30–50 mg Zn^{2+} per day, but larger quantities may be required.

Bhutta ZA: The role of zinc in child health in developing countries: Taking the science where it matters. Indian Pediatr 2004; 41:429 [PMID: 15181293].

Black RE: Zinc deficiency, infectious disease and mortality in the developing world. J Nutr 2003;133:1485S [PMID: 12730449].

Jalla S et al: Zinc homeostasis in premature infants does not differ between those fed preterm formula or fortified human milk. Pediatr Res 2004;56:615 [PMID: 15295087].

Krebs NF, Westcott J: Zinc and breastfed infants: If and when is there a risk of deficiency? Adv Exp Med Biol 2002;503:69 [PMID: 12026029].

Copper

A. FUNCTION

Copper is a vital component of several oxidative enzymes: cytochrome c oxidase, the terminal oxidase in the electron transport chain; cytosolic and mitochondrial superoxide dismutase, which have key roles in the body defense against free radicals; lysyl oxidase, which is necessary for the cross-linking of elastin and collagen; and ferroxidases (including ceruloplasmin) necessary for the oxidation of ferrous storage iron to ferric iron prior to attachment to transferrin for transport to the red cell precursors in the bone marrow. Cu^{2+} is highly reactive and must be transported in the circulation bound to ceruloplasmin so that its oxidative potential can be contained.

B. DEFICIENCY

Copper deficiency occurs in the following circumstances: in premature infants fed milk preparations low in copper; in association with prolonged feeding with unmodified cow's milk; in association with generalized malnutrition; in patients maintained on prolonged total parenteral nutrition (TPN) without copper supplementation; and in patients with intestinal malabsorption or prolonged diarrhea.

Osteoporosis is an early finding of copper deficiency. Later, enlargement of costochondral cartilages, cupping and flaring of long-bone metaphyses, and spontaneous rib fractures may occur. The radiologic findings must be distinguished from child abuse (asymmetrical fractures), rickets, and scurvy. Neutropenia and hypochromic anemia are other early manifestations. The anemia is unresponsive to iron therapy. Very severe central nervous system disease is present in Menkes steely (kinky) hair syndrome, in which a profound copper deficiency state results from an X-linked defect in cellular metabolism of copper.

A low plasma copper or ceruloplasmin level helps confirm the diagnosis of copper deficiency. However, these levels are normally very low in the young infant, especially the premature infant, and are higher than adult values in later infancy and early childhood. Hence, age-matched normal data are necessary for comparison. Interleukin-1 grossly elevates both ceruloplasmin and copper levels; the levels are also high in pregnancy.

C. TREATMENT

Copper deficiency can be treated with a 1% copper sulfate solution (2 mg of the salt or 500 μg of elemental copper per day for infants).

Araya M et al: Copper deficiency and excess: Developing a research agenda. J Pediatr Gastroenterol Nutr 2003;37:422 [PMID: 14508211].

Hurwitz M et al: Copper deficiency during parenteral nutrition: A report of four pediatric cases. Nutr Clin Pract 2004;19:305 [PMID: 16215119].

Selenium

A. FUNCTION

Selenium is an essential component of glutathione peroxidase, which catalyzes the reduction of hydrogen per-oxide to water in the cell cytosol by the addition of reducing equivalents derived from glutathione. Hence, selenium plays an important role in protection against free-radical injury.

B. DEFICIENCY

Selenium deficiency is the major causal factor in Keshan disease, an often fatal cardiomyopathy primarily affecting infants, children, and young women in a large area of China where there is a severe geochemical selenium deficiency. Similar cases have been identified in the United States in patients maintained on long-term TPN without adequate selenium supplement, in whom symptoms also include skeletal muscle pain and tenderness. Macrocytosis and loss of hair pigment occur in milder selenium deficiency. Premature infants have exceptionally low serum selenium levels, which decline further without supplementation. The minimum recommended selenium content for full-term infant formulas is 1.5 μg/100 kcal, and that for preterm infant formulas is 1.8 μg/100 kcal.

A plasma selenium level less than 0.5 μmol/L (< 40 μg/L) suggests mild selenium deficiency. A level less than 0.12 μmol/L (< 10 μg/L) indicates a possible severe selenium deficiency.

Iodine

A. FUNCTION

Iodine functions as an essential component of thyroid hormones and regulates metabolism, growth, and mental development.

B. DEFICIENCY

Endemic goiter resulting from environmental iodine deficiency has been eradicated in North America by prophylactic measures but continues to be a health problem in many developing countries. Goiter occurs when iodine intake is less than 20 μg/d. Most persons with endemic goiter are clinically euthyroid. Maternal iodine deficiency causes endemic neonatal hypothyroidism in about 5–15% of neonates who may have goiter at birth.

Neurologic endemic cretinism, seen in most parts of the world, is characterized by severe mental retardation, deaf–mutism, spastic diplegia, and strabismus. Evidence of hypothyroidism is usually absent, and it is thought that the neurologic damage is due to a direct effect of fetal iodine deficiency or to an imbalance between thyroxine (low) and triiodothyronine (normal or elevated). Myxedematous endemic cretinism occurs in some central African countries. Signs of congenital hypothyroidism are present. Milder neurologic damage occurs in some cases of endemic neonatal goiter.

The use of iodized salt has been highly effective in preventing goiter. In areas where endemic goiter occurs,

Table 10–4. Supplemental fluoride recommendations (mg/d).

Age	Concentration of Fluoride in Drinking Water		
	< 0.3 ppm	0.3–0.6 ppm	> 0.6 ppm
6 months to 3 years	0.25	0	0
3–6 years	0.5	0.25	0
6–16 years	1	0.5	0

Reproduced, with permission, from Centers for Disease Control and Prevention: Recommendations for using fluoride to prevent and control dental caries in the United States. MMWR Morb Mortal Wkly Rep 2001;50(RR-14):8.

intramuscular depot injections of iodized oil have also been used for prevention.

Andersson M et al: Current global iodine status and progress over the last decade towards the elimination of iodine deficiency. Bull World Health Org 2005;83(7):518 [PMID: 16175826].

Fluoride

A. FUNCTION

Fluoride is incorporated into the hydroxyapatite matrix of dentin and effectively reduces the incidence of dental caries. Fluoride is most effectively administered as an additive to drinking water, but in infancy and childhood, fluoride vitamin preparations serve the same purpose. Ready-made formulas contain less than 0.3 ppm of fluoride.

B. DEFICIENCY

Inadequate fluoride intake can lead to increased incidences of dental caries. However, the recognized benefits of topical fluoride supplementation in preventing caries must be weighed against the increasing incidence of fluorosis in children in the United States. Fluorosis is characterized by an increased porosity (underminiralization) of the enamel and is evident clinically as discoloration of the teeth. Recommendations for fluoride supplementation are provided in Table 10–4. The American Academy of Pediatrics Committee on Nutrition, recommends withholding fluoride supplementation until age 6 months.

Bader JD et al: Physicians' roles in preventing dental caries in preschool children: A summary of the evidence for the U.S. Preventive Services Task Force. Am J Prev Med 2004;26(4):315 [PMID: 15110059].

VITAMINS

1. Fat-Soluble Vitamins

Because they are insoluble in water, the fat-soluble vitamins require digestion and absorption of dietary fat and a carrier system for transport in the blood. Deficiencies in these vitamins develop more slowly than deficiencies in water-soluble vitamins because the body accumulates stores of fat-soluble vitamins. Excessive intakes carry a considerable potential for toxicity (Table 10–5).

Table 10–5. Effects of vitamin toxicity.

Thiamin
 (Very rare.) Anaphylaxis; respiratory depression
Riboflavin
 None
Pyridoxine
 Sensory neuropathy at doses > 500 mg/d
Niacin
 Histamine release → cutaneous vasodilation; cardiac arrhythmias; cholestatic jaundice; gastrointestinal disturbance; hyperuricemia; glucose intolerance
Pantothenic acid
 Diarrhea
Biotin
 None
Folic acid
 May mask B_{12} deficiency, hypersensitivity
Cobalamin
 None
Vitamin C
 Interference with copper absorption; decreased tolerance to hypoxia, increased oxalic acid excretion
Carnitine
 None recognized
Vitamin A
 (> 20,000 IU/d): Vomiting, increased intracranial pressure (pseudotumor cerebri); irritability; headaches; insomnia; emotional lability; dry, desquamating skin; myalgia and arthralgia; abdominal pain; hepatosplenomegaly; cortical thickening of bones of hands and feet
Vitamin D
 (> 40,000 IU/d): Hypercalcemia; vomiting; constipation; nephrocalcinosis
Vitamin E
 (> 25–100 mg/kg/d intravenously): Necrotizing enterocolitis and liver toxicity (but probably due to polysorbate 80 used as a solubilizer)
Vitamin K
 Lipid-soluble vitamin K: Very low order of toxicity.
 Water-soluble, synthetic vitamin K: Vomiting, porphyrinuria; albuminuria; hemolytic anemia; hemoglobinuria; hyperbilirubinemia (do not give to neonates)

Vitamin A

A. DIETARY SOURCES

Dietary sources of vitamin A include dairy products, fortified margarine, eggs, liver, meats, fish oils, and corn. The vitamin A precursor β-carotene is abundant in yellow and green vegetables.

B. ABSORPTION/METABOLISM

Dietary retinyl palmitate requires hydrolysis by pancreatic and intestinal hydrolases. Beta-carotene is cleaved in the intestinal mucosal cells by dioxygenase to yield two molecules of retinal (retinaldehyde), which is then reduced to retinol (vitamin A alcohol). Carotene appears to have an important role in its own right as an antioxidant.

Retinol is reesterified in the intestinal mucosa and transported in chylomicrons to the liver for storage. From the liver, vitamin A is exported to the body attached to retinol-binding protein and prealbumin. Retinol-binding protein may be decreased in liver disease or in protein-energy malnutrition. Circulating retinol-binding protein may be increased in chronic renal failure.

Vitamin A has a critical role in the photochemical basis of vision. The photosensitive pigment rhodopsin is formed from retinal and a protein called opsin. Vitamin A also modifies differentiation and proliferation of epithelial cells, especially in the respiratory tract. Vitamin A is necessary for glycoprotein synthesis. Retinol can be irreversibly oxidized to retinoic acid, which is effective in glycoprotein synthesis but is ineffective for vision.

C. DEFICIENCY

Vitamin A deficiency occurs in premature infants, in association with IV nutrition with inadequate vitamin A supplement, and in protein-energy malnutrition. During the latter state, manifestations are made more severe by measles. Other causes of deficiency are dietary insufficiency and fat malabsorption.

The features of vitamin A deficiency are primarily ocular. Vitamin A deficiency is the leading cause of childhood blindness worldwide. Night blindness progresses to xerosis (dryness of cornea and conjunctiva), xerophthalmia (extreme dryness of the conjunctiva), Bitot spots, keratomalacia (clouding and softening of the cornea), ulceration and perforation of the cornea, prolapse of the lens and iris, and eventually blindness. Other features of vitamin A deficiency include follicular hyperkeratosis (dry, thickened, rough skin), pruritus, growth retardation, increased susceptibility to infection, anemia, and hepatosplenomegaly. Administration of vitamin A to children with measles in developing countries has been associated with reduction in morbidity and mortality.

Serum retinol levels below 20 μg/dL are low, and levels less than 10 μg/dL indicate deficiency. A ratio of retinol to retinol-binding protein below 0.7 is also indicative of vitamin A deficiency.

Suggested intakes of vitamin A are summarized in Table 10–6. Therapy of xerophthalmia requires 5000–10,000 international units (IU)/kg/d for 5 days orally or intramuscularly. The standard maintenance dose in fat malabsorption syndromes is 2500–5000 IU (800–1600 μg). Doses as high as 25,000–50,000 IU/d may be needed, but monitoring to avoid toxicity is essential. The effects of vitamin A toxicity are summarized in Table 10–5.

Ambalavanan N et al: Vitamin A supplementation for extremely low birth weight infants: Outcome at 18 to 22 months. Pediatrics 2005;115(3):e249 [PMID: 15713907].

Vitamin D

A. DIETARY SOURCES

The primary dietary source is fortified milk and formulas. Egg yolk and fatty fish contain some vitamin D. Vitamin D requirements are normally met primarily from cholecalciferol (vitamin D_3) produced by ultraviolet radiation of dehydrocholesterol in the skin. Similarly, ergocalciferol (vitamin D_2) is derived from ultraviolet irradiation of ergosterol in the skin. Vitamin D is transported from the skin to the liver attached to a specific carrier protein.

B. ABSORPTION/METABOLISM

Vitamin D is a fat-soluble substance and is transported to the liver in chylomicrons. Vitamins D_2 and D_3 undergo 25-hydroxylation in the liver and then 1α-hydroxylation in kidney proximal tubules to yield 1,25-dihydroxycholecalciferol (calcitriol) and calcitriol, respectively. PTH activates the 1α-hydroxylase enzyme in the kidney. 25-Hydroxycholecalciferol (calcidiol) is the major circulating form of vitamin D. Calcitriol is the biologically active form of vitamin D. Calcitriol stimulates intestinal absorption of calcium and phosphate, renal reabsorption of filtered calcium, and mobilization of calcium and phosphorus from bone.

C. DEFICIENCY

Vitamin D deficiency usually results from a combination of inadequate sunlight exposure and low dietary intake. An infant with light skin pigmentation requires only about 30 minutes per week of total body sun exposure or 2 hours per week of head exposure to maintain adequate vitamin D status. Adequate sun exposure for infants with more darkly pigmented skin is difficult to quantify. Dermatologists advise caution in exposure to sun, even for young infants. Vitamin D content of human milk is low. In the United States, cow's milk and infant formulas are routinely supplemented with

Table 10–6. Summary of dietary reference intakes for select vitamins.

	0–6 mo	7–12 mo	1–3 yr	4–8 yr	9–13 yr	14–18 yr male	14–18 yr female
Thiamin (mg/d)	0.2[a]	0.3[a]	0.5	0.6	0.9	1.2	1.0
Riboflavin (mg/d)	0.3[a]	0.4[a]	0.5[a]	0.6[a]	0.9[a]	1.3[a]	1.0[a]
Pyridoxine (mg/d)	0.1[a]	0.3[a]	0.5	0.6	1.0	1.3	1.2
Niacin (mg/d)	2[a]	4[a]	6	8	12	16	14
Pantothenic Acid (mg/d)	1.7[a]	1.8[a]	2[a]	3[a]	4[a]	5[a]	5[a]
Biotin (μg/d)	5[a]	6[a]	8[a]	12[a]	20[a]	25[a]	25[a]
Folic Acid (μg/d)	65[a]	80[a]	150	200	300	400	400
Cobalamin (μg/d)	0.4[a]	0.5[a]	0.9	1.2	1.8	2.4	2.4
Vitamin C (mg/d)	40[a]	50[a]	15	25	45	75	65
Vitamin A (μg/d)	400[a]	500[a]	300	400	600	900	700
Vitamin D (IU/d)	200[a]	200[a]	200[a]	200[a]	200[a]	200[a]	200[a]
Vitamin E (mg/d)	4[a]	5[a]	6	7	11	15	15
Vitamin K (μg/d)	2[a]	2.5[a]	30[a]	55[a]	60[a]	75[a]	75[a]

[a]Adequate Intakes (AI). All other values represent the recommended Dietary Allowances (RDA). Both the RDA and AI may be used as goals for individual intakes.

Reproduced, with permission, from National Academy of Sciences, Food and Nutritional Board, Institute of Medicine: *Dietary Reference Intakes, Applications in Dietary Assessment.* National Academy Press, 2000:287. Available online at: http://www.nap.edu

vitamin D. The American Academy of Pediatrics recommends vitamin D supplementation (200 IU/d) for all breast-fed infants until they are receiving at least 500 mL/d of vitamin D-fortified formula or milk. Supplementation should be initiated during the first 2 months of life.

Vitamin D deficiency also occurs in fat malabsorption syndromes. Use of CYP-450–stimulating drugs may decrease hydroxylated vitamin D, which can also be decreased by hepatic and renal disease and by inborn errors of metabolism. End-organ unresponsiveness to calcitriol may also occur.

The clinical effects of vitamin D deficiency are osteomalacia (adults) or rickets (children), in which osteoid (matrix) with reduced calcification accumulates in bone. Cartilage fails to mature and calcify. Clinical findings include craniotabes, rachitic rosary, pigeon breast, bowed legs, delayed eruption of teeth and enamel defects, Harrison groove, scoliosis, kyphosis, dwarfism, painful bones, fractures, anorexia, and weakness. Radiographic findings include cupping, fraying, and flaring of metaphyses. The loss of sharp definition of bone trabeculae accounts for the general decrease in skeletal radiodensity. The diagnosis is supported by characteristic radiologic abnormalities of the skeleton, low serum phosphorus, high serum alkaline phosphatase, and high serum PTH. The diagnosis can be confirmed by a low level of serum 25-hydroxycholecalciferol.

Rickets is treated with 1600–5000 IU/d of vitamin D_3 (1 IU = 0.025 μg). If this is poorly absorbed, calcidiol, 25 μg/d (1000 IU), or calcitriol, 0.05–0.2 μg/kg/d, is given. Renal osteodystrophy is treated with calcitriol.

Suggested dietary intakes for vitamin D are summarized in Table 10–6. The toxic effects are given in Table 10–5.

Gartner LM, Greer FR, Section on Breastfeeding and Committee on Nutrition, American Academy of Pediatrics: Prevention of rickets and vitamin D deficiency: New guidelines for vitamin D intake. Pediatrics 2003;111(4):908 [PMID: 12671133].

Pettifor JM. Rickets and vitamin D deficiency in children and adolescents. Endocrinol Metab Clin North Am 2005;34(3):537 [PMID: 16085158].

Vitamin E

A. DIETARY SOURCES

Vegetable oils are the main dietary source of vitamin E. Coconut and olive oils, however, are low in vitamin E. Some vitamin E is present in cereals, dairy products, and eggs. Vitamin activity may decrease with processing, storage, or heating.

B. FUNCTIONS

Vitamin E is a family of tocopherols with four major forms: alpha, gamma, beta, and delta. Alpha-tocopherol has the highest biologic activity. Vitamin E can donate an electron to a free-radical molecule to stop oxidation reactions. Oxidized vitamin E is then reduced by ascorbic acid or glutathione. The reduced tocopherol is able to scavenge another free radical. Nutrients participating in antioxidant defense include β-carotene, vitamin C, selenium, copper, manganese, and zinc. Vitamin E is located at specific sites in the cell to protect polyunsaturated fatty acids in the membrane from peroxidation and to protect thiol groups and nucleic acids. Vitamin E also functions as a cell membrane stabilizer, may function in the electron transport chain, and may modulate chromosomal expression.

C. DEFICIENCY

Vitamin E deficiency may occur in the following circumstances: prematurity; cholestatic liver disease, pancreatic insufficiency, abetalipoproteinemia, and short bowel syndrome; as an isolated inborn error of vitamin E metabolism; and perhaps as a result of increased consumption during oxidant stress.

Vitamin E deficiency shortens red cell half-life and may cause hemolytic anemia. Chronic vitamin E deficiency results in a progressive neurologic disorder with loss of deep tendon reflexes, loss of coordination, vibratory and position sensation, nystagmus, weakness, scoliosis, and retinal degeneration.

Vitamin E nutritional status can be partially assessed by measuring serum vitamin E (normal range for children is 3–15 mg/mL). The ratio of serum vitamin E to total serum lipid is normally more than 0.8 mg/g. Sensitivity of erythrocytes to hydrogen peroxide-induced hemolysis is also used as a test of vitamin E status.

Suggested dietary intakes of vitamin E are summarized in Table 10–6. Requirements increase if dietary polyunsaturated fatty acids increase. Between 0.4 mg and 0.5 mg of vitamin E is needed per gram of polyunsaturated fatty acids in the diet (1 IU = 1 mg of DL-α-tocopherol acetate).

Large oral doses (up to 100 IU/kg/d) of vitamin E correct the deficiency resulting from most malabsorption syndromes. For abetalipoproteinemia, 100–200 IU/kg/d of vitamin E are needed. Vitamin E therapy in ischemia-reperfusion injury and in the prevention of intracranial hemorrhage in the preterm infant remains controversial. Toxic effects of intravenously administered vitamin E are summarized in Table 10–5.

Vitamin K

A. DIETARY SOURCES

Vitamin K_1 (phylloquinone) is found in leafy vegetables, soybean oil, fruits, seeds, and cow's milk. Vitamin K_2 (menaquinone), which has 60% of the activity of K_1, is synthesized by intestinal bacteria. K_2 may be a major source of vitamin K in infants and young children, but less is produced in the intestine of breast-fed infants.

B. FUNCTION

Vitamin K is necessary for the post-translational carboxylation of glutamic acid residues of the vitamin K–dependent coagulation proteins. Carboxylation allows these proteins to bind calcium, leading to activation of the clotting factors. Thus, vitamin K is necessary for the maintenance of normal plasma levels of coagulation factors II (prothrombin), VII, IX, and X and is also necessary for maintenance of normal levels of the anticoagulation protein C.

C. DEFICIENCY

Vitamin K deficiency occurs in newborns, especially those who are breast-fed and who have not received vitamin K prophylaxis at delivery. Deficiency may result in hemorrhagic disease of the newborn. Later, vitamin K deficiency may result from fat malabsorption syndromes and the use of nonabsorbed antibiotics and anticoagulant drugs (eg, warfarin). Clinical features are bruising or bleeding in the GI tract, genital urinary tract, gingiva, lungs, joints, and brain. Vitamin K status can be assessed with plasma levels of protein-induced vitamin K absence or by prothrombin time.

Vitamin K requirements are summarized in Table 10–6. Newborns require prophylactic intramuscular vitamin K (0.5–1.0 mg). For older children with acute bleeding, 3–10 mg of vitamin K is given intramuscularly or intravenously. For chronic malabsorption syndromes, 2.5 mg twice weekly to 5 mg/d is given orally. To reverse warfarin effect, 25–50 mg of IV vitamin K is given. Toxic effects of vitamin K are summarized in Table 10–5.

Miller CA, Committee on Fetus and Newborn, American Academy of Pediatrics: Controversies concerning vitamin K and the newborn. Pediatrics 2003;112(1):191 [PMID: 12837888].

2. Water-Soluble Vitamins

Deficiencies of water-soluble vitamins are uncommon in the United States because of the abundant food supply and fortification of prepared foods. Most bread and wheat products are fortified with B vitamins, including the mandatory addition of folic acid to enriched grain products since January 1998. There is conclusive evidence that folic acid supplements (400 μg/d) during the periconceptional period protect against neural tube defects. Dietary intakes of folic acid from natural foods and enriched products also are protective. Recommended intakes of folic acid during the periconceptional period may also afford protection later against neuroectodermal brain tumors in young children.

The risk of toxicity from water-soluble vitamins is not as great as that associated with fat-soluble vitamins because excesses are excreted in the urine. However, deficiencies of these vitamins develop more quickly than deficiencies in fat-soluble vitamins because of limited stores.

Additional salient details are summarized in Tables 10–6 through 10–11. Although dietary intake of the water-soluble vitamins on a daily basis is not necessary, these vitamins, with the exception of vitamin B_{12}, are not stored in the body.

Carnitine is synthesized in the liver and kidneys from lysine and methionine. In certain circumstances (see Table 10–10) synthesis is inadequate, and carnitine can then be considered a vitamin. A dietary supply of other organic compounds, such as inositol, may also be required in certain circumstances.

Bryan J et al: Nutrients for cognitive development in school-aged children. Nutr Rev 2004;62:295 [PMID: 15478684].

■ INFANT FEEDING

BREAST FEEDING

Breast feeding provides optimal nutrition for the normal infant during the early months of life. The World

Table 10–7. Summary of biologic roles of water-soluble vitamins.

B vitamins involved in production of energy
Thiamin (B_1)
  Thiamin pyrophosphate is a coenzyme in oxidative decarboxylation (pyruvate dehydrogenase, α-ketoglutarate dehydrogenase, and transketolase).
Riboflavin (B_2)
  Coenzyme of several flavoproteins (eg, flavin mononucleotide [FMN] and flavin adenine dinucleotide [FAD]) involved in oxidative/electron transfer enzyme systems.
Niacin
  Hydrogen-carrying coenzymes: nicotinamide-adenine dinucleotide (NAD), nicotinamide-adenine dinucleotide phosphate (NADP); decisive role in intermediary metabolism.
Pantothenic acid
  Major component of coenzyme A.
Biotin
  Component of several carboxylase enzymes involved in fat and carbohydrate metabolism.
Hematopoietic B vitamins
Folic acid
  Tetrahydrofolate has essential role in one-carbon transfers. Essential role in purine and pyramidine synthesis; deficiency → arrest of cell division (especially bone marrow and intestine).
Cobalamin (B_{12})
  Methyl cobalamin (cytoplasm): synthesis of methionine with simultaneous synthesis of tetrahydrofolate (reason for megaloblastic anemia in B_{12} deficiency). Adenosyl cobalamin (mitochondria) is coenzyme for mutases and dehydratases.
Other B vitamins
Pyridoxine (B_6)
  Prosthetic group of transaminases, etc, involved in amino acid interconversions; prostaglandin and hemesynthesis; central nervous system function; carbohydrate metabolism; immune development.
Other water-soluble vitamins
L-Ascorbic acid (C)
  Strong reducing agent—probably involved in all hydroxylations. Roles include collagen synthesis; phenylalanine → tyrosine; tryptophan → 5-hydroxytryptophan; dopamine → norepinephrine; Fe^{3+}; folic acid → folinic acid; cholesterol → bile acids; leukocyte function; interferon production; carnitine synthesis. Copper metabolism; reduces oxidized vitamin E.
Carnitine
  Transfer of long-chain fatty acids from cytosol to mitochondria (necessary for β-oxidation).

Health Organization recommends exclusive breast feeding for approximately the first 6 months of life, with continued breast feeding along with appropriate complementary foods through the first 2 years of life. Numer-

Table 10–8. Major dietary sources of water-soluble vitamins.

Thiamin
Whole grains, cereals (including fortification), lean pork, legumes

Riboflavin
Dairy products, meat, poultry, wheat germ, leafy vegetables

Pyridoxine
All foods

Niacin
Meats, poultry, fish, legumes, wheat, all foods except fats; synthesized in body from tryptophan

Pantothenic acid
Ubiquitous

Biotin
Yeast, liver, kidneys, legumes, nuts, egg yolks (synthesized by intestinal bacteria)

Folic acid
Leafy vegetables (lost in cooking), fruits, whole grains, wheat germ, orange juice, beans, nuts

Cobalamin
Eggs, dairy products, liver, meats; none in plants

Vitamin C
Fresh fruits and vegetables

Carnitine
Meats, dairy products; none in plants

Table 10–9. Circumstances in which the possibility of vitamin deficiencies merits consideration.

Circumstance	Possible Deficiency
Prematurity	All vitamins
Protein-energy malnutrition	B_1, B_2, folate, A
Synthetic diets (including total parenteral nutrition)	All vitamins
Inherited disorders	Folate, B_{12}, D, carnitine
Vitamin–drug interactions	B_6, biotin, folate, B_{12}, carnitine, fat-soluble vitamins
Fat malabsorption syndrome	Fat-soluble vitamins
Breast-feeding	B_1,[a] folate,[b] B_{12},[c] D,[d] K[e]
Periconceptional	Folate

[a]Alcoholic or malnourished mother.
[b]Folate-deficient mother.
[c]Vegan mother or maternal pernicious anemia.
[d]Infant not exposed to sunlight and mother's vitamin D status suboptimal.
[e]Maternal status poor; neonatal prophylaxis omitted.

Table 10–10. Causes of deficiencies in water-soluble vitamins.

Thiamin
Infantile beriberi; seen in infants breast-fed by mothers with history of alcoholism or poor diet; has been described as complication of total parenteral nutrition (TPN); protein–energy malnutrition; prematurity

Riboflavin
General undernutrition; prematurity; inactivation in TPN solutions exposed to light

Pyridoxine
Prematurity (these infants may not convert pyridoxine to pyridoxal-5-P); B_6 dependency syndromes; drugs (isoniazid); heat-treated formulas (historical)

Niacin
Maize or millet diets (high leucine and low tryptophan intakes); prematurity

Pantothenic acid
None

Biotin
Suppressed intestinal flora and impaired intestinal absorption

Folic acid
Prematurity; seen in term breast-fed infants whose mothers are folate-deficient and in term infants fed unsupplemented processed cow's milk or goat's milk; kwashiorkor; chronic overcooking; malabsorption of folate because of a congenital defect; sprue; celiac disease; drugs (phenytoin)
Increased requirements: chronic hemolytic anemias, diarrhea, malignancies, hypermetabolic states, infections, extensive skin disease, cirrhosis, pregnancy

Cobalamin
Rare; seen in breast-fed infants of mothers with latent pernicious anemia or who are on an unsupplemented strict vegetarian diet; absence of luminal proteases; congenital malabsorption of B_{12}

Vitamin C
Prematurity; maternal megadoses during pregnancy → deficiency in infants; lack of fresh fruits or vegetables; seen in infants fed formula and pasteurized cow's milk (historical)

Carnitine
Seen in premature infants fed unsupplemented formula or fed intravenously; dialysis; inherited deficits in carnitine synthesis; organic acidemias; valproic acid

Table 10–11. Clinical features of deficiencies in water-soluble vitamins.

Thiamin
Infantile beriberi (cardiac; aphonic; pseudomeningitic)
Riboflavin
Cheilosis; angular stomatitis; glossitis; soreness and burning of lips and mouth; dermatitis of nasolabial fold and genitals; ± ocular signs (photophobia → indistinct vision)
Pyridoxine
Listlessness; irritability; seizures; gastrointestinal disturbance; anemia; cheilosis; glossitis
Niacin
Pellagra (weakness; lassitude; dermatitis of exposed areas; diarrhea; dementia)
Pantothenic acid
Weakness; gastrointestinal disturbance; burning feet.
Biotin
Scaly dermatitis; alopecia; irritability; lethargy
Folic acid
Megaloblastic anemia; neutropenia; thrombocytopenia; growth retardation; delayed maturation of central nervous system in infants; diarrhea (mucosal ulcerations); glossitis; jaundice; mild splenomegaly; neural tube defects
Cobalamin
Megaloblastic anemia; neurologic degeneration
Vitamin C
Anorexia, irritability, apathy, pallor; fever; tachycardia; diarrhea; failure to thrive; increased susceptibility to infections; hemorrhages under skin, mucous membranes, into joints and under periosteum; long-bone tenderness; costochondral beading
Carnitine
Increased serum triglycerides and free fatty acids; decreased ketones; fatty liver; hypoglycemia; progressive muscle weakness, cardiomyopathy, hypoglycemia

ous immunologic factors in breast milk (including secretory IgA, lysozyme, lactoferrin, bifidus factor, and macrophages) provide protection against GI and upper respiratory infections. In developing countries, lack of refrigeration and contaminated water supplies make formula feeding hazardous. Although formulas have improved progressively and are made to resemble breast milk as closely as possible, it is impossible to replicate the nutritional or immune composition of human milk. Additional differences of physiologic importance continue to be identified. Furthermore, the relationship developed through breast feeding can be an important part of early maternal interactions with the infant and provides a source of security and comfort to the infant.

Breast feeding has been reestablished as the predominant mode of feeding young infants in the United States. Unfortunately, breast-feeding rates remain low among several subpopulations, including low-income,

minority, and young mothers. Many mothers face obstacles in maintaining lactation once they return to work, and rates of breast feeding at 6 months are considerably less than the goal of 50%. Skilled use of a breast pump, particularly an electric one, can help to maintain lactation in these circumstances.

Absolute contraindications to breast feeding are rare. They include tuberculosis (in the mother) and galactosemia (in the infant). Breast feeding is associated with maternal-to-child transmission of human immunodeficiency virus (HIV), but the risk is influenced by duration and pattern of breast feeding and maternal factors, including immunologic status and presence of mastitis. Complete avoidance of breast feeding by HIV-infected women is presently the only mechanism to ensure prevention of maternal–infant transmission. Current recommendations are that HIV-infected mothers in developed countries refrain from breast feeding if safe alternatives are available. In developing countries, the benefits of breast feeding, especially the protection of the child against diarrheal illness and malnutrition outweigh the risk of HIV infection via breast milk. In such circumstances, mixed feeding should be avoided because of the apparent increased risk of HIV transmission with mixed feeds.

In newborns less than 1500 g, human milk should be fortified to increase protein, calcium, phosphorus, and micronutrient content as well as caloric density. Breast-fed infants with cystic fibrosis can be breast-fed successfully if exogenous pancreatic enzymes are provided. If normal growth rates are not achieved in breast-fed infants with cystic fibrosis, energy or specific macronutrient supplements may be necessary. All infants with cystic fibrosis should receive supplemental vitamins A, D, E, K, and sodium chloride.

Coutsoudis A, Rollins N: Breast-feeding and HIV transmission: The jury is still out. J Pediatr Gastroenterol Nutr 2003; 26(4):434 [PMID: 12658031].

Gartner LM et al: Breastfeeding and the use of human milk. Pediatrics 2005;115:496 [PMID: 15687461].

Ryan AS et al: Breastfeeding continues to increase into the new millennium. Pediatrics 2002;110(6):1103 [PMID: 12456906].

Management of Breast Feeding

In developed countries, health professionals are now playing roles of greater importance in supporting and promoting breast feeding. Organizations such as the American Academy of Pediatrics and La Leche League have initiated programs to promote breast feeding and provide education for health professionals and mothers.

Perinatal hospital routines and early pediatric care have a great influence on the successful initiation of breast feeding by promoting prenatal and postpartum education, frequent mother–baby contact after delivery, one-on-one advice about breast-feeding technique, demand feeding, rooming-in, avoidance of bottle supplements, early follow-up after delivery, maternal confidence, family support, adequate maternity leave, and advice about common problems such as sore nipples. Breast feeding is undermined by mother and baby separations, bottle-feeding babies in the nursery at night, routine supplemental bottle feedings, conflicting advice from staff, incorrect infant positioning and latch-on, scheduled feedings, lack of maternal support, delayed follow-up, early return to employment, and inaccurate advice for common breast-feeding difficulties.

Very few women are unable to nurse their babies. The newborn is generally fed ad libitum every 2–3 hours, with longer intervals (4–5 hours) at night. Thus a newborn infant nurses at least 8 to 10 times a day, so that a generous milk supply is stimulated. This frequency is not an indication of inadequate lactation. In neonates, a loose stool is often passed with each feeding; later (at age 3–4 months), there may be an interval of several days between stools. Failure to pass several stools a day in the early weeks of breast feeding suggests inadequate milk intake and supply.

Expressing milk may be indicated if the mother returns to work or if the infant is premature, cannot suck adequately, or is hospitalized. Electric breast pumps are very effective and can be borrowed or rented.

Technique of Breast Feeding

Breast feeding can be started after delivery as soon as both mother and baby are stable. Correct positioning and breast-feeding technique are necessary to ensure effective nipple stimulation and optimal breast emptying with minimal nipple discomfort.

If the mother wishes to nurse while sitting, the infant should be elevated to the height of the breast and turned completely to face the mother, so that their abdomens touch. The mother's arms supporting the infant should be held tightly at her side, bringing the baby's head in line with her breast. The breast should be supported by the lower fingers of her free hand, with the nipple compressed between the thumb and index fingers to make it more protractile. The infant's initial licking and mouthing of the nipple helps make it more erect. When the infant opens its mouth, the mother should rapidly insert as much nipple and areola as possible.

The most common early cause of poor weight gain in breast- fed infants is poorly managed mammary engorgement, which rapidly decreases milk supply. Unrelieved engorgement can result from inappropriately long intervals between feeding, improper infant suckling, a nondemanding infant, sore nipples, maternal or infant illness, nursing from only one breast, and latching difficulties. Poor maternal feeding technique, inappropriate feeding routines, and inadequate amounts of fluid and rest all can be factors. Some infants are too sleepy to do well on an ad libitum regimen and may need waking to feed at night. Primary lactation failure occurs in less than 5% of women.

A sensible guideline for duration of feeding is 5 minutes per breast at each feeding the first day, 10 minutes on each side at each feeding the second day, and 10–15 minutes per side thereafter. A vigorous infant can obtain most of the available milk in 5–7 minutes, but additional sucking time ensures breast emptying, promotes milk production, and satisfies the infant's sucking urge. The side on which feeding is commenced should be alternated. The mother may break suction gently after nursing by inserting her finger between the baby's gums.

Follow-Up

Individualized assessment before discharge should identify mothers and infants needing additional support. All mother–infant pairs require early follow-up. The onset of copious milk secretion between the second and fourth postpartum days is a critical time in the establishment of lactation. Failure to empty the breasts during this time can cause engorgement, which quickly leads to diminished milk production.

Common Problems

Nipple tenderness requires attention to proper positioning of the infant and correct latch-on. Ancillary measures include nursing for shorter periods, beginning feedings on the less sore side, air drying the nipples well after nursing, and use of lanolin cream. Severe nipple pain and cracking usually indicate improper infant attachment. Temporary pumping may be needed.

Breast-feeding jaundice is exaggerated physiologic jaundice associated with inadequate intake of breast milk, infrequent stooling, and unsatisfactory weight gain. (See Chapter 1.) If possible, the jaundice should be managed by increasing the frequency of nursing and, if necessary, augmenting the infant's sucking with regular breast pumping. Supplemental feedings may be necessary, but care should be taken not to decrease breast milk production further.

In a small percentage of breast-fed infants, breast milk jaundice is caused by an unidentified property of the milk that inhibits conjugation of bilirubin. In severe cases, interruption of breast feeding for 24–36 hours may be necessary. The mother's breast should be emptied with an electric breast pump during this period.

The symptoms of mastitis include flulike symptoms with breast tenderness, firmness, and erythema. Antibiotic therapy covering β-lactamase-producing organisms should be given for 10 days. Analgesics may be necessary, but breast feeding should be continued. Breast pumping may be helpful adjunctive therapy.

American Academy of Pediatrics Subcommittee on Hyperbilirubine-mia: Management of hyperbilirubinemia in the newborn infant 35 of more weeks of gestation. Pediatrics 2004;114:297-316 [PMID: 15231951]. Erratum: Pediatrics 2004;114:1138.

Dann MH: The lactation consult: Problem solving, teaching, and support for the breastfeeding family. J Pediatr Health Care 2005;19(1):12 [PMID: 15662357].

Maternal Drug Use

Factors playing a role in the transmission of drugs in breast milk, include the route of administration, dosage, molecular weight, pH, and protein binding. Generally, any drug prescribed to a newborn can be consumed by the breast-feeding mother without ill effect. Very few drugs are absolutely contraindicated in breast-feeding mothers; these include radioactive compounds, antime-tabolites, lithium, diazepam, chloramphenicol, antithy-roid drugs, and tetracycline. For up-to-date information, a regional drug center should be consulted.

Maternal use of illicit or recreational drugs is a contra-indication to breast feeding. Expression of milk for a feed-ing or two after use of a drug is not an acceptable compro-mise. The breast-fed infants of mothers taking methadone (but not alcohol or other drugs) as part of a treatment pro-gram have generally not experienced ill effects when the daily maternal methadone dose is less than 40 mg.

Case Western Reserve University. http://www.breastfeedingbasics.org

Dr. Hale's Breastfeeding Pharmacology Page. http://neonatal.ttuhsc.edu/lact/

Hale TW: Maternal medications during breastfeeding. Clin Obstet Gynecol 2004;47(3):696 [PMID: 15326432].

Nutrient Composition

The nutrient composition of human milk is summarized and compared with that of cow's milk and formulas in Table 10–12. Outstanding characteristics include (1) rela-tively low but highly bioavailable protein content, which is adequate for the normal infant; (2) generous but not exces-sive quantity of essential fatty acids; (3) long-chain unsat-urated ω3 fatty acids, of which DHA is thought to be especially important; (4) relatively low sodium and solute load; and (5) lower concentration of highly bioavailable calcium, iron, and zinc, which are adequate for the needs of normal breast-fed infants for approximately 6 months.

Weaning and Complementary Foods

The American Academy of Pediatrics and the World Health Organization recommend the introduction of solid foods in normal infants at about 6 months of age. Gradual introduction of a variety of foods including enriched cereals, fruits, vegetables, and meats should complement the breast milk diet. Although the order of introduction is not critical, single-ingredient comple-mentary foods are introduced one at a time at weekly intervals before a new food is given. Fruit juice is not an essential part of an infant diet. Juice should not be introduced until after 6 months; should only be offered in a cup; and the amount should be limited to 4 oz/d. Breast feeding should ideally continue for at least 12 months, and thereafter for as long as mutually desired. Infants who are not breast-fed should receive standard iron-fortified infant formula. Whole cow's milk can be introduced after the first year of life.

Kramer MS et al: Infant growth and health outcomes associated with 3 compared with 6 months of exclusive breastfeeding. Am J Clin Nutr 2003;78:291 [PMID: 12885711].

SPECIAL DIETARY PRODUCTS FOR INFANTS

Soy Protein Formulas

A common rationale for the use of soy protein formulas is transient lactose intolerance after acute gastroenteri-tis. In such cases it is reasonable to recommend a soy protein formula for a period of 2–4 weeks. These for-mulas are also useful for infants with galactosemia and hereditary lactase deficiency. Lactose-free cow's milk protein-based formulas are also available. Soy protein formulas are often used in cases of suspected intolerance to cow's milk protein. Although infants with true cow's milk protein intolerance may also be intolerant of soy protein, those with documented IgE-mediated allergy to cow's milk protein usually do well on soy formula.

Semielemental & Elemental Formulas

Semielemental formulas include protein hydrolysate formulas. The major nitrogen source of most of these products is casein hydrolysate, supplemented with selected amino acids, but partial hydrolysates of whey are also available. These formulas contain an abundance of EFA from vegetable oil; certain brands also provide substantial amounts of MCTs. Elemental formulas are available with free amino acids and varying levels and types of fat components.

Semielemental and elemental formulas are invalu-able for infants with a wide variety of malabsorption syndromes. They are also effective in infants who can-not tolerate cow's milk and soy protein. Controlled tri-als suggest that for infants with a family history of atopic disease, partial hydrolysate formulas may delay or prevent atopic disease. For specific product informa-tion, consult standard pediatric reference texts, formula manufacturers, or a pediatric dietitian.

Hays T, Wood RA: A systematic review of the role of hydrolyzed infant formulas in allergy prevention. Arch Pediatr Adolesc Med 2005;159:810 [PMID: 15143739].

Table 10–12. The composition of milk (per 100 kcal).

Nutrient (unit)	Minimal Level Recommended[a]	Mature Human Milk	Typical Commercial Formula	Cow's Milk (mean)
Protein (g)	1.8[b]	1.3–1.6	2.3	5.1
Fat (g)	3.3[c]	5	5.3	5.7
Carbohydrate (g)	—	10.3	10.8	7.3
Linoleic acid (mg)	300	560	2300	125
Vitamin A (IU)	250	250	300	216
Vitamin D (IU)	40	3	63	3
Vitamin E (IU)	0.7/g linoleic acid	0.3	2	0.1
Vitamin K (µg)	4	2	9	5
Vitamin C (mg)	8	7.8	8.1	2.3
Thiamin (µg)	40	25	80	59
Riboflavin (µg)	60	60	100	252
Niacin (µg)	250	250	1200	131
Vitamin B_6 (µg)	15 µg of protein	15	63	66
Folic acid (µg)	4	4	10	8
Pantothenic acid (µg)	300	300	450	489
Vitamin B_{12} (µg)	0.15	0.15	0.25	0.56
Biotin (µg)	1.5	1	2.5	3.1
Inositol (mg)	4	20	5.5	20
Choline (mg)	7	13	10	23
Calcium (mg)	5	50	75	186
Phosphorus (mg)	25	25	65	145
Magnesium (mg)	6	6	8	20
Iron (mg)	1	0.1	1.5 in fortified	0.08
Iodine (µg)	5	4–9	10	7
Copper (µg)	60	25–60	80	20
Zinc (mg)	0.5	0.1–0.5	0.65	0.6
Manganese (µg)	5	1.5	5–160	3
Sodium (mEq)	0.9	1	1.7	3.3
Potassium (mEq)	2.1	2.1	2.7	6
Chloride (mEq)	1.6	1.6	2.3	4.6
Osmolarity (mOsm)	—	11.3	16–18.4	40

[a]Committee on Nutrition, American Academy of Pediatrics.
[b]Protein of nutritional quality equal to casein.
[c]Includes 300 mg of essential fatty acids.

Hernell O, Lonnerdal B: Nutritional evaluation of protein hydrolysate formulas in healthy term infants: Plasma amino acids, hematology, and trace elements. Am J Clin Nutr 2003;78:296 [PMID: 12885712].

Formula Additives

Occasionally it may be necessary to increase the caloric density of an infant feeding to provide more calories or restrict fluid intake. Concentrating formula to 24–26 kcal/oz is usually well tolerated, delivers an acceptable renal solute load, and increases the density of all the nutrients. Beyond this, individual macronutrient additives (Table 10–13) are usually employed to achieve the desired caloric density (up to 30 kcal/oz) based on the infant's needs and underlying condition(s). A pediatric nutrition specialist can be helpful in formulating calorically dense infant formula feedings. The caloric density of breast milk can be increased by adding infant formula powder or any of the additives used with infant formula. Human milk fortifiers are generally used only for premature infants because of their specialized nutrient composition.

Table 10–13. Common infant formula additives.

Additive	Kcal/g	Kcal/Tbsp	Kcal/mL	Comments
Dry rice cereal	3.75	15	—	Thickens formula but not breast milk
Polycose (Ross)	3.8	23	2	Glucose polymers
Moducal (Mead Johnson)	3.75	30	—	Maltodextrin
MCT oil (Mead Johnson)	8.3	116	7.7	Not a source of essential fatty acids
Microlipid (Mead Johnson)	9	68.5	4.5	Safflower oil emulsion with 0.4 g linoleic acid/mL
Vegetable oil	9	124	8.3	Does not mix well
Promod (Ross)	4.3	16.8 (3 g protein)	—	Whey protein concentrate
Casec (Mead Johnson)	3.8	16.7 (4 g protein)	—	Calcium caseinate
Duocal (SHS)	4.9	42	—	Protein-free mix of hydrolyzed corn starch (60% kcal) and fat (35% MCT)

MCT, medium-chain triglyceride.

Special Formulas

Special formulas are those in which one component, often an amino acid, is reduced in concentration or removed for the dietary management of a specific inborn metabolic disease. Also included under this heading are formulas designed for the management of specific disease states, such as hepatic failure, pulmonary failure with chronic carbon dioxide retention, and renal failure. These condition-specific formulas were formulated primarily for critically ill adults and are even used sparingly in those populations; thus their use in pediatrics should only be undertaken with clear indication and caution.

Complete information regarding the composition of these special formulas, the standard infant formulas, specific metabolic disease formulas, and premature infant formulas can be found in standard reference texts and in the manufacturers' literature.

▓ NUTRITION FOR THE OLDER CHILD

Because of the association of diet with the development of such chronic diseases as diabetes, obesity, and cardiovascular disease, learning a healthy eating behavior at a young age is an important preventative measure.

Salient features of the diet for children older than 2 years include the following:

1. Consumption of three regular meals per day, and two or three healthful snacks according to appetite, activity, and growth needs.
2. Inclusion of a variety of foods. Diet should be nutritionally complete and promote optimal growth and activity.
3. Fat less than 35% of total calories (though severe fat restriction may result in an energy deficit and growth failure). Saturated fats and polyunsaturated fats each should provide less than 10% of total calories. Monounsaturated fats should provide 10% or more of caloric intake. Consumption of trans fatty acids, found in stick margarine and shortening, and in many processed foods, should be kept as low as possible.
4. Cholesterol intake less than 100 mg/1000 kcal/d, to a maximum of 300 mg/d.
5. Carbohydrates should provide 45–65% of daily caloric intake, with no more than 10% in the form of simple sugars. A high-fiber, whole-grain-based diet is recommended.
6. Limitation of grazing behavior, eating while watching television, and the consumption of soft drinks and other sweetened beverages.
7. Limitation of sodium intake by choosing fresh over highly processed foods.

The consumption of lean cuts of meats, poultry, and fish should be encouraged. Skim or low-fat milk, soft margarine, and vegetable oils (especially canola or olive oil) should be used. Whole-grain bread and cereals and plentiful amounts of fruits and vegetables are recommended. The consumption of processed foods, soft drinks, desserts, and candy should be limited.

A prudent diet should be only one component of counseling on lifestyles for children. Other aspects are the maintenance of a desirable body weight and body mass index (BMI), regular physical activity, avoidance of smoking, and screening for hypertension. Universal screening for total cholesterol is controversial. Current recommendations are to routinely screen those children who have a positive family history of premature cardiovascular disease, although this approach will identify only about 50% of those with significantly elevated cholesterol levels. If the result is high ($\geq$ 200 mg/dL), a fasting lipoprotein analysis should be obtained.

Gidding SS et al: Dietary Recommendations for Children and Adolescents: A Guide for Practitioners, Consensus Statement from the American Heart Association. Circulation 2005;112:2061 [PMID: 16186441].

Kavey RE et al: American Heart Association guidelines for primary prevention of atherosclerotic cardiovascular disease beginning in childhood. J Pediatr 2003;142(4):368 [PMID: 12712052].

■ PEDIATRIC UNDERNUTRITION

Failure to thrive is a term used to describe infants and young children whose weight curve has fallen by two major percentile channels from a previously established rate of growth. (See Chapter 8.) The acute loss of weight, or failure to gain weight at the expected rate, produces a condition of reduced weight for height known as **wasting.** The reduction in height for age, as is seen with more chronic malnutrition, is termed **stunting.**

The typical pattern for mild pediatric undernutrition is decreased weight, with normal height and head circumference. In more chronic malnutrition, height and eventually head circumference growth will slow relative to the standard for age. Significant calorie deprivation produces severe wasting, called **marasmus.** Significant protein deprivation in the face of adequate energy intake, possibly with additional insults such as infection, may produce edematous malnutrition called **kwashiorkor.**

Pediatric undernutrition is usually multifactorial in origin, and successful treatment depends on accurate identification and management of those factors. The terms "organic" and "nonorganic" failure to thrive, though still used by many medical professionals, are not helpful because any systemic illness or chronic condition can cause growth impairment and yet may also be compounded by psychosocial problems.

A discussion of the multiple medical conditions that can cause pediatric undernutrition are beyond the scope of this chapter. However, the most common cause is inadequate dietary intake. Inappropriate formula mixing or a family's dietary beliefs may lead to hypocaloric or unbalanced dietary intakes. Diets restricted because of suspected food allergies or intolerances may result in inadequate intake of calories, protein, or specific micronutrients. Iron and zinc are micronutrients that are often marginal in many young children with undernutrition. Zinc deficiency can depress appetite and affect growth, and can easily be corrected with oral zinc supplements given over 1–2 months. Cases of severe malnutrition and kwashiorkor have occurred in infants of well-intentioned parents who substitute "health food" milk alternatives (eg, rice milk or unfortified soy milk) for infant formula.

Poor eating is often a learned behavior. Families should be counseled regarding choices of foods that are appropriate for the age and developmental level of the child. Children should have structured meal times (eg, three meals and two to three snacks during the day), ideally at the same time other family members eat. Consultation with a pediatric dietitian can be helpful for educating the families. Estimates of calorie needs should be based on the need for catch-up growth rather than on the usual RDA for age. Poor feeding may be related to family dysfunction. Children whose households are chaotic and children who are abused, neglected, or exposed to poorly controlled mental illness may be described as poor eaters, and may fail to gain. Careful assessment of the social environment of such children is critical, and disposition options may include support services, close medical follow-up visits, family counseling, and even foster placement while a parent receives therapy.

Block RW, Krebs NF: Failure to thrive as a manifestation of child neglect. Pediatrics 2005;116:1234 [PMID: 16264015].

Shah MD: Failure to thrive in children. J Clin Gastroenterol 2002;35(5):371 [PMID: 12394222].

■ PEDIATRIC OVERWEIGHT/ OBESITY (See Also Chapter 3 for Specifics on Adolescent Obesity.)

BACKGROUND

The prevalence of childhood and adolescent obesity has increased rapidly in the United States and many other parts of the world. Currently in the United States, approximately 15% of 6- to 19-year-olds are overweight, with even higher rates among subpopulations of minority and economically disadvantaged children. The increasing incidence of childhood obesity is related to a complex combination of genetic, environmental, psychosocial, biologic, and socioeconomic factors.

Overweight status in the pediatric population is associated with significant comorbidities which, if untreated, are likely to persist into adulthood. The probability of obesity persisting into adulthood increases from 20% at 4 years to 80% by adolescence. Obesity is associated with cardiovascular and endocrine abnormalities (eg, dyslipidemia, insulin resistance, and type II diabetes), orthopedic problems, pulmonary complications (eg, obstructive sleep apnea), and mental health problems.

DEFINITIONS

BMI is the standard measure of obesity in adults. Its use in children provides a consistent measure across age groups. BMI is correlated with more accurate measures of body fatness and is calculated with readily available information: weight and height (kg ÷ m^2). Routine plotting of the BMI on age- and gender-appropriate charts (http://www.cdc.gov/growthcharts) can identify those with excess weight gain relative to linear growth. BMI between the 85th and 95th percentile for age and sex identifies those at risk of being overweight. Overweight or obese is defined as BMI at or above 95% and is associated with increased risk of secondary complications. An upward change in BMI percentiles in any range should prompt an evaluation and possible treatment. Although the degree of change that indicates risk has not been defined, an annual increase of 3–4 BMI units is almost always an indicator of a rapid increase in body fat. For children younger than 2 years, weight for length greater than 95th percentile indicates overweight and warrants further assessment, especially of energy intake and feeding behaviors.

RISK FACTORS

There are multiple risk factors for developing obesity, reflecting the complex relationships between genetic and environmental factors. Family history is a strong risk factor. If one parent is obese, the odds ratio is approximately 3 for obesity in adulthood, but if both parents are obese, the odds ratio increases to greater than 10.

Environmental risk factors offer potential areas to target for intervention. The absence of family meals, excessive consumption of sweetened beverages, large portion sizes, frequent consumption of foods prepared outside the home, excessive television viewing, and sedentary lifestyle are all associated with a greater prevalence of obesity.

ASSESSMENT

Early recognition of high-risk patterns of weight gain or high-risk behaviors is essential, as it is likely that antici-

patory guidance or intervention before weight gain becomes severe will be more successful. Routine evaluation at well-child visits should include:

1. Measurement of weight and height, calculation of BMI, and plotting all three parameters on age- and sex-appropriate growth charts (http://www.cdc.gov/growthcharts). Evaluate for upward crossing of BMI percentile channels.

2. History regarding diet and activity patterns (Table 10–14). Physical exam: Blood pressure, assess distribution of adiposity (central vs generalized); markers of comorbidities, such as acanthosis nigricans, hirsutism, hepatomegaly, orthopedic abnormalities; physical stigmata of genetic syndrome (eg, Prader–Willi syndrome).

3. Laboratory studies are generally reserved for children with BMI in overweight category (> 95th percentile) or those who have evidence of comorbidities; may include fasting lipid profile, insulin and glucose, liver function tests, thyroid function (if evidence of plateau in linear growth). Other studies should be guided by findings in the history and physical.

TREATMENT

Therapy should be based on risk factors, including age, severity of obesity, and comorbidities, as well as family history and support. For all children with uncomplicated obesity, the primary goal is to achieve healthy eating and activity patterns, not necessarily to achieve ideal body weight. For children with a secondary complication, improvement of the complication is an important goal. For children 2–7 years old with BMI at 95% or modestly above and without complications, the goal should generally be maintenance of baseline weight, allowing the child to "grow into" his or her height, with a gradual normalization of BMI. For children 2–7 years old with BMI at

Table 10–14. Suggested areas for assessment of diet and activity patterns.

Diet
  Meal and snack pattern: structured vs grazing, skipping meals
  Portion sizes: adult portions for young children?
  Frequency of meals away from home (restaurants or take out)
  Frequency/amounts of caloric beverages (soda, juice, milk)
  Frequency of eating fruits and vegetables
  Frequency of family meals?
Activity
  Time spent in sedentary activity: television, video games
  Time spent in vigorous activity: organized sports, physical education, free play
  Activities of daily living: walking to school, chores, yard work

---

95% or above and secondary complications, weight loss is indicated. For children older than 7 years with BMI between 85th and 95th percentile, without complications, weight maintenance is an appropriate goal. If secondary complications are present, weight loss is recommended; an appropriate goal is 1 pound weight loss/month until a BMI less than 85% is achieved. Excessive acute weight loss should be avoided, as this may contribute to nutrient deficiencies and linear growth stunting.

There are few studies of the long-term effects of weight control programs for children. Treatment focused on behavior changes in the context of family involvement has been associated with sustained weight loss and decreases in BMI. Clinicians should assess the family's readiness to take action (transtheoretical model and motivational interviewing). Concurrent changes in dietary patterns and increasing physical activity are most likely to provide success. The whole family should be encouraged to adopt healthy eating patterns, with parents modeling healthy food choices, controlling foods brought into the home, and guiding appropriate portion sizes. Limiting sedentary activity has been found to be more effective than specifically promoting increased physical activity. The American Academy of Pediatrics recommends no television for children younger than 2 years old, and a maximum of 2 h/d of television and video games for older children.

Treatment may be considered at three different levels depending on the severity of overweight, the age of the child, the ability of the family to implement changes, the preferences of the parents and child, and the skills of the health care provider.

1. *General:* Counseling regarding problem areas identified by screening questions (see Table 10–14); emphasis on guidelines around healthy eating and physical activity patterns. This is especially appropriate for preventing further weight gain or for mildly overweight children.

2. *Structured:* Provide more specific and structured dietary pattern, such as meal planning, exercise prescription, behavior change goals. This may be done in the primary care setting or, if resources are available, referred to more specialized treatment program.

3. *Group treatment:* Generally best for the older child or adolescent, with varying level of parental involvement depending on age of child. Several published programs are available. The Weight Information Network (WIN) is a service available through the National Institutes of Health, which disseminates information on weight control programs and is available online: http://win.niddk.nih.gov/index.htm

No single prescription is effective for all patients. The physician will do his or her best to assess the severity of the problem, treatment needs in context of the family's preferences and abilities, and local resources, including availability of registered dietitians with expertise in pediatric weight management and behaviorists or family therapists.

Pharmacotherapy can be an adjunct to dietary, activity, and behavioral treatment, but by itself it is unlikely to result in significant or sustained weight loss. Two medications are approved for obesity treatment in adolescents: sibutramine, a selective serotonin reuptake inhibitor, is approved for patients over 16 years; orlistat, a lipase inhibitor, is approved for patients over 12 years. For severe obesity in adolescents, particularly with comorbidities, bariatric surgery is being performed in some centers. This is still considered experimental, and there is an urgent need for long-term outcome, safety, and efficacy data. However, there is limited evidence that in carefully selected and closely monitored patients, medications or surgery (or both) can result in significant weight loss with a reduction in comorbidities for those who are severely afflicted.

Baker S et al: Overweight children and adolescents: A clinical report of the North American Society for Pediatric Gastroenterology, Hepatology and Nutrition. J Pediatr Gastroenterol Nutr 2005;40:533 [PMID: 15861011].

Daniels SR et al: Overweight in children and adolescents. Pathophysiology, consequences, prevention, and treatment. Circulation 2005;111:1999 [PMID: 15837955].

Dietz WH, Robinson TN: Overweight children and adolescents. N Engl J Med 2005;353:2100 [PMID: 15901863].

Krebs NF: Screening for overweight in children and adolescents: A call to action. Pediatrics 2005;116(1):238 [PMID: 15995062].

Krebs NF, Jacobson MS, Committee on Nutrition, American Academy of Pediatrics: Prevention of Pediatric Overweight and Obesity Policy Statement. Pediatrics 2003;112(2):1 [PMID: 12897303].

NUTRITION SUPPORT

1. Enteral

Indications

Enteral nutrition support is indicated when a patient cannot adequately meet nutritional needs by oral intake alone and has a functioning GI tract. This method of support can be used for short- and long-term delivery of nutrition. Even when the gut cannot absorb 100% of nutritional needs, some enteral feedings should be attempted. Enteral nutrition, full or partial, has many benefits:

1. Maintaining gut mucosal integrity
2. Preserving gut-associated lymphoid tissue
3. Stimulation of gut hormones and bile flow

The nutritional needs of most patients requiring enteral nutrition can be met with standard enteral formulations. Specialized formulas are available for patients

Table 10–15. Guidelines for the initiation and advancement of tube feedings.

Age	Drip Feeds		Bolus Feeds	
	Initiation	Advancement	Initiation	Advancement
Preterm	1–2 mL/kg	1 mL as tolerated	5–20 mL	5–10 mL as tolerated
Birth–12 mo	5–10 mL/h	5–10 mL q 2–8 h	10–60 mL	20–40 mL q 3–4 h
1–6 yr	10–15 mL/h	10–15 mL q 2–8 h	30–90 mL	30–60 mL q feed
6–14 yr	15–20 mL/h	10–20 mL q 2–8 h	60–120 mL	60–90 mL q feed
> 14 yr	20–30 mL/h	20–30 mL q 2–8 h	60–120 mL	60–120 mL q feed

of all ages with severe milk protein allergy, single- or multiple-nutrient malabsorption, renal failure, and hepatic failure. The decision to use such specialized formulas must be made in the context of the patient's condition and nutritional needs.

Access Devices

Nasogastric feeding tubes can be used for supplemental enteral feedings, but generally are not used for more than 6 months because of the complications of otitis media and sinusitis. Initiation of nasogastric feeding usually requires a brief hospital stay to ensure tolerance to feedings and to allow for parental instruction in tube placement and feeding administration.

If long-term feeding support is anticipated, a more permanent feeding device, such as a gastrostomy tube, may be considered. Unfortunately, many insurance carriers do not cover the cost of formula for tube feedings. Referral to a home care company is necessary for equipment and other services such as nursing visits and dietitian follow-up.

Table 10–15 suggests appropriate timing for initiation and advancement of drip and bolus feedings, according to a child's age. Clinical status and tolerance to feedings should ultimately guide their advancement.

Monitoring

Monitoring the adequacy of enteral feeding depends on nutritional goals. Growth should be frequently assessed, especially for young infants and malnourished children. Hydration status should be monitored carefully at the initiation of enteral feeding. Either constipation or diarrhea can be problems, and attention to stool frequency, volume, and consistency can help guide management. When diarrhea occurs, factors such as infection, hypertonic enteral medications, antibiotic use, and alteration in normal gut flora should be addressed before making formula changes.

It is important to determine whether the feeding schedule is developmentally appropriate. This will not be possible for all patients, especially those who are critically ill. However, for children who are more stable, tube-feeding schedules should mimic as closely as possible an age-appropriate feeding schedule (eg, six small feedings per day for a toddler). When night drip feedings are used in conjunction with daytime feeds, it is suggested that less than 50% of goal calories be delivered at night so as to maintain a daytime sense of hunger and satiety. This will be especially important once a transition to oral intake begins. Children who are satiated by tube feedings will be less likely to take significant amounts of food by mouth, thus possibly delaying the transition from tube to oral nutrition.

2. Parenteral Nutrition

Indications

A. PERIPHERAL PARENTERAL NUTRITION

Peripheral parenteral nutrition is indicated when complete enteral feeding is temporarily impossible or undesirable. Short-term partial IV nutrition via a peripheral vein is a preferred alternative to administration of dextrose and electrolyte solutions alone. Because of the osmolality of the solutions required, it is usually impossible to achieve total calorie and protein needs with parenteral nutrition via a peripheral vein.

B. TOTAL PARENTERAL NUTRITION

TPN should be provided only when clearly indicated. Apart from the expense, numerous risks are associated with this method of feeding (see section on Complications). Even when TPN is indicated, every effort should be made to provide at least a minimum of nutrients enterally to help preserve the integrity of the GI mucosa and of GI function.

The primary indication for TPN is the loss of function of the GI tract that prohibits the provision of more than a small proportion of required nutrients by the enteral route. Important examples include short bowel syndrome, some congenital defects of the GI tract, and prematurity.

Catheter Selection & Position

An indwelling central venous catheter is preferred for long-term IV nutrition. For periods of up to 3–4 weeks, a percutaneous central venous catheter threaded into the superior vena cava from a peripheral vein can be used. For the infusion of dextrose concentrations higher than 12.5%, the tip of the catheter should be located in the superior vena cava. Catheter positioning in the right atrium has been associated with complications, including arrhythmias and right atrial thrombus. After placement, a chest radiograph must be obtained to check catheter position. If the catheter is to be used for nutrition and medications, a double-lumen catheter is preferred.

Complications

A. MECHANICAL COMPLICATIONS

1. Related to catheter insertion or to erosion of catheter through a major blood vessel—Complications include trauma to adjacent tissues and organs, damage to the brachial plexus, hydrothorax, pneumothorax, hemothorax, and cerebrospinal fluid penetration. The catheter may slip during dressing or tubing changes, or the patient may manipulate the line.

Chaturvedi A et al: Catheter malplacement during central venous cannulation through arm veins in pediatric patients. J Neurosurg Anesthes 2003;15(3):170 [PMID: 12826963].

2. Clotting of the catheter—Addition of heparin (1000 U/L) to the solution is an effective means of preventing this complication. If an occluded catheter does not respond to heparin flushing, filling the catheter with recombinant tissue plasminogen activator or sterile 95% ethanol may be effective.

3. Related to composition of infusate—Calcium phosphate precipitation may occur if excess amounts of calcium or phosphorus are administered. Factors that increase the risk of calcium phosphate precipitation include increased pH and decreased concentrations of amino acids. Precipitation of medications incompatible with TPN or lipids can also cause clotting.

Freytes CO: Thromboembolic complications related to indwelling central venous catheters in children. Curr Opin Oncol 2003;15:289 [PMID: 12874506].

B. SEPTIC COMPLICATIONS

Septic complications are the most common cause of nonelective catheter removal, but strict use of aseptic technique and limiting entry into the catheter can reduce the rates of line sepsis.

Fever over 38–38.5 °C in a patient with a central catheter should be considered a line infection until proved otherwise. Cultures should be obtained and IV antibiotics empirically initiated. Removing the catheter may be necessary with certain infections (eg, fungal), and catheter replacement may be deferred until infection is treated.

C. METABOLIC COMPLICATIONS

Many of the metabolic complications of IV nutrition are related to deficiencies or excesses of nutrients in administered fluids. These complications are less common as a result of experience and improvements in nutrient solutions. However, specific deficiencies still occur, especially in the premature infant. Avoidance of deficiencies and excesses and of metabolic disorders requires attention to the nutrient balance, electrolyte composition, and delivery rate of the infusate and careful monitoring, especially when the composition or delivery rate is changed.

Currently the most challenging metabolic complication is cholestasis, particularly common in premature infants of very low birth weight. The cause of cholestasis associated with TPN is unknown. Patient and medical risk factors include prematurity, sepsis, hypoxia, major surgery (especially GI surgery), absence of enteral feedings, and small bowel bacterial overgrowth. Risk factors related to IV nutrition include amino acid excess or imbalance and prolonged duration of administration. Amino acid solutions with added cysteine decrease cholestasis. Practices that may minimize cholestasis include initiating even minimal enteral feedings as soon as feasible, avoiding sepsis by meticulous line care, avoiding overfeeding, using cysteine- and taurine-containing amino acid formulations designed for infants, preventing or treating small bowel bacterial overgrowth, protecting TPN solutions from light, and avoiding hepatotoxic medications.

Forchielli ML, Walker WA: Nutritional factors contributing to the development of cholestasis during parenteral nutrition. Adv Pediatr 2003;50:245 [PMID: 14626490].

NUTRIENT REQUIREMENTS & DELIVERY

Energy

When patients are fed intravenously, no fat and carbohydrate intakes are unabsorbed, and no energy is used in nutrient absorption. These factors account for at least 7% of energy in the diet of the enterally fed patient. The intravenously fed patient usually expends less energy in physical activity because of the impediment to mobility. Average energy requirements may therefore be lower in children fed intravenously, and the decrease in activity probably increases this figure to a total reduction of 10–15%. Caloric guidelines for the IV feeding of infants and young children are outlined below.

Age (months)	Requirements (kcal/kg/d)
0–1	100–110
2–4	90–100
5–60	70–90
> 5 years	1500 kcal for 1st 20 kg + 25 kcal for each additional kg/d

The guidelines are averages, and individuals vary considerably. Factors significantly increasing the energy requirement estimates include exposure to cold environment, fever, sepsis, burns, trauma, cardiac or pulmonary disease, and catch-up growth after malnutrition.

With few exceptions, such as some cases of respiratory insufficiency, at least 50–60% of energy requirements are provided as glucose. Up to 40% of calories may be provided by IV fat emulsions.

Dextrose

The energy density of IV dextrose (monohydrate) is 3.4 kcal/g. Dextrose is the main exogenous energy source provided by total IV feeding. IV dextrose suppresses gluconeogenesis and provides a substrate that can be oxidized directly, especially by the brain, red and white blood cells, and wounds. Because of the high osmolality of dextrose solutions ($D_{10}W$ yields 505 mOsm/kg H_2O), concentrations greater than 10–12.5% cannot be delivered via a peripheral vein or improperly positioned central line.

Dosing guidelines: The standard initial quantity of dextrose administered will vary by age (Table 10–16). Tolerance to IV dextrose normally increases rapidly, due primarily to suppression of hepatic production of endogenous glucose. Dextrose can be increased by 2.5 g/kg/d; by 2.5–5%/day; or by 2–3 mg/kg/min/d if there is no glucosuria or hyperglycemia. Standard final infusates for infants via a properly positioned central venous line usually range from 15–25% dextrose, though concentrations of up to 30% dextrose may be used at low flow rates. Tolerance to IV dextrose loads is markedly diminished in the premature neonate and in hypermetabolic states.

Problems associated with IV dextrose administration include hyperglycemia, hyperosmolality, and glucosuria (with osmotic diuresis and dehydration). Possible causes of unexpected hyperglycemia include the following: (1) inadvertent infusion of higher glucose concentrations than ordered, (2) uneven flow rate, (3) sepsis, (4) a stress situation, and (5) pancreatitis. IV insulin reduces hyperglycemia but does not increase glucose oxidation rates; it may also decrease the oxidation of fatty acids, resulting in less energy for metabolism. Hence, insulin should be used very cautiously. A stan-

Table 10–16. Pediatric macronutrient guidelines for total parenteral nutrition.

Age	Dextrose		Amino acids	Lipid
	mg/kg/min	g/kg/d	g/kg/d	g/kg/d
	50–60% kcal		10–20% kcal	30–40% kcal
Preterm	Initial 5–8 Max 11–12.5	Initial 7–11 Max 16–18	Initial 1.5–2 Max 3–4	Initial 0.5–1 Max 2.5–3.5
Birth–12 mo	Initial 6–8 Max 11–15	Initial 9–11 Max 16–21.5	Initial 1.5–2 Max 3	Initial 1 Max 2.5–3.5
1–6 yr	Initial 6–7 Max 10–12	Initial 8–10 Max 14–17	Initial 1–1.5 Max 2–2.5	Initial 1 Max 2.5–3.5
> 6 yr	Initial 5–7 Max 9	Initial 8–10 Max 13	Initial 1 Max 1.5–2	Initial 1 Max 3
> 10 yr	Initial 4–5 Max 6–7	Initial 5–7 Max 8–10	Initial 1 Max 1.5–2	Initial 1 Max 2–3
Adolescents	Initial 2–3 Max 5–6	Initial 3–4 Max 7–8	Initial 1 Max 1.5–2	Initial 0.5–1 Max 2

dard IV dose is 1 U/4 g of carbohydrate, but much smaller quantities may be adequate and, usually, one starts with 0.2–0.3 U/4 g of carbohydrate.

Hypoglycemia may occur after an abrupt decrease in or cessation of IV glucose. When cyclic IV nutrition is provided, the IV glucose load should be decreased steadily for 1–2 hours prior to discontinuing the infusate. If the central line must be removed, the IV dextrose should be tapered gradually over several hours.

Maximum oxidation rates for infused dextrose decrease with age. It is important to note that the ranges for dextrose administration provided in Table 10–16 are guidelines and that individual patient tolerance and clinical circumstances may warrant administration of either less or more dextrose. Quantities of exogenous dextrose in excess of maximal glucose oxidation rates are used initially to replace depleted glycogen stores; hepatic lipogenesis occurs thereafter. Excess hepatic lipogenesis may lead to a fatty liver. Lipogenesis results in release of carbon dioxide, which when added to the amount of carbon dioxide produced by glucose oxidation (which is 40% greater than that produced by lipid oxidation) may elevate the $PaCO_2$ and aggravate respiratory insufficiency or impede weaning from a respirator.

Lipids

The energy density of lipid emulsions (20%) is 10 kcal/g of lipid or 2 kcal/mL of infusate. The lipids are derived from either soybean or safflower oil. All consist of more than 50% linoleic acid and 4–9% linolenic acid. It is recognized that this high level of linoleic acid is not ideal, except when small quantities of lipid are being given to prevent an EFA deficiency. Ultimately, improved emulsions are anticipated. Because 10% and 20% lipid emulsions contain the same concentrations of phospholipids, a 10% solution delivers more phospholipid per gram of lipid than a 20% solution. Twenty percent lipid emulsions are preferred.

The level of lipoprotein lipase (LPL) activity is the rate-limiting factor in the metabolism and clearance of fat emulsions from the circulation. LPL activity is inhibited or decreased by malnutrition, leukotrienes, immaturity, growth hormone, hypercholesterolemia, hyperphospholipidemia, and theophylline. LPL activity is enhanced by glucose, insulin, lipid, catecholamines, and exercise. Heparin releases LPL from the endothelium into the circulation and enhances the rate of hydrolysis and clearance of triglycerides. In small premature infants, low-dose heparin infusions may increase tolerance to IV lipid emulsion.

The advantages of using fat emulsions to provide up to 40% of caloric intake include the following:

1. The high energy density allows more energy to be provided when fluid volume is restricted.

2. The low osmolality (280 mOsm/kg H_2O) is of special value when using a peripheral line.

3. EFA deficiencies can be prevented.

4. The production of CO_2 is 40% lower per unit of energy, an important consideration in cases of pulmonary insufficiency.

5. The energy cost of fat storage is negligible.

6. The risk of fatty liver is decreased because of decreased hepatic lipogenesis from dextrose.

Potential disadvantages of fat emulsions include the following:

1. Impairment of function of neutrophils, macrophages, and the reticuloendothelial system.

2. Coagulation defects, including thrombocytopenia, elevated prothrombin time, and partial thromboplastin time.

3. Decrease in pulmonary oxygen diffusion.

4. Competition by free fatty acids with bilirubin and drugs for albumin-binding sites.

5. Increase in low-density lipoprotein cholesterol.

In general, these adverse effects can be avoided by starting with modest quantities and advancing cautiously in light of results of triglyceride monitoring and clinical circumstances. In cases of severe sepsis, special caution is required to ensure that the lipid is metabolized effectively. Monitoring with long-term use is also essential.

IV lipid dosing guidelines: Check serum triglycerides before starting and after increasing the dose. Commence with 1 g/kg/d, given over 12–20 hours or 24 hours in small preterm infants. Advance by 0.5–1.0 g/kg/d, every 1–2 days, up to goal (see Table 10–16).

As a general rule, do not increase the dose if the serum triglyceride level is above 250 mg/dL during infusion (150 mg/dL in neonates) or if the level is greater than 150 mg/dL 6–12 hours after cessation of the lipid infusion.

Serum triglyceride levels above 400–600 mg/dL may precipitate pancreatitis. In patients for whom normal amounts of IV lipid are contraindicated, 4–8% of calories as IV lipid should be provided (300 mg linoleic acid/100 kcal) to prevent essential fatty acid deficiency. Neonates and malnourished pediatric patients receiving lipid-free parenteral nutrition are at high risk for EFA deficiency because of limited adipose stores.

Nitrogen

One gram of nitrogen is yielded by 6.25 g of protein (1 g of protein contains 16% nitrogen). Caloric density of protein is equal to 4 kcal/g.

A. PROTEIN REQUIREMENTS

Protein requirements for IV feeding are the same as those for normal oral feeding (see Table 10–2).

B. PROTEIN–ENERGY INTERACTIONS

There are important interactions between protein and energy requirements. A positive nitrogen balance cannot be achieved on a hypocaloric diet, because protein will be catabolized for energy. When energy intakes are low, the administration of some amino acid does, however, lessen the severity of the negative nitrogen balance. Conversely, when nitrogen intake is low, the provision of calories improves nitrogen balance to some extent. In infants, the energy necessary to minimize nitrogen loss associated with an amino acid-free diet is approximately 70 kcal/kg/d. At this level of energy intake, positive nitrogen balance depends on the level of nitrogen intake and is independent of further increase in energy intake.

In infants receiving about 50 kcal/kg/d, increasing protein intake up to 3 g/kg/d improves the nitrogen balance. In these circumstances, therefore, a ratio of grams of nitrogen per kilocalorie as low as 1:100 can be advantageous. However, at higher levels of energy intake, ratios of 1:250 to 1:150 or more are optimal. Although these ratios provide a useful crude check, they are not usually the best means of determining protein requirements.

C. INTRAVENOUS AMINO ACID SOLUTIONS

Nitrogen requirements can be met by one of the commercially available amino acid solutions. For older children and adults, none of the standard preparations has a clear advantage over the others as a source of amino acids. For infants, however, including premature infants, accumulating evidence suggests that the use of TrophAmine (McGaw) is associated with a normal plasma amino acid profile, superior nitrogen retention, and a lower incidence of cholestasis. TrophAmine contains 60% essential amino acids, is relatively high in branched-chain amino acids, contains taurine, and is compatible with the addition of cysteine within 24–48 hours after administration. The dose of added cysteine is 40 mg/g of TrophAmine. The relatively low pH of TrophAmine is also advantageous for solubility of calcium and phosphorus.

D. DOSING GUIDELINES

Amino acids can be started at 1–2 g/kg/d in most patients (see Table 10–16). In severely malnourished infants, the initial amount should be 1 g/kg/d. Even in infants of very low birth weight, there is evidence that higher initial amounts of amino acids are tolerated with little indication of protein "toxicity." Larger quantities of amino acids in relation to calories can minimize the degree of negative nitrogen balance when the infusate is hypocaloric. Amino acid intake can be advanced by 0.5–1.0 g/kg/d toward the goal. Normally the final infusate will contain 2–3% amino acids, depending on the rate of infusion. Concentration should not be advanced beyond 2% in peripheral vein infusates due to osmolality.

E. MONITORING

Monitoring for tolerance of the IV amino acid solutions should include routine blood urea nitrogen. Serum alkaline phosphatase, γ-glutamyltransferase, and bilirubin should be monitored to detect the onset of cholestatic liver disease.

F. SPECIAL AMINO ACID PREPARATIONS

Some solutions are designed to provide high concentrations of branched-chain amino acids. These solutions are expensive and should not be ordered without a specific reason, which does not include their routine use in liver disease. They may be indicated in hepatic failure, especially in the presence of encephalopathy, and are also undergoing experimental use in multisystem organ failure. In this circumstance, the branched-chain amino acids are given as a source of metabolizable energy, providing up to 25% of energy intake. Solutions containing only essential amino acids have shown no benefit in decreasing blood urea nitrogen or forestalling the need for dialysis in acute renal failure, and thus should be used with caution, if at all.

G. ALBUMIN

Albumin can be added to the infusate when clinically indicated to restore blood volume or oncotic pressure. If the origin of hypoalbuminemia is considered to be primarily nutritional, however, the hypoalbuminemia should be managed by careful nutritional rehabilitation rather than by IV administration of albumin. Albumin is deficient in isoleucine and tryptophan and has too long a half-life (15–20 days) to be considered a useful nutritional source of amino acids. Potential adverse effects of IV albumin administration include loss of albumin from the circulation into interstitial fluid of the lungs and elsewhere due to increased capillary permeability, coagulation defects secondary to volume expansion and dilution of clotting factors, inhibition of platelet aggregation, increases in prothrombin time and partial thromboplastin time, increased sodium intake in the albumin infusate, and increased binding to serum calcium resulting in decreased ionized calcium.

Albumin is a poor nutritional marker because of the number of nonnutritional factors that contribute to hypoalbuminemia.

Dosing guidelines: When clinical circumstances warrant, albumin can be added to parenteral nutrition in the amount of 0.5–1.0 g/kg/d. The half-life of IV albumin in critical illness can be as short as under 12 hours.

Minerals & Electrolytes

A. CALCIUM, PHOSPHORUS, AND MAGNESIUM

Intravenously fed premature and full-term infants should be given relatively high amounts of calcium and phosphorus. Current recommendations are as follows: calcium, 500–600 mg/L; phosphorus, 400–450 mg/L; and magnesium, 50–70 mg/L. After 1 year of age, the recommendations are as follows: calcium, 200–400 mg/L; phosphorus, 150–300 mg/L; and magnesium, 20–40 mg/L. The ratio of calcium to phosphorous should be 1.3:1.0 by weight or 1:1 by molar ratio. These recommendations are deliberately presented as milligrams per liter of infusate to avoid inadvertent administration of concentrations of calcium and phosphorus that are high enough to precipitate in the tubing. During periods of fluid restriction, care must be taken not to inadvertently increase the concentration of calcium and phosphorus in the infusate. These recommendations assume an average fluid intake of 120–150 mL/kg/d and an infusate of 25 g of amino acid per liter. With lower amino acid concentrations, the concentrations of calcium and phosphorus should be decreased.

B. ELECTROLYTES

Standard recommendations are given in Table 10–17. After chloride requirements are met, the remainder of the anion required to balance the cation should be given as acetate to avoid the possibility of acidosis resulting from excessive chloride. The required concentrations of electrolytes depend to some extent on the flow rate of the infusate and must be modified if flow rates are unusually low or high and if there are specific indications in individual patients. IV sodium should be administered sparingly in the severely malnourished patient because of impaired membrane function and high intracellular sodium levels. Conversely, generous quantities of potassium are indicated. Replacement electrolytes and fluids should be delivered via a separate infusate.

C. TRACE ELEMENTS

Recommended IV intakes of trace elements are as follows: zinc 100 μg/kg, copper 20 μg/kg, manganese 1 μg/kg, chromium 0.2 μg/kg, selenium 2 μg/kg, and iodide 1 μg/kg. Of note, IV zinc requirements may be as high as 400 μg/kg for premature infants and can be up to 250 μg/kg for infants with short bowel syndrome and significant GI losses of zinc. When IV nutrition is supplemental or limited to fewer than 2 weeks, and pre-existing nutritional deficiencies are absent, only zinc need routinely be added.

IV copper requirements are relatively low in the young infant because of the presence of hepatic copper stores. These are significant even in the 28-week fetus. Circulating levels of copper and manganese should be monitored in the presence of cholestatic liver disease. If monitoring is not feasible, temporary withdrawal of added copper and manganese is advisable. Copper and manganese are excreted primarily in the bile, but selenium, chromium, and molybdenum are excreted primarily in the urine. These trace elements, therefore, should be administered with caution in the presence of renal failure.

Although low doses of iron are routinely added in some centers to the IV infusate for infants and children, no official recommendation has been made because of the lack of adequate published data regarding compatibility. Iron added to the infusate should be in a diluted form of iron dextran in a concentration of 1 mg/L. After age 2 months, maintenance IV iron requirements for the full-term infant are approximately 100 μg/kg/d. After the first month, the premature infant requires up to 200 μg/kg/d intravenously. Although overload is unlikely to occur during short-term parenteral nutrition, a surreptitious accumulation of extra iron could occur if parenteral nutrition is prolonged. This risk is enhanced if the patient has received blood transfusions. A second concern is that the potential for free iron is increased in malnourished infants with low transferrin levels. Excess iron is thought to enhance the risk of gram-negative septicemia. Iron has powerful oxidant properties and can enhance the demand for antioxidants, especially vitamin E. None of these concerns appear to preclude the routine use of iron supplements during IV nutrition, but they do emphasize the need for a conservative approach in determining dosage schedules.

Vitamins

Two vitamin formulations are available for use in pediatric parenteral nutrition: MVI Pediatric and MVI-12 (AstraZeneca). MVI Pediatric contains the following: vitamin A, 0.7 mg; vitamin D, 400 IU; vitamin E, 7 mg; vitamin K, 200 μg; ascorbic acid, 80 mg; thiamin, 1.2 mg; riboflavin,

Table 10–17. Electrolyte requirements for parenteral nutrition.

Electrolyte	Preterm Infant	Full-Term Infant	Child	Adolescent
Sodium	2–5 mEq/kg	2–3 mEq/kg	2–3 mEq/kg	60–150 mEq/d
Chloride	2–5 mEq/kg	2–3 mEq/kg	2–3 mEq/kg	60–150 mEq/d
Potassium	2–3 mEq/kg	2–3 mEq/kg	2–3 mEq/kg	70–180 mEq/d

Table 10–18. Routine total parenteral nutrition monitoring summary.

Variables	Acute Stage	Long-Term[b]
Growth		
Weight	Daily	Weekly
Length	Weekly	
Head circumference	Weekly	
Urine		
Glucose (dipstick)	With each void	With changes in intake or status
Specific gravity	Void	
Volume	Daily	
Blood		
Glucose	4 hours after changes,[a] then daily × 2 days	Weekly
Na^+, K^+, Cl^-, CO_2, blood urea nitrogen	Daily for 2 days after changes,[a] then twice weekly	Weekly
Ca^{2+}, Mg^{2+}, P	Initially, then twice weekly	Weekly
Total protein, albumin, bilirubin, aspartate transaminase, and alkaline phosphatase	Initially, then weekly	Every other week
Zinc and copper	Initially according to clinical indications	Monthly
Triglycerides	Initially, 1 day after changes,[a] then weekly	Weekly
Compete blood count	Initially, then twice weekly; according to clinical indications (see text)	Twice weekly

[a]Changes include alterations in concentration or flow rate.
[b]Long-term monitoring can be tapered to monthly or less often, depending on age, diagnosis, and clinical status of patient.

1.4 mg; niacinamide, 17 mg; pyridoxine, 1 mg; vitamin B_{12}, 1 µg; folic acid, 140 µg; pantothenate, 5 mg; and biotin, 20 µg. This formulation is suboptimal, with too little vitamin A and excessive amounts of water-soluble vitamins, but it is the best one available. Recommended dosing is as follows: 5 mL for children weighing more than 3 kg, 3.25 mL for infants 1–3 kg, and 1.5 mL for infants weighing less than 1 kg. Children older than 11 years can receive 10 mL of the adult formulation, MVI-12, which contains the following: vitamin A, 1 mg; vitamin D, 200 IU; vitamin E, 10 mg; ascorbic acid, 100 mg; thiamin, 3 mg; riboflavin, 3.6 mg; niacinamide, 40 mg; pyridoxine, 4 mg; vitamin B_{12}, 5 µg; folic acid, 400 µg; pantothenate, 15 mg; and biotin, 60 µg. MVI-12 contains no vitamin K.

IV lipid preparations contain enough tocopherol to affect total blood tocopherol levels. The majority of tocopherol in soybean oil emulsion is α-tocopherol, which has substantially less biologic activity than the α-tocopherol present in safflower oil emulsions.

A dose of 40 IU/kg/d of vitamin D (maximum 400 IU/d) is adequate for both full-term and preterm infants.

Fluid Requirements

The initial fluid volume and subsequent increments in flow rate are determined by basic fluid requirements, the patient's clinical status, and the extent to which additional fluid administration can be tolerated and may be required to achieve adequate nutrient intake. Calculation of initial fluid volumes to be administered should be based on standard pediatric practice. Tolerance of higher flow rates must be determined on an individual basis. If replacement fluids are required for ongoing abnormal losses, these should be administered via a separate line.

Monitoring

Vital signs should be checked on each shift. With a central catheter in situ, a fever of more than 38.5 °C requires that peripheral and central-line blood cultures, urine culture, complete physical examination, and examination of the IV entry point be made. Instability of vital signs, elevated white blood cell count with left shift, and glycosuria suggest sepsis. Removal of the central venous catheter should be considered if the patient is toxic or unresponsive to antibiotics.

A. Physical Examination

Monitor especially for hepatomegaly (differential diagnoses include fluid overload, congestive heart failure, steatosis, and hepatitis) and edema (differential diagnoses include fluid overload, congestive heart failure, hypoalbuminemia, and thrombosis of superior vena cava).

B. Intake and Output Record

Calories and volume delivered should be calculated from the previous day's intake and output records (that which was delivered rather than that which was ordered). The following entries should be noted on flow sheets: IV, enteral, and total fluid (mL/kg/d); dextrose (g/kg/d or mg/kg/min); protein (g/kg/d); lipids (g/kg/d); energy (kcal/kg/d); and percent of energy from enteral nutrition.

C. Growth, Urine, and Blood

Routine monitoring guidelines are given in Table 10–18. These are minimum requirements, except in the very long-term stable patient. Individual variables should be

monitored more frequently as indicated, as should additional variables or clinical indications. For example, a blood ammonia analysis should be ordered for an infant with lethargy, pallor, poor growth, acidosis, azotemia, or abnormal liver test results.

Greene HL et al: Guidelines for the use of vitamins, trace elements, calcium, magnesium, and phosphorus in infants and children receiving total parenteral nutrition: Report of the Subcommittee on Pediatric Parenteral Nutrient Requirements from the Committee on Clinical Practice Issues of the American Society for Clinical Nutrition. Am J Clin Nutr 1988;48:1324 [PMID: 3142247].

Shulman RJ, Phillips S: Parenteral nutrition in infants and children. J Pediatr Gastroenterol Nutr 2003;36(5):587 [PMID: 12717082].

Emergencies & Injuries

Glenn Faries, MD, & F. Keith Battan, MD

■ I. EMERGENCIES & INJURIES

ADVANCED LIFE SUPPORT FOR INFANTS & CHILDREN

When faced with a seriously ill or injured child, a systematic approach and rapid determination of the child's physiologic status with concurrent initiation of resuscitative measures is imperative. Initial management must be directed at correcting any physiological derangement. Specifically, one must evaluate the airway for any obstruction, assess ventilatory status, and evaluate for shock. Intervention to correct any abnormalities in these three parameters must be undertaken immediately. Following this initial intervention the provider must then carefully consider the underlying cause, focusing on those that are treatable and/or reversible. Specific diagnoses can then be made, and targeted therapy (eg, intravenous [IV] glucose for hypoglycemia) can be initiated.

Progressive deterioration may lead to bradycardia and ultimately to asystole, with significant hypoxic and ischemic insult to the brain and other vital organs making neurologic recovery extremely unlikely, even in the doubtful event that the child survives the arrest. Children who respond to rapid intervention with ventilation and oxygenation alone or to less than 5 minutes of advanced life support are much more likely to survive neurologically intact. Therefore, it is essential to recognize the child who is at risk for progressing to cardiopulmonary arrest and to provide aggressive intervention before asystole occurs.

Note: Standard precautions (personal protective equipment) must be maintained during resuscitation efforts.

THE ABCs OF RESUSCITATION

Any severely ill child should be rapidly evaluated in a deliberate sequence of *a*irway patency, *b*reathing adequacy, and *c*irculation integrity. Derangement at each point must be corrected before proceeding. Thus, if a child's airway is obstructed, the airway must be opened (eg, by head positioning and the chin lift maneuver) before breathing and circulation are assessed.

Airway

Look, listen, and feel for upper airway patency: *Look* for signs of obstruction such as increased work of breathing. Significant airway obstruction will often be associated with altered level of consciousness, including agitation or lethargy. *Listen* for adventitious breath sounds such as stridor, stertor, or gurgling. *Feel* for air movement with your face near the child's mouth and nose.

The airway is managed initially by noninvasive means such as oxygen administration, chin lift, jaw thrust, suctioning, or bag–valve–mask ventilation. Invasive maneuvers such as endotracheal intubation, laryngeal mask insertion, or rarely, cricothyroidotomy are required if the above maneuvers are not successful. If neck injury is suspected, the cervical spine must be immobilized and kept from extension or flexion. (See Approach to the Pediatric Trauma Patient section.) The following discussion assumes that basic life support has been instituted.

Knowledge of pediatric anatomy is important for airway management. Children's tongues are large relative to their oral cavities, and the larynx is high and anteriorly located. Infants are obligate nasal breathers; therefore, secretions or blood in the nasopharynx can cause significant distress.

A. Place the head in the sniffing position (Figure 11–1). The neck should be slightly flexed and the head gently extended so as to bring the face forward. This position aligns the oral, pharyngeal, and tracheal planes (Figure 11–2). Reposition the head if airway obstruction persists after head tilt and jaw thrust. In infants, the relatively large occiput puts the head in a sniffing position when supine; in an older child, more head extension is necessary. Avoid hyperextension of the neck, especially in infants.

B. Perform the chin lift or jaw thrust maneuver (Figure 11–3). Lift the chin upward while avoiding pressure on the submental triangle, or lift the jaw by traction upward on the angle of the jaw. **Head tilt must not be done if cervical spine injury is possible.**

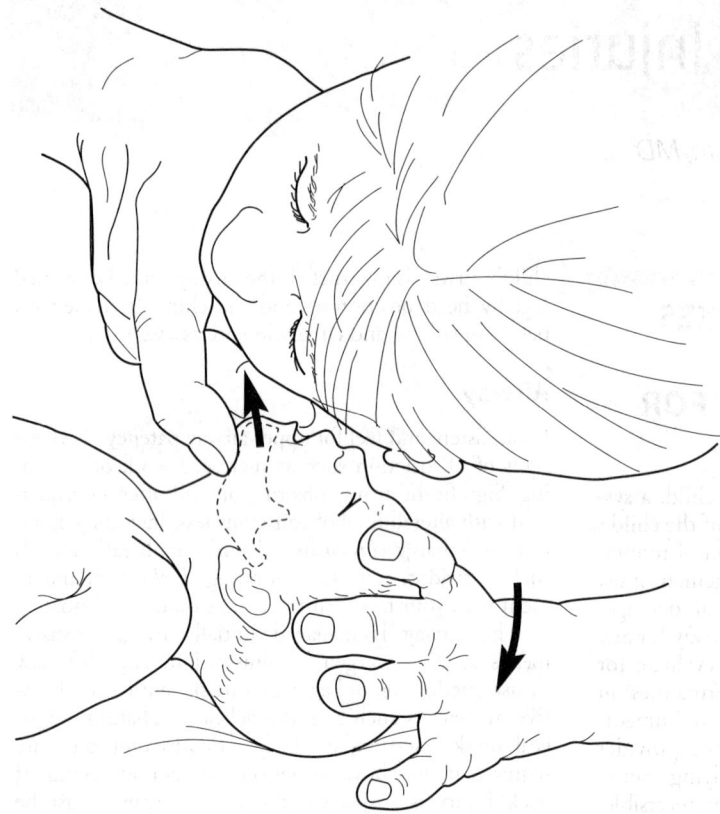

Figure 11–1. Opening the airway with the head tilt/chin lift. Gently lift the chin with one hand and push down on the forehead with the other hand. (Reproduced, with permission, from *Textbook of Pediatric Life Support.* American Heart Association, 1997.)

C. Suction the mouth of any foreign material.

D. Remove visible foreign bodies, using fingers or a Magill forceps. Visualize by means of a laryngoscope if necessary. Blind finger sweeps should not be done.

E. Insert an oropharyngeal airway (nasopharyngeal in a conscious patient) to relieve upper airway obstruction due to prolapse of the tongue into the posterior pharynx (Figures 11–4 and 11–5). This is the most common cause of airway obstruction in unconscious children. Correct size for an oropharyngeal airway is obtained by measuring from the upper central gumline to the angle of the jaw. Nasopharyngeal airways should fit snugly within the nares and should be equal in length to the distance from the nares to the tragus.

Breathing

Assessment of respiratory status is largely accomplished by inspection. *Look* for adequate and symmetrical chest rise and fall, rate and work of breathing (eg, retractions, flaring, and grunting), accessory muscle use, skin color, and tracheal deviation. Cyanosis can be a late finding in children owing to their relative anemia; pulse oximetry determination is highly desirable. Note mental status.

Listen for adventitious breath sounds such as wheezing. Auscultate for air entry, symmetry of breath sounds, and rales. *Feel* for subcutaneous crepitus.

If spontaneous breathing is inadequate, initiate positive-pressure ventilation with bag–mask ventilation and 100% oxygen and coordinate bagging with the patient's efforts, if present. Adequacy of ventilation is reflected in adequate chest movement and auscultation of good air entry bilaterally. If the chest does not rise and fall easily with bagging, reposition the airway as previously described. Perform airway foreign body extraction maneuvers if the airway remains obstructed, including visualizing the airway with a laryngoscope and using Magill forceps. The presence of asymmetrical breath sounds in a child in cardiac arrest or in severe distress suggests pneumothorax and is an indication for needle thoracostomy. In small children, the transmission of breath sounds throughout the chest may impair the ability to auscultate the presence of a pneumothorax. Bag–mask ventilation is effective in the *vast* majority of cases.

Note: Effective oxygenation and ventilation are the keys to successful resuscitation.

Using cricoid pressure (Sellick maneuver) during all positive-pressure ventilation, intubate the trachea in

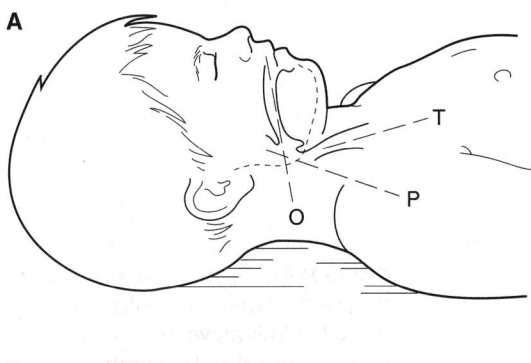

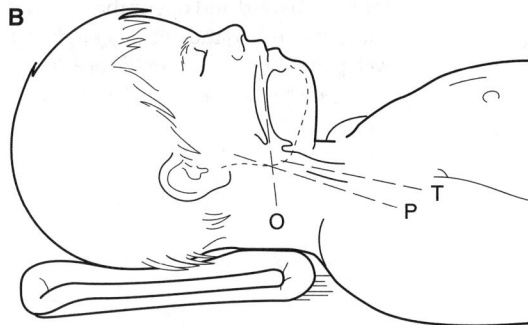

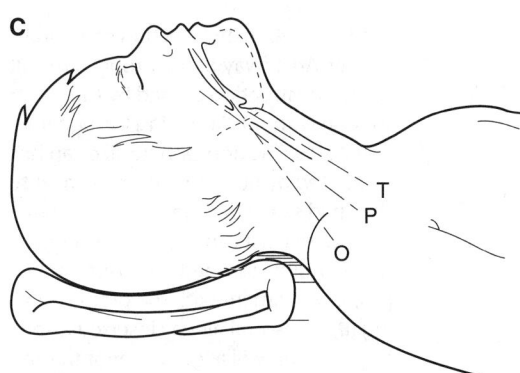

Figure 11–2. Correct positioning of the child older than 2 years of age for ventilation and tracheal intubation. **A:** With the patient on a flat surface (eg, bed or table), the oral (O), pharyngeal (P), and tracheal (T) axes pass through three divergent planes. **B:** A folded sheet or towel placed under the occiput of the head aligns the pharyngeal and tracheal axes. **C:** Extension of the atlanto-occipital joint results in alignment of the oral, pharyngeal, and tracheal axes. (Reproduced, with permission, from *Textbook of Pediatric Life Support.* American Heart Association, 1997.)

patients unresponsive to bag–mask ventilation, those in coma, those who require airway protection, or those who will require prolonged ventilation. Cricothyroidotomy is rarely necessary. Advanced airway management techniques are described in the references accompanying this section. (See also Approach to the Pediatric Trauma Patient section.)

Circulation

The diagnosis of shock can and should be made by clinical examination, and must be done rapidly. Clinical assessments A–F aid in assessing perfusion.

A. PULSES

Check adequacy of peripheral pulses. Pulses become weak and thready only with severe hypovolemia. Compare peripheral pulses to central pulses.

B. HEART RATE

Compare with age-specific norms. Tachycardia can be a nonspecific sign of distress; bradycardia for age is a pre-arrest sign and necessitates aggressive resuscitation.

C. EXTREMITIES

As shock progresses, extremities become cooler, from distal to proximal. A child whose extremities are cool distal to the elbows and knees is in severe shock.

D. CAPILLARY REFILL TIME

This is an important indicator of perfusion; longer than 2 seconds is abnormal unless the child is cold.

E. MENTAL STATUS

Hypoxia, hypercapnia, or ischemia will result in altered mental status. Other important treatable conditions may also result in altered mental status, such as intracranial hemorrhage, meningitis, and hypoglycemia.

F. SKIN COLOR

Pallor, gray, mottled, or ashen skin colors all indicate compromised circulatory status.

G. BLOOD PRESSURE

It is important to remember that shock (inadequate perfusion of vital organs) may be present before the blood pressure falls below the normal limits for age. As intravascular volume falls, peripheral vascular resistance increases. Blood pressure is maintained until there is 35–40% depletion of blood volume, followed by precipitous and often irreversible deterioration (Figure 11–6). Shock that occurs with any signs of decreased perfusion but normal blood pressure is **compensated** shock. When blood pressure also falls, **decompensated** shock is present. Blood pressure determination should be done

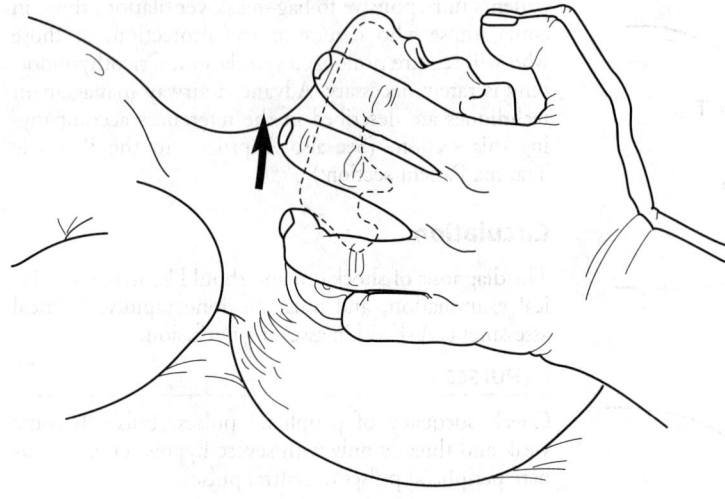

Figure 11–3. Opening the airway with the jaw thrust. Lift the angles of the mandible. This moves the jaw and tongue forward and opens the airway **without bending the neck.** (Reproduced, with permission, from *Textbook of Pediatric Life Support*. American Heart Association, 1997.)

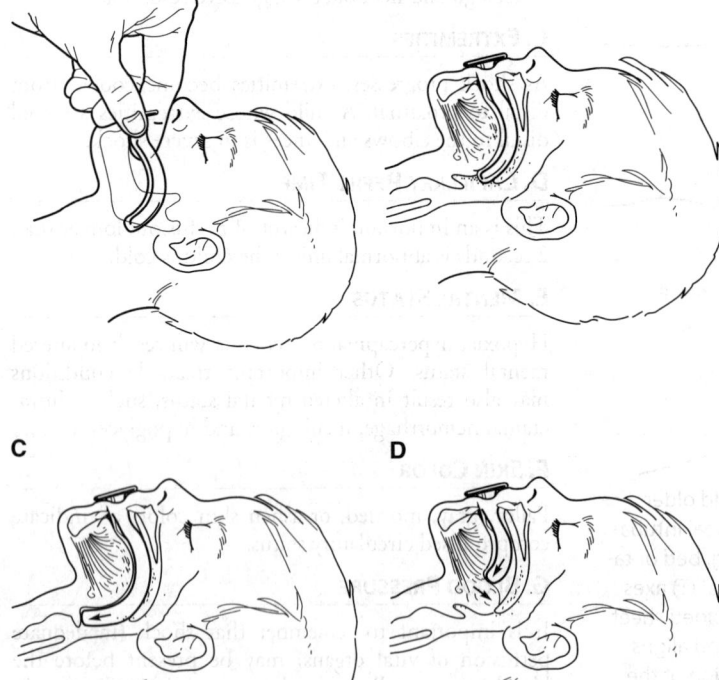

Figure 11–4. A–D: Selection of an oral airway. An airway of the proper size will relieve obstruction caused by the tongue without damaging laryngeal structures. The appropriate size can be estimated by holding the airway next to the child's face (**A**). The tip of the airway should end just cephalad to the angle of the mandible (dashed line), resulting in proper alignment with the glottic opening (**B**). If the oral airway inserted is too large, the tip will align posterior to the angle of the mandible (**C**) and obstruct the glottic opening by pushing the epiglottis down (arrow). If the oral airway is too small, the tip will align well above the angle of the mandible (**D**) and exacerbate airway obstruction by pushing the tongue into the hypopharynx (arrows). (Adapted, with permission, from *Textbook of Pediatric Life Support*. American Heart Association, 1997.)

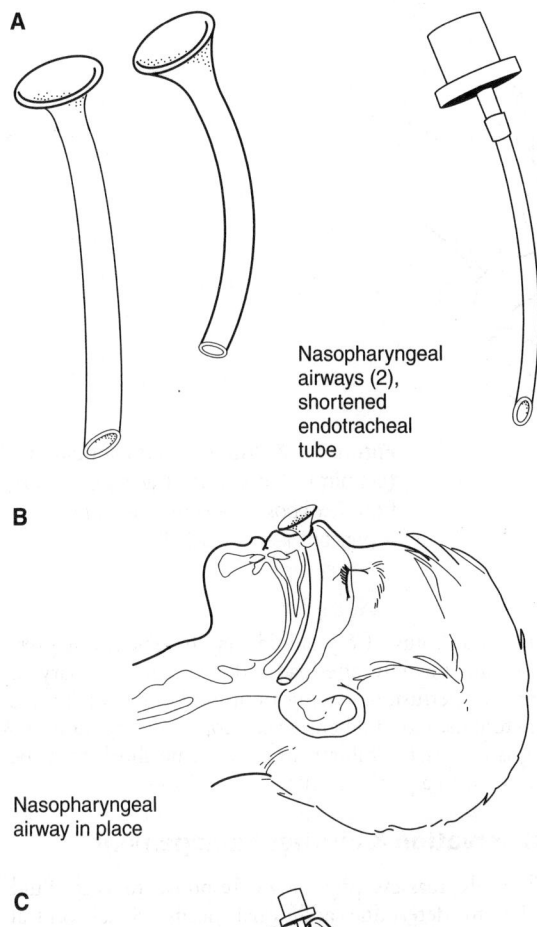

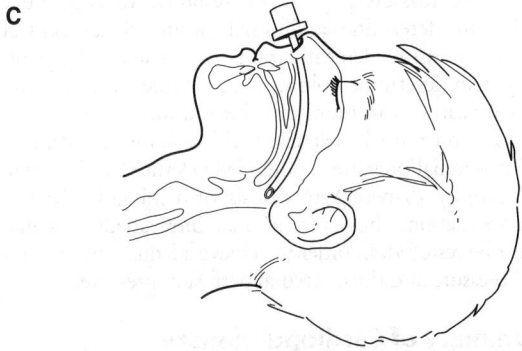

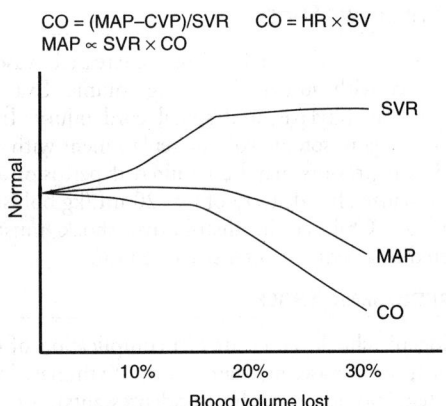

manually, using an appropriately sized cuff, because automated machines can give erroneous readings in children.

MANAGEMENT OF SHOCK

Intravenous (IV) access is essential but can be difficult to establish in children with shock. Peripheral access, especially the antecubital veins, should be attempted first, but central cannulation should follow quickly if peripheral access is unsuccessful. Alternatives are percutaneous cannulation of femoral, subclavian, or internal or external jugular veins; cutdown at antecubital, femoral, or saphenous sites; or intraosseous (IO) lines (Figure 11–7). Consider IO needle placement in any severely ill child when venous access cannot be established rapidly. Decisions on more invasive access should be based on individual expertise as well as urgency of obtaining access. Use short, wide-bore catheters to allow maximal flow rates. Two IV lines should be started in severely ill children. In newborns, the umbilical veins may be cannulated. Consider arterial access if beat-to-beat monitoring or frequent laboratory tests will be needed.

Differentiation of Shock States & Initial Therapy

Therapy for inadequate circulation is determined by the cause of circulatory failure.

A. HYPOVOLEMIC SHOCK

The most common type of shock in the pediatric population is hypovolemia. Frequent causes include dehydration,

Figure 11–5. **A:** Nasopharyngeal airways. A shortened tracheal tube may be substituted (to reduce resistance). **B:** Placement of a nasopharyngeal airway. **C:** Shortened (cut) tracheal tube used as a nasopharyngeal airway. Note that the standard 15-mm adapter must be firmly reinserted into the tracheal tube. (Reproduced, with permission, from *Textbook of Pediatric Life Support.* American Heart Association, 1997.)

Figure 11–6. Model for cardiovascular response to hypovolemia from hemorrhage (based on normative data). (Reproduced, with permission, from *Pediatric Advanced Life Support Provider Manual.* American Heart Association, 2002.)

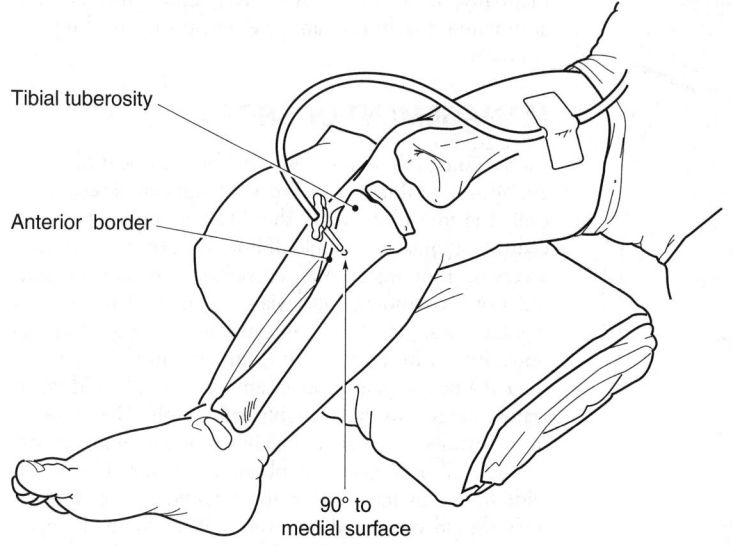

Tibial tuberosity

Anterior border

90° to
medial surface

Figure 11–7. Interosseous cannulation technique. (Reproduced, with permission, from *Textbook of Pediatric Life Support.* American Heart Association, 1997.)

diabetes, heat illness, hemorrhage, and burns. Normal saline or lactated Ringer solution (isotonic crystalloid) is given as initial therapy. Give 20 mL/kg body weight, repeated as necessary, with frequent reassessments, until perfusion normalizes. Children tolerate large volumes of fluid replacement. Typically, in hypovolemic shock, no more than 50 mL/kg is needed, but more may be required if ongoing losses are severe. Appropriate monitoring and reassessment will guide your therapy. Packed red blood cell transfusion is indicated in trauma patients not responding to two boluses of crystalloid solution. Pressors are not required in simple hypovolemic states.

B. DISTRIBUTIVE SHOCK

Distributive shock results from increased vascular capacitance with normal circulating volume. Examples are sepsis, anaphylaxis, and spinal cord injury. Initial therapy is again isotonic volume replacement with crystalloid, but pressors may be required if perfusion does not normalize after delivery of two 20 mL/kg boluses of crystalloid. Children in distributive shock must be admitted to a pediatric intensive care unit.

C. CARDIOGENIC SHOCK

Cardiogenic shock can occur as a complication of congenital heart disease, myocarditis, dysrhythmias, ingestions (eg, clonidine, cyclic antidepressants), or as a complication of prolonged shock due to any cause. The diagnosis is suggested by any of the following signs: abnormal cardiac rhythm, distended neck veins, rales, abnormal heart sounds such as an S_3 or S_4, friction rub, narrow pulse pressure, or hepatomegaly. Chest radiographs may show cardiomegaly and pulmonary edema.

An initial bolus of crystalloid may be given, but pressors, and possibly afterload reducers, are necessary to improve perfusion. Giving multiple boluses of fluid is deleterious. Comprehensive cardiopulmonary monitoring is essential. Children in cardiogenic shock must be admitted to a pediatric intensive care unit.

Observation & Further Management

Clinically reassess physiologic response to each fluid bolus to determine additional needs. Serial central venous pressure determinations or a chest radiograph may help determine volume status. Place an indwelling urinary catheter to monitor urine output.

Caution must be exercised with volume replacement if intracranial pressure is potentially elevated, as in severe head injury, diabetic ketoacidosis, or meningitis. Even in such situations, however, normal intravascular volume must be restored, in order to achieve adequate mean arterial pressure and thus, cerebral perfusion pressure.

Summary of Cardiopulmonary Resuscitation

Assess the ABCs in sequential fashion and, before assessing the next system, immediately intervene if physiologic derangement is detected. It is essential that each system be reassessed after each intervention to ensure improvement and prevent failure to recognize clinical deterioration.

Gausche-Hill M, Fuchs S: *APLS: The Pediatric Emergency Medicine Resource.* American College of Emergency Physicians/American Academy of Pediatrics, 2004.

Table 11–1. Emergency drugs that can be given by endotracheal tube.

Lidocaine
Epinephrine
Atropine
Naloxone

http://www.aap.org/apls/aplsmain.htm

Hazinski MF et al (editors): *PALS Provider Manual.* American Heart Association, 2002.

McNiece WL, Dierdorf SF: The pediatric airway. Semin Pediatr Surg 2004;13(3):152 [PMID: 15272423].

EMERGENCY PEDIATRIC DRUGS

Though careful attention to airway and breathing remains the mainstay of pediatric resuscitation, medications are often needed. Rapid delivery to the central circulation, which can be via peripheral IV catheter, is essential. Infuse medications close to the catheter's hub and flush in with saline to achieve the most rapid systemic effects. If no IV or IO access is achievable, some drugs may be given by endotracheal tube (Table 11–1). The use of length-based emergency measuring tapes that contain preprinted drug dosages, equipment sizes, and IV fluid amounts (Broselow tapes) or preprinted resuscitation drug charts is much more accurate than estimation formulas and helps minimize dosing errors. Selected emergency drugs used in pediatrics are summarized in Table 11–2.

APPROACH TO THE SERIOUSLY ILL CHILD

An unstable patient may present with a known diagnosis (asthma with status asthmaticus and respiratory failure; complications of known congenital heart disease) or in cardiorespiratory failure of unknown cause. The initial approach must rapidly identify and reverse life-threatening conditions. Children with chronic disease may present with an acute exacerbation or secondary to a new, unrelated problem.

Preparation for Emergency Management

Resuscitation occurs simultaneously at two levels: rapid cardiopulmonary assessment, with indicated stabilizing measures, while venous access is gained and cardiopulmonary monitoring initiated. The technique of accomplishing these concurrent goals is outlined as follows:

A. If advance notice of the patient's arrival has been received, prepare a resuscitation room and summon appropriate personnel as needed, such as a neurosurgeon for an unresponsive child after severe head injury or a radiology technician for imaging studies.

B. Assign team responsibilities, including a team leader plus others designated to manage the airway, perform chest compressions, achieve access, draw blood for laboratory studies, place monitors, gather additional historical data, and provide family support. The team approach is invaluable.

C. Age-appropriate equipment (including laryngoscope blade, endotracheal tubes, naso- or orogastric tubes, IV lines, and an indwelling urinary catheter) and monitors (cardiorespiratory monitor, pulse oximeter, and appropriate blood pressure cuff) should be assembled and readily available. Use a length-based emergency tape if available. See Table 11–3 for sizes.

Reception & Assessment

Upon patient arrival, the team leader begins a rapid assessment as team members perform their preassigned tasks. If the patient is received from prehospital care providers, careful attention must be paid to their report, which contains information that they alone have observed. Interventions and medications should be ordered only by the team leader to avoid confusion. The leader should refrain from personally performing procedures, which may distract him or her from optimal direction of the resuscitation. A complete timed record should be kept of events, including medications, interventions, and response to intervention.

A. ALL CASES

In addition to cardiac compressions and ventilation, ensure that the following are instituted:

1. 100% high-flow oxygen.
2. Cardiorespiratory monitoring, pulse oximetry, and end-tidal CO_2 if the patient is intubated.
3. Vascular (peripheral, IO, or central) access. Two lines preferred.
4. Blood drawn and sent. Bedside blood glucose determination is essential.
5. Full vital signs.
6. Clothes removed.
7. Foley catheter and naso- or orogastric tube inserted.
8. Complete history.
9. Notify needed consultants.
10. Family support.
11. Consider law enforcement/security activation and emergency unit lockdown for cases involving potential terrorism, gang violence, or threats to staff or family.

B. AS APPROPRIATE

1. Immobilize neck.
2. Obtain chest radiograph (line and tube placement).
3. Insert central venous pressure and arterial line.

Table 11–2. Emergency pediatric drugs.

Drug	Indications	Dosage and Route	Comment
Atropine	1. Bradycardia, especially cardiac in origin 2. Vagally mediated bradycardia, eg, during laryngoscopy and intubation 3. Anticholinesterase poisoning	0.01–0.02 mg/kg (minimum, 0.1 mg; maximum, 2 mg) IV, IO, ET. May repeat every 5 min.	Atropine may be useful in hemodynamically significant primary cardiac-based bradycardias. Because of paradoxic bradycardia sometimes seen in infants, a minimum dose of 0.1 mg is recommended by the American Heart Association. Epinephrine is the first-line drug in pediatrics for bradycardia caused by hypoxia or ischemia.
Bicarbonate	1. Documented metabolic acidosis 2. Hyperkalemia	1 mEq/kg IV or IO; by arterial blood gas: $0.3 \times$ kg $\times$ base deficit. May repeat every 5 min.	Infuse slowly. Sodium bicarbonate will be effective only if the patient is adequately oxygenated, ventilated, and perfused. Some adverse side effects.
Calcium chloride 10%	1. Documented hypocalcemia 2. Calcium channel blocker overdose 3. Hyperkalemia, hypermagnesemia	10–30 mg/kg slowly IV, preferably centrally, or IO with caution.	Calcium is no longer indicated for asystole. Potent tissue necrosis results if infiltration occurs. Use with caution.
Epinephrine	1. Bradycardia, especially hypoxic–ischemic 2. Hypotension (by infusion) 3. Asystole 4. Fine ventricular fibrillation refractory to initial defibrillation 5. Pulseless electrical activity 6. Anaphylaxis	Bradycardia and first dose in arrests: 0.01 mg/kg of 1:10,000 solution IV or IO. Second and subsequent doses in arrests: 0.1–0.2 mg/kg of 1:1000 solution IV or IO. Repeat every 3–5 min. ET: 10x intended IV dose SC: 0.01 mg/kg of 1:1000 solution (= 0.01 mL/kg) (anaphylactic shock). Maximum dose: 0.3–0.5 mL. Constant infusion by IV drip: 0.1–1 µg/kg/min.	Epinephrine is the single most important drug in pediatric resuscitation. Evidence from animal studies and small series of human subjects indicates that the present recommended dose may be insufficient, and some clinicians use doses of 0.1–0.3 mg/kg IV. A randomized controlled trial has not been done.
Glucose	1. Hypoglycemia 2. Altered mental status (empirical) 3. With insulin, for hyperkalemia	0.5–1 g/kg IV or, IO. May repeat as necessary.	Neonates: 1 mL/kg $D_{10}W$. Older children: 2–4 mL/kg $D_{25}W$, 6–10 mL/kg $D_{10}W$.
Naloxone	1. Opioid overdose 2. Altered mental status (empirical)	0.1 mg/kg IV, IO, or ET; maximum dose, 2 mg. May repeat as necessary.	Side effects are few. A dose of 2 mg may be given in young children. Repeat as necessary, or give as constant infusion in opioid overdoses.

ET, endotracheally, IO, intraosseously, IV, intravenously, SC, subcutaneously.

Table 11–3. Equipment sizes and estimated weight by age.

Age (years)	Weight (kg)	Endotracheal Tube Size (mm)[a]	Laryngoscope Blade (Size)	Chest Tube (Fr)	Foley (Fr)
Premature	1–2.5	2.5 uncuffed	0	8	5
Term newborn	3	3.0	0–1	10	8
1	10	3.5–4.0	1	18	8
2	12	4.5	1	18	10
3	14	4.5	1	20	10
4	16	5.0	2	22	10
5	18	5.0–5.5	2	24	10
6	20	5.5	2	26	12
7	22	5.5–6.0	2	26	12
8	24	6.0 cuffed	2	28	14
10	32	6.0–6.5 cuffed	2–3	30	14
Adolescent	50	7.0 cuffed	3	36	14
Adult	70	8.0 cuffed	3	40	14

[a]Internal diameter.

Brown K, Bocock J: Update in pediatric resuscitation. Emerg Med Clin North Am 2002;20(1):1 [PMID: 11826630].

Parker M et al: Pediatric considerations. Crit Care Med 2004; 32(11 Suppl):S591 [PMID: 15542968].

APPROACH TO THE PEDIATRIC TRAUMA PATIENT

Injuries, including motor vehicle crashes, falls, burns, and immersions, account for the greatest number of deaths among children older than age 1 year. All providers of pediatric care must be cognizant of this sobering statistic. Cooperative efforts between injury prevention specialists, prehospital providers, and emergency, critical care and rehabilitation physicians and nurses will help reduce these terrible losses.

A team approach to the severely injured child, using assigned roles as outlined in the preceding section, will optimize outcomes. A calm atmosphere in the receiving area will contribute to thoughtful care. Conscious children are terribly frightened by serious injury; reassurance can help alleviate anxiety. Analgesia and sedation must be given to stable patients. It is unconscionable to let children suffer pain needlessly. Treat pain expeditiously with oral or parenteral analgesics with ongoing monitoring. Parents are often anxious, angry or guilty, requiring ongoing support from staff, social workers, or child life workers (therapists knowledgeable about child development). To provide optimal multidisciplinary care, regional pediatric trauma centers provide dedicated teams of pediatric specialists in emergency pediatrics, trauma surgery, orthopedics, neurosurgery, and critical care. Most children with severe injuries are not seen in these centers. Primary care providers must be able to provide initial assessment and stabilization of the child with life-threatening injuries before transport to a verified pediatric trauma center.

Mechanism of Injury

Document the time of occurrence, the type of energy transfer (eg, hit by a car, rapid deceleration), secondary impacts (if the child was thrown by the initial impact), appearance of the child at the scene, interventions performed, and clinical condition during transport. The report of emergency service personnel is invaluable. Forward all of this information with the patient to the referral facility if secondary transport occurs.

Trauma in children is predominantly blunt, with penetrating trauma occurring in 10% of cases. Head and abdominal injuries are particularly common and important.

Initial Assessment & Management

The vast majority of children who reach a hospital alive survive to discharge. As most deaths from trauma in children are due to head injuries, cerebral resuscitation must be the foremost consideration when treating children with serious injuries. The ultimate measure of outcome is the child's eventual level of functioning. Strict attention to the ABCs ensures optimal oxygenation, ventilation, and perfusion, and ultimately, cerebral perfusion.

The primary and secondary survey is a method for evaluating and treating injured patients in a systematic way that provides a rapid assessment and stabilization phase, followed by a head-to-toe examination and definitive care phase.

PRIMARY SURVEY

The primary survey is designed to immediately identify and treat all physiologic derangements resulting from trauma. It is the resuscitation phase. Priorities are still airway, breathing, and circulation, but with important further considerations in the trauma setting:

Airway, with cervical spine control

Breathing

Circulation, with hemorrhage control

Disability (neurologic deficit)

Exposure (maintain a warm *Environment*, undress the patient completely, and *Examine*)

Evaluation and treatment of the ABCs are discussed earlier in this chapter. Modifications in the trauma setting are added in the sections that follow.

Airway

Failure to manage the airway appropriately is the most common cause of **preventable** morbidity and death. Administer 100% high-flow oxygen to all patients. During assessment and management of the airway, provide cervical spine protection, initially by manual in-line immobilization, not traction. A hard cervical spine collar is then applied. The head and body are secured to a backboard, surrounded by a lightweight means of cushioning (eg, rolled blankets) to further immobilize the head and body and allow log-rolling of the child in case of vomiting. Assess the airway for patency. Use jaw thrust rather than chin lift during intubation to avoid flexion or extension of the neck. Suction the mouth and pharynx free of blood, foreign material, or secretions, and remove loose teeth. Insert an oropharyngeal airway if upper airway noises are heard or obstruction from posterior prolapse of the tongue occurs. A child with a depressed level of consciousness, a need for prolonged ventilation or hyperventilation, or operative intervention requires endotracheal intubation after bag–mask preoxygenation. Orotracheal intubation is the route of choice and is possible without cervical spine manipula-

tion. Nasotracheal intubation may be possible in children 12 years of age or older who have spontaneous respirations—if not contraindicated by midfacial injury with the possibility of cribriform plate disruption. Rarely, if tracheal intubation cannot be accomplished—particularly in the setting of massive facial trauma—cricothyroidotomy may be necessary. Needle cricothyroidotomy using a large-bore catheter through the cricothyroid membrane is the procedure of choice in patients younger than age 12 years. Operative revision will be needed for formal controlled tracheostomy.

Breathing

Most ventilatory problems are resolved adequately by the airway maneuvers described earlier in this chapter and by positive-pressure ventilation. Breathing assessment is as described previously: Assess for an adequate rate and for symmetrical chest rise, work of breathing, color, tracheal deviation, crepitus, flail segments, deformity, or penetrating wounds. Sources of traumatic pulmonary compromise include pneumothorax, hemothorax, pulmonary contusion, flail chest, and central nervous system (CNS) depression. Asymmetrical breath sounds, particularly with concurrent tracheal deviation, cyanosis, or bradycardia, suggest pneumothorax, possibly under tension. To evacuate a tension pneumothorax, insert a large-bore catheter-over-needle assembly attached to a syringe through the second intercostal space in the midclavicular line into the pleural cavity and withdraw air. If a pneumothorax or hemothorax is present, place a chest tube in the fourth intercostal space in the anterior axillary line. Connect to water seal. Insertion should be over the rib to avoid the neurovascular bundle that runs below the rib margin. Open pneumothoraces can be treated temporarily by taping petrolatum-impregnated gauze on three sides over the wound, creating a flap valve.

Circulation

After airway and breathing interventions have begun, hemodynamic status may be addressed. Ongoing hemorrhage, external or internal, gives pediatric trauma some of its anxiety-provoking character. During the assessment of circulation, IV access should be achieved, preferably at two sites. If peripheral access is not readily available, a central line, cutdown, or IO line is established. A cardiorespiratory monitor and oximeter should be applied early in the resuscitation. Peripheral perfusion and blood pressure should be assessed and recorded at frequent intervals. Determine hematocrit, blood type and cross-match, and serum amylase. Consider blood and urine toxicologic screening.

External hemorrhage can be controlled by direct pressure. To avoid damage to adjacent neurovascular structures, avoid placing hemostats on vessels, except in the scalp.

Determination of the site of internal hemorrhage can be challenging. Sites include the chest, abdomen, retroperitoneum, pelvis, and thighs. Bleeding into the intracranial vault rarely causes shock in children except in infants. Evaluation by an experienced clinician with adjunctive computed tomography (CT) or ultrasound will localize the site of internal bleeding.

Suspect cardiac tamponade after penetrating or blunt injuries to the chest if shock, pulseless electrical activity, narrowed pulse pressure, distended neck veins, hepatomegaly, or muffled heart sounds are present. Ultrasound may be diagnostic if readily available. Diagnose and treat with pericardiocentesis and rapid volume infusion.

Treat signs of poor perfusion vigorously: A tachycardic child with a capillary refill time of 3 seconds, or other evidence of diminished perfusion, is in *shock* and is sustaining vital organ insults. Remember that hypotension is a late finding. Volume replacement is initially accomplished by rapid infusion of normal saline or lactated Ringer solution at 20 mL/kg of body weight, followed by 10 mL/kg of packed red blood cells if perfusion does not normalize after two crystalloid bolus infusions.

Rapid reassessment must follow each bolus. If clinical signs of perfusion have not normalized, repeat the bolus. Lack of response or later/recurring signs of hypovolemia suggest the need for blood transfusion and possible surgical exploration. For every milliliter of external blood loss 3 mL of crystalloid solution should be administered.

A common problem is the brain-injured child who is at risk for intracranial hypertension and who is also hypovolemic. In such cases, circulating volume must be restored to ensure adequate cerebral perfusion; therefore, fluid replacement is required until perfusion normalizes. Thereafter provide maintenance fluids with careful serial reassessments. **Do not restrict fluids** for children with head injuries.

Disability–Neurologic Deficit

Assess pupillary size and reaction to light and the level of consciousness. The level of consciousness can be reproducibly characterized by the AVPU system (Table 11–4). Pediatric Glasgow Coma Scale assessments can be done as part of the secondary survey (Table 11–5).

Exposure and Environment

Significant injuries can be missed unless the child is completely undressed and examined fully, front and back. Cutting away clothing can minimize movement. Because of their high ratio of surface area to body mass, infants and children cool rapidly. Because hypothermia compromises outcome except with isolated head injuries, it is necessary to continuously monitor the body temperature and to use warming techniques vigorously as necessary. Hyperthermia

Table 11–4. AVPU system for evaluation of level of consciousness.

A	Alert
V	Responsive to Voice
P	Responsive to Pain
U	Unresponsive

can adversely affect outcomes in children with acute brain injuries, so maintain normal body temperatures.

Monitoring

Cardiopulmonary monitors, pulse oximetry, and end-tidal CO_2 monitors should be put in place immediately. At the completion of the primary survey, additional "tubes" should be placed.

A. NASOGASTRIC OR OROGASTRIC TUBE

Children's stomachs should be assumed to be full, and gastric distention from positive-pressure ventilation increases the chance of vomiting and aspiration. The nasogastric route should be avoided in patients with significant midface injuries.

B. URINARY CATHETER

An indwelling urinary bladder catheter should be placed to monitor urine output. Contraindications are based on the risk of urethral transection; signs include blood at the

Table 11–5. Glasgow Coma Scale.[a]

Eye opening response	
Spontaneous	4
To speech	3
To pain	2
None	1
Verbal response	
Oriented	5
Confused conversation	4
Inappropriate words	3
Incomprehensible sounds	2
None	1
Best upper limb motor response	
Obeys	6
Localizes	5
Withdraws	4
Flexion in response to pain	3
Extension in response to pain	2
None	1

[a]The appropriate number from each section is added to total between 3 and 15. A score less than 8 usually indicates central nervous system depression requiring positive pressure ventilation.

meatus or in the scrotum or a displaced prostate detected on rectal examination. Urine should be tested for blood. Urine output should exceed 1 mL/kg/h.

SECONDARY SURVEY

After the resuscitation phase, a head-to-toe examination should be performed to reveal all injuries and determine priorities for definitive care.

Skin

Search for lacerations, hematomas, swelling, and abrasions. Remove foreign material, and cleanse as necessary. Cutaneous findings may indicate underlying pathology (eg, a flank hematoma overlying a renal contusion), although surface signs may be absent even with significant internal injury. Make certain the child's tetanus immunization status is current. Consider tetanus immune globulin for incompletely immunized children.

Head

Check for hemotympanum and for clear or bloody cerebrospinal fluid leak from the nares. Battle sign (hematoma over the mastoid) and raccoon eyes are late signs of basilar skull fracture. Explore wounds, evaluating for foreign bodies and defects in galea or skull. CT scan of the head is an integral part of evaluation for altered level of consciousness, post-traumatic seizure, or focal neurologic findings (see Head Injury section). Pneumococcal vaccine is indicated for basilar skull fractures.

Spine

Cervical spine injury must be excluded in all children. This can be done clinically in children with normal neurologic findings on examination (including voluntary movement of all extremities) who are able to deny midline neck pain or midline tenderness on palpation of the neck and who have no other painful injuries that might obscure the pain of a cervical spine injury. If radiographs are indicated, a cross-table lateral neck view is obtained initially, followed by anteroposterior, odontoid, and in some cases, oblique views. Normal studies do not exclude significant injury, either bony or ligamentous, or involving the spinal cord itself. Therefore, an obtunded child should be maintained in cervical spine immobilization until the child has awakened and an appropriate neurologic examination can be performed. The entire thoracolumbar spine must be palpated and areas of pain or tenderness examined by radiography.

Chest

Pneumothoraces are detected and decompressed during the primary survey. Hemothoraces can occur with rib fractures or with injury to intercostal vessels, large pulmonary vessels, or lung parenchyma. Tracheobronchial disruption is suggested by large continued air leak despite chest tube decompression. Pulmonary contusions may require ventilatory support. Myocardial contusions and aortic injuries are unusual in children.

Abdomen

Blunt abdominal injury is common in multisystem injuries. Significant injury may exist without cutaneous signs or instability of vital signs. Tenderness, guarding, distention, diminished or absent bowel sounds, or poor perfusion mandates immediate evaluation by a pediatric trauma surgeon. Injury to solid viscera frequently can be managed nonoperatively in stable patients; however, intestinal perforation or hypotension necessitates operative treatment. Serial examinations, ultrasound, and CT scan provide diagnostic help. Elevated liver function tests have good specificity but only fair sensitivity for hepatic injury. Serum amylase will rise progressively with pancreatic injury, which may not be easily visualized by initial CT.

Pelvis

Pelvic fractures are classically manifested by pain, crepitus, and abnormal motion. Pelvic fracture is a relative contraindication to urethral catheter insertion. Perform a rectal examination, noting tone, tenderness, and in boys, prostate position. Stool should be tested for blood.

Genitourinary System

If urethral transection is suspected (see earlier discussion), perform a urethrogram before catheter placement. Diagnostic imaging of the child with hematuria includes CT scan, or occasionally IV urograms. Management of kidney injury is largely nonoperative except for renal pedicle injuries.

Extremities

Long bone fractures are common but rarely life-threatening. Test for pulses, perfusion, and sensation. Neurovascular compromise requires immediate orthopedic consultation. Delayed diagnosis of fracture may occur when children are comatose; reexamination is necessary to avoid overlooking previously missed fractures.

Central Nervous System

Most deaths in children with multisystem trauma are from head injuries, so optimal neurointensive care is important. Significant injuries include diffuse axonal injury, cerebral edema, subdural, subarachnoid and epidural hematomas, and parenchymal hemorrhages. Spinal cord injury occurs less commonly. A full sensorimotor examination should be performed. Deficits require immediate neurosurgical consultation. Extensor or flexor posturing represents intracranial hypertension, not seizure activity, until proven otherwise, and should be treated with mild hyperventilation ($PaCO_2$ in the mid-30s mm Hg), and adequate but not excessive volume resuscitation. If accompanied by a fixed, dilated pupil a herniation syndrome is present, and hyperventilation should be to a $PaCO_2$ in the mid-20s. Mannitol should be given if perfusion is normal and signs of herniation are present. Normal peripheral perfusion **must** be ensured to optimize cerebral perfusion. Level of consciousness by the AVPU system (see Table 11–4) or Glasgow Coma Scale (see Table 11–5) should be assessed serially. Seizure activity warrants exclusion of significant intracranial injury. In the trauma setting, seizures are frequently treated with fosphenytoin. Acute spinal cord injury may benefit from high-dose methylprednisolone therapy. Corticosteroids are not indicated for head trauma.

American College of Surgeons, Committee on Trauma: *Advanced Trauma Life Support Program for Doctors: ATLS.* American College of Surgeons, 1997.

http://www.facs.org/trauma/atls/information.html

Cirak B et al: Spinal injuries in children. J Pediatr Surg 2004; 39(4):607 [PMID: 15065038].

Gaines BA, Ford HR: Abdominal and pelvic trauma in children. Crit Care Med 2002;30(11 Suppl):S416 [PMID: 12528783].

Hendey GW et al: Spinal cord injury without radiologic abnormality: Results of the National Emergency X-radiography Utilization Study in blunt cervical study. J Trauma 2002;53:1 [PMID: 12131380].

Holmes JF et al: Identification of children with intra-abdominal injuries after blunt trauma. Ann Emerg Med 2002;39:500 [PMID: 11973557].

Tenney-Soeiro R, Wilson C: An update on child abuse and neglect. Curr Opin Pediatr 2004;16(2):233 [PMID: 15021210].

Viccellio P et al: A prospective multicenter study of cervical spine injury in children. Pediatrics 2001;108(2):E20 [PMID: 11483830].

HEAD INJURY

Closed head injuries range in severity from minor asymptomatic trauma without sequelae, to those leading to death. Head injury, including the shaken-baby syndrome, is common in cases of child abuse. Even following minor closed head injury, neuropsychiatric sequelae can occur.

Assessment

The considerations discussed earlier in the Approach to the Pediatric Trauma Patient section apply here as well. The history should include the time and mechanism of injury. How far, and onto what surface, did the child fall? Was there loss of consciousness? Is there antegrade or retrograde amnesia? What have been the child's levels of consciousness and activity since the injury? Has there been vomiting, headache, ataxia, seizures, or visual disturbance?

The physical examination, including a detailed neurologic examination, should be complete and mindful of the mechanism of injury. Look for associated injuries such as mandibular fracture, scalp or skull injury, or cervical spine injury. Cerebrospinal fluid leak from the ears or nose or the later appearance of periorbital hematomas (raccoon eyes) or Battle sign, imply basilar skull fracture, and indicate the need for pneumococcal vaccine. Obtain vital signs and assess the child's level of consciousness by the AVPU system (see Table 11–4) or Glasgow Coma Scale (see Table 11–5), noting irritability or lethargy, pupillary equality, size, and reaction to light, funduscopic examination, reflexes, body posture, and rectal tone. Always consider child abuse; the injuries observed should be consistent with the history and the child's developmental level.

Radiographic studies may be indicated. Plain films are useful only in cases of penetrating head trauma or for assessing depressed skull fractures and ruling out foreign bodies. Major morbidity does not follow from skull fracture per se but rather from the associated intracranial injury. Though a skull fracture can be associated with an increased likelihood of an intracranial injury, CT scan should be performed based on clinical findings in the child with persistent vomiting or an abnormal or lateralizing neurologic examination, including an abnormal mental status that does not quickly return to normal. In infants, a normal neurologic exam does not exclude significant intracranial hemorrhage; in the setting of an appropriate mechanism, and if scalp findings such as large hematomas are found, consider performing CT.

CONCUSSION

A concussion injury is defined as a brief loss or alteration of consciousness followed by a return to normal. Brain tissue is not damaged, and there are no focal findings on detailed neurologic examination. There may be pallor, amnesia, or several episodes of vomiting. Disposition is based on the clinical course and suitability of follow-up. The patient may be discharged when neurologically normal after a period of observation. Parents should closely observe the child at home and return if the child exhibits altered level of consciousness, persistent vomiting, gait disturbances, unequal pupils, seizures, or increasing headache, or if the parents have any concerns.

CONTUSION

A bruise of the brain matter is a contusion. The child's level of consciousness decreases, and focal findings, if any, correspond to the area of the brain that is injured. These patients require CT scan, a period of observation, and consideration of neurorehabilitation follow-up for post-traumatic brain injury sequelae.

DIFFUSE AXONAL INJURY

Diffuse axonal injury is a potentially severe form of traumatic brain injury characterized by coma without focal signs on neurologic examination. No external signs of trauma may be apparent. The initial CT scan is normal or may demonstrate only scattered small areas of cerebral contusion and areas of low density. Prolonged disability may follow diffuse axonal injury.

ACUTE INTRACRANIAL HYPERTENSION

Close observation will detect early signs and symptoms of intracranial pressure elevation. Early recognition is essential to avoid disastrous outcomes. In addition to traumatic causes, intracranial pressure elevation with or without herniation syndromes may be seen in spontaneous intracranial hemorrhage, CNS infection, hydrocephalus, ruptured arteriovenous malformation, metabolic derangement (eg, diabetic ketoacidosis), ventriculoperitoneal shunt obstruction, or tumor. Symptoms include headache, vision changes, vomiting, gait difficulties, and a progressively decreasing level of consciousness. Other signs may include stiff neck, cranial nerve palsies, and progressive hemiparesis. Cushing triad (bradycardia, hypertension, and irregular respirations) is a late and ominous finding. Papilledema is also a late finding. Consider CT scan before lumbar puncture if there is concern about intracranial pressure elevation because of the risk of precipitating herniation. Lumbar puncture should be deferred if the patient is unstable.

Therapy for intracranial pressure elevation must be swift and aggressive. Strict attention to adequate oxygenation, ventilation, and perfusion is paramount. Controlled rapid sequence intubation with appropriate sedation, muscle relaxation, and agents to reduce the intracranial pressure elevation that accompanies intubation is followed by mild hyperventilation ($PaCO_2$ lowered to 35–38 mm Hg) and avoidance of hypoperfusion and hypoxemia. Mannitol (0.5 g/kg intravenously), an osmotic diuretic, will reduce brain water, as will furosemide (0.1–0.2 mg/kg intravenously). These measures may acutely lower intracranial pressure. Fluid infusion and, ultimately, pressors should be used to maintain normal arterial blood pressure and peripheral perfusion, if necessary. Adjunctive measures include elevating the head of the bed 30 degrees, treating hyperpyrexia and pain, and maintaining the head in a midline position. Obtain immediate neurosurgical evaluation. Further details about management of intracranial hypertension (cerebral edema) are presented in Chapter 13.

DISPOSITION FOR CHILDREN WITH CLOSED HEAD INJURY

After a period of observation patients with mild head injury may be discharged with detailed written instructions, if the examination remains normal and parental supervision and follow-up are appropriate. Children with persistent deficits require admission or prolonged observation. In patients responding to voice commands whose mental status is improving gradually over time, observation may be done without further radiographic studies. If mental status deteriorates, however, CT scan and neurosurgical consultation are indicated. If the CT scan is normal and the neurologic findings normalize, these children may be discharged after a period of observation. Patients with severe head injury require cerebral resuscitation, evaluation by a neurosurgeon, and admission to hospital.

Dias MS: Traumatic brain and spinal cord injury. Pediatr Clin North Am 2004;51(2):271 [PMID: 15062672].

Khoshyomn S, Tranmer BI: Diagnosis and management of pediatric closed head injury. Semin Pediatr Surg 2004 May;13(2):80 [PMID: 15362277].

BURNS

Thermal injury is a major cause of accidental death and disfigurement in children. Pain, morbidity, the association with child abuse, and the preventable nature of burns constitute an area of major concern in pediatrics. Common causes include hot water or food, appliances, flames, grills, vehicle-related burns, and curling irons. Burns occur commonly in toddlers—in boys more frequently than in girls.

ELECTRICAL BURNS

Even brief contact with a high-voltage source will result in a contact burn. When an infant or toddler bites an electric cord, burns to the commissure of the lips occur that appear gray and necrotic, with surrounding erythema. If an arc is created with passage of current through the body, the pattern of the thermal injury will depend on the path of the current; therefore, search for an exit wound and internal injuries. Extensive damage to deep tissues may occur. Current traversing the heart may cause nonperfusing arrhythmias. Neurologic effects of electrical burns can be immediate (eg, confusion, disorientation, peripheral nerve injury), delayed (eg, nerve damage in the thrombosed limb after compartment syndrome), or late (eg, impaired concentration or memory).

EVALUATION OF THE BURNED PATIENT

Classification

Burns are classified clinically according to the nature of the burn and the extent and thickness; associated injuries are ascertained in the initial evaluation.

Superficial (first-degree) burns are easily recognized and treated. They are painful, dry, red, and hypersensitive. Sunburn is a common example. Healing occurs with minimal damage to epidermis. Full-thickness (third-degree) burns affect all epidermal and dermal elements, leaving devascularized skin. The wound is dry, depressed, leathery in appearance, and without sensation. Unless skin grafting is provided, the scar will be hard, uneven, and fibrotic. Partial-thickness (second-degree) burns are further classified as superficial or deep, depending on appearance and healing time, with each subgroup treated differently. Superficial partial-thickness burns are red and may blister. Deep partial-thickness burns are white and dry, blanch with pressure, and the involved skin has decreased sensitivity to pain.

Management

Management also depends on the depth and extent of injury. Burn extent can be classified as major or minor. Minor burns are less than 10% of the body surface area for superficial and partial-thickness burns, or less than 2% for full-thickness burns. Partial- or full-thickness burns of the hands, feet, face, eyes, ears, and perineum are considered major.

A. SUPERFICIAL AND PARTIAL-THICKNESS BURNS

These injuries can generally be treated in the outpatient setting. It is *mandatory* that effective analgesia be rapidly provided, and redosed as indicated by the child. Oral codeine or parenteral narcotics are indicated. Superficial burns are treated with cool compresses and analgesia. Treatment of partial-thickness burns with blisters consists of antiseptic cleansing, topical antimicrobial coverage, and observation for infection. Blisters appear early in deeper partial-thickness burns and, if open, may be debrided. Alternatively, the blister may be used as a protective flap after cleaning and dressing. After debridement, the wound should be cleansed with dilute (1–5%) povidone–iodine solution, thoroughly washed with normal saline, and covered with topical antibiotic. The wound should be protected with a bulky dressing and reexamined within 24 hours and serially thereafter. Wounds with a potential for causing disfigurement or functional impairment—especially wounds of the hand or digits—should be referred promptly to a burn surgeon. Outpatient analgesia should be provided on discharge.

B. FULL-THICKNESS AND DEEP OR EXTENSIVE PARTIAL-THICKNESS BURNS

Major burns place particular importance on the ABCs of trauma management. Early establishment of an artificial airway is critical with oral or nasal burns because of their association with inhalation injuries and critical airway narrowing.

The protocol for the Primary Survey should be followed. There may be inhalation injury from carbon monoxide, cyanide, or other toxic products. A nasogastric tube and bladder catheter should be placed. The secondary survey should ascertain whether any other injuries are present, including those suggestive of abuse.

Fluid administration is based on several principles. Capillary permeability is markedly increased. Fluid needs are based on examination findings, percentage of body surface area burned, depth, and age. Maintaining normal intravascular pressure and replacing fluid losses are essential. Figure 11–8 shows percentages of body surface area by body part in infants and children. The Parkland formula for fluid therapy is 4 mL/kg/% body surface area burned for the first 24 hours, with half in the first 8 hours, **in addition to maintenance rates.** Acutely, however, fluid resuscitation should be based on clinical assessment of volume status.

Indications for admission include major burns as previously defined, uncertainty of follow-up, suspicion of abuse, presence of upper airway injury, explosion, inhalation, electrical or chemical burns, burns associated with fractures or the need for parenteral pain control. Children with chronic metabolic or connective tissue diseases and infants deserve hospitalization.

Foglia RP et al: Evolving treatment in a decade of pediatric burn care. J Pediatr Surg 2004;39:957 [PMID: 15185233].

Procedural Sedation and Analgesia (PSA)

Relief of pain and anxiety are paramount concepts in the provision of acute care pediatrics, and should be considered at all times. Many agents also have amnestic properties. Parenteral agents can be effective and safe and produce few side effects if used judiciously.

Conditions such as fracture reduction, laceration repair, burn care, sexual assault examinations, lumbar puncture, and diagnostic procedures such as CT and magnetic resonance imaging may all be performed more effectively and compassionately if effective sedation or analgesia is used. The clinician should decide whether procedures will require either sedation or analgesia alone, or both, and then choose agents accordingly.

Safe and effective sedation requires thorough knowledge of the selected agent and its side effects, as well as suitable monitoring devices, resuscitative medications, equipment, and personnel. Appropriate informed con-

Infant Less Than One Year of Age

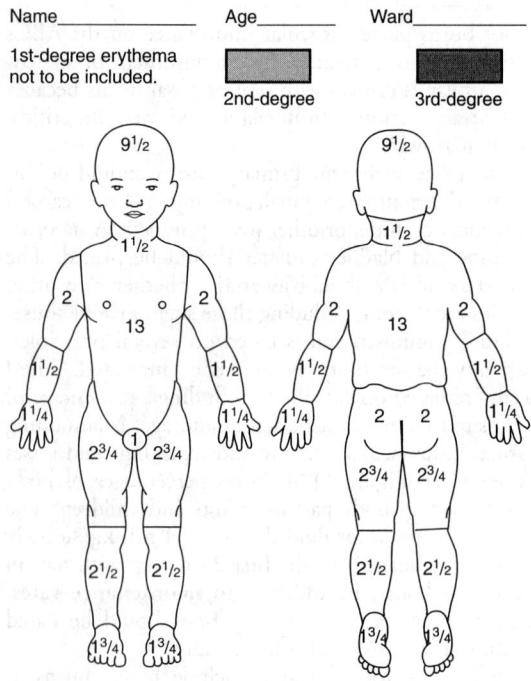

Name_____ Age_____ Ward_____

1st-degree erythema not to be included.

2nd-degree

3rd-degree

Variations From Adult Distribution in Infants and Children (in Percent).

	New-born	1 Year	5 Years	10 Years
Head	19	17	13	11
Both thighs	11	13	16	17
Both lower legs	10	10	11	12
Neck	2			
Anterior trunk	13			
Posterior trunk	13			
Both upper arms	8		These percentages	
Both lower arms	6		remain constant at	
Both hands	5		all ages	
Both buttocks	6			
Both feet	7			
Genitalia	1			
	100			

Figure 11–8. Lund and Browder modification of Berkow scale for estimating extent of burns. (The table under the illustration is after Berkow.)

sent from the parents must be obtained. PSA proceeds as follows:

1. Choose the appropriate medication(s).
2. Discuss risks and benefits of the proposed PSA and obtain verbal informed consent from the parents.
3. Ensure appropriate NPO (nothing-by-mouth) status for 4–6 hours. For certain emergency proce-

dures, suboptimal NPO status may be allowed, with attendant risks identified.

4. Establish vascular access as required.
5. Ensure that resuscitative equipment and personnel are readily available.
6. Attach appropriate monitoring devices, as indicated.
7. Give the agent selected, with continuous monitoring for side effects. A dedicated observer, usually a nurse, should monitor the patient at all times. Respiratory effort, perfusion, and mental status should be assessed and documented serially.
8. Titrate the medication to achieve the desired sedation level. The ideal level is that of "conscious" or "light" sedation—that is, the patient's sensorium is slightly dulled, but eyes are generally open and airway reflexes are preserved.
9. Continue monitoring the patient after finishing the procedure. Once a painful stimulus has been corrected, mental status can decrease.
10. Criteria for discharge include the child's ability to sit unassisted, take oral fluids, and answer verbal commands. A PSA discharge handout should be given, with precautions for close observation and avoidance of potentially dangerous activities.

The following are some commonly used sedatives and analgesics:

1. Midazolam—This agent has particular usefulness in pediatrics due to its safety, rapid onset, and short half-life. Administration may be oral, rectal, intranasal, intramuscular, or IV. When given slowly intranasally the drug's kinetics are similar as when given intravenously. Many children report a burning sensation with intranasal administration. Oral or rectal administration results in relatively delayed onset, and titration is difficult. Intramuscular injections can be combined with opioid analgesics if systemic analgesia is desired. IV administration allows optimal ability to titrate dosing to the desired sedation level. Complicated or prolonged procedures are best facilitated by IV placement to facilitate redosing, which also provides IV access if resuscitation becomes necessary. Potential side effects of midazolam include cardiorespiratory depression.

2. Barbiturates—This class of agents (eg, pentobarbital) has the advantage of minimizing movement during procedures, which makes them advantageous for diagnostic studies such as CT or magnetic resonance imaging. Rectal administration of thiopental is safe and effective. Onset of action with IV administration is rapid. Potential side effects, although uncommon, include respiratory and cardiac depression and laryngospasm.

3. Narcotics—Agents such as fentanyl and morphine have powerful analgesic and sedative effects and can be combined with anxiolytics such as benzodiazepines.

Desired and adverse effects, such as respiratory depression, are potentiated when benzodiazepines and narcotics or barbiturates are given together. Therefore, sedative doses should be reduced when sedatives and analgesics are given together.

4. Ketamine—Now commonly used in emergency departments, this agent has the advantage of being a sympathomimetic, thus increasing heart rate and blood pressure. *It also allows the patient to maintain his or her own respiratory drive and airway protective reflexes.* It is a potent analgesic and anxiolytic with amnestic properties. Side effects include salivation (therefore, it is usually given with glycopyrrolate as an antisalivation agent), laryngospasm (rarely), nystagmus, emergence reactions, and vomiting. With comprehensive knowledge of this medication, its use can be a significant advantage to children.

5. Propofol—Propofol is a nonopioid, nonbarbiturate sedative that is highly effective. It is finding increased use as an adjunct to analgesia for painful procedures in the emergency department. Onset of action and recovery are rapid. Side effects include transient hypotension and dose-dependent respiratory depression or apnea. Careful monitoring is essential.

American Academy of Pediatrics, Committee on Drugs: Guidelines for monitoring and management of pediatric patients during and after sedation for diagnostic and therapeutic procedures: An addendum. Pediatrics 2002;110:836 [PMID: 12359805].

Bassett KE et al: Propofol for procedural sedation in children in the emergency department. Ann Emerg Med 2003;42(6):773 [PMID: 14634602].

Bauman BH, McManus JG Jr: Pediatric pain management in the emergency department. Emerg Med Clin North Am 2005; 23(2):393. [PMID: 15829389].

Berde CB, Sethna NF: Analgesics for the treatment of pain in children. N Engl J Med 2002;347:1094 [PMID: 12362012].

Green SM, Krauss B: Clinical practice guideline for emergency department ketamine dissociative sedation in children. Ann Emerg Med 2004;44(5):460. [PMID: 15520705].

Roback MG et al: Adverse events associated with procedural sedation and analgesia in a pediatric emergency department: A comparison of common parenteral drugs. Acad Emerg Med 2005;12(6):508 [PMID: 15930401].

Singer AJ et al: Parents and practitioners are poor judges of young children's pain severity. Acad Emerg Med 2002;9:609 [PMID: 12045074].

DISORDERS DUE TO HIGH ENVIRONMENTAL TEMPERATURE

Heat-related illnesses range from mild cramps to life-threatening heat stroke. Heat *cramps* are characterized by brief, severe cramping (not rigidity) of skeletal or abdominal muscles following exertion. Core body temperature is normal or only slightly elevated. There may be associated relative sodium deficiency. Mild cases can be treated with oral salt-containing solutions; more severe cases require IV infusion of normal saline solution. Heat *exhaustion* is manifested by constitutional symptoms after exposure to heat and humidity. Patients continue to sweat, and core temperature is normal or only slightly increased. Patients with heat exhaustion have varying proportions of salt and water depletion. Presenting symptoms and signs include weakness, fatigue, headache, disorientation, pallor, thirst, nausea and vomiting, and occasionally muscle cramps. Shock may be present. No major CNS dysfunction is present. Treat with IV fluids, guided by serum electrolyte levels. Both heat cramps and heat exhaustion can be prevented by acclimatization and liberal water and salt intake during exercise.

Heat *stroke* represents failure of thermoregulation and is life-threatening. Diagnosis is based on a rectal temperature of over 40° C with associated neurologic signs in a patient with an exposure history. Lack of sweating is **not** a necessary criterion. Symptoms are similar to those of heat exhaustion, but CNS dysfunction is more prominent. Patients with heat stroke are often incoherent and combative. In more severe cases, vomiting, shivering, coma, seizures, nuchal rigidity, and posturing may be present. Cardiac output may be high, low, or normal. Cellular hypoxia, enzyme dysfunction, and disrupted cell membranes lead to global end-organ derangements: rhabdomyolysis, myocardial necrosis, electrolyte abnormalities, acute tubular necrosis and renal failure, hepatic degeneration, adult respiratory distress syndrome, and disseminated intravascular coagulation. Consider sepsis, malignant hyperthermia, and neuroleptic malignant syndrome in the differential diagnosis.

Heat Stroke Management

1. Immediately cool the patient with cool water mist, ice, fans, or other cooling device.

2. Administer 100% oxygen. If patient is unresponsive, manage the airway.

3. Administer IV fluids: isotonic crystalloid for hypotension, 5% dextrose normal saline for maintenance. Consider central venous pressure monitoring.

4. Place monitors, check rectal temperatures continuously, and place a Foley catheter and nasogastric tube.

5. Obtain laboratory tests: complete blood count; electrolytes; glucose; creatinine; prothrombin time and partial thromboplastin time; creatine kinase; liver function tests; arterial blood gases; urinalysis; and serum calcium, magnesium, and phosphate.

6. Admit to pediatric intensive care unit.

Malignant Hyperthermia

Malignant hyperthermia is a rare but life-threatening syndrome characterized by a hypermetabolic state including high fever, diaphoresis, malaise, rhabdomyolysis, disseminated intravascular coagulation, hyperreflexia, and psychosis. Most often associated with anesthetic agents, it can also be seen in the outpatient setting in the neuroleptic-malignant syndrome. Drugs such as atropine, lidocaine, meperidine, nonsteroidal anti-inflammatory agents, tricyclic antidepressants, cocaine, and antipsychotics can induce a central hyperthermic syndrome. Treatment includes cooling, rectal acetaminophen, seizure treatment with a benzodiazepine, and, in the case of malignant hyperthermia caused by neuromuscular blockers, dantrolene sodium.

HYPOTHERMIA

Seriously ill children should have core temperature quickly determined. Hypothermia in children, defined as core body temperature less than 35° C, is frequently associated with cold water submersion incidents. Other disorders cause incidental hypothermia, including sepsis, metabolic derangements, ingestions, CNS disorders, and endocrinopathies. Neonates, trauma victims, intoxicated patients, and the chronically disabled are particularly at risk. Mortality rates are high and are related to the underlying disorder. Conversely, mild therapeutic hypothermia following hypoxic–ischemic CNS insult and isolated traumatic brain injury may be a recommendation in the near future.

As core temperature falls, a variety of mechanisms begin to conserve and produce heat. Peripheral vasoconstriction allows optimal maintenance of core temperature. Heat production can be increased by a hypothalamic-mediated increase in muscle tone and metabolism. Shivering increases heat production to two to four times basal levels.

Clinical Findings

Clinical manifestations of hypothermia vary with severity of body temperature depression. Severe cases (< 28° C) mimic death: Patients are pale or cyanotic, pupils may be fixed and dilated, muscles are rigid, and there may be no palpable pulses. Heart rates as low as 4–6/min may provide adequate perfusion, because of the lowered metabolic needs in severe hypothermia. If these findings are a result of primary hypothermia and not postmortem changes, the fact of death cannot be ascertained until the patient has been rewarmed and remains unresponsive to resuscitative efforts. Children with a core temperature as low as 19° C have survived neurologically intact.

Treatment

A. GENERAL SUPPORTIVE MEASURES

Management of hypothermia is largely supportive. Core body temperature must be continuously documented; monitor with a low-reading indwelling rectal thermometer. Patients must be handled gently, because the hypothermic myocardium is exquisitely sensitive and prone to arrhythmias. Ventricular fibrillation may occur spontane-

ously or as a result of minor handling or invasive procedures. If asystole or ventricular fibrillation is present on the cardiac monitor, perform chest compressions and use standard pediatric advanced life support techniques and medications. Spontaneous reversion to sinus rhythm at 28–30° C may occur as rewarming proceeds.

B. REWARMING

1. Passive rewarming, such as covering with blankets, is appropriate only for mild cases (> 33° C).
2. Active external rewarming methods include warming lights, thermal mattresses or electric warming blankets, immersion in warm baths, and hot water bottles or warmed bags of IV solutions. One must be aware of the potential for core temperature depression after rewarming is begun; vasodilation allows cooler peripheral blood to be distributed to the core circulation.

   Active core rewarming techniques are optimal and include the delivery of warmed, humidified oxygen and the use of warmed (to 40° C) fluids for IV replacement, peritoneal dialysis, and mediastinal lavage. Bladder and bowel irrigation are not generally effective because of low surface areas for temperature exchange. Extracorporeal blood rewarming achieves controlled core rewarming, can stabilize volume and electrolyte disturbances, and is maximally effective (Table 11–6).

Table 11–6. Management of hypothermia.

General measures
Administer warmed and humidified 100% oxygen.
Monitor core temperature, heart and respiratory rates, and blood pressure continuously.
Consider central venous pressure determination for severe hypothermia.

Laboratory studies
Complete blood count and platelets
Serum electrolytes, glucose, creatinine, amylase
Prothrombin time, partial thromboplastin time
Arterial blood gases
Consider toxicology screen

Treatment
Correct hypoxemia, hypercapnia, pH < 7.2, clotting abnormalities, and glucose and electrolyte disturbances.
Start rewarming techniques: passive, active (core and external), depending on degree of hypothermia.
Replace intravascular volume with warmed intravenous crystalloid infusion at 42° C.
Treat asystole and ventricular fibrillation per PALS protocols. Cardiac massage should be continued at least until core temperature reaches 30° C, when defibrillation is more likely to be effective.

PALS, pediatric advanced life support.

SUBMERSION INJURIES

Drowning is the second most common cause of death by unintentional injury among children. Water hazards are ubiquitous and include lakes and streams, swimming pools, bathtubs, and even toilets, buckets, and washing machines. Risk factors include epilepsy, alcohol, and lack of supervision. Males predominate in submersion deaths, as in most other nonintentional deaths. Prevention is paramount.

Major morbidity stems from CNS and pulmonary insult. Laryngospasm or breath-holding may lead to loss of consciousness and cardiovascular collapse before aspiration can occur (dry drowning).

Anoxia from laryngospasm or aspiration leads to irreversible CNS damage after only 4–6 minutes. A child must fall through ice or directly into icy water for cerebral metabolism to be slowed sufficiently by hypothermia to provide protection from anoxic damage.

Cardiovascular changes include myocardial depression and arrhythmias. Electrolyte alterations are generally slight. Unless hemolysis occurs, hemoglobin concentrations also change only slightly.

Assessment & Management

Depending on the duration of submersion and any protective hypothermia effects, children may appear clinically dead or completely normal. Observation over time assists with prognosis. The child who has been rewarmed to at least 33° C, and is still apneic and pulseless, will probably not survive to discharge or will be left with severe neurologic deficits. Until a determination of brain death can be made, however, aggressive resuscitation should be continued in a patient with return of circulation.

One should keep in mind possible associated injuries, including head or neck trauma. For children who appear well initially, observation for 8–12 hours will detect late pulmonary compromise or changes in neurologic status. Respiratory distress, an abnormal chest radiograph, abnormal arterial blood gases, or hypoxemia by pulse oximetry indicates the need for treatment with supplemental oxygen, cardiopulmonary monitoring, and frequent reassessment. Serially assess respiratory distress and mental status. Signs of pulmonary infection may appear many hours after the submersion event.

Patients who are in coma and who require mechanical ventilation have a high risk of anoxic encephalopathy. The value of therapy with hyperventilation, corticosteroids, intentional hypothermia, and barbiturates remains unproved.

BITES: ANIMAL & HUMAN

Bites account for a large number of visits to the emergency department. Most fatalities are due to dog bites. However, the majority of infected bite wounds are from human and cat bites.

DOG BITES

Boys are bitten more frequently than girls, and the dog is known by the victim in most cases. Younger children have a higher incidence of head and neck wounds, whereas school-age children are bitten most often on the upper extremities.

Dog bites are treated similarly to other wounds: high-pressure, high-volume irrigation with normal saline, debridement of any devitalized tissue, removal of foreign matter, and tetanus prophylaxis. The risk of rabies from dogs is low in developed countries, but rabies prophylaxis should be considered when appropriate. Wounds should be sutured only if necessary for cosmetic reasons because wound closure increases the risk of infection. Prophylactic antibiotics have not been proven to decrease rates of infection in low-risk dog bite wounds not involving the hands or feet. If a bite involves a joint, periosteum, or neurovascular bundle, prompt orthopedic surgery consultation should be obtained.

Pathogens that infect dog bites include *Pasteurella multocida,* streptococci, staphylococci, and anaerobes. Infected dog bites can be treated with penicillin for *P multocida,* and broad-spectrum coverage can be provided by amoxicillin and clavulanic acid or cephalexin (see dose for cat bites in the next section). Complications of dog bites include scarring, CNS infections, septic arthritis, osteomyelitis, endocarditis, and sepsis.

CAT BITES

Cat-inflicted wounds occur more frequently in girls, and their principal complication is infection. The infection risk is higher in cat bites than dog bites because cat bites produce a puncture wound. Management is similar to that for dog bites. Cat wounds should **not** be sutured except when absolutely necessary for cosmetic reasons. *P multocida* is the most common pathogen. Cat bites create a puncture-wound inoculum, and prophylactic antibiotics (penicillin plus cephalexin, or amoxicillin and clavulanic acid) are recommended. The dose of amoxicillin trihydrate and clavulanic acid should be on the high side of recommended dosage in order to ensure adequate tissue penetration both in dog and cat bites. The dosage of the amoxicillin component should be 80 mg/kg/24 h in three divided doses. The maximum dosage is 2 g/24 h. Scratches or bites from cats may also result in cat scratch fever.

HUMAN BITES

Most human bites occur during fights. *P multocida* is not a known pathogen in human bites; cultures most com-

Pediatric Emergency Medicine

Pediatric emergency medicine is a subspecialty with fellowship and subboard certification that provides resuscitation urgent care of ill or injured infants, children, and adolescents. The body of emergency research literature is substantial and growing. EMS-C (Emergency Medical Services for Children) programs to enhance the spectrum of care of the severely ill or injured through, for example, community injury prevention, prehospital by emergency medical technicians and paramedics, emergency based stabilization and critical care, and rehabilitation. Emergency medicine physicians are intimately involved in the care of injured patients, because trauma is the leading cause death among children over age 1 year.

monly grow streptococci, anaerobes, staphylococci, and *Eikenella corrodens*. Hand wounds and deep wounds should be treated with antibiotic coverage against *E corrodens* and gram-positive pathogens by a penicillinase-resistant antibiotic. Wound management is the same as for dog bites. Only severe lacerations involving the face should be sutured. Other wounds can be managed by delayed primary closure or healing by second intention.

A major complication of human bite wounds is infection of the metacarpophalangeal joints. A hand surgeon should evaluate clenched-fist injuries from human bites. Operative debridement is followed in many cases by IV antibiotics.

Capellan O, Hollander JE: Management of lacerations in the emergency department. Emerg Med Clin North Am 2003;21(1):205 [PMID: 12630738].

Knapp JF: Updates in wound management for the pediatrician. Pediatr Clin North Am 1999 46(6):1201 [PMID: 10629682].

Poisoning

Richard C. Dart, MD, PhD, & Barry H. Rumack, MD

Poisonings result from the complex interaction of the agent, the child, and the family environment. The peak incidence is at age 2 years. Most ingestions occur in children younger than age 5 years as a result of insecure storage of drugs, household chemicals, and the like. Twenty-five percent of children will have a second episode of ingestion within 1 year following the first one. Repeated poisonings may require intervention on the child's behalf. Accidental poisonings are unusual after age 5 years. Poisonings in older children and adolescents usually represent manipulative behavior, chemical or drug abuse, or genuine suicide attempts.

Watson WA et al: 2004 annual report of the American Association of Poison Control Centers Toxic Exposure Surveillance System. Am J Emerg Med 2005;23:589 [PMID: 16140178].

PREVENTING CHILDHOOD POISONINGS

Each year, children are accidentally poisoned by medicines, polishes, insecticides, drain cleaners, bleaches, household chemicals, and materials commonly stored in the garage. It is the responsibility of adults to make sure that children are not exposed to potentially toxic substances.

You may wish to obtain pamphlets from your local poison control center to hand out at the 6-month checkup. Here are some suggestions for parents:

1. Insist on packages with safety closures and learn how to use them properly.
2. Keep household cleaning supplies, medicines, garage products, and insecticides out of the reach and sight of your child. Lock them up whenever possible.
3. Never store food and cleaning products together. Store medicine and chemicals in original containers and never in food or beverage containers.
4. Avoid taking medicine in your child's presence. Children love to imitate. Never suggest that medicine is candy.
5. Read the label on all products and heed warnings and cautions. Never use medicine from an unlabeled or unreadable container. Never pour medicine in a darkened area where the label cannot be seen clearly.

6. If you are interrupted while using a product, take it with you—it takes only a few seconds for your child to get into it.
7. Know what your child can do physically. For example, if you have a crawling infant, keep household products stored above floor level, not beneath the kitchen sink.
8. Keep the phone numbers of your doctor, poison control center, hospital, police department, and emergency medical system near the phone.

PHARMACOLOGIC PRINCIPLES OF TOXICOLOGY

In the evaluation of the poisoned patient, it is important to compare the anticipated pharmacologic or toxic effects with the patient's clinical presentation. If the history is that the patient ingested a tranquilizer 30 minutes ago, but the clinical examination reveals dilated pupils, tachycardia, dry mouth, absent bowel sounds, and active hallucinations—clearly anticholinergic toxicity—diagnosis and therapy should proceed accordingly.

LD_{50}

Estimates of the LD_{50} (the amount per kilogram of body weight of a drug required to kill 50% of a group of experimental animals) or median lethal dose are of little clinical value in humans. It is usually impossible to determine with accuracy the amount swallowed or absorbed, the metabolic status of the patient, or in which patients the response to the agent will be atypical. Furthermore, these values are often not valid in humans even if the history is accurate.

Half-Life ($t_{1/2}$)

The $t_{1/2}$ of an agent must be interpreted carefully. Most published $t_{1/2}$ values are for therapeutic dosages. The $t_{1/2}$ may increase as the quantity of the ingested substance increases for many common intoxicants such as salicylates, acetaminophen, and phenytoin. One cannot rely on the published $t_{1/2}$ for salicylate (2 hours) to assume rapid elimination of the drug. In an acute salicylate overdose (150 mg/kg), the apparent $t_{1/2}$ is prolonged to 24–30 hours.

Volume of Distribution

The volume of distribution (Vd) of a drug is determined by dividing the amount of drug absorbed by the blood level. With theophylline, for example, the Vd is 0.46 L/kg body weight, or 32 L in an average adult. In contrast, digoxin distributes well beyond total body water. Because the calculation produces a volume above body weight this figure is referred to as an "apparent volume of distribution" (Table 12–1).

The Vd can be useful in predicting which drugs will be removed by dialysis or exchange transfusion. When a drug is differentially concentrated in body lipids or is heavily tissue- or protein-bound and has a high volume of distribution, only a small proportion of the drug will be in the free form and thus accessible to diuresis, dialysis, or exchange transfusion. A drug that is water-soluble and has a low volume of distribution may cross the dialysis membrane well and also respond to diuresis. In general, methods of extracorporeal elimination are not effective for toxic agents with a Vd greater than 1 L/kg.

Metabolism & Excretion

The route of excretion or detoxification is important for planning treatment. Methanol, for example, is metabolized to the toxic product, formic acid. This metabolic step may be blocked by the antidote fomepizole or ethanol.

Blood Levels

Care of the poisoned patient should never be guided solely by laboratory measurements. Treatment should be directed first by the clinical signs and symptoms, fol-lowed by more specific therapy based on laboratory determinations. Clinical information may speed the identification of a toxic agent by the laboratory.

GENERAL TREATMENT OF POISONING

The telephone is often the first contact in pediatric poisoning. Proper telephone management can reduce morbidity and prevent unwarranted or excessive treatment. The decision to refer the patient is based on the identity and dose of the ingested agent, the age of the child, the time of day, the reliability of the parent, and whether child neglect or endangerment is suspected. Poison control centers are the source of expert telephone advice and have excellent follow-up programs to manage patients in the home.

Initial Telephone Contact

Basic information obtained at the first telephone contact includes the patient's name, age, weight, address and telephone number, the agent and amount of agent ingested, the patient's present condition, and the time elapsed since ingestion or other exposure.

Use the history to evaluate the urgency of the situation and decide whether immediate emergency transportation to a health facility is indicated. An emergency exists if the ingestant is high risk (caustic solutions, hydrogen fluoride, drugs of abuse, or medications such as a calcium channel blocker, opioid, hypoglycemic agent, or antidepressant) or if the self-poisoning was intentional. If immediate danger does not exist, obtain more details about the suspected toxic agent. It may be difficult to obtain an accurate history. Obtain names of drugs or ingredients, manufacturers, prescription num-

Table 12–1. Some examples of pK_a and Vd.

Drug	pK_a	Diuresis	Dialysis	Apparent Vd
Amobarbital	7.9	No	No	200–300% body weight
Amphetamine	9.8	No	Yes	60% body weight
Aspirin	3.5	Alkaline	Yes	15–40% body weight
Chlorpromazine	9.3	No	No	40–50 L/kg (2800–3500% body weight)
Codeine	8.2	No	No	5–10 L/kg (350–700% body weight)
Desipramine	10.2	No	No	30–40 L/kg (2100–2800% body weight)
Ethchlorvynol	8.7	No	No	5–10 L/kg (350–700% body weight)
Glutethimide	4.5	No	No	10–20 L/kg (700–1400% body weight)
Isoniazid	3.5	Alkaline	Yes	61% body weight
Methadone	8.3	No	No	5–10 L/kg (350–700% body weight)
Methicillin	2.8	No	Yes	60% body weight
Phenobarbital	7.4	Alkaline	Yes	75% body weight
Phenytoin	8.3	No	No	60–80% body weight
Tetracycline	7.7	No	No	200–300% body weight

bers, names and phone numbers of prescribing physician and pharmacy, and so on. Find out whether the substance was shared among several children, whether it had been recently purchased, who had last used it, how full the bottle was, and how much was spilled. If unsure of the significance of an exposure, consult with a certified poison control center.

FIRST AID FOR POISONING (Advice for Parents)

Induction of vomiting is no longer recommended in most cases; activated charcoal is used to bind poisons. Use syrup of ipecac and activated charcoal only as advised by your poison control center. Poison control centers no longer recommend keeping ipecac in the home.

Inhaled Poisons

If smoke, gas, or fumes have been inhaled, immediately drag or carry the victim to fresh air. Then call 911, the poison control center, or your doctor. Do not enter an area where poisonous fumes are present that have caused loss of consciousness. Too often the rescuer becomes a victim as well.

Poisons on the Skin

If the poison has been spilled on the skin or clothing, remove the clothing and flood the involved parts with water. Wash with soapy water and rinse thoroughly.

Swallowed Poisons

If the substance swallowed is a medicine, give nothing. Milk or water should be administered immediately to any patient who has ingested a strongly acid or alkaline agent. Do not give more than 15 mL/kg (250 mL maximum in a child weighing 16 kg or more). Do not induce vomiting in patients who are comatose, convulsing, or who have lost the gag reflex. Induce emesis with ipecac or administer charcoal **only** if advised to do so by a health care professional. *Caution:* Antidote labels on products may be incorrect. Do not give salt, vinegar, or lemon juice. Call the poison control center before doing anything else.

Poisons in the Eye

Rinse out the eye with plain water before the patient arrives at the emergency room. Use plain tap water—do not try to neutralize acids or bases. Pour water into the eye from a drinking glass or pitcher for 15–20 minutes or fill a basin with water and have the patient put his or her face into the water and open the eyes to dilute. Then transport the patient to the hospital.

Bring the Poison to the Hospital

Everything in the vicinity of the patient that may be a cause of poisoning should be brought to the health care facility.

OBTAINING INFORMATION ABOUT POISONS

Current data on ingredients of commercial products and medications can be obtained from a certified regional poison center. All poison control centers can be reached by dialing 1-800-222-1222 and the call will be automatically routed to the correct regional center. It is important to have the actual container at hand when calling. *Caution:* Antidote information on labels of commercial products or in the *Physicians' Desk Reference* may be incorrect or inappropriate.

FOLLOW-UP

In over 95% of cases of ingestion of potentially toxic substances by children, a trip to the hospital is not required. In these cases, it is important to call the parent at 1 and 4 hours after an ingestion. If the child has ingested an additional unknown agent and develops symptoms, a change in management may be needed, including transportation to the hospital. An additional call should be made 24 hours after the ingestion to begin the process of poison prevention.

PREVENTION OF POISONING

A major goal of pediatricians is to reduce the number of accidental ingestions in the high-risk age group (ie, < 5 years). A systematic poison education effort should be part of the routine care of every patient. Parents of very young children should be encouraged to search the house and identify all hazardous substances that should be removed from the home or locked up. All poison centers can be reached by dialing 1-800-222-1222 and the call will be automatically routed to the correct regional center. Pediatric or medical office staff can help families with poison prevention by telephone by asking a few simple questions about storage of hazardous substances in the home. The following is a partial list of potentially poisonous substances that must be stored safely if small children are in the home: drain-cleaning crystals or liquid, dishwasher soap and cleaning supplies, paints and paint thinners, garden spray and other insecticide materials, automobile products (antifreeze, windshield wiper fluid, gasoline), and all medications.

Syrup of ipecac is not recommended for use in the home. Reinforcement should occur at the 1-year checkup to make certain that adequate poison-proofing measures have been instituted and maintained.

Poison treatment in the home. American Academy of Pediatrics Committee on Injury, Violence, and Poison Prevention. Pediatrics 2003;112:1182 [PMID: 14595067].

INITIAL EMERGENCY DEPARTMENT CONTACT

Make Certain the Patient Is Breathing

As in all emergencies, the principles of treatment are attention to airway, breathing, and circulation. These are sometimes overlooked under the stressful conditions of a pediatric poisoning.

Treat Shock

Initial therapy of the hypotensive patient should consist of laying the patient flat and administering intravenous isotonic solutions. Vasopressors should be reserved for poisoned patients in shock who do not respond to these standard measures.

Treat Burns

Burns may occur following exposure to strong acid or strong alkaline agents or petroleum distillates. Burned areas should be decontaminated by flooding with sterile saline solution or water. A burn unit should be consulted if more than minimal burn damage has been sustained. Skin decontamination should be performed in a patient with cutaneous exposure. Emergency department personnel in contact with a patient who has been contaminated (with an organophosphate insecticide, for example) should themselves be decontaminated if their skin or clothing becomes contaminated.

Take a Pertinent History

The history should be taken from the parents and all individuals present at the scene. It may be crucial to determine all of the kinds of poisons in the home. These may include drugs used by family members, chemicals associated with the hobbies or occupations of family members, or the purity of the water supply. Unusual dietary or medication habits or other clues to the possible cause of poisoning should also be investigated.

DEFINITIVE THERAPY OF POISONING

Prevention of Absorption

A. EMESIS

Induced vomiting is contraindicated in patients who have ingested a minimally toxic substance (eg, most antibiotics), who are comatose or convulsing, or who have lost the gag reflex or ingested strong acids, strong bases, some hydrocarbons, or sharp objects. The use of ipecac has decreased dramatically over the past 10 years and is reserved for those instances when medications have been taken within 30–60 minutes prior to contact. It is not recommended for use at home.

1. Ipecac method—This may be effective if administered within an hour of ingestion but should only be used under the supervision of a health care professional. Adult dose, 30 mL; pediatric dose, 15 mL. Give orally (PO) and repeat once in 20 minutes if necessary.

2. Other emetics—The only approved oral emetic agent is syrup of ipecac. Use of sodium chloride may lead to lethal hypernatremia. Apomorphine, mustard, soap, and other emetics should not be used.

B. LAVAGE

Lavage is rarely performed in pediatric patients. Emesis and lavage recover an average of about 30% of the stomach contents if performed soon after ingestion. Although these procedures may be helpful in reducing the amount of material available for absorption, approximately 70% of an ingested dose will remain. Additional measures such as charcoal should be instituted to prevent further absorption.

C. CHARCOAL

The dose of charcoal is 1–2 g/kg (maximum, 100 g) per dose. Repeating the dose of activated charcoal may be useful for those agents that slow passage through the gastrointestinal (GI) tract. When multiple doses of activated charcoal are given, repeated doses of sorbitol or saline cathartics must not be given. Repeated doses of cathartics may cause electrolyte imbalances and fluid loss. Charcoal dosing is repeated every 2–6 hours until charcoal is passed through the rectum.

D. CATHARSIS

Despite their widespread use, cathartics do not improve outcome. The use of cathartics should therefore be avoided.

E. WHOLE GUT LAVAGE

Whole bowel lavage uses an orally administered, nonabsorbable hypertonic solution such as CoLyte or GoLYTELY. The use of this procedure in poisoned patients remains controversial. Preliminary recommendations for use of whole bowel irrigation include poisoning with sustained-release preparations, mechanical movement of items through the bowel (eg, cocaine packets, iron tablets), and poisoning with substances poorly absorbed by charcoal (eg, lithium, iron). Underlying bowel pathology and intestinal obstruction are relative contraindications to its use. Consultation with a certified regional poison center is recommended.

American Academy of Clinical Toxicology, European Association of Poisons Centers and Clinical Toxicologists: Position paper: Ipecac syrup. J Toxicol Clin Toxicol 2004;42:133 [PMID: 15214617].

American Academy of Clinical Toxicology, European Association of Poisons Centers and Clinical Toxicologists: Position statement and practice guidelines on the use of multidose activated charcoal in the treatment of acute poisoning. J Toxicol Clin Toxicol 1999;37:731 [PMID: 10584586].

Gielen AC et al: Effects of improved access to safety counseling, products, and home visits on parents' safety practices: Results of a randomized trial. Arch Pediatr Adolesc Med 2002; 156:33 [PMID: 11772188].

Hoffman RJ, Nelson L: Rational use of toxicology testing in children. Curr Opin Pediatr 2001;13:183 [PMID: 11317063].

Vale JA: Position statement: Gastric lavage. American Academy of Clinical Toxicology; European Association of Poisons Centres and Clinical Toxicologists. J Toxicol Clin Toxicol 1997;35:711 [PMID: 9482426].

Enhancement of Excretion

Excretion of certain substances can be hastened by urinary alkalinization or dialysis. It is important to make certain that the patient is not volume-depleted. Volume-depleted patients should receive a normal saline bolus of 10–20 mL/kg, followed by sufficient intravenous (IV) fluid administration to maintain urine output at 2–3 mL/kg/h.

A. URINARY ALKALINIZATION

1. Alkaline diuresis——Urinary alkalinization should be chosen on the basis of the substance's pK_a, so that ionized drug will be trapped in the tubular lumen and not reabsorbed (see Table 12–1). Thus, if the pK_a is less than 7.5, urinary alkalinization is appropriate; if it is over 8.0, this technique is not usually beneficial. The pK_a is sometimes included along with general drug information. Urinary alkalinization is achieved with sodium bicarbonate. It is important to observe for hypokalemia, caused by the shift of potassium intracellularly. Follow serum K^+ and observe for electrocardiogram (ECG) evidence of hypokalemia. If complications such as renal failure or pulmonary edema are present, hemodialysis or hemoperfusion may be required.

B. DIALYSIS

Hemodialysis (or peritoneal dialysis if hemodialysis is unavailable) is useful in the poisonings listed below. Dialysis should be considered part of supportive care if the patient satisfies any of the following criteria:

1. Clinical criteria——

a. Potentially life-threatening toxicity that is caused by a dialyzable drug and cannot be treated by conservative means.

b. Hypotension threatening renal or hepatic function that cannot be corrected by adjusting circulating volume.

c. Marked hyperosmolality or severe acid–base or electrolyte disturbances not responding to therapy.

d. Marked hypothermia or hyperthermia not responding to therapy.

2. Immediate dialysis—Immediate dialysis should be considered in ethylene glycol and methanol poisoning only if acidosis is refractory, the patient does not respond to fomepizole treatment, or blood levels of ethanol of 100 mg/dL are consistently maintained.

3. Dialysis indicated on basis of condition of patient—In general, dialyze if the patient is in a coma deeper than level 3. Peritoneal dialysis or exchange transfusion may be more useful than hemodialysis in small children—as much for ease of achieving fluid and electrolyte homeostasis as for poison removal. Other drugs not listed here may be dialyzable. Information should be verified prior to institution of dialysis.

■ MANAGEMENT OF SPECIFIC COMMON POISONINGS

ACETAMINOPHEN (Paracetamol)

Overdosage of acetaminophen is the most common pediatric poisoning and can produce severe hepatotoxicity. The incidence of hepatotoxicity in adults and adolescents has been reported to be 10 times higher than in children younger than age 5 years. In the latter group, less than 0.1% develop hepatotoxicity after acetaminophen overdose. In children, toxicity most commonly results from repeated overdosage arising from confusion about the age-appropriate dose, use of multiple products that contain acetaminophen, or use of adult suppositories.

Acetaminophen is normally metabolized in the liver. A small percentage of the drug goes through a pathway leading to a toxic metabolite. Normally, this electrophilic reactant is removed harmlessly by conjugation with glutathione. In overdosage, the supply of glutathione becomes exhausted, and the metabolite may bind covalently to components of liver cells to produce necrosis. Some authors have proposed that therapeutic doses of acetaminophen may be toxic to children with depleted glutathione stores. However, there is no evidence that administration of therapeutic doses can cause toxicity, and only a few inadequate case reports have been made in this regard.

Treatment

Treatment is to administer acetylcysteine. It may be administered either orally or intravenously. Consultation on difficult cases may be obtained from any poison control center or the Rocky Mountain Poison & Drug Center (http://www.rmpdc.org/). Blood levels should

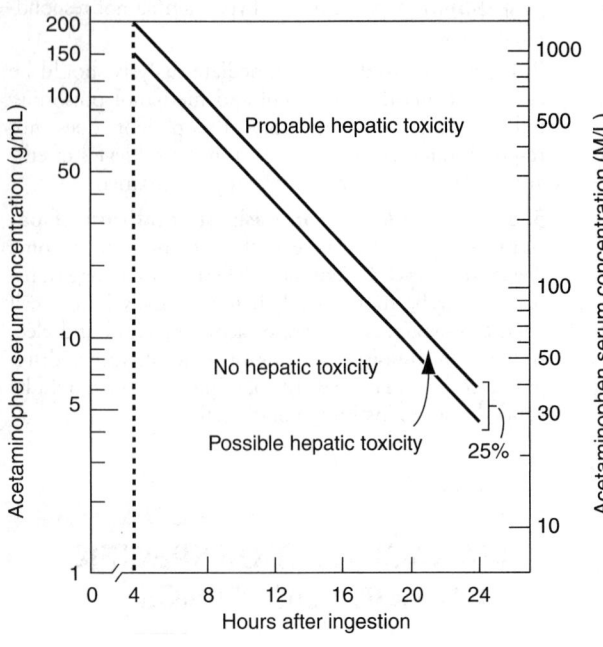

Figure 12–1. Semi-logarithmic plot of plasma acetaminophen levels versus time. (Modified and reproduced, with permission, from Rumack BH, Matthew H: Acetaminophen poisoning and toxicity. Pediatrics 1975;55:871.)

be obtained 4 hours after ingestion or as soon as possible thereafter and plotted on Figure 12–1. The nomogram is used only for acute ingestion, not repeated supratherapeutic ingestions. If the patient has ingested acetaminophen in a liquid preparation, blood levels obtained 2 hours after ingestion will give an accurate reflection of the toxicity to be expected relative to the standard nomogram (see Figure 12–1). Acetylcysteine is administered to patients whose acetaminophen levels plot in the toxic range on the nomogram. Acetylcysteine is effective even when given more than 24 hours after ingestion although it is most effective when given within 8 hours postingestion.

The oral dose of acetylcysteine is 140 mg/kg, diluted to a 5% solution in sweet fruit juice or carbonated soft drink. The primary problems associated with administration are nausea and vomiting. After this loading dose, 70 mg/kg should be administered PO every 4 hours for 72 hours.

For children weighing 40 kg or more, IV acetylcysteine (Acetadote) should be administered as a loading dose of 150 mg/kg administered over 15–60 minutes; followed by a second infusion of 50 mg/kg over 4 hours, and then a third infusion of 100 mg/kg over 16 hours (dosage calculator is available at http://www.acetadote.com) (Table 12–2).

For patients less than 40 kg, IV acetylcysteine must have less dilution to avoid hyponatremia (Table 12–3).

Aspartate aminotransferase, alanine aminotransferase, serum bilirubin, and plasma prothrombin time should be followed daily. Significant abnormalities of liver function may not peak until up to 72 hours after ingestion.

Repeated miscalculated overdoses given by parents to treat fever are the major source of toxicity in children younger than age 10 years, and parents are often unaware of the significance of symptoms of toxicity, thus delaying its prompt recognition and therapy.

Bond GR: Reduced toxicity of acetaminophen in children: It's the liver. J Toxicol Clin Toxicol 2004;42:149 [PMID: 15214619].

Marzullo L: An update of *N*-acetylcysteine treatment for acute acetaminophen toxicity in children. Curr Opin Pediatr 2005;17:239 [PMID: 15800420].

Rumack BH: Acetaminophen hepatotoxicity: The first 35 years. J Toxicol Clin Toxicol 2002;40:3 [PMID: 11990202].

Smilkstein M et al: Efficacy of oral *N*-acetylcysteine in the treatment of acetaminophen overdose. N Engl J Med 1988;319:1557 [PMID: 0003059186].

ALCOHOL, ETHYL (Ethanol)

Alcoholic beverages, tinctures, cosmetics, and rubbing alcohol are common sources of poisoning in children. Concomitant exposure to other depressant drugs increases the seriousness of the intoxication. (Blood levels cited here are for adults; comparable figures for children are not available.) In most states, alcohol levels of 50–80 mg/dL are considered compatible with impaired faculties, and levels of 80–100 mg/dL are considered evidence of intoxication.

Complete absorption of alcohol requires 30 minutes to 6 hours, depending on the volume, the presence of food, and the time spent in consuming the alcohol. The rate of metabolic degradation is constant

Table 12–2. Intravenous acetylcysteine administration for children weighing 40 kg or more.

Body Weight		FIRST 150 mg/kg in 200 mL 5% Dextrose in 15 min	SECOND 50 mg/kg in 500 mL 5% Dextrose in 4 h	THIRD 100 mg/kg in 1000 mL 5% Dextrose in 16 h
(kg)	(lb)	Acetadote (mL)	Acetadote (mL)	Acetadote (mL)
100	220	75	25	50
90	198	67.5	22.5	45
80	176	60	20	40
70	154	52.5	17.5	35
60	132	45	15	30
50	110	37.5	12.5	25
40	88	30	10	20

Table 12–3. Intravenous acetylcysteine administration for children weighing less than 40 kg.

Body Weight		Loading Infusion (15 min)—150 mg/kg		
kg	lb	NAC 20% (mL)	Diluent Volume D$_5$W (mL)	Final Volume (mL)
30	66	22.5	90	112.5
25	55	18.75	75	93.75
20	44	15	60	75
15	33	11.25	45	56.25
10	22	7.5	30	37.5
Body Weight		Second Infusion (4 h)—50 mg/kg		
kg	lb	NAC 20% (mL)	Diluent Volume D$_5$W (mL)	Final Volume (mL)
30	66	7.5	30	37.5
25	55	6.25	25	31.25
20	44	5	20	25
15	33	3.75	15	18.75
10	22	2.5	10	12.5
Body Weight		Third Infusion (16 h)—100 mg/kg		
kg	lb	NAC 20% (mL)	Diluent Volume D$_5$W (mL)	Final Volume (mL)
30	66	15	60	75
25	55	12.5	50	62.5
20	44	10	40	50
15	33	7.5	30	37.5
10	22	5	20	25

(about 20 mg/h in an adult). Absolute ethanol, 1 mL/kg, results in a peak blood level of about 100 mg/dL in 1 hour after ingestion. Acute intoxication and chronic alcoholism increase the risk of subarachnoid hemorrhage.

Treatment

Management of hypoglycemia and acidosis is usually the only measure required. Start an IV drip of D_5W or $D_{10}W$ if blood glucose is under 60 mg/dL. Fructose has been suggested as an accelerator of metabolism, but it may cause vomiting, intensify lactic acidosis, and decrease blood volume via osmotic diuresis. Glucagon does not correct the hypoglycemia, because hepatic glycogen stores are reduced. Death is usually caused by respiratory failure. In severe cases, cerebral edema should be treated with IV dexamethasone, 0.1 mg/kg every 4–6 hours. Dialysis is indicated in life-threatening intoxication.

Ernst AA et al: Ethanol ingestion and related hypoglycemia in a pediatric and adolescent emergency department population. Acad Emerg Med 1996;3:46 [PMID: 8749967].

Roy M et al: What are the adverse effects of ethanol used as an antidote in the treatment of suspected methanol poisoning in children? J Toxicol Clin Toxicol 2003;41:155 [PMID: 12733853].

AMPHETAMINES & RELATED DRUGS (Methamphetamine)

Clinical Presentation

A. ACUTE POISONING

Amphetamine and methamphetamine poisoning is common because of the widespread availability of "diet pills" and the use of "speed," "crank," "crystal," and "ice" by adolescents. (Care must be taken in the interpretation of slang terms because they have multiple meanings.) A new cause of amphetamine poisoning is drugs for treating attention deficit hyperactivity disorder, such as methylphenidate. Symptoms include central nervous system (CNS) stimulation, anxiety, hyperactivity, hyperpyrexia, hypertension, abdominal cramps, nausea and vomiting, and inability to void urine. Severe cases often include rhabdomyolysis. A toxic psychosis indistinguishable from paranoid schizophrenia may occur. Methamphetamine laboratories in homes are a potential cause of childhood exposure to a variety of hazardous and toxic substances.

B. CHRONIC POISONING

Chronic amphetamine users develop tolerance; more than 1500 mg of IV methamphetamine can be used daily. Hyperactivity, disorganization, and euphoria are followed by exhaustion, depression, and coma lasting 2–3 days. Heavy users, taking more than 100 mg/d, have restlessness, incoordination of thought, insomnia,

nervousness, irritability, and visual hallucinations. Psychosis may be precipitated by the chronic administration of high doses. Depression, weakness, tremors, GI complaints, and suicidal thoughts occur frequently.

Treatment

Standard decontamination procedures should be used: gastric emptying followed by charcoal in recent ingestions; activated charcoal alone if ingestion occurred hours earlier. The treatment of choice is diazepam, titrated in small increments to effect. Very large total doses may be needed. In case of extreme agitation or hallucinations, droperidol (0.1 mg/kg/dose) or haloperidol (up to 0.1 mg/kg) parenterally has been used. When combinations of amphetamines and barbiturates (diet pills) are used, the action of the amphetamines begins first, followed by a depression caused by the barbiturates. In these cases, treatment with additional barbiturates is contraindicated because of the risk of respiratory failure.

Chronic users may be withdrawn rapidly from amphetamines. If amphetamine–barbiturate combination tablets have been used, the barbiturates must be withdrawn gradually to prevent withdrawal seizures. Psychiatric treatment should be provided.

Kolecki P: Inadvertent methamphetamine poisoning in pediatric patients. Pediatr Emerg Care 1998;14:385 [PMID: 9881979].

Schwartz RH, Miller NS: MDMA (ecstasy) and the rave: A review. Pediatrics 1997;100:705 [PMID: 9310529].

ANESTHETICS, LOCAL

Intoxication from local anesthetics may be associated with CNS stimulation, acidosis, delirium, ataxia, shock, convulsions, and death. Methemoglobinuria has been reported following local dental analgesia. The maximum recommended dose for subcutaneous (SQ) infiltration is 4.5 mg/kg. The temptation to exceed this dose in procedures lasting a long time is great and may result in inadvertent overdosage. PO application of viscous lidocaine may produce toxicity. Hypercapnia may lower the seizure threshold to locally injected anesthetics.

Local anesthetics used in obstetrics cross the placental barrier and are not efficiently metabolized by the fetal liver. Mepivacaine, lidocaine, and bupivacaine can cause fetal bradycardia, neonatal depression, and death. Prilocaine causes methemoglobinemia, which should be treated if levels in the blood exceed 40% or if the patient is symptomatic.

Accidental injection of mepivacaine into the head of the fetus during paracervical anesthesia has caused neonatal asphyxia, cyanosis, acidosis, bradycardia, convulsions, and death.

Treatment

If the anesthetic has been ingested, mucous membranes should be cleansed carefully and activated charcoal may be administered. Oxygen administration is indicated, with assisted ventilation if necessary. Methemoglobinemia is treated with methylene blue, 1%, 0.2 mL/kg (1–2 mg/kg/dose, IV) over 5–10 minutes; this should promptly relieve the cyanosis. Acidosis may be treated with sodium bicarbonate, seizures with diazepam, and bradycardia with atropine. Therapeutic levels of mepivacaine, lidocaine, and procaine are less than 5 mg/mL.

Bozynski MEA et al: Lidocaine toxicity after maternal pudendal anesthesia in a term infant with fetal distress. Am J Perinatol 1987;4:164 [PMID: 3566884].

Spiller HA et al: Multi-center retrospective evaluation of oral benzocaine exposure in children. Vet Hum Toxicol 2000;42:228 [PMID: 10928690].

ANTIHISTAMINES

Although antihistamines typically cause CNS depression, children often react paradoxically with excitement, hallucinations, delirium, ataxia, tremors, and convulsions followed by CNS depression, respiratory failure, or cardiovascular collapse. Anticholinergic effects such as dry mouth, fixed dilated pupils, flushed face, fever, and hallucinations may be prominent.

Antihistamines are widely available in allergy, sleep, cold, and antiemetic preparations, and many are supplied in sustained-release forms, which increase the likelihood of dangerous overdoses. They are absorbed rapidly and metabolized by the liver, lungs, and kidneys. A potentially toxic dose is 10–50 mg/kg of the most commonly used antihistamines, but toxic reactions have occurred at much lower doses.

Treatment

Activated charcoal should be used to reduce drug absorption. Emetics may be ineffective if the antihistamine is structurally related to phenothiazines. Whole bowel irrigation may be useful for sustained-release preparations. Physostigmine, 0.5–2.0 mg IV slowly administered, dramatically reverses the central and peripheral anticholinergic effects of antihistamines, but it should be used only for diagnostic purposes. Diazepam, 0.1–0.2 mg/kg IV, can be used to control seizures. Forced diuresis is not helpful. Exchange transfusion was reported to be effective in one case.

Cetaruk EW, Aaron CK: Hazards of nonprescription medications. Emerg Med Clin North Am 1994;12:483 [PMID: 8187693].

Skare JA: Antihistamine-containing cough/cold medications present a low hazard in pediatric accidental exposure incidents: Analysis of Poison Control Center data. Vet Hum Toxicol 1997;39:367 [PMID: 9397509].

Ten Eick AP et al: Safety of antihistamines in children. Drug Saf 2001;24:119 [PMID: 11235817].

ARSENIC

Arsenic is used in some insecticides (fruit tree or tobacco sprays), rodenticides, weed killers, and wood preservatives. It is well absorbed primarily through the GI and respiratory tracts, but skin absorption may occur. Arsenic can be found in the urine, hair, and nails by laboratory testing.

Highly toxic soluble derivatives of this compound, such as sodium arsenite, are frequently found in liquid preparations and can cause death in as many as 65% of victims. The organic arsenates found in persistent or preemergence weed killers are relatively less soluble and less toxic. Poisonings with a liquid arsenical preparation that does not contain alkyl methanearsonate compounds should be considered potentially lethal. Patients exhibiting clinical signs other than gastroenteritis should receive treatment until laboratory tests indicate that treatment is no longer necessary.

Clinical Presentation

A. ACUTE POISONING

Abdominal pain, vomiting, watery and bloody diarrhea, cardiovascular collapse, paresthesias, neck pain, and garlic odor on the breath occur as the first signs of acute poisoning. Convulsions, coma, anuria, and exfoliative dermatitis are later signs. Inhalation may cause pulmonary edema. Death is the result of cardiovascular collapse.

B. CHRONIC POISONING

Anorexia, generalized weakness, giddiness, colic, abdominal pain, polyneuritis, dermatitis, nail changes, alopecia, and anemia often develop.

Treatment

In acute poisoning, empty the stomach and administer activated charcoal. Then immediately give dimercaprol (commonly known as BAL), 3–5 mg/kg intramuscularly (IM), and follow with 2 mg/kg IM every 4 hours. The dimercaprol–arsenic complex is dialyzable. A second choice is succimer. The initial dose is 10 mg/kg every 8 hours for 5 days. A third choice is penicillamine, 100 mg/kg PO to a maximum of 1 g/d in four divided doses.

Chronic arsenic intoxication should be treated with succimer or penicillamine. Collect a 24-hour baseline urine specimen and then begin chelation. If the 24-hour urine arsenic level is greater than 50 mg, continue chelation for 5 days. After 10 days, repeat the 5-day cycle once or twice depending on how soon the urine arsenic level falls below 50 mg/24 h.

Abernathy CO et al: Arsenic: Health effects, mechanisms of actions, and research issues. Environ Health Perspect 1999;107:593 [PMID: 10379007].

Cullen MN et al: Pediatric arsenic ingestion. Am J Emerg Med 1995;13:432 [PMID: 7605532].

BARBITURATES

The toxic effects of barbiturates include confusion, poor coordination, coma, miotic or fixed dilated pupils, and respiratory depression. Respiratory acidosis is commonly associated with pulmonary atelectasis, and hypotension occurs frequently in severely poisoned patients. Ingestion of more than 6 mg/kg of long-acting or 3 mg/kg of short-acting barbiturates is usually toxic.

Treatment

Activated charcoal should be administered. Careful, conservative management with emphasis on maintaining a clear airway, adequate ventilation, and control of hypotension is critical. Urinary alkalinization and the use of multiple-dose charcoal may decrease the elimination half-life of phenobarbital but have not been shown to alter the clinical course. Hemodialysis is not useful in the treatment of poisoning with short-acting barbiturates. Analeptics are contraindicated.

Amitai Y, Degani Y: Treatment of phenobarbital poisoning with multiple dose activated charcoal in an infant. J Emerg Med 1990;8:449 [PMID: 2212564].

Cote CJ et al: Adverse sedation events in pediatrics: Analysis of medications used for sedation. Pediatrics 2000;4:633 [PMID: 11015502].

BELLADONNA ALKALOIDS
(Atropine, Jimsonweed, Potato Leaves, Scopolamine, Stramonium)

The effects of anticholinergic compounds include dry mouth; thirst; decreased sweating with hot, dry, red skin; high fever; and tachycardia that may be preceded by bradycardia. The pupils are dilated, and vision is blurred. Speech and swallowing may be impaired. Hallucinations, delirium, and coma are common. Leukocytosis may occur, confusing the diagnosis.

Atropinism has been caused by normal doses of atropine or homatropine eye drops, especially in children with Down syndrome. Many common plants and over-the-counter medications contain belladonna alkaloids.

Treatment

Emesis or lavage should be followed by activated charcoal. Gastric emptying is slowed by anticholinergics, so that gastric decontamination may be useful even if delayed. Physostigmine, 0.5–2.0 mg IV, administered slowly, dramatically reverses the central and peripheral signs of atropinism but should be used only as a diagnostic agent. High fever must be controlled. Catheterization may be needed if the patient cannot void.

Burns MJ et al: A comparison of physostigmine and benzodiazepines for the treatment of anticholinergic poisoning. Ann Emerg Med 2000;35:374 [PMID: 10736125].

Schultz U et al: Central anticholinergic syndrome in a child undergoing circumcision. Acta Anesthesiol Scand 2002;46:224 [PMID: 11942877].

CARBON MONOXIDE

The degree of toxicity correlates well with the carboxyhemoglobin level taken soon after acute exposure but not after oxygen has been given or when there has been some time since exposure. Onset of symptoms may be more rapid and more severe if the patient lives at a high altitude, has a high respiratory rate (ie, infants), is pregnant, or has myocardial insufficiency or lung disease. Normal blood may contain up to 5% carboxyhemoglobin (10% in smokers).

The most prominent early symptom is headache. Other effects include confusion, unsteadiness, and coma. Proteinuria, glycosuria, elevated serum aminotransferase levels, or ECG changes may be present in the acute phase. Permanent cardiac, liver, renal, or CNS damage occurs occasionally. The outcome of severe poisoning may be complete recovery, vegetative state, or any degree of mental injury between these extremes. The primary mental deficits are neuropsychiatric.

Treatment

The biologic half-life of carbon monoxide on room air is approximately 200–300 minutes; on 100% oxygen, it is 60–90 minutes. Hyperbaric oxygen therapy at 2.0–2.5 atm of oxygen shortens the half-life to 30 minutes. After the level has been reduced to near zero, therapy is aimed at the nonspecific sequelae of anoxia. Dexamethasone, 0.1 mg/kg IV or IM every 4–6 hours, should be added if cerebral edema develops.

Chou KJ: Characteristics and outcome of children with carbon monoxide poisoning with and without smoke exposure referred for hyperbaric oxygen therapy. Pediatr Emerg Care 2000;3:151 [PMID: 10888449].

Walker AR: Emergency department management of house fire burns and carbon monoxide poisoning in children. Curr Opin Pediatr 1996;8:239 [PMID: 8814401].

CAUSTICS

1. Acids (Hydrochloric, Hydrofluoric, Nitric, & Sulfuric Acids; Sodium Bisulfate)

Strong acids are commonly found in metal and toilet bowl cleaners, batteries, and other products. Hydrofluoric acid is the most toxic and hydrochloric acid the least toxic of these household substances. However, even a few drops can be fatal if aspirated into the trachea.

Painful swallowing, mucous membrane burns, bloody emesis, abdominal pain, respiratory distress due to edema of the epiglottis, thirst, shock, and renal failure can occur. Coma and convulsions sometimes are seen terminally. Residual lesions include esophageal, gastric, and pyloric strictures as well as scars of the cornea, skin, and oropharynx.

Hydrofluoric acid is a particularly dangerous poison. Dermal exposure creates a penetrating burn that can progress for hours or days. Large dermal exposure or ingestion may produce life-threatening hypocalcemia abruptly as well as burn reactions.

Treatment

Emetics and lavage are contraindicated. Water or milk (< 15 mL/kg) is used to dilute the acid, because a heat-producing chemical reaction does not occur. Take care not to induce emesis by excessive fluid administration. Alkalies should not be used. Burned areas of the skin, mucous membranes, or eyes should be washed with copious amounts of warm water. Opioids for pain may be needed. An endotracheal tube may be required to alleviate laryngeal edema. Esophagoscopy should be performed if the patient has significant burns or difficulty in swallowing. Acids are likely to produce gastric burns or esophageal burns. Evidence is not conclusive, but corticosteroids have not proved to be of use.

Hydrofluoric acid burns on skin are treated with 10% calcium gluconate gel or calcium gluconate infusion. Severe exposure may require large doses of IV calcium. Therapy should be guided by calcium levels, the ECG, and clinical signs.

2. Bases (Clinitest Tablets, Clorox, Drano, Liquid-Plumr, Purex, Sani-Clor)

Alkalies produce more severe injuries than acids. Some substances, such as Clinitest tablets or Drano, are quite toxic, whereas the chlorinated bleaches (3–6% solutions of sodium hypochlorite) are usually not toxic. When sodium hypochlorite comes in contact with acid in the stomach, hypochlorous acid, which is very irritating to the mucous membranes and skin, is formed. Rapid inactivation of this substance prevents systemic toxicity. Chlorinated bleaches, when mixed with a strong acid (toilet bowl cleaners) or ammonia, may produce irritating chlorine or chloramine gas, which can cause serious lung injury if inhaled in a closed space (eg, bathroom).

Alkalies can burn the skin, mucous membranes, and eyes. Respiratory distress may be due to edema of the epiglottis, pulmonary edema resulting from inhalation of fumes, or pneumonia. Mediastinitis or other intercurrent infections or shock can occur. Perforation of the esophagus or stomach is rare.

Treatment

The skin and mucous membranes should be cleansed with copious amounts of water. A local anesthetic can be instilled in the eye if necessary to alleviate blepharospasm. The eye should be irrigated for at least 20–30 minutes. Ophthalmologic consultation should be obtained for all alkaline eye burns.

Ingestions should be treated with water as a diluent. Routine esophagoscopy is no longer indicated to rule out burns of the esophagus due to chlorinated bleaches unless an unusually large amount has been ingested or the patient is symptomatic. The absence of oral lesions does not rule out the possibility of laryngeal or esophageal burns following granular alkali ingestion. The use of corticosteroids is controversial, but has not been shown to improve long-term outcome except possibly in partial-thickness esophageal burns. Antibiotics may be needed if mediastinitis is likely, but they should not be used prophylactically. (See Caustic Burns of the Esophagus section in Chapter 20.)

Hamza AF et al: Caustic esophageal strictures in children: 30 years' experience. J Pediatr Surg 2003;338:828 [PMID: 12778375].

Lamireau T et al: Accidental caustic ingestion in children: Is endoscopy always mandatory? J Pediatr Gastroenterol Nutr 2001;33:81 [PMID: 11479413].

Lovejoy FH Jr: Corrosive injury of the esophagus in children: Failure of corticosteroid treatment reemphasizes prevention. N Engl J Med 1990;323:668 [PMID: 2385270].

Tiryaki T et al: Early bougienage for relief of stricture formation following caustic esophageal burns. Pediatr Surg Intl 2005;21:78 [PMID: 15619090].

COCAINE

Cocaine is absorbed intranasally or via inhalation or ingestion. Effects are noted almost immediately when the drug is taken intravenously or smoked. Peak effects are delayed for about an hour when the drug is taken orally or nasally. Cocaine prevents the reuptake of endogenous catecholamines, thereby causing an initial sympathetic discharge, followed by catechol depletion after chronic abuse.

Clinical Findings

A local anesthetic and vasoconstrictor, cocaine is also a potent stimulant to both the CNS and the cardiovascular system. The initial tachycardia, hyperpnea, hypertension, and stimulation of the CNS are often followed by coma, seizures, hypotension, and respiratory depression. In severe cases of overdose, various dysrhythmias may be seen, including sinus tachycardia, atrial arrhythmias, premature ventricular contractions, bigeminy, and ventricular fibrillation. If large doses are taken intravenously, cardiac failure, dysrhythmias, rhabdomyolysis, or hyperthermia may result in death.

In addition to those poisoned through recreational use of cocaine, others are at risk of overdose. A "body stuffer" is one who quickly ingests the drug, usually poorly wrapped, to avoid discovery. A "body packer" wraps the drug carefully for prolonged transport. A stuffer typically manifests toxicity within hours of ingestion; a packer is asymptomatic unless the package ruptures, usually days later.

Treatment

Except in cases of body stuffers or body packers, decontamination is seldom possible. Activated charcoal should be administered, and whole bowel irrigation may be useful in selected cases. Testing for cocaine in blood or plasma is generally not clinically useful, but a qualitative analysis of the urine may aid in confirming the diagnosis. For severe cases, an ECG is indicated. In suspected cases of body packing, radiographs of the GI tract may show multiple packets. X-ray films are usually not helpful for identifying stuffers. Seizures are treated with IV diazepam titrated to response. Hypotension is treated with standard agents. Because cocaine abuse may deplete norepinephrine, an indirect agent such as dopamine may be less effective than a direct agent such as norepinephrine. Agitation is best treated with a benzodiazepine.

Delaney-Black V: Prenatal cocaine exposure as a risk factor for later developmental outcomes. JAMA 2001;286:46 [PMID: 11434823].

King TA et al: Neurologic manifestations of in utero cocaine exposure in near-term and term infants. Pediatrics 1995;96: 259 [PMID: 7630680].

Mott SH et al: Neurologic manifestations of cocaine exposure in childhood. Pediatrics 1994;93:557 [PMID: 8134208].

Qureshi AI et al: Cocaine use and the likelihood of nonfatal myocardial infarction and stroke: Data from the Third National Health and Nutrition Examination Survey. Circulation 2001;103:502 [PMID: 11157713].

CONTRACEPTIVE PILLS

The only known toxic effects following acute ingestion of oral contraceptive agents are nausea, vomiting, and vaginal bleeding in girls.

COSMETICS & RELATED PRODUCTS

The relative toxicities of commonly ingested products in this group are listed in Table 12–4. Permanent wave neutralizers may contain bromates, peroxides, or perborates. Bromates have been removed from most products because they can cause nausea, vomiting, abdominal pain, shock, hemolysis, renal failure, and convulsions.

Table 12–4. Relative toxicities of cosmetics and similar products.

High toxicity	Low toxicity
Permanent wave neutralizers	Perfume
	Hair removers
Moderate toxicity	Deodorants
Fingernail polish	Bath salts
Fingernail polish remover	**No toxicity**
Metallic hair dyes	Liquid makeup
Home permanent wave lotion	Vegetable hair dye
Bath oil	Cleansing cream
Shaving lotion	Hair dressing (nonalcoholic)
Hair tonic (alcoholic)	
Cologne, toilet water	Hand lotion or cream
	Lipstick

Perborates can cause boric acid poisoning. Four grams of bromate salts is potentially lethal.

Poisoning is treated by gastric lavage with 1% sodium thiosulfate followed by demulcents to relieve gastric irritation. Sodium bicarbonate, 2%, in the lavage fluid may reduce hydrobromic acid formation. Sodium thiosulfate, 25%, 1.65 mL/kg, can be given intravenously, but methylene blue should not be used to treat methemoglobinemia in this situation because it increases the toxicity of bromates. Dialysis is indicated in renal failure but does not enhance excretion of bromate.

Fingernail polish removers used to contain toluene, but now usually have an acetone base, which does not require specific treatment other than monitoring CNS status.

Cobalt, copper, cadmium, iron, lead, nickel, silver, bismuth, and tin are sometimes found in metallic hair dyes. In large amounts they can cause skin sensitization, urticaria, dermatitis, eye damage, vertigo, hypertension, asthma, methemoglobinemia, tremors, convulsions, and coma. Treatment for ingestions is to administer demulcents and, only with large amounts, the appropriate antidote for the heavy metal involved.

Home permanent wave lotions, hair straighteners, and hair removers usually contain thioglycolic acid salts, which cause alkaline irritation and perhaps CNS depression.

Shaving lotion, hair tonic, hair straighteners, cologne, and toilet water contain denatured alcohol, which can cause CNS depression and hypoglycemia.

Deodorants usually consist of an antibacterial agent in a cream base. Antiperspirants are aluminum salts, which frequently cause skin sensitization. Zirconium oxide can cause granulomas in the axilla with chronic use.

CYCLIC ANTIDEPRESSANTS

Cyclic antidepressants (eg, amitriptyline, imipramine) have a very low ratio of toxic to therapeutic doses, and even a moderate overdose can have serious effects.

Cyclic antidepressant overdosage causes dysrhythmias, coma, convulsions, hypertension followed by hypotension, and hallucinations. These effects may be life-threatening and require rapid intervention. One agent, amoxapine, differs in that it causes fewer cardiovascular complications, but it is associated with a higher incidence of seizures.

Treatment

Decontamination should include gastric lavage and administration of activated charcoal.

An ECG should be taken in all patients. A QRS interval greater than 100 ms specifically identifies patients at risk to develop dysrhythmias. If dysrhythmias are demonstrated, the patient should be admitted and monitored until free of irregularity for 24 hours. Another indication for monitoring is persistent tachycardia of more than 110 beats/min. The onset of dysrhythmias is rare beyond 24 hours after ingestion.

Alkalinization with sodium bicarbonate, 0.5–1.0 mEq/kg IV, or hyperventilation may dramatically reverse ventricular dysrhythmias and narrow the QRS interval. Lidocaine may be added for treatment of arrhythmias. Bolus administration of sodium bicarbonate is recommended for all patients with QRS widening to above 120 ms and for those with significant dysrhythmias, to achieve a pH of 7.5–7.6. Forced diuresis is contraindicated. A benzodiazepine should be given for convulsions.

Hypotension is a major problem. Cyclic antidepressants block the reuptake of catecholamines, thereby producing initial hypertension followed by hypotension. Treatment with physostigmine is contraindicated. Vasopressors are generally effective. Dopamine is the agent of choice because it is readily available. If dopamine is ineffective, norepinephrine (0.1–1 µg/kg/min, titrated to response) should be added. Diuresis and hemodialysis are not effective.

Kerr GW et al: Tricyclic antidepressant overdose: A review. Emerg Med J 2001;18:236 [PMID: 11435353].

McKinney PE et al: Reversal of severe tricyclic antidepressant-induced cardiotoxicity with intravenous hypertonic saline solution. Ann Emerg Med 2003;42:20 [PMID: 12827118].

DIGITALIS & OTHER CARDIAC GLYCOSIDES

Toxicity is typically the result of incorrect dosing or unrecognized renal insufficiency. Clinical features include nausea, vomiting, diarrhea, headache, delirium, confusion, and, occasionally, coma. Cardiac dysrhythmias typically involve bradydysrhythmias, but every type of dysrhythmia has been reported in digitalis intoxication, including atrial fibrillation, paroxysmal atrial tachycardia, and atrial flutter. Death usually is the result of ventricular fibrillation. Transplacental intoxication by digitalis has been reported.

Treatment

If vomiting has not occurred, induce emesis or provide lavage followed by charcoal. Potassium is contraindicated in acute overdosage unless there is laboratory evidence of hypokalemia. In acute overdosage, hyperkalemia is more common. Hypokalemia is common in chronic toxicity.

The patient must be monitored carefully for ECG changes. The correction of acidosis better demonstrates the degree of potassium deficiency present. Bradycardias have been treated with atropine. Phenytoin, lidocaine, magnesium salts (not in renal failure), amiodarone, and bretylium have been used to correct arrhythmias.

Definitive treatment is with digoxin immune Fab (ovine) (Digibind). Indications for its use include hypotension or any dysrhythmia, typically ventricular dysrhythmias and progressive bradydysrhythmias that produce clinical concern. Elevated T waves indicate high potassium and may be an indication for digoxin immune Fab (Digibind, DigiFab) use. Techniques of determining dosage and indications related to levels, when available are described in product literature.

Woolf AD et al: The use of digoxin-specific Fab fragments for severe digitalis intoxication in children. N Engl J Med 1992;326:1739 [PMID: 1997016].

DIPHENOXYLATE WITH ATROPINE (Lomotil)

Lomotil contains diphenoxylate hydrochloride, a synthetic narcotic, and atropine sulfate. Loperamide (Imodium) has largely replaced Lomotil and does not produce toxicity. Small amounts are potentially lethal in children; it is contraindicated in children younger than age 2 years. Early signs of intoxication with this preparation result from its anticholinergic effect and consist of fever, facial flushing, tachypnea, and lethargy. However, the miotic effect of the narcotic predominates. Later, hypothermia, increasing CNS depression, and loss of the facial flush occur. Seizures are probably secondary to hypoxia.

Treatment

Prolonged monitoring (24 hours) with pulse oximetry and careful attention to airway is sufficient in most cases.

Naloxone hydrochloride (0.4–2.0 mg IV in children and adults) should be given. Repeated doses may be required because the duration of action of diphenoxylate is considerably longer than that of naloxone.

McCarron MM et al: Diphenoxylate-atropine (Lomotil) overdose in children: An update. Pediatrics 1991;87:694 [PMID: 2020516].

DISINFECTANTS & DEODORIZERS

1. Naphthalene

Naphthalene is commonly found in mothballs, disinfectants, and deodorizers. Naphthalene's toxicity is often not fully appreciated. It is absorbed not only when ingested but also through the skin and lungs. It is potentially hazardous to store baby clothes in naphthalene, because baby oil is an excellent solvent that may increase dermal absorption. *Note:* Most mothballs contain *para*-dichlorobenzene and not naphthalene (see next section). Metabolic products of naphthalene may cause severe hemolytic anemia, similar to that due to primaquine toxicity, 2–7 days after ingestion. Other physical findings include vomiting, diarrhea, jaundice, oliguria, anuria, coma, and convulsions. The urine may contain hemoglobin, protein, and casts.

Treatment

Induced vomiting should be followed by activated charcoal. Urinary alkalinization may prevent blocking of the renal tubules by acid hematin crystals. Anuria may persist for 1–2 weeks and still be completely reversible.

Ostlere L et al: Haemolytic anaemia associated with ingestion of naphthalene-containing anointing oil. Postgrad Med J 1988;64:444 [PMID: 3211822].

Siegel E, Wason S: Mothball toxicity. Pediatr Clin North Am 1986;33:369 [PMID: 3515301].

2. P-Dichlorobenzene, Phenolic Acids, & Others

Disinfectants and deodorizers containing *p*-dichlorobenzene or sodium sulfate are much less toxic than those containing naphthalene. Disinfectants containing phenolic acids are highly toxic, especially if they contain a borate ion. Phenol precipitates tissue proteins and causes respiratory alkalosis followed by metabolic acidosis. Some phenols cause methemoglobinemia.

Local gangrene occurs after prolonged contact with tissue. Phenol is readily absorbed from the GI tract, causing diffuse capillary damage and, in some cases, methemoglobinemia. Pentachlorophenol, which has been used in terminal rinsing of diapers, has caused infant fatalities.

The toxicity of alkalies, quaternary ammonium compounds, pine oil, and halogenated disinfectants varies with the concentration of active ingredients. Wick deodorizers are usually of moderate toxicity. Iodophor disinfectants are the safest. Spray deodorizers are not usually toxic, because a child is not likely to swallow a very large dose.

Signs and symptoms of acute quaternary ammonium compound ingestion include diaphoresis, strong irritation, thirst, vomiting, diarrhea, cyanosis, hyperactivity, coma, convulsions, hypotension, abdominal pain, and pulmonary edema. Acute liver or renal failure may develop later.

Treatment

Activated charcoal may be used prior to gastric lavage. Castor oil dissolves phenol and may retard its absorption. This property of castor oil, however, has not been proved clinically. Mineral oil and alcohol are contraindicated because they increase the gastric absorption of phenol. The metabolic acidosis must be managed carefully. Anticonvulsants or measures to treat shock may be needed.

Because phenols are absorbed through the skin, exposed areas should be irrigated copiously with water. Undiluted polyethylene glycol may be a useful solvent as well.

Mucklow ES: Accidental feeding of dilute antiseptic solution (chlorhexidine 0.05% with cetrimide 1%) to five babies. Hum Toxicol 1988;7:567 [PMID: 3229768].

Van Berkel M, de Wolff FA: Survival after acute benzalkonium chloride poisoning. Hum Toxicol 1988;7:191 [PMID: 3378808].

DISK-SHAPED BATTERIES

Small, flat, smooth disk-shaped batteries measure between 10 and 25 mm in diameter. About 69% of them pass through the GI tract in 48 hours and 85% in 72 hours. Some may become entrapped. These batteries contain caustic materials and heavy metals.

Batteries impacted in the esophagus may cause symptoms of refusal to take food, increased salivation, vomiting with or without blood, and pain or discomfort. Aspiration into the trachea may also occur. Fatalities have been reported in association with esophageal perforation.

When a history of disk battery ingestion is obtained, radiographs of the entire respiratory tract and GI tract should be taken so that the battery can be located and the proper therapy determined.

Treatment

If the disk battery is located in the esophagus, it must be removed immediately. If the battery has been in the esophagus for more than 24 hours, the risk of caustic burn is greater.

Location of the disk battery below the esophagus has been associated with tissue damage, but the course is benign in most cases. Perforated Meckel diverticulum has been the major complication. It may take as long as 7 days for spontaneous passage to occur, and lack of movement in the GI tract may not require removal in an asymptomatic patient.

Some researchers have suggested repeated radiographs and surgical intervention if passage of the battery pauses, but this approach may be excessive. Batteries that have opened in the GI tract have been associated with some toxicity due to mercury, but the patients have recovered.

Emesis is ineffective. Asymptomatic patients may simply be observed and stools examined for passage of the battery. If the battery has not passed within 7 days or if the patient becomes symptomatic, radiographs should be repeated. If the battery has come apart or appears not to be moving, a purgative, enema, or nonabsorbable intestinal lavage solution should be administered. If these methods are unsuccessful, surgical intervention may be required. Levels of heavy metals (mainly mercury) should be measured in patients in whom the battery has opened or symptoms have developed.

Dane S: A truly emergent problem: Button battery in the nose. Acad Emerg Med 2000;7:204 [PMID: 10691084].

Litovitz TL, Schmitz BF: Ingestion of cylindrical and button batteries: An analysis of 2382 cases. Pediatrics 1992;89:747 [PMID: 2304794].

GAMMA-HYDROXYBUTYRATE, GAMMA-BUTYROLACTONE, & BUTANEDIOL

Gamma-hydroxybutyrate (GHB), γ-butyrolactone (GBL), and butanediol have become popular drugs of abuse in adolescents and adults. GHB is a CNS depressant that is structurally similar to the inhibitory neurotransmitter γ-aminobutyric acid. GBL and butanediol are converted in the body to GHB. These drugs cause deep but short-lived coma; the coma often lasts only 1–4 hours. Treatment consists of supportive care with close attention to airway and endotracheal intubation if respiratory depression or decreased gag reflex complicates the poisoning. Atropine has been used successfully for symptomatic bradycardia.

Withdrawal from GHB, GBL, or butanediol can cause several days of extreme agitation, hallucination, or tachycardia. Treatment with high doses of benzodiazepines or with butyrophenones (eg, haloperidol or droperidol) or secobarbital may be needed for several days.

Dyer JE et al: Gamma-hydroxybutyrate withdrawal syndrome. Ann Emerg Med 2001;37:147 [PMID: 11174231].

Sporer KA et al: Gamma-hydroxybutyrate serum levels and clinical syndrome after severe overdose. Ann Emerg Med 2003;42:3 [PMID: 12827115].

HYDROCARBONS (Benzene, Charcoal Lighter Fluid, Gasoline, Kerosene, Petroleum Distillates, Turpentine)

Ingestion of hydrocarbons may cause irritation of mucous membranes, vomiting, blood-tinged diarrhea, respiratory distress, cyanosis, tachycardia, and fever. Although a small amount (10 mL) of certain hydrocarbons is potentially fatal, patients have survived ingestion of several ounces of other petroleum distillates. The more aromatic a hydrocarbon is and the lower its viscosity rating, the more potentially toxic it is. Benzene, gasoline, kerosene, and red seal oil furniture polish are the most dangerous. A dose exceeding 1 mL/kg is likely to cause CNS depression. A history of coughing or choking, as well as vomiting, suggests aspiration with resulting hydrocarbon pneumonia. This is an acute hemorrhagic necrotizing disease that usually develops within 24 hours of the ingestion and resolves without sequelae in 3–5 days. However, several weeks may be required for full resolution of a hydrocarbon pneumonia. Pneumonia may be caused by the aspiration of a few drops of petroleum distillate into the lung or by absorption from the circulatory system. Pulmonary edema and hemorrhage, cardiac dilatation and dysrhythmias, hepatosplenomegaly, proteinuria, and hematuria can occur following large overdoses. Hypoglycemia is occasionally present. A chest radiograph may reveal pneumonia within hours after the ingestion. An abnormal urinalysis in a child with a previously normal urinary tract suggests a large overdose.

Treatment

Both emetics and lavage should be avoided when only a small amount has been ingested. Mineral oil should not be given, because it can cause a low-grade lipoid pneumonia.

Epinephrine should not be used with halogenated hydrocarbons because it may affect an already sensitized myocardium. The usefulness of corticosteroids is debated, and antibiotics should be reserved for patients with infections. Oxygen and mist are helpful. Extracorporeal membrane oxygenation has been successful in at least two cases of failure with standard therapy.

Anas N et al: Criteria for hospitalizing children who have ingested products containing hydrocarbons. JAMA 1981;246:840 [PMID: 7253158].

Bysani GK et al: Treatment of hydrocarbon pneumonitis. High frequency jet ventilation as an alternative to extracorporeal membrane oxygenation. Chest 1994;106:300 [PMID: 8020296].

Lifshitz M et al: Hydrocarbon poisoning in children: A 5-year retrospective study. Wilderness Environ Med 2003;14:78 [PMID: 12825880].

Lorenc JD: Inhalant abuse in the pediatric populations: A persistent challenge. Curr Opin Pediatr 2003;15:204 [PMID: 12640280].

Sheridan RL: Burns with inhalation injury and petrol aspiration in adolescents seeking euphoria through hydrocarbon inhalation. Burns 1996;22:566 [PMID: 8909762].

IBUPROFEN

Most exposures in children do not produce symptoms. In one study, for example, children ingesting up to 2.4 g remained asymptomatic. When symptoms occur, the most common are abdominal pain, vomiting, drowsiness, and lethargy. In rare cases, apnea (especially in young children), seizures, metabolic acidosis, and CNS depression leading to coma have occurred.

Treatment

If a child has ingested less than 100 mg/kg, dilution with water or milk may be all that is necessary to minimize the GI upset. In children, the volume of liquid used for dilution should be less than 4 oz. When the ingested amount is more than 400 mg/kg, seizures or CNS depression may occur; therefore, gastric lavage may be preferred to emesis. Activated charcoal may also be of value. There is no specific antidote. Neither alkalinization of the urine nor hemodialysis is helpful.

Cuzzolin L et al: NSAID-induced nephrotoxicity from the fetus to the child. Drug Safety 2001;242:9 [PMID: 11219488].

Hall AH et al: Ibuprofen overdose in adults. J Toxicol Clin Toxicol 1992;30:23 [PMID: 1542147].

Lesko SM: The safety of ibuprofen suspension in children. Intl J Clin Pract (Suppl) 2003;135:50 [PMID: 12723748].

Oker EE et al: Serious toxicity in a young child due to ibuprofen. Acad Emerg Med 2000;7:821 [PMID: 10917334].

INSECT STINGS (Bee, Wasp, & Hornet)

Insect stings are painful but not usually dangerous; however, death from anaphylaxis may occur. Bee venom has hemolytic, neurotoxic, and histamine-like activities that can on rare occasion cause hemoglobinuria and severe anaphylactoid reactions. Massive envenomation from numerous stings may cause hemolysis, rhabdomyolysis, and shock leading to multiple organ failure.

Treatment

The physician should remove the stinger, taking care not to squeeze the attached venom sac. For allergic reactions, epinephrine 1:1000 solution, 0.01 mL/kg, should be administered IV or SQ above the site of the sting. Three to four whiffs from an isoproterenol aerosol inhaler may be given at 3- to 4-minute intervals as needed. Corticosteroids (hydrocortisone), 100 mg IV, and diphenhydramine, 1.5 mg/kg IV, are useful ancillary drugs but have no immediate effect. Ephedrine or antihistamines may be used for 2 or 3 days to prevent recurrence of symptoms.

A patient who has had a potentially life-threatening insect sting should be desensitized against the Hymenoptera group, because the honey bee, wasp, hornet, and yellow jacket have common antigens in their venom. For the more usual stings, cold compresses, aspirin, and diphenhydramine 1 mg/kg PO, are sufficient.

Reisman RE, Livingstone A: Late-onset allergic reactions, including serum sickness after insect stings. J Allergy Clin Immunol 1989;84:331 [PMID: 2778239].

Ross RN et al: Effectiveness of specific immunotherapy in the treatment of hymenoptera venom hypersensitivity: A meta-analysis. Clin Ther 2000;22:351 [PMID: 10963289].

Vetter RS et al: Mass envenomations by honey bees and wasps. West J Med 1999;170:223 [PMID: 10344177].

INSECTICIDES

The petroleum distillates or other organic solvents used in these products are often as toxic as the insecticide itself. Decontamination may be performed by aspirating the stomach with a nasogastric tube.

1. Chlorinated Hydrocarbons (eg, Aldrin, Carbinol, Chlordane, DDT, Dieldrin, Endrin, Heptachlor, Lindane, Toxaphene)

Signs of intoxication include salivation, GI irritability, abdominal pain, vomiting, diarrhea, CNS depression, and convulsions. Inhalation exposure causes irritation of the eyes, nose, and throat; blurred vision; cough; and pulmonary edema.

Chlorinated hydrocarbons are absorbed through the skin, respiratory tract, and GI tract. Decontamination of skin with soap and evacuation of the stomach contents are critical. All contaminated clothing should be removed. Castor oil, milk, and other substances containing fats or oils should not be left in the stomach because they increase absorption of the chlorinated hydrocarbons. Convulsions should be treated with diazepam, 0.1–0.3 mg/kg IV. Epinephrine should not be used because it may cause cardiac arrhythmias.

2. Organophosphate (Cholinesterase-Inhibiting) Insecticides (eg, Chlorothion, Co-Ral, DFP, Diazinon, Malathion, Paraoxon, Parathion, Phosdrin, TEPP, Thio-TEPP)

Dizziness, headache, blurred vision, miosis, tearing, salivation, nausea, vomiting, diarrhea, hyperglycemia, cyanosis, sense of constriction of the chest, dyspnea, sweating, weakness, muscular twitching, convulsions, loss of reflexes and sphincter control, and coma can occur.

The clinical findings are the result of cholinesterase inhibition, which causes an accumulation of acetylcholine. The onset of symptoms occurs within 12 hours of the exposure. Red cell cholinesterase levels should be measured as soon as possible. (Some normal individuals have a low serum cholinesterase level.) Normal values vary in different laboratories. In general, a decrease of red cell cholinesterase to below 25% of normal indicates significant exposure.

Repeated low-grade exposure may result in sudden, acute toxic reactions. This syndrome usually occurs after repeated household spraying rather than agricultural exposure.

Although all organophosphates act by inhibiting cholinesterase activity, they vary greatly in their toxicity. Parathion, for example, is 100 times more toxic than malathion. The toxicity is influenced by the specific compound, the type of formulation (liquid or solid), the vehicle, and the route of absorption (lungs, skin, or GI tract).

Treatment

Decontamination of skin, nails, hair, and clothing with soapy water is extremely important. Atropine plus a cholinesterase reactivator, pralidoxime, is an antidote for organophosphate insecticide poisoning. After assessment and management of the ABCs, atropine should be given and repeated every few minutes until airway secretions diminish. An appropriate starting dose of atropine is 2–4 mg IV in an adult and 0.05 mg/kg in a child. The patient should receive enough atropine to stop secretions (mydriasis in not an appropriate stopping point). Severe poisoning may require gram quantities of atropine administered over 24 hours.

Because atropine antagonizes the muscarinic parasympathetic effects of the organophosphates but does not affect the nicotinic receptor, it does not improve muscular weakness. Pralidoxime should also be given immediately in more severe cases and repeated every 6–12 hours as needed (25–50 mg/kg diluted to 5% and infused over 5–30 minutes at a rate of no more than 500 mg/min). Pralidoxime should be used in addition to—not in place of—atropine if red cell cholinesterase is less than 25% of normal. Pralidoxime is most useful within 48 hours after the exposure but has shown some effects 2–6 days later. Morphine, theophylline, aminophylline, succinylcholine, and tranquilizers of the reserpine and phenothiazine types are contraindicated. Hyperglycemia is common in severe poisonings.

Eisenstein EM, Amitai Y: Index of suspicion: Case 1. Organophosphate intoxication. Pediatr Rev 2000;21:205 [PMID: 10854316].

Lifshitz M et al: Carbamate and organophosphate; poisoning in young children. Pediatr Emerg Care 1999;15:102 [PMID: 10220078].

3. Carbamates (eg, Carbaryl, Sevin, Zectran)

Carbamate insecticides are reversible inhibitors of cholinesterase. The signs and symptoms of intoxication are similar to those associated with organophosphate poisoning but are generally less severe. Atropine titrated to effect is sufficient treatment. Pralidoxime should not be used with carbaryl poisoning but is of value with other carbamates. In combined exposures to organophosphates, give atropine but reserve pralidoxime for cases in which the red cell cholinesterase is depressed below 25% of normal or marked effects of nicotinic receptor stimulation are present.

4. Botanical Insecticides (eg, Black Flag Bug Killer, Black Leaf CPR Insect Killer, Flit Aerosol House & Garden Insect Killer, French's Flea Powder, Raid)

Allergic reactions, asthma-like symptoms, coma, and convulsions have been reported. Pyrethrins, allethrin, and rotenone do not commonly cause signs of toxicity. Antihistamines, short-acting barbiturates, and atropine are helpful as symptomatic treatment.

IRON

Five stages of intoxication may occur in iron poisoning: (1) Hemorrhagic gastroenteritis, which occurs 30–60 minutes after ingestion and may be associated with shock, acidosis, coagulation defects, and coma. This phase usually lasts 4–6 hours. (2) Phase of improvement, lasting 2–12 hours, during which patient looks better. (3) Delayed shock, which may occur 12–48 hours after ingestion. Metabolic acidosis, fever, leukocytosis, and coma may also be present. (4) Liver damage with hepatic failure. (5) Residual pyloric stenosis, which may develop about 4 weeks after the ingestion.

Once iron is absorbed from the GI tract, it is not normally eliminated in feces but may be partially excreted in the urine, giving it a red color prior to chelation. A reddish discoloration of the urine suggests a serum iron level greater than 350 mg/dL.

Treatment

GI decontamination is based on clinical assessment. Syrup of ipecac may be administered at home, with appropriate follow-up, provided the history does not warrant an emergency department visit. The patient should be referred to a health care facility if symptomatic or if the history indicates toxic amounts. Gastric lavage and whole bowel irrigation should be considered in these patients.

Shock is treated in the usual manner. Sodium bicarbonate and Fleet Phospho-Soda left in the stomach to form the insoluble phosphate or carbonate have not shown clinical benefit and have caused lethal hypernatremia or hyperphosphatemia. Deferoxamine, a specific chelating agent for iron, is a useful adjunct in the treatment of severe iron poisoning. It forms a soluble complex that is excreted in the urine. It is contraindicated in patients with renal failure unless dialysis can be used. IV deferoxamine chelation therapy should be instituted if the patient is symptomatic and a serum iron determination cannot be obtained readily, or if the peak serum iron exceeds 400 μg/dL (62.6 μmol/L) at 4–5 hours after ingestion.

Deferoxamine should not be delayed until serum iron levels are available in serious cases of poisoning. IV administration is indicated if the patient is in shock, in which case it should be given at a dosage of 15 mg/kg/h. Infusion rates up to 35 mg/kg/h have been used in life-threatening poisonings. Rapid IV administration can cause hypotension, facial flushing, urticaria, tachycardia, and shock. Deferoxamine, 90 mg/kg IM every 8 hours (maximum, 1 g), may be given if IV access cannot be established, but the procedure is painful. The indications for discontinuation of deferoxamine have not been clearly delineated. Generally, it can be stopped after 12–24 hours if the acidosis has resolved and the patient is improving.

Hemodialysis, peritoneal dialysis, or exchange transfusion can be used to increase the excretion of the dialyzable complex. Urine output should be monitored and urine sediment examined for evidence of renal tubular damage. Initial laboratory studies should include blood typing and cross-matching; total protein; serum iron, sodium, potassium, and chloride; pCO_2; pH; and liver function tests. Serum iron levels fall rapidly even if deferoxamine is not given.

After the acute episode, liver function studies and an upper GI series are indicated to rule out residual damage.

Black J et al: Child abuse by intentional iron poisoning presenting as shock and persistent acidosis. Pediatrics 2003;111:197 [PMID: 12509576].

Juurlink DN et al: Iron poisoning in young children: Association with the birth of a sibling. CMAJ 2003;165:1539 [PMID: 12796332].

Morris CC: Pediatric iron poisonings in the United States. South Med J 2000;93:352 [PMID: 11142463].

LEAD

Lead poisoning (plumbism) causes vague symptoms, including weakness, irritability, weight loss, vomiting, personality changes, ataxia, constipation, headache, and colicky abdominal pain. Late manifestations consist of retarded development, convulsions, and coma associated with increased intracranial pressure, which is a medical emergency.

Plumbism usually occurs insidiously in children younger than age 5 years. The most likely sources of lead include flaking leaded paint, artist's paints, fruit tree sprays, solder, brass alloys, home-glazed pottery, and fumes from burning batteries. Only paint containing less than 1% lead is safe for interior use (eg, furniture, toys). Repetitive ingestions of small amounts of lead are far more serious than a single massive exposure. Toxic effects are likely to occur if more than 0.5 mg of lead per day is absorbed.

Blood lead levels are used to assess the severity of exposure. A complete blood count and serum ferritin concentration should be obtained; iron deficiency increases absorption of lead. Glycosuria, proteinuria, hematuria, and aminoaciduria occur frequently. Blood lead levels usually exceed 80 μg/dL in symptomatic patients. Abnormal blood lead levels should be repeated in asymptomatic patients to rule out laboratory error. Specimens must be meticulously obtained in acid-washed containers. A normocytic, slightly hypochromic anemia with basophilic stippling of the red cells and reticulocytosis may be present in plumbism. Stippling of red blood cells is absent in cases involving only recent ingestion.

The cerebrospinal fluid (CSF) protein is elevated, and the white cell count is usually less than 100 cells/mL. CSF pressure may be elevated in patients with encephalopathy; lumbar punctures must be performed cautiously to prevent herniation.

Treatment

Standard GI decontamination is indicated if an acute ingestion has occurred or lead is noted on the abdominal radiograph. Succimer is an orally administered chelator approved for use in children and reported to be as efficacious as calcium edetate. Treatment for blood lead levels of 20–45 μg/dL in children has not been determined. Succimer should be initiated at blood lead levels over 45 μg/dL. The initial dose is 10 mg/kg (350 mg/m²) every 8 hours for 5 days. The same dose is then given every 12 hours for 14 days. At least 2 weeks should elapse between courses. Blood lead levels increase somewhat (ie, rebound) after discontinuation of therapy. Courses of dimercaprol (4 mg/kg/dose) and calcium edetate may still be used but are no longer the preferred method, except in cases of lead encephalopathy.

Anticonvulsants may be needed. Mannitol or corticosteroids and volume restriction are indicated in patients with encephalopathy. A high-calcium, high-phosphorus diet and large doses of vitamin D may remove lead from the blood by depositing it in the bones. A public health team should evaluate the source of the lead. Necessary corrections should be completed before the child is returned home.

American Academy of Pediatrics Committee on Drugs: Treatment guidelines for lead exposure in children. Pediatrics 1995;96:155 [PMID: 7596706].

Markowitz M: Lead poisoning. Pediatr Rev 2000;21:327 [PMID: 11010979].

Rogan WJ et al: Exposure to lead in children—How low is low enough? N Engl J Med 2003;16:1515 [PMID: 12700370].

Rogan WJ et al: Treatment of Lead-Exposed Children Trial Group: The effect of chelation therapy with succimer on neuropsychological development in children exposed to lead. N Engl J Med 2001;344:1421 [PMID: 11346806].

MUSHROOMS

Toxic mushrooms are often difficult to distinguish from edible varieties. Contact a poison control center to obtain identification assistance. Symptoms vary with the species ingested, time of year, stage of maturity, quantity eaten, method of preparation, and interval since ingestion. A mushroom that is toxic to one individual may not be toxic to another. Drinking alcohol and eating certain mushrooms may cause a reaction similar to that seen with disulfiram and alcohol. Cooking destroys some toxins but not the deadly one produced by *Amanita phalloides,* which is responsible for 90% of deaths due to mushroom poisoning. Mushroom toxins are absorbed relatively slowly. Onset of symptoms within 2 hours of ingestion suggests muscarinic toxin, whereas a delay of symptoms for 6–48 hours after ingestion strongly suggests *Amanita* (amanitin) poisoning. Patients who have ingested *A phalloides* may relapse and die of hepatic or renal failure following initial improvement.

Mushroom poisoning may produce muscarinic symptoms (salivation, vomiting, diarrhea, cramping abdominal pain, tenesmus, miosis, and dyspnea), coma, convulsions, hallucinations, hemolysis, and delayed hepatic and renal failure.

Treatment

Induce vomiting and follow with activated charcoal. If the patient has muscarinic signs, give atropine, 0.05 mg/kg IM (0.02 mg/kg in toddlers), and repeat as needed (usually every 30 minutes) to keep the patient atropinized. Atropine, however, is used only when cholinergic effects are present and not for all mushrooms. Hypoglycemia is most likely to occur in patients with delayed onset of symptoms. Try to identify the mushroom if the patient is symptomatic. Consultation with a certified poison center is recommended. Local botanical gardens, university departments of botany, and societies of mycologists may be able to help. Supportive care is usually all that is needed; however, in the case of *A phalloides,* penicillin, silibinin, or hemodialysis may be indicated.

Lampe KF, McCann MA: Differential diagnosis of poisoning by North American mushrooms, with particular emphasis on *Amanita phalloides*-like intoxication. Ann Emerg Med 1987; 16:956 [PMID: 3631682].

Michelot D et al: *Amanita muscaria:* Chemistry, biology, toxicology and ethnomycology. Mycol Res 2003;107:131 [PMID: 12747324].

Pawlowska J et al: Liver transplantation in three family members after *Amanita phalloides* mushroom poisoning. Transplant Proc 2002;34:3313 [PMID: 12493457].

NITRITES, NITRATES, ANILINE, PENTACHLOROPHENOL, & DINITROPHENOL

Nausea, vertigo, vomiting, cyanosis (methemoglobinemia), cramping abdominal pain, tachycardia, cardiovascular collapse, tachypnea, coma, shock, convulsions, and death are possible manifestations of nitrite or nitrate poisoning.

Nitrite and nitrate compounds found in the home include amyl nitrite, butyl nitrates, isobutyl nitrates, nitroglycerin, pentaerythritol tetranitrate, sodium nitrite, nitrobenzene, and phenazopyridine. Pentachlorophenol and dinitrophenol, which are found in wood preservatives, produce methemoglobinemia and high fever because of uncoupling of oxidative phosphorylation. Headache, dizziness, and bradycardia have been reported. High concentrations of nitrites in well water or spinach have been the most common cause of nitrite-induced methemoglobinemia. Symptoms do not usually occur until 15–50% of the hemoglobin has been converted to methemoglobin. A rapid test is to compare a drop of normal blood with the patient's blood on a dry filter paper. Brown discoloration of the patient's blood indicates a methemoglobin level of more than 15%.

Treatment

Induce vomiting and administer activated charcoal. Decontaminate affected skin with soap and water. Oxygen and artificial respiration may be needed. If the blood methemoglobin level exceeds 30%, or if levels cannot be obtained and the patient is symptomatic, give a 1% solution of methylene blue, 0.2 mL/kg IV over 5–10 minutes. Avoid perivascular infiltration, because it causes necrosis of the skin and subcutaneous tissues. A dramatic change in the degree of cyanosis should occur. Transfusion is occasionally necessary. Epinephrine and other vasoconstrictors are contraindicated. If reflex bradycardia occurs, atropine should be used.

Herman MI et al: Methylene blue by intraosseous infusion for methemoglobinemia. Ann Emerg Med 1999;33:111 [PMID: 9867898].

Kennedy N et al: Faulty sausage production causing methaemoglobinaemia. Arch Dis Child 1997;76:367 [PMID: 9166036].

OPIOIDS (Codeine, Heroin, Methadone, Morphine, Propoxyphene)

Opioid-related medical problems may include drug addiction, withdrawal in a newborn infant, and accidental overdoses. Unlike other narcotics, methadone is absorbed readily from the GI tract. Most opioids, including heroin, methadone, meperidine, morphine, and codeine, are excreted in the urine within 24 hours and can be detected readily.

Narcotic-addicted adolescents often have other medical problems, including cellulitis, abscesses, thrombophlebitis, tetanus, infective endocarditis, HIV infection, tuberculosis, hepatitis, malaria, foreign body emboli, thrombosis of pulmonary arterioles, diabetes mellitus, obstetric complications, nephropathy, and peptic ulcer.

Treatment of Overdosage

Opioids can cause respiratory depression, stridor, coma, increased oropharyngeal secretions, sinus bradycardia, and urinary retention. Pulmonary edema rarely occurs in children; deaths usually result from aspiration of gastric contents, respiratory arrest, and cerebral edema. Convulsions may occur with propoxyphene overdosage.

Although suggested doses for naloxone hydrochloride range from 0.01–0.1 mg/kg, it is generally unnecessary to calculate the dosage on this basis. This extremely safe antidote should be given in sufficient quantity to reverse opioid binding sites. For children under age 1 year, 1 ampoule (0.4 mg) should be given initially; if there is no response, five more ampoules (2 mg) should be given rapidly. Older children should be given 0.4–0.8 mg, followed by 2–4 mg if there is no response. An improvement in respiratory status may be followed by respiratory depression, because the antagonist's duration of action is less than 1 hour. Neonates poisoned in utero may require 10–30 mg/kg to reverse the effect.

Withdrawal in the Addict

Diazepam, 10 mg every 6 hours PO, has been recommended for the treatment of mild narcotic withdrawal in ambulatory adolescents. Management of withdrawal in the confirmed addict may be accomplished with the administration of clonidine, by substitution with methadone, or with reintroduction of the original addicting agent, if available through a supervised drug withdrawal program. A tapered course over 3 weeks will accomplish this goal. Death rarely, if ever, occurs. The abrupt discontinuation of narcotics (cold turkey method) is not recommended and may cause severe physical withdrawal signs.

Withdrawal in the Newborn

A newborn infant in opioid withdrawal is usually small for gestational age and demonstrates yawning, sneezing, decreased Moro reflex, hunger but uncoordinated sucking action, jitteriness, tremor, constant movement, a shrill protracted cry, increased tendon reflexes, convulsions, vomiting, fever, watery diarrhea, cyanosis, dehydration, vasomotor instability, seizure, and collapse.

The onset of symptoms commonly begins in the first 48 hours but may be delayed as long as 8 days depending on the timing of the mother's last fix and her predelivery medication. The diagnosis can be confirmed easily by identifying the narcotic in the urine of the mother and the baby.

Several treatment methods have been suggested for narcotic withdrawal in the newborn. Phenobarbital, 8 mg/kg/d IM or PO in 4 doses for 4 days and then reduced by one-third every 2 days as signs decrease, may be continued for as long as 3 weeks. Methadone may be necessary in those infants with congenital methadone addiction who are not controlled in their withdrawal by large doses of phenobarbital. Dosage should be 0.5 mg/kg/d in two divided doses but can be increased gradually as needed. After control of the symptoms is achieved, the dose may be tapered over 4 weeks.

It is unclear whether prophylactic treatment with these drugs decreases the complication rate. The mortality rate of untreated narcotic withdrawal in the newborn may be as high as 45%.

American Academy of Pediatrics Committee on Drugs: Naloxone dosage and route of administration for infants and children: Addendum to emergency drug doses for infants and children. Pediatrics 1990;86:484 [PMID: 2388800].

Traub SJ et al: Pediatric "body packing". Arch Pediatr Adolesc Med 2003;157:174 [PMID: 12580688].

PHENOTHIAZINES (Chlorpromazine, Prochlorperazine, Trifluoperazine)

Clinical Presentations

A. Extrapyramidal Crisis

Episodes characterized by torticollis, stiffening of the body, spasticity, poor speech, catatonia, and inability to communicate although conscious are typical manifestations. These episodes usually last a few seconds to a few minutes but have rarely caused death. Extrapyramidal crises may represent idiosyncratic reactions and are aggravated by dehydration. The signs and symptoms occur most often in children who have received prochlorperazine. They are commonly mistaken for psychotic episodes.

B. Overdose

Lethargy and deep prolonged coma commonly occur. Promazine, chlorpromazine, and prochlorperazine are the drugs most likely to cause respiratory depression and precipitous drops in blood pressure. Occasionally, paradoxic hyperactivity and extrapyramidal signs as well as hyperglycemia and acetonemia are present. Seizures are uncommon.

C. Neuroleptic malignant syndrome

Neuroleptic malignant syndrome is a rare idiosyncratic complication of phenothiazine use that may be lethal. It is a syndrome involving mental status change (confusion, coma), motor abnormalities (lead pipe rigidity, clonus), and autonomic dysfunction (tachycardia, hyperpyrexia).

Treatment

Extrapyramidal signs are alleviated within minutes by the slow IV administration of diphenhydramine, 1–2 mg/kg (maximum, 50 mg), or benztropine mesylate, 1–2 mg IV (1 mg/min). No other treatment is usually indicated.

Patients with overdoses should receive conservative supportive care. Activated charcoal should be administered. Hypotension may be treated with standard agents, starting with isotonic saline administration. Agitation is best treated with diazepam. Neuroleptic malignant syndrome is treated by discontinuing the drug, giving aggressive supportive care, and administering dantrolene or bromocriptine.

Baker PB et al: Hyperthermia, hypertension, hypertonia, and coma in massive thioridazine overdose. Am J Emerg Med 1988; 6:346 [PMID: 3390252].

Dyer KS et al: Use of phenothiazines as sedatives in children: What are the risks? Drug Saf 1999;21:81 [PMID: 10456377].

O'Malley GF et al: Olanzapine overdose mimicking opioid intoxication. Ann Emerg Med 1999;34:279 [PMID: 10424936].

PLANTS

Many common ornamental, garden, and wild plants are potentially toxic. Only in a few cases will small amounts of a plant cause severe illness or death. Table 12–5 lists the most toxic plants, symptoms and signs of poisoning, and treatment. Contact your poison control center for assistance with identification.

PSYCHOTROPIC DRUGS

Psychotropic drugs consist of four general classes: stimulants (amphetamines, cocaine), depressants (eg, narcotics, barbiturates), antidepressants and tranquilizers, and hallucinogens (eg, LSD, PCP).

Clinical Presentations

The following clinical findings are commonly seen in patients abusing drugs. See also other entries discussed in alphabetic order in this chapter.

A. Stimulants

Agitation, euphoria, grandiose feelings, tachycardia, fever, abdominal cramps, visual and auditory hallucinations, mydriasis, coma, convulsions, and respiratory depression.

B. Depressants

Emotional lability, ataxia, diplopia, nystagmus, vertigo, poor accommodation, respiratory depression, coma, apnea, and convulsions. Dilatation of conjunctival blood vessels suggests marijuana ingestion. Narcotics cause miotic pupils and, occasionally, pulmonary edema.

C. Antidepressants and Tranquilizers

Hypotension, lethargy, respiratory depression, coma, and extrapyramidal reactions.

D. Hallucinogens and Psychoactive Drugs

Belladonna alkaloids cause mydriasis, dry mouth, nausea, vomiting, urinary retention, confusion, disorientation, paranoid delusions, hallucinations, fever, hypotension, aggressive behavior, convulsions, and coma. Psychoactive drugs such as LSD cause mydriasis, unexplained bizarre behavior, hallucinations, and generalized undifferentiated psychotic behavior.

Management of the Patient Who Abuses Drugs

Only a small percentage of the persons using drugs come to the attention of physicians; those who do are usually experiencing adverse reactions such as panic states, drug psychoses, homicidal or suicidal thoughts, or respiratory depression.

Even with cooperative patients, an accurate history is difficult to obtain. A drug history is most easily obtained in a quiet spot by a gentle, nonthreatening, honest examiner, and without the parents present. The user often does not really know what drug has been taken or how much. Street drugs are almost always adulterated with one or more other compounds. Multiple drugs are often taken together. Friends may be a useful source of information.

The patient's general appearance, skin, lymphatics, cardiorespiratory status, GI tract, and CNS should be focused on during the physical examination, because they often provide clues suggesting drug abuse.

Hallucinogens are not life-threatening unless the patient is frankly homicidal or suicidal. A specific diagnosis is usually not necessary for management; instead, the presenting signs and symptoms are treated. Does the patient appear intoxicated? In withdrawal? "Flashing back?" Is some illness or injury (eg, head trauma) being masked by a drug effect? (Remember that a known drug user may still have hallucinations from meningoencephalitis.)

Table 12–5. Poisoning due to plants.[a]

	Symptoms and Signs	Treatment
Arum family: *Caladium, Dieffenbachia,* calla lily, dumbcane (oxalic acid)	Burning of mucous membranes and airway obstruction secondary to edema caused by calcium oxalate crystals.	Accessible areas should be thoroughly washed. Corticosteroids relieve airway obstruction. Apply cold packs to affected mucous membranes.
Castor bean plant (ricin—a toxalbumin) Jequinty bean (abrin—a toxalbumin)	Mucous membrane irritation, nausea, vomiting, bloody diarrhea, blurred vision, circulatory collapse, acute hemolytic anemia, convulsions, uremia.	Fluid and electrolyte monitoring. Saline cathartic. Forced alkaline diuresis will prevent complications due to hemagglutination and hemolysis.
Foxglove, lily of the valley, and oleander[b]	Nausea, diarrhea, visual disturbances, and cardiac irregularities (eg, heart block).	See treatment for digitalis drugs in text.
Jimsonweed: See Belladonna Alkaloids section in text	Mydriasis, dry mouth, tachycardia, and hallucinations.	Activated charcoal.
Larkspur (ajacine, *Delphinium,* delphinine)	Nausea and vomiting, irritability, muscular paralysis, and central nervous system depression.	Symptomatic. Atropine may be helpful.
Monkshood (aconite)	Numbness of mucous membranes, visual disturbances, tingling, dizziness, tinnitus, hypotension, bradycardia, and convulsions.	Activated charcoal, oxygen. Atropine is probably helpful.
Poison hemlock (coniine)	Mydriasis, trembling, dizziness, bradycardia. Central nervous system depression, muscular paralysis, and convulsions. Death is due to respiratory paralysis.	Symptomatic. Oxygen and cardiac monitoring equipment are desirable. Assisted respiration is often necessary. Give anticonvulsants if needed.
Rhododendron (grayanotoxin)	Abdominal cramps, vomiting, severe diarrhea, muscular paralysis. Central nervous system and circulatory depression. Hypertension with very large doses.	Atropine can prevent bradycardia. Epinephrine is contraindicated. Antihypertensives may be needed.
Yellow jessamine (active ingredient, geisemine, is related to strychnine)	Restlessness, convusions, muscular paralysis, and respiratory depression.	Symptomatic. Because of the relation to strychnine, activated charcoal and diazepam for seizures are worth trying.

[a]Many other plants cause minor irritation but are not likely to cause serious problems unless large amounts are ingested. See Lampe KF, McCann MA: *AMA Handbook of Poisonous and Injurious Plants.* American Medical Association, 1985. See also Rumack BH, Spoerke DG (editors): POISINDEX Information System. Micromedex, Inc., published quarterly.
[b]Done AK: Ornamental and deadly. Emerg Med 1973;5:255.

The signs and symptoms in a given patient are a function not only of the drug and the dose but also of the level of acquired tolerance, the "setting," the patient's physical condition and personality traits, the potentiating effects of other drugs, and many other factors.

A common drug problem is the "bad trip," which is usually a panic reaction. This is best managed by "talking the patient down" and minimizing auditory and visual stimuli. Allowing the patient to sit with a friend while the drug effect dissipates may be the best treatment. This may take several hours. The physician's job is not to terminate the drug effect but to help the patient through the bad experience.

Drug therapy is often unnecessary and may complicate the clinical course of a drug-related panic reaction.

Although phenothiazines have been commonly used to treat bad trips, they should be avoided if the specific drug is unknown, because they may enhance toxicity or produce unwanted side effects. Diazepam is the drug of choice if a sedative effect is required. Physical restraints are rarely indicated and usually increase the patient's panic reaction.

For treatment of life-threatening drug abuse, consult the section on the specific drug elsewhere in this chapter and the section on general management at the beginning of the chapter.

After the acute episode, the physician must decide whether psychiatric referral is indicated; in general, patients who have made suicidal gestures or attempts and adolescents who are not communicating with their families should be referred.

Dar KJ, McBrien ME: MDMA induced hyperthermia: Report of a fatality and review of current therapy. Intensive Care Med 1996;22:995 [PMID: 8905441].

Weir E: Raves: A review of the culture, the drugs and the prevention of harm. CMAJ 2000;162:1843 [PMID: 10906922].

SALICYLATES

The use of childproof containers and publicity regarding accidental poisoning have reduced the incidence of acute salicylate poisoning. Nevertheless, serious intoxication still occurs and must be regarded as an emergency. In recent years, the frequency of poisoning has begun to rise again.

Salicylates uncouple oxidative phosphorylation, leading to increased heat production, excessive sweating, and dehydration. They also interfere with glucose metabolism and may cause hypoglycemia or hyperglycemia. Respiratory center stimulation occurs early.

Patients usually have signs of hyperventilation, sweating, dehydration, and fever. Vomiting and diarrhea sometimes occur. In severe cases, disorientation, convulsions, and coma may develop.

The severity of acute intoxication can, in some measure, be judged by serum salicylate levels. High levels are always dangerous irrespective of clinical signs, and low levels may be misleading in chronic cases. Other laboratory values usually indicate metabolic acidosis despite hyperventilation, low serum K^+ values, and often abnormal serum glucose levels.

In mild and moderate poisoning, stimulation of the respiratory center produces respiratory alkalosis. In severe intoxication (occurring in severe acute ingestion with high salicylate levels and in chronic toxicity with lower levels), respiratory response is unable to overcome the metabolic overdose.

Once the urine becomes acidic, progressively smaller amounts of salicylate are excreted. Until this process is reversed, the half-life will remain prolonged, because metabolism contributes little to the removal of salicylate.

Chronic severe poisoning may occur as early as 3 days after a regimen of salicylate is begun. Findings usually include vomiting, diarrhea, and dehydration.

Treatment

Charcoal binds salicylates well, and, after emesis or lavage, it should be given for acute ingestions. Mild poisoning may require only the administration of oral fluids and confirmation that the salicylate level is falling. Moderate poisoning involves moderate dehydration and depletion of potassium. Fluids must be administered at a rate of 2–3 mL/kg/h to correct dehydration and produce urine with a pH of greater than 7.0. Initial IV solutions should be isotonic, with sodium bicarbonate constituting half the electrolyte content. Once the patient is rehydrated, the solution can contain more free water and approximately 40 mEq of K^+ per liter.

Severe toxicity is marked by major dehydration. Symptoms may be confused with those of Reye syndrome, encephalopathy, and metabolic acidosis. Salicylate levels may even be in the therapeutic range. Major fluid correction of dehydration is required. Once this has been accomplished, hypokalemia must be corrected and sodium bicarbonate given. Usual requirements are sodium bicarbonate, 1–2 mEq/kg/h over the first 6–8 hours, and K^+, 20–40 mEq/L. A urine flow of 2–3 mL/kg/h should be established. Despite this treatment some patients will develop the paradoxical aciduria of salicylism. This is due to hypokalemia and the saving of K^+ and excretion of H^+ in the renal tubule. Correction of K^+ will allow the urine to become alkaline and ionize the salicylate, resulting in excretion rather than reabsorption of nonionized salicylate in acid urine.

Renal failure or pulmonary edema is an indication for dialysis. Hemodialysis is most effective and peritoneal dialysis is relatively ineffective. Hemodialysis should be used in all patients with altered mental status or deteriorating clinical status. Acetazolamide should not be used.

Yip L et al: Concepts and controversies in salicylate toxicity. Emerg Med Clin North Am 1994;12:351 [PMID: 8187688].

SCORPION STINGS

Scorpion stings are common in arid areas of the southwestern United States. Scorpion venom is more toxic than most snake venoms, but only minute amounts are injected. Although neurologic manifestations may last a week, most clinical signs subside within 24–48 hours.

The most common scorpions in the United States are *Vejovis, Hadrurus, Androctonus,* and *Centruroides* species. Stings by the first three produce edema and pain. Stings by *Centruroides* (the Bark scorpion) cause tingling or burning paresthesias that begin at the site of the sting; other findings include hypersalivation, restlessness, muscular fasciculation, abdominal cramps, opisthotonos, convulsions, urinary incontinence, and respiratory failure.

Treatment

Sedation is the primary therapy. Antivenom is reserved for severe poisoning. In severe cases, the airway may become compromised by secretions and weakness of respiratory muscles. Endotracheal intubation may be required. Patients may require treatment for seizures, hypertension, or tachycardia.

The prognosis is good as long as the patient's airway is managed appropriately.

Gibly R et al: Continuous intravenous midazolam infusion for *Centruroides exilicauda* scorpion envenomation. Ann Emerg Med 1999;34:620 [PMID: 10533010].

LoVecchio F et al: Incidence of immediate and delayed hypersensitivity to *Centruroides* antivenom. Ann Emerg Med 1999;34:615 [PMID: 10533009].

SNAKEBITE

Despite the lethal potential of venomous snakes, human morbidity and mortality rates are surprisingly low. The outcome depends on the size of the child, the site of the bite, the degree of envenomation, the type of snake, and the effectiveness of treatment.

Nearly all poisonous snakebites in the United States are caused by pit vipers (rattlesnakes, water moccasins, and copperheads). A few are caused by elapids (coral snakes), and occasional bites occur from cobras and other nonindigenous exotic snakes kept as pets. Snake venom is a complex mixture of enzymes, peptides, and proteins that may have predominantly cytotoxic, neurotoxic, hemotoxic, or cardiotoxic effects but other effects as well. Up to 25% of bites by pit vipers do not result in venom injection. Pit viper venom causes predominantly local injury with pain, discoloration, edema, and hemorrhage.

Swelling and pain occur soon after rattlesnake bite and are a certain indication that envenomation has occurred. During the first few hours, swelling and ecchymosis extend proximally from the bite. The bite is often obvious as a double puncture mark surrounded by ecchymosis. Hematemesis, melena, hemoptysis, and other manifestations of coagulopathy develop in severe cases. Respiratory difficulty and shock are the ultimate causes of death. Even in fatal rattlesnake bite, a period of 6–8 hours usually elapses between the bite and death; as a result, there is usually enough time to start effective treatment.

Coral snake envenomation causes little local pain, swelling, or necrosis; and systemic reactions are often delayed. The signs of coral snake envenomation include bulbar paralysis, dysphagia, and dysphoria; these signs may appear in 5–10 hours and may be followed by total peripheral paralysis and death in 24 hours.

Treatment

Children in snake-infested areas should wear boots and long trousers, should not walk barefoot, and should be cautioned not to explore under ledges or in holes.

A. EMERGENCY (FIRST AID) TREATMENT

The most important first aid measure is transportation to a medical facility. Splint the affected extremity and minimize the patient's motion. Tourniquets and ice packs are contraindicated. Incision and suction are not useful for either crotalid or elapid snake bite.

B. DEFINITIVE MEDICAL MANAGEMENT

Blood should be drawn for hematocrit, clotting time and platelet function, and serum electrolyte determinations. Establish two secure IV sites for the administration of antivenom and other medications.

Specific antivenom is indicated when signs of progressive envenomation are present. Two antivenoms are available for treating pit viper envenomation: polyvalent pit viper antivenom and polyvalent Crotalidae Fab (CroFab). Both are effective, but their indications differ. For coral snake bites, an eastern coral snake antivenom (Wyeth Laboratories) is available. Patients with pit viper bites should receive antivenom if progressive local injury, coagulopathy, or systemic signs (eg, hypotension, confusion) are present. (Antivenom should not be given IM or SQ.) See package labeling or call your certified poison center for details of use. Hemorrhage, pain, and shock diminish rapidly with adequate amounts of antivenom. For coral snake bites, give three to five vials of antivenom in 250–500 mL of isotonic saline solution. An additional three to five vials may be required.

To control pain, administer a narcotic analgesic, such as meperidine, 0.6–1.5 mg/kg/dose, given PO or IM. Cryotherapy is contraindicated because it commonly causes additional tissue damage. Early physiotherapy minimizes contractures. In rare cases, fasciotomy to relieve pressure within muscular compartments is required. The evaluation of function and of pulses will better predict the need for fasciotomy. Antihistamines and corticosteroids (hydrocortisone, 1 mg/kg, given PO for a week) are useful in the treatment of serum sickness or anaphylactic shock. Antibiotics are not needed unless clinical signs of infection occur. Tetanus status should be evaluated and the patient immunized, if needed.

Bond GR: Snake, spider, and scorpion envenomation in North America. Pediatr Rev 1999;20:147 [PMID: 10233171].

Dart RC, McNally J: Efficacy, safety, and use of snake antivenoms in the United States. Ann Emerg Med 2001;37:181 [PMID: 11174237].

SOAPS & DETERGENTS

1. Soaps

Soap is made from salts of fatty acids. Some toilet soap bars contain both soap and detergent. Ingestion of soap bars may cause vomiting and diarrhea, but they have a low toxicity. Induced emesis is unnecessary.

2. Detergents

Detergents are nonsoap synthetic products used for cleaning purposes because of their surfactant properties. Commercial products include granules, powders, and liquids. Dishwasher detergents are very alkaline and can cause caustic burns. Low concentrations of bleaching and antibacterial agents as well as enzymes are found in many preparations. The pure compounds are moderately toxic, but the concentration used is too small to alter the product's toxicity significantly, although occasional primary or allergic irritative phenomena have been noted in persons who frequently use such products and in employees manufacturing these products.

Cationic Detergents (Ceepryn, Diaperene, Phemerol, Zephiran)

Cationic detergents in dilute solutions (0.5%) cause mucosal irritation, but higher concentrations (10–15%) may cause caustic burns to mucosa. Clinical effects include nausea, vomiting, collapse, coma, and convulsions. As little as 2.25 g of some cationic agents have caused death in an adult. In four cases, 100–400 mg/kg of benzalkonium chloride caused death. Cationic detergents are rapidly inactivated by tissues and ordinary soap.

Because of the caustic potential and rapid onset of seizures, emesis is not recommended. Activated charcoal should be administered. Anticonvulsants may be needed.

Anionic Detergents

Most common household detergents are anionic. Laundry compounds have water softener (sodium phosphate) added, which is a strong irritant and may reduce ionized calcium. Anionic detergents irritate the skin by removing natural oils. Although ingestion causes diarrhea, intestinal distention, and vomiting, no fatalities have been reported.

The only treatment usually required is to discontinue use if skin irritation occurs and replace fluids and electrolytes. Induced vomiting is not indicated following ingestion of automatic dishwasher detergent, because of its alkalinity. Dilute with water or milk.

Nonionic Detergents (Brij Products; Tritons X-45, X-100, X-102, & X-144)

These compounds include lauryl, stearyl, and oleyl alcohols and octyl phenol. They have a minimal irritating effect on the skin and are almost always nontoxic when swallowed.

Klasaer AE et al: Marked hypocalcemia and ventricular fibrillation in two pediatric patients exposed to a fluoride-containing wheel cleaner. Ann Emerg Med 1996;28:713 [PMID: 8953969].

Lovejoy FH Jr, Woolf AD: Corrosive ingestions. Pediatr Rev 1995;16:473 [PMID: 8559706].

Vincent JC, Sheikh A: Phosphate poisoning by ingestion of clothes washing liquid and fabric conditioner. Anesthesiology 1998;53:1004 [PMID: 9893545].

SPIDER BITES

Most medically important bites in the United States are caused by the black widow spider (*Latrodectus mactans*) and the North American brown recluse (violin) spider (*Loxosceles reclusa*). Positive identification of the spider is helpful, because many spider bites may mimic those of the brown recluse spider.

Black Widow Spider

The black widow spider is endemic to nearly all areas of the United States. The initial bite causes sharp fleeting pain. Local and systemic muscular cramping, abdominal pain, nausea and vomiting, and shock can occur. Convulsions occur more commonly in small children than in older children. Systemic signs of black widow spider bite may be confused with other causes of acute abdomen. Although paresthesias, nervousness, and transient muscle spasms may persist for weeks in survivors, recovery from the acute phase is generally complete within 3 days. In contrast to popular opinion, death is extremely rare.

Most authors recommend calcium gluconate as initial therapy (50 mg/kg IV per dose, up to 250 mg/kg/24 h), although it is often not effective and the effects are of short duration. Methocarbamol (15 mg/kg PO) or diazepam titrated to effect is useful. Morphine or barbiturates may occasionally be needed for control of pain or restlessness, but they increase the possibility of respiratory depression. Antivenom is available but should be reserved for severe cases in which the above therapies have failed. Local treatment of the bite is not helpful.

Brown Recluse Spider (Violin Spider)

The North American brown recluse spider is most commonly seen in the central and Midwestern areas of the United States. Its bite characteristically produces a localized reaction with progressively severe pain within 24 hours. The initial bleb on an erythematous ischemic base is replaced by a black eschar within 1 week. This eschar separates in 2–5 weeks, leaving an ulcer that heals slowly. Systemic signs include cyanosis, morbilliform rash, fever, chills, malaise, weakness, nausea and vomiting, joint pains, hemolytic reactions with hemoglobinuria, jaundice, and delirium. Fatalities are rare. Fatal disseminated intravascular coagulation has been reported.

Although of unproved efficacy, the following therapies have been used: dexamethasone, 4 mg IV four times a day, during the acute phase; polymorphonuclear leukocyte inhibitors, such as dapsone or colchicine, and oxygen applied to the bite site; and total excision of the lesion to the fascial level.

Clark RF et al: Clinical presentation and treatment of black widow spider envenomation: A review of 163 cases. Ann Emerg Med 1992;21:782 [PMID: 1351707].

Sams HH et al: Nineteen documented cases of *Loxosceles reclusa* envenomation. J Am Acad Dermatol 2001;44:603 [PMID: 11260528].

THYROID PREPARATIONS (Thyroid Desiccated, Sodium Levothyroxine)

Ingestion of the equivalent of 50–150 g of desiccated thyroid can cause signs of hyperthyroidism, including irritability, mydriasis, hyperpyrexia, tachycardia, and diarrhea. Maximal clinical effect occurs about 9 days after ingestion—several days after the protein-bound iodine level has fallen dramatically.

Induce vomiting. If the patient develops clinical signs of toxicity, propranolol, 0.01–0.1 mg/kg (maximum, 1 mg), is useful because of its antiadrenergic activity.

Brown RS et al: Successful treatment of massive acute thyroid hormone poisoning with iopanoic acid. J Pediatr 1998;132: 903 [PMID: 9602214].

Golightly LK et al: Clinical effects of accidental levothyroxine ingestion in children. Am J Dis Child 1987;141:1025 [PMID: 2887106].

TOXIC ALCOHOLS

Ethylene glycol and methanol are the toxic alcohols. The primary source of ethylene glycol is antifreeze, while methanol is present in windshield wiper fluid and also as an ethanol denaturant. Ethylene glycol causes severe metabolic acidosis and renal failure. Methanol causes metabolic acidosis and blindness. Onset of symptoms with both agents occurs within several hours after ingestion, longer if ethanol was ingested simultaneously.

Treatment

The primary treatment is to block the enzyme alcohol dehydrogenase which converts both agents to their toxic metabolites. This is accomplished with fomepizole (loading dose of 15 mg/kg) or ethanol. Fomepizole is preferred for children, due to its reduced side effects in this age group.

Barceloux DG et al: American Academy of Clinical Toxicology Practice Guidelines on the Treatment of Methanol Poisoning. J Toxicol Clin Toxicol 2002;40:415 [PMID: 12216995].

Brent J et al: Fomepizole for the treatment of ethylene glycol poisoning: Methylpyrazole for toxic alcohols study group. N Engl J Med 1999;40:832 [PMID: 10080845].

VITAMINS

Accidental ingestion of excessive amounts of vitamins rarely causes significant problems. Occasional cases of hypervitaminosis A and D do occur, however, particularly in patients with poor hepatic or renal function. The fluoride contained in many multivitamin preparations is not a realistic hazard, because a 2- or 3-year-old child could eat 100 tablets, containing 1 mg of sodium fluoride per tablet, without experiencing serious symptoms. Iron poisoning has been reported with multivitamin tablets containing iron. Pyridoxine abuse has caused neuropathies; nicotinic acid has resulted in myopathy.

Dean BS, Krenzelok EP: Multiple vitamins and vitamins with iron: Accidental poisoning in children. Vet Hum Toxicol 1988; 30:23 [PMID: 3354178].

Fraser DR: Vitamin D. Lancet 1995;345:104 [PMID: 7815853].

WARFARIN

Warfarin is used as a rodenticide. It causes hypoprothrombinemia and capillary injury. It is absorbed readily from the GI tract but is absorbed poorly through the skin. A dose of 0.5 mg/kg of warfarin may be toxic in a child. A prothrombin time is helpful in establishing the severity of the poisoning.

If bleeding occurs or the prothrombin time is prolonged, give 1–5 mg of vitamin K_1 (phytonadione) IM or SQ. For large ingestions with established toxicity, 0.6 mg/kg may be given.

Another group of long-acting anticoagulant rodenticides (brodifacoum, difenacoum, bromadolone, diphacinone, pinene, valone, and coumatetralyl) have been a more serious toxicologic problem than warfarin. They also cause hypoprothrombinemia and a bleeding diathesis that responds to phytonadione, although the anticoagulant activity may persist for periods ranging from 6 weeks to several months. Treatment with vitamin K_1 may be needed for weeks.

Isbister GK, Whyte IM: Management of anticoagulant poisoning. Vet Hum Toxicol 2001;43:117 [PMID: 11308119].

Mullins ME et al: Unintentional pediatric superwarfarin exposures: Do we really need a prothrombin time? Pediatrics 2000;105:402 [PMID: 10654963].

Critical Care

13

Todd C. Carpenter, MD, Emily L. Dobyns, MD, Eva N. Grayck, MD, Peter M. Mourani, MD, Margaret A. Ferguson, MD, & Kurt R. Stenmark, MD

Caring for critically ill children remains one of the most demanding and challenging aspects of the field of pediatrics. The care of patients with life-threatening conditions, from serious medical illness to traumatic injuries and recovery from major surgery, requires a detailed understanding of the physiology of the body and the pathophysiology of major illnesses, as well as an understanding of and experience with the rapidly changing technologies available in a modern intensive care unit (ICU). In addition, the science of caring for the critically ill patient has evolved rapidly over the last decade, as the molecular mediators of illness have become better defined and new therapies have been devised based on those advances. As a result, critical care is more than ever a multidisciplinary field that requires a team-oriented approach, including critical care physicians and nursing staff, pharmacists, referring physicians, consulting specialists, and social services specialists.

The intensivist plays an essential role in coordinating and directing the care provided by the ICU team, and in so doing stands at the crossroads of the various participating disciplines. There are two primary models of ICU organization: "open" units, where primary responsibility for the patient remains with the referring physician and secondary responsibility lies with the intensivist as consultant; and "closed" units, where only the on-site intensivist is allowed to write orders directing the patient's care. Although the merits of these organizational approaches are debated, a substantial and growing body of evidence from studies conducted in adult medical, surgical, and pediatric ICUs suggests that the closed ICU model lead to significant reductions in ICU length of stay and resource use, and to reductions in mortality of as much as 15%.

An additional factor to consider in the provision of critical care services for children is the cost of those services in relation to the outcomes achieved. Critical care services in the United States are estimated to account for 30% of all acute-care hospital costs; some estimates run as high as 1% of the gross national product. One study examining the cost-effectiveness of pediatric ICU care, compared with adult ICU care, found that the short- and long-term

mortality among pediatric patients was three times lower than it was among adult ICU patients, despite similar ICU costs and length of stay. These findings suggest that pediatric critical care services are relatively cost-effective.

Brilli RJ et al: Critical care delivery in the intensive care unit: Defining clinical roles and the best practice model. Crit Care Med 2001;29:2007 [PMID: 11588472].

Epstein D, Brill JE. A history of pediatric critical care medicine. Pediatr Res 2005;58:987 [PMID: 16183804].

Seferian EG et al: Comparison of resource utilization and outcome between pediatric and adult intensive care unit patients. Pediatr Crit Care Med 2001;2:2 [PMID: 12797880].

Tilford JM et al: Volume-outcome relationships in pediatric intensive care units. Pediatrics 2000;106:289 [PMID: 10920153].

Young MP, Birkmeyer JD: Potential reduction in mortality rates using an intensivist model to manage intensive care units. Eff Clin Pract 2000;3:284 [PMID: 11151525].

ACUTE RESPIRATORY FAILURE

Acute respiratory failure, defined as the inability of the respiratory system to adequately deliver oxygen or remove CO_2, contributes significantly to the morbidity and mortality of critically ill children. This condition accounts for approximately 50% of deaths in children younger than age 1 year. Anatomic and developmental differences place infants at higher risk than adults for respiratory failure. An infant's thoracic cage is more compliant than that of the adult or older child. The intercostal muscles are poorly developed and unable to achieve the "bucket-handle" motion characteristic of adult breathing. Furthermore, the diaphragm is shorter and relatively flat with fewer type I muscle fibers, and therefore less effective and more easily fatigued. The infant's airways are smaller in caliber than those in older children and adults, resulting in greater resistance to inspiratory and expiratory airflow and greater susceptibility to occlusion by mucus plugging and mucosal edema. Compared with adults, the alveoli of children are smaller and have less collateral ventilation, resulting in a greater tendency to collapse and develop atelectasis. Finally, young infants may have an especially reactive pulmonary vascular bed, impaired immune system, or residual effects from prematurity, all of which increase the risk of respiratory failure.

Respiratory failure can be classified into two types, which usually coexist in variable proportion. The partial arterial oxygen pressure (PaO_2) is low in both, whereas the partial arterial carbon dioxide pressure ($PaCO_2$) is high only in patients with type II respiratory failure (Table 13–1). Type I respiratory failure is a failure of oxygenation and occurs in three situations: (1) **ventilation-perfusion mismatch,** or V/Q mismatch, which occurs when blood flows to parts of the lung that are inadequately ventilated, or when ventilated areas of the lung are inadequately perfused; (2) **diffusion defects,** caused by thickened alveolar membranes or excessive interstitial fluid at the alveolar-capillary junction; and (3) **intrapulmonary shunt,** which occurs when structural anomalies in the lung allow blood to flow through the lung without participating in gas exchange. Type II respiratory failure generally results from alveolar hypoventilation and is usually secondary to situations such as central nervous system (CNS) dysfunction, oversedation, or neuromuscular disorders (see Table 13–1).

Table 13–1. Types of respiratory failure.

Findings	Causes	Examples
Type I Hypoxia Decreased PaO_2 Normal $PaCO_2$	Ventilation/perfusion defect	Positional (supine in bed), acute respiratory distress syndrome (ARDS), atelectasis, pneumonia, pulmonary embolus, bronchopulmonary dysplasia
	Diffusion impairment	Pulmonary edema, ARDS, interstitial pneumonia
	Shunt	Pulmonary arteriovenous malformation, congenital adenomatoid malformation
Type II Hypoxia Hypercapnia Decreased PaO_2 Increased $PaCO_2$	Hypoventilation	Neuromuscular disease (polio, Guillain–Barré syndrome), head trauma, sedation, chest wall dysfunction (burns), kyphosis, severe reactive airways

Table 13–2. Clinical features of respiratory failure.

> **Respiratory**
> Wheezing
> Expiratory grunting
> Decreased or absent breath sounds
> Flaring of alae nasi
> Retractions of chest wall
> Tachypnea, bradypnea, or apnea
> Cyanosis
> **Neurologic**
> Restlessness
> Irritability
> Headache
> Confusion
> Convulsions
> Coma
> **Cardiac**
> Bradycardia or excessive tachycardia
> Hypotension or hypertension
> **General**
> Fatigue
> Sweating

Clinical Findings

A. SYMPTOMS AND SIGNS

The clinical findings in respiratory failure are caused by the low PaO_2, high $PaCO_2$, and pH changes affecting the lungs, heart, kidneys, and brain. The clinical features of progressive respiratory failure are summarized in Table 13–2. Hypercapnia depresses the CNS, and also results in acidemia that depresses myocardial function. Patients in respiratory failure can exhibit significant changes in CNS and cardiac function. Features of respiratory failure are not always clinically evident, however, and some signs or symptoms may have nonrespiratory causes. Furthermore, a strictly clinical assessment of arterial hypoxemia or hypercapnia is not reliable. As a result, the precise assessment of the adequacy of oxygenation and ventilation must be based on both clinical and laboratory data.

B. LABORATORY FINDINGS

Laboratory findings are helpful in assessing the severity and acuity of respiratory failure and in determining specific treatment. Arterial oxygen saturation can be measured continuously and noninvasively by **pulse oximetry,** a technique that should be used in the assessment and treatment of all patients with suspected respiratory failure. **End-tidal CO_2 monitoring** provides a continuous noninvasive means of assessing arterial PCO_2. Because carbon dioxide diffuses freely across the alveolar-capillary barrier,

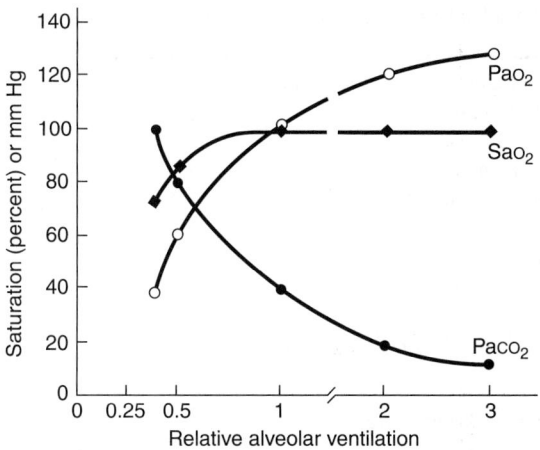

Figure 13-1. Relationship between alveolar ventilation, arterial oxygen saturation (SaO_2), and partial pressures of oxygen and CO_2 in the arterial blood (PaO_2 and $PaCO_2$, respectively). (Reproduced, with permission, from Pagtakhan RD, Chernick V: Respiratory failure in the pediatric patient. Pediatr Rev 1982;3:244.)

the exhaled end-tidal CO_2 ($ETCO_2$) level approximates the alveolar pCO_2, which should equal the arterial pCO_2. Though useful for following trends in ventilation, this technique is susceptible to significant error, particularly with patients who have rapid, shallow breathing or increased dead space ventilation. **Arterial blood gas (ABG) analysis** remains the gold standard for assessment of acute respiratory failure. ABGs give information on the patient's acid-base status (with a measured pH and calculated bicarbonate level) as well as PaO_2 and $PaCO_2$ levels. The PaO_2 is a critical determinant of oxygen delivery to the tissues, and the $PaCO_2$ is a sensitive measure of ventilation related inversely to the minute ventilation (Figure 13-1). Although measurement of capillary or venous blood gases may provide some reassurance regarding ventilatory function if blood gas results are normal, these tests yield virtually no useful information regarding oxygenation and may generate highly misleading information about the ventilatory status of patients who have poor perfusion or who had blood draws that were difficult. As a result, ABG analysis is important for all patients with suspected respiratory failure, particularly those with abnormal venous or capillary gases.

Knowing the ABG values and the inspired oxygen concentration also enables one to calculate the difference between alveolar oxygen concentration and the arterial oxygen value, known as the **alveolar-arterial oxygen difference** ($A-aDO_2$, or A-a gradient). The A-a gradient is less than 15 mm Hg under normal conditions, though it widens with increasing inspired oxygen concentrations to

about 100 mm Hg in normal patients breathing 100% oxygen. This number has prognostic value in severe hypoxemic respiratory failure, with A-a gradients over 400 mm Hg being strongly associated with mortality. Diffusion impairment, shunts, and V/Q mismatch all increase the $A-aDO_2$ (Table 13-3).

In addition to the calculation of the $A-aDO_2$, assessment of intrapulmonary shunting (the percentage of pulmonary blood flow that passes through nonventilated areas of the lung) may be helpful. Normal individuals have less than a 5% physiologic shunt from bronchial, thebesian, and coronary circulations. Shunt fractions greater than 15% usually indicate the need for aggressive respiratory support. When intrapulmonary shunt reaches 50% of pulmonary blood flow, PaO_2 does not increase regardless of the amount of supplemental oxygen used.

Treatment

A. OXYGEN SUPPLEMENTATION

Patients with hypoxemia induced by respiratory failure may respond to **supplemental oxygen** administration alone (Table 13-4). Those with hypoventilation and diffusion defects respond better than do patients with shunts or V/Q mismatch. Severe V/Q mismatch generally responds only to aggressive airway management and mechanical ventilation. Patients with severe hypoxemia, hypoventilation, or apnea require assistance with bag and mask ventilation until the airway is successfully intubated and controlled artificial ventilation can be provided. Ventilation may be maintained for some time with a mask of the proper size, but gastric distention, emesis, and inadequate tidal volumes are possible complications. An artificial airway may be life-saving for patients who fail to respond to simple oxygen supplements.

B. INTUBATION

Intubation of the trachea in infants and children requires experienced personnel and the right equipment. A patient in respiratory failure whose airway must be stabilized should first be positioned properly to facilitate air exchange while supplemental oxygen is given. The sniffing position is used in infants. Head extension with jaw thrust is used in older children without neck injuries. If obstructed by secretions or vomitus, the airway must be cleared by suction. When not obstructed, the airway should open easily with proper positioning and placement of an oral or nasopharyngeal airway of the correct size. Patients with a normal airway may be intubated under intravenous (IV) anesthesia by experienced personnel (Table 13-5). Patients with obstructed upper airways (eg, patients with croup, epiglottitis, foreign bodies, or subglottic stenosis) should be awake when intubated unless trained airway specialists decide otherwise.

Table 13–3. Key equations describing pulmonary function and oxygen delivery.

Pio_2 = (barometric pressure – 47) × % inspired oxygen concentration
$A–aDo_2$ = $Pio_2 – (Paco_2/R) – Pao_2$ (normal = 5–15 mm Hg)
CO_2 = $(1.34 \times$ hemoglobin $\times Sao_2) + (0.003 \times Pao_2)$
Do_2 = $Cao_2 \times CI \times 10$ (normal 620 + 50 mL/min/m^2)
Oxygen consumption $(Vo_2) = (Cao_2 – Cvo_2) \times CI \times 10$ (normal 120–200 mL/min/m^2)

$$\frac{Qs}{Qt} = \frac{Cco_2 – Cao_2}{Cco_2 – Cvo_2} \qquad (normal < 5\%)$$

$$Vd = \frac{(Paco_2 – Peco_2)}{Pcco_2} \qquad (normal\ approximately\ 2\ mL/kg)$$

$$Compliance = \frac{Volume\ (tidal\ volume)}{Pressure\ (PIP – PEEP)} \qquad (normal\ varies\ with\ age)$$

$A–aDo_2$	=	Alveolar–arterial oxygen difference (mm Hg)
Cao_2	=	Oxygen content of arterial blood (mL/dL)
Cco_2	=	Oxygen content of pulmonary capillary blood (mL/dL)
CI	=	Cardiac index (L/min)
CO_2	=	Oxygen content of the blood (mL/dL)
Cvo_2	=	Oxygen content of mixed venous blood (mL/dL)
Do_2	=	Oxygen delivery (mL/min)
$Paco_2$	=	Partial pressure of carbon dioxide in arterial blood (mm Hg)
Pao_2	=	Partial pressure of oxygen in arterial blood (mm Hg)
$Pcco_2$	=	Partial pressure of carbon dioxide in capillary blood (mm Hg)
$Peco_2$	=	Partial pressure of carbon dioxide in expired air (mm Hg)
Pio_2	=	Partial pressure of oxygen in inspired air (mm Hg)
PIP	=	Peak inspiratory pressure
Qs/Qt	=	Intrapulmonary shunt (in patients without cardiac shunt) (%)
R	=	Respiratory quotient (usually 0.8)
Sao_2	=	Arterial oxygen saturation (fractional)
Vd	=	Physiologic dead space (anatomic dead space + alveolar dead space) (mL)
Ve	=	Expiratory minute volume (L/min)
Vo_2	=	Oxygen consumption per minute

The size of the endotracheal tube is of critical importance in pediatrics (see Table 11–3 for sizes). An inappropriately large endotracheal tube can cause pressure necrosis of the tissues in the subglottic region, leading in some cases to scarring and permanent stenosis of the subglottic region that can require surgical repair. An inappropriately small endotracheal tube can result in inadequate pulmonary toilet and excessive air leak around the endotracheal tube, making optimal ventilation and oxygenation difficult. Two useful methods for calculating the correct size of endotracheal tube for a child are (1) measuring the child's height with a Broselow tape and then reading the corresponding endotracheal tube size on the tape, or (2) in children older than age 2 years, choosing a tube size equal to the simple computation (16 + age in years) ÷ 4.

Correct placement of the endotracheal tube should be confirmed by auscultation for the presence of equal bilateral breath sounds and if using a colorimetric filter (pH-sensitive indicator that changes from purple to yellow when exposed to carbon dioxide) by the detection of carbon dioxide. An assessment of air leakage around the endotracheal tube is also important. To do this, connect an anesthesia bag and pressure manometer to the endotracheal tube and allow it to inflate, creating positive pressure. Check for the leak by auscultating over the throat, noting the pressure at which air escapes around the endotracheal tube. Leaks at pressures of 15–20 cm H$_2$O are acceptable. Leaks at lower pressures may lead to ineffective ventilation, and the endotracheal tube should be upsized if continued mechanical ventilation is needed. Leaks at higher pressures are

Table 13–4. Supplemental oxygen therapy.

Source	Maximum % O_2	Range of Rates	Advantages	Disadvantages
Nasal cannula	35–40%	0.125–4 L/min	Easily applied, relatively comfortable	Uncomfortable at higher flow rates, requires open nasal airways, easily dislodged, lower % O_2, nosebleeds
Simple mask	50–60%	5–10 L/min	Higher % O_2, good for mouth breathers	Uncomfortable, dangerous for patients with poor airway control and at risk for emesis, hard to give airway care, unsure of % O_2
Face tent	40–60%	8–10 L/min	Higher % O_2, good for mouth breathers, less restrictive	Uncomfortable, dangerous for patients with poor airway control and at risk for emesis, hard to give airway care, unsure of % O_2
Rebreathing mask	80–90%	5–10 L/min	Higher % O_2, good for mouth breathers, highest O_2 concentration	Uncomfortable, dangerous for patients with poor airway control and at risk for emesis, hard to give airway care, unsure of % O_2
Oxyhood	90–100%	5–10 L/min (mixed at wall)	Stable and accurate O_2 concentration	Difficult to maintain temperature, hard to give airway care

Table 13–5. Drugs commonly used for controlled intubation.

Drug	Class of Agent	Dose	Advantages	Disadvantages
Atropine	Anticholinergic	0.02 mg/kg, minimum of 0.1 mg	Prevents bradycardia, dries secretions	Tachycardia, fever; seizures and coma with high doses
Fentanyl	Narcotic (sedative)	1–3 µg/kg IV	Rapid onset, hemodynamic stability	Respiratory depression, chest wall rigidity with rapid administration in neonates
Midazolam	Benzodiazepine (sedative)	0.1–0.2 mg/kg IV	Rapid onset, amnestic	Respiratory depression, hypotension
Thiopental	Barbiturate (anesthetic)	3–5 mg/kg IV	Rapid onset, lowers intracranial pressure (ICP)	Hypotension, decreased cardiac output, no analgesia provided
Ketamine	Dissociative anesthetic	1–2 mg/kg IV 2–4 mg/kg IM	Rapid onset, bronchodilator, hemodynamic stability	Increases oral and airway secretions, may increase ICP and pulmonary artery pressure
Rocuronium	Nondepolarizing muscle relaxant	1 mg/kg	Rapid onset, suitable for rapid sequence intubation, lasts 30 minutes	Requires refrigeration
Pancuronium	Nondepolarizing muscle relaxant	0.1 mg/kg	Longer duration of action (40–60 min)	Tachycardia, slow onset (2–3 min)

IV, intravenously, IM, intramuscularly.

acceptable only with patients who have severe lung disease and poor compliance and who thus require high pressures to ventilate and oxygenate. A chest radiograph is necessary for final assessment of endotracheal tube placement.

Artigas A et al: The American-European Consensus Conference on ARDs, Part 2. Am J Respir Crit Care Med 1998;157:1332 [PMID: 9563759].

Bateman ST, Arnold JH: Acute respiratory failure in children. Curr Opin Pediatr 2000;12:233 [PMID: 10836159].

Green KE, Peters JI: Pathophysiology of acute respiratory failure. Clin Chest Med 1994;15:1 [PMID: 8200186].

Hedenstierna G, Lattuada M: Gas exchange in the ventilated patient. Curr Opin Crit Care 2002;8:39 [PMID: 12205405].

Sagarin MJ et al; National Emergency Airway Registry (NEAR) investigators: Pediatr Emerg Care 2002;18:417 [PMID: 12488834].

Shapiro MB et al: Respiratory failure. Conventional and high-tech support. Surg Clin North Am 2000;80:871 [PMID: 10897266].

Sigillito RJ, DeBlieux PM: Evaluation and initial management of the patient in respiratory distress. Emerg Med Clin North Am 2003;21:239 [PMID: 12793613].

Weiss IK et al: Clinical use of continuous arterial blood gas monitoring in the pediatric intensive care unit. Pediatrics 1999; 103:440 [PMID: 9925838].

MECHANICAL VENTILATION

The increased compliance of an infant's chest wall, the relative alveolar hypoplasia in early childhood, the small caliber of the airways, and the small tidal volumes of young children make mechanical ventilation of the pediatric patient challenging. The goals of mechanical ventilation are to facilitate the movement of gas into and out of the lungs (ventilation) and to improve oxygen uptake into the bloodstream (oxygenation). Modern mechanical ventilators can accomplish these objectives in a variety of ways. Depending on the mode of ventilation selected, the ventilator can deliver a machine-controlled breath (control ventilation), or can assist the patient's own spontaneous respiratory efforts (support ventilation), or can do both (mixed mode ventilation). Additionally, ventilator breaths can be delivered as a targeted tidal volume (volume ventilation) or as a targeted airway pressure (pressure ventilation). This section will describe the modes of mechanical ventilation most commonly used in pediatric intensive care units.

Pressure Ventilation

In pressure-controlled modes of ventilation, air flow is begun at the start of the inspiratory cycle and continues until a preset airway pressure is reached. That airway pressure is then maintained until, at the end of the set inspiratory time, the exhalation valve on the ventilator opens and gas exits into the machine. Because airway pressure is the controlling variable with this mode of ventilation, changes in the compliance of the respiratory system will lead to fluctuations in the actual tidal volume delivered to the patient. The advantage of pressure-controlled ventilation lies primarily in the avoidance of high airway pressures that might cause lung injury or barotrauma, particularly in those patients with fragile lung parenchyma, such as premature infants. The main disadvantage of pressure-controlled ventilation is the possibility of delivering either inadequate or excessive tidal volumes during periods of changing lung compliance, as described earlier.

Volume Ventilation

Volume-controlled ventilation is the most commonly used mode of mechanical ventilation in most pediatric intensive care units (PICUs). Volume ventilation delivers a preset tidal volume to the patient. Changes in lung compliance will lead to fluctuations in the airway pressure generated by the tidal volume. The main advantage of volume ventilation is more reliable delivery of the desired tidal volume and thus better control of ventilation. More reliable tidal volume delivery may also help prevent atelectasis due to hypoventilation. Disadvantages of volume ventilation include the risk of barotrauma from excessive airway pressures and difficulties overcoming leaks in the ventilator circuit. Older volume ventilators also suffered from a lack of continuous gas flow through the circuit, thus increasing the patient's work of breathing on spontaneous breaths. Most modern machines have overcome that problem by providing a continuous flow through the circuit and by improved triggering mechanisms to deliver the breaths in synchrony with the patient's demands.

Modes of Ventilation

Most modern ventilators can deliver either a pressure-controlled or a volume-controlled breath in several manners. **Assist-control** modes deliver breaths at a selected rate and duration (inspiratory time) and can be targeted for either volume or pressure set by the clinician (as opposed to the patient). Spontaneous breaths are not assisted, and the patient's own respiratory efforts are not considered. **Synchronized intermittent mandatory ventilation** is a mode in which the rate, inspiratory time, and volume or pressure settings are set by the clinician. But the ventilator allows a window of time around each breath in which it waits for the patient to make an inspiratory effort. The machine breath is then synchronized with the patient's effort, to improve the comfort of those who are breathing spontaneously. In **pressure-support ventilation,** the patient's own efforts are assisted by the delivery of gas flow to achieve a certain airway pressure. This mode of ventilation allows the patient to determine the rate and inspiratory time of breaths, thus improving patient comfort and decreasing the work of breathing. Perhaps the most common mode of ventilation in PICUs is **synchronized intermittent mandatory ventilation with pressure support,** a mixed mode allowing pressure-supported breaths between the synchronized machine breaths. Whether such mixed modes of ventilation provide any measurable advantage over single modes remains unclear.

Setting the Ventilator

When initiating mechanical ventilation, the clinician will vary the parameters according to the mode of ventilation selected. Volume-controlled modes of ventilation generally require a set tidal volume, inspiratory time, rate, and level of positive end-expiratory pressure (PEEP). A typical initial tidal volume is 8–12 mL/kg, as long as that volume does not cause excessive airway pressures. The inspiratory time is typically set at 1 second or 33% of the respiratory cycle, whichever is shorter. Rate can be adjusted to patient comfort and blood gas measurements of ventilation, but generally patients starting on mechanical ventilation will require full support at least initially with a rate of 20–30 breaths/min.

Pressure-controlled ventilation is set up in a similar fashion, though the sufficiency of the inspiratory pressure to provide an adequate tidal volume is assessed by observing the patient's chest rise and by measuring the returned tidal volume. Typically, patients without lung disease will require pressures of 15–20 cm H_2O, and patients with respiratory illnesses will initially require 20–30 cm H_2O pressure to provide adequate ventilation.

Positive End-Expiratory Pressure

The PEEP level is the final major setting required to initiate mechanical ventilation. All mechanical ventilators open their expiratory limbs at the end of inspiration until a preset pressure is achieved; this is the PEEP value. During ventilation of normal lungs, physiologic PEEP is in the range of 2–4 cm H_2O pressure. This pressure helps to prevent the end-expiratory collapse of open lung units, thus preventing atelectasis and shunting. In disease states such as pulmonary edema, pneumonia, or acute respiratory distress syndrome (ARDS), a higher PEEP may increase the patient's functional residual capacity, help to keep open previously collapsed alveoli, increase mean airway pressure, and improve oxygenation. Conceptually, it is important to remember that PEEP is an expiratory pressure. As a result, high PEEP levels do not open lung units in and of themselves, but rather prevent the collapse of units opened during lung inflation. Indeed, some evidence suggests that elevated levels of PEEP are most effective at improving oxygenation when used together with specific lung recruiting maneuvers. High levels of PEEP,

although often valuable in improving oxygenation, may also cause CO_2 retention, barotrauma with resultant air leaks, decreased central venous return and resulting decline in cardiac output, and increased intracranial pressure (ICP). In general, PEEP should be set at 3–5 cm H_2O initially and titrated up to maintain adequate oxygenation at an acceptable fractional inspiratory oxygen (FIO_2), while watching carefully for the adverse effects listed earlier.

Monitoring the Ventilated Patient

Ventilated patients must be monitored carefully for respiratory rate and activity, chest wall movement, and quality of breath sounds. Oxygenation should be measured either by ABGs or by continuous pulse oximetry. Ventilation should be assessed by blood gas analysis or by noninvasive means, such as transcutaneous monitoring or end-tidal sampling. Transcutaneous pO_2 or pCO_2 measurements are most useful with younger patients who have good skin perfusion, but they become problematic with poorly perfused or obese patients. End-tidal CO_2 monitoring is done by placing a gas-sampling port on the endotracheal tube and analyzing expired gas for CO_2. This technique appears to be more valuable for patients with large tidal volumes, lower respiratory rates, and without leaks around the endotracheal tube. In practice, end-tidal CO_2 values may differ significantly from measured $PaCO_2$ values and thus are most useful for following relative fluctuations in ventilation. Frequent, preferably continuous, blood pressure monitoring is also necessary for patients receiving oxygen at a high PEEP, given the risk of adverse cardiovascular effects.

Adjusting the Ventilator

Mechanical ventilation can assist with both ventilation (pCO_2) and oxygenation (pO_2). Ventilation is most closely associated with the delivered minute volume, or the tidal volume multiplied by the respiratory rate. Abnormal pCO_2 values can be most effectively addressed by changes in the respiratory rate or the tidal volume. Increased rate or tidal volume should increase minute volume and thus decrease PCO_2 levels; decreases in rate or tidal volume should act in the opposite fashion. In some circumstances, additional adjustments may also be necessary. For example, for patients with disease characterized by extensive alveolar collapse, increasing PEEP may improve ventilation by helping to keep open pre~ ously collapsed lung units. Also, for patients with d~ characterized by significant airway obstruction, ~ in respiratory rate may allow more time fo~ and improve ventilation despite an appar~ the minute volume provided.

The variables most closely associa~ are the inspired oxygen concentration way pressure during the respiratory cycle. Increases in inspired oxygen concentration will generally increase arterial oxygenation, unless right-to-left intracardiac or intrapulmonary shunting is a significant component of the patient's illness. Concentrations of inspired oxygen above 60–65%, however, may lead to hyperoxic lung injury. Patients with hypoxemic respiratory failure requiring those levels of oxygen or higher to maintain adequate arterial saturations should have their hypoxemia addressed by increases in mean airway pressure.

Mean airway pressure is affected by PEEP, peak inspiratory pressure, and inspiratory time. Increases in any one of those factors will increase mean airway pressure and should improve arterial oxygenation. It is important to bear in mind, however, that increases in mean airway pressure may also lead to decreases in cardiac output. In this circumstance, raising mean airway pressure may increase arterial oxygenation but actually compromise oxygen delivery to the tissues. For patients with severe hypoxemic respiratory failure, these trade-offs highlight the need for careful monitoring of these variables by experienced personnel.

High-frequency oscillatory ventilation (HFOV) is an alternate mode of mechanical ventilation in which the ventilator provides very small, very rapid tidal volumes. Respiratory rates used during oscillatory ventilation typically range from 5–10 Hz (rates of 300–600 breaths/min) in most PICU patients. This mode of ventilation has been used successfully for neonates, older pediatric patients, and adults; and for diseases as diverse as pneumonia, pulmonary contusion, ARDS, and asthma. HFOV is increasingly being used as initial therapy in severe, diffuse lung diseases, such as ARDS, which require high mean airway pressures to maintain oxygenation. The advantage of HFOV is that these high levels of mean airway pressure can be achieved without high peak inspiratory pressures or large tidal volumes, thus theoretically protecting the lung from ventilator-induced lung injury. Disadvantages of HFOV include generally poor tolerance by patients who are not heavily sedated or even paralyzed, the risk of cardiovascular compromise due to high mean airway pressures, and the risk of barotrauma in patients with heterogeneous lung disease. Although HFOV clearly may be useful for selected patients, it remains unsettled whether HFOV provides a clear benefit compared with carefully managed conventional modes of ventilation.

Managing the Ventilated Patient

Patients undergoing mechanical ventilation require the same meticulous supportive care given to all PICU patients. Since mechanical ventilation is often frightening and uncomfortable for patients, leading to dyssynchrony with the ventilator and impaired ventilation and oxygenation, they deserve careful attention directed toward opti-

mizing comfort and decreasing anxiety. Sedative-anxiolytics are typically provided as intermittent doses of benzodiazepines, with or without opioids. Some patients respond better to the steady state of sedation provided by continuous infusion of these agents, although oversedation of the ventilated patient may lead to longer durations of ventilation and difficulties with weaning from the ventilator.

For a patient with severe respiratory illnesses, even small movements by the patient may compromise ventilation and oxygenation. In such cases, muscle paralysis may facilitate oxygenation and ventilation. Nondepolarizing neuromuscular blocking agents are most commonly used for this purpose, and they may be given as intermittent doses or as continuous infusions. When muscle relaxants are given, extra care must be taken to ensure that levels of sedation are adequate, as many of the usual signs of patient discomfort are masked by the paralytics.

Cheifetz IM: Invasive and noninvasive pediatric mechanical ventilation. Respir Care 2003;48:442 [PMID: 12667269].

Flaatten H et al: Outcome after acute respiratory failure is more dependent on dysfunction in other vital organs than on the severity of the respiratory failure. Crit Care 2003;7:R72 [PMID: 12930559].

Frank JA, Matthay MA: Science review: mechanisms of ventilator-induced injury. Crit Care 2003;7:233 [PMID: 12793874].

Gattinoni L et al: Physiologic rationale for ventilator setting in acute lung injury/acute respiratory distress syndrome patients. Crit Care Med 2003;31:S300 [PMID: 12682456].

Marini JJ, Gattinoni L: Ventilatory management of acute respiratory distress syndrome: a consensus of two. *Crit Care Med* 2004; 32:250.

ACUTE RESPIRATORY DISTRESS SYNDROME

ARDS is a syndrome of acute respiratory failure characterized by increased pulmonary capillary permeability and pulmonary edema that results in refractory hypoxemia, decreased lung compliance, and bilateral diffuse alveolar infiltrates on chest radiography. Statistics of ARDS reflect one of the true successes of current ICU management, as mortality has decreased over the past decade from approximately 50–60% to less than 40%.

An international consensus conference was convened in 1997 to establish the current guidelines defining diagnostic criteria for ARDS. The diagnosis of ARDS rests on four features: (1) an underlying illness or injury that predisposes to ARDS; (2) bilateral infiltrates on chest radiograph; (3) an absence of evidence of heart failure, and in particular left ventricular (LV) failure; and most importantly, (4) severe hypoxemic respiratory failure. Hypoxemia is assessed using the ratio of the arterial oxygen level (PaO_2) to the inspired oxygen concentration (FIO_2). When the PaO_2:FIO_2 ratio is less than 200, and the other criteria are met, the case is defined as ARDS. When the

PaO_2:FIO_2 ratio is between 200 and 300, and the other criteria are met, the case is defined as acute lung injury. This definition is debated, however, particularly since the current criteria do not include any assessment of the airway pressure needed to oxygenate the patient. Numerous other diagnostic systems have been proposed.

In addition, because the clinical disorder or disorders that led to the development of acute lung injury clearly influence the patient's prognosis for recovery, precise definition of the underlying problem is important. Although the average mortality in this population is 40%, the rate is dependent on the associated clinical disorder. Mortality can be as high as 90% among adult ARDS patients with underlying liver failure, and less than 10% among pediatric ARDS associated with respiratory syncytial virus infection. The development of multisystem organ failure is a frequent complicating factor in the care of the patient with ARDS, and the failure of organs outside the lung has a large role in determining the prognosis. In fact, nonpulmonary organ failures are the leading cause of death in the most recent studies of adult or pediatric ARDS patients.

Clinical Presentation & Pathophysiology

ARDS may be precipitated by a variety of insults (Table 13–6), of which infection is the most common. Despite the diversity of causes, the clinical presentation is remarkably similar in most cases. ARDS can be divided roughly into four clinical phases (Table 13–7). In the earliest phase, the patient may have dyspnea and tachypnea with a relatively normal PO_2 and a hyperventilation-induced respiratory alkalosis. No significant abnormalities are noted on physical or radiologic examination of the chest. Experimental studies suggest that neutrophils accumulate in the lungs at this stage and that their products damage lung endothelium.

Table 13–6. Acute respiratory distress syndrome risk factors.

Direct Lung Injury	Indirect Lung Injury
Aspiration of gastric contents	Sepsis
Hydrocarbon ingestion or aspiration	Shock
	Pancreatitis
Inhalation injury (heat or toxin)	Burns
Pulmonary contusion	Trauma
Pneumonia	Fat embolism
Near-drowning	Drug overdoses (including aspirin, opioids, barbiturates, tricyclic antidepressants)
	Transfusion of blood products

Over the next few hours, hypoxemia increases and respiratory distress becomes clinically apparent, with cyanosis, tachycardia, irritability, and dyspnea. Radiographic evidence of early parenchymal change is noted by "fluffy" alveolar infiltrates initially appearing in dependent lung fields, indicative of pulmonary edema. The edema fluid typically has a high concentration of protein (75–95% of plasma protein concentration), which is characteristic of an increased permeability-type edema and differentiates it from cardiogenic or hydrostatic pulmonary edema. Protein in the air spaces acts to inactivate surfactant, which, combined with damage to type 2 alveolar pneumocytes, leads to a marked deficiency in surfactant content in the lung. As a result, the lung is particularly prone to collapse and to shearing injuries due to the high surface tension required to open collapsed alveoli.

Alveolar epithelial injury in ARDS lowers the threshold for alveolar edema formation and impairs gas exchange. The functional integrity of the alveolar epithelium, as measured by the ability of the alveoli to clear liquid out of the air spaces, has prognostic importance in ARDS. Those patients who still show evidence of functional alveolar liquid clearance mechanisms during the first day of their illness have a much higher survival rate than those with evidence of severe epithelial impairment.

Pulmonary hypertension, decrease in lung compliance, and increase in airway resistance are also commonly noted. Clinical studies suggest that airway resistance may be increased in 50% of patients with ARDS.

Computed tomography studies of adult patients in the acute phases of ARDS have established that this illness is characterized by heterogeneous collapse of the lung, with typical areas of dependent consolidation, overinflation in the upper zones, and relatively small areas of normally expanded lung. These findings have suggested that the lung in ARDS is best viewed as "small" rather than stiff, prompting a shift toward ventilating these patients with smaller tidal volumes and tolerating the relative hypercarbia that may ensue. In addition, a large body of research has shown that ventilation with large tidal volumes and low PEEP levels allows a pattern of cyclic alveolar overdistention and collapse, which causes a lung injury histologically similar to ARDS, even in normal lungs. This phenomenon is now called ventilator-induced lung injury. Taken together, these findings have given rise to the view that acute ARDS can best be treated by rerecruiting those areas of dependent collapse and minimizing the stretch-induced injury, or volutrauma, in the nondependent areas of the lung. This approach has been termed the open-lung strategy and has been the subject of intense scrutiny in recent years (see below).

The subacute phase of ARDS (5–10 days after lung injury) is characterized by type II cell and fibroblast pro-

Table 13–7. Pathophysiologic changes of modern acute respiratory distress syndrome (low-pressure pulmonary edema).

	Symptoms	Laboratory Findings	Pathophysiology
Phase 1 (early changes)			
Normal radiograph	Dyspnea, tachypnea, normal chest examination	Mild pulmonary hypertension, normoxemic or mild hypoxemia, hypercapnia.	Neutrophil sequestration, no clear tissue damage
Phase 2 (onset of parenchymal changes)[a]			
Patchy alveolar infiltrates beginning in dependent lung No perivascular cuffs (unless a component of high pressure edema is present) Normal heart size	Dyspnea, tachypnea, cyanosis, tachycardia, coarse rales	Pulmonary hypertension, normal wedge pressure, increased lung permeability, increased lung water, increasing shunt, progressive decrease in compliance, moderate to severe hypoxemia.	Neutrophil infiltration, vascular congestion, fibrin strands, platelet clumps, alveolar septal edema, intraalveolar protein, white cells, type I epithelial damage
Phase 3 (acute respiratory failure with progression, 2–10 days)			
Diffuse alveolar infiltrates Air bronchograms Decreased lung volume No bronchovascular cuffs Normal heart	Tachypnea, tachycardia, hyperdynamic state, sepsis syndrome, signs of consolidation, diffuse rhonchi	Phase 2 changes persist. Progression of abnormalities, increasing shunt fraction, further decrease in compliance, increased minute ventilation, impaired oxygen extraction of hemoglobin.	Increased interstitial and alveolar inflammatory exudate with neutrophil and mononuclear cells, type II cell proliferation, beginning fibroblast proliferation, thromboembolic occlusion
Phase 4 (pulmonary fibrosis, pneumonia with progression, > 10 days)[b]			
Persistent diffuse infiltrates Superimposed new pneumonic infiltrates Recurrent pneumothorax Normal heart size Enlargement with cor pulmonale	Symptoms as above, recurrent sepsis, evidence of multiple organ system failure	Phase 3 changes persist. Recurrent pneumonia, progressive lung restriction, impaired tissue oxygenation, impaired oxygen extraction. Multiple organ system failure.	Type II cell hyperplasia, interstitial thickening; infiltration of lymphocytes, macrophages, fibroblasts; loculated pneumonia or interstitial fibrosis; medial thickening and remodeling of arterioles

[a]The process is readily reversible at this stage if the initiating factor is controlled.
[b]Multiple organ system failure is common. The mortality rate is greater than 80% at this stage, since resolution is more difficult.
Modified slightly and reproduced, with permission, from Demling RH: Adult respiratory distress syndrome: Current concepts. New Horizons 1993;1:388.

liferation in the interstitium of the lung. This results in decreased lung volumes and signs of consolidation that are noted clinically and radiographically. Worsening of the hypoxemia with an increasing shunt fraction, as well as a further decrease in lung compliance, are noted. Some patients develop an accelerated fibrosing alveolitis in which fibroblasts and collagen formation in the interstitium are markedly increased. The mechanisms responsible for these changes are unclear. Current investigation centers on the role of growth and differentiation factors, such as transforming growth factor-β and platelet-derived growth factor released by resident and nonresident lung cells such as alveolar macrophages, mast cells, neutrophils, alveolar type II cells, and fibroblasts.

During the chronic phase of ARDS (10–14 days after lung injury), fibrosis, emphysema, and pulmonary vascular obliteration occur. During this phase of the illness, oxygenation defects generally improve, and the lung becomes more fragile and susceptible to barotrauma. Air leak is common among patients still ventilated with high levels of airway pressure at this late stage in their illness. Also, patients have increased amounts of dead space, and difficulties with ventilation are common. Airway compliance remains low, perhaps because of ongoing pulmonary fibrosis and insufficient surfactant production.

Secondary infections are common in the subacute and chronic phases of ARDS and significantly influence the outcome. The mechanisms responsible for increased host susceptibility to infection during this phase are not well understood.

Mortality in the late phase of ARDS exceeds 80%. Death is usually caused by multiple organ failure and systemic hemodynamic instability rather than by hypoxemia.

Treatment

A. MONITORING

Multiorgan system monitoring is mandatory for patients with ARDS. ABG analysis is required for accurate assessment of oxygenation and ventilation and for the rational titration of ventilator strategies that may have profound adverse effects. Hemodynamic monitoring should include, at a minimum, central venous pressure (CVP) measurements to help determine the level of cardiac preload, and an indwelling arterial catheter for continuous blood pressure measurements and ABG sampling. For patients with severe disease or concurrent cardiac dysfunction, consideration can be given to pulmonary artery catheterization to help with fluid management and to allow assessment of mixed venous blood saturation as an index of overall tissue oxygenation. Obtaining chest films daily is important for patients receiving vigorous support because severe ARDS is associated with a 40–60% incidence of air leaks. Since secondary infections are common and increase mortality rates strikingly, surveillance for infection is important, requiring appropriate cultures and following the temperature curve and white blood cell count. Renal, liver, and gastrointestinal (GI) function should be watched closely because of the great likelihood of multiple organ dysfunction.

B. FLUID MANAGEMENT

Given the increases in pulmonary capillary permeability in ARDS, pulmonary edema accumulation is likely with any elevation in pulmonary hydrostatic pressures. In this setting, most clinicians reduce intravascular volume to the lowest level that is still compatible with an adequate cardiac output and adequate oxygen delivery to the tissues.

C. HEMODYNAMIC SUPPORT

Hemodynamic support is directed toward increasing perfusion and oxygen delivery. In those circumstances when volume expansion is necessary to improve oxygen delivery, this can best be achieved by giving packed red blood cells to maintain the hematocrit between 35% and 40%, and by giving colloid or crystalloid solutions to nonanemic volume-depleted patients. Inotropes should be used as needed to optimize oxygen delivery to the tissues.

D. VENTILATORY SUPPORT

In addition to the basic principles of ventilator management described earlier (see section on Adjusting the Ven-

tilator), current ventilatory management of ARDS is directed at the rerecruitment of areas of dependent alveolar collapse and the protection of noncollapsed areas from overdistention. Since an FIO_2 greater than 60% over 24 hours can cause additional injury to the lung, mean airway pressure should be increased to provide an adequate PaO_2 (> 55 mm Hg) at an FIO_2 of 60% or less. In general, this can be accomplished by incremental increases in PEEP every 15–30 minutes until adequate oxygenation is achieved or until a limiting side effect of the PEEP is reached. Ventilation with high levels of PEEP acts by helping to prevent dependent collapse of edematous lung units. PEEP levels of 12–14 cm H_2O are not unusual, and levels as high as 20–25 cm H_2O have been used successfully in these patients. Before increasing PEEP significantly, the physician should optimize conditions by making sure that the patient's intravascular volume is appropriate, the endotracheal tube does not leak, and the patient is heavily sedated and paralyzed.

The actual mode of ventilation employed (volume or pressure) with an ARDS patient is probably unimportant. However, recent work from a large multicenter trial sponsored by the National Institutes of Health suggests that the tidal volumes used may be important. Using a PEEP strategy similar to that described in the preceding paragraph, the investigators compared the effects of a low (6 mL/kg) tidal volume versus a normal (12 mL/kg) tidal volume in 861 adult ARDS patients. Those patients ventilated with the lower tidal volume demonstrated fewer extrapulmonary organ failures and an overall 25% decrease in mortality. In keeping with these findings and with experimental data demonstrating ventilator-induced lung injury at alveolar pressures greater than 30 cm H_2O, we suggest that current practice for pediatric ARDS patients should consist of ventilation with tidal volumes in the 6- to 8-mL/kg range, or at least with tidal volumes small enough to keep alveolar pressures below 30–35 cm H_2O.

E. OTHER THERAPIES

As previously described, HFOV is an increasingly popular technique that has been used successfully in pediatric patients with ARDS. When used as part of a strategy of aggressive increases in mean airway pressure to rerecruit deflated areas of the lung and to prevent cyclic overdistention and collapse, HFOV is a physiologically rational approach to this illness. It has not yet been determined whether HFOV provides additional benefits compared with open-lung strategy ventilation with conventional ventilator modes.

Prone positioning is a technique of changing the patient's position in bed from supine to prone, with the goal of allowing postural drainage and improving ventilation of collapsed dependent lung units. This technique often dramatically improves oxygenation, particularly for patients early in the course of ARDS. The oxygenation improvements are often not sustained, however, necessitating repeated position changes to maintain the effect. Whether prone positioning contributes to improved outcomes for patients with ARDS remains uncertain.

Based on the ability of inhaled **nitric oxide** (iNO) to reduce pulmonary artery pressure and to improve the matching of ventilation with perfusion without producing systemic vasodilation, iNO has been proposed as a beneficial therapy for ARDS. Several recent multicenter trials of iNO in the treatment of ARDS, both in adults and in children, have shown acute improvements in oxygenation in subsets of patients but no significant improvement in overall survival. As a result, the current role of iNO in the treatment of ARDS remains unclear. Additional studies are now focusing on the anti-inflammatory role (by reducing neutrophil adhesion and activation) iNO may play in ARDS. Studies to evaluate the combined effects of several of these alternative therapies are also being planned.

Surfactant replacement therapy has been tried with some success in patients with ARDS. In some instances surfactant replacement improves lung compliance and oxygenation, and hastens weaning from mechanical ventilation. In randomized trials of surfactant replacement, there were no differences in outcome (death, length of ventilation, or hospitalization), but there was some evidence of decreased inflammation. A multicenter trial of surfactant treatment for pediatric ARDS is currently in progress.

Although **corticosteroids** have not been found to be beneficial in early-stage ARDS, these agents may reduce the inflammation and fibrosis associated with later-stage ARDS. Indeed, the use of methylprednisolone in adults whose lung injury was not improving after 7 days of ARDS was associated with an improvement of lung injury and multiple organ dysfunction. Mortality was also reduced, when compared with control subjects receiving placebo. A large multicenter trial is under way to further evaluate the use of steroids in the late phase of ARDS.

Extracorporeal membrane oxygenation (ECMO) has been used in pediatric patients with severe ARDS. In older studies, patients who received ECMO had better survival rates than did control subjects. ECMO has not been studied in comparison with current conventional ventilation strategies. In addition, recent improvements in outcome for pediatric ARDS patients receiving conventional therapies have made the role of ECMO less clear and have made further prospective randomized studies of ECMO difficult to complete. For now, ECMO remains a rescue therapy for patients with severe ARDS unresponsive to other modalities.

F. Follow-Up

Information regarding the long-term outcome of pediatric patients with ARDS remains limited. One report of 10 children followed 1–4 years after severe ARDS showed three still symptomatic and seven with hypoxemia at rest. Until further information is available, all patients with a history of ARDS need close follow-up of pulmonary function.

Acute Respiratory Distress Syndrome Network: Ventilation with lower tidal volumes as compared with traditional tidal volumes for acute lung injury and the acute respiratory distress syndrome. N Engl J Med 2000;342:1301 [PMID: 10793162].

Anderson MR: Update on pediatric acute respiratory distress syndrome. Respir Care 2003;48:261 [PMID: 1266727].

Burns SM: Mechanical ventilation of patients with acute respiratory distress syndrome and patients requiring weaning; the evidence guiding practice. Crit Care Nurse 2005;25:14 [PMID: 16034030].

Calfee CS, Matthay MA: Recent advances in mechanical ventilation. Am J Med 205;118:584 [PMID: 15922687].

Gattinoni L, Eleonara C, Caironi P: Monitoring of pulmonary mechanics in acute respiratory distress syndrome to titrate therapy. Curr Opin Crit Care 2005;11:252 [PMID: 15928475].

Krishnan JA, Brower RG: High-frequency ventilation for acute lung injury and ARDS. Chest 2000;118:795 [PMID: 10988205].

Lewandowski K: Extracorporeal membrane oxygenation for severe acute respiratory failure. Crit Care 2000;4:156 [PMID: 11094500].

Matthay MA, Zimmerman GA: Acute lung injury and the acute respiratory distress syndrome: four decades of inquiry into pathogenesis and rational management. Am J Respir Cell Mol Biol 2005;33:319 [PMID: 16272252].

Meduri GU et al: Effect of prolonged methylprednisolone therapy in unresolving acute respiratory distress syndrome: A randomized controlled trial. JAMA 1998;280:159 [PMID: 9669790]. (Classic)

Santos CC, Zhang H, Liu M, Slutsky AS: Bench-to-bedside review: biotrauma and modulation of the innate immune response. Crit Care 2005;9:280 [PMID: 15987418].

Schwarz MA: Acute lung injury: cellular mechanism and derangements. Pediatr Respir Rev 2001;2:3. [PMID: 16263475].

Shorr AF et al: D-Dimer correlates with proinflammatory cytokine levels and outcomes in critically ill patients. Chest 2002;121:1262 [PMID: 11948062].

Sokol J et al: Inhaled nitric oxide for acute hypoxemic respiratory failure in children and adults. Cochrane Database Syst Rev 2000;4:CD002787 [PMID: 11914763].

Vincent JL: New management strategies in ARDS: Immunomodulation. Crit Care Clin 2002;18:69 [PMID: 11910733].

ASTHMA (Life-Threatening)

Status asthmaticus may be defined as reversible small airway obstruction that is refractory to sympathomimetic and anti-inflammatory agents and that may progress to respiratory failure without prompt and aggressive intervention. Life-threatening asthma is caused by severe bronchospasm, excessive mucus secretion, inflammation, and edema of the airways (see Chapter 18). Reversal of these mechanisms is the key to successful treatment. Status asthmaticus remains a common diagnosis among children admitted to the PICU, and asthma is associated with surprisingly high mortality rates.

The physical examination helps determine the severity of illness. Accessory muscle use (sternocleidomastoid) correlates well with a forced expiratory volume in 1 second and peak expiratory flow rates less than 50% of normal predicted values. A pulsus paradoxus of over 22 mm Hg has been correlated with elevated $PaCO_2$ levels. The absence of wheezing may be misleading because, in order to produce a wheezing sound, the patient must take in a certain amount of air. The ABG analysis remains the single most important laboratory determination in the evaluation of a child in severe status asthmaticus. Patients with severe respiratory distress, signs of exhaustion, alterations in consciousness, elevated $PaCO_2$, or acidosis should be admitted to the PICU.

Treatment

Much of the morbidity associated with the treatment of severe asthma is related to the complications of mechanical ventilation that occur in patients with severe airflow obstruction. As a result, the goal of initial treatment of the patient with life-threatening status asthmaticus is to improve the patient's ability to ventilate without resorting to intubation and mechanical ventilation. The medical therapies described in the following discussion should be undertaken swiftly and aggressively with the goal of reversing the bronchospasm before respiratory failure necessitates invasive ventilation.

Due to inadequate minute ventilation and V/Q mismatching, patients with severe asthma are almost always hypoxemic and should receive supplemental **humidified oxygen** immediately.

Inhaled β₂-agonist therapy with agents such as albuterol remains first-line therapy to reverse acute bronchoconstriction. If the patient is in severe distress and has poor inspiratory flow rates, thus preventing adequate delivery of nebulized medication, subcutaneous injection of epinephrine or terbutaline may be considered. The frequency of β₂-agonist administration varies according to the severity of the patient's symptoms and the occurrence of adverse side effects. Nebulized albuterol may be given intermittently at a dose of 0.1 mg/kg per nebulization up to 2.5 mg, or it can be administered continuously at a dose of 0.5 mg/kg/h to a maximum of 20 mg/h, usually without serious side effects. The heart rate and blood pressure of these patients should be monitored closely, because excessive tachycardia and ventricular ectopy may occur.

Systemic **corticosteroids** are the mainstay of therapy for the inflammatory component of asthma. Corticosteroids act by decreasing inflammation, stabilizing mast cells, and increasing β₂-receptor expression. These agents speed the resolution of severe asthma exacerbations and should be given to all patients admitted to the hospital with severe asthma. The anti-inflammatory effect is generally observed 6–12 hours after administration. It is preferable to administer the corticosteroid by the intravenous route due to the risk of vomiting or difficulty swallowing. A typical pediatric dose is 1 mg/kg of IV methylprednisolone every 6 hours, with the adult dose between 40 and 250 mg. The acute complications of corticosteroid use include GI bleeding, hyperglycemia, and hypertension.

Inhaled **anticholinergic bronchodilators** may also improve lung function when administered to patients with severe asthma along with albuterol. Nebulized ipratropium bromide is the drug of choice, and is given at a dose of 250–500 µg/dose. It has variable effectiveness though and, as it has few side effects, should be considered along with albuterol in patients with severe asthma, especially when they have chronic high use of β-agonists.

Intravenous β-agonists should be considered in patients with severe bronchospasm unresponsive to inhaled bronchodilators. The agent most commonly used in the United States is terbutaline, a relatively specific β₂-agonist, which can be given as a bolus dose or as a continuous infusion. Owing to its relative specificity for β₂-receptors, terbutaline has fewer cardiac side effects than previously available IV β-agonists like isoproterenol. Terbutaline is given as a bolus or loading dose of 10 µg/kg followed by a continuous infusion of 0.5–5 µg/kg/min. In general, patients receiving IV β₂-agonist therapy should have indwelling arterial lines for continuous blood pressure and blood gas monitoring.

Theophylline is a methylxanthine which remains a controversial agent in the management of severe asthma. Clinical studies yield mixed results on its benefit when given with steroids and β₂-agonists for children with asthma. The theoretical advantage of this medication is that it relaxes airway smooth muscle by a separate mechanism from β₂-agonists by preventing degradation of cyclic guanosine monophosphate. Besides causing bronchodilation, this agent decreases mucociliary inflammatory mediators and reduces microvascular permeability. However, the pharmacokinetics of theophylline are erratic and therapeutic levels can be difficult to manage, and serious side effects can occur with high drug levels such as seizures and cardiac arrhythmias. Theophylline is given IV as aminophylline. Each 1 mg/kg of aminophylline given as a loading dose will increase the serum level by approximately 2 mg/dL. For a patient who has not previously received aminophylline or oral theophylline preparations, load with 7–8 mg/kg of aminophylline in an attempt to achieve a level of 10–15 mg/dL; then start a continuous infusion of aminophylline at a dosage of 0.8–1 mg/kg/h. A post-bolus level and steady-state level should be drawn with the initiation of the medication as well as continued monitoring of steady-state levels. Watch closely for toxicity (gastric upset, tachycardia, and seizures) and follow serum levels closely, trying to maintain steady-state levels of 12–16 mg/dL.

Magnesium sulfate has been reported to be an effective bronchodilator in adult patients with severe status asthmaticus when given in conjunction with steroids and β_2-agonists, and may be considered for patients in danger of worsening respiratory failure. The mechanism of action of magnesium is unclear, but its smooth muscle relaxation properties are probably caused by interference with calcium flux in the bronchial smooth muscle cell. Magnesium sulfate is given IV at a dose of 25–50 mg/kg/dose. Though it is usually well tolerated, hypotension and flushing are side effects.

Heliox is a mixture of helium and oxygen which is less viscous than ambient air and can improve airway delivery of albuterol. A 2003 meta-analysis of heliox did not report a benefit in the initial treatment of acute asthma, although it may be considered in refractory asthma. The caveat for use of heliox is that it requires at least 60–70% helium to decrease airway resistance, limiting its use in patients requiring higher concentrations of supplemental oxygen.

While **leukotriene antagonists** are used for maintenance asthma therapy, their use in the intensive care setting has not been yet demonstrated.

If the previously described aggressive management fails to result in significant improvement, **mechanical ventilation** may be necessary. In general, if there is steady deterioration (increased acidosis and rising $PaCO_2$) despite intensive therapy for asthma, the patient should be intubated and ventilated mechanically. Mechanical ventilation for patients with asthma is difficult because the severe airflow obstruction often leads to very high airway pressures, air trapping, and resultant barotrauma. The goal of mechanical ventilation with an intubated asthmatic patient is to maintain adequate oxygenation and ventilation with the least amount of barotrauma until other therapies become effective. Worsening hypercarbia after intubation should be anticipated and aggressive efforts to normalize blood gases should be moderated, as such efforts may only lead to complications. Due to the severe airflow obstruction, these patients will require long inspiratory times to deliver a breath and long expiratory times to avoid air trapping. In general, the ventilator rate should be decreased until the expiratory time is long enough to allow emptying prior to the next machine breath. Ventilator rates of 8–12 breaths/min are typical initially. Either volume- or pressure-targeted modes of ventilation can be used effectively in these patients, though tidal volumes and pressure limits should be closely monitored. As a patient moves towards extubation, a support mode of ventilation is useful, as the patient can set his or her own inspiratory time and flow rate. Due to air trapping, patients can have significant auto-PEEP. The level of PEEP on the ventilator is usually set relatively low (3–5 cm H_2O) to minimize high peak pressures. Isolated reports have noted patients who respond to greater PEEP, but these cases are the exception. The acute ventilator strategies and the resulting hypercarbia typically are uncomfortable, requiring that patients be heavily sedated and often medically paralyzed. Fentanyl and midazolam are good choices for sedation. Ketamine, a dissociative anesthetic, should be considered for its sedative properties, although it also increases bronchial secretions, which can complicate management. Barbiturates should be avoided as well as morphine, which increases histamine release. Most patients, at least initially, will also require neuromuscular blockade to optimize ventilation and minimize airway pressures. In intubated patients who are failing all the above strategies, **inhaled anesthetics,** such as isoflurane, can be considered. These agents can cause significant hypotension due to vasodilation.

Monitoring

Severely asthmatic patients should be monitored for heart rate, blood pressure, O_2 saturation, and arterial pH and $PaCO_2$. Continuous blood pressure monitoring is necessary because air trapping can lead to increased levels of occult PEEP (auto-PEEP), an effect that can impair venous return and decrease cardiac output. Close ventilator monitoring is necessary because increases in inspiratory pressure or decreases in pulmonary compliance may signal worsening bronchoconstriction, mucus plugging, or an extrapleural air leak. Chest films of ventilated asthmatic patients should be obtained daily and immediately with sudden changes in patient condition, due to the risk of pneumothorax and pneumomediastinum. In addition, if the patient is receiving neuromuscular blocking agents, the degree of nerve block should be monitored closely because nondepolarizing agents such as pancuronium, when given with corticosteroids, can cause prolonged paralysis and muscle weakness.

Supplement to Circulation: Part 10.5 Near-Fatal Asthma. Circulation 2005;112:IV-139 to IV-142.

DiNicola LK et al: Drug therapy approaches in the treatment of acute severe asthma in hospitalized children. Paediatr Drugs 2001;3:509 [PMID: 11513282].

McFadden ER Jr.: Acute severe asthma. Am J Respir Crit Care Med 2003;168:740.

Rodrigo GJ et al: Use of helium-oxygen mixtures in the treatment of acute asthma: a systematic review. Chest 2003;123:891 [PMID: 12628893].

Werner HA: Status asthmaticus in children: A review. Chest 2001; 119:1913 [PMID: 11399724].

SHOCK

Shock may be defined as failure of the cardiovascular system to deliver critical substrates and to remove toxic metabolites. This failure leads to anaerobic metabolism in cells and ultimately to irreversible cellular damage. Shock has been categorized into a series of recognizable stages: compensated, uncompensated, and irreversible. Patients in compensated shock have relatively normal cardiac output and normal blood pressures, but they have alterations in the microcirculation that increase flow to some organs and reduce flow to others. In infants, compensatory increases in cardiac output are achieved primarily by tachycardia rather than by increases in stroke volume. Heart rates of 190–210/min are common in infants with compensated shock, but heart rates over 220/min raise the possibility of supraventricular tachycardia. In older patients, cardiac contractility (stroke volume) and heart rate increase to improve cardiac output. Blood pressure remains normal initially because of peripheral vasoconstriction and increased systemic vascular resistance. Thus hypotension occurs late and is more characteristic of the uncompensated stage of shock. In the uncompensated stage, the oxygen and nutrient supply to the cells deteriorates further with subsequent cellular breakdown and release of toxic substances, causing further redistribution of flow. At this point, the patient is hypotensive, with poor cardiac output.

Shock can be classified by mechanism into hypovolemic (including distributive), cardiogenic, and septic. Often, two or three of these occur together.

A. HYPOVOLEMIC SHOCK

Hypovolemic shock is caused by decreased circulating blood volume or preload. This may result from loss of whole blood or plasma or from fluid loss from the kidney or gut. These patients usually have intact compensatory mechanisms that maintain normal blood pressure by increasing cardiac output and shunting blood away from certain organs. These responses protect blood flow to the heart and brain. Untreated, hypovolemic shock can progress to an irreversible stage. Additionally, a relative hypovolemia occurs when arterial and capillary shunting past tissue beds occurs with an increase in venous capacitance, causing blood to pool—so-called distributive shock. This results from anaphylaxis or vasodilating drugs.

B. CARDIOGENIC SHOCK/FAILURE

Age-dependent differences occur in myocardial physiology that are relevant to therapy. Neonatal myocardium has reduced systolic performance and contractility. The sarcolemma, sarcoplasmic reticulum, and T-tubules are less well developed, resulting in a greater dependency on transsarcolemma Ca^{2+} flux (ie, extracellular serum Ca^{2+}) for contraction. A high resting state of myocardial contractility occurs that limits the response to inotropic agents. Relatively minor increases in afterload can result in diminished stroke volume. Diastolic compliance is diminished, and small changes in volume result in large changes in ventricular wall tension. Consequently preload reserve is limited, and maximization of the Frank-Starling curve occurs relatively quickly (10–15 mm Hg in animal models). Aggressive volume resuscitation beyond this is often ineffective and not tolerated. Stroke volume is relatively fixed, and greater increases in cardiac output are seen through increased heart rate.

Central to the understanding of cardiogenic failure are the progressive nature of ventricular dysfunction and the compensatory mechanisms that occur in the presence of excessive hemodynamic demands. Inadequate cardiac output activates the renin-angiotensin system. The consequent sodium and water retention augments intravascular volume and increases cardiac output through increased preload. With progression, cardiac compliance is decreased and preload augmentation via the Frank-Starling mechanism is maximized. Subsequently, small changes in ventricular volume can lead to large increases in ventricular pressure, and therefore pulmonary venous pressure, with resultant pulmonary edema. Thus, fluids should be cautiously administered in this setting and should possibly be guided by central venous pressure or left atrial/pulmonary artery capillary wedge pressure monitoring. The atrial distention that occurs in the failing heart leads to increased production and release of atrial natriuretic peptide, a vasodilator that augments sodium and water excretion.

Heart failure also induces autonomic nervous system changes, including increased activation of the adrenergic sympathetic system and decreased parasympathetic stimulation. Increased adrenergic tone is associated with elevated circulating norepinephrine levels and increased vasoconstriction and afterload. These combined factors in turn lead to a cycle of increased afterload, increased energy expenditure, decreased cardiac output, myocyte death, and progressive ventricular dysfunction. The cardiomyocyte effects of prolonged adrenergic stimulation include downregulation of β-receptors, decreased norepinephrine stores, and therefore potentially decreased responses to sympathetic stimulation. Increased cellular concentrations of cyclic adenosine monophosphate and inositol triphosphate lead to increased inward Ca^{2+} flux and at least transient increases in contractility. Subsequently, excessive unremoved calcium impairs lusitropy and augments the propensity for arrhythmias. Blood flow is redistributed away from the splanchnic system, skin, and muscles and toward the heart, brain, adrenal glands, and diaphragm. Endothelial dysfunction is common and contributes to the abnormal vascular tone. Endothelin-1 production is elevated in the lung and increases pulmonary vascular resistance and systemic vascular resistance (SVR). The release of endothelial-derived nitric oxide is also impaired. Circulating arginine vasopressin and tumor necrosis factor-α (TNF-α) levels have also been reported to be elevated. In the later stages of heart failure, cardiomyocyte hypertrophy, fibroblast hyperplasia, and increases in altered production and accumulation occur in extracellular matrix, leading to impaired myocardial function.

Signs and symptoms of cardiac failure are produced by the body's attempts to compensate for the decreased pump function. The body compensates by activating the sympathetic nervous and renin-angiotensin-aldosterone systems. The child in acute heart failure will present with hypotension and such evidence of poor perfusion as metabolic acidosis and organ dysfunction. In response to the poor output, tachycardia and vasoconstriction will be manifest as cool and mottled extremities. Although the extremities are cool, the child's core temperature will be elevated. To improve cardiac output, the body will retain fluid and sodium, resulting in generalized edema. Pulmonary edema will cause tachypnea, and rales can be heard on auscultation. The pulmonary edema may be severe enough to compromise respiration and lead to hypoxemia and respiratory failure.

The work-up can be performed at the same time treatment is initiated, and should include an echocardiogram to evaluate cardiac anatomy and function. Serial echocardiograms may also be helpful to specifically assess the improvement in function with treatment. A chest radiograph can reveal the amount of cardiomegaly, pulmonary edema, and the presence of any effusions. Laboratory tests should include electrolyte measurements and renal and liver function tests.

Management of cardiogenic failure in the pediatric patient is complicated by the varied underlying causes that often require disparate therapies. Cardiac output is a product of stroke volume and heart rate. The factors that influence cardiac output are preload, afterload, contractility, and cardiac rhythm. An analysis of a low cardiac output state should consider the specific cardiac lesion and should use these factors as a framework for therapy.

Cardiogenic failure results from an imbalance of systemic oxygen delivery and demand. Therapy is aimed at restoring oxygen delivery and reducing demand. Sedation, reduced environmental stress, temperature regulation, supplemental O_2, red cell transfusion, and augmentation of cardiac output all have roles. The overall goal of increasing cardiac output should include restoring an appropriate sinus rate and rhythm, optimizing preload, augmenting myocardial contractility with minimal increases in myocardial O_2 consumption, and maximizing afterload reduction. If bradycardia is excessive, temporary pacing with transthoracic, transesophageal, or intracardiac methods should be considered. Excessive tachycardia is to be avoided, as it shortens ventricular diastole, leading to a reduction in diastolic filling, shortened diastolic coronary perfusion, and increased myocardial O_2 consumption.

Cardiogenic failure is associated with elevated ventricular filling pressures (> 20 mm Hg). Thus, although increasing preload can result in augmented cardiac output (to a degree), volume should be administered cautiously—the Frank-Starling curve may remain flat with little further improvement possible, occurring at the expense of elevating pulmonary venous pressure with resultant pulmonary edema. Diuretics can be administered to reduce pulmonary edema and to improve pulmonary compliance, the work of breathing, and oxygenation. Contractility can be augmented through inotropic stimulation of myocardial β_1-receptors (Table 13–8). Dopamine is an α- and β-agonist, which, at moderate doses (3–10 µg/kg/min), improves myocontractility. Low doses (< 3 µg/kg/min) may increase blood flow to the renal, coronary, and splanchnic beds, via D_1 receptors. Newer agents (eg, fenoldopam) are selective for the dopaminergic receptors and are being used to selectively improve renal blood flow and urine output. At higher doses (generally > 10 µg/kg/min) the α-receptor effects predominate, with vasoconstriction increasing SVR and pulmonary vascular resistance. As a first-line pharmacotherapy single agent, low-dose dopamine is often beneficial by improving contractility without increasing afterload and by limiting chronotropic effect. Dobutamine is predominantly a β-agonist that additionally effects a dose-dependent vasodilation (β_2-receptor) and has been shown to shift the ventricular pressure-volume loop toward normal, reducing LV filling pressure and hence pulmonary venous pressure. Its use in infants may be limited by its chronotropic effects leading to impaired ventricular filling. Many institutes use dobutamine as an alternative first-line agent. Isoproterenol is a pure β-agonist that causes significant tachycardia, increased myocardial O_2 consumption, and systemic and pulmonary arterial vasodilation. Though limited by its tachycardic effects as an inotrope, it is useful in instances of associated bradycardia, such as occur in heart transplantation and heart block. Epinephrine is an α- and β-agonist that causes the greatest increase in myocardial O_2 consumption of all inotropes. At a low dose (< 0.05 µg/kg/min) it increases heart rate and contractility and decreases SVR (β_2-receptor). At higher doses the α-effects predomi-

Table 13–8. Pharmacologic support of the shock patient.

Drug	Dose	Alpha-Adrenergic Effect[a]	Beta-Adrenergic Effect[a]	Vasodilator Effect	Actions and Advantages	Disadvantages
Dopamine	1–20 µg/kg/min	+ to +++ (dose-related)	+ to +++ (dose-related)	At low doses, renal vasodilation occurs (dopaminergic receptors)	Moderate inotrope, wide and safe dosage range, short half-life.	May cause worsening of pulmonary vasoconstriction
Dobutamine	1–10 µg/kg/min	0	+++		Moderate inotrope, less chronotropic, fewer dysrhythmias than with isoproterenol or epinephrine.	Marked variation among patients
Epinephrine	0.05–1 µg/kg/min	++ to +++ (dose-related)	+++		Significant increases in inotropy, chronotropy, and SVR.	Tachycardia, dysrhythmias, renal ischemia, systemic and PVR
Isoproterenol	0.05–1 µg/kg/min	0	+++	Peripheral vasodilation	Significant increase in inotropy and chronotropy. SVR can drop, and PVR should not increase and may decrease.	Significant myocardial oxygen consumption increases, tachycardia, dysrhythmias
Norepinephrine	0.05–1 µg/kg/min	+++	+++		Powerful vasoconstrictor (systemic and pulmonary); rarely used except possibly in patients with very low SVR or in conjunction with vasodilator.	Reduced cardiac output if afterload is too high, renal ischemia
Nitroprusside	0.05–8 µg/kg/min	0	0	Arterial and venous dilation (smooth muscle relaxation)	Decreases SVR and PVR, very short-acting. Blood pressure returns to previous levels within 1–10 minutes after infusion is stopped.	Toxicities (thiocyanates and cyanide), increased intracranial pressure and ventilation/perfusion mismatch, methemoglobinemia, increased intracranial pressure
Milrinone	0.25–0.75 µg/kg/min	0	0		Phosphodiesterase III inhibition. Decreases VR and PVR, increases myocardial contractility with only mild increase in myocardial O_2 consumption. Usually used with low-dose dopamine or dobutamine.	

[a]0, no effect; +, small effect; ++, moderate effect; +++, potent effect.
SVR, systemic vascular resistance; PVR, pulmonary vascular resistance.

nate, increasing afterload. Despite these drawbacks, epinephrine can be useful as a second-line agent in cases unresponsive to low-dose dopamine. It is often administered in combination with a vasodilator to off-set the α effects. Milrinone (0.25–0.75 µg/kg/min) is a useful agent in the class of phosphodiesterase inhibitors, preventing degradation of both cyclic guanosine monophosphate and cyclic adenosine monophosphate. Its beneficial effects include a limited increase in myocardial O_2 consumption, decreased SVR and pulmonary vascular resistance, increased contractility, and improved lusiotropy. It is frequently used as a first-line drug, often in combination with low-dose dopamine or epinephrine.

Afterload reduction is an important additional therapy that increases stroke volume and decreases myocardial O_2 consumption. Agents commonly used are nitroprusside, hydralazine, and the angiotensin-converting enzyme inhibitors. Nitroprusside is a rapid-acting IV agent, which is readily titratable and causes venodilation and arteriolar dilation, resulting in decreased SVR and pulmonary vascular resistance. Venodilation can decrease preload, and volume may therefore need to be coadministered to restore an appropriate preload. It is limited by its toxic metabolite, cyanide, which will accumulate over days of treatment and inhibit mitochondrial function, leading to metabolic acidosis. Angiotensin-converting enzyme inhibitors are the agents of choice for oral afterload reduction and have been shown to improve survival and functional status in adults. Patients should be switched to angiotensin-converting enzyme inhibitors as soon as indicated. LV afterload is a function of systolic transmural pressure (aortic pressure/intrapleural pressure), and mechanical afterload reduction can be attained by delivering positive airway pressure through mechanical ventilation or through continuous positive airway pressure/bilevel positive airway pressure. This must be taken into account when weaning a patient with significant LV dysfunction from mechanical ventilation. If cardiac output cannot be augmented sufficiently despite aggressive medical therapy, consideration should be given to mechanical circulatory support as a bridge to cardiac transplantation. Such support is provided by ECMO, a ventricular access device, or intra-aortic balloon pump counterpulsation.

Congenital heart defects pose special concerns. **Aortic stenosis,** for instance, obstructs flow across the LV outflow tract, elevates intraventricular pressure, and increases systolic workload and LV hypertrophy. Due to the outflow tract gradient and hypertrophy, diastolic flow in the coronaries is decreased, which can result in subendocardial ischemia. Dopamine is indicated for inotropic support. Afterload reduction is relatively contraindicated, as it may further compromise coronary flow.

Hypertrophic cardiomyopathy is associated with a hypertrophied nondilated left ventricle, often with dynamic left or biventricular outflow tract obstruction. Coronary abnormalities with luminal compromise are frequent. Systolic function is elevated, ejection fraction is increased, and diastolic dysfunction is evident. Inotropes are avoided due to increased dynamic gradient, coronary compromise, and subendocardial ischemia. Cardiac output is optimized by providing sufficient preload and pharmacotherapy with β-blockers and calcium channel antagonists.

Aortic insufficiency is associated with retrograde flow into the left ventricle during diastole. The amount of regurgitation depends in part on the pressure gradient across the aortic valve and on the heart rate. With increasing heart rates, diastole is shortened and regurgitation limited. Therapy should include inotropic support to improve overall cardiac output and aggressive afterload reduction to reduce the regurgitant fraction. Heart rate can be increased with isoproterenol or transesophageal pacing.

In **mitral regurgitation,** blood is forced back into the low-pressure left atrium during systole. The regurgitant fraction depends partly on the relative resistance to flow across the mitral and aortic valves during systole. Therapy includes inotropic support to improve total cardiac output, and aggressive afterload reduction to improve antegrade aortic flow.

Patients with **anomalous left coronary artery** exhibit myocardial dysfunction secondary to myocardial ischemia. The anomalous coronary artery typically arises from the pulmonary artery. In this scenario, blood flow to the right coronary artery is diverted to the left coronary artery and into the pulmonary artery, resulting in a "steal" phenomenon in the left coronary distribution and ischemia. Medical therapy is futile, though dopamine and milrinone may be use to temporize the situation while awaiting urgent surgical correction. Prior to surgery, care must be exercised not to reduce pulmonary arterial pressure (and increase steal) or excessively increase myocardial O_2 consumption.

Cardiopulmonary bypass (high- or low-flow) and deep hypothermic circulatory arrest are frequently required to facilitate surgical correction of congenital defects. These techniques are associated with widespread organ system effects, including increased total body water, transient myocardial dysfunction, gas exchange abnormalities, coagulation abnormalities, and hormonal and stress responses. Impairment in myocardial contractility is predictable 6–12 hours following surgery. The myocardium can be supported with increased preload, inotropes, and afterload reduction. The use of perioperative steroids and modified ultrafiltration are tools that appear to limit post-bypass–induced myocardial and vascular dysfunction.

C. SEPTIC SHOCK

Septic shock has components of both cardiogenic and hypovolemic shock. Septic shock is only indirectly caused by microorganisms. Rather, septic shock is the direct result of the production and secretion of inflammatory mediators. Proinflammatory mediators (TNF-α, interleukin-1, interleukin-6, interleukin-8, and platelet-activating factor) are produced and released in excess of the anti-inflammatory mediators (interleukin-10, glucocorticoids, and catecholamines), resulting in a proinflammatory cascade that initiates a number of pathophysiologic responses.

Septic shock caused by gram-negative organisms appears to be mediated by endotoxins (lipopolysaccharides) and the subsequent release of cytokines (TNF, interleukin-1, and interleukin-10), eicosanoid products, bradykinin, and endorphins. These agents can directly mediate many of the manifestations of septic shock and also act to amplify the injury by attracting granulocytes and macrophages—cells that cause further cellular injury. Vasodilators (prostaglandin I_2 and endorphins) predominate early, causing a drop in systemic vascular resistance. Cardiac output generally is increased to compensate for the decreased systemic vascular resistance. This phase has been described as warm shock, because the skin remains well perfused and warm. As septic shock progresses, the heart is no longer able to maintain such a high output, and vasoconstrictors (thromboxane, leukotrienes, and endothelin) predominate, with resultant decreased peripheral perfusion. Extremities become cool, urine output decreases, and oxygen delivery falls.

Shock caused by gram-positive organisms is becoming more common in the PICU. This may be due to use of broad-spectrum empiric antibiotics, the increasing use of long-term intravascular catheters and other surgically implanted foreign bodies, the changing epidemiology of gram-positive pathogens, and antibiotic resistance among gram-positive organisms. It is important to realize that the pathogenesis of gram-positive septic shock is different from that of gram-negative sepsis. Gram-positive infections most often arise from skin wounds, soft tissues, and catheter sites, rather than the GI and genitourinary sources associated with gram-negative infections. Gram-negative bacteria have an outer membrane composed of endotoxin that plays a key role in the pathogenesis of gram-negative infection, but the cell wall of gram-positive bacteria is embedded with molecules of lipoteichoic acid that are able to mimic some properties of endotoxin. Additionally, gram-positive bacteria make a range of soluble extracellular toxins, including the pyrogenic toxin superantigens of staphylococci and streptococci.

These superantigens are unusual because they do not require previous processing and specific presentation by antigen-presenting cells. These superantigens are able to bind and activate more lymphocytes than conventionally processed antigens. It is hypothesized that in gram-positive septic shock, toxins are released, resulting in a massive lymphocyte activation with a release of T-cell cytokines, which then causes cellular injury and organ failure.

The host response to gram-positive sepsis is also different from that to gram-negative sepsis. Gram-negative endotoxin induces a rapid (1–5 hours) release of proinflammatory cytokines. Gram-positive toxins induce a more delayed response (50–75 hours) dominated by TNF-α and interferon-α.

Other Organ Involvement

Organ dysfunction during and after an episode of shock is common. Systems most often affected include the kidney, the blood coagulation system, the lungs, the CNS, the liver, and the GI tract. The kidney responds to hypotension by increasing plasma renin and angiotensin concentrations, thereby decreasing glomerular filtration rate and urine output. This can progress to damage of the energy-consuming renal parenchyma, causing acute tubular necrosis. Coagulopathies may exist in any type of shock, but are especially common in septic shock. They result from the release of mediators that activate the clotting cascade, leading ultimately to a consumptive coagulopathy (ie, disseminated intravascular coagulation). The CNS dysfunction is related to decreased cerebral perfusion pressure and thus to decreased substrate delivery to the brain. Liver dysfunction commonly occurs after shock and may be manifested by increases in liver enzymes and decreased production of clotting factors leading to a bleeding diathesis. GI problems include ileus, bleeding (eg, gastritis and ulcers), and necrosis with sloughing of intestinal mucosa. Evaluation of multiorgan system dysfunction is mandatory in the work-up of shock. Multiple organ system failure secondary to shock greatly increases the mortality of the disease.

Monitoring

Both noninvasive and invasive monitoring of the patient in shock provides information on the severity, progression, and response to treatment. Extremely valuable information can be derived from examination of the cardiovascular, mucocutaneous, musculoskeletal, renal, and central nervous systems.

A. CLINICAL FINDINGS

1. Cardiovascular system—Tachycardia is not always present even when hypotension is profound. Hypotension occurs late in pediatric shock (median systolic blood pressure for a child older than age 2 years can be estimated by adding 90 mm Hg to twice the age in years). An important part of the cardiovascular examination is simultaneous palpation of distal and proximal pulses. An increase in the amplitude difference of pulses between proximal arteries (carotid, brachial, and femoral) and distal arteries (radial, posterior tibial, and dorsalis pedis) can be palpated in early shock and reflects increased systemic vascular resistance. Distal pulses may be thready or absent even in the presence of normal blood pressure because of poor stroke volume compensated by tachycardia and increased systemic vascular resistance. In uncompensated shock, hypotension is present and proximal pulses are also diminished. Early shock causes peripheral cutaneous vasoconstriction, which preserves flow to vital organs.

2. Skin—Because of peripheral vasoconstriction, the skin is gray or ashen in newborns and pale and cold in older patients. Capillary refilling after blanching is slow (> 3 seconds). Mottling of the skin may also be observed.

3. Musculoskeletal system—Decreased oxygen delivery to the musculoskeletal system produces hypotonia. Decreased spontaneous motor activity, flaccidity, and prostration are observed.

4. Urinary output—Urine output is directly proportionate to renal blood flow and the glomerular filtration rate and therefore is a good reflection of cardiac output. Catheterization of the bladder is necessary to give accurate and continuous information. (Normal urine output is > 1 mL/kg/h; outputs < 0.5 mL/kg/h are considered significantly decreased.)

5. Central nervous system—The patient's level of consciousness reflects the adequacy of cortical perfusion. When cortical perfusion is severely impaired, the infant or child fails to respond first to verbal stimuli, then to light touch, and finally to pain. Lack of motor response and failure to cry in response to venipuncture or lumbar puncture should alert the clinician to the severity of the situation. In uncompensated shock in the presence of hypotension, brainstem perfusion may be decreased. Poor thalamic perfusion can result in loss of sympathetic tone. Finally, poor medullary flow produces irregular respirations followed by gasping, apnea, and respiratory arrest.

B. INVASIVE MONITORING

Patients with poor cardiac output who are hypovolemic often need invasive monitoring for diagnostic and therapeutic reasons. Arterial catheters give constant blood pressure readings, and to an experienced interpreter, the shape of the waveform is helpful in evaluating cardiac output. CVP monitoring gives useful information about relative changes in volume status as therapy is given. CVP monitoring does not provide information about absolute volume status, as decreased right ventricular compliance will produce a higher CVP for the same volume status as a normally compliant ventricle. Intravascular volume can be assessed more accurately by monitoring pulmonary capillary wedge pressure or left atrial pressure using a pulmonary artery catheter. The pulmonary artery catheter also provides valuable information on cardiac status and vascular resistance and enables calculations of oxygen delivery and consumption (Table 13–9), but is associated with a higher complication rate than CVP lines. Most patients can be managed using alternative strategies to monitor clinical status. Measurements of arterial and mixed venous oxygen saturations and arterial and central venous pressures, along with echocardiography, are useful in assessing cardiac function and oxygen consumption. Newer technologies are under investigation to monitor cardiac output via a peripheral artery.

Treatment

Early stabilization of hemodynamics with fluid and inotropes is similar in either gram-positive or gram-negative sepsis.

Table 13–9. Hemodynamic parameters.[a]

Parameter	Formula	Normal Values	Units
Cardiac output	$CO = HR \times SV$	Wide age-dependent range	L/min
Cardiac index	$CI = CO/BSA$	3.5–5.5	L/min/m^2
Stroke index	$SI = SV/BSA$	30–60	mL/m^2
Systemic vascular resistance	$SVR = 79.9 \dfrac{(MAP - CVP)}{CI}$	800–1600	dyne s/cm^{-5}/m^2
Pulmonary vascular resistance	$PVR = 79.9 \dfrac{(MPAP - PCWP)}{CI}$	80–240	dyne s/cm^{-5}/m^2

[a]Formulas and normals from Katz RW, Pollack M, Weibley R: Pulmonary artery catheterization in pediatric intensive care. Adv Pediatr 1983;30:169.

HR, heart rate; SV, stroke volume; BSA, body surface area; MAP, mean arterial pressure; CVP, central venous pressure; MPAP, mean pulmonary artery pressure; PCWP, pulmonary capillary wedge pressure.

A. Fluid Resuscitation

Fluid infusion should start with 20-mL/kg boluses titrated to clinical monitors of cardiac output, heart rate, urine output, capillary refill, and level of consciousness. Patients who do not respond rapidly to a 30- to 60-mL/kg fluid bolus should be monitored in an intensive care setting and considered for invasive hemodynamic monitoring (placement of a CVP monitor, arterial line, and occasionally pulmonary artery catheter).

Initially, most patients tolerate crystalloid (salt solution), which is readily available and inexpensive. However, 4 hours after a crystalloid infusion, only 20% of the solution remains in the intravascular space. Patients with serious capillary leaks and ongoing plasma losses (eg, burn cases) should initially receive crystalloid, because in these cases colloid (protein and salt solution) leaks into the interstitium. The protein draws intravascular fluid into the interstitium, thus increasing ongoing losses. Patients with hypoalbuminemia or those with intact capillaries who need to retain volume in the intravascular space (eg, patients at risk for cerebral edema) probably benefit from colloid infusions. Experience with dextran (a starch compound dissolved in salt solution) is limited. Patients with normal heart function tolerate increased volume better than those with poor function. Additionally, large volumes of fluid for acute stabilization in children with shock have not been shown to increase the incidence of ARDS or cerebral edema. Increased fluid requirements may persist for several days.

B. Pharmacotherapy

Empiric antibiotics are chosen according to the most likely cause of infection. Inotropic support should be considered for patients who continue to have clinical evidence of decreased cardiac output after receiving 60 mL/kg of fluid resuscitation. Dopamine remains the first-line vasopressor although there is ongoing interest in norepinephrine as an early agent in patients with low SVR and hypotension. Dopamine causes vasoconstriction by stimulating the release of norepinephrine from sympathetic nerves. Infants younger than 6 months of age may not have fully developed sympathetic vesicles and may therefore be resistant to dopamine and more responsive to norepinephrine. As discussed earlier in the section on cardiogenic shock, dopamine can increase myocardial contractility and renal, coronary, and cerebral blood flow by its action on β-receptors and dopaminergic receptors. At higher doses (10–15 mg/kg/min), α-vasoconstrictor actions predominate. Dobutamine may be added to dopamine; however, children younger than 12 months of age may be less responsive. For septic patients with hypotension and low-output states, epinephrine is another front-line agent that can be used alone or in conjunction with dopamine (see Table 13–8). Hypocalcemia is often a contributor to cardiac dysfunction in shock. Calcium replacement should be given to normalize ionized calcium levels.

The role of inflammatory mediators in the pathogenesis of septic shock continues to be defined. Drugs that block some of these mediators appear to be beneficial when given early to animals. Human studies of these same blockers have failed to demonstrate a clear benefit. The differences in pathogenesis and host response to gram-positive or gram-negative sepsis may explain some of the differential responsiveness to anti-inflammatory agents seen in past clinical trials. Additionally, the discrepancies may result from low-affinity binding by these antibodies. The molecular mechanisms by which lipopolysaccharide activates cells are becoming better understood, which may assist in the development of more effective therapies. Modulation of T cells (with glucocorticoids, cyclosporine, and antibodies directed at cytokines) in models of superantigen-induced injury have proven beneficial, but remain experimental. Ibuprofen, because of its ability to block cyclooxygenase (cyclooxygenase metabolites are potent modulators of cell function), was also extensively studied in patients with septic shock, although the evidence does not support the use of ibuprofen for septic shock. Excess production of nitric oxide by the inducible isoform of nitric oxide synthase in inflammatory cells contributes to the hypotension and poor perfusion occurring in shock. Analogs of N-methyl-L-arginine (L-NMA), however, while useful in animal models of septic shock, worsened outcome in studies of adults with severe septic shock, presumably due to broad deleterious effects of total blockade of nitric oxide production.

Protein C is a primary regulator of coagulation, fibrinolysis, and coagulation-induced inflammation. Deficits in protein C activation correlate with morbidity and mortality in septic shock. Deficiencies of protein C have been found in children and adults with sepsis. Recombinant activated protein C reduced mortality rates in an animal model of sepsis. A large randomized, double-blind, placebo-controlled trial of recombinant activated protein C in adults with severe sepsis showed a significant reduction in mortality rates in treated patients. A similarly designed clinical trial of activated protein C in pediatric patients with severe sepsis was halted due to concern over hemorrhagic complications without an observed clear benefit.

Corticosteroids, by virtue of their action on many mediators, are thought to play a role in shock, and based on positive results in animal models of septic shock, have been advocated for treatment of shock in humans. Children with meningococcal meningitis and patients with the acquired immunodeficiency syndrome who have *Pneumocystis carinii* pneumonia have shown improvement in oxygenation and a trend toward improved survival when treated with corticosteroids. The use of hydrocortisone in adults with relative adrenal insufficiency and septic shock was shown to improve short-term outcome. Importantly, a low aldosterone state may be more common in children with septic shock than previously thought. Hydrocortisone (50 mg/kg) should be considered for children at risk for adrenal insufficiency—those with purpura fulminans or pituitary or adrenal abnormalities, those receiving steroids for chronic illness, and those with septic shock and multi-organ system dysfunction not responding well to traditional inotropic therapy. The studies do not currently support a definitive need for an adrenal stimulation test prior to initiating corticosteroid therapy due to the difficulty in interpreting the results.

Vasopressin is currently under investigation as an additional agent to treat refractory septic shock. Early studies indicate that it can improve organ perfusion and decrease the doses of epinephrine required to maintain organ perfusion.

ECMO has been considered in the treatment of shock in patients with recoverable cardiac and pulmonary function who require both pulmonary and cardiac support.

Annane D, Bellissant E, Cavaillon JM: Septic shock. Lancet 2005; 365:63.

Beale RJ et al: Vasopressor and inotropic support in septic shock: an evidence-based review. Crit Care Med 2004;32:S455.

Bochud PY et al: Antimicrobial therapy for patients with severe sepsis and septic shock: an evidence-based review. Crit Care Med 2004;32:S495.

Carcillo JA: Pediatric septic shock and multiple organ failure. Crit Care Clin 2003;19:413 [PMID: 1284813].

Goldestein B, Giroir B, Randolph A: International pediatric sepsis consensus conference: definitions for sepsis and organ dysfunction in pediatrics. Pediatr Crit Care Med 2005;6:2.

Holmes CL, Walley KR: Vasopressin in the ICU. Curr Opin Crit Care 2004;10:442.

Keh D, Sprung CL: Use of corticosteroid therapy in patients with sepsis and septic shock: an evidence-based review. Crit Care Med 2004;32:S527.

McCarthy RE III et al: Long term outcome of fulminant myocarditis as compared with acute (nonfulminant) myocarditis. N Engl J Med 2000;342:690 [PMID: 10706898].

Proft T, Fraser JD: Bacterial superantigens. Clin Exp Immunol 2003;133:299 [PMID: 12930353].

Rhodes A, Bennett ED: Early goal-directed therapy: an evidence-based review. Crit Care Med 2004;32:S448.

Vincent JL et al and the Recombinant Human Activated Protein C Worldwide Evaluation in Severe Sepsis (PROWESS) Study Group: Effects of drotrecogin alfa (activated) on organ dysfunction in the PROWESS trial. Crit Care Med 2003;31:834 [PMID: 12626993].

Vincent JL, Gerlach H: Fluid resuscitation in severe sepsis and septic shock: an evidence-based review. Crit Care Med 2004;32:S451.

INDICATIONS FOR CENTRAL VENOUS & ARTERIAL CANNULATION

Placement of catheters into the central venous or arterial circulation may be justified for continuous assessment of intravascular volume or cardiac function; blood drawing for lab work; or administration of volume, drugs, or hyperalimentation. One should always weigh the risks of bleeding, infection, and clotting against the expected benefits before placing any indwelling catheter.

General Rules for Equipment Selection & Technique

1. Set up and examine all equipment needed before getting started. Use of a limited number of kits and equipment will provide greater consistency and success.

2. Apply EMLA cream (eutectic mixture of local anesthetics, lidocaine 2.5% and prilocaine 2.5%) to the area of puncture (45 minutes before the procedure) or infiltrate with local anesthetic before prepping the skin.

3. The remainder of the procedure should occur under aseptic technique (including gown, mask, and hair cover for operator and assistant).

4. Sterilize and drape the area around the point of entry.

5. When searching for the vessel, make straight passes while maintaining slight negative pressure. Advance and withdraw the needle at the same speed. Frequently, the blood return will occur during withdrawal.

6. Once there is free flow of venous blood into the syringe, remove the syringe without moving the needle, and if using the Seldinger technique, pass the J wire through the needle. When appropriate, watch the electrocardiogram for arrhythmias, because they frequently occur when the J wire touches the right side of the heart.

7. Withdraw the needle over the J wire and clean the wire of blood.

8. Make a nick with a no. 11 blade at the point where the J wire enters the skin. Pass the introducer or the intravascular catheter (or both) over the J wire.

9. With the catheters in place, remove the wire along with the introducer.

10. Check to make sure that blood can be drawn easily through the new line.

11. Verify the position of the line on radiograph.

Points of Entry for Venous Line Placement

A. EXTERNAL JUGULAR VEIN

Place a soft cloth roll beneath the patient's shoulder and turn the head to the contralateral side (Figure 13–2). The Valsalva maneuver, Trendelenburg position, and occlusion of the vessel at the clavicular level are ways of temporarily increasing jugular distention and visibility.

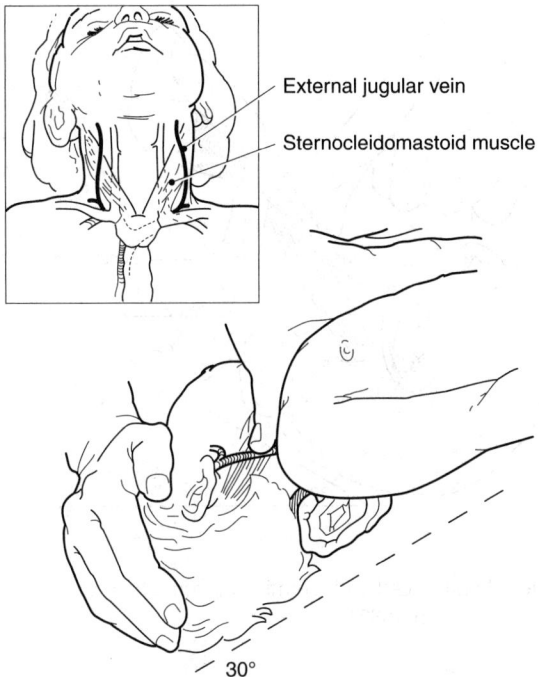

Figure 13–2. External jugular vein technique. (Reproduced, with permission, from Chameides L: *Textbook of Pediatric Advanced Life Support.* American Heart Association, 1988.)

To overcome the problems of this vessel's mobility and thick wall, apply cephalic retraction of the skin over the vessel superior to the point of needle entry. Maintain gentle negative pressure in the syringe attached to the needle as it is advanced toward the vessel. Needle entry into the vessel lumen is usually signaled by a change in resistance followed by appearance of venous blood in the hub of the needle. Remove the syringe without moving the needle and pass a soft J wire to the vessel lumen. Remove the needle and pass the central line over the J wire.

B. INTERNAL JUGULAR VEIN

Once the patient has been prepped, draped, and positioned as shown in Figure 13–3, feel for the trachea halfway between the angle of the jaw and the suprasternal notch and then feel lateral to the trachea for the carotid pulse. Just lateral to the carotid pulse, at a 30-degree angle from horizontal, insert a finder needle (25-gauge), aiming between the ipsilateral nipple and shoulder. Once venous return is established, remove the finder needle and repeat the procedure with the appropriate-size larger needle.

C. SUBCLAVIAN VEIN

After the patient has been prepped, draped, and positioned (Figure 13–4), move the needle flat along the chest, entering along the inferior edge of the clavicle just lateral to the midclavicular line and aiming for the

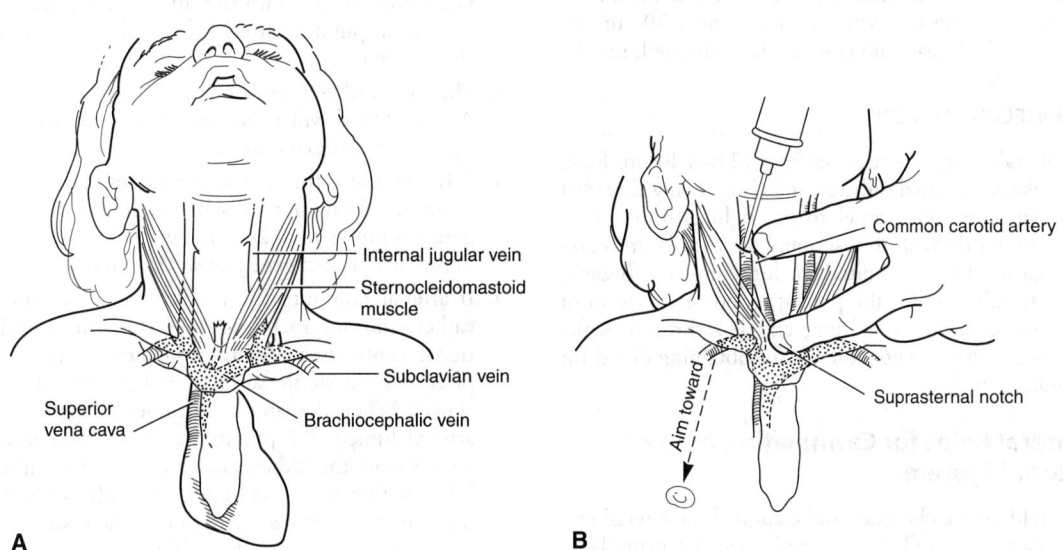

A   **B**

Figure 13–3. **A:** The internal jugular vein and its relationship to the surrounding anatomy. **B:** Technique of anterior internal jugular cannulation. (Reproduced, with permission, from Chameides L: *Textbook of Pediatric Advanced Life Support.* American Heart Association, 1988.)

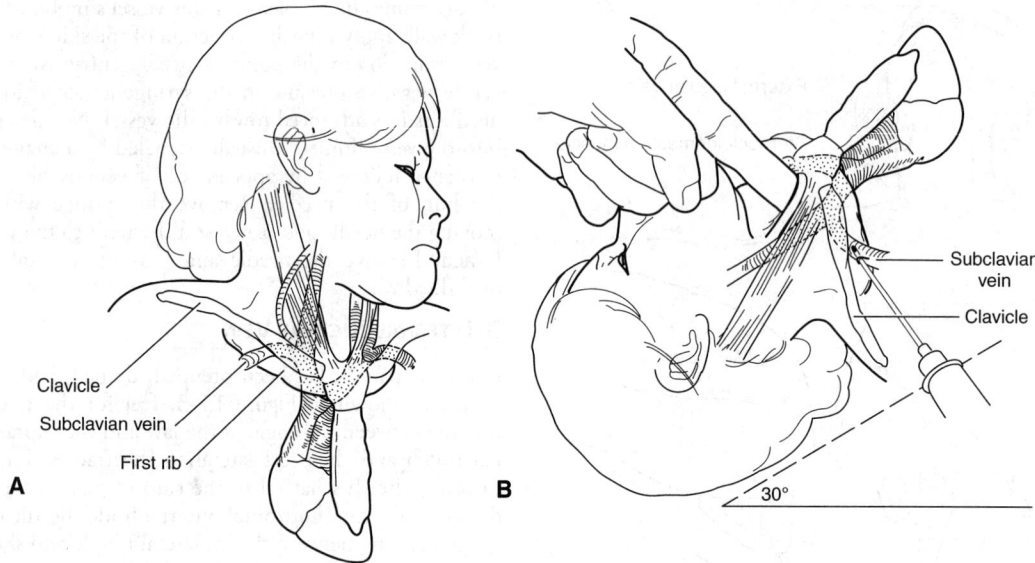

Figure 13–4. Subclavian artery. **A:** Anatomy. **B:** Technique. (Reproduced, with permission, from Chameides L: *Textbook of Pediatric Advanced Life Support.* American Heart Association, 1988.)

suprasternal notch. Once venous return is established, use the Seldinger technique.

D. FEMORAL VEIN

With the patient's leg slightly abducted (Figure 13–5), find the femoral artery 3–4 cm below the inguinal ligament. The femoral vein is just medial and parallel to the femoral artery. Insert the needle at a 30- to 45-degree angle. Once venous return is established, use the Seldinger technique.

E. ANTECUBITAL VEIN

Peripherally inserted catheter lines (2.8–4 F) are long, soft, Silastic, styletted catheters most commonly threaded from an antecubital vessel to the right atrium. These lines are not difficult to insert and are easy to dress and keep clean. They are suited for long-term use because they are tolerable for the patient, good for infusion of hyperalimentation and drugs, and less thrombogenic. In general, they are not suitable for obtaining blood for laboratory analysis.

General Rules for Cannulation of the Arterial System

The Seldinger technique can be applied for arterial tree cannulation as well. Most arteries can be cannulated percutaneously.

1. Puncture the skin at the insertion site to eliminate any drag or resistance on the catheter advancement.

2. Insert the cannula at a 30-degree angle to the skin surface, advancing at a slow rate toward the arterial pulse. Watch the hub of the cannula for a flash of arterial blood.

3. When arterial flash is seen, lower the catheter to a 10-degree angle with the surface of the skin and advance the catheter into the lumen of the artery. If successful, pulsatile arterial flow will continue into the catheter.

4. Hold the catheter while removing the needle stylet. Arterial blood will pulse out of the catheter if the tip is in the arterial lumen.

5. Advance the catheter into the lumen; attach a syringe containing normal saline with 1 U/mL of heparin; aspirate to make certain that there are no bubbles; and then gently flush the catheter.

6. If arterial flow into the needle stylet stops during catheter advancement, advance this unit an additional centimeter. Remove the needle stylet and place it on a sterile surface. Pull the catheter out slowly. When the tip of the catheter flips into the arterial lumen, the pulsatile arterial blood flow is seen. Rotate the catheter to ensure that the catheter is free within the vessel lumen, then advance the remainder of the catheter length into the vessel.

7. Suture the catheter in place while ensuring that the arterial trace is not damped.

8. Dress the insertion site with sterile gauze, and tape it to the skin.

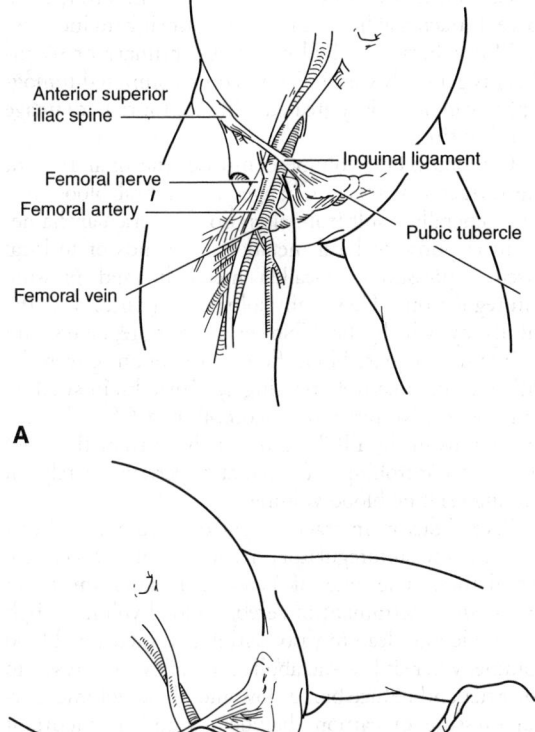

A

B

Figure 13–5. Femoral vein. **A:** Anatomy. **B:** Technique. (Reproduced, with permission, from Chameides L: *Textbook of Pediatric Advanced Life Support.* American Heart Association, 1988.)

Points of Entry for Arterial Line Placement

Always consider whether collateral arterial blood is flowing to the structures distal to the insertion point. The Allen test must be done prior to radial or ulnar artery cannulation.

Arterial sites, listed in order of preference, include:

1. Radial artery (nondominant arm first)
2. Femoral artery (morbidity is the same as for the radial artery beyond the newborn period)
3. Posterior tibial artery
4. Dorsalis pedis artery
5. Ulnar artery (if distal radial filling is present in that hand)
6. Axillary artery
7. Brachial artery (poor collateral flow, used only during cardiac surgery in newborn-sized patients with arterial access limitations)

Final Considerations

1. Patient benefit should outweigh any risks from central venous or arterial cannulation.
2. Coagulation status of the patient at the time of placement and throughout the time of use must be considered, because deep venous and arterial thrombus formation is partially related to the patient's coagulation status.
3. The incidence of catheter colonization and infection increases if central venous and arterial lines are left in for more than 6 days.

Stovroff M, Teague WG: Intravenous access in infants and children. Pediatr Clin North Am 1998;45:1373 [PMID: 9889758].

Odetola FO et al: Nosocomial catheter-related bloodstream infections in a pediatric intensive care unit: risk and rates associated with various intravascular technologies. Pediatr Crit Care Med 2003;4:432 [PMID: 14525637].

O'Grady NP et al: Guidelines for the prevention of intravascular catheter-related infections. The Hospital Infection Control Practices Advisory Committee, Center for Disease Control and Prevention, U.S. Pediatrics. 2002;110:e51 [PMID: 12415057].

BRAIN INJURY/CEREBRAL EDEMA

Intracranial hypertension is a common feature of many illnesses treated in the PICU (Table 13–10). The early signs and symptoms of intracranial hypertension (Table 13–11) tend to be nonspecific. The classic Cushing triad of bradycardia, hypertension, and apnea occurs late and is often incomplete in children.

Accurate assessment and treatment of elevations in ICP requires an understanding of the basic pathophysiology of intracranial hypertension, as well as the current evidence supporting the various treatment options. Most of our current understanding and approach to treatment is based on studies of patients with traumatic brain injuries. Whether those concepts are directly relevant to the pathophysiologic processes involved in more global CNS injuries, such as hypoxia and metabolic disorders, remains a matter of debate.

Within the constraints of a closed skull, an enlargement of brain tissue, an increased volume of cerebrospinal fluid (CSF), or an increased volume of blood (or the presence of a space-occupying lesion such as a tumor or an abscess) will reduce the size of the other compart-

Table 13–10. Pediatric illnesses commonly associated with intracranial hypertension.

Diffuse processes
Trauma
Hypoxic-ischemic
Near-drowning
Cardiorespiratory arrest
Infectious
Encephalitis
Meningitis
Metabolic
Reye syndrome
Liver failure
Inborn error metabolism
Toxic
Lead
Vitamin A
Focal processes
Trauma
Hypoxic-ischemic
Trauma
Stroke
Infectious
Abscess
Mass lesions
Tumors
Hematomas

ments or increase pressure. The factors contributing to intracranial hypertension can be understood by considering each of these three primary compartments.

The brain occupies about 80% of the volume of the skull. Apart from solid tumors, increases in the brain compartment are generally a result of cerebral edema. Cerebral edema can be divided into three forms: vasogenic, hydrostatic, and cytotoxic. **Vasogenic** edema occurs in areas of inflamed tissue characterized by increased capillary permeability, and is most typical around CNS tumors, abscesses, and infarcts. This form of edema is thought to be at least partially responsive to corticosteroid therapy. **Hydrostatic,** or interstitial, edema is a result of elevated CSF hydrostatic pressures. It occurs primarily in lesions associated with obstruction to CSF flow, and in a typical periventricular distribution. This form of edema is best treated by CSF drainage. The third form of cerebral edema, **cytotoxic** edema, is the most common of the three forms seen in the PICU and is, unfortunately, the least easily treated. Cytotoxic edema occurs as a result of direct injury to brain cells, often leading to irreversible cell swelling and death. This form of cerebral edema is typical of traumatic brain injuries as well as hypoxic-ischemic injuries and metabolic disease.

CSF occupies an estimated 10% of the intracranial space. Intracranial hypertension due primarily to increases in CSF volume (eg, hydrocephalus, primary or secondary) is generally easily diagnosed by computed tomography scan and easily treated with appropriate drainage and shunting.

Cerebral blood volume comprises the final 10% of the intracranial space. Changes in cerebral blood volume generally result from alterations in vascular diameter in response to local metabolic demands or to local vascular pressures—so-called metabolic and pressure autoregulation. These physiologic responses are the means by which the CNS circulation regulates and maintains adequate blood flow to the brain. Given the difficulty in effectively treating cytotoxic brain swelling and the relative rarity of uncomplicated CSF obstructive lesions in the PICU, most of the current therapies aimed at controlling intracranial hypertension rely on altering cerebral blood volume.

Several factors interact to control cerebral blood volume via the autoregulatory responses of the cerebral vasculature. The rate of cerebral metabolism is an important determinant of cerebral blood volume. High metabolic rates lead to vasodilation and increased blood volume, whereas low metabolic rates allow the vessels to constrict and reduce blood flow and blood volume. Partial pressure of carbon dioxide is another important determinant of cerebral blood volume, as elevations in blood pCO_2 lead to cerebral vasodilation and decreases in pCO_2 lead to vasoconstriction. Finally, cerebral blood volume is linked to cerebral blood flow through the phenomenon of pressure autoregulation. As shown in Figure 13–6, at low systolic blood pressures, the cerebral vessels are maximally dilated and blood flow is only increased by increasing blood pressure. Within the range of autoregulation, the cerebral vessels attempt to

Table 13–11. Signs and symptoms of intracranial hypertension in children.

Early
Poor feeding, vomiting
Irritability, lethargy
Seizures
Hypertension
Late
Coma
Decerebrate responses
Cranial nerve palsies
Abnormal respirations
Bradycardia
Hypertension
Apnea

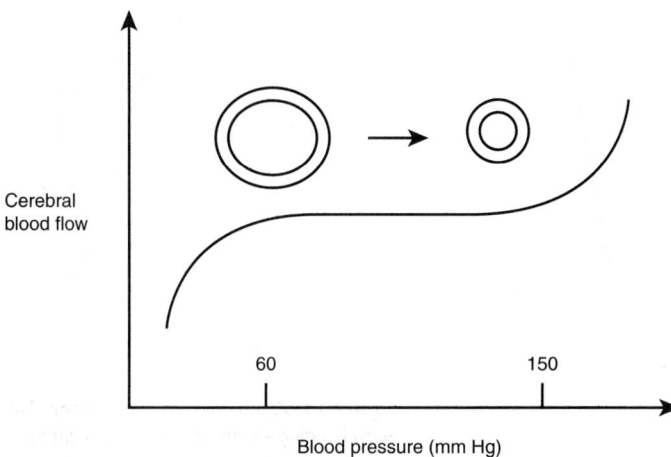

Figure 13–6. Pressure autoregulation in the cerebral vasculature.

maintain a constant flow rate over a range of blood pressures; increased blood pressure results in vasoconstriction, in turn reducing cerebral blood volume. Once the cerebral vessels are maximally constricted, continued increases in pressure may further increase cerebral blood flow and volume.

Treatments for intracranial hypertension are largely derived from experience with traumatic brain injury. An important concept in this regard is that of a "primary" as opposed to a "secondary" brain injury. In this context, primary injury refers to direct damage to brain tissue resulting from the original insult to the CNS, such as physical damage from trauma. This injury is complete before the patient reaches the health care system. As the injured brain swells due to cytotoxic edema, intracranial hypertension develops, potentially limiting cerebral blood flow to portions of the brain and leading to extension of the initial injury (ie, secondary injury). Medical treatment of the patient with intracranial hypertension aims to prevent or reduce secondary injuries.

The primary goal of treatment is to optimize perfusion of areas of the brain that are salvageable. This can be accomplished by reducing ICP and by ensuring adequate perfusion. Rational guidance of treatment requires invasive monitoring so that it can be effectively titrated. Although a complete discussion of the indications for ICP monitoring is beyond the scope of this chapter, the topic can be briefly summarized with the suggestion that an ICP monitor be used for patients at significant risk for intracranial hypertension, in whom the treatment of elevated CNS pressures is planned. Monitoring other parameters of CNS oxygen delivery (ie, blood pressure, ABGs, and intravascular volume) generally mandates the placement of arterial and central venous catheters. Little evidence exists to support the utility of ICP-directed therapies in conditions associated with global CNS injuries (eg, anoxic brain injuries).

Maintenance of adequate cardiac output and oxygen delivery to the CNS is critical in treating patients with intracranial hypertension. Studies in both adult and pediatric head injury patients show that even a single episode of hypotension or arterial hypoxemia is associated with a marked increase in mortality rates. Although studies have not delineated clear age-appropriate thresholds for blood pressure and arterial pO_2 in this setting, a rational starting point for therapy would seem to be maintenance of an adequate circulating blood volume, a blood pressure at least well within the normal range for age, and an arterial pO_2 of at least 60 mm Hg. Hypotension and hypoxemia should be treated urgently and aggressively.

In general, the threshold at which treatment for intracranial hypertension should be started is in the range of 15–20 cm H_2O pressure. Above this pressure, the compliance of the skull worsens dramatically (Figure 13–7), and very minor increases in intracranial contents lead to large increases in ICP. Initial therapy for intracranial hypertension should always consist of securing the airway and providing adequate sedation. Additional measures would include the removal of any mass lesions (eg, tumors, abscesses, and hematomas) and adequate ventricular drainage. Further efforts are then largely directed at reducing cerebral blood volume.

Osmotic diuretics such as mannitol are often used to treat intracranial hypertension. They are thought to act first by decreasing blood viscosity, allowing for increased flow and subsequent autoregulatory vasoconstriction. The osmotic effects on the cells and interstitium of the brain prolong the reduction in ICP. Although mannitol has never been subjected to a placebo-controlled trial, it has been shown to lead to better outcomes than barbiturate therapy in patients with refractory ICP elevations. Current guidelines suggest the use of mannitol in doses of 0.25–0.5 g/kg for intracranial hypertension

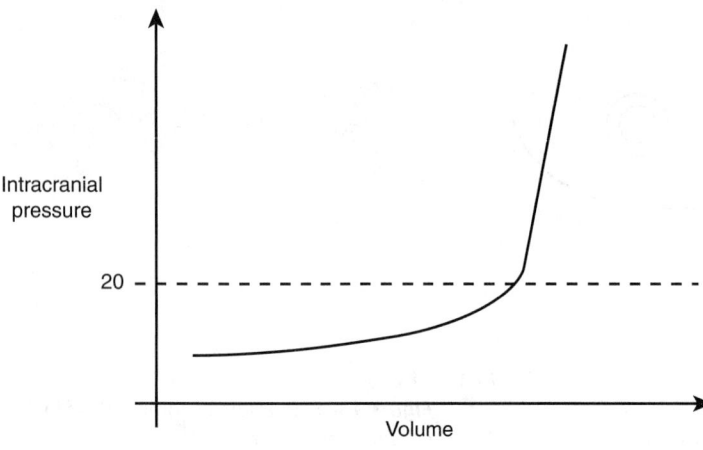

Figure 13–7. Compliance curve of the skull with changing volume of intracranial contents.

unresponsive to sedation. Renal failure due to acute tubular necrosis can be a treatment-limiting side effect, particularly if serum osmolarity is allowed to rise above 320 mmol and intravascular volume depletion occurs.

Hyperventilation—long a mainstay in the treatment of intracranial hypertension—is controversial. Although acutely effective in causing cerebral vasoconstriction, hyperventilation leads to much larger decreases in blood flow than in blood volume, such that hyperventilation to the point necessary to control ICP may actually compromise CNS perfusion and lead to worsened secondary injury. This concept has been confirmed by studies showing worse outcomes in head-injured patients consistently hyperventilated to a pCO_2 of 25 mm Hg or less. Current guidelines suggest that moderate hyperventilation (pCO_2 of 30–35 mm Hg) may be used for mild to moderate intracranial hypertension, but that extreme hyperventilation ($pCO_2 < 30$ mm Hg) should be reserved for patients with ICP elevations unresponsive to other measures, including sedation, paralysis, ventricular drainage, and osmotic diuretics. Due to the risks of worsened CNS ischemia, monitoring cerebral perfusion by blood flow studies or jugular bulb saturation is recommended for patients undergoing extreme hyperventilation.

The use of barbiturates in this setting is based on their suppression of cerebral metabolism and the subsequent metabolic autoregulation effects on cerebral blood volume. Although effective in many instances for ICP elevations, these agents are potent cardiac depressants, and their use often leads to hypotension, necessitating the use of a pressor to maintain perfusion. In addition, plasma barbiturate levels correlate poorly with effect on ICP, suggesting that monitoring of CNS electrical activity by electroencephalography is necessary to accurately titrate the use of these agents. Current guidelines suggest the use of barbiturates for treating intra-

cranial hypertension refractory to sedation, paralysis, ventricular drainage, and osmotic diuretics.

Another important concept in the management of intracranial hypertension is that of the cerebral perfusion pressure. The cerebral perfusion pressure is the driving pressure across the cerebral circulation and is defined as mean arterial pressure – CVP (or ICP, whichever is higher). Some authors have suggested that careful attention to maintenance of a supranormal cerebral perfusion pressure may lead to better outcomes for head-injured patients. Although there are no well-controlled trials to draw from (particularly for pediatric patients), current guidelines suggest that maintenance of a "normal" cerebral perfusion pressure for age (50–70 mm Hg) is a valid secondary goal of treatment, as long as it is included in a plan to use the other ICP-directed therapies discussed earlier.

A suggested treatment algorithm for patients with documented intracranial hypertension is presented in Figure 13–8. As mentioned earlier, this algorithm represents the current best evidence for the management of intracranial hypertension. The information is largely drawn from experience with traumatic brain injuries, and the direct applicability of these concepts to other illnesses associated with intracranial hypertension remains unclear.

Bayir H et al: Traumatic brain injury in infants and children: Mechanisms of secondary damage and treatment in the intensive care unit. Crit Care Clin 2003;19:529 [PMID: 12848319].

Carney NA et al: Guidelines for the acute medical management of severe traumatic brain injury in infants, children, and adolescents. Pediatr Crit Care Med 2003;4:S1 [PMID: 12847355].

Heimann A et al: Effects of hypertonic/hyperoncotic treatment after rat cortical vein occlusion. Crit Care Med 2003;31:2495 [PMID: 14530757].

Khoshyomn S, Tranmer BI: Diagnosis and management of pediatric closed head injury. Semin Pediatr Surg 2004;13:2004 [PMID: 153662277].

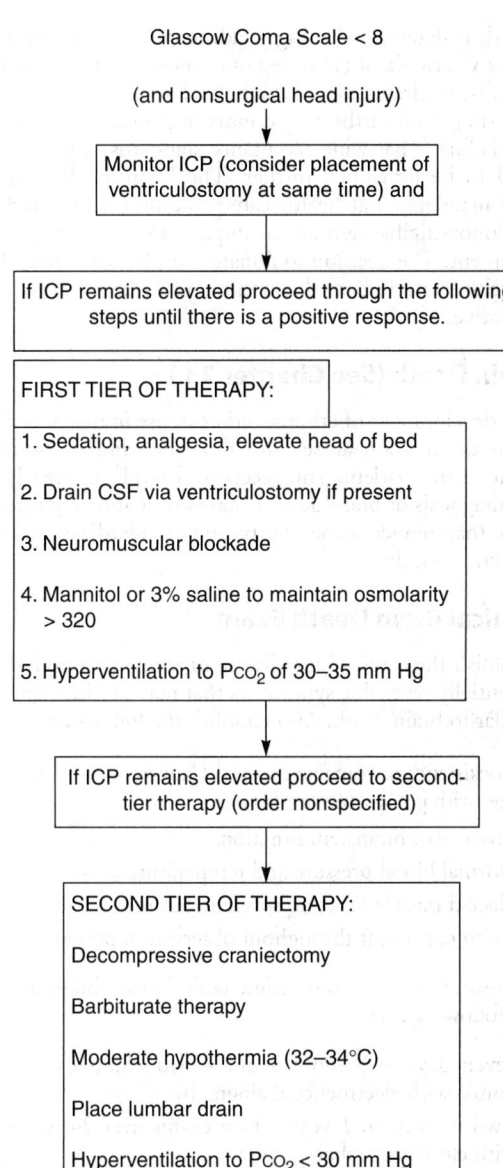

Glasgow Coma Scale < 8

(and nonsurgical head injury)

Monitor ICP (consider placement of ventriculostomy at same time) and

If ICP remains elevated proceed through the following steps until there is a positive response.

FIRST TIER OF THERAPY:

1. Sedation, analgesia, elevate head of bed

2. Drain CSF via ventriculostomy if present

3. Neuromuscular blockade

4. Mannitol or 3% saline to maintain osmolarity > 320

5. Hyperventilation to P_{CO_2} of 30–35 mm Hg

If ICP remains elevated proceed to second-tier therapy (order nonspecified)

SECOND TIER OF THERAPY:

Decompressive craniectomy

Barbiturate therapy

Moderate hypothermia (32–34°C)

Place lumbar drain

Hyperventilation to P_{CO_2} < 30 mm Hg

Figure 13–8. Proposed treatment algorithm for intracranial hypertension in head injury. CSF, cerebrospinal fluid; ICP, intracranial pressure; P_{CO_2}, partial pressure of arterial CO_2.

Littlejohns LR et al: Brain tissue oxygen monitoring in severe brain injury: I. Research and usefulness in critical care. Crit Care Nurse 2003;23:17 [PMID: 12961780].

McArthur DL, Chute DJ, Villablanca JP: Moderate and severe traumatic brain injury: epidemiologic, imaging and neuro-pathologic perspectives. Brain Pathol 2004;14:185 [PMID: 15193031].

McIntyre LA et al: Prolonged therapeutic hypothermia after traumatic brain injury in adults: A systematic review. JAMA 2003;289:2992 [PMID: 12799408].

Noppens R, Brambrink AM: Traumatic brain injury in children—clinical implications. Exp Toxicol Pathol 2004;56:113 [PMID: 15581282].

Okonkwo DO, Stone JR: Basic science of closed head injuries and spinal cord injuries. Clin Sports Med 2003;22:467 [PMID: 12852680].

Phillis JW, O'Regan MH: The role of phospholipases, cyclooxygenases, and lipoxygenases in cerebral ischemic/traumatic injuries. Crit Rev Neurobiol 2003;15:61 [PMID: 14513863].

ETHICAL DELIBERATION & END-OF-LIFE CARE IN THE PICU

Bioethics Consultation in the PICU

Advances in critical care medicine give PICU practitioners the ability to prolong life without being able to ensure a reasonable quality of life. Health care professionals in this setting are often called on to help patients and families wrestle with questions of medical futility. As conflict surrounding care and decision making has arisen, the introduction of ethics consultation in the ICU setting has served to improve the process by helping to identify, analyze, and resolve ethical problems. Ethics consultation can independently clarify views and allow the health care team, patient, and family to make decisions that respect patient autonomy and promote maximum benefit and minimal harm to the patient.

Managed Withdrawal of Treatment

With increasing frequency, PICU deaths are predictable and result from the withholding or withdrawing of life-sustaining medical therapy (LSMT). Discussions with patients and families regarding the decision to limit resuscitation or to withdraw LSMT should respect the following basic principles:

- Deliberations begin with a clear statement that the patient's good is the goal.
- With the assistance of the health care team, the patient and family can make reasonable decisions about limitation or withdrawal of LSMT based on goals of care for the patient.
- The burden of continued life (pain and suffering) should outweigh any potential benefit from continued therapy.
- Discussions with the patient and family are conducted by experienced personnel with the ability to communicate in a clear and compassionate manner at an appropriate time and place.
- It should be emphasized that decisions are not irrevocable; if at any time the family or health care provid-

ers wish to reconsider the decision, full medical therapy should be reinstituted until the situation is clarified.

Palliative Care

Helping a patient experience a dignified and pain-free death is one of the many unique challenges facing caregivers in the PICU. Pediatric death is characterized by its relative infrequency, by the prognostic uncertainties of many pediatric illnesses, and by the fine line between congenital disorder and incurable disease. When a predictable early death is likely, intensivists are often called on to care for the patient and family during the final days and hours of the patient's life.

In the past several years, palliative medicine has developed as a specialized field of practice to address the needs of dying children. The practice of providing supportive care at end of life in pediatrics is fundamentally different from that in adult medicine. In-hospital deaths in pediatrics encompass a more heterogeneous patient population with developmental issues and family dynamics that complicate the process.

Once the inclusive decision is made to limit or withdraw LSMT, a palliative care plan should be agreed on and instituted. The plan should address the following basic principles:

- Adequate pain control and sedation
- Provision of warmth and cleanliness
- Nutrition
- Ongoing patient and family support

The decision to withhold or withdraw LSMT from a pediatric patient does not suggest a plan to hasten the death. The goal of palliative care remains optimization of the patient's and family's experience prior to and following the death.

Tissue & Organ Donation

Organ transplantation has become standard therapy. Although the demand for tissue and solid organs has increased, donations have remained largely unchanged. The prospect of organ or tissue donation should be considered with all patients dying in the PICU. To be a solid organ donor, the patient must be clinically brain dead and have no conditions contraindicating donation. With patients from whom life-support must be withdrawn, tissue (heart valves, corneas, skin, and bone) can be obtained after cardiac death. The need for new donor organs has led to the re-emergence of procuring organs from nonheartbeating (asystolic) donors. In these cases the family or patient has refused life-sustaining therapy and has chosen to have life-support withdrawn, and donate their organs after death.

Death is determined using "traditional" or "cardiopulmonary" criteria of (1) unresponsiveness, (2) apnea, and (3) absent circulation. A high level of scrutiny exists regarding nonheartbeating donors in pediatric patients, and before it has wide acceptance standards of practice need to be developed further. The Required Request Law mandates that health care professionals approach all donor-eligible families to inquire about organ procurement. The decision to donate must be made free of coercion, with informed consent, and without financial incentive.

Brain Death (See Chapter 23.)

The development of criteria and expertise in the clinical brain death exam arose out of the demand for solid organs from patients still receiving LSMT. Currently, the diagnosis of brain death is based on national guidelines that render some clarity and standardization to this critical task.

Clinical Brain Death Exam

Establish the cause of the disease or injury and exclude potentially reversible syndromes that may produce signs similar to brain death. Also establish the following:

- Coexistence of coma and apnea[1] ("apnea test" ~ 3 minutes with $pCO_2 > 60$ mm Hg)
- Absence of brainstem function
- Normal blood pressure and temperature
- Flaccid muscle tone, no spontaneous movements
- Exam consistent throughout observation period

Recommended observation periods for children of the following ages:

- Seven days to 2 months old—Two exams over 48 hours; with electroencephalography
- Two months to 1 year—Two exams over 24 hours; with electroencephalography
- Over 1 year—Two exams over 12–24 hours

A position paper by the Ethics Committee, American College of Critical Care Medicine, Society of Critical Care Medicine: Recommendations for nonheartbeating organ donation. Crit Care Med 2001;29:1826.

Deray M: Brain death and persistent vegetative state. International Pediatr 2005;20:113.

Goh AY-T, Mok Q: Clinical course and determination of brainstem death in a children's hospital. Acta Paediatr 2004;93:47.

---

[1]Cerebral angiography, radionuclide scanning, or transcranial Doppler ultrasonography can be used to assess brain function if apnea testing cannot be performed or if there is need for corroborative studies.

Kopelman LM: Are the 21-year-old Baby Doe rules misunderstood or mistaken? Pediatrics 2005;116:797.

Solomon MZ, Sellers DE, Heller KS, et al: New and lingering controversies in pediatric end-of-life care. Pediatrics 2005;116:872.

Troug RD, Cist AFM, Brackett SE, et al: Recommendations for end-of-life care in the intensive care unit: the Ethics Committee of the Society of Critical Care Medicine. Crit Care Med 2001;29:2332.

NUTRITIONAL SUPPORT OF THE CRITICALLY ILL CHILD

Metabolic & Physiologic Responses

When severely ill pediatric patients are admitted to the intensive care unit, the initial therapy is directed at the primary or underlying problem and at providing cardiorespiratory and hemodynamic support. Although this management is critical to sustaining life in these patients, provision of adequate nutritional support is often overlooked early in the course of therapy. As increasing evidence demonstrates that nutritional status and support affect the morbidity and mortality of critically ill patients, it is vital that this aspect of care be addressed early in the hospital course.

Trauma, surgery, burns, and sepsis impose metabolic and physiologic disturbances that vary in degree, but have many similarities. The insult triggers the afferent limb of the neurophysiologic reflex, which is composed of pain and neurosensory pathways. In response, the efferent limb consisting of neurologic and endocrine pathways, increases autonomic sympathetic activity with norepinephrine and epinephrine secretions and increases pituitary release of a host of hormones including adrenocorticotropic hormone, growth hormone, and antidiuretic hormone. Release of catecholamines inhibits insulin secretion and activity, and stimulates glucagon and adrenocorticotropic hormone production. Adrenocorticotropic hormone and antidiuretic hormone increase corticosteroid release, inhibit insulin activity, and increase aldosterone. The overall effect is to direct an end-organ increase in metabolic rate and to provide increased substrate availability for energy use (Table 13–12). In addition, the body has a cellular response to tissue injury. Cells migrate to the damaged area to facilitate wound healing and aid in infection control with the release of inflammatory mediators. These cells are mainly dependent on glucose for their energy source, which is an important reason the hypermetabolic state is necessary. These events initiate a hypermetabolic response that influences the mobilization and use of nutrients as substrates. Although all substrates undergo increased use, the fraction of calories derived from glucose is reduced, and the fraction derived from protein and lipid breakdown is increased.

Hyperglycemia and glucose intolerance are characteristic traits of the hypermetabolic state. Although glucose use is increased, serum glucose levels are elevated, reflecting neuroendocrine stimulation of glycogenolysis and gluco-

Table 13–12. Metabolic and physiologic responses to severe illness.

Physiologic
Cardiovascular
 Increased cardiac output
 Peripheral vasodilatation and capillary leak
 Expansion of vascular compartment
Pulmonary
 Increased minute ventilation
 Ventilation/perfusion mismatch
 Inefficient gas exchange
 Increased carbon dioxide responsiveness
Skeletal muscle
 Easier fatigability
 Slower relaxation
 Altered force-frequency pattern
Renal
 Salt and water retention
 Impaired concentrating ability

Metabolic
Hormone and hormone-like levels
 Increased insulin
 Increased glucocorticoids
 Increased catecholamines
 Increased interleukin-1
 Increased tumor necrosis factor
Carbohydrate metabolism
 Increased blood glucose
 Increased gluconeogenesis
 Increased glucose turnover
 Glucose intolerance
Fat metabolism
 Increased lipid turnover and utilization
 Insuppressible lipolysis
 Decreased ketogenesis
Protein metabolism
 Increased muscle protein catabolism
 Increased muscle branched-chain amino acid oxidation
 Increased serum amino acids
 Increased mitogen losses

neogenesis. Gluconeogenesis occurs primarily from lactate, alanine, glutamine, and other amino acids derived from muscle breakdown and from glycerol derived from lipolysis. The hepatic production of glucose is increased, and fails to respond to increased plasma concentrations of glucose or insulin when these substances are infused intravenously. Hyperglycemia and secondary hyperinsulinemia also inhibit ketosis despite the increased rate of lipolysis. The hyperglycemia does, however, maintain glucose supply to the brain. An elevated glucagon:insulin ratio and increased secretion and plasma concentrations of catecholamines produce relative peripheral insulin resistance. Inefficient glucose and fatty acid uptakes are inadequate to meet increased energy needs, leading to increased oxidation of branched-chain amino acids. Because branched-chain amino acids are essential amino acids, their oxidation depletes a valuable pool of precursors for protein synthesis. Administration of excess glucose can lead to hyperosmolar complications, excess energy expenditure, increased CO_2 production, cholestasis, and fatty infiltration of the liver.

Lipids are the major source of energy used during periods of stress starvation. Thus, lipolysis is increased and lipogenesis is decreased despite high levels of glucose and insulin. During stress starvation, peripheral tissues, such as skeletal muscle, myocardium, and respiratory muscles are able to use lipids as their primary energy source. Turnover of medium- and long-chain fatty acids is increased, although the clearance rate of long-chain fatty acids and triglycerides is reduced, primarily through a reduction in peripheral lipoprotein lipase activity that is inhibited by TNF. If excess lipids are administered, complications such as hyperlipidemia, bacteremia, and suppression of in vitro tests of polymorphonuclear and lymphocyte function may occur.

Protein catabolism is the hallmark of the metabolic stress response. Although the rate of protein synthesis is actually increased in the hypermetabolic state, it is significantly inadequate compared with the rate of protein breakdown. Protein is broken down mainly to provide carbon skeletons for use in gluconeogenesis, but amino acids are also used to support the cellular inflammatory response, the hepatic synthesis of acute-phase reactant proteins, and wound healing. Thus, the contribution of protein to total caloric expenditure increases from 10% in normal children to 15–20% in critically ill children. The discrepancy between protein catabolism and synthesis leads to a negative nitrogen balance and loss of lean body mass. This condition can be reduced or even reversed with increased nonprotein calorie and protein nutrition. Increased nutrient intake appears to make a difference in the ability of the patient to tolerate stress.

Nutritional Assessment

The pediatric patient is at a marked disadvantage compared with adults during periods of stress starvation. The child is a growing organism with little metabolic reserve to compensate for the metabolic stresses created by surgery, trauma, and sepsis. Preexisting nutritional status and the degree of stress imposed by the disease process are important factors in estimating nutritional requirements of the critically ill patient. Accurate assessment of nutritional requirements is important as both overfeed-

ing and underfeeding can lead to increased morbidity. One way to estimate nutritional requirements is to apply U.S. recommended dietary allowances. However, since these recommendations are based on populations of normal healthy subjects, applying recommended dietary allowances to critically ill patients significantly overestimates their caloric requirements. Therefore, several equations have been formulated in an attempt to predict basal energy needs of the critically ill patient. Some of these formulas estimate the basal metabolic rate, which is the energy requirement for a fasting (10–12 hours) person who recently awoke from sleep and is at rest with a normal body temperature in the absence of any stress. Other formulas estimate the resting energy expenditure (REE), which is the energy expenditure of a person at rest with a normal body and ambient temperature, but not necessarily fasting. The basal metabolic rate and REE are similar, usually differing by less than 10%. Harris-Benedict and the World Health Organization have recommended formulas that are among the most commonly used (Table 13–13). Once the basal metabolic demand has been estimated, it is then multiplied by a stress factor correlated to the underlying disease process to determine the ultimate energy requirements for the patient (Table 13–14). Compared with recommended dietary allowances, these formulas better estimate energy requirements in sick patients. However, recent evidence suggests that even they may not be accurate enough to use in critically ill children.

Table 13–13. Estimating needs for critically ill pediatric patients.

	Age	Resting Energy Expenditure (REE) kcal/kg	Average Range of Energy Needs kcal/kg	Average Range of Protein Needs g/kg
Infants	0–6 mo	55	90–120	2–3.5
	6–12 mo	55	90–120	1.5–2.5
Children	1–3 y	55	75–100	1.5–2.5
	4–6 y	45	65–90	1.5–2.0
	7–10 y	40	55–70	1.0–2.0
Males	11–14 y	30	40–55	1.0–2.0
	15–18 y	30	40–45	1.0–1.5
	19–24 y	25	30–40	1.0–1.5
Females	11–14 y	30	40–55	1.0–2.0
	15–18 y	25	30–40	1.0–1.5
	19–24 y	25	30–40	1.0–1.5

Based on World Health Organization formulas for protein and energy requirements.

Table 13–14. Activity and stress factors (× REE).

Condition	Factor
ICU on ventilation	Activity 1.0–1.15
Confined to bed	Activity 1.1–1.2
Light activity	Activity 1.2–1.3
Fever, per 1 °C	Stress 1.12–1.13
Major surgery	Stress 1.2–1.3
Multiple fractures	Stress 1.2–1.35
Peritonitis	Stress 1.2–1.5
Cardiac failure	Stress 1.25–1.5
Head injury	Stress 1.3–1.4
Liver failure	Stress 1.4–1.5
Sepsis	Stress 1.4–1.5
Burns	Stress 1.5–2.0

ICU, intensive care unit; REE, resting energy expenditure.

Indirect calorimetry has been used to measure patients' REE and appears to reflect a more accurate method of determining nutritional requirements. Indeed, indirect calorimetry measurements were used to derive the stress factors used with prediction formulas. Though this method was once used strictly for research, technology has enabled the production of portable, accurate devices that can be used anywhere in the hospital. Indirect calorimetry measures the amount of oxygen absorbed across the lung. This value is assumed to be equal to the amount of oxygen consumed in metabolic processes. The metabolic rate determined in milliliters of oxygen consumed per minute can be converted to calories per hour, thereby providing a measure of REE. Carbon dioxide production is also measured. The ratio of CO_2 production to O_2 consumption yields the respiratory quotient, which is a measure of substrate use. Inefficiencies in substrate use can be discovered and corrected by modification of the respiratory quotient through alteration of energy substrates that are provided to the patient. A recent study with 55 critically ill children was performed comparing two well-known prediction formulas with indirect calorimetry. The data suggest that prediction methods are unreliable for clinical use, and that indirect calorimetry is the only useful way of determining REE in sick children.

Provision of Nutrition

Once energy requirements are determined, the practitioner must decide to deliver nutritional support through either the enteral or the parenteral route. Enteral feeding is preferred because it is more physiologic, associated with fewer complications, and in some cases the only way to safely deliver some nutrients. More knowledge exists about enteral feeding in relation to both energy requirements and utilization; and practically, it is less expensive than parental nutrition.

Patients should be screened shortly after admission for nutritional requirements and preferred route of administration. Over the years, many practice patterns have been developed that list specific conditions or therapies in which enteral feeding may not be well tolerated by patients. Recent studies are proving that these may not be based on true physiologic differences and that a majority of patients who are critically ill can tolerate enteral feedings. The list of absolute contraindications for enteral feeding is shrinking and now may include just diseases of the GI tract.

Because it provides for a more physiologic digestive process, direct gastric feeding is preferable to the intestinal route. Patients supported with gastric feeds can usually tolerate higher osmotic loads and larger volumes, and have a lower frequency of diarrhea. Gastric acid also has a bactericidal effect that may decrease a patient's susceptibility to infection. However, for severely ill patients sedated and on mechanical ventilation, the high risk of reflux and aspiration becomes an increasing concern with this manner of feeding. Therefore, transpyloric feeding has been instituted in these patients and in any patient at high risk for aspiration. Although transpyloric feeding may limit reflux and aspiration, it does not entirely eliminate it. A suggested enteral feeding algorithm for critically ill children is presented in Figure 13–9.

The choice of formulas must be based on age, GI function, history of feeding tolerance, nutrient requirements, and route of feeding. The osmolality, nutrient complexity, caloric density, and cost are all factors that should be taken into consideration. An increasing number of commercially made formulas and additives are now available to meet the nutritional needs of the critically ill patient (Table 13–15).

Parenteral nutrition is indicated for patients who are unable to meet nutritional needs with enteral feeds. It consists of the IV delivery of nutrients, fluid, carbohydrates, protein, fat, electrolytes, vitamins, minerals, and trace elements. The proportions of these elements are individualized to suit the patient's specific nutritional needs. Parenteral nutrition often requires central venous access, and thus this method also carries the risks associated with central venous catheters (infection, clots, and insertion-related complications).

Parenteral nutrition can be ordered in many ways, as nutrients can be ordered based on a child's weight or per liter, or a combination of both. Standard ranges and guidelines are usually provided on order forms. Parenteral energy

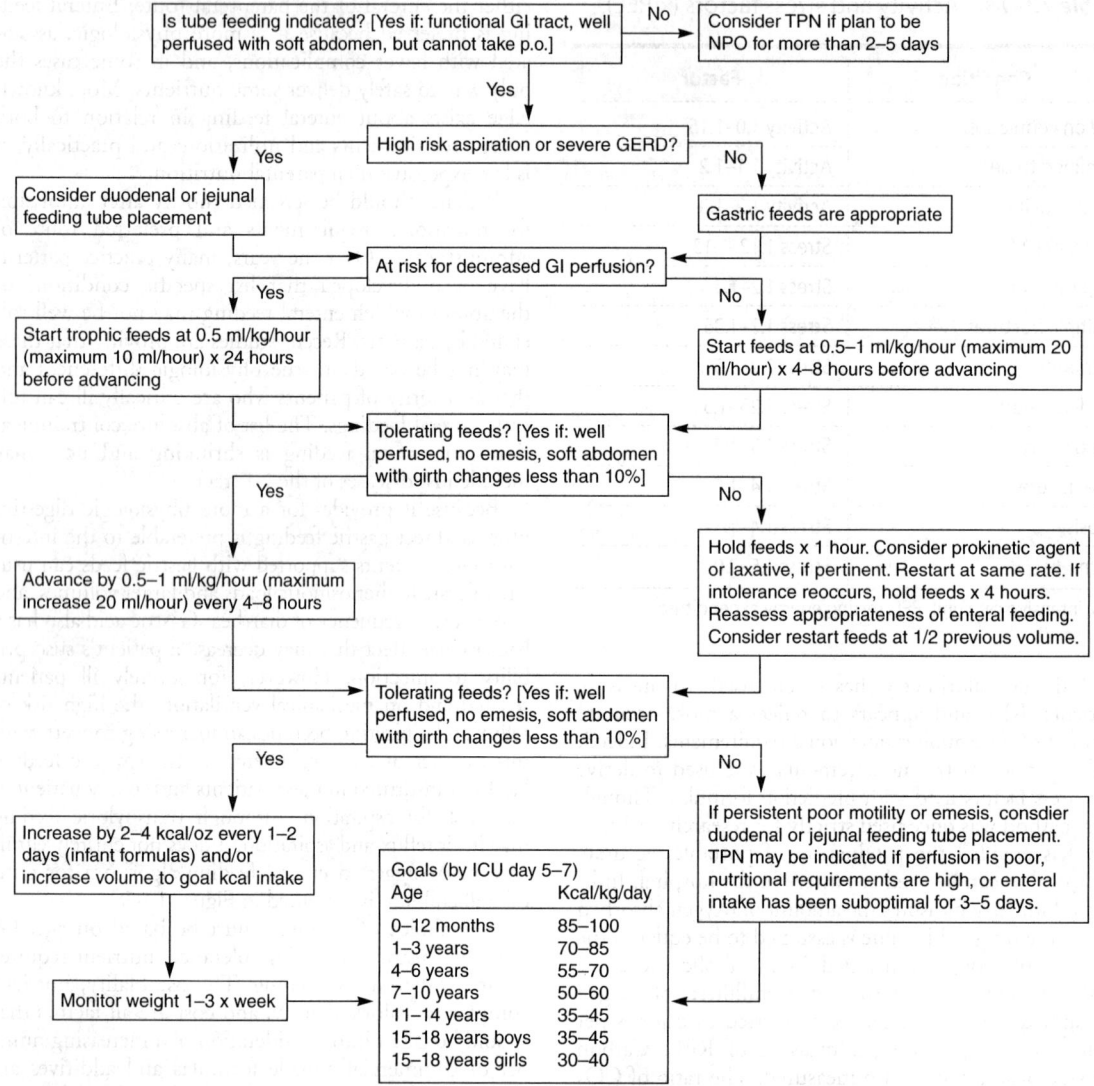

Figure 13–9. Proposed enteral feeding algorithm for critically ill children.

needs can be approximately 10–15% lower than estimated enteral needs due to reduced energy required for digestion, absorption, and fecal losses. The percentage of protein, carbohydrate, and fat that contributes to ideal total energy intake varies with the individual and the disease condition. General guidelines for energy distribution are 8–15% protein, 45–60% carbohydrate, and 25–40% fat. Solutions should be instituted slowly and advanced gradually over several days as tolerated by the patient. Guidelines for the administration of a balanced parenteral diet are provided in Chapter 10. A constant flow rate is important to maintaining steady glucose delivery. If parenteral nutrition must be stopped abruptly, a 10% glucose solution should be started

to prevent hypoglycemia. Administration of high glucose and amino acid concentrations in total parenteral nutrition requires central venous access.

Immunonutrition is an area of growing interest and research. The term describes a point of view that dietary factors can confer an advantage to the immune system or other adaptive functions in infants and children. The claims of health benefits ascribed to foods or dietary supplements are not new, but until recently these claims have not been supported by scientific review. Breast milk, the model for infant formula manufacturers, has long been recognized for its immunonutritive properties, containing such nutrients as secretory immunoglobulins,

Table 13–15. Pediatric enteral formulas.

Formula Category	Formula Examples	Typical Uses
Standard, milk protein-based	Pediasure Pediasure with Fiber Kindercal (with/without fiber) Nutren Junior	Nutritionally complete for ages 1–10 years. Can be used for tube feeds or oral supplements.
Food based	Compleat Pediatric	Made with beef protein, fruits, and vegetables—does contain lactose. Fortified with vitamins/minerals.
Semielemental	Peptamen Jr.	Indicated for impaired gut function with peptides as protein source, and high MCT content with lower total fat % than standard pediatric formulas.
Elemental	Pediatric Vivonex (24 kcal/oz) Elecare Neocate One Plus	Indicated for impaired gut function or protein allergy, and contains free amino acids and lower fat with majority as MCT.

MCT, medium-chain triglycerides.

lysozymes, interferon, and growth factors. However, the contribution of specific components to a positive outcome has yet to be elucidated. Growing evidence supports the immunomodulatory effects of minerals (eg, iron, zinc, selenium, and vitamin A), amino acids (arginine and glutamine), and nucleotides. Evidence also points to the emergence of prebiotics, nondigestable food components that favor the colonization and growth of bacteria normally resident in the colon; and probiotics, live microbial feed supplements with beneficial effects to the host. Although some of these concepts hold promise, it is still too early to advocate any specific guidelines, because some of these nutrients used in high doses have been reported to produce possible harmful effects.

Briassoulis G et al: Early enteral administration of immunonutrition in critically ill children: results of a blinded randomized controlled clinical trial. Nutrition 2005;21(7-8):799 [PMID: 15975487].

Coss-Bu JA et al: Energy metabolism, nitrogen balance and substrate utilization in critically ill children. Am J Clin Nutr 2001;74:664 [PMID: 11684536].

Dominguez-Cherit G et al: Total parenteral nutrition. Curr Opin Crit Care 2002;8:285 [PMID: 12386487].

Griffiths RD: Specialized nutrition support in critically ill patients. Curr Opin Crit Care 2003;9:249 [PMID: 12883278].

Irving SY et al: Nutrition for the critically ill child: Enteral and parenteral support. AACN Clin Issues 2000;11:541 [PMID: 11288418].

King W et al: Enteral nutrition and cardiovascular medications in the pediatric intensive care unit. JPEN J Parenter Enteral Nutr 2004;28:334 [PMID: 15449573].

Lafeber HN: The art of using indirect calorimetry for nutritional assessment of sick infants and children. Nutrition 2005;21:280 [PMID: 15723759].

Suchner U et al: Immune-modulatory actions of arginine in the critically ill. Br J Nutr 2002;87:S121 [PMID: 11895148].

Wernerman J: Glutamine and acute illness. Curr Opin Crit Care 2003;9:279 [PMID: 12883282].

PAIN & ANXIETY CONTROL

Anxiety control and pain relief are important responsibilities of the critical care physician. It is well recognized that infants and children experience pain and require pain relief. Indeed, outcomes are improved in children receiving appropriate pain control. A child's anxiety in the PICU may heighten perception of pain to a level that causes deterioration of his or her condition. It is important to distinguish between anxiety and pain, because pharmacologic therapy may be directed at one or both of these symptoms (Table 13–16). Furthermore, before initiating or increasing sedative drugs, it is important to exclude or address physiologic causes of agitation, such as hypoxemia, hypercapnia, and cerebral hypoperfusion caused by low cardiac output.

Sedation

Sedative (anxiolytic) drugs are used to induce calmness without producing sleep—although at high doses, all anxiolytics will cause drowsiness and sleep. The five indications for the use of sedative drugs are (1) to allay fear and anxiety; (2) to manage acute confusional states; (3) to facilitate treatment or diagnostic procedures; (4) to facilitate mechanical ventilation; and (5) to obtund physiologic responses to stress—that is, reduce tachycardia, hypertension, or increases in ICP. Parenteral administration (bolus or infusion) allows titration of response in the critically ill child. Sedatives fall into several

Table 13–16. Pain and anxiety control.

Drug	Dose and Method of Administration[a]	Advantages	Disadvantages	Usual Duration of Effect
Morphine	IV, 0.1 mg/kg; continuous infusion, 0.01–0.05 mg/kg/h	Excellent pain relief, reversible	Respiratory depression, hypotension, nausea, suppression of intestinal motility, histamine release	2–4 h
Meperidine	IV, 1 mg/kg	Good pain relief, reversible	Respiratory depression, histamine release, nausea, suppression of intestinal motility	2–4 h
Fentanyl	IV, 1–2 μg/kg; continuous infusion, 0.5–2 μg/kg/h	Excellent pain relief, reversible, short half-life	Respiratory depression, chest wall rigidity, severe nausea and vomiting	30 min
Diazepam	IV, 0.1 mg/kg	Sedation and seizure control	Respiratory depression, jaundice, phlebitis	1–3 h
Lorazepam	IV, 0.1 mg/kg	Longer half-life, sedation and seizure control	Nausea and vomiting, respiratory depression, phlebitis	2–4 h
Midazolam	IV, 0.1 mg/kg	Short half-life, only benzodiazepine given as continuous infusion	Respiratory depression	30–60 min

[a]Intravenous (IV) administration is most common in the ICU. The effects of morphine, meperidine, and fentanyl are reversible by administration of naloxone (opioid antagonist).

classes, with the opioid and benzodiazepine classes serving as the mainstay of anxiety treatment in the ICU.

A. BENZODIAZEPINES

Benzodiazepines possess anxiolytic, hypnotic, anticonvulsant, and skeletal muscle relaxant properties. Although their exact mode of action is unknown, it appears to be located within the limbic system of the CNS and to involve the neuroinhibitory transmitter γ-aminobutyric acid. Most benzodiazepines are metabolized in the liver, with their metabolites subsequently excreted in the urine; thus, patients in liver failure are likely to have long elimination times.

Benzodiazepines can cause respiratory depression if given rapidly in high doses, and they potentiate the analgesic and respiratory depressive effects of opioids and barbiturates. Therefore, it is important to monitor cardiorespiratory status and have resuscitation equipment available. Three benzodiazepines with differing half-lives are presently used in the ICU setting:

1. Midazolam—Midazolam has the shortest half-life (1½–3½ hours) of the benzodiazepines and is the only benzodiazepine that should be administered as a continuous IV infusion. It produces excellent retrograde amnesia lasting for 20–40 minutes after a single IV

dose. Therefore, it can be used either for short-term sedation or for "awake" procedures such as endoscopy or as a continuous infusion in the anxious, restless patient. The single IV dose is 0.1 mg/kg, whereas a continuous infusion should be started at a rate of 0.1 mg/kg/h after an initial loading dose of 0.1 mg/kg. The midazolam infusion dosage must be titrated upward to achieve the desired effect. Midazolam is not an analgesic; therefore, small doses of an analgesic such as morphine or fentanyl may be needed.

2. Diazepam—Diazepam has a longer half-life than midazolam and can be given orally as well as by the IV route. Its disadvantage in the ICU is its intermediary metabolite, nordazepam, which has a very long half-life and may accumulate, prolonging sedation. It produces excellent anxiolysis and amnesia. Additionally, it is used to treat acute status epilepticus. The IV dose is 0.1 mg/kg and can be repeated every 15 minutes to achieve the desired effect or until undesirable side effects (somnolence and respiratory depression) occur.

3. Lorazepam—Lorazepam possesses the longest half-life of the three benzodiazepines discussed here and can be used to achieve sedation for as long as 6–8 hours. It has less effect on the cardiovascular and respiratory systems than other benzodiazepines and can be given orally, IV, or intramuscularly (IM). The IV route is the most common. The IV dosage is 0.1 mg/kg. Lorazepam can also be used to treat acute status epilepticus.

B. OTHER DRUGS

1. Chloral hydrate—Chloral hydrate is an enteral sedative and hypnotic agent frequently used in children. After administration, it is rapidly metabolized by the liver to its active form trichloroethanol, which has an 8-hour half-life. A sedative dose is 6–20 mg/kg per dose, usually given every 6–8 hours, whereas the hypnotic dose is up to 50 mg/kg with a maximum dose of 1 g. The hypnotic dose is frequently used to sedate young children for outpatient radiologic procedures such as computed tomographic scanning and magnetic resonance imaging. There is little effect on respiration or blood pressure with therapeutic doses of chloral hydrate. The drug is irritating to mucous membranes, however, and may cause gastric upset if administered on an empty stomach.

2. Ketamine—Ketamine is a phencyclidine derivative that produces a trancelike state of immobility and amnesia known as dissociative anesthesia. After IM or IV administration, it causes central sympathetic nervous system stimulation with resultant increases in heart rate, blood pressure, and cardiac output. Respiration is not depressed at therapeutic doses. Because salivary and tracheobronchial mucous gland secretions are increased, atropine should be administered 20 minutes prior to the ketamine. A disadvantage of ketamine use is the occurrence of unpleasant dreams or hallucinations. The incidence is less in children than in adults, and it can be reduced even further by the concurrent administration of a benzodiazepine. Because of its inotropic properties, ketamine is useful for the sedation of certain critically ill patients whose conditions are unstable. Additionally, its bronchodilator effects make it the induction agent of choice for patients with status asthmaticus requiring intubation. It is given as an IV injection of 1–2 mg/kg over 60 seconds, with supplementary doses of 0.5 mg/kg being required every 10–30 minutes to maintain an adequate level of anesthesia. Alternatively, it can be administered as an IM injection of 3–7 mg/kg, which usually produces the desired level of anesthesia within 3–4 minutes. If prolonged anesthesia is required, ketamine can be administered by IV infusion at doses of 3–20 mg/kg/h.

3. Antihistamines—The antihistamines diphenhydramine and hydroxyzine can be used as sedatives but are not as effective as the benzodiazepines. Diphenhydramine produces sedation in only 50% of those patients receiving it. It can be given IV, IM, or PO at a dose of 1 mg/kg. Hydroxyzine can be given either IM or PO. It is frequently used concurrently with morphine or meperidine, adding anxiolysis and potentiating the effects of the opioid. The sedative effects of both drugs can last from 4–6 hours following a single dose.

4. Propofol—Propofol is an anesthetic induction agent whose main advantages are a rapid recovery time and no cumulative effects resulting from its rapid hepatic metabolism. It has no analgesic properties and frequently causes pain on injection. Dose-related hypotension and metabolic acidosis have been reported in pediatric patients, and the FDA recommends against the use of propofol in pediatric patients outside the controlled environment of the operating room.

5. Barbiturates—Barbiturates (phenobarbital and thiopental) can cause direct myocardial and respiratory depression and are, in general, poor choices for sedation of seriously ill patients. Phenobarbital has a very long half-life (up to 4 days), and recovery from thiopental, although it is a short-acting barbiturate, can be prolonged because remobilization of tissue stores occurs.

Analgesia

A. OPIOID ANALGESICS

Opioid analgesics (morphine, fentanyl, codeine, and meperidine) are the mainstays of therapy for most forms of acute severe pain as well as chronic cancer pain management. They possess both analgesic and dose-related sedative effects, although a range of plasma concentrations produce analgesia without sedation. In addition, opioids can cause respiratory depression, nausea, pruritus, slowed intestinal motility, miosis, urinary retention, cough suppression, biliary spasm, and vasodilation. The dose of opioid required to produce adequate analgesia varies greatly from one individual to the next. Therefore, in the intensive care setting, a continuous infusion of morphine or fentanyl allows dosages to be easily titrated to achieve the desired effect.

In general, infants younger than age 3 months are more susceptible than older children to the respiratory depressant effects of opioids. Starting dosages for these patients should be about one-third to one-half the usual pediatric dose. Most opioids (except meperidine) have minimal cardiac depressive effects, and critically ill patients generally tolerate them well. Fentanyl does not cause the histamine release that morphine does and thus produces less vasodilation and drop in systemic blood pressure. Opioids are metabolized in the liver, with metabolites excreted in the urine. Thus patients with hepatic or renal impairment may have a prolonged response to their administration. Long-term (> 7 days) administration and high doses (> 1.5–2.5 mg/kg cumulative fentanyl dose) of continuous infusions of opioids and/or benzodiazepines can lead to tolerance and physical dependence with the development of withdrawal symptoms (agitation, tachypnea, tachycardia, sweating, and diarrhea) upon acute termination of these drugs. In these patients, gradual tapering of the opioid dosage over a 5- to 10-day period will prevent withdrawal symptoms. The mechanism of opioid tolerance is related to conformational changes in the drug-receptor interaction. The use of continuous infusions and synthetic opioids is associated with the faster development of tolerance. As with any potent sedative or analgesic used in the ICU setting, appropriate patient monitoring (pulse oximetry, cardiorespiratory monitoring, and blood pressure monitoring) should be used during the period of opioid administration, and equipment should be available to support prompt intervention if undesired side effects occur.

The ICU regimen for sedation and analgesia must be carefully modified when the patient is transferred to the ward or a lower vigilance area. Patients with baseline respiratory, hepatic, or renal insufficiencies are most predisposed to respiratory insufficiency from sedatives or opioid analgesics.

Advantages of continuous infusions of sedatives are that it provides a more constant level of sedation, increases patient comfort, and allows better tolerance of newer approaches to mechanical ventilation. Prolongation of mechanical ventilation, hospitalization, and inability to assess neurologic function and mental status have been recognized as disadvantages of continuous infusions. Daily interruption of continuous sedation, allowing adult patients to "wake up," has been associated with a decrease in duration of mechanical ventilation and length of stay in the ICU. Currently, similar data are not available for pediatric patients.

Frequently pediatric patients will require relatively deep levels of sedation while undergoing a procedure (eg, vascular line placement or radiographic studies). Often these patients are not intubated and are not expected to require intubation and ventilatory support—so called conscious sedation. (New American Academy of Pediatrics guidelines will recommend a change in terminology to "moderate sedation/analgesia.") A systematic approach should include the following:

1. Pertinent history to elicit underlying illnesses
2. Physical exam focusing on the anatomy and adequacy of the child's airway (ie, large tonsils or facial deformity)
3. Informed consent
4. Appropriate patient fasting from solids (6 hours) and liquids (2 hours)
5. Age- and size-appropriate equipment
6. Drug dosages calculated on a milligram per kilogram basis
7. Monitoring and documentation of vital signs (including continuous pulse oximetry, respiratory rate and pattern, and level of arousability)
8. Separate observer to monitor deeply sedated patients
9. Practitioner capable of intubating and treating patients who enter a deeper state of sedation than initially anticipated
10. Discharge criteria ensuring that the patient has recovered to his or her baseline level of consciousness

Short-acting agents are preferred. Agents typically used include an opioid (usually fentanyl or morphine) and a benzodiazepine (most often midazolam). Another option is ketamine and midazolam. It is important to select and become comfortable with a specific combination; learn the indications and potential complications. Using a familiar agent and following the systematic approach outlined earlier have reduced anesthetic complications in this population of patients.

Patient-controlled analgesia is a done via a computer-governed infusion pump for constant infusion or patient-regulated bolus infusion of opioid analgesics. The basal infusion mode is intended to provide a constant serum level of analgesic. The bolus mode allows the patient, by pushing a button, to self-administer additional doses for breakthrough pain. The patient is usually permitted six boluses an hour, with 10-minute lockouts. If the patient is using allotted hourly boluses, this usually means that the basal infusion rate is too low. The patient must understand the concept of patient-controlled analgesia in order to be a candidate for its use. In some circumstances in pediatrics it is more appropriate for the nurse or parent to administer the bolus dose.

Naloxone reverses the analgesic, sedative, and respiratory depressive effects of opioid agonists. Its administration should be titrated to achieve the desired effect (eg, reversal of respiratory depression) because full reversal using $1–10\ \mu g/kg$ may cause acute anxiety, dysphoria, nausea, and vomiting. Furthermore, because the duration of effect of naloxone is shorter (30 minutes) than that of most opioids, the patient must be observed carefully for reappearance of the undesired effect.

B. NONOPIOID ANALGESICS

Nonopioid analgesics used in the treatment of mild to moderate pain include acetaminophen, aspirin, and other nonsteroidal anti-inflammatory drugs (NSAIDs) such as ibuprofen and naproxen.

1. Acetaminophen—Acetaminophen is the most commonly used analgesic in pediatrics in the U.S. and is the drug of choice for mild to moderate pain because of its low toxicity and lack of effect on bleeding time. It is metabolized by the liver. Suggested doses are 10–15 mg/kg orally to approximately 10–20 mg/kg per rectum every 4 hours.

2. Aspirin—Aspirin is also an effective analgesic for mild to moderate pain at doses of 10–15 mg/kg orally every 4 hours. However, its prolongation of bleeding time, association with Reye syndrome, and propensity to cause gastric irritation limit its usefulness in pediatric practice. Aspirin and other NSAIDs are still useful, especially for pain of inflammatory origin, bone pain, and pain associated with rheumatic conditions.

3. Other NSAIDs—Ibuprofen and naproxen are NSAIDs whose use has been limited in pediatrics to date. Naproxen is FDA-approved for children aged 2–12 years (5–7 mg/kg PO every 8–12 hours), whereas ibuprofen requires more frequent dosing intervals (4–10 mg/kg PO every 6–8 hours).

All of the NSAIDs have a therapeutic ceiling after which no increase occurs in analgesic potency above the recommended dose. They all can cause gastritis and should be given with antacids or with meals, and they should be used with caution in people at risk for renal compromise. In addition, the analgesic effects of acetaminophen, aspirin, and other NSAIDs are additive to those of opioids. Thus, if additional analgesia is required,

their use should be continued and an appropriate oral opioid (codeine or morphine) or parenteral opioid (morphine or fentanyl) begun.

Cray SH et al: Lactic acidemia and bradyarrhythmia in a child sedated with propofol. Crit Care Med 1998;26:2087 [PMID: 9875925].

Gehlbach BK, Kress JP: Sedation in the intensive care unit. Curr Opin Crit Care 2002;8:290 [PMID: 12386488].

Greco C, Berde C: Pain management for the hospitalized pediatric patient. Pediatr Clin North Am 2005;52:995 [PMID: 16009254].

Tobias JD: Sedation and analgesia in the pediatric intensive care unit. Pediatr Ann 2005;34:636 [PMID: 16149752].

Turner HN: Complex pain consultations in the pediatric intensive care unit. AACN Clin Issues 2005;16:388 [PMID: 16082240].

Roback MG, Wathen JE, Bajaj L, Bothner JP: Adverse events associated with procedural sedation and analgesia in a pediatric emergency department: a comparison of common parenteral drugs. Acad Emerg Med 2005;12:508 [PMID: 15930401].

Skin

14

Joseph G. Morelli, MD, & Joanna M. Burch, MD

■ GENERAL PRINCIPLES OF DIAGNOSIS OF SKIN DISORDERS

Examination of the skin requires that the entire surface of the body be palpated and inspected in good light. The onset and duration of each symptom should be recorded, together with a description of the primary lesion and any secondary changes, using the terminology set forth in Table 14–1. In practice, the characteristics of skin lesions are described in an order opposite that shown in the table. Begin with distribution, then configuration, color, secondary changes, and primary changes. For example, guttate psoriasis could be described as generalized, discrete, red, scaly papules.

■ GENERAL PRINCIPLES OF TREATMENT OF SKIN DISORDERS

TOPICAL THERAPY

Treatment should be simple and aimed at preserving normal skin physiology. Topical therapy is often preferred because medication can be delivered in optimal concentrations to the desired site.

Water is an important therapeutic agent, and optimally hydrated skin is soft and smooth. This occurs at approximately 60% environmental humidity. Because water evaporates readily from the cutaneous surface, skin hydration (stratum corneum of the epidermis) is dependent on the water concentration in the air, and sweating contributes little. However, if sweat is prevented from evaporating (eg, in the axilla, groin), local humidity and hydration of the skin are increased. As humidity falls below 15–20%, the stratum corneum shrinks and cracks; the epidermal barrier is lost and

allows irritants to enter the skin and induce an inflammatory response. Replacement of water will correct this condition if evaporation is prevented. Therefore, dry and scaly skin is treated by soaking the skin in water for 5 minutes and then adding a barrier to evaporation (Table 14–2). Oils and ointments prevent evaporation for 8–12 hours, so they must be applied once or twice a day. In areas already occluded (axilla, diaper area), creams or lotions are preferred, but more frequent application may be necessary.

Overhydration (maceration) can also occur. As environmental humidity increases to 90–100%, the number of water molecules absorbed by the stratum corneum increases and the tight lipid junctions between the cells of the stratum corneum are gradually replaced by weak hydrogen bonds; the cells eventually become widely separated, and the epidermal barrier falls apart. This occurs in immersion foot, diaper areas, axillae, and the like. It is desirable to enhance evaporation of water in these areas by air drying.

WET DRESSINGS

By placing the skin in an environment where the humidity is 100% and allowing the moisture to evaporate to 60%, pruritus is relieved. Evaporation of water stimulates cold-dependent nerve fibers in the skin, and this may prevent the transmission of the itching sensation via pain fibers to the central nervous system. It also is vasoconstrictive, thereby helping to reduce the erythema and also decreasing the inflammatory cellular response.

The simplest form of wet dressing consists of one set of wet underwear (eg, long johns) worn under dry pajamas. The underwear should be soaked in warm (not hot) water and wrung out until no more drops come out. This should be done overnight for a few days up to 1 week. When the condition has improved, the wet dressings are discontinued.

TOPICAL GLUCOCORTICOIDS

Twice-daily application of topical steroids is the mainstay of treatment for all forms of dermatitis (Table 14–3). Topical steroids can also be used under wet dressings. After wet dressings are discontinued, topical steroids

Table 14–1. Examination of the skin.

Clinical Appearance	Description and Examples
Primary lesions (first to appear)	
Macule	Any circumscribed color change in the skin that is flat. Examples: white (vitiligo), brown (café au lait spot), purple (petechia).
Papule	A solid, elevated area less than 1 cm in diameter whose top may be pointed, rounded, or flat. Examples: acne, warts, small lesions of psoriasis.
Plaque	A solid, circumscribed area more than 1 cm in diameter, usually flat-topped. Example: psoriasis.
Vesicle	A circumscribed, elevated lesion less than 1 cm in diameter and containing clear serous fluid. Example: blisters of herpes simplex.
Bulla	A circumscribed, elevated lesion more than 1 cm in diameter and containing clear serous fluid. Example: bullous impetigo.
Pustule	A vesicle containing a purulent exudate. Examples: acne, folliculitis.
Nodule	A deep-seated mass with indistinct borders that elevates the overlying epidermis. Examples: tumors, granuloma annulare. If it moves with the skin on palpation, it is intradermal; if the skin moves over the nodule, it is subcutaneous.
Wheal	A circumscribed, flat-topped, firm elevation of skin resulting from tense edema of the papillary dermis. Example: urticaria.
Secondary changes	
Scales	Dry, thin plates of keratinized epidermal cells (stratum corneum). Examples: psoriasis, ichthyosis.
Lichenification	Induration of skin with exaggerated skin lines and a shiny surface resulting from chronic rubbing of the skin. Example: atopic dermatitis.
Erosion and oozing	A moist, circumscribed, slightly depressed area representing a blister base with the roof of the blister removed. Examples: burns, impetigo. Most oral blisters present as erosions.
Crusts	Dried exudate of plasma on the surface of the skin following acute dermatitis. Examples: impetigo, contact dermatitis.
Fissures	A linear split in the skin extending through the epidermis into the dermis. Example: angular cheilitis.
Scars	A flat, raised, or depressed area of fibrotic replacement of dermis or subcutaneous tissue. Examples: acne scar, burn scar.
Atrophy	Depression of the skin surface caused by thinning of one or more layers of skin. Example: lichen sclerosis.
Color	The lesion should be described as red, yellow, brown, tan, or blue. Particular attention should be given to the blanching of red lesions. Failure to blanch suggests bleeding into the dermis (petechiae).
Configuration of lesions	
Annular (circular)	Annular nodules represent granuloma annulare; annular scaly papules are more apt to be caused by dermatophyte infections.
Linear (straight lines)	Linear papules represent lichen striatus; linear vesicles, incontinentia pigmenti; linear papules with burrows, scabies.
Grouped	Grouped vesicles occur in herpes simplex or zoster.
Discrete	Discrete lesions are independent of each other.
Distribution	Note whether the eruption is generalized, acral (hands, feet, buttocks, face), or localized to a specific skin region.

Table 14–2. Bases used for topical preparations.

Base	Combined With	Uses
Foam		Cosmetically eloquent; at this time, only available for two topical steroid preparations
Liquids		Wet dressings: relieve pruritus, vasoconstrict
	Powder	Shake lotions, drying pastes: relieve pruritus, vasoconstrict
	Grease and emulsifier; oil in water	Cream: penetrates quickly (10–15 min) and thus allows evaporation
	Excess grease and emulsifier; water in oil	Emollient cream: penetrates more slowly and thus retains moisture on skin
Grease		Ointments: occlusive (hold material on skin for prolonged time) and prevent evaporation of water
Gel		Transparent, colorless, semisolid emulsion: nongreasy, more drying and irritating than cream
Powder		Enhances evaporation

Characteristics of bases for topical preparations:

1. Thermolabile, low-residue foam vehicle is more cosmetically acceptable and uses novel permeability pathway for delivery.
2. Most greases are triglycerides (eg, Aquaphor, petrolatum, Eucerin).
3. Oils are fluid fats (eg, Alpha Keri, olive oil, mineral oil).
4. True fats (eg, lard, animal fats) contain free fatty acids that cause irritation.
5. Ointments (eg, Aquaphor, petrolatum) should not be used in intertriginous areas such as the axillae, between the toes, and in the perineum, because they increase maceration. Lotions or creams are preferred in these areas.
6. Oils and ointments hold medication on the skin for long periods and are therefore ideal for barriers or prophylaxis and for dried areas of skin. Medication gets into the skin more slowly from ointments.
7. Creams carry medication into skin and are preferable for intertriginous dermatitis.
8. Solutions, gels, or lotions should be used for scalp treatments.

should be applied only to areas of active disease. They should never be applied to normal skin to prevent recurrence. Only low-potency steroids (see Table 14–3) are applied to the face or intertriginous areas.

Table 14–3. Topical glucocorticoids.

Glucocorticoid	Concentrations
Low potency[a] = 1–9	
Hydrocortisone	0.5% and 1%
Desonide	0.05%
Moderate potency = 10–99	
Mometasone furoate	0.1%
Hydrocortisone valerate	0.2%
Fluocinolone acetonide	0.025%
Triamcinolone acetonide	0.01%
Amcinonide	0.1%
High potency = 100–499	
Desoximetasone	0.25%
Fluocinonide	0.05%
Halcinonide	0.1%
Super potency = 500–7500	
Betamethasone dipropionate	0.05%
Clobetasol propionate	0.05%

[a]1% hydrocortisone is defined as having a potency of 1.

Isaksson M, Bruze M Corticosteroids. Dermatitis 2005;16:3 [PMID: 15996344].

Kraft JN, Lynde CW Moisturizers: What they are and a practical approach to product selection. Skin Therapy Lett 2005;10:1 [PMID 15986082].

Schnopp C et al. Topical steroids under wet-wrap dressings in atopic dermatitis—A vehicle controlled trial. Dermatology 2002;204(1):56 [PMID: 11834851].

■ DISORDERS OF THE SKIN IN NEWBORNS

TRANSIENT DISEASES IN NEWBORNS

Milia

Milia are tiny epidermal cysts filled with keratinous material. These 1–2 mm white papules occur predominantly on the face in 40% of newborns. Their intraoral counterparts are called Epstein pearls and occur in up to 60–85% of neonates. These cystic structures spontaneously rupture and exfoliate their contents.

Sebaceous Gland Hyperplasia

Prominent white to yellow papules at the opening of pilosebaceous follicles without surrounding erythema—especially over the nose—represent overgrowth of sebaceous glands in response to maternal androgens. They occur in more than half of newborns and spontaneously regress in the first few months of life.

Neonatal Acne

Inflammatory papules and pustules with occasional comedones predominantly on the face occur in as many as 20% of newborns. Although neonatal acne can be present at birth, it most often occurs between 2–4 weeks of age. Spontaneous resolution occurs over a period of 6 months to 1 year. A recently recognized entity that is often confused with neonatal acne is **neonatal cephalic pustulosis.** This is a more monomorphic eruption with red papules and pustules on the head and neck that appears in the first month of life. There is associated neutrophilic inflammation and yeasts of the genus *Malassezia.* This eruption will resolve spontaneously, but responds to topical anti-yeast preparations.

Harlequin Color Change

A cutaneous vascular phenomenon unique to neonates in the first week of life occurs when the infant (particularly one of low birth weight) is placed on one side. The dependent half develops an erythematous flush with a sharp demarcation at the midline, and the upper half of the body becomes pale. The color changes usually subside within a few seconds after the infant is placed supine but may persist for as long as 20 minutes.

Mottling

A lace-like pattern of bluish, reticular discoloration representing dilated cutaneous vessels appears over the extremities and often the trunk of neonates exposed to lowered room temperature. This feature is transient and usually disappears completely on rewarming.

Erythema Toxicum

Up to 50% of full-term infants develop erythema toxicum. Usually at 24–48 hours of age, blotchy erythematous macules 2–3 cm in diameter appear, most prominently on the chest but also on the back, face, and extremities. These are occasionally present at birth. Onset after 4–5 days of life is rare. The lesions vary in number from a few up to as many as 100. Incidence is much higher in full-term versus premature infants. The macular erythema may fade within 24–48 hours or may progress to formation of urticarial wheals in the center of the macules or, in 10% of cases, pustules. Examination of a Wright-stained smear of the lesion will reveal numerous eosinophils. No organisms are seen on Gram stain. This may be accompanied by peripheral blood eosinophilia of up to 20%. All of the lesions fade and disappear within 5–7 days. Transient neonatal pustular melanosis is a pustular eruption in newborns of African American descent. The pustules rupture leaving a collarette of scale surrounding a macular hyperpigmentation. Unlike erythema toxicum, the pustules contain mostly neutrophils and often involve the palms and soles.

Sucking Blisters

Bullae, either intact or as an erosion (the blister base) without inflammatory borders, may occur over the forearms, wrists, thumbs, or upper lip. These presumably result from vigorous sucking in utero. They resolve without complications.

Miliaria

Obstruction of the eccrine sweat ducts occurs often in neonates and produces one of two clinical pictures. Superficial obstruction in the stratum corneum causes miliaria crystallina, characterized by tiny (1- to 2-mm), superficial grouped vesicles without erythema over intertriginous areas and adjacent skin (eg, neck, upper chest). More commonly, obstruction of the eccrine duct deeper in the epidermis results in erythematous grouped papules in the same areas and is called miliaria rubra. Rarely, these may progress to pustules. Heat and high humidity predispose the patient to eccrine duct pore closure. Removal to a cooler environment is the treatment of choice.

Subcutaneous Fat Necrosis

This entity presents in the first 7 days of life as reddish or purple, sharply circumscribed, firm nodules occurring over the cheeks, buttocks, arms, and thighs. Cold injury is thought to play an important role. These lesions resolve spontaneously over a period of weeks, although in some instances they may calcify.

Conlon J, Drolet B: Skin lesions in the neonate. Pediatr Clin North Am 2004;51:863 [PMID: 15275979].

PIGMENT CELL BIRTHMARKS, NEVI, & MELANOMA

Birthmarks may involve an overgrowth of one or more of any of the normal components of skin (eg, pigment cells, blood vessels, lymph vessels). A nevus is a hamartoma of highly differentiated cells that retain their normal function.

Mongolian Spot

A blue-black macule found over the lumbosacral area in 90% of infants of Native American, African American, and Asian descent is called a mongolian spot. These spots are occasionally noted over the shoulders and back and may extend over the buttocks. Histologically, they consist of spindle-shaped pigment cells located deep in the dermis. The lesions fade somewhat with time as a result of darkening of the overlying skin, but some traces may persist into adult life.

Café au Lait Macule

A café au lait macule is a light brown, oval macule (dark brown on brown or black skin) that may be found anywhere on the body. Café au lait spots over 1.5 cm in greatest diameter are found in 10% of white and 22% of black children. These lesions persist throughout life and may increase in number with age. The presence of six or more such lesions over 1.5 cm in greatest diameter may be a clue to neurofibromatosis 1 (NF-1). Patients with McCune–Albright syndrome (see Chapter 30) have a large, unilateral café au lait macule.

Spitz Nevus

A reddish brown solitary nodule appearing on the face or upper arm of a child represents a Spitz nevus. Histologically, it consists of pigment-producing cells of bizarre shape with numerous mitoses. Although these lesions can look concerning histologically, they have a benign clinical course.

ACQUIRED MELANOCYTIC NEVI (Common Moles)

Well-demarcated, brown to brown-black macules represent junctional nevi. They can begin to appear in the first years of life and increase with age. Histologically, these lesions are clones of melanocytes at the junction of the epidermis and dermis. Approximately 20% may progress to compound nevi—papular lesions with melanocytes both in junctional and intradermal locations. Intradermal nevi are often lighter in color and can be fleshy and pedunculated. Melanocytes in these lesions are located purely within the dermis. Nevi look dark blue (blue nevi) when they contain more deeply situated melanocytes in the dermis.

Melanoma

Melanoma in prepubertal children is very rare. Pigmented lesions with variegated colors (red, white, blue), notched borders, asymmetric shape, and very irregular or ulcerated surfaces should arouse a suspicion of mela-

noma. Ulceration and bleeding are advanced signs of melanoma. If melanoma is suspected, wide local excision sent for pathologic examination should be done as the treatment of choice.

Congenital Melanocytic Nevi

One in 100 babies is born with a congenital nevus. Congenital nevi tend to be larger and darker brown than acquired nevi and may have many terminal hairs. If the pigmented plaque covers more than 5% of the body surface area, it is considered a giant or large congenital nevus and occurs in 1 in 20,000 infants. Often the lesions are so large they cover the entire trunk (bathing trunk nevi). Histologically, they are compound nevi with melanocytes often tracking around hair follicles and other adnexal structures deep in the dermis. The risk of malignant melanoma in small congenital nevi is controversial in the literature, but most likely very low. Transformation to malignant melanoma in giant congenital nevi has been estimated in the best studies to be between 1–5%. Two-thirds of melanoma in children with giant congenital nevi develop in areas other than the skin.

Fishman C et al: Diagnosis and management of nevi and cutaneous melanoma in infants and children. Clin Dermatol 2002;20:44 [PMID: 11849894].

Makkar HS, Frieden IJ: Congenital melanocytic nevi: An update for the pediatrician. Curr Opin Pediatr 2002;14:397 [PMID: 12130901].

Turchin I, Barankin B, Morelli J: Myths and misconceptions: The risk of melanoma in small congenital nevi. Skinmed 2004;3:228 [PMID: 15249787].

VASCULAR BIRTHMARKS
Capillary Malformations

Capillary malformations are an excess of capillaries in localized areas of skin. The degree of excess is variable. The color of the lesions range from light red/pink to dark red.

Light red macules are found over the nape of the neck, upper eyelids, and glabella of newborns. Fifty percent of infants have such lesions over their necks. Eyelid and glabellar lesions usually fade completely within the first year of life. Lesions that occupy the total central forehead area usually do not fade. Those on the neck persist into adult life.

Port-wine stains are dark red macules appearing anywhere on the body. A bilateral facial port-wine stain or one covering the entire half of the face may be a clue to Sturge–Weber syndrome, which is characterized by seizures, mental retardation, glaucoma, and hemiplegia. (See Chapter 23.) Most infants with smaller, unilateral facial port-wine stains do not have Sturge–Weber syndrome. Similarly, a port-wine stain over an extremity may be associated with hypertrophy of the soft tissue and bone of that extremity (Klippel–Trénaunay syndrome). The pulsed dye laser is the treatment of choice for infants and children with port-wine stains.

Lanigan SW, Taibjee SM: Recent advances in laser treatment of port-wine stains. Br J Dermatol 2004;151:527 [PMID: 15377336].

Hemangioma

A red, rubbery nodule is a hemangioma. The lesion is often not present at birth but is represented by a permanent blanched area on the skin that is supplanted at age 2–4 weeks by red nodules. Histologically, these are benign tumors of capillary endothelial cells. Hemangiomas may be superficial, deep, or mixed. The terms strawberry and cavernous are misleading and should not be used. The biologic behavior of a hemangioma is the same despite its location. Fifty percent resolve spontaneously by age 5 years, 70% by age 7 years, and 90% by age 9 years, leaving redundant skin, hypopigmentation, and telangiectasia. Local complications include superficial ulceration and secondary pyoderma.

Complications that require immediate treatment are (1) airway obstruction (hemangiomas of the head and neck may be associated with subglottic hemangiomas), (2) visual obstruction (with resulting amblyopia), and (3) cardiac decompensation (high-output failure). In these instances, the treatment of choice is with prednisolone, 2–3 mg/kg orally daily for 6–12 weeks. Interferon alfa-2a has been used to treat serious hemangiomas unresponsive to prednisone. Ten percent of patients with hemangiomas treated with interferon alfa-2a have developed spastic diplegia. Therefore, interferon alfa-2a therapy should be reserved for truly life-threatening hemangiomas. If the lesion is ulcerated or bleeding, pulsed dye laser treatment may be helpful. The Kasabach–Merritt syndrome, which is platelet trapping with consumption coagulopathy, does not occur with solitary cutaneous hemangiomas. It is seen only with internal hemangiomas or the very rare vascular tumors called hemangioendotheliomas and tufted angiomas.

Bruckner AL, Frieden IJ: Hemangiomas of infancy. J Am Acad Dermatol 2003;48:477 [PMID: 12664009].

Chang MW: Updated classification of hemangiomas and other vascular anomalies. Lymphat Res Biol 2003;1:259 [PMID: 15624554].

Lymphatic Malformations

Lymphatic malformations may be superficial or deep. Superficial lymphatic malformations present as fluid-filled vesicles often described as looking like frog spawn. Deep lymphatic malformations are rubbery, skin-colored nodules occurring in the parotid area (cystic hygromas) or on the tongue. They often result in grotesque enlargement of soft tissues. Histologically, they can be either macrocystic or microcystic. Therapy includes injection of picibanil or surgery.

Smith RJ: Lymphatic malformations. Lymphat Res Biol 2004;2:25 [PMID: 15609924].

EPIDERMAL BIRTHMARKS
Epidermal Nevus

The majority of these birthmarks present in the first year of life but can first appear in adulthood. They are hamartomas of the epidermis that are warty to papillomatous plaques often in a linear array. They range in color from skin-colored to dirty yellow to brown. Histologically they have a thickened epidermis with hyperkeratosis. The condition of widespread epidermal nevi associated with other developmental anomalies (central nervous system, eye, and skeletal), is called the epidermal nevus syndrome. Treatment once or twice daily with topical calcipotriene may flatten some lesions. The only definitive cure is surgical excision.

Happle R, Rogers M: Epidermal nevi. Adv Dermatol 2002;18:175 [PMID: 12528406].

Vujevich J, Mancini A: The epidermal nevus syndromes: Multisystem disorders. J Am Acad Dermatol 2004;50:957 [PMID: 15153903].

Nevus Sebaceus

This is a hamartoma of sebaceous glands and underlying apocrine glands that is diagnosed by the appearance at birth of a yellowish, hairless plaque in the scalp or on the face. The lesions can be contiguous with an epidermal nevus on the face and widespread lesions can constitute part of the epidermal nevus syndrome.

Histologically, nevus sebaceus represents an overabundance of sebaceous glands without hair follicles. At puberty, with androgenic stimulation, the sebaceous cells in the nevus divide, expand their cellular volume, and synthesize sebum, resulting in a warty mass. Because 15% of these lesions become basal cell carcinomas after puberty, excision is recommended before puberty.

Cribier B et al: Tumors arising in nevus sebaceous: A study of 596 cases. J Am Acad Dermatol 2000;42:263 [PMID: 10642683].

CONNECTIVE TISSUE BIRTHMARKS (Juvenile Elastoma, Collagenoma)

Connective tissue nevi are smooth, skin-colored papules 1–10 mm in diameter that are grouped on the trunk. A solitary, larger (5–10 cm) nodule is called a shagreen

Table 14–4. Four major types of ichthyosis.

Name	Age at Onset	Clinical Features	Genetic Defect	Inheritance
Ichthyosis with normal epidermal turnover				
Ichthyosis vulgaris	Childhood	Fine scales, deep palmar and plantar markings	Filaggrin/profilaggrin	Autosomal-dominant
X-linked ichthyosis	Birth	Palms and soles spared; thick scales that darken with age; corneal opacities in patients and carrier mothers	Cholesterol sulfatase	X-linked
Ichthyosis with increased epidermal turnover				
Epidermolytic hyperkeratosis	Birth	Verrucous, yellow scales in flexural areas and palms and soles	Keratins 1 and 10	Autosomal-dominant
Lamellar ichthyosis	Birth; collodion baby	Erythroderma, ectropion, large coarse scales; thickened palms and soles	Transglutaminase 1	Autosomal-recessive

patch and is histologically indistinguishable from other connective tissue nevi that show thickened, abundant collagen bundles with or without associated increases of elastic tissue. Although the shagreen patch is a cutaneous clue to tuberous sclerosis (Chapter 23), the other connective tissue nevi occur as isolated events. These nevi remain throughout life and need no treatment.

HEREDITARY SKIN DISORDERS

Ichthyosis

Ichthyosis is a term applied to several heritable diseases characterized by the presence of excessive scales on the skin. Major categories are listed in Table 14–4. Treatment consists of controlling scaling with lactic acid with ammonium hydroxide (Lac-Hydrin or AmLactin) 12% applied once daily. Daily lubrication and a good dry skin care regimen are important for these patients.

DiGiovanni JJ, Robinson-Bostom L: Ichthyosis: Etiology, diagnosis and management. Am J Clin Dermatol 2003;4:81 [PMID: 12553849].

Epidermolysis Bullosa

This is a group of heritable disorders characterized by skin fragility with blistering. Depending on the genetic defect, and therefore where the blister occurs, these disorders can be divided into scarring and nonscarring types (Table 14–5).

For the severely effected, a good deal of the surface area of the skin may have blisters and erosions, requiring daily wound care and dressings. These children are prone to frequent skin infections, have anemia, growth problems, mouth erosions and esophageal strictures and chronic pain issues, among many others.

Treatment consists of protection of the skin with topical emollients as well as nonstick dressings. The other medical needs and potential complications of the severe forms of epidermolysis bullosa require a multidisciplinary approach. For the less severe types, protecting areas of most trauma with padding and dressings as well as intermittent topical or oral antibiotics for superinfection are appropriate treatments. If hands and feet are involved, reducing skin friction with 5% glutaraldehyde every 3 days is helpful.

Fine JD et al: Revised classification system for inherited epidermolysis bullosa: Report of the Second International Consensus Meeting on etiology and classification of epidermolysis bullosa. J Am Acad Dermatol 2000;42:1051 [PMID: 10827412].

Pai S, Marinkovich MP: Epidermolysis bullosa: New and emerging trends. Am J Clin Dermatol 2002;3:371 [PMID: 12113646].

COMMON SKIN DISEASES IN INFANTS, CHILDREN, & ADOLESCENTS

ACNE

Acne affects 85% of adolescents. The onset of adolescent acne is between ages 8 and 10 years in 40% of children. The early lesions are usually limited to the face and are primarily closed comedones (whiteheads; see following discussion).

Clinical Findings

Acne is a disease of the sebaceous follicles which are follicles associated with sebaceous glands that usually lack ter-

Table 14–5. Types of epidermolysis bullosa.

Name	Age at Onset	Clinical Features	Genetic Defect	Inheritance
Nonscarring types				
Epidermolysis bullosa simplex	Birth–first few years of life	Hemorrhagic blisters over the lower legs; cooling prevents blisters; blisters brought out by walking	Keratins 5 and 14	Autosomal-dominant
Junctional bullous dermolysis (Herlitz disease)	Birth	Erosions on legs, oral mucosa; severe peri-oral involvement	Laminin V	Autosomal-recessive
Scarring types				
Epidermolysis bullosa dystrophica, dominant	Infancy	Numerous blisters on hands and feet; milia formation	Type VII collagen	Autosomal-dominant
Epidermolysis bullosa dystrophica, recessive	Birth	Repeated episodes of blistering, secondary infection and scarring—"mitten hands and feet"	Type VII collagen	Autosomal-recessive

minal hair. They are located primarily on the face, upper chest, back, and penis. Obstruction of the sebaceous follicle opening produces the clinical lesion of acne. If the obstruction occurs at the follicular mouth, the clinical lesion is characterized by a wide, patulous opening filled with a plug of stratum corneum cells. This is the open comedo, or blackhead. Open comedones are the predominant clinical lesion in early adolescent acne. The black color is caused not by dirt but by oxidized melanin within the stratum corneum cellular plug. Open comedones do not often progress to inflammatory lesions. Closed comedones, or whiteheads, are caused by obstruction just beneath the follicular opening in the neck of the sebaceous follicle, which produces a cystic swelling of the follicular duct directly beneath the epidermis. Most authorities believe that closed comedones are precursors of inflammatory acne lesions (red papules, pustules, nodules and cysts). If open or closed comedones are the predominant lesions on the skin in adolescent acne, the condition is called comedonal acne.

In typical adolescent acne, several different types of lesions are present simultaneously. Severe, chronic, inflammatory lesions may rarely occur as interconnecting, draining sinus tracts. Adolescents with cystic acne require prompt medical attention, because ruptured cysts and sinus tracts result in severe scar formation. New acne scars are highly vascular and have a reddish or purplish hue. Such scars return to normal skin color after several years. Acne scars may be depressed beneath the skin level, raised, or flat to the skin. In adolescents with a tendency toward keloid formation, keloidal scars can occur following acne lesions, particularly on the chest and upper back.

Differential Diagnosis

Consider rosacea, nevus comedonicus, flat warts, miliaria, molluscum contagiosum, and the angiofibromas of tuberous sclerosis.

Pathogenesis

The primary event in acne formation is obstruction of the sebaceous follicle and subsequent formation of the microcomedo (not evident clinically). This is the precursor to all future acne lesions. This phenomenon is androgen-dependent in adolescent acne. The keratinocytes of the sebaceous follicles contain an enzyme, 5α-reductase, which converts plasma testosterone to dihydrotestosterone (DHT). This androgen is a potent stimulus for cell proliferation. The four primary factors in the pathogenesis of acne are (1) plugging of the hair follicle; (2) increased sebum production; (3) proliferation of *Propionibacterium acnes* in the obstructed follicle, and (4) inflammation. Many of these factors are influenced by androgens.

Drug-induced acne should be suspected in teenagers if all lesions are in the same stage at the same time and if involvement extends to the lower abdomen, lower back, arms, and legs. Drugs responsible for acne include corticotropin (ACTH), glucocorticoids, androgens, hydantoins, and isoniazid, each of which increases plasma testosterone.

Treatment

Different treatment options are listed in Table 14–6. Recent data have indicated that combination therapy that targets multiple pathogenic factors increases the efficacy of treatment.

Table 14–6. Acne treatment.

Comedonal acne	One of the following: Retinoic acid, 0.025, 0.05, or 0.1% cream; 0.01 or 0.025% gel; or 0.1% microgel Adapalene, 0.1% gel or solution; 0.05% cream
Papular inflammatory acne	One from first grouping, plus one of the following: Topical antibiotics Benzoyl peroxide, 2.5, 4, 5, 8, or 10% gel or lotion; 4 or 8% wash Azelaic acid, 15% cream Clindamycin, 1% lotion, solution, or gel
Pustular inflammatory acne	One from first grouping, plus one of the following: Oral antibiotics Tetracycline or erythromycin, 250–500 mg, bid Minocycline or doxycycline, 50–100 mg, bid
Nodulocystic acne	Accutane, 1 mg/kg/d

A. TOPICAL KERATOLYTIC AGENTS

Topical keratolytic agents address the plugging of the follicular opening with keratinocytes and include retinoids, benzoyl peroxide, and azelaic acid. The first-line treatment for both comedonal and inflammatory acne is now topical retinoids (tretinoin [retinoic acid], adapalene, and tazarotene). These are the most effective keratolytic agents. These topical agents may be used once daily, or the combination of a retinoid applied to acne-bearing areas of the skin in the evening and a benzoyl peroxide gel or azelaic acid applied in the morning may be used. This regimen will control 80–85% of cases of adolescent acne.

B. TOPICAL ANTIBIOTICS

Topical antibiotics are less effective than systemic antibiotics and at best are equivalent in potency to 250 mg of tetracycline orally once a day. One percent clindamycin phosphate solution is the most efficacious topical antibiotic. Most *P acnes* are now resistant to topical erythromycin solutions. Topical antibiotic therapy alone should never be used. Multiple studies have shown a combination of benzoyl peroxide or a retinoid and a topical antibiotic are more effective than the antibiotic alone.

C. SYSTEMIC ANTIBIOTICS

Antibiotics that are concentrated in sebum, such as tetracycline, minocycline, and doxycycline should be reserved for moderate to severe inflammatory acne. The usual dose of tetracycline is 0.5–1.0 g divided twice a day on an empty stomach; minocycline and doxycycline 50–100 mg taken once or twice daily can be taken with food. Monotherapy with oral antibiotics should never be used. Recent recommendations are that oral antibiotics should be used for a finite time period, and then discontinued as soon as possible. The tetracycline antibiotics should not be given to children less than 8 years of age due to the effect on dentition. These antibiotics have anti-inflammatory effects in addition to decreasing *P acnes* in the follicle.

D. ORAL RETINOIDS

An oral retinoid, 13-*cis*-retinoic acid (isotretinoin; Accutane), is the most effective treatment for severe cystic acne. The precise mechanism of its action is unknown, but decreased sebum production, decreased follicular obstruction, decreased skin bacteria, and general anti-inflammatory activities have been described. The initial dosage is 40 mg once or twice daily. This therapy is reserved for severe nodulocystic acne, or acne recalcitrant to aggressive standard therapy. Side effects include dryness and scaling of the skin, dry lips, and, occasionally, dry eyes and dry nose. Fifteen percent of patients may experience some mild achiness with athletic activities. Up to 10% of patients experience mild, reversible hair loss. Elevated liver enzymes and blood lipids have rarely been described. Acute depression may occur. Isotretinoin is teratogenic in young women of childbearing age. Because of this and the other side effects, it is not recommended unless strict adherence to the FDA guidelines is ensured. The FDA has just approved a strict registration program (iPLEDGE) that will be implemented in 2006.

E. OTHER ACNE TREATMENTS

Hormonal therapy (oral contraceptives) is often an effective option for girls that have perimenstrual flares of acne, or have not responded adequately to conventional therapy. Adolescents with endocrine disorders such as polycystic ovary syndrome will also see improvement of their acne with hormonal therapy. Oral contraceptives can be added to a conventional therapeutic regimen and should always be used in females on oral isotretinoin unless absolute contraindications exist.

F. AVOIDANCE OF COSMETICS AND HAIR SPRAY

Acne can be aggravated by a variety of external factors that result in further obstruction of partially occluded sebaceous follicles. Discontinuing the use of oil-based cosmetics, face creams, and hair sprays may alleviate the comedonal component of acne within 4–6 weeks.

Patient Education & Follow-Up Visits

The multifactorial pathogenesis of acne and its role in the treatment plan must be explained to adolescent patients.

Time should be set aside at the first visit to answer questions. Acne therapy is aimed at preventing the microcomedone, so therapy takes 8–12 weeks to see improvement. This delay should be stressed to the patient. Realistic expectations should be encouraged in the adolescent patient because no therapy will prevent an adolescent from ever having another acne lesion. A written education sheet is useful.

Follow-up visits should be made every 8–12 weeks. An objective method to chart improvement should be documented by the provider, because patient's assessment of improvement tends to be inaccurate. Explain again what medications are being used and why, what the treatment is intended to achieve, and that 8–12 weeks of consistent therapy is required for improvement in most cases. Ensure on follow-up that the patient is applying the medication properly (eg, topical keratolytics are to be applied to the entire area of skin that tends to be affected, not to individual lesions already present).

Gollnick H, Cunliffe W: Management of acne: A report from a global alliance to improve outcomes in acne. J Am Acad Dermatol 2003;49:S1 [PMID: 12833004].

BACTERIAL INFECTIONS OF THE SKIN

Impetigo

Erosions covered by honey-colored crusts are diagnostic of impetigo. Staphylococci and group A streptococci are important pathogens in this disease, which histologically consists of superficial invasion of bacteria into the upper epidermis, forming a subcorneal pustule.

Impetigo should be treated with an antimicrobial agent effective against *Staphylococcus aureus* (β-lactamase-resistant penicillins or cephalosporins, clindamycin, amoxicillin–clavulanate) for 7–10 days. Topical mupirocin and fusidic acid (three times daily) are also effective.

Bullous Impetigo

All impetigo is bullous, with the blister forming just beneath the stratum corneum, but in bullous impetigo there is, in addition to the usual erosion covered by a honey-colored crust, a border filled with clear fluid. Staphylococci may be isolated from these lesions, and systemic signs of circulating exfoliatin are absent. Bullous varicella is a disorder that represents bullous impetigo as a superinfection in varicella lesions. Treatment with oral antistaphylococcal drugs for 7–10 days is effective. Application of cool compresses to debride crusts is a helpful symptomatic measure.

Konig S, Verhagen AP, van Suijlekom-Smit LW et al: Interventions for impetigo. Cochrane Database Syst Rev 2004;2:CD003261 [PMID: 15106198].

Ecthyma

Ecthyma is a firm, dry crust, surrounded by erythema that exudes purulent material. It represents deep invasion by group A β-hemolytic streptococci through the epidermis to the superficial dermis. Treatment is with systemic penicillin. This should not be confused with ecthyma gangrenosum. Lesions of ecthyma gangrenosum may be similar in appearance, but they are seen in a severely ill or immunocompromised patient and are due to systemic dissemination of bacteria, usually *Pseudomonas aeruginosa,* through the bloodstream.

Cellulitis

Cellulitis is characterized by erythematous, hot, tender, ill-defined, edematous plaques accompanied by regional lymphadenopathy. Histologically, this disorder represents invasion of microorganisms into the lower dermis and sometimes beyond, with obstruction of local lymphatics. Group A β-hemolytic streptococci and coagulase-positive staphylococci are the most common causes; pneumococci and *Haemophilus influenzae* are rare causes. Staphylococcal infections are usually more localized and more likely to have a purulent center; streptococcal infections spread more rapidly, but these characteristics cannot be used to specify the infecting agent. An entry site of prior trauma or infection (eg, varicella) is often present. Septicemia is a potential complication. Treatment is with an appropriate systemic antibiotic.

FOLLICULITIS

A pustule at a follicular opening represents folliculitis. If the pustule occurs at eccrine sweat orifices, it is correctly called poritis. Staphylococci and streptococci are the most frequent pathogens. Treatment consists of measures to remove follicular obstruction—either cool, wet compresses for 24 hours or keratolytics such as those used for acne.

Luelmo-Aguilar J, Santandreu MS: Folliculitis: Recognition and management. Am J Clin Dermatol 2004;5:301 [PMID: 15554731].

Abscess

An abscess occurs deep in the skin, at the bottom of a follicle or an apocrine gland, and is diagnosed as an erythematous, firm, acutely tender nodule with ill-defined borders. Staphylococci are the most common organisms. Treatment consists of incision and drainage and systemic antibiotics.

Scalded Skin Syndrome

This entity consists of the sudden onset of bright red, acutely painful skin, most obvious periorally, periorbitally, and in the flexural areas of the neck, the axillae, the popliteal and antecubital areas, and the groin. The slightest pressure on the skin results in severe pain and separation of the epidermis, leaving a glistening layer (the stratum granulosum of the epidermis) beneath. The disease is caused by a circulating toxin (exfoliatin) elaborated by phage group II staphylococci. Exfoliatin binds to desmoglein-1 resulting in a separation of cells in the granular layer. The causative staphylococci may be isolated not from the skin but rather from the nasopharynx, an abscess, sinus, blood culture, and so on. Treatment is with systemic antistaphylococcal drugs.

Patel GK: Treatment of staphylococcal scalded skin syndrome. Expert Rev Anit Infect 2004;2:575 [PMID: 15482221].

Hedrick J: Acute bacterial skin infections in pediatric medicine: Current issues in presentation and treatment. Paedriatr Drugs 2003;5[Suppl 1]:35 [PMID: 14632104].

FUNGAL INFECTIONS OF THE SKIN

1. Dermatophyte Infections

Dermatophytes become attached to the superficial layer of the epidermis, nails, and hair, where they proliferate. They grow mainly within the stratum corneum and do not invade the lower epidermis or dermis. Release of toxins from dermatophytes, especially those whose natural hosts are animals or soil, for example, *Microsporum canis* and *Trichophyton verrucosum*—results in dermatitis. Fungal infection should be suspected with any red and scaly lesion.

Classification & Diagnosis

A. Tinea Capitis

Thickened, broken-off hairs with erythema and scaling of underlying scalp are the distinguishing features (Table 14–7). In endemic ringworm, hairs are broken off at the surface of the scalp, leaving a "black dot" appearance. Pustule formation and a boggy, fluctuant mass on the scalp occur in *M canis* and *T tonsurans* infections. This mass, called a kerion, represents an exaggerated host response to the organism. Diffuse scaling of the scalp may also be seen. Fungal culture should be performed in all cases of suspected tinea capitis.

B. Tinea Corporis

Tinea corporis presents either as annular marginated papules with a thin scale and clear center or as an annular confluent dermatitis. The most common organisms are *Trichophyton mentagrophytes* and *M canis*. The diagnosis is made by scraping thin scales from the border of the lesion, dissolving them in 20% KOH, and examining for hyphae.

Table 14–7. Clinical features of tinea capitis.

Most Common Organisms	Clinical Appearance	Microscopic Appearance in KOH
Trichophyton tonsurans (90%)	Hairs broken off 2–3 mm from follicle; "black dot"; diffuse pustule; seborrheic dermatitis-like; no fluorescence	Hyphae and spores within hair
Microsporum canis (10%)	Thickened broken-off hairs that fluoresce yellow-green with Wood's lamp	Small spores outside of hair; hyphae within hair

C. Tinea Cruris

Symmetrical, sharply marginated lesions in inguinal areas occur with tinea cruris. The most common organisms are *Trichophyton rubrum, T mentagrophytes,* and *Epidermophyton floccosum.*

D. Tinea Pedis

The diagnosis of tinea pedis is becoming more common in the prepubertal child, although it is still most commonly seen in postpubertal males. Presentation is with red scaly soles, blisters on the instep of the foot, or fissuring between the toes.

E. Tinea Unguium (Onychomycosis)

Loosening of the nail plate from the nail bed (onycholysis), giving a yellow discoloration, is the first sign of fungal invasion of the nails. Thickening of the distal nail plate then occurs, followed by scaling and a crumbly appearance of the entire nail plate surface. *T rubrum* and *T mentagrophytes* are the most common causes. The diagnosis is confirmed by KOH examination and fungal culture. Usually only one or two nails are involved. If every nail is involved, psoriasis, lichen planus, or idiopathic trachyonychia is a more likely diagnosis than fungal infection.

Treatment

The treatment of dermatophytosis is quite simple: If hair is involved, griseofulvin is the treatment of choice. Topical antifungal agents do not enter hair or nails in sufficient concentration to clear the infection. The absorption of griseofulvin from the gastrointestinal tract is enhanced by a fatty meal; thus, whole milk or ice cream taken with the medication increases absorption. The dosage of griseofulvin is 20 mg/kg/d. With hair infections, cultures should be done every 4 weeks, and treatment should be continued for 4 weeks following a negative culture. The side effects are few, and the drug has been used successfully in the newborn period. Itraconazole and terbinafine have been used when response to griseofulvin is unsatisfactory. For nails, daily administration of topical ciclopirox 8% (Penlac nail lacquer) can be considered, as can pulsed-dose itraconazole given in three 1-week pulses separated by 3 weeks.

Tinea corporis, tinea pedis, and tinea cruris can be treated effectively with topical medication after careful inspection to make certain that the hair and nails are not involved. Treatment with any of the imidazoles, allylamines, benzylamines, or ciclopirox applied twice daily for 3–4 weeks is recommended.

2. Tinea Versicolor

Tinea versicolor is a superficial infection caused by *Pityrosporum orbiculare* (also called *Malassezia furfur*), a yeast-like fungus. It characteristically causes polycyclic connected hypopigmented macules and very fine scales in areas of sun-induced pigmentation. In winter, the polycyclic macules appear reddish brown.

Treatment consists of application of selenium sulfide (Selsun), 2.5% suspension, or topical antifungals. Selenium sulfide should be applied to the whole body and left on overnight. Treatment can be repeated again in 1 week and then monthly thereafter. It tends to be somewhat irritating, and the patient should be warned about this difficulty.

Gupta AK, Cooper EA, Ryder JE et al: Optimal management of fungal infections of the skin, hair, and nails. Am J Clin Dermatol 2004;5:225 [PMID: 15301570].

3. Candida albicans *Infections* *(See Also Chapter 39)*

In addition to being a frequent invader in diaper dermatitis, *Candida albicans* also infects the oral mucosa, where it appears as thick white patches with an erythematous base (thrush); the angles of the mouth, where it causes fissures and white exudate (perlêche); and the cuticular region of the fingers, where thickening of the cuticle, dull red erythema, and distortion of growth of the nail plate suggest the diagnosis of candidal paronychia. *Candida* dermatitis is characterized by sharply defined erythematous patches, sometimes with eroded areas. Pustules, vesicles, or papules may be present as satellite lesions. Similar infections may be found in other moist areas, such as the axillae and neck folds. This infection is more common in children who have recently received antibiotics.

A topical imidazole cream is the drug of first choice for *C albicans* infections. In diaper dermatitis, the cream form can be applied every 3–4 hours. In oral thrush, nystatin suspension should be applied directly to the mucosa with the parent's finger or a cotton-tipped applicator, because it is not absorbed and acts topically. In candidal paronychia, the antifungal agent is applied over the area, covered with occlusive plastic wrapping, and left on overnight after the application is made airtight. Refractory candidiasis will respond to a brief course of oral fluconazole.

Kyle AA, Dahl MV: Topical therapy for fungal infections. Am J Clin Dermatol 2004;5:443 [PMID: 15663341].

VIRAL INFECTIONS OF THE SKIN (See Chapter 36.)

Herpes Simplex

Painful, grouped vesicles or erosions on a red base suggest herpes simplex. Rapid immunofluorescent tests for herpes simplex virus (HSV) and varicella-zoster virus (VZV) are available. A Tzanck smear is done by scraping a vesicle base with a No. 15 blade, smearing on a glass slide, and staining the epithelial cells with Wright stain. This is positive if there are epidermal multinucleated giant cells visualized. A positive Tzanck indicates herpesvirus infection (HSV or VZV). In infants and children, lesions resulting from herpes simplex type 1 are seen most commonly on the gingiva, lips, and face. Involvement of a digit (herpes whitlow) will occur if the child sucks the thumb or fingers. Herpes simplex type 2 lesions are seen on the genitalia and in the mouth in adolescents. Cutaneous dissemination of herpes simplex occurs in patients with atopic dermatitis (eczema herpeticum) and appears clinically as very tender, punched out erosions among the eczematous skin changes. The treatment of HSV infections is discussed in Chapter 36.

Waggoner-Fountain LA, Grossman LB: Herpes simplex virus. Pediatr Rev 2004;25:86 [PMID: 14993516].

Whitley RJ: Herpes simplex virus in children. Curr Treat Options Neurol 2002;4:231 [PMID: 11931730].

Varicella-Zoster

Grouped vesicles in a dermatome, usually on the trunk or face, suggest varicella-zoster reactivation. Zoster in children may not be painful and usually has a mild course. In patients with compromised host resistance, the appearance of an erythematous border around the vesicles is a good prognostic sign. Conversely, large bullae without a tendency to crusting and systemic illness imply a poor host response to the virus. Varicella-zoster and herpes simplex lesions undergo the same series of changes: papule, vesicle, pustule, crust, slightly depressed scar. Lesions of primary varicella appear in crops, and many different stages of lesions are present at the same time (eg, papules), eccentrically placed vesicles on an erythematous base ("dew drop" on a rose petal), erosions, and crusts.

Antihistamines may be used for pruritus, cool baths or drying lotions such as calamine lotion are usually sufficient to relieve symptoms. In immunosuppressed children, intravenous or oral acyclovir should be used.

Chen TM et al: Clinical manifestations of varicella-zoster virus infection. Dermatol Clin 2002;20:267 [PMID: 12120440].

Feder HM Jr, Hoss DM: Herpes zoster in otherwise healthy children. Pediatr Infect Dis J 2004;23:451 [PMID: 15131470].

Human Immunodeficiency Virus Infection (See also Chapter 37.)

The average time of onset of skin lesions after perinatally acquired human immunodeficiency virus (HIV) infection is 4 months; after transfusion-acquired infection, it is 11 months. Persistent oral candidiasis and recalcitrant candidal diaper rash are the most frequent cutaneous features of infantile HIV infection. Severe or recurrent herpetic gingivostomatitis, varicella-zoster infection, and molluscum contagiosum infection occur. Recurrent staphylococcal pyodermas, tinea of the face, and onychomycosis are also observed. A generalized dermatitis with features of seborrhea (severe cradle cap) is extremely common. In general, persistent, recurrent, or extensive skin infections should make one suspicious of HIV infection.

Garman ME, Tyring SK: The cutaneous manifestations of HIV infection. Dermatol Clin 2002;20:193 [PMID: 12120434].

Stefanaki C et al: Skin manifestations of HIV-1 infection in children. Clin Dermatol 2002;20:74 [PMID: 11849897].

Wananukul S et al: Mucocutaneous findings in pediatric AIDS related to degree of immunosuppression. Pediatr Dermatol 2003;20:289 [PMID: 1286945].

Virus-Induced Tumors

A. MOLLUSCUM CONTAGIOSUM

Molluscum contagiosum is a poxvirus that induces the epidermis to proliferate, forming a pale papule. Molluscum contagiosum consists of umbilicated, white or whitish yellow papules in groups on the genitalia or trunk. They are common in infants and preschool children, as well as sexually active adolescents. Treatment for molluscum includes topical imiquimod, topical cantharidin, oral cimetidine, cryotherapy with liquid nitrogen, and curettage. Left untreated, they will resolve over months to years.

Silverberg NB: Warts and molluscum in children. Adv Dermatol 2004;20:23 [PMID: 15544196].

Smith KJ, Skelton H: Molluscum contagiosum: Recent advances in pathogenic mechanisms and new therapies. Am J Clin Dermatol 2002;3:535 [PMID: 12358555].

B. WARTS

Warts are skin-colored papules with irregular (verrucous) surfaces. They are intraepidermal tumors caused by infection with human papillomavirus (HPV). There are over 100 types of this DNA virus which induces the epidermal cells to proliferate, thus resulting in the warty growth. Flat warts are smoother and smaller than common warts and are often seen on the face. Certain types of HPV are associated with certain types of warts (eg, flat warts) or location of warts (eg, genital warts).

No therapy for warts is ideal and 30% of warts will clear in 6 months irrespective of the therapy chosen.

The gold standard of therapy for the common (vulgaris) wart is liquid nitrogen. The treated lesion should stay white for 20 seconds. Aggressive treatment with prolonged freeze times and too much pressure applied with a cotton applicator can lead to blistering and scarring. The patient should be seen at treatment intervals of 2–3 weeks. Longer times between treatments result in lower efficacy. Large mosaic plantar warts are treated most effectively by applying 40% salicylic acid plaster cut with a scissors to fit the lesion. The adhesive side of the plaster is placed against the lesion and taped securely in place with duct, electrician's, or athletic tape. The plaster and tape should be placed on Monday and removed on Friday. Over the weekend, the patient should soak the skin in warm water for 30 minutes to soften it. Then the white, macerated tissue should be pared with a pumice stone, cuticle scissors, or a nail file. This procedure is repeated every week, and the patient is seen every 4 weeks. Most plantar warts resolve in 6–8 weeks when treated in this way. Vascular pulsed dye lasers are a useful adjunct therapy for the treatment of plantar warts.

For flat warts, a good response to 0.05% tretinoin cream or topical imiquimod (Aldara) cream, applied once daily for 3–4 weeks, has been reported.

Surgical excision, electrosurgery, and nonspecific burning laser surgery should be avoided; these modalities do not have higher cure rates and result in scarring.

Venereal warts (condylomata acuminata) (see Chapter 40) may be treated with imiquimod, 25% podophyllum resin (podophyllin) in alcohol, or podofilox, a lower concentration of purified podophyllin which is applied at home. Podophyllin should be painted on the lesions in the practitioner's office and then washed off after 4 hours. Re-treatment in 2–3 weeks may be necessary. Podofilox is applied by the patient daily, whereas imiquimod is used 3 times a week on alternating days. Lesions not on the vulvar mucous membrane but on the adjacent skin should be treated as a common wart and frozen.

For periungual warts, a blistering agent called cantharidin is effective and painless in children. An undesirable complication is the appearance of warts along the margins of the cantharidin blister (ring wart). Cantharidin is applied to the skin, allowed to dry, and covered with occlusive tape or a bandage for 24 hours.

No wart therapy is immediately and definitively successful. Realistic expectations should be set and appropriate follow-up treatments scheduled.

Silverberg NB: Human papillomavirus infections in children. Curr Opin Pediatr 2004;16:402 [PMID: 15273501].

Smolinski KN, Yan AC: How and when to treat molluscum contagiosum and warts in children. Pediatr Ann 2005;34:211 [PMID: 15792113].

INSECT INFESTATIONS

Scabies

Scabies is suggested by linear burrows about the wrists, ankles, finger webs, areolas, anterior axillary folds, genitalia, or face (in infants). Often there are excoriations, honey-colored crusts, and pustules from secondary infection. Identification of the female mite or her eggs and feces is necessary to confirm the diagnosis. Scrape an unscratched papule or burrow with a No. 15 blade and examine microscopically in immersion oil to confirm the diagnosis. In a child who is often scratching, scrape under the fingernails. Examine the parents for unscratched burrows. Permethrin 5% is now the treatment of choice for scabies. It should be applied as a single overnight application. The need for re-treatment is rare.

McCarthy JS et al: Scabies: More than just an irritation. Postgrad Med J 2004;80:382 [PMID: 15254301].

Pediculoses (Louse Infestations)

The presence of excoriated papules and pustules and a history of severe itching at night suggest infestation with the human body louse. This louse may be discovered in the seams of underwear but not on the body. In the scalp hair, the gelatinous nits of the head louse adhere tightly to the hair shaft. The pubic louse may be found crawling among pubic hairs, or blue-black macules may be found dispersed through the pubic region (maculae cerulea). The pubic louse is often seen on the eyelashes of newborns. Initial treatment of head lice is often instituted by parents with an over-the-counter pyrethrin or permethrin. If head lice are not eradicated after 2 applications 7 days apart with these products, 5% permethrin should be used. Malathion 0.5% is highly effective, but is toxic if ingested, and flammable. It should only be used in resistant cases.

Frankowski BL: American Academy of Pediatrics guidelines for the prevention and treatment of head lice. Am J Manag Care 2004;10:S269 [PMID: 15515631].

Papular Urticaria

Papular urticaria is characterized by grouped erythematous papules surrounded by an urticarial flare and distributed over the shoulders, upper arms, and buttocks in infants. Although not a true infestation, these lesions represent delayed hypersensitivity reactions to stinging or biting insects and can be reproduced by patch testing with the offending insect. Fleas from dogs and cats are the usual offenders. Less commonly, mosquitoes, lice, scabies, and bird and grass mites are involved. The sensitivity is transient, lasting 4–6 months. Usually no other family members are affected. It is often difficult for the parents to understand why no one else is affected. The logical therapy is to remove the offending insect, although in most cases it is very difficult to identify the exact cause. Topical corticosteroids and oral antihistamines will control symptoms.

Demain JG: Papular urticaria and things that bite in the night. Curr Allergy Asthma Rep 2003;3:291 [PMID: 12791206].

DERMATITIS (Eczema)

The terms *dermatitis* and *eczema* are currently used interchangeably in dermatology, although the term *eczema* truly denotes an acute weeping dermatosis. All forms of dermatitis, regardless of cause, may present with acute edema, erythema, and oozing with crusting, mild erythema alone, or lichenification. Lichenification is diagnosed by thickening of the skin with a shiny surface and exaggerated, deepened skin markings. It is the response of the skin to chronic rubbing or scratching.

Although the lesions of the various dermatoses are histologically indistinguishable, clinicians have nonetheless divided the disease group called dermatitis into several categories based on known causes in some cases and differing natural histories in others.

1. Atopic Dermatitis

Atopic dermatitis is a general term for chronic superficial inflammation of the skin that can be applied to a heterogeneous group of patients. Many (not all) patients go through three clinical phases. In the first, infantile eczema, the dermatitis begins on the cheeks and scalp and frequently expresses itself as oval patches on the trunk, later involving the extensor surfaces of the extremities. The usual age at onset is 2–3 months, and this phase ends at age 18 months to 2 years. Only one-third of all infants with infantile eczema progress to phase 2 childhood or flexural eczema in which the predominant involvement is in the antecubital and popliteal fossae, the neck, the wrists, and sometimes the hands or feet. This phase lasts from age 2 years to adolescence. Some children will have involvement only of the soles of the feet, with cracking, redness, and pain, so-called atopic feet. Only one-third of children with typical flexural eczema will progress to adolescent eczema, which is usually manifested by the continuation of chronic flexural eczema alone with hand dermatitis. Atopic dermatitis is quite unusual after age 30 years.

Atopic dermatitis results from an interaction between susceptibility genes, the host environment, skin barrier defects, pharmacologic abnormalities and immunologic response. The case for food and inhalant allergens as specific causes of atopic dermatitis is not strong. However, since the cause of atopic dermatitis remains unknown, there is debate between dermatologists and allergists on the exact role of allergy in atopic dermatitis. (See Chapter 34.)

A few patients with atopic dermatitis have immunodeficiency with recurrent pyodermas, unusual susceptibility to herpes simplex viruses, hyperimmunoglobulinemia E, defective neutrophil and monocyte chemotaxis, and impaired T-lymphocyte function. (See Chapter 29.)

A faulty epidermal barrier may predispose the patient with atopic dermatitis to itchy skin. Inability to hold water within the stratum corneum results in rapid evaporation of water, shrinking of the stratum corneum, and cracks in the epidermal barrier. Such skin forms an ineffective barrier to the entry of various irritants—and, indeed, it may be clinically useful to regard atopic dermatitis as a primary-irritant contact dermatitis and simply tell the patient, you have sensitive skin. Chronic atopic dermatitis is frequently infected secondarily with *Staphylococcus aureus* or *Streptococcus pyogenes*. Patients with atopic dermatitis have a deficiency of antimicrobial peptides in their skin which may account for the susceptibility to recurrent skin infection.

Treatment

A. ACUTE STAGES

Application of wet dressings and topical corticosteroids is the treatment of choice for acute, weeping atopic eczema. A topical steroid preparation is applied two times daily and covered with wet dressings as outlined at the beginning of this chapter. Superinfection or colonization with *S aureus* is common, and appropriate systemic antibiotics may be necessary. If the expected improvement is not seen, bacterial cultures should be obtained to identify the possibility of an organism resistant to standard therapy.

B. CHRONIC STAGES

Treatment is aimed at avoiding irritants and restoring water to the skin. No soaps or harsh shampoos should be used, and the patient should avoid woolen or any rough clothing. Bathing is minimized to every second or third day. Twice-daily lubrication of the skin is very important.

Nonperfumed lotions or creams are suitable lubricants. Plain petrolatum is an acceptable lubricant, but some people find it too greasy and during hot weather it may also cause considerable sweat retention. Liberal use of Cetaphil lotion as a soap substitute four or five times a day is also satisfactory as a means of lubrication. A bedroom humidifier is often helpful. Topical corticosteroids should be limited to medium strength (see Table 14–3). There is never any reason to use super- or high-potency corticosteroids in atopic dermatitis. In superinfected atopic dermatitis, systemic antibiotics for 10–14 days are necessary.

Topical tacrolimus and pimecrolimus are topical immunosuppressive agents that are effective in atopic dermatitis. Due to concerns about the development of malignancies, tacrolimus and pimecrolimus should be reserved for children older than 2 years of age with atopic dermatitis unresponsive to medium-potency topical steroids. It has been argued that an increased risk of malignancy has not been seen in immunologically normal individuals using these products. Recommendations for usage likely will change with time. Treatment failures in chronic atopic dermatitis are most often the result of patient noncompliance. This is a frustrating disease for parent and child. Return to a normal lifestyle for the parent and child is the ultimate goal of therapy.

Beck LA: The efficacy and safety of tacrolimus ointment: A clinical review. J Am Acad Dermatol 2005;53:S165 [PMID: 16021171].

Izadpanah A, Gallo RL: Antimicrobial peptides. J Am Acad Dermatol 2005;52:381 [PMID: 15761415].

Williams HC: Atopic dermatitis. N Engl J Med 2005;353:2314 [PMID: 15930422].

2. Nummular Eczema

Nummular eczema is characterized by numerous symmetrically distributed coin-shaped patches of dermatitis, principally on the extremities. These may be acute, oozing, and crusted or dry and scaling. The differential diagnosis should include tinea corporis, impetigo, and atopic dermatitis.

The same topical measures should be used as for atopic dermatitis, although treatment is often more difficult.

3. Primary Irritant Contact Dermatitis (Diaper Dermatitis)

Contact dermatitis is of two types: primary irritant and allergic eczematous. Primary irritant dermatitis develops within a few hours, reaches peak severity at 24 hours, and then disappears. Allergic eczematous contact dermatitis (described in the next section) has a delayed onset of 18 hours, peaks at 48–72 hours, and often lasts as long as 2–3 weeks even if exposure to the offending antigen is discontinued.

Diaper dermatitis, the most common form of primary irritant contact dermatitis seen in pediatric practice, is caused by prolonged contact of the skin with urine and feces, which contain irritating chemicals such as urea and intestinal enzymes. The diagnosis of diaper dermatitis is based on the picture of erythema and scaling of the skin in the perineal area and the history of prolonged skin contact with urine or feces. This is frequently seen in the "good baby" who sleeps many hours through the night without waking. In 80% of cases of diaper dermatitis lasting more than 3 days, the affected area is colonized with *C albicans* even before appearance of the classic signs of a beefy red, sharply marginated dermatitis with satellite lesions.

Treatment consists of changing diapers frequently. Because rubber or plastic pants prevent evaporation of the contactant and enhance its penetration into the skin, they should be avoided as much as possible. Air drying is useful. Streptococcal perianal cellulitis and infantile psoriasis should be included in the differential diagnosis. Treatment of long-standing diaper dermatitis should include application of nystatin or an imidazole cream with each diaper change.

Gupta AK, Skinner AR: Management of diaper dermatitis. Intl J Dermatol 2004;43:830 [PMID: 15533067].

4. Allergic Eczematous Contact Dermatitis (Poison Ivy Dermatitis)

Plants such as poison ivy, poison sumac, and poison oak cause most cases of allergic contact dermatitis in children. Allergic contact dermatitis has all the features of delayed-type (T-lymphocyte–mediated) hypersensitivity. Many substances may cause such a reaction; nickel sulfate, potassium dichromate, and neomycin are the most common causes. Nickel is found to some degree in all metals. Nickel allergy is commonly seen on the ears secondary to the wearing of earrings, and near the umbilicus from pants snaps and belt buckles. The true incidence of allergic contact dermatitis in children is unknown. Children often present with acute dermatitis with blister formation, oozing, and crusting. Blisters are often linear and of acute onset.

Treatment of contact dermatitis in localized areas is with topical corticosteroids. In severe generalized involvement, prednisone, 1–2 mg/kg/d orally for 10–14 days, can be used.

Bruckner AL, Weston WL: Allergic contact dermatitis in children: A practical approach to management. Skin Therapy Lett 2002;7:3 [PMID: 12548328].

5. Seborrheic Dermatitis

Seborrheic dermatitis is an erythematous scaly dermatitis accompanied by overproduction of sebum occurring in areas rich in sebaceous glands (ie, the face, scalp, and perineum). This common condition occurs predominantly in the newborn and at puberty, the ages at which hormonal stimulation of sebum production is maximal. Although it is tempting to speculate that overproduction of sebum causes the dermatitis, the exact relationship is unclear.

Seborrheic dermatitis on the scalp in infancy is clinically similar to atopic dermatitis, and the distinction may become clear only after other areas are involved. Psoriasis also occurs in seborrheic areas in older children and should be considered in the differential diagnosis.

Seborrheic dermatitis responds well to low-potency topical corticosteroids.

Gupta AK, Kogan N: Seborrheic dermatitis: Current treatment practices. Expert Opin Pharmacother 2004;5:1755 [PMID: 15264990].

6. Dandruff

Physiologic scaling or mild seborrhea, in the form of greasy scalp scales, may be treated by medicated dandruff shampoos. The cause is unknown.

7. Dry Skin Dermatitis (Asteatotic Eczema, Xerosis)

Newborns and older children who live in arid climates are susceptible to dry skin, characterized by large cracked scales with erythematous borders. The stratum corneum is dependent on environmental humidity for its water, and below 30% environmental humidity the stratum corneum loses water, shrinks, and cracks. These cracks in the epidermal barrier allow irritating substances to enter the skin, predisposing the patient to dermatitis.

Treatment consists of increasing the water content of the skin in the immediate external environment. House humidifiers are very useful. Minimize bathing to every second or third day.

Frequent soaping of the skin impairs its water-holding capacity and serves as an irritating alkali, and all soaps should therefore be avoided. Frequent use of emollients (eg, Cetaphil, Eucerin, Lubriderm) should be a major part of therapy.

8. Keratosis Pilaris

Follicular papules containing a white inspissated scale characterize keratosis pilaris. Individual lesions are discrete and may be red. They are prominent on the extensor surfaces of the upper arms and thighs and on the buttocks and cheeks. In severe cases, the lesions may be generalized. Such lesions are seen frequently in children with dry skin and have also been associated with atopic dermatitis and ichthyosis vulgaris.

Treatment is with keratolytics such as urea creams, lactic acid, or topical retinoic acid followed by skin hydration.

9. Pityriasis Alba

White, scaly macular areas with indistinct borders are seen over extensor surfaces of extremities and on the cheeks in children with pityriasis alba. Suntanning exaggerates these lesions. Histologic examination reveals a mild dermatitis. These lesions may be confused with tinea versicolor. Low-potency topical steroids may help decrease any inflammatory component and may lead to faster return of normal pigmentation.

Blessman-Weber M et al: Pityriasis alba: A study of pathogenic factors. J Eur Acad Dermatol Venereol 2002;16:463 [PMID: 12428838].

COMMON SKIN TUMORS

If the skin moves with the nodule on lateral palpation, the tumor is located within the dermis; if the skin moves over the nodule, it is subcutaneous. Seventy-five percent of lumps in childhood will be either epidermal inclusion cysts (60%) or pilomatrichomas (15%).

Epidermoid Cysts

These are the most common type of cutaneous cyst. Other names for epidermoid cysts are epidermal cysts, epidermal inclusion cysts, and "sebaceous" cysts. This last term is a misnomer since they contain neither sebum nor sebaceous glands. Epidermoid cysts can occur anywhere, but are most common on the face and upper trunk. They usually arise from and are lined by the stratified squamous epithelium of the follicular infundibulum. Clinically, epidermoid cysts are dermal nodules with a central punctum, representing the follicle associated with the cyst. They can reach several centimeters in diameter. These lesions can rupture, causing a foreign-body inflammatory reaction, or become infected. Infectious complications should be treated with antibiotics and drainage. Definitive treatment is surgical excision. **Dermoid cysts** are areas of sequestration of skin along embryonic fusion lines. They are present at birth and occur most commonly on the lateral eyebrow. Treatment, if desired, is surgical excision.

Pilomatrichomas are benign tumors of the hair matrix. They are most commonly seen on the face and upper trunk. They are firm and may be irregular. Their color varies from flesh-colored to pink or blue. The firmness is secondary to calcification of the tumor. Treatment is by surgical excision.

Granuloma Annulare

Circles or semicircles of nontender intradermal nodules found over the lower legs and ankles, the dorsum of the hands and wrists, and the trunk, in that order of frequency, suggest granuloma annulare. Histologically, the disease appears as a central area of tissue death (necrobiosis) surrounded by macrophages and lymphocytes. No treatment is necessary. Lesions resolve spontaneously within 1–2 years in most children.

Pyogenic Granuloma

These lesions appear over 1–2 weeks following skin trauma as a dark red papule with an ulcerated and crusted surface that may bleed easily even with minor trauma. Histologically, this represents excessive new vessel formation with or without inflammation (granulation tissue). It should be regarded as an abnormal healing response. Pulsed dye laser for very small lesions or curettage followed by electrocautery are the treatments of choice.

Keloids

Keloids are scars of delayed onset that continue for up to several years to progress beyond the initial wound margins. The tendency to keloid is inherited. They are often found on the face, earlobes, neck, chest, and back. Treatment includes intralesional injection with triamcinolone acetonide, 20 mg/mL, or excision and injection with corticosteroids. A recent study suggested that ear piercing before age 11 is associated with a decreased risk of keloid formation.

Lane JE, Waller JL, Davis LS: Relationship between age of ear piercing and keloid formation. Pediatrics 2005;115:1312 [PMID: 15867040].

Luba MC et al: Common benign skin tumors. Am Fam Physician 2003;67:729 [PMID: 12613727].

PAPULOSQUAMOUS ERUPTIONS

Papulosquamous eruptions (Table 14–8) comprise papules or plaques with varying degrees of scale.

1. Pityriasis Rosea

Pink to red, oval plaques with fine scales that tend to align with their long axis parallel to skin tension lines (eg, "Christmas tree pattern" on the back) are characteristic lesions of pityriasis rosea. In 20–80% of cases the generalized eruption is preceded for up to 30 days by a solitary, larger, scaling plaque with central clearing and a scaly border (the herald patch). The herald patch is clinically similar to ringworm and can be confused. In whites, the lesions are primarily on the trunk; in

Table 14–8. Papulosquamous eruptions in children.

Psoriasis
Pityriasis rosea
Tinea corporis
Lichen planus
Pityriasis lichenoides (acute or chronic)
Dermatomyositis
Lupus erythematosus
Pityriasis rubra pilaris
Secondary syphilis

---

blacks, lesions are primarily on the extremities and may be accentuated in the axillary and inguinal areas. This disease is common in school-age children and adolescents and is presumed to be viral in origin. The role of human herpes virus 7 in the pathogenesis of pityriasis rosea is debated. The condition lasts 6 weeks and may be pruritic. The major differential diagnosis is secondary syphilis, and a VDRL test should be done if syphilis is suspected, especially in high-risk patients with palm and/or sole involvement. Pityriasis rosea that lasts more than 12 weeks should be referred to a dermatologist for evaluation.

Exposure to natural sunlight may help hasten the resolution of lesions. Oral antihistamines can be used for pruritus. Often, no treatment is necessary.

Karnath B et al: Pityriasis rosea. Appearance and distribution of macules aid diagnosis. Postgrad Med 2003;113:94 [PMID: 12764899].

2. Psoriasis

Psoriasis is characterized by erythematous papules covered by thick white scales. Guttate (drop-like) psoriasis is a common form in children that often follows an episode of streptococcal pharyngitis by 2–3 weeks. The sudden onset of small papules (3–8 mm), seen predominantly over the trunk and quickly covered with thick white scales, is characteristic of guttate psoriasis. Chronic psoriasis is marked by thick, large scaly plaques (5–10 cm) over the elbows, knees, scalp, and other sites of trauma. Pinpoint pits in the nail plate are seen, as well as yellow discoloration of the nail plate resulting from onycholysis. Psoriasis occurs frequently on the scalp, elbows, knees, periumbilical area, ears, sacral area, and genitalia. It should always be in the differential of "dermatitis" on the scalp or genitalia of children.

The pathogenesis of psoriasis is complex and incompletely understood. It is a familial condition and there is increased epidermal turnover and inflammation. Psoriatic epidermis has a turnover time of 3–4 days versus

28 days for normal skin. These rapidly proliferating epidermal cells are producing excessive stratum corneum, giving rise to thick, opaque scales. Papulosquamous eruptions that present problems of differential diagnosis are listed in Table 14–8.

Treatment

Topical steroids are the initial treatment of choice. Penetration of topical corticosteroids through the enlarged epidermal barrier in psoriasis requires that more potent preparations be used, for example, fluocinonide 0.05% (Lidex) or clobetasol 0.05% (Temovate) ointment twice daily.

The second line of therapy is topical calcipotriene (Dovonex) applied twice daily or the combination of a superpotent topical steroid twice daily on weekends and calcipotriene twice daily on weekdays for 8 weeks.

Topical retinoids such as tazarotene (0.1%, 0.5% cream, gel) can be used in combination with topical corticosteroids to help restore normal epidermal differentiation and turnover time. However, these treatments can cause skin to become dry.

Anthralin therapy is also useful. Anthralin is applied to the skin for a short contact time (eg, 20 minutes once daily) and then washed off with a neutral soap (eg, Dove). A 6-week course of treatment is recommended. This can be used in combination with topical corticosteroids.

Crude coal tar therapy is messy and stains bedclothes. The newer tar gels (Estar, PsoriGel) cause less staining and are most efficacious. They are applied twice daily for 6–8 weeks. These preparations are sold over the counter and are not usually covered by insurance plans.

Scalp care using a tar shampoo requires leaving the shampoo on for 5 minutes, washing it off, and then shampooing with commercial shampoo to remove scales. It may be necessary to shampoo daily until scaling is reduced. More severe cases of psoriasis are best treated by a dermatologist.

Marcoux D, Prost Y: Pediatric psoriasis revisited. J Cutan Med Surg 2002;6:22 [PMID: 11976986].

Rogers M: Childhood psoriasis. Curr Opin Pediatr 2002;14:404 [PMID: 12130902].

HAIR LOSS (Alopecia)

Hair loss in children (Table 14–9) imposes great emotional stress on the patient and the parent. A 60% hair loss in a single area is necessary before hair loss can be detected clinically. Examination should begin with the scalp to determine whether there are inflammation, scale, or infiltrative changes. Hairs should be examined microscopically for breaking and structural defects and to see whether growing or resting hairs are being shed. Placing removed hairs in mounting fluid (Permount) on a glass microscope slide makes them easy to examine. Three dis-

Table 14–9. Other causes of hair loss in children.

Hair loss with scalp changes
Atrophy:
Lichen planus
Lupus erythematosus
Nodules and tumors:
Epidermal nevus
Nevus sebaceus
Thickening:
Burn
Hair loss with hair shaft defects (hair fails to grow out enough to require haircuts)
Monilethrix—alternating bands of thin and thick areas
Pili annulati—alternating bands of light and dark pigmentation
Pili torti—hair twisted 180 degrees, brittle
Trichorrhexis invaginata (bamboo hair)—intussusception of one hair into another
Trichorrhexis nodosa—nodules with fragmented hair

eases account for most cases of hair loss in children: alopecia areata, tinea capitis (described earlier in this chapter), and hair pulling.

Alopecia Areata

Loss of every hair in a localized area is called alopecia areata. This is the most common cause of hair loss in children. An immunologic pathogenic mechanism is suspected because dense infiltration of lymphocytes precedes hair loss. Ninety-five percent of children with alopecia areata completely regrow their hair within 12 months, although as many as 40% may have a relapse in 5–6 years. A rare and unusual form of alopecia areata begins at the occiput and proceeds along the hair margins to the frontal scalp. This variety, called ophiasis, often eventuates in total scalp hair loss (alopecia totalis). The prognosis for regrowth in ophiasis is poor.

Treatment of alopecia areata is difficult. Systemic corticosteroids given to suppress the inflammatory response will result in hair growth, but the hair may fall out again when the drug is discontinued. Superpotent topical steroids, minoxidil (Rogaine), and anthralin are treatment options. In children with alopecia totalis, a wig is most helpful.

Tan E et al: A clinical study of childhood alopecia areata in Singapore. Pediatr Dermatol 2002;19:298 [PMID: 12220271].

Hair Pulling

Traumatic hair pulling causes the hair shafts to be broken off at different lengths, with an ill-defined area of hair loss, petechiae around follicular openings, and a wrinkled hair shaft on microscopic examination. This behavior may be merely habit, an acute reaction to severe stress, or a sign of a psychiatric disorder (trichotillomania). Eyelashes and eyebrows rather than scalp hair may be pulled out. If the behavior has a long history, psychiatric evaluation may be helpful. Oiling the hair to make it slippery is an aid to behavior modification.

Harrison S, Sinclair R: Optimal management of hair loss (alopecia) in children. Am J Clin Dermatol 2003;4:757 [PMID: 14572298].

REACTIVE ERYTHEMAS

Erythema Multiforme

Erythema multiforme begins with papules that later develop a dark center and then evolve into lesions with central bluish discoloration or blisters and the characteristic target lesions (iris lesions) that have three concentric circles of color change. Primary injury is to endothelial cells, with later destruction of epidermal basal cells. Erythema multiforme has sometimes been diagnosed in patients with severe mucous membrane involvement, but Stevens–Johnson syndrome is the usual diagnosis when severe involvement of conjunctiva, oral cavity, and genital mucosa also occur.

Many causes are suspected, particularly concomitant herpes simplex virus, drugs, especially sulfonamides, and *Mycoplasma* infections. Recurrent erythema multiforme is usually associated with reactivation of herpes simplex virus. In the mild form, spontaneous healing occurs in 10–14 days, but Stevens–Johnson syndrome may last 6–8 weeks.

Treatment is symptomatic in uncomplicated erythema multiforme. Removal of offending drugs is an obvious measure. Oral antihistamines such as hydroxyzine, 2 mg/kg/d orally, are useful. Cool compresses and wet dressings will relieve pruritus. Steroids have not been demonstrated to be effective. Chronic acyclovir therapy has been successful in decreasing attacks in those patients with herpes-associated recurrent erythema multiforme.

Forman R et al: Erythema multiforme, Stevens–Johnson syndrome and toxic epidermal necrolysis in children: A review of 10 years' experience. Drug Saf 2002;25:965 [PMID: 12381216].

Drug Eruptions

Drugs may produce urticarial, morbilliform, scarlatiniform, pustular, bullous, or fixed skin eruptions. Urticaria may appear within minutes after drug administration, but most reactions begin 7–14 days after the drug is first administered. These eruptions may occur in patients who have received these drugs for long periods, and eruptions continue for days after the drug has been discontinued. Drug eruptions with fever, eosinophilia, and systemic symptoms (DRESS syndrome) is most commonly seen with anticonvulsants, but may be seen with other drugs. Drugs commonly implicated in skin reactions are listed in Table 14–10.

Table 14–10. Common drug reactions.

Urticaria
Barbiturates
Opioids
Penicillins
Sulfonamides
Morbilliform eruption
Anticonvulsants
Cephalosporins
Penicillins
Sulfonamides
Fixed drug eruption/erythema multiforme/toxic epidermal necrolysis/Stevens-Johnson syndrome
Anticonvulsants
Nonsteroidal anti-inflammatory drugs
Sulfonamides
DRESS syndrome
Anticonvulsants
Photodermatitis
Psoralens
Sulfonamides
Tetracyclines
Thiazides

DRESS syndrome = drug eruptions with fever, eosinophilia, and systemic symptoms.

Millikan LE, Feldman M: Pediatric drug allergy. Clin Dermatol 2002;20:29 [PMID: 11849892].

Roujeau JC: Clinical heterogeneity of drug hypersensitivity. Toxicology 2005;209:123 [PMID: 15767024].

MISCELLANEOUS SKIN DISORDERS ENCOUNTERED IN PEDIATRIC PRACTICE

Aphthous Stomatitis

Recurrent erosions on the gums, lips, tongue, palate, and buccal mucosa are often confused with herpes simplex. A smear of the base of such a lesion stained with Wright stain will aid in ruling out herpes simplex by the absence of epithelial multinucleate giant cells. A culture for herpes simplex is also useful in differential diagnostics. The cause remains unknown, but T-cell–mediated cytotoxicity to various viral antigens has been postulated.

There is no specific therapy for this condition. Rinsing the mouth with liquid antacids will provide relief in most patients. Topical corticosteroids in a gel base may provide some relief. In severe cases that interfere with eating, prednisone, 1 mg/kg/d orally for 3–5 days, will suffice to abort an episode. Colchicine, 0.2–0.5 mg/d, sometimes reduces the frequency of attacks.

Akintoye SO, Greenberg MS: Recurrent aphthous stomatitis. Dent Clin North Am 2005;49:31 [PMID: 15567359].

Vitiligo

Vitiligo is characterized clinically by the development of areas of depigmentation. These are often symmetrical and occur mainly on extensor surfaces. The depigmentation results from a destruction of melanocytes. The basis for this destruction is unknown, but immunologically mediated damage is likely and vitiligo sometimes occurs in individuals with autoimmune endocrinopathies, selective IgA deficiency, or graft-versus-host disease. Treatment is not very effective. Potent topical steroids, tacrolimus, or both for 4 months are the initial treatment. Topical calcipotriene has also been used. Narrow-band ultraviolet B waves (UVB 311 nm) may be used in severe cases.

Handa S, Dogra S: Epidemiology of childhood vitiligo: A study of 625 patients from north India. Pediatr Dermatol 2003;20:207 [PMID: 12787267].

Silverberg NB et al: Tacrolimus ointment promotes repigmentation of vitiligo in children: A review of 57 cases. J Am Acad Dermatol 2004;51:760 [PMID: 15523355].

Eye

Rebecca Sands, MD, & Arlene Drack, MD

Normal vision is a sense that develops during infancy and childhood. To become adept requires a normal visual environment. The child must experience equally good visual inputs from well-aligned eyes during this period while the visual nervous system is still exhibiting plasticity. Thus, pediatric ophthalmology emphasizes early diagnosis and treatment of pediatric eye diseases in order to obtain the best possible visual outcome. But eye disease in children does not always originate in the ocular system. Abnormal eye findings in a child may be a sign of systemic disease.

COMMON NONSPECIFIC SIGNS & SYMPTOMS

Nonspecific signs and symptoms commonly occur as the chief complaint or as an element of the history of a child with eye disease. Five of these findings are presented in the following sections with a sixth—leukocoria—which is less common, but often has serious implications. Do not hesitate to seek the help of a pediatric ophthalmologist when you believe the diagnosis and treatment of these signs and symptoms requires in-depth clinical experience.

Redness

Redness (injection) of the bulbar conjunctiva or deeper vessels is a common presenting complaint. It may be mild and localized or diffuse and bilateral. Causes include superficial or penetrating foreign bodies, infection, allergy, and conjunctivitis associated with systemic entities such as Stevens-Johnson syndrome or Kawasaki disease. Irritating noxious agents also cause injection. Subconjunctival hemorrhage may be traumatic or spontaneous or may be associated with hematopoietic disease, vascular anomalies, or inflammatory processes. Uncommonly, an injected eye can be due to an intraocular or orbital tumor.

Tearing

Tearing in infants is usually due to nasolacrimal obstruction, but may also be associated with congenital glaucoma, in which case photophobia and blepharospasm may also be present. Inflammation, allergic and viral dis-

eases, or conjunctival and corneal irritation can also cause tearing.

Discharge

Purulent discharge is usually associated with bacterial conjunctivitis. In infants and toddlers with nasolacrimal obstruction, a mucopurulent discharge may be present with low-grade, chronic dacryocystitis. Watery discharge occurs with viral infection, iritis, superficial foreign bodies, and nasolacrimal obstruction. Mucoid discharge may be a sign of allergic conjunctivitis or nasolacrimal obstruction. A mucoid discharge due to allergy typically contains eosinophils; a purulent bacterial discharge will contain polymorphonuclear leukocytes.

Pain & Foreign Body Sensation

Pain in or around the eye may be due to foreign bodies, corneal abrasions, lacerations, acute infections of the globe or ocular adnexa, iritis, and angle-closure glaucoma. Large refractive errors, poor accommodative ability, and sinus disease may manifest as headaches. Trichiasis (inturned lashes) and contact lens problems also cause ocular discomfort.

Photophobia

Acute aversion to light may occur with corneal abrasions, foreign bodies, and iritis. Squinting of one eye in bright light is a common sign of intermittent exotropia. Photophobia is present in infants with glaucoma, albinism, aniridia, and retinal dystrophies such as achromatopsia. Photophobia is common after ocular surgery and after dilation of the pupil with mydriatic and cycloplegic agents. Photophobia in individuals with no ocular pathology may be due to migraine headache, meningitis, and retrobulbar optic neuritis.

Leukocoria

Although not a common sign or complaint, leukocoria (a white pupil) is associated with serious diseases and requires prompt ophthalmologic consultation. Causes of leukocoria include retinoblastoma, retinopathy of prematurity, pupillary membrane, cataract, vitreous

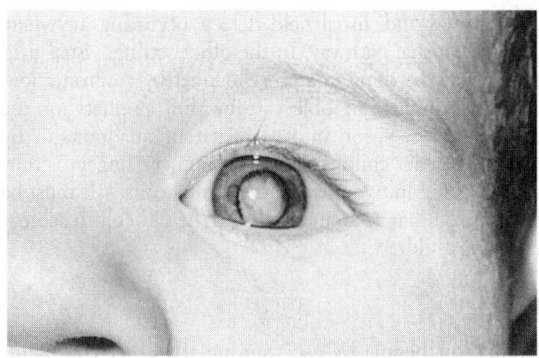

Figure 15–1. Leukocoria of the left eye caused by retrolental membrane (persistent hyperplastic primary vitreous or persistent fetal vasculature).

opacities, retinal detachment, *Toxocara* infection, and retinal dysplasia (Figure 15–1).

REFRACTIVE ERRORS

Refractive error refers to the optical state of the eye (Figure 15–2). It is a physical characteristic like height or weight and can be quantitated. Not all refractive errors require correction, but severe errors can cause amblyopia (reduced vision with or without an organic lesion) (see section on amblyopia and strabismus). Those that do can usually be corrected with glasses. Less often, contact lenses are required, usually for very high or asymmetrical refractive errors, or for adolescents who do not want to wear spectacles. Laser refractive surgery is not currently indicated for most children. There are three common refractive errors: myopia, hyperopia, and astigmatism. Inequality of the refractive state between the two eyes (anisometropia) can cause amblyopia. Children at particular risk for refractive errors requiring correction with spectacles include those who were born prematurely, those with Down syndrome, those who are offspring of parents with refractive errors, and those who have certain systemic conditions such as Stickler, Marfan, or Ehlers-Danlos syndrome.

Myopia (Nearsightedness)

For the myopic or nearsighted individual, objects nearby are in focus; those at a distance are blurred. This is because the plane of focus is anterior to the retina. The onset is typically at about age 8 years and may progress throughout adolescence and young adulthood. A myopic person may squint to produce a pinhole effect, which improves distance vision. Divergent lenses provide clear distance vision. Many studies have been done attempting to slow or stop myopic progression. Atropine eye drops have shown some effect, but

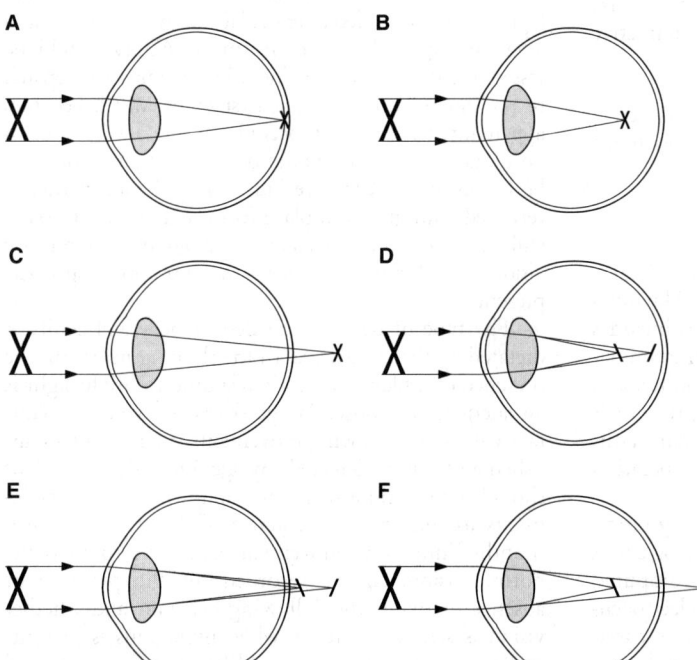

Figure 15–2. Different refractive states of the eye. **A:** Emmetropia. Image plane from parallel rays of light falls on retina. **B:** Myopia. Image plane focuses anterior to retina. **C:** Hyperopia. Image plane focuses posterior to retina. **D:** Astigmatism, myopic type. Images in horizontal and vertical planes focus anterior to retina. **E:** Astigmatism, hyperopic type. Images in horizontal and vertical planes focus posterior to retina. **F:** Astigmatism, mixed type. Images in horizontal and vertical planes focus on either side of the retina.

produce many side effects. A newer drug, pirenzepine, has shown promise in animal studies, and human studies are underway.

Tan DT et al, and Asian Pirenzepine Study Group: One-year multicenter, double-masked, placebo-controlled, parallel safety and efficacy study of 2% pirenzepine ophthalmic gel in children with myopia. Ophthalmology 2005;112:84 [PMID: 15629825].

Hyperopia (Farsightedness)

Saying that the hyperopic child is sighted for far (not near) is somewhat misleading, because the child can focus on near objects if the hyperopia is not excessive. Large amounts of uncorrected hyperopia can cause esotropia (inward deviation, or crossing, of the eyes) and amblyopia (see section on amblyopia and strabismus). Most infants have a hyperopic refraction that begins to diminish during the toddler years and does not require correction.

Astigmatism

When either the cornea or the crystalline lens is not perfectly spherical, an image will not be sharply focused in one plane. Schematically, there will be two planes of focus. Both of the planes can be either in front of or behind the retina, or one of the planes can be in front of the retina and the other behind it. This refractive state is described as astigmatism. Large amounts of astigmatism not corrected at an early age can cause decreased vision from amblyopia, but proper refractive correction can prevent this.

Harvey EM et al: Prescribing eyeglass correction for astigmatism in infancy and early childhood: a survey of AAPOS members. J AAPOS 2005;9:189 [PMID: 15838450].

EXAMINATION

Ophthalmic examination of the pediatric patient begins with a calm demeanor and reassuring voice. Having a parent present is invaluable. The examination includes a history, assessment of visual acuity, external examination, observation of ocular alignment and motility, and ophthalmoscopic examination. Intraocular pressure is less frequently measured. Testing of binocular status and near point is desirable when age and cooperation permit.

Circumstances will dictate the use of ancillary procedures such as instilling fluorescein dye and radiologic tests (magnetic resonance imaging [MRI] and computed tomography scan). Electroretinography and electrooculography test retinal function. Visual evoked response testing assesses the function of the cortical visual pathways. Visual field testing demonstrates the presence or absence of scotomas and visual field defects occurring anywhere along the visual pathway. In the office setting, visual field testing may be done in a gross manner by confrontation, that is, bringing an object from the periphery of the child's field of vision into each of four quadrants or by having an older child count the examiner's fingers as they are presented in two quadrants simultaneously. It must be emphasized that accurate results can be difficult to achieve in young children.

History

Evaluation begins by ascertaining the chief complaint and taking a history of the present illness. Elements of the history include onset of the complaint, its duration, whether it is monocular or binocular, treatment received thus far, and associated systemic symptoms. If an infectious disease is suspected, ask about possible contact with others having similar findings. The ocular history is obtained, as is the perinatal and developmental history and any history of allergy. The family history should be explored for ocular disorders that may be familial or inherited.

Visual Acuity

Visual acuity testing is the single most important test of visual function and should be part of every general physical examination. This is the non-ophthalmologist's most definitive test for amblyopia, refractive errors, and lesions along the optic pathways. The child's visual acuity should be tested and recorded after ocular trauma and before and after any ophthalmologic treatment. Acuity should be tested in each eye individually, using an adhesive eyepatch to prevent peeking. If latent nystagmus, which becomes apparent when one eye is occluded, is present (see section on nystagmus), vision should be tested simultaneously in both eyes and in each eye individually. Vision is usually recorded with glasses in place (corrected vision). In older children who can cooperate, use of a pinhole will improve vision in children not wearing the appropriate spectacle prescription.

The type of test used to determine visual acuity is dictated by the child's age. In the sleeping newborn, the presence of a blepharospastic response to bright light is an adequate response. At age 6 weeks, eye-to-eye contact with slow following movements is becoming established and can be detected. By age 3 months, the infant should demonstrate fixing and following ocular movements for objects at a distance of 2–3 feet. At age 6 months, interest in movement across the room is the norm. Vision can be recorded for the presence or absence of fixing and following behavior and whether vision is steady (unsteady when nystagmus is present) and maintained. Vision should be tested and recorded for each eye. Visual acuity can be quantified in infants using other techniques, such as the 15-diopter prism test, preferential looking technique, or the pattern visual evoked response.

In the verbal child, the use of familiar icons will allow for a quantitative test. Allen or Lea symbols with familiar pictures can be used to test children age ≤ 2–3 years. Four-year-old children are often ready to play the tumbling E game (in which the child identifies the orientation of the letter E, which is turned in one of four directions) or the HVOT letters game (in which these four letters are shown individually at a distance and matched on a board that the child is holding). Literate children are tested with letters. Typical acuity levels in developmentally appropriate children are approximately 20/60 or better in children ≤ 2–3 years old, 20/40–20/30 in 3-year-old children, 20/30–20/25 in 4-year-old children, and 20/20 in literate children 5–6 years old. Perhaps more important than the absolute visual acuity is the presence of a difference of acuity between the two eyes, which might be a sign of amblyopia, uncorrected refractive error, or disease. As little as one line difference in acuity should be considered significant.

The practitioner should be aware of two situations complicated by nystagmus. Children who require a face turn or torticollis (in which the head is tilted to the right or left) to quiet the nystagmus will have poor visual acuity results when tested in the absence of the compensatory head posture.

When latent nystagmus is present, acuity testing is particularly challenging (see section on nystagmus). Nystagmus appears or worsens when an eye is occluded, degrading central vision. To minimize the nystagmus, the occluder should be held about 12 inches in front of the eye not being tested. Testing both eyes simultaneously without occlusion often gives a better visual acuity measurement than when either eye is tested individually.

Becker R et al: Examination of young children with Lea symbols. Br J Ophthalmol 2002;86:513 [PMID: 11973243].

Kvarnstrom G, Jakobsson P: Is vision screening in 3-year-old children feasible? Comparison between the Lea Symbol chart and the HVOT (LM) chart. Acta Ophthalmol Scand 2005;83:76 [PMID: 15715562].

External Examination

Inspection of the anterior segment of the globe and its adnexa requires adequate illumination and often magnification. A penlight provides good illumination and should be used in both straight-ahead and oblique illumination. A Wood lamp or a blue filter cap placed over a penlight is needed for evaluation after applying a fluorescent stain. Immobilization of the child may be necessary. A drop of topical anesthetic may facilitate the examination. Assessment of the entire anterior segment except the trabecular meshwork, and to a lesser extent the lens, is possible.

In cases of suspected foreign body, pulling down on the lower lid provides excellent visualization of the inferior cul-de-sac (palpebral conjunctiva). Visualizing the upper cul-de-sac and superior bulbar conjunctiva is possible by having the patient look inferiorly while the upper lid is pulled away from the globe and the examiner peers into the upper recess. Illumination with a penlight is necessary. The upper lid should be everted to evaluate the superior tarsal conjunctiva (Figure 15–3).

When indicated for further evaluation of the cornea, a small amount of fluorescein solution should be instilled into the lower cul-de-sac. Blue light will stain defects yellow-green. Disease-specific staining patterns may be observed. For example, herpes simplex lesions of the corneal epithelium produce a dendrite or branch-like pattern. A foreign body lodged beneath the upper lid shows one or more vertical lines of stain on the cornea due to the constant movement of the foreign body over the cornea. Contact lens overwear produces a central staining pattern. A fine, scattered punctate pattern may be a sign of viral keratitis or medication toxicity. Punctate erosions of the inferior third of the cornea can be seen with staphylococcal blepharitis or exposure keratitis secondary to incomplete lid closure.

Pupils

The child's pupils should be evaluated for reaction to light, regularity of shape, and equality of size as well as for the presence of afferent pupillary defect. This defect,

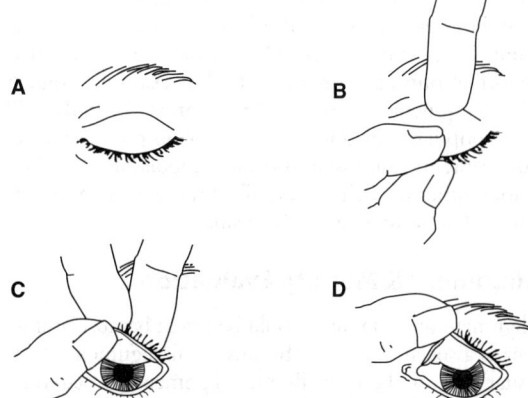

Figure 15–3. Eversion of the upper lid. **A:** The patient looks downward. **B:** The fingers pull the lid down, and an index finger or cotton tip is placed on the upper tarsal border. **C:** The lid is pulled up over the finger. **D:** The lid is everted.

Table 15–1. Function and innervation of each of the extraocular muscles.

Muscle	Function	Innervation
Medial rectus	Adductor	Oculomotor (third)
Lateral rectus	Abductor	Abducens (sixth)
Inferior rectus	Depressor Adductor Extorter	Oculomotor
Superior rectus	Elevator Adductor Intorter	Oculomotor
Inferior oblique	Elevator Abductor Extorter	Oculomotor
Superior oblique	Depressor Abductor Intorter	Trochlear (fourth)

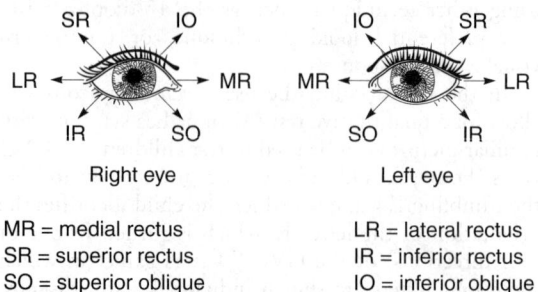

MR = medial rectus   LR = lateral rectus
SR = superior rectus   IR = inferior rectus
SO = superior oblique   IO = inferior oblique

Figure 15–4. Cardinal positions of gaze and muscles primarily tested in those fields of gaze. Arrow indicates position in which each muscle is tested.

occurring in optic nerve disease, is evaluated by the swinging flashlight test (see section on diseases of the optic nerve). Irregular pupils are associated with iritis, trauma, pupillary membranes, and structural defects such as iris coloboma (see section on iris coloboma).

Pupils vary in size due to lighting conditions and also age. In general, infants have miotic (constricted) pupils. Children have larger pupils than either infants or adults, whereas the elderly have miotic pupils.

Anisocoria, a size difference between the two pupils, may be physiologic if the size difference is within 1 mm and is the same in light and dark. Anisocoria occurs with Horner syndrome, third nerve palsy, Adie tonic pupil, iritis, and trauma. Medication could also cause abnormal pupil size or reactivity. For example, contact with atropinelike substances (belladonna alkaloids) will cause pupillary dilation with little or no pupillary reaction. Systemic antihistamines and scopolamine patches, among other medicines, can dilate the pupils and interfere with accommodation (focusing).

Alignment & Motility Evaluation

Alignment and motility should be tested because amblyopia is associated with strabismus, a misalignment of the visual axes of the eyes. Besides alignment, ocular rotations should be evaluated in the six cardinal positions of gaze (Table 15–1; Figure 15–4). A small toy is an interesting target for testing ocular rotations in infants; a penlight works well in older children.

Alignment can be assessed in several ways. In order of increasing accuracy, these methods are observation, the corneal light reflex test, and cover testing. Observation includes an educated guess about whether the eyes are properly aligned. Corneal light reflex evaluation (Hirschberg test) is performed by shining a light beam at the patient's eyes, observing the reflections off each cornea, and estimating whether these "reflexes" appear to be positioned properly. If the reflection of light is noted temporally on the cornea, esotropia is suspected (Figure 15–5). Nasal reflection of the light suggests exotropia (outward deviation). Accuracy of these tests increases with increasing angles of misalignment.

Another way of evaluating alignment is with the cover test, in which the patient fixes on a target while one eye is covered. If an esotropia or an exotropia is present, the deviated eye will make a corrective movement to fixate on the target when the previously fixating eye is occluded. The other eye is tested similarly. When the occluder is removed from the eye just uncovered, a refixation movement of that eye indicates a phoria, or latent deviation if alignment is reestablished. If the uncovered eye picks up fixation and strabismus is still present, then that eye can be presumed to be dominant and the nonpreferred eye possibly amblyopic. If the eye remains deviated after the occluder is removed, a tropia is noted to be present (Figure 15–6). A deviated eye that is blind or has very poor vision will not fixate on a tar-

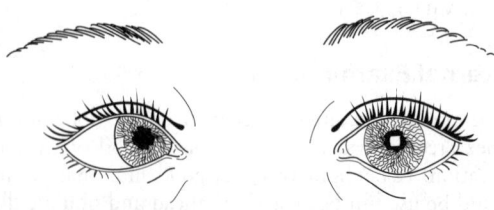

Figure 15–5. Temporal displacement of light reflection showing esotropia (inward deviation) of the right eye. Nasal displacement of the reflection would show exotropia (outward deviation).

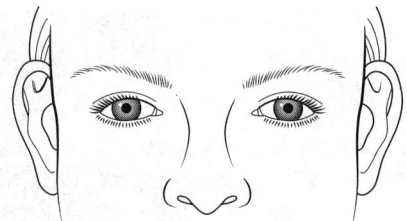

Eyes straight (maintained in position by fusion).

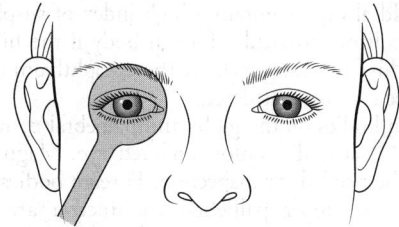

Position of eye under cover in orthophoria (fusion-free position). The right eye under cover has not moved.

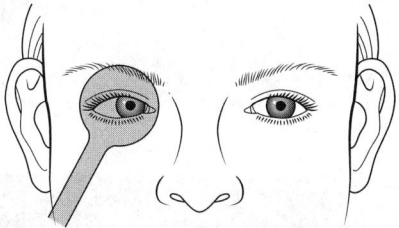

Position of eye under cover in esophoria (fusion-free position). Under cover, the right eye has deviated inward. Upon removal of cover, the right eye will immediately resume its straight-ahead position.

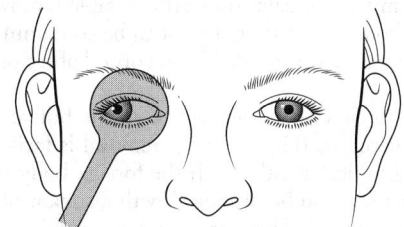

Position of eye under cover in exophoria (fusion-free position). Under cover, the right eye had deviated outward. Upon removal of the cover, the right eye will immediately resume its straight-ahead position.

Figure 15–6. Cover testing. The patient is instructed to look at a target at eye level 20 feet away. Note that in the presence of constant strabismus (ie, a tropia rather than a phoria), the deviation will remain when the cover is removed. (Reproduced, with permission, from *General Ophthalmology*, 15th ed. Originally published by Appleton & Lange. Copyright © 2003 by the McGraw-Hill Companies, Inc.)

get. Consequently, spurious results to cover testing may occur, as can happen with disinterest on the part of the patient, small-angle strabismus, and inexperience in administering cover tests.

Ophthalmoscopic Examination

A handheld direct ophthalmoscope allows visualization of the ocular fundus. As the patient's pupil becomes more constricted, viewing the fundus becomes more difficult. Although it is taught that pupillary dilation can precipitate an attack of closed-angle glaucoma in the predisposed adult, children are very rarely predisposed to angle closure. Exceptions include those with a dislocated lens, past surgery, or an eye previously compromised by a retrolental membrane, such as in retinopathy of prematurity. Therefore, if an adequate view of the fundus is precluded by a miotic pupil, use of a dilating agent (eg, 1 drop in each eye of 2.5% phenylephrine or 0.5% or 1% tropicamide) should provide adequate mydriasis (dilation). In infants, 1 drop of a combination of 1% phenylephrine with 0.2% cyclopentolate (Cyclomydril) is safer. Structures to be observed during ophthalmoscopy include the optic disk, blood vessels, the macular reflex, and retinal changes if present, as well as the clarity of the vitreous

media. By increasing the amount of plus lens dialed into the instrument, the point of focus moves anteriorly from the retina to the lens and finally to the cornea.

Ophthalmoscopy should include assessment of the clarity of the ocular media, that is, the quality of the red reflex. The practitioner should take the time to become familiar with this reflex. The red reflex test (Brückner test) is useful for identifying disorders such as media opacities (eg, cataracts), large refractive errors, tumors such as retinoblastoma, and strabismus. A difference in quality of the red reflexes between the two eyes constitutes a positive Brückner test and requires referral to an ophthalmologist.

The red reflex of each eye can be compared simultaneously when the observer is approximately 4 feet away from the patient. The largest diameter of light is shown through the ophthalmoscope, and no correction (zero setting) is dialed in the ophthalmoscope unless it is to compensate for the examiner's uncorrected refractive error. A red reflex chart is available through the American Academy of Pediatrics.

OCULAR TRAUMA

A foreign body of the globe or adnexa may be difficult to visualize due to its small size or location. The clinician should always maintain a high index of suspicion for an occult or intraocular foreign body if the history suggests this. In cases such as these, ophthalmologic referral needs to be considered.

Foreign bodies on the globe and palpebral conjunctiva usually cause discomfort and red eye. Magnification may be needed for inspection. Foreign bodies that lodge on the upper palpebral conjunctiva are best viewed by everting the lid on itself and removing the foreign body with a cotton applicator. The conjunctival surface (palpebral conjunctiva) of the lower lid presents no problem with visualization. After simple removal of a foreign body that is thought not to be contaminated, no other treatment is needed if no corneal abrasion has occurred.

When foreign bodies are noted on the bulbar conjunctiva or cornea (Figure 15–7), removal is facilitated by using a topical anesthetic. If the foreign body is not too adherent, it can be dislodged with a stream of irrigating solution (Dacriose or saline) or with a cotton applicator after instillation of a topical anesthetic. Otherwise, a foreign body spud or needle is used to undermine the foreign body. This must be done with adequate magnification and illumination. An antibiotic ointment is then instilled. Ferrous corneal bodies often have an associated rust ring, which may be removed under slitlamp visualization in cooperative children or under anesthesia if necessary.

Corneal abrasions are evaluated with fluorescein dye and treated with a topical antibiotic, but not necessarily a pressure patch. Patching is not advised for corneal abrasions caused by contact lens wear, and it is used less frequently for corneal abrasions and after removal of corneal foreign bodies since the moist, hypoxic environment predisposes to bacterial infection. One drop of topical cycloplegic agent such as 5% homatropine, 1% atropine (with appropriate warnings to parents about systemic side effects), or 0.25% scopolamine is useful to relieve the discomfort of ciliary spasm and iritis. Daily follow-up is required until healing is complete.

Suspected intraocular foreign bodies and corneal and scleral lacerations require emergency referral to an ophthalmologist. In cases of suspected perforation of the globe, it may be best to keep the child at rest, gently shield the eye with a metal shield or cut-down paper cup, and keep the extent of examination to a necessary minimum to prevent expulsion of intraocular contents. In this setting, the child should be given nothing by mouth in case eye examination under anesthesia or surgical repair is required. The diagnosis may be difficult if the obvious signs of corneal perforation (shallow anterior chamber with hyphema and irregular pupil) are not present (Figure 15–8). Furthermore, nonradiopaque materials such as glass will not be seen on x-ray film. A computed tomographic scan may be useful in evaluating ocular trauma, including bony injury and for-

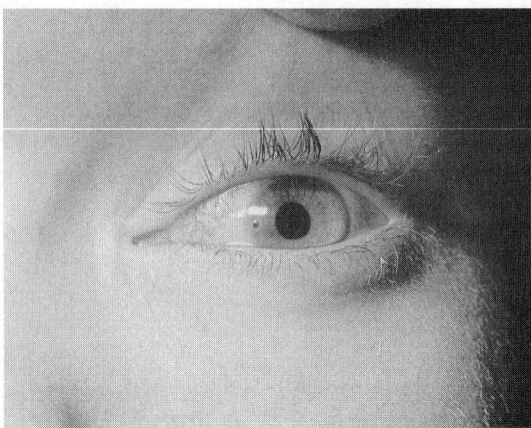

A

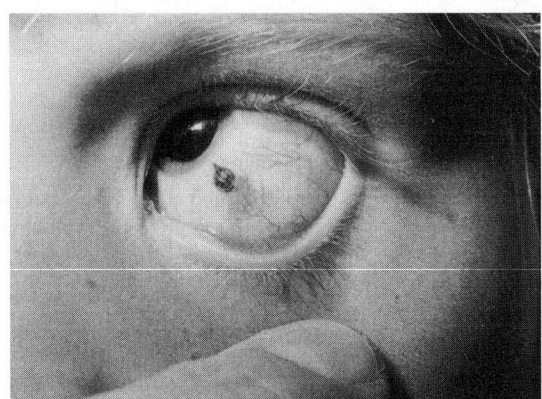

B

Figure 15–7. **A:** Corneal foreign body at the nasal edge of the cornea. **B:** Subconjunctival foreign body of graphite.

eign body wound. MRI will not provide bony detail and must be avoided if a magnetic foreign body is suspected.

Sarrazin L et al: Traumatic pediatric retinal detachment: a comparison between open and closed globe injuries. Am J Ophthalmol 2004;137:1042 [PMID: 15183788].

INJURIES TO THE EYELIDS

Ecchymosis

Orbital and soft tissue trauma may produce so-called black eye or ecchymosis (blue or purplish hemorrhagic areas) of the eyelids. The extent of the injury to the eye and orbit may not correlate fully with its appearance. Blowout fracture, which occurs from blunt trauma fracturing the walls of the orbit, must be suspected. Ocular motility must be assessed, the globe examined, and

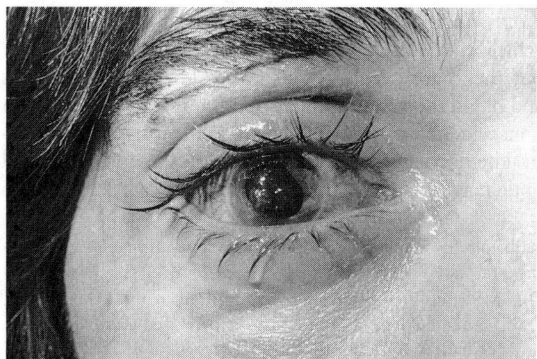

Figure 15–8. Corneal laceration with irregular pupil and vitreous loss.

intraocular pressure measured, usually by an ophthalmologist. Cold compresses or ice packs for brief periods (eg, 10 minutes at a time) are recommended in older children in the first 24 hours after injury to reduce hemorrhage and swelling. Abuse needs to be considered when orbital injury is poorly explained.

Lacerations

The lids and lacrimal apparatus are susceptible to laceration. Except for superficial lacerations away from the globe, repair in children is best performed in the operating room under general anesthesia. Special consideration must be given to lacerations involving the lid margin, to through-and-through lacerations, to lacerations that may involve the levator muscle in the upper lid, and to those that may involve the canaliculus (Figure 15–9). These injuries are best repaired by an ophthalmologist.

Burns

Eyelid burns can occur in toddlers from contact with a lighted cigarette. The cornea is often involved as well. Curling irons can cause similar burns. These burns usually heal following application of antibiotic ointment. Severe thermal or chemical burns can cause scars resulting in ectropion or entropion of the lid and scarring of the conjunctiva and cul-de-sac.

Burns of the conjunctiva and cornea may be thermal, radiant, or chemical. Superficial thermal burns cause pain, tearing, and injection. Management is with topical antibiotics and patching. Add a cycloplegic agent if corneal involvement is present, because pain from ciliary spasm and iritis may accompany the injury.

Radiant energy causes ultraviolet keratitis. Typical examples are welder's burn and burns associated with skiing without goggles in bright sunlight. The fluorescein dye pattern will show a uniformly stippled appearance of the corneal epithelium. Antibiotic ointment, pressure patches, and a cycloplegic agent such as 5% homatropine are usually followed by recovery within 24 hours.

Chemical burns with strong acidic and alkaline agents can be blinding and constitute a true ocular emergency. Examples are burns caused by exploding batteries, spilled drain cleaner, and bleach. Alkali burns may not cause significant injection because the conjunctival vessels become damaged. Alkalis tend to penetrate deeper than acids into ocular tissue. Immediate treatment consists of copious irrigation and removal of precipitates as soon as possible after the injury. The patient should be referred to an ophthalmologist after immediate first aid has been given.

Lee HJ et al: CT of orbital trauma. Emerg Radiol 2004;10:168 [PMID: 15290482].

Hyphema

Blunt trauma to the globe may cause hyphema, or bleeding within the anterior chamber from a ruptured vessel located near the root of the iris or in the anterior chamber angle. Bleeding may be microscopic or may fill the entire anterior chamber (Figure 15–10). Blunt trauma severe enough to cause hyphema may be associated with additional ocular injury, including iritis, lens subluxation, retinal edema or detachment, and glaucoma. In patients with sickle cell anemia or trait, even moderate elevations of intraocular pressure may quickly lead to optic atrophy and permanent vision loss. Therefore, all African Americans whose sickle cell status is unknown should be tested if hyphema is observed. These patients require extra vigilance in diagnosing and treating hyphema.

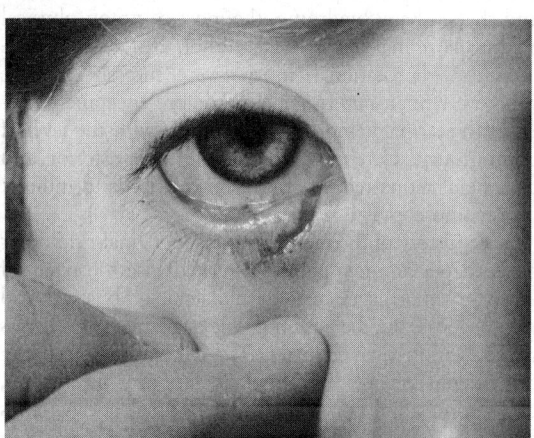

Figure 15–9. Laceration involving right lower lid and canaliculus.

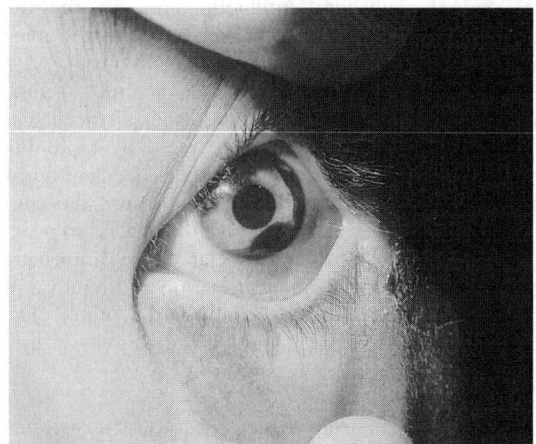

Figure 15–10. Hyphema filling approximately 20% of the anterior chamber.

Management of hyphema in an otherwise uninjured patient should include testing of visual acuity and assessment of the integrity of the globe and orbit. A shield should be placed over the eye, the head elevated, and arrangements made for ophthalmologic referral.

Nontraumatic causes of hyphema include juvenile xanthogranuloma and blood dyscrasias. Rarely, hyphema is noted in the newborn after a stressful birth.

Rocha KM et al: Outpatient management of traumatic hyphema in children: prospective evaluation. J AAPOS 2004;8:357 [PMID: 15314597].

Nonaccidental Trauma & Shaken Baby Syndrome

From an ocular standpoint, in both nonaccidental trauma and shaken baby syndrome, the most common physical finding is retinal hemorrhage, although it need not be present with rotational injury severe enough to cause subdural hematoma. In general, the presence and severity of the retinal hemorrhages correlates with the level of brain injury. Careful evaluation of the posterior and peripheral retina requires pupillary dilation and indirect ophthalmoscopy.

The history of the injuries leading to retinal findings is often vague and often poorly correlated with the extent of injury. Hemorrhages may be unilateral or bilateral and may be located in the posterior pole or periphery. Whereas retinal hemorrhages tend to resolve fairly quickly, those in the vitreous do not. If a blood clot lies over the macula, deprivation amblyopia may occur. Retinal and vitreous hemorrhages associated with intracranial hemorrhage from skull injury comprise the Terson syndrome. Retinal hemorrhages are rarely associated with cardiopulmonary resuscitation or seizures. Retinal hemorrhages do not com-

monly occur from major accidental trauma such as motor vehicle crashes unless a compressive chest injury is present, but they have been associated with low fibrinogen levels and blood dyscrasias. Other ocular findings associated with nonaccidental trauma include lid ecchymosis, subconjunctival hemorrhage, hyphema, retinal folds, retinoschisis, and optic nerve edema. Acute-onset esotropia can also occur.

Carbaugh SF: Understanding shaken baby syndrome. Adv Neonatal Care 2004;4:105 [PMID: 15138993].

Dias MS et al: Preventing abusive head trauma among infants and young children: a hospital-based, parent education program. Pediatrics 2005;115:e470 [PMID: 15805350].

Minns RA, Busuttil A: Patterns of presentation of the shaken baby syndrome: four types of inflicted brain injury predominate. BMJ 2004;328:766 [PMID: 15044297].

Wagner RS: Inflicted childhood neurotrauma: new name and new information. J Pediatr Ophthalmol Strabismus 2004;41:79 [PMID: 15089061].

Prevention of Ocular Injuries

Air rifles, paintballs, and fireworks are responsible for many serious eye injuries in children. Golf injuries can be very severe. Bungee cords have been associated with multiple types of severe ocular trauma, including corneal abrasion, iris tears, hyphema, vitreous hemorrhage, retinal detachment, and blindness. These activities should be avoided or very closely supervised. Safety goggles should be used in laboratories and industrial arts classes and when operating snow blowers, power lawn mowers, and power tools, or when using hammers and nails. Sports-related eye injuries can be prevented with protective eyewear. Sports goggles and visors of polycarbonate plastic will prevent injuries in games using fast projectiles such as tennis or racquet balls, or where opponents may swing elbows or poke at the eye.

The one-eyed individual should be specifically advised to always wear polycarbonate eyeglasses and goggles for all sports. High-risk activities such as boxing and the martial arts should be avoided by one-eyed children.

American Academy of Pediatrics, Committee on Sports Medicine and Fitness; American Academy of Ophthalmology, Eye Health and Public Information Task Force: Protective eyewear for young athletes. Ophthalmology 2004;111:600 [PMID: 15019343].

Listman DA: Paintball injuries in children: more than meets the eye. Pediatrics 2004;113(1 Pt 1):e15 [PMID: 14702489].

Thompson CG et al: The aetiology of perforating ocular injuries in children. Br J Ophthalmol 2002;86:920 [PMID: 12140216].

DISORDERS OF THE OCULAR STRUCTURES

Diseases of the Eyelids

Blepharitis is inflammation of the lid margin characterized by crusty debris at the base of the lashes; varying degrees of erythema at the lid margins; and in severe cases, secondary corneal changes such as punctate erosions, vascularization, and ulcers. When conjunctival injection accompanies blepharitis, the condition is known as blepharoconjunctivitis. *Staphylococcus* is the most common bacterial cause. Treatment includes lid scrubs with a nonburning baby shampoo several times a week and application of a topical antibiotic ointment such as erythromycin or bacitracin at bedtime.

Rosacea can also occur in the pediatric age group and cause chronic blepharoconjunctivitis with corneal changes that decrease vision. Systemic antibiotics and local treatment are required.

Pediculosis of the lids (phthiriasis palpebrarum) is caused by *Pthirus pubis*. Nits and adult lice can be seen on the eyelashes when viewed with appropriate magnification. Mechanical removal and application to the lid margins of phospholine iodide or 1% mercuric oxide ointment can be effective. Other bodily areas of involvement must also be treated if involved. Family members and contacts may also be infected (see Chapter 14).

Papillomavirus may infect the lid and conjunctiva. Warts may be recurrent, multiple, and difficult to treat. Treatment modalities include cryotherapy, cautery, carbon dioxide laser, and surgery.

Localized staphylococcal infections of the glands of Zeis within the lid cause a sty (hordeolum) (Figure 15–11). When the infection coalesces and points internally or externally, it may discharge itself or require incision. The lesion is tender and red. Warm compresses help to hasten the acute process. Some practitioners prescribe a topical antibiotic ointment. Any coexisting blepharitis should be treated.

A chalazion is an inflammation of the meibomian glands, which may produce a tender nodule over the tarsus of the upper or lower lid. In addition to localized erythema of the corresponding palpebral conjunctiva, there may be a yellow lipogranuloma (Figure 15–12). Treatment includes warm compresses for 10–15 min-

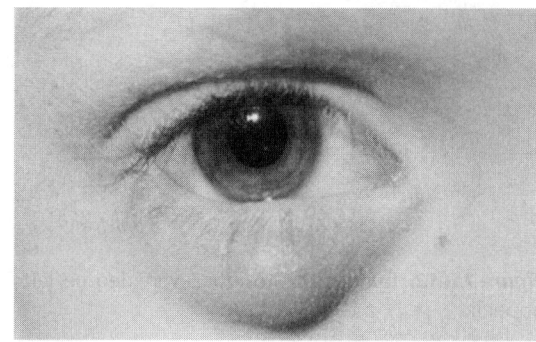

A

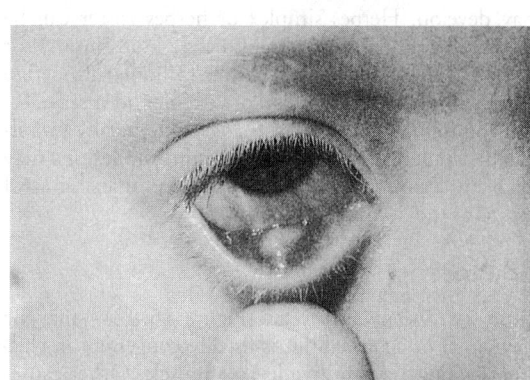

B

Figure 15–12. Chalazion. **A:** Right lower lid, external view. **B:** Right lower lid conjunctival surface.

utes four times a day for up to 6 weeks. If incision and curettage are needed because the lesion is slow to resolve, the child will require a general anesthetic.

Viral Lid Disease

Herpes simplex virus may involve the lids at the time of primary herpes simplex infection. Vesicular lesions with an erythematous base occur. Primary herpes simplex blepharoconjunctivitis should be treated with systemic acyclovir (a liquid formulation is available), valacyclovir, or famciclovir. When either the conjunctiva or the cornea is involved, treatment should include topical 1% trifluridine or 3% vidarabine.

Herpes zoster causes vesicular disease in association with a skin eruption in the dermatome of the ophthalmic branch of the trigeminal nerve. In older children, treatment of ophthalmic herpes zoster with oral acyclovir, valacyclovir, or famciclovir within 5 days after onset may reduce the morbidity. When vesicles are present on the tip of the nose with herpes zoster (Hutchinson sign), ocular involvement, including iritis,

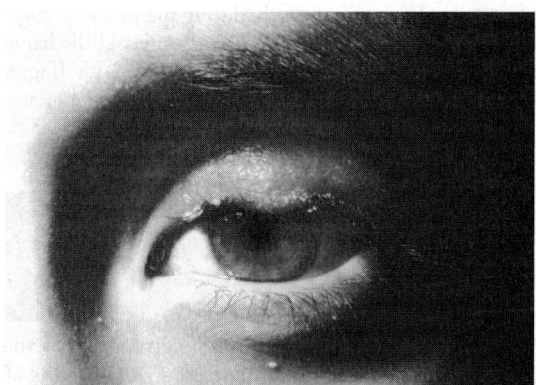

Figure 15–11. Hordeolum and blepharitis, left upper lid.

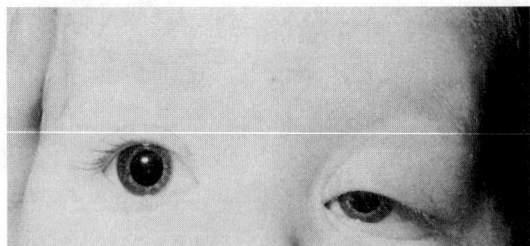

Figure 15–13. Congenital ptosis of severe degree, left upper lid.

may develop. Herpes simplex or herpes zoster can be diagnosed by rapid viral culture (24–48 hours) or detection of antigen in skin lesions (3 hours). Impetigo is in the differential diagnosis of vesicular lid disease.

Molluscum contagiosum lesions are typically umbilicated papules. If near the lid margin, the lesions may shed and cause conjunctivitis. Cautery or excision of lesions at the lid margin is useful.

Lid Ptosis

Ptosis—a droopy upper lid (Figure 15–13)—may be congenital or acquired but is usually congenital in children owing to a defective levator muscle. Other causes of ptosis are myasthenia gravis, lid injuries, third nerve palsy, and Horner syndrome (see next section). Surgical correction is indicated for moderate to severe ptosis. Mild cases less often require operative management. Cosmesis may be better if surgery is delayed until most of the facial growth has occurred, usually around 5 years old. Ptosis may be associated with astigmatism and amblyopia.

An association sometimes seen with congenital ptosis is the Marcus Gunn jaw-winking phenomenon. Intermittent reduction of the ptosis occurs during mastication or sucking, due to a synkinesis or simultaneous firing of either the external or internal pterygoid muscle (innervated by the trigeminal nerve) and the levator muscle (innervated by the oculomotor nerve).

Horner Syndrome

Horner syndrome, which may be congenital or acquired, is the triad of miosis, ptosis, and anhidrosis. The ptosis is usually mild with a well-defined upper lid crease. This differentiates it from congenital ptosis, which typically has a poorly defined lid crease. Another key finding of congenital Horner syndrome is heterochromia of the two irides, with the lighter colored iris occurring on the same side as the lesion (Figure 15–14). Anhidrosis can occur in congenital and acquired cases. Of note, not all of the three signs must be present to make the diagnosis. The

syndrome is caused by an abnormality or lesion to the sympathetic chain. The congenital variety is most commonly the result of birth trauma. Acquired cases may occur in children who have had cardiothoracic surgery, trauma, or brainstem vascular malformation. Most worrisome is a Horner syndrome caused by neuroblastoma of the sympathetic chain in the apical lung region. An excellent screening test for this is the spot urine vanillylmandelic acid:creatinine ratio.

Pharmacologic assessment of the pupils with topical cocaine and hydroxyamphetamine or epinephrine will help determine whether the Horner syndrome is due to a preganglionic or postganglionic lesion of the sympathetic chain. There are preliminary studies that suggest that topical apraclonidine may also be useful in the diagnosis of Horner syndrome. Physical examination, including palpation of the neck and abdomen for masses, and MRI of structures in the head, neck, chest, and abdomen should be considered.

Bacal DA, Levy SR: The use of apraclonidine in the diagnosis of Horner syndrome in pediatric patients. Arch Ophthalmol 2004;122:276 [PMID: 14769608].

Eyelid Tics

Eyelid tics may occur as a transient phenomenon lasting several days to months. Although a tic may be an isolated finding in an otherwise healthy child, it may also occur in children with multiple tics, attention-deficit/hyperactivity disorder, or Tourette syndrome. Caffeine consumption may cause or exacerbate eyelid tics. If the disorder is a short-lived annoyance, no treatment is needed.

DISORDERS OF THE NASOLACRIMAL SYSTEM

Nasolacrimal Duct Obstruction

Nasolacrimal obstruction occurs in up to 6% of infants. Most cases clear spontaneously during the first year. Signs and symptoms include a wet eye with mucoid discharge, erythema of one or both lids, and conjunctivitis (Figure 15–15). Obstruction in any part of the drainage system

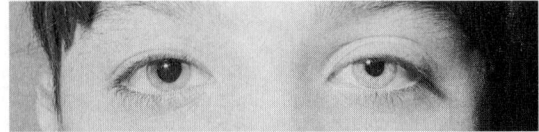

Figure 15–14. Congenital Horner syndrome. Ptosis, miosis, and heterochromia. Lighter colored iris is on the affected left side.

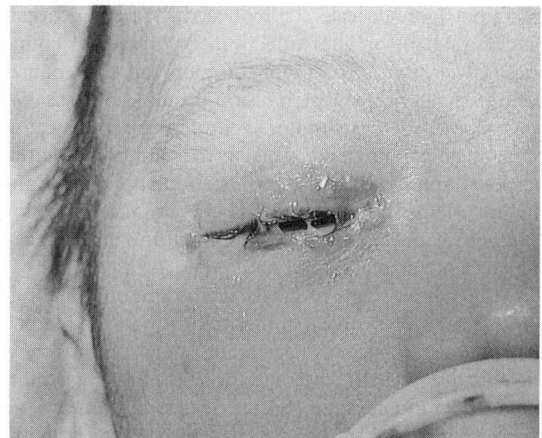

Figure 15–15. Nasolacrimal obstruction, right eye. Mattering on upper and lower lids.

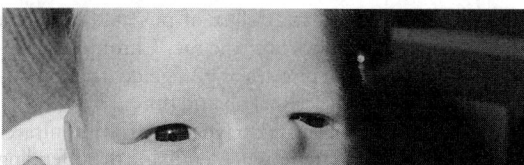

Figure 15–16. Congenital dacryocystocele on the left side. Raised, bluish discolored mass of enlarged nasolacrimal sac. Note superiorly displaced medial canthus.

may result from incomplete canalization of the duct or membranous obstructions. Nasolacrimal obstruction may also occur in individuals with craniofacial abnormalities or amniotic band syndrome. Differential diagnosis of tearing includes congenital glaucoma, foreign bodies, nasal disorders, and in older children, allergies.

Massage over the nasolacrimal sac may empty debris from the nasolacrimal sac and may clear the obstruction, although the efficacy of massage in clearing nasolacrimal obstruction is debated. Cleansing the lids and medial canthal area decreases the likelihood of infection and irritation. Superinfection may occur, and treatment with topical antibiotics may help decrease the discharge. The mainstay of surgical treatment is probing, which is successful 80% or more of the time, but the success rate may decrease after the infant reaches age 1 year. Other surgical procedures, including infraction of the inferior nasal turbinate, balloon dilation, and silicone tube intubation, may be necessary if probing fails. Much less often, dacryocystorhinostomy is required.

Lee DH et al: Success of simple probing and irrigation in patients with nasolacrimal duct obstruction and otitis media. J AAPOS 2005;9:192 [PMID: 15838451].

Yuksel D et al: Balloon dilatation for treatment of congenital nasolacrimal duct obstruction. Eur J Ophthalmol 2005;15:179 [PMID: 15812757].

Congenital Dacryocystocele

Congenital dacryocystocele is thought to result from obstructions proximal and distal to the nasolacrimal sac. An intranasal duct cyst may be present beneath the inferior turbinate at the valve of Hasner. These cysts may be associated with respiratory distress. At birth, the nasolacrimal sac is distended and has a bluish hue that often leads to an erroneous diagnosis of hemangioma. The tense and swollen sac displaces the medial canthus superiorly (Figure 15–16). Massage and warm compresses are sometimes effective, but probing of the nasolacrimal system often is necessary. Repeated probing and endoscopic marsupialization of the intranasal cyst under general anesthesia may be required. Dacryocystitis and sepsis can result from dacryocystocele.

Levin AV et al: Nasal endoscopy in the treatment of congenital lacrimal sac mucoceles. Int J Pediatr Otorhinolaryngol 2003; 67:255 [PMID: 12633925].

Dacryocystitis

Acute and chronic dacryocystitis are typically caused by bacteria that colonize the upper respiratory tract, such as *Staphylococcus aureus*, *Streptococcus pneumoniae*, *Streptococcus pyogenes*, *Streptococcus viridans*, *Moraxella catarrhalis*, and *Haemophilus* species. Acute dacryocystitis presents with inflammation, swelling, tenderness, and pain over the lacrimal sac (located inferior to the medial canthal tendon). Fever may be present. The infection may point externally (Figure 15–17). A purulent discharge and tearing can be expected, because the cause of infection is almost always nasolacrimal obstruction.

Signs of chronic dacryocystitis are mucopurulent debris on the lids and lashes, tearing, injection of the

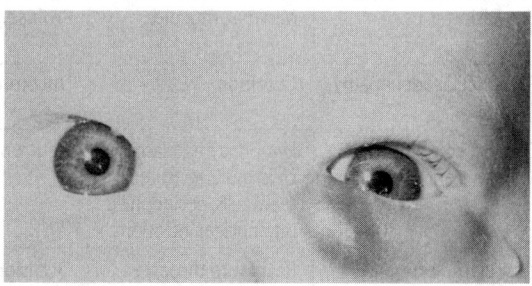

Figure 15–17. Acute dacryocystitis in an 11-week-old infant.

palpebral conjunctiva, and reflux of pus at the puncta when pressure is applied over the sac. Chronic dacryocystitis and recurrent episodes of low-grade dacryocystitis are caused by nasolacrimal obstruction.

Treatment of severe acute dacryocystitis is with intravenous antibiotics after attempts at identifying the offending organism by culture and staining. Oral antibiotics can be tried in milder cases. Topical antibiotic administration is adjunctive and is also used with recurrent chronic infections. Warm compresses are beneficial. After the acute episode subsides—and in chronic cases—the nasolacrimal obstruction must be relieved surgically. If it cannot be drained via the intranasal portion of the nasolacrimal duct, external drainage may be necessary. This should be done as a last resort since a fistula may develop.

DISEASES OF THE CONJUNCTIVA

Conjunctivitis may be infectious, allergic, or associated with systemic disease. Trauma, irritation of the conjunctiva, and intraocular inflammation also can cause injection of conjunctival vessels that can be confused with conjunctivitis (Table 15–2).

Ophthalmia Neonatorum

Ophthalmia neonatorum (conjunctivitis in the newborn) occurs during the first month of life. It is characterized by redness and swelling of the lids and conjunctiva and by discharge (Figure 15–18). Ophthalmia neonatorum may be due to inflammation resulting from silver nitrate prophylaxis given at birth, bacterial infection (gonococcal, staphylococcal, pneumococcal, or chlamydial), or viral infection. In developed countries, *Chlamydia* is the most common cause. Neonatal conjunctivitis may threaten vision if caused by *Neisseria gonorrhoeae*. Herpes simplex is a rare but serious cause of neonatal conjunctivitis, since it may indicate systemic herpes simplex infection. Gram staining, Giemsa staining for elementary bodies, enzyme immunoassay for *Chlamydia,* and bacterial and viral cultures aid in making an etiologic diagnosis.

Although no single prophylactic medication can eliminate all cases of neonatal conjunctivitis, povidone-iodine may provide broader coverage against the organisms causing this disease than silver nitrate or erythromycin ointment. Silver nitrate is not effective against *Chlamydia.* The choice of prophylactic agent is often dictated by local epidemiology and cost considerations.

Treatment of these infections requires specific systemic antibiotics because they can cause serious infections in other organs. Specifically, *Chlamydia* can cause a delayed-onset pneumonitis. Parents should be examined and receive treatment when a sexually associated pathogen is present.

Bacterial Conjunctivitis

In general, bacterial conjunctivitis is accompanied by a purulent discharge and viral infection by a watery discharge. One or both eyes may be involved. Regional lymphadenopathy is not a common finding in bacterial conjunctivitis except in cases of oculoglandular syndrome due to *S aureus,* group A β-hemolytic streptococci, *Mycobacterium tuberculosis* or atypical mycobacte-

Table 15–2. Clinical and laboratory features of conjunctivitis.

	Viral	Bacterial	Chlamydial	Allergic
Itching	Minimal	Minimal	Minimal	Severe
Hyperemia	Generalized	Generalized	Generalized	Generalized
Tearing	Profuse	Moderate	Moderate	Moderate
Exudation	Minimal, mucoid	Profuse, purulent	Profuse; mucoid or mucopurulent	Minimal, slight mucus
Preauricular adenopathy	Common	Uncommon	Common in inclusion conjunctivitis	None
Stained conjunctival smears and scrapings	Lymphocytes, plasma cells, multinucleated giant cells, eosinophilic intranuclear inclusions	Neutrophils, bacteria	Neutrophils, plasma cells, basophilic intracytoplasmic inclusions	Eosinophils
Associated sytemic signs and symptoms	Rash, sore throat, fever in some patients	Occasional fever, sore throat	Pneumonia in neonates	Variable—may or may not be present

Modified from Vaughan D, Asbury T, Riordan-Eva P (eds): *General Ophthalmology,* 15th ed. Appleton & Lange, 2003.

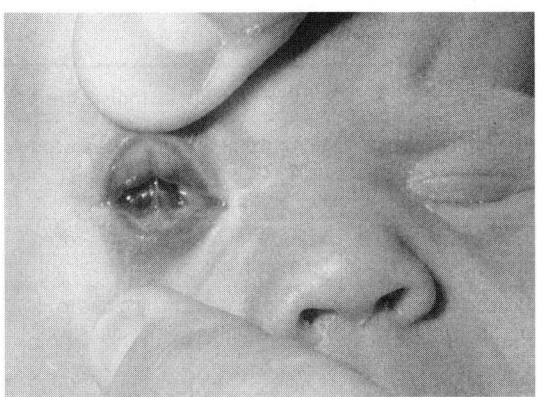

Figure 15-18. Ophthalmia neonatorum due to *Chlamydia trachomatis* infection in a 2-week-old infant. Note marked lid and conjunctival inflammation.

ria, *Francisella tularensis* (the agent of tularemia), and *Bartonella henselae* (the agent of cat-scratch fever).

Common bacterial causes of conjunctivitis in older children include nontypable *Haemophilus* species, *S pneumoniae, M catarrhalis,* and *S aureus.* If conjunctivitis is not associated with systemic illness, topical antibiotics such as erythromycin, polymyxin-bacitracin, sulfacetamide, tobramycin, and fluoroquinolones are adequate. Systemic therapy is recommended for conjunctivitis associated with *Chlamydia trachomatis, N gonorrhoeae,* and *N meningitidis.*

Viral Conjunctivitis

Adenovirus infection is often associated with pharyngitis, a follicular reaction of the palpebral conjunctiva, and preauricular adenopathy (pharyngoconjunctival fever). Epidemics of adenoviral keratoconjunctivitis occur. Treatment is supportive. Children with presumed adenoviral keratoconjunctivitis are considered contagious 10–14 days from the day of onset. They should stay out of school and group activities as long as their eyes are red and tearing. Strict hand-washing precautions are recommended.

During the prodromal period of measles infection, conjunctivitis occurs; this is preceded by a transverse marginal line of conjunctival injection across the lower lids.

Herpes simplex virus may cause conjunctivitis or blepharoconjunctivitis. Treatment is with topical trifluridine 1% drops or 3% vidarabine ointment. Oral acyclovir may be used prophylactically in children to reduce recurrence of herpes simplex ocular disease.

Teoh DL, Reynolds S: Diagnosis and management of pediatric conjunctivitis. Pediatr Emerg Care 2003;19:48. [PMID: 12592117].

Allergic Conjunctivitis

In hay fever conjunctivitis, the eyes are red and itchy, with mucoid discharge. Topical ophthalmic solutions that combine both antihistamine and mast cell stabilizers, including olopatadine 0.1%, epinastine HCl 0.05%, and ketotifen fumarate 0.025%, are very effective at treating allergic conjunctivitis. Other agents available include a combination topical vasoconstrictor plus an antihistamine (naphazoline-antazoline); a nonsteroidal anti-inflammatory drug such as ketorolac tromethamine 0.5%; a mast cell stabilizer such as lodoxamide tromethamine 0.1%; or a corticosteroid like prednisolone 0.125% (Table 15–3). Corticosteroids should be used with caution because their extended use causes glaucoma and or cataracts in some patients.

Vernal conjunctivitis is a seasonal form of allergic conjunctivitis associated with tearing, itching, and a stringy discharge. It is more common in males. In the palpebral form, dramatic changes of the superior palpebral conjunctiva occur, with cobblestone papillae (Figure 15–19). Corneal ulcers can occur. Topical treatments include a mast cell stabilizer such as 4% cromolyn sodium or 0.1% lodoxamide tromethamine and limited use of a topical corticosteroid. One form of vernal conjunctivitis (limbal vernal) presents with nodules at the limbus (the corneal-conjunctival junction). Contact lens wear may induce a conjunctivitis that appears similar to the palpebral form of vernal conjunctivitis.

Mucocutaneous Diseases

Conjunctivitis and conjunctival changes are associated with a number of systemic syndromes. Examples are erythema multiforme (Stevens-Johnson syndrome; see Chapter 14), Reiter syndrome (Chapter 40), and Kawasaki disease (Chapter 19). The latter is also associated with iritis. With Stevens-Johnson syndrome, conjunctival changes include erythema, vesicular lesions that frequently rupture, and symblepharon (adhesions) between the raw edges of the bulbar and palpebral (lid) conjunctivae. Management may include artificial tears and lubricants to provide comfort and a topical corticosteroid to prevent adhesions and dry eye in severe cases. Lysis of adhesions or use of a scleral ring by an ophthalmologist may be required. Surgical treatment of severe cases of symblepharon with amniotic membrane grafts are under investigation. Cycloplegic agents and topical corticosteroids are prescribed for iritis in Kawasaki disease.

Meallet MA et al: Amniotic membrane transplantation with conjunctival limbal autograft for total limbal stem cell deficiency. Ophthalmology 2003;110:1585 [PMID: 12917178].

Table 15–3. Common ocular allergy medications.

Generic Name	Brand Name	Mechanism of Action	Side Effects	Dosage	Indications
Lodoxamide tromethamine 0.1%	Alomide	Mast-cell stabilizer	Transient burning or stinging	1 drop 4 times daily—taper	Vernal keratoconjunctivitis
Cromolyn Na 4%	Crolom, Opticrom	Mast-cell stabilizer	Transient burning or stinging	1 drop 4–6 times daily	Vernal keratoconjunctivitis
Olopatidine	Patanol	Mast-cell stabilizer, H_1-receptor antagonist	Headache, burning or stinging	Twice daily (interval 6–8 h)	Itching due to allergic conjunctivitis
Ketorolac tromethamine 0.5%	Acular	Nonsteroidal anti-inflammatory drug	Transient burning or stinging	1 drop 4 times daily	Itching due to seasonal allergic conjunctivitis
Levocobastine HCl 0.05%	Livostin	H_1-receptor antagonist	Transient burning or stinging, headache	1 drop 4 times daily	Relief of symptoms of seasonal allergic conjunctivitis
Naphazoline HCl 0.1%	AK-Con, Naphcon, Opcon, Vasocon	Ocular decongestant, vasoconstrictor	Mydriasis, increased redness, irritation, discomfort, punctate keratitis, increased intraocular pressure, dizzy, headache, nausea, nervousness, hypertension, weakness, cardiac effects, hyperglycemia	Varies by preparation	Temporary relief of redness due to minor eye irritants
Pheniramine maleate	Component in AK-Con A, Opcon-A, Naphcon-A	Antihistamine		1 drop every 3–4 h, as needed	Relief of symptoms of seasonal allergic conjunctivitis

DISORDERS OF THE IRIS

Iris Coloboma

Iris coloboma is a developmental defect due to incomplete closure of the anterior embryonal fissure. The child's pupil will have an elongated shape reminiscent of a keyhole or cat's eye (Figure 15–20). The affected area is located inferonasally, but may extend posteriorly, involving the retina and choroid. The effect on visual acuity is variable. Iris coloboma may be an isolated defect or may be associated with a number of chromosomal abnormalities and syndromes. Variable genetic expression of coloboma can include a broad spectrum, from iris coloboma, to microphthalmia-with-cyst, and clinical anophthalmia.

Aniridia

Aniridia is a bilateral disorder that includes macular hypoplasia and absence of almost all of the iris (Figure 15–21). Cataract, corneal changes, and glaucoma are often seen. Photophobia and nystagmus occur. Aniridia may occur as an autosomal dominant disease or in a sporadic form associated with Wilms tumor. Repeated examination and abdominal ultrasonography are indicated. The aniridia gene has been isolated to the 11p13 chromosome region. Aniridia, genitourinary abnormalities, and mental retardation have been linked to an 11p deletion.

Albinism

Albinism is caused by defective melanogenesis, usually as an autosomal recessive disease, but an X-linked form does occur. Tyrosinase is an essential enzyme in the production of melanin. Many cases of complete albinism are caused by mutations of the tyrosinase gene. Albinism with some pigment production, especially in people of African descent, is more commonly caused by mutations of the *p* gene.

Affected individuals are usually legally blind and have nystagmus (see section on nystagmus). Iris, skin, and hair

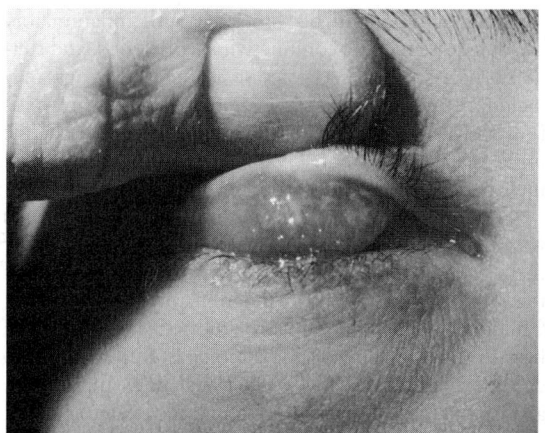

Figure 15–19. Vernal conjunctivitis. Cobblestone papillae in superior tarsal conjunctiva.

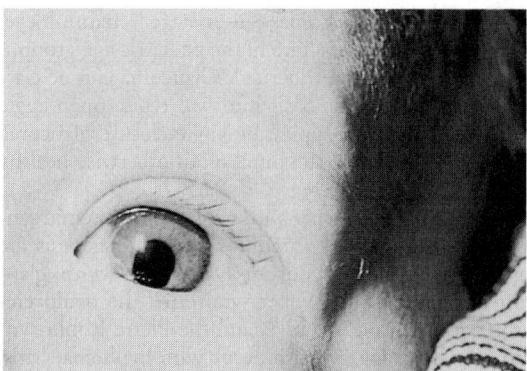

Figure 15–20. Iris coloboma located inferiorly.

color vary with the type and severity of albinism as well as the individual's race. Iris transillumination is abnormal transmission of light through an iris with decreased pigment. This may be obvious or may require slitlamp examination with retroillumination to detect focal areas of transillumination. Other ocular abnormalities include foveal hypoplasia, abnormal optic pathway projections, strabismus, and poor stereoacuity. Children with albinism should be evaluated by a pediatric ophthalmologist in order to optimize their visual function.

Albinism may be associated with other systemic manifestations. Bleeding problems occur in individuals with Hermansky-Pudlak syndrome (chromosome 10q23 or 5q13), in which oculocutaneous albinism is associated with a platelet abnormality. Chédiak-Higashi syndrome (chromosome 1q42–44) is characterized by neutrophil defects, recurrent infections, and oculocutaneous albinism. Other conditions associated with albinism are Waardenburg, Prader-Willi, and Angelman syndromes.

The risk of skin cancer is much higher in individuals with albinism. Parents and patients must be advised to use sunscreen and wear protective clothing.

Dorey SE et al: The clinical features of albinism and their correlation with visual evoked potentials. Br J Ophthalmol 2003;87:767 [PMID: 12770978].

Other Iris Conditions

Heterochromia, or a difference in iris color, can occur in congenital Horner syndrome, after iritis, or with tumors and nevi of the iris and use of topical prostaglandins. Malignant melanoma of the iris may also cause iris heterochromia. Acquired iris nodules (Lisch nodules), which occur in type I neurofibromatosis, usually become apparent by age 8 years. When seen on slit-

lamp examination, Lisch nodules are 1–2 mm in diameter and often beige in color, although their appearance can vary. Iris xanthogranuloma occurring with juvenile xanthogranuloma can cause hyphema and glaucoma. Patients with juvenile xanthogranuloma should be evaluated by an ophthalmologist for ocular involvement.

Ward et al: Neurofibromatosis 1: from lab bench to clinic. Pediatr Neurol 2005;32:221 [PMID: 15797177].

GLAUCOMA

Glaucoma is increased intraocular pressure, which causes damage to ocular structures and loss of vision. Signs of glaucoma presenting within the first year of life include buphthalmos (enlargement of the globe due to low scleral rigidity in the infant eye) as well as tearing, photophobia, blepharospasm, corneal clouding due to edema, and optic nerve cupping. After age 3 years, usually only optic nerve changes occur.

Pediatric glaucoma can be congenital or acquired, papillary block or angle closure, and unilateral or bilateral. In general, do not expect to see a red, inflamed eye with congenital or infantile glaucoma. Although acute

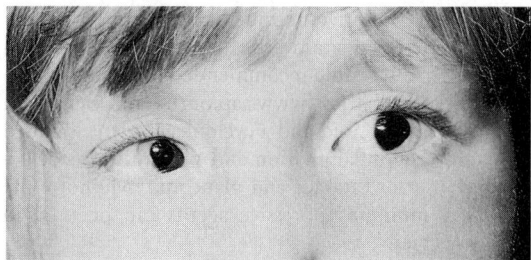

Figure 15–21. Bilateral aniridia. Iris remnants present temporally in each eye.

pupillary block glaucoma causes a red, painful eye, pupillary block is quite rare in the pediatric age group.

Glaucoma may be inherited. Glaucoma can be classified on an anatomic basis into two types: open-angle and closed-angle. Precipitating angle-closure glaucoma in a child by dilating the pupil of an otherwise healthy eye is a very rare occurrence.

Glaucoma also occurs with ocular and systemic syndromes. Aniridia and anterior segment dysgenesis are examples. Systemic syndromes associated with glaucoma include Sturge-Weber syndrome, the oculocerebrorenal syndrome of Lowe, and the Pierre Robin syndrome. Glaucoma can also occur with hyphema, iritis, lens dislocation, intraocular tumor, and retinopathy of prematurity. Treatment depends on the cause, but surgery is often the choice unless the rise in intraocular pressure is transient, in which case medical treatment is indicated.

Be aware that some individuals are "steroid responders" who develop increased intraocular pressure when challenged with exogenous steroids. The optic nerve of African Americans is probably prone to damage with acute increases in intraocular pressure.

UVEITIS

Inflammation of the uveal tract can be subdivided according to the uveal tissue primarily involved (iris, choroid, or retina) or by location, that is, anterior, intermediate, or posterior uveitis. Perhaps the most commonly diagnosed form of uveitis in childhood is traumatic iridocyclitis (iritis).

Anterior Uveitis

Injection, photophobia, pain, and blurred vision usually accompany iritis (anterior uveitis or iridocyclitis). An exception to this is iritis associated with juvenile rheumatoid arthritis (Chapter 26), when the eye is quiet and asymptomatic, but slitlamp examination will reveal anterior chamber inflammation with inflammatory cells and protein flare.

Iridocyclitis associated with juvenile rheumatoid arthritis occurs most often in girls with pauciarticular arthritis and a positive antinuclear antibody. Children with juvenile rheumatoid arthritis need to be screened according to a schedule recommended by the American Academy of Pediatrics (www.aap.org). Treatment with a topical corticosteroid and a cycloplegic agent is aimed at quieting the inflammation and preventing or delaying the onset of cataract and glaucoma. Methotrexate and other immunosuppressive agents can be used in refractory cases.

Inflammatory bowel disease is also associated with iritis—perhaps more commonly with Crohn disease than with ulcerative colitis. Other ocular findings of the anterior segment that can be associated with inflammatory bowel disease include conjunctivitis, episcleritis, and sterile corneal infiltrates. Posterior segment findings may include central serous retinochoroidopathy, panuveitis (inflammation of all uveal tissue), choroiditis, ischemic optic neuropathy, retinal vasculitis, neuroretinitis, and intermediate uveitis (see section on intermediate uveitis).

Posterior subcapsular cataracts can develop in patients with or without ocular inflammation. Most, if not all, of these patients have been taking corticosteroids as part of the long-term treatment of inflammatory bowel disease. Children with Crohn disease or ulcerative colitis should have routine periodic ophthalmologic examinations to detect ocular inflammation, which may be asymptomatic, and cataracts associated with systemic corticosteroids.

Other causes of anterior uveitis in children include syphilis, tuberculosis, sarcoidosis, relapsing fever (borreliosis), and Lyme disease, all but the last also causing posterior uveitis. Juvenile spondyloarthropathies, including ankylosing spondylitis, Reiter syndrome, and psoriatic arthritis, are also associated with anterior uveitis. A substantial percentage of cases are of unknown origin.

Foster CS: Diagnosis and treatment of juvenile idiopathic arthritis-associated uveitis. Curr Opin Ophthalmol 2003;14:395 [PMID: 14615646].

Petty et al: Arthritis and uveitis in children. A pediatric rheumatology perspective. Am J Ophthalmol 2003;135:879 [PMID: 12788129].

Posterior Uveitis

The terms choroiditis, retinitis, and retinochoroiditis denote the tissue layer primarily involved in posterior uveitis. Characteristic features occur with posterior uveitis as a result of certain organisms. Active toxoplasmosis (see Chapter 39) produces a white lesion appearing as a "headlight in the fog" owing to the overlying vitritis. Inactive lesions have a hyperpigmented border. Contiguous white satellite lesions suggest reactivation of disease. Congenital infections must be treated with a triple drug regimen (pyrimethamine, sulfadiazine, and leucovorin) for 1 year. Studies have shown improved ophthalmic and neurologic outcomes with prolonged treatment. A granular "salt and pepper" retinopathy is characteristic of congenital rubella. In infants, the TORCH complex (toxoplasmosis, other infections, rubella, cytomegalovirus [CMV], and herpes simplex virus) and syphilis must be suspected in congenital infections that cause chorioretinitis.

Congenital lymphocytic choriomeningitis virus may also present with chorioretinitis. The virus is transmitted to humans by consumption of food contaminated with rodent urine or feces. It most closely resembles congenital toxoplasmosis in presentation. Diagnosis is made by immunofluorescent antibody or enzyme-linked immunosorbent assay serologic testing. If possible, pregnant women should avoid exposure to rodents.

Ocular candidiasis occurs typically in an immunocompromised host or an infant in the intensive care nursery receiving hyperalimentation. Candidal chorioretinitis appears as multifocal, whitish yellow, fluffy retinal lesions that may spread into the vitreous and produce a so-called cotton/fungus ball vitritis.

Acute retinal necrosis syndrome is caused most often by varicella-zoster virus and occasionally by herpes simplex virus. Patients may present with a red and painful eye. Ophthalmoscopy may show unilateral or bilateral patchy white areas of retina, arterial sheathing, vitreous haze, atrophic retinal scars, retinal detachment, and optic nerve involvement.

CMV infection must be considered as a cause of retinitis in immunocompromised and human immunodeficiency virus–infected children. CMV retinitis appears as a white retinal lesion, typically but not always associated with hemorrhage, or as a granular, indolent-appearing lesion with hemorrhage and a white periphery. Cotton-wool spots (nerve fiber layer infarcts) also commonly occur in human immunodeficiency virus–positive patients.

In toddlers and older youngsters, *Toxocara canis* or *T cati* infections (ocular larva migrans; see Chapter 39) occur from ingesting soil contaminated with parasite eggs. The disease is usually unilateral. Common signs and symptoms include a red injected eye, leukocoria, and decreased vision. Fundus examination may show endophthalmitis (vitreous abscess) or localized granuloma. Diagnosis is based on the appearance of the lesion and serologic testing using enzyme-linked immunosorbent assay for *T canis* and *T cati*. Treatment options include periocular corticosteroid injections and vitrectomy.

Bresin AP et al: Ophthalmic outcomes after prenatal and postnatal treatment of congenital toxoplasmosis. Am J Ophthalmol 2003; 135:779 [PMID: 12788116].

Sevilla N et al: Infection of dendritic cells by lymphocytic choriomeningitis virus. Curr Top Microbiol Immunol 2003;276:125 [PMID: 12797446].

Intermediate Uveitis

Pars planitis, often of uncertain cause, can be associated with vitreous floaters. The inflammation is described as snowbanking because a heaped-up white precipitate is located in the far anterior periphery of the retina and vitreous base. Pupillary dilation and indirect ophthalmoscopy are required for observation. Macular edema and decreased vision can result.

Toxocara infections with peripheral granuloma can be associated with intermediate uveitis, as can inflammatory bowel disease, multiple sclerosis, and sarcoidosis. Retinoblastoma and other neoplasms can imitate uveitis, causing a so-called masquerade syndrome.

ACQUIRED IMMUNODEFICIENCY SYNDROME & THE EYE

Ocular infections are important manifestations of acquired immunodeficiency syndrome (see Chapter 37). As CD4 T-lymphocyte counts fall below 200/μL, opportunistic infections increase in these patients. Pathogens commonly causing eye infection include *Toxoplasma gondii* and CMV. Especially when CD4+ counts fall below 50/μL, the patient is at high risk for CMV retinitis, the leading cause of vision loss in patients with the acquired immunodeficiency syndrome (see section on posterior uveitis) and blindness. Active CMV retinitis must be treated with intravenous antiviral therapy. Ganciclovir is the usual initial therapy; foscarnet may be required if resistance develops. Intravitreal ganciclovir or ganciclovir implants in conjunction with oral valganciclovir may be required in severe cases or in individuals intolerant to intravenous therapy. The incidence of CMV retinitis has fallen dramatically with the use of multidrug antiretroviral therapy.

Acute retinal necrosis syndrome (see section on posterior uveitis) is a severe necrotizing retinitis that often results in blindness in patients with the acquired immunodeficiency syndrome. Most cases are thought to be caused by varicella-zoster virus. Other implicated agents are herpes simplex types 1 and 2 and occasionally CMV. Therapy with antiviral agents is required, but the prognosis is poor. A specific human immunodeficiency virus retinopathy not associated with other known infectious agents also occurs. Various retinal abnormalities include cotton-wool spots, retinal hemorrhages, microaneurysms, perivasculitis, and decreased visual acuity from ischemic maculopathy.

Cvetkovic RS et al: Valganciclovir: a review of its use in the management of CMV infection and disease in immunocompromised patients. Drugs 2005;65:859 [PMID: 15819597].

Jabs DA et al: Characteristics of patients with cytomegalovirus retinitis in the era of highly active antiretroviral therapy. Am J Ophthalmol 2002;133:48 [PMID: 11755839].

DISORDERS OF THE CORNEA
Conditions Causing Corneal Clouding

The differential diagnosis of corneal clouding in a newborn infant includes forceps trauma, congenital glaucoma, infection, congenital malformation, and tumor. In older children, corneal clouding is associated with mucopolysaccharidoses, Wilson disease, and cystinosis. Infiltrates occur with viral infections, staphylococcal lid disease, corneal dystrophies, and interstitial keratitis due to congenital syphilis.

Microcornea & Megalocornea

Microcornea—a corneal diameter less than 10 mm in a full-term infant or older child—may be associated with other anterior segment malformations or a microphthalmic globe. Megalocornea—diameter of 12.5 mm or greater—should be regarded as due to congenital glaucoma until proved otherwise.

Keratitis

Both herpes simplex and herpes zoster can infect the cornea. When the epithelium breaks down, a dendritic or ameboid pattern can be seen with fluorescein staining. Corneal involvement with herpes simplex can be recurrent and lead to blindness. Topical antivirals such as trifluridine and vidarabine are indicated when herpes simplex infection is limited to the corneal epithelium, although additional systemic therapy is required in newborns. Topical corticosteroids may be a useful addition to antiviral therapy when stromal disease is present. The use of corticosteroids in the presence of herpetic disease should be undertaken only by an ophthalmologist because of the danger of worsening the disease. Oral acyclovir started in the early phase (first 5 days) may be helpful in treating herpes zoster eye disease. Acyclovir prophylaxis is helpful in preventing recurrent herpetic epithelial keratitis (see section on viral conjunctivitis) and stromal keratitis caused by herpes simplex.

Adenovirus conjunctivitis may progress to keratitis 1–2 weeks after onset. Slitlamp examination reveals white infiltrates beneath the corneal epithelium. Vision may be decreased. In most cases no treatment is necessary because adenovirus keratitis is most often self-limiting. However, adenovirus is highly contagious and easily spread (see section on conjunctivitis).

Contact lens wearers are at risk for severe vision-threatening *Acanthamoeba* keratitis from contaminated contact lens solutions. Treatment is difficult and may require corneal transplantation (see Chapter 39).

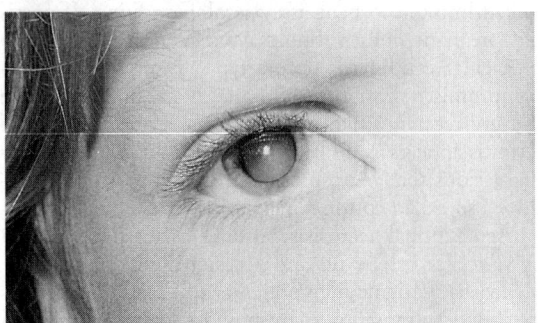

Figure 15–23. Cataract causing leukocoria.

Chong et al: Herpes simplex virus keratitis in children. Am J Ophthalmol 2004;138:474 [PMID: 15364233].

Corneal Ulcers

Bacterial corneal ulcers in healthy children who are not contact lens wearers are usually secondary to corneal trauma from corneal abrasion or a penetrating foreign body. Decreased vision, pain, injection, a white corneal infiltrate or ulcer (Figure 15–22), and hypopyon (pus in the anterior chamber) may all be present. Prompt referral to an ophthalmologist is necessary for culture and antibiotic treatment.

DISORDERS OF THE LENS

Lens disorders involve abnormality of clarity or position. Lens opacification–cataract can affect vision depending on its density, size, and position. Visual potential is also influenced by age at onset and the success of amblyopia treatment.

Cataracts

Cataracts in children may be unilateral or bilateral, may exist as isolated defects, or may be accompanied by other ocular disorders or systemic disease (Figure 15–23). Congenital and infantile cataracts may also be part of a chromosomal syndrome. Leukocoria, poor fixation, and strabismus or nystagmus (or both) may be the presenting complaints. In the newborn, absence of a red reflex should suggest the possibility of cataract, especially if the infant's pupil has been dilated for the examination. This requires an urgent referral to an ophthalmologist.

The appearance of the cataract may sometimes suggest its cause. Anterior capsular cataracts are developmental, that is, not related to infection or metabolic problems. Laboratory investigation for infectious and metabolic causes is often indicated. Such investigation would include cultures or serologic tests for toxoplasmosis, rubella, CMV, herpes simplex virus, and syphi-

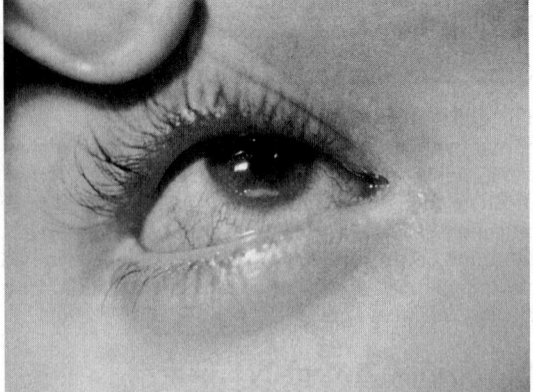

Figure 15–22. Corneal ulcer. Note white infiltrate located on inferior cornea.

lis, as well as evaluation for metabolic errors, such as may occur with galactosemia or Lowe syndrome.

Early diagnosis and treatment are necessary to prevent deprivation amblyopia in children younger than age 9 years, because they are visually immature. Cataracts that are visually significant require removal. Visually significant cataracts in infants are usually removed prior to 6 weeks of age to prevent deprivation amblyopia. Rehabilitation with an intraocular lens is commonplace, especially with cataracts removed after the age of 2 years. But contact lenses and glasses still play a role, as does occlusion of the better-seeing eye to treat the amblyopia.

Ellis FJ: Management of pediatric cataract and lens opacities. Curr Opin Ophthalmol 2002;13:33 [PMID: 11807387].

Wilson ME et al: Paediatric cataract blindness in the developing world: Surgical techniques and intraocular lenses in the new millennium. Br J Ophthalmol 2003;87:14 [PMID: 12488254].

Dislocated Lenses

Nontraumatic lens dislocation is usually bilateral. Subluxation causes refractive errors of large magnitude that are difficult to correct. Another ophthalmologic concern is pupillary block glaucoma, in which a malpositioned unstable lens interferes with the normal flow of aqueous humor from the ciliary body (posterior to the pupil) where it is produced into the trabecular meshwork (anterior to the pupillary plane).

Dislocated lenses are associated with systemic diseases, including Marfan syndrome, homocystinuria, Weill-Marchesani syndrome, sulfite oxidase deficiency, hyperlysinemia, syphilis, and Ehlers-Danlos syndrome. Work-up and treatment are multidisciplinary endeavors.

DISORDERS OF THE RETINA

Retinal Hemorrhages in the Newborn

Retinal hemorrhages are commonly seen in the otherwise healthy newborn. Although they occur most often after vaginal delivery, they can also be present after suction delivery or cesarean section. The hemorrhages may be unilateral or bilateral and be located anywhere in the retina. They may appear as dot, blot, subretinal, or preretinal hemorrhages. They may also break into the vitreous.

In general, retinal hemorrhages of the newborn disappear quickly, usually within the first month of life, which may help differentiate this condition from retinal hemorrhages that occur in the shaken baby syndrome. Retinal hemorrhages also occur in association with coagulopathy.

Retinopathy of Prematurity

Retinopathy of prematurity (ROP) continues to be an important cause of blindness, especially for infants born at less than 28 weeks' gestation and weighing less than 1250 g. Premature infants with incomplete retinal vascularization are at risk for developing abnormal peripheral retinal vascularization, which may lead to retinal detachment. However, most cases of ROP do not progress to retinal detachment and require no treatment.

The Cryotherapy for Retinopathy of Prematurity (CRYO-ROP) study outlined a standard nomenclature to describe the progression and severity of ROP (Table 15–4). Since retinal blood vessels emanate from the optic nerve, and do not fully cover the developing retina until term, the optic nerve is used as the central landmark. The most immature zone of retina, zone 1, is the most posterior concentric imaginary circle around the optic nerve. Further out is zone 2, and beyond that is zone 3. Zone 1 disease is by definition more high-risk than disease in more anterior zones. Similarly, the stages of the abnormal vessels are numbered from zero, or simply incomplete vascularization, through stages I–V. When five contiguous or eight noncontiguous clock hours of stage 3 disease occur, "threshold" has been reached. At this stage in the CRYO-ROP study, 50% of eyes had a bad outcome without treatment, progressing to stage IV or V. This was therefore chosen as the stage for mandatory treatment. "Plus disease" (+) refers to dilation and tortuosity of the vessels around the optic nerve, and is an ominous sign of active, worsening ROP. "Rush disease" refers to cases in which the disease skips intervening stages and goes rapidly to retinal detachment.

The risk of developing visually threatening ROP is inversely proportional to birth weight and gestational age. Infants weighing less than 1500 g at birth or born at less than 33 weeks' gestation may develop visually threatening ROP. The cause of this disorder—including the role of supplemental oxygen in the neonatal period—is still not fully understood. During the first epidemic of ROP in the 1960s, delivery of high levels of oxygen without arterial monitoring appeared to contribute significantly to the development of ROP. Pulse

Table 15–4. Stages of retinopathy of prematurity.

Stage I	Demarcation line or border dividing the vascular from the avascular retina.
Stage II	Ridge. Line of stage I acquires volume and rises above the surface retina to become a ridge.
Stage III	Ridge with extraretinal fibrovascular proliferation.
Stage IV	Subtotal retinal detachment.
Stage V	Total retinal detachment.

oximetry and better oxygen regulation led to a decline in cases, but better survival for the smallest, sickest infants has increased the numbers of affected infants once again, leading to speculation that low birth weight and gestational age may be more important than oxygen in etiology. Anecdotal reports of improvement in near-threshold ROP with high oxygen saturations led to the Supplemental Therapeutic Oxygen for Prethreshold Retinopathy of Prematurity (STOP-ROP) study, which investigated whether keeping partial arterial oxygen pressure high at this critical stage reduced the need for laser. The results did not show a benefit. A study in which infants were kept at relatively low oxygen saturation from birth did show a reduction in severe ROP cases and showed no increase in cerebral palsy at 18 months follow-up, which had been reported in the past with oxygen curtailment. Further study and follow-up of this method is needed. Other risk factors for severe ROP are bronchopulmonary dysplasia, intraventricular hemorrhage, sepsis, apnea and bradycardia, and mutations of the Norrie disease gene. White males, infants with zone 1 disease, and infants with very low birth weight and gestational age have a higher risk of reaching threshold.

Ambient light in the nursery as a cofactor was ruled out by the multicenter Light Reduction in Retinopathy of Prematurity (LIGHT-ROP) trial. Recent studies suggest that vascular endothelial growth factor may play a key role in ROP development, and methods of modulating it are being investigated.

Screening guidelines and a uniform classification system have been adopted, but alternative screening paradigms have also been suggested. The first retinal examination is recommended at age 4–6 weeks after birth, or 31 weeks postmenstrual age, whichever is earlier. The frequency of follow-up examinations depends on the findings and the risk factors for developing the disease, but for most infants will be every 1–2 weeks. Acute-phase ROP begins to involute at a mean postmenstrual age of 38.6 weeks, but the range for onset of involution is wide. Examinations can be discontinued when the retinas are fully vascularized, or when the baby is 45 weeks' gestational age and has never had prethreshold disease or worse, or is vascularized out to zone 3 and never had zone 1 or 2 disease. The treatment of threshold ROP within 72 hours of diagnosis with cryotherapy reduced the occurrence of bad visual outcomes by 50%. Diode laser treatment has largely replaced cryotherapy because it provides better access for treating zone 1 disease and causes less inflammation. Reported success rates are higher than with cryotherapy. However, some patients still progress to a retinal detachment which can have a very poor prognosis for vision. Surgical treatment for a retinal detachment involves scleral buckling or a lens-sparing vitrectomy by an ophthalmologist specializing in vitreoretinal surgery.

With smaller, sicker infants surviving, treatment guidelines have been amended to treat earlier than threshold in some infants. The Early Treatment for Retinopathy of Prematurity (ETROP) studies have shown that early treatment of high-risk prethreshold ROP significantly reduced unfavorable outcomes. Infants with zone 1 ROP are at the highest risk for complications from ROP. Studies investigating oxygen management and its influence on the progression of ROP are underway.

Children with a history of ROP require lifelong management by an ophthalmologist. They are at a much higher risk of developing strabismus, amblyopia, myopia, and glaucoma than the average child.

Chow LC et al: CSMC Oxygen Administration Study Group: Can changes in clinical practice decrease the incidence of severe retinopathy of prematurity in very low birth weight infants? Pediatrics 2003;111:339 [PMID: 12563061].

Early Treatment for Retinopathy of Prematurity Cooperative Group: Revised indications for the treatment of retinopathy of prematurity. Arch Ophthalmol 2003;121:1684 [PMID: 14662586].

Ellis A, Hicks M, Fielden M, Ingram A: Severe retinopathy of prematurity: longitudinal observation of disease and screening implications. Eye 2005;19:138 [PMID: 15218516].

Good WV et al: The incidence and course of retinopathy of prematurity: findings from the early treatment for retinopathy of prematurity study. Pediatrics 2005;116:15 [PMID: 15995025].

Hartnett ME et al: Comparison of retinal outcomes after scleral buckle or lens-sparing vitrectomy for stage 4 retinopathy of prematurity. Retina 2004;24:753 [PMID: 15492630].

Hubbard GB 3rd et al: Lens-sparing vitrectomy for stage 4 retinopathy of prematurity. Ophthalmology 2004;111:2274 [PMID: 15582086].

Karna P et al: Retinopathy of prematurity and risk factors: a prospective cohort study. BMC Pediatr 2005;5:18 [PMID: 15985170].

The International Committee for the Classification of Retinopathy of Prematurity: The international classification of retinopathy of prematurity revisited. Arch Ophthalmol 2005;123:991 [PMID: 16009843].

Vannay A et al: Association of genetic polymorphisms of vascular endothelial growth factor and risk for proliferative retinopathy of prematurity. Pediatr Res 2005;57:396 [PMID: 15635051].

Retinoblastoma

Retinoblastoma is the most common primary intraocular malignancy of childhood, with an incidence estimated between 1:17,000 and 1:34,000 live births (see Chapter 28). Most patients present before age 3 years; children with hereditary or bilateral retinoblastoma usually present earlier than those with unilateral, sporadic disease.

Inherited forms of retinoblastoma are autosomal dominant with high penetrance. The disease may consist of a solitary mass or multiple tumors in one or both eyes. All bilateral cases and some unilateral cases are caused by germinal mutations; however, most unilateral cases are caused by a somatic retinal mutation. In both situations, the mutation occurs in the retinoblastoma gene (*Rb*) at chromosome 13q14. This is a tumor suppressor gene. One mutated copy may be inherited in an autosomal dominant fashion (germline mutation). If a second mutation spontaneously occurs in any cell, tumorigenesis is likely. Individuals with a germinal mutation are at risk for the development of tumors other than retinoblastoma (pineal tumors, osteosarcoma, and other soft tissue sarcomas). All children with unilateral or bilateral retinoblastoma must be presumed to have the germline form, and followed expectantly for other tumors in the remaining eye and at extra-ocular sites. Approximately 15% of patients with unilateral disease have germline mutations.

The most common presenting sign in a child with previously undiagnosed retinoblastoma is leukocoria (see Figure 15–1). Evaluation of the pupillary red reflex is important, although a normal red reflex does not rule out retinoblastoma. Examination requires indirect ophthalmoscopy with scleral depression and pupillary dilation, performed by an ophthalmologist. Other children present with strabismus, red eye, glaucoma, or pseudo-hypopyon (appearance of puslike material in the anterior chamber).

Treatment of unilateral cases, especially of large tumors, often requires enucleation, because at the time of presentation the eye is filled with tumor. Vision and eyes can be salvaged in some cases. Chemoreduction of intraocular tumors is a newer treatment technique used to reduce initial tumor volume. In conjunction with local treatment such as laser photocoagulation, cryotherapy, plaque radiotherapy, and thermotherapy, combined therapy can often preserve vision and spare the patient enucleation and radiation that may lead to disfigurement and the induction of secondary tumors, especially in eyes classified with less extensive disease. Agents used in chemoreduction include carboplatin, etoposide, and vincristine. Eradication of tumor before infiltration into the optic nerve or choroid carries a good prognosis for survival.

Genetic testing is available for patients with retinoblastoma. Once the causative mutation is found in an affected individual, unaffected members of the family should be tested to determine their personal and reproductive risk. This will avoid many unnecessary examinations under anesthesia for young relatives of patients with retinoblastoma.

Chan HS et al: Chemotherapy for retinoblastoma. Ophthalmol Clin North Am 2005;18:55 [PMID: 15763191].

Curnyn KM et al: The eye examination in the pediatrician's office. Pediatr Clin North Am 2003;50:25 [PMID: 12713102].

Linn Murphree A: Intraocular retinoblastoma: the case for a new group classification. Ophthalmol Clin North Am 2005;18:41 [PMID: 15763190].

Richter S et al: Sensitive and efficient detection of *RB1* gene mutations enhances care for families with retinoblastoma. Am J Hum Genet 2003;72:253 Epub 2002 Dec 18 [PMID: 12541220].

Sussman DA et al: Comparison of retinoblastoma reduction for chemotherapy vs external beam radiotherapy. Arch Ophthalmol 2003;121:979 [PMID: 12860801].

Retinal Detachment

Retinal detachment occurs infrequently in children. Common causes are trauma and high myopia. Other causes are ROP, Marfan syndrome, and Stickler syndrome.

Symptoms of detachment are floaters, flashing lights, and loss of visual field; however, children often cannot appreciate or verbalize their symptoms. A detachment may not be discovered until the child is referred after failing a vision screening examination, strabismus supervenes, or leukocoria is noted. Treatment of retinal detachment is surgical. For children with conditions predisposing to retinal detachment, or a strong family history, examinations under anesthesia by an ophthalmologist, with prophylactic laser treatment, are often recommended.

Diabetes Mellitus

Diabetic retinopathy is a specific vascular complication of diabetes mellitus. Patients with type 1, or insulin-dependent, diabetes are at higher risk of developing severe proliferative retinopathy leading to visual loss than are those with type 2, or non-insulin-dependent, diabetes. The American Diabetes Association recommends annual screening for retinopathy 5 years after onset of diabetes in adults. In children older than age 9 years, referral to an ophthalmologist for screening of retinopathy should be begun 3–5 years after the onset of diabetes. Acute onset of diabetes may be accompanied by sudden myopia and by cataracts. Both conditions may be reversible with systemic glucose control. Young children with type 1 diabetes should be followed for the Wolfram, or DIDMOD, syndrome, in which diabetes mellitus occurs in conjunction with diabetes insipidus, optic atrophy, and deafness.

Harvey JN et al: The long-term renal and retinal outcome of childhood-onset type 1 diabetes. Diabet Med 2004;21:26 [PMID: 14706050].

Henricsson M et al: The incidence of retinopathy 10 years after diagnosis in young adult people with diabetes: results from the nationwide population-based Diabetes Incidence Study in Sweden (DISS). Diabetes Care 2003;26:349 [PMID: 12547861].

DISEASES OF THE OPTIC NERVE

Optic nerve function is evaluated by checking visual acuity, color vision, pupillary response, and visual fields.

Poor optic nerve function results in decreased central or peripheral vision, decreased color vision, strabismus, and nystagmus.

The swinging flashlight test is used to assess function of each optic nerve. It is performed by shining a light alternately in front of each pupil to check for an afferent pupillary defect or Marcus Gunn pupillary defect. An abnormal response in the affected eye is pupillary dilation when the light is directed into that eye after having been shown in the other eye with its healthy optic nerve. This results from poorer conduction along the optic nerve of the affected eye, which in turn results in less pupillary constriction of both eyes than occurs when the light is shined into the noninvolved eye. Hippus—rhythmic dilating and constricting movements of the pupil—can be confused with an afferent pupillary defect.

The optic nerve is evaluated as to size, shape, color, and vascularity. Occasionally, myelinization past the entrance of the optic nerve head occurs. It appears white, with a feathered edge (Figure 15–24). Myelinization onto the retina can be associated with myopia and amblyopia. Anatomic defects of the optic nerve include colobomatous defects and pits.

Optic nerve hypoplasia may be associated with absence of the septum pellucidum and hypothalamic-pituitary dysfunction, which is known as septo-optic dysplasia, or de Morsier syndrome. Children with septo-optic dysplasia and hypocortisolism are at risk for sudden death during febrile illness from thermoregulatory disturbance and dehydration from diabetes insipidus.

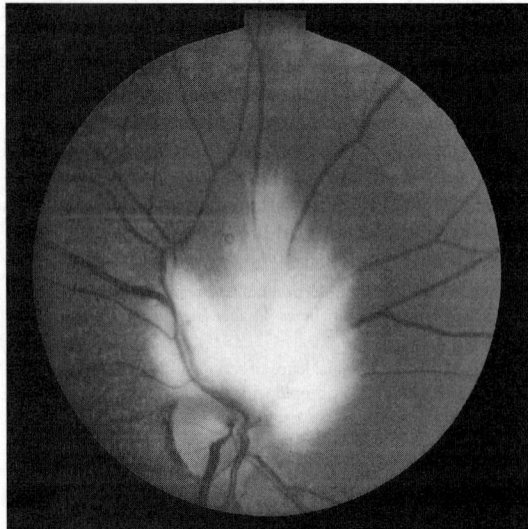

Figure 15–24. Myelinization extending from optic nerve superiorly onto the retina.

Optic nerve hypoplasia may occur in infants of diabetic mothers and has also been associated with alcohol use or ingestion of quinine or phenytoin during pregnancy. Anatomically, the size of the involved optic nerve may range from absent (aplasia) to almost full size, with a segmental defect. However, the nerve often appears larger than it is because it is surrounded by a depigmented halo. Visual function with optic nerve hypoplasia ranges from mildly decreased to absent light perception. If only one eye is involved, the child usually presents with strabismus. If both eyes are affected, nystagmus is usually the presenting sign.

Because the optic nerve is an outgrowth of the brain, changes in this structure often reflect central nervous system (CNS) disease and defects of central midline structures.

Papilledema

Papilledema (optic disc edema or choked disc) is associated with increased intracranial pressure due to any cause, such as tumor or intracranial infection. This dysfunction appears as an elevated disc with indistinct margins, increased vessel diameter, and increased capillarity, giving the disc a hyperemic appearance with surrounding hemorrhages and exudates in more severe cases. Observed changes may be subtle to striking. Optic nerve head changes are bilateral and generally symmetrical.

Besides known causes such as hydrocephalus and intracranial tumor, papilledema is associated with so-called benign intracranial hypertension, also known as pseudotumor cerebri or idiopathic intracranial hypertension. Papilledema occurs almost equally in boys and girls and sometimes is associated with obesity or upper respiratory tract infection. Other associated causes are viral infections, corticosteroid use and withdrawal, sinus infection, trauma, tetracycline use, growth hormone, and venous sinus thrombosis. Early in the course of the disorder, the patient may not notice a change in vision, although the blind spot may be enlarged. Transient obscurations of vision (amaurosis fugax) may occur as the process becomes more long-standing. Further effects on vision will occur as the papilledema becomes chronic and ultimately leads to optic atrophy. Work-up and treatment are directed toward finding the underlying systemic or CNS cause. Treatment of idiopathic intracranial hypertension may be pharmacologic—for example, using acetazolamide, a carbonic anhydrase inhibitor, or a corticosteroid. Diagnostic lumbar puncture may also be curative. Optic nerve sheath fenestration and lumboperitoneal shunt are surgical interventions.

Rekate HL et al: Lumboperitoneal shunts in children. Pediatr Neurosurg 2003;38:41 [PMID: 12476026].

Ng YT et al: Idiopathic intracranial hypertension in the pediatric population. J Child Neurol 2003;18:440 [PMID: 12886985].

Thuente DD et al: Pediatric optic nerve sheath decompression. Ophthalmology 2005;112:724 [PMID: 15808268].

Papillitis

Papillitis is a form of optic neuritis seen on ophthalmoscopic examination as an inflamed optic nerve head. Optic neuritis in the pediatric age group may be idiopathic, or associated with multiple sclerosis, acute disseminated encephalomyelitis, Devic disease, or cat-scratch disease.

Papillitis may have the same appearance as papilledema. However, papillitis may be unilateral, whereas papilledema is almost always bilateral. Papillitis can be differentiated from papilledema by an afferent pupillary defect (Marcus Gunn pupil), by its greater effect in decreasing visual acuity and color vision, and by the presence of a central scotoma. Papilledema that is not yet chronic will not have as dramatic an effect on vision. Because increased intracranial pressure can cause both papilledema and a sixth (abducens) nerve palsy, papilledema can be differentiated from papillitis if esotropia and loss of abduction are also present. However, esotropia may also develop secondarily in an eye that has lost vision from papillitis. In pseudopapilledema, a normal variant of the optic disc, the disc appears elevated, with indistinct margins and a normal vascular pattern. Pseudopapilledema sometimes occurs in hyperopic individuals. Retrobulbar neuritis, an inflamed optic nerve but with a normal-appearing nerve head, is associated with pain and the other findings of papillitis.

Work-up of the patient with papillitis includes lumbar puncture and cerebrospinal fluid analysis. *Bartonella henselae* can be detected by serology. MRI is the preferred imaging study. An abnormal MRI is associated with a worse visual outcome. Treatment with corticosteroids is frequently used.

Optic Atrophy

Optic atrophy, noted as pallor of the nerve head with loss of capillarity, occurs in children most frequently after neurologic compromise during the perinatal period. An example would be a premature infant who develops an intraventricular hemorrhage. Hydrocephalus, glioma of the optic nerve, craniosynostosis, certain neurologic diseases, and toxins such as methyl alcohol can cause optic atrophy, as can certain inborn errors of metabolism, long-standing papilledema, or papillitis.

DISEASES OF THE ORBIT

Periorbital & Orbital Cellulitis

The fascia of the eyelids joins with the fibrous orbital septum to isolate the orbit from the lids. This septum serves as a barrier to the posterior spread of infection from preseptal infection. Infections arising anterior to the orbital septum are termed preseptal. Preseptal (periorbital) cellulitis, which indicates infection of the structures of the eyelid, is characterized by lid edema, erythema, swelling, pain, and mild fever. It usually arises from a local exogenous source such as an abrasion of the eyelid, from other infections (hordeolum, dacryocystitis, or chalazion), or from infected varicella or insect bite lesions. *Staphylococcus aureus* and *Streptococcus pyogenes* are the most common pathogens cultured from these sources. Preseptal infections in children younger than age 3 years also occur from bacteremia, although this is much less common since *Haemophilus influenzae* immunization became available. *Streptococcus pneumoniae* bacteremia is still an occasional cause of this infection. Children with periorbital cellulitis from presumed bacteremia must be examined for additional foci of infection.

Infection of the orbit almost always arises from contiguous sinus infection, because the walls of three sinuses make up portions of the orbital walls and infection can breach these walls or extend by way of a richly anastomosing venous system. The orbital contents can develop a phlegmon (orbital cellulitis), or frank pus can develop in the orbit (orbital abscess). When the orbit is infected, the signs of periorbital disease are joined by proptosis (a protruding eye), restricted eye movement, and pain with eye movement. Fever is usually high. Computed tomography scanning or MRI is required to establish the extent of the infection within the orbit. Sinus imaging should be obtained at the same time. The pathogenic agents are those of acute or chronic sinusitis—respiratory flora and anaerobes. *S aureus* is also frequently implicated.

Therapy for preseptal and orbital cellulitis infection is with systemic antibiotics. Treatment of orbital infections may require surgical drainage for subperiosteal abscess in conjunction with intravenous antibiotics. Drainage of infected sinuses is often part of the therapy.

Herrmann BW et al: Simultaneous intracranial and orbital complications of acute rhinosinusitis in children. Int J Pediatr Otorhinolaryngol 2004;68:619 [PMID: 15081240].

Karkos PD et al: Recurrent periorbital cellulitis in a child. A random event or an underlying anatomical abnormality? Int J Pediatr Otorhinolaryngol 2004;68:1529 [PMID: 15533566].

Craniofacial Anomalies

Craniofacial anomalies can affect the orbit and visual system. Examples of changes associated with craniofacial disease involving the orbits are proptosis, corneal exposure, hypertelorism (widely spaced orbits), strabismus, amblyopia, lid coloboma, papilledema, and optic atrophy. Craniofacial anomalies occur with craniosynostoses and midface syndromes such as Treacher Collins and Pierre Robin syndrome. Fetal alcohol syndrome is associated with similar changes of the ocular adnexa.

Orbital Tumors

Both benign and malignant orbital lesions occur in children. The most common tumor is capillary hemangioma (Figure 15–25). This type of tumor may be located superficially in the lid or deep in the orbit and can cause ptosis, refractive errors, and amblyopia. Deeper lesions may cause proptosis. Capillary hemangiomas in infants initially increase in size before involuting at about age 2–4 years. Therapy with intralesional or systemic corticosteroids is indicated if the lesion is large enough to cause amblyopia.

Orbital dermoid cysts vary in size and are usually found temporally at the brow and orbital rim or supranasally. These lesions are firm, well encapsulated, and mobile. Rupture of the cyst causes a severe inflammatory reaction. Treatment is by excision. Lymphangioma occurring in the orbit is typically poorly encapsulated, increases in size with upper respiratory infection, and is susceptible to hemorrhage. Other benign tumors of the orbit are orbital pseudotumor, neurofibroma, teratoma, and tumors arising from bone, connective tissue, and neural tissue.

Of grave concern is orbital rhabdomyosarcoma, the most common primary orbital malignancy in childhood (see Chapter 28). This tumor grows rapidly and displaces the globe. The average age at onset is 6–7 years. The tumor is often initially mistaken for orbital swelling due to insignificant trauma. Radiation and chemotherapy are the mainstays of treatment after biopsy confirms the diagnosis. With expeditious diagnosis and proper treatment, the survival rate of patients with orbital rhabdomyosarcoma confined to the orbit approaches 90%.

Tumors metastatic to the orbit also occur; neuroblastoma is the most common. The patient may exhibit proptosis, orbital ecchymosis (raccoon eyes), Horner syndrome, or opsoclonus (dancing eyes). Ewing sarcoma, leukemia, Burkitt lymphoma, and the histiocytosis X group of diseases may involve the orbit.

Castillo BV Jr et al: Pediatric tumors of the eye and orbit. Pediatr Clin North Am 2003;50:149 [PMID: 12713110].

NYSTAGMUS

Nystagmus is a rhythmic oscillation or jiggling of the eyes. It may be unilateral or bilateral, more pronounced in one eye, or gaze-dependent. Nystagmus may be associated with esotropia or may occur with ocular lesions that cause deprivation amblyopia (eg, cataract and eyelid ptosis) or conditions in which the visual pathways are hypoplastic, sometimes referred to as "sensory nystagmus." Both optic nerve hypoplasia and macular hypoplasia, the latter occurring with aniridia or albinism, are associated with nystagmus. Nystagmus can also occur with normal ocular structures and seemingly normal CNS development, sometimes referred to as "motor nystagmus." In the latter instance, the nystagmus may be blocked in certain positions of gaze, in which case a face turn or torticollis may develop. Latent nystagmus occurs when one eye is occluded. This type of nystagmus occurs in patients with congenital esotropia. An associated amblyopia may be present.

Most nystagmus occurring in childhood is of ocular origin, but CNS disease, and less frequently inner ear disease, are other causes. A CNS cause is likely when the nystagmus is acquired. The clinician should evaluate the fundus for optic nerve abnormalities and the quality of the macular reflex, because both optic nerve hypoplasia and macular hypoplasia can cause nystagmus.

Evaluation of nystagmus begins with the pediatric ophthalmologist. Careful evaluation for iris transillumination defects caused by albinism should be performed. An electroretinogram is usually required to rule out retinal pathology as the cause. Some types of nystagmus, usually motor nystagmus, can be treated, generally with surgery; less frequently, prisms are useful. Spasmus nutans, in which a rapid, shimmering, dysconjugate nystagmus occurs with head bobbing and torticollis, is said to improve with time. Glioma of the hypothalamus can mimic spasmus nutans. Neuroimaging may be necessary to determine if the cause of the nystagmus is due to a CNS disease.

AMBLYOPIA & STRABISMUS

Visual development is a learned function. For it to proceed normally, a child must experience a normal visual environment with well-aligned eyes that are free of vision-threatening disease and significant refractive errors. The consequences of not meeting these requirements during the sensitive period of visual development

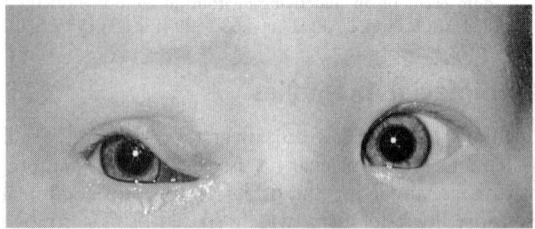

Figure 15–25. Right upper lid hemangioma causing ptosis.

in the first decade of life are strabismus and decreased vision, or amblyopia.

Amblyopia

Amblyopia is a unilateral or bilateral reduction in central visual acuity due to the sensory deprivation of a well-formed retinal image that occurs with or without a visible organic lesion commensurate with the degree of visual loss. Amblyopia can occur only during the critical period of visual development in the first decade of life when the visual nervous system is plastic. Approximately 3% of the population is amblyopic. Screening for amblyopia should be a component of periodic well-child examinations. The single best screening technique to discover amblyopia is obtaining visual acuity in each eye. In preverbal children unable to respond to visual acuity assessment, amblyogenic factors are sought, including strabismus; media opacities; unequal Brückner reflexes (pupillary red reflexes); and a family history suggestive of strabismus, amblyopia, or ocular disease occurring in childhood (see section on examination).

Amblyopia is classified according to its cause. Strabismic amblyopia can occur in the nondominant eye of a strabismic child. Refractive amblyopia can occur in both eyes if significant refractive errors are untreated (ametropic or refractive amblyopia). Another type of refractive amblyopia can occur in the eye with the worse refractive error when imbalance is present between the eyes (anisometropic amblyopia). Deprivation amblyopia occurs when dense cataracts or complete ptosis prevents formation of a formed retinal image. Of the three types of amblyopia, this form of amblyopia results in the worst vision.

The earlier treatment is begun, the better the chance of improving visual acuity. Treatment is usually discontinued after age 9 years. Amblyogenic factors such as refractive errors are addressed. Because of the extreme sensitivity of the visual nervous system in infants, congenital cataracts and media opacities must be diagnosed and treated within the first few weeks of life. Visual rehabilitation and amblyopia treatment must then be started in order to foster visual development.

After eradicating amblyogenic factors, the mainstay of treatment is patching the sound eye, which causes the visual nervous system to process input from the amblyopic eye and in that way permits the development of useful vision. Other treatment modalities include "fogging" the sound eye with cycloplegic drops (atropine), lenses, and filters.

Repka MX et al: A randomized trial of patching regimens for treatment of moderate amblyopia in children. Arch Ophthalmol 2003;121:603 [PMID: 12742836].

Repka MX et al: Pediatric Eye Disease Investigator Group. Two-year follow-up of a 6-month randomized trial of atropine vs patching for treatment of moderate amblyopia in children. Arch Ophthalmol 2005;123:149 [PMID: 15710809].

Strabismus

Strabismus is misalignment of the visual axes of the two eyes. Its prevalence in childhood is about 2–3%. Strabismus is categorized by the direction of the deviation and its frequency. Early diagnosis of strabismus and amblyopia, which often coexist, provides the best chance of reaching full visual potential. Strabismus may cause or be due to amblyopia.

Misdiagnosis of strabismus when the eyes are well aligned—pseudostrabismus—can occur when relying on the gross observation of the appearance of the two eyes. If the child has prominent epicanthal folds, pseudoesotropia may be diagnosed erroneously. Observation of the reflection of a penlight on the cornea, the corneal light reflex, is a more accurate means of determining if the eyes are straight. If strabismus is present, the corneal light reflex will not be centered in both eyes.

An infant whose eyes are destined to be well aligned may appear intermittently esotropic, but this should occur less frequently over the first few months of life. By age 5 or 6 months, the baby's eyes should be constantly well aligned.

Besides its effect on visual development, strabismus may be a marker of other ocular or systemic disease. Twenty percent of patients with retinoblastoma exhibit strabismus. Patients with CNS disorders such as hydrocephalus, space-occupying lesions, and an amaurotic (blind) eye can also exhibit strabismus. In children younger than age 3 or 4 years, blind eyes tend to assume a position of esodeviation, but after about age 4 years an amaurotic eye tends to show an exotropic shift.

A. ESOTROPIA

In esotropia, the visual axes of the eyes are excessively convergent. In terms of cause and treatment, esotropia can be categorized by age at onset. Congenital esotropia (infantile esotropia) has its onset in the first year of life in healthy infants. The deviation is large and obvious. Surgery is the mainstay of treatment. Controversy exists as to how young the child should be when surgery is performed so that the child can obtain an optimal binocular result. The age range is from younger than 6 months to 2 years. Esotropia beginning in the first year also occurs in premature infants or in children with a complicated perinatal history associated with CNS problems such as intracranial hemorrhage and periventricular leukomalacia. Esotropia is associated with certain syndromes. In Möbius' syndrome (congenital facial diplegia), a sixth nerve palsy causing esotropia is associated with palsies of the seventh and twelfth cranial nerves and limb deformities. Duane syndrome can affect the medial or lateral rectus muscles (or both). It may be an isolated defect or may be associated with a multitude of systemic defects (eg, Goldenhar syndrome). Duane syndrome is often misdiagnosed as a sixth (abducens) nerve palsy. The left eye is involved more commonly than the right, but both eyes can be involved. Girls are affected more frequently than boys. Children with unilateral paretic or restrictive causes of esotropia may develop face turns toward the affected eye in order to maintain binocularity.

The most frequent type of acquired esotropia is the accommodative type (Figure 15–26). Onset is usually between ages 2 and 5 years. The deviation is variable in magnitude and constancy and is often accompanied by amblyopia. One type of accommodative esotropia is associated with a high hyperopic refraction. In another type, the deviation is worse with near than with distant vision. This type of esodeviation is usually associated with lower refractive errors. Management includes

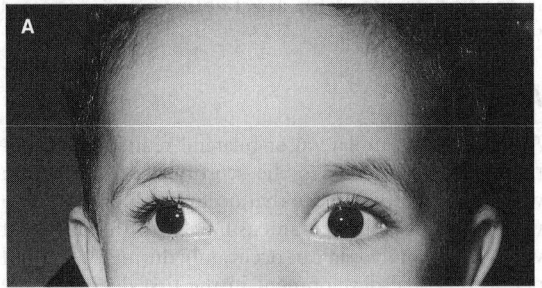

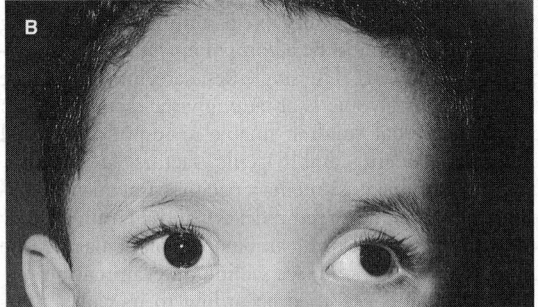

Figure 15–27. Exotropia. **A:** Fixation with left eye. **B:** Fixation with right eye.

glasses with or without bifocals, amblyopia treatment, and in some cases surgery. After age 5 years, any esotropia of recent onset should arouse suspicion of CNS disease. Infratentorial masses, hydrocephalus, demyelinating diseases, and idiopathic intracranial hypertension are causes of abducens palsy, which appears as an esotropia, lateral rectus paralysis or paresis, and face turn. The face turn is an attempt to maintain binocularity away from the field of action of the paretic muscle. Papilledema is often but not invariably present with increased intracranial pressure. Besides the vulnerability of the abducens nerve to increased intracranial pressure, it is susceptible to infection and inflammation. Otitis media and Gradenigo syndrome (inflammatory disease of the petrous bone) can cause sixth nerve palsy. Less commonly, migraine and diabetes mellitus are considerations in children with sixth nerve palsy. Work-up includes imaging studies and neurologic examination.

B. EXOTROPIA

Exotropia does not usually offer as many diagnostic pitfalls as esotropia. The visual axes of the two eyes are deviated in a divergent position (Figure 15–27). The deviation most often begins intermittently and occurs after age 2 years. Congenital (infantile) exotropia is extremely rare in an otherwise healthy infant. Early-onset exotropia may occur in infants and children with severe neurologic problems. All children with constant,

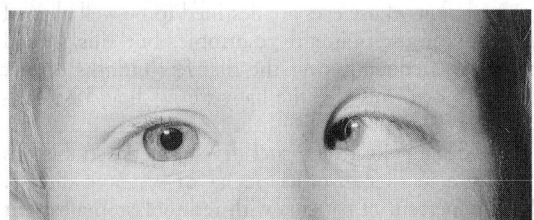

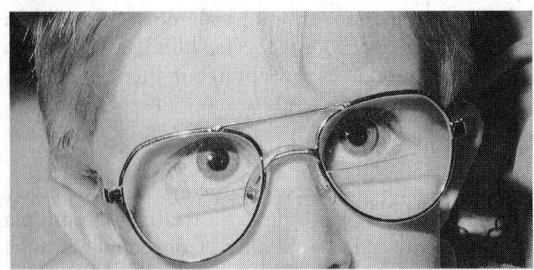

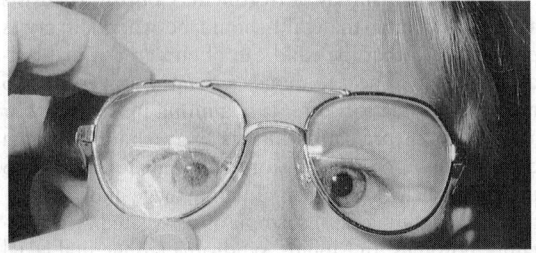

Figure 15–26. Accommodative esotropia. Without glasses, esotropic (**A**). With glasses, well-aligned at distance (**B**), and at near with bifocal correction (**C**).

congenital exotropia require CNS neuroimaging. Treatment of exotropia is with surgery, orthoptic exercises, patching, and occasionally glasses.

Archer SM et al: Social and emotional impact of strabismus surgery on quality of life in children. J AAPOS 2005;9:148 [PMID: 15838442].

Birch EE et al: Measurement of stereoacuity outcomes at ages 1 to 24 months: Randot Stereocards. J AAPOS 2005;9:31 [PMID: 15729278].

Ing MR et al: Outcome study of the development of fusion in patients aligned for congenital esotropia in relation to duration of misalignment. J AAPOS 2004;8:35 [PMID: 14970797].

Mohney BG et al: Common forms of childhood exotropia. Ophthalmology 2003;110:2093 [PMID: 14597514].

UNEXPLAINED DECREASED VISION IN INFANTS & CHILDREN

Some infants with delayed visual development during the first few months of life who are otherwise normal neurologically will reach an appropriate level of visual maturation. Occult causes of poor vision and blindness in children are those for which there are no obvious ocular defects: they include Leber congenital amaurosis, a childhood form of retinitis pigmentosa; achromatopsia, the absence of functioning cones in the retina; and optic nerve abnormalities, including optic nerve hypoplasia and atrophy.

Cerebral visual impairment, also known as cortical blindness, is manifested as decreased visual attentiveness of varying degree. Cerebral visual impairment can be congenital or acquired. Insults to the optic pathways and higher cortical visual centers are responsible. Asphyxia, trauma, intracranial hemorrhage, and periventricular leukomalacia are some of the causes of cortical visual impairment.

Besides an ophthalmologic work-up, electroretinogram and visual evoked response testing may be required in children with decreased vision of unexplained etiology. Imaging studies of the brain and a pediatric neurologic evaluation may be useful. A low-vision assessment may be indicated. Low-vision aids enhance remaining vision. Devices used include magnifiers for both distance and near vision, closed-circuit television, and large-print reading materials.

Hoyt CS: Visual function in the brain-damaged child. Eye 2003;17:369 [PMID: 12724701].

THE BLIND CHILD

Vision is the principal route of sensory input. A child's development will therefore be affected profoundly by blindness or very poor vision. There are psychological consequences for the child blind from birth, as well as for the family. It can be devastating to a young family to find out that their newborn is blind. Although acquired blindness may give an individual time to grow as a sighted person and make preparations for life as a nonsighted person if loss of vision is slow and predicted, psychological consequences for the child and family must be addressed. The child blind from birth or from very early childhood has had little or no opportunity to form visual impressions of the physical world. Blind children and their families should receive the benefit of knowledgeable therapists and support groups.

Blind infants reach developmental landmarks on a different schedule from that of sighted children. In addition, some blind children are multiply handicapped. For example, the premature child who is blind from ROP may also have cerebral palsy. Children with Usher syndrome become both deaf and blind.

Leading causes of blindness in the pediatric age group differ among regions of the world and between industrialized nations and developing countries. The most common causes of blindness in the pediatric age group are thought to be cerebral visual impairment, ROP, and optic nerve hypoplasia. Albinism, optic atrophy, cataract, retinitis pigmentosa, microphthalmia or anophthalmia, aniridia, and glaucoma are other diseases causing blindness.

Thompson L et al: The visually impaired child. Pediatr Clin North Am 2003;50:225 [PMID: 12713115].

LEARNING DISABILITIES & DYSLEXIA

Visits to the physician because of educational difficulties are common. Evaluation of the child with learning disabilities and dyslexia should include ophthalmologic examination to identify any ocular disorders that could cause or contribute to poor school performance. Most children with learning difficulties have no demonstrable problems on ophthalmic examination.

A multidisciplinary approach as suggested by the American Academy of Pediatrics, the American Association for Pediatric Ophthalmology and Strabismus, and the American Academy of Ophthalmology is recommended in evaluating children with learning disabilities. Although many therapies directed at "training the eyes" exist, scientific support for such approaches is weak.

Smith LA et al: Developmental differences in understanding the causes, controllability and chronicity of disabilities. Child Care Health Dev 2005;31:479 [PMID: 15948885].

VISION SCREENING

Vision screening in the pediatric age group is a challenge, especially in younger and developmentally delayed children. Accuracy of the screening test being administered to a particular population and expense in terms of time, equipment, and personnel are some of the factors that must be considered in screening individuals and groups. Vision screening is consistent with the recommendations of the American Academy of Pediatrics (www.aap.org). Risk factors that should be screened for because they interfere with normal visual development and are amblyogenic include media opacities, strabismus, and refractive errors that are different in the two eyes (anisometropia) or of large magnitude in both eyes.

The practitioner should have an understanding of the limitations of the screening test being administered. For example, one study cites the sensitivity and specificity of visual acuity screening in preschool children as 90% and 44%, respectively. When possible, visual acuity of each eye and alignment of the two eyes should be assessed (see section on visual acuity for acceptable acuities at different ages). Two caveats are to be observed when testing monocular visual acuity. First, in an amblyopic patient who demonstrates the crowding phenomenon, an amblyopic eye may score better when presented with single, isolated targets than with multiple targets on a line. Second, monocular visual acuity is worse in a patient with latent nystagmus. Preschool and young school-age children often test better when looking at a visual acuity chart at a 10-foot distance than at one placed at 20 feet or when looking into the type of machine typically used at a motor vehicle licensing department.

When it is not possible to measure visual acuity or assess alignment in the preschool-age group, random dot stereopsis testing (for depth perception) is effective in screening for manifest strabismus and amblyopia, but this test may miss some cases of anisometropic (unequal refractive error) amblyopia and small-angle strabismus. This test is not designed to detect refractive errors.

An innovative technique that is being used more frequently in the pediatric age group and may prove useful for developmentally delayed children and perhaps infants is photoscreening. Photoscreening relies on the Brückner test of corneal light reflexes. Photoscreening does not screen directly for amblyopia but for amblyogenic factors, which include strabismus, media opacities, and refractive errors. Automated methods of photoscreening are still being validated. Problems exist with sensitivity and specificity of the instruments, and the role of their use in the pediatric population remains a controversy.

Arnold RW et al: The cost and yield of photoscreening: impact of photoscreening on overall pediatric ophthalmic costs. J Pediatr Ophthalmol Strabismus 2005;42:103 [PMID: 15825747].

Salcido AA et al: Predictive value of photoscreening and traditional screening of preschool children. J AAPOS 2005;9:114 [PMID: 15838437].

Oral Medicine & Dentistry

William A. Mueller, DMD

The American Academy of Pediatric Dentistry and the American Academy of Pediatrics recommend that a child's first oral examination be performed no later than age 12 months, and optimally within 6 months after eruption of the first tooth. This recommendation is especially important for low-income children and others in the high-risk group who are most susceptible to early disease. It is intended to establish the child's dental home and provide an opportunity to implement preventive dental health habits. Because the bacterial infection causing dental caries can be acquired as early as age 14 months, waiting until age 3 years, which was the prior recommendation, allows for significant disease before treatment. Pediatric dentists, or other dentists who focus on the high-risk child, are knowledgeable about early childhood caries. Their familiarity with the effectiveness of sealants, fluorides, and cariology makes them the parents' best resource for help in rearing caries-free children. Some experts have suggested that infant oral health begin with prenatal oral health counseling. This recommendation becomes more critical when we consider the emerging evidence of an association between maternal periodontal disease and preterm birth.

Most oral disease in children is preventable. Oral evaluation of a child should consist of infant risk assessment and anticipatory guidance. This approach advances dental care past tooth monitoring to health promotion. Infant risk assessment determines the danger for each child of developing oral disease. Anticipatory guidance is directed toward individualized cost-effective use of dental services. Because pediatricians and other pediatric health care professionals are far more likely to encounter new mothers and infants than are dentists, it is essential that they be aware of the infectious pathophysiology and associated risk factors of early childhood dental caries in order to guide effective intervention. The foremost risk factor for childhood oral disease is poverty.

The primary goals for an infant oral health program are (1) to establish with parents the goals of oral health, (2) to inform parents of their role in reaching these goals, (3) to motivate parents to learn and practice good preventive dental care, and (4) to initiate a long-term dental care relationship with parents. Pediatri-cians should incorporate oral health into anticipatory guidance either by providing this information in their offices or by referring the child to a pediatric dental colleague.

ORAL EXAMINATION OF THE NEWBORN & INFANT

The mouth of the normal newborn is lined with an intact, smooth, moist, and shiny mucosa (Figure 16–1). The alveolar ridges are continuous and relatively smooth. Within the alveolar bone are numerous tooth buds, which at birth are mostly primary teeth.

Teeth

The primary teeth begin to form at approximately 6 weeks of gestation, and their calcification starts in the second trimester. The permanent teeth are just beginning to develop at birth. There is enough development of permanent teeth to permit their damage by perinatal or antenatal insults, such as anoxia, severe jaundice, or infection.

The primary teeth usually begin to erupt at approximately age 6–7 months. However, on rare occasions (1:2000), teeth are present at birth (natal teeth) or erupt within the first month (neonatal teeth). These are most common in the anterior mandible and can be "real" primary teeth or supernumerary teeth. These can be differentiated radiographically. On occasion, these teeth must be removed to facilitate nursing, heal persistent ulceration of the tongue, or eliminate the risk of aspiration.

Frena

Noticeable but small maxillary and mandibular labial frena should be present (Figure 16–2). Several small accessory frena may also be present farther posteriorly. The extreme is multiple thick tightly bound frena, as in oral-facial-digital syndrome. Decisions about if and when a labial frenum should be reduced surgically are best left until adolescence. Many thick frena need not be corrected.

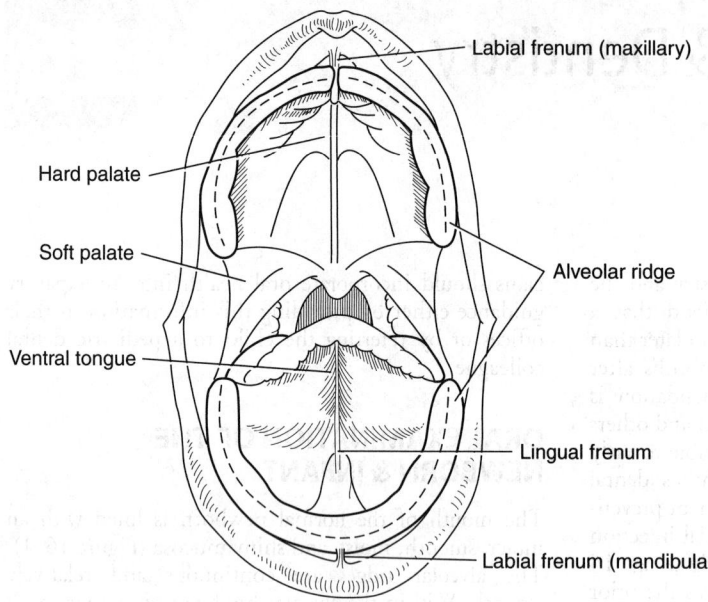

Figure 16–1. Normal anatomy of the newborn mouth.

The tongue is connected to the floor of the mouth by the lingual frenum (Figures 16–1 and 16–3). This connection should not impede the free movement of the tongue. If the attachment is tight and high up on the alveolar ridge (Figure 16–4), it may restrict movement and cause periodontal damage. This condition is called ankyloglossia (tongue-tie). If it needs to be corrected surgically, earlier (at age 3–4 years) is better than later, but there is usually no urgency for surgery in the neonatal period.

Palate

The palate of the newborn should be intact and continuous from the alveolar ridge anteriorly to the uvula (see Figure 16–1). Cleft lip and palate are common defects

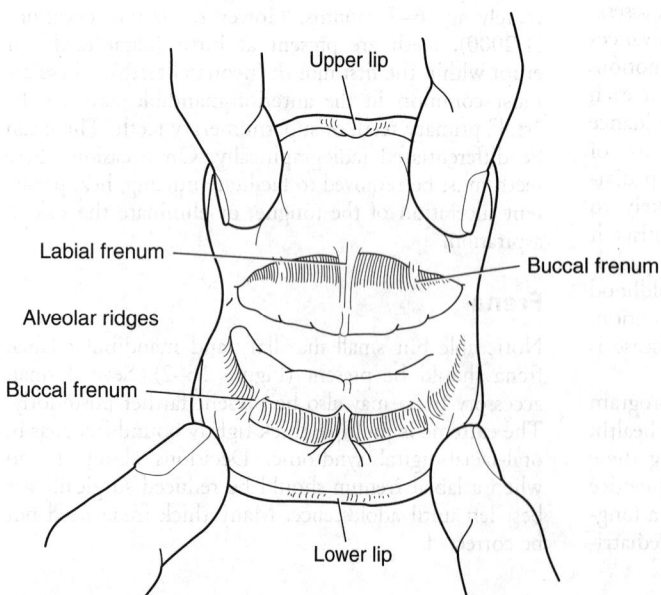

Figure 16–2. The frena.

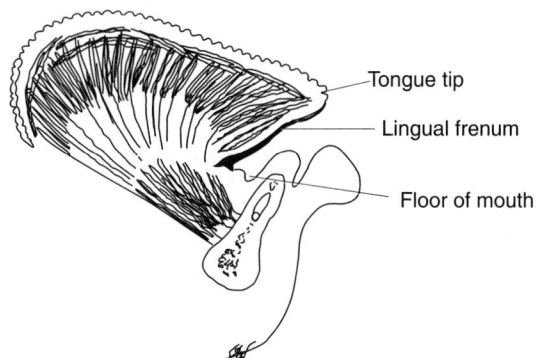

Figure 16–3. Normal position of lingual frenum.

(1:700 live births). The cleft of the palate can be unilateral or bilateral (Figure 16–5). The cleft can involve just the alveolar ridge, or the ridge and entire palate. Clefts can also be isolated soft palate defects. This is common in the Pierre Robin syndrome. Cleft palate may also present a submucous cleft, which may be detected by passing a finger posteriorly along the midline of the palate. Normally the posterior nasal spine is detectable, but if a submucous cleft is present, a bony notch will be found. Affected children sometimes have a bifid uvula.

Cleft lip and palate rehabilitation requires an extensive program involving many specialties and can be a lifelong endeavor. Children with cleft palate are best treated by a cleft palate team which coordinates care from relevant specialties. Cleft lip and palate treatment may begin immediately after birth with fabrication of a palatal obturator as a feeding aid. This appliance also helps approximate the alveolar segments in order to facilitate the initial lip repair. In the case of bilateral cleft lip and palate, the dentist may apply extraoral orthopedic traction to guide the protruding premaxilla back into the oral cavity to facilitate surgical lip closure.

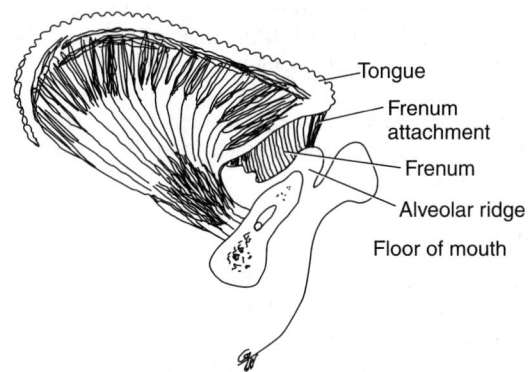

Figure 16–4. Ankyloglossia (tongue-tie).

Dental involvement in children with cleft palate is extensive and is coordinated by the cleft palate team.

Other Soft Tissue Variations

Other minor soft tissue variations can exist in the newborn mouth. Small (1–2 mm), round, smooth, whitish bumps can appear on the alveolar ridges or the palate. These are keratin cysts, called Epstein pearls or dental lamina cysts, that are benign and require no treatment because they usually disappear.

Some newborns may have small intraoral lymphangiomas on the alveolar ridge or the floor of the mouth. These and any other soft tissue variations that are more noticeable or larger than those just described should be evaluated by a dentist familiar with neonates.

ERUPTION OF THE TEETH

Normal Eruption

As the child grows, problems of teething may occur. Primary teeth generally begin to erupt at about age 6 months. They are usually mandibular incisors, but can be maxillary, and appear as early as age 3–4 months or as late as age 12–16 months. Many side effects are ascribed to teething, such as diarrhea, drooling, fever, and rash. But any real correlation is doubtful.

Common treatment for teething pain has been application of a topical anesthetic or "teething gel." Most of these agents contain benzocaine, or less commonly lidocaine. They can cause numbness of the entire oral cavity and pharynx, and suppression of the gag reflex can be a serious side effect. Systemic analgesia (acetaminophen or ibuprofen) is safer and more effective. Solid rubber or chilled fluid-filled teething toys are beneficial, if only for distraction purposes. Massaging the gums can be very soothing.

Occasionally, swelling of the gingiva is seen during teething. This condition can appear as red to purple, round, raised, smooth lesions that may be symptomatic but usually are not. They appear in the anterior or posterior alveolar ridge and on the crest. These so-called eruption cysts or eruption hematomas are fluid-filled areas immediately overlying an erupting tooth and generally disappear spontaneously.

Delayed Eruption

Premature loss of a primary tooth can either accelerate or delay eruption of the underlying secondary tooth. Early eruption occurs when the permanent tooth is beginning its active eruption and the overlying primary tooth is removed. This generally occurs when the primary tooth is within 1 year of its normal exfoliation. If, however, loss of the primary tooth occurs more than 1 year before expected exfoliation, the permanent tooth

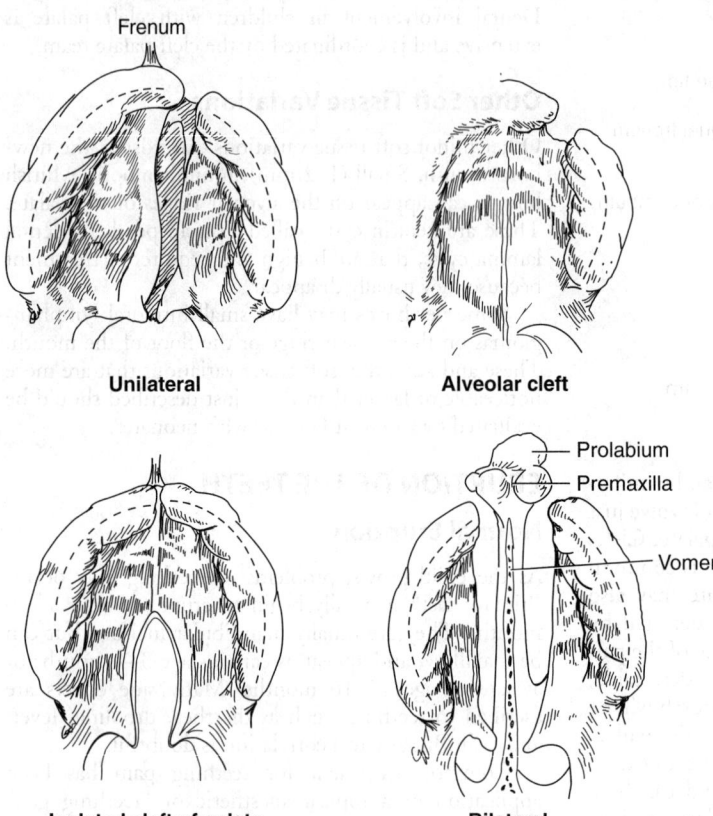

Frenum

Unilateral

Alveolar cleft

Prolabium
Premaxilla
Vomer

Isolated cleft of palate

Bilateral

Figure 16–5. Types of clefts.

will probably be delayed in eruption owing to healing that results in filling in of bone and gingiva over the permanent tooth. The loss of a primary tooth may cause adjacent teeth to tip into the space and lead to impaction of the underlying permanent tooth. A space maintainer should be placed by a dentist to avoid this.

Other local factors delaying or preventing eruption include supernumerary teeth, cysts, tumors, overretained primary teeth, ankylosed primary teeth, and impaction. A generalized delay in eruption may be due to endocrinopathies (hypothyroidism or hypopituitarism) or other systemic conditions (cleidocranial dysplasia, rickets, or trisomy 21).

Ectopic Eruption

Ectopic eruption occurs when the position of an erupting tooth is abnormal. In severe instances, the order in which teeth erupt is affected. If the dental arch provides insufficient room, permanent teeth may erupt abnormally. In the mandible, lower incisors may be lingually placed to such an extent that the primary incisors do not exfoliate. The parents' concern about a "double row of teeth" may be the reason for the child's first dental

visit. If the primary teeth are not loose, they may be removed by the dentist; if they are loose, they are generally allowed to exfoliate naturally. In the maxilla, inadequate room for eruption of the permanent first molar may cause abnormal resorption of the distal root structures of the second primary molar. If the problem is severe, the permanent molar may even become caught under the unresorbed enamel crown of the deciduous molar and thus require extraction of the primary tooth and orthodontic repositioning of the permanent first molar after it has erupted. If the first molar is not repositioned, the second premolar is likely to become impacted. If problems are detected early, the dentist may be able to redirect the permanent molar's eruption pathway so that it erupts correctly and the second primary molar is not lost.

Impaction

Impaction occurs when a tooth is prevented from erupting for any reason. The teeth most often affected are the third molars (wisdom teeth) and the maxillary canines. Patients with impacted third molars are at risk for developing odontogenic tumors or dentigerous cysts. The impacted third molar (along with its opposing third molar) may be removed after it has been determined that eruption cannot occur, but this decision may not be possible until the late teens. Impacted maxillary canines should not be extracted because of their aesthetic importance and key role in facial development and dental occlusion. They can often be brought into correct alignment through surgical exposure and orthodontic treatment.

Other Variations

Failure of teeth to develop—a condition sometimes called congenitally missing teeth—is rare in the primary dentition. However, it occurs in about 5% of permanent dentitions, with one or more of the third molars missing in about 25% of all individuals. The ones most frequently missing are maxillary lateral incisors and mandibular second premolars. The incidence of congenitally missing teeth varies among different genetic groups.

Occasionally, extra teeth are present, most typically an extra (fourth) molar or extra (third) bicuspid. Mesiodens, which are peg-shaped supernumerary teeth situated at the maxillary midline that occur in about 5% of individuals, may interfere with eruption of permanent incisors. Mesiodens should be considered for removal even if they do not erupt.

DENTAL CARIES & PERIODONTAL DISEASE

The process of tooth decay (caries) and periodontal disease are among the most common and easily preventable of all infectious diseases. Current research is changing the traditional view of dental caries as the manifestation of caries activity (eg, "holes in the teeth"). Practitioners are now pursuing the more practical objective of diagnosing and treating the caries process in the context of a life continuum, rather than only as cavitated teeth. The traditional "cavity" is irreversible and requires surgical correction. Filling cavities does nothing to address the underlying pathologic process that caused them. Prevention, early diagnosis, and prompt intervention offer greater efficiency and better health outcomes with lower costs.

The basic tenets of cariology are

1. Caries is the most common chronic disease of childhood.
2. Caries is an infectious disease that is transmissible and caused by colonization with *Streptococcus mutans.*
3. *S mutans* is transmitted from a mother to her child and detectable by 26 months on average, with a range of 12–36 months.
4. Caries is a process present in all individuals. The expression of cavities depends on its level of activity and the host's resistance.

5. After establishment of *S mutans* in the oral cavity, caries is a dietary disease.
6. Control of caries before age 3 years is aimed at limiting the establishment of *S mutans* by reducing the number of episodes of direct transmission from highly infectious mothers; reducing dietary support for *S mutans* (refined carbohydrates); and ensuring proper levels of fluoride exposure topically and systemically.
7. Control of caries after age 3 years is aimed at limiting the acidogenesis of oral flora by reducing the frequency of carbohydrate ingestion and maintaining a high frequency of fluoride exposures.
8. There is a threshold of caries activity below which clinical disease does not develop.
9. Caries is largely a disease of poverty; the 29 million children and adolescents in low-income families account for 80% of tooth decay. The greatest impact physicians can have on this disease is through early referral of low-income, high-risk children to dental practitioners.

Teeth can be attacked by acidogenic bacteria, especially *S mutans*. Dental plaque accumulates on the surface of the teeth as an adherent film. As plaque grows, bacteria accumulate within it in close proximity to the tooth. An equally important factor is a substrate for the bacteria. Carbohydrate—especially a refined carbohydrate such as sucrose—is the most effective substrate for caries, since bacteria readily metabolize sucrose to produce acid. The acidic environment causes the enamel of the teeth to dissolve, which is the beginning of caries. After the decay process has penetrated the enamel, there is very little to keep it from affecting the vital tissues (nerve) of the tooth. The tooth subsequently becomes necrotic, and an abscess occurs (Figure 16–6). This process is not always symptomatic, but it can lead to severe pain, fever, and swelling.

In the early stages of decay, the tooth may be sensitive to temperature changes, or especially to sweets. At this point, the tooth can be repaired by removing the caries and filling the defect. As the decay progresses, more pain may be involved, and root canal therapy may be necessary for both primary or permanent teeth. Once an abscess has formed, with or without swelling, a choice must be made between root canal therapy and removal of the tooth. In the presence of cellulitis or facial space abscess, extraction is usually the treatment of choice.

Many people question the importance of the primary dentition. However, baby teeth allow the child to eat properly, speak properly, have a good self-image, and preserve the space for the permanent dentition. Premature loss of primary teeth can cause major orthodontic and dental growth and development problems.

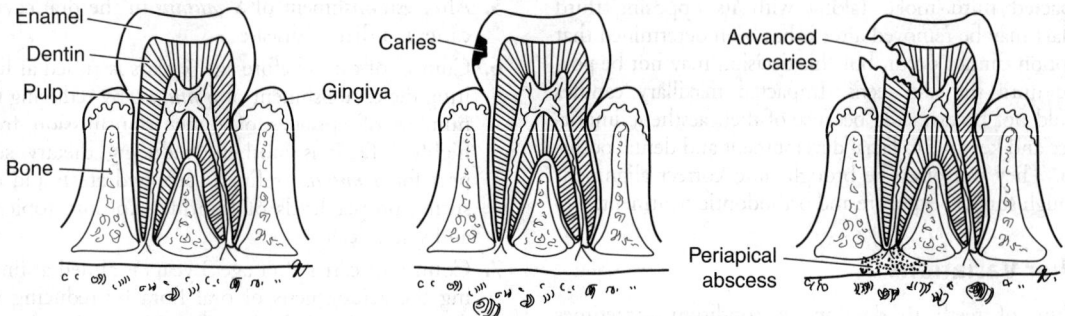

Figure 16–6. Tooth anatomy and progression of caries.

Preventing Dental Caries

To prevent dental caries, it is necessary to remove the bacteria on a regular basis. Oral hygiene for the infant should start at birth. The gums can be cleaned gently with a moist, soft cloth. Once the teeth begin to erupt, oral hygiene must be practiced in earnest. Again, a moist, soft cloth can be used after feeding to gently rub the teeth. A very small, very soft toothbrush can be used as well. Toothpaste at the start is not necessary but should be added by age 2 years. Prior to age 6 years parents may need to be involved in brushing and flossing. Brushing with a fluoride-containing toothpaste (at least twice daily) and flossing the teeth regularly will minimize the oral flora. A second step is to decrease the amount of substrate available to the bacteria. Eliminating refined carbohydrates is very effective (low-sugar diets), but limiting exposure to them is also beneficial because each exposure produces an acidic environment for up to 30 minutes. The form of the substrate is important. Caramels, licorice, raisins, and gummy bears contain concentrated sugar with a sticky texture that will remain on the teeth much longer than the same sugar in liquid form. The primary care physician can play an invaluable role in disseminating this information and reinforcing these ideas.

Fluoride

Fluoride prevents dental caries predominantly after eruption of the tooth into the mouth. Its actions are primarily topical for both children and adults. The mechanisms of action include inhibition of demineralization, enhancement of remineralization, and inhibition of bacterial activity in dental plaque. Table 16–1 sets forth the current systemic fluoride dosages to be administered to children as recommended by the American Academy of Pediatrics and the American Academy of Pediatric Dentistry. It is important not to exceed these recommendations because doing so may lead to fluorosis, which is unsightly staining of the permanent teeth. Children from low-income families residing in areas with fluoridated water incur treatment costs one-half that for such children in nonfluoridated areas, and they require less hospitalization for treatment.

Daily topical fluoride therapy is used in addition to all other oral hygiene measures in certain high-risk children. Children allowed to take their bottle to bed and those who nurse at will and fall asleep nursing are at

Table 16–1. Fluoride dosages administered to children based on tap water fluoride supply.

Age	Dose of Fluoride Administered		
	If < 0.3 ppm F in Drinking Water	If 0.3–0.6 ppm F in Drinking Water	If > 0.6 ppm F in Drinking Water
6 months to 3 years	0.25 mg/d	0	0
3–6 years	0.5 mg/d	0.25 mg/d	0
6–16 years	1 mg/d	0.5 mg/d	0

higher risk for early childhood caries. This particular type of decay typically involves the maxillary incisors and any other teeth present. When a child is lying in bed sucking on a bottle, the contents of the bottle are "trapped" between the backs of the front teeth and the tongue. This allows for more concentrated damage to the teeth as the acid produced by bacteria fails to dissipate. In addition, as the child falls asleep, salivary function decreases dramatically. This further endangers the teeth by eliminating the buffering capacity of saliva and its remineralizing potential. Topical fluoride may slow the decay process and, combined with elimination of high-risk nursing practices and institution of good oral hygiene, can prevent serious dental problems in these infants. The single most important oral care advice the physician can give to a new mother is to brush the child's teeth daily starting as soon as a tooth is present.

Patients with chronically low oral pH may benefit from daily topical fluoride. This includes those with gastroesophageal reflux, bulimia, or salivary dysfunction from radiation, graft-versus-host disease, or autoimmune disease. Saliva is a very effective oral cavity buffer. It also helps remineralize minor enamel dissolution. Xerostomia can lead to rampant caries. These children need dental care more frequently than healthy children. Multiply handicapped children who cannot maintain proper oral hygiene can also benefit from additional topical fluoride. Any child with a serious medical problem or disability should be referred to a pediatric dentist as early as possible, usually before age 1 year.

Periodontal Disease

Periodontal disease involves the supporting structures: bone, gums, and ligaments. It begins as inflammation of the gum tissue adjacent to the tooth. Bacterial accumulation in the space between the tooth and gum (gingival sulcus) causes irritation that leads to inflamed tissue. This beginning phase is called gingivitis. As the inflammation spreads through the sulcus, it involves more soft tissue. Eventually soft tissue destruction and loss of bone occur as disease spreads toward the apex of the tooth. This is called periodontitis and requires professional cleaning and often medication or surgery for correction. Figure 16–7 shows the different stages and progression of periodontal disease.

The prevention and initial management of periodontal disease in children involves removal of bacteria from the teeth with proper oral hygiene. An association between maternal periodontal disease and preterm birth has been established. It is currently unclear whether this association involves causation or it is a marker for another etiology.

OROFACIAL TRAUMA

Orofacial trauma often consists only of abrasions or lacerations of the lips, gingiva, tongue, or mucosa, includ-

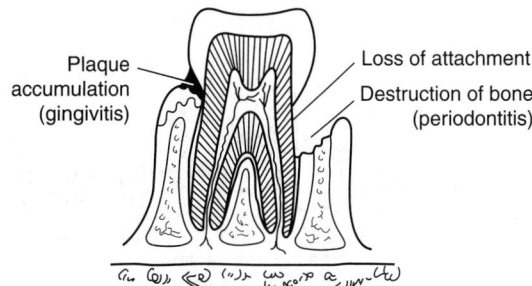

Figure 16–7. Periodontal disease.

ing the frena, without damage to the teeth. Lacerations should be cleansed and inspected for foreign bodies and sutured if necessary. Occasionally, radiographs of the tongue, lips, or cheeks are used to detect tooth fragments or other foreign bodies.

Tooth-related trauma can result in displacement (luxation), fracture, or loss of teeth (avulsion). Figure 16–8 demonstrates the different luxation injuries, and Figure 16–9 shows the different degrees of tooth fracture.

The least problematic luxation injury is mobility without displacement (subluxation). Unless mobility is extensive, this condition can be followed without active intervention. An intrusive luxation in the primary dentition is usually observed for a period of time to discern whether the tooth or teeth will reerupt (see Figure 16–8). If this has not occurred after several months or if the area

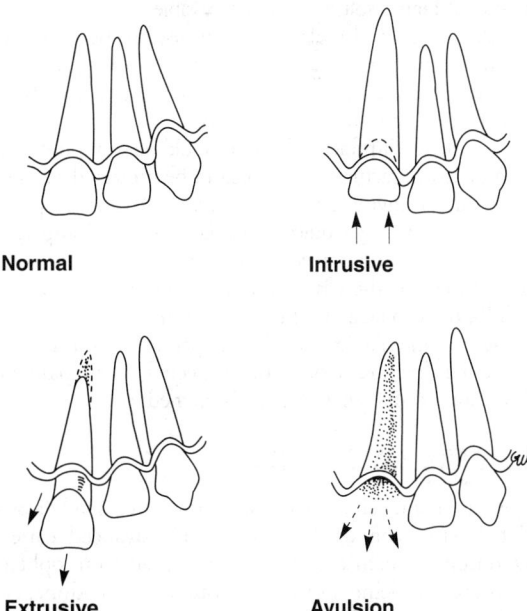

Figure 16–8. Patterns of luxation injuries.

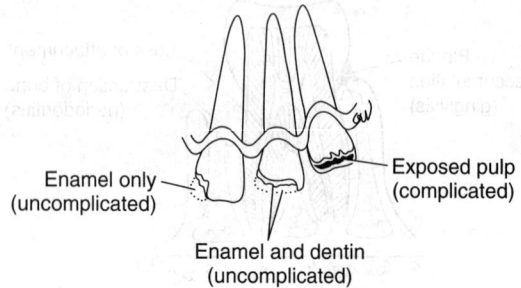

Enamel only
(uncomplicated)

Enamel and dentin
(uncomplicated)

Exposed pulp
(complicated)

Figure 16–9. Patterns of crown fractures.

becomes infected, the teeth are usually removed. Permanent teeth may be damaged with any intrusive injury of primary teeth. Permanent teeth intrusions are corrected with surgical or orthodontic repositioning of teeth and placement of a splint for 10–14 days. Root canal treatment may be necessary later. Lateral and extrusive luxations of permanent teeth are generally repositioned and splinted. Severe luxations in any direction in primary teeth are treated with extraction.

Avulsed primary dentition is not replanted. The area is investigated for fractured roots or foreign bodies. Avulsed permanent teeth are gently cleansed and replanted with splinting. If replaced into the alveolar bone within 1 hour, the prognosis for these teeth is good. The prognosis worsens rapidly with increased time outside of the mouth. Hanks solution is the best storage and transport medium for avulsed teeth that will be replanted. Milk or saline can be used if Hanks solution is not accessible.

All luxated and replanted teeth need to be followed carefully and regularly by a dentist. These teeth can become abscessed or fused to the bone (ankylosed) at any time during the healing process.

A patient with fractured teeth should be seen promptly by a dentist. Fractured teeth need to be protected quickly to avoid sensitivity, pain, or infection of exposed pulp. Severe fracture may require immediate root canal surgery.

All facial trauma needs to be evaluated for jaw fracture. Blows to the chin are among the most common childhood orofacial traumas. They are also a leading cause of condylar fracture in the pediatric population. Condylar fracture should be suspected when pain or deviation occurs when the jaw is opened.

DENTAL EMERGENCIES

Dental emergencies other than trauma are usually associated with pain or swelling due to advanced caries. Odontogenic pain usually responds to acetaminophen, ibuprofen, codeine, or in severe cases, hydrocodone. As with teething, topical application of medicaments is of limited value.

Swelling confined to the gum tissue above or below the tooth is usually not an urgent situation. This "gumboil" or parulis represents infection that has spread outward from the root of the tooth through the bone and periosteum into the gum. Usually it will begin to drain and leave a fistulous tract. If the infection invades the facial spaces, cellulitis can occur. Swelling of the midface—especially the bridge of the nose and the lower eyelid—should be urgently evaluated as a potential dental infection. Extraction of teeth or root canal therapy combined with antibiotics is the usual treatment. With extensive facial cellulitis, many young children require hospitalization and intravenous antibiotics.

ANTIBIOTICS IN PEDIATRIC DENTISTRY

The antibiotics of choice for odontogenic infection are amoxicillin and clindamycin. Several patient groups require prophylactic antibiotic coverage prior to any invasive dental manipulation, including tooth cleaning. Children with heart diseases that place them at risk for subacute bacterial endocarditis head this list. Some immunosuppressed patients also receive coverage during dental procedures. Although there is some controversy regarding the need for antibiotics in children with indwelling central venous catheters (eg, Broviac, Quinton, Hickman, and other lines), some experts medicate them prior to invasive dental treatment.

Children with a ventriculoperitoneal shunt should not receive prophylaxis because there is no circulatory connection to such a shunt. The guidelines for prophylaxis are regularly updated by the American Heart Association. Current recommendations for dentistry are located on the AAPD.org website.

SPECIAL PATIENT POPULATIONS

Children with Cancer

Children with cancer should be evaluated by a dentist knowledgeable about pediatric oncology soon after diagnosis. The aim is to eliminate all existing and potential sources of infection before the child receives chemotherapy and becomes neutropenic. Areas of concern include abscessed teeth, teeth with extensive caries, teeth that will soon exfoliate, ragged or broken teeth or fillings, and orthodontic appliances. Once chemotherapy begins, there is a brief interval before its myelosuppressive effects reach their nadir (7–14 days). Once the child becomes neutropenic, abscessed, infected, or severely carious teeth can no longer be considered innocent, even if asymptomatic. A loose tooth that will soon exfoliate can become a nidus for infection as well as a cause of bleeding in a thrombocytopenic patient. Sharp, ragged teeth can irritate the mucosa and lead to infection. Chemotherapeutic drugs and local irradiation are cytotoxic to the oral mucosa, which becomes atrophic and ulcerates with ease (mucositis). This is painful and often leads to inadequate oral intake and nutrition. Once the mucosal barrier is breached by ulceration, the patient can become septic, especially with α-hemolytic streptococci and other mouth flora. Herpes simplex virus is another pathogen that can enhance drug-induced mucositis. Friction and damage to the mucosa is the main concern with braces. Therefore, all orthodontic hardware is removed prior to chemotherapy.

The pediatric oncology patient should be monitored throughout therapy to screen for infection, manage oral bleeding, and control oral pain. They can experience spontaneous oral hemorrhage, especially when the platelet count is below 20,000/mL. Poor oral hygiene or areas of irritation can increase the chances of bleeding.

Children receiving radiation therapy to the head and neck are prone to develop extensive salivary dysfunction (xerostomia) when salivary tissue is in the path of the primary beam of radiation. Xerostomia should be managed aggressively to avoid rapid extensive destruction of dentition. Customized fluoride applicators are used in this situation in combination with close follow-up.

Children undergoing bone marrow transplantation may have an acute graft-versus-host reaction that contributes to severe oral mucositis. Long-term follow-up includes managing salivary dysfunction from total body radiation and treatment of oral graft-versus-host disease.

The pediatric oncology patient also needs to be followed by a dentist who is familiar with young children and their growth and development. Oral and maxillofacial growth disturbances can occur after therapy. Late effects of therapy include morphologic changes in tooth development (microdontia or extensive hypocalcification), disturbances in eruption (blunted roots or delayed eruption), or alterations in facial bone growth.

Children with Hematologic Problems

The child with hemophilia needs to have the appropriate clotting factor provided before and after any invasive dental procedures (including the administration of local anesthesia, even for simple fillings) (see Chapter 27). Some patients with very mild factor VIII deficiency or von Willebrand disease may respond to desmopressin acetate. Antifibrinolytic medications such as aminocaproic acid and tranexamic acid are used successfully after dental treatment. Postoperative bleeding can also be treated with a wide variety of topical medicaments, such as Gelfoam and thrombin. The pediatric patient receiving anticoagulant therapy must undergo dosage adjustment before invasive dental treatment. This is a relatively simple matter when dealing with heparin, with its short half-life of 4–6 hours. It is a much more difficult problem with warfarin, which has a half-life of 40–70 hours.

Children with Diabetes

Children who are insulin-dependent are at higher risk for dental problems. They have an impaired capacity to heal, a higher incidence of periodontal disease, and a higher caries rate. These children need to be followed carefully on a routine basis. Care must be taken not to disturb the regular cycle of eating and insulin dosage. Anxiety associated with dental appointments can cause a major upset in the diabetic child's routine. Postoperative pain or pain from dental abscess can prevent them from eating. Insulin levels must be adjusted to conform to treatment needs and vice versa.

MATERNAL-FETAL RELATIONSHIP

In addition to the discovery that childhood caries is an infectious disease transmitted by bacteria from the mother to the child, a number of other maternal-fetal relationships related to the oral cavity have been identified. A large prospective study has shown a significant association between maternal periodontitis at 21–24 weeks' gestation and preterm birth. It is unknown whether treatment of periodontitis will reduce the risk of preterm birth.

The risk of preterm birth is elevated if a mother smokes and is of low socioeconomic status, both of which also increase the risk for periodontitis. Secondhand or passive smoke increases the risk of caries in children. This association is independent of age, family income, geographic region, and frequency of dental visits.

Given the known association between maternal periodontitis and preterm birth, passive smoke and children's dental caries, and the knowledge of maternal transmission of caries-causing bacteria, it is important to advise expectant teenage mothers about these risk factors.

Moreover, low-birth-weight preterm children have a greater predisposition to many oral developmental anomalies than normal-birth-weight children. These include generalized enamel hypoplasia associated with increased predisposition to early childhood caries, localized enamel hypoplasia, crown dilaceration of the maxillary left incisors, and palatal deformations associated with laryngoscopy and endotracheal intubation. Dental development in preterm infants is retarded in the eruption of the primary dentition and in the development of the permanent teeth. Information about the association between maternal oral disease and low-birth-weight children, as well as about the infectious transmission of caries-causing bacteria from mother to child, provide a role for physicians to educate expectant mothers and new mothers about efforts critical to the reduction of oral disease and its side effects.

DENTAL AND ORTHODONTIC REFERRAL

Referral to a dentist is appropriate whenever there is a question about a child's oral and maxillofacial health and development. Most pediatric dentists will want to see a child for a first visit by age 12 months. Any child with additional risk factors should be seen earlier.

Orthodontic referral is usually made by the dentist. Generally early referral is indicated for any child with a craniofacial growth disorder. Other children may be referred at any time between age 6 and 12 years, depend-

ing on their growth and oral development. Orthodontists differ in when to begin treatment. Many pediatric dentists provide early or even complete orthodontic management as a part of their practices.

REFERENCES

Hale KJ, American Academy of Pediatrics Section on Pediatric Dentistry: Oral health risk assessment timing and establishment of the dental home. Pediatrics 2003;111:1113 [PMID: 1272810].

Ear, Nose, & Throat

17

Peggy E. Kelley, MD, Norman R. Friedman, MD, Candice E. Johnson, MD, & Patricia J. Yoon

▓ I. THE EAR

INFECTIONS OF THE EAR

The spectrum of infectious ear diseases includes the structures of the outer ear (otitis externa), the middle ear (acute otitis media), the mastoid bone (mastoiditis), and the inner ear (labyrinthitis).

1. Otitis Externa

Otitis externa is inflammation of the skin lining the ear canal and surrounding soft tissue. The most common cause is loss of the protective function of cerumen, leading to maceration of the underlying skin such as occurs with swimming. Other causes are trauma to the ear canal from using cotton-tipped applicators for cleaning or from using poorly fitted ear plugs while swimming; contact dermatitis due to hair sprays, perfumes, or self-administered ear drops; secondary infection of the canal from otitis media with a patent tympanostomy tube; and chronic drainage from a perforated tympanic membrane (TM). Infections due to *Staphylococcus aureus* or *Pseudomonas aeruginosa* are the most common.

Symptoms include pain and itching in the ear, especially with chewing or pressure on the tragus. Movement of the pinna or tragus causes considerable pain. Drainage may be minimal unless the otitis externa is from a draining pressure equalization tube or TM perforation. The ear canal is typically grossly swollen, and the patient may resist any attempt to insert an ear speculum. Debris is noticeable in the canal. It is often impossible to visualize the TM. Hearing is normal unless complete occlusion has occurred.

Treatment

Topical treatment usually suffices. Fluoroquinolone drops may be more effective than traditional combination drops and are safer to use. If the TM cannot be seen, then a perforation may be presumed to exist. Children with otitis externa secondary to draining tubes or perforations should be treated with topical therapy only in the absence of systemic symptoms. The topical therapy chosen must be safe for the inner ear because the perforation or the patent tube allows the drops access to the middle and inner ear. If the ear canal is open, ototopical antibiotics are placed and prescribed for 5–7 days as indicated. If the canal is too edematous to allow the ear drop to get in, a Pope ear wick is needed for the first few days to assure antibiotic delivery. Oral antibiotics are indicated if any signs of invasive infection, such as fever, cellulitis of the auricles, or tender postauricular lymph nodes, are present. In such cases, prescribe an antistaphylococcal antibiotic while awaiting the results of the cultured ear canal discharge. Systemic antibiotics alone without topical treatment will not successfully treat otitis externa. Narcotic analgesics may be required until the infection begins to resolve in 2–3 days.

During the acute phase, the patient should avoid swimming. A cotton ear plug is not helpful and may prolong the infection. Schedule a follow-up visit in 1 week to document an intact tympanic membrane (Figure 17–1). Children who have intact TMs and are predisposed to external otitis should receive 2 or 3 drops of a 1:1 solution of white vinegar and 70% ethyl alcohol into the ears before and after swimming.

Manolidis S et al: Comparative efficacy of aminoglycoside versus fluoroquinolone topical antibiotic drops. Otolaryngol Head Neck Surg 2004;130:S83 [PMID: 15054366].

Roland PS et al: Consensus panel on role of potentially ototoxic antibiotics for topical middle ear use: introduction, methodology and recommendations. Otolaryngol Head Neck Surg 2004;130:S51 [PMID: 15543836].

2. Acute Otitis Media

Classification & Clinical Findings

Otitis media is an infection associated with middle ear effusion (a collection of fluid in the middle ear space) or with otorrhea (a discharge from the ear through a perforation in the TM or a ventilating tube). Otitis media can be further classified by its associated clinical symptoms, otoscopic findings, duration, frequency, and complica-

Right Tympanic Membrane

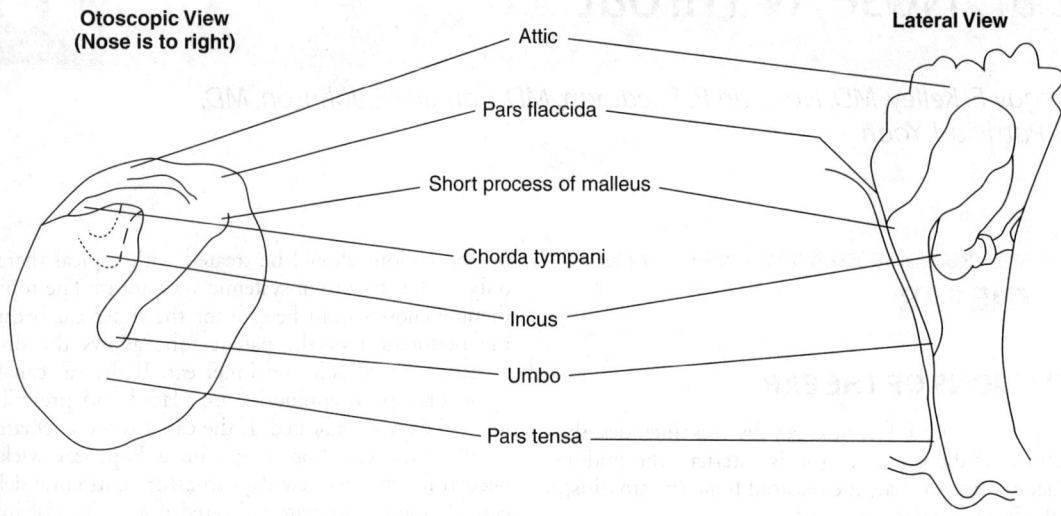

Figure 17–1. Tympanic membrane.

tions. These more specific classifications are acute otitis media, otitis media with effusion, and chronic suppurative otitis media.

Acute otitis media (AOM) is commonly defined as inflammation of the middle ear resulting in an effusion and associated with rapid onset of symptoms such as otalgia, fever, irritability, anorexia, or vomiting. The 2004 Guidelines from the American Academy of Pediatrics and of the American Academy of Family Physicians specified three criteria which must be present (Table 17–1). The presence of an ear effusion is best determined by either pneumatic otoscopy or tympanometry. To distinguish AOM from otitis media with effusion (OME), signs of inflammation of the TM and symptoms of acute infection must be present. Otoscopic findings specific for AOM are a bulging TM; impaired visibility of the ossicular landmarks; a yellow, white, or bright red color; opacification of the eardrum; and squamous exudate or bullae on the eardrum. OME is associated with a nonbulging eardrum, which may be retracted or neutral, but always has decreased mobility, may have opacification, and may have white or amber discoloration. Children with OME may develop superimposed acute infection, but they will then exhibit inflammation of the eardrum as described for AOM.

Factors that make otitis media more common in children than in adults include bacterial nasopharyngeal colonization in the absence of antibody, frequent upper respiratory infections (URIs), exposure to parental cigarette smoke, unfavorable eustachian tube function, and allergies.

A. BACTERIAL COLONIZATION

Nasopharyngeal colonization with *Streptococcus pneumoniae, Haemophilus influenzae,* or *Moraxella catarrhalis* increases the risk of otitis media, whereas colonization with normal flora such as viridans streptococci may prevent otitis episodes by inhibiting the growth of these pathogens. Colonization usually occurs sequentially with different pathogen serotypes present for about 2

Table 17–1. Definition of acute otitis media (AOM).

A diagnosis of AOM requires (1) a history of acute onset of signs and symptoms, (2) the presence of MEE, and (3) signs and symptoms of middle-ear inflammation.
Elements of the definition of AOM are all of the following:
1. Recent, usually abrupt, onset of signs and symptoms of middle-ear inflammation and MEE
2. The presence of MEE that is indicated by any of the following:
   a. Bulging of the tympanic membrane
   b. Limited or absent mobility of the tympanic membrane
   c. Air-fluid level behind the tympanic membrane
   d. Otorrhea
3. Signs or symptoms of middle ear inflammation as indicated by either
   a. Distinct erythema of the tympanic membrane or
   b. Distinct otalgia (discomfort clearly referable to the ear[s]) that results in interference with or precludes normal activity or sleep

MEE, middle ear effusion.

months, and there is a risk of AOM with each new serotype acquired. Infants in day care acquire these serotypes at a younger age than those in home care. Since younger children are at higher risk of AOM, the increased number of children in day care over the last 3 decades has undoubtedly played a major role in the increase in AOM in the United States.

B. Viral Upper Respiratory Infections

These infections increase the colonization of the nasopharynx with otitis pathogens. Viral infection also impairs eustachian tube function by causing both adenoidal swelling and edema of the tube. Therefore, factors that increase the frequency of viral respiratory infections, such as child care attendance, smoke exposure, later birth order, and absence of breast feeding, promote colonization with otitis pathogens and predispose to otitis media.

C. Smoke Exposure

Passive smoking increases the risk of persistent middle ear effusion by enhancing colonization, prolonging the inflammatory response, and impeding drainage through the eustachian tube. For infants age 12–18 months, exposure to each additional pack of cigarettes smoked at home is associated with an 11% increase in the duration of a middle ear effusion.

D. Eustachian Tube Dysfunction

Infants born with craniofacial disorders, such as Down syndrome or a cleft palate, are often affected by AOM and OME. The patency of the tube allows aeration of the middle ear. When the tube is obstructed, a vacuum develops in the middle ear, which can pull nasopharyngeal secretions and pathogens into the middle ear.

E. Host Immune Defenses

Immunocompromised children such as those with selective IgA deficiency usually experience recurrent AOM, sinusitis, and pneumonia. However, most children who experience recurrent or persistent otitis only have selective impairments of immune defenses against specific otitis pathogens. For example, a recent study showed some children have low-to-absent IgG2 or IgA pneumococcal polysaccharide antibody responses (or both) after vaccination, despite normal serum levels of total IgG2 and IgA.

F. Breast Feeding

Breast feeding reduces the incidence of acute respiratory infections, provides IgA antibodies that reduce colonization with otitis pathogens, and decreases the aspiration of contaminated secretions into the middle ear space when a bottle is propped in the crib.

G. Genetic Susceptibility

Although we know AOM to be multifactorial, and no gene for susceptibility has yet been identified, recent studies of twins and triplets suggest that as much as 70% of the risk is genetically determined. This has implications for the subsequent offspring of parents with a child experiencing recurrent AOM. These families might wish to consider breast feeding and home child care for later children.

Microbiology of Acute Otitis Media

The role of respiratory viral infection in precipitating otitis media is unquestionable, yet fewer than 12% of ear effusions culture positive for viruses. Recent studies with sensitive viral antigen or nucleic acid tests have detected virus in over 40% of infected ears. The viral infection usually precedes the bacterial otitis media by 3–14 days and presumably causes adenoid hypertrophy and eustachian tube dysfunction. The two viruses most clearly shown to precipitate otitis media are respiratory syncytial virus and influenza, accounting for the annual surge in otitis media cases from January to May in temperate climates.

Historically, over 50% of AOM in the Midwestern and northeastern U.S. was due to *S pneumoniae,* while the hotter, drier climates of southern Israel and Denver reported a preponderance of nontypable *H influenzae* (Table 17–2). However, since widespread use of the pneumococcal conjugate vaccine (Prevnar; PCV-7) in children under 2 years of age, the incidence of *H influenzae* may be on the rise and that of *S pneumoniae* may be declining. The pattern of infection in Kentucky now resembles that seen before PCV-7 in Colorado. (No data are available for Denver in the post-Prevnar era.) More importantly, Prevnar has increased the percentage of cases due to non-PCV serotypes nationally from 12% in 1999 to 32% in 2002. The clinical significance of this change is to decrease the overall percentage of drug-resistant pneumococci, since the serotypes included in the vaccine are the most multiply resistant.

The third most common pathogen in some studies is *Moraxella catarrhalis,* which causes up to 25% of AOM in the United States, accounting for about 10% of the disease. The fourth organism found is *Streptococcus pyogenes,* which is more common in school-aged children than in infants. This organism and *S pneumoniae* are the predominant causes of mastoiditis. Contrary to earlier teaching, the etiology of AOM in early infancy differs only little from that in adult life. The only difference is that the risk of gram-negative enteric infection is slightly increased in infants less than age 4 weeks of age who are or have been hospitalized in a neonatal intensive care nursery.

Table 17–2. Bacteriology of acute otitis media.

	Denver (Author)	Kentucky[a] Pre-PCV7 (Prevnar)	Kentucky[a] Post-PCV7
Streptococcus pneumoniae	32	48	31
Haemophilus influenzae	50	41	56
Moraxella catarrhalis	8	9	11
Streptococcus pyogenes	4	2	2
S pneumoniae + H influenzae	5	Not reported	Not reported

[a]Data used, with permission, from Block SL et al: Community-wide vaccination with the heptavalent pneumococcal conjugate significantly alters the microbiology of acute otitis media. Pediatr Infect Dis J 2004;23:829.

Drug-resistant *S pneumoniae* is a common pathogen in acute otitis media and strains may be resistant to only one drug (ie, penicillin or macrolides) or to multiple classes. Children with resistant strains tend to be younger and to have had more unresponsive infections. Antibiotic treatment in the preceding 3 months also increases the risk of harboring resistant pathogens. Penicillin resistance develops through stepwise mutations in the structure of the three penicillin-binding proteins. Strains for which minimum inhibitory concentrations of penicillin range between 0.12 and 1.0 μg/mL are said to exhibit "intermediate" resistance. Strains for which minimum inhibitory concentrations are equal to or higher than 2 μg/mL are said to have a "high-level resistance." The prevalence of resistant strains no longer varies significantly among geographic areas within the U.S., but it does vary worldwide. Lower incidences are found in countries using fewer courses of antibiotic per person. These strains are also resistant to many other drug classes. Nationwide resistance rates include: 63% for trimethoprim-sulfamethoxazole, 32% for macrolides, and 2% for amoxicillin (dosed at 90 mg/kg/d). Oral cephalosporins vary widely in efficacy, with the highest resistance rates for cefixime and cefaclor and lowest rates (about 35%) for cefuroxime, cefprozil, cefpodoxime, and cefdinir. Over 90% of highly penicillin-resistant strains are still susceptible to clindamycin, rifampin, and fluoroquinolones. Unfortunately, fluoroquinolones are not yet approved for children younger than 16 years; however, studies are under way to assess their safety and efficacy in this age group.

Diagnosis

A. PNEUMATIC OTOSCOPY

Acute otitis media is overdiagnosed. Contributing to errors in diagnosis are the temptation to accept the diagnosis without removing enough cerumen to adequately visualize the eardrum, and the mistaken belief that a red eardrum establishes the diagnosis. In fact, redness of the eardrum is often a vascular flush caused by either fever, crying, or even efforts to remove cerumen. Failure to achieve an adequate seal with the otoscope, poor visualization due to low light intensity, and mistaking the ear canal wall for the membrane can make it impossible to assess eardrum mobility.

A pneumatic otoscope with a rubber suction bulb and tube is used to assess mobility of the TM. The speculum inserted into the patient's ear canal must be large enough to provide an airtight seal. Placing a piece of rubber tubing 0.25–0.5 cm wide near the end of the ear speculum helps to create an adequate pneumatic seal. The tubing should fit snugly on the speculum at a distance about 0.5 cm from its end. The largest possible speculum (usually 3 or 4 mm) should be used to maximize the field of view. When the rubber bulb is squeezed, the TM will move freely to and fro if no fluid is present; if fluid is present in the middle ear space, the mobility of the TM will be absent or resemble a fluid wave. The ability to assess mobility is compromised by low light intensity; a halogen source is necessary. These bulbs dim, but rarely ever burn out, so they must be replaced on a schedule.

Disposable ear specula have become popular but are not needed for infection control, because reusable specula can be easily disinfected. The disposable specula are sharp at the tip and often cause pain when pushed to get an airtight seal.

B. CERUMEN REMOVAL

Cerumen removal is an essential skill for anyone who cares for children. Impacted cerumen pushed against the TM can cause itching, otalgia, or hearing loss. Parents should be advised that earwax protects the ear (cerumen contains lysozymes and immunoglobulins that inhibit infection) and will usually come out by itself; therefore parents should never put anything solid into the ear canal to remove the earwax.

The physician may safely remove cerumen under direct visualization through the operating head of an otoscope, provided two adults are present to hold the child. A plastic disposable ear size 0 curette should be used. It should not be pointed or sharp.

Irrigation can also be used to remove hard or flaky cerumen. Asian children may have an ear wax variant that is flaky, called "rice bran wax." This type of wax can be softened with 1% sodium docusate solution, carbamyl peroxide solutions, mineral oil, or a few drops of detergent before irrigation is attempted. After 20 minutes, irrigation with a soft bulb syringe can be started with water warmed to 35–38 °C to prevent vertigo. A commercial jet tooth cleanser (eg, Water Pik) is also an excellent device for removing cerumen, but it is important to set it at low power (2 or less) to prevent damage to the TM. A perforated TM or patent tympanostomy tube is a contraindication to any form of irrigation.

C. TYMPANOMETRY

Tympanometry can rapidly identify an effusion in infants over about 6 months, and it requires little training. It should be preceded by pneumatic otoscopy to assure that 50% or more of the canal is wax-free. Because it does not identify inflammation, it cannot differentiate acute OM and OM with effusion. Tympanometry measures TM compliance and displays it in graphic form (along the y axis, expressed in mm H_2O). Compliance is determined as air pressures are varied from +200 to –400 mm H_2O in the sealed external ear canal.

Tympanograms can be classified into four major patterns, as shown in Figure 17–2. The pattern shown in Figure 17–2A, characterized by maximum compliance at normal atmospheric pressure, indicates a normal TM, good eustachian tube function, and absence of effusion. The height and sharpness of the peak is not important when using the Welch-Allyn tympanometer. The pattern shown in Figure 17–2B identifies a nonmobile TM, which indicates middle ear effusion. The pattern shown in Figure 17–2C indicates an intact mobile TM with poor eustachian tube function and excessive negative pressure (> –300 mm H_2O air pressure) in the middle ear. Figure 17–2D shows a flat tracing, which would have a very large middle ear volume on the printout, due to a patent tube or large perforation.

D. ACOUSTIC REFLECTOMETRY

Acoustic reflectometry measures the spectral gradient of the TM using a handheld instrument, without requiring an airtight seal. However, recent data suggest that this method cannot reliably distinguish negative middle ear pressure from effusion. The instrument is not commercially available at present.

Treatment

A. PAIN MANAGEMENT

Children with pain related to AOM may obtain relief from acetaminophen or ibuprofen, accompanied by a topical anesthetic drop. In a randomized controlled trial, Auraglan (benzocaine and antipyrine) ear drops were superior to olive oil in reducing pain. When severe pain is present, tympanocentesis should be considered for pain relief and to diagnose the causative pathogen.

B. THE OBSERVATION OPTION (WATCHFUL WAITING)

Few issues are as controversial as the necessity of immediate antibiotic treatment of otitis media. Doctors must balance the desire of the parents for symptom relief against the risk of selecting for drug-resistance by overuse of antibiotics. In two recent editorials, Dr. Ellen Wald has pointed out that the major overuse of antibiotics is for the treatment of viral colds and viral pharyngitis, not otitis media. The second reason for antibiotic overuse is overdiagnosis of acute otitis media by providers. The natural history of untreated AOM is to improve through host defenses or by perforation of the TM; but mastoiditis was not an infrequent complication before the use of antibiotics. In Dr. Howie's classic studies in the 1970s in which he randomized children to placebo or various antibiotics, bacteriologic cure rates determined by a second tympanocentesis while on therapy were only 32% in the placebo group. The spontaneous cure rate varied greatly by organism, 16% for *S pneumoniae*, 50% for nontypable *H influenzae* and about 84% for *M catarrhalis*, which he considered a contaminant. Several authors have correlated clinical cure rates at the end of therapy with bacteriologic cure on day 4 to 6, and clinical cure rates are always higher than bacteriologic cure rates. However, the children who are bacteriologic failures at the end of treatment have an extremely high likelihood of also experiencing clinical failure. This has important implications for study design, which has led the Food and Drug Administration to start requiring new antibiotics to be studied for proof of bacteriologic cure in a subset of patients. In 2004 the two academies (Family Physicians and Pediatrics) issued a clinical practice guideline which suggested nontreatment of limited groups of children with AOM (Table 17–3). Key points are that children over 2 years of age with nonsevere disease were recommended for nontreatment for the first 48–72 hours after onset of symptoms. Those under 2 years of age and older children with severe pain or fever were always recommended to receive immediate antibiotics. Children failing observation were to begin antibiotics after 48–72 hours. Although, not mentioned, a prescription can be given at the first visit, with instructions to fill if no

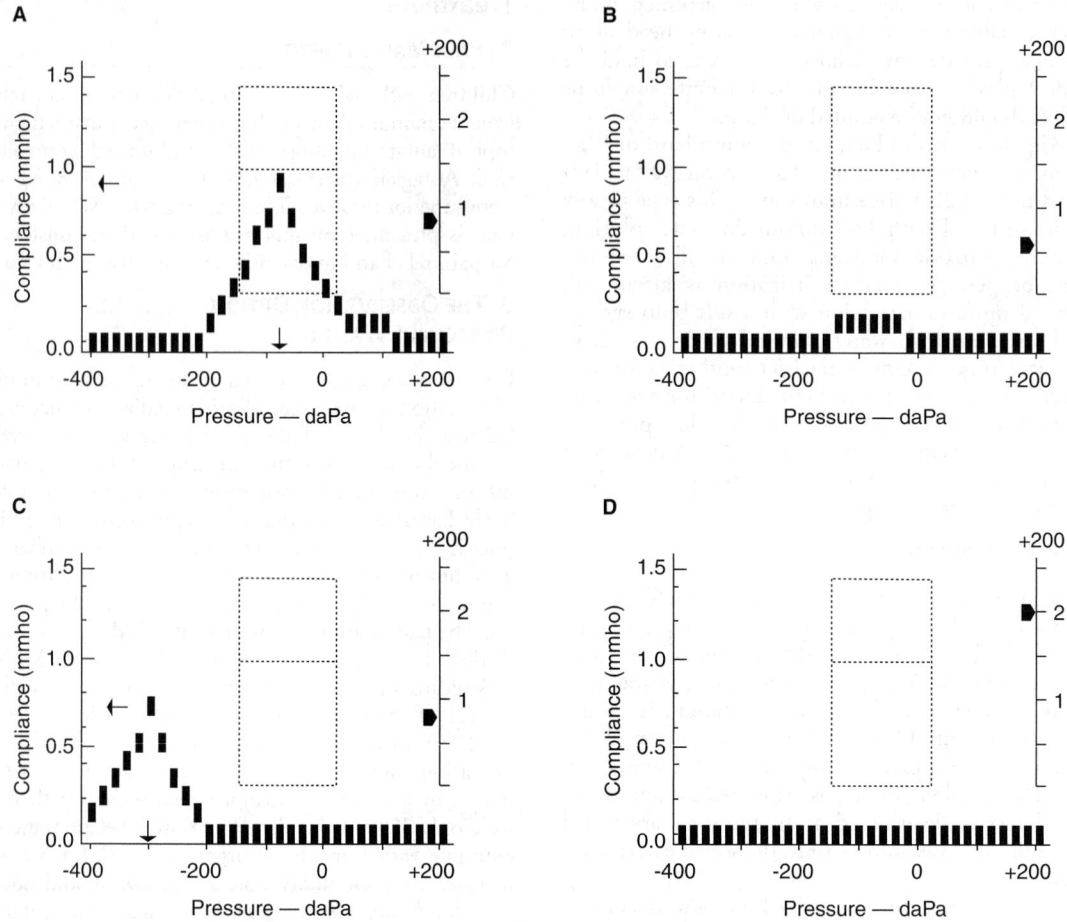

Figure 17–2. Four types of tympanograms obtained with Welch-Allyn MicroTymp 2. **A:** Normal middle ear. **B:** Otitis media with effusion or acute otitis media. **C:** Negative middle ear pressure due to eustachian tube dysfunction. **D:** Patent tympanostomy tube or perforation in the tympanic membrane. Same as B except for a very large middle ear volume.

improvement is seen after the specified observation period. The guidelines offer different recommendations for "certain" versus "uncertain" diagnosis, but the clinician should be able to see the eardrum and make a correct diagnosis if they master cerumen removal and pneumatic otoscopy. An "uncertain" diagnosis should only occur when pus, blood, or cerumen obscure the eardrum. For infants under 6 months of age, antibiotics are always recommended on the first visit, regardless of the certainty of diagnosis. The guidelines also emphasize the importance of using pneumatic otoscopy or tympanometry to establish the presence of effusion, and the importance of differentiating OME from AOM by the absence of acute signs and symptoms of inflammation (see Table 17–3). Everyone agrees that overtreatment of OME by well-meaning providers has led to

overuse of antibiotics for no discernible benefit. AOM requires the recent onset of otalgia, which may be harder to diagnose in infants, but often presents as night-awakening, ear tugging, anorexia due to pain on swallowing, and unexplained crying. Although most clinicians routinely treat acute otitis with antibiotics, it is also reasonable to involve parents in the decision. There is a trade-off for the individual child between the risks of antibiotic treatment (cost, allergic reactions, side effects, and colonization with an antibiotic-resistant pathogen) and the benefit of a possibly more rapid clinical response. More rapid pain relief alone may justify treatment in older children. Children younger than age 2 years should be immediately treated with antibiotics because studies show an advantage over placebo, and they are more likely to develop complications.

Table 17–3. Criteria for initial antibiotic treatment in children with acute otitis media.

Age	Certain Diagnosis	Uncertain Diagnosis
< 6 mo	Antibacterial therapy	Antibacterial therapy
6 mo to 2 yr	Antibacterial therapy	Antibacterial therapy if severe illness; observation option[a] if nonsevere illness
≥ 2 yr	Antibacterial therapy if severe illness; observation option[a] if nonsevere illness	Observation option[a]

[a]Nonsevere illness is mild otalgia and fever < 39° C in the past 24 hours.

C. ANTIBIOTIC THERAPY

Amoxicillin remains the first-line antibiotic for treating otitis media, even with a high prevalence of drug-resistant *S pneumoniae*, because resistance to β-lactam antibiotics, such as amoxicillin, develops as a stepwise process over many years. A bacterial strain resistant to low levels of amoxicillin will usually be eradicated by a higher dosage. Amoxicillin dosage may be raised considerably without toxicity; for example, a dosage of 200 mg/kg/d has been used to treat meningitis in children, and a maximum daily dose of 4 g has been used in adults. Studies have shown that increasing the dosage from 40 mg/kg to 90 mg/kg yields a drug concentration in middle ear fluid that surpasses the minimal level needed to inhibit 98% of all pneumococcal otitis media. A second advantage is that dosing amoxicillin at these higher levels may help delay stepwise emergence of resistance. In recognition of this new pharmacodynamic data, the federal government in June 1999 doubled the minimum inhibitory concentration used to define resistance to amoxicillin to 8 μg/mL or greater. Because otitis media is not a life-threatening disease, it is not necessary for a first-line antibiotic to achieve 100% cure. High-dose amoxicillin will usually eradicate the most invasive pathogen, *S pneumoniae,* and if no improvement occurs, a second-line antibiotic may be chosen to cover *M catarrhalis* and β-lactamase–producing *H influenzae.*

Amoxicillin-clavulanate enhanced strength, with 90 mg/kg/d of amoxicillin dosing (14:1 ratio of amoxicillin to clavulanate) is an appropriate choice when a child is clinically failing after 48–72 hours on amoxicillin (Table 17–4). In this situation, the most likely pathogen is *H influenzae,* and the addition of clavulanate to amoxicillin will broaden the coverage while retaining efficacy against *S pneumoniae.* The older 200- and 400-mg/teaspoon formulations of amoxicillin-clavulanate (7:1 ratio) should never be doubled in dosage, since the amount of clavulanate will be too high and may cause diarrhea.

Three oral cephalosporins (cefuroxime, cefpodoxime, and cefdinir) are more β-lactamase-stable and these are alternative choices for second-line therapy in children who develop papular rashes with amoxicillin (see Table 17–4). Unfortunately, the coverage of highly penicillin-resistant pneumococci with these agents is poor and only the intermediate-resistance classes are covered. Of these three drugs, cefdinir is quite palatable in the liquid form while the other two drugs have a bitter aftertaste which is difficult, but not impossible, to conceal. Newer flavoring agents may be helpful here. A second-line antibiotic is also indicated when a child experiences symptomatic infection within 1 month of stopping amoxicillin; however, repeat use of high-dose amoxicillin is indicated if more than 4 weeks have passed without symptoms, because a new pathogen is usually present. Macrolides such as azithromycin and clarithromycin are not recommended as second-line agents for two reasons. First, the national *S pneumoniae* resistance rate to macrolides is approximately 30% in respiratory isolates. Second, double tympanocentesis studies have demonstrated eradication of *H influenzae,* regardless of β-lactamase produc-

Table 17–4. Treatment of acute otitis media in an era of drug resistance.

First-line therapy
1. Amoxicillin 90 mg/kg/d, up to 4 g/d. For children over 2 years of age, give for 5 days; under 2 years of age, for 10 days.
2. If amoxicillin has caused a rash, give cefuroxime (Ceftin), cefdinir (Omnicef), or cefpodoxime (Vantin).
3. If urticaria or other IgE-mediated events have occurred, give trimethoprim-sulfamethoxazole or azithromycin (Zithromax).
4. If the child is unable to take oral medication, give single intramuscular dose of ceftriaxone (Rocephin).

Second-line therapy
This is for clinical failure after 48–72 hours of treatment, or for recurrences within 4 weeks.
1. Amoxicillin-clavulanate (Augmentin ES-600), given so that the patient receives amoxicillin at 90 mg/kg/d.
2. If amoxicillin has caused allergic symptoms, see recommendations above.

Third-line therapy
1. Tympanocentesis is recommended to determine the cause.
2. Ceftriaxone (Rocephin), two doses given intramuscularly, 48 hours apart, with the option of a third dose.

Recurrences > 4 weeks after the first episode
1. A new pathogen is likely, so restart first-line therapy.
2. Be sure the diagnosis is not OM with effusion, which may be observed for 3–6 months without treatment.

tion. Virtually all strains of *H influenzae* have an intrinsic macrolide efflux pump, which pumps antibiotic out of the bacterial cell. In a recent double tympanocentesis study, the on-therapy eradication rate of all pathogens was 94.2% for high-dose amoxicillin-clavulanate and 70.3% for azithromycin (*p* <0.001).

If a child remains symptomatic longer than 3 days while taking a second-line agent, a tympanocentesis is useful to identify the causative pathogen. The tap may be sterile or the organism may be sensitive. Reasons for failure to eradicate a sensitive pathogen may be noncompliance, poor drug absorption, or vomiting of drug. If a highly resistant pneumococcus is found or if tympanocentesis is not feasible, intramuscular ceftriaxone at 50 mg/kg/d for 3 consecutive days is probably the best choice based on a study performed in Israel. Further study is needed to see if one or two daily doses may equal three doses, which is a major time and financial commitment for parents. Table 17–4 also lists alternative drugs for penicillin-allergic children. If the child has experienced anaphylaxis to amoxicillin, cephalosporins should not be substituted. However, the maculopapular rash frequently seen with amoxicillin is not IgE-mediated, and cephalosporins may be used.

With the emergence of *S pneumoniae* with minimum inhibitory concentration values of 4 μg/mL, high-dose amoxicillin will undoubtedly fail to cure. Therefore, two new classes of antibiotics are in active clinical trials for AOM: fluoroquinolones and ketolides. Fluoroquinolones are divided into two classes; the older class includes ciprofloxacin, ofloxacin, and levofloxacin. The newer class is the 8-methoxy-fluoroquinolones, which include gatifloxacin and moxifloxacin. The difference between the two classes is that the newer drugs have a lower tendency to select resistant *S pneumoniae,* because two mutations are required. Pneumococcal resistance has been seen in countries where fluoroquinolones were widely used in adults. Levofloxacin was evaluated in a double tympanocentesis trial and found to be highly efficacious, but the manufacturers have chosen not to apply to the FDA for use in AOM at this time. In a double tympanocentesis study of high-risk children, gatifloxacin was shown to eradicate 96% of pathogens. Cartilage toxicity has been seen only in juvenile laboratory animals, and no increased incidence of arthropathy has been seen during the compassionate use of any fluoroquinolone.

Telithromycin (Ketek) is the first ketolide antibiotic to be licensed in adults in the United States, and it is currently under study for AOM in children. Ketolides are related to macrolides and bind to the ribosome, but they are active against pneumococci resistant to macrolides. These new antibiotics may be useful in multiple-drug–resistant pneumonia and refractory AOM, but they are not indicated for first- or second-line use, to protect against selecting for resistance.

Figure 17–3 shows the recommended follow-up of AOM that resolves with a residual effusion at 3–4 weeks. Children, particularly those young enough to still be developing language skills, should be seen monthly for otoscopic exams to determine if the effusion is persistent or occurs only with symptomatic infections. Prophylactic antibiotics and corticosteroids are no longer recommended for OME. An audiology evaluation should be performed after approximately 3 months of continuous bilateral effusion in children younger than 3 years and those at risk of language delay due to poverty or craniofacial anomalies. Children with hearing loss or speech delay should be referred to an otolaryngologist for possible ventilation tubes. Older children may have periodic hearing testing in the primary provider's office (see section on OME).

D. DURATION OF THERAPY

The duration of antibiotic treatment is controversial. Only three recent trials have used stringent entry and outcome criteria. Success rates were higher following 10 days of therapy in all three studies, particularly for children younger than 2 years of age, and for those in day care. At this time, short-course (5-day) therapy can only be recommended for children older than 2 years and not in day care.

A recent study of preschoolers demonstrated that drug-resistant pneumococcal carriage at day 28 post-therapy was lower in a short-course high-dose amoxicillin group compared with a group given a standard course of therapy. This is an important finding, because we now know that the nasopharyngeal flora influences the pathogen of the next AOM.

E. TYMPANOCENTESIS

Tympanocentesis is performed by placing a needle through the TM and aspirating the middle ear fluid. Indications for tympanocentesis are (1) AOM in a patient with compromised host resistance, (2) research studies, (3) evaluation for presumed sepsis or meningitis, such as in a neonate, (4) unresponsive otitis media despite courses of two appropriate antibiotics, and (5) acute mastoiditis or other suppurative complications. The technique of tympanocentesis is as follows:

1. Premedication—In the conditions mentioned, the pain associated with tympanocentesis is only slightly greater than the pain of existing acute inflammation of the TM. Therefore, no premedication is used, but the provider should perform the procedure rapidly and return the child immediately to the parent's arms.

2. Restraint—A papoose board or a sheet can be used to immobilize the patient's body, and an extra attendant is required to hold the child's head steady. It is helpful to have the parent remain in sight of the child for reassurance.

Acute Otitis Media (AOM)

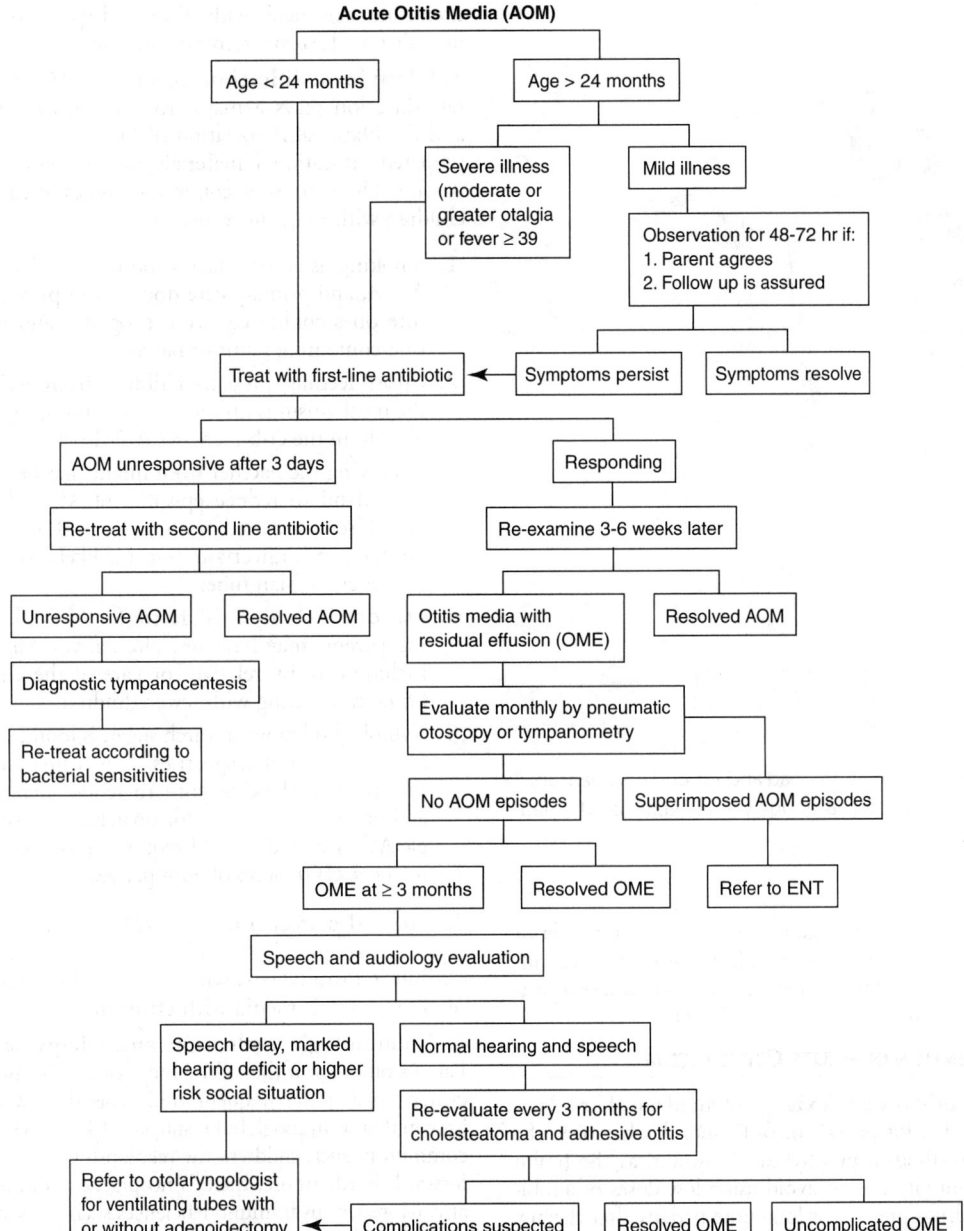

Figure 17–3. Algorithm for acute otitis media. ENT, ear, nose, and throat consult.

3. Site selection—With an open-headed operating otoscope (Figure 17–4), the operator carefully selects a target. This is best done in the anteroinferior quadrant, although the posteroinferior quadrant is a safe but shallower alternative. These sites avoid damage to the ossicles during the procedure.

4. Aspiration—An 8.8-cm spinal needle (no. 18 or no. 20) with a short bevel is attached to a 3-mL syringe. Alternatively, either an Alden-Senturia trap (Storz Instrument Co., St. Louis, Mo.) or the Tymp-Tap aspirator (Xomed Surgical Products, Jackson, Fl.) is attached to a suction pump. The operator then aspi-

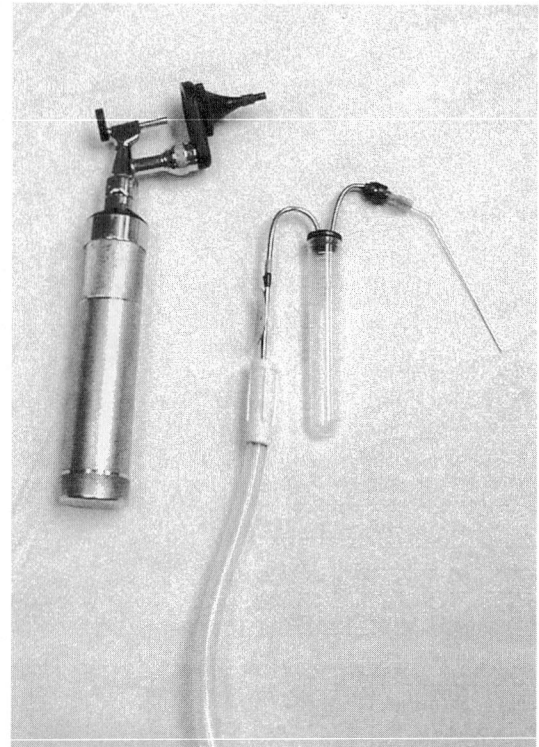

Figure 17–4. Operating head and Alden-Senturia trap for tympanocentesis. 18-gauge spinal needle is attached and bent.

rates the middle ear effusion from the anterior inferior quadrant. Aspirate should be placed directly onto culture plates for maximum recovery, and chocolate agar is adequate to grow all common pathogens.

F. PREVENTION OF ACUTE OTITIS MEDIA

1. Antibiotic prophylaxis—Prolonged use of low doses of antibiotics, for periods of 6–12 months, has been the primary method of prophylaxis. However, as the health care community tries to avoid using low doses of antibiotics (or drugs present for long time periods after therapy such as azithromycin), this method should be reserved for unusual situations. Amoxicillin is the drug most studied. A situation in which prophylaxis might still be recommended is a child being considered for tympanostomy tube placement for recurrent infections who presents in late spring. A 1–2 month course of amoxicillin might prevent infection until the low-risk summer season when AOM is uncommon. Another recommendation for prophylaxis is in the child with patent tympanostomy tubes who experiences recurrent AOM on more than one occasion. Antibiotic prophylaxis is not recommended for chil-

dren with otitis media with effusion, despite earlier guidelines that made such a recommendation.

2. Lifestyle modifications to prevent AOM—Parental education plays a major role in decreasing AOM, and the National Association of Daycare Providers has prepared educational materials for its centers and its parents. Here are some counseling topics to consider in children with frequent recurrences:

1. Smoking is a risk factor both for URI and for AOM, and primary care doctors can provide literature on smoking cessation programs and on nicotine-containing gums or patches.
2. Breast feeding protects children from AOM, but the mechanism is unknown. Also, propping a bottle of milk in the crib increases AOM risk.
3. Removing the pacifier from infants has been shown in Finland to reduce episodes of AOM by about one-third compared with a control group. The mechanism is uncertain, but it is likely to be effects on the eustachian tube.
4. Day care is clearly a risk factor for AOM, but working parents may have few alternatives. Suggestions include care by relatives or care of the child in a home care setting with fewer children.
5. Xylitol, also known as birch sugar, is found in plums, strawberries, and raspberries. It was first studied in Europe as a chewing gum to reduce dental caries, and proved effective. Unfortunately, to prevent a single AOM episode would require a group of children to chew 4100 pieces of gum per year.

3. Surgical prevention of AOM—Tympanostomy tubes are an effective, albeit expensive, alternative to antibiotic prophylaxis, which will be discussed in the section on otitis media with effusion.

4. Immunologic evaluation and allergy testing—Parents often ask if their child may have an immune deficiency causing the frequent otitis episodes. While it is known that immunoglobulin subclass deficiencies are more common in such children, the relationship is not straightforward. Furthermore, there is no practical immune therapy. More serious immunodeficiences such as selective IgA deficiency should be sought in children with a combination of recurrent AOM, sinusitis, and pneumonia. Parents may also inquire about the role of allergy, since a generation ago many children with recurrent AOM were placed on milk elimination diets. No benefits were seen. In the school-aged child or the preschooler with an atopic background, skin-testing may be beneficial in identifying allergens that predispose to AOM.

5. Vaccines for the prevention of acute otitis media—With the increasing problems of antibiotic therapy and prophylaxis, vaccines are increasingly important. The seven-valent pnuemococcal vaccine PCV7 was designed to prevent meningitis and sepsis, not AOM. However, it did produce a 55% reduction in AOM due to the seven serotypes found in the vaccine, and these strains include the serotypes most likely to be penicillin and macrolide resistant. Overall PCV7 reduced AOM by 6% in California, compared to a control group. More impressively, it reduced pressure equalization tube placements by 20% and greatly reduced AOM incidence in those children having six or more episodes per year. Furthermore, studies are showing a herd immunity effect on the older siblings of vaccinated children, which may further reduce drug-resistant serotype circulation. The vaccine should be used as a single dose for children 2–5 years old with a history of either recurrent AOM or OME with superimposed AOM episodes.

In recent studies, intranasal influenza vaccine reduced the number of influenza-associated cases of AOM by 92%. For children older than 6 months with recurrent AOM, it seems prudent to recommend yearly influenza vaccine, although this is not yet an official recommendation.

Vaccines currently being studied in animals that hold promise for AOM prevention include a respiratory syncytial virus vaccine and a nontypeable *H influenzae* vaccine. Studies of pregnant women in the third trimester have shown that their pneumococcal antibody levels are raised by a heptavalent pneumococcal vaccine, which may also raise antibody levels in the offspring. A recent study showed that low cord blood pneumococcal antibody is a risk factor for AOM and OME, so passive transfer from the mother is a logical next step to study.

Dagan R, Arguedas A, Schaad UB: Potential role of fluoroquinolone therapy in childhood otitis media. Pediatr Infect Dis J 2004;23:390 [PMID: 15131460].

Dagan R, McCracken Jr GH: Flaws in design and conduct of clinical trials in acute otitis media. Pediatr Infect Dis J 2002;21:894 [PMID: 12394809].

Finkelstein JA, Stille CJ, Rifas-Shiman SL et al: Watchful waiting for acute otitis media: are parents and physicians ready? Pediatrics 2005;115:1466 [PMID: 15930205].

Hoberman A, Dagan R, Leibovitz E et al: Large dosage amoxicillin/clavulanate, compared with azithromycin, for the treatment of bacterial acute otitis media in children. Pediatr Infect Dis J 2005;24:525 [PMID: 15933563].

Jacobs MR, Johnson CE: Macrolide resistance: an increasing concern for treatment failure in children. Pediatr Infect Dis J 2003;22:S131 [PMID: 14566999].

McCormick DP, Chonmaitree T, Pittman C et al: Nonsevere acute otitis media: a clinical trial comparing outcomes of watchful waiting versus immediate antibiotic treatment. Pediatrics 2005;115:1455 [PMID: 15930204].

McEllistrem MC, Adams JM, Patel K et al: Acute otitis media due to penicillin-nonsusceptible *Streptococcus pneumoniae*

before and after the introduction of the pneumococcal conjugate vaccine. Clin Infect Dis 2005;40:1738 [PMID: 15909260].

Pelton SI: Otitis media: re-evaluation of diagnosis and treatment in the era of antimicrobial resistance, pneumococcal conjugate vaccine, and evolving morbidity. Pediatr Clin North Am 2005;52:711 [PMID: 15925659].

Ruohola A, Heikkinen T, Meurman O et al: Antibiotic treatment of acute otorrhea through tympanostomy tube: randomized double-blind placebo-controlled study with daily follow-up. Pediatrics 2003;111:1061 [PMID: 12728089].

Siegel RM, Bien JP: Acute otitis media in children: a continuing story. Pediatr Rev 2004;25:187 [PMID: 15173451].

Subcommittee on Management of Acute Otitis Media: Diagnosis and management of acute otitis media. Pediatrics 2004;113:1451 [PMID: 15121972].

Wald ER: Acute otitis media: more trouble with the evidence. Pediatr Infect Dis J 2003;22:103 [PMID: 12586970].

Wald ER: To treat or not to treat. Pediatrics 2005;115:1087 [PMID: 15805394].

Websites

American Academy of Pediatrics (www.aap.org/otitismedia/www/): This is a website on diagnosis and treatment of acute otitis media, written for the American Academy of Pediatrics. It features video clips of tympanic membranes being insufflated, to help clinicians learn normal landmarks and pathologic states. It requires Apple QuickTime to run.

Centers for Disease Control and Prevention: Appropriate Antibiotic Use (www.cdc.gov/drugresistance): This is a Centers for Disease Control and Prevention site with excellent advice for clinicians on (1) distinguishing OME from AOM, (2) careful antibiotic use for respiratory infections, and (3) patient education material on these two topics.

www.pedisurg.com/pteducent/otitis_media.htm: Information for parents on AOM and tympanostomy tubes, with graphics.

The Ear Treatment Group at the University of Texas Medical Branch (www.atc.utmb.edu/aom/home.htm): This is an interactive site for medical students, residents, and physicians to learn about otitis media and to test their knowledge. The site contains links to other otitis media–related resources as well as parent educational material.

G. MANAGEMENT OF OTITIS MEDIA WITH RESIDUAL AND PERSISTENT EFFUSIONS

OME has been treated primarily to avoid any prolonged conductive hearing loss. Available data show a causal relationship between severe sensorineural hearing loss and language delay, but not between conductive hearing loss due to OME and language delay. Studies looking at middle ear effusion (MEE) and its effects on language development do not show differences at age 3 years. But auditory processing disorders are not testable until age 5–7 years, so final results of these studies are still pending. Two-thirds of children with AOM have an MEE or high negative middle ear pressure 2 weeks after diagnosis and one-third at 1 month after diagnosis regardless of antibiotic therapy. The management options for otitis media with residual effusion at 6 weeks to 4 months include observation and corticosteroid therapy. Corticosteroids (prednisone, 1 mg/kg/d) can be administered for 7 days. Unvaccinated children with no clear history of varicella infection who have been exposed in the preceding month should not receive prednisone because of the potential risk of disseminated varicella-zoster viral disease. Short courses of prednisone increase appetite and cause fluid retention, occasional vomiting, and rarely, marked behavioral changes.

If the patient clears the persistent MEE unilaterally or bilaterally, the physician should follow the patient monthly. Because of the increase in antibiotic resistance, the use of prophylaxis, even intermittently, must be restricted to carefully selected patients. The guideline recommendation developed by the Agency for Health Care Policy and Research for the management of OME is that ventilating tubes should be placed after the effusion has persisted for 4 months and is accompanied by a bilateral hearing impairment of 20 dB or greater. Earlier placement of ventilating tubes should depend on the child's developmental and behavioral status as well as on parental preference. The value of ventilating tubes for treating unilateral effusions in otherwise healthy children is unclear.

Children with otitis media and persistent effusion have an increased incidence of cholesteatoma, adhesive otitis, retraction pockets, membrane atrophy, and persistent membrane perforation. As there is no way to identify the small proportion of candidate children for whom insertion of ventilating tubes will prevent the damage, and close follow-up of abnormal ears may be best accomplished by an otolaryngologist.

Berman S: Management of otitis media and functional outcomes related to language, behavior, and attention: Is it time to change our approach? Pediatrics 2001;107:1175 [PMID: 11331703].

Paradise JL et al: Effect of early or delayed insertion of tympanostomy tubes for persistent otitis media on developmental outcomes at the age of three years. N Engl J Med 2001;344:1179 [PMID: 11309632].

Paradise JL et al: Language, speech sound production, and cognition in three-year-old children in relation to otitis media in their first three years of life. Pediatrics 2000;105:1119 [PMID: 10890473].

3. Mastoiditis

Mastoiditis is a spectrum of disease that ranges from inflammation of the mastoid periosteum to bony destruction of the mastoid air system (coalescent mastoiditis) or abscess development. Infection of the periosteum of the mastoid bone is a rare complication of AOM in the post-antibiotic era. Mastoiditis can occur in any age group, but more than 60% of the patients are younger than age 2 years. Many children do not have a prior history of recurrent acute otitis media. The most common pathogens are *Streptococcus pneumoniae* and *S pyogenes,* with *Staphylococcus aureus* and *H influenzae* occasionally seen. Rarely gram-negative bacilli and anaerobes are isolated. Antibiotics may affect the incidence and morbidity of acute mastoiditis. However, acute mastoiditis does occur in children who are on antibiotics for an acute ear infection. In the Netherlands, where only 31% of AOM patients receive antibiotics, the incidence of acute mastoiditis is 4.2 per 100,000 person-years. In the United States, where more than 96% of patients with AOM receive antibiotics, the incidence of acute mastoiditis is 2 per 100,000 person-years. The higher antibiotic usage in the United States correlates with a higher rate of resistant organisms and more adverse drug interactions. Moreover, despite the routine use of antibiotics, the incidence of acute mastoiditis has been rising in some cities. The pattern change may be secondary to the emergence of resistant *S pneumoniae.*

Clinical Findings

The principal complaints of patients with mastoiditis are usually postauricular pain, fever, and outwardly displaced pinna. On examination, the mastoid area often appears swollen and reddened. In the late stage, it may be fluctuant. The earliest finding is severe tenderness on mastoid palpation.

AOM, by otoscopy, is almost always present. Late findings are a pinna that is pushed forward by postauricular swelling and an ear canal that is narrowed in the posterosuperior wall because of pressure from the mastoid abscess. In infants younger than age 1 year, the swelling occurs superior to the ear and pushes the pinna downward rather than outward. In the acute phase, diffuse inflammatory clouding of the mastoid cells occurs, as in every case of AOM. In more severe cases, bony destruction and resorption of the mastoid air cells may occur. The best way to determine the extent of disease is by computed tomography (CT) scan.

Meningitis is a complication of acute mastoiditis and should be suspected when a child has associated high fever, stiff neck, severe headache, or other meningeal signs. Lumbar puncture should be performed for diagnosis. Brain abscess occurs in 2% of patients and may be associated with persistent headaches, recurring fever, or changes in sensorium. Facial palsy, cavernous sinus thrombosis, and thrombophlebitis may be encountered.

Treatment for noncoalescent mastoiditis is typically myringotomy, with or without tube placement, in order to obtain material for culture. Hospitalization for intravenous therapy follows. Reasonable initial therapy is ceftriaxone plus nafcillin or clindamycin until culture results are returned. If clinical improvement does not occur after 24–48 hours of intravenous or intramuscular therapy, or if any signs or symptoms of intracranial complications exist, immediate surgery to drain the mastoid abscess is indicated. The primary management for coalescent mastoiditis is cortical mastoidectomy. A recent review from the University of Texas–Southwestern revealed that 39% of patients required a mastoidectomy. After significant clinical improvement is achieved with parenteral therapy, oral antibiotics are begun and should be continued for 3 weeks. If the child has an isolated subperiosteal abscess and not coalescent mastoiditis, either needle aspiration or incision and drainage with an associated myringotomy has produced good clinical outcomes.

4. Otitis Media with Complications

Complications of otitis media may involve damage to the middle ear structures, such as tympanosclerosis, retraction pockets, adhesions, ossicular erosion, cholesteatoma, perforations, and intratemporal and intracranial injury.

A. TYMPANOSCLEROSIS

A white plaquelike appearance on the TM is caused by chronic inflammation or trauma that produces granulation tissue and hyalinization. The appearance of a small defect in the posterosuperior area of the pars tensa or in the pars flaccida suggests a retraction pocket. Retraction pockets occur when chronic inflammation and negative pressure in the middle ear space produce atrophy and atelectasis of the TM.

Continued inflammation can cause adhesions between the retraction pocket and the ossicles. This condition, referred to as adhesive otitis, predisposes to formation of a cholesteatoma or fixation and erosion of the ossicles (Figure 17–5). Erosion of the ossicles results from osteitis and compromise of the blood supply. Ossicular discontinuity may produce a maximal hearing loss with a 50-dB threshold. A tympanogram with very high compliance suggests ossicular discontinuity.

B. CHOLESTEATOMA

A greasy-looking mass or pearly white debris seen in a retraction pocket or perforation suggests a cholesteatoma, whether or not there is discharge (see Figure 17–5). A perforation is usually painless. If infection is absent, the middle ear cavity generally contains normal mucosa. If infection is superimposed, serous or purulent drainage will be seen, and the middle ear cavity may contain granulation tissue or even polyps. Persistent or recurrent otorrhea following appropriate medical management should make one suspect a cholesteatoma.

C. TYMPANIC MEMBRANE PERFORATION

Occasionally, an episode of AOM is associated with otorrhea. An aural discharge indicates that the TM has

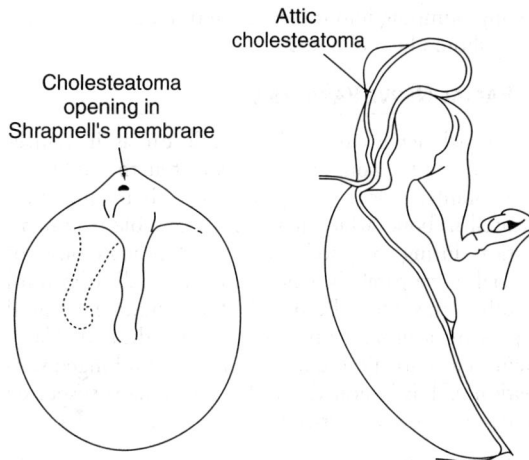

Figure 17–5. Attic cholesteatoma, formed from an indrawing of an attic retraction pocket.

perforated. Most likely the perforation will heal spontaneously. If the perforation has not healed within 3 months, surgical intervention will be necessary. A conductive hearing loss is usually present, depending on the size and location of the perforation. The site of perforation is important. Central perforations surrounded by intact TM are usually relatively safe from cholesteatoma formation. With a peripheral perforation, especially in the pars flaccida, the perforation extends to the canal wall without any intervening TM. Peripheral perforations create a risk for cholesteatoma because the ear canal epithelium may invade the perforation.

Most perforations with AOM heal within 2 weeks. When perforations fail to heal after 3–6 months, surgical repair may be needed. Repair of the defect in the TM is generally delayed until the child is older and eustachian tube function has improved. Procedures include paper patch, fat myringoplasty, and tympanoplasty. Tympanoplasty is generally deferred until age 7–9 years. In otherwise healthy children without any craniofacial anomalies, some surgeons repair the perforated TM earlier if the contralateral nonperforated drum remains free of infection and effusion for 1 year. This policy does not guarantee success. The age of the child when repair is performed is the more probable indicator of success. Occasionally, a perforation is closed in a child of younger age if recurrent otorrhea is thought to be secondary to water contamination or nasopharyngeal reflux. Earlier closure of the perforation will seal the middle ear space and reestablish the air cushion provided by the mastoid air system. An older child is more likely to have a successful outcome from closure of the perforation. Water activities should be limited to surface swimming, preferably with the use of an ear mold.

Diving, jumping into the water, and underwater swimming should be prohibited.

D. FACIAL NERVE PARALYSIS

The facial nerve crosses the middle ear as it courses through the temporal bone to its exit at the stylomastoid foramen. Occasionally, the nerve is incompletely encased in bone, which makes it susceptible to inflammation during an episode of AOM. The acute onset of a facial nerve paralysis is not idiopathic Bell palsy until all other causes have been excluded. If middle ear fluid is present, a prompt myringotomy is indicated. Placement of a ventilation tube will allow for prolonged ventilation. CT is indicated if a cholesteatoma is suspected or acute coalescent mastoiditis is present.

E. CHRONIC SUPPURATIVE OTITIS MEDIA

Chronic suppurative otitis media is present when persistent otorrhea occurs in a child with tympanostomy tubes or TM perforations. Occasionally, it is an accompanying sign of cholesteatoma. Visualization of the TM, meticulous cleaning with culture of the drainage, and appropriate antimicrobial therapy are keys to management of cases not related to cholesteatoma. The successful treatment of chronic suppurative otitis usually requires therapy with an antibiotic that covers *Pseudomonas* and anaerobes. Oral quinolone antibiotics effective against *Pseudomonas* infection are not yet approved for use in growing children. Recent studies suggest that topical quinolones for 14 days may be effective. It is very important to clean the ear canal by suction to allow penetration of drops, and it is often useful to culture the secretions. An ear wick should be inserted and drops placed on the wick several times daily. The child should be seen in 7 days, the wick removed, and suction repeated if necessary. When a cholesteatoma is associated with chronic suppurative otitis media, medical therapy is not effective (see Figure 17–5). If the discharge does not respond to 2 weeks of aggressive therapy, mastoiditis, cholesteatoma, tuberculosis, or fungal infection should be suspected. Serious central nervous system (CNS) complications such as extradural abscess, subdural abscess, brain abscess, meningitis, labyrinthitis, or lateral sinus thrombophlebitis can occur with extension of this process. Therefore, patients with facial palsy, vertigo, or other CNS signs should be immediately referred to an otolaryngologist.

Lahav J et al: Postauricular needle aspiration of subperiosteal abscess in acute mastoiditis. Ann Otol Rhinol Laryngol 2005; 114:323 [PMID: 15895789].

Leskinen K: Complications of acute otitis media in children. Curr Allergy Asthma Rep 2005;5:308 [PMID: 15967073].

Leskinen K, Jero J: Complications of acute otitis media in children in southern Finland. Int J Pediatr Otorhinolaryngol 2004; 68:317 [PMID: 15129942].

Oestreicher-Kedem Y et al: Complications of mastoiditis in children at the onset of a new millennium. Ann Otol Rhinol Laryngol 2005;114:147 [PMID: 15757196].

Zapalac JS et al: Suppurative complications of acute otitis media in the era of antibiotic resistance. Arch Otolaryngol Head Neck Surg 2002;128:660 [PMID: 12049560].

Website

www.entnet.org: This is the official website of the American Academy of Otolaryngology and Head and Neck Surgery. The site contains patient information, clinical indications for common surgical procedures, and links to other ear, nose and throat sites.

ACUTE TRAUMA TO THE MIDDLE EAR

Head injuries, a blow to the ear canal, sudden impact with water, blast injuries, or the insertion of pointed instruments into the ear canal can lead to perforation of the TM or hematoma of the middle ear. One study reported that 50% of serious penetrating wounds of the TM were due to parental use of a cotton-tipped swab.

Treatment of middle ear hematomas consists mainly of watchful waiting. Antibiotics are not necessary unless signs of infection appear. The prognosis for unimpaired hearing depends on whether the ossicles are dislocated or fractured in the process. The patient needs to be followed with audiometry or an otolaryngologist until hearing has returned to normal, which is expected within 6–8 weeks.

Traumatic perforations of the TM often do not heal spontaneously, in which case the patient should be referred to an otolaryngologist. Perforations caused by a foreign body must be attended to immediately, especially if accompanied by vertigo.

EAR CANAL FOREIGN BODY

Numerous objects can be inserted into the ear canal by a child. If the object is large, wedged into place, or difficult to remove with available instruments, the patient should be referred to an otolaryngologist early rather than risk traumatizing the child or the ear canal or causing edema that will require removal under anesthesia. An emergency condition exists if the foreign body is a disk-type battery used in clocks, watches, and hearing aids. An electric current is generated in the moist canal, and a severe burn with resulting scarring can occur in less than 4 hours.

Lin VY, Daniel SJ, Papsin BC: Button batteries in the ear, nose and upper aerodigestive tract. Int J Pediatr Otorhinolaryngol 2004;68:473 [PMID: 15013616].

HEMATOMA OF THE PINNA

Trauma to the ear can result in a hematoma between the perichondrium and cartilage. The hematoma appears as a boggy purple swelling of the upper half of the ear. If this is not treated, it can cause pressure necrosis of the underlying cartilage and result in "cauliflower ear." To prevent this cosmetic deformity, physicians should urgently refer patients to an otolaryngologist for aspiration and application of a carefully molded pressure dressing. Recurrent or persistent hematoma of the ear may require surgical drainage.

CONGENITAL EAR MALFORMATIONS

Agenesis of the external ear canal results in conductive hearing loss that requires evaluation in the first month of life by hearing specialists and an otolaryngologist.

"Lop ears," folded down or protruding ears (so-called "Dumbo" ears), are a source of much teasing and ridicule. In the past, surgical correction at age 5 or 6 years was offered. Taping the ears into a correct anatomic position is very effective if performed in the first 72–96 hours of life. Tape is applied over a molding of wax and continued for 2 weeks. Another alternative for the ear that can be molded solely by finger pressure into a normal configuration is an incisionless otoplasty, which can be performed at a much earlier age and is associated with little postoperative morbidity. Because no cartilage destruction is associated with this technique, future growth is unaffected.

An ear is low-set if the upper pole is below eye level. This condition is often associated with renal malformations (eg, Potter syndrome), and renal ultrasound examination is suggested.

Preauricular tags, ectopic cartilage, fistulas, sinuses, and cysts require surgical correction, mainly for cosmetic reasons. Children exhibiting any of these findings should have their hearing tested. Most preauricular pits cause no symptoms. If one should become infected, the patient should receive antibiotic therapy and be referred to an otolaryngologist for eventual excision.

Fritsch MH: Incisionless otoplasty. Facial Plast Surg 2004;20:267 [PMID: 15778913].

Yotsuyanagi T et al: Nonsurgical treatment of various auricular deformities. Clin Plast Surg 2002;29:327 [PMID: 12120687].

IDENTIFICATION AND MANAGEMENT OF HEARING LOSS

Hearing loss is classified as being conductive, sensorineural, or mixed in nature. Conductive hearing loss occurs when there is a blockage of sound transmission between the opening of the external ear and the cochlear receptor cells. The most common cause of conductive hearing loss in children is fluid in the middle ear. Sensorineural hearing loss is due to a defect in the neural transmission of sound, arising from a defect in the cochlear hair cells or the auditory nerve. Mixed hearing loss is characterized by elements of both conductive and sensorineural loss.

Hearing is measured in decibels (dB). The threshold, or 0 dB, refers to the level at which a sound is perceived in normal subjects 50% of the time. Hearing is considered normal if an individual's thresholds are within 15 dB of normal. In children, severity of hearing loss is graded as follows: 5–30 dB mild, 31–60 dB moderate, 61–90 dB severe, and 91+ dB profound.

Hearing loss can significantly impair a child's ability to communicate, and hinder academic, social, and emotional development. Studies suggest that periods of auditory deprivation may have enduring effects on auditory processing, even after normal hearing is restored. In the past, the effects of unilateral hearing loss were thought to be of little consequence, but studies have shown that even a unilateral loss is associated with difficulties in school and behavioral issues. Early identification and management of any hearing impairment is therefore critical.

Conductive Hearing Loss

The most common cause of childhood conductive hearing loss is otitis media and related conditions such as middle ear effusion and eustachian tube dysfunction. Other causes of conductive hearing loss may include external auditory canal atresia or stenosis, tympanic membrane perforation, cerumen impaction, cholesteatoma, and middle ear abnormalities, such as ossicular fixation or discontinuity. Often, a conductive loss may be corrected with surgery.

Middle ear effusions may be serous, mucoid, or purulent, as in acute otitis media. Effusions are generally associated with a mild conductive hearing loss that usually normalizes once the effusion is gone. The American Academy of Pediatrics recommends that hearing and language skills be assessed in children who have recurrent acute otitis media or middle ear effusions lasting longer than 3 months.

Sensorineural Hearing Loss

Sensorineural hearing loss (SNHL) arises due to a defect in the cochlear receptor cells or the auditory nerve (cranial nerve VIII). The loss may be congenital (present at birth) or acquired. In both the congenital and acquired categories, the hearing loss may be either hereditary (due to a genetic mutation) or nonhereditary. It is estimated that SNHL affects 2–3 out of every 1000 live births, making this the most common congenital sensory impairment. The incidence is thought to be considerably higher among the neonatal intensive care unit population. Well-recognized risk factors for SNHL in neonates include positive family history of childhood SNHL, birthweight less than 1500 grams, low Apgar scores (0–4 at 1 minute or 0–6 at 5 minutes), craniofacial anomalies, hypoxia, in utero infections (eg, TORCH syndrome), hyperbilirubinemia requiring exchange transfusion, and mechanical ventilation for greater than 5 days.

A. CONGENITAL HEARING LOSS

Nonhereditary causes account for approximately 50% of congenital hearing loss. These include prenatal infections, teratogenic drugs, and perinatal injuries. The other half of cases are attributed to genetic factors. Among children with hereditary hearing loss, approximately one-third of cases are thought to be due to a known syndrome, while the other two-thirds are considered nonsyndromic.

Syndromic hearing impairment is associated with malformations of the external ear or other organs, or with medical problems involving other organ systems. Over 400 genetic syndromes that include hearing loss have been described. All patients being evaluated for hearing loss should also be evaluated for features commonly associated with these syndromes. These include branchial cleft cysts or sinuses, preauricular pits, ocular abnormalities, white forelock, café au lait spots, and craniofacial anomalies. Some of the more frequently mentioned syndromes associated with congenital hearing loss include the following: Waardenberg, branchio-oto-renal, Usher, Pendred, Jervell and Lange-Nielsen, and Alport.

Over 70% of hereditary hearing loss is nonsyndromic (ie, there are no associated visible abnormalities or related medical problems). The most common mutation associated with nonsyndromic hearing loss is in the *GJB2* gene, which encodes the protein connexin 26. The *GJB2* mutation has a carrier rate of about 3% in the general population. Most nonsyndromic hearing loss, including that due to the *GJB2* mutation, is autosomal recessive, but gene loci for autosomal dominant and X-linked hearing loss have also been identified.

B. ACQUIRED HEARING LOSS

Hereditary hearing loss may be delayed in onset, as in Alport syndrome and most types of autosomal dominant nonsyndromic hearing loss. Vulnerability to aminoglycoside-induced hearing loss has also been linked to a mitochondrial gene defect.

Nongenetic etiologies for delayed-onset SNHL include exposure to ototoxic medications, meningitis, autoimmune or neoplastic conditions, noise exposure, and trauma. Infections such as syphilis or Lyme disease have been associated with hearing impairment. Hearing loss associated with congenital cytomegalovirus infection may be present at birth, or may have a delayed onset. The loss is progressive in approximately half of all patients with congenital cytomegalovirus-associated hearing loss. Other risk factors for delayed-onset, progressive loss include a history

of persistent pulmonary hypertension and extracorporeal membrane oxygenation therapy

Identification of Hearing Loss

A. OFFICE CLINICAL ASSESSMENT

In the past, the parents' report of their infant's behavior was considered an adequate assessment of hearing. However, a deaf infant's behavior can appear normal and mislead the parents as well as the professional, especially if the infant has autosomal recessive deafness and is the first-born child of carrier parents. The following office screening techniques should identify gross hearing losses but may not detect less severe losses due to otitis media.

1. Birth to 4 months—In response to a sudden loud sound (70 dB or more) produced by a horn, clacker, or special electronic device, the infant should show a startle reflex or blink the eyes.

2. 4 months to 2 years—While the infant is distracted with a toy or bright object, a noisemaker is sounded softly outside the field of vision at the child's waist level. Normal responses are as follows: at 4 months, there is widening of the eyes, interruption of other activity, and perhaps a slight turning of the head in the direction of the sound; at 6 months, the head turns toward the sound; at 9 months or older, the child is usually able to locate a sound originating from below as well as turn to the appropriate side; after 1 year, the child is able to locate sound whether it comes from below or above.

After responses to soft sounds are noted, a loud horn or clacker should be used to produce an eye blink or startle reflex. This latter maneuver is necessary because deaf children are often visually alert and able to scan the environment so actively that their scanning can be mistaken for an appropriate response to the softer noise test. A deaf child will not blink in response to the loud sound. Consonant sounds such as "mama," "dada," and "baba" should be present in speech by age 11 months. Children who fail to respond appropriately should be referred for audiologic assessment.

B. NEWBORN HEARING SCREENING

Prior to the institution of universal screening programs, the average age at identification of hearing loss was 30 months. Recognizing the importance of early detection, in 1993, a National Institutes of Health Consensus Panel recommended that all newborns be screened for hearing impairment prior to hospital discharge. Today, universal newborn hearing screening is mandated in a majority of states, with a goal of hearing loss identification by 3 months of age, and appropriate intervention by the age of 6 months. Subjective testing is not reliable in infants, and therefore objective, physiologic methods are used for screening. Auditory brainstem response and otoacoustic emission testing are the two commonly employed screening modalities.

C. AUDIOLOGIC EVALUATION OF INFANTS AND CHILDREN

Audiometry subjectively evaluates hearing. There are several different methods used, based on patient age:

- Behavioral observational audiometry: Birth to 6 months. Sounds are presented at various intensity levels, and the audiologist watches closely for a reaction, such as change in respiratory rate, starting or stopping of activity, startle, head turn, or muscle tensing. This method is highly tester-dependent and error-prone.
- Visual reinforcement audiometry: 6 months to 2.5 years. Auditory stimulus is paired with positive reinforcement. For example, when a child reacts appropriately by turning toward a sound source, the behavior is rewarded by activation of a toy which lights up. After a brief conditioning period, the child localizes toward the tone, if audible, in anticipation of the lighted toy.
- Conditioned play audiometry: 2.5 to 5 years. The child responds to sound stimulus by performing an activity, such as putting a peg into a board.
- Conventional audiometry: Age 5 and up. The child indicates when he or she hears a sound.

Objective methods such as auditory brainstem response and otoacoustic emission testing may be used if a child cannot be reliably tested using the above methods.

Referral

A child who fails newborn hearing screening or has a suspected hearing loss should be referred for further audiologic evaluation, and any child with hearing loss should be referred to an otolaryngologist for further work-up and treatment. In addition to the infants who fall into the high-risk categories for SNHL as outlined above, hearing should be tested in children with a history of developmental delay, bacterial meningitis, ototoxic medication exposure, neurodegenerative disorders, or a history of infection such as mumps or measles. Even if a newborn screening was passed, all infants who fall into a high-risk category for progressive or delayed-onset hearing loss should receive ongoing audiologic monitoring for 3 years and at appropriate intervals thereafter to avoid a missed diagnosis.

Prevention

Appropriate care may treat or prevent conditions causing hearing deficits. Aminoglycosides and diuretics, particularly in combination, are potentially ototoxic

and should be used judiciously and monitored carefully. Given the association of a mitochondrial gene defect and aminoglycoside ototoxicity, use should be avoided, if possible, in patients with a known family history of aminoglycoside-related hearing loss. Reduction of repeated exposure to loud noises may help prevent high frequency hearing loss associated with acoustic trauma. Any sudden-onset sensorineural hearing loss should be seen by an otolaryngologist immediately, as in some cases, steroid therapy may reverse the loss if initiated right away.

Downs MP, Yoshinaga-Itano C: The efficacy of early identification and intervention for children with hearing impairment. Pediatr Clin North Am 1999;46:79 [PMID: 10079791].

Grose JH, Hall JW: Auditory development. In: Lalwani AK, Grundfast KM (editors): *Pediatric Otology and Neurotology*. Philadelphia: Lippincott-Raven; 1998:29.

Grundfast KM, Siparsky NF. Hearing loss. In: Bluestone CD, Stool, SE, Alper CM et al (editors): *Pediatric Otolaryngology*, Vol. 1. Philadelphia: Saunders; 2003:306.

Joint Committee on Infant Hearing: Year 2000 position statement: principles and guidelines for early hearing detection and intervention programs. Pediatrics 2000;106:798 [PMID: 11015525].

Lieu JE: Speech-language and educational consequences of unilateral hearing loss in children. Arch Otolaryngol Head Neck Surg 2004;130:524 [PMID: 15148171].

Smith RJH, Green GE, Van Camp G: Deafness and hereditary hearing loss overview. Last revision 2/18/2005. www.geneclinics.org/profiles/deafness-overview/details.html

■ II. THE NOSE & PARANASAL SINUSES

ACUTE VIRAL RHINITIS (Common Cold; See Also Chapter 36.)

The common cold is the most common pediatric infectious disease, and the incidence is higher in early childhood than in any other period of life. Children younger than age 5 years have 6–12 colds per year, of which 30% are caused by rhinoviruses, 15% influenza or parainfluenza, 10% coronavirus, and 5% enterovirus.

Clinical Findings

The patient usually experiences a sudden onset of clear or mucoid rhinorrhea, nasal congestion, and fever. Mild sore throat and cough may develop. Although the fever is usually low-grade in older children, in the first 5 or 6 years of life it can be as high as 40.6 °C without superinfection. The nose, throat, and TM can appear red and inflamed. Figure 17–6 shows the duration of cough, sore throat, and

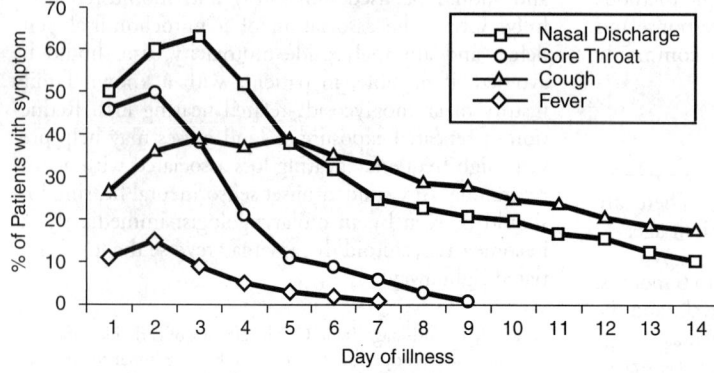

Figure 17–6. Duration of symptoms in the common cold in adults. (Reproduced, with permission, from Gwaltney JM: Rhinovirus infections in an industrial population. II. Characteristics of illness and antibody response. JAMA 1967;202:494.)

rhinorrhea in adults with rhinovirus-proven infections. Note that one-quarter are still symptomatic at 14 days, although they may be improving.

Treatment

An algorithm for the management of acute nasal congestion and sinusitis is presented in Figure 17–7. Treatment for the common cold should be purely symptomatic; however, a recent study showed that diagnostic uncertainly or white blood cell count elevation may support the use of antibiotics. Acetaminophen or ibuprofen is helpful for fever, sore throat, or muscle aches. A stuffy, congested nose can be treated with normal saline nose drops (mix ¹/₂ tsp table salt with 6 oz of water), 3 drops in each nostril. After several minutes, a suction bulb can be used to remove the secretions if the infant is unable to blow his or her nose. If this procedure fails after several attempts and the stuffy nose still interferes with feeding or sleep, consider long-acting xylometazoline or oxymetazoline 0.05% nose drops twice daily. Drops should be used only when the nose is congested and discontinued within 3 days to prevent rebound chemical rhinitis.

Antihistamines are not effective in relieving cold symptoms. In rhinoviral colds, increased levels of histamine are not observed. Antibiotics do not prevent superinfection and should not be used. Cough suppression at night is the number one goal of many parents; however, the effectiveness of dextromethorphan is unclear. It is believed by most experts to be effective in adults and adolescents, but it has not been studied adequately in children with colds. Use of codeine should be discouraged because it has caused fatal respiratory distress. A cool mist vaporizer or humidifier may help the cough, but the device should have antibacterial solution added to the water or be washed every 3 days or less, to prevent mold growth. Parents should be instructed that fast breathing or difficult breathing with retraction is a sign of lower respiratory infection such as

bronchiolitis or pneumonia. Prolonged fever may indicate otitis media or sinusitis.

Arnold SR et al: Antibiotic prescribing for upper respiratory tract infection: the importance of diagnostic uncertainty. Pediatrics 2005;146:222 [PMID: 15689913].

Casey JR et al: White blood cell count can aid judicious antibiotic prescribing in acute upper respiratory infections in children. Clin Pediatr (Phila) 2003;42:113 [PMID: 12659383].

RHINOSINUSITIS

The use of the term rhinosinusitis has replaced sinusitis. Rhinosinusitis acknowledges that the nasal and sinus mucosa are involved in similar and concurrent inflammatory processes.

1. Acute Bacterial Rhinosinusitis

The diagnosis of acute bacterial rhinosinusitis (ABRS) was revised by the Sinus and Allergy Health Partnership in 2004. The general recommendation is to make the diagnosis of ABRS when a child with a viral URI does not improve after 10 days or worsens after 5–7 days. The maxillary and ethmoidal sinuses are most commonly involved when mucociliary clearance and drainage are impaired by a URI or allergic rhinitis. Both the ethmoid and maxillary sinuses are present at birth, forming in the third to fourth gestational month. The sphenoid sinuses pneumatize as an extension of a posterior ethmoid cell by age 5 years, and the frontal sinuses form from an anterior ethmoid cell appearing about age 7–8 years. Frontal sinusitis is unusual before age 10 years.

A combination of anatomic, mucosal, microbial, and immune pathogenic processes is believed to underlie sinusitis in children. Both viral and bacterial infections have integral roles in the pathogenesis of sinusitis. Viral URIs commonly cause sinus mucosal injury and swelling, resulting in osteomeatal obstruction, loss of ciliary activity, and mucus hypersecretion. The bacterial pathogens that cause acute

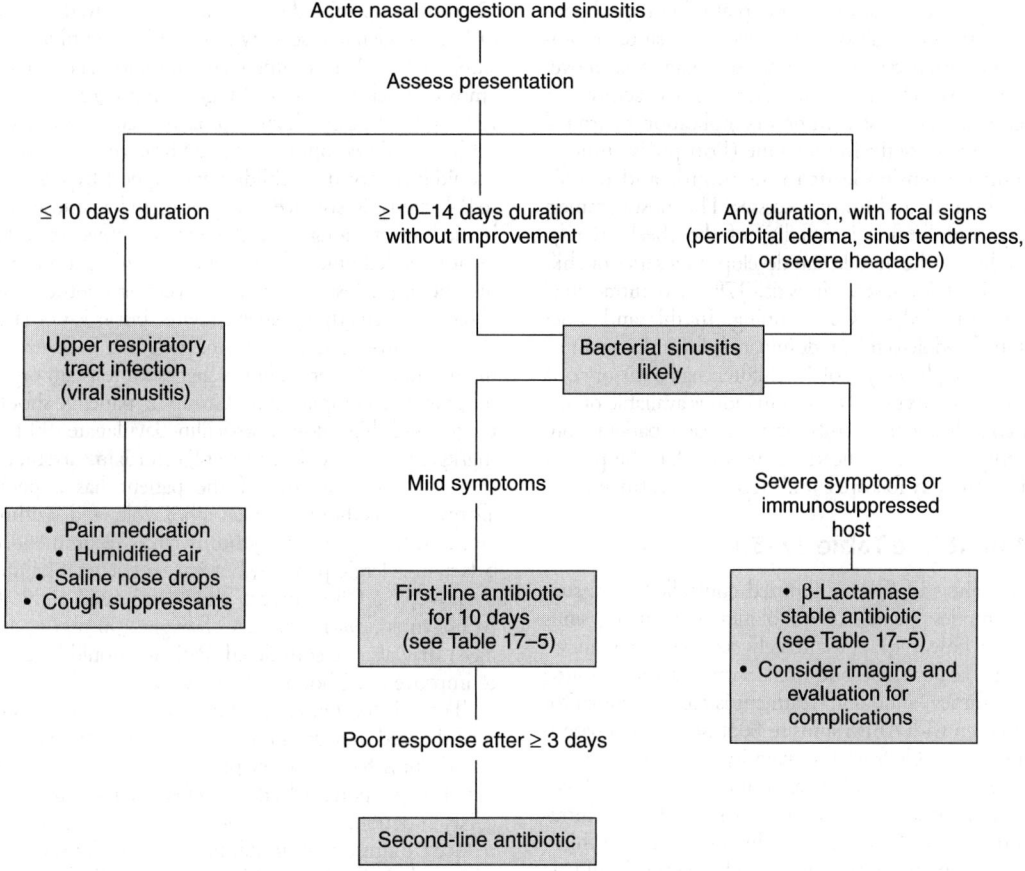

Figure 17–7. Algorithm for acute nasal congestion and sinusitis.

sinusitis are usually *S pneumoniae, H influenzae* (nontypable), *M catarrhalis,* and β-hemolytic streptococci. Rarely, anaerobic bacterial infections can cause fulminant frontal sinusitis.

Clinical Findings

The development of symptoms in acute sinusitis in children may be gradual or sudden. According to the Sinus and Allergy Health Partnership, common symptoms are nasal drainage, nasal congestion, facial pressure/pain, postnasal drainage, hyposmia/anosmia, fever, cough, fatigue, maxillary dental pain, and ear pressure/fullness. The physical examination is rarely helpful in making a diagnosis of acute bacterial sinusitis, as the findings will be nearly the same as those in a child with viral rhinosinusitis. Occasionally percussion tenderness overlying the sinus is present, but this is a finding typical only of the older child and is unreliable when compared with antral irrigation results. Transillumination

of the sinuses is difficult to perform and not very helpful unless the sinuses are grossly asymmetrical.

The physician should consider sinus aspiration by an otolaryngologist for diagnostic purposes in patients with complications and in immunocompromised patients. Gram stain or culture of nasal discharge does not correlate with cultures of sinus aspirates. If the patient is hospitalized because of complications, a blood culture should be obtained.

Imaging studies of the paranasal sinuses during acute illness are not indicated except for evaluation of complications. Because of the lack of specificity between abnormal CTs or plain films, the Sinus and Allergy Health Partnership (see references) does not recommend any imaging study to diagnose uncomplicated cases of acute bacterial sinusitis in any age group.

Complications

Complications are most apt to develop with ethmoiditis. These complications represent a continuum beginning with preseptal cellulitis, then postseptal cellulitis, subperiosteal abscess, orbital abscess, and cavernous sinus thrombosis. They are associated with decreased extraocular movement, proptosis, chemosis, and altered visual acuity (see Chapter 15). The most common complication of frontal sinusitis is osteitis of the frontal bone (Pott puffy tumor). Intracranial extension leads to meningitis and to epidural, subdural, and brain abscesses. The most common maxillary complication is cellulitis of the cheek. Rarely, osteomyelitis of the maxilla can develop. In a series of children admitted for severe sinusitis, 17% had intracranial abscesses identified on CT scanning. In this and other studies, male adolescents predominated, for unknown reasons. Interestingly, only 1 of 13 children had a history of a previous sinus infection. No information is available on the rate of complications in ambulatory sinusitis patients, but the severity of the complications suggests that the patient should be carefully followed while receiving treatment.

Treatment (see Table 17–5.)

A meta-analysis of five randomized controlled trials suggested a modest benefit of antibiotics in reducing sinus symptoms; however, approximately six children required therapy to achieve one additional cure. Despite limited proof of efficacy, antibiotic treatment is recommended for most children with ABRS sinusitis because bacterial pathogens are recoverable from the majority of affected sinuses. Patients with evidence of invasive infection or any CNS complications should be hospitalized immediately. Intravenous therapy with nafcillin or clindamycin plus a third-generation cephalosporin such as cefotaxime should be initiated until culture results become available. For uncomplicated sinus infections, the guidelines divide patients into two groups: (1) those with mild symptoms who have not received antibiotics within the past 4–6 weeks and

(2) those with mild disease who have received antibiotics, or have moderate disease with or without antibiotic exposure. Group 1 recommended antibiotics are high-dose amoxicillin-clavulanate (90 mg/6.4 mg/kg/d), amoxicillin (90 mg/kg/d), cefpodoxime proxetil, cefuroxime axetil, or cefdinir. Trimethoprim-sulfamethoxazole and macrolides should be reserved for children with type 1 hypersensitivity to β-lactams. Resistance to any of these bacteriostatic antibiotic is great enough that these medications are no longer recommended unless the patient is allergic to both penicillin and cephalosporin. Clindamycin is another possible choice, particularly in older patients, but it is not effective against gram-negative organisms such as *H influenzae*. Failure to improve after 72 hours suggests a resistant organism or potential complication. Group 2 patients should be treated with high-dose amoxicillin-clavulanate (90 mg/6.4 mg/kg/d). Cefpodoxime proxetil, cefuroxime axetil, or cefdinir are recommended if the patient has a penicillin allergy. Trimethoprim-sulfamethoxazole and azithromycin, clarithromycin, or erythromycin is recommended for β-lactam–allergic patients, but have a bacterial failure rate of 20–25%. Clindamycin should be used only if the pathogen is *S pneumoniae*. Cefriaxone (50 mg/kg/d for 5 days) may also be considered. Patients should be expected to improve in 72 hours or be reassessed.

Topical decongestants and oral combinations are frequently used in acute sinusitis to promote drainage. Their effectiveness has not been proved, and concern has been raised about potential adverse effects related to impaired ciliary function, decreased blood flow to the mucosa, and reduced diffusion of antibiotic into the sinuses. Patients with underlying allergic rhinitis may benefit from intranasal cromolyn or corticosteroid nasal spray. Vasoconstrictor nose drops and spray are associated with rebound edema if used for more than 3 days.

The patient may require acetaminophen, ibuprofen, or even codeine to permit sleep until drainage is achieved. The application of ice over the sinus may help to relieve pain.

McAlister WH et al: Sinusitis in the pediatric population: American College of Radiology. ACR appropriateness criteria. Radiology 2000;215(Suppl):811 [PMID: 11037504].

Sinus and Allergy Health Partnership: Antimicrobial treatment guidelines for acute bacterial rhinosinusitis. Otolaryngol Head Neck Surg 2004;13:1 [PMID: 14726904].

2. Recurrent or Chronic Rhinosinusitis

As the definition of acute bacterial rhinosinusitis (ABRS) changed, so has the diagnosis of patients with recurrent or chronic rhinosinusitis. Recurrent rhinosinusitis occurs when episodes of ABRS clear with antibiotic treatment but recur with each or most URIs. Chronic rhinosinusitis is diagnosed when the child has not cleared in the expected time but has not developed acute complications. Both symptoms and physical findings are required to support the

Table 17–5. Antibiotic treatment of acute sinusitis.

First-line therapy
1. Amoxicillin-clavulanate 90 mg/6.4 mg/kg/d or amoxicillin 90 mg/kg/d
2. Cefpodoxime proxetil, cefuroxime axetil, or cefdinir
3. Trimethoprim-sulfa-methoxazole and macrolides if β-lactam allergic
4. Clindamycin if known to be strep
Second-line therapy
1. High dose amoxicillin-clavulanate 90 mg/6.4 mg/kg/d
2. Cefpodoxime proxetil, cefuroxime axetil, or cefdinir if penicillin allergy
3. Trimethoprim-sulfa-methoxazole and macrolides if β-lactam allergic
4. Clindamycin for *S pneumoniae*
5. Ceftriaxone 50 mg/kg/d for 5 days
Reassess in 72 hours if not improved

diagnosis and CT scan may be a useful adjuvant in making the diagnosis. Although recent meta-analysis evaluations have resulted in recommendations for acute sinusitis, there is a paucity of data for the treatment of recurrent or chronic rhinosinusitis. Important factors to consider include allergies, anatomic variations, and disorders in host immunity. Mucosal inflammation leading to obstruction is most commonly caused by allergic rhinitis and occasionally by nonallergic rhinitis. Gastroesophageal reflux has also been found to be associated with chronic sinusitis, and treatment of reflux may result in dramatic improvements in sinus symptoms. Rarely, chronic sinusitis is caused by anatomic variations, such as septal deviation, polyp, or foreign body. Allergic polyps are unusual in children younger than age 10 years and therefore indicate a work-up for cystic fibrosis. In cases of chronic or recurrent pyogenic pansinusitis, poor host resistance (eg, an immune defect, Kartagener syndrome, or cystic fibrosis)—though rare—must be ruled out by immunoglobulin studies, microscopic studies of respiratory cilia, and a sweat chloride test. Anaerobic and staphylococcal organisms are often responsible for chronic sinusitis. Evaluation by an allergist and an otolaryngologist may be useful in determining the underlying causes.

Medical Treatment

Antibiotic therapy is similar to that used for acute sinusitis, but the duration is longer. Antimicrobial choice should include drugs effective against staphylococcal organisms. Adjuvant therapies such as saline nasal irrigation, decongestants, antihistamines, and topical intranasal steroids may be helpful depending on the underlying cause.

Surgical Treatment

A. ANTRAL LAVAGE

Antral lavage, generally regarded as a diagnostic procedure, may have some therapeutic value. An aspirate or a sample irrigated from the maxillary sinus is retrieved under anesthesia, either with a spinal needle or a curved-tip instrument. In the very young child, this may be the only procedure that should be performed.

B. ENDOSCOPIC SINUS SURGERY

No data are available comparing the outcome of this procedure with traditional surgical drainage procedures. There are large variations in the reported uses of this procedure by otolaryngologists, especially in younger patients.

C. EXTERNAL DRAINAGE

External drainage procedures are reserved for complications arising from ethmoid and frontal sinusitis.

Chan KH et al: Chronic rhinosinusitis in young children differs from adults: a histopathology study. J Pediatr 2004;144:206 [PMID: 14760263].

Jailwala JA, Shaker R: Oral and pharyngeal complications of gastroesophageal reflux disease: Globus, dental erosions, and chronic sinusitis. J Clin Gastroenterol 2000;30(3 Suppl):S35 [PMID: 10777170].

Phipps CD et al: Gastroesophageal reflux contributing to chronic sinus disease in children: A prospective analysis. Arch Otolaryngol Head Neck Surg 2000;126:831 [PMID: 10888994].

CHOANAL ATRESIA

Choanal atresia occurs in approximately 1 in 7000 live births. The female:male ratio is 2:1, and unilateral:bilateral ratio is also 2:1. Bilateral atresia results in severe respiratory distress at birth and requires immediate placement of an oral airway. Unilateral atresia usually appears later as a unilateral chronic nasal discharge that can be confused with chronic sinusitis. Diagnosis may be suspected if a 6F catheter cannot be passed through the nose and is confirmed by axial CT scan. CHARGE association (**c**oloboma, **h**eart disease, **a**tresia of the choanae, **r**etarded growth and retarded development and/or CNS anomalies, **g**enital hypoplasia, and **e**ar anomalies and/or deafness) (see Chapter 33) or other congenital anomalies are present in 50% of patients. An oral airway should be used when a newborn has been diagnosed with bilateral choanal atresia until more definitive treatment by an otolaryngologist has been accomplished.

Keller JL, Kacker A: Choanal atresia, CHARGE association, and congenital nasal stenosis. Otolaryngol Clin North Am 2000; 33:1343 [PMID: 11449791].

RECURRENT RHINITIS

Recurrent rhinitis is frequently seen in the office practice of pediatrics. The child is brought in with the chief complaint of having "one cold after another," "constant colds," or "always being sick." Approximately two-thirds of these children have recurrent colds, and the remainder have either allergic rhinitis or recurrent sinusitis.

Allergic Rhinitis

Allergic rhinitis has significant morbidity and may contribute to the development of sinusitis and asthma exacerbations. Symptoms of frequent sneezing, rubbing of the nose, and clear drainage interfere with concentration at school. Nighttime nasal congestion interferes with sleep and causes daytime somnolence and hyperactivity. On physical examination the nasal turbinates are swollen, but may be red or pale pink. Treatment with nasal steroids is effective in decreasing the airway obstruction and rhinorrhea. Sneezing and clear drainage are controlled with nonsedating antihistamines. Recently, montelukast, a leukotriene antagonist, has been shown to be effective in reducing nasal congestion. However, it is less likely to improve the symptoms of itching, sneezing, and rhinorrhea, which are related to histamine release. Ipratropium can be used as an adjunctive therapy.

Pullerits T et al: Comparison of a nasal glucocorticoid, antileukotriene, and a combination of antileukotriene and antihistamine in the treatment of seasonal allergic rhinitis. J Allergy
Clin Immunol 2002;109:949 [PMID: 12063523].

Weinstein SF et al: Onset of efficacy of montelukast in seasonal allergic
rhinitis. Allergy Asthma Proc 2005;26:41 [PMID: 15813287].

http://www.aaaai.org/patients/allergic_conditions/rhinitis.stm

Vasomotor Rhinitis

Some children react to sudden changes in environmental
temperature with prolonged congestion and rhinorrhea.
Air pollution (especially tobacco smoke) may be a factor.
Oral decongestants or nasal steroids can be used to give
symptomatic relief.

EPISTAXIS

The nose is an extremely vascular structure. In most cases,
epistaxis (nosebleed) is due to mild trauma to the anterior
portion of the nasal septum (Kiesselbach area), usually due
to vigorous nose rubbing, nose blowing, or nose picking. If
a patient has been using a nasal steroid spray, check the
patient's technique to make sure he or she is directing the
nozzle at the lateral canthus of the eye and not the septum.
If this does not reduce the nosebleeds, then the steroid
spray should be discontinued. Examination of the Kiesselbach area usually reveals a red, raw surface with fresh clots
or old crusts. Also look for telangiectasia, hemangiomas, or
varicosities.

Less than 5% of epistaxis is caused by a bleeding disorder such as von Willebrand disease. Patients need a hematologic work-up if any of the following is present: a family
history of a bleeding disorder; a medical history of easy
bleeding, particularly with circumcision or dental extraction; spontaneous bleeding at any site; bleeding that lasts
for over 30 minutes or blood that will not clot with direct
pressure by the physician; onset before age 2 years; or a
drop in hematocrit due to epistaxis. High blood pressure
may rarely predispose to prolonged nosebleeds.

A nasopharyngeal angiofibroma may be manifested by
recurrent epistaxis. Adolescent boys are affected almost
exclusively. CT scan of the nasal cavity and nasopharynx is
diagnostic.

Treatment

The following approach can be carried out in the office or
offered as phone advice: The patient should sit up and lean
forward so as not to swallow the blood. Swallowed blood
may cause nausea, and hematemesis alarms the family. The
nasal cavity should be cleared of clots by gentle blowing.
The soft part of the nose below the nasal bones is pinched
firmly enough to prevent arterial blood flow, with pressure
over the bleeding site being maintained for 5 minutes by
the clock. For persistent bleeding, a one time only application of oxymetazoline (Afrin) into the nasal cavity may be
helpful. If bleeding continues, the bleeding site needs to be
visualized. A small piece of gelatin sponge (Gelfoam) or
collagen sponge (Surgicel) can be inserted over the bleeding site and held in place by the parent.

Friability of the nasal vessels can be decreased with
daily application of water-based ointment by cotton-
tipped applicator. The lubricant is applied daily until 5
days have passed without a nosebleed, then weekly for 1
month. Twice-daily nasal saline irrigation and humidification of the patient's bedroom may also be helpful.
Aspirin and ibuprofen should be avoided, as should vigorous blowing of the nose.

NASAL INFECTION

A nasal furuncle is an infection of a hair follicle in the anterior nares. Hair plucking or nose picking can provide a
route of entry. The most common organism is S aureus.
The diagnosis is made by finding an exquisitely tender,
firm, red lump in the anterior nares. Treatment includes
dicloxacillin or cephalexin orally for 5 days to prevent
spread. The lesion should be gently incised and drained as
soon as it points, usually with a needle. Topical bacitracin
ointment may be of additional value. Because this lesion is
in the drainage area of the cavernous sinus, the patient
should be followed closely until healing is complete. Parents should be advised never to pick or squeeze a furuncle
in this location—and neither should the physician. Associated cellulitis or spread requires hospitalization for administration of intravenous antibiotics.

A nasal septal abscess usually follows nasal trauma or a
nasal furuncle. Examination reveals a fluctuant gray septal
swelling, usually bilateral. The possible complications are
the same as for nasal septum hematoma (see following discussion). In addition, spread of the infection to the CNS is
possible. Treatment consists of immediate hospitalization
and incision and drainage by an otolaryngologist.

NASAL TRAUMA

Newborn infants rarely present with subluxation of the
quadrangular cartilage of the septum. In this disorder,
the top of the nose deviates to one side, the inferior septal
border deviates to the other side, the columella leans, and
the nasal tip is unstable. This disorder must be distinguished from the more common transient flattening of
the nose caused by the birth process. In the past, physicians were encouraged to reduce all subluxations in the
nursery. Otolaryngologists are more likely to perform the
reduction under anesthesia for more difficult cases.

Most blows to the nose result in swallowing of blood
and hematoma formation without fracture. A persistent
nosebleed after trauma, crepitus or instability of the bones
in the nasal bridge, and marked deviation of the nose to
one side indicate fracture. However, septal injury can be
ruled out only by careful intranasal examination, not radiologically. Patients with suspected nasal fractures should be

referred to an otolaryngologist for definitive therapy. Since the nasal bones may start healing within 7 days, the child should be seen by an otolaryngologist within 48–72 hours.

After nasal trauma, it is essential to examine the inside of the nose with a nasal speculum. Hematoma of the nasal septum imposes a considerable risk of pressure necrosis and resorption of the cartilage, leading to septal perforation or a saddle-back nose in adulthood. This diagnosis is confirmed by the abrupt onset of nasal obstruction following trauma and the presence of a boggy, widened nasal septum. The normal nasal septum is only 2–4 mm thick, and the back end of a cotton swab may be helpful for palpation. Treatment consists of immediate referral to an otolaryngologist for evacuation of the hematoma and packing of the nose.

FOREIGN BODIES IN THE NOSE

The most common foreign bodies in the nose are seeds or beads. If the diagnosis is delayed, unilateral rhinorrhea, foul smell, halitosis, bleeding, or nasal obstruction may occur. The leading cause of halitosis in children is a nasal foreign body, and not dental disease as in adults.

There are many ways to remove nasal foreign bodies. The obvious first maneuver is vigorous nose blowing if the child is old enough. The next step in removal requires topical anesthesia, nasal decongestion, good lighting, correct instrumentation, and physical restraint. Topical tetracaine or lidocaine can be used in young children. Nasal decongestion can be achieved by topical pseudoephedrine or oxymetazoline. When the child is properly restrained, most nasal foreign bodies can be removed using a pair of alligator forceps through an operating head otoscope. If the object seems unlikely to be removed on the first attempt, is wedged in, or is quite large, the patient should be referred to an otolaryngologist rather than worsening the situation through futile attempts at removal.

Because the nose is a moist cavity, the electrical current generated by disk-type batteries—such as those used in clocks, watches, and hearing aids—can cause necrosis of mucosa and cartilage destruction in less than 4 hours. This constitutes a true foreign body emergency.

Kelley PE: Foreign bodies in the nose and pharynx. In: Burg FD et al (editors): *Gellis and Kagan's Current Pediatric Therapy,* 16th ed. WB Saunders, 1999.

III. THE THROAT & ORAL CAVITY

ACUTE STOMATITIS

Recurrent Aphthous Stomatitis

Also referred to as canker sores, these small ulcers (3–10 mm) are usually found on the inner aspect of the lips or on the tongue; rarely they may appear on the tonsils or palate. There is usually no associated fever and no cervical adenopathy. The ulcers may be painful and last 1–2 weeks. They may recur numerous times throughout life. The cause is unknown, although an allergic or autoimmune basis is suspected.

Treatment consists of coating the lesions with betamethasone valerate ointment twice daily, because unlike other topical steroids, it adheres to the mucosa. Pain can also be reduced by eating a bland diet, avoiding salty or acidic foods and juices, and giving acetaminophen or ibuprofen.

Other less common causes of recurrent oral ulcers include Behçet disease, familial Mediterranean fever, and the FAPA syndrome (**f**ever, **a**phthous stomatitis, **p**haryngitis, and cervical **a**denopathy). FAPA syndrome was first described in 1987, and its cause is unknown. It usually begins before a child is 5 years of age and continues through adolescence, then resolves. It recurs at 4- to 6-week intervals, and an episode may be dramatically improved with prednisone bursts, but recurrences continue. In one case report it resolved totally with a 6-month course of cimetidine, suggesting an immune etiology. FAPA may also resolve with tonsillectomy (see section on tonsillectomy), and an otolaryngology referral is appropriate. The ulcers in all of these syndromes respond to betamethasone valerate application. A diagnosis of Behçet disease requires two of the following: genital ulcers, uveitis, and erythema nodosum–like lesions. Patients with Mediterranean fever usually have a positive family history, serosal involvement, and recurrent fever.

Dahn KA, Glode MP, Chan KH: Periodic fever and pharyngitis in young children: A new disease for the otolaryngologist? Arch Otolaryngol Head Neck Surg 2000;126:1146 [PMID: 10979131].

Herpes Simplex Gingivostomatitis (See also Chapter 36.)

Children having their first infection with the herpes simplex virus develop 10 or more small ulcers (1–3 mm) of the buccal mucosa, anterior pillars, inner lips, tongue, and especially the gingiva. The lesions are often associated with fever, tender cervical nodes, and generalized inflammation of the mouth. Affected children are commonly younger than 3 years of age. Gingivostomatitis lasts 7–10 days. Treatment is symptomatic, as described earlier for recurrent aphthous stomatitis, with the exception that corticosteroids are contraindicated because they may cause spread of the infection. If seen early in the course, the physician should prescribe oral acyclovir suspension (200 mg/5 mL), 20 mg/kg/dose, four times daily for 5 days. The patient must be followed closely because dehydration occasionally develops, requiring hospitalization. Herpetic laryngotracheitis is a rare complication.

Thrush (See also Chapter 39.)

Oral candidiasis mainly affects infants and occasionally older children in a debilitated state. *Candida albicans* is a saprophyte that normally is not invasive unless the mouth is abraded or the patient is immunocompromised. The use of broad-spectrum antibiotics and systemic or inhaled steroids may be contributing factors. The symptoms include soreness of the mouth and refusal of feedings. Lesions consist of white curd-like plaques predominantly on the buccal mucosa which cannot be washed away after a feeding.

Specific treatment consists of nystatin oral suspension, 2 mL four times daily for 1 week. Treatment should begin by removing large plaques with a moistened cotton-tipped applicator and half the nystatin may be rubbed on the lesions with an applicator. Gentian violet is probably also effective, but it can severely stain clothing and skin.

Traumatic Oral Ulcers

Mechanical trauma most commonly occurs on the buccal mucosa secondary to accidentally biting with the molars. Thermal trauma, from very hot foods, can also cause ulcerative lesions. Chemical ulcers can be produced by mucosal contact with aspirin, caustics, and the like. Oral ulcers can also occur with leukemia or on a recurrent basis with cyclic neutropenia.

ACUTE VIRAL PHARYNGITIS & TONSILLITIS

Figure 17–8 is an algorithm for the management of a sore throat.

Over 90% of cases of sore throat and fever in children are due to viral infections. The findings seldom give any clue to the particular viral agent, but six types of viral pharyngitis are sufficiently distinctive to support an educated guess about the specific cause and are listed below.

Clinical Findings

A. INFECTIOUS MONONUCLEOSIS

The findings are exudative tonsillitis, generalized cervical adenitis, and fever, usually in a patient older than 5 years of age. A palpable spleen or axillary adenopathy increases the likelihood of the diagnosis. The presence of more than 10% atypical lymphocytes on a peripheral blood smear or a positive mononucleosis spot test supports the diagnosis, although these tests are often falsely negative in children younger than age 5 years. Epstein-Barr virus serology showing an elevated IgM-capsid antibody is definitive.

B. HERPANGINA

Herpangina ulcers are classically 3 mm in size and surrounded by a halo, and are found on the anterior pillars, the soft palate, and the uvula, but not the anterior mouth or tonsils. Herpangina is caused by several members of the coxsackie A group of viruses, and a patient may have several bouts of herpangina. Enteroviral polymerase chain reaction testing is now widely available, but is not necessary, since it is a self-limiting illness.

C. HAND, FOOT, AND MOUTH DISEASE

This entity is caused by several entreoviruses, only one of which (enterovirus 71) can rarely cause encephalitis. Ulcers occur anywhere in the mouth. Vesicles, pustules, or papules may be found on the palms, soles, interdigital areas, and buttocks. In younger children lesions may be seen on the distal extremities and even the face.

D. PHARYNGOCONJUNCTIVAL FEVER

This disorder is caused by an adenovirus and often is epidemic. Exudative tonsillitis, conjunctivitis, lymphadenopathy, and fever are the main findings, and treatment is symptomatic.

ACUTE BACTERIAL PHARYNGITIS

Approximately 10% of children with sore throat and fever have a group A streptococcal infection (GAS). Less common causes of bacterial pharyngitis are *Mycoplasma pneumoniae*, *Chlamydia pneumoniae*, groups C and G streptococci, and *Arcanobacterium hemolyticum*. Of the five, *M pneumoniae* is by far the most common and may cause over one-third of all pharyngitis cases in adolescents and adults.

Untreated streptococcal pharyngitis can result in acute rheumatic fever, glomerulonephritis, and suppurative complications (eg, cervical adenitis, peritonsillar abscess, otitis media, cellulitis, and septicemia). Anterior cervical nodes, palatal petechiae, a beefy-red uvula, and a tonsillar exudate suggest streptococcal infection; however, the only way to make a definitive diagnosis is by throat culture or rapid antigen test. Rapid antigen tests are very specific, but have a sensitivity of only 85–95%. Therefore, a positive test indicates *S pyogenes* infection, but a negative result requires confirmation by performing a culture.

The physician should treat cases of suspected or proven group A streptococcal infection with a 10-day course of oral penicillin V potassium, a cephalosporin, or intramuscularly injected penicillin G benzathine LA (Table 17–6). Penicillin VK is equally effective if given in two or three divided doses in school-aged children. However, in adolescents, three doses are recommended. Amoxicillin and azithromycin may be used once daily if compliance is a concern; however, both are broad-spectrum drugs that select for resistant nasopharyngeal flora. The American Heart Association guidelines continue to recommend penicillin, with erythromycin for

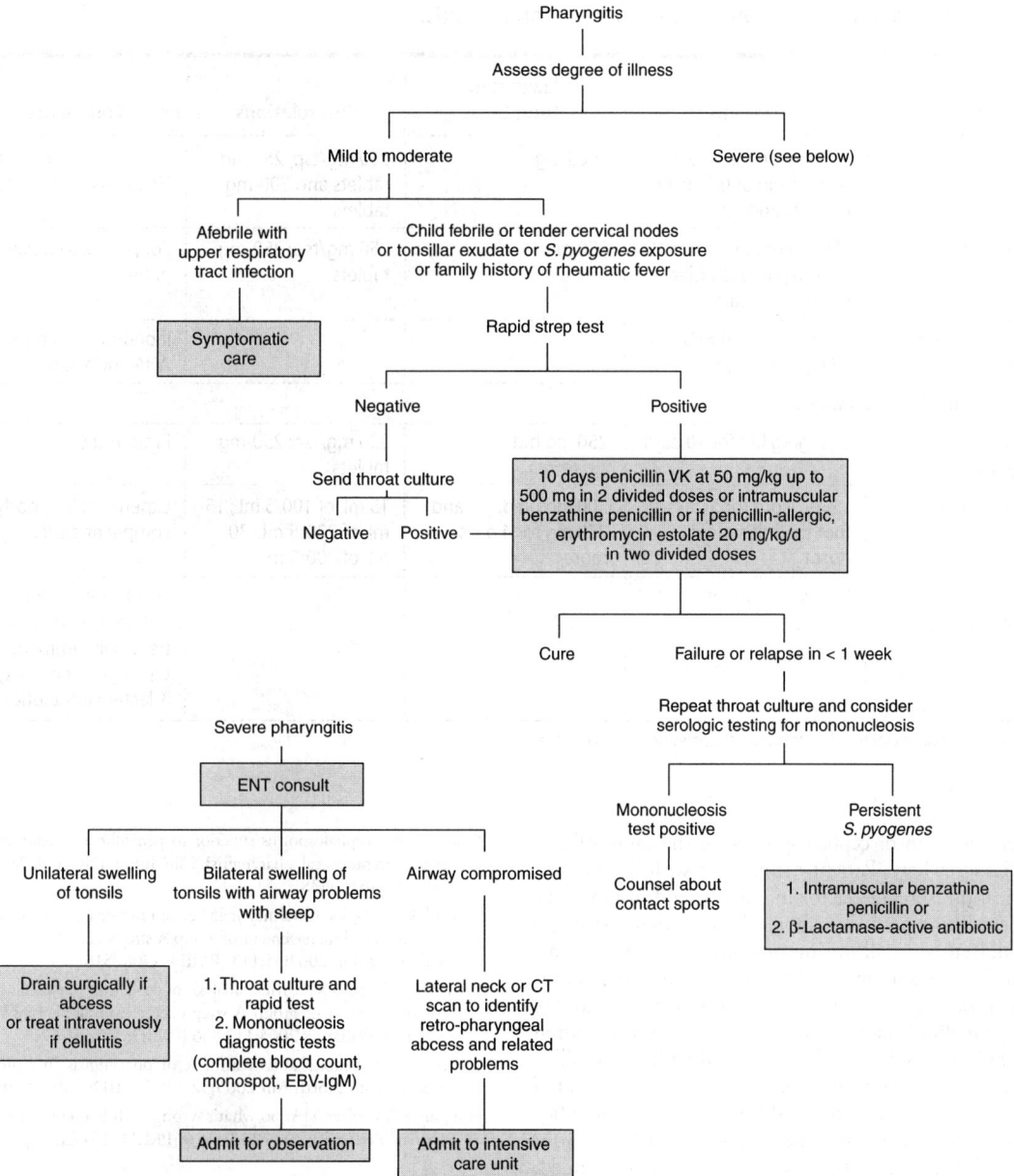

Figure 17–8. Algorithm for pharyngitis. CT, computed tomography; ENT, ear, nose, and throat; EBV, Epstein-Barr virus.

penicillin-allergic patients. A recent meta-analysis of trials of oral cephalosporins for streptococcal pharyngitis has concluded that penicillin should no longer be used. Just as in the case of otitis media meta-analyses, the quality of the trials included biases the results. In this case, inclusion of children who are carriers may bias certain of these trials. For further analysis of this controversy, the 2005 review by Gerber is highly recommended. The treatment failure rate after 10 days of penicillin VK administered three times daily varies from 6–23%. However, over 50 years of treatment with penicillin, no GAS species have developed resistance to

Table 17–6. Treatment of group A streptococcal pharyngitis.

Drug	Dosage	Maximum Adult Dose	Formulations	Comments
Penicillin VK	250 mg bid for 10 days, 500 mg bid or tid for adolescents and adults	1000 mg	250 mg/tsp; 250 mg tablets and 500-mg tablets	Preferred by American Heart Association (AHA)
Amoxicillin[a]	750 mg once daily for 10 days in patients older than age 3 years	750 mg	250 mg/tsp; 250-mg tablets	For poorly compliant patients
IM benzathine penicillin	If < 27 kg, 600,000 U; if > 27 kg, 1.2 million U			If preferred by parent; AHA endorsed
For penicillin-allergic patients				
Erythromycin estolate (250/5)	20 mg/kg bid for 10 days	250 mg bid	250 mg/tsp; 250-mg tablets	Preferred by AHA
Azithromycin	12 mg/kg/d for 5 days (not the otitis media dose)	500 mg on day 1 and 250 mg for 4 days more	15 mL of 100/5 mL; 15 mL of 200/5 mL; 30 mL of 200/5 mL	Expensive; for poorly compliant patients
First-generation cephalosporins	Varies with agent			These agents should not be used to treat patients with immediate-type hypersensitivity to β-lactam antibiotics

[a]Preferred by some doctors for younger children because of taste.

either penicillin or cephalosporins, so the cause of failure lies elsewhere. Patient compliance with 20 doses of medication is a large factor in failures, and intramuscular benzathine penicillin should be considered strongly in children who fail during or immediately after treatment. It has been suggested that the presence of β-lactamase–producing organisms in the pharynx may inactivate penicillin, but this has not been proven. Children who fail treatment may also be treated with amoxicillin-clavulanate or azithromycin. Approximately 5% of *S pyogenes* are resistant to erythromycin, and trimethoprim-sulfamethoxazole is ineffective against GAS. Routine culturing after treatment is not recommended, since children may be carriers.

In general, the carrier state is harmless, self-limited (2–6 months), and not contagious. An attempt to eradicate the carrier state is warranted only if the patient or another family member has frequent streptococcal infections or when a family member or patient has a history of rheumatic fever or glomerulonephritis. If eradication is chosen, a course of clindamycin for 10 days or of rifampin for 5 days should be used.

In the past, daily penicillin prophylaxis was occasionally recommended; however, to prevent development of drug resistance, tonsillectomy is now preferred.

Bisno AL: Are cephalosporins superior to penicillin for treatment of acute streptococcal pharyngitis? Clin Infect Dis 2004;38:1535 [PMID: 15156438].

Bisno Al, Gerber MA, Gwaltney Jr JM et al: Practice guidelines for the diagnosis and management of group A streptococcal pharyngitis. Clin Infect Dis 2002;35:113 [PMID: 12087516].

Casey JR, Pichichero ME: Meta-analysis of cephalosporin versus penicillin treatment of group A streptococcal tonsillopharyngitis in children. Pediatrics 2004;113:866 [PMID: 15156437].

Gerber MA: Diagnosis and treatment of pharyngitis in children. Pediatr Clin North Am 2005;52:729 [PMID: 15925660].

Shulman ST, Gerber MA: So what's wrong with penicillin for strep throat? Pediatrics 2004;113:1816 [PMID: 15173515].

PERITONSILLAR CELLULITIS OR ABSCESS (Quinsy)

Tonsillar infection occasionally penetrates the tonsillar capsule, spreads to the surrounding tissues, and causes peritonsillar cellulitis. If untreated, necrosis occurs and a tonsillar abscess forms. This can occur at any age. The most common cause is β-hemolytic streptococcal infection. Other pathogens are group D streptococci, β-hemolytic streptococci, *S pneumoniae,* and anaerobes.

The patient complains of a severe sore throat even before the physical findings become marked. A high fever is usually present, and the process is almost always unilateral. The tonsil bulges medially, and the anterior tonsillar pillar is prominent. The soft palate and uvula on the involved side are edematous and displaced toward the uninvolved side. In cases of abscess formation, trismus, ear pain, dysphagia, and eventually drooling occur. The most serious complication of inadequately treated peritonsillar abscess is a lateral pharyngeal abscess. This causes fullness and tenderness of the lateral neck as well as torticollis. Without intervention, the lateral pharyngeal abscess threatens life by airway obstruction or carotid artery erosion. If airway symptoms are present, an immediate otolaryngology consultation is indicated.

It is often difficult to differentiate peritonsillar cellulitis from abscess. In some children, it is possible to aspirate the peritonsillar space to diagnose and treat an abscess. However, it is reasonable to admit a child for 12–24 hours of intravenous antimicrobial therapy, because aggressive treatment in early cases of peritonsillar cellulitis usually prevents suppuration. Therapy with penicillin or clindamycin is appropriate. Failure to respond to therapy during the first 12–24 hours indicates a high probability of abscess formation. An otolaryngologist should be consulted for incision and drainage or for aspiration under local or general anesthesia.

Recurrent peritonsillar abscesses are so uncommon (7%) that routine tonsillectomy for a single bout is not indicated unless other tonsillectomy indications exist. Hospitalized patients can be discharged on oral antibiotics when fever has resolved for 24 hours and dysphagia has improved.

Schraff S, McGinn JD, Derkay CS: Peritonsillar abscess in children: a 10-year review of diagnosis and management. Int J Pediatr Otorhinolaryngol 2001;57:213 [PMID: 11223453].

RETROPHARYNGEAL ABSCESS

Retropharyngeal nodes drain the adenoids, nasopharynx, and paranasal sinuses and can become infected. The most common causes are β-hemolytic streptococci and *S aureus*. If this pyogenic adenitis goes untreated, a retropharyngeal abscess forms. The process occurs most commonly during the first 2 years of life. Beyond this age, retropharyngeal abscess usually results from superinfection of a penetrating injury of the posterior wall of the oropharynx.

The diagnosis of retropharyngeal abscess should be strongly suspected in an infant with fever, respiratory symptoms, and neck hyperextension. Dysphagia, drooling, dyspnea, and gurgling respirations are also found and are due to impingement by the abscess. Prominent swelling on one side of the posterior pharyngeal wall confirms the diagnosis. Swelling usually stops at the midline because a medial raphe divides the prevertebral space. Lateral neck soft tissue films show the retropharyngeal space to be wider than the C4 vertebral body.

Although retropharyngeal abscess is a surgical emergency, frequently it cannot be distinguished from retropharyngeal adenitis. Immediate hospitalization and intravenous antimicrobial therapy with a semisynthetic penicillin or clindamycin is the first step for most cases. Immediate surgical drainage is required when a definite abscess is seen radiographically or when the airway is compromised markedly. In most instances, a period of 12–24 hours of antimicrobial therapy will help to differentiate the two entities. In the child with adenitis, fever will decrease and oral intake will increase. A child with retropharyngeal abscess will continue to deteriorate. A surgeon should incise and drain the abscess under general anesthesia to prevent its extension.

LUDWIG ANGINA

Ludwig angina is a rapidly progressive cellulitis of the submandibular space that can cause airway obstruction and death. The submandibular space extends from the mucous membrane of the floor of the mouth to the muscular and fascial attachments of the hyoid bone. This infection is encountered infrequently in infants and children. The initiating factor in over 50% of cases is dental disease, including abscesses and extraction. Some patients have a history of lacerations and injuries to the floor of the mouth. Group A streptococci are the most common organism identified, but other pathogens cause the infection.

The manifestations are fever and tender swelling of the floor of the mouth. The tongue can become enlarged as well as tender and erythematous. Upward displacement of the tongue may cause dysphagia, drooling, and airway obstruction.

Treatment consists of giving high doses of intravenous clindamycin or ampicillin plus nafcillin until the results of cultures and sensitivity tests are available. Because the most common cause of death in Ludwig angina is sudden airway obstruction, the patient must be monitored closely in the intensive care unit and intubation provided for progressive respiratory distress. An otolaryngologist should be consulted to identify and perform a drainage procedure.

Britt JC et al: Ludwig's angina in the pediatric population: Report of a case and review of the literature. Int J Pediatr Otorhinolaryngol 2000;52:79.

ACUTE CERVICAL ADENITIS

Local infections of the ear, nose, and throat can infect a regional node and form an abscess. The typical case involves a unilateral, solitary, anterior cervical node. About 70% of these cases are due to β-hemolytic streptococcal infection, 20% to staphylococci, and the remainder to viruses, atypical mycobacteria, and *Bartonella henselae*. For the past several years methicillin-resistant *Staphylococcus aureus* must also be considered.

The initial evaluation of cervical adenitis should generally include a rapid GAS test, a complete blood count with differential looking for atypical lymphocytes, and a purified protein derivative skin test, looking for nontuberculous mycobacteria. If multiple enlarged nodes are found in addition to the sentinel node, a rapid mononucleosis test is useful. Early treatment with antibiotics prevents many cases of adenitis from progressing to suppuration. However, once fluctuation occurs, antibiotic therapy alone is often insufficient and needle aspiration may promote resolution.

Cat-scratch disease is caused by *Bartonella henselae* and is the most frequently cause of indolent ("cold") adenopathy. The diagnosis is aided by the finding of a primary papule at the scratch site on the face. In over 90% of patients, there is a history of contact with kittens. The node is usually only mildly tender, but may over a month or more suppurate and drain. About one-third of children have fever and malaise, and rarely neurologic sequelae and prolonged fever occur. Cat-scratch disease can be diagnosed by serologic testing available at commercial laboratories, but testing is not always confirmatory. Blood should be drawn 2–8 weeks after onset of symptoms. Because most nodes caused by this pathogen spontaneously resorb within 1–3 months, the benefit of antibiotics is controversial. In a placebo-controlled trial, azithromycin for 5 days caused a more rapid decrease in node size. Other drugs likely to be effective include rifampin, trimethoprim-sulfamethoxazole, erythromycin, clarithromycin, doxycycline, ciprofloxacin, and gentamicin.

Cervical lymphadenitis can be caused by nontuberculous mycobacterial species or *Mycobacterium avium* complex. Mycobacterial disease is unilateral and may involve several matted nodes, and poor dentition may provide an entry portal. A characteristic violaceous appearance may develop over a prolonged period of time without systemic signs or much local pain. Atypical mycobacterial infections are often associated with positive purified protein derivative skin test reactions less than 10 mm in diameter, and a second-strength (250-test-unit) purified protein derivative skin test is virtually always positive.

A chest radiograph should be done to rule out mediastinal adenopathy. Nodes may recur, usually within 3 months of surgery. In such cases, a newer macrolide in combination with a second drug (rifampin or ethambutol) is given for 3–6 months.

Differential Diagnosis

A. Neoplasms and Cervical Nodes

Malignant tumors usually are not suspected until the adenopathy persists despite antibiotic treatment. Classically,

the nodes are painless, nontender, and firm to hard in consistency. They may be fixed to underlying tissues. These nodes may occur as a single node, as unilateral nodes in a chain, bilateral cervical nodes, or generalized adenopathy. Common malignancies that may present in the neck include Hodgkin disease, non-Hodgkin lymphoma, rhabdomyosarcoma, and thyroid carcinoma.

B. Imitators of Adenitis

Several structures in the neck can become infected and resemble a node. The first three masses are of congenital origin and are listed in order of frequency.

1. Thyroglossal duct cyst—When superinfected, this congenital malformation can become acutely swollen. Helpful findings are the fact that it is in the midline, located between the hyoid bone and suprasternal notch, and moves upward when the tongue is stuck out or during swallowing. Occasionally, the cyst develops a sinus tract and opening just lateral to the midline.

2. Branchial cleft cyst—When superinfected, this malformation can become a tender mass 3–5 cm in diameter. Aids to diagnosis are the fact that the mass is located along the anterior border of the sternocleidomastoid muscle and is smooth and fluctuant. Occasionally it is attached to the overlying skin by a small dimple or a draining sinus tract.

3. Lymphatic malformation (cystic hygroma)—Most of these lymphatic cysts are located in the posterior triangle just above the clavicle. The mass is soft and compressible and can be transilluminated. Over 60% of hygromas are noted at birth, and the remainder are usually seen by the time the child is age 2 years. If cysts become large enough, they can compromise the patient's ability to swallow and breathe.

4. Parotitis—The most common pitfall is mistaking parotitis for cervical adenitis. However, a swollen parotid crosses the angle of the jaw, is associated with preauricular percussion tenderness, and is bilateral in 70% of cases. There may be a history of exposure to mumps, but in the U.S. viruses such as parainfluenza are now the main cause. An amylase level will be elevated in parotitis.

5. Ranula—A ranula is a cyst in the floor of the mouth caused by obstruction of the ducts of the sublingual gland. A plunging ranula extends below the mylohyoid muscle and can appear as a neck mass.

6. Sternocleidomastoid muscle hematoma—This cervical mass is noted at age 2–4 weeks. On close examination, it is found to be part of the muscle body and not movable. An associated torticollis usually confirms the diagnosis.

Fennelly GJ: *Mycobacterium bovis* versus *Mycobacterium tuberculosis* as a cause of acute cervical lymphadenitis without pulmonary disease. Pediatr Infect Dis J 2004;23:590 [PMID: 15194851].

Peters TR, Edwards KM: Cervical lymphadenopathy and adenitis. Pediatr Rev 2000;21:399 [PMID: 11121496].

SNORING, MOUTH BREATHING, & UPPER AIRWAY OBSTRUCTION

In April 2002, the American Academy of Pediatrics published a clinical practice guideline for the diagnosis and management of uncomplicated childhood obstructive sleep apnea syndrome. The guideline emphasizes that pediatricians should screen all children for snoring and that complex high-risk patients should be referred to a specialist.

When parents report that their child has nightly snoring and is a mouth breather even during the day, one should be suspicious of obstructive sleep apnea (OSA). Figure 17–9 is an algorithm for management of these complaints. The pathway relies on clinical symptoms and tonsil size. Low muscle tone also contributes to one's propensity to experience sleep-disordered breathing (SDB). However, measurement of muscle tone is not straightforward. Although the pathway states an asymptomatic child with markedly enlarged tonsils (4+) should undergo an overnight polysomnographic study, a period of observation is reasonable. One's clinical suspicion of SDB should be heightened in the presence of enlarged tonsils, especially if the parents cannot provide a reliable history. If the child has no clinical symptoms and the tonsils are only moder-

ately enlarged (3+), observation is appropriate. Educating the parents of the risks of SDB and what to look for is paramount. A polysomnographic study is recommended for a child who has no adenotonsillar hypertrophy with a patent nose but significant daytime symptoms of SDB. Other conditions, especially a periodic limb movement disorder, may mimic SDB. If the polysomnogram does detect SDB in a child with no adenotonsillar hypertrophy, a complete evaluation of the upper airway by flexible laryngoscopy should be performed to look for other possible sites of obstruction: base of tongue, lingual tonsils, hypopharynx or larynx. The adenoids can also be assessed by radiographic studies. Either adenoid hypertrophy or nasal obstruction can be assumed when a child has hyponasal speech. The consonants "m," "n," and "ng" rely on the palate not touching the posterior pharyngeal wall. By having a child repeat the word "banana" or "ninety-nine" with the nose open or pinched closed, one may assess the nasal and nasopharyngeal airways. If the voice does not change with occlusion of the nostrils, then either adenoid or nasal obstruction is present.

Although nasal obstruction is usually due to allergic rhinitis and can be diagnosed by a careful allergy history, there are other less common causes. Nasal polyps appear as glistening, gray to pink, jellylike masses that are prominent just inside the anterior nares and occur singly or in clusters. They occur in cystic fibrosis and severe allergic rhinitis. Persistent mouth breathing may

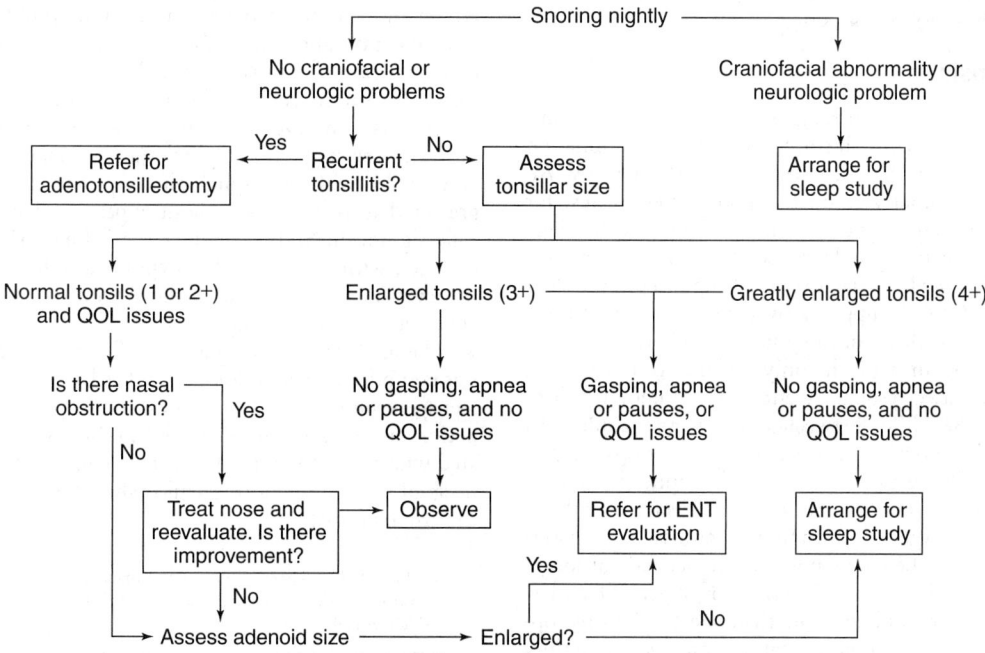

Figure 17–9. Algorithm for snoring. ENT, ear, nose and throat; QOL, quality of life.

Tonsil Grade

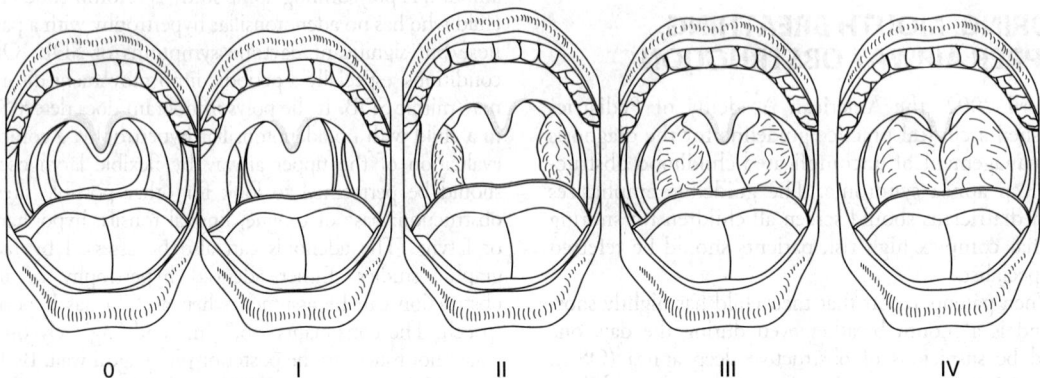

0   I   II   III   IV

Figure 17–10. A grading scale for tonsil size that ranges from 0 to IV. With grade 0 the tonsils are small and contained within the tonsillar fossa; in grade IV the tonsils are so large they almost touch ("kissing"). (Reprinted, with permission, from Brodksy L: Modern assessment of tonsils and adenoids. Pediatr Clin North Am 1989;36:1551 [PMID: 2685730].)

also rarely be due to a nasopharyngeal tumor, or to a meningocele herniated into the nasal cavity. For male patients, if unilateral nasal obstruction and epistaxis occur frequently, juvenile angiofibroma should be suspected. If allergic rhinitis is the suspected cause of snoring, a trial of intranasal corticosteroid spray is indicated. If enlarged tonsils (Figure 17–10) or adenoids are present, a referral to an otolaryngologist or a pediatric sleep laboratory is in order.

Diagnosis

The gold standard for diagnosis of OSA is a polysomnogram. A patient's history and clinical examination cannot predict the presence or severity of OSA. An overnight oximetry study is a poor screening test for OSA. The test may detect those patients with severe disease but miss the milder cases. OSA is part of a spectrum of disorders that occur during sleep. A milder form of OSA is upper airway resistance syndrome. Patients with this syndrome have an otherwise normal polysomnogram with the only evidence of obstruction being increased respiratory effort. The criteria for diagnosing OSA differ between children and adults. An obstructive event occurs when airflow stops despite persistence of respiratory effort. A hypopnea is counted when airflow and respiratory effort decrease with an associated oxygen desaturation or arousal. Normative values are just being established. The second edition of the International Classification of Sleep Disorders states that for children, more than one apnea or hypopnea an hour with duration of at least two respiratory cycles is abnormal. However, the committee qualified

its recommendation, stating that the criteria may be modified once more comprehensive data become available. An investigation of sleep-disordered breathing in children between the ages of 6 and 11 years is the first study to evaluate clinical relevance using full polysomnograms. The study demonstrated that a respiratory disturbance index of at least one event an hour when associated with a 3% oxygen desaturation was associated with daytime sleepiness and learning problems. If oxygen desaturations were absent, an respiratory disturbance index of five was associated with clinical symptoms. In summary, an obstructive apnea index of greater than one event may be statistically significant, but whether it is clinically relevant remains unclear. Any child with an apnea-plus-hypopnea index of greater than five events an hour appears to have clinically significant SDB. The dilemma is how to manage children with an apnea-plus-hypopnea index > 1 but < 5 events an hour. Some of these children do experience neurocognitive symptoms.

The importance of diagnosing OSA in children cannot be underestimated. Recent studies have shown that teenagers who are loud snorers exhibit impaired school performance, and that behavioral problems are associated with OSA. One should strongly consider the diagnosis of OSA in a snoring child who otherwise meets the criteria for ADHD.

Clinical Practice Guideline: Diagnosis and management of childhood obstructive sleep apnea syndrome. Pediatrics 2002;109:704 [PMID: 11927718].

Goodwin JL et al: Clinical outcomes associated with sleep-disordered breathing in Caucasian and Hispanic children—the

Tucson Children's Assessment of Sleep Apnea study (Tu-CASA). Sleep 2003;26:587 [PMID: 12853523].

Montgomery-Downs HE, et al: Snoring and sleep-disordered breathing in young children: subjective and objective correlates. Sleep 2004;27:87 [PMID: 14998242].

O'Brien LM et al: Neurobehavioral implications of habitual snoring in children. Pediatrics 2004;114:44 [PMID: 15231906].

Schechter MS: Technical report: Diagnosis and management of childhood obstructive sleep apnea syndrome. Pediatrics 2002;109:e69 [PMID: 11927742].

Websites

National Sleep Foundation: http://www.sleepfoundation.org/

Child friendly website: http://www.sleepforkids.org/

Children's Hospital website: http://www.thechildrenshospital.org/public/cs/detail.cfm?RecordID=407

TONSILLECTOMY & ADENOIDECTOMY

Tonsillectomy

A tonsillectomy with or without adenoidectomy is typically performed for either hypertrophy or recurrent infections. Nowadays, the most common indication for an adenotonsillectomy is adenotonsillar hypertrophy that is associated with an obstructed breathing pattern at night. OSA is associated with loud snoring during sleep with periods of respiratory pauses terminated with gasping and agitated arousal. The American Academy of Pediatrics technical report on OSA (http://www.pediatrics.org/cgi/content/full/109/4/e69) suggests that primary snoring may also have developmental consequences. Other symptoms of OSA include ADHD, failure to thrive, and nocturnal enuresis. Besides producing airway obstruction, adenotonsillar hypertrophy may produce dysphagia or dental malocclusion. Rarely, the size may produce pulmonary hypertension or cor pulmonale. Recurrent infections are present when a child has seven or more documented *S pyogenes* infections in 1 year, five per year for 2 years, or three per year for 3 years. A tonsillectomy is reasonable if fewer infections are present but the child has missed multiple school days or has a complicated course. Recurrent peritonsillar abscesses and persistent streptococcal carrier state are other indications, as well as unilateral tonsil hypertrophy that appears neoplastic.

A possible new indication is FAPA syndrome (see previous discussion), in which the fever is predictable and commonly occurs every 4–8 weeks. Removal of the tonsils was shown to relieve the symptoms in five children in one recent study.

Recently, a proliferation of new surgical techniques has occurred that can potentially reduce the morbidity associated with an adenotonsillectomy.

Dahn KA et al: Periodic fever and pharyngitis in young children. Arch Otolaryngol Head Neck Surg 2000;126:1146 [PMID: 10979131].

Darrow DH, Siemens C: Indications for tonsillectomy and adenoidectomy. Laryngoscope 2002;112(8 Pt 2 Suppl 100):6.

Derkay CS, Maddern BR: Innovative techniques for adenotonsillar surgery in children Laryngoscope 2002;112(8 Pt 2):2 [PMID: 12172227].

Gigante J: Tonsillectomy and adenoidectomy. Pediatr Rev 2005; 26:199 [PMID: 15930327].

Website

Website dedicated to children and sponsored by the American Academy of Otolaryngology/Head and Neck Surgery: http://www.entnet.org/kidsent/

Adenoidectomy

The adenoids, composed of lymphoid tissue in the nasopharynx, are a component of the Waldeyer ring of lymphoid tissue with the palatine tonsils and lingual tonsils. Enlargement of the adenoids with or without infection can obstruct the upper airway, alter normal orofacial growth, and interfere with speech, swallowing, or eustachian tube function. Most children with prolonged mouth breathing eventually develop dental malocclusion and what has been termed an adenoidal facies. The face is pinched and the maxilla narrowed because the molding pressures of the orbicularis oris and buccinator muscles are unopposed by the tongue. The role of hypertrophy and chronic infection in the pathogenesis of sinusitis is unclear, but adenoidectomy has been shown to be effective in some patients with chronic rhinosinusitis.

Indications for adenoidectomy with or without tonsillectomy include pulmonary conditions such as chronic hypoxia related to upper airway obstruction; orofacial conditions such as mandibular growth abnormalities, dental malocclusion, and swallowing disorders; speech abnormalities; persistent middle ear effusion; recurrent and chronic otitis media; and chronic sinusitis.

Complications of Tonsillectomy & Adenoidectomy

The reported mortality rates associated with tonsillectomy and adenoidectomy now approximate that of general anesthesia alone. The rate of hemorrhage varies between 0.1% and 8.1% depending on the definition of hemorrhage; the rate of postoperative transfusion is 0.04%. Other complications include hypernasal speech (< 0.01%), and more rarely nasopharyngeal stenosis, atlantoaxial subluxation, mandible condyle fracture, and psychological trauma.

Contraindications to Tonsillectomy & Adenoidectomy

A. SHORT PALATE

Adenoids should not be removed completely in a child with a cleft palate or submucous cleft palate because of the risk of aggravating the velopharyngeal incompetence and causing hypernasal speech and nasal regurgitation. A superior or partial adenoidectomy can be performed in a child with marked obstructive sleep apnea who has a submucous cleft palate or ongoing conductive hearing loss from middle ear effusion.

B. BLEEDING DISORDER

If a chronic bleeding disorder is present, it must be diagnosed and treated before tonsillectomy and adenoidectomy.

C. ACUTE TONSILLITIS

An elective tonsillectomy and adenoidectomy can often be postponed until acute tonsillitis is resolved. Urgent tonsillectomy may be required for tonsillitis unresponsive to medical therapy.

DISORDERS OF THE LIPS

Labial Sucking Tubercle

A young baby may present with a small callus in the mid-upper lip. It usually is asymptomatic and disappears after cup feeding is initiated.

Cheilitis

Dry, cracked, scaling lips are usually caused by sun or wind exposure. Contact dermatitis from mouthpieces or various woodwind or brass instruments has also been reported. Licking the lips accentuates the process, and the patient should be warned of this. Liberal use of lip balms gives excellent results.

Inclusion Cyst

Inclusion (retention) cysts are due to the obstruction of mucous glands or other mucous membrane structures. In the newborn, they occur on the hard palate or gums and are called Epstein pearls. These small cysts resolve spontaneously in 1–2 months. In older children, inclusion cysts usually occur on the palate, uvula, or tonsillar pillars. They appear as taut yellow sacs varying in size from 2–10 mm. Inclusion cysts that do not resolve spontaneously may undergo incision and drainage. Occasionally a mucous cyst on the lower lip (mucocele) requires excision for cosmetic reasons. Mucoceles pathologically are a blocked minor salivary gland.

DISORDERS OF THE TONGUE

Geographic Tongue (Benign Migratory Glossitis)

This condition of unknown cause occurs in 1–2% of the population with no age, sex, or racial predilection and is characterized by irregularly shaped areas on the tongue that are devoid of papillae and surrounded by parakeratotic reddish borders. The pattern changes as alternating regeneration and desquamation occurs. The lesions are generally asymptomatic and require no treatment.

Fissured Tongue (Scrotal Tongue)

This condition is marked by numerous irregular fissures on the dorsum of the tongue. It occurs in approximately 1% of the population and is usually a dominant trait. It is also frequently seen in children with trisomy 21 and other developmentally delayed patients who have the habit of chewing on a protruded tongue.

Coated Tongue (Furry Tongue)

The tongue normally becomes coated if mastication is impaired and the patient is taking a liquid or soft diet. Mouth breathing, fever, or dehydration can accentuate the process.

Macroglossia

Tongue hypertrophy and protrusion may be a clue to trisomy 21, Beckwith-Wiedemann syndrome, glycogen storage disease, cretinism, mucopolysaccharide storage disease, lymphangioma, or hemangioma. Tongue reduction procedures should be considered in otherwise healthy subjects when macroglossia affects airway patency.

HALITOSIS

Bad breath is usually due to acute stomatitis, pharyngitis, sinusitis, a nasal foreign body, or dental hygiene problems. In older children and adolescents, halitosis can be a manifestation of chronic sinusitis, gastric bezoar, bronchiectasis, or lung abscess. The presence of orthodontic devices or dentures can cause halitosis if good dental hygiene is not maintained. Halitosis can also be caused by decaying food particles embedded in cryptic tonsils. In adolescents, tobacco use is a common cause. Mouthwashes and chewable breath fresheners give limited improvement. Treatment of the underlying cause is indicated, and a dental referral may be in order.

Cicek Y et al: Effect of tongue brushing on oral malodor in adolescents. Pediatr Int 2003;45:719 [PMID: 14651548].

SALIVARY GLAND DISORDERS

Parotitis

A first episode of parotitis may safely be considered to be of viral origin, unless fluctuance is present. The leading cause was mumps until adoption of vaccination; now the leading viruses are parainfluenza and Epstein-

Barr virus. Human immunodeficiency virus should be considered if the child is known to be at risk.

Suppurative Parotitis

Suppurative parotitis is an uncommon clinical disorder occurring chiefly in newborns and debilitated elderly patients. The parotid gland is swollen, tender, and often reddened and is usually a unilateral process. The diagnosis is made by expression of purulent material from the Stensen duct. The material should be smeared and cultured. Fever and leukocytosis may be present.

Treatment includes hospitalization and intravenous nafcillin because the most common causative organism is *S aureus.*

Recurrent Idiopathic Parotitis

Some children experience repeated episodes of parotid swelling that last 1–2 weeks and then resolve spontaneously, or can become infected and require antibiotics for resolution. There is usually pain and often no fever. The process is most often unilateral, suggesting some sort of obstructive process, but can be associated with Sjögren syndrome, another autoimmune process, human immunodeficiency virus infection, or a calculus in the parotid duct. Serum amylase levels are normal, which speaks against a diagnosis of viral parotitis. Recently increased IgA levels have been found in these children. Many episodes occur from age 2 years on. The problem often resolves spontaneously at puberty.

Treatment includes analgesics if pain is present and an antistaphylococcal antibiotic for prophylaxis of infection and quicker resolution at the onset of symptoms. A second attack of parotid swelling without fever should result in referral to an otolaryngologist to make the diagnosis.

Fazekas T: Selective IgA deficiency in children with recurrent parotitis of childhood. Pediatr Infect Dis J 2005;24:461 [PMID: 15876950].

Tumors of the Parotid Gland

Mixed tumors, hemangiomas, sarcoidosis, and leukemia can be manifested in the parotid gland as a hard or persistent mass. A cystic mass or multiple cystic masses may represent an HIV infection. Work-up may require consultation with oncology, infectious diseases, hematology, and otolaryngology.

Ranula

A ranula is a retention cyst of a sublingual salivary gland. It occurs on the floor of the mouth to one side of the lingual frenulum. Ranula has been described as resembling a frog's belly because it is thin-walled and contains a clear bluish fluid. Referral to an otolaryngologist for excision of the cyst and associated sublingual gland is the treatment of choice.

CONGENITAL ORAL MALFORMATIONS

Tongue-Tie (Ankyloglossia)

The tightness of the lingual frenulum varies greatly among normal people. A short frenulum prevents both protrusion and elevation of the tongue. Puckering of the midline of the tongue occurring with tongue movement is noted on physical examination.

When mild, treatment consists of reassurance. If the tongue cannot protrude past the teeth or alveolar ridge or move between the gums and cheek, referral to an otolaryngologist or dentist for evaluation is indicated. Frenulectomy may be recommended if there is a question of suckling difficulties, dental health (related to the inability to clear food from around the teeth), or articulation problems.

Messner AH, Lalakea ML: Ankyloglossia: Controversies in management. Int J Pediatr Otorhinolaryngol 2000;54:123 [PMID: 10967382].

Messner AH, Lalakea ML: The effect of ankyloglossia on speech in children. Otolaryngol Head Neck Surg 2002;127:539 [PMID: 12501105].

Torus Palatini

Hard midline masses on the palate are called torus palatini. They are bony protrusions that form at suture lines of bone. Usually they are asymptomatic and require no therapy. They can be surgically reduced if necessary.

Cleft Lip & Cleft Palate (See Chapter 33.)

A. SUBMUCOUS CLEFT PALATE

A bifid uvula is present in 3% of healthy children. However, a close association exists (as high as 75%) between bifid uvula and submucous cleft palate. A submucous cleft can be diagnosed by noting a translucent zone in the middle of the soft palate (zona pellucida). Palpation of the hard palate reveals absence of the posterior bony protrusion. Affected children have a 40% risk of developing persistent middle ear effusion. They are at risk also of incomplete closure of the palate, resulting in hypernasal speech. During feeding, some of these infants experience nasal regurgitation of food. Children with submucous cleft palate causing abnormal speech or nasal regurgitation of food require referral for surgical repair.

B. HIGH-ARCHED PALATE

A high-arched palate is usually a genetic trait of no consequence. It also occurs in children who are chronic mouth breathers and in premature infants who undergo prolonged oral intubation. Some rare causes of high-arched palate are congenital disorders such as Marfan syndrome, Treacher Collins syndrome, and Ehlers-Danlos syndrome.

C. PIERRE ROBIN SEQUENCE

This group of congenital malformations is characterized by the triad of micrognathia, cleft palate, and glossoptosis. Affected children present as emergencies in the newborn period because of infringement on the airway by the tongue. The main objective of treatment is to prevent asphyxia until the mandible becomes large enough to accommodate the tongue. In some cases, this objective can be achieved by leaving the child in a prone position while unattended. Other airway manipulations such as a nasal trumpet may be necessary. Recently distraction osteogenesis has been used to avoid tracheostomy. In severe cases, a tracheostomy is required. The child requires close observation and careful feeding until the problem is outgrown.

Denny A, Amm C: New technique for airway correction in neonates with severe Pierre Robin sequence. J Pediatr 2005; 147:97 [PMID: 16027704].

Respiratory Tract & Mediastinum 18

Gwendolyn S. Kerby, MD, Frank J. Accurso, MD, Robin R. Deterding, MD, Vivek Balasubramaniam, MD, Scott D. Sagel, MD, & Keith L. Cavanaugh, MD

■ RESPIRATORY TRACT

Pediatric pulmonary diseases account for almost 50% of deaths in children younger than age 1 year and about 20% of all hospitalizations of children younger than age 15 years. Approximately 7% of children have some sort of chronic disorder of the lower respiratory system. Understanding the pathophysiology of many pediatric pulmonary diseases requires an appreciation of the normal growth and development of the lung.

GROWTH & DEVELOPMENT

The lung has its origins from an outpouching of the foregut during the fourth week of gestation. The development of the lung is divided into five overlapping stages. The first stage is the embryonic stage (3–7 weeks gestation) during which the primitive lung bud undergoes asymmetrical branching and then subsequent dichotomous branching, leading to the development of the conducting airways. This stage of lung development is dependent on a complex interaction of various growth factors originating in both the pulmonary epithelium and the splanchnic mesenchyme. This stage also sees the development of the large pulmonary arteries from the sixth aortic arch and the pulmonary veins as outgrowths of the left atrium. Abnormalities during this stage result in congenital abnormalities such as lung aplasia, tracheoesophageal fistula, and congenital pulmonary cysts. The embryonic stage overlaps with the next stage: the pseudoglandular stage (5–17 weeks gestation). During this stage the lung has a glandular appearance and witnesses the completion of the conducting airways (bronchi and bronchioles). The respiratory epithelium of these airways begins to differentiate, and the presence of cartilage, smooth muscle cells, and mucus glands are first seen. In addition, the pleuroperitoneal cavity divides into two distinct compartments. Abnormalities during this stage lead to pulmonary sequestration, cystic ade-

nomatoid malformation, and congenital diaphragmatic hernia. The next stage witnesses the delineation of the pulmonary acinus: the canalicular stage (16–26 weeks gestation). During this stage the alveolar type II cells differentiate into type I cells, the pulmonary capillary network develops, and the alveolar type I cells closely approximate with the developing capillary network. Abnormalities of development during this stage include neonatal respiratory distress syndrome and lung hypoplasia. The next stage is the saccular stage (26–36 weeks gestation), during which further branching of the terminal saccules takes place as well as a thinning of the interstitium and fusion of the type I cell and capillary basement membrane in preparation for the lungs' function as a gas-exchange organ. The final stage of lung development is the alveolar stage (36 weeks gestation to 3–8 years of age). Controversy surrounds the length of this stage of lung development. This stage witnesses secondary septal formation, further sprouting of the capillary network, and the development of true alveoli. Abnormalities during this stage lead to lung hypoplasia and can result in the development of bronchopulmonary dysplasia.

At birth, the lung assumes the gas-exchanging function served by the placenta in utero, placing immediate stress on all components of the respiratory system. Abnormalities in the lung, respiratory muscles, chest wall, airway, respiratory controller, or pulmonary circulation may therefore be present at birth. Survival after delivery depends, for example, on the development of the surfactant system to maintain airspace stability and allow gas exchange. Immaturity of the surfactant system, often seen in infants born at less than 35 weeks gestational age, can result in severe respiratory morbidity in the immediate neonatal period as well as subsequent chronic lung disease. A lethal form of lung disease has been recognized in infants homozygous for abnormalities in the gene for surfactant protein B. Persistent pulmonary hypertension of the newborn (failure of the normal transition to a low-resistance pulmonary circulation at birth) can complicate a number of neonatal respiratory diseases. There is mounting evidence that abnormalities during fetal and neonatal growth and development of the lung have long-standing effects into adulthood, such as reduced gas exchange,

493

exercise intolerance, asthma, and an increased risk of chronic obstructive pulmonary disease.

Barker DJ: The intrauterine origins of cardiovascular and obstructive lung disease in adult life: The Marc Daniels Lecture 1990. J R Coll Physicians Lond 1991;25:129 [PMID: 2066923].

Bogue CW: Genetic and molecular basis of airway and lung development. In: Haddad GG et al (editors): *Basic Mechanisms of Pediatric Respiratory Disease.* BC Decker, 2002.

Burri P: Structural aspects of prenatal and postnatal development and growth of the lung. In: McDonald JA (editor): *Lung Growth and Development.* BC Dekker, 1997.

Wharburton D et al: Molecular mechanisms of early lung specification and branching morphogenesis. Pediatr Res 2005;57(5 Pt 2)26R [PMID: 15817505].

DIAGNOSTIC AIDS

PHYSICAL EXAMINATION OF THE RESPIRATORY TRACT

The four components of a complete pulmonary examination include: inspection, palpation, auscultation, and percussion. *Inspection* of respiratory rate, depth, ease, symmetry, and rhythm of respiration is critical to the detection of pulmonary disease. In young children, an elevated respiratory rate may be an initial indicator of pneumonia or hypoxemia. In a study of children with respiratory illnesses, abnormalities of attentiveness, consolability, respiratory effort, color, and movement had a good diagnostic accuracy in detecting hypoxemia. *Palpation* of tracheal position, symmetry of chest wall movement, and vibration with vocalization can help in identifying intrathoracic abnormalities. A shift in tracheal position can suggest pneumothorax or significant atelectasis. Tactile fremitus may change with the presence of consolidation or air in the pleural space. Other helpful noise transmission tests include whispered pectoriloquy, bronchophony, and egophony. While chest x-ray has replaced the utility of these tests, they can be helpful when imaging is not available. *Auscultation* should assess the quality of breath sounds and detect the presence of abnormal sounds such as fine or coarse crackles, wheezing, or rhonchi. It is important to know the lung anatomy in order to identify the location of abnormal findings (Figure 18–1). In older patients, unilateral crackles are the most valuable examination finding in pneumonia. *Percussion* may identify tympanic or dull sounds that can help define an intrathoracic process. However, its usefulness can prove challenging with young children. Extrapulmonary manifestations of pulmonary disease include growth failure, altered mental status (from hypoxemia or hypercapnia), cyanosis, clubbing, and osteoarthropathy. Evidence of cor pulmonale (loud pulmonic component

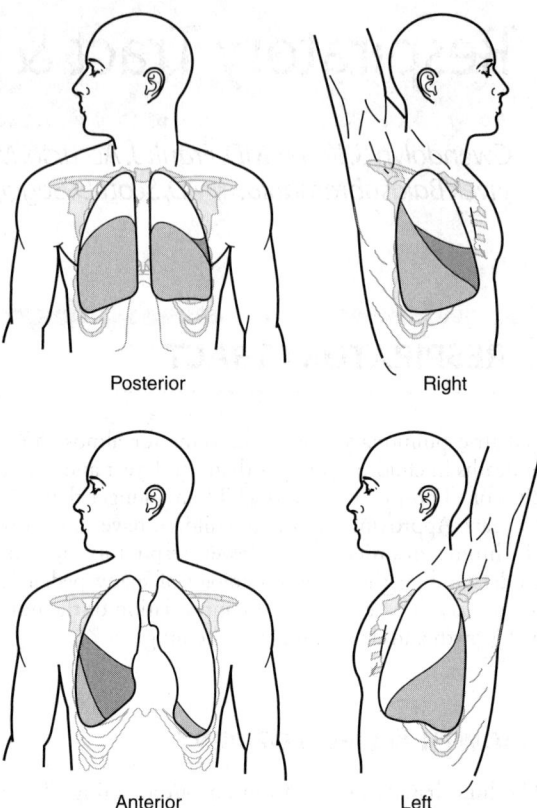

Posterior   Right

Anterior   Left

Figure 18–1. Projections of the pulmonary lobes on the chest surface. The upper lobes are white, the right-middle lobe is black, and the lower lobes are dotted.

of the second heart sound, hepatomegaly, elevated neck veins, and rarely peripheral edema) signifies advanced lung disease.

Respiratory disorders can be secondary to disease in other systems. It is therefore important to look for other conditions such as congenital heart disease (murmur or gallop), neuromuscular disease (muscle wasting or scoliosis), immunodeficiency (rash or diarrhea), and autoimmune disease or occult malignancy (arthritis or hepatosplenomegaly).

Palafox M et al: Diagnostic value of tachypnea in pneumonia defined radiologically. Arch Dis Child 2000;82:41 [PMID: 10630911].

Wipf JE et al: Diagnosing pneumonia by physical examination: Relevant or relic? Arch Intern Med 1999;159:1082 [PMID: 10335685].

PULMONARY FUNCTION TESTS

Lung function tests can help to differentiate obstructive from restrictive lung diseases, measure disease severity, define precipitants of symptoms, and evaluate response to therapy. They can help define the risks of anesthesia and surgery and assist in the planning of respiratory care in the postoperative period. However, the range of normal values for a test may be wide, and the predicted normal values change dramatically with growth. For this reason, serial determinations of lung function are often more informative than a single determination. Patient cooperation is essential for almost all physiologic assessments. Some children are not able to perform the necessary maneuvers before age 5 years and benefit from a well-trained technician, visual incentives, and interactive computer-animated systems. Lung functions in infants and toddlers are available at specialized centers. Despite these problems, tests of lung function are valuable in the care of children.

Spirometers are available on which forced vital capacity can be recorded either as a volume-time tracing (spirogram) or a flow-volume curve. The patient inhales maximally, holds his or her breath for a short period, and then exhales as fast as possible for at least 3 seconds. The tracing produced by the exhalation shows forced vital capacity (FVC), which is the total amount of air that is exhaled from maximum inspiration, and the forced expiratory volume in the first second of the exhalation (FEV_1). The maximum midexpiratory flow rate is the mean flow rate during the middle portion of the FVC maneuver. The FEV_1:FVC ratio is calculated from these absolute values; a ratio greater than 0.85 in children and young adults shows unlimited normal airflow.

These basic tests of lung function differentiate obstructive from restrictive processes. Examples of obstructive processes include asthma, chronic bronchitis, and cystic fibrosis (CF); restrictive problems include chest wall deformities that limit lung expansion and interstitial processes due to collagen-vascular diseases, hypersensitivity pneumonitis, and interstitial fibrosis. Classically, diseases that obstruct airflow decrease the FEV_1 more than the FVC, so that the FEV_1:FVC ratio is low. In restrictive problems, however, the decreases in the FEV_1 and FVC are proportionate; thus, the ratio of FEV_1 to FVC is either normal or high. Clinical suspicion of a restrictive disease is usually an indication for referral to a specialist for evaluation.

The peak expiratory flow rate, the maximal flow recorded during an FVC maneuver, can be assessed by handheld devices. The records of the peak expiratory flow rate can be helpful in following the course of pulmonary disorders that are difficult to control and require multiple medications (eg, asthma). These devices can also be used to give patients with poor perception of their disease an awareness of a decrease in lung function, thus facilitating earlier treatment.

Blonshine SB: Pediatric pulmonary function testing. Respir Care Clin North Am 2000;6:27 [PMID: 10639555].

Hammer J, Eber E (editors): *Paediatric Pulmonary Function Testing.* Karger, 2005.

Pellegrino R et al: Interpretative strategies for lung function tests. Eur Respir J 2005;26:948 [PMID: 16264058].

ASSESSMENT OF OXYGENATION AND VENTILATION

Arterial blood gas determination defines the balance between respiration at the tissue level and that in the lungs. Assessment of blood gases is essential in critically ill children and may be used also for determining the severity of lung involvement in chronic conditions. Blood gas measurements are affected by abnormalities of respiratory control, gas exchange, respiratory mechanics, and the circulation. In pediatrics, hypoxemia (low partial pressure of arterial oxygen [PaO_2]) most commonly results from mismatching of ventilation and perfusion. Hypercapnia (elevated partial pressure of arterial carbon dioxide [$PaCO_2$]) results from inadequate alveolar ventilation (ie, inability to clear the CO_2 produced). This is termed *hypoventilation.* Causes include decreased central respiratory drive, paralysis of respiratory muscles, and low-tidal-volume breathing as seen in restrictive lung diseases, severe scoliosis, or chest wall trauma. Table 18–1 gives normal values for arterial pH, PaO_2, and $PaCO_2$ at sea level and at 5000 feet.

Exhaled or end-tidal CO_2 monitoring can be used to estimate arterial CO_2 content. It is used to monitor alveolar ventilation and is most accurate in patients without significant lung disease, particularly those with a good match of ventilation and perfusion and without airway obstruction. Monitoring of exhaled or end-tidal CO_2 is increasingly being used to confirm endotracheal tube placement and ensure endotracheal rather than esophageal intubation. This assessment is accurate in children who weigh more than 2 kg and have a perfusing rhythm. Exhaled CO_2 can be monitored by attaching a CO_2 detector to an endotracheal tube or to a nasal cannula. Qualitative CO_2 monitors use a chemical detector in a strip of paper that changes color when CO_2 is present. Capnography devices are quantitative and measure the

Table 18–1. Normal arterial blood gas values on room air.

	pH	PaO_2 (mm Hg)	$PaCO_2$ (mm Hg)
Sea level	7.38–7.42	85–95	36–42
5000 feet	7.36–7.40	65–75	35–40

$PaCO_2$, partial pressure of arterial carbon dioxide; PaO_2, partial pressure of arterial oxygen.

concentration of CO_2 by infrared absorption detectors. These display continuous exhaled CO_2 concentration as a waveform and with a digital display of end-tidal CO_2.

Transcutaneous gas monitoring is a noninvasive assessment of PaO_2 and $PaCO_2$ using electrodes that measure gas tension at the skin surface. Transcutaneous monitoring can underestimate the PaO_2 and overestimate the $PaCO_2$ unless skin perfusion is maximal. Thus heating of the skin site is required, and cardiac function should be stable.

Pulse oximetry (measuring light absorption by transilluminating the skin) is the most reliable and easiest form of noninvasive monitoring of oxygenation. Oxygenated hemoglobin absorbs red light at certain wavelengths. Measurement during a systolic pulse allows estimation of arterial oxygen saturation as the machine corrects for the light absorbed at the tissue level between pulses. No heating of the skin is necessary. Values of oxygen saturation are reliable as low as 80%. The pulse oximeter has reduced reliability during conditions causing reduced arterial pulsation such as hypothermia, hypotension, or infusion of vasoconstrictor drugs. Carbon monoxide bound by hemoglobin results in falsely high oxygen saturation readings.

Bhende MS: End-tidal carbon dioxide monitoring in pediatrics—clinical applications. J Postgrad Med 2001;47:215 [PMID: 11832630].

Hay WW Jr: Pulse oximetry: As good as it gets? J Perinatol 2000;20:181 [PMID: 10802844].

Hazinski MF (editor): *Pediatric Advanced Life Support Provider Manual.* American Heart Association and the American Academy of Pediatrics, 2002.

Soubani AO: Noninvasive monitoring of oxygen and carbon dioxide. Am J Emerg Med 2001;19:141 [PMID: 11239260].

CULTURE OF MATERIAL FROM THE RESPIRATORY TRACT

Spontaneously expectorated sputum is the easiest and most convenient sample to culture though it is rarely available from patients younger than age 6 years. In young children, especially those with cystic fibrosis, a deep pharyngeal throat swab may be obtained in an attempt to try to identify a predominant bacterial pathogen. Cultures from the lower respiratory tract can be obtained invasively by tracheal aspiration through an endotracheal tube or rigid bronchoscope, or by performing a bronchoalveolar lavage through a flexible bronchoscope. Sputum induction, performed by inhaling aerosolized hypertonic saline, is a relatively safe noninvasive means of obtaining lower airway secretions. Other less commonly employed means of obtaining lung specimens include computed tomography–guided needle aspiration and lung biopsy, either open or thoracoscopic. Thoracentesis should be considered when pleural fluid is present.

McIntosh K: Community-acquired pneumonia in children. N Engl J Med 2002;346:429 [PMID: 11832532].

IMAGING OF THE RESPIRATORY TRACT

The plain chest radiograph remains the foundation for investigating the pediatric thorax. Both frontal and lateral views should be obtained. The radiograph is useful for evaluating air trapping caused by airway obstruction, opacification caused by pneumonia, and interstitial problems such as pulmonary edema. Hyperinflation is best demonstrated in lateral views as flattening of the diaphragm. It is often seen because young children commonly develop small-airway obstruction and asthma. Parenchymal changes may cause increased interstitial markings, consolidation, air bronchograms, or loss of diaphragm or heart contours. When pleural fluid is suspected, lateral decubitus radiographs may be helpful in determining the extent and mobility of the fluid. When a foreign body is suspected, forced expiratory radiographs may show focal air trapping and shift of the mediastinum to the contralateral side. Lateral neck radiographs can be useful in assessing the size of adenoids and tonsils and also in differentiating croup from epiglottitis, the latter being associated with the "thumbprint" sign.

Barium swallow is indicated for patients with suspected aspiration to detect swallowing dysfunction, tracheoesophageal fistula, gastroesophageal reflux, and achalasia. This technique is also important in detecting vascular rings and slings, because most of these abnormalities compress the esophagus. Airway fluoroscopy is another important tool for assessing both fixed airway obstruction (eg, tracheal stenosis) and dynamic airway obstruction (eg, tracheomalacia). Fluoroscopy or ultrasound of the diaphragm can detect paralysis by demonstrating paradoxic movement of the involved hemidiaphragm.

High-resolution computed tomography (CT) scanning is useful to evaluate parenchymal changes caused by interstitial lung disease and airway abnormalities including bronchiectasis. Characteristic patterns seen in interstitial lung disease (eg, ground-glass opacification) or airway disease (eg, bronchiectasis) are often missed on chest radiographs. Magnetic resonance imaging (MRI) is useful for defining subtle or complex abnormalities and vascular rings. Ventilation-perfusion scans can provide information about regional ventilation and perfusion and can help detect vascular malformations and pulmonary emboli (rare in children). Pulmonary angiography is occasionally necessary to define the pulmonary vascular bed more precisely.

Brody AS: Imaging considerations: interstitial lung disease in children. Radiol Clin North Am 2005;43:391 [PMID: 15737375].

Williams HJ, Alton HM: Imaging of paediatric mediastinal abnormalities. Paediatr Respir Rev 2003;4:55 [PMID: 12615033].

LARYNGOSCOPY & BRONCHOSCOPY

The indications for laryngoscopy include undiagnosed hoarseness, stridor, symptoms of obstructive sleep apnea, and laryngeal wheezing consistent with a diagnosis of vocal cord dysfunction; indications for bronchoscopy include wheezing, suspected foreign body, pneumonia, atelectasis, chronic cough, hemoptysis, and placement of an endotracheal tube and assessment of patency. In general, the more specific the indication, the higher the diagnostic yield.

Pediatric bronchoscopy instruments are of either the flexible fiberoptic or the rigid open tube type. Flexible bronchoscopy has the following advantages:

1. With conscious sedation and topical anesthetics, the procedure can be done at the bedside.
2. Evaluation of the upper airway can be done with little risk in patients who are awake.
3. The distal airways of intubated patients can be examined without removing the endotracheal tube.
4. The instrument can be used as an obturator to intubate a patient with a difficult upper airway.
5. Endotracheal tube placement and patency can be checked.
6. Assessment of airway dynamics is generally better.
7. It is possible to examine more distal airways.

Improvements in digital optics have greatly enhanced the image quality. The advantages of using a rigid instrument are (1) easier removal of foreign bodies (so rigid bronchoscopy is preferred for suspected foreign body aspiration); and (2) better airway control, allowing the patient to be ventilated through the bronchoscope. In addition, this approach to the airway allows better assessment of the subglottic space for stenosis. The choice of procedures depends largely on the expertise available.

Bronchoalveolar lavage through a flexible bronchoscope is used to detect infection. Aspiration and hemorrhage can be suspected in the presence of lipid- and hemosiderin-laden macrophages, respectively, though lipid-laden macrophages can also be found in other conditions. Analysis of lavage fluid can also be completed for cell counts, surfactant proteins, and inflammatory mediators. Transbronchial biopsy in children is limited to evaluation for infection and rejection in transplant patients due to poor diagnostic yield in most conditions. Transbronchial biopsy may have a role in diagnosing diffuse lung diseases such as sarcoidosis.

Schellhase DE: Pediatric flexible airway endoscopy. Curr Opin Pediatr 2002;14:327 [PMID: 12011674].

Naguib ML et al: Use of laryngeal mask airway in flexible bronchoscopy in infants and children. Pediatr Pulmonol 2005;39:56 [PMID: 15558607].

GENERAL THERAPY OF PEDIATRIC LUNG DISEASES

OXYGEN THERAPY

Oxygen therapy in children with respiratory disease can reduce the work of breathing, resulting in fewer respiratory symptoms; relax the pulmonary vasculature, lessening the potential for pulmonary hypertension and congestive heart failure; and improve feeding. Patients breathing spontaneously can be treated by nasal cannula, head hood, or mask (including simple, rebreathing, nonrebreathing, or Venturi masks). The general goal of oxygen therapy is to achieve an arterial oxygen tension of 65–90 mm Hg or an oxygen saturation above 92%. The actual oxygen concentration achieved by nasal cannula or mask depends on the flow rate, the type of mask used, and the patient's age. Small changes in flow rate during oxygen administration by nasal cannula can lead to substantial changes in inspired oxygen concentration in young infants. The amount of oxygen required to correct hypoxemia may vary according to the child's activity. It is not unusual, for example, for an infant with chronic lung disease to require 0.75 L/min while awake but 1 L/min while asleep or feeding.

Although the head hood is an efficient device for delivery of oxygen in young infants, the nasal cannula is used more often because it allows the infant greater mobility. The cannula has nasal prongs that are inserted in the nares. Flow through the nasal cannula should generally not exceed 3 L/min to avoid excessive drying of the mucosa. Even at high flow rates, oxygen by nasal cannula rarely delivers inspired oxygen concentrations greater than 40–45%. In contrast, partial rebreathing and nonrebreathing masks or head hoods achieve inspired oxygen concentrations as high as 90–100%.

Because the physical findings of hypoxemia are subtle, the adequacy of oxygenation should be measured as the arterial oxygen tension, or oxygen saturation can be determined by oximetry. The advantages of the latter noninvasive method include the ability to obtain continuous measurements during various normal activities and to avoid artifacts caused by crying or breath-holding during attempts at arterial puncture. For children with chronic cardiopulmonary disorders that may require supplemental oxygen therapy (eg, bronchopulmonary dysplasia or CF), frequent noninvasive assessments are essential to ensure the safety and adequacy of treatment.

Hazinski MF (editor): *Pediatric Advanced Life Support Provider Manual.* American Heart Association and the American Academy of Pediatrics, 2002.

INHALATION OF BRONCHODILATORS

Airway obstruction that is at least partially reversed by a bronchodilator can be seen in CF, bronchiolitis, and bronchopulmonary dysplasia, as well as in acute and chronic asthma.

The β-adrenergic agonists may be delivered by metered-dose inhaler, dry powder inhaler, or nebulizer. Metered-dose inhalers are convenient and best combined with valved holding chambers, especially for children who lack the ability to coordinate actuation of the metered-dose inhaler with inhalation. In contrast, the nebulizer is an effective method of delivering medication to infants and young children. Long-acting inhaled β_2-adrenergic agents that are relatively selective for the respiratory tract are described in Chapter 34. Inhaled bronchodilators are as effective as injected agents for treating acute episodes of airway obstruction and have fewer side effects. These drugs can be safely administered at home as long as both the physician and the family realize that a poor response may signify the need for corticosteroids to help restore β-adrenergic responsiveness.

Anticholinergic agents may also acutely decrease airway obstruction. Furthermore, they may yield a longer duration of bronchodilation than do many adrenergic agents. Selected patients may benefit from receiving both β-adrenergic and anticholinergic agents. In general, this class of drugs is most effective in the treatment of chronic bronchitis.

Rubin BK, Fink JB: The delivery of inhaled medication to the young child. Pediatr Clin North Am 2003;50:717 [PMID: 12877243].

AIRWAY CLEARANCE THERAPY

Chest physical therapy, with postural drainage, percussion, and forced expiratory maneuvers, has been widely used to improve the clearance of lower airway secretions even though there are limited data on the efficacy of these techniques. Children with cystic fibrosis have been shown to benefit from routine airway clearance. Many airway clearance techniques exist, but only a few long-term studies have compared the various options. The various techniques currently available include chest physiotherapy, autogenic drainage, positive expiratory pressure (Flutter or Acapella), intrapulmonary percussive ventilation, or high-frequency chest compression. The decision about which technique to use should be based on the patient's age and preference after trying different approaches. Often bronchodilators or mucolytic medications are given prior to or during airway clearance therapy. Inhaled corticosteroids and inhaled antibiotics should be given after airway clearance therapy so that the airways are first cleared of secretions, allowing the medications to maximally penetrate into the lung.

Perrotta C et al: Chest physiotherapy for acute bronchiolitis in paediatric patients between 0 and 24 months old. Cochrane Database Syst Rev 2005:CD004873 [PMID: 15846736].

Wagener JS, Headley AA: Cystic fibrosis: Current trends in respiratory care. Respir Care 2003;48:234; discussion 246 [PMID: 12667274].

AVOIDANCE OF ENVIRONMENTAL HAZARDS

All parents or other caregivers should be counseled about environmental hazards to the lung. The list of potential hazards includes small objects that may be aspirated, allergens that can precipitate respiratory symptoms in atopic children, and cigarette smoke. The harmful effects of smoking in the home deserve special emphasis. Children from families where the parents and others smoke have decreased lung growth as well as decreased pulmonary function in comparison with children raised in smoke-free homes. Exposure of children to tobacco smoke also leads to an increased frequency of lower respiratory tract infections and an increased incidence of respiratory symptoms, including recurrent wheezing. Health care providers must increase their efforts to educate patients and their families about the hazards of smoking.

Bradley JP et al: Severity of respiratory syncytial virus bronchiolitis is affected by cigarette smoke exposure and atopy. Pediatrics 2005;115:e7 [PMID: 15629968].

DiFranza JR et al: Prenatal and postnatal environmental tobacco smoke exposure and children's health. Pediatrics 2004;113:1007 [PMID: 15060193].

DISORDERS OF THE CONDUCTING AIRWAYS

The conducting airways (the nose, mouth, pharynx, larynx, trachea, bronchi, and bronchioles) direct inspired air to the gas-exchange units of the lung; they do not participate in gas exchange themselves. Airflow obstruction in the conducting airways occurs by (1) external compression (eg, vascular ring or tumor), (2) abnormalities of the airway structure itself (eg, congenital defects or thickening of an airway wall due to inflammation), or (3) material in the airway lumen (eg, foreign body or mucus).

Airway obstruction can be fixed (airflow limited in both the inspiratory and the expiratory phases) or variable (airflow limited more in one phase of respiration than in the other). Variable obstruction is common in children because their airways are more compliant and susceptible to dynamic compression. With variable extrathoracic airway obstruction (eg, croup), airflow limitation is greater during inspiration, leading to inspiratory stridor. With variable intrathoracic obstruction (eg, bronchomalacia), limitation is greater during expiration, producing expiratory wheezing. Thus determining the phase of respiration in which obstruction is greatest may be helpful in localizing the site of obstruction.

EXTRATHORACIC AIRWAY OBSTRUCTION

Patients with abnormalities of the extrathoracic airway may present with snoring and other symptoms of obstructive apnea, hoarseness, brassy cough, or stridor. The course of the illness may be acute (eg, infectious croup), recurrent (eg, spasmodic croup), chronic (eg, subglottic stenosis), or progressive (eg, laryngeal papillomatosis). Significant risk factors are difficult delivery, ductal ligation, and intubation. Examination should determine if obstructive symptoms are present at rest or with agitation, if they are positional, or if they are related to sleep. The presence of agitation, air hunger, severe retractions, cyanosis, lethargy, or coma should alert the physician to a potentially life-threatening condition that may require immediate airway intervention. Helpful diagnostic studies in the evaluation of upper airway obstruction include chest and lateral neck radiographs, airway fluoroscopy, and barium swallow. In patients who have symptoms of severe chronic obstruction, an electrocardiogram should be obtained to evaluate for right ventricular hypertrophy and pulmonary hypertension. Patients with obstructive sleep apnea should have polysomnography (measurements during sleep of the motion of the chest wall, airflow at the nose and mouth, heart rate, oxygen saturation, and selected electroencephalographic leads to stage sleep) to determine severity and to evaluate the need for tonsillectomy and adenoidectomy, oxygen, or continuous or biphasic positive airway pressure. In older children, pulmonary function tests can differentiate fixed from variable airflow obstruction and identify the site of variable obstruction. If noninvasive studies are unable to establish the cause, direct laryngoscopy and bronchoscopy remain the procedures of choice to establish the precise diagnosis. Treatment should be directed at relieving airway obstruction and correcting the underlying condition if possible.

INTRATHORACIC AIRWAY OBSTRUCTION

Intrathoracic airway obstruction usually causes expiratory wheezing. The history should include the following:

1. Age at onset
2. Precipitating factors (eg, exercise, upper respiratory illnesses, allergens, or choking while eating)
3. Course—acute (bronchiolitis or foreign body), chronic (tracheomalacia or vascular ring), recurrent (asthma), or progressive (CF or bronchiolitis obliterans)
4. Presence and nature of cough
5. Production of sputum
6. Previous response to bronchodilators
7. Symptoms with positional changes (vascular rings)
8. Involvement of other organ systems (malabsorption in CF)

Physical examination should include growth measurements and vital signs. The examiner should look for cyanosis or pallor, barrel-shaped chest, retractions and use of accessory muscles, and clubbing. Auscultation should define the pattern and timing of respiration, detect the presence of crackles and wheezing, and determine whether findings are localized or generalized.

Routine tests include plain chest radiographs, a sweat test, and pulmonary function tests in older children. Other diagnostic studies are dictated by the history and physical findings. Treatment should be directed toward the primary cause of the obstruction, but generally includes a trial of bronchodilators.

STRIDOR & NOISY BREATHING FROM CONGENITAL DISORDERS OF THE EXTRATHORACIC AIRWAY: PRESENTATION FROM BIRTH OR WITHIN THE FIRST FEW MONTHS OF LIFE

LARYNGOMALACIA

Laryngomalacia is a benign congenital disorder in which the cartilaginous support for the supraglottic structures is underdeveloped. It is the most common cause of persistent stridor in infants and usually is seen in the first 6 weeks of life. Stridor has been reported to be worse in the supine position, with increased activity, with upper respiratory infections, and during feeding; however, the clinical presentation can be variable. Patients may have slight oxygen desaturation during sleep. Gastroesophageal reflux may also be associated with laryngomalacia requiring treatment. The condition usually improves with age and resolves by age 2 years, but in some cases symptoms persist for years. The diagnosis is established by direct laryngoscopy, which shows inspiratory collapse of an omega-shaped epiglottis (with or without long, redundant arytenoids). In mildly affected patients with a typical presentation (those without stridor at rest or retractions), this procedure may not be necessary. No treatment is usually needed. However, in patients with severe symptoms of airway obstruction associated with feeding difficulties, failure to thrive, obstructive sleep apnea, or severe dyspnea, surgical epiglottoplasty may be necessary.

O'Sullivan BP et al: Use of nasopharyngoscopy in the evaluation of children with noisy breathing. Chest 2004;125:1265 [PMID: 15078733].

Toynton SC et al: Aryepiglottoplasty for laryngomalacia: 100 consecutive cases. J Laryngol Otol 2001;115:35 [PMID: 11233619].

OTHER CONGENITAL PROBLEMS

Other rare congenital lesions of the larynx (laryngeal atresia, laryngeal web, laryngocele and cyst of the larynx, subglottic hemangioma, and laryngeal cleft) are best evaluated by direct laryngoscopy. Laryngeal atresia presents immediately after birth with severe respiratory distress and is usually fatal. Laryngeal web, representing fusion of the anterior portion of the true vocal cords, is associated with hoarseness, aphonia, and stridor. Surgical correction may be necessary depending on the degree of airway obstruction.

Congenital cysts and laryngoceles are believed to have similar origin. Cysts are more superficial, whereas laryngoceles communicate with the interior of the larynx. Cysts are generally fluid-filled, whereas laryngoceles may be air- or fluid-filled. Airway obstruction is usually prominent and requires surgery or laser therapy.

Subglottic hemangiomas are seen in infancy with signs of upper airway obstruction and can be associated with similar lesions of the skin (but not always). Although these lesions tend to regress spontaneously, airway obstruction may require surgical treatment or even tracheostomy.

Laryngeal cleft is a very rare condition resulting from failure of posterior cricoid fusion. Patients with this condition may have stridor but always aspirate severely, resulting in recurrent or chronic pneumonia and failure to thrive. Barium swallow is always positive for severe aspiration, but diagnosis can be very difficult even with direct laryngoscopy. Patients often require tracheostomy and gastrostomy, because success with surgical correction can be mixed.

Bitar MA et al: Management of congenital subglottic hemangioma: trends and success over the past 17 years. Otolaryngol Head Neck Surg 2005;132:226 [PMID: 15692531].

Dinwiddie R: Congenital upper airway obstruction. Paediatr Respir Rev 2004;5:17 [PMID: 15222950].

Johnson LB et al: Acquired subglottic cysts in preterm infants. J Otolaryngol 2005;34:75 [PMID: 16076404].

STRIDOR & NOISY BREATHING FROM ACQUIRED DISORDERS OF THE EXTRATHORACIC AIRWAY: PATIENTS GENERALLY PRESENT WITH ACUTE OR SUBACUTE SYMPTOMS

CROUP SYNDROME

Croup describes acute inflammatory diseases of the larynx, including viral croup (laryngotracheobronchitis), epiglottitis (supraglottitis), and bacterial tracheitis. These are the main entities in the differential diagnosis for patients presenting with acute stridor, although spasmodic croup, angioneurotic edema, laryngeal or esophageal foreign body, and retropharyngeal abscess should be considered as well.

1. Viral Croup

Viral croup generally affects younger children in the fall and early winter months and is most often caused by parainfluenza virus serotypes. Other organisms causing croup include respiratory syncytial virus (RSV), influenza virus, rubeola virus, adenovirus, and *Mycoplasma pneumoniae*. Although inflammation of the entire airway is usually present, edema formation in the subglottic space accounts for the predominant signs of upper airway obstruction.

Clinical Findings

A. SYMPTOMS AND SIGNS

Usually a prodrome of upper respiratory tract symptoms is followed by a barking cough and stridor. Fever is usually absent or low-grade but may on occasion be high-grade. Patients with mild disease may have stridor when agitated. As obstruction worsens, stridor occurs at rest, accompanied in severe cases by retractions, air hunger, and cyanosis. On examination, the presence of cough and the absence of drooling favor the diagnosis of viral croup over epiglottitis.

B. IMAGING

Lateral neck radiographs can be diagnostically supportive by showing subglottic narrowing and a normal epiglottis. This is not done routinely in the child with a classic presentation.

Treatment

Treatment of viral croup is based on the symptoms. Mild croup, signified by a barking cough and no stridor at rest, requires supportive therapy with oral hydration and minimal handling. Mist therapy is used by some physicians, although clinical studies demonstrating its effectiveness are lacking. Conversely, patients with stridor at rest require active intervention. Oxygen should be administered to patients with oxygen desaturation. Nebulized racemic epinephrine (2.25% solution; 0.05 mL/kg to a maximum of 1.5 mL diluted in sterile saline) is commonly used because it has a rapid onset of action within 10–30 minutes. Both racemic epinephrine and epinephrine hydrochloride are effective in alleviating symptoms and decreasing the need for intubation. Once controversial, the efficacy of glucocorticoids in croup is now more firmly established. Dexamethasone, 0.6 mg/kg intramuscularly as one dose, improves symptoms, reduces the duration of hospitalizations and frequency of intubations, and permits earlier discharge from the emergency department. Oral dexamethasone appears equally effective, and limited data suggest that lower doses of oral dexamethasone (0.15 mg/kg) may be as effective as the higher dose. Inhaled budesonide (2–4 mg) also improves symptoms and decreases hospital stay. Onset of action occurs within 2 hours, and this agent may be as effective as dexamethasone; however, dexamethasone is still the most cost-effective steroid of choice. If symptoms resolve within 3 hours of glucocorticoids and nebulized epinephrine, patients can safely be discharged without fear of a sudden rebound in symptoms. If, however, recurrent nebulized epinephrine treatments are required or if respiratory distress persists, patients require hospitalization for close observation, supportive care, and nebulization treatments as needed. In patients with impending respiratory failure, an airway must be established (see following paragraph). Hospitalized patients with persistent symptoms over 3–4 days despite treatment should initiate consideration of another underlying cause.

Patients with impending respiratory failure require an artificial airway. Intubation with an endotracheal tube of slightly smaller diameter than would ordinarily be used is reasonably safe. Extubation should be accomplished within 2–3 days to minimize the risk of laryngeal injury. If the patient fails extubation, tracheostomy may be required.

Prognosis

Most children with viral croup have an uneventful course and improve within a few days. Some evidence suggests that patients with a history of croup associated with wheezing may have airway hyperreactivity. It is not clear if this was present prior to the croup episode or if the croup episode itself altered airway function. Recurrence of croup occurs in some instances, implying airway hyperreactivity.

Russell K et al: Glucocorticoids for croup. Cochrane Database Syst Rev 2004;1:CD001955 [PMID: 14973975].

Wright RB et al: New approaches to respiratory infections in children: Bronchiolitis and croup. Emerg Med Clin North Am 2002;20:93 [PMID: 11826639].

2. Epiglottitis

Epiglottitis is a true medical emergency. In published case series, it is almost always caused by *Haemophilus influenzae* type B, although other organisms such as nontypable *H influenzae, Streptococcus pneumoniae,* groups A and C *Streptococcus pyogenes, Neisseria meningitidis,* and staphylococci have been implicated. Resulting inflammation and swelling of the supraglottic structures (epiglottis and arytenoids) can develop rapidly and lead to life-threatening upper airway obstruction. The incidence has decreased dramatically since *H influenzae* conjugate vaccine was introduced, indicating that the best treatment strategy is prevention.

Clinical Findings

A. SYMPTOMS AND SIGNS

Typically, patients present with a sudden onset of fever, dysphagia, drooling, muffled voice, inspiratory retractions, cyanosis, and soft stridor. They often sit in the so-called sniffing dog position, which gives them the best airway possible under the circumstances. Progression to total airway obstruction may occur and result in respiratory arrest. The definitive diagnosis is made by direct inspection of the epiglottis, a procedure that should be done by an experienced airway specialist under controlled conditions (usually the operating room). The typical findings are cherry-red and swollen epiglottis and arytenoids.

B. IMAGING

Diagnostically, lateral neck radiographs may be helpful in demonstrating a classic "thumbprint" sign. Obtaining radiographs, however, may delay important airway intervention.

Treatment

Once the diagnosis of epiglottitis is made, endotracheal intubation must be performed immediately. Most anesthesiologists prefer general anesthesia (but not muscle relaxants) to facilitate intubation. After an airway is established, cultures of the blood and epiglottis should be obtained and the patient started on appropriate intravenous antibiotics to cover *H influenzae* (ceftriaxone sodium or equivalent cephalosporin). Extubation can usually be accomplished in 24–48 hours, when direct inspection shows significant reduction in the size of the epiglottis. Intravenous antibiotics should be continued for 2–3 days, followed by oral antibiotics to complete a 10-day course.

Prognosis

Prompt recognition and appropriate treatment usually results in rapid resolution of swelling and inflammation. Recurrence is unusual.

Rotta AT, Wiryawan B: Respiratory emergencies in children. Respir Care 2003;48:248 [PMID: 12667275].

3. Bacterial Tracheitis

Bacterial tracheitis (pseudomembranous croup) is a severe life-threatening form of laryngotracheobronchitis. The organism most often isolated is *Staphylococcus aureus,* but organisms such as *H influenzae,* group A *Streptococcus pyogenes, Neisseria* species, *Moraxella catarrhalis,* and others have been reported. The disease probably represents localized mucosal invasion of bacteria in patients with primary viral croup, resulting in inflammatory edema, purulent secretions, and pseudomembranes. Although cultures of the tracheal secretions are frequently positive, blood cultures are almost always negative.

Clinical Findings

A. Symptoms and Signs

The early clinical picture is similar to that of viral croup. However, instead of gradual improvement, patients develop higher fever, toxicity, and progressive or intermittent severe upper airway obstruction that is unresponsive to standard croup therapy. The incidence of sudden respiratory arrest or progressive respiratory failure is high; in such instances, airway intervention is required. Findings of toxic shock and the acute respiratory distress syndrome may also be seen. Recently, subsets of patients with tracheal membranes have been reported with a less severe clinical presentation. Aggressive medical treatment and debridement still must occur in these patients. A higher index of suspicion is required for this life-threatening condition.

B. Laboratory Findings

The white cell count is usually elevated, with left shift. Cultures of tracheal secretions usually demonstrate one of the causative organisms.

C. Diagnosis

Lateral neck radiographs show a normal epiglottis but often severe subglottic and tracheal narrowing. Irregularity of the contour of the proximal tracheal mucosa can frequently be seen radiographically and should elicit concern. Bronchoscopy showing a normal epiglottis and the presence of copious purulent tracheal secretions and membranes confirm the diagnosis.

Treatment

Suspected bacterial tracheitis should be managed in a fashion similar to that for epiglottitis. The incidence of respiratory arrest or progressive respiratory failure is high, necessitating intubation. Patients often have thick, purulent tracheal secretions requiring debridement, and humidification, frequent suctioning, and intensive care monitoring are required to prevent endotracheal tube obstruction. Intravenous antibiotics to cover *Staphylococcus aureus, H influenzae,* and the other organisms are indicated. Thick secretions persist for several days, usually resulting in longer periods of intubation for bacterial tracheitis than for epiglottitis or croup. Despite the severity of this illness, the reported mortality rate is very low if recognized and treated promptly.

Salamone FN et al: Bacterial tracheitis reexamined: is there a less severe manifestation? Otolaryngol Head Neck Surg 2004;131:871 [PMID: 15577783].

VOCAL CORD PARALYSIS

Unilateral or bilateral vocal cord paralysis may be congenital, or more commonly may result from injury to the recurrent laryngeal nerves. Risk factors for acquired paralysis include difficult delivery (especially face presentation), neck and thoracic surgery (eg, ductal ligation or repair of tracheoesophageal fistula), trauma, mediastinal masses, and central nervous system disease (eg, Arnold-Chiari malformation). Patients usually present with varying degrees of hoarseness, aspiration, or high-pitched stridor. Unilateral cord paralysis is more likely to occur on the left because of the longer course of the left recurrent laryngeal nerve and its proximity to major thoracic structures. Patients with unilateral paralysis are usually hoarse but rarely have stridor. With bilateral cord paralysis, the closer to midline the cords are positioned, the greater the airway obstruction; the more lateral the cords are positioned, the greater the tendency to aspirate and experience hoarseness or aphonia. If partial function is preserved (paresis), the adductor muscles tend to operate better than the abductors, with a resultant high-pitched inspiratory stridor and normal voice. Airway intervention (tracheostomy) is rarely indicated in unilateral paralysis but is often necessary for bilateral paralysis. Recovery is related to the severity of nerve injury and the potential for healing.

Miyamoto RC et al: Bilateral congenital vocal cord paralysis: a 16-year institutional review. Otolaryngol Head Neck Surg 2005; 133:241 [PMID: 16087022].

Parikh SR: Pediatric unilateral vocal fold immobility. Otolaryngol Clin North Am 2004;37:203 (Review) [PMID: 15062694].

SUBGLOTTIC STENOSIS

Subglottic stenosis may be congenital, or more commonly may result from endotracheal intubation. Neonates and infants are particularly vulnerable to subglottic injury from intubation: The subglottis is the narrowest part of an infant's airway, and the cricoid cartilage, which supports the subglottis, is the only cartilage that completely encircles the airway. The clinical presentation may vary from totally asymptomatic to the typical picture of severe upper airway obstruction. Patients with signs of stridor who repeatedly fail extubation are likely to have subglottic stenosis. Subglottic stenosis should also be suspected in children with multiple, prolonged, or severe episodes of croup. Diagnosis is made by direct laryngoscopy and bronchoscopy to size the airway. Tracheostomy is often required when airway compromise is severe. Surgical intervention is ultimately required to correct the stenosis. Depending on the type of stenosis, a cricoid split in which the cricoid cartilage is surgically opened (better for acquired than for congenital lesions) may be tried. Laryngotracheal reconstruction in which a cartilage graft from another source (eg, rib) is used to expand the airway has become the standard procedure for symptomatic subglottic stenosis in children.

Khariwala SS et al: Laryngotracheal consequences of pediatric cardiac surgery. Arch Otolaryngol Head Neck Surg 2005;131:336 [PMID: 15837903].

White DR et al: Pediatric cricotracheal resection: surgical outcomes and risk factor analysis. Arch Otolaryngol Head Neck Surg 2005;131:896 [PMID: 16230593].

LARYNGEAL TRAUMA

Injury to the larynx may result from external trauma, such as automobile accidents, snowmobile accidents (clothesline injury), and hanging; or internal trauma, such as noxious inhalation (burns and caustic substances) and intubation. Laryngeal trauma frequently requires emergent airway management to prevent death.

Myer CM: Trauma of the larynx and craniofacial structures: airway implications. Paediatr Anaesth 2004;14:103 (Review) [PMID: 14717882].

LARYNGEAL PAPILLOMATOSIS

Papillomas of the larynx are benign, warty growths that are difficult to treat and are the most common laryngeal neoplasm in children. Human papillomaviruses 6, 11, and 16 have been implicated as causative agents. A substantial percentage of mothers of patients with laryngeal papillomas have a history of genital condylomas at the time of delivery, so the virus may be acquired during passage through an infected birth canal.

The age at onset is usually 2–4 years, but juvenile-onset recurrent respiratory papillomatosis is well documented. A younger age of onset may be a worse prognostic indicator. Patients usually develop hoarseness, voice changes, croupy cough, or stridor that can lead to life-threatening airway obstruction. Diagnosis is by direct laryngoscopy. The larynx was involved at the time of diagnosis in over 95% of patients, most of whom had only one site involved.

Treatment is directed toward relieving airway obstruction, usually by surgical removal of the lesions. Tracheostomy is necessary when life-threatening obstruction or respiratory arrest occurs. Various surgical procedures (laser, cup forceps, or cryosurgery) have been used to remove papillomas, but recurrences are the rule, and frequent reoperation may be needed. The lesions occasionally spread down the trachea and bronchi, making surgical removal more difficult. The use of interferon therapy remains controversial. Fortunately, spontaneous remissions do occur, usually by puberty, so that the goal of therapy is to maintain an adequate airway until remission occurs.

Reeves WC et al: National registry for juvenile-onset recurrent respiratory papillomatosis. Arch Otolaryngol Head Neck Surg 2003;129:976 [PMID: 12975271].

Wiatrak BJ et al: Recurrent respiratory papillomatosis: a longitudinal study comparing severity associated with human papilloma viral types 6 and 11 and other risk factors in a large pediatric population. Laryngoscope 2004;114:1 [PMID: 15514560].

CONGENITAL DISORDERS OF THE INTRATHORACIC AIRWAYS

MALACIA OF AIRWAYS

Tracheomalacia or bronchomalacia exists when the cartilaginous framework of the airway is inadequate to maintain airway patency. Because cartilage of the infant airway is normally soft, all infants may have some degree of dynamic collapse of a central airway when pressure outside the airway exceeds intraluminal pressure. In tracheomalacia, whether congenital or acquired, dynamic collapse leads to airway obstruction. The congenital variety may be isolated or associated with another developmental defect, such as tracheoesophageal fistula, vascular ring, or various syndromes. It may be localized to part of the trachea, or more commonly may involve the entire trachea as well as the remainder of the conducting airways. In severe cases, cartilage in the involved area may be missing or underdeveloped. The acquired variety has been associated with long-term ventilation of premature newborns that results in chronic tracheal injury.

Coarse wheezing, cough, stridor, or radiographic changes are common findings. Symptoms classically present insidiously over the first few months of life and can increase with agitation, upper respiratory tract infections, or with the use of bronchodilators. Diagnosis can be made by fluoroscopy or bronchoscopy. Barium swallow may be indicated to rule out coexisting conditions. Conservative treatment is usually indicated for the isolated condition, which generally improves over time with growth. Coexisting lesions such as tracheoesophageal fistulas and vascular rings need primary repair. In severe cases of tracheomalacia, intubation or tracheostomy may be necessary. However, this alone is seldom satisfactory because airway collapse continues to exist below the tip of the artificial airway. Positive pressure ventilation may be required to stent the collapsing airway. Surgical approaches to the problem (tracheopexy or aortopexy) may be considered as alternatives prior to or in an effort to wean off of ventilatory support.

Austin J, Ali T: Tracheomalacia and bronchomalacia in children: Pathophysiology, assessment, treatment and anaesthesia management. Paediatr Anaesth 2003;13:3 [PMID: 12535032].

Carden KA et al: Tracheomalacia and tracheobronchomalacia in children and adults. Chest 2005;127:984.

VASCULAR RINGS & SLINGS

The most common vascular anomalies to compress the trachea or esophagus are a double aortic arch, right aortic arch with left ligamentum arteriosum or patent ductus arteriosus, pulmonary sling, anomalous innominate or left carotid artery, and aberrant right subclavian artery. All but the latter can cause tracheal compression and present in infancy with symptoms of chronic airway obstruction (stridor, coarse wheezing, and croupy cough). Symptoms are often worse in the supine position. Respiratory compromise is most severe with double aortic arch and may lead to apnea, respiratory arrest, or even death. Esophageal compression, present in all but anomalous innominate or carotid artery, may result in feeding difficulties, including dysphagia and vomiting. Barium swallow showing esophageal compression is the mainstay of diagnosis. Chest x-ray and echocardiogram may miss abnormalities. Anatomy can be further defined by angiography, CT, MRI or MR angiography, or bronchoscopy.

Patients with significant symptoms require surgical correction, especially those with double aortic arch. Patients usually improve following correction but may have persistent but milder symptoms of airway obstruction due to associated tracheomalacia.

Masters IB et al: Series of laryngomalacia, tracheomalacia, and bronchomalacia disorders and their associations with other conditions in children. Pediatr Pulmonol 2002;34:189 [PMID: 12203847].

Turner A et al: Vascular rings—presentation, investigation and outcome. Eur J Pediar 2005;164:266.

BRONCHOGENIC CYSTS

Bronchogenic cysts generally occur in the middle mediastinum (see section on mediastinal masses) near the carina and adjacent to the major bronchi but can be found elsewhere in the lung. They range in size from 2–10 cm. Cyst walls are thin and may contain pus, mucus, or blood. Cysts develop from abnormal lung budding of the primitive foregut. They can be seen in involvement with other congenital pulmonary malformations such as sequestration or lobar emphysema.

Clinically, respiratory distress can appear acutely in early childhood, and present as chronic wheezing, chronic cough, tachypnea, recurrent pneumonia, or stridor, depending on the location and size of the cysts and the degree of airway compression, or they may remain asymptomatic into adulthood. However, all asymptomatic cysts will eventually become symptomatic with chest pain being the most common presenting complaint. On examination, the trachea may deviate from the midline, breath sounds over such areas will be decreased, and percussion over involved lobes may be hyperresonant. Diagnostic studies of bronchogenic cysts are controversial. Chest radiograph can show air trapping and hyperinflation of the affected lobes or may show a spherical lesion with or without an air-fluid level. Yet, early detected or smaller lesions may not be seen on chest radiographs. CT scan is the preferred imaging study and can differentiate solid versus cystic mediastinal masses and define the cyst's relationship to the rest of the lung. A barium swallow can help determine whether the lesion communicates with the gastrointestinal tract. MRI and ultrasound are other imaging modalities utilized.

Treatment is surgical resection. Postoperatively, vigorous pulmonary physiotherapy is required to prevent complications (atelectasis or infection of the lung distal to the site of resection of the cyst).

McAdams HP et al: Bronchogenic cyst: Imaging features with clinical and histopathologic correlation. Radiology 2000;217:441 [PMID: 11058643].

Stewart B et al: Unusual case of stridor and wheeze in an infant: Tracheal bronchogenic cyst. Pediatric Pulmonol 2002;34:320 [PMID: 12205574].

ACQUIRED DISORDERS OF THE INTRATHORACIC AIRWAYS

FOREIGN BODY ASPIRATION

Aspiration of a foreign body into the respiratory tract is rarely observed, so it is the abrupt onset of cough, choking, or wheezing—especially in children who have access to high-risk objects such as peanuts, hard candy, and small toys—that suggests the diagnosis. Children age 6 months to 4 years are at highest risk, and many deaths are caused by respiratory obstruction each year.

1. Foreign Bodies in the Upper Respiratory Tract

The diagnosis is established by acute onset of choking along with *inability* to vocalize or cough and cyanosis with marked distress (complete obstruction), or with drooling, stridor, and *ability* to vocalize (partial obstruction).

Foreign bodies that lodge in the esophagus may compress the airway and cause respiratory distress. More typically, the foreign body lodges in the supra-glottic airway, triggering protective reflexes that result in laryngospasm. Onset is generally abrupt, with a history of the child running with food in the mouth or playing with seeds, small coins, toys, and the like. Poor child-proofing in the home and cases in which an older sibling feeds age-inappropriate foods (eg, peanuts, hard candy, or carrot slices) to the younger child are typical. Without treatment, progressive cyanosis, loss of consciousness, seizures, bradycardia, and cardiopulmonary arrest follow.

Treatment

The emergency treatment of upper airway obstruction due to foreign body aspiration is somewhat controversial. If *complete* obstruction is present, then one must intervene immediately. If partial obstruction is present, then the choking subject should be allowed to use their own cough reflex to extrude the foreign body. If after a brief observation period the obstruction increases or the airway becomes completely obstructed, acute intervention is required. The American Academy of Pediatrics and the American Heart Association distinguish between children younger than and older than age 1 year. A choking infant younger than age 1 year should be placed face down over the rescuer's arm, with the head positioned below the trunk. Five measured back blows are delivered rapidly between the infant's scapulas with the heel of the rescuer's hand. If obstruction persists, the infant should be rolled over and five rapid chest compressions performed (similar to cardiopulmonary resuscitation). This sequence is repeated until the obstruction is relieved. In a choking child older than age 1 year, abdominal thrusts (Heimlich maneuver) may be performed, with special care in younger children because of concern about possible intra-abdominal organ injury.

Blind finger sweeps should *not* be performed in infants or children because the finger may actually push the foreign body further into the airway causing further

obstruction. The airway may be opened by jaw thrust, and if the foreign body can be directly visualized, careful removal with the fingers or instruments (Magill forceps) can be attempted. Patients with persistent apnea and inability to achieve adequate ventilation may require emergency intubation, tracheostomy, or needle cricothyrotomy, depending on the setting and the rescuer's skills.

Hazinski MF (editor): *Pediatric Advanced Life Support Provider Manual.* American Heart Association and the American Academy of Pediatrics, 2002.

2. Foreign Bodies in the Lower Respiratory Tract

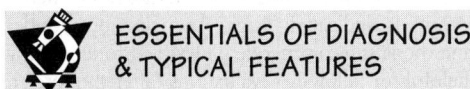

ESSENTIALS OF DIAGNOSIS & TYPICAL FEATURES

- *Sudden onset of coughing, wheezing, or respiratory distress.*
- *Asymmetrical physical findings of decreased breath sounds or localized wheezing.*
- *Asymmetrical radiographic findings, especially with forced expiratory view.*

Clinical Findings

A. SYMPTOMS AND SIGNS

Respiratory symptoms and signs vary depending on the site of obstruction and the duration following the acute episode. For example, a large or central airway obstruction may cause marked distress. The acute cough or wheezing caused by a foreign body in the lower respiratory tract may diminish over time only to recur later and present as chronic cough or persistent wheezing. Foreign body aspiration should be suspected in children with chronic cough, persistent wheezing, or recurrent pneumonia. Long-standing foreign bodies may lead to bronchiectasis or lung abscess. Hearing asymmetrical breath sounds or localized wheezing also suggests a foreign body.

B. IMAGING

Inspiratory and forced expiratory (obtained by manually compressing the abdomen during expiration) chest radiographs should be obtained if foreign body aspiration is suspected. Chest radiographs may be normal up to 25% of the time. If abnormal, the initial inspiratory view may show localized hyperinflation due to the ball-valve effect of the foreign body, causing distal air trapping or aeration within an area of atelectasis. A positive forced expiratory study shows a mediastinal shift away from the affected side. If airway obstruction is complete, atelectasis and related volume loss will be the major radiologic findings. Lateral decubitus views may be helpful if the child is too young to cooperate. Chest fluoroscopy is an alternative approach for detecting air trapping and mediastinal shift.

Treatment

When a foreign body is highly suspected, a normal chest radiograph should not rule out the possibility of an airway foreign body. If clinical suspicion persists based on two of three findings: history of possible aspiration, focal abnormal lung exam, or an abnormal chest radiograph, then a bronchoscopy is indicated. Rigid bronchoscopy under general anesthesia is recommended. Flexible bronchoscopy may be helpful for follow-up evaluations (after the foreign object has been removed).

Children with suspected acute foreign body aspiration should be admitted to the hospital for evaluation and treatment. Chest postural drainage is no longer recommended because the foreign body may become dislodged and obstruct a major central airway. Bronchoscopy should not be delayed in children with respiratory distress but should be performed as soon as the diagnosis is made—even in children with more chronic symptoms. Following the removal of the foreign body, β-adrenergic nebulization treatments followed by chest physiotherapy are recommended to help clear related mucus or treat bronchospasm. Failure to identify a foreign body in the lower respiratory tract can result in bronchiectasis and lung abscess. This risk justifies an aggressive approach to suspected foreign bodies in suspicious cases.

Chiu CY et al: Factors predicting early diagnosis of foreign body aspiration in children. Pediatr Emerg Care 2005;21:161.

Dunn GR et al: Management of suspected foreign body aspiration in children. Clin Otolaryngol 2002;27:384 [PMID: 12383302].

Girardi B et al: Two new radiographic findings to improve the diagnosis of bronchial foreign body aspiration in children. Pediatr Pulmonol 2004;38:261.

Rovin JD, Rodgers BM: Pediatric foreign body aspiration. Pediatr Rev 2000;21:86 [PMID: 10702322].

BRONCHIOLITIS

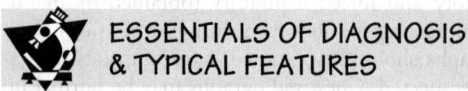

ESSENTIALS OF DIAGNOSIS & TYPICAL FEATURES

- Clinical syndrome characterized by coughing, tachypnea, labored breathing, and/or hypoxia.

- Irritability, poor feeding, vomiting.
- Wheezing and crackles on chest auscultation.

Bronchiolitis is the most common serious acute respiratory illness in infants and young children. One to three percent of infants with bronchiolitis will require hospitalization, especially during the winter months. The typical presentation is acute onset of tachypnea, cough, rhinorrhea, and expiratory wheezing. RSV is by far the most common viral cause of acute bronchiolitis. Parainfluenza, influenza, adenovirus, *Mycoplasma, Chlamydia, Ureaplasma,* and *Pneumocystis* are less common causes of bronchiolitis during early infancy. Major concerns include not only the acute effects of bronchiolitis but also the possible development of chronic airway hyperreactivity (asthma). Bronchiolitis due to RSV infection contributes substantially to morbidity and mortality in children with underlying medical disorders, including chronic lung disease of prematurity, cystic fibrosis, congenital heart disease, and immunodeficiency.

Clinical Findings

A. SYMPTOMS AND SIGNS

The usual course of RSV bronchiolitis is 1–2 days of fever, rhinorrhea, and cough, followed by wheezing, tachypnea, and respiratory distress. Typically the breathing pattern is shallow, with rapid respirations. Nasal flaring, cyanosis, retractions, and rales may be present, along with prolongation of the expiratory phase and wheezing, depending on the severity of illness. Some young infants present with apnea and few findings on auscultation but may subsequently develop rales, rhonchi, and expiratory wheezing.

B. LABORATORY FINDINGS

A viral nasal wash may be performed to identify the causative pathogen. The peripheral white blood cell count may be normal or may show a mild lymphocytosis.

C. IMAGING

Chest radiographic findings are generally nonspecific and typically include hyperinflation, peribronchial cuffing, increased interstitial markings, and subsegmental atelectasis.

Prevention & Treatment

The most effective prevention against RSV infection is to use proper hand-washing techniques and to reduce exposure to potential environmental risk factors. Major challenges have impeded the development of an RSV vaccine, but a licensed product may be expected in the near future. Prophylaxis with a monoclonal antibody (palivizumab) has proven effective in reducing the rate of hospitalization and associated morbidities in high-risk premature infants and those with chronic cardiopulmonary conditions.

Although most children with RSV bronchiolitis are readily treated as outpatients, hospitalization is frequently required in young infants (younger than 6 months of age) and in patients with hypoxemia on room air, a history of apnea, moderate tachypnea with feeding difficulties, marked respiratory distress with retractions, or underlying chronic cardiopulmonary disorders. Supportive strategies including frequent suctioning and providing adequate fluids to maintain hydration form the mainstays of treatment for bronchiolitis. If hypoxemia is present, supplemental oxygen should be administered. Although bronchodilators and corticosteroids may attenuate airway obstruction, their use remains controversial and empiric, and patients should be assessed individually to determine responsiveness.

In immunocompromised patients, especially bone marrow transplant recipients, a combination of RSV intravenous immune globulin and the antiviral ribavirin has been tried. Therapy for RSV, however, remains limited, controversial, and mostly supportive.

Prognosis

The prognosis for the majority of infants with acute bronchiolitis is very good. With improved supportive care and prophylaxis with palivizumab, the mortality rate among high-risk infants has decreased substantially.

Domachowske JB, Rosenberg HF: Advances in the treatment and prevention of severe viral bronchiolitis. Pediatr Ann 2005; 34:35 [PMID: 15693214].

Martinez FD: Respiratory syncytial virus bronchiolitis and the pathogenesis of childhood asthma. Pediatr Infect Dis J 2003;22(2 Suppl):S76 [PMID: 12671456].

Paes BA: Current strategies in the prevention of respiratory syncytial virus disease. Paediatr Respir Rev 2003;4:21 [PMID: 12615029].

DISORDERS OF MUCOCILIARY CLEARANCE

OVERVIEW OF MUCOCILIARY CLEARANCE

Mucociliary clearance is the primary defense mechanism for the lung. Inhaled particles including microbial pathogens are entrapped in mucus on the airway surface, then cleared by the coordinated action of cilia. The volume and composition of airway surface liquid influence the efficiency of ciliary function and mucus clearance. The two main genetic diseases of mucociliary clearance include disorders of ion transport (cystic fibrosis, CF), and disorders in ciliary function (primary ciliary dyskinesia, PCD).

CYSTIC FIBROSIS

ESSENTIALS OF DIAGNOSIS & TYPICAL FEATURES

- *Greasy, bulky, malodorous stools; failure to thrive.*
- *Recurrent respiratory infections.*
- *Digital clubbing on examination.*
- *Bronchiectasis on chest imaging.*
- *Sweat chloride > 60 mmol/L.*

General Considerations

Cystic fibrosis (CF), an autosomal recessive disease, is one of the most common lethal genetic diseases in the United States, with an incidence of approximately 1:3000 among whites. It is a major cause of pulmonary and gastrointestinal morbidity in children and a leading cause of death in early adulthood. Although CF is characterized by abnormalities in the hepatic, gastrointestinal, and male reproductive systems, lung disease is the major cause of morbidity and mortality. Almost all patients develop obstructive lung disease associated with chronic infection that leads to progressive loss of pulmonary function.

The cause of CF is a defect in a single gene on chromosome 7 that encodes a cyclic adenosine monophosphate–regulated chloride channel called the cystic fibrosis transmembrane conductance regulator. This regulator functions as an ion channel and controls the movement of salt and water into and out of epithelial cells lining the airways, biliary tree, intestines, vas deferens, sweat ducts, and pancreatic ducts. Over 1000 mutations in the CF gene have been identified. The most common mutation, ΔF508, is a deletion of three base pairs. This and other gene mutations lead to defects or deficiencies in the cystic fibrosis transmembrane conductance regulator, causing problems in salt and water movement across cell membranes, resulting in abnormally thick secretions in various organ systems.

Clinical Findings

A. SYMPTOMS AND SIGNS

Approximately 15% of newborns with CF present at birth with meconium ileus, a severe intestinal obstruction resulting from inspissation of tenacious meconium in the terminal ileum. Meconium ileus is virtually diagnostic of

CF, so the infant should be treated presumptively as having CF until a sweat test or genotyping can be obtained.

During infancy and beyond, a common presentation of CF is failure to thrive. These children fail to gain weight despite good appetite and typically have frequent, bulky, foul-smelling, oily stools. These symptoms are the result of severe exocrine pancreatic insufficiency, the failure of the pancreas to produce sufficient digestive enzymes to allow breakdown and absorption of fats and protein. Pancreatic insufficiency occurs in over 85% of persons with CF. Infants with undiagnosed CF may also present with hypoproteinemia with or without edema, anemia, and deficiency of the fat-soluble vitamins A, D, E, and K, because of ongoing steatorrhea.

Persons with CF frequently have respiratory symptoms that include a chronic productive cough, wheezing, and exercise intolerance. It is not uncommon for CF children to have recurrent pneumonias and/or bronchitis. Rales may be heard on physical examination. Digital clubbing also develops as the lung disease progresses. Older persons with CF intermittently experience pulmonary exacerbations consisting of signs and symptoms of increased cough and sputum production, increased dyspnea, poor appetite, weight loss, occasionally fever, fatigue, reduction in pulmonary function, increased hemoptysis, change in chest radiographic findings, or change in chest physical examination findings (increased rales or rhonchi, decreased air exchange, and increased use of accessory muscles of respiration). Such symptoms should prompt intensification of the antibiotic regimen.

CF lung disease is characterized by a cycle of chronic, persistent infections with CF-related pathogens and an excessive inflammatory response that progressively damages the airways and lung parenchyma. This results in a characteristic airflow obstruction on lung function testing and bronchiectasis on chest imaging (best demonstrated by high-resolution computed tomography scans). Airway infection with bacteria including *Staphylococcus aureus* and *Haemophilus influenzae* often begins in the first few months of life, even in asymptomatic infants. Eventually, *Pseudomonas aeruginosa* becomes the predominant pathogen. Acquisition of the characteristic mucoid *Pseudomonas* is associated with a more rapid decline in pulmonary function. In addition, infection with *Burkholderia cepacia* has been associated with rapid deterioration and death.

CF should also be considered in infants and children who present with severe dehydration and hypochloremic alkalosis. Other findings that should prompt a diagnostic evaluation for CF include unexplained bronchiectasis, rectal prolapse, nasal polyps, chronic sinusitis, and unexplained pancreatitis or cirrhosis.

B. DIAGNOSIS

The diagnosis of CF is made by a sweat chloride concentration greater than 60 mmol/L in the presence of some appropriate clinical manifestation (chronic pulmonary disease, pancreatic insufficiency, or both) or an appropriate family history (sibling or first cousin who has CF). The most acceptable type of sweat test is performed by iontophoresis of pilocarpine into the skin to stimulate sweating. Sweat then is collected and analyzed for chloride. This test should be performed at a CF Foundation–accredited laboratory. A diagnosis can also be confirmed by genotyping that reveals two alleles that have CF-causing mutations. Several states are now doing newborn screening for CF by measuring immunoreactive trypsin in blood. Most infants who have CF have elevated immunoreactive trypsin, but there are also many false-positive results. Therefore, diagnosis must be confirmed by sweat test or by genotyping.

Treatment

It is strongly recommended that individuals with CF be followed at a CF Foundation–accredited CF care center (www.cff.org).

The cornerstone of gastrointestinal treatment is pancreatic enzyme supplementation. Persons with CF are required to take pancreatic enzyme capsules immediately prior to each meal and with snacks. Occasionally, enzyme supplementation alone does not control the malabsorption, and antacids are added to the regimen. Individuals should also take daily multivitamins that contain vitamins A, D, E, and K. Moreover, caloric supplements are often added to the patient's diet to optimize growth.

Airway clearance therapy and aggressive antibiotic use form the mainstays of treatment for CF lung disease. Antibiotic therapy appears to be one of the primary reasons for the increased life expectancy of persons with CF. Three evidence-based medications that are now routinely used in many persons with CF are an inhaled mucolytic agent, recombinant human DNase (Pulmozyme), inhaled tobramycin (TOBI), and oral azithromycin for those with chronic *Pseudomonas* infection. These therapies have been shown to maintain lung function and reduce the need for hospitalizations and intravenous antibiotics. Bronchodilators and anti-inflammatory therapies are also frequently used.

Prognosis

A few decades ago, CF was fatal in early childhood. Now the median life expectancy is around 34 years of age. The rate of progression of lung involvement usually determines survival. Lung transplantation may be performed in those with end-stage lung disease. In addition, new treatments, including gene therapy trials and agents that modulate cystic fibrosis transmembrane conductance regulator protein function, are being developed based on improved understanding of the disease at the cellular and molecular levels.

Gibson RL et al: Pathophysiology and management of pulmonary infections in cystic fibrosis. Am J Respir Crit Care Med 2003;168:918 [PMID: 14555458].

Ratjen F, Doring G: Cystic fibrosis. Lancet 2003;361:681 [PMID: 12606185].

PRIMARY CILIARY DYSKINESIA

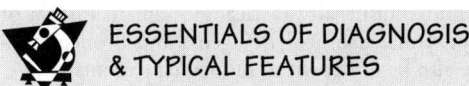

ESSENTIALS OF DIAGNOSIS & TYPICAL FEATURES

- *Chronic bronchitis, sinusitis, and otitis.*
- *Situs inversus in ~ 50% of cases.*
- *Respiratory distress in the newborn period.*
- *Consistent ultrastructural defect of cilia demonstrated by electron microscopy.*

General Considerations

Primary ciliary dyskinesia (PCD), also known as immotile cilia syndrome or Kartagener syndrome, is a human genetic disease associated with abnormal ciliary structure and function. Occurring in approximately 1 in 15,000 births, PCD is an inherited disease that causes impaired clearance of bacteria from the lung, paranasal sinuses, and middle ear. Half of the patients with PCD have their internal organs reversed (situs abnormalities), and men are usually infertile.

Clinical Findings

A. SYMPTOMS AND SIGNS

Children with PCD have a variety of clinical features including chronic productive cough, wheezing, nasal congestion and rhinorrhea, chronic sinusitis, bronchitis and pneumonias. Recurrent, chronic otitis media is a serious problem, and hearing loss is common. A history of transient neonatal respiratory distress and unexplained atelectasis is frequently elicited. Approximately 50% of PCD patients have situs inversus totalis, which suggests a role for embryonic cilia in the rotation of internal organs. The diagnosis of PCD should also be considered in any patients with unexplained bronchiectasis or in males with infertility issues.

B. DIAGNOSIS

The diagnosis of PCD currently requires a compatible clinical phenotype and abnormal ciliary ultrastructure by electron microscopy. Cilia samples are usually obtained from either the upper airways (nasal passage) or lower airways (trachea) and then examined by trans-

mission electron micrography. Significant expertise is required to produce high-quality transmission electron micrographs of cilia, and to interpret primary versus secondary defects in ciliary ultrastructure. Functional assessments of cilia consist of crude measures of nasal mucociliary clearance (the saccharin test), or measures of lung mucociliary clearance, using radioisotopic techniques. The current limitations in diagnosis of PCD provide a compelling case for an extensive effort to define disease-causing genetic mutations, which will allow great improvement in the identification and diagnosis of PCD through genetic testing.

Treatment

At present, no specific therapies are available to correct the ciliary dysfunction in PCD. Management at present includes aggressive airway clearance therapy, and frequent courses of antibiotics to treat bacterial infections in the airways, sinuses, and middle ear. No randomized clinical trials have been conducted in this disease because it is so rare and most centers follow only a few PCD patients. In order to better define the pathogenesis of PCD and study treatments in this population, a consortium of four national sites has been created through funding from the National Institutes of Health and Office of Rare Diseases (www.rarediseasesnetwork.org).

Prognosis

The progression of lung disease in PCD is quite variable and for most affected individuals is less severe than in CF. Importantly, though, persons with PCD are at risk for chronic lung disease with bronchiectasis. With monitoring and aggressive treatment during times of illness, most individuals with PCD should experience a normal or near-normal lifespan.

Bush A, O'Callaghan C: Primary ciliary dyskinesia. Arch Dis Child 2002;87:363 [PMID: 12390901].

Noone PG et al: Primary ciliary dyskinesia: diagnostic and phenotypic features. Am J Respir Crit Care Med 2004;169:459 [PMID: 14656747].

BRONCHIECTASIS

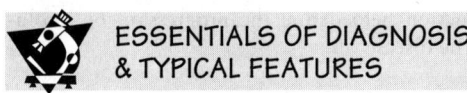

ESSENTIALS OF DIAGNOSIS & TYPICAL FEATURES

- *Chronic cough with sputum production.*
- *Rhonchi and/or wheezes on chest auscultation.*
- *Diagnosis confirmed by high-resolution CT scan.*

General Considerations

Bronchiectasis is the permanent dilation of bronchi. The dilation may be regular, with the airway continuing to have a smooth outline (cylindric bronchiectasis); irregular, with areas of dilation and constriction (varicose bronchiectasis); or marked, with destruction of structural components of the airway wall (saccular or cystic bronchiectasis).

Bronchiectasis results from airway obstruction by retained mucus secretions or inflammation in response to chronic or repeated infection. It occurs either as a consequence of a preceding illness (severe pneumonia or foreign body aspiration) or as a manifestation of an underlying systemic disorder (cystic fibrosis, primary ciliary dyskinesia, or immunodeficiency).

Clinical Findings

A. SYMPTOMS AND SIGNS

Persons with bronchiectasis will typically have chronic cough, purulent sputum, fever, and weight loss. Recurrent respiratory infections and dyspnea on exertion are also common. Hemoptysis occurs less frequently in children than in adults with bronchiectasis. On physical examination, finger clubbing may be seen. Rales, rhonchi, and decreased air entry are often noted over the bronchiectatic areas.

B. LABORATORY FINDINGS AND IMAGING

Cultures from the lower respiratory tract usually reveal normal oropharyngeal flora. These include *Streptococcus pneumoniae, Staphylococcus aureus,* and nontypable *H influenzae. Pseudomonas aeruginosa* can also be found in children with bronchiectasis, even in those without CF.

Chest radiographs may be mildly abnormal with slightly increased bronchovascular markings or areas of atelectasis, or they may demonstrate cystic changes in one or more areas of the lung. The extent of bronchiectasis is best defined by high-resolution CT scan of the lung, which often reveals far wider involvement of lung than expected from the plain chest radiograph. Pulmonary function testing often reveals airflow obstruction. Evaluation of lung function after use of a bronchodilator is helpful in assessing the benefit a patient may have from bronchodilators. Serial assessments of lung function help define the progression or resolution of the disease.

Differential Diagnosis

Bronchiectasis has numerous causes. It can occur following severe respiratory tract infections by bacteria (*Bordetella pertussis*), viruses (adenovirus), or other organisms (*Mycobacterium tuberculosis*). Bronchiectasis is commonly seen in persons with CF, PCD, immuno-

deficiency, and collagen vascular conditions. Other diagnostic considerations include foreign body aspiration, chronic aspiration of gastric or oropharyngeal contents, and allergic bronchopulmonary aspergillosis.

Treatment

Aggressive antibiotic therapy during pulmonary exacerbations and routine airway clearance are mainstays of treatment. Inhaled mucolytic agents and bronchodilators may also be of benefit in individual patients.

Surgical removal of an area of lung affected with severe bronchiectasis is considered when the response to medical therapy is poor. Other indications for operation include severe localized disease, repeated hemoptysis, and recurrent pneumonia in one area of lung. If bronchiectasis is widespread, surgical resection offers little advantage.

Prognosis

The prognosis depends on the underlying cause and severity of bronchiectasis, the extent of lung involvement, and the response to medical management. Good pulmonary hygiene and avoidance of infectious complications in the involved areas of lung may reverse cylindric bronchiectasis.

Barker AF: Bronchiectasis. N Engl J Med 2002;346:1383 [PMID: 11986413].

Chang AB et al: Non-CF bronchiectasis: Clinical and HRCT evaluation. Pediatr Pulmonol 2003;35:477 [PMID: 12746947].

BRONCHIOLITIS OBLITERANS

Bronchiolitis obliterans is characterized by obstruction of bronchi and bronchioles by fibrous tissue. The disorder follows damage to the lower respiratory tract, such as inhalation of toxic gases, infections (adenovirus, influenza virus, rubeola virus, *Bordetella,* or *Mycoplasma*), connective tissue diseases, transplantation, and aspiration. Bronchiolitis obliterans may also develop in children who have Stevens-Johnson syndrome with pulmonary involvement. Many cases of bronchiolitis obliterans are idiopathic. Adenovirus-induced bronchiolitis obliterans occurs more frequently in the Native American population.

Clinical Findings

A. SYMPTOMS AND SIGNS

Bronchiolitis obliterans should be considered when persistent cough, wheezing, or sputum production is present after an episode of acute pneumonia. Prolonged rales or wheezing or persistent exercise intolerance following a pulmonary insult should also suggest this disease.

B. Laboratory Findings and Imaging

Chest radiograph abnormalities include evidence of localized or generalized air trapping as well as (in some cases) nodular densities and alveolar opacification. Scattered areas of matched decreases in ventilation and perfusion are seen when the lung is scanned. Pulmonary angiograms reveal decreased vasculature in involved lung, and bronchograms show marked pruning of the bronchial tree. An assessment of lung function demonstrates an obstructive process that may be combined with evidence of restriction. Inhaled bronchodilators or corticosteroids provide little improvement in lung function.

Differential Diagnosis

Poorly treated asthma, CF, and bronchopulmonary dysplasia must be considered in children with persistent airway obstruction. A trial of medications (including bronchodilators and corticosteroids) may help to determine the reversibility of the process when the primary differential is between asthma and bronchiolitis obliterans. Although the results of imaging and pulmonary function testing are very suggestive, the most definitive way to establish a diagnosis is by lung biopsy.

Complications

Sequelae of bronchiolitis obliterans include persistent airway obstruction, recurrent wheezing, bronchiectasis, chronic atelectasis, recurrent pneumonia, and unilateral hyperlucent lung syndrome.

Treatment

Supplemental oxygen should be given to patients with oxygen desaturation during normal activities or sleep. In addition, early treatment should be directed at preventing ongoing airway damage due to problems such as aspiration, which may be either the primary insult or an acquired problem secondary to marked hyperinflation. The effectiveness of other forms of treatment may be more difficult to evaluate. Oral and inhaled bronchodilators may reverse airway obstruction if the disease has a reactive component. Many children also receive at least one course of corticosteroid treatment in an attempt to reverse the obstruction or prevent ongoing damage. Antibiotics should be used as indicated for pneumonia.

Prognosis

Prognosis may depend in part on the underlying cause as well as the age at which the insult occurred. The course varies from mild asthma-like symptoms to rapidly fatal deterioration despite therapy.

Kurland G, Michelson P: Bronchiolitis obliterans in children. Pediatr Pulmonol 2005;39:193 [PMID: 15635614].

BRONCHOPULMONARY DYSPLASIA

 **ESSENTIALS OF DIAGNOSIS & TYPICAL FEATURES**

- *Acute respiratory distress in the first week of life.*
- *Required oxygen therapy or mechanical ventilation, with persistent oxygen requirement at 36 weeks gestational age.*
- *Persistent respiratory abnormalities, including physical signs and radiographic findings.*

General Considerations

Bronchopulmonary dysplasia (BPD) remains one of the most significant sequelae of acute respiratory distress in the neonatal intensive care unit, with an incidence of about 30% for infants with a birth weight of less than 1000 g. This disease was first characterized in 1967 when Northway and coworkers reported the clinical, radiologic, and pathologic findings in a group of premature newborns that required prolonged mechanical ventilation and oxygen therapy to treat hyaline membrane disease. The progression from acute hyaline membrane disease to chronic lung disease was divided into four stages: acute respiratory distress shortly after birth, usually hyaline membrane disease (stage I); clinical and radiographic worsening of the acute lung disease, often due to increased pulmonary blood flow secondary to a patent ductus arteriosus (stage II); and progressive signs of chronic lung disease (stages III and IV). The pathologic findings and clinical course of BPD in recent years have changed due to a combination of new therapies (surfactants, prenatal glucocorticoids, and different ventilation strategies) and increased survival of infants born at earlier gestational ages. Although the incidence of BPD has not changed, the severity of the lung disease has decreased. Pathologically this "new" BPD is characterized by a reduction in inflammation, decreased alveolar number, and a dysmorphic vascular structure.

A recent summary of a National Institutes of Health workshop on BPD proposes a definition of the disease that includes oxygen requirement for more than 28 days, a history of positive pressure ventilation or continuous positive airway pressure, and gestational age. The new definition accommodates several key observations regarding the disease, including: (1) although most of these children were premature and had hyaline membrane disease, full-term newborns with such disorders as meconium aspiration or persistent pulmonary hypertension can also develop bronchopulmonary dysplasia; (2) some extremely preterm newborns require minimal ventilator support yet subsequently develop a prolonged oxygen requirement despite the absence of severe acute manifestations of respiratory failure; (3) newborns dying within the first weeks of life can already have the aggressive, fibroproliferative pathologic lesions that resemble bronchopulmonary dysplasia; and (4) physiologic abnormalities (increased airway resistance) and biochemical markers of lung injury (altered protease:antiprotease ratios, and increased inflammatory cells and mediators), which may be predictive of bronchopulmonary dysplasia, are already present in the first week of life.

The precise mechanism that results in the development of BPD is unclear. The premature lung makes insufficient functional surfactant; furthermore, the antioxidant defense mechanisms are not sufficiently mature to protect the lung from the toxic oxygen metabolites generated from therapeutic hyperoxia treatment. Lungs destined to develop BPD show early inflammation and hypercellularity followed by healing with fibrosis. Thus abnormal lung mechanics due to structural immaturity, surfactant deficiency, atelectasis, and pulmonary edema—plus lung injury secondary to hyperoxia and mechanical ventilation—lead to further abnormalities of lung function, causing increases in ventilator and oxygen requirements and resulting in a vicious cycle that compounds the progression of lung injury. Excessive fluid administration, patent ductus arteriosus, pulmonary interstitial emphysema, pneumothorax, infection, pulmonary hypertension, and inflammatory stimuli secondary to lung injury or infection also play important roles in the pathogenesis of the disease. Although the exact mechanisms leading to chronic lung disease are not completely understood, bronchopulmonary dysplasia represents the consequences of lung injury caused by oxygen toxicity, barotrauma, and inflammation superimposed on a susceptible, generally immature lung.

Differential Diagnosis

The radiologic appearance of BPD is changing, and severe chronic lung findings of fibrosis with infiltrate are less common. The changes in severe BPD necessitate ruling out meconium aspiration syndrome, congenital infection (eg, with cytomegalovirus or *Ureaplasma*), cystic adenomatoid malformation, recurrent aspiration, pulmonary lymphangiectasia, total anomalous pulmonary venous return, overhydration, and idiopathic pulmonary fibrosis.

Clinical Course & Treatment

The clinical course of infants with bronchopulmonary dysplasia ranges from a mild increased oxygen require-

ment that gradually resolves over a few months to more severe disease requiring chronic tracheostomy and mechanical ventilation for the first 2 years of life. In general, patients show slow, steady improvements in oxygen or ventilator requirements but can have frequent respiratory exacerbations leading to frequent and prolonged hospitalizations. Clinical management generally includes careful attention to growth, nutrition (caloric requirements of infants with oxygen dependence and respiratory distress are quite high), metabolic status, developmental and neurologic status, and related problems, along with the various cardiopulmonary abnormalities described in a later discussion.

Short courses of postnatal glucocorticoid therapy have been helpful in increasing the success of weaning from the ventilator. This therapy is controversial, however, because data show decreased alveolarization in preterm and postnatal animals given long courses of corticosteroids. Longer courses of postnatal glucocorticoids have been linked to an increased incidence of cerebral palsy. Inhaled glucocorticoids may help reduce the need for systemic steroids, but the overall incidence of bronchopulmonary dysplasia has not been affected. Early use of surfactant therapy with adequate lung recruitment increases the chance for survival without bronchopulmonary dysplasia and can decrease the overall mortality and reduce the need for ventilation. Thus early interventions are important prior to the development of bronchopulmonary dysplasia to decrease morbidity and mortality. Ongoing studies of the imbalance of proteolytic enzymes, elastolytic lung damage, and the role of specific anti-inflammatory medications during the early development of bronchopulmonary dysplasia are needed.

Because increased airway resistance and bronchial hyperreactivity are common in affected infants, inhaled corticosteroids together with occasional use of β-adrenergic agonists are commonly part of the treatment plan. Part of the rationale for the use of corticosteroids is to decrease lung inflammation and enhance responsiveness to β-adrenergic drugs, as in the treatment of severe asthma. β-Adrenergic agonists followed by chest physiotherapy are often used for the thick secretions that may contribute to airway obstruction or recurrent atelectasis.

Although bronchial hyperreactivity in affected infants is well recognized, structural lesions (eg, subglottic stenosis, vocal cord paralysis, tracheal stenosis, tracheomalacia, bronchial stenosis, and granulomatous bronchial polyps) often contribute to airflow limitation. Children with significant stridor, sleep apnea, chronic wheezing, or excessive respiratory distress need diagnostic bronchoscopy. In addition, the contribution of gastroesophageal reflux and aspiration should be considered in the face of worsening chronic lung disease.

Infants often have recurrent pulmonary edema, which may be due to increased permeability of the injured pulmonary circulation or to increases in hydrostatic pressure if left ventricular dysfunction is present. Salt and water retention secondary to chronic hypoxemia, hypercapnia, or other stimuli may be present. Chronic or intermittent diuretic therapy is commonly used if rales or signs of persistent pulmonary edema are present and clinical studies show acute improvement in lung function. Unfortunately, diuretics often have adverse effects, including severe volume contraction, hypokalemia, alkalosis, and hyponatremia. Potassium and arginine chloride supplements are commonly required.

Infants with BPD are at risk of developing pulmonary hypertension, and in many of these children even mild hypoxemia can cause significant elevations of pulmonary arterial pressure. To minimize the harmful effects of hypoxemia, the arterial oxygen saturation should be kept above 93%, with care to avoid hyperoxia during retinal vascular development. Electrocardiographic and echocardiographic studies should be performed to monitor for the development of right ventricular hypertrophy. If hypertrophy persists or if it develops where it was not previously present, intermittent hypoxemia should be considered and further assessments of oxygenation pursued, especially while the infant sleeps. Even intermittent hypoxia contributes to the development or progression of pulmonary hypertension and cor pulmonale; therefore, noninvasive assessments of oxygenation must be made during all activities, including the infant's waking, sleeping, and feeding periods. Infants with a history of intubation can develop obstructive sleep apnea secondary to a high-arched palate or subglottic narrowing. Barium swallow, esophageal pH probe studies, bronchoscopy, and cardiac catheterization will diagnose unsuspected cardiac or pulmonary lesions that contribute to the underlying pathophysiology, such as aspiration, tracheomalacia, obstructive sleep apnea, and anatomic cardiac lesions. Long-term care should include monitoring for systemic hypertension and the development of left ventricular hypertrophy.

Nutritional problems in infants may be due to increased oxygen consumption, feeding difficulties, gastroesophageal reflux, and chronic hypoxemia. Hypercaloric formulas and gastrostomies are often required to ensure adequate intake while avoiding overhydration. Influenza vaccination is recommended. With the onset of acute wheezing secondary to suspected viral infection, rapid diagnostic testing for RSV infection may facilitate early treatment. Immune prophylaxis of RSV reduces the morbidity of bronchiolitis in infants with bronchopulmonary dysplasia.

For children who remain ventilator-dependent, attempts should be made to maintain $PaCO_2$ below 60 mm Hg—even when pH is normal—because of the potential adverse effects of hypercapnia on salt and water retention, cardiac function, and perhaps pulmonary vascular tone. Changes in ventilator settings in children with severe lung disease should be slow, because the effects of many of the changes may not be apparent for days. These signs may include poor feeding, irritability, weight loss, vomiting, increased retractions, wheezing, increased somnolence, and CO_2 retention. Medical staff should meet frequently with the parents to review progress and changes in treatment plans and thereby ease some of the family stresses involved in caring for a child who has a chronic disease. Patience, continued family support, attention to developmental issues, and speech and physical therapy help to improve the long-term outlook.

Prognosis

Surfactant replacement therapy has had a significant effect on reducing morbidity and mortality from bronchopulmonary dysplasia. Infants of younger gestational age are surviving in greater numbers. Surprisingly, the effect of neonatal care has not decreased the incidence of bronchopulmonary dysplasia significantly, as half the survivors go on to develop this diagnosis. The disorder typically develops in the most immature infants, but the long-term outlook for most survivors is generally favorable. Long-term follow-up studies suggest that lung function may be altered for life. Hyperinflation and damage to small airways has been reported in children 10 years out from the first signs of bronchopulmonary dysplasia. In addition, these infants are at a higher risk for developing such sequelae as persistent airway hyperreactivity, exercise intolerance, pulmonary hypertension, increased risk for chronic obstructive pulmonary disease, and perhaps abnormal lung growth. As smaller, more immature infants survive, abnormal neurodevelopmental outcomes become more likely. The incidence of cerebral palsy, hearing loss, vision abnormalities, spastic diplegia, and developmental delays is increased. Feeding abnormalities, behavior difficulties, and increased irritability have all been reported. Finally, children with bronchopulmonary dysplasia frequently develop airway obstruction, hyperreactive airways, and decreased oxygen saturation during exercise. This should be taken into account for children residing at higher altitudes. A focus on good nutrition, prophylaxis against respiratory pathogens and airway hyperreactivity, and attention to school performance continue to provide the best outcomes.

Allen J et al and the American Thoracic Society: Statement on the care of the child with chronic lung disease of infancy and childhood. Am J Respir Crit Care Med 2003;168:356 [PMID: 12888611].

Bancalari E et al: Bronchopulmonary dysplasia: Changes in pathogenesis, epidemiology and definition. Semin Neonatol 2003;8:63 [PMID: 12667831].

Coalson JJ: Pathology of new bronchopulmonary dysplasia. Semin Neonatol 2003;8:73 [PMID 12667832].

Cole CH: Inhaled glucocorticoid therapy in infants at risk for neonatal chronic lung disease. J Asthma 2000;37:533 [PMID: 11060660].

Jobe AH, Bancalari E: Bronchopulmonary dysplasia. Am J Respir Crit Care Med 2001;163:1723 [PMID: 11401896].

Jobe AH, Ikegami M: Prevention of bronchopulmonary dysplasia. Curr Opin Pediatr 2001;13:124 [PMID: 11317052].

Kresch MJ, Clive JM: Meta-analysis of surfactant replacement therapy of infants with birth weights less than 2000 grams. J Perinatol 1998;18:276 [PMID: 9730197].

Northway WH et al: Pulmonary disease following respiratory therapy of hyaline membrane disease: Bronchopulmonary dysplasia. N Engl J Med 1967;276:357 [PMID: 5334613].

Parker TA, Abman SH: The pulmonary circulation in bronchopulmonary dysplasia. Semin Neonatol 2003;8:51 [PMID: 12667830].

Saugstad OD: Bronchopulmonary dysplasia—Oxidative stress and antioxidants. Semin Neonatol 2003;8:39 [PMID: 12667829].

Speer CP: Inflammation and bronchopulmonary dysplasia. Semin Neonatol 2003;8:29 [PMID: 12667828].

CONGENITAL MALFORMATIONS OF THE LUNG

What follows is a brief description of selected congenital pulmonary malformations.

PULMONARY AGENESIS & HYPOPLASIA

With unilateral pulmonary agenesis (complete absence of one lung), the trachea continues into a main bronchus and often has complete tracheal rings. The left lung is affected more often than the right. With compensatory postnatal growth, the remaining lung often herniates into the contralateral chest. Chest radiographs show a mediastinal shift toward the affected side, and vertebral abnormalities may be present. Absent or incomplete lung development may be associated with other congenital abnormalities, such as absence of one or both kidneys or fusion of ribs, and the outcome is primarily related to the severity of associated lesions. About 50% of patients survive; the mortality rate is higher with agenesis of the right lung than of the left lung. This difference is probably not related to the higher incidence of associated anomalies but rather to a greater shift in the mediastinum that leads to tracheal compression and distortion of vascular structures.

Pulmonary hypoplasia is incomplete development of one or both lungs, characterized by a reduction in alveolar number and a reduction in airway branches. Pulmonary hypoplasia is present in up to 10–15% of perinatal autopsies. The hypoplasia can be a result of an intrathoracic mass, resulting in lack of space for the lungs to grow; decreased size of the thorax; decreased fetal breathing movements; decreased blood flow to the lungs; or possibly a primary mesodermal defect affecting multiple organ systems. Congenital diaphragmatic hernia is the most common cause, with an incidence of 1:2200 births. Other causes include extralobar sequestration, diaphragmatic eventration or hypoplasia, thoracic neuroblastoma, fetal hydrops, and fetal hydrochylothorax. Chest cage abnormalities, diaphragmatic elevation, oligohydramnios, chromosomal abnormalities, severe musculoskeletal disorders, and cardiac lesions may also result in hypoplastic lungs. Postnatal factors may play important roles. For example, infants with advanced bronchopulmonary dysplasia can have pulmonary hypoplasia.

Clinical Findings

A. SYMPTOMS AND SIGNS

The clinical presentation is highly variable and is related to the severity of hypoplasia as well as associated abnormalities. Lung hypoplasia is often associated with pneumothorax. Some newborns present with perinatal stress, severe acute respiratory distress, and persistent pulmonary hypertension of the newborn secondary to primary pulmonary hypoplasia (without associated anomalies). Children with lesser degrees of hypoplasia may present with chronic cough, tachypnea, wheezing, and recurrent pneumonia.

B. LABORATORY FINDINGS AND IMAGING

Chest radiographic findings include variable degrees of volume loss in a small hemithorax with mediastinal shift. Pulmonary agenesis should be suspected if tracheal deviation is evident on the chest radiograph. The chest CT scan is the optimal diagnostic imaging procedure if the chest radiograph is not definitive. Ventilation-perfusion scans, angiography, and bronchoscopy are often helpful in the evaluation, demonstrating decreased pulmonary vascularity or premature blunting of airways associated with the maldeveloped lung tissue. The degree of respiratory impairment is defined by analysis of arterial blood gases.

Treatment & Prognosis

Treatment is supportive. The outcome is determined by the severity of underlying medical problems, the extent of the hypoplasia, and the degree of pulmonary hypertension.

Chinoy MR: Pulmonary hypoplasia and congenital diaphragmatic hernia: Advances in the pathogenetics and regulation of lung development. J Surg Res 2002;106:209 [PMID: 12127828].

Laudy JA, Wladimiroff JW: The fetal lung. 2: Pulmonary hypoplasia. Ultrasound Obstet Gynecol 2000;16:482 [PMID: 11169336].

Nowotny T et al: Right-sided pulmonary aplasia: longitudinal lung function studies in two cases and comparison to results from term healthy neonates. Pediatr Pulmonol 1998;26:138 [PMID: 9727767].

Winn HN et al: Neonatal pulmonary hypoplasia and perinatal mortality in patients with midtrimester rupture of amniotic membranes—a critical analysis. Am J Obstet Gynecol 2000;182:1638 [PMID: 10871491].

PULMONARY SEQUESTRATION

Pulmonary sequestration is nonfunctional pulmonary tissue that does not communicate with the tracheobronchial tree and receives its blood supply from one or more anomalous systemic arteries. This abnormality originates during the embryonic period of lung development. It is classified as either extralobar or intralobar. Extralobar sequestration is a mass of pulmonary parenchyma anatomically separate from the normal lung, with a distinct pleural investment. Its blood supply derives from the systemic circulation (more typical), from pulmonary vessels, or from both. Rarely it communicates with the esophagus or stomach. Pathologically, extralobar sequestration appears as a solitary thoracic lesion near the diaphragm. Abdominal sites are rare. Size varies from 0.5–12 cm. The left side is involved in over 90% of cases. In contrast to intralobar sequestrations, venous drainage is usually through the systemic or portal venous system.

Histologic findings include uniformly dilated bronchioles, alveolar ducts, and alveoli. Occasionally the bronchial structure appears normal; however, often the cartilage in the wall is deficient, or no cartilage-containing structures can be found. Lymphangiectasia is sometimes found within the lesion. Extralobar sequestration can be associated with other anomalies, including bronchogenic cysts, heart defects, and diaphragmatic hernia, the latter occurring in over half of cases.

Intralobar sequestration is an isolated segment of lung within the normal pleural investment that often receives blood from one or more arteries arising from the aorta or its branches. Intralobar sequestration is usually found within the lower lobes (98%), two-thirds are found on the left side, and it is rarely associated with other congenital anomalies (less than 2% versus 50% with extralobar sequestration). It rarely presents in the newborn period (unlike extralobar sequestration). Some researchers have hypothesized that intralobar sequestration is an acquired lesion secondary to chronic infection. Clinical presentation includes chronic cough, wheezing, or recurrent pneumonias. Rarely, patients with intralobar sequestration can present with hemoptysis. Diagnosis is often made by angiography, which shows large systemic arteries perfusing the lesion. Recently, spiral CT scans with contrast or magnetic resonance angiography have proven useful in identifying anomalous systemic arterial supply to the lung. Treatment is usually by surgical resection.

Alton H: Pulmonary vascular imaging. Paediatr Respir Rev 2001; 2:227 [PMID: 12052324].

Blesovsky A: Pulmonary sequestration. A report of an unusual case and a review of the literature. Thorax 1967;22:351 [PMID: 6035799].

Conran RM, Stocker JT: Extralobar sequestration with frequently associated congenital cystic adenomatoid malformation, type 2: Report of 50 cases. Pediatr Dev Pathol 1999;2:454 [PMID: 10441623].

Halkic N et al: Pulmonary sequestration: A review of 26 cases. Eur J Cardiothorac Surg 1998;14:127 [PMID: 9754996].

Salmons S: Pulmonary sequestration. Neonatal Netw 2000;19:27 [PMID: 11949021].

Zylak CJ et al: Developmental lung anomalies in the adult: Radiologic-pathologic correlation. Radiographics 2002;22(Spec No):S25 [PMID: 12376599].

CONGENITAL LOBAR EMPHYSEMA

Patients with congenital lobar emphysema—also known as infantile lobar emphysema, congenital localized emphysema, unilobar obstructive emphysema, congenital hypertrophic lobar emphysema, or congenital lobar overinflation—present most commonly with severe neonatal respiratory distress or progressive respiratory impairment during the first year of life. Rarely the mild or intermittent nature of the symptoms in older children or young adults results in delayed diagnosis. Most patients are white males. Although the cause of congenital lobar emphysema is not well understood, some lesions show bronchial cartilaginous dysplasia due to abnormal orientation or distribution of the bronchial cartilage. This leads to expiratory collapse, producing obstruction and the symptoms outlined in the following discussion.

Clinical Findings

A. SYMPTOMS AND SIGNS

Clinical features include tachypnea, cyanosis, wheezing, retractions, and cough. Breath sounds are reduced on the affected side, perhaps with hyperresonance to percussion, mediastinal displacement, and bulging of the chest wall on the affected side.

B. IMAGING

Radiologic findings include overdistention of the affected lobe (usually an upper or middle lobe; > 99%), with wide separation of bronchovascular markings, collapse of adjacent lung, shift of the mediastinum away from the affected side, and a depressed diaphragm on the affected side. The radiographic diagnosis may be confusing in the newborn because of retention of alveolar fluid in the affected lobe causing the appearance of a homogeneous density. Other diagnostic studies include chest radiograph with fluoroscopy, ventilation-perfusion study, and chest CT scan followed by bronchoscopy, angiography, and exploratory thoracotomy.

Differential Diagnosis

The differential diagnosis of congenital lobar emphysema includes pneumothorax, pneumatocele, atelectasis with compensatory hyperinflation, diaphragmatic hernia, and congenital cystic adenomatoid malformation. The most common site of involvement is the left upper lobe (42%) or right middle lobe (35%). Evaluation must differentiate regional obstructive emphysema from lobar hyperinflation secondary to an uncomplicated ball-valve mechanism due to extrinsic compression from a mass (ie, bronchogenic cyst, tumor, lymphadenopathy, foreign body, pseudotumor or plasma cell granuloma, or vascular compression) or intrinsic obstruction from a mucus plug due to infection and inflammation from various causes.

Treatment

When respiratory distress is marked, a segmental or complete lobectomy is usually required. Less symptomatic older children may do equally well with or without lobectomy.

Al-Bassam A et al: Congenital cystic disease of the lung in infants and children (experience with 57 cases). Eur J Pediatr Surg 1999;9:364 [PMID: 10661844].

Babu R et al: Prenatal sonographic features of congenital lobar emphysema. Fetal Diagn Ther 2001;16:200 [PMID: 11399878].

Horak E et al: Congenital cystic lung disease: Diagnostic and therapeutic considerations. Clin Pediatr 2003;42:251 [PMID: 12739924].

Mandelbaum I et al: Congenital lobar obstructive emphysema: Report of eight cases and literature review. Ann Surg 1965;162:1075 [PMID: 5845589].

Ozcelik U et al: Congenital lobar emphysema: Evaluation and long-term follow-up of thirty cases at a single center. Pediatr Pulmonol 2003;35:384 [PMID: 12687596].

CONGENITAL CYSTIC ADENOMATOID MALFORMATION

Patients with congenital cystic adenomatoid malformations, which are unilateral hamartomatous lesions, generally present with marked respiratory distress within the first days of life. This disorder accounts for 95% of cases of congenital cystic lung disease.

Right and left lungs are involved with equal frequency. These lesions originate during the first 4–6 weeks of gestation during the embryonic period of lung development. These lesions appear as glandlike space-occupying masses or have an increase in terminal respiratory structures, forming intercommunicating cysts of various sizes, lined by cuboidal or ciliated pseudostratified columnar epithelium. They may have polypoid formations of mucosa, with focally increased elastic tissue in the cyst wall beneath the bronchial type of epithelium. Air passages appear malformed and tend to lack cartilage.

There are three types of such malformations. Type 1 is most common (55%) and consists of single or multiple large cysts (> 2 cm in diameter) with features of mature lung tissue. Type 1 is amenable to surgical resection. A mediastinal shift is evident on examination or chest radiograph in 80% of patients and can mimic infantile lobar emphysema. Approximately 75% of type 1 lesions are on the right side. A survival rate of 90% is generally reported.

Type 2 lesions (40% of cases) consist of multiple small cysts (< 2 cm) resembling dilated simple bronchioles and are often (60%) associated with other anomalies, especially renal agenesis or dysgenesis, cardiac malformations, and intestinal atresia. Approximately 60% of type 2 lesions are on the left side. Mediastinal shift is evident less often (10%) than in type 1, and the survival rate is worse (40%).

Type 3 lesions consist of small cysts (< 0.5 cm). They appear as bulky, firm masses. The reported survival rate is 50%.

Recently, two additional types have been described: type 0, a malformation of the proximal tracheobronchial tree (incompatible with life), and type 4, a malformation of the distal acinus. Both types are extremely uncommon.

Clinical Findings

A. SYMPTOMS AND SIGNS

Clinically, respiratory distress is noted soon after birth. Expansion of the cysts occurs with the onset of breathing and produces compression of normal lung areas with mediastinal herniation. Breath sounds are decreased. With type 3 lesions, dullness to percussion may be present. Older patients can present with a spontaneous pneumothorax or with pneumonia-like symptoms.

B. IMAGING

With type 1 lesions, chest radiograph shows an intrapulmonary mass of soft tissue density with scattered radiolucent areas of varying sizes and shapes, usually with a mediastinal shift and pulmonary herniation. Placement of a radiopaque feeding tube into the stomach helps in the differentiation from diaphragmatic hernia. Type 2 lesions appear similar except that the cysts are smaller. Type 3 lesions may appear as a solid homogeneous mass filling the hemithorax and causing a marked mediastinal shift. Differentiation from sequestration is not difficult because congenital cystic adenomatoid malformations have no systemic blood supply.

Treatment

Treatment of types 1 and 3 lesions involves surgical removal of the affected lobe. Resection is often indicated because of the risk of infection and air trapping, since the malformation communicates with the tracheobronchial tree but mucous clearance is compromised. Because type 2 lesions are often associated with other severe anomalies, management may be more complex. Segmental resection is not feasible because smaller cysts may expand after removal of the more obviously affected area. Cystic adenomatoid malformations have been reported to have malignant potential; therefore, expectant management with observation alone should proceed with caution. Recent development of intrauterine surgery for congenital malformations has led to promising results.

Breckenridge RL et al: Congenital cystic adenomatoid malformation of the lung. J Pediatr 1965;67:863 [PMID: 5845450].

Duncombe GJ et al: Prenatal diagnosis and management of congenital cystic adenomatoid malformation of the lung. Am J Obstet Gynecol 2002;187:950 [PMID: 12388984].

MacSweeney F et al: An assessment of the expanded classification of congenital cystic adenomatoid malformations and their relationship to malignant transformation. Am J Surg Pathol 2003;27:1139 [PMID: 12883247].

ACQUIRED DISORDERS INVOLVING ALVEOLI

BACTERIAL PNEUMONIA

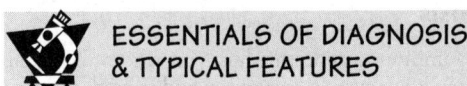

ESSENTIALS OF DIAGNOSIS & TYPICAL FEATURES

- *Fever, cough, dyspnea.*
- *Abnormal chest examination (rales or decreased breath sounds).*
- *Abnormal chest radiograph (infiltrates, hilar adenopathy, pleural effusion).*

General Considerations

Bacterial pneumonia is inflammation of the lung classified according to the infecting organism. Patients with the following problems are particularly predisposed to this disease: aspiration, immunodeficiency or immunosuppression, congenital anomalies (intrapulmonary sequestration, tracheoesophageal fistula, or cleft palate), abnormalities in clearance of mucus (CF, ciliary dysfunction, tracheomalacia, or bronchiectasis), congestive heart failure, and perinatal contamination.

Clinical Findings

A. SYMPTOMS AND SIGNS

The bacterial pathogen, severity of the disease, and age of the patient may cause substantial variations in the presentation of acute bacterial pneumonia. Infants may have few or nonspecific findings on history and physical examination. Immunocompetent older patients may not be extremely ill. Some patients may present with fever only or only with signs of generalized toxicity. Others may have additional symptoms or signs of lower respiratory tract disease (respiratory distress, cough, and sputum production), pneumonia (rales, decreased breath sounds, dullness to percussion, and abnormal tactile or vocal fremitus), or pleural involvement (splinting, pain, friction rub, and dullness to percussion). Some patients may have additional extrapulmonary findings, such as meningismus or abdominal pain, due to pneumonia itself. Others may have evidence of infection at other sites due to the same organism causing their pneumonia: meningitis, otitis media, sinusitis, pericarditis, epiglottitis, or abscesses.

B. LABORATORY FINDINGS

Elevated white blood cell counts (> 15,000/μL) frequently accompany bacterial pneumonia. However, a low white blood count (< 5000/μL) can be an ominous finding in this disease.

C. IMAGING

Chest radiographic findings (lateral and frontal views) define bacterial pneumonia. Patchy infiltrates, atelectasis, hilar adenopathy, or pleural effusion may be observed. Radiographs should be taken in the lateral decubitus position to identify pleural fluid. Complete lobar consolidation is not a common finding in infants and children. Severity of disease may not correlate with radiographic findings. Clinical resolution precedes resolution apparent on chest radiograph.

D. SPECIAL EXAMINATIONS

Invasive diagnostic procedures (bronchial brushing or washing, lung puncture, or open or thoracoscopic lung biopsy) should be undertaken in critically ill patients when other means do not adequately identify the cause (see section earlier on culture of material from the respiratory tract).

Differential Diagnosis

The differential diagnosis of pneumonia varies with the age and immunocompetence of the host. The spectrum of potential pathogens to be considered includes aerobic, anaerobic, and acid-fast bacteria as well as *Chlamydia trachomatis, C pneumoniae, C psittaci, Coxiella burnetii* (Q fever), *Pneumocystis jiroveci, Bordetella pertussis, Myco-*

plasma pneumoniae, Legionella pneumophila, and respiratory viruses. *Streptococcus pneumoniae* is the most prevalent bacterial pathogen. Vaccination with pneumococcal vaccine will aid in the prevention of pneumonia.

Noninfectious pulmonary disease (including gastric aspiration, foreign body aspiration, atelectasis, congenital malformations, congestive heart failure, malignant growths, tumors such as plasma cell granuloma, chronic interstitial lung diseases, and pulmonary hemosiderosis) should be considered in the differential diagnosis of localized or diffuse infiltrates. When effusions are present, additional noninfectious disorders such as collagen diseases, neoplasm, and pulmonary infarction should also be considered.

Complications

Empyema may occur frequently with staphylococcal, pneumococcal, and group A β-hemolytic streptococcal disease. Distal sites of infection—meningitis, otitis media, sinusitis (especially of the ethmoids), and septicemia—may be present, particularly with disease due to *S pneumoniae* or *H influenzae.* Certain immunocompromised patients, such as those who have undergone splenectomy or who have hemoglobin SS or SC disease or thalassemia, are especially prone to overwhelming sepsis with these organisms. Distal infection of the bones, joints, or other organs (eg, liver abscess) may occur in certain hosts with specific organisms.

Treatment

Antimicrobial therapy should be guided by Gram stain of sputum, tracheobronchial secretions, or pleural fluid if available; radiographic findings; age and known or suspected immunocompetence of the host; and local epidemiologic information. Reasonable coverage for pneumonia in the sick, immunocompromised, or debilitated patient, pending the results of bronchoalveolar lavage or thoracoscopic biopsy, should include ceftazidime, clindamycin, vancomycin, a macrolide for *Legionella* and *Mycoplasma,* and possibly trimethoprim-sulfamethoxazole for *P jiroveci.* Depending on the circumstances and the level of illness, empiric antifungal or antiviral therapy may be considered. In specific circumstances such as aspiration due to neurologic impairment or in patients with tracheostomies, clindamycin is indicated, pending culture and sensitivity studies, owing to the likely presence of resistant anaerobes.

Less severe pneumonias can often be treated with oral antibiotics based on the patient's age and suspected organism. Lobar pneumonias presumed to be due to *S pneumoniae* can be treated initially with oral β-lactams, including cefuroxime axetil, amoxicillin, or amoxicillin-clavulanate. However, persistence or worsening of symptoms within 3–5 days suggests the presence of a resistant organism, and newer quinolones, clindamycin, or vancomycin may be required. When possible, therapy can be guided by the antibiotic sensitivity pattern of the organisms isolated.

Whether a child should be hospitalized depends on his or her age, the severity of illness, the suspected organism, and the anticipated reliability of compliance at home. Home treatment is adequate for most older children. With febrile pneumonias, infants generally—and toddlers often—require admission. Moderate to severe respiratory distress, apnea, hypoxemia, poor feeding, clinical deterioration on treatment, or associated complications (large effusions, empyema, or abscess) indicate the need for immediate hospitalization. Careful follow-up within 12 hours to 5 days is often indicated in those not admitted. Cefuroxime or a macrolide, depending on the clinical picture, may be appropriate initial therapy for patients in this category.

Additional therapeutic considerations include oxygen, humidification of inspired gases, hydration and electrolyte supplementation, and nutrition. Removal of pleural fluid for diagnostic purposes is indicated initially to guide antimicrobial therapy. Many feel that early chest tube drainage of empyema fluid is indicated. Repeat pleural taps should be considered in the patient who has persistent high fever and respiratory symptoms in association with significant pleural effusions. The persistence of organisms in this fluid or the persistence of toxicity, malaise, anorexia, and wasting in the patient suggests the potential need for pleural decortication, a procedure that can be made less morbid by thoracoscopy in skilled hands.

Endotracheal intubation or mechanical ventilation may be indicated in patients with respiratory failure or in those too debilitated or overwhelmed to handle their secretions.

Prognosis

For the immunocompetent host in whom bacterial pneumonia is adequately recognized and treated, the survival rate is high. For example, the mortality rate from uncomplicated pneumococcal pneumonia is less than 1%. If the patient survives the initial illness, persistently abnormal pulmonary function following empyema is surprisingly uncommon, even when treatment has been delayed or inappropriate.

McIntosh K: Community-acquired pneumonia in children. N Engl J Med 2002;346:429 [PMID: 11832532].

Sinaniotis CA, Sinaniotis AC: Community-acquired pneumonia in children. Curr Opin Pulm Med 2005;11:218 [PMID: 15818183].

VIRAL PNEUMONIA

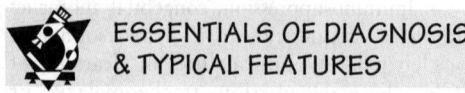

ESSENTIALS OF DIAGNOSIS & TYPICAL FEATURES

• *Upper respiratory infection prodrome (fever, coryza, cough, hoarseness).*

- *Wheezing or rales.*
- *Myalgia, malaise, headache (older children).*

General Considerations

Most pneumonias in children are caused by viruses. RSV, parainfluenza (1, 2, and 3) viruses, influenza (A and B) viruses, and human metapneumovirus are responsible for the large majority of cases. Severity of disease, severity of fever, radiographic findings, and the characteristics of cough or lung sounds do not reliably differentiate viral from bacterial pneumonias. Furthermore, such infections may coexist. However, substantial pleural effusions, pneumatoceles, abscesses, lobar consolidation with lobar volume expansion, and "round" pneumonias are generally inconsistent with viral disease.

Clinical Findings

A. SYMPTOMS AND SIGNS

An upper respiratory infection frequently precedes the onset of lower respiratory disease due to viruses. Although wheezing or stridor may be prominent in viral disease, cough, signs of respiratory difficulty (retractions, grunting, and nasal flaring), and physical findings (rales and decreased breath sounds) may not be distinguishable from those in bacterial pneumonia.

B. LABORATORY FINDINGS

The peripheral white blood cell count can be normal or slightly elevated and is not useful in distinguishing viral from bacterial disease. A markedly elevated neutrophil count, however, indicates that viral disease is less likely.

Rapid viral diagnostic methods—such as fluorescent antibody tests or enzyme-linked immunosorbent assay for RSV or other viruses—should be performed on nasopharyngeal secretions to confirm this diagnosis in high-risk patients and for epidemiology or infection control. Rapid diagnosis of RSV infection does not preclude the possibility of concomitant infection with other pathogens.

C. IMAGING

Chest radiographs frequently show perihilar streaking, increased interstitial markings, peribronchial cuffing, or patchy bronchopneumonia. Lobar consolidation may occur, however, as in bacterial pneumonia. Patients with adenovirus disease may have severe necrotizing pneumonias, resulting in the development of pneumatoceles. Hyperinflation of the lungs may occur when involvement of the small airways is prominent.

Differential Diagnosis

The differential diagnosis of viral pneumonia is the same as for bacterial pneumonia. Patients with prominent wheezing may have asthma, airway obstruction caused by foreign body aspiration, acute bacterial or viral tracheitis, or parasitic disease.

Complications

Bronchiolitis obliterans or severe chronic respiratory failure may follow adenovirus pneumonia. Bronchiolitis or viral pneumonia may contribute to persistent asthma in some patients. Bronchiectasis, chronic interstitial lung diseases, and unilateral hyperlucent lung (Sawyer-James syndrome) may follow measles, adenovirus, and influenzal pneumonias. Viral pneumonia or laryngotracheobronchitis may predispose the patient to subsequent bacterial tracheitis or pneumonia as immediate sequelae. Plasma cell granuloma may develop as a rare sequela to viral or bacterial pneumonia.

Treatment

General supportive care for viral pneumonia does not differ from that for bacterial pneumonia. Patients can be quite ill and should be hospitalized according to the level of their illness. Because bacterial disease often cannot be definitively excluded, antibiotics may be indicated.

Patients at risk for life-threatening RSV infections (eg, those with bronchopulmonary dysplasia or other severe pulmonary conditions, congenital heart disease, or significant immunocompromise) should be hospitalized and ribavirin should be considered. Rapid viral diagnostic tests may be a useful guide for such therapy (see bronchiolitis section regarding prevention). These high-risk patients and all children 6–23 months of age should be immunized annually against influenza A and B viruses. Despite immunization, however, influenza can still occur. When available epidemiologic data indicate an active influenza A infection in the community, rimantadine, amantadine hydrochloride, or oseltamivir phosphate should be considered early for high-risk infants and children who appear to be infected. Children with suspected viral pneumonia should be placed in respiratory isolation.

Prognosis

Although most children with viral pneumonia recover uneventfully, worsening asthma, abnormal pulmonary function or chest radiographs, persistent respiratory insufficiency, and even death may occur in high-risk patients such as newborns or those with underlying lung, cardiac, or immunodeficiency disease. Patients with adenovirus infection or those concomitantly infected with RSV and second pathogens such as influenza, adenovirus, cytomegalovirus, or *P jiroveci* also have a poorer prognosis.

Klig JE, Chen L: Lower respiratory infections in children. Curr Opin Pediatr 2003;15:121 [PMID: 12544283].

Klig JE: Current challenges in lower respiratory infections in children. Curr Opin Pediatr 2004;16:107 [PMID: 14758123].

CHLAMYDIAL PNEUMONIAS

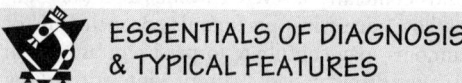

ESSENTIALS OF DIAGNOSIS & TYPICAL FEATURES

- *Cough, pharyngitis, tachypnea, rales, few wheezes, fever.*
- *Inclusion conjunctivitis, eosinophilia, and elevated immunoglobulins in some cases.*

General Considerations

Pulmonary disease due to *C trachomatis* usually evolves gradually as the infection descends the respiratory tract. Infants may appear quite well despite the presence of significant pulmonary illness. Infant infections are now at epidemic proportions in urban environments worldwide. *C pneumoniae* is now recognized as a common cause of respiratory infections in adults and children.

Clinical Findings

A. SYMPTOMS AND SIGNS

About 50% of infants with *C trachomatis* pneumonia have active inclusion conjunctivitis or a history of it. Rhinopharyngitis with nasal discharge or otitis media may have occurred or may be currently present. Female patients may have vulvovaginitis. Cough is usually present. It can have a staccato character and resemble the cough of pertussis. The infant is usually tachypneic. Scattered inspiratory rales are commonly heard, but wheezes rarely. Significant fever suggests a different or additional diagnosis.

In children *C pneumoniae* is a common respiratory pathogen and may cause 5–20% of all community-acquired pneumonias. Often these lower respiratory tract illnesses are mild or asymptomatic, though this can occasionally be a serious pathogen.

B. LABORATORY FINDINGS

Although patients may frequently be hypoxemic, CO_2 retention is not common. Peripheral blood eosinophilia (400 cells/μL) has been observed. Serum immunoglobulins are usually abnormal. IgM is virtually always elevated, IgG is high in many, and IgA is less frequently abnormal.

C trachomatis can usually be identified in nasopharyngeal washings using fluorescent antibody or culture techniques. *C pneumoniae* isolation can be difficult and the diagnosis is often made by serology.

C. IMAGING

Chest radiographs may reveal diffuse interstitial and patchy alveolar infiltrates, peribronchial thickening, or focal consolidation. A small pleural reaction can be present. Despite the usual absence of wheezes, hyperexpansion is commonly present.

Differential Diagnosis

Bacterial, viral, and fungal (*P jiroveci*) pneumonias should be considered. Premature infants and those with bronchopulmonary dysplasia may also have chlamydial pneumonia. *C pneumoniae* is often accompanied by coinfection with other pathogens, particularly *S pneumoniae* and *M pneumoniae*.

Treatment

Erythromycin or sulfisoxazole therapy should be administered for 14 days. Hospitalization may be required for children with significant respiratory distress, coughing paroxysms, or posttussive apnea. Oxygen therapy may be required for prolonged periods in some patients.

Prognosis

An increased incidence of obstructive airway disease and abnormal pulmonary function tests may occur for at least 7–8 years following infection.

Darville T: *Chlamydia trachomatis* infections in neonates and young children. Semin Pediatr Infect Dis 2005;16:235 [PMID: 16210104].

Hammerschlag MR: Pneumonia due to *Chlamydia pneumoniae* in children: epidemiology, diagnosis, and treatment. Pediatr Pulmonol 2003;36:384 [PMID: 14520720].

Principi N, Esposito S: Emerging role of *Mycoplasma pneumoniae* and *Chlamydia pneumoniae* in paediatric respiratory tract infections. Lancet Infect Dis 2001;1:334 [PMID: 11871806].

MYCOPLASMAL PNEUMONIA

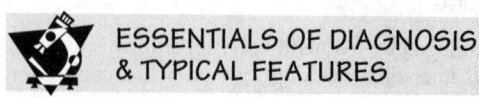

ESSENTIALS OF DIAGNOSIS & TYPICAL FEATURES

- *Fever.*
- *Cough.*
- *Most common age: older than 5 years.*

General Considerations

M pneumoniae is a common cause of symptomatic pneumonia in older children though it can be seen in children under 5. Endemic and epidemic infection can occur. The incubation period is long (2–3 weeks), and the onset of symptoms is slow. Although the lung is the primary infection site, extrapulmonary complications sometimes occur.

Clinical Findings

A. SYMPTOMS AND SIGNS

Fever, cough, headache, and malaise are common symptoms as the illness evolves. Although cough is usually dry at the onset, sputum production may develop as the illness progresses. Sore throat, otitis media, otitis externa, and bullous myringitis may occur. Rales are frequently present on chest examination; decreased breath sounds or dullness to percussion over the involved area may be present.

B. LABORATORY FINDINGS

The total and differential white blood cell counts are usually normal. The cold hemagglutinin titer can be determined and may be elevated during the acute presentation. A titer of 1:64 or higher supports the diagnosis. Acute and convalescent titers for *M pneumoniae* demonstrating a fourfold or greater rise in specific antibodies confirm the diagnosis. Diagnosis of mycoplasma pneumonia by polymerase chain reaction is becoming more readily available.

C. IMAGING

Chest radiographs usually demonstrate interstitial or bronchopneumonic infiltrates, frequently in the middle or lower lobes. Pleural effusions are extremely uncommon.

Complications

Extrapulmonary involvement of the blood, central nervous system, skin, heart, or joints can occur. Direct Coombs-positive autoimmune hemolytic anemia, occasionally a life-threatening disorder, is the most common hematologic abnormality that can accompany *M pneumoniae* infection. Coagulation defects and thrombocytopenia can also occur. Cerebral infarction, meningoencephalitis, Guillain-Barré syndrome, cranial nerve involvement, and psychosis all have been described. A wide variety of skin rashes, including erythema multiforme and Stevens-Johnson syndrome, can occur. Myocarditis, pericarditis, and a rheumatic fever–like illness can also occur.

Treatment

Antibiotic therapy with a macrolide for 7–10 days usually shortens the course of illness. Ciprofloxacin is a possible alternative. Supportive measures, including hydration, antipyretics, and bed rest, are helpful.

Prognosis

In the absence of the less common extrapulmonary complications, the outlook for recovery is excellent. The extent to which *M pneumoniae* can initiate or exacerbate chronic lung disease is not well understood.

Hammerschlag MR: *Mycoplasma pneumoniae* infections. Curr Opin Infect Dis 2001;14:181 [PMID: 11979130].

Waites KB: New concepts of *Mycoplasma pneumoniae* infections in children. Pediatr Pulmonol 2003;36:267 [PMID: 12950038].

TUBERCULOSIS

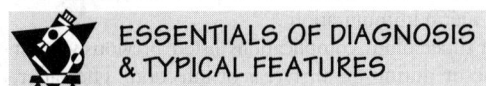

ESSENTIALS OF DIAGNOSIS & TYPICAL FEATURES

- *Positive tuberculin skin test or anergic host.*
- *Positive culture for Mycobacterium tuberculosis.*

General Considerations

There is a resurgence of tuberculosis in all age groups, including children. The clinical spectrum of tuberculosis includes a positive tuberculin skin test without evident disease, asymptomatic primary infection, the Ghon complex, bronchial obstruction with secondary collapse or obstructed airways, segmental lesions, calcified nodules, pleural effusions, progressive primary cavitating lesions, contiguous spread into adjacent thoracic structures, acute miliary tuberculosis, acute respiratory distress syndrome, overwhelming reactivation infection in the immunocompromised host, occult lymphohematogenous spread, and metastatic extrapulmonary involvement at almost any site. Symptoms of airway obstruction, sometimes with secondary bacterial pneumonia resulting from hilar adenopathy, are common presenting features in children.

Clinical Findings

A. SYMPTOMS AND SIGNS

The most important aspect of the history is contact with an individual with tuberculosis—often an elderly relative, a caregiver, or a person previously residing in a region where tuberculosis is endemic—or a history of travel to or residence in such an area. Homeless and extremely impoverished children are also at high risk, as are those in contact with high-risk adults (acquired immunodeficiency syndrome patients, residents or employees of correctional institutions or nursing homes, drug users, and health care workers). Once exposed, pediatric patients at risk for developing active disease include infants and those with malnutrition, acquired immunodeficiency syndrome, diabetes mellitus, or immunosuppression (cancer chemotherapy or corticosteroids). In suspected cases, the patient, immediate family, and suspected carriers should be tuberculin-tested. Spread is mainly respiratory, so isolated pulmonary parenchymal tuberculosis constitutes more than 95% of presenting cases. The primary focus (usually single) and associated nodal involvement may not be seen radiographically. Because healing—rather than progression—is the usual course in the uncompromised host, a positive tuberculin test may be the only manifestation. However, for patients born outside the United States, a positive test may indicate only a previous bacillus Calmette-Guérin immunization.

The tuberculous complications listed previously most often occur during the first year of infection. Thereafter, infection remains quiescent until adolescence, when reactivation of pulmonary tuberculosis is common. At any stage, chronic cough, anorexia, weight loss or failure to gain weight, and fever are useful clinical signs if present. Except in cases with complications or advanced disease, physical findings are few. Most children with pulmonary tuberculosis are asymptomatic.

B. LABORATORY FINDINGS

A positive tuberculin skin test is defined by the size of induration as defined by risk factors for TB. This is read 48–72 hours after intradermal injection of 5 tuberculin units of purified protein derivative. Tine tests should not be used. Appropriate control skin tests, such as those for hypersensitivity to diphtheria-tetanus, mumps, or *Candida albicans,* should be applied in patients with suspected or proven immunosuppression or in those with possible severe disseminated disease. If the patient fails to respond to purified protein derivative, the possibility of tuberculosis is not excluded.

Anteroposterior and lateral chest radiographs should be obtained in all suspected cases. Culture for *M tuberculosis* is critical for proving the diagnosis and for defining drug susceptibility. Early morning gastric lavage following an overnight fast should be performed on three occasions in infants and children with suspected active pulmonary tuberculosis before treatment is started, when the severity of illness allows. Although stains for acid-fast bacilli on this material are of little value, this is the ideal culture site. Despite the increasing importance of isolating organisms because of multiple drug resistance, only 40% of children will yield positive cultures.

Sputum cultures from older children and adolescents are similarly useful. Stains and cultures of bronchial secretions are useful if bronchoscopy is performed as part of the patient's evaluation. When pleural effusions are present, pleural biopsy for cultures and histopathologic examination for granulomas or organisms provide diagnostic information. Meningeal involvement is a possibility in young children, and lumbar puncture should be considered in their initial evaluation.

Differential Diagnosis

Fungal diseases that affect mainly the lungs, such as histoplasmosis, coccidioidomycosis, cryptococcosis, and North American blastomycosis, may resemble tuberculosis and in doubtful cases should be excluded by appropriate serologic studies. Atypical tuberculous organisms may involve the lungs, especially in the immunocompromised patient. Depending on the presentation, diagnoses such as lymphoreticular and other malignancies, collagen-vascular disorders, or other pulmonary infections may be considered.

Complications

In addition to those complications listed in the sections on general considerations and clinical findings, lymphadenitis, meningitis, osteomyelitis, arthritis, enteritis, peritonitis, and renal, ocular, middle ear, and cutaneous disease may occur. The infant born to tuberculous parents is at great risk for developing illness. The possibility of life-threatening airway compromise must always be considered in patients with large mediastinal or hilar lesions.

Treatment

Because the risk of hepatitis due to isoniazid is extremely low in children, this drug is indicated in those with a positive tuberculin skin test. This greatly reduces the risk of subsequent active disease and complications with minimal morbidity. Isoniazid plus rifampin treatment for 6 months, plus pyrazinamide during the first 2 months, is indicated when the chest radiograph is abnormal or when extrapulmonary disease is present. Without pyrazinamide, isoniazid plus rifampin must be given for 9 months. In general, the more severe tuberculous complications are treated with a larger number of drugs. Enforced, directly-observed therapy (twice or three times weekly) is indicated when nonadherence is suspected. Recommendations for antituberculosis chemotherapy based on disease stage are continuously being updated. The most current edition of the American Academy of Pediatrics *Red Book* is a reliable source for these protocols.

Corticosteroids are used to control inflammation in selected patients with potentially life-threatening airway compression by lymph nodes, acute pericardial effusion, massive pleural effusion with mediastinal shift, or miliary tuberculosis with respiratory failure.

Prognosis

In patients with an intact immune system, modern anti-tuberculous therapy offers good potential for recovery. The outlook for patients with immunodeficiencies, organisms resistant to multiple drugs, poor drug compliance, or advanced complications is guarded. Organisms resistant to multiple drugs are increasingly common. Resistance emerges either because the physician prescribes an inadequate regimen or because the patient discontinues medications. When resistance to or intolerance of isoniazid and rifampin prevents their use, cure rates are 50% or less.

Feja K, Saiman L: Tuberculosis in children. Clin Chest Med 2005;26:295 [PMID: 15837112].

Mandalakas AM, Starke JR: Current concepts of childhood tuberculosis. Semin Pediatr Infect Dis 2005;16:93 [PMID: 15825140].

ASPIRATION PNEUMONIA

Patients whose anatomic defense mechanisms are impaired are at risk of aspiration pneumonia (Table 18–2). Acute disease is commonly caused by bacteria present in the mouth (especially gram-negative anaerobes). Chronic aspiration often causes recurrent bouts of acute febrile pneumonia. It may also lead to chronic focal infiltrates, atelectasis, illness resembling asthma or interstitial lung disease, or failure to thrive.

Clinical Findings

A. SYMPTOMS AND SIGNS

Acute onset of fever, cough, respiratory distress, or hypoxemia in a patient at risk suggests aspiration pneumonia. Chest physical findings, such as rales, rhonchi, or decreased breath sounds, may initially be limited to the lung region into which aspiration occurred. Although any region may be affected, the right side—especially the right

Table 18–2. Risk factors for aspiration pneumonia.

Seizures
Depressed sensorium
Recurrent gastroesophageal reflux, emesis, or gastrointestinal obstruction
Neuromuscular disorders with suck-swallow dysfunction
Anatomic abnormalities (laryngeal cleft, tracheoesophageal fistula, vocal cord paralysis)
Debilitating illnesses
Occult brainstem lesions
Near-drowning
Nasogastric, endotracheal, or tracheostomy tubes
Severe periodontal disease

upper lobe in the supine patient—is commonly affected. In patients with chronic aspiration, diffuse wheezing may occur. Generalized rales may also be present. Such patients may not develop acute febrile pneumonias.

B. LABORATORY FINDINGS AND IMAGING

Chest radiographs may reveal lobar consolidation or atelectasis and focal or generalized alveolar or interstitial infiltrates. In some patients with chronic aspiration, perihilar infiltrates with or without bilateral air trapping may be seen.

In severely ill patients with acute febrile illnesses, a bacteriologic diagnosis should be made. In addition to blood cultures, cultures of tracheobronchial secretions and bronchoalveolar lavage specimens may be desirable (see section on culture of material from the respiratory tract).

In patients with chronic aspiration pneumonitis, solid documentation of aspiration as the cause of illness may be elusive. Barium contrast studies may provide evidence of suck-swallow dysfunction, laryngeal cleft, occult tracheoesophageal fistula, or gastroesophageal reflux. Overnight or 24-hour esophageal pH probe studies may also help establish the latter. Although radionuclide scans are commonly used, the yield from such studies is disappointingly low. Rigid bronchoscopy in infants or flexible bronchoscopy in older children can be useful in more definitively excluding tracheoesophageal fistula and obtaining bronchoalveolar lavage specimens to search for lipid-laden macrophages, which can suggest chronic aspiration.

Differential Diagnosis

In the acutely ill patient, bacterial and viral pneumonias should be considered. In the chronically ill patient, the differential diagnosis may include disorders causing recurrent pneumonia (eg, immunodeficiencies, ciliary dysfunction, or foreign body), chronic wheezing, or interstitial lung disorders (see section on interstitial lung diseases), depending on the presentation.

Complications

Empyema or lung abscess may result from acute aspiration pneumonia. Chronic aspiration may result in bronchiectasis.

Treatment

Antimicrobial therapy for acute aspiration pneumonia includes coverage for gram-negative anaerobic organisms. In general, clindamycin is appropriate initial coverage. However, in some hospital-acquired infections, additional coverage for multiply resistant *P aeruginosa*, streptococci, and other organisms may be required.

Treatment of recurrent and chronic aspiration pneumonia may include the following: surgical correction of anatomic abnormalities; improved oral hygiene; improved hydration; and inhaled bronchodilators, chest physical therapy, and suctioning. In patients with compromise of the central nervous system, exclusive feeding by gastrostomy and (in some) tracheostomy may be required to control airway secretions. Gastroesophageal reflux, often requiring surgical correction, is commonly present in such patients.

Prognosis

The outlook is directly related to the disorder causing aspiration.

Brook I: Anaerobic pulmonary infections in children. Pediatr Emerg Care 2004;20:636 [PMID: 15599270].

Colombo JL, Hallberg TK: Pulmonary aspiration and lipid-laden macrophages: In search of gold (standards). Pediatr Pulmonol 1999;28:79 [PMID: 10423305].

PNEUMONIA IN THE IMMUNOCOMPROMISED HOST

Pneumonia in an immunocompromised host may be due to any common bacteria (streptococci, staphylococci, or *M pneumoniae*) or less common pathogens such as *Toxoplasma gondii*, *P jiroveci*, *Aspergillus* species, *Mucor, Candida* species, *Cryptococcus neoformans,* gram-negative enteric and anaerobic bacteria, *Nocardia, Legionella pneumophila,* mycobacteria, and viruses (cytomegalovirus, varicella-zoster, herpes simplex, influenza virus, RSV, metapneumovirus, or adenovirus). Multiple organisms are commonly present.

Clinical Findings

A. SYMPTOMS AND SIGNS

Patients often present with subtle signs such as mild cough, tachypnea, or low-grade fever that can rapidly progress to high fever, respiratory distress, and hypoxemia. An obvious portal of infection, such as an intravascular catheter, may predispose to bacterial or fungal infection.

B. LABORATORY FINDINGS AND IMAGING

Fungal, parasitic, or bacterial infection, especially with antibiotic-resistant bacteria, should be suspected in the neutropenic child. Cultures of peripheral blood, sputum, tracheobronchial secretions, urine, nasopharynx or sinuses, bone marrow, pleural fluid, biopsied lymph nodes, or skin lesions or cultures through intravascular catheters should be obtained as soon as infection is suspected.

Invasive methods are commonly required to make a diagnosis. Appropriate samples should be obtained soon after a patient with pneumonia fails to respond to initial treatment. The results of these procedures usually lead to important changes in empiric preoperative therapy. Sputum is often unavailable. Bronchoalveolar lavage

frequently provides the diagnosis of one or more organisms and should be done early in evaluation. The combined use of a wash, brushing, and lavage has a high yield. In patients with rapidly advancing disease, lung biopsy becomes more urgent. The morbidity and mortality of this procedure can be reduced by a surgeon skilled in video-assisted thoracoscopic surgical (VATS) techniques. Because of the multiplicity of organisms that may cause disease, a comprehensive set of studies should be done on lavage and biopsy material. These consist of rapid diagnostic studies, including fluorescent antibody studies for *Legionella;* rapid culture and antigen detection for viruses; Gram, acid-fast, and fungal stains; cytologic examination for viral inclusions; cultures for viruses, anaerobic and aerobic bacteria, fungi, mycobacteria, and *Legionella;* and rapid immunofluorescent studies for *P jiroveci.*

Chest radiographs may be useful. In *P jiroveci* pneumonia, dyspnea and hypoxemia may be marked despite minimal radiographic abnormalities.

Differential Diagnosis

The organisms causing disease vary with the type of immunocompromise present. For example, the splenectomized patient may be overwhelmed by infection with *S pneumoniae* or *H influenzae*. The infant receiving adrenocorticotropic hormone therapy may be more likely to have *P jiroveci* infection. The febrile neutropenic child who has been receiving adequate doses of intravenous broad-spectrum antibiotics may have fungal disease. The key to diagnosis is to consider all possibilities of infection.

Depending on the form of immunocompromise, perhaps only one-half to two-thirds of new pulmonary infiltrates in such patients represents infection. The remainder are caused by pulmonary toxicity of radiation, chemotherapy, or other drugs; pulmonary disorders, including hemorrhage, embolism, atelectasis, aspiration, idiopathic pneumonia syndrome in bone marrow transplant patients, or acute respiratory distress syndrome; recurrence or extension of primary malignant growths or immunologic disorders; transfusion reactions, leukostasis, or tumor cell lysis; or interstitial lung disease, such as lymphocytic interstitial pneumonitis with human immunodeficiency virus infection.

Complications

Progressive respiratory failure, shock, multiple organ damage, disseminated infection, and death commonly occur in the infected immunocompromised host if the primary etiology is not treated effectively.

Treatment

Broad-spectrum intravenous antibiotics are indicated early in febrile, neutropenic, or immunocompromised children. Trimethoprim-sulfamethoxazole (for *Pneumocystis*) and macrolides (for *Legionella*) are also indicated early in the treatment of immunocompromised children before an organism is identified. Further therapy should be based on studies of specimens obtained from bronchoalveolar lavage or lung biopsy. Recently, data suggest use of noninvasive ventilation strategies early in the course of pulmonary insufficiency or respiratory failure may decrease mortality.

Prognosis

Prognosis is based on the severity of the underlying immunocompromise, appropriate early diagnosis and treatment, and the infecting organisms. Intubation and mechanical ventilation have been associated with high mortality rates, especially in bone marrow transplant patients.

Ferrer M et al: Noninvasive ventilation in severe hypoxemic respiratory failure: a randomized clinical trial. Am J Respir Crit Care Med 2003;168:1438 [PMID: 14500259].

Neville K et al: Pneumonia in the immunocompromised pediatric cancer patient. Semin Respir Infect 2002;17:21 [PMID: 11891516].

Perez Mato S et al: Pulmonary infections in children with HIV infection. Semin Respir Infect 2002;17:33 [PMID: 11891517].

HYPERSENSITIVITY PNEUMONIA

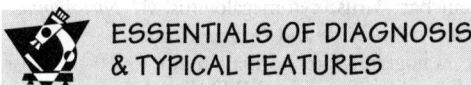

ESSENTIALS OF DIAGNOSIS & TYPICAL FEATURES

- *History of exposure (eg, birds, organic dusts, drug therapy, hot tubs, molds).*
- *Interstitial infiltrates on chest radiograph or diffuse rales.*
- *Recurrent cough, fever, wheezing, or weight loss can occur.*

General Considerations

Hypersensitivity pneumonitis, or extrinsic allergic alveolitis, is a T-cell–mediated disease involving the peripheral airways, interstitium, and alveoli. Both acute and chronic forms may occur. In children, the most common forms are brought on by exposure to domestic and occasionally wild birds or bird droppings (eg, pigeons, parakeets, parrots, or doves). However, inhalation of almost any organic dust (moldy hay, compost, logs or tree bark, sawdust, or aerosols from humidifiers or hot tubs) can cause disease. Methotrexate-induced hypersensitivity has also been described in a child with juvenile rheumatoid arthritis. Hot tub lung can be caused

by exposure to aerosolized *Mycobacterium avium complex*. A high level of suspicion and a thorough history are required for diagnosis.

Clinical Findings

A. SYMPTOMS AND SIGNS

Episodic cough and fever can occur with acute exposures. Chronic exposure results in weight loss, fatigue, dyspnea, cyanosis, and ultimately, respiratory failure.

B. LABORATORY FINDINGS

Acute exposure may be followed by polymorphonuclear leukocytosis with eosinophilia and evidence of airway obstruction on pulmonary function testing. Chronic disease results in a restrictive picture on lung function tests. Arterial blood gases may reveal hypoxemia with a decreased $PaCO_2$ and normal pH.

The serologic key to diagnosis is the finding of precipitins (precipitating IgG antibodies) to the organic material that contain avian proteins or fungal or bacterial antigens. Ideally, to identify avian proteins, the patient's sera should be tested with antigens from droppings of the suspected species of bird. However, exposure may invoke precipitins without causing disease.

Bronchoscopy with bronchoalveolar lavage findings of lymphocytosis or *Mycobacterium avium complex* may be suggestive. Normal cell counts may help rule out acute hypersensitivity pneumonitis.

Differential Diagnosis

Patients with mainly acute symptoms must be differentiated from those with atopic asthma. Patients with chronic symptoms must be distinguished from those with collagen-vascular, immunologic, or primary interstitial pulmonary disorders.

Complications

Prolonged exposure to offending antigens may result in pulmonary hypertension due to chronic hypoxia, cor pulmonale, irreversible restrictive lung disease due to pulmonary fibrosis, or respiratory failure.

Treatment

Complete elimination of exposure to the offending antigens is required. If drug-induced hypersensitivity pneumonitis is suspected, discontinuation is required. Corticosteroids may hasten recovery.

Prognosis

With appropriate early diagnosis and identification and avoidance of offending antigens, the prognosis is excellent.

Fan LL: Hypersensitivity pneumonitis in children. Curr Opin Pediatr 2002;14:323 [PMID: 12011673].

Fink JN et al: Needs and opportunities for research in hypersensitivity pneumonitis. Am J Respir Crit Care Med 2005;171:792 [PMID: 15657460].

Marras TK et al: Hypersensitivity pneumonitis reaction to *Mycobacterium avium* in household water. Chest 2005;127:664 [PMID: 15706013].

CHILDREN'S INTERSTITIAL LUNG DISEASE SYNDROME

Key Features

Presence of three to five of the following criteria in the absence of any identified primary etiology:

1. Symptoms of impaired respiratory function (cough, tachypnea, retractions, exercise intolerance)
2. Evidence for impaired gas exchange (resting hypoxemia or hypercarbia, desaturation with exercise)
3. Diffuse infiltrates on imaging
4. Presence of adventitious sounds (crackles, wheezing)
5. Abnormal spirometry, lung volumes, or carbon monoxide diffusing capacity

General Considerations

children's **I**nterstitial **L**ung **D**isease (chILD) syndrome is a constellation of signs and symptoms and not a specific diagnosis. Once recognized, chILD syndrome should elicit a search for a more specific rare interstitial lung disease (ILD). Known disorders can present as chILD syndrome and must be excluded as the primary cause of symptoms. These disorders include: cystic fibrosis, cardiac disease, asthma, acute infection, immunodeficiency, neuromuscular disease, scoliosis, thoracic cage abnormality, typical BPD or premature respiratory distress syndrome, and confirmed significant aspiration on a swallow study. However, if patients present with symptoms out of proportion to the diagnosis, a consideration of other ILD disorders should be given.

Clinical Findings

A. Symptoms and Signs

chILD syndrome may present acutely in the newborn period with respiratory failure or gradually over time with a chronic dry cough or a history of dyspnea on exertion. The child with more advanced disease may have increased dyspnea, tachypnea, retractions, cyanosis, clubbing, failure to thrive, or weight loss.

B. Differential Diagnosis

chILD syndrome is composed of a group of diverse conditions that can be different from adult ILD conditions. Common adult causes of ILD such as usual interstitial pneumonitis also known as idiopathic pulmonary fibrosis, which is associated with a high mortality rate, and respiratory bronchiolitis, associated with smoking, have not been found in children. Conversely, newly identified conditions unique to infancy such as neuroendocrine cell hyperplasia of infancy or pulmonary interstitial glycogenosis, have not been described in adults. Other chILD conditions include the genetically recognized surfactant dysfunction mutations SP-B, SP-C, and ABCA3, developmental abnormalities, and growth disorders, especially in younger children. Older children are more likely to have SP-C or ABCA3 surfactant mutations, hypersensitivity pneumonitis, or collagen-vascular disease. Other known conditions must also be ruled out.

C. Evaluation

Once chILD syndrome is recognized, initial evaluations should be directed to rule out known conditions. The initial evaluations should include the following diagnostic studies: radiographs, barium swallow, pulmonary function tests, and skin tests (see section on tuberculosis); complete blood count and erythrocyte sedimentation rate; sweat chloride test for CF; electrocardiogram or echocardiogram; serum immunoglobulins and other immunologic evaluations; sputum studies (see section on pneumonia in the immunocompromised host); and possibly studies for Epstein-Barr virus, cytomegalovirus, *M pneumoniae*, *Chlamydia*, *Pneumocystis*, and *U urealyticum*.

Chest radiographs are normal in up to 10–15% of patients. Frequently, specific chILD disorders can be suspected by findings on inspiratory and expiratory high-resolution computerized tomography, which should be considered early in the course of evaluation. Infants and young children under 5 years of age require sedation, which allows either infant pulmonary function testing or bronchoscopy evaluations to be completed at the same time.

On pulmonary function testing, multiple patterns can be seen depending on the specific ILD condition such as (1) a restrictive pattern of decreased lung volumes, compliance, and carbon monoxide diffusing capacity, (2) an obstructive pattern with hyperinflation, or (3) a mixed obstructive/restrictive pattern. Infant pulmonary function testing can provide insight into pulmonary mechanics and different chILD disorders. Exercise-induced or nocturnal hypoxemia is often the earliest detectable abnormality of lung function in children.

During the second phase, perform bronchoscopy to exclude anatomic abnormalities, obtain multiple bronchial brushings to examine cilia if cilial dysfunction is considered a possibility, and obtain bronchoalveolar lavage for microbiologic and cytologic testing.

In patients with static or slowly progressing disease, one can then await results of bronchoscopic studies. In patients with acute, rapidly progressive disease, this stage should be combined with video-assisted thoracoscopic biopsy. Lung biopsy is the most reliable method for definitive diagnosis when analyzed by pathologists experienced in chILD disorders. A new chILD histology classification is being proposed to improve diagnostic yields. Tissue should be processed in a standard manner for special stains and cultures, electron microscopy, and immunofluorescence for immune complexes if indicated. Although transbronchial biopsy may be useful in diagnosing a few diffuse disorders and graft rejection in transplant (eg, sarcoidosis), its overall usefulness in chILD is limited at this time.

Genomic mutational analysis of tissue or blood for SP-B, SP-C, and ABCA3 is not offered in clinical laboratories and should be considered in most patients with diffuse lung disease or a strong family history of ILD.

Complications

Respiratory failure or pulmonary hypertension with cor pulmonale may occur. Mortality and morbidity can be significant in some chILD disorders.

Treatment

Therapy for known causes of ILD such as infection, aspiration, or cardiac disorders should be directed toward the primary disorder. It must be recognized that treatment for chILD conditions are anecdotal and based on case reports and small case series. chILD conditions such as surfactant dysfunction mutations, pulmonary interstitial glycogenosis, hypersensitivity pneumonitis, and systemic collagen-vascular disease are frequently treated initially with oral (2 mg/kg per day for 6 weeks) or monthly pulse glucocorticoids (IV doses of 10–30 mg/kg for 1–3 days). Many patients require even more protracted therapy with alternate-day prednisone. Chloroquine (5–10 mg/kg/d) may be useful in selected disorders such as desquamative interstitial pneumonitis, surfactant dysfunction mutations, or refractory disease. In noninflammatory chILD syndrome conditions like neuroendocrine cell hyperplasia of infancy or developmental or growth abnormalities, treatment is supportive and may not require steroids. In refractory cases, azathioprine and cyclophosphamide may be tried. Newer antifibrotic agents such as interferon-γ, which are being investigated in adult patients with interstitial pulmonary fibrosis, have not been tried in children to date. Finally, some patients with severe disease may require long-term mechanical ventilation or lung transplantation for survival. chILD disorders should be evaluated and cared for by a multidisciplinary team experienced in chILD.

Prognosis

The prognosis is guarded in children with interstitial lung disease due to collagen-vascular disease, surfac-

tant dysfunction mutations, and developmental disorders (eg, alveolar-capillary dysplasia). Other conditions such as neuroendocrine cell hyperplasia of infancy and pulmonary interstitial glycogenosis have not had deaths reported.

Fan LL et al: Pediatric interstitial lung disease revisited. Pediatr Pulmonol 2004;38:369 [PMID: 15376335].

Whitsett JA: Genetic disorders of surfactant homeostasis. Biol Neonate 2005;87:283 [PMID: 15985750].

EOSINOPHILIC PNEUMONIA

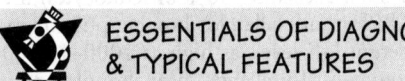

ESSENTIALS OF DIAGNOSIS
& TYPICAL FEATURES

- *Pulmonary infiltrates, often migratory, seen on chest radiograph.*
- *Persistent cough; wheezes or rales on chest auscultation.*
- *Increased eosinophils in peripheral blood or in lung biopsy specimens.*

General Considerations

A spectrum of diseases should be considered under this heading: (1) allergic bronchopulmonary helminthiosis (ABPH), (2) pulmonary eosinophilia with asthma (allergic bronchopulmonary aspergillosis and related disorders), (3) hypereosinophilic mucoid impaction, (4) bronchocentric granulomatosis, and (5) collagen-vascular disorders. The old term, Löffler syndrome (transient migratory pulmonary infiltrates and eosinophilia), is no longer used because most patients had undiagnosed ABPH, medication reactions (www.pneumotox.com), or allergic bronchopulmonary aspergillosis. Many of these disorders occur in children with personal or family histories of allergies or asthma. ABPH may be related to hypersensitivity to migratory parasitic nematodes (*Ascaris, Strongyloides, Ancylostoma, Toxocara,* or *Trichuris*) and larval forms of filariae (*Wuchereria bancrofti*). Allergic bronchopulmonary aspergillosis is related to hypersensitivity to the fungus *Aspergillus.* Hypersensitivity to other fungi has also been documented. Eosinophilic pneumonias are rare but can be associated with drug hypersensitivity, sarcoidosis, Hodgkin disease or other lymphomas, and bacterial infections, including brucellosis and those caused by *M tuberculosis* and atypical mycobacteria.

Clinical Findings

A. Symptoms and Signs

Cough, wheezing, and dyspnea are common presenting complaints. In allergic bronchopulmonary helminthiosis, fever, malaise, sputum production, and rarely hemoptysis may be present. In allergic bronchopulmonary aspergillosis, patients may present with all of these findings and occasionally produce brown mucus plugs. Anorexia, weight loss, night sweats, and clubbing can also occur.

B. Laboratory Findings and Imaging

Elevated absolute peripheral blood eosinophil counts (3000/μL and often exceeding 50% of leukocytes) are present in ABPH and allergic bronchopulmonary aspergillosis. Serum IgE levels as high as 1000–10,000 IU/mL are common. In allergic bronchopulmonary aspergillosis, the serum IgE concentration appears to correlate with activity of the disease. Stools should be examined for ova and parasites—often several times—to clarify the diagnosis. Isohemagglutinin titers are often markedly elevated in ABPH.

In allergic bronchopulmonary aspergillosis and related disorders, patients may show central bronchiectasis on chest radiograph (so-called tramlines) or CT scan. Saccular proximal bronchiectasis of the upper lobes is pathognomonic. Although the chest radiograph may be normal, peribronchial haziness, focal or platelike atelectasis, or patchy to massive consolidation can occur. Positive immediate skin tests, serum IgG precipitating antibodies, or IgE specific for the offending fungus is present.

Differential Diagnosis

These disorders must be differentiated from exacerbations of asthma, CF, or other underlying lung disorders that cause infiltrates to appear on chest radiographs. Allergic bronchopulmonary aspergillosis can occur in patients with CF.

Complications

Delayed recognition and treatment of allergic bronchopulmonary aspergillosis may cause progressive lung damage and bronchiectasis. Lesions of the conducting airways in bronchocentric granulomatosis can extend into adjacent lung parenchyma and pulmonary arteries, resulting in secondary vasculitis.

Treatment

Therapy for the specific parasite causing ABPH should be given, and corticosteroids may be required when illness is severe. Treatment of disease due to microfilariae is both diagnostic and therapeutic. Allergic bronchopul-monary aspergillosis and related disorders are treated with prolonged courses of oral corticosteroids, bronchodilators, and chest physical therapy. In patients with CF, itraconazole may decrease steroid doses for those with allergic bronchopulmonary aspergillosis. Pulmonary vasculitis associated with collagen-vascular disease is usually treated with high-dose steroids or cytotoxic agents.

Oermann CM et al: Pulmonary infiltrates with eosinophilia syndromes in children. J Pediatr 2000;136:351 [PMID: 10700692].

Wubbel C et al: Chronic eosinophilia pneumonia. Chest 2003; 123:1763 [PMID: 12740299].

LUNG ABSCESS

Lung abscesses are most likely to occur in immunocompromised patients; in those with severe infections elsewhere (embolic spread); or in those with recurrent aspiration, malnutrition, or blunt chest trauma. Although organisms such as *S aureus, H influenzae, S pneumoniae,* and viridans streptococci more commonly affect the previously normal host, anaerobic and gram-negative organisms as well as *Nocardia, Legionella* species, and fungi (*Candida* and *Aspergillus*) should also be considered in the immunocompromised host.

Clinical Findings

A. Symptoms and Signs

High fever, malaise, and weight loss are often present. Symptoms and signs referable to the chest may or may not be present. In infants, evidence of respiratory distress can be present.

B. Laboratory Findings and Imaging

Elevated peripheral white blood cell count with a neutrophil predominance or an elevated erythrocyte sedimentation rate may be present. Blood cultures are rarely positive except in the overwhelmed host.

Chest radiographs usually reveal single or multiple thick-walled lung cavities. Air-fluid levels can be present. Local compressive atelectasis, pleural thickening, or adenopathy may also occur. Chest CT scan may provide better localization and understanding of the lesions.

In patients producing sputum, stains and cultures may provide the diagnosis. Direct percutaneous aspiration of material for stains and cultures guided by fluoroscopy or ultrasonography should be considered in the severely compromised or ill.

Differential Diagnosis

Loculated pyopneumothorax, an *Echinococcus* cyst, neoplasms, plasma cell granuloma, and infected congenital cysts and sequestrations should be considered.

Complications

Although complications due to abscesses are now rare, mediastinal shift, tension pneumothorax, and spontaneous rupture can occur. Diagnostic maneuvers such as lung puncture may also cause complications (pneumothorax).

Treatment

Because of the risks of lung puncture, uncomplicated abscesses are frequently conservatively treated in the uncompromised host with appropriate broad-spectrum antibiotics directed at *S aureus, H influenzae,* and streptococci. Additional coverage for anaerobic and gram-negative organisms should be provided for others. Prolonged therapy (3 weeks or more) may be required. Attempts to drain abscesses via bronchoscopy have caused life-threatening airway compromise. Surgical drainage or lobectomy is occasionally required, primarily in immunocompromised patients. However, such procedures may themselves cause life-threatening complications.

Prognosis

Although radiographic resolution may be very slow, resolution occurs in most patients without risk factors for lower respiratory tract infections or loss of pulmonary function. In the immunocompromised host, the outlook depends on the underlying disorder.

Chan PC et al: Clinical management and outcome of childhood lung abscess: a 16-year experience. J Microbiol Immunol Infect 2005;38:183 [PMID: 15986068].

Wali SO et al: Percutaneous drainage of pyogenic lung abscess. Scand J Infect Dis 2002;34:673 [PMID: 12374359].

Diseases of the Pulmonary Circulation

PULMONARY HEMORRHAGE

Pulmonary hemorrhage is caused by a spectrum of disorders affecting the large and small airways and alveoli. It can occur as an acute or chronic process. Hemorrhage involving the alveoli is termed diffuse alveolar hemorrhage. If pulmonary hemorrhage is subacute or chronic, hemosiderin-laden macrophages are found in the sputum and tracheal or gastric aspirate. Many cases are secondary to infection (bacterial, mycobacterial, parasitic, viral, or fungal), lung abscess, bronchiectasis (CF or other causes), foreign body, coagulopathy (often with overwhelming sepsis), or elevated pulmonary venous pressure (secondary to congestive heart failure or anatomic heart lesions). Other causes include lung contusion from trauma, arteriovenous fistula, multiple telangiectasias, pulmonary sequestration, agenesis of a single pulmonary artery, and esophageal duplication or bronchogenic cyst. Rarer causes are tumors (eg, bronchial adenoma or left atrial myxoma) and pulmonary infarction secondary to pulmonary embolus.

Diffuse alveolar hemorrhage may be idiopathic or drug-related or may occur in Goodpasture syndrome, rapidly progressive glomerulonephritis, and systemic vasculitides (often associated with such collagen-vascular diseases as systemic lupus erythematosus, rheumatoid arthritis, Wegener granulomatosis, polyarteritis nodosa, Henoch-Schönlein purpura, and Behçet disease). Idiopathic pulmonary hemosiderosis refers to the accumulation of hemosiderin in the lung, especially the alveolar macrophage, as a result of chronic or recurrent hemorrhage (usually from pulmonary capillaries) that is not associated with the previously listed causes. Children and young adults are mainly affected, with the age at onset ranging from 6 months to 20 years. This group of disorders includes milk allergy in young infants (Heiner syndrome).

Several cases of pulmonary hemorrhage and pulmonary hemosiderosis have been reported in infants exposed to a toxigenic mold, *Stachybotrys chartarum,* and other fungi. This association was initially noted in Cleveland, Ohio. The infants were primarily African American, living in older homes, and often the homes had recent water damage. Environmental tobacco smoke was also frequently present in the environment. Other forms of hypersensitivity pneumonitis have also been reported to cause pulmonary bleeding.

Clinical Findings

A. Symptoms and Signs

Pulmonary hemorrhage has as many symptoms as it has causes. Large airway hemorrhage presents with hemoptysis and symptoms of the underlying cause, such as infection, foreign body, or bronchiectasis in CF. Hemoptysis from larger airways is often bright red or contains clots. Idiopathic pulmonary hemosiderosis usually presents with nonspecific respiratory symptoms (cough, tachypnea, and retractions) with or without hemoptysis, poor growth, and fatigue. Some children or young adults may present with massive hemoptysis, marked respiratory distress, stridor, or a pneumonia-like syndrome. Fever, abdominal pain, digital clubbing, and chest pain may be reported. Jaundice and hepatosplenomegaly may be present with chronic bleeding. Physical examination often reveals decreased breath sounds, rales, rhonchi, or wheezing.

B. Laboratory Findings and Imaging

Laboratory studies vary depending on the cause of hemorrhage. Following long-standing idiopathic pulmonary hemorrhage, iron deficiency anemia and heme-positive sputum are present. Nonspecific findings may include lymphocytosis and an elevated erythrocyte sedimentation rate. Peripheral eosinophilia is present in up to 25% of patients. Chest radiographs demonstrate a range of findings, from transient perihilar infiltrates to large, fluffy alveolar infiltrates with or without atelectasis and mediastinal adenopathy. Pulmonary function testing generally reveals restrictive impairment, with low lung volumes, poor compliance, and an increased diffusion capacity. Hemosiderin-laden macrophages are found in bronchial or gastric aspirates. The diagnostic usefulness of lung biopsy is controversial.

Diffuse alveolar hemorrhage with underlying systemic disease such as systemic lupus erythematosus, Wegener granulomatosis, and occasionally Goodpasture syndrome can occur with the histologic entity known as necrotizing pulmonary capillaritis. On lung biopsy the alveolar septa are infiltrated with neutrophils, and alveolar hemorrhage is acute or chronic. The septa can fill with edema or fibrinoid necrosis. Idiopathic pulmonary hemosiderosis may represent a mild form of capillaritis associated with alveolar hemorrhage. It might represent a process that waxes and wanes, and capillaritis may be focal or mild. Likewise, an immune-mediated process may cause idiopathic pulmonary hemosiderosis, although no serologic marker has yet been identified. Although capillaritis has been described without evidence of underlying systemic disease, the search for collagen-vascular disease, vasculitis, or pulmonary fibrosis should be exhaustive.

The investigation should include serologic studies such as circulating antineutrophilic cytoplasmic autoantibodies for Wegener granulomatosis, perinuclear antineutrophilic cytoplasmic autoantibodies for microscopic polyangiitis, antinuclear antibodies for systemic lupus erythematosus, and anti–basement membrane antibodies for Goodpasture syndrome. α_1-Antitrypsin deficiency has been associated with vasculitides and should be considered.

Suspected cases of cow's milk–induced pulmonary hemosiderosis can be confirmed by laboratory findings that include high titers of serum precipitins to multiple constituents of cow's milk and positive intradermal skin tests to various cow's milk proteins. Improvement after an empiric trial of a diet free of cow's milk also supports the diagnosis.

Differential Diagnosis

The search for the site of respiratory bleeding, underlying systemic illness, and cardiac or vascular abnormalities will help define the diagnosis. When gross hemoptysis is present, large airway bronchiectasis, epistaxis, foreign body, and arteriovenous or pulmonary malformations should be ruled out. MRI or CT-assisted angiography can localize abnormal or systemic arterial flow.

Alveolar bleeding with hemoptysis is often frothy and pink. The differential diagnosis includes the disorders causing diffuse alveolar hemorrhage listed earlier. In contrast to idiopathic pulmonary hemosiderosis, Goodpasture syndrome occurs in a slightly older age group (15–35 years), tends to have a more aggressive pulmonary course, and has renal involvement (crescentic proliferative glomerulonephritis and circulating antiglomerular basement membrane antibody). Wegener granulomatosis also has renal involvement (granulomatous glomerulitis with necrotizing vasculitis, but renal biopsy may be nonspecific) and other systemic manifestations, especially with upper and lower respiratory tract inflammation. Upper tract involvement includes sinusitis, rhinitis, recurrent epistaxis, otitis media, saddle-nose deformity, and subglottic stenosis. Wegener granulomatosis may occur without renal involvement early in the course of the disease. The diagnosis can be made by biopsy or an elevated circulating antineutrophilic cytoplasmic autoantibody titer.

Treatment

Therapy should be aimed at direct treatment of the underlying disease. Supportive measures, including iron therapy, supplemental oxygen, and blood transfusions, may be needed. A diet free of cow's milk should be tried in infants. Systemic corticosteroids have been used for various causes of diffuse alveolar hemorrhage and have been particularly successful in those secondary to collagen-vascular disorders and vasculitis. Case reports have been published on the variable effectiveness of steroids, chloroquine, cyclophosphamide, and azathioprine for idiopathic pulmonary hemosiderosis.

Prognosis

The outcome of idiopathic pulmonary hemosiderosis is variable, characterized by a waxing and waning course of intermittent intrapulmonary bleeds and the gradual development of pulmonary fibrosis over time. The severity of the underlying renal disease contributes to the mortality rates associated with Goodpasture syndrome and Wegener granulomatosis. Diffuse alveolar hemorrhage is considered a lethal pulmonary complication of systemic lupus erythematosus.

Ben-Abraham R et al: Diffuse alveolar hemorrhage following allogeneic bone marrow transplantation in children. Chest 2003; 124:660 [PMID: 12907557].

Bull TM et al: Pulmonary vascular manifestations of mixed connective tissue disease. Rheum Dis Clin North Am 2005;31:451 [PMID: 16084318].

Etzel RA et al: Acute pulmonary hemorrhage in infants associated with exposure to *Stachybotrys atra* and other fungi. Arch Pediatr Adolesc Med 1998;152:757 [PMID: 9701134].

Etzel RA: *Stachybotrys.* Curr Opin Pediatr 2003;15:103 (Review) [PMID: 12544280].

Godfrey S: Pulmonary hemorrhage/hemoptysis in children. Pediatr Pulmonol 2004;37:476 [PMID: 15114547].

Ioachimescu OC et al: Idiopathic pulmonary haemosiderosis revisited. Eur Respir J 2004;24:162. [PMID: 15293620].

Kiper N et al: Long-term clinical course of patients with idiopathic pulmonary hemosiderosis (1979–1994): Prolonged survival with low-dose corticosteroid therapy. Pediatr Pulmonol 1999;27:180 [PMID: 10213256].

Update: Pulmonary hemorrhage/hemosiderosis among infants–Cleveland, Ohio, 1993–1996. MMWR Morb Mortal Wkly Rep 2000;49:180 (erratum in: MMWR Morb Mortal Wkly Rep 2000;49:213) [PMID: 11795499].

PULMONARY EMBOLISM

Although pulmonary embolism is apparently rare in children, the incidence is probably underestimated because it is often not considered in the differential diagnosis of respiratory distress. It occurs most commonly in children with sickle cell anemia as part of the acute chest syndrome and with rheumatic fever, infective endocarditis, schistosomiasis, bone fracture, dehydration, polycythemia, nephrotic syndrome, atrial fibrillation, and other conditions. A recent report suggests that a majority of children with pulmonary emboli referred for hematology evaluation have coagulation regulatory protein abnormalities and antiphospholipid antibodies. Emboli may be single or multiple, large or small, with clinical signs and symptoms dependent on the severity of pulmonary vascular obstruction.

Clinical Findings

A. Symptoms and Signs

Pulmonary embolism usually presents clinically as an acute onset of dyspnea and tachypnea. Heart palpitations or a sense of impending doom may be reported.

Pleuritic chest pain and hemoptysis may be present (not common), along with splinting, cyanosis, and tachycardia. Massive emboli may be present with syncope and cardiac arrhythmias. Physical examination is usually normal (except for tachycardia and tachypnea) unless the embolism is associated with an underlying disorder. Mild hypoxemia, rales, focal wheezing, or a pleural friction rub may be found.

B. Laboratory Findings and Imaging

Radiographic findings may be normal, but a peripheral infiltrate, small pleural effusion, or elevated hemidiaphragm can be present. If the emboli are massive, differential blood flow and pulmonary artery enlargement may be appreciated. The electrocardiogram is usually normal unless the pulmonary embolus is massive. Echocardiography is useful in detecting the presence of a large proximal embolus. A negative D-dimer has a > 95% negative predictive value for an embolus. Ventilation-perfusion scans show localized areas of ventilation without perfusion.

Spiral CT with contrast may be helpful, but pulmonary angiography is the gold standard. Further evaluation may include Doppler ultrasound studies of the legs to search for deep venous thrombosis. Coagulation studies, including assessments of antithrombin III and protein C or S deficiencies or defective fibrinolysis may be indicated. Antiphospholipid antibodies and other coagulation regulatory proteins (proteins C and S, and factor V Leiden) should be checked, as abnormalities have been demonstrated in 70% of the hematology referrals in one pediatric institution.

Treatment

Acute treatment includes supplemental oxygen, sedation, and anticoagulation. Current recommendations include heparin administration to maintain an activated partial thromboplastin time that is one and one-half or more times the control value for the first 24 hours. Urokinase (2000–4000 U/kg for 36 hours) can be used to help dissolve the embolus. Tissue plasminogen activator is another option via central or peripheral administration. These therapies should be followed by warfarin therapy for at least 6 weeks with an International Normalized Ratio > 2. In patients with identifiable deep venous thrombosis of the lower extremities and significant pulmonary emboli (with hemodynamic compromise despite anticoagulation), inferior vena caval interruption may be necessary. Long-term prospective data regarding this latter therapy are lacking, however.

Bounameaux H: Review: ELISA D-dimer is sensitive but not specific in diagnosing pulmonary embolism in an ambulatory clinical setting. ACP J Club 2003;138:24 [PMID: 12511136].

Kearon C: Duration of therapy for acute venous thromboembolism. Clin Chest Med 2003;24:63 [PMID: 12685057].

Konstantinides S et al: Heparin plus alteplase compared with heparin alone in patients with submassive pulmonary embolism. N Engl J Med 2002;347:1143 [PMID: 12374874].

Rahimtoola A et al: Acute pulmonary embolism: an update on diagnosis and management. Curr Probl Cardiology 2005;30:61 [PMID: 15650680].

Remy-Jardin M et al: Pulmonary embolus imaging with multislice CT. Radiol Clin North Am 2003;41:507 [PMID: 12797603].

PULMONARY EDEMA

Pulmonary edema is excessive accumulation of extravascular fluid in the lung. This occurs when fluid is filtered into the lungs faster than it can be removed, leading to changes in lung mechanics such as decreased lung compliance, worsening hypoxemia from ventilation-perfusion mismatch, bronchial compression, and if advanced, decreased surfactant function. There are two basic types of pulmonary edema: increased pressure (cardiogenic or hydrostatic) and increased permeability (noncardiogenic or primary). Hydrostatic pulmonary edema is usually due to excessive increases in pulmonary venous pressure, which is most commonly due to congestive heart failure from multiple causes. In contrast, many lung diseases, especially acute respiratory distress syndrome, are characterized by the development of pulmonary edema secondary to changes in permeability due to injury to the alveolocapillary barrier. In these settings, pulmonary edema occurs independently of the elevations of pulmonary venous pressure.

Clinical Findings

A. SYMPTOMS AND SIGNS

Cyanosis, tachypnea, tachycardia, and respiratory distress are commonly present. Physical findings include rales, diminished breath sounds, and (in young infants) expiratory wheezing. More severe disease is characterized by progressive respiratory distress with marked retractions, dyspnea, and severe hypoxemia.

B. IMAGING

Chest radiographic findings depend on the cause of the edema. Pulmonary vessels are prominent, often with diffuse interstitial or alveolar infiltrates. Heart size is usually normal in permeability edema but enlarged in hydrostatic edema.

Treatment

Although specific therapy depends on the underlying cause, supplemental oxygen therapy, and if needed, ventilator support for respiratory failure are indicated. Diuretics, digoxin, and vasodilators may be indicated for congestive heart failure along with restriction of salt and water. Recommended interventions for permeability edema are reduction of vascular volume and maintenance of the lowest central venous or pulmonary arterial wedge pressure possible without sacrificing cardiac output or causing hypotension (see following discussion). β-Adrenergic agonists such as terbutaline have been shown to increase alveolar clearance of lung water, perhaps through the action of a sodium-potassium channel pump. Maintaining normal albumin levels and a hematocrit > 30 maintains the filtration of lung liquid toward the capillaries, avoiding low oncotic pressure.

Cotter G et al: Pulmonary edema: new insight on pathogenesis and treatment. Curr Opin Cardiol 2001;16:159 [PMID: 11357010].

Redding GJ: Current concepts in adult respiratory distress syndrome in children. Curr Opin Pediatr 2001;13:261 [PMID: 11389362].

Van Kooy MA, Gargiulo RF: Postobstructive pulmonary edema. Am Fam Physician 2000;62:401 [PMID: 10929702].

CONGENITAL PULMONARY LYMPHANGIECTASIA

Structurally, congenital pulmonary lymphangiectasia appears as dilated subpleural and interlobular lymphatic channels and may present as part of a generalized lymphangiectasis (in association with obstructive cardiovascular lesions—especially total anomalous pulmonary venous return) or as an isolated idiopathic lesion. Pathologically, the lung appears firm, bulky, and noncompressible, with prominent cystic lymphatics visible beneath the pleura. On cut section, dilated lymphatics are present near the hilum, along interlobular septa, around bronchovascular bundles, and beneath the pleura. Histologically, dilated lymphatics have a thin endothelial cell lining overlying a delicate network of elastin and collagen.

Clinical Findings

Congenital pulmonary lymphangiectasia is a rare, usually fatal disease that generally presents as acute or persistent respiratory distress at birth. Although most patients do not survive the newborn period, some survive longer, and there are isolated case reports of its diagnosis later in childhood. It may be associated with features of Noonan syndrome, asplenia, total anomalous pulmonary venous return, septal defects, atrioventricular canal, hypoplastic left heart, aortic arch malformations, and renal malformations. Chylothorax has been reported. Chest radiographic findings include a ground-glass appearance, prominent interstitial markings suggesting lymphatic distention, diffuse hyperlucency of the pulmonary parenchyma, and hyperinflation with depression of the diaphragm.

Prognosis

Although the onset of symptoms may be delayed for as long as the first few months of life, prolonged survival is extremely rare. Most deaths occur within weeks after birth. Rapid diagnosis is essential in order to expedite the option of pulmonary transplant.

Esther CR et al: Pulmonary lymphangiectasia: diagnosis and clinical course. Pediatr Pulmonol 2004;38:308 [PMID: 15334508].

Huber A et al: Congenital pulmonary lymphangiectasia. Pediatr Pulmonol 1991;10:310 [PMID: 1896243].

DISORDERS OF THE CHEST WALL

EVENTRATION OF THE DIAPHRAGM

Eventration of the diaphragm occurs when striated muscle is replaced with connective tissue and is demonstrated on radiograph by elevation of part or all of the diaphragm. There are two types: congenital and acquired. The congenital type is thought to represent incomplete formation of the diaphragm in utero. The acquired type is related to atrophy of diaphragm muscles secondary to prenatal or postnatal phrenic nerve injury. The differential diagnosis of eventration includes phrenic nerve injury and partial diaphragmatic hernia. Small eventrations may be an incidental finding on a chest radiograph, commonly seen on the right side. Ultrasound provides useful information to further define a suspected eventration. When defects are small, there is no paradoxical movement of the diaphragm and little symptomatology. When defects are large, paradoxical movement of the diaphragm may be present. The degree of respiratory distress depends in large part on the amount of paradoxical motion of the diaphragm. When the diaphragm moves upward during inspiration, instability of the inferior border of the chest wall increases the work of breathing and can lead to respiratory muscle fatigue and potential failure when stressed. Symptoms include persistent increased work of breathing, particularly with feeding or failure to extubate. Treatment is based on severity of symptoms. If symptoms persist for 2–4 weeks, the diaphragm is surgically plicated, which stabilizes it. Function returns to the diaphragm in about 50% of cases of phrenic nerve injury whether or not plication was performed. Recovery periods of up to 100 days have been reported in these cases.

Clements BS: Congenital malformations of the lungs and airways. In: Taussig LM, Landau LI (editors): *Pediatric Respiratory Medicine.* Mosby, 1999.

Eren S et al: Congenital diaphragmatic eventration as a cause of anterior mediastinal mass in children: imaging modalities and literature review. Eur J Radiol 2004;51:85.

SCOLIOSIS

Scoliosis is defined as lateral curvature of the spine and is commonly categorized as idiopathic, congenital, or neuromuscular. No pulmonary impairment is typically seen with a Cobb angle showing thoracic curvature of less than 35 degrees. Most cases of idiopathic scoliosis occur in adolescent girls and are corrected before significant pulmonary impairment occurs. Congenital scoliosis of severe degree or with other major abnormalities carries a more guarded prognosis. Patients with progressive neuromuscular disease, such as Duchenne muscular dystrophy, can be at risk for respiratory failure due to severe scoliosis. Timing of treatment is debatable, with observation alone if thoracic curvature is less than 15 degrees, bracing considered between 25 and 45 degrees, and surgery considered if greater than 45 degrees. Severe scoliosis can lead to impaired lung function and possible death from cor pulmonale if uncorrected.

Greiner KA: Adolescent idiopathic scoliosis: Radiologic decision-making. Am Fam Physician 2002;65:1817.

Kearon C et al: Factors determining pulmonary function in adolescent idiopathic thoracic scoliosis. Am Rev Respir Dis 1993;148:288 [PMID: 8342890].

PECTUS EXCAVATUM

Pectus excavatum is anterior depression of the chest wall that may be symmetrical or asymmetrical with respect to the midline. Its presence can be psychologically difficult for the patient. Whether or not it is cause for cardiopulmonary limitations is controversial. While subjective exertional dyspnea can be reported and may improve with repair, objective cardiopulmonary function may not change postoperatively. Therefore, the decision to repair the deformity may be based on cosmetic or physiologic considerations. Surgical literature is providing more information regarding long-term outcomes following repair. Timing of repair is also critical in light of growth plate maturation. It may be associated with congenital heart disease.

Borowitz D et al: Pulmonary function and exercise response in patients with pectus excavatum after Nuss repair. J Pediatr Surg 2003;38:544 [PMID: 12677562].

Lawson ML et al: Impact of pectus excavatum on pulmonary function before and after repair with the Nuss procedure. J Pediatr Surg 2005;40:174 [PMID: 15868581].

Malek MH et al: Ventilatory and cardiovascular responses to exercise in patients with pectus excavatum. Chest 2003;124:870 [PMID: 12970011].

PECTUS CARINATUM

Pectus carinatum is a protrusion of the upper or lower (more common) portion of the sternum, more commonly seen in males. Once again, psychological impact may be present, but impedance of pulmonary function is debated. The decision to repair this deformity is often based on cosmetic grounds, but research has shown that those with reduced endurance or dyspnea with mild exercise experienced marked improvement within 6 months following repair, suggesting possible physiologic indications. It may be associated with systemic diseases such as the mucopolysaccharidoses and congenital heart disease.

Fonkalsrud EW, Anselmo DM: Less extensive techniques for repair of pectus carinatum: the undertreated chest deformity. J Am Coll Surg 2004;198:898.

Williams AM, Crabbe DC: Pectus deformities of the anterior chest wall. Paediatr Respir Rev 2003;4:237 [PMID: 12880759].

NEUROMUSCULAR DISORDERS

Weakness of the respiratory and pharyngeal muscles leads to chronic or recurrent pneumonia secondary to aspiration and infection, atelectasis, hypoventilation, and respiratory failure in severe cases. Scoliosis, which frequently accompanies long-standing neuromuscular disorders, may further compromise respiratory function. Typical physical findings are a weak cough, decreased air exchange, crackles, wheezing, and dullness to percussion. Signs of cor pulmonale (loud pulmonary component to the second heart sound, hepatomegaly, and elevated neck veins) may be evident in advanced cases. Chest radiographs generally show small lung volumes. If chronic aspiration is present, increased interstitial infiltrates and areas of atelectasis or consolidation may be present. Arterial blood gases demonstrate hypoxemia in the early stages and compensated respiratory acidosis in the late stages. Typical pulmonary function abnormalities include low lung volumes and decreased inspiratory force generated against an occluded airway. Treatment is supportive and includes vigorous pulmonary toilet, antibiotics with infection, and oxygen to correct hypoxemia. Consideration of bi-level positive airway pressure and mechanical airway clearance support, like mechanical in-exsufflation, should be introduced before respiratory failure is present. Unfortunately, despite aggressive medical therapy, many neuromuscular conditions progress to respiratory failure and death. The decision to intubate and ventilate is a difficult one; it should be made only when there is real hope that deterioration, though acute, is potentially reversible or when chronic ventilation is wanted. Chronic mechanical ventilation using either noninvasive or invasive techniques is being used more frequently in patients with chronic respiratory insufficiency.

Birnkrant DJ: The assessment and management of the respiratory complications of pediatric neuromuscular diseases. Clin Pediatr 2002;41:301 [PMID: 12086195].

Mallory GB: Pulmonary complications of neuromuscular disease. Pediatr Pulmonol 2004;(Suppl 26):138 [PMID: 15029630].

Miske LJ et al: Use of the mechanical in-exsufflator in pediatric patients with neuromuscular disease and impaired cough. Chest 2004;125:1406 [PMID: 15078753].

Simonds AK: Nocturnal ventilation in neuromuscular disease—When and how? Monaldi Arch Chest Dis 2002;57:273 [PMID: 12814040].

DISORDERS OF THE PLEURA & PLEURAL CAVITY

The visceral pleura covers the outer surface of the lungs, and the inner surface of the chest wall is the parietal pleura. Disease processes can lead to accumulation of air or fluid in the pleural space. Pleural effusions are classified as transudates or exudates. Transudates occur when there is imbalance between hydrostatic and oncotic pressure, so that fluid filtration exceeds reabsorption (eg, congestive heart failure). Exudates form as a result of inflammation of the pleural surface leading to increased capillary permeability (eg, parapneumonic effusions). Other pleural effusions include chylothorax and hemothorax.

Thoracentesis is helpful in characterizing the fluid and providing definitive diagnosis. Recovered fluid is considered an exudate (as opposed to a transudate) if

any of the following are found: a pleural fluid:serum protein ratio greater than 0.5, a pleural fluid:serum lactate dehydrogenase ratio greater than 0.6, or a pleural fluid lactate dehydrogenase greater than 200 U/L. Important additional studies on pleural fluid include cell count; pH and glucose; Gram, acid-fast, and fungal stains; cultures; counterimmunoelectrophoresis for specific organisms; and occasionally, amylase concentration. Cytologic examination of pleural fluid should be performed to rule out leukemia or other neoplasm.

Hilliard TN et al: Management of parapneumonic effusion and empyema. Arch Dis Child 2003;88:915 [PMID: 14500314].

PARAPNEUMONIC EFFUSION & EMPYEMA

Bacterial pneumonia is often accompanied by pleural effusion. Some of these effusions harbor infection, and others are inflammatory reactions to pneumonia. The nomenclature in this area is somewhat confusing. Some use the term *empyema* for grossly purulent fluid and *parapneumonic effusion* for nonpurulent fluid. It is clear, however, that some nonpurulent effusions will also contain organisms and represent either partially treated or early empyema. It is probably best to refer to all effusions associated with pneumonia as parapneumonic effusions, some of which are infected and some not.

The most common organism associated with empyema is *S pneumoniae*. Other common organisms include *H influenzae* and *S aureus*. Less common causes are group A streptococci, gram-negative organisms, anaerobic organisms, and *M pneumoniae*. Effusions associated with tuberculosis are almost always sterile and constitute an inflammatory reaction.

Clinical Findings

A. SYMPTOMS AND SIGNS

Patients usually present with typical signs of pneumonia, including fever, tachypnea, and cough. They may have chest pain, decreased breath sounds, and dullness to percussion on the affected side and may prefer to lie on the affected side. With large effusions, there may be tracheal deviation to the contralateral side.

B. LABORATORY FINDINGS

The white blood cell count is often elevated, with left shift. Blood cultures are sometimes positive. The tuberculin skin test is positive in most cases of tuberculosis. Thoracentesis reveals findings consistent with an exudate. Cells in the pleural fluid are usually neutrophils in bacterial disease and lymphocytes in tuberculous effusions. In bacterial disease, pleural fluid pH and glucose are often low. pH < 7.2 suggests active bacterial infection. The pH of the specimen should be determined in a blood gas syringe sent to the laboratory on ice. Extra heparin should not be used in the syringe since it can falsely lower the pH. Although in adults the presence of low pH and glucose necessitates aggressive and thorough drainage procedures, the prognostic significance of these findings in children is unknown. Gram stain, cultures, and counterimmunoelectrophoresis are often positive for the offending organism.

C. IMAGING

The presence of pleural fluid is suggested by a homogeneous density that obscures the underlying lung on chest radiograph. Large effusions may cause a shift of the mediastinum to the contralateral side. Small effusions may only blunt the costophrenic angle. Lateral decubitus radiographs may help to detect freely movable fluid by demonstrating a layering-out effect. If the fluid is loculated, no such effect is perceived. Ultrasonography can be extremely valuable in localizing the fluid and detecting loculations, especially when thoracentesis is contemplated, but availability may be limited. Chest CT can help determine if loculations are present and direct further care of complicated pneumonias.

Treatment & Prognosis

After initial thoracentesis and identification of the organism, appropriate intravenous antibiotics and adequate drainage of the fluid remain the mainstay of therapy, but the approach is debated. Although there is a trend toward managing smaller pneumococcal empyemas without a chest tube, most larger effusions require chest tube drainage. Often the empyema has been present for more than 7 days, increasing the chance for loculation of fluid. Evidence of early decortication using thoracoscopic techniques like video-assisted thoracoscopic surgery (VATS) may reduce morbidity and has been shown to shorten length of hospital stay when done by an experienced surgeon. While there is growing use of VATS as first-line therapy, it is not standard of care. Aggressive management with drainage of pleural cavity fluid and release of adhesions with fibrinolytics is often sought in many institutions where the chest tube is placed in the operating room under anesthesia. The decision on therapeutic choice will vary depending on the resources available to the clinician. The prognosis is related to the severity of disease but is generally excellent, with complete or nearly complete recovery expected in most instances.

Efrati O et al: Pleural effusions in the pediatric population. Pediatr Rev 2002;23:417.

Gates RL et al: Drainage, fibrinolytics, or surgery: A comparison of treatment options in pediatric empyema. J Pediatr Surg 2004;39:1638.

Quadri A, Thomson AH: Pleural fluids associated with chest infection. Paediatr Respir Rev 2002;3:349 [PMID: 12457606].

Rodgers BM: The role of thoracoscopy in pediatric surgical practice. Semin Pediatr Surg 2003;12:62 [PMID: 12520474].

HEMOTHORAX

Accumulation of blood in the pleural space can be caused by surgical or accidental trauma, coagulation defects, and pleural or pulmonary tumors. With blunt trauma, hemopneumothorax may be present. Symptoms are related to blood loss and compression of underlying lung parenchyma. There is some risk of secondary infection, resulting in empyema. Drainage of a hemothorax is required when significant compromise of pulmonary function is present, as with hemopneumothorax. In uncomplicated cases, observation is indicated because blood is readily absorbed spontaneously from the pleural space.

VATS has been used successfully in the management of hemothorax. Chest CT scan is helpful to select patients who may require surgery, as identification of blood and the volume of blood may be more predictive by this method than by chest radiograph.

Bliss D, Silen M: Pediatric thoracic trauma. Crit Care Med 2002;30(11 Suppl):S409 [PMID: 12528782].

CHYLOTHORAX

The accumulation of chyle, fluid of intestinal origin containing fat digestion products, in the pleural space usually results from accidental or surgical trauma to the thoracic duct. In the newborn, chylothorax can be congenital or secondary to birth trauma. This condition also occurs as a result of superior vena caval obstruction secondary to central venous lines and following Fontan procedures for tricuspid atresia. Symptoms of chylothorax are related to the amount of fluid accumulation and the degree of compromise of underlying pulmonary parenchyma. Thoracentesis reveals typical milky fluid (unless the patient has been fasting) containing chiefly T lymphocytes.

Treatment should be conservative because many chylothoraces resolve spontaneously. Oral feedings with medium-chain triglycerides reduce lymphatic flow through the thoracic duct. Recent literature has shown somatostatin as a viable therapeutic option. Drainage of chylous effusions should be performed only for respiratory compromise because the fluid often rapidly reaccumulates. Repeated or continuous drainage may lead to protein malnutrition and T-cell depletion, rendering the patient relatively immunocompromised. If reaccumulation of fluid persists, surgical ligation of the thoracic duct or sclerosis of the pleural space can be attempted, though the results may be less than satisfactory.

Beghetti M et al: Etiology and management of pediatric chylothorax. J Pediatr 2000;136:653 [PMID: 10802499].

Romero S: Nontraumatic chylothorax. Curr Opin Pulm Med 2000;6:287 [PMID: 10912634].

PNEUMOTHORAX & RELATED AIR LEAK SYNDROMES

Pneumothorax can occur spontaneously in newborns and in older children, or more commonly, as a result of birth trauma, positive pressure ventilation, underlying obstructive or restrictive lung disease, and rupture of a congenital or acquired lung cyst. Pneumothorax can also occur as an acute complication of tracheostomy. Air usually dissects from the alveolar spaces into the interstitial spaces of the lung. Migration to the visceral pleura ultimately leads to rupture into the pleural space. Associated conditions include pneumomediastinum, pneumopericardium, pneumoperitoneum, and subcutaneous emphysema. These conditions are more commonly associated with dissection of air into the interstitial spaces of the lung with retrograde dissection along the bronchovascular bundles toward the hilum.

Clinical Findings

A. SYMPTOMS AND SIGNS

The clinical spectrum can vary from asymptomatic to severe respiratory distress. Associated symptoms include cyanosis, chest pain, and dyspnea. Physical examination may reveal decreased breath sounds and hyperresonance to percussion on the affected side with tracheal deviation to the opposite side. When pneumothorax is under tension, cardiac function may be compromised, resulting in hypotension or narrowing of the pulse pressure. Pneumopericardium is a life-threatening condition that presents with muffled heart tones and shock. Pneumomediastinum rarely causes symptoms by itself.

B. IMAGING

Chest radiographs usually demonstrate the presence of free air in the pleural space. If the pneumothorax is large and under tension, compressive atelectasis of the underlying lung and shift of the mediastinum to the opposite side may be demonstrated. Cross-table lateral and lateral decubitus radiographs can aid in the diagnosis of free air. Pneumopericardium is identified by the presence of air completely surrounding the heart, whereas in patients with pneumomediastinum, the heart and mediastinal structures may be outlined with air, but the air does not involve the diaphragmatic cardiac border. Chest CT may be helpful with recurrent spontaneous pneumothoraces to look for subtle pulmonary disease not seen on chest radiograph, but this is debated.

Differential Diagnosis

Acute deterioration of a patient on a ventilator can be caused by tension pneumothorax, obstruction or dislodgment of the endotracheal tube, or ventilator failure. Radiographically, pneumothorax must be distinguished from diaphragmatic hernia, lung cysts, congenital lobar emphysema, and cystic adenomatoid malformation, but this task is usually not difficult.

Treatment

Small or asymptomatic pneumothoraces usually do not require treatment and can be managed with close observation. Larger or symptomatic ones usually require drainage, although inhalation of 100% oxygen to wash out blood nitrogen can be tried.

Needle aspiration should be used to relieve tension acutely, followed by chest tube or pigtail catheter placement. Pneumopericardium requires immediate identification, and if clinically symptomatic, needle aspiration to prevent death, followed by pericardial tube placement.

In older patients with spontaneous pneumothorax, recurrences are common; sclerosing and surgical procedures are often required.

Baumann MH et al: Management of spontaneous pneumothorax: An American College of Chest Physicians Delphi Consensus Statement. ACCP Pneumothorax Consensus Group. Chest 2001;119:590 [PMID: 11171742].

Damore DT, Dayan PS: Medical causes of pneumomediastinum in children. Clin Pediatr 2001;40:87 [PMID: 11261455].

Panitch HB et al: Abnormalities of the pleural space. In: Taussig LM, Landau LI (editors): *Pediatric Respiratory Medicine.* Mosby, 1999.

DISORDERS OF SLEEP

Sleep apnea is recognized as a major public health problem in adults, with the risk of excessive daytime sleepiness, driving accidents, poor work performance, and effects on mental health. Pediatric sleep disorders are less commonly recognized because of a lack of training in sleep problem recognition and the presentation, risks, and outcome all differ from those in adults. The spectrum of sleep-disordered breathing includes obstructive sleep apnea, upper airway resistance disorder, and primary snoring. Sleep apnea is defined as cessation of breathing and can be classified as obstructive (the attempt to breathe through an obstructed airway) or central (the lack of effort to breathe).

OBSTRUCTIVE SLEEP APNEA

Obstructive sleep apnea occurs in normal children with an incidence of about 2%, increasing in children with craniofacial abnormalities, neuropathies, or other medical problems. The incidence also increases when children are medicated with hypnotics, sedatives, or anticonvulsants. While not all children who snore have sleep apnea, there is recent literature that raises concerns that snoring without apnea has neurobehavioral consequences. (See Chapter 17.) Obstructive sleep apnea should be suspected whenever a child presents with nightly snoring, witnessed apnea, labored breathing, frequent nighttime arousals, failure to thrive, oxygen desaturations, life-threatening events, behavior abnormalities, obesity, or craniofacial abnormalities. Upper airway resistance syndrome is characterized by the presence of daytime fatigue or sleepiness in the presence of a normal polysomnogram and oxygen saturations. Symptoms are similar to obstructive sleep apnea, including change in appetite, poor performance in school, and problems with behavior.

CENTRAL SLEEP APNEA

Central apneas are common in infants and children. They are considered significant if longer than 20 seconds or associated with bradycardia or desaturations. Clinical significance is uncertain, but may be relevant if they occur frequently or gas exchange problems exist. Healthy children have been shown to have central apneas lasting 25 seconds without clear consequences. In comparison, central hypoventilation syndrome patients have intact voluntary control of ventilation, but lack automatic control. During sleep, they will hypoventilate to the point at which they need ventilatory support that may require treatment with positive airway pressure and a rated tidal volume via tracheostomy. Central sleep apnea may be present with this syndrome, but is not usually noted.

When sleep apnea is suspected, the polysomnogram is the diagnostic test of choice. This test measures sleep state with electroencephalogram leads and electromyography, airflow at the nose, heart rate and rhythm, gas exchange (CO_2 and oxygenation), and leg movements, along with other potential data including esophageal pH, end-tidal CO_2, body position, muscle activity, and other optional additions. Polysomnography allows diagnosis of various forms of apnea, sleep fragmentation, periodic limb movement disorder, or other sleep disorders of children.

First-line therapy for obstructive sleep apnea in children is adenotonsillectomy, which improves the clinical status for most children with normal craniofacial structure. Even children with craniofacial anomalies or neuromuscular disorders may benefit, although additional treatment with continuous positive airway pressure may be indicated. With Down syndrome, up to half of these children can still have obstructive sleep apnea despite adenotonsillectomy. Treatment of young or developmentally delayed children with apnea also presents several challenges.

Because the differential diagnosis of sleepiness is quite varied among children, pediatric sleep disorder centers are the referral of choice for testing and initiation of therapy.

Carroll JL: Obstructive sleep-disordered breathing in children: New controversies, new directions. Clin Chest Med 2003; 24:261 [PMID: 12800783].

Marcus CL: Sleep-disordered breathing in children. Am J Respir Crit Care Med 2001;164:16 [PMID: 11435234].

Sateia MJ (editor): *The International Classification of Sleep Disorders,* 2nd ed. American Academy of Sleep Medicine, 2005.

Schechter MS et al: Technical report: Diagnosis and management of childhood obstructive sleep apnea syndrome. Pediatrics 2002;109:e69 [PMID: 11927742].

Section on Pediatric Pulmonology, Subcommittee on Obstructive Sleep Apnea Syndrome, American Academy of Pediatrics: Clinical practice guideline: Diagnosis and management of childhood obstructive sleep apnea syndrome. Pediatrics 2002;109:704 [PMID: 11927718].

APPARENT LIFE-THREATENING EVENTS IN INFANCY

Apparent life-threatening events (ALTEs) are characterized as being frightening to the observer and commonly include some combination of apnea, color change (usually cyanosis or pallor), a marked change in muscle tone (usually extreme limpness), choking, or gagging. The observer sometimes fears the infant has died. The most frequent problems associated with an ALTE are gastrointestinal (about 50%), neurologic (30%), respiratory (20%), cardiovascular (5%), metabolic and endocrine (under 5%), or diverse other problems, including child abuse. Up to 50% of ALTEs remain unexplained and are referred to as apnea of infancy. The relationship between ALTE and future risk of sudden infant death syndrome (SIDS) is not clear. The term ALTE replaced "near-miss SIDS" in order to distance the event from a direct association with SIDS. Literature has reported an increased risk when extreme cardiopulmonary events were present at the time of the ALTE. Fewer than 10% of SIDS victims have had a prior history of ALTE.

The mechanism for ALTEs is unknown, but because they do not occur after infancy, immaturity is felt to play a major role. Indeed, classic studies on the nervous system, reflexes, and responses to apnea or hypoxia during sleep show profound cardiovascular compromise in infants during stimulation of the immature autonomic nervous system; adults would not be affected.

The following section describes an approach to the patient who has undergone an ALTE, taking note of the very broad differential diagnosis and uncertainties in both evaluation and treatment.

Differential Diagnosis

Table 18–3 classifies disorders associated with ALTEs. A careful history is often the most helpful part of the evaluation. It is useful to determine whether the infant has been chronically ill or essentially well. A history of several days of poor feeding, temperature instability, or respiratory or gastrointestinal symptoms suggests an infectious process. Reports of "struggling to breathe" or "trying to breathe" imply airway obstruction. Association of the episodes with feeding implies discoordinated swallowing, gastroesophageal reflux, or airway obstruction. Episodes that typically follow crying may be related to breath-holding. Association of episodes with sleeping may also suggest gastroesophageal reflux, apnea of infancy, or sleep-disordered breathing. Attempts should be made to determine the duration of the episode, but this is often difficult. It is helpful to role-play the episode with the family. Details regarding the measures taken to resuscitate the infant and the infant's recovery from the episode are often useful in determining severity.

The physical examination provides further direction in pursuing the diagnosis. Fever or hypothermia suggests infection. An altered state of consciousness implies a postictal state or drug overdose. Respiratory distress implies cardiac or pulmonary lesions.

Most patients are hospitalized for observation in order to reduce stress on the family and allow prompt completion of the evaluation. Laboratory evaluation includes a complete blood count for evidence of infection. Serum electrolytes are usually obtained. Elevations in serum bicarbonate suggest chronic hypoventilation, whereas decreases suggest acute acidosis, perhaps due to hypoxia during the episode. Chronic acidosis suggests an inherited metabolic disorder. The chest radiograph is examined for infiltrates suggesting acute infection or chronic aspiration and for cardiac size as a clue to intrinsic cardiac disease. Arterial blood gas studies provide an initial assessment of oxygenation and acid-base status, and low PaO_2 or elevated $PaCO_2$ (or both) implies cardiorespiratory disease. A significant base deficit suggests that the episode was accompanied by hypoxia or circulatory impairment. Oxygen saturation measurements in the hospital assess oxygenation status during different activities and are more comprehensive than a single blood gas sample.

Because apnea has been associated with respiratory infections, diagnostic studies for RSV and other viruses, pertussis, and *Chlamydia* may help with diagnosis. The apnea occurring with infection often precedes other physical findings. If the episode might have involved airway obstruction, the airway should be examined either directly, by fiberoptic bronchoscopy, or radiographically, by CT or barium swallow. Barium swallow is a useful tool to rule out the possibility of anatomic abnormalities such as vascular ring and tracheoesophageal fistula. This study may also demonstrate reflux and aspiration. If reflux is suspected, it should be documented by esophageal pH monitoring coupled with respiratory pattern recording. Most infants with reflux and apnea can be given medical antireflux treatment. Infants with reflux and repeated episodes of apnea may benefit from a surgical antireflux procedure.

ALTEs occur in the same age group as infants who die of sudden death (2–4 months is the peak age). Sleep-disordered breathing has been implicated as a possible cause of ALTEs and perhaps sudden death. Depending on the discretion of the clinician in appropriate scenarios, polysomnograms can be useful to determine abnormalities of cardiorespiratory function, sleep state, oxygen saturation, CO_2 retention, and seizure activity. They can be used in conjunction with pH monitoring to determine the contribution of reflux to apnea. Esophageal pressure manometry can be useful to detect subtle changes in respiratory effort related to partial obstructive breathing (hypopnea). Infants may be at more risk of adverse events from sleep-disordered breathing due to their immature nervous system.

There are several neurologic causes of ALTEs. Apnea as the sole manifestation of a seizure disorder is unusual

Table 18–3. Potential causes of apparent life-threatening events.

Infectious	Viral: respiratory syncytial virus and other respiratory viruses
	Bacterial: sepsis, pertussis, chlamydia
Gastrointestinal	Gastroesophageal reflux with or without obstructive apnea
Respiratory	Airway abnormality; vascular rings, pulmonary slings, tracheomalacia
	Pneumonia
Neurologic	Seizure disorder
	Central nervous system infection: meningitis, encephalitis
	Vasovagal response
	Leigh encephalopathy
	Brain tumor
Cardiovascular	Congenital malformation
	Dysrhythmias
	Cardiomyopathy
Nonaccidental trauma	Battering
	Drug overdose
	Münchausen syndrome by proxy
No definable cause	Apnea of infancy

but may occur. In cases of repeated episodes, 24-hour electroencephalographic monitoring may be helpful in detecting a seizure disorder. Leigh disease, a brainstem disorder characterized pathologically by neuronal dropout, may present with apneic episodes.

Apneic episodes have been linked to child abuse in several ways. Head injury following nonaccidental trauma may be first brought to medical attention because of apnea. Other signs of abuse are usually immediately apparent in such cases. Drug overdose, either accidental or intentional, may also present with apnea. Several series document that apneic episodes may be falsely reported by parents seeking attention (ie, Münchhausen syndrome by proxy). Parents may physically interfere with a child's respiratory efforts, in which case pinch marks on the nares are sometimes found.

Treatment

Therapy is directed at the underlying cause if one is found. After blood cultures are taken, antibiotics should be given to infants who appear toxic. Seizure disorders are treated with anticonvulsants. Gastroesophageal reflux should be treated, but may not prevent future episodes of ALTE. Vascular rings and pulmonary slings must be corrected surgically because of severe morbidity and high mortality rates when untreated.

The approach to care of infants with ALTEs where no definable cause can be ascertained is controversial. Home monitoring has been used in the past as treatment, but the efficacy of monitoring has not been demonstrated in controlled trials. The rationale for use of monitors is that infants at risk for subsequent severe episodes can be identified. With over 20 years of home monitoring, the sudden infant death rate did not change due to this intervention. Although monitors can detect apnea or bradycardia, they do not predict which children will have future ALTEs. Parents should be taught cardiopulmonary resuscitation prior to discharge. They should also be aware of the possibility of frequent false alarms. It must be noted that many parents cannot handle the stress associated with having a monitor in the home.

The decision to monitor these infants involves the participation of the family. Infants with severe initial episodes or repeated severe episodes are now thought to be at significantly increased risk and should probably be monitored in the home. Episodes in these children are so severe that the parents want to know the infant's condition at all times. The decision to discontinue monitoring is usually based on the infant's ability to go several months without triggering the alarm.

Oxygen has been used as therapy for ALTEs for several reasons. First, it reduces periodic breathing of infancy, an immature pattern of breathing that can cause some degree of oxygen desaturation. Second, infants have small chest capacities with increased chest wall compliance that reduces lung volume. Oxygen can increase the baseline saturation, reducing the severity of desaturation with short apneas. Respiratory stimulants such as caffeine and aminophylline have been used in specific cases of central apnea or periodic breathing.

Davies F, Gupta R: Apparent life threatening events in infants presenting to an emergency department. Emerg Med J 2002;19:11 [PMID: 11777863].

Farrell PA et al: SIDS, ALTE, apnea, and the use of home monitors. Pediatr Rev 2002;23:3 [PMID: 11773587].

Kahn A: Recommended clinical evaluation of infants with an apparent life-threatening event. Consensus document of the European Society for the Study and Prevention of Infant Death, 2003. Eur J Pediatr 2004;163:108.

SUDDEN INFANT DEATH SYNDROME

SIDS is defined as the sudden death of an infant younger than age 1 year that remains unexplained after a thorough case investigation, including performance of a complete autopsy, examination of the death scene, and review of the clinical history. The postmortem examination is an important feature of the definition because approximately 20% of cases of sudden death can be explained by autopsy findings. The incidence of SIDS in the United States has declined to less than 1:1000 live births. The part of the decline that has occurred since 1994 is likely due to alterations of risk factors (see following discussion).

Epidemiologic and pathologic data constitute most of what is known about SIDS. The number of deaths peaks between ages 2 and 4 months, and most deaths occur in infants a few weeks to 6 months of age. Most deaths occur between midnight and 8 AM, while the infant and often the caregiver are sleeping. In fact, the only unifying features of all SIDS cases are age and sleep. Previous studies showed a peak in SIDS during the respiratory virus season, but the association becomes weaker when the data are controlled for risk factors such as tobacco exposure. SIDS is more common among ethnic and racial minorities and socioeconomically disadvantaged populations. Racial disparity in the prevalence of prone positioning may also be contributing to the continued disparity in SIDS rates between black and white infants. There is a 3:2 male predominance in most series. Other risk factors include low birth weight, teenage or drug-addicted mothers, maternal smoking, and a family history of SIDS. Most of these risk factors are associated with a two- to threefold elevation of incidence but are not specific enough to be useful in predicting which infants will die unexpectedly. Recent immunization is not a risk factor.

Since 1990, SIDS rates have declined more than 60% worldwide. Population studies in New Zealand and

Europe identified risk factors, which when changed had a major effect on the incidence of SIDS. Since 1994 the American Academy of Pediatrics' "Back-to-Sleep" campaign has promoted education about SIDS risk factors in the U.S. Modifiable risk factors include sleeping position, bottle feeding, maternal smoking, and infant overheating; sleeping position and smoke exposure may have the largest influence. The prone sleep position could contribute to SIDS through decreased arousal during sleep or during hypoxia, rebreathing of exhaled gases, or effects on the immature autonomic nervous system. The side position, often used in hospitals and then mimicked at home, also shows increased risk of SIDS compared with the supine position. Maternal smoking, especially prenatal maternal smoking, increases the risk of SIDS. Investigations of tobacco effects on the autonomic nervous system of the developing fetus, pulmonary growth and function of the newborn, or its combination with viral infection all point to differences in SIDS compared with control subjects. Although the mechanism is not known, recent literature review has shown a reduced risk of SIDS associated with pacifier use. While beneficial for many reasons, breast feeding is debated regarding decreasing SIDS risk.

The most consistent pathologic findings are intrathoracic petechiae and mild inflammation and congestion of the respiratory tract. Subtler pathologic findings include brainstem gliosis, extramedullary hematopoiesis, and increases in periadrenal brown fat. These latter findings suggest that infants who succumb to SIDS have had intermittent or chronic hypoxia before death.

The mechanism or mechanisms of death in SIDS are unknown. For example, it is unknown whether the initiating event at the time of death is cessation of breathing, cardiac arrhythmia, or asystole. Hypotheses have included upper airway obstruction, catecholamine excess, and increased fetal hemoglobin. However, maldevelopment or delay in maturation of the brainstem, which is responsible for arousal remains the predominant theory. It has been recognized that some infants who presented with apneic episodes subsequently died from SIDS; however, study of these infants and prospective studies of large numbers of newborns have indicated that most infants with apnea do not die from SIDS and that most infants with SIDS have no identifiable episodes of apnea. The American Academy of Pediatrics has recommended that infant home monitoring not be used as a strategy to prevent SIDS, but may be useful in some infants who have had an ALTE (see section on apparent life-threatening events, above).

A history of mild symptoms of upper respiratory infection before death is not uncommon, and SIDS victims are sometimes seen by physicians a day or so before death. When infants are discovered blue, cold, and motionless by parents or caregivers, they are most commonly taken to the emergency department, where resus-

Table 18–4. American Academy of Pediatrics recommendations regarding sudden infant death syndrome (SIDS) risk reduction.

"Back-to-Sleep" (supine sleeping position)
Firm sleep surface
Soft objects/loose bedding out of crib
Do not smoke during pregnancy
Separate but proximate sleeping environment
Consider offering a pacifier at nap and bed time
Avoid overheating
Avoid commercial devices marketed to reduce the risk of SIDS
Do not use home monitors as a strategy to reduce the risk of SIDS
Avoid development of positional plagiocephaly

Reproduced, with permission, from American Academy of Pediatrics Task Force on Sudden Infant Death Syndrome: The changing concept of sudden infant death syndrome: diagnostic coding shifts, controversies regarding the sleeping environment, and new variables to consider in reducing risk. Pediatrics 2005;116:1245 (Epub 2005 Oct 10) [PMID: 16216901].

citation usually fails. Families must then be supported following the death. The National SIDS Resource Center (www.sidscenter.org) provides information about psychosocial support groups and counseling for families of SIDS victims. The postmortem examination is essential for the diagnosis of SIDS and may help the family by excluding other possible causes of death. A death scene investigation is also important in determining the cause of sudden unexpected deaths in infancy.

The health care provider is instrumental in parental education regarding the modifiable risk factors for SIDS (Table 18–4). Education includes promotion of the supine sleeping position, firm sleep surface, avoidance of overheating, smoking cessation, pacifier use, and identification of child care settings, as many parents rely on others to watch their children, where the importance of infant sleep position may not recognized. Hospitals should set an example by placing infants in the supine position. With education, the mortality rate may continue to decline.

American Academy of Pediatrics Task Force on Sudden Infant Death Syndrome: The changing concept of sudden infant death syndrome: diagnostic coding shifts, controversies regarding the sleeping environment, and new variables to consider in reducing risk. Pediatrics 2005;116:1245 (Epub 2005 Oct 10) [PMID: 16216901].

Committee on the fetus and newborn, American Academy of Pediatrics: Apnea, sudden infant death syndrome, and home monitoring. Pediatrics 2003;111:914 [PMID: 12671135].

Hunt CE: Sudden infant death syndrome and other causes of infant mortality: Diagnosis, mechanisms, and risk for recurrence in siblings. Am J Respir Crit Care Med 2001;164:346 [PMID: 11500332].

Nagler J: Sudden infant death syndrome. Curr Opin Pediatr 2002;14:247 [PMID: 11981299].

Ramanathan R et al: Cardiorespiratory events recorded on home monitors: Comparison of healthy infants with those at increased risk for SIDS. JAMA 2001;285:2199 [PMID: 11325321].

Toomey S, Bernstein H: Sudden infant death syndrome. Curr Opin Pediatr 2001;13:207 [PMID: 11317067].

■ MEDIASTINUM

MEDIASTINAL MASSES

Mediastinal masses may present because of symptoms produced by pressure on the esophagus, airways, nerves, or vessels within the mediastinum, or may be discovered on a routine chest radiograph. Once the mass is identified, localization to one of four mediastinal compartments aids in the differential diagnosis. The superior mediastinum is the area above the pericardium that is bordered inferiorly by an imaginary line from the manubrium to the fourth thoracic vertebra. The anterior mediastinum is bordered by the sternum anteriorly and the pericardium posteriorly, and the posterior mediastinum is defined by the pericardium and diaphragm anteriorly and the lower eight thoracic vertebrae posteriorly. The middle mediastinum is surrounded by these three compartments.

Clinical Findings

A. SYMPTOMS AND SIGNS

Respiratory symptoms, when present, are due to pressure on an airway (cough or wheezing) or an infection (unresolving pneumonia in one area of lung). Hemoptysis can also occur but is an unusual presenting symptom. Dysphagia may occur secondary to compression of the esophagus. Pressure on the recurrent laryngeal nerve can cause hoarseness due to paralysis of the left vocal cord. Superior vena caval obstruction can lead to dilation of neck vessels and other signs and symptoms of obstruction of venous return from the upper part of the body (superior mediastinal syndrome).

B. LABORATORY FINDINGS AND IMAGING

The mass is initially defined by frontal and lateral chest radiographs together with thoracic CT scans and perhaps MRI. A barium swallow may also help define the extent of a mass. Other studies that may be required include angiography (to define the blood supply to large tumors), electrocardiography, echocardiography, ultrasound of the thorax, fungal and mycobacterial skin tests, and urinary catecholamine assays. MRI or myelography may be necessary in children suspected of having a neurogenic tumor in the posterior mediastinum.

Differential Diagnosis

The differential diagnosis of mediastinal masses is determined by their location. Within the superior mediastinum, one may find cystic hygromas, vascular or neurogenic tumors, thymic masses, teratomas, intrathoracic thyroid tissue, and esophageal lesions. A mediastinal abscess may also be found in this region. Within the anterior mediastinum, thymic tissue (thymomas, hyperplasia, and cysts) and teratomas, vascular tumors, and lymphatic tissue (lymphomas or reactive lymphadenopathy) give rise to masses. An intrathoracic thyroid and a pleuropericardial cyst may also be found in this region. Within the middle mediastinum one may again find lymphomas and hypertrophic lymph nodes, granulomas, bronchogenic or enterogenous cysts, metastases, and pericardial cysts. Abnormalities of the great vessels and aortic aneurysms may also present as masses in this compartment. Within the posterior mediastinum, neurogenic tumors, enterogenous cysts, thoracic meningoceles, or aortic aneurysms may be present.

In some series, more than 50% of mediastinal tumors occur in the posterior mediastinum and are mainly neurogenic tumors or enterogenous cysts. Most neurogenic tumors in children younger than age 4 years are malignant (neuroblastoma or neuroganglioblastoma), whereas a benign ganglioneuroma is the most common histologic type in older children. In the middle and anterior mediastinum, tumors of lymphatic origin (lymphomas) are the primary concern. Bulky anterior mediastinal tumors that compress the trachea and the great vessels can lead to a superior mediastinal syndrome, which presents a diagnostic problem because of anesthesia hazards. Definitive diagnosis in most instances relies on surgery to obtain the mass or a part of the mass for histologic examination. In cases of lymphoma, the scalene nodes may also contain tumor, and a biopsy should be performed in an attempt to establish a diagnosis.

Treatment & Prognosis

The appropriate therapy and the response to therapy depend on the cause of the mediastinal mass.

Franco A et al: Imaging evaluation of pediatric mediastinal masses. Radiol Clin North Am 2005;43:325 [PMID: 15737372].

Williams HJ, Alton HM: Imaging of paediatric mediastinal abnormalities. Paediatr Respir Rev 2003;4:55 [PMID: 12615033].

Cardiovascular Diseases

Henry M. Sondheimer, MD, Anji T. Yetman, MD, & Shelley D. Miyamoto, MD

Cardiovascular disease is a significant cause of death and chronic illness in childhood. In North America, 8 in 1000 infants are born with a congenital heart defect. Acquired heart disease, including Kawasaki disease, myocarditis, rheumatic heart disease, and others, is also a significant cause of pediatric morbidity and mortality. With advances in medical and surgical care, more than 85% of children with congenital heart defects will live into adulthood. It is therefore important that attention be paid not only to the diagnosis and treatment of congenital cardiac lesions but also to the prevention of secondary comorbidities such as hyperlipidemia and atherosclerosis. Pediatric health maintenance visits must focus on diagnosis and prevention of hypercholesterolemia and hypertension. Counseling on the hazards of smoking and the benefits of exercise should be part of routine care. Subspecialty clinics that address the needs of young adults with congenital heart disease are needed to serve this growing patient population. Previously rare clinical issues, including the impact of pregnancy on patients with congenital cardiac lesions, the risks of anticoagulation during pregnancy, and vocational choices must be addressed.

■ DIAGNOSTIC EVALUATION

The presence of a heart murmur suggests the possibility of heart disease. Murmurs, however, may be functional or innocent, and not all serious cardiovascular disorders are accompanied by an easily detectable murmur.

Sequence of Evaluation

1. History
2. Physical examination
3. Electrocardiogram
4. Chest radiograph
5. Echocardiogram
6. Other studies, including cardiopulmonary stress testing, 24-hour Holter or other ambulatory electrocardiographic (ECG) monitoring, cardiac catheteriza-

tion, angiocardiography, nuclear imaging studies, and cardiac magnetic resonance imaging (MRI)

HISTORY

Most congenital defects lead either to decreased pulmonary blood flow or increased pulmonary blood flow with pulmonary congestion (see Table 19–1). Symptoms vary according to the alteration in pulmonary blood flow (Table 19–1). The presence of other cardiovascular symptoms such as palpitations and chest pain should also be determined by history in the older child, paying particular attention to the timing (at rest or activity-related), onset, and termination (gradual versus sudden), and precipitating and relieving factors.

PHYSICAL EXAMINATION

General

The examination should begin with a visual assessment of activity (agitation or lethargy), skin perfusion, and skin color. Heart rate, respiratory rate, blood pressure (in all four extremities), and oxygen saturation are required. Many congenital cardiac defects occur as part of a genetic syndrome (Table 19–2), and overall assessment includes an evaluation for dysmorphic features that may be clues to the associated cardiac defect.

1. Cardiovascular Examination

Inspection & Palpation

Chest conformation should be noted by observing the supine patient from the end of the examining table. A left precordial bulge indicates long-standing cardiomegaly. Palpation may reveal increased precordial activity, right ventricular lift, or left-sided heave; a diffuse point of maximal impulse; or a precordial thrill caused by a grade IV/VI murmur. The thrill of aortic stenosis should be sought in the suprasternal notch. In patients with severe pulmonary hypertension, palpable pulmonary closure (P_2) is frequently noted at the upper left sternal border. A palpable fourth heart sound may be seen in association with a hypertrophied, noncompliant ventricle as in hypertrophic cardiomyopathy.

Table 19–1. Symptoms of increased and decreased pulmonary blood flow.

Decreased Pulmonary Blood Flow	Increased Pulmonary Blood Flow
Infant/Toddler:	
Cyanosis	Tachypnea with activity/feeds
Squatting	Diaphoresis
Loss of consciousness	Poor weight gain
Older child:	
Dizziness	Exercise intolerance
Syncope	Dyspnea on exertion, diaphoresis

Auscultation

A. HEART SOUNDS

The first heart sound (S_1) is the sound of atrioventricular (AV) valve closure. It is best heard at the lower left sternal border and is usually medium-pitched. Although S_1 has multiple components, usually only one of these (M_1) is audible.

The second heart sound (S_2) is the sound of semilunar valve closure. It is best heard at the upper left sternal border. S_2 has two component sounds, A_2 and P_2 (aortic and pulmonary valve closure). Splitting of S_2 varies with respiration, widening with inspiration and narrowing with expiration. Abnormal splitting of S_2 may be an indication of cardiac disease (Table 19–3).

The third heart sound (S_3) is the sound of rapid filling of the left ventricle (LV). It occurs in early diastole, after S_2, and is medium- to low-pitched. In healthy children,

Table 19–2. Cardiac defects in common syndromes.

Genetic Syndrome	Commonly Associated Cardiac Defect
Down syndrome	AVSD
Turner syndrome	Bicuspid aortic valve, coarctation
Noonan syndrome	Dysplastic pulmonic valve, HCM
Williams-Beuren syndrome	Supravalval aortic stenosis, PPS
Marfan syndrome	MVP, MR, dilated aortic root
Fetal alcohol syndrome	VSD, ASD
Maternal rubella	PDA, PPS

AVSD, atrioventricvular septal defect; HCM, hypertrophic cardiomyopathy; MVP, mitral valve prolapse; MR, mitral regurgitation; VSD, ventricular septal defect; ASD, atrial septal defect; PDA, patent ductus arteriosus; PPS, peripheral pulmonary stenosis.

Table 19–3. Abnormal splitting of S_2.

Causes of wide split S_2
RV volume overload: ASD, anomalous pulmonary venous return, PI
RV pressure overload: Pulmonary valve stenosis
Delayed RV conduction: RBBB
Causes of narrow split S_2
Pulmonary hypertension
Single semilunar valve (aortic atresia, pulmonary atresia, truncus arteriosus)

RV, right ventricle; ASD, atrial septal defect; PI, pulmonic insufficiency; RBBB, right bundle branch block.

S_3 diminishes or disappears when going from supine to sitting or standing. A persistent S_3 is often heard in the presence of a dilated LV caused by a cardiomyopathy or large left-to-right shunt. The fourth heart sound (S_4) is associated with atrial contraction and increased atrial pressure and has a low pitch similar to that of S_3. It occurs just prior to S_1 and is not normally audible. It is heard in the presence of atrial contraction into a noncompliant ventricle as in hypertrophic or restrictive cardiomyopathy or hypertrophied LV from other causes.

Ejection clicks are high-pitched and are usually related to dilated great vessels or valve abnormalities. They can be heard throughout ventricular systole and are classified as early, mid, or late. Early ejection clicks at the mid left sternal border are from the pulmonic valve. Aortic clicks are typically best heard at the apex. In contrast to aortic clicks, pulmonic clicks vary with respiration, becoming louder during inspiration. A mid to late ejection click at the apex is most typically caused by mitral valve prolapse. Early clicks may also be heard with a closing ventricular septal defect (VSD).

B. MURMURS

Murmurs are the most common cardiovascular finding leading to a cardiology referral. Innocent or functional heart murmurs are common, and 40–45% of children have an innocent murmur at some time during childhood.

1. Characteristics—All murmurs should be described based on the following characteristics:

a. Location and radiation—Where the murmur is best heard and where the sound extends.

b. Relationship to cardiac cycle and duration—Systolic ejection (immediately following S_1 with a crescendo/decrescendo change in intensity), pansystolic (occurring throughout most of systole and of constant intensity), diastolic, and continuous. The timing of the murmur provides valuable clues as to underlying pathology (Table 19–4).

Table 19–4. Pathologic murmurs.

Systolic Ejection	Pansystolic	Diastolic	Continuous
Semilunar valve stenosis (AS/PS/truncal stenosis) ASD Coarctation	VSD AVVR (MR/TR)	Semilunar valve regurgitation (AI/PI/truncal insufficiency) AV valve stenosis (MS/TS)	Runoff lesions (PDA/AVM/aortopulmonary collaterals)

VSD, ventricular septal defect; AS/PS, aortic stenosis/pulmonic stenosis; MR/TR, mitral regurgitation/tricuspid regurgitation; AI/PI, aortic insufficiency/pulmonic insufficiency; PDA/AVM, patent ductus arteriosus/arteriovenous malformation; ASD, atrial septal defect; AV, atrioventricular; MS/TS, mitral stenosis/tricuspid stenosis; AVVR, atrioventricular valve regurgitation.

c. Intensity—Grade I describes a soft murmur heard with difficulty; grade II, soft but easily heard; grade III, loud but without a thrill; grade IV, loud and associated with a precordial thrill; grade V, loud, with thrill, and audible with the edge of the stethoscope; grade VI, very loud and audible with the stethoscope off the chest.

d. Quality—Harsh, musical, or rough; high, medium, or low in pitch.

e. Variation with position—Audible when the patient is supine, sitting, standing, or squatting.

2. Functional murmurs—The six most common functional murmurs of childhood are:

a. Newborn murmur—Heard in the first few days of life, this murmur is at the lower left sternal border, without significant radiation. It has a soft, short, vibratory grade I–II/VI quality that often subsides when mild pressure is applied to the abdomen. It usually disappears by age 2–3 weeks.

b. Functional murmur of peripheral arterial pulmonary stenosis—This murmur, often heard in newborns, is caused by the normal branching of the pulmonary artery. It is heard with equal intensity at the upper left sternal border, at the back, and in both axillae. It is a soft, short, high-pitched, grade I–II/VI systolic ejection murmur and usually disappears by age 2. This murmur must be differentiated from true peripheral pulmonary stenosis (Williams syndrome, Alagille syndrome, or rubella syndrome), coarctation of the thoracic aorta, valvular pulmonary stenosis, and atrial septal defect (ASD).

c. Still murmur—This is the most common innocent murmur of early childhood. It is typically heard between 2 and 7 years of age. It is loudest midway between the apex and the lower left sternal border and often is transmitted to the remainder of the precordium. Still murmur is a musical or vibratory, short, high-pitched, grade I–III early systolic murmur. It is loudest when the patient is supine; it diminishes or disappears with inspiration, when the patient stands, or during Valsalva maneuver. Still murmur is louder in patients with fever, anemia, or sinus tachycardia from any reason.

d. Pulmonary ejection murmur—This is the most common innocent murmur in older children. It is heard from age 3 years onward. It is usually a soft systolic ejection murmur, grade I–II in intensity and well localized to the upper left sternal border. The murmur is louder when the patient is supine or when cardiac output is increased. The pulmonary ejection murmur must be differentiated from murmurs associated with pulmonary stenosis, coarctation of the aorta, ASD, and peripheral pulmonary artery stenosis.

e. Venous hum—This murmur is usually heard after age 2 years. It is located in the infraclavicular areas and is usually louder on the right. It is a continuous musical hum of grade I–II intensity and may be accentuated in diastole and with inspiration. It is best heard in the sitting position. Turning the child's neck, placing the child supine, and compressing the jugular vein obliterates the venous hum. Venous hum is produced by turbulence at the confluence of the subclavian and jugular veins.

f. Innominate or carotid bruit—This murmur is more common in the older child and adolescent. It is heard in the right supraclavicular area. It is a long systolic ejection murmur, somewhat harsh and of grade II–III intensity. The bruit can be accentuated by light pressure on the carotid artery and must be differentiated from all types of aortic stenosis.

When functional murmurs are found in a child, the physician should assure the parents that these are normal heart sounds of the developing child and that they do not represent structural cardiac abnormalities.

2. Extracardiac Examination

Arterial Pulse

A. RATE AND RHYTHM

Cardiac rate and rhythm vary greatly during infancy and childhood, so multiple determinations should be

Table 19–5. Resting heart rates.

Age	Low	High
< 1 month	80	160
1–3 months	80	200
2–24 months	70	120
2–10 years	60	90
11–18 years	40	90

made. This caution is particularly important for infants (Table 19–5) whose heart rate varies with activity. In children, the rhythm may be regular, or there may be a phasic variation with respiration (sinus arrhythmia), which is normal.

B. QUALITY AND AMPLITUDE OF PULSE

The pulses of the upper and lower extremities should be compared. A bounding pulse is characteristic of run-off lesions, including patent ductus arteriosus (PDA), aortic regurgitation, arteriovenous malformation (AVM), or any condition with a low diastolic pressure (fever, anemia, or septic shock). These conditions may also be associated with palpable palmar pulses, which otherwise are not normally present. Narrow or thready pulses occur in patients with conditions reducing cardiac output such as cardiomyopathy, myocarditis, pericardial tamponade, or severe aortic stenosis. A reduction in pulse amplitude or blood pressure (> 10 mm Hg) with inspiration is referred to as pulsus paradoxus and is a telltale sign of pericardial tamponade. With inspiration, venous return is increased to the right side of the heart. Because of a fixed pericardial constraint, an increase in right heart volume must be accompanied by a reduction in left heart volume and thus a reduction in cardiac output during the inspiratory phase of respiration. The femoral pulse should be palpable and equal in amplitude and simultaneous with the brachial pulse. A femoral pulse that is absent or weak, or that is delayed in comparison with the brachial pulse, suggests coarctation of the aorta.

C. ARTERIAL BLOOD PRESSURE

Blood pressures should be obtained in the upper and lower extremities. Systolic pressure in the lower extremities should be greater than or equal to that in the upper extremities. The cuff must cover the same relative area of the arm and leg. Measurements should be repeated several times.

D. EXTREMITIES

1. Cyanosis—Cyanosis results from an increased concentration (4–5 g/dL) of reduced hemoglobin in the blood. Bluish skin color is usually, but not always, a sign.

Anemic patients may not appear blue, and patients with polycythemia may appear cyanotic, even though blood oxygen content is normal. Visible cyanosis accompanies low cardiac output, hypothermia, and systemic venous congestion, even in the presence of adequate oxygenation. Cyanosis should be judged only by the color of the mucous membranes (lips). Bluish discoloration around the mouth (acrocyanosis) is a feature of skin that has not been exposed to sun, and it does not correlate with cyanosis.

2. Clubbing of fingers and toes—Clubbing is often associated with severe cyanotic congenital heart disease. It usually appears after age 1 year. Hypoxemia producing cyanosis is the most common cause of digital clubbing, but it also occurs in patients with endocarditis, chronic liver disease, inflammatory bowel diseases, chronic pulmonary insufficiency (PI), and lung abscess. Digital clubbing may be a benign genetic variant.

3. Edema—Edema of dependent areas (lower extremities in the older child and the face and sacrum in the younger child) is characteristic of elevated right heart pressure, which may be seen with tricuspid valve pathology or right ventricle (RV) dysfunction (right heart failure) from a variety of causes including LV dysfunction.

E. ABDOMEN

Hepatomegaly is the cardinal sign of right heart failure in the infant and child. Apparent hepatomegaly may also be seen in the child with pulmonary edema from lesions causing left-to-right shunting or left heart failure. Splenomegaly may be present in patients with long-standing congestive heart failure (CHF), and is characteristic of infective endocarditis. Ascites is also a feature of chronic right heart failure. Examination of the abdomen may reveal shifting dullness or a fluid wave.

Advani N et al: The diagnosis of innocent murmurs in childhood. Cardiol Young 2000;10:340 [PMID: 10950330].

Murphy DJ: The patient population and requirements for optimal care: Adult congenital heart disease. Prog Pediatr Cardiol 2003;17:1.

Williams CL et al: Cardiovascular health in childhood: A statement for health professionals. Circulation 2002;106:143 [PMID: 12093785].

ELECTROCARDIOGRAPHY

The electrocardiogram (ECG) is essential in the evaluation of the cardiovascular system. A consistent approach to the ECG will allow for interpretation of even the most complex and initially confusing ECG recording. The heart rate should first be determined, then the cardiac rhythm (Is the patient in a normal sinus rhythm or other rhythm as evidenced by a P wave with a consistent PR interval before every QRS complex?), and then the axis (Are the P and QRS axes normal for the patient's age?). Once this initial assessment of rate, rhythm, and axis is

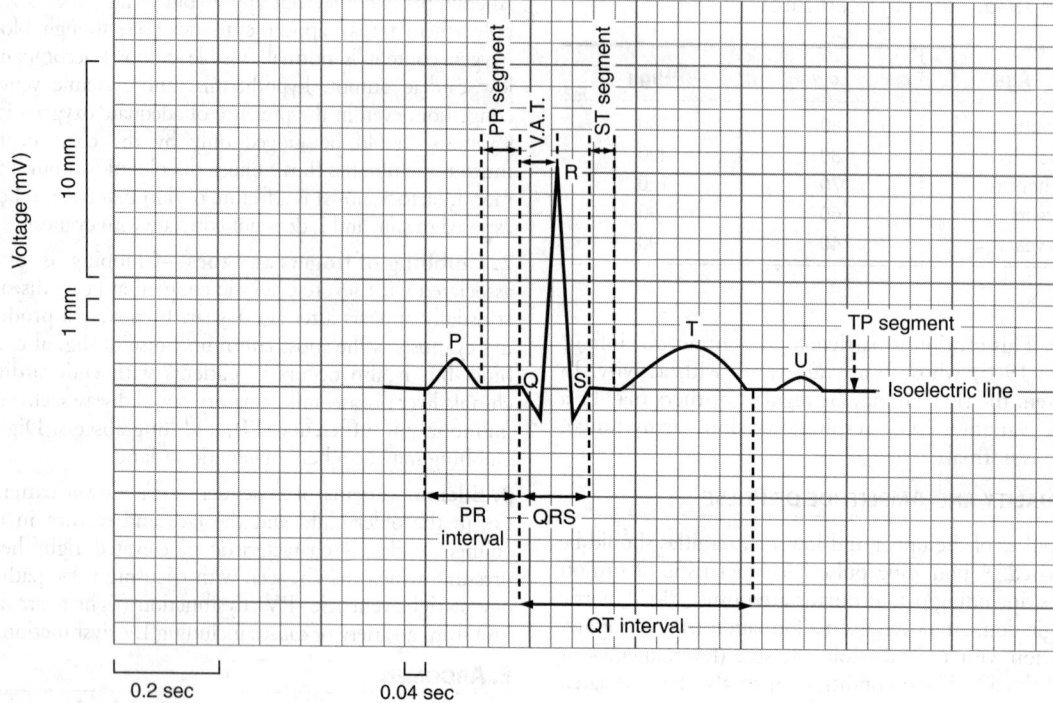

Figure 19–1. Complexes and intervals of the electrocardiogram.

performed, attention can be directed toward assessment of chamber enlargement and finally to assessment of cardiac intervals and ST segments.

Age-Related Variations

The ECG evolves with age. The rate decreases and intervals increase with age. RV dominance in the newborn changes to LV dominance in the older infant, child, and adult. The normal ECG of the 1-week-old infant is abnormal for a 1-year-old child, and the ECG of a 5-year-old child is abnormal for an adult.

Electrocardiographic Interpretation

Figure 19–1 defines the events recorded by the ECG.

A. RATE

Heart rate varies markedly in the child depending on age, activity, and state of emotional and physical well-being. For most infants and younger children, the heart rate will range from 70–200 beats per minute depending on the above.

B. RHYTHM

Sinus rhythm should always be present in normal children. In contrast to adults, premature atrial and ventricular contractions are uncommon during childhood.

C. AXIS

P wave axis: The P wave is generated from atrial contraction beginning in the high right atrium at the site of the sinus node. The impulse proceeds leftward and inferiorly, thus leading to a positive deflection in all left-sided and inferior leads (II, III, and aVF). Conversely, the P wave in patients in normal sinus rhythm should be negative in lead aVR.

QRS axis: The net voltage should be positive in leads I and aVF in children with a normal axis. In the young child, RV dominance may persist, leading to a negative net deflection in lead I. Several congenital cardiac lesions are associated with alterations in the normal QRS axis (Table 19–6).

D. P WAVE

In the pediatric patient, the amplitude of the P wave is normally no greater than 3 mm and the duration no more than 0.08 second. The P wave is best seen in leads II and V_1.

E. PR INTERVAL

The PR is measured from the beginning of the P wave to the beginning of the QRS complex. It increases with age and with slower rates. The PR interval ranges from a minimum of 0.10 second in infants to a maximum of 0.18 second in older children with slow rates. The PR

Table 19–6. QRS axis deviation.

Right Axis Deviation	Left Axis Deviation
Tetralogy of Fallot	Atrioventricular septal defect
Dextro transposition of the great arteries	Pulmonary atresia with intact ventricular septum
Total anomalous pulmonary venous return	Tricuspid atresia
Atrial septal defect	

interval is commonly prolonged in patients who have rheumatic heart disease and by digitalis.

F. QRS COMPLEX

This represents ventricular depolarization, and its amplitude and direction of force (axis) reveal the relative size of (viable) ventricular mass in hypertrophy, hypoplasia, and infarction. Abnormal ventricular conduction (ie, right or left bundle-branch block) is also revealed.

G. QT INTERVAL

This interval is measured from the beginning of the QRS complex to the end of the T wave. The QT duration may be prolonged as a primary condition or secondarily due to drugs or electrolyte imbalances (Table 19–7). The normal QT duration is rate-related and must be corrected using the Bazett formula:

$$QTc = \frac{QT\ interval(s)}{\sqrt{R - R\ interval(s)}}$$

The normal QTc is less than or equal to 0.44 second.

Table 19–7. Causes of QT prolongation.[a]

Cardiac medications
  Antiarrhythmics: IA (quinidine, procainamide, disopyramide) class III (amiodarone, sotalol)
  Inotropic agents: dobutamine, dopamine, epinephrine, isoproterenol
Noncardiac medications
  Antibiotics/antivirals: azithromycin, clarithromycin, levofloxacin, amantadine
  Antipsychotics: risperidol, thioridazine, lithium, haloperidol
  Other: albuterol, levalbuterol, ondansetron, phenytoin, pseudoephedrine
Sedatives: chloral hydrate, methadone
Electrolyte disturbances: hypokalemia, hypomagnesemia, hypocalcemia

[a]Partial list only.

H. ST SEGMENT

This segment, lying between the end of the QRS complex and the beginning of the T wave, is affected by drugs, electrolyte imbalances, or myocardial injury.

I. T WAVE

The T wave represents myocardial repolarization and is altered by electrolytes, myocardial hypertrophy, and ischemia.

J. IMPRESSION

The ultimate impression of the ECG is derived from a systematic analysis of the features described earlier as compared with expected normal values for the child's age.

Al-Khatib SM et al: What clinicians should know about the QT interval. JAMA 2003;289:2120 [PMID: 12709470].

Benson DW Jr: The normal electrocardiogram. In: Emmanouilides GC et al (editors): *Moss and Adams Heart Disease in Infants, Children, and Adolescents,* 5th ed. Williams & Wilkins, 1995.

Viskin S et al: Long QT syndrome caused by noncardiac drugs. Prog Cardiovasc Dis 2003;45:415 [PMID: 12704598].

CHEST RADIOGRAPH

Evaluation of the chest radiograph for cardiac disease should focus on: (1) position of the cardiac apex, (2) position of the abdominal viscera, (3) cardiac size, (4) cardiac configuration, and (5) character of the pulmonary vasculature.

A segmental approach is used when evaluating cardiac anatomy, either by chest radiograph or by echocardiography. The position of the heart should be noted as either levocardia (heart predominantly in the left chest), dextrocardia (heart predominantly in the right chest), or mesocardia (midline heart). The position of the liver and stomach bubble should be noted as either in the normal position (abdominal situs solitus), in reverse position with stomach bubble on the right (abdominal situs inversus), or a variable stomach position with midline liver (abdominal situs ambiguous). The heart appears relatively large in normal newborns and decreases on the chest radiograph with age. The heart size should be less than 50% of the chest diameter in children older than age 1 year. The cardiac configuration on chest x-ray may provide useful diagnostic information, as certain cardiac lesions have a characteristic radiographic appearance (Tables 19–8 and 19–9). The pulmonary vasculature should be assessed. The presence of increased or decreased pulmonary blood flow provides a clue to cardiac diagnosis, particularly in the cyanotic infant (Table 19–10).

Table 19–8. Radiographic changes with cardiac chamber enlargement.

Chamber Enlarged	Change in Cardiac Silhouette on Anteroposterior Film
Right ventricle	Apex of the heart is tipped upward
Left ventricle	Apex of the heart is tipped downward
Left atrium	Double shadow behind cardiac silhouette
	Increase in subcarinal angle
Right atrium	Prominence of right atrial border of the heart

The standard posteroanterior and left lateral chest radiographs are used (Figure 19–2).

Dextrocardia

Dextrocardia is a radiographic term used when the heart is on the right side of the chest. When dextrocardia occurs with reversal of position of the other important organs of the chest and abdomen (eg, liver, lungs, and spleen), the condition is called situs inversus totalis, and the heart is usually normal. When dextrocardia occurs with otherwise normal organs (situs solitus), the heart usually has severe defects.

Rarely, the abdominal organs and lungs are in situs ambiguous. The liver is central and anterior in the upper abdomen, with the stomach pushed posteriorly. Bilateral right-sidedness (asplenia syndrome) or bilateral left-sidedness (polysplenia syndrome) may occur, but in virtually all cases of situs ambiguous, congenital heart disease is present.

Table 19–9. Lesion-specific chest radiographic findings.

Diagnosis	Chest Radiograph Appearance
Dextrotransposition of the great arteries	Egg on a string
Tetralogy of Fallot	Boot-shaped heart
Unobstructed total anomalous pulmonary venous drainage	Snowman
Obstructed total anomalous pulmonary venous drainage	Small heart with congested lungs
Coarctation	Figure 3 sign + rib notching

Table 19–10. Alterations in pulmonary blood flow in cyanotic cardiac lesions.

Increased Pulmonary Blood Flow	Decreased Pulmonary Blood Flow
Total anomalous pulmonary venous return	Pulmonic stenosis
TA/large ventricular septal defect	Tricuspid atresia/restrictive ventricular septal defect
Complete transposition of the great arteries	Tetralogy of Fallot
Truncus arteroisus	Pulmonary atresia with intact ventricular septum
	Hypoplastic left heart syndrome

Burrows PE et al: Imaging of the neonate with congenital heart disease. In: Freedom RM (editor): *Neonatal Heart Disease.* Springer-Verlag, 1992.

ECHOCARDIOGRAPHY

Echocardiography is a central noninvasive method for diagnosing congenital heart defects and is used to define anatomy and to evaluate function, chamber size, vessel size, and valve abnormalities. In most cases two-dimensional echocardiography is sufficient for the accurate diagnosis of congenital cardiac lesions, and no further testing is required prior to initial medical or surgical intervention. Two-dimensional echocardiography with Doppler ultrasonography (color, pulsed, or continuous-wave ultrasound measurements) is used to assess cardiac output, magnitude of regurgitant and stenotic lesions, diastolic LV relaxation, and pulmonary artery pressure. Stress echocardiography allows for quantification of ventricular systolic and diastolic function and assessment of myocardial wall motion abnormalities in patients after exercise or pharmacologic stress with dobutamine infusion.

Two-dimensional echocardiography should be performed with a systematic series of steps to define the intracardiac anatomy:

1. Position of the cardiac apex
2. Position of the abdominal vessels (inferior vena cava [IVC] and aorta)
3. Relationship between the atria and ventricles
4. Relationship between the ventricles and great vessels
5. Evaluation of intracardiac defects

The relationship between the atria and ventricles is noted. If the morphologic right atrium empties into a morphologic RV, and similarly the morphologic left atrium empties into a morphologic LV, atrioventricular concordance is present. If the atria correspond to the

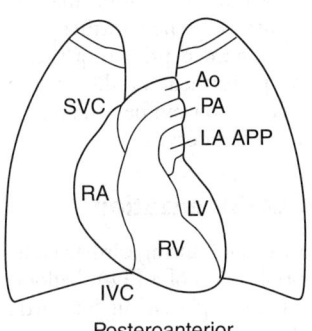
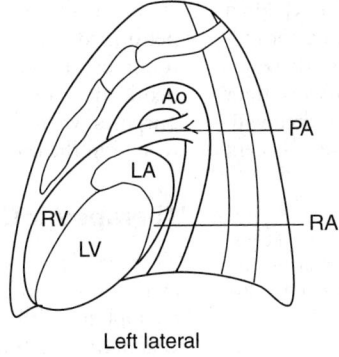

Posteroanterior

Left lateral

Figure 19–2. Position of cardiovascular structures in principal radiograph views. Ao, aorta; IVC, inferior vena cava; LA, left atrium; LA APP, left atrial appendage; LV, left ventricle; PA, pulmonary artery; RA, right atrium; RV, right ventricle; SVC, superior vena cava.

wrong ventricle (eg, right atrium emptying into the LV), atrioventricular discordance is present. Other possible AV relationships include double-inlet LV (both atria empty into the LV), double-inlet RV, and atresia of a right or left AV valve with associated single inlet (eg, tricuspid atresia). Similarly, the relationship between the ventricles and great vessels is noted. Normally, the pulmonary artery (PA) arises from the RV and the aorta from the LV and ventriculoarterial concordance is present. If the relationships are reversed (ie, aorta from the RV and PA from the LV), then ventriculoarterial discordance is present (as in transposition of the great arteries [TGA]). Other possible ventriculoarterial relationships include double-outlet RV, double-outlet LV, and atresia of one outlet (eg, pulmonary or aortic atresia). If both AV discordance and ventriculoarterial discordance are present, the patient has what is referred to as congenitally corrected transposition.

Pahl E et al: The role of stress echocardiography in children. Echocardiography 2000;17:507 [PMID: 10979027].

Snider AR et al: *Echocardiography in Congenital Heart Disease.* Mosby, 1997.

NUCLEAR CARDIOLOGY

Nuclear imaging may be useful as an adjunct to cardiopulmonary exercise testing in assessing both fixed and reversible areas of myocardial ischemia. This testing is valuable in evaluating myocardial perfusion in patients with Kawasaki disease, repaired anomalous left coronary artery or other coronary anomalies, myocardial bridging in the setting of hypertrophic cardiomyopathy, or chest pain in association with ECG changes with exercise.

MAGNETIC RESONANCE IMAGING

MRI is a valuable tool in the evaluation and noninvasive follow-up of many congenital heart defects. It is particularly useful in imaging the vascular structures of the thorax, which are difficult to image by transthoracic echocardio-

gram. The addition of cardiac gated imaging allows dynamic evaluation of the structure and blood flow in the heart and great vessels. MRI is invaluable in the initial assessment and long-term follow-up of coarctation of the aorta, in following the progression of aortic dilation in patients with Marfan syndrome, in quantification of regurgitant lesions such as PI following repair of tetralogy of Fallot (ToF), and in quantification of ventricular function in patients whose echocardiographic images are inadequate. Because it allows the operator to move the heart and great vessels on the computer screen, three-dimensional MRI is an ideal method of noninvasive reconstruction of the entire heart and useful for both assessing intracardiac anatomy and analyzing great vessel anatomy and relationships. If a cardiac MRI is performed in a child under the age of 8 years, general anaesthesia is most often required.

Boxt LM, Rozenshtein A: MR imaging of congenital heart disease. Magn Reson Imaging Clin North Am 2003;11:27 [PMID: 12797509].

Cardiopulmonary Stress Testing

Most children with heart disease are capable of normal activity, and data on cardiac function after exercise are essential to preventing the unnecessary restriction of activities. The response to exercise is valuable in determining the timing of, and need for, cardiovascular surgery as well as a useful objective outcome measure for the evaluation of medical and surgical interventions.

Bicycle ergometers or treadmills can be used to test children as young as age 5 years. The addition of a metabolic cart enables one to assess whether exercise impairment is secondary to cardiac limitation, pulmonary limitation, deconditioning, or lack of effort. Exercise variables include the ECG, blood pressure response to exercise, oxygen saturation, ventilation, maximal oxygen consumption, and peak work load attained. Cardiopulmonary stress testing is routine in children with congenital cardiac lesions to ascertain limitations, develop exercise prescriptions, assess the effect of therapies, and decide on the need for cardiac transplantation. Stress testing is also employed in children with structurally normal hearts to rule out cardiac or pulmonary pathology in children with symptoms during exertion. Significant stress ischemia or dysrhythmias warrant physical restrictions or appropriate therapy. Children with poor performance due to suboptimal conditioning benefit from a planned exercise program.

McManus A, Leung M: Maximizing the clinical use of exercise gaseous exchange testing in children with repaired cyanotic congenital heart defects: The development of an appropriate test strategy. Sports Med 2000;29:229 [PMID: 10783899].

ARTERIAL BLOOD GASES

Quantitating the partial oxygen pressure (PO_2) or O_2 saturation (eg, by pulse oximetry) during the administration of 100% oxygen is the most useful method of distinguishing cyanosis produced primarily by heart disease or by lung disease in sick infants. In cyanotic heart disease, the partial arterial oxygen pressure (PaO_2) increases very little when 100% oxygen is administered over the values obtained while breathing room air. However, PaO_2 usually increases very significantly when oxygen is administered to a patient who has lung disease. Table 19–11 illustrates the responses seen in patients with heart or lung disease during the hyperoxic test. Routine pulse oximetry has been advocated as an adjunct to the current newborn screening evaluation, as it is a simple, cost-effective means of screening for major cardiac defects prior to hospital discharge.

Koppel RI et al. Effectiveness of pulse oximetry screening for congenital heart disease in asymptomatic newborns. Pediatrics 2003;111:451 [PMID: 12612220].

CARDIAC CATHETERIZATION & ANGIOCARDIOGRAPHY

Cardiac catheterization precisely defines the anatomic and physiologic abnormalities in simple and complex

Table 19–11. Examples of responses to 10 minutes of 100% oxygen in lung disease and heart disease.

	Lung Disease		Heart Disease	
	Room Air	100% O_2	Room Air	100% O_2
Color	Blue →	Pink	Blue →	Blue
Oximetry	60% →	99%	60% →	62%
PaO_2 (mm Hg)	35 →	120	35 →	38

PaO_2, partial arterial oxygen pressure.

cardiac malformations. Cardiac catheterization may be performed for diagnostic purposes when further anatomic or physiologic data are needed prior to a therapeutic decision or may be performed for therapeutic purposes when the cardiac condition can be palliated or treated in the catheterization laboratory.

Therapeutic Cardiac Catheterization

Therapeutic procedures performed during cardiac catheterization include coil embolization of a PDA, balloon angioplasty with or without stent placement for aortic coarctation or branch pulmonary artery stenoses, balloon atrial septostomy, valvuloplasty of stenotic aortic or pulmonic valves, and placement of ASD and VSD devices. Cardiac catheterization is also performed to evaluate the effects of pharmaceutical therapy. An example of this use of catheterization is monitoring changes in pulmonary vascular resistance during the administration of nitric oxide or prostacyclin in a child with primary pulmonary hypertension. Electrophysiologic evaluation and ablation of abnormal electrical pathways in children can be performed by qualified personnel in the pediatric catheterization laboratory.

The risks of cardiac catheterization (morbidity and mortality) must be explained to the patient's family. Although the risks are very low for elective studies in older children (< 0.1%), the risk of major complications in distressed infants is about 2%. Interventional procedures such as balloon valvuloplasty increase these risks further.

Cardiac Catheterization Data

Figure 19–3 shows oxygen saturation (in percent) and pressure (in millimeters of mercury) values obtained at cardiac catheterization from the chambers and great arteries of the heart. These values are within the normal range for a child.

A. OXYGEN CONTENT AND SATURATION; PULMONARY (Q_P) AND SYSTEMIC (Q_S) BLOOD FLOW (CARDIAC OUTPUT)

In most laboratories, left-to-right shunting is determined by changes of blood oxygen content or saturation during sampling through the right side of the heart. A significant increase in oxygen saturation between one right chamber and the other indicates the presence of a left-to-right shunt at the site of the increase. The oxygen saturation of the peripheral arterial blood should always be determined during cardiac catheterization. Normal arterial oxygen saturation is 95–97% at sea level and 92–94% at 5280 feet. Subnormal saturations suggest the presence of a right-to-left shunt, underventilation, or pulmonary disease.

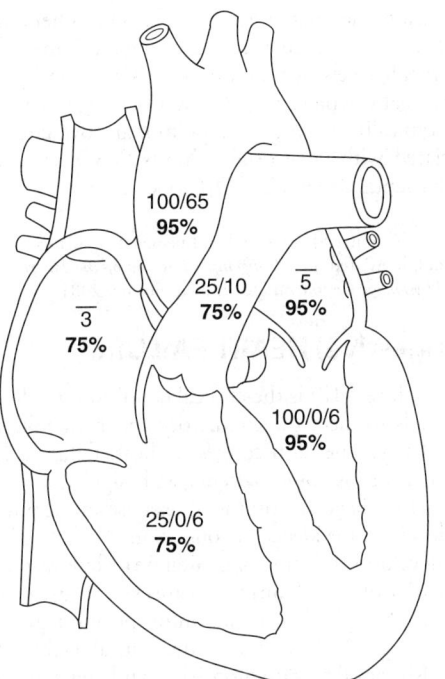

Figure 19–3. Pressures (in millimeters of mercury) and oxygen saturation (in percent) obtained by cardiac catheterization in a healthy child. 3, mean pressure of 3 mm Hg in the right atrium; 5, mean pressure of 5 mm Hg in the left atrium.

The size of a left-to-right shunt is usually expressed as a ratio of pulmonary to systemic blood flow (Q_p/Q_s) or as liters per minute as determined by the Fick principle:

$$\frac{\text{Cardiac output}}{(L/min)} = \frac{\text{Oxygen consumption (mL/min)}}{\text{Arteriovenous difference (mL/L)}}$$

B. PRESSURES

Pressures should be determined in all chambers and major vessels entered. It is not normal for systolic pressure in the ventricles to exceed systolic pressure in the great arteries, or mean diastolic pressure in the atria to exceed end-diastolic pressure in the ventricles. If a gradient in pressure exists, an obstruction is present, and the severity of the gradient is one criterion for the necessity of operative repair or catheter intervention. An RV systolic pressure of 100 mm Hg and a pulmonary artery systolic pressure of 20 mm Hg yield a gradient of 80 mm Hg. In this case, the patient would be classified as having severe pulmonary stenosis requiring balloon dilation of the pulmonic valve or surgery if valvuloplasty fails to significantly reduce the gradient.

C. PULMONARY AND SYSTEMIC VASCULAR RESISTANCE

The vascular resistance is calculated from the following formula and reported in units or in dynes $\times$ cm^{-5}/m^2:

$$\text{Resistance} = \frac{\text{Pressure}}{\text{Flow}}$$

The pressure drop used to determine pulmonary vascular resistance is calculated by subtracting the mean pulmonary artery wedge or left atrial pressure from the mean pulmonary artery pressure. This pressure drop is divided by pulmonary blood flow per square meter of body surface area. (Pulmonary blood flow is determined by thermodilution or from the Fick principle, as noted earlier.) Similarly, systemic vascular resistance is determined by subtracting the mean central venous pressure from the mean systemic arterial pressure and dividing this pressure drop by systemic blood flow.

Normally, the pulmonary vascular resistance ranges from 1–3 U/m^2, or from 80–240 dynes $\times$ cm^{-5}/m^2. Systemic vascular resistance ranges from 15–20 U/m^2, or from 1200–1600 dynes $\times$ cm^{-5}/m^2. If pulmonary resistance is greater than 10 units or the ratio of pulmonary to systemic resistance is greater than 0.5, the child may have pulmonary vascular disease and therefore be inoperable.

Freedom RM et al: *Congenital Heart Disease: Textbook of Angiography.* Futura, 1997.

Simpson JM et al: Cardiac catheterization of low birth weight infants. Am J Cardiol 2001;87:1372 [PMID: 11397356].

PERINATAL & NEONATAL CIRCULATION

At birth, two events occur that affect the cardiovascular and pulmonary system: (1) the umbilical cord is clamped, removing the placenta from the maternal circulation; and (2) breathing commences. As a result, marked changes in the circulation occur. During fetal life, the placenta offers low resistance to blood flow. In contrast, the pulmonary arterioles are markedly constricted and offer high resistance to the flow of blood into the lungs. Pulmonary blood flow accounts for only 7–10% of the combined in utero ventricular output. At birth, pulmonary blood flow dramatically increases with the fall in pulmonary vascular resistance and pressure. The etiology of prolonged high pulmonary vascular resistance includes physical factors (lack of an adequate air-liquid interface or ventilation), low oxygen tension, and vasoactive mediators such as elevated endothelin peptide levels or leukotrienes. Clamping the cord causes an immediate increase in resistance to flow in the systemic circuit. As the lung becomes the organ of respiration, the PO_2 increases in the small pulmonary arterioles, resulting in a decrease in their constriction and a decrease in the pulmonary vascular resistance. Increased oxygen tension, rhythmic lung distention, and production of nitric oxide as well as prostacyclin play major roles in the fall in pulmonary vascular resistance at birth. The pulmonary vascular resistance falls below that of the systemic circuit, resulting in a change in blood flow across the ductus arteriosus to left to right.

Functional closure of the ductus arteriosus begins to develop shortly after birth. The ductus arteriosus usually remains patent for 3–5 days. During the first hour after birth, a small right-to-left shunt is present (as in the fetus). However, after 1 hour, bidirectional shunting occurs, with the left-to-right direction predominating. In most cases, right-to-left shunting disappears completely by 8 hours. In patients with severe hypoxia (eg, in the syndrome of persistent pulmonary hypertension of the newborn), the pulmonary vascular resistance remains elevated, resulting in a continued right-to-left shunt. Increased PO_2 of the arterial blood causes spasm of the ductus. Although flow through the ductus arteriosus usually is gone within 5 days, the vessel does not close anatomically for 7–14 days.

In fetal life, the foramen ovale serves as a one-way valve to shunt blood from the inferior vena cava through the right atrium into the left atrium. At birth, because of the changes in the pulmonary and systemic vascular resistance and the increase in the quantity of blood returning from the pulmonary veins to the left atrium, the left atrial pressure rises above that of the right atrium. This functionally closes the flap of the foramen ovale, preventing flow of blood across the septum. The foramen ovale remains probe patent in 10–15% of adults.

Persistent pulmonary hypertension is a clinical syndrome that occurs in full-term infants. The neonate develops tachypnea, cyanosis, and clinical evidence of pulmonary hypertension during the first 8 hours after delivery. These infants have massive right-to-left ductal or foramen shunting (or both) for 3–7 days because of high pulmonary vascular resistance. The clinical course is one of progressive hypoxia and acidosis, terminating in early death unless the pulmonary resistance can be lowered. Instituting appropriate means to increase alveolar PO_2—hyperventilation, alkalosis, paralysis, surfactant administration, high-frequency ventilation, and cardiac pressors—can usually reverse the resistance. Inhaled nitric oxide is a selective pulmonary vasodilator that produces a sustained improvement in oxygenation and reduces the use of extracorporeal membrane oxygenation. Postmortem findings include increased thickness of the pulmonary arteriolar media.

In the normal newborn, pulmonary vascular resistance and the pulmonary arterial pressure continue to fall during the first weeks of life. This phenomenon results from demuscularization of the pulmonary arterioles. Adult levels of pulmonary resistance and pressure are normally achieved by 4–6 weeks of age. It is at this time typically that signs of pulmonary overcirculation associated with left-to-right shunts (VSD or atrioventricular septal defect [AVSD]) appear.

Fineman JR, Soifer SJ: The fetal and neonatal circulations. In: Rudolph AR (editor): *Congenital Diseases of the Heart: Clinical Physiologic Considerations,* 2nd ed. Futura, 2001.

(Congestive) HEART FAILURE

Heart failure (HF) is the clinical condition in which the heart fails to meet the circulatory and metabolic needs of the body. The term congestive heart failure is falling out of favor, as some patients with significant cardiac dysfunction have symptoms of exercise intolerance and fatigue without evidence of congestion. Almost all infants who develop HF from congenital heart lesions do so by 6 months of age. Common causes of HF in infants include VSD, PDA, coarctation of the aorta, AV septal defect, large AVMs, and chronic atrial tachyarrhythmias. Metabolic, mitochondrial, and neuromuscular disorders with an associated cardiomyopathy present at various ages depending on the specific diagnosis. HF due to acquired cardiac conditions, such as myocarditis, may occur at any age. Children with HF may present with irritability, diaphoresis with feeds, fatigue, exercise intolerance, or evidence of pulmonary congestion as noted in Table 19–1.

Treatment

The therapy of HF should be directed toward the underlying cause as well as the symptoms. Regardless of the cause, neurohormonal activation occurs early when ventricular systolic dysfunction is present. Plasma catecholamine levels (eg, norepinephrine) increase and result in tachycardia, diaphoresis, and indirectly through activation of the renin-angiotensin system, peripheral vasoconstriction and salt and water retention. There is no gold standard diagnostic or therapeutic approach to heart failure in the pediatric population. Treatment must be individualized and therapies should be aimed at improving cardiac performance by targeting the three determinants of cardiac performance: (1) preload, (2) afterload, and (3) contractility.

Inpatient Management of Congestive Heart Failure

Patients with cardiac decompensation may require hospitalization for initiation or augmentation of HF therapy. Table 19–12 demonstrates intravenous inotropic agents used to augment cardiac output and their rela-

Table 19–12. Intravenous inotropic agents.

Drug	Dose	Renal Perfusion	Heart Rate	Cardiac Index	SVR
Dopamine	2–5 µg/kg/min	↑ via vasodilation	0	0	0
	5–10	↑ via ↑ cardiac index	↑	↑	0
	> 10	↓	↑	↑	↑
Dobutamine	2.5–10 µg/kg/min	↑ via ↑ cardiac index	↑	↑	↑↓
Epinephrine	0.2–2.0 µg/kg/min	↓	↑	↑	↑
Norepinephrine	0.05–0.1 µg/kg/min	↓	0	↑	↑↑
Isoproterenol	0.05–2.0 µg/kg/min	0	↑↑	↑	↓↓

SVR, systemic vascular resistance.

tive effect on heart rate, systemic vascular resistance, and cardiac index. The drug used will depend in part on the cause of the HF.

A. INTRAVENOUS INOTROPIC SUPPORT

1. Afterload reduction

a. Milrinone—This selective phosphodiesterase inhibitor increases the level of cyclic adenosine monophosphate, thereby improving the inotropic state of the heart. In addition to a dose-dependent increase in cardiac contractility, milrinone is a systemic and pulmonary vasodilator and thus an effective agent in cases of right or left ventricular systolic dysfunction. Milrinone has been shown to reduce the incidence of low cardiac output syndrome following open heart surgery. The usual dosage range is 0.25–0.75 µg/kg/min.

b. Nitroglycerin—Nitroglycerin functions primarily as a dilator of venous capacitance vessels and causes a reduction of right and left atrial pressure. Systemic blood pressure may also fall, and reflex tachycardia may occur. Nitroglycerin is used to improve coronary blood flow and may be especially useful in the setting of low cardiac output secondary to coronary underperfusion following congenital heart surgery. The usual intravenous dosage range is 1–3 µg/kg/min.

2. Enhancement of contractility

a. Dopamine—This naturally occurring catecholamine increases myocardial contractility primarily via cardiac β-adrenergic activation. Dopamine also directly acts on renal dopamine receptors to improve renal perfusion. The usual dose range for CHF is 3–10 µg/kg/min.

b. Dobutamine—This synthetic catecholamine increases myocardial contractility secondary to cardiospecific β-adrenergic activation while resulting in little peripheral vasoconstriction. Dobutamine administration does not usually result in a marked tachycardic response, which is a distinct advantage. However, the drug does not selectively improve renal perfusion as does dopamine. The usual dose range is essentially the same as for dopamine.

3. Mechanical circulatory support—Mechanical support is indicated in children with severe, refractory myocardial failure secondary to cardiomyopathy, myocarditis, or following cardiac surgery. Mechanical support is used for a limited time while cardiac function improves, or as a bridge to cardiac transplantation.

a. Extracorporeal membrane oxygenation (ECMO)—ECMO functions as a temporary means of providing oxygenation, carbon dioxide removal, and hemodynamic support in patients with cardiac or pulmonary failure that is refractory to conventional therapy. Flow from a catheter positioned within the patient's venous system (eg, right atrium) passes through a membrane oxygenator and then is delivered back to the patient via a catheter positioned within the arterial system (eg, aorta or common carotid artery). Flow rates are adjusted to maintain adequate systemic perfusion, as judged by mean arterial blood pressure, acid-base status, end-organ function, and mixed venous oxygen saturation. The patient is monitored closely for improvement in cardiac contractility. Risks are significant and include severe internal and external bleeding, infection, thrombosis, and pump failure.

b. Ventricular assist devices—Currently pulsatile assist device use is limited in children by patient size, availability and institution-dependent expertise. These devices allow hemodynamic support in a less invasive fashion than with ECMO. A device cannula is positioned within the apex of the ventricular chamber and via a battery-operated pump blood is removed from the ventricle. Blood is then returned to the patient through a separate cannula positioned within the aorta or pulmonary artery, depending on the ventricle being supported. There is lower risk of bleeding and pump failure than with ECMO, but the risk of infection and thrombosis remain.

Outpatient Congestive Heart Failure Management

A. MEDICATIONS

1. Afterload-reducing agents—Oral afterload-reducing agents improve cardiac output by decreasing systemic vascular resistance. Angiotensin-converting enzyme (ACE) inhibitors (captopril, enalapril, and lisinopril) are first-line therapy in patients with HF requiring long-term treatment. These agents, which block angiotensin II–mediated systemic vasoconstriction, are particularly useful in children with structurally normal hearts but reduced LV myocardial function (ie, myocarditis or dilated cardiomyopathies). These agents are also useful in ameliorating mitral and aortic insufficiency and have a role in controlling refractory HF in patients with large left-to-right shunts in whom systemic vascular resistance is elevated.

2. Beta blockade—β-Blockers may be a useful adjunctive therapy in children with refractory HF already taking ACE inhibitors. Excessive circulating catecholamines are present due to the activation of the sympathetic nervous system that results from heart failure. Although this compensatory response is beneficial acutely, over time myocardial fibrosis, myocyte hypertrophy, and myocyte apoptosis may contribute to the progression of heart failure. β-Blockers (eg, carvedilol and metoprolol) antagonize this sympathetic activation and may offset these deleterious effects. Side effects of β-blockers are not benign and include symptomatic bradycardia and hypotension, and worsening heart failure may occur in some patients.

3. Diuretics—Diuretic therapy may be necessary in the treatment of HF in order to maintain the patient in a euvolemic state.

a. Furosemide—This rapidly acting loop diuretic may be given intravenously or orally. Furosemide removes large amounts of potassium and chloride from the body, producing hypochloremic metabolic alkalosis when used chronically. Electrolytes should be monitored during long-term therapy.

b. Thiazides—The thiazides are distal tubular diuretics used to complement furosemide in severe cases of HF.

c. Spironolactone—Spironolactone is a potassium-sparing aldosterone inhibitor diuretic. It is used frequently in conjunction with furosemide or thiazides for its enhanced diuretic function. Because it spares potassium, supplemental potassium may be avoided. Spironolactone may also be used as a neurohormonal antagonist with potential benefit in HF regardless of its diuretic effect. In adults with advanced HF, the addition of spironolactone to the standard medical regimen has been associated with LV remodeling and improved life expectancy.

4. Digitalis—Digitalis is a cardiac glycoside that has a positive inotropic effect on the heart with an associated

Table 19–13. Digoxin dosing schedule.

Age	Parenteral	Oral
Premature	0.035 mg/kg	0.04 mg/kg
1 week to 2 years	0.05 mg/kg	0.06 mg/kg
< 1 week or > 2 years	0.04 mg/kg	0.05 mg/kg

decrease in systemic vascular resistance. The standard preparation of digitalis used in clinical practice is digoxin. Large studies in adult patients with HF have demonstrated no mortality benefit of digoxin, but treatment results in reduced hospitalization rates for HF exacerbations.

a. Dosing—The routine schedule consists of giving one-half of the total digitalizing dose initially, then one-quarter of the total digitalizing dose at 6 and 12 hours of therapy (Table 19–13). Twenty-four hours after the last digitalizing dose, maintenance therapy is started. Serum digoxin levels are not routinely monitored unless there are concerns regarding compliance or toxicity.

b. Digitalis toxicity—Any dysrhythmia that occurs during digoxin therapy should be attributed to the drug until proven otherwise. Ventricular bigeminy and first-, second-, or third-degree AV block are characteristic of digoxin toxicity. A trough level should be obtained if digoxin toxicity is suspected.

c. Digitalis poisoning—This is an acute emergency that must be treated without delay. Digoxin poisoning most commonly occurs in toddlers who have taken their parents' or grandparents' medications. The child's stomach should be emptied immediately by gastric lavage even if several hours have passed since ingestion. Patients who have ingested massive amounts of digoxin should receive large doses of activated charcoal. In advanced heart block, atropine or temporary ventricular pacing may be needed. Digoxin immune Fab can be used to reverse potentially life-threatening intoxication. Antiarrhythmic agents may be useful.

5. Fluid restriction—Fluid restriction is rarely used in pediatric cardiology today due to the effectiveness of diuretics. Ensuring the adequacy of caloric intake to allow normal growth velocity is a more important goal in children suffering from heart failure.

Azeka E et al: Delisting of infants and children from the heart transplantation waiting list after carvedilol treatment. J Am Coll Cardiol 2002;40:2034 [PMID: 12475466].

Fiser WP et al: Pediatric arteriovenous ECMO as a bridge to cardiac transplantation. J Heart Lung Transplant 2003;22:770 [PMID: 12873545].

Hoffman TM et al: Efficacy and safety of milrinone in preventing low cardiac output syndrome in infants and children after corrective surgery for congenital heart disease. Circulation 2003;107:996 [PMID: 12600913].

Rosenthal D et al: International Society for Heart and Lung Transplantation: Practice guidelines for management of heart failure in children. J Heart Lung Transplant 2004;23:1313 [PMID: 15607659].

CONGENITAL HEART DISEASE

Congenital heart disease occurs in 0.8% of North American and European populations, making this the most common category of congenital structural malformation. Curative or palliative surgical correction is now available for virtually all patients with congenital heart disease.

Etiology

Congenital heart disease often has a genetic basis. The most common abnormality now recognized is a microdeletion in the long arm of chromosome 22 (22q11) associated with DiGeorge syndrome. These children tend to have either interrupted aortic arch or other conotruncal abnormalities such as truncus arteriosus, ToF, or double-outlet RV. Intrauterine factors such as maternal diabetes, alcohol consumption, progesterone use, viral infection, and other maternal teratogen exposure are associated with an increased incidence of malformations. Even acquired heart diseases, such as rheumatic fever, appear to be under strong genetic control. Atherosclerosis clearly occurs in families, although in some circumstances it can also be influenced by diet, drugs, or lifestyle. Genetic diagnosis may allow for a more accurate prediction of the risk of recurrence of a congenital heart disease in a subsequent pregnancy.

Boneva RS et al: Mortality associated with congenital heart defects in the United States, trends and racial disparities. Circulation 2001;103:2376 [PMID: 11352887].

NONCYANOTIC CONGENITAL HEART DISEASE

1. Atrial Septal Defect of the Ostium Secundum Variety

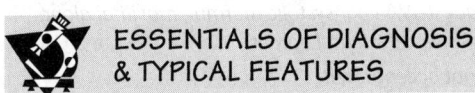

ESSENTIALS OF DIAGNOSIS & TYPICAL FEATURES

- *RV heave.*
- *S_2 widely split and usually fixed.*
- *Grade I–III/VI ejection systolic murmur at the pulmonary area.*
- *Systolic ejection murmur loudest at the left upper sternal edge.*
- *Diastolic flow murmur at the lower left sternal border (if the shunt is significant in size).*
- *ECG with rsR' in lead V_1.*

General Considerations

An ASD is an opening in the atrial septum permitting the shunting of blood between the atria. There are three major types: (1) the ostium secundum type (discussed here) is the most common and is in the middle of the septum in the region of the foramen ovale; (2) the sinus venosus type is positioned high in the atrial septum, is the least common, and is frequently associated with partial anomalous pulmonary venous return; (3) the ostium primum type is low in position and is a form of an atrioventricular septal defect. It is discussed in that section.

ASD of the ostium secundum variety occurs in 10% of patients with congenital heart disease and is twice as common in females as in males. It most commonly occurs on a sporadic basis but may be familial in nature, associated with conduction disturbances (heterozygous NKX2-5 mutation) or upper extremity malformations (Holt-Oram syndrome). Diagnosis in infancy is becoming more common. Pulmonary hypertension and growth failure are uncommon but occur occasionally in infancy and childhood. After the third decade, atrial arrhythmias and/or pulmonary vascular disease may develop; in the setting of pulmonary vascular disease, left-to-right shunting decreases, and right-to-left shunting becomes the major clinical abnormality.

Clinical Findings

A. SYMPTOMS AND SIGNS

Infants with an ASD rarely present with CHF. Children often have no cardiovascular symptoms. Some patients remain asymptomatic throughout life; others develop easy fatigability as older children or adults. Cyanosis does not occur unless pulmonary hypertension develops.

The peripheral pulses are normal and equal. The heart is usually hyperactive, with an RV heave felt best at the mid to lower left sternal border. No thrills are usually present. S_2 at the pulmonary area is widely split and often fixed. The pulmonary component is normal in intensity. A grade I–III/VI ejection-type systolic murmur is heard best at the left sternal border in the second intercostal space. This murmur is caused by increased flow across the pulmonic valve. No murmur is heard from the flow across the ASD. A mid-diastolic murmur can often be heard in the fourth intercostal space at the left sternal border. This murmur is caused by increased flow across the tricuspid valve during diastole. The presence of this murmur suggests a high flow with a pulmonary to systemic blood flow ratio greater than 2:1.

B. Imaging

Radiographs show cardiac enlargement. The main pulmonary artery may be dilated and pulmonary vascular markings increased owing to the increased pulmonary blood flow.

C. Electrocardiography

The usual ECG shows right axis deviation. In the right precordial leads, an rsR' pattern is usually present. In patients with a mutation in the cardiac homeobox gene (NKX2-5), atrioventricular heart block may be present.

D. Echocardiography

Echocardiography shows a dilated right atrium and right ventricle. Direct visualization of the ASD by two-dimensional echocardiography, plus demonstration of a left-to-right shunt through the defect by color-flow Doppler, confirms the diagnosis and has eliminated the need for cardiac catheterization prior to open-heart surgery or catheter closure of the defect. During the echocardiogram careful assessment of all of the pulmonary veins is made to rule out associated anomalous pulmonary venous return.

E. Cardiac Catheterization

Oximetry reveals a significant increase in oxygen saturation at the atrial level. The pulmonary artery pressure is usually normal, as is pulmonary vascular resistance. The ratio of pulmonary to systemic blood flow may vary from 1.5:1 to 4:1. Cardiac catheterization is rarely needed for diagnostic purposes; however, placement of a device to close the ostium secundum ASD during cardiac catheterization is becoming increasingly common.

Treatment

Surgical or catheterization laboratory closure is generally recommended for symptomatic children with a large atrial level defect and associated right heart dilation. In the asymptomatic child with a large hemodynamically significant defect, closure is performed electively between ages 1 and 3 years. The mortality rate for surgical closure is less than 1%. When closure is performed by age 3 years, late complications of RV dysfunction and significant dysrhythmias are avoided. Sur-

gical repair can now be safely performed via a "mini" median sternotomy or posterior thoracotomy approach. Many defects are amenable to nonoperative device closure in the cardiac catheterization laboratory, but the defect must have adequate tissue rims on all sides on which to anchor the device.

Course and Prognosis

Patients usually tolerate an ASD well in the first two decades of life. Pulmonary hypertension and reversal of the shunt are rare late complications. Infective endocarditis is uncommon. Spontaneous closure occurs, most frequently in children with a defect originally measured by echo as less than 4 mm in diameter. Exercise tolerance and oxygen consumption in surgically corrected children are generally normal, and restriction of physical activity is unnecessary. Of all the forms of congenital heart disease, ostium secundum ASD is the most likely to present in middle to late adulthood, either with increased fatigue or with atrial tachyarrhythmias.

Elliott DA et al: Cardiac homeobox gene NKX2-5 mutations and congenital heart disease: associations with atrial septal defect and hypoplastic left heart syndrome. J Am Coll Cardiol 2003;41:2072 [PMID: 12798584].

Fredriksen PM et al: Aerobic capacity in adults with various congenital heart diseases. Am J Cardiol 2001;87:310 [PMID: 11165966].

Lopez L et al: Echocardiographic considerations during deployment of the Helex Septal Occluder for closure of atrial septal defects. Cardiol Young 2003;13:290 [PMID: 12903878].

Roos-Hesselink JW et al: Excellent survival and low incidence of arrhythmias, stroke and heart failure long-term after surgical ASD closure at a young age: A prospective follow-up study of 21–33 years. Eur Heart J 2003;24:190 [PMID: 12573276].

Ryan WH et al: Safety and efficacy of minimally invasive atrial septal defect closure. Ann Thorac Surg 2003;75:1532 [PMID: 12735575].

2. Ventricular Septal Defect

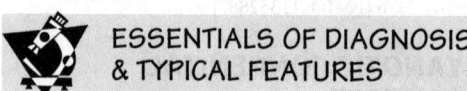

ESSENTIALS OF DIAGNOSIS & TYPICAL FEATURES

Small- to moderate-sized left-to-right shunt without pulmonary hypertension:

- *Acyanotic, relatively asymptomatic.*
- *Grade II–IV/VI pansystolic murmur, maximal along the lower left sternal border.*
- *P₂ not accentuated.*

Large left-to-right shunt:

- *Acyanotic.*
- *Easy fatigability.*

- *CHF in infancy (often).*
- *Hyperactive heart; biventricular enlargement.*
- *Grade II–IV/VI pansystolic murmur, maximal at the lower left sternal border.*
- *P_2 usually accentuated.*
- *Diastolic flow murmur at the apex.*

Insignificant left-to-right shunt or bidirectional shunt with pulmonary hypertension:

- *Quiet precordium with RV lift.*
- *Palpable P_2.*
- *Short ejection systolic murmur along the left sternal border; single accentuated S_2.*
- *Systemic arterial oxygen desaturation may be present; pulmonary arterial pressure and systemic arterial pressures are equal; little or no oxygen saturation increase at the RV level by catheterization.*

General Considerations

Simple VSD is the most common congenital heart malformation, accounting for about 30% of all cases of congenital heart disease. Defects in the ventricular septum occur both in the membranous portion of the septum (most common) and in the muscular portion. VSDs follow one of four courses:

A. SMALL, HEMODYNAMICALLY INSIGNIFICANT VENTRICULAR SEPTAL DEFECTS

Between 80% and 85% of all VSDs are small (< 3 mm in diameter) at birth, and will close spontaneously. In general, small defects in the muscular interventricular septum will close sooner than those in the membranous septum. In most cases, a small VSD never requires surgical closure. Fifty percent of small VSDs will close by age 2 years, and 90% will close by age 6 years. The remaining 10% will close during the school years, and parents should be told at the time of diagnosis and echocardiographic confirmation that all small VSDs will eventually close.

B. MODERATE VENTRICULAR SEPTAL DEFECTS

Asymptomatic patients with moderate VSDs (3–5 mm in diameter) account for only 3–5% of children with VSDs. In general these children do not have CHF or pulmonary hypertension, the two indicators for surgical closure. In those who have cardiac catheterization, the ratio of pulmonary to systemic blood flow is usually less than 2:1, and serial cardiac catheterizations demonstrate that the shunts get progressively smaller. If there is neither CHF nor pulmonary hypertension, these defects can be followed until spontaneous closure.

C. LARGE VENTRICULAR SEPTAL DEFECTS WITH NORMAL PULMONARY VASCULAR RESISTANCE

These defects are usually 6–10 mm in diameter. Unless they become markedly smaller within a few months after birth, they will require surgery. The timing of surgery depends on the clinical situation. Many infants with large VSDs and normal pulmonary vascular resistance will develop CHF and failure to thrive by age 3–6 months, and require correction at that time. In all cases, surgery before age 2 years is required so that the risk of pulmonary vascular disease can be minimized.

D. LARGE VENTRICULAR SEPTAL DEFECTS WITH PULMONARY VASCULAR OBSTRUCTIVE DISEASE

The vast majority of patients with inoperable pulmonary hypertension develop the condition progressively. The combined data of the multicenter National History Study indicate that almost all cases of irreversible pulmonary hypertension can be prevented by surgical repair of a large VSD before age 2 years.

Clinical Findings

A. SYMPTOMS AND SIGNS

Patients with small or moderate left-to-right shunts usually have no cardiovascular symptoms. Patients with large left-to-right shunts are usually ill early in infancy. Such patients have frequent upper and lower respiratory infections. They gain weight slowly. Dyspnea, diaphoresis, exercise intolerance, and fatigue are common. CHF develops between 1 and 6 months of age. After the first year, symptoms usually improve, although easy fatigability may persist. Over time, in the face of a large left-to-right shunt, the pulmonary vascular bed may undergo structural changes, leading to increased pulmonary vascular resistance and a reversal of the shunt from left to right, to right to left (Eisenmenger syndrome). Cyanosis will be present.

1. Small left-to-right shunt—No lifts, heaves, or thrills are present. The first sound at the apex is normal, and the second sound at the pulmonary area is split physiologically. The pulmonary component is normal. A grade II–IV/VI, medium- to high-pitched, harsh pansystolic murmur is heard best at the left sternal border in the third and fourth intercostal spaces. The murmur radiates over the entire precordium. No diastolic murmurs are heard.

2. Moderate left-to-right shunt—Slight prominence of the precordium is common. Moderate LV heave is evident. A systolic thrill may be palpable at the lower left sternal border between the third and fourth intercostal spaces. The second sound at the pulmonary area is most often split but may be single. A grade III–IV/

VI, harsh pansystolic murmur is heard best at the lower left sternal border in the fourth intercostal space. A mitral diastolic flow murmur indicates that the pulmonary venous return is large and that the pulmonary to systemic blood flow ratio is at least 2:1.

3. Large ventricular septal defects with pulmonary hypertension—The precordium is prominent, and the sternum bulges. An LV thrust and an RV heave are palpable. S_2 may be felt at the pulmonary area. A thrill may be present at the lower left sternal border. S_2 is usually single or narrowly split, with accentuation of the pulmonary component. The murmur ranges from grade I to grade IV/VI and is usually harsh and pansystolic. Occasionally, when the defect is large, a murmur is difficult to hear. A diastolic flow murmur may be heard, depending on the size of the shunt.

B. IMAGING

In patients with small shunts, the radiograph may be normal. Patients with large shunts usually show significant cardiac enlargement involving both the left and right ventricles and the left atrium. The aorta is small to normal in size, and the main pulmonary artery segment is dilated. The pulmonary vascular markings are increased in patients with large shunts.

C. ELECTROCARDIOGRAPHY

The ECG is normal in patients with small left-to-right shunts. Left ventricular hypertrophy (LVH) usually occurs in patients with large left-to-right shunts and normal pulmonary vascular resistance (moderate-sized defects). Combined ventricular enlargement (both right and left) occurs in patients with pulmonary hypertension caused by increased flow, increased resistance, or both. Pure RV hypertrophy occurs in patients with pulmonary hypertension secondary to pulmonary vascular obstruction (Eisenmenger syndrome).

D. ECHOCARDIOGRAPHY

Two-dimensional echocardiography can reveal defects that are 2 mm or larger and often can be used to pinpoint the anatomic location of the defect. Color-flow Doppler allows detection of even the smallest VSDs. Multiple defects can be detected by combining two-dimensional and color-flow imaging. Doppler can aid in the evaluation of VSDs by estimating the pressure difference between the left and right ventricles. A pressure difference greater than 50 mm Hg indicates the absence of severe pulmonary hypertension. The combination of excellent visualization of the VSD using echocardiography and Doppler, plus the ability to estimate pulmonary artery pressures on the basis of the gradient across the VSD, allows for the vast majority of isolated defects to be repaired surgically without cardiac catheterization and angiocardiography.

E. CARDIAC CATHETERIZATION AND ANGIOCARDIOGRAPHY

The pulmonary artery pressure may vary from normal to systemic levels (equal to the aortic pressure). Left atrial pressure (pulmonary wedge pressure) may be normal to increased. Pulmonary vascular resistance varies from normal to markedly increased. Angiocardiographic examination defines the number, size, and location of the defects.

Treatment

A. MEDICAL MANAGEMENT

Patients who develop CHF should receive vigorous treatment with anticongestive measures (see section on heart failure). If the patient does not respond to anticongestive measures, or if he or she shows signs of progressive pulmonary hypertension, surgery is indicated without delay. Transcatheter closure of muscular VSDs is currently being used in selected cases.

B. SURGICAL TREATMENT

The indications for surgical closure of a VSD are CHF, failure to thrive and/or pulmonary hypertension. Primary closure of the defect with a synthetic patch is used. The age at which elective surgery is performed has decreased and most defects are closed in infancy. Patients with cardiomegaly, poor growth, poor exercise tolerance, or other clinical abnormalities who have a significant shunt (> 2:1) without significant pulmonary hypertension typically undergo surgical repair at age 3–6 months. Patients with pulmonary artery pressures equal to systemic pressure (pulmonary hypertension) undergo surgical repair well before age 2 years to avoid pulmonary vascular disease. In most centers these children have surgery before age 1 year. As a result of this management, the incidence of VSD with pulmonary vascular disease and right-to-left shunting (Eisenmenger syndrome) has been virtually eliminated. In all cases of VSD, the surgical mortality rate is below 2%.

Course & Prognosis

Significant late dysrhythmias are uncommon. Functional exercise capacity and oxygen consumption are usually normal, and physical restrictions are unnecessary. Adults with corrected defects have a normal quality of life. With complete VSD closure, antibiotic prophylaxis for bacterial endocarditis can be discontinued 6 months after surgery.

Thanopoulous B et al: Transcatheter closure of muscular ventricular septal defects with the Amplatzer ventricular septal defect occluder: Initial clinical applications in children. J Am Coll Cardiol 1999;33:1395 [PMID: 10193744].

Thanopoulous B et al: Transcatheter closure of perimembranous ventricular septal defects with the Amplatzer asymmetric ventricular septal defect occluder: Preliminary experience in children. Heart 2003;89:918 [PMID: 12860872].

3. Atrioventricular Septal Defect

ESSENTIALS OF DIAGNOSIS & TYPICAL FEATURES

- *Murmur often inaudible in neonates.*
- *Loud pulmonary component of S$_2$.*
- *Common in infants with Down syndrome.*
- *ECG with left axis deviation.*

General Considerations

AV septal defect is a congenital cardiac abnormality resulting from incomplete fusion of the embryonic endocardial cushions. The endocardial cushions help to form the lower portion of the atrial septum, the membranous portion of the ventricular septum, and the septal leaflets of the tricuspid and mitral valves. These defects are not very common. They account for about 4% of all cases of congenital heart disease. Forty-five percent of children with Down syndrome have congenital heart disease. Of these, 35–40% have AV septal defects.

AV septal defects are divided into partial and complete forms. The complete form consists of a posterior-inlet VSD, an ostium primum ASD that is continuous with the ventricular defect, and a cleft in the anterior leaflet of the mitral valve. In the partial form, any one of these components may be present. The most common partial form of AV septal defect is the ostium primum type of ASD with a cleft in the mitral valve and little or no VSD.

The complete form results in large left-to-right shunts at both the ventricular and atrial levels, tricuspid and mitral regurgitation, and pulmonary hypertension, usually with some increase in pulmonary vascular resistance. When pulmonary hypertension is present, the shunts may be bidirectional. The hemodynamics in the partial form depend on the lesions present.

Clinical Findings

A. SYMPTOMS AND SIGNS

The clinical picture varies depending on the severity of the defect. In the partial form, patients may be clinically indistinguishable from children with ostium secundum ASDs. They are often asymptomatic. Patients with complete AV septal defect usually are severely affected. CHF often develops in infancy, and recurrent bouts of pneumonia are common.

In the neonate with the complete form, the murmur may be inaudible. After 4–6 weeks, a nonspecific systolic murmur develops. The murmur is usually not as harsh as that of an isolated VSD. The heart is significantly enlarged (both the right and left sides). S$_2$ is loud. A pronounced diastolic flow murmur may be heard at the apex and the lower left sternal border.

When severe pulmonary vascular obstructive disease is present, dominant RV enlargement usually occurs. S$_2$ can be palpated at the pulmonary area. No thrill is felt. A nonspecific short systolic murmur is heard at the lower left sternal border. No diastolic flow murmurs are heard. Cyanosis is detectable in severe cases with predominant right-to-left shunts.

The physical findings in the incomplete form depend on the lesions. In the most common variety (ostium primum ASD with mitral regurgitation), the findings are similar to those of ostium secundum ASD with or without findings of mitral regurgitation.

B. IMAGING

Cardiac enlargement is always present. In the complete form, all four chambers are enlarged. The pulmonary vascular markings are increased. In patients with pulmonary vascular obstructive disease, only the main pulmonary artery segment and its branches are prominent. The peripheral pulmonary vascular markings are usually decreased.

C. ELECTROCARDIOGRAPHY

In all forms of AV septal defect, left axis deviation with a counterclockwise loop in the frontal plane is present. The mean axis varies from approximately –30 to –90 degrees. The ECG is an important diagnostic tool. Only 5% of isolated VSDs have this ECG abnormality. First-degree heart block is present in over 50% of patients. Right, left, or combined ventricular hypertrophy is present depending on the particular type of defect and the presence or absence of pulmonary hypertension.

D. ECHOCARDIOGRAPHY

Echocardiography is the diagnostic technique of choice. The anatomy can be very well visualized by two-dimensional echocardiography, noting both AV valves to be at the same level. A primum ASD and an inlet VSD are present. AV valve regurgitation may be present. The LV outflow tract is elongated and has been likened to a gooseneck. The LV outflow tract may be obstructed.

E. CARDIAC CATHETERIZATION AND ANGIOCARDIOGRAPHY

Cardiac catheterization is not routinely used in the diagnostic assessment of AV septal defects but may be of value in assessing pulmonary artery pressures in the older infant with Down syndrome, as this patient group is predisposed to early-onset pulmonary hypertension, which may prohibit surgical closure. The results of cardiac catheterization vary with the type of defect. The catheter is easily passed across the lower atrial septum and frequently enters the LV directly from the right atrium. This catheter course is a result of the very low ASD and the cleft in the mitral valve. Increased oxygen saturation in the RV or the right atrium identifies the level of the shunt. Angiocardiography reveals the characteristic gooseneck deformity of the LV outflow tract in the complete form.

Treatment

Since spontaneous improvement does not occur, surgery is always required. In the partial form, surgery carries a low mortality rate (1–2%), but patients require ongoing follow-up because of the risk of late-occurring LV outflow tract obstruction and mitral valve dysfunction. The complete form is associated with a somewhat higher mortality rate, but complete correction in the first year of life, prior to the onset of irreversible pulmonary hypertension, is obligatory. Patients with Down syndrome tend to have a lower incidence of associated mitral valve dysplasia and have a lower risk of reoperation. Primary correction should be performed when the child is well, and if possible, weighs more than 5 kg. At corrective surgery, transesophageal echocardiography is useful in assessing the adequacy of repair in the operating room at the completion of cardiopulmonary bypass.

Al-Hay AA et al: Complete atrioventricular septal defect, Down syndrome and surgical outcome: Risk factors. Ann Thorac Surg 2003;75:412 [PMID: 12607648].

El-Najdawi EK et al: Operation for partial atrioventricular septal defect: A forty year review. J Thorac Cardiovasc Surg 2000; 119:880 [PMID: 10788807].

PATENT DUCTUS ARTERIOSUS

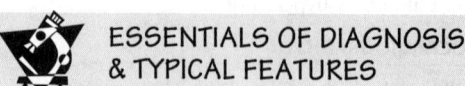

ESSENTIALS OF DIAGNOSIS & TYPICAL FEATURES

- *Variable murmur, with active precordium and full pulses, in newborn premature infants.*
- *Continuous murmur and full pulses in older infants.*

General Considerations

PDA is the persistence of the normal fetal vessel that joins the pulmonary artery to the aorta. It closes spontaneously in normal full-term infants at 3–5 days of age. It is a common abnormality, accounting for 10% of all cases of congenital heart disease. The incidence of PDA is higher in infants born at high altitudes (over 10,000 ft). It is twice as common in females as in males. In preterm infants weighing less than 1500 g, the frequency of PDA ranges from 20–60%.

The defect occurs as an isolated abnormality, but associated lesions sometimes occur. Coarctation of the aorta and VSD are commonly associated with PDA. Even more important to recognize are those patients with murmurs of PDA, but without readily apparent findings of other associated lesions, who are being kept alive by the patent ductus (eg, a patient with PDA with unsuspected pulmonary atresia).

Clinical Findings

A. Symptoms and Signs

The clinical findings and the clinical course depend on the size of the shunt and the degree of pulmonary hypertension.

1. Typical patent ductus arteriosus—The pulses are bounding, and pulse pressure is widened. S_1 is normal and S_2 is usually narrowly split. Rarely, in large shunts, S_2 is paradoxically split; that is, S_2 closes on inspiration and splits on expiration. The paradoxical splitting is caused by the volume overload of the LV and the prolonged ejection of blood from this chamber.

The murmur is quite characteristic. It is a very rough machinery murmur that is maximal at the second left intercostal space. It begins shortly after S_1, rises to a peak at S_2, and passes through the S_2 into diastole, where it becomes a decrescendo murmur and fades before the S_1. The murmur tends to radiate fairly well over the lung fields anteriorly, but relatively poorly over the lung fields posteriorly. A diastolic flow murmur is often heard at the apex.

2. Patent ductus arteriosus with pulmonary hypertension—If pulmonary hypertension is primarily the result of an increase in blood flow and only a slight increase in pulmonary vascular resistance, the physical findings are similar to those listed earlier. The significant difference is the presence of an accentuated pulmonary component of S_2. Bounding pulses and a loud continuous heart murmur are present. In patients with increased pulmonary vascular resistance, the findings are very different. S_2 is single and accentuated, and no significant heart murmur is present. The pulses are normal rather than bounding.

3. Patent ductus arteriosus in the premature neonate with associated respiratory distress syndrome—A preterm neonate during or after respiratory distress syndrome may have a significant PDA that is difficult to detect by auscultation but which may still be clinically significant. A soft, nonspecific systolic murmur or no murmur is heard rather than the classic continuous murmur. Increase in peripheral pulses is a helpful sign. Increasing oxygen requirement and increased need for respiratory support or CHF may be signs that a PDA is causing significant left-to-right shunting. The chest radiograph will show cardiomegaly. Echocardiography is used to confirm the presence or absence of a PDA in the premature infant with lung disease.

B. Imaging

In simple PDA, the radiographic appearance depends on the size of the shunt. If the shunt is relatively small, the heart is not enlarged. If the shunt is large, both left atrial and LV enlargement may be present. The aorta and the main pulmonary artery segment may be prominent.

C. Electrocardiography

The ECG may be normal or may show LVH, depending on the size of the shunt. In patients with pulmonary hypertension caused by increased blood flow, biventricular hypertrophy usually occurs. In those with pulmonary vascular obstructive disease, pure right ventricular hypertrophy (RVH) occurs.

D. Echocardiography

Echocardiography provides direct visualization of the ductus and confirmation of the direction and degree of shunting. Preterm infants with a suspected PDA may undergo echocardiography to confirm the diagnosis, assess the magnitude of the left-to-right shunt, and rule out any ductal-dependent lesions.

E. Cardiac Catheterization and Angiocardiography

Children with PDA never require a cardiac catheterization for diagnostic purposes. However, children > 5 kg with a PDA routinely have the ductus closed in the catheterization laboratory. Device closure is the sole indication for cardiac catheterization in PDA.

Treatment

Treatment is surgical when the PDA is large, except in patients with pulmonary vascular obstructive disease. Patients with large left-to-right shunts and pulmonary hypertension should be operated on by age 1 year to prevent the development of progressive pulmonary vascular obstructive disease. A symptomatic PDA with normal pulmonary artery pressure can be safely coil-occluded in the catheterization lab after the child has reached 5 kg.

Patients with nonreactive pulmonary vascular obstruction who have resistance greater than 10 units and a ratio of pulmonary to systemic resistance greater than 0.7 despite vasodilator therapy (eg, nitric oxide) should not be operated on. These patients are made worse by closure of the ductus, because the ductus serves as an escape route for their pulmonary hypertension.

Symptomatic PDA is a common problem in preterm infants. Indomethacin, a prostaglandin synthesis inhibitor, is routinely used to close the PDA in premature infants. Indomethacin does not close the PDA of full-term infants or children. The success of indomethacin therapy is as high as 80–90% in premature infants with a birth weight over 1200 g, but it is less successful in smaller infants. Indomethacin (0.1–0.3 mg/kg orally every 8–24 hours or 0.1–0.3 mg/kg parenterally every 12 hours) can be used if adequate renal, hematologic, and hepatic function is demonstrated. Management during indomethacin therapy includes fluid restriction with or without diuretics and close observation of the urinary output because of its tendency to decrease renal function. If indomethacin is not successful and the ductus remains hemodynamically significant, surgical ligation should be performed. If the ductus closes substantially so that it is no longer hemodynamically significant, even with some residual flow from left to right, surgery is not needed, and a second course of indomethacin may be used. Recent studies from Europe indicate that ibuprofen may be as effective as indomethacin for the medical closure of the preterm PDA.

Course & Prognosis

Patients with simple PDA and small-to-moderate shunts usually do well without surgery. However, in the third or fourth decade of life, symptoms of easy fatigability, dyspnea on exertion, and exercise intolerance appear, usually as a consequence of the development of pulmonary hypertension or CHF.

Spontaneous closure of a PDA may occur up to age 1 year. This is especially true in preterm infants. After age 1 year, spontaneous closure is rare. Because infective endocarditis is a potential complication, closure is recommended if the defect persists beyond age 1 year.

The prognosis for patients with large shunts or pulmonary hypertension is not as good. Poor growth and development, frequent episodes of pneumonia, and the development of CHF occur in these children. Therefore, patients with PDA and large shunts who are beyond the newborn period should have immediate surgical ligation of their PDA.

Liang CD et al: Echocardiographic guidance for transcatheter coil occlusion of patent ductus arteriosus in the catheterization laboratory. J Am Soc Echocardiogr 2003;16:476 [PMID: 12724658].

Overmeire BV et al: A Comparison of ibuprofen and indomethacin for closure of patent ductus arteriosus. N Engl J Med 2000; 343:674 [PMID: 10974130].

MALFORMATIONS ASSOCIATED WITH OBSTRUCTION TO BLOOD FLOW ON THE RIGHT SIDE OF THE HEART

1. Valvular Pulmonary Stenosis with Intact Ventricular Septum

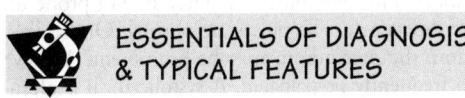

ESSENTIALS OF DIAGNOSIS & TYPICAL FEATURES

• *No symptoms with mild and moderately severe cases.*

- Cyanosis and a high incidence of right-sided CHF in very severe cases in infancy.
- RV lift; systolic ejection click at the pulmonary area in mild to moderately severe cases.
- S_2 widely split with soft to inaudible P_2; grade I–VI/VI obstructive systolic murmur, maximal at the pulmonary area.
- Dilated pulmonary artery on posteroanterior chest radiograph.

General Considerations

Pulmonic valve stenosis accounts for 10% of all cases of congenital heart disease. In the usual case, the cusps of the pulmonary valve are fused to form a membrane or diaphragm with a hole in the middle that varies from 2–10 mm in diameter. Occasionally, only two cusps may fuse, producing a bicuspid pulmonary valve. In the more severe cases, a secondary infundibular stenosis is present. The pulmonary valve annulus is usually small. Moderate to marked poststenotic dilation of the main and left pulmonary arteries is usually evident.

Obstruction to blood flow across the pulmonary valve results in an increase in right ventricular pressure. Pressures greater than systemic are potentially life-threatening and are associated with critical obstruction. Because of the increased work required of the RV, severe RVH and eventual RV failure can occur. In contrast to patients with severe pulmonic valve stenosis, patients with this obstruction who also have a large VSD (ie, ToF) are not at risk for heart failure. In this situation, the septal defect limits the pressure developed in the RV to systemic pressure, making heart failure extremely uncommon.

When obstruction is severe and the ventricular septum is intact, a right-to-left shunt will often occur at the atrial level through a patent foramen ovale. Thus, patients with this condition will have cyanosis which necessitates immediate intervention.

Clinical Findings

A. Symptoms and Signs

Patients with mild or even moderate valvular pulmonary stenosis are acyanotic and completely asymptomatic. Patients with more severe valvular obstruction may develop cyanosis very early—even as neonates.

Patients with mild to moderate obstruction are usually well developed and well nourished. They are not prone to pulmonary infections. The pulses are normal. On cardiac examination, the precordium may be prominent. An RV heave can frequently be palpated. A systolic thrill is often present in the pulmonary area. S_1 is normal. In patients with mild to moderate stenosis, a prominent ejection click of pulmonary origin is heard best at the third left intercostal space. This click varies with respiration. It is much more prominent during expiration than inspiration. In patients with severe stenosis, the click tends to merge with S_1. S_2 varies with the degree of stenosis. In mild pulmonic stenosis, S_2 is normal. In moderate pulmonic stenosis, S_2 is more widely split and the pulmonary component is softer. In severe pulmonary stenosis, S_2 is single because the pulmonary component cannot be heard. A rough ejection systolic murmur is best heard at the second left interspace. It radiates very well to the back. With severe obstruction of the valve, the murmur is usually short. No diastolic murmurs are audible.

B. Imaging

The heart size is normal. Poststenotic dilation of the main pulmonary artery and the left pulmonary artery often occurs.

C. Electrocardiography

The ECG is usually normal in patients with mild obstruction. RVH is present in patients with moderate to severe pulmonic stenosis. In severe obstruction, RV hypertrophy with a RV strain pattern (deep inversion of the T wave) are seen in the right precordial leads. Right atrial enlargement may be present. Right axis deviation also occurs in the moderate to severe forms.

D. Echocardiography

The pulmonary valve is unusually thickened with reduced valve leaflet excursion. The transvalvular pressure gradient can be estimated accurately by Doppler.

E. Cardiac Catheterization and Angiocardiography

In severe cases, a right-to-left shunt occurs at the atrial level. Pulmonary artery pressure is normal. RV pressure is always higher than pulmonary artery pressure. The gradient across the pulmonary valve varies from 10–200 mm Hg. In severe cases, the right atrial pressure is often elevated, with a predominant 'a' wave. Angiocardiography in the RV shows thickening of the pulmonary valve and its narrow opening. This produces a jet of contrast into the pulmonary artery. Infundibular hypertrophy may be present. Catheterization is performed for therapeutic intervention rather than for diagnostic purposes, as pulmonic stenosis is easily diagnosed by physical examination, the ECG, and echocardiography. Catheterization is reserved for balloon pulmonic valvuloplasty.

Treatment

Relief of pulmonic stenosis is recommended for children with RV systolic pressures greater than two-thirds of systemic pressure. Immediate correction is indicated for patients with systemic or suprasystemic RV pressure. Percutaneous balloon valvuloplasty is the procedure of choice. It is as effective as surgery in relieving obstruction and causes less valve insufficiency. Surgery is needed to treat pulmonic valve stenosis only when balloon pulmonic valvuloplasty is unsuccessful.

Course & Prognosis

Patients with mild pulmonary stenosis live normal lives. Occasionally, children diagnosed with mild pulmonic valve stenosis will have their valves improve to normal without intervention. Those with stenosis of moderate severity are rarely symptomatic. Those with severe valvular obstruction may develop severe cyanosis in infancy.

After balloon pulmonic valvuloplasty or surgery, most patients have good voluntary maximum exercise capacity unless they have significant PI. Patients with isolated PI, a common occurrence after surgical pulmonary valvotomy, may be significantly limited in exercise performance. Severe PI leads to progressive RV dilation and dysfunction, which may precipitate ventricular arrhythmias or right heart failure in adulthood. Patients with severe PI may benefit from replacement of the pulmonic valve. If relief of valvular obstruction occurs before age 20 years, longevity is normal. Limitation of physical activity is unwarranted. The quality of life of adults with successfully treated pulmonary stenosis and minimal PI is normal.

Yetman AT et al: Comparison of exercise performance in patients after pulmonary valvulotomy for pulmonary stenosis and tetralogy of Fallot. Am J Cardiol 2002;90:1412 [PMID: 12480060].

2. Infundibular Pulmonary Stenosis without Ventricular Septal Defect

Pure infundibular pulmonary stenosis is rare. Infundibular hypertrophy may occur, often in association with a small perimembranous VSD, and lead to a "double chambered RV" wherein there is significant obstruction from the inflow to the outflow portion of the RV. One should suspect such an abnormality if there a prominent precordial thrill, no audible pulmonary ejection click, and a murmur that is maximal in the third and fourth intercostal spaces rather than in the second intercostal space. The clinical picture is otherwise identical to that of pulmonic valve stenosis. Intervention, if indicated, is always surgical because this condition does not improve with balloon catheter dilation.

3. Distal Pulmonary Stenosis

Supravalvular Pulmonary Stenosis

Supravalvular pulmonary stenosis, a relatively rare condition, is caused by narrowing of the main pulmonary artery. The clinical picture may be identical to that of valvular pulmonary stenosis, although the murmur is maximal in the first intercostal space at the left sternal border and in the suprasternal notch. No ejection click is audible. The murmur radiates into the neck and over the lung fields. This condition occurs most often in children with Noonan syndrome.

Peripheral Pulmonary Branch Stenosis

In peripheral pulmonary branch stenosis, multiple narrowings of the branches of the pulmonary artery occur at the bifurcation of the main pulmonary artery or in the periphery of the lung. Systolic murmurs may be heard over both lung fields, both anteriorly and posteriorly. Transient pulmonary branch stenosis murmurs of infancy are innocent. The three most common causes of significant pulmonary artery branch stenosis are Williams syndrome, Alagille syndrome, and congenital rubella syndrome. Surgery is often unsuccessful. Transvenous balloon angioplasty is currently being used to treat this condition, with moderate success. In many instances, the stenoses improve with age.

4. Other Congenital Right Heart Lesions

Ebstein Malformation of the Tricuspid Valve

In Ebstein malformation of the tricuspid valve, the tricuspid valve is displaced downward so that the septal leaflet of the valve is attached to the RV wall (inside the RV) rather than at the tricuspid annulus. As a result, the upper portion of the RV is physiologically within the right atrium. The so-called atrialized portion of the RV is thin-walled and does not contribute to RV output. The portion of the ventricle below the displaced tricuspid valve is diminished in volume and represents the functioning RV. This is an uncommon condition.

Clinical Findings

A. Symptoms and Signs

The degree of displacement of the tricuspid valve is variable, and the clinical picture of Ebstein malformation varies with this displacement. In the most extreme form, the septal leaflet is markedly displaced into the RV outflow tract, leading to obstruction of antegrade flow to the pulmonary artery. Patients are cyanotic shortly after birth because of poor pulmonary artery flow. At the opposite extreme, symptoms may not develop until adulthood when tachyarrhythmias in association with right atrial dilation or an associated reentrant pathway occur. These older patients typically have a lesser degree of displacement of the septal leaflet of the tricuspid valve.

B. Imaging

The chest radiograph usually shows cardiomegaly with prominence of the right heart border. The degree of cardiomegaly is influenced by the degree of tricuspid valve displacement and by the presence and size of the atrial level shunt. Massive cardiomegaly with a "wall-to-wall heart" occurs in the setting of severe displacement and a restrictive atrial level defect.

C. ELECTROCARDIOGRAM

ECG may be normal but more typically shows right atrial enlargement. Right bundle-branch block (RBBB) and LV enlargement may be found. A delta wave from coexisting Wolff-Parkinson-White (WPW) syndrome may be seen.

D. ECHOCARDIOGRAPHY

Echocardiography is necessary to confirm the diagnosis and may aid in predicting outcome. The degree of displacement, the size of the right atrium, the presence of an associated atrial level shunt, and LV systolic function all affect outcome. The size of the atrialized portion of the RV is determined by echo.

E. COURSE AND PROGNOSIS

In cyanotic neonates, prostaglandin E infusion is used to maintain pulmonary blood flow until pulmonary vascular resistance decreases, facilitating antegrade pulmonary artery flow. If the patient remains significantly cyanotic, surgical intervention is required in the neonatal period.

Surgical repair consists of an annuloplasty to modify the level of the tricuspid orifice and diminish tricuspid insufficiency. The success rate of this procedure is highly variable. Late arrhythmias are common. Postoperative exercise tolerance increases but remains lower than that for age-related normals. If a significant Ebstein malformation is not treated, atrial tachyarrhythmias will frequently begin during adolescence.

Absence of a Pulmonary Artery

Absence of a pulmonary artery (left or right) may be an isolated malformation or may occur in association with other congenital heart diseases. It occurs occasionally in patients with ToF.

Absence of the Pulmonary Valve

Absence of the pulmonary valve is a rare abnormality usually associated with VSD. In about 50% of cases, infundibular pulmonary stenosis is also present (ToF with absent pulmonary valve).

Driscoll DJ et al: Spectrum of exercise intolerance in 45 patients with Ebstein's anomaly and observations on exercise tolerance in 11 patients after surgical repair. J Am Coll Cardiol 1988; 11:831 [PMID: 3351151].

Yetman AT et al: Outcome in cyanotic neonates with Ebstein's anomaly. Am J Cardiol 1998;81:1 [PMID: 9527086].

MALFORMATIONS ASSOCIATED WITH OBSTRUCTION TO BLOOD FLOW ON THE LEFT SIDE OF THE HEART

1. Coarctation of the Aorta

 ESSENTIALS OF DIAGNOSIS & TYPICAL FEATURES

- *Pulse lag in lower extremities.*
- *Systolic blood pressure 20 mm Hg or more higher in the upper than in the lower extremities.*
- *Blowing systolic murmur in the left axilla.*

General Considerations

Coarctation is common, accounting for about 6% of all congenital heart disease. Three times as many males as females are affected. Many affected females have 45 XO Turner syndrome. Coarctation usually occurs in the thoracic portion of the descending aorta distal to the takeoff of the left subclavian artery in the juxtaductal region. The abdominal aorta is rarely involved. The term "Shone syndrome" refers to multiple levels of left heart obstructive disease, including mitral stenosis, bicuspid aortic valve with or without aortic stenosis, tubular hypoplasia of the aortic isthmus, and coarctation of the aorta. The incidence of an associated bicuspid aortic valve with coarctation is 80–85%.

Clinical Findings

A. SYMPTOMS AND SIGNS

The cardinal physical finding is decrease or absence of femoral pulses. Infants with severe coarctation have equal upper and lower extremity pulses from birth to 2 days of age. Unequal pulses and clinical symptoms develop between 4 and 10 days of age as the ductus arteriosus closes. Approximately 40% of children with coarctation will present at this young age. Coarctation alone, or in combination with VSD, ASD, or other congenital cardiac anomalies, is the leading cause of CHF in the first month of life.

Coarctation presents more insidiously in the 60% of children with no symptoms in infancy. Their coarctation is diagnosed by a pulse discrepancy between the arms and legs on physical exam or by arm hypertension on blood pressure measurement. The level of blood pressure in the arms may be elevated only moderately, even in severe coarctation, or it may be elevated significantly. In any case, the pulses in the legs are diminished or absent in affected infants. The left subclavian artery is occasionally involved in the coarctation, in which case the left brachial pulse is also weak. An ejection systolic murmur of grade II/VI intensity is often heard at the aortic area and the lower left sternal border along with an apical ejection click from the bicuspid aortic valve. The pathognomonic murmur of coarctation is heard in the left axilla and the left back. The murmur is usually systolic but may spill into diastole. If the coarctation is complicated by other malformations, murmurs associated with these other abnormalities will be audible.

B. IMAGING

In the older child, radiographic findings may show a normal sized heart, although there is usually some evidence of LV enlargement. The aorta proximal to the coarctation is prominent. The aortic outline indents at the level of the coarctation. The poststenotic segment is dilated. This combination of abnormalities results in the "figure 3" sign on chest radiograph. Notching of the ribs caused by marked enlargement of the intercostal collaterals can be seen. MRI has become extremely useful for determining noninvasively the anatomy of the coarctation. In patients with a severe coarctation and associated CHF, marked cardiac enlargement and pulmonary venous congestion occur.

C. ELECTROCARDIOGRAPHY

ECGs in older children may be normal or may show LVH. ECGs usually shows RVH in infants with severe coarctation.

D. ECHOCARDIOGRAPHY

Two-dimensional echocardiography and color-flow Doppler are used to visualize the coarctation directly, and continuous-wave Doppler estimates the degree of obstruction. Diastolic run-off flow is found by continuous-wave Doppler if the obstruction is severe. If the ductus arteriosus is patent, echocardiography may not detect the coarctation. Associated lesions such as a bicuspid aortic valve or mitral abnormalities may suggest the presence of a coarctation. In the face of poor LV systolic function, the coarctation may be difficult to visualize.

E. CARDIAC CATHETERIZATION AND ANGIOCARDIOGRAPHY

These studies demonstrate the position, anatomy, and severity of the coarctation and assess the adequacy of collateral circulation. Cardiac catheterization and angiocardiography are rarely performed for infants or children with coarctation unless dilation of the coarct during catheter study is planned.

Treatment

Infants with coarctation of the aorta and CHF may present in extremis secondary to LV dysfunction and associated low cardiac output. Resuscitative measures include initiation of prostaglandin infusion (0.025–0.1 μg/kg/min) to reopen the ductus arteriosus and inotropic support. Once stabilized, the infant should undergo corrective repair. Some centers perform primary balloon aortoplasty in infants with coarctation, but this is not universal. Surgery, either the modified end-to-end anastomosis technique or the left subclavian approach, has a high success rate, but there is a 10–15% rate of recoarctation after repair. Fortunately, recurrent coarctation is treatable with balloon aortoplasty in the catheterization laboratory. Coarctation of the aorta in infants who do not have CHF is corrected electively. In elective repairs, either surgery or balloon aortoplasty can be used. In the older patient, particularly when of adult size, aortic stent placement is effective.

Course & Prognosis

Children with coarctation of the aorta who survive the neonatal period without developing CHF do quite well through childhood and adolescence. Fatal complications (eg, hypertensive encephalopathy or intracranial bleeding) are uncommon in childhood. Infective endocarditis (actually endarteritis in this condition) is rare before adolescence.

Children with coarctation corrected after age 5 years are at increased risk for systemic hypertension and myocardial dysfunction even with successful surgery. Exercise testing is mandatory for these children prior to their participation in athletic activities.

Hamdan MA et al: Endovascular stents for coarctation of the aorta: Initial results and intermediate-term follow-up. J Am Coll Cardiol 2001;38:1518 [PMID: 11691533].

Ovaert C et al: Balloon angioplasty of native coarctation: Clinical outcomes and predictors of success. J Am Coll Cardiol 2000; 35:988 [PMID: 10732899].

2. Aortic Stenosis

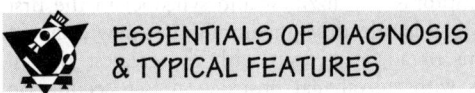

ESSENTIALS OF DIAGNOSIS
& TYPICAL FEATURES

- *Systolic ejection murmur at the upper right sternal border.*
- *Thrill in the carotid arteries.*
- *Systolic click at the apex.*
- *Dilation of the ascending aorta on chest radiograph.*

General Considerations

Aortic stenosis is defined as obstruction to outflow from the LV at or near the aortic valve that produces a systolic pressure gradient of more than 10 mm Hg between the LV and the aorta. Aortic stenosis accounts for approximately 7% of congenital heart disease. There are three anatomic types of congenital aortic stenosis.

A. VALVULAR AORTIC STENOSIS (75%)

In critical aortic stenosis presenting in infancy, the aortic valve is usually a unicuspid diaphragmlike structure without well-defined commissures. Preschool and school-age children more commonly have a bicuspid aortic valve. Teenagers and young adults characteristically have a tricuspid valve with partially fused leaflets. This lesion is more common in males than in females.

B. SUBVALVULAR AORTIC STENOSIS (23%)

In this type, a membranous or fibrous ring occurs just below the aortic valve. The ring forms a diaphragm with a hole in the middle and causes obstruction to LV outflow. The aortic valve itself and the anterior leaflet of the mitral valve are often deformed.

C. SUPRAVALVULAR AORTIC STENOSIS (1–2%)

In this type, constriction of the ascending aorta occurs just above the coronary arteries. The condition is often familial, and two different genetic patterns are found, one with an abnormal facies and mental retardation (Williams syndrome) and one with normal facies and no developmental delay.

Clinical Findings

A. SYMPTOMS AND SIGNS

Most patients with aortic stenosis have no cardiovascular symptoms. Except in the most severe cases, the patient may do well until the third to fifth decades of life. Some patients have mild exercise intolerance and fatigability. A small percentage of patients have significant symptoms (ie, dizziness and syncope) in the first decade. Sudden death is uncommon but may occur in all forms of aortic stenosis with the greatest risk in patients with subvalvular obstruction (see section on hypertrophic cardiomyopathy).

Although isolated valvular aortic stenosis seldom causes symptoms in infancy, severe heart failure occasionally occurs when critical obstruction is present at birth. Response to medical therapy is poor; therefore, an aggressive approach using interventional catheterization or surgery is required. The physical findings vary depending on the anatomic type of lesion:

1. Valvular aortic stenosis—Affected patients are well developed and well nourished. Pulses are usually normal and equal throughout. If the stenosis is severe and a gradient of greater than 80 mm Hg exists, the pulses are diminished with a slow upstroke. Cardiac examination reveals an LV thrust at the apex. A systolic thrill at the right base, the suprasternal notch, and both carotid arteries may accompany moderate disease.

S_1 is normal. A prominent aortic ejection click is best heard at the apex. The click corresponds to the opening of the aortic valve. It is separated from S_1 by a short but appreciable interval. It does not vary with respiration. S_2 at the pulmonary area is normal. The aortic component of S_2 is of good intensity. A grade III–V/VI, rough, medium- to high-pitched ejection-type systolic murmur is evident, loudest at the first and second intercostal spaces, radiating well into the suprasternal notch and along the carotids. The grade of the murmur correlates well with the severity of the stenosis.

2. Discrete membranous subvalvular aortic stenosis—The findings are essentially the same as those of valvular aortic stenosis except for the absence of a click. The murmur and thrill are usually somewhat more intense at the left sternal border in the third and fourth intercostal spaces than at the aortic area. Frequently, however, the murmur is equally intense at both sites. A diastolic murmur of aortic insufficiency is commonly heard after age 5 years.

3. Supravalvular aortic stenosis—The thrill and murmur are characteristically best heard in the suprasternal notch and along the carotids but are well transmitted over the aortic area and near the mid left sternal border. A difference in pulses and blood pressure between the right and left arms may be found, with more prominent pulse and pressure in the right arm (Coanda effect).

B. IMAGING

In most cases the heart is not enlarged. The LV, however, is slightly prominent. In valvular aortic stenosis, dilation of the ascending aorta is frequently seen.

C. ELECTROCARDIOGRAPHY

Patients with mild aortic stenosis have normal ECGs. Some patients with severe obstruction have ECG evidence of LVH and LV strain but many do not. In about 25% of severe cases, the ECG is normal. Progressive increase in LVH on serial ECGs indicates a significant degree of obstruction. LV strain is an indication for surgery.

D. ECHOCARDIOGRAPHY

This is a reliable noninvasive technique for the evaluation of all forms of aortic stenosis. Doppler accurately estimates the transvalvular gradient.

E. CARDIAC CATHETERIZATION AND ANGIOCARDIOGRAPHY

Left heart catheterization demonstrates the pressure differential between the LV and the aorta and the level at which the gradient exists. Echocardiography is now the standard method for following the severity of aortic valve stenosis, and catheterization is reserved for patients whose resting gradient has reached 60–80 mm Hg and in whom intervention is planned. For those with valvular aortic stenosis, balloon valvuloplasty is usually the first option. In subvalvular or supravalvular aortic stenosis, interventional catheterization is not effective and surgery is required.

Treatment

Surgery should be considered only in patients with symptoms, a high resting gradient (60–80 mm Hg) despite balloon angioplasty, or coexisting aortic insufficiency. In many cases, the gradient cannot be significantly diminished without producing aortic insufficiency. Percutaneous balloon valvuloplasty is now accepted as standard initial treatment. Patients who develop significant aortic insufficiency will require surgical intervention to repair or replace the valve with either a prosthetic valve or with the patient's own pulmonic valve (Ross procedure). In the Ross procedure, an RV-to-PA conduit is used to replace the pulmonic valve. Discrete subvalvular aortic stenosis is usually surgically repaired at a lesser gradient because continued trauma to the aortic valve by the subvalvular jet may damage the valve and produce aortic insufficiency. Unfortunately, simple resection is followed by recurrence in more than 25% of patients with subvalvular aortic stenosis. All patients should have close follow-up, and those older than age 6 years should undergo yearly exercise testing. If exercise testing is normal, restriction of physical activity may not be necessary in patients with mild to moderate aortic stenosis.

Course & Prognosis

All forms of LV outflow tract obstruction tend to be progressive. Pediatric patients with LV outflow tract obstruction—with the exception of those with critical aortic stenosis of infancy—are usually asymptomatic. Symptoms accompanying severe unoperated obstruction (angina, syncope, or CHF) are rare because of detection and surgical or catheter intervention. Preoperative or postoperative children whose obstruction is mild to moderate appear to have normal oxygen consumption and maximum voluntary working capacity. Children in this category with normal heart size and normal resting and exercising ECG may safely participate in vigorous physical activity, including nonisometric competitive sports. Children with severe aortic stenosis may demonstrate ventricular dysrhythmias.

Mitchell BM et al: Serial exercise performance in children with surgically corrected congenital aortic stenosis. Pediatr Cardiol 2003;24:319 [PMID: 12632225].

Rao PS: Long-term follow-up results after balloon dilation of pulmonic stenosis, aortic stenosis and coarctation of the aorta: A review. Prog Cardiovasc Dis 1999;42:59 [PMID: 10505493].

3. Mitral Valve Prolapse

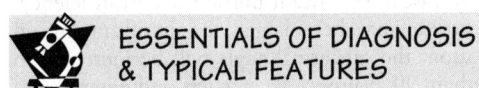

ESSENTIALS OF DIAGNOSIS & TYPICAL FEATURES

- *Midsystolic click best heard with the patient in the standing position or during the Valsalva maneuver.*
- *Late systolic "whooping" or "honking" murmur.*

General Considerations

Mitral valve prolapse (MVP) is a common entity associated with abnormal auscultatory findings in older pediatric patients. It results from redundant valve tissue or abnormal tissue comprising the mitral valve apparatus. The mitral valve prolapses, moving posteriorly or superiorly into the left atrium during ventricular systole as the mitral valve closes. A midsystolic click occurs at the time of this movement and is the clinical hallmark of this entity. Mitral insufficiency may occur late in systole, causing an atypical, short, late systolic murmur with variable radiation. MVP occurs in about 2% of thin adolescent females, a minority of whom have concomitant mitral insufficiency. Although MVP is most commonly an isolated lesion, it can occur in association with Marfan syndrome and Ehlers-Danlos syndrome. These coexisting conditions should be ruled out by clinical examination.

Clinical Findings

A. SYMPTOMS AND SIGNS

Most patients with MVP are asymptomatic. Chest pain, palpitations, and dizziness may be reported, but it is unclear whether these symptoms are more common in affected patients than in the normal population. Significant dysrhythmias have been reported, including increased ventricular ectopy and nonsustained ventricular tachycardia. If significant mitral regurgitation is present, atrial arrhythmias may also occur. Standard auscultation technique must be modified to diagnose MVP. Clicks, with or without systolic murmur, are elicited best in the standing position due to the decrease in left ventricular volume. Conversely, maneuvers that increase LV volume, such as squatting or handgrip exercise, will cause delay or obliteration of the click-murmur complex. The systolic click usually is heard at the apex, but may be audible at the left sternal border. A systolic murmur after the click implies mitral insufficiency and is much less common than isolated prolapse. The murmur is unlike rheumatic mitral insufficiency in that it is not pansystolic.

B. IMAGING

In the rare case of significant mitral valve insufficiency, the left atrium may be enlarged. In significant mitral regurgitation, the subcarinal angle will be increased to greater than 90 degrees. Most chest radiographs are normal and are not indicated in this condition.

C. ELECTROCARDIOGRAPHY

The ECG may be normal. Diffuse flattening or inversion of T waves may occur in the precordial leads. U waves are prominent. Chest pain on exertion is rare and should be assessed with cardiopulmonary stress testing.

D. ECHOCARDIOGRAPHY

Significant posterior systolic movement of the mitral valve leaflets to the atrial side of the mitral annulus is diagnostic. Echocardiography assesses the degree of myxomatous change of the mitral valve and the degree of mitral insufficiency.

E. OTHER TESTING

Invasive procedures are rarely indicated. Holter monitoring or event recorders may be useful in establishing the presence of ventricular dysrhythmias in patients with palpitations.

Treatment & Prognosis

Propranolol may be effective in treatment of coexisting arrhythmias. Prophylaxis for infectious endocarditis is indicated only in individuals with significant myxomatous change on echocardiography or those with mitral insufficiency.

The natural course of this condition is not well defined. Twenty years of observation indicate that isolated MVP in childhood is usually a benign entity. Surgery for mitral insufficiency is rarely needed.

Bobkowski W et al: A prospective study to determine the significance of ventricular late potentials in children with mitral valve prolapse. Cardiol Young 2002;12:333 [PMID: 12206555].

Freed LA et al: Prevalence and clinical outcome of mitral valve prolapse. N Engl J Med 1999;341:1 [PMID: 10387935].

4. Other Congenital Left Heart Valvular Lesions

Congenital Mitral Stenosis

Congenital mitral stenosis is a rare disorder in which the valve leaflets are thickened and fused, producing a diaphragmlike or funnel-like structure with a central opening. When mitral stenosis occurs with other left-sided obstructive lesions, such as subaortic stenosis and coarctation of the aorta, the complex is known as Shone syndrome. Most patients develop symptoms early in life with tachypnea, dyspnea, and failure to thrive. Physical examination reveals an accentuated S_1 and a loud pulmonary closure sound. No opening snap can be heard. In most cases, a presystolic crescendo murmur is heard at the apex. Occasionally, only a mid-diastolic murmur can be heard. Rarely, no murmur is present. ECG shows right axis deviation, biatrial enlargement, and RVH. Radiograph reveals left atrial enlargement and frequently pulmonary venous congestion. Echocardiography shows abnormal mitral valve structures with reduced excursion and left atrial enlargement. Cardiac catheterization reveals an elevated pulmonary capillary wedge pressure and pulmonary hypertension.

Mitral valve repair or mitral valve replacement with a prosthetic mitral valve may be performed even in young infants. Mitral valve repair is the preferred surgical option, as valve replacement has a poor outcome in very young children.

Cor Triatriatum

Cor triatriatum is a rare abnormality in which the pulmonary veins join together at their confluence but the confluence is not completely incorporated into the left atrium. The confluence communicates with the left atrium through an opening of variable size. The consequences of this condition are similar to those of mitral stenosis. Clinical findings depend on the size of the opening. If the opening is small, symptoms develop early in life. If the opening is larger, patients may be asymptomatic for a considerable time. Echocardiography reveals a linear density in the left atrium with a gradient between the pulmonary venous chamber and the true left atrium. Cardiac catheterization may be needed if the diagnosis is in doubt. A high pulmonary wedge pressure and a low left atrial pressure (with the catheter passed through the foramen ovale into the true left atrium) confirms the diagnosis. Angiocardiography identifies both the proximal and distal left atria. Surgical repair is always required in the presence of an obstructive membrane, and long-term results are good. Coexisting mitral valve abnormalities may be noted, including a supravalvular mitral ring or a dysplastic mitral valve.

Congenital Mitral Regurgitation

Congenital mitral regurgitation is a rare abnormality usually associated with other congenital heart lesions, such as congenitally corrected TGA, AV septal defect, and anomalous left coronary artery. Isolated congenital mitral regurgitation is very rare. It is sometimes present in patients with Marfan syndrome, usually associated with a myxomatous prolapsing mitral valve.

Congenital Aortic Regurgitation

Congenital aortic regurgitation is rare. The most common causes are bicuspid aortic valve, with or without coarctation of the aorta; VSD with aortic cusp prolapse and aortic insufficiency; and fenestration of the aortic valve cusp (one or more holes in the cusp).

Eble BK et al: Mitral valve replacement in children: Predictors of long-term outcome. Ann Thorac Surg 2003;76:853 [PMID: 12963215].

DISEASES OF THE AORTA

Aortic dilation and dissection may occur in childhood. Although the aorta may not be dilated at birth, the structural abnormality that predisposes to dilation is presumed to be congenital in origin. Patients at risk for progressive aortic dilation and possible dissection include those with isolated bicuspid aortic valve, Marfan syndrome, Turner syndrome, and type IV Ehlers-Danlos syndrome.

Bicuspid Aortic Valve

Patients with bicuspid aortic valves have an increased incidence of aortic dilation and dissection, regardless of the presence of aortic stenosis. Histologic examination demonstrates cystic medial degeneration of the aortic wall, similar to that seen in patients with Marfan syndrome. Patients with isolated bicuspid aortic valve require regular follow-up even in the absence of aortic insufficiency or aortic stenosis. Significant aortic root dilation requiring surgical intervention typically does not occur until adulthood.

Marfan Syndrome

Marfan syndrome is an autosomal dominant disorder of connective tissue caused by a mutation in the fibrillin-1 gene. The incidence of spontaneous mutations is 25%, and thus family history is not always helpful. Patients are diagnosed by the Ghent criteria and must have at a minimum, major involvement of two body systems plus involvement of a third body system or a positive family history. Body systems involved include cardiovascular, ocular, musculoskeletal, pulmonary, and integumentary. Cardiac manifestations include aortic root dilation and MVP, which may be present at birth. Patients are at risk for aortic dilation and dissection and are restricted from competitive athletics, contact sports, and isometric activities. β-Blockers or ACE inhibitors are used to lower blood pressure and slow the rate of aortic dilation. Elective surgical intervention is performed in patients of adult size

when the aortic root dimension reaches 50 mm. The ratio of actual to expected aortic root dimension is used to determine the need for surgery in the young child. Surgical options include replacement of the dilated aortic root with a composite valve graft (Bentall technique) or a David procedure in which the patient's own aortic valve is spared and a Dacron tube graft is used to replace the dilated ascending aorta. Young age at diagnosis was previously thought to confer a poor prognosis; however, early diagnosis with close follow-up and early medical therapy has been associated with more favorable outcome in most patients. Ventricular dysrhythmias may contribute to the increased mortality seen in these patients.

Turner Syndrome

Cardiovascular abnormalities are common in patients with Turner syndrome. Patients are at risk for aortic dissection, typically during adulthood. Risk factors include hypertension regardless of cause, aortic dilation, bicuspid aortic valve, and coarctation of the aorta. There are rare reports of aortic dissection in adult Turner syndrome patients in the absence of any risk factors. Patients with Turner syndrome require routine follow-up from adolescence onward to monitor this potentially lethal complication.

Bonderman D et al: Mechanisms underlying aortic dilation in congenital aortic valve malformation. Circulation 1999;99:2138 [PMID: 10217654].

Bordeleau L et al: Aortic dissection and Turner's syndrome: A review of the literature. J Emerg Med 1998;16:593 [PMID: 9696176].

Yetman AT et al: Comparison of outcome of the Marfan's syndrome in patients diagnosed at < or > 6 years of age. Am J Cardiol 2003;91:102 [PMID: 12505586].

Yetman AT et al: Long-term outcome in patients with Marfan's syndrome: Is aortic dissection the only cause of sudden death? J Am Coll Cardiol 2003;41:329 [PMID: 12535830].

CORONARY ARTERY ABNORMALITIES

A number of anomalies involve the origin, course, and distribution of the coronary arteries. The only abnormality seen with regularity, and which has disastrous consequences if unrecognized, is anomalous origin of the left coronary artery.

1. Anomalous Origin of the Left Coronary Artery

The left coronary artery arises from the pulmonary artery rather than the aorta. In neonates, who have relatively high pulmonary arterial pressure, the perfusion of the left coronary artery is adequate and the child is asymptomatic. By age 2 months the pulmonary arterial pressure falls, causing a progressive decrease in myocardial perfusion supplied by the left coronary artery. Ischemia and then infarction of the LV occur. Affected infants present at age 2–4 months with severe CHF due to LV dysfunction and mitral insufficiency. Immediate surgery is needed to reimplant the left coronary artery and restore adequate myocardial perfusion. The surgery is relatively high-risk, especially if infarction of the papillary muscles supporting the mitral apparatus has occurred. Mitral valve replacement is sometimes needed.

Clinical Findings

A. SYMPTOMS AND SIGNS

Patients appear healthy at birth. Growth and development are relatively normal for a few months, although detailed questioning often discloses a history of intermittent abdominal pain, pallor, and sweating, especially during or after feeding. These episodes, often thought to be colic, in fact are attacks of angina.

On physical examination, the patients are usually well developed and well nourished. The pulses are typically weak but equal. A prominent left precordial bulge is present. The pansystolic murmur of mitral regurgitation is frequently present, although a murmur need not be present.

B. IMAGING

Chest radiographs show cardiac enlargement and left atrial enlargement and may show pulmonary venous congestion.

C. ELECTROCARDIOGRAPHY

The ECG is very helpful. There are T-wave inversions in leads I and aVL. The precordial leads show T-wave inversions from V_4–V_7. Deep, and often wide, Q waves are present in leads I, aVL, and sometimes in V_4–V_6. These findings of myocardial infarction are similar to those in adults.

D. ECHOCARDIOGRAPHY

The diagnosis can be made with two-dimensional echo techniques by visualizing a single large right coronary artery arising from the aorta, LV dysfunction with mitral insufficiency, and visualization of the anomalous left coronary artery arising from the main pulmonary artery. Flow reversal in the left coronary confirms the diagnosis.

E. CARDIAC CATHETERIZATION AND ANGIOCARDIOGRAPHY

A small left-to-right shunt (a result of the flow of blood from the right through the left coronary artery and into the pulmonary artery) can sometimes be detected. Aortogram fails to show the origin of the left coronary

artery. A large right coronary artery fills directly from the aorta and contrast flows from the right coronary system via collaterals into the left coronary arteries and finally into the pulmonary artery.

Treatment & Prognosis

Medical management with anticongestives and afterload reduction cannot correct the anatomic defect and surgical intervention should not be delayed. Surgery is required to give a two-coronary system. Simple ligation of the left coronary artery or subclavian to coronary artery anastomosis (without cardiopulmonary bypass) have poor long-term results. Because survival after coronary surgery is dependent on the degree of mitral insufficiency, a decision must be made prior to bypass whether to replace the mitral valve. Anomalous left coronary artery is a high-risk diagnosis. The prognosis is guarded at best.

Michielon G et al: Anomalous coronary artery origin from the pulmonary artery: Correlation between surgical timing and left ventricular function recovery. Ann Thorac Surg 2003;76:581 [PMID: 12902108].

CYANOTIC CONGENITAL HEART DISEASE

Tetralogy of Fallot

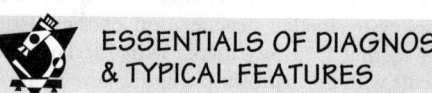

ESSENTIALS OF DIAGNOSIS & TYPICAL FEATURES

- *Cyanosis after the neonatal period.*
- *Hypoxemic spells during infancy.*
- *Right-sided aortic arch in 25% of patients.*
- *Systolic ejection murmur at the upper left sternal border.*

General Considerations

In ToF, a VSD is present and obstruction to RV outflow occurs so that intracardiac shunt is typically from right to left. This is the most common cyanotic cardiac lesion, accounting for 10% of all cases of congenital heart disease. The VSD is usually located in the membranous ventricular septum but may be surrounded completely by muscular tissue. The defect is usually large. Obstruction to RV outflow may be primarily at the infundibular level (in 25–50% of cases), at the valvular level alone (rarely), or at both levels (most commonly). The primary embryologic abnormality is in the septation of the conus and truncus arteriosus with anterior deviation of the conus into the RV outflow tract, which produces an enlarged overriding aorta and hypoplasia of the pulmonary outflow. The term "tetralogy" has been used to describe this combination of lesions, because RVH is always present and a varying degree of overriding of the aorta occurs in addition to the VSD and pulmonic and subpulmonic stenosis. A right-sided aortic arch is present in 25% of cases, and an ASD occurs in 15%.

Obstruction to RV outflow plus a large VSD results in a right-to-left shunt at the ventricular level and arterial desaturation. The degree of desaturation depends on the resistance to RV outflow and systemic vascular resistance. The greater the obstruction and the lower the systemic vascular resistance, the greater the right-to-left shunt. Although the patient may be deeply cyanotic, the amount of pressure the RV can develop is limited to that of the systemic (aortic) pressure because the VSD is unrestrictive. The RV is able to maintain this level of pressure without developing heart failure. An association between ToF and deletions in the long arm of chromosome 22 (22q11) has now been established in as many as 15% of children with tetralogy.

Clinical Findings

A. SYMPTOMS AND SIGNS

Clinical findings vary with the degree of RV outflow obstruction. Patients with mild obstruction are minimally cyanotic or even acyanotic. Those with maximal obstruction are deeply cyanotic from birth. Few children are asymptomatic. Most have cyanosis by age 4 months, and the cyanosis usually is progressive. Growth and development are not typically delayed, but easy fatigability and dyspnea on exertion are common. When children with ToF begin walking, they frequently squat to increase systemic vascular resistance and thus ward off cyanotic spells.

Hypoxemic spells, also called cyanotic or Tet spells, are one of the hallmarks of severe ToF and are characterized by: (1) sudden onset of cyanosis or deepening of cyanosis; (2) sudden dyspnea; (3) alterations in consciousness, in a spectrum from irritability to syncope; and (4) decrease or disappearance of the systolic murmur. These episodes most commonly start at age 4–6 months. Acute treatment of cyanotic spells is administration of oxygen and placing the patient in the knee-chest position. Acidosis, if present, should be corrected with intravenous sodium bicarbonate. Morphine should be administered cautiously by a parenteral route in a dosage of 0.1 mg/kg. Propranolol, 0.1–0.2 mg/kg IV, is useful. Chronic oral prophylaxis of cyanotic spells with propranolol, 1 mg/kg orally every 4 hours, may be useful to delay surgery but the onset of Tet spells usually leads to surgery. The fingers and toes show varying degrees of clubbing depending on the age of the child and the severity of cyanosis.

An RV lift is palpable. S_1 is normal; occasionally, an ejection click is heard at the apex that is aortic in origin.

S_2 is predominantly aortic and single. A grade II–IV/VI, rough, ejection-type systolic murmur is present that is maximal at the left sternal border in the third intercostal space and that radiates well to the back.

B. LABORATORY FINDINGS

Hemoglobin, hematocrit, and red blood cell count are usually elevated secondary to arterial desaturation.

C. IMAGING

Chest radiographs show a heart of normal size. The RV is hypertrophied, which is often shown in the posteroanterior projection by an upturning of the apex (boot-shaped heart). The main pulmonary artery segment is usually concave, and when there is a right aortic arch the aortic knob is to the right of the trachea. The pulmonary vascular markings are usually decreased.

D. ELECTROCARDIOGRAPHY

The QRS axis is rightward, ranging from +90 to +180 degrees. The P waves are usually normal. RVH is always present, but RV strain patterns are rare.

E. ECHOCARDIOGRAPHY

Two-dimensional imaging is diagnostic, revealing thickening of the RV wall, overriding of the aorta and a large subaortic VSD. Furthermore, obstruction at the level of the infundibulum and pulmonary valve can be identified, and the size of the proximal pulmonary arteries can be measured. The anatomy of the coronary arteries should be visualized.

F. CARDIAC CATHETERIZATION AND ANGIOCARDIOGRAPHY

Cardiac catheterization reveals a right-to-left shunt at the ventricular level in most cases. Arterial desaturation of varying degrees is present. The RV pressure is at systemic levels and the pressure tracing in the RV is identical to that in the LV. The pulmonary artery pressure is low. Pressure gradients may be noted at the valvular level, the infundibular level, or both. Angiography is helpful. RV injection reveals RV outflow obstruction and right-to-left shunt at the ventricular level. The major indications for cardiac catheterization are to establish coronary artery and distal pulmonary artery anatomy. Some patients may be palliated by balloon dilation of the RV outflow tract during infancy to improve the pulmonary blood flow, thereby delaying surgical intervention.

Treatment

A. PALLIATIVE TREATMENT

Palliative treatment is performed at some centers for small infants with severe symptoms (severe cyanosis or frequent severe hypoxic spells) and in whom complete correction is too risky. Medical palliation with chronic oral β-blocking agents, or more often, surgical palliation by creation of a systemic arterial to pulmonary arterial anastomosis, is used. Balloon angioplasty is being used for palliation in some centers. The pulmonic valve and the entire RV outflow tract are balloon dilated in order to reduce RV outflow tract obstruction and improve pulmonary artery growth. The most common surgical palliation is the insertion of a GoreTex shunt from the subclavian artery to the ipsilateral pulmonary artery (modified Blalock-Taussig shunt). This operation has a very low likelihood of mortality or pulmonary artery distortion.

B. TOTAL CORRECTION

The timing of open-heart surgery for repair of ToF ranges from birth to age 2 years, varying with the experience of each center. The current surgical trend is toward earlier repair based on the severity of symptoms. Patients may be repaired in the neonatal period, although if asymptomatic, surgery is deferred until 6 months of age. During surgery, the VSD is closed and the obstruction to RV outflow removed. Surgical mortality varies from 1–2%. The major limiting anatomic feature of total correction is the size of the pulmonary arteries.

Course & Prognosis

Infants with severe ToF are usually deeply cyanotic at birth. These children require early surgery, either a Blalock-Taussig shunt or primary correction.

All children with ToF require open-heart surgery. Complete repair before age 2 years usually produces fair to good function, although patients occasionally die as a result of ventricular dysrhythmias. A competent pulmonary valve without a dilated RV appears to diminish arrhythmias and enhance exercise performance.

Bacha EA et al: Long-term results after early primary repair of tetralogy of Fallot. J Thorac Cardiovasc Surg 2001;122:154 [PMID: 11436019].

Botto LD et al: A population-based study of the 22q11.2 deletion: Phenotype, incidence and contribution to major birth defects in the population. Pediatrics 2003;112(1 Pt 1):101 [PMID: 12837874].

Mulder TJ et al: A multicenter analysis of the choice of initial surgical procedure in tetralogy of Fallot. Pediatr Cardiol 2002;23:580 [PMID: 12530488].

Therrien J et al: Impact of pulmonary valve replacement on arrhythmia propensity late after repair of tetralogy of Fallot. Circulation 2001;103:2489 [PMID: 11369690].

PULMONARY ATRESIA WITH VENTRICULAR SEPTAL DEFECT

This condition consists of complete atresia of the pulmonary valve in association with VSD. It is essentially an extreme form of ToF. Because there is no antegrade flow from the RV to the pulmonary artery, pulmonary blood flow must be derived from a PDA or from aortopulmonary collateral arteries. The clinical picture depends entirely on the size of the ductus or collateral channels. If they are large, patients may be quite stable. If pulmonary blood flow is low, there is severe hypoxia and immediate palliation is required. Newborns are stabilized with intravenous prostaglandin E_1 (PGE_1) to maintain patency of the ductus arteriosus while being prepared for surgery. Once stabilized, a decision must be made between palliative Blalock-Taussig shunt or primary correction. In most centers, a shunt is performed in the newborn period and open-heart surgery planned for age 9–18 months.

Echocardiography or cardiac catheterization and angiocardiography are diagnostic. One corrective surgical procedure that has been successful in patients with adequate-sized pulmonary arteries consists of closing the VSD and inserting a homograft from the RV to the main pulmonary artery. Success depends on precise definition of pulmonary arterial and collateral blood supply to the lung, and if needed, prior unifocalization of segments with dual arterial blood supply into a single pulmonary arterial tree.

Mair DD, Puga FJ: Management of pulmonary atresia with ventricular septal defect. Curr Treat Options Cardiovasc Med 2003;5:409 [PMID: 12941209].

PULMONARY ATRESIA WITH INTACT VENTRICULAR SEPTUM

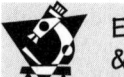 ESSENTIALS OF DIAGNOSIS & TYPICAL FEATURES

- *Cyanosis at birth.*
- *Chest radiograph with a concave pulmonary artery segment and the apex tilted upward.*

General Considerations

In this uncommon condition, the pulmonary valve is atretic. The pulmonic annulus usually has a small diaphragm consisting of the fused valve cusps. The ventricular septum is intact. The main pulmonary artery segment is usually present but is somewhat hypoplastic. Although the RV is always reduced in size, the degree of reduction is variable. The size of the RV is critical to the success of surgical repair. Some children with pulmonic atresia may have an RV that is adequate for ultimate two-ventricular repair. The RV has three component parts (inlet, trabecular, and outlet). The absence of any one of the components makes adequate RV function extremely unlikely. Even with all three components, some RVs are inadequate.

Following birth, the pulmonary circulation is maintained by the PDA. Although a bronchial-pulmonary collateral network may be present, it is usually insufficient to maintain pulmonary circulation. A continuous infusion of PGE_1 must be started as soon as possible after birth to maintain ductal patency.

Clinical Findings

A. SYMPTOMS AND SIGNS

Although patients may be normal at birth, they are usually cyanotic. Cyanosis progresses as the ductus arteriosus closes. A blowing systolic murmur resulting from the associated PDA may be heard at the pulmonary area. A pansystolic murmur is often heard at the lower left sternal border, as many children develop significant tricuspid insufficiency.

B. IMAGING

The heart size varies from small to markedly enlarged depending on the degree of tricuspid insufficiency. With severe tricuspid insufficiency, right atrial enlargement may be massive and the cardiac silhouette may fill the chest on x-ray.

C. ELECTROCARDIOGRAPHY

ECG reveals a left axis for age (45–90 degrees) in the frontal plane. Findings of right atrial enlargement are usually striking. There is LV dominance for age with reduced RV forces.

D. ECHOCARDIOGRAPHY

Echocardiography shows absence of the pulmonary valve with varying degrees of RV cavity tricuspid annulus hypoplasia. The severity of tricuspid regurgitation correlates with RV size.

E. CARDIAC CATHETERIZATION AND ANGIOCARDIOGRAPHY

RV pressure is high and is almost always suprasystemic. An angiogram in the RV reveals no filling of the pulmonary artery. It also demonstrates the size of the RV chamber, relative hypoplasia of the three components of the RV, and the presence or absence of tricuspid regurgitation. Approximately 15% of children with pulmonary atresia and intact ventricular septum have sinusoids between the RV and the coronary arteries. The presence of sinusoids indicates that the coronary circulation may depend on RV flow. This situation is associated with a high risk of sudden death.

Treatment & Prognosis

As in pulmonary atresia with VSD, PGE_1 is used to stabilize the patient and maintain patency of the ductus until

surgery can be performed. Surgery should be undertaken as soon as possible. A Rashkind balloon atrial septostomy is performed, depending on RV size, to open communication across the atrial septum. If the RV is tripartite and an eventual two-chamber repair is planned, the pulmonary valve plate is opened during cardiac catheterization in the newborn period to allow antegrade flow from the RV to the pulmonary artery and to encourage RV cavity growth. If the RV is inadequate, significant sinusoids are present, or the pulmonic valve cannot be opened successfully in the catheterization laboratory, an immediate Blalock-Taussig shunt is performed to establish pulmonary blood flow. Later in infancy, a communication between the RV and pulmonary artery can be created to stimulate RV cavity growth. If either RV dimension or function is inadequate for two-ventricular repair, a one-ventricular systemic venous to pulmonary artery palliation is indicated (Fontan procedure). Children with significant sinusoids receive a Blalock-Taussig shunt as immediate treatment, but they are often considered for cardiac transplantation if they are felt to be at risk for coronary insufficiency and sudden death.

The prognosis in this condition is guarded. Our overall experience strongly favors opening the atretic valve in the catheterization laboratory in the newborn period if possible. If this is not possible, a Blalock-Taussig shunt should be placed. Ultimate plans for two-ventricular repair, Fontan procedure, or cardiac transplantation depend on the anatomy.

Humpl T et al: Percutaneous balloon valvotomy in pulmonary atresia with intact ventricular septum: Impact on patient care. Circulation 2003;108:826 [PMID: 12885744].

Minnich LL et al: Usefulness of the preoperative tricuspid/mitral valve ratio for predicting outcome in pulmonary atresia with intact ventricular septum. Am J Cardiol 2000;85:1325 [PMID: 10831948].

Powell AJ et al: Outcome in infants with pulmonary atresia, intact ventricular septum, and right ventricular-dependent coronary circulation. Am J Cardiol 2000;86:1272 [PMID: 11090809].

TRICUSPID ATRESIA

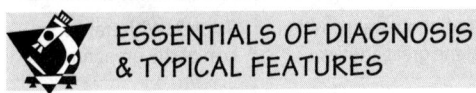

ESSENTIALS OF DIAGNOSIS & TYPICAL FEATURES

- *Marked cyanosis present from birth.*
- *ECG with left axis deviation, right atrial enlargement, and LVH.*

General Considerations

This rare condition (< 1% of cases of congenital heart disease) is characterized by complete atresia of the tricuspid valve. No direct communication exists between the right atrium and the RV. Tricuspid atresia is divided into two types based on the relationship of the great arteries (Table 19–14).

Because no direct communication exists between the right atrium and the RV, the entire systemic venous return flows through the atrial septum (either ASD or patent foramen ovale) into the left atrium. The left atrium receives both systemic venous return and pulmonary venous return. Complete mixing occurs in the left atrium, resulting in variable degrees of arterial desaturation.

Because of the lack of direct communication, the development of the RV depends on the presence of a ventricular left-to-right shunt. Severe hypoplasia of the RV occurs when there is no VSD or when the VSD is small.

Clinical Findings

A. Symptoms and Signs

In most patients symptoms develop early in infancy. Except in patients whose pulmonary blood flow is high, cyanosis is present at birth. Growth and development are poor, and the infant usually exhibits exhaustion during feedings, tachypnea, and dyspnea. Patients with an increase in pulmonary blood flow—types 1(c) and 2(b)—may develop CHF.

Digital clubbing is present in older children. S_1 is normal and S_2 is most often single. A murmur from the VSD is usually present. It ranges from grade II to grade III/VI in intensity and usually is heard best at the lower left sternal border.

B. Imaging

The heart is slightly to markedly enlarged. The main pulmonary artery segment is usually small or absent. The size of the right atrium varies from moderately to massively enlarged, depending on the size of the communication at the atrial level. The pulmonary vascular markings are usu-

Table 19–14. Tricuspid atresia.

Type 1: Without transposition of the great arteries	Type 2: With transposition of the great arteries
(a) No ventricular septal defect; hypoplasia or atresia of the pulmonary artery; patent ductus arteriosus	(a) With ventricular septal defect and pulmonary stenosis
(b) Small ventricular septal defect; pulmonary stenosis; hypoplastic pulmonary artery	(b) With ventricular septal defect but without pulmonary stenosis
(c) Large ventricular septal defect and no pulmonary stenosis; normal-sized pulmonary artery	

ally decreased, although in types 1(c) and 2(b) they are increased.

C. Electrocardiography

The ECG is usually helpful. It shows left axis deviation. The P waves are tall and peaked, indicative of right atrial hypertrophy. LVH or LV dominance is found in almost all cases. RV forces on the ECG are usually low or absent.

D. Echocardiography

Two-dimensional methods are diagnostic and show absence of the tricuspid valve, the relationship between the great arteries, and the size of the pulmonary arteries.

E. Cardiac Catheterization and Angiocardiography

Catheterization reveals a large right-to-left shunt at the atrial level. Because of mixing in the left atrium, oxygen saturations in the LV, RV, pulmonary artery, and aorta are identical to the left atrium. Right atrial pressure is increased. LV and systemic pressures are normal. The catheter cannot be passed through the tricuspid valve from the right atrium to the RV. A balloon atrial septostomy is performed if a restrictive foramen ovale is present.

Treatment & Prognosis

In infants with high pulmonary artery flow, conventional anticongestive therapy should be given until the infant begins to outgrow the VSD. Rarely, a pulmonary artery band is needed to protect the pulmonary bed in preparation for a Fontan procedure.

In infants with diminished pulmonary blood flow, PGE_1 is given until an aortopulmonary shunt can be performed. The Fontan procedure is usually performed in stages. A Glenn procedure (superior vena cava to pulmonary artery anastomosis) is done with concomitant ligation of the aortopulmonary shunt at 3–9 months when saturations begin to fall, and completion of the Fontan procedure (redirection of IVC and SVC to pulmonary artery) is performed when the child reaches 15 kg.

The prognosis for patients with tricuspid atresia depends on the achievement of a balance of pulmonary blood flow that permits adequate oxygenation of the tissues without producing CHF. The long-term prognosis for children treated by the Fontan procedure is unknown. In the short term, the best results for the Fontan procedure occur in children with low pulmonary artery pressures prior to open-heart surgery.

Fogel MA et al: Caval contribution to flow in the branch pulmonary arteries of Fontan patients with a novel application of magnetic resonance presaturation pulse. Circulation 1999;99: 1215 [PMID: 10069790].

Mair DD et al: The Fontan procedure for tricuspid atresia: Early and late results of a 25-year experience with 216 patients. J Am Coll Cardiol 2001;37:933 [PMID: 11693773].

HYPOPLASTIC LEFT HEART SYNDROME

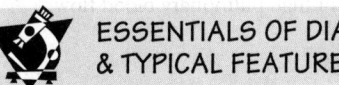

ESSENTIALS OF DIAGNOSIS & TYPICAL FEATURES

- *Mild cyanosis at birth. Minimal auscultatory findings.*
- *Rapid onset of shock with ductal closure.*

General Considerations

Hypoplastic left heart syndrome includes a number of conditions in which lesions of the left heart result in hypoplasia of the LV. The syndrome occurs in 1.4–3.8% of infants with congenital heart disease.

The most common abnormalities in this syndrome are mitral atresia, aortic atresia, or both. In the neonate, survival depends on a PDA because antegrade flow into the systemic circulation is inadequate and the ductus arteriosus provides flow to the aorta. Children with hypoplastic left heart syndrome are usually stable at birth, but they deteriorate rapidly as the ductus starts to close in the first week of life. Untreated, the average age at death is 5–7 days. Rarely, the ductus remains patent on its own and infants may survive for months without PGE_1 therapy.

Clinical Findings

A. SYMPTOMS AND SIGNS

Neonates with hypoplastic left heart syndrome appear stable at birth because the ductus is patent. They deteriorate rapidly when the ductus closes with CHF first, followed almost immediately by shock and acidosis secondary to inadequate systemic perfusion.

B. IMAGING

Chest radiograph at presentation shows cardiac enlargement with severe pulmonary venous congestion.

C. ELECTROCARDIOGRAPHY

The ECG shows right axis deviation, right atrial enlargement, and RVH with a relative paucity of LV forces and absence of a Q wave in lead V_6. A QR pattern is often seen in lead V_1.

D. ECHOCARDIOGRAPHY

Echocardiography is diagnostic. Cardiac catheterization is not needed. A very small aorta and LV with an atretic mitral valve are diagnostic. The systemic circulation depends on the PDA. Color-flow Doppler imaging shows retrograde flow in the ascending aorta.

Treatment & Prognosis

PGE_1 is essential initially, as systemic circulation depends on a patent ductus arteriosus. Later management depends on balancing pulmonary and systemic blood flow because the RV provides both. At a few days of age the pulmonary resistance falls, favoring pulmonary overcirculation and systemic underperfusion. Therapy must be directed to increasing pulmonary vascular tone by inducing hypoxia or hypercapnic ventilation. Nitrogen is used to decrease inspired oxygen to < 21%. This therapy must be carefully monitored but results in increased pulmonary arterial tone and systemic perfusion. Nitrogen is blended with room air, and the delivered O_2 content is monitored continuously. Adequate systemic perfusion can usually be obtained by keeping systemic O_2 saturation between 65% and 80%.

Shortly after birth a decision must be made between several treatment options. In the Norwood procedure, the RV is used as the systemic ventricle while an aortopulmonary shunt is created for pulmonic flow. Alternatively, the child can be listed for orthotopic cardiac transplantation. Children who have a Norwood procedure (and subsequent Glenn anastomosis and completion of a Fontan procedure) or who are listed for receipt of a donor heart have a 50–60% chance for 5-year survival at the best centers. Although this is a major improvement over nonsurgical intervention, hypoplastic left heart syndrome remains one of the most challenging lesions in pediatric cardiology.

Mahle WT et al: Impact of prenatal diagnosis on survival and early neurologic morbidity in neonates with the hypoplastic left heart syndrome. Pediatrics 2001;107:1277 [PMID: 11389243].

Mosca RS et al: Early results of the Fontan procedure in one hundred consecutive patients with hypoplastic left heart syndrome. J Thorac Cardiovasc Surg 2000;119:1110 [PMID: 10838526].

Tworetzky W et al: Improved surgical outcome after fetal diagnosis of hypoplastic left heart syndrome. Circulation 2001;103:1269 [PMID: 11238272].

TRANSPOSITION OF THE GREAT ARTERIES

ESSENTIALS OF DIAGNOSIS & TYPICAL FEATURES

- *Cyanotic newborn without respiratory distress.*
- *More common in males.*

General Considerations

Transposition of the great arteries (dextroposed TGA or complete TGA) is the second most common cyanotic congenital heart disease, accounting for 5% of all

Table 19–15. Complete (D) transposition of the great arteries.

Type 1: With intact ventricular septum	Type 2: With ventricular septal defect
(a) Without pulmonary stenosis (b) With pulmonary stenosis subvalvular or valvular (or both)	(a) With pulmonary stenosis (b) With pulmonary vascular obstruction (c) Without pulmonary vascular obstruction (normal pulmonary vascular resistance)

cases of congenital heart disease. The male:female ratio is 3:1. The disorder is caused by an embryologic abnormality in the spiral division of the truncus arteriosus in which the aorta arises from the RV and the pulmonary artery from the LV. In 60% of cases only the two usual newborn cardiac connections (patent foramen ovale and PDA) are present, but VSDs, pulmonic stenosis, coarctation of the aorta, or aortic stenosis occur in a significant number of patients. Left unrepaired, transposition is associated with a high incidence of early pulmonary vascular obstructive disease. TGA can be classified into two types (Table 19–15).

Because the aorta arises directly from the RV, survival is impossible without mixing between the systemic and pulmonary circulations. Oxygenated blood from the pulmonary veins must reach the systemic arterial circuit. In patients with an intact ventricular septum, mixing occurs at the atrial and ductal levels. However, in most patients, these communications are small and the ductus closes shortly after birth. These patients are therefore severely cyanotic. Patients with a VSD have better mixing and less cyanosis. Patients with a VSD and pulmonary stenosis (types 2[a] and 2[b]) are usually severely cyanotic because of the limited blood flow to the lungs. Patients with a VSD and normal pulmonary vascular resistance (type 2[c]) have the least cyanosis but often develop heart failure early because of high pulmonary blood flow.

Clinical Findings

A. SYMPTOMS AND SIGNS

Many neonates are large, some weighing 4 kg at birth, and most are severely cyanotic. Infants with an intact ventricular septum are striking in appearance because of their large size, profound cyanosis (unresponsive to increasing the ambient O_2) without respiratory distress, and the absence of a significant murmur. Only infants with a large VSD will be less cyanotic and they usually have a prominent murmur. The findings on cardiovascular examination depend on the intracardiac defects. Patients with type 1(a)

defects have only soft murmurs or none at all. S_1 is usually normal in these patients. S_2 is single and accentuated as the aortic valve is anterior. Patients with type 1(b) defects have loud obstructive systolic murmurs that are maximal at the second and third intercostal spaces and the left sternal border, radiating well to the first and second intercostal spaces. Patients with type 2(a) defects have a murmur of pulmonary stenosis (obstructive systolic murmur at the base of the heart, best heard to the right of the sternum). Those with type 2(c) defects have a systolic murmur along the lower sternal border and a mitral diastolic flow murmur at the apex.

B. IMAGING

The chest radiograph in transposition is usually nondiagnostic. Sometimes, however, there is an "egg on a string" appearance because the aorta is directly anterior to the main pulmonary artery, giving the image of a narrow mediastinum.

C. ELECTROCARDIOGRAPHY

Because the newborn ECG normally has RV predominance, the ECG in transposition is of little help.

D. ECHOCARDIOGRAPHY

Two-dimensional imaging and Doppler evaluation demonstrate the anatomy and physiology of transposition. The aorta arises from the RV and the pulmonary artery arises from the LV. If clinically indicated, a balloon atrial septostomy may be performed during the echo.

E. CARDIAC CATHETERIZATION AND ANGIOCARDIOGRAPHY

When complete transposition of the great arteries is present a Rashkind balloon atrial septostomy is performed to open the atrial septum unless a true ASD exists. The coronary anatomy is delineated by ascending aortography.

Treatment

Early corrective surgery is recommended for transposition. The arterial switch operation (ASO) is performed at age 4–7 days. The arteries are switched in the anterior chest, and the coronaries are reimplanted into the neoaorta. Small associated VSDs may be left to close on their own, but large VSDs are always closed at this time. The atrial septum is also closed. The ASO has replaced the previously performed atrial switch procedures (Mustard and Senning operations). Because the ASO must be performed while the LV musculature can still support systemic blood pressure, it is rarely delayed beyond age 14 days in infants with an intact ventricular septum or small VSD. If a large, unrestrictive VSD is present that maintains LV pressure at systemic levels, corrective surgery can be delayed for a few months. Surgery should still be performed by age 3–4 months because of the high risk of early pulmonary vascular disease associated with transposition.

Survival after the ASO is now greater than 95% in major centers. In addition, the switch procedure greatly shortens the time that the child remains severely cyanotic before corrective surgery. Early relief of cyanosis may improve the developmental outcome for children with transposition. Finally, the switch procedure leaves the LV as the systemic ventricle. The older atrial corrective procedures left the RV in this role and there was a significant incidence of late RV failure. Since the LV is designed for systemic pressures, late failure of the LV after the ASO is unlikely and it has not been reported.

Bellinger DC et al: Developmental and neurological status of children at 4 years of age after heart surgery with hypothermic circulatory arrest or low flow cardiopulmonary bypass. Circulation 1999;100:526 [PMID: 10430767].

Singh TP et al: Assessment of progressive changes in exercise performance in patients with a systemic right ventricle following atrial switch repair. Pediatr Cardiol 2001;22:210 [PMID: 11343144].

Wernovsky G et al: Factors influencing early and late outcome of the arterial switch operation for transposition of the great arteries. J Thorac Cardiovasc Surg 1995;109:289 [PMID: 7583882].

CONGENITALLY CORRECTED TRANSPOSITION OF THE GREAT ARTERIES

Congenitally corrected transposition of the great arteries (ccTGA or l-TGA) is a relatively uncommon congenital heart disease that may present with cyanosis, depending on the associated lesions. In ccTGA, both AV and VA discordance occurs so that the right atrium connects to a morphologic LV, which supports the pulmonary artery. Conversely, the left atrium empties via a tricuspid valve into a morphologic RV, which supports the aorta. Commonly associated lesions include VSDs and pulmonary stenosis. A dysplastic left-sided tricuspid valve is almost always present. Previously, surgical repair was directed at VSD closure and relief of pulmonary outflow tract obstruction. This surgical technique maintained the RV as the systemic ventricle supporting the aorta. It is now recognized that these patients have a reduced lifespan, and thus other surgical techniques have been advocated. The double-switch procedure is one such technique in which an atrial level switch (Mustard or Senning technique) is performed, and an arterial switch operation then restores the morphologic LV to its position as systemic ventricle. In the absence of associated lesions, patients with ccTGA are often undiagnosed until adulthood when they present with

left-sided AV valve insufficiency or arrhythmias. Patients with ccTGA have an increased incidence of complete heart block with an estimated risk of 1% per year and an overall frequency of 50%.

Graham TP et al: Long-term outcome in congenitally corrected transposition of the great arteries. J Am Coll Cardiol 2000; 36:255 [PMID: 10898443].

DOUBLE-OUTLET RIGHT VENTRICLE

In this uncommon malformation, both great arteries arise from the RV. There is always a VSD that allows blood to exit the LV. The presentation depends on the relationship of the VSD to the semilunar valves. The VSD may be subaortic, subpulmonary, remote, or doubly committed. If the VSD is subaortic, pulmonary stenosis may or may not be present. If there is no pulmonary stenosis, a large left-to-right shunt exists and the clinical picture resembles that of a large VSD. Early primary correction, with the VSD patch fashioned to the anterior aortic root, is usually successful. If pulmonic or subpulmonic stenosis is present, the physiology and the clinical management are the same as in ToF. If the VSD is subpulmonic, aortic outflow tract obstruction is common (Taussig-Bing malformation), and the presentation and management are similar to transposition, unrestrictive VSD, and left ventricular outflow obstruction.

In all forms of double-outlet RV, echocardiography with Doppler flow assessment is useful in clarifying the anatomy and physiology. Preoperative cardiac catheterization and angiocardiography are used if questions remain about the pulmonary or coronary arteries, or in children with the Taussig-Bing malformation who have severe cyanosis requiring balloon atrial septostomy for atrial mixing.

Dearani JA et al: Late follow-up of 1095 patients undergoing operation for complex congenital heart disease utilizing pulmonary ventricle to pulmonary artery conduits. Ann Thorac Surg 2003;75:399 [PMID: 12607647].

Sondheimer HM et al: Double outlet right ventricle: Clinical spectrum and prognosis. Am J Cardiol 1977;39:709 [PMID: 67796].

TOTAL ANOMALOUS PULMONARY VENOUS RETURN WITH OR WITHOUT OBSTRUCTION

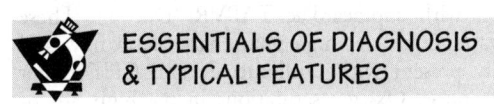

ESSENTIALS OF DIAGNOSIS & TYPICAL FEATURES

- *Cyanosis.*
- *Systolic ejection murmur with lower left sternal border flow rumble and accentuated P$_2$.*

• *Right atrial and RVH.*
• *Abnormal pulmonary venous connection.*

General Considerations

This malformation accounts for 2% of all congenital heart lesions. The pulmonary venous blood drains into a confluence behind the left atrium, but the confluence is not connected to the left atrium. The pulmonary venous blood finds another route to rejoin the circulation via the systemic veins. This leads to complete mixing at the level of the right atrium. The clinical presentation of total anomalous pulmonary venous return (TAPVR) depends on the method of return to the systemic circulation and whether the return is unrestricted or restricted.

The malformation is classified by the site of entry of the pulmonary veins into the right side of the heart. Although the most common form of TAPVR is unobstructed via the left superior vena cava, other types exist:

• Type 1 (50%): Entry into the left superior vena cava (persistent anterior cardinal vein) or right superior vena cava, unobstructed or obstructed

• Type 2 (20%): Entry into the right atrium directly or via the coronary sinus, unobstructed

• Type 3 (20%): Entry below the diaphragm (usually into the portal vein), almost always obstructed

• Type 4 (10%): Multiple sites of entry (mixed TAPVR)

Because the entire venous drainage from the body comes to the right atrium, a right-to-left shunt is always present at the atrial level, either an ASD or a patent foramen ovale. Occasionally the atrial septum is restrictive and balloon septostomy is needed at birth to allow filling of the left heart. Complete mixing of systemic and pulmonary venous return occurs in the right atrium, so that left atrial and systemic arterial saturation levels are equal to right atrial saturation.

Clinical Findings

A. WITH UNOBSTRUCTED PULMONARY VENOUS RETURN

This large group includes all children with pulmonary venous return to the right atrium (type 2) and most children with supracardiac TAPVR (type 1). These patients tend to have high pulmonary blood flow and typically present with cardiomegaly and CHF rather than cyanosis. Oxygen saturations in the high 80s or low 90s are common. Most patients in this group have mild to moderate elevation of pulmonary artery pressure owing to elevated pulmonary blood flow. In most instances, PA pressure does not reach systemic levels.

1. Symptoms and signs—Patients may have mild cyanosis in the neonatal period and during early infancy. Thereafter, they do relatively well except for frequent respiratory infections. They are usually small and thin resembling patients with other large left-to-right shunts. Examination discloses dusky nail beds and mucous membranes but overt cyanosis and digital clubbing are usually absent. The arterial pulses are normal. An RV heave is palpable.

The pulmonary component of the second sound is usually increased. A grade II–III/VI ejection-type systolic murmur is heard at the pulmonary area. It radiates over the lung fields anteriorly and posteriorly. A mid-diastolic flow murmur is often heard at the lower left sternum from increased tricuspid diastolic flow.

2. Imaging—Chest radiography reveals cardiomegaly involving the right heart and pulmonary artery. Pulmonary vascular markings are increased. A characteristic cardiac contour called a "snowman" or "figure of 8" is often seen when the anomalous veins drain via a persistent left superior vena cava to the innominate vein and then the right superior vena cava. This radiographic appearance is not present until approximately 3 months of age because it requires time for the vertical vein and innominate vein to dilate.

3. Electrocardiography—ECG shows right axis deviation and varying degrees of right atrial and right ventricular hypertrophy. A QR pattern is often seen over the right precordial leads.

4. Echocardiography—Demonstration by echocardiography of a chamber posterior to the left atrium is strongly suggestive of the diagnosis. However, echocardiographic discrimination between anomalies of pulmonary venous return and persistence of pulmonary fetal circulation can be challenging. The availability of two-dimensional echocardiography plus color-flow Doppler has increased diagnostic accuracy such that diagnostic cardiac catheterization is rarely required.

B. WITH OBSTRUCTED PULMONARY VENOUS RETURN

This group includes all patients with subdiaphragmatic TAPVR and a few of the patients in whom venous drainage is into a systemic vein above the diaphragm.

1. Symptoms and signs—These infants usually present shortly after birth with severe cyanosis and require early corrective surgery. Cardiac examination discloses a striking RV impulse. S_1 is accentuated and S_2 is markedly accentuated and single. A grade I–III/VI ejection-type systolic murmur is frequently heard over the pulmonary area with radiation over the lung fields. Diastolic murmurs are uncommon. In many cases, no murmur is heard at all.

2. Imaging—In the most severe cases, the heart is small and pulmonary venous congestion is severe with associated air bronchograms. The appearance of the chest x-ray may lead to an erroneous diagnosis of severe lung disease. In less severe cases, the heart size may be normal or slightly enlarged with mild pulmonary venous congestion.

3. Electrocardiography—The ECG shows right axis deviation, right atrial hypertrophy, and RVH.

4. Echocardiography—Echocardiography shows a combination of a small left atrium and LV and a vessel lying parallel and anterior to the descending aorta and to the left of the inferior vena cava. Color-flow Doppler echocardiography is useful to establish the diagnosis. Right-to-left atrial shunting occurs.

5. Cardiac catheterization and angiocardiography—Cardiac catheterization and cineangiocardiography demonstrate TAPVR and show the site of entry of the anomalous veins. They also demonstrate the ratio of pulmonary to systemic blood flow and the degree of pulmonary hypertension and pulmonary vascular resistance.

Treatment

Surgery is always required for TAPVR. If pulmonary venous return is obstructed, surgery must be performed immediately. In infants with unobstructed TAPVR, surgery may be delayed for weeks to months. The timing of surgery can be determined by the child's weight gain and the risk of pulmonary infection. If early surgery is not needed and the atrial septum is restrictive, a balloon atrial septostomy should be performed in the newborn period. The results of surgery are excellent.

Course & Prognosis

Most children with TAPVR do well after surgery. Approximately 5% of surgical survivors develop late stenosis of the pulmonary veins. This condition is difficult to treat either with interventional catheterization or surgery and has a very poor prognosis. Pulmonary vein stenosis, when it occurs, is most often seen in children who initially had obstructed total veins, but it occurs occasionally in children whose initial presentation was unobstructed. A new surgical technique of sutureless in situ pericardial repair of recurrent pulmonary venous obstruction holds great promise. By avoiding direct suturing at the pulmonary venous ostia, the chance of recurrent stenosis at the anastomotic site is lessened.

Lacour-Gayet F et al: Surgical management of progressive pulmonary venous obstruction after repair of total anomalous pulmonary venous connection. J Thorac Cardiovasc Surg 1999; 117:679 [PMID: 10096962].

Monro JL et al: Reoperations and survival after primary repair of congenital heart defects in children. J Thorac Cardiovasc Surg 2003;126:511 [PMID: 12928652].

TRUNCUS ARTERIOSUS

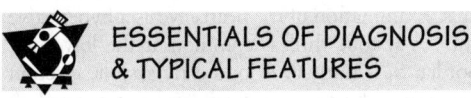

ESSENTIALS OF DIAGNOSIS & TYPICAL FEATURES

- *Early CHF.*
- *Mild or no cyanosis.*
- *Systolic ejection click.*

General Considerations

Truncus arteriosus accounts for less than 1% of congenital heart malformations. A single great artery arises from the heart, giving rise to the systemic, pulmonary, and coronary circulations. Truncus develops embryologically as a result of failure of the division of the common truncus arteriosus into the aorta and the pulmonary artery. A VSD is always present. The number of truncal valve leaflets varies from two to six, and the valve may be sufficient, insufficient, or stenotic.

Truncus arteriosus is divided into distinct subtypes by the anatomy of the pulmonary circulation:

- Type 1: A single main pulmonary artery arises from the base of the trunk just above the semilunar valve and then branches into left and right pulmonary arteries.
- Type 2: Two pulmonary arteries arise side by side from the posterior aspect of the truncus.
- Type 3: Two pulmonary arteries arise independently from either side of the trunk.

In patients with truncus, blood from both ventricles leaves the heart through a single exit. Thus, the oxygen saturation in the pulmonary artery is equal to that in the systemic arteries. The degree of systemic arterial oxygen saturation depends on the ratio of pulmonary to systemic blood flow. If pulmonary vascular resistance is normal, the pulmonary blood flow is greater than the systemic blood flow and the saturation is relatively high. If pulmonary vascular resistance is elevated because of pulmonary vascular obstructive disease or small pulmonary arteries, pulmonary blood flow is reduced and oxygen saturation is low. The systolic pressures are systemic in both ventricles.

Clinical Findings

A. SYMPTOMS AND SIGNS

The clinical picture depends on the degree of pulmonary blood flow.

1. High pulmonary blood flow—This is the most common presentation of truncus arteriosus. Patients with high pulmonary blood flow are usually acyanotic and their clinical presentation in CHF is similar to that of patients with large VSDs. Examination of the heart reveals a hyperactive precordium. A systolic thrill is common at the lower left sternal border. S_1 is normal. A loud early systolic ejection click is commonly heard. S_2 is single and accentuated. A grade III–IV/VI pansystolic murmur is audible at the lower left sternal border. A diastolic flow murmur can often be heard at the apex (mitral flow murmur). A diastolic murmur of truncal insufficiency may be present.

2. Low pulmonary blood flow—Patients with decreased pulmonary blood flow are cyanotic early and do poorly. The most common manifestations are growth retardation, easy fatigability, dyspnea on exertion, and CHF. The heart is not hyperactive. S_1 and S_2 are single and loud. A systolic grade II–IV/VI murmur is heard at the lower left sternal border. No diastolic flow murmur is heard. A loud systolic ejection click is commonly heard.

B. IMAGING

The common radiographic findings are a boot-shaped heart, absence of the main pulmonary artery segment, and a large aorta that has a right arch 30% of the time. The pulmonary vascular markings vary with the degree of pulmonary blood flow.

C. ELECTROCARDIOGRAPHY

The axis is usually normal. RVH or combined ventricular hypertrophy is commonly present. LVH as an isolated finding is rare.

D. ECHOCARDIOGRAPHY

Images generally show override of a single great artery (similar to ToF). The origin of the pulmonary arteries and the degree of truncal valve abnormality can be seen. Color-flow Doppler can aid in the description of pulmonary flow and the function of the truncal valve, both of which are critical to management.

E. ANGIOCARDIOGRAPHY

Cardiac catheterization is not routinely performed but may be of value in older infants in whom pulmonary vascular disease must be ruled out. Injection of contrast material into either ventricle demonstrates the VSD and the single great artery arising from the heart. The exact type of truncus is often best imaged from an injection in the truncal root itself. This also allows for evaluation of truncal insufficiency.

Treatment

Anticongestive measures are needed for patients with high pulmonary blood flow and congestive failure. Surgery is always required in this condition. Because of CHF, surgery is usually performed in the neonatal period. The VSD is closed to allow LV egress to the truncal valve as in ToF. The pulmonary artery (type 1) or arteries (types 2–3) are separated from the truncus as a block, and a conduit is fashioned from the RV to the pulmonary circulation. The conduit may be valved or nonvalved, but most surgeons prefer a valved allograft for this repair.

Course & Prognosis

Children with truncus types 1–3 with good surgical results do well. They almost always outgrow the RV-to-pulmonary conduit placed in infancy and require revision of the conduit in later childhood. The risk of early pulmonary vascular obstructive disease is high in the unrepaired patient and a decision to delay open-heart surgery beyond age 4–6 months is not wise even in stable patients.

McElhinney DB et al: Reinterventions after repair of common arterial trunk in neonates and young infants. J Am Coll Cardiol 2000;35:1317 [PMID: 10758975].

■ ACQUIRED HEART DISEASE

RHEUMATIC FEVER

The availability of penicillin and improvements in the standard of living and hygiene have greatly reduced the incidence of rheumatic fever in the U.S. since 1950, but there has been a resurgence in the Midwest in 1984 and the intermountain West since 1987. The reason for these regional epidemics is unknown. In both Salt Lake City and Denver, 30–50 new cases are now seen each year. The character of the illness has changed somewhat.

Group A β-hemolytic streptococcal infection of the upper respiratory tract is the essential trigger in predisposed individuals. The latest attempts to define host susceptibility implicate immune response genes that are present in approximately 15% of the population. The immune response triggered by colonization of the pharynx with group A streptococci consists of (1) sensitization of B lymphocytes by streptococcal antigens, (2) formation of antistreptococcal antibody, (3) formation of immune complexes that cross-react with cardiac sarcolemma antigens, and (4) myocardial and valvular inflammatory response.

The peak age of risk in the United States is 5–15 years. The disease is slightly more common in girls and in African Americans. The annual death rate from rheumatic heart disease in school-age children (whites and nonwhites) recorded in the 1980s was less than 1:100,000.

Table 19–16. Jones criteria (modified) for diagnosis of rheumatic fever.

Major manifestations
  Carditis
  Polyarthritis
  Sydenham chorea
  Erythema marginatum
  Subcutaneous nodules
Minor manifestations
  Clinical
    Previous rheumatic fever or rheumatic heart disease
    Polyarthralgia
    Fever
  Laboratory
    Acute phase reaction: elevated erythrocyte sedimentation rate, C-reactive protein, leukocytosis
    Prolonged PR interval

Plus

Supporting evidence of preceding streptococcal infection, that is, increased titers of antistreptolysin O or other streptococcal antibodies, positive throat culture for group A *Streptococcus*

The modified Jones criteria are used to diagnose acute rheumatic fever. Two major or one major and two minor manifestations (plus supporting evidence of streptococcal infection) are needed (Table 19–16).

Sydenham Chorea

Sydenham chorea is characterized by emotional instability and involuntary movements. These symptoms become progressively worse and may be accompanied by ataxia and slurring of speech. Muscular weakness becomes apparent following the onset of the involuntary movements. The attack of chorea is self-limiting, although it may last up to 3 months. Chorea may not be apparent for months to years after the acute episode of rheumatic fever.

Polyarthritis

The large joints (knees, hips, wrists, elbows, and shoulders) are most commonly involved. Joint swelling and associated limitation of movement should be present. Arthralgia alone is not a major criterion.

Erythema Marginatum

A macular erythematous rash with a circinate border appears primarily on the trunk and the extremities. The face is usually spared.

Subcutaneous Nodules

These usually occur only in severe cases, and then most commonly over the joints, scalp, and spinal column.

They vary from a few millimeters to 2 cm in diameter and are nontender and freely movable under the skin.

Essential Manifestation

Except in cases of rheumatic fever manifesting solely as Sydenham chorea or long-standing carditis, there should be clear evidence of a streptococcal infection such as scarlet fever, a positive throat culture for group A β-hemolytic *Streptococcus,* and increased antistreptolysin O or other streptococcal antibody titers. The antistreptolysin O titer is significantly higher in rheumatic fever than in uncomplicated streptococcal infections.

Treatment & Prophylaxis

A. TREATMENT OF THE ACUTE EPISODE

1. Anti-infective therapy—Eradication of the streptococcal infection is essential. Long-acting benzathine penicillin is the drug of choice. Depending on the age and weight of the patient, give a single intramuscular injection of 0.6–1.2 million units; alternatively, give penicillin V, 125–250 mg orally four times a day for 10 days. Erythromycin, 250 mg orally four times a day, may be substituted if the patient is allergic to penicillin.

2. Anti-inflammatory agents—

  a. Aspirin—30–60 mg/kg/d is given in four divided doses. This dose is usually sufficient to effect dramatic relief of arthritis and fever. Higher dosages carry a greater risk of side effects and there are no proven short- or long-term benefits of high doses that produce salicylate blood levels of 20–30 mg/dL. The duration of therapy is tailored to meet the needs of the patient, but 2–6 weeks of therapy with reduction in dose toward the end of the course is usually sufficient. Other nonsteroidal anti-inflammatory agents used because of concerns about Reye syndrome are less effective than aspirin.

  b. Corticosteroids—Corticosteroids are rarely indicated except in the rare patient with severe carditis and CHF where they may be life-saving. Steroids are given as follows: prednisone, 2 mg/kg/d orally for 2 weeks; reduce prednisone to 1 mg/kg/d during the third week, and begin aspirin, 50 mg/kg/d; stop prednisone at the end of 3 weeks, and continue aspirin for 8 weeks or until the C-reactive protein is negative and the sedimentation rate is falling.

3. Therapy of congestive heart failure—See section on congestive heart failure.

4. Bed rest and ambulation—Bed rest is not required for patients with arthritis and carditis without CHF. Indoor activity followed by modified outdoor activity may be ordered when symptoms have disappeared but clinical and laboratory evidence of rheumatic activity remains. Modified bed rest for 2–6 weeks is generally adequate. Children should not return to school while there is clear evidence of rheumatic activity. Most acute episodes of rheumatic fever are managed on an outpatient basis.

B. TREATMENT AFTER THE ACUTE EPISODE

1. Prevention—The patient who has had rheumatic fever is at great risk of a recurrence after the next inadequately treated group A β-hemolytic streptococcal infection. Prevention is thus critical. Follow-up visits after the acute episode are not so much to evaluate mitral or aortic insufficiency as to reinforce the necessity for prophylaxis with regular long-acting benzathine penicillin. The physician should stress that protection is better with intramuscular than oral medication and that failure to comply with regular medication increases the risk for a recurrence of rheumatic fever. If myocardial or valvular disease persists, antibacterial prophylaxis is a lifelong commitment. More commonly with transient or no cardiac involvement, 3–5 years of therapy or discontinuance at adolescence is an effective approach.

The following preventive regimens are in current use:

a. Penicillin G benzathine—1.2 million units intramuscularly every 21–28 days is the drug of choice.

b. Sulfadiazine—500 mg daily as a single oral dose for patients weighing over 27 kg is the drug of second choice. Blood dyscrasias and a lesser effectiveness in reducing streptococcal infections make this drug less satisfactory than penicillin benzathine G.

c. Penicillin V—250,000 units orally twice daily offers approximately the same protection afforded by sulfadiazine but is much less effective than intramuscular penicillin benzathine G (5.5 versus 0.4 streptococcal infections per 100 patient-years).

d. Erythromycin—250 mg orally twice a day may be given to patients who are allergic to both penicillin and sulfonamides.

2. Residual valvular damage—Chronic CHF may follow a single severe episode of acute rheumatic carditis, or more commonly, after repeated episodes. In the U.S., the typical manifestations of residual valvular damage in children are mitral and aortic insufficiency. Murmurs are not accompanied by CHF in most children as long as repeated attacks are prevented.

Methods of managing CHF have been discussed previously. Children with valvular damage that cannot be managed adequately on a medical regimen must be considered for valve replacement before the myocardium is irreversibly damaged.

Ayoub EM: Resurgence of rheumatic fever in the United States: The changing picture of a preventable illness. Postgrad Med 1992;92:139 [PMID: 1518750].

Dajani AS et al: Guidelines for the diagnosis of rheumatic fever: Jones criteria, updated 1992. Circulation 1993;87:302.

Veasey LG: Time to take soundings in acute rheumatic fever? Lancet 2001;357:1994 [PMID: 11438128].

RHEUMATIC HEART DISEASE

Mitral Insufficiency

Mitral insufficiency is the most common valvular residua of acute rheumatic carditis. There are reports from all over the world of silent mitral insufficiency with echocardiographic findings characteristic of acute rheumatic fever.

Mitral Stenosis

Mitral stenosis after acute rheumatic fever is rarely encountered in the United States until 5–10 years after the first episode. Thus, mitral stenosis is much more commonly seen in adults than in children. Interventional cardiovascular balloon dilation of mitral stenosis is now being used in many patients prior to consideration of mitral valve replacement.

Aortic Insufficiency

This early decrescendo diastolic murmur is occasionally encountered as the sole valvular manifestation of rheumatic carditis. It is the second most common valve affected in polyvalvular as well as in single-valve disease. It appears that the aortic valve is involved more often in males and in African Americans.

Aortic Stenosis

Dominant aortic stenosis of rheumatic origin does not occur in pediatric patients. In one large study, the shortest length of time observed for a patient to develop dominant aortic stenosis secondary to rheumatic heart disease was 20 years.

KAWASAKI DISEASE

Kawasaki disease was first described in Japan in 1967 and was initially called mucocutaneous lymph node syndrome. The cause is unclear and there is no specific diagnostic test. Kawasaki disease is the leading cause of acquired heart disease in children in the U.S. Eighty percent of patients are < 5 years old (median age at diagnosis is 2 years), and the male-to-female ratio is 1.5:1. Diagnostic criteria are fever for more than 5 days and at least four of the following features: (1) bilateral, painless, nonexudative conjunctivitis, (2) lip or oral cavity changes (eg, lip cracking and fissuring, strawberry tongue, and inflammation of the oral mucosa), (3) cervical lymphadenopathy (≥ 1.5 cm in diameter

Table 19–17. Noncardiac manifestations of Kawaski disease.

System	Associated Signs and Symptoms
Gastrointestinal	Vomiting, diarrhea, gallbladder hydrops, elevated transaminases
Blood	Elevated ESR or CRP, leukocytosis, hypoalbuminemia, mild anemia in acute phase and thrombocytosis in subacute phase (usually second to third week of illness)
Renal	Sterile pyuria, proteinuria
Respiratory	Cough, rhinorrhea, infiltrate on chest radiograph
Joint	Arthralgia and arthritis
Neurologic	Mononuclear pleocytosis of cerebrospinal fluid, irritability, facial palsy

ESR, erythrocyte sedimentation rate; CRP, C-reactive protein.

and usually unilateral), (4) polymorphous exanthema, and (5) extremity changes (redness and swelling of the hands and feet with subsequent desquamation). Clinical features not part of the diagnostic criteria, but frequently associated, are shown in Table 19–17.

The potential for cardiovascular complications is the most serious aspect of Kawasaki disease. Complications during the acute illness include myocarditis, pericarditis, valvular heart disease (usually mitral or aortic regurgitation), and coronary arteritis. Patients with fever for at least 5 days but fewer than four of the diagnostic features can be diagnosed with atypical Kawasaki disease if they have coronary artery abnormalities detected by echocardiography.

Coronary artery lesions range from mild transient dilation of a coronary artery to large aneurysms. Aneurysms rarely form before day 10 of illness. Untreated patients have a 15–25% risk of developing coronary aneurysms. Those at greatest risk of aneurysm are males, young children (< 6 months), and those not treated with intravenous immunoglobulin (IVIG).

Two-dimensional echocardiography is very sensitive in detecting coronary abnormalities and is the recommended screening test in children with Kawasaki disease. Most coronary artery aneurysms resolve within 5 years of diagnosis; however, as aneurysms resolve, associated obstruction or stenosis (19% of all aneurysms) may develop, which may result in coronary ischemia. Giant aneurysms (> 8 mm) are less likely to resolve, and nearly 50% eventually become stenotic. Of additional concern, acute thrombosis of an aneurysm can occur, resulting in myocardial infarction that is be fatal in approximately 20% of cases.

Immediate management of Kawasaki disease is IVIG and high-dose aspirin. This therapy is effective in decreasing the incidence of coronary artery dilation and aneurysm formation. The currently recommended regimen is 2 g/kg of IVIG administered over 10–12 hours and 80–100 mg/kg/d of aspirin in four divided doses. The duration of high-dose aspirin is institution-dependent: many centers reduce the dose once the patient is afebrile for 48–72 hours; others continue through day 14 of the illness. Once high-dose aspirin is discontinued, low-dose aspirin (3–5 mg/kg daily) is given through the subacute phase of the illness (6–8 weeks) or until coronary artery abnormalities resolve. If fever recurs within 48–72 hours of the initial treatment course and no other source of the fever is detected, a second dose of IVIG is often recommended; however, the effectiveness of this approach has not been clearly demonstrated. Corticosteroids are only recommended for patients who have persistent fever despite at least two infusions of IVIG. The effect of steroids on the development of coronary artery abnormalities is unknown.

Follow-up of patients with treated Kawasaki disease depends on the degree of coronary involvement. In those with no or minimal coronary disease at the time of diagnosis, an echocardiogram 2 weeks and again 6–8 weeks after diagnosis is sufficient. Repeat echocardiography > 8 weeks after diagnosis in those with no coronary abnormalities is optional. In 2004, the American Heart Association published updated guidelines for the long-term management of Kawasaki disease based on the risk level of the patient. The risk stratification and recommended follow-up can be reviewed in Table 19–18.

American Heart Association: Diagnostic guidelines for Kawasaki disease. Circulation 2004;26;110:2747 [PMID: 15505111].

Burns JC et al: Intravenous gamma-globulin treatment and retreatment in Kawasaki disease. Pediatr Infect Dis J 1998;17):1144 [PMID: 9877364].

McMorrow Tuohy AM et al: How many echocardiograms are necessary for follow-up evaluation of patients with Kawasaki disease? Am J Cardiol 2001;88:328 [PMID: 11472722].

CARDIOMYOPATHY

As in adults, three patterns of cardiomyopathy are recognized in children: (1) dilated, (2) hypertrophic, and (3) restrictive.

1. Dilated Cardiomyopathy

This most frequent of the childhood cardiomyopathies occurs with an annual incidence of 4–8 cases per 100,000 population in the United States and Europe. Although usually idiopathic, diagnosable causes include acute or chronic myocarditis, long-standing untreated tachyarrhythmias, left heart obstructive lesions, congenital abnormalities of the coronary arteries, anthracycline toxicity, and genetic and metabolic diseases (inborn errors of fatty acid oxidation and mitochondrial oxida-

Table 19–18. Long-term management in Kawasaki disease.

Risk Level	Definition	Management Guidelines
I	No coronary artery changes at any stage of the illness	No ASA is needed beyond the subacute phase (6–8 weeks). No follow-up beyond the first year
II	Transient ectasia of coronary arteries during the acute phase	Same as above, or clinical follow-up ± ECG every 3–5 years
III	Single small to medium coronary aneurysm	ASA until abnormality resolves. Annual follow-up with ECG and echo if < 10 years old and every-other-year stress testing if > 10 years
IV	Giant aneurysm or multiple small to medium aneurysms without obstruction	Long term ASA ± warfarin. Annual follow-up with ECG, echo, and stress testing (in those > 20 years)
V	Coronary artery obstruction	Long-term ASA ± warfarin ± calcium channel blocker to reduce myocardial oxygen consumption. Echo and ECG every 6 months. Stress testing and Holter exam annually

ASA, acetyl salicylic acid; ECG, electrocardiogram; Echo, echocardiogram.

tive phosphorylation defects). Genetic causes include abnormalities of the dystrophin gene as occur in Duchenne and Becker muscular dystrophy.

Clinical Findings

A. SIGNS AND SYMPTOMS

As the heart dilates, cardiac output falls, and affected children develop heart failure (HF) with decreased exercise tolerance, failure to thrive, diaphoresis, and tachypnea. As the heart deteriorates, pulses and perfusion become weaker, hepatomegaly and rales develop, and the cardiac examination shows a prominent gallop. The initial diagnosis in a previously healthy child can be difficult, as presenting symptoms can resemble a viral respiratory infection, pneumonia, or asthma.

B. IMAGING

Chest radiograph shows generalized cardiomegaly with or without pulmonary venous congestion.

C. ELECTROCARDIOGRAPHY

Sinus tachycardia with ST-T segment changes is commonly seen on ECG. The criteria for right and left ventricular hypertrophy may also be met. One must ensure that a narrow complex tachycardia is in fact sinus tachycardia with a normal P-wave axis as opposed to an atrial or junctional tachyarrhythmia that may be the underlying cause of the cardiomyopathy.

D. ECHOCARDIOGRAPHY

The echocardiogram shows LV and left atrial enlargement with decreased LV shortening fraction and ejec-

tion fraction. The calculated end-diastolic and end-systolic dimensions are increased. With more advanced disease, mitral insufficiency will occur as the LV dilates. A careful evaluation for evidence of structural abnormalities (especially coronary artery anomalies) must be performed in infant patients.

E. OTHER TESTING

Cardiac catheterization is useful to evaluate the hemodynamic status and the coronary artery anatomy. Endomyocardial biopsies can be obtained in those with idiopathic disease. Biopsy specimens may show acute myocarditis, abnormal myocyte architecture, and myocardial fibrosis. Electron micrographs may reveal evidence of mitochondrial or other metabolic disorders. Polymerase chain reaction testing may be performed on biopsies to detect viral genome products in infectious myocarditis. Skeletal muscle biopsy may be helpful in those with evidence of possible skeletal muscle myopathy. Cardiopulmonary stress testing is useful in cardiomyopathy for measuring response to medical therapy and as an objective assessment of the cardiac limitations to exercise.

Treatment & Prognosis

Patients with dilated cardiomyopathy may require in-hospital management of HF—either on initial presentation or with a heart failure exacerbation. As outpatients they are treated with various combinations of digoxin, diuretics, and afterload-reducing agents (see section on heart failure). There is an ongoing multicenter, placebo-controlled, double-blind trial of carvedilol use in children with heart failure that will help determine the efficacy of β-blocker therapy as an adjunct in these patients. Aspirin or warfarin may be used to prevent thrombus formation in the dilated and poorly contractile cardiac chambers. Arrhythmias are more common in dilated hearts. Antiarrhythmic agents that do not suppress myocardial contractility, such as digoxin and amiodarone, may be used. Internal defibrillators are used in some patients with dilated cardiomyopathy and life-threatening ventricular arrhythmias.

Therapy directed at the cause of cardiomyopathy is always indicated if available. Treatment of carnitine deficiency may result in improved cardiac function. Antiarrhythmic therapy in patients with arrhythmia-induced cardiomyopathy is often curative. Unfortunately despite complete evaluation, a diagnosis is discovered in less than 30% of patients with dilated cardiomyopathy. If medical management is unsuccessful, cardiac transplantation is considered.

2. Hypertrophic Cardiomyopathy

The most common cause of hypertrophic cardiomyopathy (HCM) is familial hypertrophic cardiomyopathy, which is found 1 in 500 individuals. It is the leading cause of sudden cardiac death. It most commonly presents in the older child, adolescent, or adult, although it may be seen in the neonatal period. Other causes of HCM in neonates and children include glycogen storage disease, Noonan syndrome, Friedreich ataxia, mitochondrial disorders, and other metabolic disorders.

Familial Hypertrophic Cardiomyopathy

In the familial form, HCM is most commonly caused by a mutation in several genes that encode proteins of the cardiac sarcomere (B-myosin heavy chain, cardiac troponin T or I, A-tropomyosin, and myosin-binding protein C).

Clinical Findings

Patients may be asymptomatic despite having significant hypertrophy, or may present with symptoms of inadequate coronary perfusion such as angina, syncope, palpitations, or exercise intolerance. Patients may experience sudden cardiac death, often precipitated by sporting activities. Although the cardiac examination may be normal early, eventually patients develop a left precordial bulge with a diffuse point of maximal impulse. LV heave may be present. A palpable or audible S_4 may be present. If outflow tract obstruction is present, a systolic ejection murmur will be audible. A murmur may not be audible at rest but is easily provoked with exercise or positional maneuvers that decrease left ventricular volume (standing) thereby increasing the outflow tract obstruction. Although the older

patient with HCM typically has disease primarily in the LV, right ventricular hypertrophy, either alone or in association with LVH, may be seen in the neonate. Affected neonates may be cyanotic if RV outflow tract obstruction is significant.

A. ECHOCARDIOGRAPHY

The diagnosis of HCM is usually made by echocardiography that demonstrates asymmetrical septal hypertrophy. Young patients may have concentric hypertrophy, which makes the diagnosis less obvious. Systolic anterior motion of the mitral valve leaflet may occur and contribute to LV outflow tract obstruction. The mitral valve leaflet may become distorted and cause mitral insufficiency. LV outflow tract obstruction may be present at rest. Provocable outflow tract obstruction can be assessed with either amyl nitrate or monitored exercise. Systolic function is most often hypercontractile in young children but may deteriorate over time, often in association with a change in morphology as hypertrophy develops into LV dilation. Diastolic function is often impaired. Patients are at risk for myocardial ischemia, possibly as a result of systolic compression of the intramyocardial septal perforators, myocardial bridging of epicardial coronary arteries, or an imbalance of coronary artery supply and demand due to the presence of massive myocardial hypertrophy.

B. ELECTROCARDIOGRAPHY

The ECG may be normal, but more typically demonstrates deep Q waves in the inferolateral leads (II, III, aVF, V_5, and V_6) secondary to the increased mass of the hypertrophied septum. ST segment abnormalities may be seen in the same leads. Age-dependent criteria for LVH are often present as are criteria for left atrial enlargement.

C. OTHER TESTING

Cardiopulmonary stress testing is a valuable tool to check for provocable LV outflow tract obstruction, ischemia, and arrhythmias, and to determine prognosis. A blunted blood pressure response and ventricular arrhythmias with exercise have both been associated with increased mortality in children. Nuclear stress testing allows for assessment of myocardial perfusion defects.

D. CARDIAC CATHETERIZATION

Cardiac catheterization should be performed in patients with HCM who have angina, syncope, resuscitated sudden death, or a worrisome stress test. Hemodynamic findings include elevated left atrial pressure secondary to impaired diastolic filling. If midcavity LV outflow tract obstruction is present, an associated pressure gradient will be evident. Provocation of LV outflow tract obstruction with either rapid atrial pacing or isoproterenol may be sought. Angiography demonstrates a "ballerina slipper" configuration of the LV secondary to the midcavitary LV obliteration during systole. Coronary angiography should be performed to evaluate possible associated myocardial bridging, which may be an important source of myocardial ischemia in these patients. Angiography will show systolic obliteration, typically of the middle left anterior descending coronary artery.

Treatment & Prognosis

The prognosis depends on the degree of hypertrophy, the degree of outflow tract obstruction, the particular genetic defect, and the presence of coronary compression. Patients may be restricted from strenuous athletics and isometric exercise. Patients with resting or latent LV outflow tract obstruction may be treated with either β-blockers, verapamil, or disopyramide with good, albeit temporary, relief of obstruction. Patients with persistent symptoms despite medical therapy and an LV outflow tract gradient greater than 30 mm Hg may require additional intervention. Surgical myectomy with resection of part of the hypertrophied septum has been used with good results. At the time of myectomy, the mitral valve may require repair or replacement in patients with a long history of systolic anterior motion of the mitral valve. Ethanol ablation is being used with increasing frequency in adults with HCM and LV outflow tract obstruction. This procedure involves the selective infiltration of ethanol in a coronary septal artery branch, thereby inducing a small myocardial infarction. This leads to a reduction in septal size and improvement of obstruction. The long-term effects of this procedure are unknown and it is not currently employed in children. Surgical unroofing of a myocardial bridge may improve prognosis in those with myocardial ischemia secondary to epicardial coronary compression. Although dual-chamber pacing has been used in some children with good relief of obstruction, larger series demonstrate no significant improvement in obstruction. Internal defibrillators are being placed in patients with documented ventricular arrhythmias, resuscitated sudden death, or a strong family history of HCM with associated sudden death.

Glycogen Storage Disease of the Heart

There are at least 10 types of glycogen storage disease. The type that primarily involves the heart is Pompe disease (GSD IIa) in which acid maltase, necessary for hydrolysis of the outer branches of glycogen, is absent. There is marked deposition of glycogen within the myocardium. Affected infants are well at birth, but symptoms occur by the sixth month of life. These children experience growth and developmental delay, feeding problems, poor weight gain, and eventual heart failure. Physical examination reveals generalized muscular

weakness, a large tongue, and cardiomegaly without significant heart murmurs. Chest radiographs reveal cardiomegaly with or without pulmonary venous congestion. The ECG shows a short PR interval and LVH with ST depression and T-wave inversion over the left precordial leads. Echocardiography shows severe concentric LVH.

Children with Pompe disease usually die before age 1 year. Death may be sudden or result from progressive heart failure.

3. Restrictive Cardiomyopathy

Restrictive cardiomyopathy is a rare entity in the pediatric population, accounting for less than 5% of all cases of cardiomyopathy. Constrictive pericarditis can have a similar presentation and must be considered in the differential diagnosis of a patient with suspected restrictive cardiomyopathy.

Clinical Findings

Patients present with signs of heart failure as outlined previously. Physical examination is remarkable for a prominent S_4 and jugular venous distention.

A. ELECTROCARDIOGRAPHY

ECG demonstrates marked right and left atrial enlargement with normal ventricular voltages. ST-T–wave abnormalities may be present.

B. ECHOCARDIOGRAPHY

The diagnosis is confirmed echocardiographically by the presence of normal sized ventricles with massively dilated atria. Due to infiltration of the ventricular myocardium, the LV becomes "restrictive," and atrial emptying is impaired.

Course & Prognosis

The condition is usually idiopathic. Endocardial fibroelastosis, a histologic diagnosis, may be noted. The endocardium has marked milky white thickening, as do the subendocardial layers of the LV and left atrium. The mitral valve may be involved. Regardless of cause, the prognosis is poor. Anticongestive therapy may be tried, but many patients will require cardiac transplantation.

Hauser M et al: Diagnosis of anthracycline-induced cardiomyopathy by exercise spiroergometry and stress echocardiography. Eur J Pediatr 2001;160:607 [PMID: 11686505].

Helton E et al: Metabolic aspects of myocardial disease and a role for L-carnitine in the treatment of childhood cardiomyopathy. Pediatrics 2000;105:1260 [PMID: 10835067].

Malcic I et al: Epidemiology of cardiomyopathies in children and adolescents: A retrospective study over the last 10 years. Cardiol Young 2002;12:253 [PMID: 12365172].

Maron BJ et al: ACC/ESC clinical expert consensus document on hypertrophic cardiomyopathy. J Am Coll Cardiol 2003;42:1687 [PMID: 14607462].

Nugent AW et al: Clinical, electrocardiographic, and histologic correlations in children with dilated cardiomyopathy. J Heart Lung Transplant 2001;20:1152 [PMID: 11704474].

Yetman AT et al: Management of pediatric hypertrophic cardiomyopathy. Curr Opin Cardiol 2005;20:80 [PMID: 15711191].

Yetman AT et al: Myocardial bridging in children with hypertrophic cardiomyopathy—A risk factor for sudden death. N Engl J Med 1998;339:1201 [PMID: 9780340].

MYOCARDITIS

The most common causes of myocarditis are adenovirus, coxsackie A and B viruses, echovirus, cytomegalovirus, parvovirus, and influenza A virus. Human immunodeficiency virus can also cause myocarditis. The ability to determine the cause of myocarditis has been enhanced by polymerase chain reaction technology, which replicates identifiable segments of the viral genome from the myocardium of affected children.

Clinical Findings

A. SYMPTOMS AND SIGNS

There are two major clinical patterns: (1) Sudden-onset heart failure in a newborn who has been in relatively good health 12–24 hours previously. This is a malignant form of the disease and is usually secondary to overwhelming viremia with tissue invasion in multiple organ systems including the heart. (2) In the older child, the onset of cardiac symptoms is more gradual and there is often a history of upper respiratory tract infection or gastroenteritis in the previous month. This more insidious form of disease may have a late postinfectious or autoimmune component. It should be remembered that clinical presentation can be acute or chronic in all ages and in all types of myocarditis.

In neonates, the signs of HF are usually obvious including pale gray skin; rapid, weak, and thready pulses; edema of the face and extremities; and cardiomegaly with weak left and right ventricular impulses. The heart sounds may be muffled and distant. S_3 and S_4 are common, resulting in a gallop rhythm. Murmurs are usually absent, although a murmur of tricuspid or mitral insufficiency may be heard. Moist rales are usually present at both lung bases. The liver is enlarged and frequently tender.

B. IMAGING

Generalized cardiomegaly is seen on radiographs with moderate to marked pulmonary venous congestion.

C. ELECTROCARDIOGRAPHY

The ECG is variable. Classically, there is low-voltage QRS in all frontal and precordial leads with ST segment depression and inversion of T waves in leads I, III, and aVF (and in the left precordial leads during the acute stage). Dysrhythmias are common, and AV and intraventricular conduction disturbances may be present. In mild disease or during the recovery phase of severe disease, high-voltage QRS complexes are seen and indicate LVH.

D. ECHOCARDIOGRAPHY

Echocardiography demonstrates four-chamber dilation with poor ventricular function and AV valve regurgitation. A pericardial effusion may be present.

E. MYOCARDIAL BIOPSY

An endomyocardial biopsy may be helpful in the diagnosis of viral myocarditis. Viral polymerase chain reaction testing of the biopsy specimen may yield a positive result in 30–40% of patients suspected to have myocarditis.

Treatment

The use of digitalis in a rapidly deteriorating child with myocarditis is dangerous and should be undertaken with great caution, as it may cause ventricular dysrhythmias. The inpatient cardiac support measures outlined previously in the section on heart failure are used in the treatment of these patients also.

The administration of corticosteroids for myocarditis is controversial. If the patient's condition deteriorates despite anticongestive measures, corticosteroids are commonly used, although conclusive data supporting their effectiveness in this condition are lacking. Subsequent to the successful use of intravenous immunoglobulin for children with Kawasaki disease, there have been several trials of IVIG in presumed viral myocarditis. The therapeutic value of IVIG remains unconfirmed in many practitioners' minds.

Prognosis

The prognosis in myocarditis is related to the age at onset and to the response to therapy. In patients younger than 6 months or older than 3 years with poor response to therapy, the prognosis is poor. Many patients recover clinically but have persistent LV dysfunction with cardiomegaly. It is possible that subclinical myocarditis in childhood is the pathophysiologic basis for some of the idiopathic dilated cardiomyopathies later in life. Children with myocarditis whose ventricular function fails to return to normal may be candidates for cardiac transplantation.

Baboonian C, McKenna W: Eradication of viral myocarditis: Is there hope? J Am Coll Cardiol 2003;42:473 [PMID: 12906975].

Bowles NE et al: Detection of viruses in myocardial tissues by polymerase chain reaction. Evidence of adenovirus as a common cause of myocarditis in children and adults. J Am Coll Cardiol 2003;42:466 [PMID: 12906974].

Liu PP, Mason JW: Advances in the understanding of myocarditis. Circulation 2001;104:1076 [PMID: 11524405].

INFECTIVE ENDOCARDITIS

 **ESSENTIALS OF DIAGNOSIS & TYPICAL FEATURES**

- *Preexisting organic heart murmur.*
- *Persistent fever.*
- *Increasing symptoms of heart disease (ranging from easy fatigability to heart failure).*
- *Splenomegaly (70% of cases).*
- *Embolic phenomena (50% of cases).*
- *Leukocytosis, elevated erythrocyte sedimentation rate, hematuria, positive blood culture.*

General Considerations

Bacterial or fungal infection of the endocardium of the heart or the intimal surface of some arterial vessels (coarcted segment of aorta or ductus arteriosus) is rare and usually occurs in the setting of a preexisting abnormality of the heart or great arteries. It may occur in a normal heart during septicemia.

The frequency of infective endocarditis (IE) appears to be increasing for a number of reasons: (1) increased survival in children with congenital heart disease, (2) increase in prolonged use of central venous catheters, and (3) increased use of prosthetic material and valves. Pediatric patients without preexisting heart disease are also at increased risk for IE because of (1) increased survival rates for children with immune deficiencies, (2) long-term use of indwelling lines in critically ill newborns and patients with many chronic diseases, and (3) increased intravenous drug abuse.

Patients at greatest risk are those with aortic stenosis, bicuspid aortic valve and aorticopulmonary shunts, allograft, heterograft, or prosthetic cardiac valves. The event responsible for an episode of IE can be identified 30% of the time. These include dental procedures, nonsterile surgical procedures, and cardiovascular surgery. Common organisms causing IE are viridans streptococci (about 50% of cases), *Staphylococcus aureus* (about 30%), and fungal agents (about 10%).

Clinical Findings

A. HISTORY

Almost all patients with IE have a history of heart disease. There may or may not be an antecedent infection or surgical procedure (tooth extraction or tonsillectomy).

B. SYMPTOMS, SIGNS, AND LABORATORY FINDINGS

Findings include changing murmurs, fever, positive blood culture, weight loss, cardiomegaly, elevated erythrocyte sedimentation rate, splenomegaly, petechiae, embolism, and leukocytosis. Other findings are hematuria, CHF, digital clubbing, joint pains, and hepatomegaly. Vegetations large enough to be seen by echocardiography occur in 70% of children with endocarditis.

Prevention

Patients at risk for infective endocarditis should receive appropriate antibiotics before any dental work (tooth extraction or cleaning); before operations in the oropharynx and gastrointestinal and genitourinary tracts; and for body piercing and tattooing. Continuous antibiotic prophylaxis (as used in rheumatic fever) is not recommended for patients with congenital heart disease.

The following schedule is recommended: under 40 kg, 50 mg/kg of oral amoxicillin; over 40 kg, 2000 mg. This dose is to be given 1 hour prior to dental procedures. If the patient is allergic to amoxicillin, an alternative prophylactic antibiotic is used.

Treatment

In a patient with heart disease, the presence of an otherwise unexplained fever should alert the physician to the possibility of infective endocarditis. A positive blood culture or other major findings of IE confirms the diagnosis. If a positive blood culture is obtained and the organism identified, treatment should be started immediately. Even if blood cultures are negative after 48 hours, it is advisable to begin antibiotic therapy if other evidence of infective endocarditis is present. If CHF occurs and progresses in the face of adequate antibiotic therapy, surgical excision of the infected area and prosthetic valve replacement must be considered.

Course & Prognosis

The prognosis depends on how early treatment is instituted in the course of the infection. The prognosis is better in patients in whom the blood culture is positive. If CHF develops, the prognosis is poor. Embolization from the vegetations themselves may occur during or after treatment.

Dajani AS et al: Prevention of bacterial endocarditis: Recommendations by the American Heart Association. JAMA 1997;277:1794 [PMID: 9178793].

Friedel JM et al: Infective endocarditis after oral body piercing. Cardiol Rev 2003;11:252 [PMID: 12943601].

PERICARDITIS

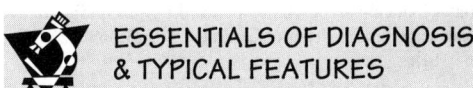

ESSENTIALS OF DIAGNOSIS & TYPICAL FEATURES

- *Retrosternal pain made worse by deep inspiration and decreased by leaning forward.*
- *Fever.*
- *Shortness of breath and grunting respirations are common.*
- *Pericardial friction rub.*
- *Tachycardia.*
- *Hepatomegaly and distention of the jugular veins.*
- *ECG with elevated ST segment.*

General Considerations

Pericarditis rarely occurs as an isolated event. In most cases, pericardial disease occurs in association with a generalized process. Common causes include rheumatic fever, viral pericarditis, purulent pericarditis, rheumatoid arthritis, uremia, and tuberculosis. Pericarditis after cardiac surgery (postpericardiotomy syndrome) is most commonly seen after surgical closure of an ASD.

In children, pericardial disease usually takes the form of acute pericarditis. In most cases, fluid effuses into the pericardial cavity. The consequences of effusion depend on the amount, type, and speed of fluid accumulation. Significant compression of the heart by pericardial effusion can lead to cardiac tamponade. Unless the pericardial fluid is evacuated in this situation, death may occur.

Clinical Findings

A. SYMPTOMS AND SIGNS

Symptoms depend to a great extent on the cause of the pericarditis. Pain is common. It is usually sharp and stabbing, located in the mid chest and in the shoulder and neck, made worse by deep inspiration, and considerably decreased by sitting up and leaning forward. Shortness of breath and grunting respirations are common.

The physical findings depend on whether there is a significant effusion: (1) In the absence of significant accumulation, the pulses are normal. The heart has a characteristic scratchy, high-pitched friction rub. The rub is often systolic and diastolic and can be located at any point between the apex and the left sternal border.

The location and timing vary considerably from time to time. The heart sounds are usually normal, and the heart is not enlarged to percussion. (2) If there is considerable pericardial fluid, the cardiovascular findings are different. The heart is enlarged to percussion, but on auscultation it is very quiet. Heart sounds are distant and muffled. A friction rub may not be present. In the absence of cardiac tamponade, the peripheral, venous, and arterial pulses are normal.

Cardiac tamponade is characterized by jugular venous distension, tachycardia, hepatomegaly, peripheral edema, and pulsus paradoxus in which systolic blood pressure drops more than 10 mm Hg during inspiration. This finding is best demonstrated with a manual blood pressure cuff. The patient with cardiac tamponade is critically ill and has the symptoms and signs of right-sided CHF.

Not all patients with cardiac compression demonstrate all of these findings. If the patient appears critically ill and pericarditis and effusion are evident, treatment should be instituted even though all the clinical signs of cardiac tamponade are not present.

B. IMAGING

In pericarditis with a significant pericardial effusion the cardiac silhouette is enlarged, often in the shape of a water bottle.

C. ELECTROCARDIOGRAPHY

The ECG is often abnormal in pericarditis. Low voltage is commonly seen with significant pericardial effusion. The ST segment is commonly elevated during the first week of involvement. The T wave is usually upright during this time. Later, the ST segment is normal and the T wave becomes flattened.

D. ECHOCARDIOGRAPHY

Echocardiography is essential in diagnosis and management of pericarditis. Serial studies allow a direct noninvasive estimate of the volume of fluid and its change over time. In addition, echocardiography will demonstrate cardiac tamponade if there is compression of the atria.

Treatment

Treatment depends on the cause of the pericarditis. Cardiac tamponade from any cause must be treated by removal of fluid. If there are findings of impending circulatory collapse, an immediate pericardiocentesis is performed. If pericardiocentesis is unsuccessful, a surgical pericardiectomy is required. Diuretics should be avoided in the patient with cardiac tamponade because they reduce ventricular preload and can exacerbate the degree of cardiac decompensation.

Prognosis

Prognosis depends to a great extent on the cause of pericardial disease. Cardiac tamponade from any cause results in death unless fluid is evacuated.

SPECIFIC DISEASES INVOLVING THE PERICARDIUM

Acute Rheumatic Fever

When pericarditis occurs during the course of acute rheumatic fever, it is almost always associated with involvement of the myocardium and the endocardium (pancarditis). Thus heart murmurs are almost always present. Pericarditis is usually of the serofibrinous variety and usually is not associated with a significant pericardial effusion. The treatment of the pericardial effusion is accomplished by treatment of the acute rheumatic fever.

Viral Pericarditis

Viral pericarditis occurs in children and young adults. The most common cause is the group of coxsackie B viruses. Influenza virus has also been implicated. There is usually a history of a protracted upper respiratory tract infection. The pericardial effusion may last for several weeks. Cardiac tamponade is rare. Constrictive pericarditis can occur late after viral pericarditis.

Purulent Pericarditis

The most common causes of purulent pericarditis are pneumococci, streptococci, staphylococci, and *Haemophilus influenzae*. In addition to signs of cardiac compression, patients are septic and extremely febrile. Purulent fluid accumulating in the pericardial sac is usually thick and filled with polymorphonuclear leukocytes. Although antibiotics sterilize the pericardial fluid, pericardial tamponade commonly develops, and surgical excision of the pericardium is frequently necessary. Acutely, pericardiocentesis may be life-saving if there is tamponade on presentation. The wide use of *H influenzae* vaccine has significantly reduced the incidence of this infection.

Postpericardiotomy Syndrome

Postpericardiotomy syndrome is characterized by fever, chest pain, friction rub, and elevation of the ST segment on ECG 1–2 weeks after open-heart surgery. The syndrome appears to be autoimmune with high titers of anti-heart antibody and evidence of fresh or reactivated viral illness. The syndrome is often self-limited and responds well to short courses of aspirin or corticosteroids. Rarely, it lasts for months to years and may require pericardiocentesis or pericardiectomy.

Cakir O et al: Purulent pericarditis in childhood: Ten years of experience. J Pediatr Surg 2002;37:1404 [PMID: 12378443].

Roodpeyma S, Sadeghian N: Acute pericarditis in childhood: A 10-year experience. Pediatr Cardiol 2000;21:363 [PMID: 10865014].

HYPERTENSION

Blood pressure should be determined at every pediatric visit beginning at 3 years. Because blood pressure is being more carefully monitored, systemic hypertension has become more widely recognized as a pediatric problem. Pediatric standards for blood pressure have been published. Blood pressures in children must be obtained when the child is relaxed and an appropriate-size cuff must always be used. The widest cuff that fits between the axilla and the antecubital fossa should be used. Most children age 10–11 years need a standard adult cuff (bladder width of 12 cm), and many high school students need a large adult cuff (width of 16 cm) or leg cuff (width of 18 cm). The 95th percentile value for blood pressure (Table 19–19) is similar for both sexes and all three major ethnic groups. Blood pressure varies more with altitude and body weight than with sex or ethnic origin. If the blood pressure taken properly exceeds the 95th percentile, it should be repeated several times over a 2- to 4-week interval. If it is elevated persistently, a search for the cause should be undertaken. Although most hypertension in children is

Table 19–19. The 95th percentile value for blood pressure (mm Hg) taken in the sitting position.[a]

Age (y)	Sea Level			10,000 ft		
	S	Dm	Dd	S	Dm	Dd
5				92	72	62
6	106	64	60	96	74	66
7	108	72	66	98	76	70
8	110	76	70	104	80	70
9	114	80	76	106	80	70
10	118	82	76	108	80	70
11	124	82	78	108	80	72
12	128	84	78	108	80	72
13	132	84	80	116	84	76
14	136	86	80	120	84	76
15	140	88	80	120	84	80
16	140	90	80	120	84	80
17	140	92	80	122	84	80
18	140	92	80	130	84	80

[a]Blood pressures: S, systolic (Korotkoff sound 1; onset of tapping); Dm, diastolic muffling (Korotkoff sound 4); Dd, diastolic disappearance (Korotkoff sound 5).

essential, there is a higher incidence of treatable conditions in children than in adults, including conditions such as coarctation of the aorta, renal artery stenosis, chronic renal disease, and pheochromocytoma. Over-the-counter and recreational drug use may cause or contribute to hypertension. If no cause is found, and hypertension is deemed essential, antihypertensive therapy should be initiated and nutritional and exercise counseling given when applicable. β-Blockers or ACE inhibitors are the usual first-line medical therapies for essential hypertension in children.

Gifford RW et al: The fifth report of the Joint National Committee on detection, evaluation, and treatment of high blood pressure. Arch Intern Med 1993;153:154 [PMID: 8422206].

Gillman MW et al: Identifying children at high risk for the development of essential hypertension. J Pediatr 1993;122:837 [PMID: 8501557].

ATHEROSCLEROSIS AS A PEDIATRIC PROBLEM

Awareness of coronary artery risk factors in general—and atherosclerosis in particular—has risen dramatically in the general population since the mid-1970s. Although coronary artery disease is still the leading cause of death in the United States, the age-adjusted incidence of death from ischemic heart disease has been decreasing as a result of improved diet, decreased smoking, awareness and treatment of hypertension, and an increase in physical activity. Since the mid-1970s, large population studies of children have been performed and a large number of serum samples from the pediatric population have been collected and analyzed for lipids. Epidemiologic studies have been performed to determine the relationship of lipid levels to coronary heart disease. The level of serum lipids in childhood usually remains the constant through adolescence. Biochemical abnormalities in the lipid profile appear early in childhood and correlate with higher risk for coronary artery disease in adulthood. High-density lipoprotein has been identified as an anti-atherogenic factor. The most common referral to lipid treatment centers is now the obese patient with high triglyceride level, modest elevation of low-density lipoprotein, and low high-density lipoprotein level with associated insulin resistance and pre-diabetes (syndrome X).

Routine lipid screening of children at age 3 years remains controversial. The National Cholesterol Education Program recommends selective screening in children with high-risk family members, defined as a parent with a total cholesterol over 240 mg/dL or a parent or grandparent with early-onset cardiovascular disease. When children have low-density lipoprotein levels greater than 130 mg/dL on two successive tests, dietary lifestyle counseling is appropriate. Dietary modification may decrease cholesterol levels by 5–20%. If the patient is unresponsive to diet change and at extreme risk (ie, a low-density lipoprotein level > 160 mg/dL, a high-density lipoprotein level < 35 mg/dL, and a history of cardiovascular disease in a first-degree relative at an age younger than 40 years), drug therapy may be indicated. Cholestyramine, a bile acid binding resin, is rarely used today due to poor compliance. Niacin and the 3-hydroxy-3-methylglutaryl coenzyme A reductase inhibitors (statins) are used in the pediatric population and may be more effective.

De Jongh S et al: Efficacy and safety of statin therapy in children with familial hypercholesterolemia: A randomized double-blind placebo-controlled trial with simvastatin. Circulation 2002;106:2231 [PMID: 12390953].

Gidding SS: Preventive pediatric cardiology: Tobacco, cholesterol, obesity, and physical activity. Pediatr Clin North Am 1999; 46:253 [PMID: 10218073].

PRIMARY PULMONARY HYPERTENSION

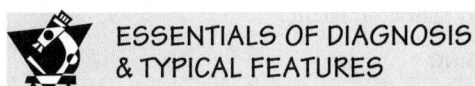

ESSENTIALS OF DIAGNOSIS & TYPICAL FEATURES

- Often subtle with symptoms of dyspnea, fatigue, chest pain, and syncope.
- Exclusion of all causes of secondary pulmonary hypertension.
- Rare, progressive, and often fatal disease without treatment.
- ECG with RVH.
- Loud pulmonary component of S_2.

General Considerations

Unexplained or primary pulmonary hypertension (PPH) in children is a rare disease with an estimated overall incidence of 1–2 persons per million worldwide. Pulmonary hypertension is defined as a mean pulmonary pressure greater than 25 mm Hg at rest or greater than 30 mm Hg during exercise. PPH is a diagnosis made after exclusion of all other causes of pulmonary hypertension. Secondary pulmonary hypertension is most commonly associated with congenital heart disease, pulmonary parenchymal disease, causes of chronic hypoxia (upper airway obstruction), thrombosis, liver disease, and collagen vascular disease. The diagnosis of PPH is difficult to make in the early stages because of its subtle manifestations. Most patients with PPH are young adults, predominantly women. The sex incidence is equal in children. Familial PPH occurs in 6% of affected individuals. The locus for familial PPH is found on chromosome 2 (2q33) and is caused by abnormalities in the transforming growth factor-β family, specifically bone morphogenetic protein receptor II. Without treatment, the median survival is 2.5 years.

Clinical Findings

A. SYMPTOMS AND SIGNS

The clinical picture varies with the severity of pulmonary hypertension. Initial symptoms may be brought on by strenuous exercise or competitive sports, and syncope may be the first symptom. Dyspnea on exertion is present in most patients; syncope occurs in approximately one-third. Palpitations or chest pain may occur with exercise. As disease progresses, patients have signs of low cardiac output and right heart failure. Right heart failure may be manifested by increasing hepatomegaly, peripheral edema, and a gallop cardiac rhythm. Murmurs of pulmonary regurgitation and tricuspid regurgitation are common. An S_3 is occasionally heard with advanced right heart failure.

B. IMAGING

The chest radiograph shows an enlarged heart with a prominent pulmonary artery and dilated proximal right and left pulmonary arteries. The peripheral pulmonary vascular markings may be normal or diminished.

C. ELECTROCARDIOGRAPHY

The ECG usually shows right atrial enlargement with RVH and right axis deviation.

D. ECHOCARDIOGRAPHY

The echocardiogram is an important tool for excluding other congenital heart diseases. It frequently shows RVH and dilation. The tricuspid and pulmonary insufficiency jets are used to estimate pulmonary artery systolic and diastolic pressures.

E. CARDIAC CATHETERIZATION AND ANGIOCARDIOGRAPHY

Cardiac catheterization carries associated risks in children with pulmonary hypertension and should be performed with caution. The procedure is done first to rule out cardiac causes of pulmonary hypertension and then to define treatment strategies. Patients who have a pulmonary vascular bed that is reactive to short-acting vasodilator agents (nitric oxide, adenosine, and prostacyclin) may receive treatment with calcium channel blockers. In contrast, patients who have a pulmonary vascular bed that does not improve with these short-acting agents often receive continuous prostacyclin therapy. Angiography may show a marked decrease in the number of small pulmonary arteries with tortuous vessels.

Treatment

The goal of therapy is to reduce pulmonary artery pressure and increase cardiac output. Cardiac catheterization data are used to define a treatment plan. Patients who respond to pulmonary vasodilators are given calcium channel blockers such as nifedipine or diltiazem. Patients unresponsive to vasodilators in the catheterization laboratory initially receive prostacyclin therapy. Patients with severe, unresponsive pulmonary hypertension may be considered for lung transplantation. Common therapies include warfarin to prevent thromboembolic events. This approach is beneficial in adults. Digoxin and diuretics may be used if signs of right heart failure are present. Receptor antagonists to the vasoconstrictor peptide endothelin show great promise in the treatment of pulmonary hypertension.

Survival rates of greater than 90% have been reported for chronic oral calcium channel blockade in patients who responded acutely to vasodilator testing. In patients in whom calcium channel blockade fails, or in those who do not respond acutely to vasodilator therapy, intravenous prostacyclin has been used with a 5-year survival rate of greater than 80%.

Archer S, Rich S: Primary pulmonary hypertension. Circulation 2000;102:2781 [PMID: 11094047].

Deng Z et al: Familial primary pulmonary hypertension (gene PPH I) is caused by mutations in the bone morphogenetic protein receptor II gene. Am J Hum Genet 2000;67:737 [PMID: 10903931].

Ivy DD: Diagnosis and treatment of severe pediatric pulmonary hypertension. Cardiol Rev 2001;9:227 [PMID: 11405903].

CHEST PAIN

Overview

Chest pain is a common complaint of pediatric patients, accounting for 6 in 1000 visits to urban emergency departments and urgent care clinics. Although children with chest pain are commonly referred for cardiac evaluation, chest pain in children is rarely cardiac. Other more likely causes of chest pain are reactive airways disease, musculoskeletal pain, esophagitis, gastritis, and functional pain.

Approach to the Work-Up

Detailed history and physical exam should guide the pediatrician through the appropriate work-up of chest pain. Rarely is there a need for laboratory tests or evaluation by a specialist. The duration, location, intensity, frequency, and radiation of the pain should be documented, and possible triggering events preceding the pain should be explored. For instance, chest pain following exertion may lead to a more elaborate evaluation for a cardiac disorder. The timing of the pain in relation to meals may suggest a gastrointestinal cause. The patient should also be asked about how pain relief is achieved. A social history to reveal psychosocial stressors and cigarette smoke exposure may assist in determining the cause. On physical exam, attention must be placed on the vital signs; general appearance of the child; the chest wall musculature; cardiac, pulmonary, and abdominal exam findings; and quality of peripheral pulses. Attempts should be made to reproduce the pain by direct palpation and through forced resistance applied to the patient's upper extremities. If the pain can be reproduced, it is almost always musculoskeletal in origin.

Clinical Considerations

Cardiac disease is a rare cause of chest pain, but if misdiagnosed it may be life-threatening. Myocardial infarction rarely occurs in healthy children. Children with underlying illnesses such as diabetes mellitus, chronic anemia, or an anomalous left coronary artery may be at increased risk for ischemia. It is also important to ask the family specifically about a history of Kawasaki disease, treated or untreated. These children are at risk for myocardial infarction secondary to thrombosis of their coronary aneurysms. More than 50% of children and adolescents who exhibit sequelae from Kawasaki disease arrive at the emergency department with chest pain.

Other cardiac causes of chest pain include arrhythmias. The most common arrhythmia in children is supraventricular tachycardia (SVT), but atrial flutter and premature ventricular contractions (PVCs) may also be associated with chest pain in children. Other structural lesions that cause chest pain include aortic stenosis, pulmonary stenosis, and mitral valve prolapse. Structural cardiac lesions are usually accompanied by significant findings on cardiac exam. Of children with mitral valve prolapse, 31% will complain of chest pain presumably caused by papillary muscle ischemia. Other cardiac lesions causing chest pain include dilated cardiomyopathy, hypertrophic obstructive cardiomyopathy, myocarditis, pericarditis, rheumatic fever, and aortic dissection. Pain from hypertrophic obstructive cardiomyopathy may be associated with exertion.

Noncardiac chest pain may be due to a respiratory illness, reactive airway disease, pneumonia, pneumothorax, or pulmonary embolism. Gastrointestinal causes of chest pain include reflux, esophagitis, and foreign body. The most common cause of chest pain (30% of children) is inflammation of musculoskeletal structures of the chest wall. Costochondritis is caused by inflammation of the costochondral joints and is usually unilateral.

The complete history and physical examination can guide the examiner to the appropriate diagnosis or, if necessary, to the appropriate laboratory tests. In most cases tests are not necessary. If a cardiac origin is suspected, a pediatric cardiologist should be consulted. Cardiac findings should first be evaluated with an ECG. Other tests including chest radiograph, echocardiogram, Holter monitor, or serum troponin levels may be required.

■ CARDIAC TRANSPLANTATION

Cardiac transplantation has become an effective therapeutic modality for infants and children with end-stage cardiac disease. Indications for transplantation include: (1) progressive heart failure despite medical therapy, (2) complex congenital heart diseases that are not amenable to surgical repair or palliation or in instances in which the surgical palliative approach has an equal or higher risk of mortality compared to transplantation, and (3) malignant arrhythmias unresponsive to medical therapy, catheter ablation, or automatic implantable cardiodefibrillator. Approximately 300–400 pediatric cardiac transplant procedures are performed annually in the United States. Infant (less than 1 year of age) transplants account for 30% of pediatric cardiac transplants. The current estimated half-life for children undergoing cardiac transplantation is approximately 13 years. This is a rapidly evolving field, and the most recent data indicate an optimistic future for the transplant recipient.

Careful evaluation of the recipient and the donor is performed prior to cardiac transplantation. Assessment of the recipient's pulmonary vascular resistance is critical, as irreversible and severe pulmonary hypertension is a risk factor for posttransplant right heart failure and early death. End-organ function of the recipient may also impact posttransplant outcome and should be evaluated closely. Donor-related factors that can impact outcome include cardiac function, amount of inotropic support needed, active infection (human immunodeficiency virus and hepatitis B and C are contraindications to donation), donor size, and ischemic time to transplantation.

Immunosuppression

The ideal posttransplant immunosuppressive regimen allows the immune system to continue to recognize and respond to foreign antigens in a productive manner while avoiding graft rejection. Although there are many different regimens, calcineurin inhibitors (eg, cyclosporine and tacrolimus) are the mainstay of maintenance immunosuppression in pediatric heart transplantation. Calcineurin inhibitors may be used in isolation. Double-drug therapy includes the addition of antimetabolite or antiproliferative medications such as azathioprine, mycophenolate mofetil, or sirolimus. Due to the significant adverse side-effects of corticosteroids in children, attempts have been made in some centers to discontinue triple-drug therapy that would include steroid use. Growth retardation, susceptibility to infection, impaired wound healing, hypertension, and a cushingoid appearance are some of the consequences of long-term steroid use.

Graft Rejection

Despite advances in immunosuppression, graft rejection remains the leading cause of death in the first 3 years after transplantation. The pathophysiologic mechanisms of rejection are not entirely known. T cells are required for rejection, but multiple cell lines and mechanisms are likely involved. Because graft rejection can present in the absence of clinical symptomatology, monitoring for and diagnosing rejection in a timely fashion can be difficult. Screening regimens include serial physical examinations, electrocardiography, echocardiography, and cardiac catheterization with endomyocardial biopsy.

Rejection Surveillance

A. SYMPTOMS AND SIGNS

Transplant recipients undergoing graft rejection are usually asymptomatic in the early stages. With progression they may develop tachycardia, tachypnea, rales, a gallop rhythm, and/or hepatosplenomegaly. Infants and young children may present with irritability, poor feeding, vomiting, or lethargy. The goal is to detect rejection prior to the development of hemodynamic compromise, as there is 50% mortality in the year following an episode of rejection resulting in cardiovascular compromise.

B. IMAGING

Chest radiographs may show cardiomegaly, pulmonary edema, or pleural effusions.

C. ELECTROCARDIOGRAPHY

Abnormalities in conduction can be present, although the most typical finding is reduced QRS voltages. Both atrial and ventricular arrhythmias occur in rejection.

D. ECHOCARDIOGRAPHY

Echocardiography is a noninvasive rejection surveillance tool in infant recipients and is helpful in all ages. Changes in ventricular compliance and function may initially be subtle, but are progressive with increasing duration of the rejection episode. A new pericardial effusion or worsening valvular insufficiency may also indicate rejection.

E. CARDIAC CATHETERIZATION AND ENDOMYOCARDIAL BIOPSY

Hemodynamic assessment including ventricular filling pressures, cardiac output, and oxygen consumption can be obtained via cardiac catheterization. The endomyocardial biopsy has been considered the gold standard for diagnosing acute graft rejection. However, because not all episodes of symptomatic rejection result in a positive biopsy, this tool is not universally reliable. The appearance of infiltrating lymphocytes with myocellular damage is the hallmark of graft rejection and is helpful if present.

Treatment of Graft Rejection

Treatment of graft rejection depends on reversing the immunologic inflammatory cascade. High-dose corticosteroids are the first line of treatment to stabilize or reverse most rejection episodes. Occasionally additional therapy with antithymocyte biologic preparations such as antithymocyte globulin or OKT-3 (a murine monoclonal antibody to the CD3 T-lymphocyte epitope) is needed to reverse rejection. Most rejection episodes can be treated effectively if diagnosed promptly. Usually graft function returns to its baseline state, although severe rejection episodes can result in graft loss and patient death even with optimal therapy.

Course & Prognosis

The course of cardiac transplantation in pediatric patients is usually quite good. The risk of infection is low after the immediate posttransplant period in spite of chronic immunosuppression. Cytomegalovirus is the most common pathogen responsible for infection-related morbidity and mortality in heart transplant recipients. Most children tolerate environmental pathogens well. Noncompliance with lifetime immunosuppression is of great concern especially in adolescent patients. Several recent studies have identified noncompliance as the leading cause of late death. Posttransplant lymphoproliferative disorder, a syndrome related to Epstein-Barr virus infection, can result in a Burkitt-like lymphoma that usually responds to a reduction in immunosuppression, but occasionally must be treated with chemotherapy. Most children are not physically limited, and they do not require restrictions related to the cardiovascular system.

The greatest long-term concern after heart transplantation is related to cardiac allograft vasculopathy. Cardiac allograft vasculopathy results from concentric intimal proliferation of the coronary arteries that can ultimately result in complete luminal occlusion. These lesions are diffuse and often involve distal vessels and thus are usually not amenable to bypass grafting, angioplasty, or stent placement. Although likely multifactorial, risk factors for cardiac allograft vasculopathy may include: older age, immunosuppressant regimen, recurrent rejection, late rejection, and noncompliance. Screening for cardiac allograft vasculopathy is by selective coronary angiography, but intravascular ultrasound may be a more sensitive tool and is utilized in combination with angiography in some centers. Overall, despite the concerns of immunosuppression, the risk of late rejection, and coronary disease, the majority of pediatric patients enjoy a good quality of life with survival rates that are improving. Currently, 10-year survival is 80% for infant recipients and 70% overall for all pediatric recipients. Newer, more specific, and more effective immunosuppressive agents are currently being tried in clinical studies or are being evaluated in preclinical studies, making the future almost certainly better for children after cardiac transplantation. Donor availability remains a major limitation to the expansion of indications for cardiac transplantation.

Boucek MM et al: Prospective evaluation of echocardiography for primary rejection surveillance after heart transplantation: comparison with endomyocardial biopsy. J Heart Lung Transplant 1994;13(1 Pt 1):66 [PMID: 8167130].

Boucek MM et al: The Registry for the International Society for Heart and Lung Transplantation: Seventh official pediatric report—2004. J Heart Lung Transplant 2004;23:933 [PMID: 15312823].

Mulla NF et al: Late rejection is a predictor of transplant coronary artery disease in children. J Am Coll Cardiol 2001;37:243 [PMID: 11153746].

Pietra BA: Transplantation immunology 2003: a simplified approach. Pediatr Clin North Am 2003;50:1233 [PMID: 14710779].

DISORDERS OF RATE & RHYTHM

As more children are surviving cardiac surgery and living with chronically altered hemodynamics there has been an increase in the incidence of arrhythmias in the pediatric population.

The introduction of invasive electrophysiology with recordings from the endocardium has greatly improved understanding of the conduction system. Cardiac ablation techniques offer some children with arrhythmias a cure rather than lifelong antiarrhythmia treatment.

Sinus Arrhythmia

Phasic variation in the heart rate (sinus arrhythmia) is normal. Typically, the sinus rate varies with the respiratory cycle, whereas P-QRS-T intervals remain stable. Marked sinus arrhythmia is defined as greater than 100% variation in heart rate. It may occur in association with respiratory distress or increased intracranial pressure, or it may be present in normal children. In isolation, it never requires treatment; however, it may be associated with sinus node dysfunction or autonomic nervous system dysfunction.

Sinus Bradycardia

Depending on age, sinus bradycardia is defined as either (1) a heart rate below the normal limit for age (neonates to 6 years, 60 beats/min; 7–11 years, 45 beats/min; older than 12 years, 40 beats/min) or (2) a heart rate inappropriately slow for the functional status of the patient (chronotropic incompetence). In critically ill patients, common causes of sinus bradycardia include hypoxia, central nervous system damage, eating disorders, and medication side effects. Only symptomatic bradycardia (syncope, low cardiac output, or exercise intolerance) requires treatment (atropine, isoproterenol. or cardiac pacing).

Sinus Tachycardia

The heart rate normally accelerates in response to stress (eg, fever, hypovolemia, anemia, or CHF). Although sinus tachycardia in the normal heart is well tolerated, symptomatic tachycardia with decreased cardiac output warrants evaluation for structural heart disease or true tachyarrhythmias. Treatment may be indicated for correction of the underlying cause of sinus tachycardia (eg, transfusion for anemia or correction of hypovolemia or fever).

PREMATURE ATRIAL CONTRACTIONS

Premature atrial contractions are triggered by an ectopic focus in the atrium. They are one of the most common premature beats occurring in pediatrics, particularly during the fetal and newborn periods. They may be conducted (followed by a QRS) or nonconducted (not followed by a QRS, as the beat has occurred so early that the AV node is still refractory) (Figure 19–4). A less-than-compensatory pause usually occurs until the next normal sinus beat. Depending on the location of the ectopic focus of the premature contraction, the P-wave morphology may be normal or abnormal. As an isolated finding, premature atrial contractions are benign and require no treatment. They need to be treated with antiarrhythmic agents only when they trigger tachyarrhythmias or produce bradycardia secondary to nonconduction.

PREMATURE JUNCTIONAL CONTRACTIONS

Premature junctional contractions arise in the AV node or the bundle of His. They usually induce a normal QRS complex with no preceding P wave. When conducted aberrantly to the ventricles, they cannot be dis-

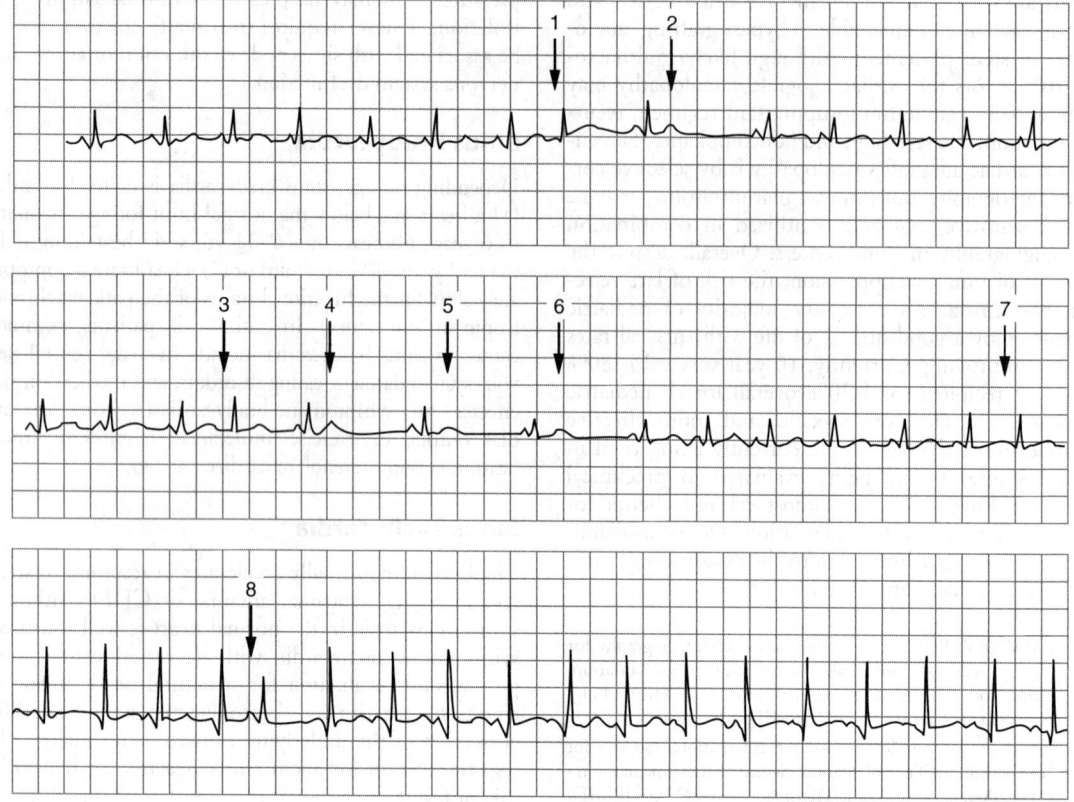

Figure 19–4. Lead II rhythm strip with premature atrial contractions. Beats 1, 3, 7, and 8 are conducted to the ventricles, whereas beats 2, 4, 5, and 6 are not.

tinguished from PVCs except by invasive electrophysiologic study. Premature junctional contractions are usually benign and require no specific therapy.

PREMATURE VENTRICULAR CONTRACTIONS

PVCs may originate in either ventricle and are characterized by an abnormal QRS of over 80 ms duration in newborns and 120 ms in adolescents and adults (Figure 19–5). PVCs originating from a single ectopic focus all have the same configuration; those of multifocal origin show varying configurations. The consecutive occurrence of two PVCs is referred to as a ventricular couplet and of three or more as ventricular tachycardia.

Most unifocal PVCs in otherwise normal patients are benign. The significance of PVCs can be confirmed by having the patient exercise. As the heart rate increases, benign PVCs usually disappear. If exercise results in an increase or coupling of contractions, underlying disease may be present. Multifocal PVCs are always abnormal and may be more dangerous. They may be associated with

drug overdose (tricyclic antidepressants or digoxin toxicity), electrolyte imbalance, myocarditis, or hypoxia. Treatment is directed at correcting the underlying disorder.

SINUS NODE DYSFUNCTION

Sinus node dysfunction, or sick sinus syndrome, is a clinical syndrome of inappropriate sinus nodal function and rate. The abnormality may be a true anatomic defect of the sinus node or its surrounding tissue, or it may be an abnormality of autonomic input. It is defined as one or more of the following:

1. Sinus bradycardia
2. Marked sinus arrhythmia
3. Chronotropic incompetence
4. Sinus pause or arrest
5. Sinoatrial exit block
6. Combined bradyarrhythmias and tachyarrhythmias
7. Sinus node reentry
8. Atrial muscle reentry tachycardia

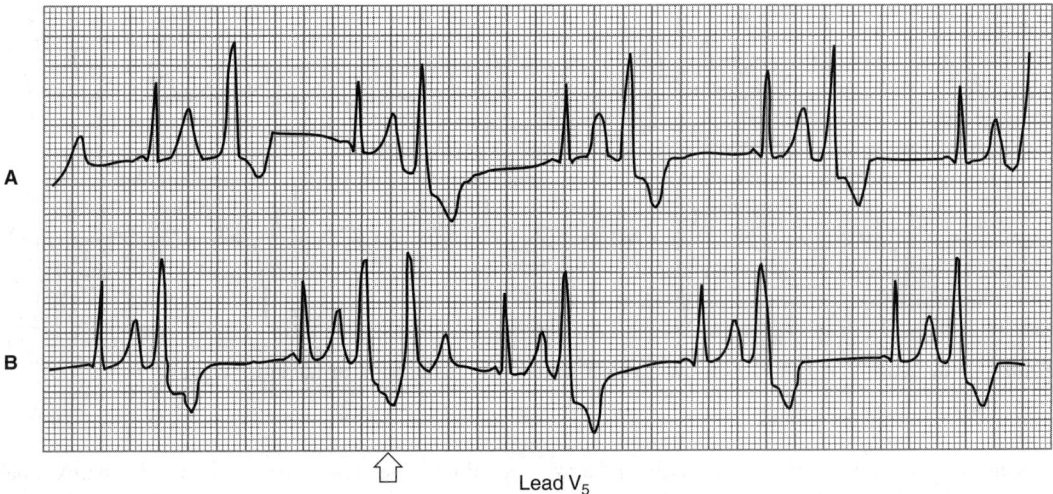

Figure 19–5. Lead V₅ rhythm strip with unifocal premature ventricular contractions in a bigeminy pattern. The arrow shows a ventricular couplet.

It is usually associated with postoperative repair of congenital heart disease (most commonly the Mustard or Senning repair for complete transposition of the great arteries or the Fontan procedure), but it is also seen in unoperated congenital heart disease, in acquired heart diseases, and in normal hearts. In some cases the disorder is inherited. Symptoms usually manifest between ages 2 and 17 years and consist of episodes of syncope, presyncope, or disorientation. Some patients may experience palpitations, pallor, or exercise intolerance.

The evaluation of sinus node dysfunction involves both surface ECG and invasive electrophysiologic testing. Exercise testing and ambulatory monitoring help define any arrhythmias and correlate rhythm changes with symptoms.

Treatment for sinus node dysfunction is indicated only in symptomatic patients. Asymptomatic patients can be observed for the onset of exercise intolerance or syncope because there is little chance of sudden death prior to the onset of such symptoms. Bradyarrhythmias are treated with vagolytic (atropine) or adrenergic (aminophylline) agents or permanent cardiac pacemakers. Antiarrhythmic treatment of tachyarrhythmias often produces or enhances bradycardia, thus requiring permanent cardiac pacing. A pacemaker is inserted prophylactically prior to the initiation of antiarrhythmic medications.

The prognosis is excellent when appropriate treatment is provided, with morbidity and mortality rates nearly equal to those of the underlying heart disease. In severe untreated cases, sinus node dysfunction may become chronic and may lead to sudden death.

Miller MS et al: Neonatal bradycardia. Prog Pediatr Cardiol 2000; 11:19 [PMID: 10822186].

SUPRAVENTRICULAR TACHYCARDIA

SVT, also known as paroxysmal SVT or paroxysmal atrial tachycardia, is defined as an abnormal arrhythmia mechanism arising above or within the bundle of His. The mode of presentation depends on the heart rate, the presence of underlying cardiac structural or functional abnormalities, coexisting illness, and patient age. Tachycardia may be poorly tolerated in a child with preexisting CHF or an underlying systemic disease such as anemia or sepsis. It may go unnoticed in an otherwise healthy child. Incessant tachycardia in an otherwise healthy individual, even if fairly slow (120–150/ min), may cause myocardial dysfunction and CHF if left untreated. The mechanisms of tachycardia are divided into three groups: reentry, enhanced automaticity, and triggered dysrhythmias.

Reentry is conduction through two or more pathways, creating a sustained repetitive circular loop. The circuit can be confined to the atrium (intra-atrial reentry, a form of atrial flutter) (Figure 19–6). It may be confined within the AV node (AV nodal reentrant tachycardia), or it may encompass an accessory connection between atria and ventricle (atrioventricular tachycardia). The arrhythmia circuit includes conduction through the normal pathway (the AV node) as well as the accessory AV connection. If during tachycardia the electrical impulse travels antegrade (from atria to ventricles) through the AV node and retrograde (from ventricle to atria) back up the accessory pathway, orthodromic reciprocating tachycardia is present. If during tachycardia the electrical impulse travels antegrade through the accessory pathway and retrograde up through the AV node, then antidromic reciprocating tachycardia is present.

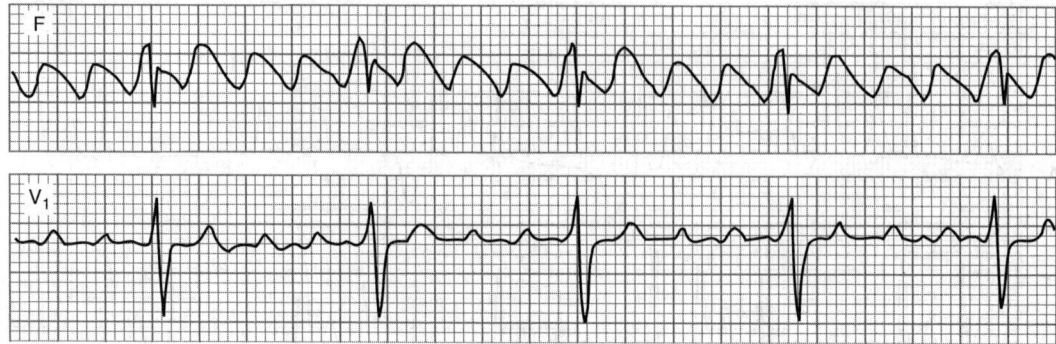

Figure 19–6. Leads aVF (F) and V$_1$, showing atrial flutter with "sawtooth" atrial flutter waves.

WPW syndrome is a subclass of reentrant tachycardia in which, during sinus rhythm, the impulse travels antegrade down the accessory connection, bypassing the AV node and creating ventricular preexcitation (early eccentric activation of the ventricle with a short PR interval and slurred upstroke of the QRS, a delta wave) (Figure 19–7). Reentrant tachycardia represents approximately 80% of pediatric arrhythmias, has a wide range of rates, and may or may not demonstrate P waves. Reentrant tachycardia initiates and terminates abruptly. Most patients with WPW have otherwise structurally normal hearts. However, WPW has been noted to occur with increased frequency in association with the following congenital cardiac lesions: tricuspid atresia, Ebstein anomaly of the tricuspid valve, HCM, and ccTGA.

Enhanced automaticity (also known as automatic or ectopic tachycardia) is created when a focus of cardiac tissue develops an abnormally fast spontaneous rate of depolarization. These arrhythmias represent approximately 20% of childhood arrhythmias and are usually under autonomic influence. ECG demonstrates a normal QRS complex preceded by an abnormal P wave (Figure 19–8). Junctional ectopic tachycardia does not have a P wave preceding the QRS waves and may be associated with AV dissociation or 1:1 retrograde conduction. Ectopic tachycardias demonstrate a gradual onset and offset and may be paroxysmal or incessant. When they are incessant, they are usually associated with CHF and a clinical picture of dilated cardiomyopathy.

Triggered dysrhythmia is extremely rare. It is caused by afterdepolarizations. These tachycardias are usually associated with diseased atrial myocardium, are triggered by premature atrial contractions or sinus tachycardia, initiate and terminate abruptly, and mimic intraatrial reentry (atrial flutter). However, they can be distinguished from atrial flutter: they terminate with the administration of adenosine, while atrial flutter does not (see section on atrial flutter and fibrillation).

Clinical Findings

A. Symptoms and Signs

Presentation varies with age. Infants tend to turn pale and mottled with onset of tachycardia and may become irritable. With long duration of tachycardia, symptoms of CHF develop. Heart rates range from 240–300 beats/min. Older children complain of dizziness, palpitations, fatigue, and chest pain. Heart rates range from 240 beats/min in the younger child to 150–180 beats/min in the teenager. CHF is less common in children than infants. Tachycardia may be associated with either

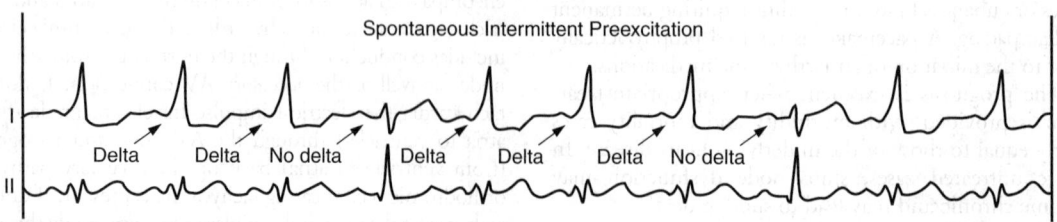

Figure 19–7. Leads I and II with spontaneous intermittent ventricular preexcitation (Wolff-Parkinson-White syndrome).

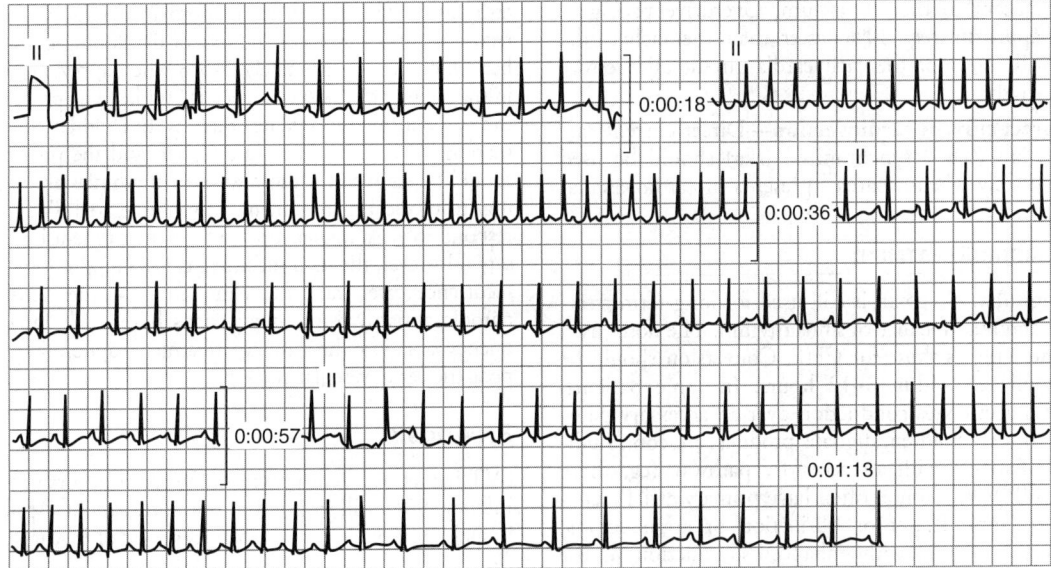

Figure 19–8. Lead II rhythm strip of ectopic atrial tachycardia. The tracing demonstrates a variable rate with a maximum of 260 beats/min, an abnormal P wave, and a gradual termination.

congenital heart defects or acquired conditions such as cardiomyopathies and myocarditis.

B. IMAGING

Chest radiographs are normal during the early course of tachycardia. If CHF is present, the heart is enlarged and pulmonary venous congestion is evident.

C. ELECTROCARDIOGRAPHY

ECG is the most important tool in the diagnosis of SVT.

1. The heart rate is rapid and out of proportion to the patient's physical status (ie, a rate of 140 beats/min with an abnormal P wave while quiet and asleep).

2. The rhythm is extremely regular. There is little variation in the rate throughout the entire tracing.

3. P waves may or may not be present. If they are present, the PR interval and appearance do not vary. P waves may be difficult to find because they are superimposed on the preceding T wave. Furthermore, if the abnormal focus is located within the AV node, the P waves will not be seen.

4. The QRS complex is usually the same as during normal sinus rhythm. However, the QRS complex is occasionally widened (SVT with aberrant ventricular conduction), in which case the condition may be difficult to differentiate from ventricular tachycardia.

Treatment

A. ACUTE TREATMENT

During the initial episodes of SVT, patients require close monitoring. Correction of acidosis and electrolyte abnormalities is also indicated.

1. Vagal maneuvers—The "diving reflex" produced by placing an ice bag on the nasal bridge for 20 seconds (for infants) or by immersing the face in ice water (for children or adolescents) will increase parasympathetic tone and terminate some tachycardias. The Valsalva maneuver, which can be performed by older compliant children, may also terminate SVT.

2. Adenosine—Adenosine transiently blocks AV conduction and terminates tachycardias that incorporate the AV node.

Adenosine does not convert tachycardias whose mechanism is confined to the atria (atrial ectopic tachycardia or intra-atrial reentry). However, it serves as a diagnostic tool in these arrhythmias by demonstrating continuation of the atrial tachycardia during AV block, implying that AV node conduction is not a crucial element of the tachycardia circuit. The dose is 50–250 µg/kg by rapid intravenous bolus. It is antagonized by aminophylline and should be used with caution in patients with sinus node dysfunction or asthma.

3. Transesophageal atrial pacing—Atrial overdrive pacing and termination can be performed from a bipolar electrode-tipped catheter positioned in the esophagus adjacent to the left atrium. Overdrive pacing at rates approximately 30% faster than the tachycardia rate will interrupt the tachycardia circuit and restore sinus rhythm.

4. Direct current cardioversion—Direct current cardioversion (0.5–2 synchronized J/kg) should be used immediately when a patient presents in cardiovascular collapse.

B. CHRONIC TREATMENT

1. Digitalis—Digoxin is still used for long-term treatment and maintenance of sinus rhythm. The doses used are the same as those for CHF. Conversion should be accomplished within 8–12 hours. In some patients, digoxin accelerates conduction over an accessory pathway. In such children, digitalis products are contraindicated. Patients with an accessory pathway (eg, those with WPW syndrome) often have primary atrial tachycardias (atrial flutter or fibrillation or atrial ectopic tachycardias), and with enhanced conduction in the accessory pathway these primary atrial tachycardias can transmit to the ventricles, causing ventricular fibrillation. Therefore, an evaluation of the effect of digoxin on the accessory pathway should be performed in the electrophysiology lab before chronic digoxin use in patients with WPW syndrome.

2. Beta-adrenergic blocking agents—Propranolol decreases sinus heart rate and AV nodal conduction. It is effective in the treatment of both reentrant and ectopic arrhythmias in doses ranging from 1–4 mg/kg/d. Long-acting β-blockers, such as atenolol and nadolol, are used because they have fewer central nervous system side effects than propranolol and may be given only once or twice a day.

3. Calcium channel antagonists—Verapamil and other calcium channel blockers markedly prolong conduction through the AV node and are effective in interrupting and preventing reentrant tachycardias that incorporate the AV node. They are ineffective in terminating atrial tachycardias but may be useful in controlling the ventricular response by producing AV blockade. Verapamil comes in short- and long-acting preparations; the dose is 3–5 mg/kg/d. It may cause myocardial dysfunction and is contraindicated in infants.

4. Other drugs—Recently introduced antiarrhythmic medications (eg, flecainide, propafenone, sotalol, and amiodarone) have increased pharmacologic actions and are extremely effective. However, these drugs also have serious side effects, including proarrhythmia (production of arrhythmias) and sudden death, and should be used only under the direction of a pediatric cardiologist.

5. Radiofrequency ablation—This is a nonsurgical transvascular catheter technique that desiccates an arrhythmia focus or accessory pathway and permanently cures an arrhythmia. The success rate is approximately 90%, with a recurrence risk of 10%. The risk of developing complete heart block is approximately 2–5% when applying burns in the vicinity of the AV node/His bundle. The procedure can be performed in infants or adults. In children younger than age 4 years, the risks are higher, and the procedure should be reserved for those whose arrhythmias are refractory to medical management. In well-tolerated SVTs that respond to vagal maneuvers, no further treatment is necessary. However, the high success rate, low complication and recurrence rates, and the elimination of the need for chronic antiarrhythmic medications have made radiofrequency ablation the primary treatment option in most pediatric cardiovascular centers.

Prognosis

SVT has an excellent prognosis. When it occurs in early infancy, 90% will respond to initial treatment. Approximately 30% will recur at an average age of 8 years.

Basson CT: A molecular basis for Wolff-Parkinson-White syndrome. N Engl J Med 2001;344:1861 [PMID: 11407351].

Dubin AM et al: Radiofrequency catheter ablation: Indications and complications. Pediatr Cardiol 2000;21:551 [PMID: 11050279].

Moak JP: Supraventricular tachycardia in the neonate and infant. Prog Pediatr Cardiol 2000;11:25 [PMID: 10822187].

ATRIAL FLUTTER & FIBRILLATION

Atrial flutter and fibrillation are rare in children and are most often associated with organic heart disease—particularly postoperative congenital heart disease and sinus node dysfunction. Atrial flutter can occur in infancy and can mimic SVT. The atrial rate is usually greater than 240 beats/min and often more than 300 beats/min. The ventricular rate depends on the rate of AV conduction and is usually slower than the atrial rate.

Treatment & Prognosis

Transesophageal atrial pacing is the treatment of choice to terminate atrial flutter. When it is not successful, antiarrhythmic medications (eg, digoxin, sotalol, and amiodarone) may succeed; however, direct current cardioversion is frequently necessary.

The prognosis in neonates without structural heart disease is excellent, and after conversion these patients may need no further treatment.

POSTOPERATIVE INCISIONAL INTRA-ATRIAL REENTRY

Improved surgical survival for patients with congenital heart disease has created a new, increasingly prevalent, chronic arrhythmia: incisional intra-atrial reentry, or postoperative atrial flutter. In these tachycardias, electrically isolated corridors of atrial myocardium (eg, the tricuspid valve–inferior vena cava isthmus, or the region between an atrial incision and the crista terminalis) act as pathways for sustained reentrant circuits of electrical activity. These tachycardias are chronic, medically refractory, and clinically incapacitating. Electromagnetic mapping permits precise localization of these corridors. Long linear radiofrequency or surgical lesions are then used to interrupt the reentrant circuits.

Delacretaz E et al: Multiple atrial macro-reentry circuits in adults with repaired congenital heart disease: Entrainment mapping combined with three-dimensional electroanatomic mapping. J Am Coll Cardiol 2001;37:1665 [PMID: 11345382].

Van Hare GF: Intra-atrial reentry tachycardia in pediatric patients. Prog Pediatr Cardiol 2001;13:41 [PMID: 11413057].

VENTRICULAR TACHYCARDIA

Ventricular tachycardia is uncommon in childhood (Figure 19–9). It is usually associated with underlying abnormalities of the myocardium (myocarditis, cardiomyopathy, myocardial tumors, or postoperative congenital heart disease) or toxicity (hypoxia, electrolyte imbalance, or drug toxicity). Sustained tachycardia is generally an unstable situation, and if left untreated will usually degenerate into ventricular fibrillation.

Accelerated idioventricular rhythm is a sustained ventricular tachycardia occurring in neonates with normal hearts. The rate is within 10% of the preceding sinus rate, and it is a self-limiting arrhythmia that requires no treatment.

Acute termination of ventricular tachycardia involves restoration of the normal myocardium when possible (correct electrolyte imbalance, drug toxicity, and so on) and direct current cardioversion (1–4 J/kg), cardioversion with lidocaine (1 mg/kg), or both. Chronic suppression of ventricular arrhythmias with antiarrhythmic drugs has many side effects (including proarrhythmia and death), and it must be initiated in the hospital under the direction of a pediatric cardiologist.

Alexander ME et al: Ventricular arrhythmias: When to worry. Pediatr Cardiol 2000;21:532 [PMID: 11050277].

Batra A et al: Ventricular arrhythmias. Prog Pediatr Cardiol 2000;11:39 [PMID: 10822188].

LONG QT SYNDROME

The congenital long QT syndromes (types 1–6) in children are arrhythmic disorders in which ventricular repolarization is irregular and prolonged (QTc > 0.44 second, or 0.46 second in postpubertal females). Some myocardial ion channelopathies predispose patients to torsade de pointes (multifocal ventricular tachycardia) and manifest as syncope, seizures, or sudden death, often in response to exercise. If untreated, they account for a very high mortality rate (5%/year). They are inherited genetically in an autosomal dominant or recessive pattern (the latter being associated with congenital deafness, the Jervell and Lange-Nielsen syndrome) or they may arise spontaneously. Treatment with β-blockade and exercise limitation is only partially successful. In recurrent, medically refractory cases, implantable cardioverter defibrillators are necessary to prevent sudden death. Congenital long QT syndrome has now been demonstrated to be one of the causes of sudden infant death syndrome.

Acquired long QT syndrome—resulting from altered ventricular repolarization secondary to myocardial toxins, ischemia, or inflammation—also predisposes a patient to ventricular arrhythmias. Numerous medications as outlined previously can also cause QT prolongation. ECGs

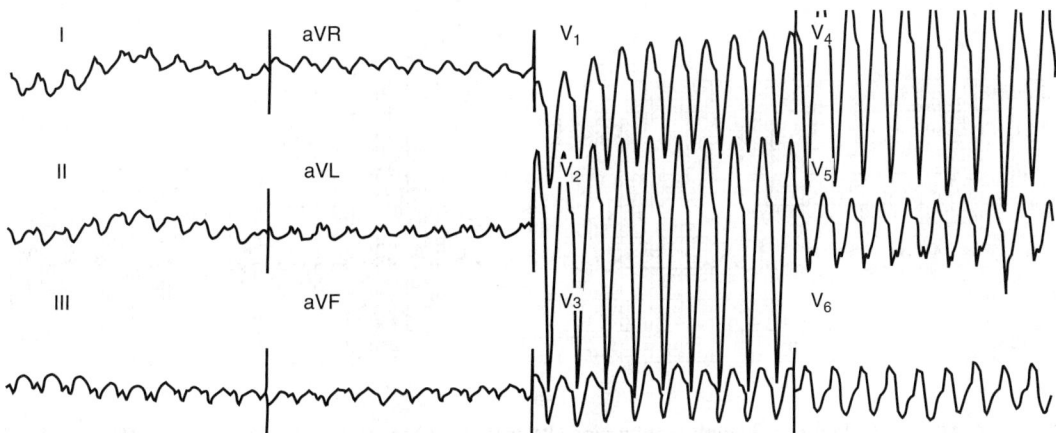

Figure 19–9. Twelve-lead ECG from a child with imipramine toxicity and ventricular tachycardia.

are recommended before therapy (for a baseline measurement) and after steady state is achieved.

Gutgesell H et al: Cardiovascular monitoring of children and adolescents receiving psychotropic drugs. A statement for healthcare professionals from the Committee on Congenital Cardiac Defects, Counsel on Cardiovascular Diseases in the Young-American Heart Association. Circulation 1999;99:979 [PMID: 10027824].

Kimbrough J et al: Clinical implications for affected parents and siblings of probands with long QT syndrome. Circulation 2001;104:557 [PMID: 11479253].

Li H et al: Current concepts in long QT syndrome. Pediatr Cardiol 2000;21:542 [PMID: 11050278].

Moss AJ et al: Effectiveness and limitations of β-blocker therapy in congenital long QT syndrome. Circulation 2000;101:616 [PMID: 10673253].

Wedekind H et al: De novo mutation in the SCN5A gene associated with early onset of sudden infant death. Circulation 2001;104:1158 [PMID: 11535573].

Zhang L et al: Spectrum of ST-T wave patterns and repolarization parameters in congenital long QT syndrome: ECG findings identify genotypes. Circulation 2000;102:2849 [PMID: 11104743].

SUDDEN DEATH

Hypertrophic cardiomyopathy (the most common cause of sudden death in young athletes) and other cardiomyopathies (dilated cardiomyopathies, restrictive cardiomyopathy, or arrhythmogenic RV dysplasia) may be hereditary and should be looked for in patients with resuscitated cardiac arrest or family members of those who have died suddenly. Congenital structural anomalies of the coronary arteries are the second most common cause of sudden death in young athletes. These anomalies are not hereditary. The coronary arteries need to be evaluated in survivors of sudden death events. Arrhythmias in patients with postoperative congenital heart disease are important causes of morbidity and mortality and may present as sudden death events. All survivors of cardiac arrest require thorough evaluation for arrhythmias, including invasive electrophysiology. Episodes of seizures, syncope, and presyncope in congenital heart disease patients should be evaluated for the possibilities of arrhythmias, and they may also require thorough electrophysiologic evaluation and treatment.

When a child dies suddenly and unexpectedly, or is resuscitated from cardiac arrest that had no apparent cause, it is necessary to conduct a detailed family history looking for seizures, syncope, or early sudden death. Family members should be examined with an arrhythmia screen, physical examination, ECG, and echocardiography to detect arrhythmias or cardiomyopathies.

Corrado D et al: Right bundle branch block, right precordial ST-segment elevation, and sudden death in young people. Circulation 2001;103:710 [PMID: 11156883].

Gatzoulis MA et al: Risk factors for arrhythmia and sudden cardiac death later after repair of tetralogy of Fallot: A Multicentre Study. Lancet 2000;356:975 [PMID: 11041398].

HEART BLOCK

1. First-Degree Heart Block

First-degree heart block is an ECG diagnosis of prolongation of the PR interval. The block does not in itself cause problems. It may be associated with structural congenital heart defects, namely AV septal defects, ccTGA, and with diseases such as rheumatic carditis. The PR interval is prolonged in patients receiving digoxin therapy.

2. Second-Degree Heart Block

Mobitz type I (Wenckebach) heart block is recognized by progressive prolongation of the PR interval until there is no QRS following a P wave (Figure 19–10). Mobitz type I heart block occurs in normal hearts at rest and is usually

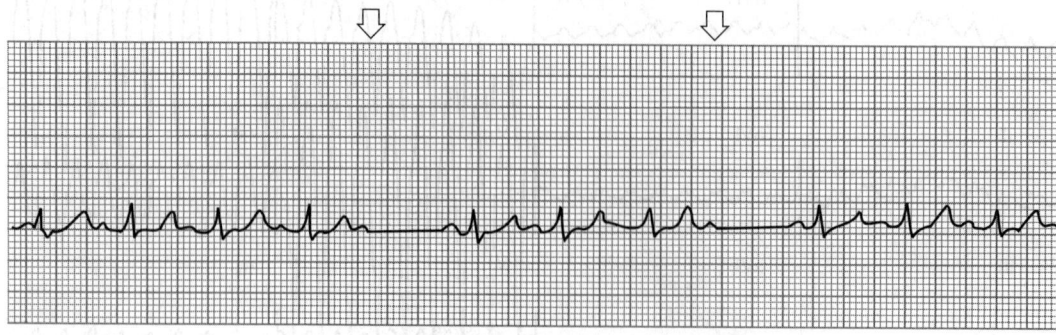

Lead I

Figure 19–10. Lead I rhythm strip with Mobitz type I (Wenckebach) second-degree heart block. There is progressive lengthening of the PR interval prior to the nonconducted P wave (*arrows*).

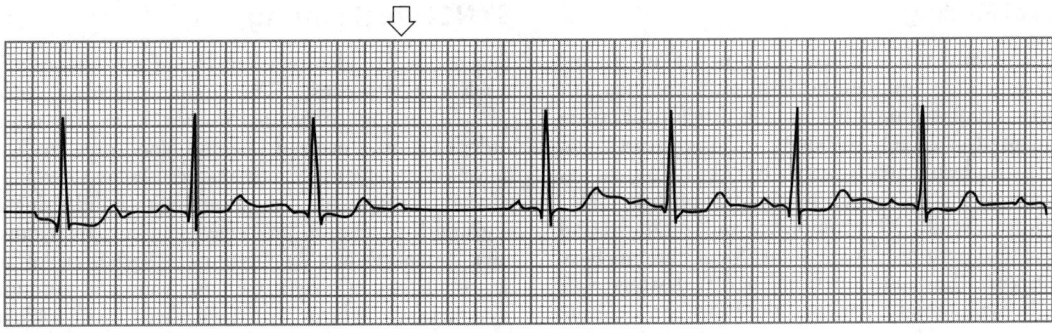

Lead III

Figure 19–11. Lead III rhythm strip with Mobitz type II second-degree heart block. There is a consistent PR interval with occasional loss of AV conduction (*arrow*).

benign. In Mobitz type II heart block, there is no progressive lengthening of the PR interval before the dropped beat (Figure 19–11). Mobitz type II heart block is frequently associated with organic heart disease, and a complete evaluation is necessary.

3. Complete Heart Block

In complete heart block, the atria and ventricles beat independently. Ventricular rates can range from 40–80 beats/min, whereas atrial rates are faster (Figure 19–12).

Congenital complete heart block, the most common form of complete heart block, has a very high association with maternal systemic lupus erythematosus antibodies. Serologic screening should be performed in the mother of an infant with complete heart block, even if she has no symptoms of collagen vascular disease. Congenital complete heart block is also associated with congenitally corrected transposition of the great vessels and AV septal defect. Acquired complete heart block may be secondary to acute myocarditis, drug toxicity, electrolyte imbalance, hypoxia, and cardiac surgery.

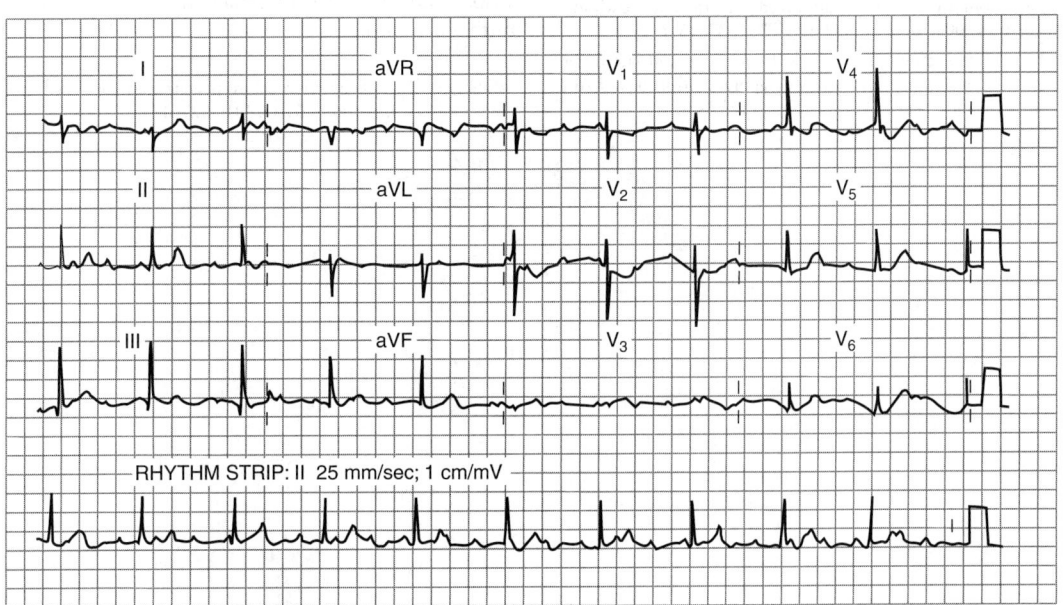

Figure 19–12. Twelve-lead ECG and lead II rhythm strip of complete heart block. The atrial rate is 150 beats/min, and the ventricular rate is 60 beats/min.

Clinical Findings

Prenatal bradycardia is frequently noted in infants with congenital complete heart block, and emergent delivery is required if hydrops fetalis develops. Postnatal adaptation largely depends on the heart rate; infants with heart rates lower than 55 beats/min are at significantly greater risk for low cardiac output, CHF, and death. Wide QRS complexes and a rapid atrial rate are also poor prognostic signs. Most patients have an innocent flow murmur from increased stroke volume. In symptomatic patients, the heart can be quite enlarged, and pulmonary edema may be present. In older patients, syncope can be the presenting symptom, or heart block may be found unexpectedly on routine physical examination. Complete cardiac evaluation, including echocardiography and Holter monitoring, is necessary to assess the patient for ventricular dysfunction and to relate any symptoms to concurrent arrhythmias.

Treatment

In patients thought to be at risk for syncope, CHF, or sudden death, the treatment of choice for complete heart block is insertion of a permanent pacemaker. Until permanent pacing can be instituted, patients can be assisted temporarily by infusions of isoproterenol or by temporary transcutaneous pacemakers.

Eronen M et al: Short- and long-term outcome of children with congenital complete heart block diagnosed in utero or as a newborn. Pediatrics 2000;106(1 Pt 1):86 [PMID: 10878154].

Moak JP et al: Congenital heart block: Development of late-onset cardiomyopathy, a previously underappreciated sequela. J Am Coll Cardiol 2001;37:238 [PMID: 11153745].

SYNCOPE (Fainting)

Syncope is a sudden transient loss of consciousness that resolves spontaneously. The common form of syncope (simple fainting) occurs in 15% of children and is a disorder of control of heart rate and blood pressure by the autonomic nervous system that causes hypotension or bradycardia. It is often associated with rapid rising and postural hypotension, prolonged standing, or hypovolemia. Patients exhibit vagal symptoms such as pallor, nausea, or diaphoresis. Syncope, also known as autonomic dysfunction, can be evaluated with head-up tilt table testing. The patient is placed supine on a tilt table, and then—under constant heart rate and blood pressure monitoring—is tilted to the upright position. If symptoms develop, they can be classified as vasodepressor (hypotension), cardioinhibitory (bradycardia), or mixed.

Syncope is usually self-limited (lasting approximately 6 months to 2 years) and can be controlled with dietary salt and volume loading to prevent hypovolemia. In refractory cases, medications to manipulate the autonomic nervous system have been useful. Fludrocortisone (0.1 mg/kg/d) is a mineralocorticoid that causes renal salt resorption and thus increases intravascular volume. β-Blockade (atenolol, 0.5–2.0 mg/kg/d) can inhibit the catecholamine surge and help prevent the rebound bradycardia and hypotension. Vagolytic agents (disopyramide 2.5 mg/kg qid) help control hypervagotonia, and the selective serotonin reuptake inhibitors have also been effective in alleviating symptoms. Syncope that occurs during exercise or stress or is associated with a positive family history is a warning sign that a serious underlying dysrhythmia may be present, calling for further investigation.

Johnsrude CL: Current approach to pediatric syncope. Pediatr Cardiol 2000;21:522 [PMID: 11050276].

Gastrointestinal Tract

Judith M. Sondheimer, MD

20

EVALUATION OF THE CHILD WITH VOMITING

Assessment of the child with recurrent vomiting starts with a complete history, physical examination, and description of the vomitus (Table 20–1). Emesis of gastric contents is characteristic of gastroesophageal (GE) reflux, gastric outlet obstruction, central nervous system masses or infection, peptic disease, urinary tract infection, otitis or sinusitis, metabolic diseases (especially those causing acidosis), rumination, and psychogenic vomiting. GE reflux should be suspected in a healthy child with effortless postprandial spitting. An upper gastrointestinal (GI) series is essential to rule out anatomic causes in young infants. A urinalysis and culture will rule out urinary tract infection or urinary obstruction especially in young infants. Serum electrolyte abnormalities, especially of sodium, potassium, magnesium, and calcium may interfere with gastric and intestinal motor function. Increased intracranial pressure may cause vomiting. The decision to obtain radiographs and scans of the central nervous system, chest, or sinuses is based on specific indications from the history or physical examination.

The infant or child with bilious emesis should be suspected of intestinal obstruction and should be evaluated immediately. Bile staining may be gold or green in color. The history and physical examination should include duration of vomiting, the presence of blood in the vomitus, the presence of abdominal pain or distention, the character of the stools, and the presence of fever. Pain localized to the right lower quadrant suggests appendicitis. Midline or diffuse abdominal pain suggests pancreatitis or generalized peritonitis. Abdominal distention suggests intestinal obstruction. Viral and bacterial gastroenteritis are associated with diarrhea and may produce ileus with bilious vomiting. Gallbladder disease is uncommon in childhood but should be suspected when there is a family or personal history of hemolytic disorders, hypercholesterolemia, or other conditions promoting gallstones. Mucus and blood in the stool suggests intussusception or bacterial or toxic colitis. Three-way abdominal radiographs are a first step in localizing the site of intestinal obstruction.

The evaluation of bloody vomitus starts by confirming that the material vomited is indeed blood. Swallowed maternal blood in newborns, oropharyngeal lesions, nosebleed, peptic disease, bleeding disorders, foreign bodies, and esophageal varices may cause hematemesis. A Mallory–Weiss mucosal tear at the GE junction is common after prolonged vomiting. If there is significant blood loss, assessment of cardiovascular stability is important before diagnostic studies. Passage of a nasogastric tube will determine whether bleeding is ongoing. The hematocrit should be measured. The most productive diagnostic test is upper intestinal endoscopy.

GASTROESOPHAGEAL REFLUX

GE reflux is common in young infants and usually resolves spontaneously by the age of walking. Postprandial regurgitation, which ranges from effortless to forceful, is the most common symptom in infants with GE reflux. The condition is usually harmless in young infants, but may rarely cause failure to thrive, esophagitis, blood loss, anemia, esophageal stricture, and inflammatory esophageal polyps. Aspiration pneumonia, chronic cough, wheezing, and asthmalike attacks are reported. Dysphagia, colic after feedings, and neck contortions (Sandifer syndrome) may occur. Rumination is sometimes a symptom. Apneic spells in young infants, especially occurring with position change after feeding, may be a result of reflux. GE reflux is common in neurologically impaired children. The underlying cause of GE reflux is unknown, but the facilitating mechanism is probably spontaneous relaxation of the lower esophageal sphincter not chronic weakness or immaturity of the sphincter.

GE reflux is a clinical diagnosis in thriving infants younger than age 6 months. An upper GI series rules out anatomic causes of vomiting, but is not an accurate test for GE reflux because of the 30% false-positive rate. Prolonged monitoring of esophageal pH is a more sensitive test which quantitates the amount of acid reflux time. Esophageal intraluminal impedance monitoring is a pH-independent means to detect fluid movement in the esophagus. Impedance studies show that nonacid reflux occurs frequently and also confirm the persistence of reflux in the presence of acid-suppressing medications. Esophagoscopy is not diagnostic, but esophagitis can be identified.

Table 20–1. Causes of vomiting and regurgitation.

GASTROINTESTINAL TRACT DISORDERS	
Esophagus	**Intestine and colon**
Achalasia	Atresia and stenosis
Gastroesophageal	Meconium ileus
reflux (chalasia)	Malrotation, volvulus
Hiatal hernia	Duplication
Esophagitis	Intussusception
Atresia with or without	Foreign body
fistula	Polyposis
Congenital vascular or	Soy or cow's milk protein
mucosal rings, webs	intolerance
Stenosis	Gluten enteropathy
Duplication and divertic-	Food allergy
ulum	Hirschsprung disease
Foreign body	Chronic intestinal pseudo-
Periesophageal mass	obstruction
Stomach	Appendicitis
Hypertrophic pyloric	Inflammatory bowel disease
stenosis	Gastroenteritis, infections
Pylorospasm	**Other abdominal organs**
Diaphragmatic hernia	Hepatitis
Peptic disease and	Gallstones
gastritis	Pancreatitis
Antral web	Peritonitis
Duodenum	
Annular pancreas	
Duodenitis and ulcer	
Duodenul stenosis/atresia	
Malrotation	
Mesenteric bands	
Superior mesenteric	
artery syndrome	

EXTRAGASTROINTESTINAL TRACT DISORDERS	
Sepsis	Adrenal insufficiency
Pneumonia	Renal tubular acidosis
Otitis media	Inborn errors
Urinary tract infection	Urea cycle disorders
Meningitis	Phenylketonuria
Subdural effusion	Maple syrup urine disease
Hydrocephalus	Organic acidemia
Brain tumor	Galactosemia
Reye syndrome	Fructose intolerance
Rumination	Tyrosinosis
Intoxications	Scleroderma
Alcohol	Epidermolysis bullosa
Aspirin	
Acetaminophen	

Treatment & Prognosis

In 85% of infants with GE reflux, the condition resolves spontaneously by 12 months, coincident with assumption of erect posture and initiation of solid feedings. Regurgitation may be reduced by offering small feedings at frequent intervals and by thickening feedings with rice cereal (2–3 tsp/oz of formula). Prethickened antireflux formulas are available. Histamine (H2)-receptor antagonists (ranitidine, 5 mg/kg/d in two doses) and proton pump inhibitors (omeprazole, 0.5–1.0 mg/kg/d in one dose) may control pain and prevent esophagitis. Prokinetic agents such as metoclopramide may hasten gastric emptying and improve esophageal motor function, but studies have not supported their efficacy in controlling symptoms.

Antireflux surgery is indicated if reflux causes (1) persistent vomiting with failure to thrive, (2) esophagitis or esophageal stricture, and (3) apneic spells or chronic pulmonary disease unresponsive to 2–3 months of medical therapy. Children older than age 18 months with large hiatal hernias or with neurologic handicaps respond less well to medical therapy.

Rudolph CD et al: Guidelines for evaluation and treatment of gastroesophageal reflux in infants and children: Recommendations of the North American Society for Pediatric Gastroenterology and Nutrition. J Pediatr Gastroenterol Nutr 2001; 23(Suppl):1 [PMID: 11525610].

ACHALASIA OF THE ESOPHAGUS

Esophageal achalasia is characterized by failure of relaxation of the lower esophageal sphincter and abnormal, nonperistaltic motor activity in the esophageal body.

Clinical Findings

A. SYMPTOMS AND SIGNS

Achalasia is uncommon in children younger than age 5 years. Symptoms include retrosternal pain and episodic sensation of food impaction. Patients eat slowly and may drink large amounts of fluid with meals. Dysphagia is relieved by repeated forceful swallowing or by vomiting. Familial cases have been described in Allgrove syndrome (alacrima, adrenal insufficiency, and achalasia) and in familial dysautonomia. Chronic cough, wheezing, recurrent aspiration pneumonitis, anemia, and poor weight gain are common.

B. IMAGING AND MANOMETRIC STUDIES

Barium esophagagram shows a dilated esophagus with a tapered "beak" at the GE junction. Esophageal dilation may not be present in infants presumably because of the short duration of obstruction. Fluoroscopy may show disordered esophageal peristalsis. Esophageal manometry may show high resting pressure in the lower esophageal sphincter, failure of the sphincter to relax with swallowing, and abnormal or absent esophageal peristalsis. The cause is unknown. Decrease in neuronal nitric oxide synthetase (nNOS) has been described in the tissues of the lower esophageal sphincter causing a local deficiency of nitric oxide that prevents normal sphincter relaxation. It is unclear whether the lack of nNOS is secondary or primary. In achalasia associated with Chagas disease nNOS is also reduced and ganglion cells may be decreased or absent in the muscular layers near the lower esophageal sphincter secondary to infection.

Differential Diagnosis

Congenital or peptic esophageal stricture, esophageal webs, and esophageal masses may mimic achalasia. Intestinal pseudoobstruction, multiple endocrine neoplasia IIb, systemic amyloidosis, and postvagotomy syndrome also cause esophageal dysmotility and symptoms similar to achalasia.

Treatment & Prognosis

Pneumatic dilation of the lower esophageal sphincter produces temporary relief of obstruction that may last weeks to years. Botulinum toxin injected into the lower esophageal sphincter may paralyze the sphincter and temporarily relieve obstruction. More long-lasting relief of obstruction is achieved by surgically dividing the lower esophageal sphincter (Heller myotomy). The procedure can be performed laparoscopically or thoracoscopically. Because of the shorter duration of esophageal obstruction with less secondary dilation of the esophagus in children, the prognosis for return of some normal esophageal motor function after surgery is better than in adults.

Hussain SZ et al: A review of achalasia in 33 children. Dig Dis Sci 2002;47:2538 [PMID: 12452392].

CAUSTIC BURNS OF THE ESOPHAGUS

Ingestion of caustic solids or liquids (pH > 12) may produce esophageal lesions ranging from superficial inflammation to coagulative necrosis with ulceration, perforation, and mediastinitis or peritonitis. The severity of immediate oral or laryngeal injury after ingestion does not always correlate with the degree of esophageal injury. Esophageal or laryngeal obstruction from edema and exudate may occur within 24 hours. Pain may be severe. Strictures of the esophagus may develop quickly or gradually over several months. Strictures develop in areas of anatomic narrowing (thoracic inlet, GE junction, or point of compression where the left bronchus crosses the esophagus), presumably where contact with the caustic agent is more prolonged. Stricture occurs only with full-thickness esophageal necrosis. Shortening of the esophagus is a late complication of long strictures that may cause hiatal hernia.

The lips, mouth, and airway should be examined in a child with suspected alkali ingestion. Vomiting should not be induced. Drooling is common and is not an accurate reflection of severity of esophageal burns. Oral injury is common with solid caustic agents. Intravenous corticosteroids (eg, methylprednisolone, 1–2 mg/kg/d) are given immediately to reduce oral swelling and laryngeal edema. Intravenous fluids are necessary if dysphagia prevents oral intake. Esophagoscopy, if needed, should be done within 24–48 hours after ingestion before liquefaction of tissues is complete. Treatment may be stopped if only first-degree burns are present. Corticosteroids may be beneficial in first- and second-degree burns, but do not prevent stricture formation from circumferential third-degree burns. Repeated esophageal dilations may be necessary as a stricture develops but are not performed acutely. When radiographs show erosion into the mediastinum or peritoneum, antibiotics are mandatory. Intraluminal esophageal stenting may be beneficial during early management. Surgical replacement of the esophagus by colon interposition or gastric tube may be needed for long strictures resistant to dilation.

Although agents such as bleach, detergents, and acids may cause esophageal irritation, it is rare for any but the strongest acids and detergents to produce full-thickness necrosis and stricture.

Del Rosario JF, Orenstein SR: Common pediatric esophageal disorders. Gastroenterologist 1998;6:104 [PMID: 9660528].

HIATAL HERNIA

Hiatal hernias are classified as paraesophageal, in which the esophagus and GE junction are normally placed with the gastric cardia herniated beside the esophagus through the diaphragmatic hiatus; or sliding, in which the GE junction and a portion of the proximal stomach are located above the diaphragmatic hiatus. Paraesophageal hernia is rare in childhood and presents with pain, esophageal obstruction, or respiratory compromise. The most common cause of paraesophageal hernia is previous fundoplication. Sliding hernia is common. GE reflux may accompany sliding hiatal hernia, although most produce no symptoms. Surgery is indicated if paraesophageal or hiatus hernia produce persistent symptoms.

PYLORIC STENOSIS

The cause of postnatal pyloric circular muscle hypertrophy with gastric outlet obstruction is unknown. The incidence is 1–8 per 1000 births, with a 4:1 male predominance. A positive family history is present in 13% of patients. Recent studies suggest that erythromycin in the neonatal period is associated with a higher incidence of pyloric stenosis in infants less than 30 days.

CLINICAL FINDINGS

A. SYMPTOMS AND SIGNS

Vomiting usually begins between 2 and 4 weeks of age and rapidly becomes projectile after every feeding. Vomiting starts at birth in about 10% of cases. Onset of symptoms may be delayed in premature infants. The vomitus is rarely bilious but may be blood-streaked. Infants are usually hungry and nurse avidly. Constipation, dehydration, weight loss, fretfulness, and finally apathy occur. The upper abdomen may be distended after feeding, and prominent gastric peristaltic waves from left to right may be seen. An olive-sized mass can be felt on deep palpation in the right upper abdomen, especially after the child has vomited.

B. LABORATORY FINDINGS

Hypochloremic alkalosis with potassium depletion occurs. Dehydration causes elevated hemoglobin and hematocrit. Mild unconjugated bilirubinemia occurs in 2–5% of cases.

C. IMAGING

An upper GI series reveals retention of contrast in the stomach and a long narrow pyloric channel with a double track of barium. The hypertrophied muscle mass produces typical semilunar filling defects in the antrum. Isolated pylorospasm is common in young infants, and by itself is insufficient to make a diagnosis of pyloric stenosis. Ultrasonography shows a hypoechoic muscle ring greater than 4-mm thick with a hyperdense center.

Treatment & Prognosis

Pyloromyotomy is the treatment of choice and consists of incision down to the mucosa along the pyloric length. The procedure can be performed laparoscopically. Treatment of dehydration and electrolyte imbalance is mandatory before surgical treatment, even if it takes 24–48 hours. The outlook after surgery is excellent. Patients often vomit postoperatively as a consequence of gastritis, esophagitis, or associated GE reflux. The postoperative barium radiograph remains abnormal despite relief of symptoms.

Fugimoto T et al: Laparoscopic extramucosal pyloromyotomy versus open pyloromyotomy for infantile hypertrophic pyloric stenosis: Which is better? J Pediatr Surg 1999;34:370 [PMID: 10052826].

Mahon BE et al: Maternal and infant use of erythromycin and other macrolide antibiotics as risk factors for infantile hypertrophic pyloric stenosis. J Pediatr 2001;139:380 [PMID: 11562617].

PEPTIC DISEASE

Peptic ulcers occur at any age but are more common between 12 and 18 years. Boys are affected more frequently than girls. Most ulcers in childhood are secondary to underlying illness, toxins, or drugs causing breakdown in normal mucosal defenses. Causes include (1) reduced mucosal protective mechanisms (aspirin, nonsteroidal anti-inflammatory drugs, hypoxia and hypoperfusion);

(2) reduced metabolic activity of the mucosal cell, which allows for diffusion of hydrogen ions into the mucosa (hypoxia, hypotension); (3) increased secretion of acid or pepsin (increased parietal cell mass, increased postprandial secretion of gastrin, increased vagal tone); (4) reflux of bile from duodenum to stomach; and (5) decreased neutralizing activity in duodenal secretions. *Helicobacter pylori* infection of the gastric antrum produces nodular antral gastritis, duodenal ulcer, and gastric ulcer. There is no evidence that *H pylori* infection causes recurrent abdominal pain of childhood or dyspepsia without gastritis. Between 10 and 20% of North American children are *H pylori*–antibody-positive. Prevalence increases with age, in areas with poor sanitation and in families with an infected member. Diagnosis of *H pylori* infection requires seeing organisms in gastric antral tissue, finding urease activity in the stomach either by testing antral tissue directly (CLO test) or indirectly (urease breath hydrogen test). Serum antibody positivity does not prove active *H pylori* infection.

Clinical Findings

A. SYMPTOMS AND SIGNS

In children younger than 6 years, vomiting and upper GI bleeding are the most common symptoms of peptic ulcer. Older children are more likely to complain of abdominal pain. Acute *H pylori* gastritis is characterized by vomiting and hematemesis. Chronically, ulcers in the pyloric channel may cause gastric outlet obstruction. Illnesses predisposing to secondary ulcers include central nervous system disease, burns, sepsis, and multiorgan system failure. Pulmonary insufficiency, Crohn disease, hepatic cirrhosis, and rheumatoid arthritis are associated with peptic disease. Upper GI bleeding requiring transfusion is more common in secondary (aspirin, alcohol, and especially nonsteroidal anti-inflammatory drug [NSAID] ingestion especially) than primary ulcers. Ulcers may occur throughout the upper GI tract secondary to NSAIDs. The use of specific cyclooxygenase-2 (COX-2) inhibitors instead of standard NSAIDs and aspirin—which inhibit both COX-1 and COX-2 enzymes—may result in a decrease in NSAID-associated complications. COX-1 regulates the production of thromboxane from arachidonic acid and decreases platelet aggregation with a resultant increase in bleeding tendency. COX-2, an inducible enzyme present in many tissues, regulates prostaglandin synthesis. COX-2 inhibition has a purer anti-inflammatory and analgesic effect with a reduced tendency to produce GI complications. Cardiac complications of COX-2 inhibitors have recently limited their use.

B. IMAGING AND ENDOSCOPY

Upper GI barium radiograph may show an ulcer crater. Soft signs suggestive of peptic disease in adults (duodenal spasticity and thick irregular folds) are not reliable indicators of peptic disease in children. Upper intestinal endoscopy is the most accurate test for peptic disease. It also allows for identification of other causes of peptic symptoms such as esophagitis, eosinophilic enteropathy, and celiac disease.

Treatment

Acid suppression or neutralization is the mainstay of peptic ulcer therapy. Liquid antacids are usually unacceptable to children in the volumes needed to neutralize gastric acid. H2-receptor antagonists and proton pump inhibitors are more effective and usually produce endoscopic healing in 4–8 weeks. Bland "ulcer diets" are not indicated in children. Foods causing pain should be avoided. Caffeine should be avoided because it increases gastric acid secretion. Aspirin and NSAIDs should not be used.

Treatment of the peptic disease associated with *H pylori* infection requires eradication of the organism. The optimal therapeutic regimen is still undetermined. The combination of amoxicillin, metronidazole, and bismuth subsalicylate for 10–14 days and omeprazole and amoxicillin, are both effective. Clarithromycin for 7 days with a proton pump inhibitor for 6 weeks is also effective. Resistance to antibiotics is common. An unresolved clinical question is whether recurrent courses of antibiotics should be used to eradicate *H pylori*. There is some epidemiologic data suggesting that the incidence of chronic GE reflux and Barrett esophagus in increasing in white males as a consequence of aggressive eradication of *H pylori*.

Crone J et al: *Helicobacter pylori* in children and adolescents: Increasing primary clarithromycin resistance 1997–2000. J Pediatr Gastroenterol Nutr 2003;36:368 [PMID: 12604976].

Suerbaum S, Michetti P: *Helicobacter pylori* infection. N Engl J Med 2002;347:1175 [PMID: 12374879].

Vakil N: Primary and secondary treatment of *Helicobacter pylori* in the United States. Rev Gastroenterol Disord 2005;5:67 [PMID: 15976737].

CONGENITAL DIAPHRAGMATIC HERNIA

Herniation of abdominal contents through the diaphragm usually occurs through a posterolateral defect in the diaphragm (foramen of Bochdalek). In about 5% of cases the diaphragmatic defect is retrosternal (foramen of Morgagni). Hernias result from failure of the diaphragmatic anlagen to fuse and divide the thoracic and abdominal cavities at 8–10 weeks gestation. All degrees of protrusion of the abdominal viscera through the diaphragmatic opening may occur. Eighty percent of posterolateral defects involve the left diaphragm. In eventration of the diaphragm, a leaf of the diaphragm with hypoplastic muscular elements balloons into the chest and leads to similar but milder symptoms.

Mild to severe respiratory distress is usually present at birth. The abdomen may be scaphoid because of displacement of the viscera. Breath sounds in the affected hemithorax are absent, and the maximal cardiac impulse is displaced. Thirty percent of newborn infants with diaphragmatic hernia die, mostly from pulmonary insufficiency. The lung on the affected side and even on the contralateral side may be hypoplastic, with decreased generations of airways, lymphatics, and pulmonary vessels. Pulmonary hypertension is present. Other complications include mediastinal shift with vascular kinking, pulmonary infection, prematurity, cardiac anomalies, and intestinal malrotation. Extracorporeal membrane oxygenation may decrease the early postoperative mortality rate in patients with poor lung compliance. Inhaled nitric oxide reduces pulmonary vascular hypertension, and it was hoped that it might improve the outcome of neonates with diaphragmatic hernia. Results in controlled trials have been disappointing. Occasionally, a diaphragmatic hernia is first identified in an older infant or child during incidental radiograph or routine physical examination. These children usually have a more favorable prognosis than neonates.

CONGENITAL DUODENAL OBSTRUCTION

Extrinsic duodenal obstruction is usually due to congenital peritoneal bands associated with intestinal malrotation, annular pancreas, or duodenal duplication. Intrinsic obstruction is caused by stenosis, mucosal diaphragm (so-called wind sock deformity), or duodenal atresia. The duodenal lumen may be obliterated by a membrane or completely interrupted with a fibrous cord between the two segments. Atresia is more often distal to the ampulla of Vater than proximal.

Clinical Findings

A. ATRESIA

Maternal polyhydramnios is common and often leads to an intrauterine diagnosis by ultrasonography. Vomiting (usually bile-stained) and epigastric distention begin within a few hours of birth. Meconium may be passed normally. Duodenal atresia is often associated with other congenital anomalies (30%), including esophageal atresia, other intestinal atresias, and cardiac and renal anomalies. Prematurity (25–50%) and Down syndrome (20–30%) are associated conditions. Abdominal radiographs show gaseous distention of the stomach and proximal duodenum (the "double-bubble" radiologic sign). With protracted vomiting, less air may be in the stomach. Absence of gas distal to the obstruction suggests atresia or severe extrinsic obstruction, whereas air scattered over the lower abdomen may indicate a partial duodenal obstruction. Barium enema may be helpful in determining the presence of malrotation or atresia lower in the GI tract.

B. DUODENAL STENOSIS

Obvious symptoms of duodenal obstruction may be delayed for weeks or years. Although the stenotic area is usually beyond the ampulla of Vater, the vomitus does not always contain bile.

Treatment & Prognosis

Duodenoduodenostomy is performed to bypass stenosis or atresia. Thorough surgical exploration is done to ensure that no anomalies are present lower in the GI tract. The mortality rate is significantly increased in infants with prematurity, Down syndrome, and associated congenital anomalies. Duodenal dilation and hypomotility from antenatal obstruction may cause functional obstructive symptoms even after surgical treatment.

CONGENITAL INTESTINAL ATRESIAS & STENOSES

Excluding anal anomalies, intestinal atresia and stenosis account for one-third of all cases of neonatal intestinal obstruction. Antenatal ultrasound can identify intestinal atresia in utero, and polyhydramnios occurs in most affected pregnancies. Prematurity and other congenital anomalies may be present. The localization and relative incidence of atresias and stenoses are listed in Table 20–2.

Bile-stained vomiting and abdominal distention usually begin in the first 48 hours of life. Atresias, stenoses, and

Table 20–2. Localization and relative frequency of congenital gastrointestinal atresias and stenoses.

	Area Involved	Type of Lesion	Relative Frequency
Pylorus		Atresia; web or diaphragm	1%
Duodenum	80% are distal to the ampulla of Vater	Atresia, stenosis; web or diaphragm	45%
Jejunoileal	Proximal jejunum and distal ileum	Atresia (multiple in 6–29%); stenosis	50%
Colon	Left colon and rectum	Atresia (usually associated with atresias of the small bowel)	5–9%

obstructing membranes may affect multiple sites. The small intestine may be shortened significantly. Radiographic features include dilated loops of small bowel and absence of colonic gas. Barium enema reveals narrow-caliber microcolon if the atresia is in the lower small bowel. In over 10% of patients with intestinal atresia the mesentery is absent, and the superior mesenteric artery cannot be identified beyond the origin of the right colic and ileocolic arteries. The ileum coils around one of these two arteries, giving rise to the so-called Christmas tree deformity. The tenuous blood supply often compromises surgical anastomoses. The differential diagnosis includes Hirschsprung disease; paralytic ileus secondary to sepsis, gastroenteritis, or pneumonia; midgut volvulus; and meconium ileus. Surgery is mandatory. Postoperative complications include short bowel syndrome and small bowel hypomotility secondary to antenatal obstruction.

ANNULAR PANCREAS

Annular pancreas is a rotational defect preventing normal fusion of the dorsal and ventral pancreatic anlage. The presentation is that of duodenal obstruction. Down syndrome and congenital anomalies of the GI tract occur frequently. Polyhydramnios is common. Symptoms may develop late in childhood if the obstruction is less than complete. Treatment consists of duodenoduodenostomy or duodenojejunostomy without operative dissection or division of the pancreatic annulus.

INTESTINAL MALROTATION WITH OR WITHOUT VOLVULUS

The midgut, which extends from the duodenojejunal junction to the mid transverse colon, is supplied by the superior mesenteric artery, which runs in the root of the mesentery. During gestation, the midgut elongates into the umbilical sac, returning to an intra-abdominal position during the 10th week of gestation. The root of the mesentery rotates in a counterclockwise direction during retraction causing the colon to cross the abdominal cavity ventrally. The cecum moves from the left to the right lower quadrant, and the duodenum crosses dorsally and becomes partly retroperitoneal. When rotation is incomplete, the dorsal fixation of the mesentery is defective and shortened, so that the bowel from the ligament of Treitz to the mid transverse colon may rotate around its narrow mesenteric root and occlude the superior mesenteric artery (volvulus).

Clinical Findings

A. SYMPTOMS AND SIGNS

Malrotation accounts for 10% of neonatal intestinal obstructions. Most infants present in the first 3 weeks of life with bile-stained vomiting or acute small bowel obstruction. Intrauterine volvulus may occur and the infant is obstructed or perforated at birth. The neonate may present with ascites. Later presenting signs include intermittent intestinal obstruction, malabsorption, protein-losing enteropathy, or diarrhea. Associated congenital anomalies, especially cardiac, occur in over 25% of symptomatic patients.

B. IMAGING

An upper GI series shows the duodenojejunal junction and the jejunum on the right side of the spine. The diagnosis of malrotation can be further confirmed by barium enema, which may demonstrate a mobile cecum located in the midline, right upper quadrant, or left abdomen.

Treatment & Prognosis

Surgical treatment of malrotation is by the Ladd procedure. In young infants the Ladd procedure should be performed even in the absence of volvulus. The duodenum is mobilized and the short mesenteric root is extended. Treatment of malrotation discovered in children older than age 12 months is uncertain. Because volvulus can occur at any age, surgical repair is usually recommended, even in asymptomatic children. Laparoscopic repair of malrotation is possible but may be technically difficult and is never performed in the presence of volvulus.

Midgut volvulus is a surgical emergency. Bowel necrosis results from occlusion of the superior mesenteric artery. When necrosis is extensive, it is recommended that a first operation include only reduction of the volvulus with lysis of mesenteric bands. Resection of necrotic bowel should be delayed if possible until a second-look operation 24–48 hours later can be undertaken in the hope that more bowel can be salvaged. The prognosis is guarded if perforation, peritonitis, or extensive intestinal necrosis is present.

Complications

If bowel necrosis is extensive, the infant may be left with an intestinal length insufficient to support normal absorption and growth. Estimates of the small bowel length of a newborn range from 150–300 cm. The commonly accepted definition of neonatal short bowel syndrome is removal of more than 50% of the small intestinal length. In these patients, it is almost certain that intravenous nutrition will be required for months to years to support growth. The most common cause of neonatal short bowel syndrome varies with the patient referral patterns of the institution, but includes necrotizing enterocolitis (45%), intestinal atresias (23%), gastroschisis (15%), volvulus (15%), and, less commonly, entities such as congenital short bowel and extensive

Hirschsprung disease. Although shortened intestine remaining after resection does not undergo compensatory increase in length, if nutrition can be maintained enterocytes will proliferate on lengthened villi and the intestine will elongate in proportion to the child's increasing height. These adaptations may eventually be sufficient for the patient's nutritional needs. Achieving independence from intravenous nutrition is less likely when less than 30 cm of small intestine remains after surgery. An intact colon and intact ileocecal sphincter are factors improving prognosis in short bowel syndrome. Liver failure, a consequence of intravenous nutrition, recurrent infection, and other injuries is the most common cause of death in patients with short bowel syndrome. Mortality among all infants with short bowel syndrome is about 10–15%.

Adzick NS, Nance ML: Pediatric surgery: First of two parts. N Engl J Med 2000;342:1651.

Adzick NS, Nance ML: Pediatric surgery: Second of two parts. N Engl J Med 2000;342:1726.

Andorsky DJ et al: Nutritional and other post operative management of neonates with short bowel syndrome correlates with clinical outcomes. J Pediatr 2001;139:27.

Sigalet DL: Short bowel syndrome in infants and children, an overview. Semin Pediatr Surg 2001;10:49.

MECKEL DIVERTICULUM & OMPHALOMESENTERIC DUCT REMNANTS

1. Meckel Diverticulum

Meckel diverticulum is the most common of the omphalomesenteric duct remnants. It is usually found on the antimesenteric border of the mid to distal ileum and is found in 1.5% of the population. It rarely causes symptoms. In addition to ileal mucosa, diverticula may contain gastric, pancreatic, jejunal, or colonic mucosa. Familial cases have been reported. Complications occur three times more frequently in males than in females, and in 50–60% of cases complications occur in the first 2 years of life. Acid secreted by heterotopic gastric tissue causes ulceration and bleeding from adjacent ileal mucosa.

Clinical Findings

A. SYMPTOMS AND SIGNS

Forty to sixty percent of symptomatic patients experience episodes of painless rectal passage of maroon or melanotic blood. Bleeding may be voluminous enough to cause shock and anemia. Occult bleeding is less common. Intestinal obstruction occurs in 25% of symptomatic patients as a result of ileocolonic intussusception. Intestinal volvulus may occur around a fibrous remnant of the vitelline duct extending from the tip of the diverticulum to the abdominal wall. In some patients, entrapment of bowel under a band running between the diverticulum and the base of the mesentery occurs. Meckel diverticula may be trapped in an inguinal hernia (Littre hernia). Diverticulitis occurs in 10–20% of symptomatic patients and is clinically indistinguishable from acute appendicitis. Perforation and peritonitis may occur. Chronic recurrent abdominal pain is rarely the only symptom.

B. IMAGING

Diagnosis of Meckel diverticulum is seldom made on barium radiograph. Radionuclide imaging uses technetium-99m (^{99m}Tc)-pertechnetate, which is taken up by the heterotopic gastric mucosa in the diverticulum. Stimulation of ^{99m}Tc-pertechnetate uptake and retention by the heterotopic gastric mucosa using pentagastrin or cimetidine before scanning can reduce the number of false-negative results. Angiography or tagged red cell scan may be useful when bleeding is brisk.

Treatment & Prognosis

Treatment is surgical. At laparoscopy or laparotomy, the ileum proximal and distal to the diverticulum may reveal ulcerations and some heterotopic gastric tissue adjacent to the neck of the diverticulum. The prognosis for Meckel diverticulum is good.

2. Other Remnants of the Omphalomesenteric Duct

Fecal discharge from the umbilicus suggests a patent omphalomesenteric duct. The duct may be completely closed forming a fibrous cord between ileum and umbilicus which may become the origin of a volvulus. Mucoid umbilical discharge may indicate a mucocele in the omphalomesenteric remnant. Mucocele may protrude through the umbilicus and be mistaken for an umbilical granuloma because it is firm and bright red. Cauterization of a mucocele is not recommended. Surgical excision of omphalomesenteric remnants is indicated.

DUPLICATIONS OF THE GASTROINTESTINAL TRACT

Duplications are congenital anomalies of the GI tract. They are spherical or tubular structures found anywhere along the GI tract, most commonly in the ileum. Duplications usually contain fluid and sometimes blood if necrosis has taken place. Most duplications do not communicate with the intestinal lumen but are attached to the mesenteric side of the gut and share a common muscular coat. The epithelial lining of the duplication is usually of the same type as that from which it originates. Some duplications (neuroenteric cysts) are attached to the spinal cord and are associated with hemivertebrae and anterior or posterior spina bifida.

Symptoms of vomiting, abdominal distention, colicky pain, rectal bleeding, partial or total intestinal obstruction, or an abdominal mass may start in infancy. Diarrhea and malabsorption may result from bacterial overgrowth in communicating duplications. Physical examination may reveal a rounded, smooth, movable mass, and barium radiograph or computed tomography of the abdomen may show a noncalcified cystic mass displacing the intestines or stomach. Scanning with ^{99m}Tc-pertechnetate may help identify duplications containing gastric mucosa. Involvement of the terminal small bowel can give rise to an intussusception. Prompt surgical treatment is indicated.

CONGENITAL AGANGLIONIC MEGACOLON (Hirschsprung Disease)

Hirschsprung disease results from an absence of ganglion cells in the mucosal and muscular layers of the colon. Neural crest cells fail to migrate into the mesodermal layers of the gut during gestation, possibly a result of abnormal end-organ cell surface receptors or local deficiency of nitric oxide synthesis. The absence of ganglion cells results in failure of the colon to relax in front of an advancing bolus. The rectum (30%) or rectosigmoid (44%) is usually affected. The entire colon may be aganglionic (8%). Segmental aganglionosis is very rare and is probably an acquired lesion. The aganglionic segment has a normal or slightly narrowed caliber with dilation of the normal colon proximal to the obstructing aganglionic segment. The mucosa of the dilated colonic segment may become thin and inflamed (enterocolitis), causing diarrhea, bleeding, and protein loss.

A familial pattern has been described, particularly in total colonic aganglionosis. The disease is four times more common in boys than girls, and 10–15% of patients have Down syndrome. Specific mutations in the *ret* protooncogene have been identified in about 15% of cases.

Clinical Findings

A. SYMPTOMS AND SIGNS

Failure of the newborn to pass meconium, followed by vomiting, abdominal distention, and reluctance to feed, suggest the diagnosis of Hirschsprung disease. Infants of diabetic mothers may have similar symptoms and, in this setting, small left colon syndrome should be suspected. Meglumine diatrizoate (Gastrografin) enema is both diagnostic and therapeutic as it reveals a meconium plug in the left colon, which is often passed during the diagnostic radiograph. The left colon is narrow but usually functional. In a small proportion of patients with small left colon, Hirschsprung disease may later be found. Enterocolitis manifested by fever, explosive diarrhea, and prostration is reported in about 50% of newborns with this disease. Enterocolitis may lead to acute inflammatory and ischemic changes in the colon, with perforation and sepsis. In some patients with Hirschsprung disease, especially those with short segment involvement, symptoms are not obvious at birth. In later infancy, alternating obstipation and diarrhea predominate. The older child is more likely complain of constipation. The stools are foul-smelling and ribbonlike, the abdomen enlarged, and the veins prominent; peristaltic waves are visible, and fecal masses palpable. Intermittent bouts of intestinal obstruction, hypochromic anemia, hypoproteinemia, and failure to thrive are common. Encopresis is rare.

On digital rectal examination, the anal canal and rectum are devoid of fecal material despite obvious retained stool on abdominal examination or radiograph. If the aganglionic segment is short, there may be a gush of flatus and stool as the finger is withdrawn.

B. LABORATORY FINDINGS

Ganglion cells are absent in both the submucosal and muscular layers of the involved bowel. Special stains may show nerve trunk hypertrophy and increased acetylcholinesterase activity. Ganglionated bowel above the aganglionic segment may be characterized by abnormal location and proliferation of ganglion cells. This finding, intestinal neuronal dysplasia, is sometimes associated with persistent mild to severe motor dysfunction of the unresected colon.

C. IMAGING

Radiographic examination of the abdomen may reveal dilated proximal colon and absence of gas in the pelvic colon. Barium enema using a catheter without a balloon and with the tip inserted barely beyond the anal sphincter usually demonstrates a narrow distal segment with a sharp transition to the proximal dilated colon. This transition zone may not be seen in neonates since the normal proximal bowel has not had time to become dilated. Retention of barium for 24–48 hours is not diagnostic of Hirschsprung disease in older children as it typically occurs in retentive constipation. Barium retention is a more reliable sign in neonates.

D. SPECIAL EXAMINATIONS

Failure of reflex relaxation of the internal anal sphincter after distention of the rectum occurs in all patients with Hirschsprung disease, regardless of the length of the aganglionic segment. In occasional patients, a nonrelaxing internal anal sphincter is the only abnormality. This condition is often called "ultrashort segment Hirschsprung disease."

Differential Diagnosis

Hirschsprung disease accounts for 15–20% of cases of neonatal intestinal obstruction. In childhood, this disease must be differentiated from retentive constipation.

In older infants and children it can be confused with celiac disease because of the striking abdominal distention and failure to thrive.

Treatment

Treatment is surgical. Diverting colostomy (or ileostomy) is performed proximal to the aganglionic segment. Resection of the aganglionic segment may be postponed until the infant is 6 months old. At the time of definitive surgery, the transition zone between ganglionated and nonganglionated bowel is identified. Aganglionic bowel is resected, and a pull-through of ganglionated bowel to the preanal rectal remnant is made. Several surgical techniques, including laparoscopic pull-through, are in use. In children with ultrashort segment disease, an internal anal sphincter myotomy or botulinum toxin injection of the internal anal sphincter may control symptoms.

Prognosis

Complications after surgery include fecal retention, fecal incontinence, anastomotic breakdown, or anastomotic stricture. Postoperative obstruction may result from inadvertent retention of a distal aganglionic colon segment or postoperative destruction of ganglion cells secondary to vascular impairment. Neuronal dysplasia of the remaining bowel may produce a pseudoobstruction syndrome. Enterocolitis occurs postoperatively in 15% of patients.

Gariepy CE: Developmental disorders of the enteric nervous system: Genetic and molecular bases. J Pediatr Gastroenterol Nutr 2004;39:5 [PMID: 15187773].

CHYLOUS ASCITES

Neonatal chylous ascites may be due to congenital infection or developmental abnormality of the lymphatic system (intestinal lymphangiectasia). If the thoracic duct is involved, chylothorax may be present. Later in life, chylous ascites may result from congenital lymphangiectasia, retroperitoneal or lymphatic tumors, peritoneal bands, abdominal trauma, or infection, or it may occur after cardiac or abdominal surgery. It may be associated with intestinal malrotation.

Clinical Findings

A. SYMPTOMS AND SIGNS

In both congenital and acquired lymphatic obstruction, chylous ascites, diarrhea, and failure to thrive occur. The abdomen is distended, with a fluid wave and shifting dullness. Unilateral or generalized peripheral edema may be present.

B. LABORATORY FINDINGS

Laboratory findings include hypoalbuminemia, hypogammaglobulinemia, and lymphopenia. Ascitic fluid contains lymphocytes and has the biochemical composition of chyle if the patient has just been fed; otherwise, it is indistinguishable from ascites secondary to cirrhosis.

Differential Diagnosis

Chylous ascites must be differentiated from ascites due to liver disease and in the older child, from constrictive pericarditis, chronic elevated right heart pressure, malignancy, infection, or inflammatory diseases causing lymphatic obstruction.

Complications & Sequelae

Chylous ascites caused by intestinal lymphatic obstruction is associated with fat malabsorption and protein loss. Intestinal loss of albumin and γ-globulin may lead to edema and increase the risk of infection. Rapidly accumulating chylous ascites may cause respiratory complications. The primary infections and malignancies causing chylous ascites may be life-threatening.

Treatment & Prognosis

Little can be done to correct congenital abnormalities due to hypoplasia, aplasia, or ectasia of the lymphatics. Treatment is supportive, consisting mainly of a very high protein diet and careful attention to infections. Shunting of peritoneal fluid into the venous system is sometimes effective. A fat-free diet supplemented with medium-chain triglycerides decreases the formation of chylous ascites. Total parenteral nutrition may rarely be necessary. Infusions of albumin generally provide only temporary relief and are rarely used for chronic management. In the neonate, congenital chylous ascites may spontaneously disappear following one or more paracenteses and a medium-chain triglyceride diet.

Chye JK et al: Neonatal chylosis ascites: Report of 3 cases and review of the literature. Pediatr Surg Int 1997;12:296 [PMID: 9099650].

CONGENITAL ANORECTAL ANOMALIES

Anorectal anomalies occur once in every 3000–4000 births. Most anomalies except for anterior anus are more common in males. Inspection of the perianal area is an essential part of the newborn physical examination.

Classification & Presentation

A. ANTERIOR DISPLACEMENT OF THE ANUS

This anomaly is more common in girls than boys. Its usual presentation is constipation and straining with stool. The diagnosis of anterior displaced anus depends on finding the anus located close to the base of the scrotum or vaginal fourchette. If the center of the anus is located less than 25% (in girls) or 33% (in boys) of the total distance from vaginal fourchette (or base of scrotum) to coccyx, there is a high likelihood of difficulty with defecation.

B. ANAL STENOSIS

In anal stenosis, the anal aperture may be very small and filled with a dot of meconium. Defecation is difficult, and there may be ribbonlike stools, passage of blood and mucus per rectum, fecal impaction, and abdominal distention. This malformation accounts for about 10% of cases of anorectal anomalies. This anomaly may not be apparent at birth and may be discovered on rectal examination of the infant with straining and mild rectal bleeding as a tight ring in the anal canal. In these cases, the anus is usually normal in appearance.

C. IMPERFORATE ANAL MEMBRANE

The infant with an imperforate anal membrane fails to pass meconium, and a greenish bulging membrane is seen in the anal aperture. After excision, bowel and sphincter function are normal.

D. ANAL AGENESIS

In the child with anal agenesis, an anal dimple is present, and stimulation of the perianal area leads to puckering, indicating that the external sphincter is present. If no associated rectoperineal fistula is present, intestinal obstruction occurs. Fistulas may also be vulvar in the female and urethral in the male.

E. ANORECTAL AGENESIS

Anorectal agenesis accounts for 75% of total anorectal anomalies. Fistulas are almost invariably present. In the female, they may be vaginal or may enter a urogenital sinus, which is a common passageway for the urethra and vagina. In the male, fistulas are rectovesical or rectourethral. Associated major congenital malformations are common. Sacral defects and absence of internal and external anal sphincters are common.

Radiologic Findings

Careful radiologic evaluation is indicated immediately so that the anal anomaly and the extent of associated anomalies of the bowel and the urogenital tract can be identified.

Treatment & Prognosis

Dilation of the anus should be performed in cases of anal stenosis. In mild cases, daily digital dilation at home for several weeks will relieve stenosis. In imperforate anus with anal membrane, treatment includes excision of the membrane and dilation. In anorectal agenesis, diverting colostomy is necessary. In patients with anal agenesis and a perineal fistula of sufficient size to pass stool, surgery can be delayed for some months. Males without a visible fistula may have a urethral fistula, and diverting colostomy is recommended.

In patients with low imperforate anus, 80–90% are continent after surgery. In those with high imperforate anus, only 30% achieve continence. Gracilis muscle transplants may improve continence. Levatorplasty may also be used as a secondary operation following surgery for anorectal agenesis. Antegrade continence enema procedures may allow children to be continent even without anal sphincter function by facilitating complete daily emptying of the colon by irrigation through a cecostomy or appendicostomy.

Endo M et al: Analysis of 1992 patients with anorectal malformations over the past two decades in Japan. J Pediatr Surg 1999;34:435 [PMID: 10211649].

ACUTE ABDOMEN

Conditions causing acute abdomen are shown in Table 20–3. Some conditions are discussed separately. Reaching a speedy and accurate diagnosis in the patient with an acute abdomen is critical and requires skill in physical diagnosis, recognition of the symptoms of a large number of conditions, and a judicious selection of laboratory and radiologic tests.

Gauderer MW: Acute abdomen. When to operate immediately and when to observe. Semin Pediatr Surg 1997;6:74 [PMID: 9159857].

PERITONITIS

Primary bacterial peritonitis accounts for less than 2% of childhood peritonitis. The most common organisms responsible are *Escherichia coli*, other enteric organisms, hemolytic streptococci, and pneumococci. Primary peritonitis occurs in patients with splenectomy, splenic dysfunction, or ascites (nephrotic syndrome, advanced liver disease, kwashiorkor). It also occurs in infants with pyelonephritis or pneumonia. Secondary peritonitis is associated with peritoneal dialysis, penetrating abdominal trauma, or ruptured viscus. The organisms associated with secondary peritonitis vary depending on the cause. Organisms not commonly pathogenic such as *Staphylococcus epidermidis* and *Candida* may be the cause of secondary peritonitis in patients on peritoneal dialysis. Multiple enteric organisms may be isolated after penetrating abdominal injury or bowel perforation. Intra-abdominal abscesses may form in pelvic, subhepatic, or subphrenic areas, but discrete localization of infection is less common in young infants than in adults.

Symptoms of peritonitis include abdominal pain, fever, nausea, and vomiting. Respirations are shallow. The abdo-

Table 20–3. Etiologic classification of acute abdomen.

Mechanical Obstruction		Inflammatory Diseases and Infections			
Intraluminal Obstruction	**Extraluminal Obstruction**	**Gastrointestinal Disease**	**Paralytic Ileus**	**Blunt Trauma**	**Miscellaneous**
Foreign body	Hernia	Appendicitis	Sepsis	Accident	Lead poisoning
Bezoar	Intussusception	Crohn disease	Pneumonia	Battered child	Sickle cell crisis
Fecalith	Volvulus	Ulcerative colitis	Pyelonephritis	syndrome	Familial Mediter-
Gallstone	Duplication	Henoch-Schönlein	Peritonitis		ranean fever
Parasites	Stenosis	purpura and	Pancreatitis		Porphyria
Distal intestinal ob-	Tumor	other causes of	Cholecystitis		Diabetic acidosis
struction syndrome	Mesenteric cyst	vasculitis	Renal and gall-		Addisonian crisis
of cystic fibrosis	Superior mesen-	Peptic ulcer	bladder stones		Torsion of testis
Tumor	teric artery syn-	Meckel diverticulitis	Pelvic inflammation		Torsion of ovarian
Fecaloma	drome	Acute gastroen-	Lymphadenitis due		pedicle
	Pyloric stenosis	teritis	to viral or bacte-		
		Pseudomembra-	rial infection		
		nous enterocolitis			

Reproduced, with permission, from Roy CC, et al: Gastrointestinal emergency problems in paediatric practice. Clin Gastroenterol 1981;10:225.

men is tender, rigid, and distended, with involuntary guarding. Bowel sounds may be absent. Diarrhea is fairly common in primary peritonitis and less so in secondary peritonitis.

The leukocyte count is high initially (> 20,000/μL), with a predominance of immature forms, and later may fall to neutropenic levels, especially in primary peritonitis. Bacterial peritonitis should be suspected if paracentesis fluid contains more than 500 leukocytes/μL or more than 32 mg/dL of lactate; if it has a pH less than 7.34; or if the pH is over 0.1 pH unit less than arterial blood pH. Diagnosis is made by Gram stain and culture, preferably of 5–10 mL of fluid for optimal yield. The blood culture is often positive in primary peritonitis.

Antibiotic treatment and supportive therapy for dehydration, shock, and acidosis are indicated. Surgical treatment of the underlying cause of secondary peritonitis is critical. Removal of infected peritoneal dialysis catheters in patients with secondary peritonitis is sometimes necessary and almost always required if *Candida* infection is present.

ACUTE APPENDICITIS

Acute appendicitis is the most common indication for emergency abdominal surgery in childhood. The frequency increases with age and peaks between 15 and 30 years. Obstruction of the appendix by fecaliths (25%) or parasites is a predisposing factor.

The incidence of perforation is high (40%) in infants and children. To avoid delay in diagnosis, it is important to maintain close communication with parents, perform a thorough physical examination and sequential examinations of the abdomen at frequent intervals over several hours, and interpret correctly the evolving symptoms and signs.

Clinical Findings

A. SYMPTOMS AND SIGNS

The typical child with appendicitis has fever and periumbilical abdominal pain, which then localizes to the right lower quadrant, accompanied by signs of peritoneal irritation. Anorexia, vomiting, constipation, and diarrhea also occur. The clinical picture is often atypical and includes generalized pain and tenderness around the umbilicus without leukocytosis. Rectal examination should always be done and may reveal localized mass or tenderness. Because many conditions cause symptoms mimicking appendicitis and because physical findings are often inconclusive, it is important to perform repeated examinations of the abdomen over several hours. In children younger than age 2 years, the pain of appendicitis is poorly localized, and perforation before surgery is common.

B. LABORATORY FINDINGS

White blood cell counts are seldom higher than 15,000/μL. Pyuria, fecal leukocytes, and guaiac-positive stool are occasionally found.

C. IMAGING

A radiopaque fecalith is reportedly present in two-thirds of cases of ruptured appendix. A positive diagnosis of nonperforated appendicitis cannot be made by barium enema. In experienced hands, ultrasonography of the acutely inflamed appendix shows a noncompressible, thickened appendix in 93% of cases. A localized fluid collection adjacent to or surrounding the appendix may also be seen. Abdominal computed tomography scan after instillation of rectal contrast with thin cuts in the area of the appendix may be diagnostic. Indium-labeled white blood cell scan may localize to an inflamed appendix. Enlarged mesenteric lymph nodes are a nondiagnostic finding.

Differential Diagnosis

The presence of intrathoracic infection (eg, pneumonia) or urinary tract infection should be kept in mind, along with other medical and surgical conditions leading to acute abdomen (see Table 20–3).

Treatment & Prognosis

Exploratory laparotomy or laparoscopy is indicated whenever the diagnosis of appendicitis cannot be ruled out after a period of close observation. Postoperative antibiotic therapy is reserved for patients with gangrenous or perforated appendix. A single intraoperative dose of cefoxitin or cefotetan is recommended for all patients to prevent postoperative complications. The mortality rate is less than 1% during childhood despite the high incidence of perforation. In uncomplicated nonruptured appendicitis, laparoscopic approach is associated with a shortened hospital stay.

Mason JD: The evaluation of acute abdominal pain in children. Emerg Med Clin North Am 1996;14:629 [PMID: 8681888].

INTUSSUSCEPTION

Intussusception is the most frequent cause of intestinal obstruction in the first 2 years of life. It is three times more common in males than in females. In most cases (85%) the cause is not apparent, although polyps, Meckel diverticulum, omphalomesenteric remnants, duplications, Henoch–Schönlein purpura, lymphoma, lipoma, parasites, foreign bodies, and viral enteritis with hypertrophy of Peyer patches are predisposing factors. Intussusception of the small intestine occurs in patients with celiac disease and cystic fibrosis related to the bulk of stool in the terminal ileum. Henoch–Schönlein purpura may also cause isolated small bowel intussusception. In children older than 6 years, lymphoma is the most common cause. Intermittent small bowel intussusception is a rare cause of recurrent abdominal pain.

The usual ileocolic intussusception starts just proximal to the ileocecal valve and extends for varying distances into the colon. Swelling, hemorrhage, incarceration, and necrosis of the intussuscepted bowel may occur. Intestinal perforation and peritonitis occur as a result of impairment of venous return.

Clinical Findings

Characteristically, a thriving infant between the ages of 3 and 12 months develops recurring paroxysms of abdominal pain with screaming and drawing up of the knees. Vomiting and diarrhea occur soon afterward (90% of cases), and bloody bowel movements with mucus appear within the next 12 hours (50%). The child is characteristically lethargic between paroxysms and may become febrile. The abdomen is tender and becomes distended. A sausage-shaped mass may be palpated, usually in the upper mid abdomen. An intussusception can persist for several days if obstruction is not complete, and patients may present with separate attacks of enterocolitis. In older children, sudden attacks of abdominal pain may be related to chronic recurrent intussusception with spontaneous reduction.

Treatment

A. CONSERVATIVE MEASURES

Barium enema and air enema are both diagnostic and therapeutic. Reduction by barium enema should not be attempted if signs of strangulated bowel, perforation, or severe toxicity are present. Air insufflation of the colon under fluoroscopic guidance is a safe alternative to barium enema with excellent diagnostic sensitivity and specificity without the risk of contaminating the abdominal cavity with barium. Care is required in performing either air or barium enema because ischemic damage to the colon secondary to vascular compromise increases the risk of perforation.

B. SURGICAL MEASURES

Surgery is required in extremely ill patients, in patients who have evidence of bowel perforation, or in those in whom hydrostatic or pneumatic reduction has been unsuccessful (25%). Surgery has the advantage of identifying a lead point such as a Meckel diverticulum. Surgical reduction of intussusception is associated with a lower recurrence rate than pneumatic reduction.

Prognosis

The prognosis relates directly to the duration of the intussusception before reduction. The mortality rate with treat-

ment is 1–2%. The patient should be observed carefully after hydrostatic or pneumatic reduction because intussusception recurs within 24 hours in 3–4% of patients.

Eshel G et al: Intussusception: A 9-year survey (1986–1995). J Pediatr Gastroenterol Nutr 1997;24:253 [PMID: 9138168].

FOREIGN BODIES IN THE ALIMENTARY TRACT

Most foreign bodies pass through the GI tract without difficulty, although objects longer than 5 cm may have difficulty negotiating the ligament of Treitz. Ingested foreign bodies tend to lodge in areas of natural constriction—valleculae, thoracic inlet, GE junction, pylorus, ligament of Treitz, and ileocecal junction. Foreign bodies lodged in the esophagus for more than 24 hours require removal. Smooth foreign bodies in the stomach, such as buttons or coins, may be monitored without attempting removal for up to several months if the child is free of symptoms. Straight pins, screws, and nails generally pass without incident. Removal of open safety pins or wooden toothpicks is recommended. Disk-shaped batteries lodged in the esophagus should be removed immediately. Disk-shaped batteries in the stomach will generally pass uneventfully. The use of balanced electrolyte lavage solutions containing polyethylene glycol may help the passage of small, smooth foreign bodies lodged in the stomach or intestine. Lavage is especially useful in hastening the passage of disk-shaped batteries or ingested tablets that may be toxic. Failure of a smooth foreign body to exit the stomach suggests the possibility of gastric outlet obstruction.

Esophagogastroscopy will permit the removal of most foreign bodies lodged in the esophagus and stomach. Under fluoroscopy, a Foley catheter with balloon inflated below the foreign body may be used to extract smooth, round esophageal foreign bodies in healthy children with no previous esophageal disease if the foreign body has been present for a short period. Only an experienced radiologist should attempt this maneuver.

Anal Fissure

Anal fissure is a slitlike tear in the squamous epithelium of the anus, usually secondary to the passage of large, hard fecal masses. Anal stenosis, anal crypt abscess, and trauma can be contributory factors. Sexual abuse must be considered in children with large, irregular, or multiple anal fissures. Anal fissures may be the presenting sign of Crohn disease in older children.

The infant or child with anal fissure typically cries with defecation and will try to hold back stools. Sparse, bright red bleeding is seen on the outside of the stool or on the toilet tissue following defecation. The fissure can often be seen if the patient is examined in a knee-chest position with the buttocks spread apart. When a fissure cannot be identified, it is essential to rule out other causes of rectal bleeding such as juvenile polyp, perianal inflammation due to group A streptococcus, or inflammatory bowel disease. Anal fissures should be treated promptly to break the constipation → fissure → retention → constipation cycle. A stool softener should be given. Anal dilation relieves sphincter spasm. Warm sitz baths after defecation may be helpful. Rarely, silver nitrate cauterization or surgery is indicated. Anal surgery should be avoided in patients with Crohn disease because of the high risk of recurrence and progression after surgery.

INGUINAL HERNIA

A peritoneal sac precedes the testicle as it descends from the genital ridge to the scrotum. The lower portion of this sac envelops the testis to form the tunica vaginalis, and the remainder normally atrophies by the time of birth. In some cases, peritoneal fluid may become trapped in the tunica vaginalis of the testis (noncommunicating hydrocele). If the processus vaginalis remains open, peritoneal fluid or an abdominal structure may be forced into it (indirect inguinal hernia).

Most inguinal hernias are of the indirect type and occur more frequently (9:1) in boys than in girls. Hernias may be present at birth or may appear at any age thereafter. The incidence in premature male infants is close to 5%. Inguinal hernia is reported in 30% of male infants weighing 1000 g or less.

Clinical Findings

No symptoms are associated with an empty processus vaginalis. In most cases, a hernia is a painless inguinal swelling. The mother of the infant may be the only person to see the mass, as it may retract when the infant is active, cold, frightened, or agitated from the physical examination. There may be a history of inguinal fullness associated with coughing or long periods of standing, or there may be a firm, globular, and tender swelling, sometimes associated with vomiting and abdominal distention. In some instances, a herniated loop of intestine may become partially obstructed, leading to pain and partial intestinal obstruction. Rarely, bowel becomes trapped in the hernia sac, and complete intestinal obstruction occurs. Gangrene of the hernia contents or testis may occur. In girls, the ovary may prolapse into the hernia sac. Inspection of the two inguinal areas may reveal a characteristic bulging or mass. Infants should be observed for evidence of swelling after crying, and older children after bearing down. A suggestive history is often the only criterion for diagnosis, along with the "silk glove" feel of the rubbing together of the two walls of the empty hernia sac.

Differential Diagnosis

Inguinal lymph nodes may be mistaken for a hernia. Nodes are usually multiple with more discrete borders. A hydrocele of the cord should transilluminate. An undescended testis is usually mobile in the canal and is associated with absence of the gonad in the scrotum.

Treatment

Manual reduction of incarcerated inguinal hernias can be attempted after the sedated infant is placed in the Trendelenburg position with an ice bag on the affected side. Manual reduction is contraindicated if incarceration has been present for more than 12 hours or if bloody stools are noted. Surgery is usually indicated if a hernia has ever incarcerated. Hydroceles frequently resolve by age 2 years. Controversy remains about exploration of the opposite side. Exploration of the unaffected groin can document the patency of the processus vaginalis, but patency does not always mean that herniation will occur, especially in patients older than age 1 year, in whom the risk of contralateral hernia is about 10%. Incarceration of an inguinal hernia is more likely to occur in boys and in children younger than 10 months of age.

Gahukamble DB, Khamage AS: Early vs delayed repair of reduced incarcerated inguinal hernias in the pediatric population. J Pediatr Surg 1996;31:1218 [PMID: 8887087].

Nicholls E: Inguino-scrotal problems in children. Practitioner 2003;247:226 [PMID: 12640831].

UMBILICAL HERNIA

Umbilical hernias are more common in premature than in full-term infants and more common in black than white infants. Small bowel may incarcerate in small-diameter umbilical hernias. Most umbilical hernias regress spontaneously if the fascial defect has a diameter of less than 1 cm. Large defects and hernias persisting after age 4 years should be treated surgically. Reducing the hernia and strapping the skin over the abdominal wall defect does not accelerate the healing process.

TUMORS OF THE GASTROINTESTINAL TRACT

1. Juvenile Polyps

Juvenile polyps are usually pedunculated and solitary. The head of the polyp is composed of hyperplastic glandular and vascular elements, often with cystic transformation. Juvenile polyps are benign, and 80% occur in the rectosigmoid. Their incidence is highest between ages 3 and 5 years, and they are rare before age 1 year and usually autoamputate by age 15 years. They are more frequent in boys. The painless passage of small amounts of bright red blood on a normal or constipated stool is the most frequent manifestation. Abdominal pain is rare, but a juvenile polyp can be the lead point for an intussusception. Low-lying polyps may prolapse during defecation.

Rarely, many juvenile polyps may be present in the colon, causing anemia, diarrhea, and protein loss. A few cases of generalized juvenile polyposis involving the stomach, small bowel, and colon have been reported. These cases are associated with a slightly increased risk of cancer.

Colonoscopy is diagnostic and therapeutic when polyps are suspected. After removal of the polyp by electrocautery, nothing further should be done if histologic findings confirm the diagnosis. There is a slight risk of developing further juvenile polyps.

Other polyposis syndromes are summarized in Table 20–4.

2. Cancers of the Esophagus, Small Intestine, & Colon

Esophageal cancer is rare in childhood. Cysts, leiomyomas, and hamartomas predominate. Caustic injury of the esophagus increases the very long-term risk of squamous cell carcinoma. Chronic peptic esophagitis is associated with Barrett esophagus, a precancerous lesion. Simple GE reflux in infancy without esophagitis is not a risk for cancer of the esophagus.

The most common gastric or small bowel cancer in children is lymphoma or lymphosarcoma. Intermittent abdominal pain, abdominal mass, intussusception, or a celiac-like picture may be present. Carcinoid tumors are usually benign and most often an incidental finding in the appendix. Metastasis is rare. The carcinoid syndrome (flushing, sweating, hypertension, diarrhea and vomiting), associated with serotonin secretion, only occurs with metastatic carcinoid tumors.

Adenocarcinoma of the colon is rare in childhood. The transverse colon and rectosigmoid are the two most commonly affected sites. The low 5-year survival rate relates to the nonspecificity of presenting complaints and the large percentage of undifferentiated types. Children with a family history of colon cancer, chronic ulcerative colitis, or familial polyposis syndromes are at greater risk.

3. Mesenteric Cysts

These rare tumors may be small or large, single or multiloculated. They are thin-walled and contain serous, chylous, or hemorrhagic fluid. They are commonly located in the small bowel mesentery but are also found in the mesocolon. Most mesenteric cysts cause no symptoms. Traction on the mesentery may lead to colicky abdominal pain, which can be mild and recurrent but may appear acutely with vomiting. Volvulus may occur around a cyst, and hemorrhage into a cyst may be mild or hemodynamically significant. A rounded mass can occasionally be palpated or seen on radiograph displacing adjacent intestine. Abdominal ultrasonography is usually diagnostic. Surgical removal is indicated.

4. Intestinal Hemangioma

Hemangiomas of the bowel may cause acute or chronic blood loss. They may also cause intestinal obstruction via intussusception, local stricture, or intramural hematoma. Thrombocytopenia and consumptive coagulopathy are occasional complications. Some lesions are telangiectasias (Rendu–Osler–Weber syndrome), and others are capillary hemangiomas. The largest group are cavernous hemangiomas, which are composed of large, thin-walled vessels arising from the submucosal vascular plexus. They may protrude into the lumen as polypoid lesions or may invade the intestine from mucosa to serosa.

ACUTE INFECTIOUS DIARRHEA (Gastroenteritis)

Viruses are the most common cause of acute gastroenteritis in developing and developed countries. Bacterial and parasitic enteric infections are discussed in Chapters 38 and 39. Of the viral agents causing enteric infection, rotavirus, a 67-nm double-stranded RNA virus with at least eight serotypes, is the most common. As with most viral pathogens, rotavirus affects the small intestine, causing voluminous watery diarrhea without leukocytes or blood. In the United States, rotavirus mainly affects infants between 3 and 15 months. Peak incidence in the United States is in the winter with sporadic cases occurring at other times. The virus is transmitted via the fecal–oral route and survives for hours on hands and for days on environmental fomites.

Diagnosis & Treatment of Rotavirus Infections

The incubation period for rotavirus is 24–48 hours. Vomiting is the first symptom in 80–90% of patients, followed within 24 hours by low-grade fever and watery diarrhea. Diarrhea usually lasts 4–8 days but may last longer in young infants or immunocompromised patients. The white blood cell count is rarely elevated. The stool sodium level is usually less than 40 mEq/L. Thus, as patients become dehydrated from unreplaced fecal water loss, they may become hypernatremic. The stool does not contain blood or white cells. Metabolic acidosis results from bicarbonate loss in the stool, ketosis from poor intake, and lactic acidemia from hypotension and hypoperfusion.

Table 20-4. Gastrointestinal polyposis syndromes.

	Location	Number	Histology	Extraintestinal Findings	Malignant Potential	Recommended Therapy
Juvenile polyps	Colon	Single (70%) Several (30%)	Hyperplastic, hamartomatous	None	None	Remove polyp for continuous bleeding or prolapse.
Familial juvenile polyposis coli[a]	Colon	More than ten	Hyperplastic with focal adenomatous change	None	10–25%; higher if familial	Remove all polyps. Consider colectomy if very numerous or adenomatous.
Generalized juvenile polyposis[a]	Stomach, small bowel, colon	Multiple	Hyperplastic with focal adenomatous change	Hydrocephaly, cardiac lesions, mesenteric lymphangioma, malrotation	10–25%	Colectomy and close surveillance.
Familial adenomatous polyposis[a]	Colon; less commonly, stomach and small bowel	Multiple	Adenomatous	None	95–100%	Colectomy by age 18 years.
Peutz–Jeghers syndrome[a]	Small bowel, stomach, colon	Multiple	Hamartomatous	Pigmented cutaneous and oral macules; ovarian cysts and tumors; bony exostoses	2–3%	Remove accessible polyps or those causing obstruction or bleeding.
Gardner syndrome	Colon; less commonly, stomach and small bowel	Multiple	Adenomatous	Cysts, tumors, and desmoids of skin and bone; ampullary tumors; other tumors, retinal pigmentations can be a screening tool in families	95–100%	Colectomy by age 18 years. Upper tract surveillance.
Cronkhite–Canada syndrome	Stomach, colon; less commonly, esophagus and small bowel	Multiple	Hamartomatous	Alopecia; onychodystrophy; hyperpigmentation	Rare	None.
Turcot syndrome[b]	Colon	Multiple	Adenomatous	Thyroid and brain tumors are the usual presentation	Possible	Central nervous system screening most important.

[a]Autosomal dominant.
[b]Autosomal recessive.

Replacement of fluid and electrolyte deficits and ongoing losses is critical, especially in small infants. (Oral and intravenous therapy are discussed in Chapter 42.) The use of oral rehydration fluid is appropriate in most cases. The use of clear liquids or hypocaloric (dilute formula) diets for more than 48 hours is not advisable in uncomplicated viral gastroenteritis because starvation depresses digestive function and prolongs diarrhea.

Intestinal lactase levels are reduced during rotavirus infection. Brief use of a lactose-free diet is associated with a shorter period of diarrhea but is not critical to successful recovery in healthy infants. Reduced fat intake during recovery may reduce nausea and vomiting.

Antidiarrheal medications are ineffective (kaolin-pectin combinations) or even dangerous (loperamide, tincture of opium, diphenoxylate with atropine). Bismuth subsalicylate preparations may reduce stool volume but are not critical to recovery. Oral immunoglobulin or specific antiviral agents have occasionally been useful in limiting duration of disease in immunocompromised patients.

Specific identification of rotavirus is not required in every case, especially in outbreaks. Rotavirus antigens can be identified in stool. The organism can be seen by scanning electron microscopy. False positives (which may actually be nonpathogenic rotavirus) are seen in neonates. Some immunity is imparted by the first episode of rotavirus infection. Serum antibodies are present, but their role in prevention of subsequent attacks is unclear. Repeat infections occur but are usually less severe. Rotavirus prevention is by good hygiene and prevention of fecal–oral contamination. In July 1999, the American Academy of Pediatrics recommended suspending oral rotavirus vaccine in the United States despite an approximately 75% protection rate of vaccinated infants because of its association with intussusception in the 3 weeks after vaccine administration. Since then a pentavalent oral rotavirus vaccine (RotaTeq) and a univalent oral vaccine (Rotarix) have been developed and appear to have an improved safety record. They have not yet been licensed in the United States.

Diagnosis & Treatment of Other Viral Infections

Other viral pathogens in stool have been identified by electron microscopy, viral culture, or enzyme-linked immunoassays in infants with diarrhea. Depending on the geographic location, enteric adenoviruses (serotypes 40 and 41) or caliciviruses are the next most common viral pathogens in infants. The symptoms of enteric adenovirus infection are similar to those produced from rotavirus, but infection is not seasonal and duration of illness may be longer. The Norwalk agent (now known as Norovirus) is a calicivirus, a small RNA virus that mainly causes vomiting but can also cause some diarrhea in older children and adults, usually in common source outbreaks. The duration of symptoms is short, usually 24–48 hours. Other potentially pathogenic viruses include astroviruses, corona-like viruses, and other small round viruses. Cytomegalovirus rarely causes diarrhea in immunocompetent children but may cause erosive colitis or enteritis in immunocompromised hosts. Cytomegalovirus enteritis is particularly common after bone marrow transplantation and in late stages of HIV infection.

Caeiro JP et al: Etiology of outpatient pediatric nondysenteric diarrhea: A multicenter study in the United States. Pediatr Infect Dis J 1999;18:94 [PMID: 10048678].

CHRONIC DIARRHEA

It is difficult to define chronic diarrhea because normal bowel habits vary greatly. Some infants normally have 5–8 soft small stools daily. A gradual or sudden increase in the number and volume of stools (> 15 g/kg/d) combined with an increase in fluidity should raise a suspicion that an organic cause of chronic diarrhea is present.

Diarrhea may result from: (1) interruption of normal cell transport processes for water, electrolytes, or nutrients; (2) decrease in the surface area available for absorption secondary to shortened bowel or mucosal disease; (3) increase in intestinal motility; (4) increase in unabsorbable osmotically active molecules in the intestinal lumen; (5) increase in intestinal permeability, leading to increased loss of water and electrolytes; and (6) stimulation of enterocyte secretion by toxins or cytokines.

Noninfectious Causes of Diarrhea

A. ANTIBIOTIC THERAPY

Diarrhea is reported in up to 60% of children receiving antibiotics. Eradication of normal gut flora and overgrowth of other organisms may cause diarrhea. Most antibiotic-associated diarrhea is watery, is not associated with systemic symptoms, and decreases when antibiotic therapy is stopped. Pseudomembranous colitis, caused by toxins produced by *Clostridium difficile,* occurs in 0.2–10% of patients taking antibiotics, especially clindamycin, cephalosporins, and amoxicillin. Patients develop fever, tenesmus, and abdominal pain with diarrhea, which contains leukocytes and sometimes gross blood up to 8 weeks after antibiotic exposure. Treatment with oral metronidazole (30 mg/kg/d) or oral vancomycin (30–50 mg/kg/d) for 7 days is recommended. Vancomycin is many times more expensive than metronidazole and no more efficacious. Relapse occurs after treatment in 10–50% of patients because of exsporulation of residual spores in the colon. Re-treatment with the same antibiotic regimen is usually effective, but multiple relapses are possible and may be a significant management problem. Ulcerative colitis may be an underlying problem in cases of recurrent *C difficile.*

B. Extraintestinal Infections

Infections of the urinary tract and upper respiratory tract (especially otitis media) are at times associated with diarrhea. The mechanism remains obscure. Antibiotic treatment of the primary infection, toxins released by infecting organisms, and local irritation of the rectum (in patients with bladder infection) may play a role.

C. Malnutrition

Malnutrition is associated with an increased frequency of enteral infections. Decreased bile acid synthesis, pancreatic enzyme output, decreased disaccharidase activity, altered motility, and changes in the intestinal flora all may cause diarrhea. Severely malnourished children are at higher risk of enteric infections because of depressed immune functions, both cellular and humoral.

D. Diet

Overfeeding may cause diarrhea, especially in young infants. Relative deficiency of pancreatic amylase in young infants may produce diarrhea after starchy foods. Fruit juices, especially those high in fructose or sorbitol, produce osmotic diarrhea because these osmotically active sugars are poorly absorbed. Intestinal irritants (spices and foods high in fiber) and histamine-containing or histamine-releasing foods (eg, citrus fruits, tomatoes, fermented cheeses, red wines, and scombroid fish) also cause diarrhea.

E. Allergic Diarrhea

Diarrhea caused by allergy to dietary proteins is a frequently entertained but rarely authenticated entity. Protein allergy is more common in infants younger than age 12 months, who may experience mild to severe colitis. A personal or family history of atopy is common in infants with enteric protein allergy. Older children may develop a celiac-like syndrome with flattening of small bowel villi, steatorrhea, hypoproteinemia, occult blood loss, and chronic diarrhea. Skin testing is not reliable. Double-blind oral challenge with the suspected food under careful observation is necessary to confirm intestinal protein allergy. Mild diarrhea with blood and mucus may occur in thriving young infants receiving either breast milk or formula. In the breast-fed infant, maternal avoidance of milk protein may be effective in reducing the signs of colitis. Feeding a protein hydrolysate formula may also reduce symptoms. Because allergic colitis in young infants is self-limited, the condition does not absolutely require treatment if the infant is thriving and the colitic symptoms are not severe. Colonoscopy is not required for diagnosis, but rectal biopsies usually show mild lymphonodular hyperplasia, mucosal edema, and slight eosinophilia. In infants, the condition usually disappears after 12 months. Allergies to fish, peanuts, and eggs are more likely to be lifelong. Multiple food allergy (more than three) is rare.

Khan S, Orenstein S: Eosinophilic gastroenteritis: Epidemiology, diagnosis and management. Paediatr Drugs 2002;4:563.

F. Chronic Nonspecific Diarrhea

Chronic nonspecific diarrhea is the most common cause of loose stools in thriving children. The typical patient is a healthy child age 6–20 months who has three to six loose mucoid stools per day during the waking hours. The diarrhea worsens with a low-residue, low-fat, or high-carbohydrate diet and during periods of stress and infection. It clears spontaneously at about age $3^1/_2$ years (usually coincident with toilet training). No organic disease is discoverable. Possible causes include abnormalities of bile acid absorption in the terminal ileum, incomplete carbohydrate absorption (excessive fruit juice ingestion seems to worsen the condition or in some cases appears to be the primary cause), and abnormal motor function. Family history of functional bowel disease is common. Stool tests for blood, white cells, fat, parasites, and bacterial pathogens are negative.

The following measures are helpful: use of a slightly high-fat (about 40% of total calories), low-carbohydrate, high-fiber diet; avoidance of between-meal snacks; and avoidance of chilled fluids, especially fruit juices. Loperamide, 0.1–0.2 mg/kg/d in two or three divided doses is often helpful. Cholestyramine, 2–4 g in divided doses, or psyllium agents, 1–2 tsp twice daily are sometimes used.

G. Secretory Diarrhea

Certain malignancies of childhood, neuroblastoma, ganglioneuroma, metastatic carcinoid, and GI neuroendocrine tumors such as pancreatic VIPoma or gastrinoma, may secrete substances such as gastrin and vasoactive intestinal polypeptide (VIP) that promote small intestine secretion of water and electrolytes. Children with these tumors may present with large volume, watery diarrhea that does not cease when they discontinue oral feedings. Fat malabsorption is not characteristic. The serum potassium level is often low because of stool losses. The hallmark of the diarrhea is that, unlike osmotic and infectious viral diarrheas, the sodium content of stool water is high, usually between 90 and 140 mEq/L of stool. Other signs and symptoms are associated with specific tumors. Neuroblastoma and ganglioneuroma produce elevations in urinary homovanillic acid and vanillylmandelic acid. Metastatic carcinoid produces characteristic flushing and sweating. Gastrinoma may produce multiple duodenal ulcers (Zollinger–Ellison syndrome). In all secretory diarrheas, a careful radiologic search for a tumor mass is indicated. Intraendoscopic ultrasound examination may discover small tumors in the bowel wall or pancreatic head. Bacterial overgrowth of the small bowel in patients with short bowel, cancer chemotherapy, or anatomic abnormalities may be associated with enterotoxins, which promote secretory diarrhea. Cholera is the best known bacterial secretory diarrhea. Its enterotoxin stimulates cyclic adenosine monophosphate in the enterocyte, which promotes salt and water secretion.

THE MALABSORPTION SYNDROMES

Malabsorption of ingested food has many causes (Table 20–5). Shortening of the small bowel (usually via sur-

Table 20–5. Malabsorption syndromes.

Intraluminal phase abnormalities	Intestinal phase abnormalities (cont'd)
Acid hypersecretion; Zollinger–Ellison syndrome	Circulatory disturbances
Gastric resection	Cirrhosis
Exocrine pancreatic insufficiency	Congestive heart failure
Cystic fibrosis	Abnormal structure of gastrointestinal tract
Chronic pancreatitis	Dumping syndrome after gastrectomy
Pancreatic pseudocysts	Malrotation
Schwachman syndrome	Stenosis of jejunum or ileum
Enterokinase deficiency	Small bowel resection; short bowel syndrome
Lipase and colipase deficiency	Polyposis
Malnutrition	Selective inborn absorptive defects
Decreased conjugated bile acids	Congenital malabsorption of folic acid
Liver production and excretion	Selective malabsorption of vitamin B_{12}
Neonatal hepatitis	Cystinuria, methionine malabsorption
Biliary atresia: intrahepatic and extrahepatic	Hartnup disease, blue diaper syndrome
Acute and chronic active hepatitis	Glucose-galactose malabsorption
Disease of the biliary tract	Primary disaccharidase deficiency
Cirrhosis	Acrodermatitis enteropathica
Fat malabsorption in the premature infant	Abetalipoproteinemia
Intestinal malabsorption of bile acids	Congenital chloridorrhea
Short bowel syndrome	Primary hypomagnesemia
Bacterial overgrowth	Hereditary fructose intolerance
Blind loop	Familial hypophosphatemic rickets
Fistula	Endocrine diseases
Strictures, regional enteritis	Diabetes mellitus
Scleroderma, intestinal pseudoobstruction	Addison disease
Intestinal phase abnormalities	Hyperthyroidism
Mucosal diseases	Hypoparathyroidism, pseudohypoparathyroidism
Infections, bacterial or viral	Neuroblastoma, ganglioneuroma
Infections, parasitic	**Vascular and lymphatic disorders**
Giardia lamblia	Whipple disease
Fish tapeworm	Intestinal lymphangiectasis
Hookworm	Congestive heart failure
Cryptosporidium	Regional enteritis with lymphangiectasis
Malnutrition	Lymphoma
Marasmus	Abetalipoproteinemia
Kwashiorkor	**Miscellaneous**
Dermatitis herpetiformis	Renal insufficiency
Folic acid deficiency	Carcinoid, mastocytosis
Drugs: methotrexate, antibiotics	Immune deficiency disorders
Crohn disease	Familial dysautonomia
Cow's milk and soy protein intolerance	Collagen–vascular disease
Secondary disaccharidase deficiency	Wolman disease
Secondary monosaccharide intolerance	Histiocytosis X
Hirschsprung disease with enterocolitis	
Tropical sprue	
Celiac disease	
Radiation enteritis	
Lymphoma	

gical resection) and mucosal damage (celiac disease) both reduce surface area. Impaired motility of the small intestine may interfere with normal propulsive movements and mixing of food with pancreatic and biliary secretions. Anaerobic bacteria proliferate under these conditions and impair fat absorption by deconjugation of bile acids (intestinal pseudoobstruction, postoperative blind loop syndrome). Impaired intestinal lymphatic (congenital lymphangiectasis) or venous drainage also causes malabsorption. Diseases reducing pancreatic exocrine function (cystic fibrosis, Shwachman syndrome) or the production and flow of biliary secretions cause nutrient malabsorption. Malabsorption of specific nutrients may be genetically determined (disaccharidase deficiency, glucose–galactose malabsorption, and abetalipoproteinemia).

Clinical Findings

GI symptoms such as diarrhea, vomiting, anorexia, abdominal pain, failure to thrive, and abdominal distension are common. Observation of the stools for abnormal color, consistency, bulk, odor, mucus, and blood is important. Microscopic examination of stools for neutral fat and fatty acids is helpful because most malabsorption syndromes involve some fat malabsorption. Pancreatic insufficiency is associated with neutral fat (triglycerides) in the stool. Fatty acids are the major fatty material found in the stool of patients with mucosal and liver disease.

Quantitation of fat absorption requires measurement of fat excreted in the feces as a proportion of fat intake for a defined period. Excretion of 5% of ingested fat is normal for a child older than age 1 year; 10–15% is normal in a younger infant. Prothrombin time and serum carotene, vitamin E, and vitamin D levels may be depressed by long-standing fat malabsorption. Accurate assessment of protein absorption is difficult and requires isotopic labeling of amino acids. Loss of serum proteins across the intestinal mucosa can be estimated by measurement of fecal α_1-antitrypsin. Malabsorption of complex carbohydrate is rarely measured. Disaccharide or monosaccharide malabsorption is estimated by reduction in stool pH, increased breath hydrogen after ingestion of carbohydrate, or decreased intestinal mucosal disaccharidase activity.

Other tests that may suggest a specific cause of malabsorption in a child include sweat chloride concentration (cystic fibrosis), intestinal mucosal biopsy (eg, celiac disease, intestinal lymphangiectasia, giardiasis, inflammatory bowel disease), liver and gallbladder function tests, and pancreatic secretion after stimulation with secretin and cholecystokinin. Some of the most common disorders associated with malabsorption in pediatric patients are detailed in the following sections.

1. Protein-Losing Enteropathies

Loss of plasma proteins into the GI tract occurs in association with intestinal inflammation, intestinal graft-versus-host disease, acute and chronic intestinal infections, venous and lymphatic obstruction/malformations, and infiltration of the intestine or its lymphatics and vasculature by malignant cells.

Clinical Findings

Signs and symptoms are mainly those related to hypoproteinemia, and in some instances to fat malabsorption. Edema, ascites, poor weight gain, and signs of specific vitamin and mineral deficiencies may all be present. Serum albumin and globulins may be decreased. Fecal α_1-antitrypsin is elevated (> 3 mg/g dry weight stool; slightly higher in breast-fed infants). Disorders associated with protein-losing enteropathy are listed in Table 20–6. In the presence of intestinal bleeding, fecal α_1-antitrypsin measurements are falsely high.

Table 20–6. Disorders associated with protein-losing enteropathy.

Vascular obstruction
 Congestive heart failure
 Constrictive pericarditis
 Atrial septal defect
 Primary myocardial disease
 Increased right atrial pressure[a]
Stomach
 Giant hypertrophic gastritis (Ménétrier disease), often secondary to cytomegalovirus infection
 Polyps
 Gastritis secondary to *Helicobacter pylori* infection
Small intestine
 Celiac disease
 Intestinal lymphangiectasia
 Blind loop syndrome
 Abetalipoproteinemia
 Chronic mucosal ischemia (eg, from chronic volvulus or radiation enteritis)
 Allergic enteropathy
 Malrotation
 Inflammatory bowel disease
Colon
 Ulcerative colitis
 Hirschsprung disease
 Pseudomembranous colitis
 Polyposis syndromes
 Villous adenoma
 Solitary rectal ulcer

[a]Children who undergo Fontan procedure for tricuspid atresia are especially prone.

Differential Diagnosis

Hypoalbuminemia may be due to an increased catabolism, poor protein intake, impaired hepatic protein synthesis, or congenital malformations of lymphatics outside the GI tract. Protein losses in the urine from nephritis and nephrotic syndrome may also cause hypoalbuminemia.

Treatment

Albumin infusions, diuretics, and a high-protein/low-fat diet may control symptoms. Treatment must be directed toward identifying and treating the underlying cause of GI protein loss if possible.

2. Celiac Disease (Gluten Enteropathy)

Celiac disease results from intestinal sensitivity to the gliadin fraction of glutens from wheat, rye, barley, and (possibly) oats. Most pediatric cases present during the second year of life, but the age at onset and the severity are variable. Up-to-date estimates of disease frequency are being revised with the widespread use of sensitive screening tests such as the tissue transglutaminase. Screening with antigliadin antibodies is not recommended because of the high frequency of false-positive tests. The frequency of celiac disease in the United States is around 1:300, a figure approaching the high incidence in European countries. It is thought that intestinal damage and villous atrophy result from a cell-mediated immune response initiated by exposure to a polypeptide fragment of gliadin, the alcohol-soluble fraction of gluten. Ten percent of first-degree relatives may be affected. The inheritance is probably polygenic, but it might result from a single gene in combination with an environmental precipitant such as intestinal viral infection. The increased incidence of celiac disease in children with type 1 diabetes mellitus, IgA deficiency, and Down syndrome is consistent with possible immunologic factors in the development of celiac disease. Individuals with HLA-DR4 and perhaps DR3 tissue types are at higher risk.

Clinical Findings

A. Symptoms and Signs

1. Diarrhea—Affected children usually have diarrhea starting 6–12 months after the introduction of grains. Initially, the diarrhea may be intermittent; subsequently it is continuous, with bulky, pale, frothy, greasy, foul-smelling stools. During celiac crises, dehydration, shock, and acidosis occur. In cases in which anorexia is severe (about 10%), diarrhea may be absent.

2. Constipation, vomiting, and abdominal pain—This triad of symptoms may occasionally dominate the clinical picture and suggest a diagnosis of intestinal obstruction. Constipation generally results from a combination of anorexia, dehydration, muscle weakness, and bulky stools.

3. Failure to thrive—The onset of diarrhea is usually accompanied by loss of appetite, failure to gain weight, and irritability. Weight loss is most marked in the limbs and buttocks. The abdomen becomes distended secondary to gas and fluid in the intestinal tract. Short stature and delayed puberty are characteristic in older children and may be the only symptoms.

4. Anemia and vitamin deficiencies—Anemia usually responds to iron supplementation and is rarely megaloblastic. Anemia is more likely to be the presenting problem of adults with celiac disease. Fat-soluble vitamin deficiency is common. Rickets can be seen when growth has not been completely halted by the disease. Osteomalacia is more common and pathologic fractures may occur. Hypoprothrombinemia secondary to vitamin K malabsorption can cause easy bleeding.

5. Silent celiac disease—Serologic screening among pediatric patients with nonspecific GI complaints, growth failure, type 1 diabetes, thyroid disease, vitiligo, IgA deficiency, Down syndrome, and family members of celiac patients is widespread. The therapy for a symptom-free child with positive serology is unclear. Intestinal biopsy specimens from children with positive serology are usually abnormal consistent with celiac disease. In these patients, the prudent response is to recommend a gluten-free diet. In patients with positive serology but normal intestinal biopsies, careful follow-up without diet therapy is the most appropriate current recommendation.

B. Laboratory Findings

1. Fat content of stools—A 3-day collection of stools usually reveals excessive fecal fat excretion. A normal child excretes 5–10% of ingested fat. In untreated celiac disease fat excretion is more than 15% of daily fat intake. Anorexia may be so severe that steatorrhea may not be present in 10–25% of patients until normal intake is established.

2. Impaired carbohydrate absorption—A low oral glucose tolerance curve is seen. Absorption of D-xylose is impaired, with blood levels lower than 20 mg/dL 60 minutes after ingestion.

3. Hypoproteinemia—Hypoalbuminemia can be severe enough to lead to edema. There is evidence of increased protein loss in the gut lumen and poor hepatic synthesis secondary to malnutrition.

C. Imaging

A small bowel series shows a malabsorptive pattern characterized by segmentation, clumping of the barium column, and hypersecretion. These changes are nonspecific and can be found in patients with other malabsorption states (see Table 20–5).

D. BIOPSY FINDINGS

Intestinal biopsy is the most reliable test for celiac disease. Jejunal biopsies observed with a hand lens lack normal slender, fingerlike villi. Under the light microscope, the celiac mucosa has shortened or absent villi, lengthened crypts of Lieberkühn, intense plasma cell infiltration of the lamina propria, and numerous intraepithelial lymphocytes. Extent of change is quantitated on the Marsh scoring system from normal to complete villous atrophy.

E. SEROLOGIC TESTS

The false-positive rate for the IgG antigliadin antibody is 10% among healthy individuals. The false-positive rate for IgA antigliadin antibodies is lower. Endomysial or tissue transglutaminase antibody assays have greater than 95% sensitivity and slightly less specificity for the diagnosis. Because both of these antibodies are of the IgA class, in a patient who is IgA-deficient results may be falsely negative. Currently, the best serologic screen is a quantitative IgA level and transglutaminase antibody assay.

Differential Diagnosis

The differential diagnosis includes disorders that cause malabsorption. Strict adherence to two diagnostic criteria is essential—the characteristic small bowel microscopic changes and clinical improvement on a gluten-free diet. Repeat mucosal biopsies to prove histologic recovery on gluten-free diet and relapse on gluten challenge are not critical in typical patients.

Treatment

A. DIET

Treatment is dietary gluten restriction for life. All sources of wheat, rye, and barley are eliminated. Some patients may be able to tolerate oats in the diet, but this should be tested only after recovery has occurred. Lactose is poorly tolerated in the acute stage because mucosal atrophy causes secondary disaccharidase deficiency. Normal amounts of fat are advisable. Supplemental calories, vitamins, and minerals are indicated in the acute phase. Clinical improvement usually starts within a week, but complete clinical recovery and histologic normality may require 3–12 months. Tissue transglutaminase titers may decrease on a gluten-free diet, but usually do not disappear.

B. CORTICOSTEROIDS

Corticosteroids can hasten clinical improvement but are indicated only in very ill patients with profound anorexia,

malnutrition, diarrhea, edema, abdominal distention, and hypokalemia.

Prognosis

Clinical and histologic recovery is the rule but may be slow. Malignant lymphoma of the small bowel occurs with increased frequency in adults with long-standing disease. Dietary treatment seems to decrease the risk of this complication.

Fasano A et al: The prevalence of celiac disease in at-risk and not-at-risk groups in the United States: A multicenter study. Arch Intern Med 2003;163:286 [PMID: 12578508].

Hill I et al: Guidelines for the diagnosis and treatment of celiac disease in children: Recommendations of the North American Society for Pediatric Gastroenterology, Hepatology and Nutrition. J Pediatr Gastroenterol Nutr 2005;40:1 [PMID: 15625418].

3. Disaccharidase Deficiency

Starches and the disaccharides sucrose and lactose are the most important dietary carbohydrates. Dietary disaccharides and oligosaccharide products of pancreatic amylase action on starch require hydrolysis by intestinal brush border disaccharidases before absorption takes place. Disaccharidase levels are higher in the jejunum and proximal ileum than in the distal ileum and duodenum.

In primary disaccharidase deficiency, a single enzyme is affected; disaccharide intolerance is permanent; intestinal histologic findings are normal; and a positive family history is common.

Because disaccharidases are located on the luminal surface of intestinal enterocytes, they are susceptible to mucosal damage. Many conditions cause secondary disaccharidase deficiency, with lactase usually most severely depressed.

Clinical Findings

A. PRIMARY (CONGENITAL)

1. Lactase deficiency—Congenital lactase deficiency is rare. Lactose ingestion causes diarrhea, gassy distention, and abdominal pain. The stools are frothy, with a pH below 4.5 owing to the presence of organic acids. Vomiting is common. Severe malnutrition may occur. Reducing substances are present in fresh stools. The blood glucose fails to rise more than 10 mg/dL after ingestion of 1 g/kg of lactose. A rise in breath hydrogen after oral administration of lactose (from hydrogen produced by normal colon flora during fermentation of unabsorbed carbohydrate) is also diagnostic.

Patients respond to a reduction of dietary lactose. Tolerance for dietary starch and sucrose is normal. Lactase extracted from *Aspergillus* and *Kluyvera* species can be added to milk products or taken with meals to enhance lactose hydrolysis. Although all human ethnic groups are lactase-sufficient at birth, genetically determined lactase deficiency may develop in certain ethnic groups after age 3–5 years. In Asians, genetic lactase deficiency develops in virtually 100%. In Africans, the incidence in most tribes is over 80%. In African Americans, the incidence is about 70%, and among European Americans, the incidence is between 30% and 60%.

2. Sucrase and isomaltase deficiency—This is a combined defect inherited as an autosomal-recessive trait. Ten percent of Alaskan natives are affected. The condition is rare in other groups. Abdominal distention, failure to thrive, and chronic diarrhea may be the presenting symptoms. Distaste for and avoidance of sucrose occurs even in young infants.

Because sucrose is not a reducing sugar, tests for reducing substances in the stool are negative unless the sucrose in the stool is hydrolyzed by colon bacteria. A sucrose tolerance test (1 g/kg) will be abnormal. Breath hydrogen will be elevated after ingestion of sucrose. Treatment of primary sucrase–isomaltase deficiency requires elimination of most sucrose. A preparation of yeast sucrase taken with meals is also effective.

B. SECONDARY (ACQUIRED)

1. Secondary lactase deficiency—The most common mechanism producing secondary lactase deficiency is small intestinal injury due to viral infection. The deficiency is usually self-limited, lasting days or, at most, weeks after recovery from infection.

2. Secondary sucrase deficiency—Intestinal mucosal damage tends to reduce the activity of all disaccharidases. Signs of sucrose intolerance are usually masked by the more striking symptoms of lactose intolerance. Infectious diarrhea is the most common cause of secondary sucrose intolerance.

Prognosis

Primary disaccharidase deficiency is a lifelong condition. However, in both lactase and sucrase deficiencies, tolerance for the disaccharide may increase with age. The prognosis in the secondary or acquired forms of disaccharidase deficiency depends on the underlying illness.

Baudon JJ et al: Sucrase-isomaltase deficiency: Changing pattern over 2 decades. J Pediatr Gastroenterol Nutr 1996;22:284 [PMID: 8708882].

Treem WR et al: Saccharosidase therapy for congenital sucrase-isomaltase deficiency. J Pediatr Gastroenterol Nutr 1999;28:137 [PMID: 9932843].

4. Glucose–Galactose Malabsorption

Glucose–galactose malabsorption is a rare disorder in which the sodium–glucose transport protein is defective.

The gene has been localized to the long arm of chromosome 22. Transport of glucose in the intestinal epithelium and renal tubule is impaired. Diarrhea begins with the first feedings, accompanied by reducing sugar in the stool and acidosis. Small bowel histologic findings are normal. Glycosuria and aminoaciduria may occur. The glucose tolerance test is flat. Fructose is well tolerated. Diarrhea subsides promptly on withdrawal of glucose and galactose from the diet. The acquired form of glucose–galactose malabsorption occurs mainly in infants younger than age 6 months, usually following acute viral or bacterial enteritis.

In the congenital disease, exclusion of glucose and galactose from the diet is mandatory. A satisfactory formula is one with a carbohydrate-free base plus added fructose. The prognosis is good if the disease is diagnosed early, because tolerance for glucose and galactose improves with age. In secondary monosaccharide intolerance, prolonged parenteral nutrition may be required until intestinal transport mechanisms for monosaccharides return.

Wright EM: Glucose galactose malabsorption. Am J Physiol 1998;275:G879 [PMID: 9815014].

5. Intestinal Lymphangiectasia

This form of protein-losing enteropathy results from a congenital ectasia of the bowel lymphatic system, often associated with abnormalities of the lymphatics in the extremities. Obstruction of lymphatic drainage of the intestine leads to rupture of the intestinal lacteals with leakage of lymph into the lumen of the bowel. Fat loss in the stool may be significant. Chronic loss of lymphocytes and immunoglobulins increases the susceptibility to infections.

Clinical Findings

Peripheral edema, diarrhea, abdominal distention, chylous effusions, and repeated infections are common. Laboratory findings are reduced serum albumin, decreased immunoglobulin levels, lymphocytopenia, and anemia. Serum calcium and magnesium are frequently depressed as these cations are lost in complex with unabsorbed fatty acids. Lymphocytes may be seen on a stool smear. Fecal α_1-antitrypsin is elevated. Radiographic studies reveal an edematous small bowel mucosal pattern, and biopsy reveals dilated lacteals in the villi and lamina propria. If only the lymphatics of the deeper layers of bowel or intestinal mesenterics are involved, laparotomy may be necessary to establish the diagnosis. Capsule (camera) endoscopy shows diagnostic brightness secondary to the fat-filled lacteals.

Differential Diagnosis

Other causes of protein-losing enteropathy must be considered, although an associated lymphedematous extremity strongly favors this diagnosis.

Treatment & Prognosis

A high protein diet (6–7 g/kg/d may be needed) enriched with medium-chain triglycerides as a fat source usually allows for adequate nutrition and growth in patients with intestinal mucosal lymphangiectasia. The serum albumin may not normalize. Vitamin and calcium supplements should be given. Parenteral nutritional supplementation may be needed temporarily. Surgery may be curative if the lesion is localized to a small area of the bowel or in cases of constrictive pericarditis or obstructing tumors. Intravenous albumin and immune globulin may also be used to control symptoms but are usually not needed chronically. The prognosis is not favorable, although remission may occur with age. Malignant degeneration of the abnormal lymphatics may occur, and intestinal lymphoma of the B-cell type may be a long-term complication.

6. Cow's Milk Protein Intolerance

Milk protein intolerance is more common in males than females and in young infants with a family history of atopy. The estimated prevalence is 0.5–1.0%. Colic, vomiting, and diarrhea are the major symptoms. Stools often contain blood and mucus. Sigmoidoscopic examination reveals a superficial colitis, often with edema, a mild eosinophilic infiltrate, and lymphonodular hyperplasia. Pneumatosis intestinalis rarely is found on x-ray. Viral gastroenteritis sometimes precedes the onset of symptoms. Less commonly, milk protein may induce eosinophilic gastroenteritis with protein-losing enteropathy, hypoalbuminemia, and hypogammaglobulinemia. A celiac-like syndrome with villous atrophy, malabsorption, hypoalbuminemia, occult blood in the stool, and anemia can occur in older children. IgE-mediated anaphylactic shock is a rare but potentially life-threatening manifestation of milk protein sensitivity in infancy. If the symptoms suggest an anaphylactic response to milk or other protein, food challenge should be performed only in a setting in which resuscitation can be carried out.

Infants who are solely breast-fed can also develop blood-streaked stools and a sigmoidoscopic picture similar to that of formula-fed infants with milk protein sensitivity. Tiny amounts of intact allergen passed in breast milk may be the cause, but other environmental allergens may play a role. Elimination of whole milk from the maternal diet sometimes relieves bloody diarrhea. A switch to a protein hydrolysate formula almost always results in improvement. Because the blood loss and diarrhea are rarely severe, it is not essential that breast feeding be stopped. If symptoms are severe or prolonged, a trial of semielemental formula is recommended. Allergic colitis in infants usually clears spontaneously by age 6–12 months.

Early reports that patients with milk protein allergy have a 30% incidence of sensitivity to soy protein, with similar symptoms, have not been uniformly confirmed.

7. Immunologic Deficiency States with Diarrhea or Malabsorption

Diarrhea is common in immune deficiency states, but the cause is often obscure. Between 50% and 60% of patients with idiopathic acquired hypogammaglobulinemia have steatorrhea and intestinal villous atrophy. Lymphonodular hyperplasia of the small intestine is prominent. Patients with congenital or Bruton-type agammaglobulinemia usually have diarrhea and abnormal intestinal morphology. Patients with isolated IgA deficiency also have chronic diarrhea, a celiac-like picture, lymphoid nodular hyperplasia, and are prone to giardiasis. Patients with isolated cellular immunity defects, combined cellular and humoral immune incompetence, and HIV infection may have severe chronic diarrhea leading to malnutrition. The cause of diarrhea may be common bacterial, viral, fungal, or parasitic pathogens, organisms usually considered nonpathogenic (*Blastocystis hominis, Candida*); or unusual organisms (cytomegalovirus, *Cryptosporidium, Isospora belli, Mycobacterium* species, microsporidia, and algal organisms such as cyanobacteria). Often the cause is not found. The incidence of disaccharidase deficiency is high. Chronic granulomatous disease may be associated with intestinal symptoms suggestive of chronic inflammatory bowel disease. A rectal biopsy may reveal the presence of typical macrophages.

Treatment must be directed toward correction of the immunologic defect. Specific treatments are available or are being developed for many of the unusual pathogens causing diarrhea in the immunocompromised host. Thus, a vigorous diagnostic search for specific pathogens is warranted in these individuals.

8. Pancreatic Insufficiency

The most common cause of pancreatic exocrine insufficiency in childhood is cystic fibrosis. Decreased secretion of pancreatic digestive enzymes is caused by obstruction of the exocrine ducts by thick secretions, which destroys pancreatic acinar cells. Destruction of acinar cells may occur antenatally. Some genotypes of cystic fibrosis have partially or completely preserved pancreatic exocrine function. Other conditions associated with exocrine pancreatic insufficiency are discussed in Chapter 21.

9. Other Genetic Disorders Causing Malabsorption

A. ABETALIPOPROTEINEMIA

Abetalipoproteinemia is an autosomal-recessive condition in which the secretion of triglyceride-rich lipopro-

Table 20–7. Causes of constipation.

Functional or retentive causes	Abnormalities of myenteric ganglion cells
Dietary causes	Hirschsprung disease
Undernutrition, dehydration	Waardenburg syndrome
Excessive milk intake	Multiple endocrine neoplasia IIa
Lack of bulk	Hypo- and hyperganglionosis
Cathartic abuse	von Recklinghausen disease
Drugs	Multiple endocrine neoplasia IIb
Narcotics	Intestinal neuronal dysplasia
Antihistamines	Chronic intestinal pseudoobstruction
Some antidepressants	Spinal cord defects
Vincristine	Metabolic and endocrine disorders
Structural defects of gastrointestinal tract	Hypothyroidism
Anus and rectum	Hyperparathyroidism
Fissure, hemorrhoids, abscess	Renal tubular acidosis
Anterior ectopic anus	Diabetes insipidus (dehydration)
Anal and rectal stenosis	Vitamin D intoxication (hypercalcemia)
Presacral teratoma	Idiopathic hypercalcemia
Small bowel and colon	Skeletal muscle weakness or incoordination
Tumor, stricture	Cerebral palsy
Chronic volvulus	Muscular dystrophy/myotonia
Intussusception	
Smooth muscle diseases	
Scleroderma and dermatomyositis	
Systemic lupus erythematosus	
Chronic intestinal pseudoobstruction	

Modified and reproduced, with permission, from Silverman A, Roy CC: *Pediatric Clinical Gastroenterology*, 3rd ed. Mosby, 1983.

teins from the small intestine (chylomicrons) and liver (very low-density lipoproteins) is abnormal. Profound steatosis of the intestinal enterocytes (and hepatocytes) and severe fat malabsorption occur. Deficiencies of fat-soluble vitamins develop with neurologic complications of vitamin E deficiency and atypical retinitis pigmentosa. Serum cholesterol level is very low, and red cell membrane lipids are abnormal, causing acanthosis of red blood cells, which may be the key to diagnosis.

B. ACRODERMATITIS ENTEROPATHICA

Acrodermatitis enteropathica is an autosomal-recessive condition in which the intestine has a selective inability to absorb zinc. The condition usually becomes obvious at the time of weaning and is characterized by rash on the extremities, rashes around the body orifices, eczema, profound failure to thrive, steatorrhea, diarrhea, and immune deficiency. Zinc supplementation by mouth results in rapid improvement.

CONSTIPATION

Chronic constipation in childhood is defined as two or more of the following characteristics for 2 months: (1) < 3 bowel movements per week; (2) > 1 episode of encopresis per week; (3) impaction of the rectum with stool; (4) passage of stool so large it obstructs the toilet; (5) retentive posturing and fecal withholding; and (6) pain with defecation. Retention of feces in the rectum results in encopresis (involuntary fecal leakage) in 60% of children with constipation. Organic causes of constipation are listed in Table 20–7. Most constipation in childhood is not organic but a result of voluntary or involuntary retentive behavior.

Clinical Findings

Infants younger than age 3 months often grunt, strain, and turn red in the face while passing normal stools. This pattern may be viewed erroneously as constipation. Failure to appreciate this normal developmental pattern may lead to the unwise use of laxatives or enemas. Infants and children may gradually develop the ability to ignore the sensation of rectal fullness and retain stool. Many factors promote and reinforce this behavior, which results in impaction of the rectum and overflow incontinence or encopresis: painful defecation; skeletal muscle weakness; psychological issues, especially those relating to control and authority; modesty and distaste for school bathrooms; medications; and others listed in Table 20–7. The dilated rectum becomes less sensitive to fullness, thus perpetuating the problem. As many as 1–2% of healthy primary school children have retentive constipation. The ratio of males to females is 4:1 in some studies.

Differential Diagnosis

Features distinguishing retentive constipation from Hirschsprung disease are summarized in Table 20–8.

Treatment of Retentive Constipation

Increased intake of fluids and high-residue foods such as bran, whole wheat, fruits, and vegetables may be sufficient therapy in mild constipation. However, the most likely response to increased fluid intake in normal children is increased urination with little effect on defecation. Barley malt extract (Maltsupex), 1–2 tsp added to feedings two or three times daily is a safe stool softener in small infants as is polyethylene glycol solution (MiraLax). Stool softeners such as dioctyl sodium sulfosuccinate, 5–10 mg/kg/d are less effective in children with voluntary stool retention. Cathartics such as standardized extract of senna fruit (Senokot syrup, Ex-Lax) can be used for short periods.

If encopresis is present, treatment should start with relieving fecal impaction. Effective stool softeners should

Table 20–8. Differentiation of retentive constipation and Hirschsprung disease.

	Retentive Constipation	Hirschsprung Disease
Onset	2–3 years	At birth
Abdominal distention	Rare	Present
Nutrition and growth	Normal	Poor
Soiling and retentive behavior	Intermittent or constant	Rare
Rectal examination	Ampulla full	Ampulla may be empty
Rectal biopsy	Ganglion cells present	Ganglion cells absent
Rectal manometry	Normal rectoanal reflex	Nonrelaxation of internal anal sphincter after rectal distention
Barium enema	Distended rectum	Narrow distal segment with proximal megacolon

thereafter be given as a maintenance medication in doses sufficient to induce two or three loose bowel movements per day. Such medications include mineral oil (2–3 mL/kg/d), a nonabsorbable osmotic agent such as polyethylene glycol (MiraLax, 1 g/kg/d), and milk of magnesia (1–2 mL/kg/d). After several weeks to months of regular loose stools, the stool softener can be tapered and stopped. Mineral oil should not be given to nonambulatory infants, physically handicapped or bed-bound children, or those with GE reflux. Aspiration of mineral oil may cause lipid pneumonia. A multiple vitamin is recommended while mineral oil is given. Recurrence of encopresis should be treated promptly with a short course of stimulant laxatives or an enema. Psychiatric consultation may be indicated for patients with resistant symptoms or severe emotional disturbances.

Benninga M et al: The Paris Consensus on Childhood Constipation Terminology (PACCT) Group. J Pediatr Gastroenterol Nutr 2005;40:273 [PMID: 15735478].

GASTROINTESTINAL BLEEDING

Vomiting blood and passing blood per rectum are alarming symptoms. The history is the key to identifying the bleeding source. The following questions should be answered:

1. Is it really blood, and is it coming from the GI tract? A number of substances simulate hematochezia or melena (Table 20–9). The presence of blood should be confirmed chemically. Coughing, tonsillitis, lost teeth, or epistaxis may cause what appears to be occult or overt GI bleeding. An adolescent female may be experiencing menarche.

2. How much blood is there and what is its color and character? Table 20–10 lists the sites of GI bleeding predicted by the appearance of the blood in the stools. Table 20–11 lists causes of rectal bleeding.

3. Is the child acutely or chronically ill? The physical examination should be thorough. Physical signs of portal hypertension, intestinal obstruction, or coagulopathy are particularly important. The nasal passages should be inspected for signs of recent epistaxis, the vagina for menstrual blood, and the anus for fissures and hemorrhoids. A systolic blood pressure below 100 mm Hg and a pulse rate above 100 beats/min in an older child suggest at least a 20% reduction of blood volume. A pulse rate increase of 20 beats/min or a drop in systolic blood pressure greater than 10 mm Hg when the patient sits up is also a sensitive index of volume depletion.

4. Is the child still bleeding? Serial determination of vital signs and hematocrit are essential to assess ongoing bleeding. Detection of blood in the gastric aspirate confirms a bleeding site proximal to the liga-

Table 20–9. Pitfalls in the diagnosis of gastrointestinal bleeding in children.

Exogenous blood
  Maternal blood[a]
  Epistaxis
  Uncooked meat
Pseudoblood
  Medications in red syrup
  Red Kool-Aid, fruit punch, red gelatin
  Tomato skin
  Tomato juice
  Cranberry juice
  Beets
  Peach skin
  Red diaper syndrome[b]
  Red cherries
Black stools
  Iron preparations[c,d]
  Pepto-Bismol
  Grape juice
  Purple grapes
  Spinach
  Chocolate

---

[a]From cracked nipples in a breast-fed baby.
[b]Red pigmentation of soiled diapers due to *Serratia marcescens* in stool.
[c]Ferrous sulfate and ferrous gluconate with guaiac and orthotolidine-based tests.
[d]High false-positive rate with orthotolidine-based tests.
Modified and reproduced, with permission, from Treem WR: Gastrointestinal bleeding in children. Gastrointest Endosc Clin North Am 1994;4:75.

ment of Treitz. However, its absence does not rule out the duodenum as the source. Testing the stool for occult blood will help in monitoring ongoing loss of blood.

Treatment

If a hemorrhagic diathesis is detected, vitamin K should be given intravenously. In severe bleeding, the need for volume replacement is monitored by measurement of central venous pressure. In less severe cases, vital signs, serial hematocrits, and gastric aspirates are sufficient.

If blood is recovered from the gastric aspirate, gastric lavage with saline should be performed until only a blood-tinged return is obtained. Upper intestinal endoscopy is then done to identify the bleeding site. Endoscopy is superior to barium contrast study for lesions such as esophageal varices, stress ulcers, and gastritis. Colonoscopy may identify the source of bright red rectal bleeding but should be performed as an emergency only if the extent of bleeding warrants immediate investigation and if plain abdominal radiographs show no signs of intestinal obstruction. Colonoscopy on an unprepped colon is often inadequate for making a diagnosis. Capsule endoscopy may help identify the site of bleeding if colonoscopy and upper endoscopy are negative. Small or large bowel lesions that bleed briskly (> 0.5 mL/min) may be localized by angiography or radionuclide scanning following injection of labeled red cells.

Persistent vascular bleeding (varices, vascular anomalies) may be relieved temporarily using intravenous octreotide, 25–30 $\mu g/m^2/h$. Sustained infusion of octreotide may be used for up to 48 hours if needed. Bleeding from esophageal varices may be stopped by compression with a Sengstaken–Blakemore tube. Endoscopic sclerosis or banding of bleeding varices is effective treatment.

If gastric decompression, acid suppressive therapy, and transfusion are ineffective in stopping ulcer bleeding, laser therapy, local injection of epinephrine, electrocautery, or emergency surgery may be necessary.

Fox VL: Gastrointestinal bleeding in infancy and childhood. Gastroenterol Clin North Am 2000;29:37 [PMID: 10752017].

RECURRENT ABDOMINAL PAIN

About 10% of healthy schoolchildren between ages 5 and 15 years will at some time experience recurrent epi-

Table 20–10. Identification of sites of gastrointestinal bleeding.

Symptom or Sign	Location of Bleeding Lesion
Effortless bright red blood from the mouth	Nasopharyngeal or oral lesions; tonsillitis; esophageal varices; lacerations of esophageal or gastric mucosa (Mallory-Weiss syndrome)
Vomiting of bright red blood or of "coffee grounds"	Lesion proximal to ligament of Treitz
Melanotic stool	Lesion proximal to ligament of Treitz, upper small bowel. Blood loss in excess of 50–100 mL/24 h
Bright red or dark red blood in stools	Lesion in the ileum or colon. (Massive upper gastrointestinal bleeding may also be associated with bright red blood in stool.)
Streak of blood on outside of a stool	Lesion in the rectal ampulla or anal canal

Table 20–11. Differential diagnosis of gastrointestinal bleeding in children by symptoms and age at presentation.

	Infant	Child (2–12 years)	Adolescent (> 12 years)
Hematemesis	Swallowed maternal blood Peptic esophagitis Mallory-Weiss tear Gastritis Gastric ulcer Duodenal ulcer Gastric, duodenal ulcer	Epistaxis Peptic esophagitis Caustic ingestion Mallory-Weiss tear Esophageal varices Gastritis Gastric ulcer Duodenal ulcer Hereditary hemorrhagic telangiectasia Hemobilia Henoch-Schönlein purpura	Esophageal ulcer Peptic esophagitis Mallory-Weiss tear Esophageal varices Gastric ulcer Gastritis Duodenal ulcer Hereditary hemorrhagic telangiectasia Hemobilia Henoch-Schönlein purpura
Painless melena	Duodenal ulcer Duodenal duplication Ileal duplication Meckel diverticulum Gastric heterotopia[a]	Duodenal ulcer Duodenal duplication Ileal duplication Meckel diverticulum Gastric heterotopia[a]	Duodenal ulcer Leiomyoma (sarcoma)
Melena with pain, obstruction, peritonitis, perforation	Necrotizing enterocolitis Intussusception[b] Volvulus	Duodenal ulcer Hemobilia[c] Intussusception[b] Volvulus Ileal ulcer (isolated)	Duodenal ulcer Hemobilia[c] Crohn disease (ileal ulcer)
Hematochezia with diarrhea, crampy abdominal pain	Infectious colitis Pseudomembranous colitis Eosinophilic colitis Hirschsprung enterocolitis	Infectious colitis Pseudomembranous colitis Granulomatous (Crohn) colitis Hemolytic-uremic syndrome Henoch-Schönlein purpura Lymphonodular hyperplasia	Infectious colitis Pseudomembranous colitis Granulomatous (Crohn) colitis Hemolytic-uremic syndrome Henoch-Schönlein purpura
Hematochezia without diarrhea or abdominal pain	Anal fissure Eosinophilic colitis Rectal gastric mucosa heterotopia Colonic hemangiomas	Anal fissure Solitary rectal ulcer Juvenile polyp Lymphonodular hyperplasia	Anal fissure Hemorrhoid Solitary rectal ulcer Colonic arteriovenous malformation

[a]Ectopic gastric tissue in jejunum or ileum without Meckel diverticulum.
[b]Classically, "currant jelly" stool.
[c]Hemobilia often accompanied by vomiting, right upper quadrant pain.
Reproduced, with permission, from Treem WR: Gastrointestinal bleeding in children. Gastrointest Endosc Clin North Am 1994;4:75.

sodes of unexplained abdominal pain severe enough to interfere with normal activities. An organic cause is found in fewer than 10% of patients.

Clinical Findings

A. SYMPTOMS AND SIGNS

Attacks of pain are characteristically of variable duration and intensity. It is not rare for the parent to report that the pain is constant, all day every day. Although the pain is usually located in the periumbilical area,

location far from the umbilicus does not rule out recurrent abdominal pain. Pain occurs both day and night. Weight loss is rare. Pain may be associated with dramatic reactions—frantic crying, clutching the abdomen, doubling over. Parents may be alarmed, and children are often taken to emergency departments, where the evaluation is negative for an abdominal crisis. School attendance may suffer, and enjoyable family events may be disrupted. The pain may be associated with pallor, nausea, vomiting, and slight temperature elevation.

The pain usually bears little relationship to bowel habits and physical activity. However, some patients have a symptom constellation suggestive of irritable bowel syndrome—bloating, postprandial pain, lower abdominal discomfort, and erratic stool habits with a sensation of obstipation or incomplete evacuation of stool. A precipitating or stressful situation in the child's life at the time the pains began can sometimes be elicited. School phobia may be a precipitant. A history of functional GI complaints is often found in family members.

A thorough physical examination is essential and usually normal. Complaints of abdominal tenderness elicited during palpation sometimes seem out of proportion to visible signs of distress.

B. Laboratory Findings

Complete blood count, sedimentation rate, urinalysis, and stool test for occult blood usually suffice. In the adolescent female patient, ultrasound of the abdomen may be helpful to detect gallbladder or ovarian pathology. If the pain is atypical, further testing suggested by symptoms and family history should be done.

Differential Diagnosis

Abdominal pain secondary to disorders of the urinary tract and extra-abdominal sources are listed in Table 20–3. Pinworms, mesenteric lymphadenitis, and chronic appendicitis are improbable causes of recurrent abdominal pain. *Helicobacter pylori* infection is rarely the cause of recurrent abdominal pain. Lactose intolerance usually causes abdominal distention, gas, and diarrhea with milk ingestion. At times, however, abdominal discomfort may be the only symptom. Abdominal migraine and abdominal epilepsy are rare conditions with an episodic character often associated with vomiting. The incidence of peptic gastritis, esophagitis, duodenitis, and ulcer disease is probably underappreciated. Upper intestinal endoscopy may be useful.

Treatment & Prognosis

Treatment consists of reassurance based on a thorough physical appraisal and a sympathetic, age-appropriate explanation of the nature of functional pain. The concept of "visceral hyperalgesia" or increased pain signaling from physiologic stimuli such as gas, acid secretion, or stool is one that parents can understand and helps them to respond appropriately to the child's complaints. Reassurance without education is rarely helpful. Regular activity should be resumed, especially school attendance. Therapy for emotional problems is sometimes required, but drugs should be avoided. In older patients, and in those with what appears to be visceral hyperalgesia, amitriptyline in low doses may occasionally be helpful. Antispasmodic medications are rarely helpful and should be reserved for patients with more typical irritable bowel complaints.

Hyams JS, Hyman PE: Recurrent abdominal pain and the biopsychosocial model of medical practice. J Pediatr 1998;133:473 [PMID: 9787683].

Hyams JS et al: Abdominal pain and irritable bowel syndrome in adolescents: A community-based study. J Pediatr 1996;129:220 [PMID: 8765619].

Van Ginkel R et al: Alterations in rectal sensitivity and motility in childhood irritable bowel syndrome. Gastroenterology 2001; 120:31 [PMID: 11208711].

INFLAMMATORY BOWEL DISEASE

Crohn disease and ulcerative colitis are the two major chronic inflammatory bowel diseases of children. They share many features resulting from bowel inflammation, such as diarrhea, pain, fever, and blood loss, but they differ in important aspects, such as distribution of disease, histologic findings, incidence and type of extraintestinal symptoms, response to medications and surgery, and prognosis. A comparison of these two conditions is shown in Table 20–12. The cause is unknown but is probably a result of inappropriate activation of the mucosal immune system fueled by luminal flora. The aberrant response appears to be facilitated by defects in the barrier function of the intestinal epithelium as well. The single greatest risk factor for inflammatory bowel disease is a positive family history (found in 15–30% of inflammatory bowel disease patients). Monozygotic twins have a 37% concordance for Crohn disease and a 10% concordance for ulcerative colitis. Recent genetic studies have identified an inflammatory bowel disease susceptibility gene on chromosome 16 (*CARD15*), the product of which is involved in the activation of the nuclear factor NFκB and also in the intestinal response to bacterial lipopolysaccharides. More genetic loci are being identified, giving some hope that basic immune mechanisms of Crohn disease and perhaps ulcerative colitis will be identified. There is no indication that emotional factors are a primary cause of these diseases.

Diagnostic Testing

A. Crohn Disease

Crohn disease can occur at any location in the GI tract from the mouth to the anus. Upper and lower endoscopy allows investigation of mouth, esophagus, duodenum, colon, and terminal ileum. Biopsy specimens from all these areas may reveal the typical histologic findings. Barium radiograph of the small intestine is still the best way to look for small bowel disease. In the absence of intestinal strictures, capsule videoendoscopy allows direct inspection of the small intestine. Computed tomography scan and magnetic resonance imaging of the small bowel can show mucosal and mural edema but are not specific enough to confirm a diagnosis. Intestinal wall thickening is often reported on computed tomography scans performed in an emergency setting to rule out appendicitis and may simply

Table 20–12. Features of Crohn disease and ulcerative colitis.

	Crohn Disease	**Ulcerative Colitis**
Age at onset	10–20 years	10–20 years
Incidence	4–6 per 100,000	3–15 per 100,000
Area of bowel affected	Oropharynx, esophagus, and stomach, rare; small bowel only, 25–30%; colon and anus only, 25%; ileocolitis, 40%; diffuse disease, 5%	Total colon, 90%; proctitis, 10%
Distribution	Segmental; disease-free skip areas common	Continuous; distal to proximal
Pathology	Full-thickness, acute, and chronic inflammation; noncaseating granulomas (50%), extraintestinal fistulas, abscesses, stricture, and fibrosis may be present	Superficial, acute inflammation of mucosa with microscopic crypt abscess
Radiographic findings	Segmental lesions; thickened, circular folds, cobblestone appearance of bowel wall secondary to longitudinal ulcers and transverse fissures; fixation and separation of loops; narrowed lumen; "string sign"; fistulas	Superficial colitis; loss of haustra; shortened colon and pseudopolyps (islands of normal tissue surrounded by denuded mucosa) are late findings
Intestinal symptoms	Abdominal pain, diarrhea (usually loose with blood if colon involved), perianal disease, enteroenteric or enterocutaneous fistula, abscess, anorexia	Abdominal pain, bloody diarrhea, urgency, and tenesmus
Extraintestinal symptoms		
Arthritis/arthralgia	15%	9%
Fever	40–50%	40–50%
Stomatitis	9%	2%
Weight loss	90% (mean 5.7 kg)	68% (mean 4.1 kg)
Delayed growth and sexual development	30%	5–10%
Uveitis, conjunctivitis	15% (in Crohn colitis)	4%
Sclerosing cholangitis	—	4%
Renal stones	6% (oxalate)	6% (urate)
Pyoderma gangrenosum	1–3%	5%
Erythema nodosum	8–15%	4%
Laboratory findings	High erythrocyte sedimentation rate; microcytic anemia; low serum iron and total iron-binding capacity; increased fecal protein loss; low serum albumin; antineutrophil cytoplasmic antibodies present in 10–20%; *Saccharomyces cerevisiae* antibodies positive in 60%.	High erythrocyte sedimentation rate; microcytic anemia, high white blood cell count with left shift; antineutrophil cytoplasmic antibodies present in 80%.

Reproduced, with permission, from Kirschner BS: Inflammatory bowel disease in children. Pediatr Clin North Am 1988;35:189.

be acute reactions to intestinal infections. Serum antibodies to *Saccharomyces cerevisiae* (ASCA) are present in 40–60% of patients with Crohn disease. ASCA is helpful for screening if positive, but it is not sensitive or specific enough to be diagnostic. Elevated fecal calprotectin, a neutrophil-associated protein, suggests the presence of an inflammatory process. It may be more useful for monitoring therapy than for diagnosis.

B. ULCERATIVE COLITIS

Colonoscopy with mucosal biopsy is the best diagnostic test for ulcerative colitis. Nearly pathognomonic signs may be seen on barium enema, but the test is being replaced in most instances by colonoscopy. The perinuclear antineutrophil cytoplasmic antibody (pANCA) is positive in 60–70% of patients with ulcerative colitis. Fecal calprotectin is high in patients with active disease.

C. INDETERMINATE COLITIS

This poorly defined entity is a diagnostic challenge and is generally a diagnosis of exclusion in patients in whom colonoscopic biopsy specimens do not seem typical of ulcerative colitis or Crohn disease. More experience is needed to determine whether this is indeed a separate disease. These patients may have superficial Crohn colitis or may have ulcerative colitis with relative rectal sparing. The same medications group is used for its treatment.

Differential Diagnosis

A. CROHN DISEASE

When extraintestinal symptoms predominate, Crohn disease can be mistaken for rheumatoid arthritis, systemic lupus erythematosus, or hypopituitarism. The acute onset of ileocolitis may be mistaken for appendicitis. Symptoms sometimes suggest celiac disease, peptic ulcer, intestinal obstruction, intestinal lymphoma, anorexia nervosa, or growth failure from endocrine causes.

B. ULCERATIVE COLITIS

In the acute stage, bacterial pathogens and toxins causing colitis must be ruled out. These include *Shigella, Salmonella, Yersinia, Campylobacter, Entamoeba histolytica*, enteroinvasive *Escherichia coli* (*E coli* 0157), *Aeromonas hydrophila*, and *Clostridium difficile* toxin. Mild ulcerative colitis sometimes mimics irritable bowel syndrome. Crohn disease of the colon is an important differential possibility.

Complications (See Table 20–12.)

A. CROHN DISEASE

Intestinal obstruction, fistula, and abscess formation are common. Perforation and hemorrhage are rare. Malnutrition is caused by anorexia compounded by malabsorption, protein-losing enteropathy, disaccharidase deficiency, and diarrhea induced by bile salt malabsorption. Other complications include perianal disease, pyoderma gangrenosum, arthritis, amyloidosis, and growth retardation. The risk of colon cancer is increased in patients with Crohn colitis although not to the extent seen in ulcerative colitis.

B. ULCERATIVE COLITIS

Arthritis, uveitis, pyoderma gangrenosum, and malnutrition all occur. Growth failure and delayed puberty are less common than in Crohn disease. Liver disease (chronic active hepatitis, sclerosing cholangitis) is more common. In patients with pancolitis, carcinoma of the colon occurs with an incidence of 1–2% per year after the first 10 years of disease. Cancer risk is a function of disease duration and not age at onset. The mortality rate from colon cancer is high because the usual signs (occult blood in stool, pain, and abnormal radiologic findings) are not specific and may be ignored in a patient with colitis. Routine cancer screening via colonoscopy, with multiple biopsies and evaluation of specimens by histology for metaplasia and by flow cytometry for aneuploidy, is recommended in pediatric patients after 10 years of pancolitis. Dysplasia that persists in absence of inflammation is an indication for colectomy, as is aneuploidy in multiple biopsies.

Treatment

A. MEDICAL TREATMENT

Medical treatment for Crohn disease and ulcerative colitis is similar and includes anti-inflammatory, antidiarrheal, and antibiotic medication. No medical therapy has proved uniformly effective.

1. Diet—A high-protein, high-carbohydrate diet with normal amounts of fat is recommended. Decreased fiber may prevent symptoms in those with active colitis or partial intestinal obstruction; however, increased fiber may be beneficial for mucosal health through bacterial production of fatty acids in patients with relatively inactive disease. Lactose is poorly tolerated when disease is active. The main concern should be ensuring adequate caloric intake. Restrictive or bland diets are counterproductive because they usually result in poor intake. Vitamin and iron supplements are recommended. Zinc levels are often low in patients with Crohn disease and should be supplemented. Supplemental calories in the form of liquid diets are well tolerated. Total parenteral nutrition for periods of 4–6 weeks may induce remission of symptoms and stimulate linear growth and sexual development. Enteral administration of low-residue or elemental liquid diets is widely used outside of the United States to induce remission in patients with Crohn disease. It is less effective in ulcerative colitis. Home programs of both enteral and parenteral nutritional support have been especially effective in patients with intractable symptoms or growth failure.

2. Nonabsorbable salicylate derivatives—Sulfasalazine is effective in mild ulcerative colitis and perhaps in cases of Crohn disease of the colon. It prevents relapse of ulcerative colitis once remission is induced. The drug is not absorbed systemically. Intact drug is hydrolyzed by colon flora into sulfapyridine and 5-aminosalicylate. The sulfonamide moiety is probably inactive but is responsible for the allergic side effects of the drug. The salicylate moiety has local anti-inflammatory activity. Side effects are common, including skin rash, nausea, headache, and abdominal pain. Rarely, serum sickness, hemolytic anemia, aplastic anemia, and pancreatitis occur. Response to therapy may be slow. Sulfasalazine inhibits folic acid absorption, and supplemental folic acid is required.

The recommended dosage is 2–3 g/d in three divided doses for children over age 10 years or 50 mg/kg/d for younger children. Half of this dosage is used as a maintenance medication for well-controlled ulcerative colitis. Salicylate polymers for oral and rectal use (olsalazine, mesalamine) are available. A variety of pH-sensitive tablet coatings and microencapsulation allow release of these products at specific locations in the GI tract, thereby improving their efficacy. They are no more effective than sulfasalazine but are used in sulfonamide-sensitive patients and have fewer side effects.

3. Corticosteroids—With more severe inflammatory bowel disease, corticosteroids are used. Methylprednisolone, 2 mg/kg/d, or hydrocortisone, 10 mg/kg/d, may be given intravenously when disease is severe. Prednisone, 1–2 mg/kg/d orally in two or three divided doses, is given for 6–8 weeks, followed by gradual tapering. Alternate-day steroids produce fewer side effects as the dosage of drug is tapered. There is no evidence that maintenance corticosteroids prevent relapse. Prednisone is often given in conjunction with sulfasalazine. The patient's varicella immunity should be confirmed by history or antibody screen and the parents counseled appropriately as to risk and therapy after varicella exposure. Serum titers against *E histolytica* and stool examination for amebic parasites must be checked before starting therapy with corticosteroids, because amebic colitis may become generalized with steroid therapy. Hydrocortisone enemas or foam can be instilled into the rectum in patients with tenesmus or ulcerative proctitis. Budesonide, which has "one pass metabolism" in the liver, is available in oral and rectal preparations. These preparations are most useful in rectal disease (enemas and suppositories) and right-sided colon disease (oral), and in appropriate doses have fewer corticoid side effects.

4. Azathioprine—Azathioprine (Imuran), 1–2 mg/kg/d orally, or 6-mercaptopurine can be used when high maintenance dose of corticosteroids is necessary to keep the inflammatory bowel disease under control (especially in Crohn disease). The optimal dose of 6-mercaptopurine depends on the patient's ability to metabolize the compound. Positive results of this therapy may be delayed weeks to months. Side effects include pancreatitis, hepatotoxicity, and bone marrow suppression. Metabolites of azathioprine should be monitored to avoid over- and underdosing in patients with variable metabolizing capacity. Testing prior to therapy to assess levels of enzymes metabolizing Imuran should be performed in order to identify patients at risk for serious side effects of Imuran.

5. Metronidazole—This drug has been used in treating Crohn disease in patients with perianal disease. Disease tends to recur when the drug is discontinued. It may also be effective in treating Crohn disease of the colon. The dosage of metronidazole is 15–30 mg/kg/d in three divided doses. Peripheral neuropathy may be a side effect with prolonged use. Ciprofloxacin may have similar therapeutic effects. Remicade has largely replaced this treatment.

6. Cyclosporine—This powerful immunosuppressant is effective in severe, steroid-resistant ulcerative colitis, but because of side effects and rapid relapse after discontinuation, it is usually used to buy time and improve severe colitis when surgical treatment is planned.

7. Methotrexate—There is encouraging experience with oral and subcutaneous methotrexate in treating Crohn disease. Liver toxicity is a risk with prolonged use.

8. Anticytokines—Tumor necrosis factor alpha (TNF-α) is a proinflammatory cytokine produced in monocytes, macrophages, and activated T cells, which among other functions stimulates production of proinflammatory cytokines such as interleukins IL-1, IL-6, IL-8, and granulocyte–macrophage colony-stimulating factor. TNF-α levels are increased in intestinal mucosa in Crohn disease. Intravenous use of a chimeric human–mouse antibody to TNF-α (infliximab) is effective in Crohn disease, especially in resistant perianal and fistulizing disease. Most patients require repeated intravenous infusions of the medication at intervals ranging from 4–12 weeks in order to remain in remission. Anaphylactic reactions to this medication have been reported but are decreasing with better "humanization" of the product. The concomitant use of azathioprine also decreases the incidence of severe allergic reactions. Treatment with the anti-inflammatory cytokine IL-10 is in the developmental stage for patients with Crohn disease. Infliximab therapy is occasionally helpful in severe colitis and in steroid-dependent colitis.

9. Thalidomide—Thalidomide has been used especially in patients with oral and vaginal ulcers secondary to Crohn disease. The mechanism of its action may be via prevention of TNF secretion or antiangiogenic activity. This medication must be used under strict supervision in postpubescent female patients because of the risk of teratogenesis.

B. SURGICAL TREATMENT

1. Crohn disease—Crohn disease is not cured by surgery. However, 70% of patients eventually require surgery to relieve obstruction, drain abscess, relieve intractable symptoms, or encourage growth and sexual maturation. Newer treatments may decrease this figure. The relapse rate 6 years after surgery is 60%. Recurrence usually occurs at the site of anastomosis within 2 years. Recurrence rate may be less in disease limited to the colon. Surgery performed to correct growth retardation must be performed before puberty.

2. Ulcerative colitis—Surgery is curative and is recommended for those with uncontrolled hemorrhage, toxic megacolon, unrelenting pain and diarrhea, growth failure, high-grade mucosal dysplasia, or malignant tumors. There are several surgical approaches (ileoanal anastomosis, Koch-type continent ileostomy) that allow a near-normal lifestyle after colectomy. Liver disease associated with ulcerative colitis (sclerosing cholangitis) is not improved by colectomy.

Prognosis

A. CROHN DISEASE

Although the mortality rate is low (2% in the first 7 years), morbidity is high. The disease is progressive in most cases. Over 50% of patients experience symptoms that affect the quality of life. About 20% have severe disabling disease, and 20% have so few symptoms that they describe themselves as healthy.

B. ULCERATIVE COLITIS

The prognosis is good. About 5% of patients present with toxic megacolon (massive colonic dilation secondary to full-thickness enterocolitis accompanied by shock and fever) and require immediate colectomy. Seventy-five percent have a relapsing and remitting course. Between 25% and 40% require colectomy—especially those with pancolitis, anemia, and hypoalbuminemia at the time of presentation.

Baldassano R et al: Infliximab (Remicade) therapy in treatment of pediatric Crohn's disease. Am J Gastroenterol 2003;98:833 [PMID: 12738464].

Bariol C et al: Early studies on the safety and effectiveness of thalidomide for symptomatic inflammatory bowel disease. J Gastroenterol Hepatol 2002;17:135 [PMID: 11966942].

Bonen DK, Cho J: The genetics of inflammatory bowel disease. Gastroenterology 2003;124:521 [PMID: 12557156].

Markowitz J et al: A multicenter trial of 6-mercaptopurine and prednisone in children with newly diagnosed Crohn's disease. Gastroenterology 2000;119:895 [PMID: 11040176].

Newman B, Siinovich KA: Recent advances in the genetics of inflammatory bowel disease. Curr Opin Gastroenterol 2005; 21:401 [PMID: 15930978].

Tamboli CP et al: Fecal calprotectin in Crohn's disease: New family ties. Gastroenterology 2003;124:1972 [PMID: 12806631].

REFERENCES

Web Resources

http://www.naspgn.org/ The website of the North American Society for Pediatric Gastroenterology, Hepatology and Nutrition (NASPGHAN) has an excellent selection of educational materials on many pediatric gastroenterologic conditions with information for parents and recommendations for evaluation and therapy.

General References

Silverman A, Roy CC: *Pediatric Clinical Gastroenterology,* 4th ed. Mosby, 1995.

Suchy FJ (editor): *Liver Disease in Children,* 2nd ed. Mosby, 2000.

Walker WA et al (editors): *Pediatric Gastrointestinal Disease,* 4th ed. BC Decker, 2003.

Wyllie R, Hyams JS (editors): *Pediatric Gastrointestinal Disease.* WB Saunders, 1993.

Liver & Pancreas

21

Ronald J. Sokol, MD, & Michael R. Narkewicz, MD

◼ LIVER

PROLONGED NEONATAL CHOLESTATIC JAUNDICE

The main clinical features of disorders causing prolonged neonatal cholestasis are (1) jaundice with elevated serum conjugated (or direct) bilirubin fraction (> 2 mg/dL or > 20% of total bilirubin), (2) variably acholic stools, (3) dark urine, and (4) hepatomegaly.

Prolonged neonatal cholestasis (conditions with decreased bile flow) has intrahepatic and extrahepatic causes. Specific clinical clues (Table 21–1) distinguish these two major categories of jaundice in 85% of cases. Histologic examination of tissue obtained by percutaneous liver biopsy increases the accuracy of differentiation to 95% (Table 21–2).

INTRAHEPATIC CHOLESTASIS

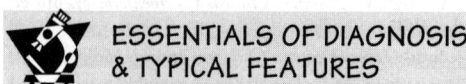

ESSENTIALS OF DIAGNOSIS & TYPICAL FEATURES

- *Elevated total and conjugated bilirubin.*
- *Hepatomegaly and dark urine.*
- *Patency of extrahepatic biliary tree.*

General Considerations

Intrahepatic cholestasis is characterized by hepatocyte dysfunction and patency of the extrahepatic biliary system. A specific cause can be identified in about 50% of cases. Patency of the extrahepatic biliary tract is suggested by pigmented stools and lack of bile duct proliferation on liver biopsy. It can be confirmed least invasively by hepatobiliary scintigraphy using technetium-99m (^{99m}Tc)-diethyliminodiacetic acid (diethyl-IDA [DIDA]). Radioactivity in the bowel within 4–24 hours is evidence of bile duct patency. Finding bilirubin in duodenal aspirates also con-

firms patency. Patency can also be determined by cholangiography carried out intraoperatively, percutaneously by transhepatic cholecystography, or endoscopic retrograde cholangiopancreatography (ERCP) using a pediatric-size side-viewing endoscope. Magnetic resonance cholangiopancreatography in infants is of limited use and highly dependent on the operator and equipment.

1. Perinatal or Neonatal Hepatitis Resulting from Infection

This diagnosis is considered in infants with jaundice, hepatomegaly, vomiting, lethargy, fever, and petechiae. It is important to identify perinatally acquired viral, bacterial, or protozoal infections (Table 21–3). Infection may occur transplacentally, by ascent through the cervix into amniotic fluid, from swallowed contaminated fluids (maternal blood, urine) during delivery, from blood transfusions administered in the early neonatal period, or from breast milk or environmental exposure. Infectious agents associated with neonatal intrahepatic cholestasis include herpes simplex virus, varicella virus, enteroviruses (coxsackievirus and echovirus), cytomegalovirus (CMV), rubella virus, adenovirus, parvovirus, human herpesvirus type 6, hepatitis B virus (HBV), human immunodeficiency virus (HIV), *Treponema pallidum,* and *Toxoplasma gondii.* Although hepatitis C may be transmitted vertically, it rarely causes neonatal cholestasis. The degree of liver cell injury caused by these agents is variable, ranging from massive hepatic necrosis (herpes simplex, enteroviruses) to focal necrosis and mild inflammation (CMV, HBV). Serum bilirubin, bile acids, alanine aminotransferase (ALT), aspartate aminotransferase (AST), and alkaline phosphatase are elevated. The infant is jaundiced, may have petechiae or rash, and generally appears ill.

Clinical Findings

A. SYMPTOMS AND SIGNS

Clinical symptoms usually appear in the first 2 weeks of life but may appear as late as age 2–3 months. Jaundice may be noted as early as the first 24 hours of life. Poor oral intake, poor sucking reflex, lethargy, and vomiting are frequent. Stools may be normal to pale in color but are seldom acholic. Dark urine stains the diaper. Hepatomegaly

638

Table 21–1. Characteristic clinical features of intrahepatic and extrahepatic neonatal cholestasis.

Intrahepatic	Extrahepatic
Preterm infant, small for gestational age, appears ill; hepatosplenomegaly, other organ or system involvement; incomplete cholestasis (stools with some color); associated cause identified (infections, metabolic, familial, etc)	Full-term infant, seems well; hepatomegaly (firm to hard); complete cholestasis (acholic stools); polysplenia syndrome, equal right and left hepatic lobes

is present, and the liver has a uniform firm consistency. Splenomegaly is variably present. Macular, papular, vesicular, or petechial rashes may occur. In less severe cases, failure to thrive may be the major complaint. Unusual presentations include neonatal liver failure, hypoproteinemia, anasarca (nonhemolytic hydrops), and hemorrhagic disease of the newborn.

B. DIAGNOSTIC STUDIES

Neutropenia, thrombocytopenia, and signs of mild hemolysis are common. Mixed hyperbilirubinemia, elevated aminotransferases with near-normal alkaline phosphatase, prolongation of clotting studies, mild acidosis, and elevated cord serum IgM suggest congenital infection. Nasopharyngeal washings, urine, stool, and cerebrospinal fluid (CSF) should be cultured for virus. Specific IgM antibody and nucleic acid tests may be useful, as are long-bone radiographs to determine the presence of "celery stalking" in the metaphyseal regions of the humeri, femurs, and tibias.

Table 21–2. Characteristic histologic features of intrahepatic and extrahepatic neonatal cholestasis.

	Intrahepatic	Extrahepatic
Giant cells	+++	+
Lobules	Disarray	Normal
Portal reaction	Inflammation/minimal fibrosis	Fibrosis
Neoductular proliferation	Rare	Marked
Other	Steatosis, extramedullary hematopoiesis	Portal bile duct plugging, bile lakes

When indicated, computed tomography (CT) and magnetic resonance imaging (MRI) scans can identify intracranial calcifications (especially CMV and toxoplasmosis). Hepatobiliary scintigraphy shows decreased hepatic clearance of the circulating isotope with excretion into the gut. Careful ophthalmologic examination may be useful for diagnosis of herpes simplex virus, CMV, toxoplasmosis, and rubella.

A percutaneous liver biopsy is useful in distinguishing intrahepatic from extrahepatic cholestasis, but may not identify a specific infectious agent (see Table 21–2). However, typical inclusions of CMV in hepatocytes or bile duct epithelial cells, the presence of intranuclear acidophilic inclusions of herpes simplex, or positive immunohistochemical stains for several viruses can be diagnostic. Variable degrees of lobular disarray characterized by focal necrosis, multinucleated giant-cell transformation, and ballooned pale hepatocytes with loss of cordlike arrangement of liver cells are usual. Intrahepatocytic and canalicular cholestasis may be prominent. Portal changes are not striking, but modest neoductular proliferation and mild fibrosis may occur. Viral cultures or polymerase chain reaction testing of biopsy material may be helpful.

Differential Diagnosis

Great care must be taken to distinguish infectious causes of intrahepatic cholestasis from genetic or metabolic disorders because the clinical presentations are similar. Galactosemia, congenital fructose intolerance, and tyrosinemia must be investigated promptly, because specific dietary therapy is available. α_1-Antitrypsin deficiency, cystic fibrosis, and neonatal iron storage disease must also be considered. Specific physical features may be helpful when considering Alagille or Zellweger syndrome. Idiopathic neonatal hepatitis may be indistinguishable from infectious causes.

Patients with intrahepatic cholestasis frequently appear ill, whereas infants with extrahepatic cholestasis do not appear ill, have stools that are usually completely acholic, and have an enlarged, firm liver. Histologic findings are described in Table 21–2.

Treatment

Most forms of viral neonatal hepatitis are treated symptomatically. However, infections with herpes simplex virus, varicella, CMV, parvovirus, adenovirus, and toxoplasmosis have specific treatments. Fluids and adequate calories are encouraged. Intravenous dextrose is needed if feedings are not well tolerated. The consequences of cholestasis are treated as indicated (Table 21–4). Vitamin K orally or by injection and vitamins D and E orally should be provided. Choleretics (ursodeoxycholic acid [UDCA] or cholestyramine) are used if cholestasis persists. Corticosteroids are contraindicated.

Table 21–3. Infectious causes of neonatal hepatitis.

Infectious Agent	Diagnostic Tests	Specimens	Treatment
Cytomegalovirus	Culture and PCR, liver histology, IgM/[a]IgG	Urine, blood, liver	?Ganciclovir (Foscarnet)[b]
Herpes simplex	PCR and culture, liver histology, Ag (skin)	Liver, blood, eye, throat, rectal, CSF, skin	Acyclovir
Rubella	Culture, IgM/[a]IgG	Liver, blood, urine	Supportive
Varicella	Culture, PCR, Ag (skin)	Skin, blood, CSF, liver	Acyclovir (Foscarnet)[b]
Parvovirus	Serum IgM/[a]IgG, PCR	Blood	Supportive, ? IVIG
Enteroviruses	Culture and PCR	Blood, urine, CSF, throat, rectal, liver	Pleconaril (investigative)
Adenovirus	Culture and PCR	Nasal/throat, rectal, blood, liver, urine	Cidofovir, ?IVIG
Hepatitis B virus (HBV)	HBsAg, HBcAg IgM	Serum	Supportive for acute infection
Hepatitis C virus (HCV)	HCV PCR, HCV-IgG	Serum	Supportive for acute infection
Treponema pallidum	Serology; dark-field exam	Serum, CSF	Penicillin
Toxoplasma gondii	IgM/[a]IgG, PCR, culture	Serum, liver	Pyrimethamine and sulfadiazine with folinic acid
Mycobacterium tuberculosis	PPD, chest radiograph, liver tissue histologic stains and culture, gastric aspirate stain and culture	Serum, liver, gastric aspirate	INH, pyrazinamide, rifampin and streptomycin

[a]IgG = positive indicates maternal infection and transfer of antibody transplacentally; negative indicates unlikelihood of infection in mother and infant.
[b]Use for resistant viruses.
Ag, viral antigen testing; CSF, cerebrospinal fluid; HBC, hepatitis B core antigen; HBsAg, hepatitis B surface antigen; INH, isoniazid; IVIG, intravenous gamma globulin; PCR, polymerase chain reaction test for viral DNA or RNA; PPD, purified protein derivative.

Penicillin for suspected syphilis or antibiotics for bacterial hepatitis need to be administered promptly.

Prognosis

Multiple organ involvement is commonly associated with neonatal infectious hepatitis and has a poor outcome. Death from hepatic or cardiac failure, intractable acidosis, or intracranial hemorrhage may occur, especially in herpesvirus or enterovirus infection and occasionally in CMV or rubella infection. HBV rarely causes fulminant neonatal hepatitis; most infected infants become asymptomatic carriers of hepatitis B. Persistent liver disease results in mild chronic hepatitis, portal fibrosis, or cirrhosis. The liver in most infants who recover from congenital viral infection is left without fibrosis. Chronic cholestasis, although rare following infections, may lead to dental enamel hypoplasia, failure to thrive, biliary rickets, severe pruritus, and xanthoma.

Specific Infectious Agents

A. Neonatal Hepatitis B Virus Disease

Infection with HBV may occur at any time during perinatal life, but the risk is higher when acute maternal disease occurs during the last trimester of pregnancy. However, most cases of neonatal disease are acquired from mothers who are asymptomatic carriers of HBV. Although HBV has been found in most body fluids, including breast milk, neonatal transmission occurs occasionally transplacentally and primarily from exposure to maternal blood at delivery. In chronic hepatitis B surface antigen (HBsAg) carrier mothers, fetal and infant acquisition risk is greatest if the mother (1) is also hepatitis B "e" antigen (HBeAg)-positive and hepatitis B "e" antibody (HBeAb)-negative, (2) has detectable levels of serum-specific hepatitis B DNA polymerase, (3) has high serum levels of hepatitis B core antibody (HBcAb), or (4) has high blood levels of HBV

Table 21–4. Treatment of complications of chronic cholestatic liver disease.

Indication	Treatment	Dose	Toxicity
Intrahepatic cholestasis	Phenobarbital	3–10 mg/kg/d	Drowsiness, irritability, interference with vitamin D metabolism
	Cholestyramine/colestipol hydrochloride	250–500 mg/kg/d	Constipation, acidosis, binding of drugs, increased steatorrhea
	Ursodeoxycholic acid	15–20 mg/kg/d	Transient increase in pruritus
Pruritus	Phenobarbital or cholestyramine/colestipol (or both)	3–10 mg/kg/d	Drowsiness, irritability, interference with vitamin D metabolism
	Antihistamines: diphenhydramine hydrochloride	5–10 mg/kg/d	Drowsiness
	Hydroxyzine	2–5 mg/kg/d	
	Ultraviolet light B	Exposure as needed	Skin burn
	Carbamazepine	20–40 mg/kg/d	Hepatotoxicity, marrow suppression, fluid retention
	Rifampin	10 mg/kg/d	Hepatotoxicity, marrow suppression
	Ursodeoxycholic acid	15–20 mg/kg/d	Transient increase in pruritus
Steatorrhea	Formula containing medium-chain triglycerides (eg, Pregestimil)	120–150 calories/kg/d for infants	Expensive
	Oil supplement containing medium-chain triglycerides	1–2 mL/kg/d	Diarrhea, aspiration
Malabsorption of fat-soluble vitamins	Vitamin A	10,000–25,000 units/d	Hepatitis, pseudotumor cerebri, bone lesions
	Vitamin D	800–5000 units/d	Hypercalcemia, hypercalciuria
	25-Hydroxycholecalciferol (vitamin D)	3–5 µg/kg/d	Hypercalcemia, hypercalciuria
	1,25-Dihydroxycholecalciferol (vitamin D)	0.05–0.2 µg/kg/d	Hypercalcemia, hypercalciuria
	Vitamin E (oral)	25–200 IU/kg/d	Potentiation of vitamin K deficiency
	Vitamin E (oral, TPGS[a])	15–25 IU/kg/d	Potentiation of vitamin K deficiency
	Vitamin E (intramuscular)	1–2 mg/kg/d	Muscle calcifications
	Vitamin K (oral)	2.5 mg twice per week to 5 mg/d	
	Vitamin K (intramuscular)	2–5 mg each 4 wk	
Malabsorption of other nutrients	Multiple vitamin	1–2 times the standard dose	
	Calcium	25–100 mg/kg/d	Hypercalcemia, hypercalciuria
	Phosphorus	25–50 mg/kg/d	Gastrointestinal intolerance
	Zinc	1 mg/kg/d	Interference with copper and iron absorption

[a]D-α-Tocopheryl polyethylene glycol-1000 succinate.

DNA. These findings are markers for circulating infectious virus; however, hepatitis B can be transmitted even if HBsAg is the only marker present.

Neonatal liver disease resulting from HBV is extremely variable. The infant has a 70–90% chance of acquiring HBV at birth from an HBsAg-positive mother if the infant does not receive prophylaxis. Most infected infants become prolonged asymptomatic carriers of HBV. Fulminant hepatic necrosis has rarely been reported. In such cases, progressive jaundice, stupor, shrinking liver size, and coagulation abnormalities dominate the clinical picture. Respiratory, circulatory, and renal failure usually follow. Histologically, the liver shows massive hepatocyte necrosis, collapse of the reticulum framework, minimal inflammation, and occasional pseudoacinar structures. Survival without liver transplantation is rare but is associated with reasonable repair of liver architecture.

In less severe cases, focal hepatocyte necrosis occurs with a mild portal inflammatory response. Cholestasis is intracellular and canalicular. Chronic hepatitis may be present for many years, with serologic evidence of persisting antigenemia (HBsAg) and mildly elevated serum aminotransferases. Chronic hepatitis may rarely progress to cirrhosis within 1–2 years. Most infected infants have only mild evidence, if any, of liver injury.

To prevent perinatal transmission, all infants of mothers who are HBsAg-positive (regardless of HBeAg status) should receive hepatitis B immunoglobulin (HBIG) and hepatitis B vaccine within the first 24 hours after birth and vaccine again at ages 1 and 6 months. (See Chapter 9.) This prevents HBV infection in 85–95% of infants. HBIG can provide some protection when given as late as 72 hours after birth. If not given at birth it can be administered as late as 7 days postpartum as long as the infant has received the vaccine.

B. NEONATAL BACTERIAL HEPATITIS

Most bacterial liver infections in newborns are acquired by transplacental invasion from amnionitis with ascending spread from maternal vaginal or cervical infection. Onset is abrupt, usually within 48–72 hours after delivery, with signs of sepsis and often shock. Jaundice appears early and is of the mixed type. The liver enlarges rapidly, and the histologic picture is that of diffuse hepatitis with or without microabscess. The most common organisms involved are *Escherichia coli, Listeria monocytogenes,* and group B streptococci. Isolated neonatal liver abscess caused by *E coli* or *Staphylococcus aureus* is associated with omphalitis or umbilical vein catheterization. Bacterial hepatitis and neonatal liver abscesses require specific antibiotics in large doses and, rarely, surgical or radiologic interventional drainage. Deaths are common, but survivors show no long-term consequences of liver disease.

C. NEONATAL JAUNDICE WITH URINARY TRACT INFECTION

Jaundice in affected infants—usually males—typically appears between the second and fourth weeks of life. This disorder causes lethargy, fever, poor appetite, jaundice, and hepatomegaly. Except for mixed hyperbilirubinemia, other liver function tests (LFTs) are mildly abnormal. Leukocytosis is present, and infection is confirmed by culture. The mechanism for the liver impairment is the inhibitory action on bile secretion of bacterial products (endotoxins) and inflammatory cytokines.

Treatment of the infection leads to prompt resolution of the cholestasis without hepatic sequelae. Metabolic liver diseases, such as galactosemia and tyrosinemia, may present with gram-negative bacterial urinary tract infection.

Broderick AL, Jonas MM: Hepatitis B in children. Semin Liver Dis 2003;23(1):59 [PMID: 12616451].

Kane MA: Hepatitis viruses and the neonate. Clin Perinatol 1997;24:181 [PMID: 9099509].

Kesson AM: Management of neonatal herpes simplex virus infection. Paediatr Drugs 2001;3:81 [PMID: 11269641].

Rosenthal P: Neonatal hepatitis and congenital infections. In: Suchy FJ et al (editors): *Liver Disease in Children.* Lippincott, Williams & Wilkins, 2001:239.

2. Intrahepatic Cholestasis Resulting from Inborn Errors of Metabolism, Familial, & "Toxic" Causes

These cholestatic syndromes caused by specific enzyme deficiencies, other genetic disorders, or certain precipitants associated with neonatal liver disease feature intrahepatic cholestasis (ie, jaundice, hepatomegaly, and normal to completely acholic stools). Some of the specific clinical conditions have characteristic clinical signs.

Enzyme Deficiencies & Other Inherited Disorders

Early specific diagnosis is important because dietary or pharmacologic treatment may be available (Table 21–5). Reversal of liver disease and clinical symptoms is prompt and permanent in several disorders as long as the diet is maintained. As with other genetic disorders, parents of the affected infant should be offered genetic counseling. For some disorders, prenatal genetic diagnosis is available.

Cholestasis caused by metabolic diseases such as galactosemia, fructose intolerance, and tyrosinemia may be accompanied by vomiting, lethargy, poor feeding, hypoglycemia, and irritability. Hepatomegaly is a constant finding. The infants often appear septic; gram-negative bacteria can be cultured from blood in 25–50% of cases, especially in patients with galactosemia. Neonatal screening programs for galactosemia usually

Table 21–5. Metabolic and genetic causes of neonatal cholestasis.

Disease	Inborn Error	Hepatic Pathology	Diagnostic Studies
Galactosemia	Galactose-1-phosphate uridylyltransferase	Cholestasis, steatosis, necrosis, pseudoacini, fibrosis	Galactose-1-phosphate uridylyltransferase assay of red blood cells
Fructose intolerance	Fructose-1-phosphate aldolase	Steatosis, necrosis, pseudoacini, fibrosis	Liver fructose-1-phosphate aldolase assay or leukocyte DNA analysis
Tyrosinemia	Fumarylacetoacetase	Necrosis, steatosis, pseudoacini, portal fibrosis	Urinary succinylacetone, fumarylacetoacetase assay of red blood cells
Cystic fibrosis	Cystic fibrosis transmembrane conductance regulator gene	Cholestasis, neoductular proliferation, excess bile duct mucus, portal fibrosis	Sweat test and leukocyte DNA analysis
Hypopituitarism	Deficient production of pituitary hormones	Cholestasis, giant cells	Thyroxine, TSH, cortisol levels
α_1-Antitrypsin deficiency	Abnormal α_1-antitrypsin molecule (Pi ZZ phenotype)	Giant cells, cholestasis, steatosis, neoductular proliferation, fibrosis, PAS-diastase-resistant cytoplasmic granules	Serum α_1-antitrypsin phenotype
Gaucher disease	β-Glucosidase	Cholestasis, cytoplasmic inclusions in Kupffer cells (foam cells)	β-Glucosidase assay in leukocytes
Niemann-Pick disease	Lysosomal sphingomyelinase	Cholestasis, cytoplasmic inclusions in Kupffer cells	Sphingomyelinase assay of leukocytes or liver or fibroblasts (type C); leukocyte DNA analysis
Glycogen storage disease type IV	Branching enzyme	Fibrosis, cirrhosis, PAS-diastase-resistant cytoplasmic inclusions	Branching enzyme analysis of leukocytes or liver
Neonatal hemochromatosis	Unknown	Giant cells, portal fibrosis, hemosiderosis, cirrhosis	Histology, iron stains, lip biopsy, abdominal MRI
Peroxisomal disorders (eg, Zellweger syndrome)	Deficient peroxisomal enzymes or assembly	Cholestasis, necrosis, fibrosis, cirrhosis, hemosiderosis	Plasma very long chain fatty acids, qualitative bile acids, plasmalogen, pipecolic acid, liver electron microscopy
Abnormalities in bile acid metabolism	Several enzyme deficiencies defined	Cholestasis, necrosis, giant cells	Urine, serum, duodenal fluid analyzed for bile acids by fast atom bombardment-mass spectroscopy
Byler disease (familial progressive intrahepatic cholestasis)	*FIC-1* and BSEP genes	Cholestasis, necrosis, giant cells, fibrosis	Histology, family history, normal cholesterol, low or normal γ-glutamyl transpeptidase, DNA analysis
MDR_3 deficiency	MDR_3 gene	Cholestasis, bile duct proliferation, portal fibrosis	Bile phospholipid level, DNA analysis
Alagille syndrome (syndromic paucity of interlobular bile ducts)	*Jagged 1* gene mutations	Cholestasis, paucity of interlobular bile ducts, increased copper levels	Three or more clinical features, liver histology, DNA analysis

PAS, periodic acid-Schiff; TSH, thyroid-stimulating hormone.

detect the disorder before cholestasis develops. Other inherited conditions associated with neonatal intrahepatic cholestasis are outlined in Table 21–5. Treatment of these disorders is discussed in Chapter 32.

"Toxic" Causes of Neonatal Cholestasis

A. NEONATAL ISCHEMIC–HYPOXIC CONDITIONS

Perinatal events that result in hypoperfusion of the gastrointestinal system are sometimes followed within 1–2 weeks by cholestasis. This occurs in premature infants with respiratory distress, severe hypoxia, hypoglycemia, shock, and acidosis. When these perinatal conditions develop in association with gastrointestinal lesions such as ruptured omphalocele, gastroschisis, or necrotizing enterocolitis, a subsequent cholestatic picture is common (25–50% of cases). Liver function studies reveal mixed hyperbilirubinemia, elevated alkaline phosphatase and γ-glutamyl transpeptidase (GGT) values, and variable elevation of the aminotransferases. Stools are seldom persistently acholic.

Choleretics (UDCA or cholestyramine), introduction of enteral feedings as soon as possible, and nutritional support are the mainstays of treatment until the cholestasis resolves (see Table 21–4). In some cases, this resolution may take 3–6 months. As long as no severe intestinal problem is present (eg, short gut syndrome), complete resolution of the hepatic abnormalities is the rule. But portal fibrosis with periportal scarring is occasionally found on follow-up biopsy.

B. PROLONGED PARENTERAL NUTRITION

Cholestasis may develop after 1–2 weeks in premature newborns receiving total parenteral nutrition. Even full-term infants with significant intestinal disease, resections, or dysmotility may develop total parenteral nutrition-related cholestasis. Contributing factors may include toxicity of intravenous amino acids, diminished stimulation of bile flow from prolonged absence of feedings, small intestinal bacterial overgrowth with translocation of intestinal bacteria and their cell wall products, missing nutrients or antioxidants, photooxidation of amino acids, infusion of lipid hydroperoxides, and the "physiologic cholestatic" propensity of the premature infant. Histology of the liver may resemble that of extrahepatic biliary obstruction. Early introduction of feedings has reduced the frequency of this disorder. The prognosis is generally good. Occasional cases of cirrhosis, liver failure, and hepatoma may develop, particularly in infants with intestinal resections or anomalies.

C. INSPISSATED BILE SYNDROME

This syndrome is the result of accumulation of bile in canaliculi and in the small- and medium-size bile ducts in hemolytic disease of the newborn (Rh, ABO) and in

some infants receiving total parenteral nutrition. The same mechanisms may cause intrinsic obstruction of the common bile duct. An ischemia–reperfusion injury may also contribute to cholestasis in Rh incompatibility. In extreme hemolysis, the cholestasis may be seemingly complete, with acholic stools. Levels of bilirubin may reach 40 mg/dL, primarily conjugated. If inspissation of bile occurs within the extrahepatic biliary tree, differentiation from biliary atresia may be difficult. A trial of choleretics is indicated. Once stools show a return to normal color or ^{99m}Tc-DIDA scanning shows biliary excretion into the duodenum, patency of the extrahepatic biliary tree is ensured. Although most cases improve slowly over 2–6 months, persistence of complete cholestasis for more than 2 weeks requires further studies (ultrasonography, DIDA scanning, liver biopsy) with possible cholangiographic or magnetic resonance imaging of the extrahepatic biliary tree. Irrigation of the common bile duct is sometimes necessary to dislodge the obstructing inspissated biliary material.

Balistreri WF et al: Intrahepatic cholestasis: Summary of an American Association for the Study of Liver Diseases single-topic conference. Hepatology 2005;42:222 [PMID: 15898074].

Heubi JE et al: Tauroursodeoxycholic acid (TUDCA) in the prevention of total parenteral nutrition-associated liver disease. J Pediatr 2002;141(2):237 [PMID: 12183720].

Teitelbaum DH et al: Use of cholecystokinin-octapeptide for the prevention of parenteral nutrition-associated cholestasis. Pediatrics 2005;115:1332 [PMID: 15867044].

3. Idiopathic Neonatal Hepatitis (Giant-Cell Hepatitis)

This type of cholestatic jaundice of unknown cause presents with features of cholestasis and a typical liver biopsy appearance; it accounts for 25–50% of cases of neonatal intrahepatic cholestasis. The degree of cholestasis is variable, and the disorder may be indistinguishable from extrahepatic causes in 10% of cases. Viral infections, α_1-antitrypsin deficiency, Alagille syndrome, Niemann–Pick type C disease (NPC), progressive familial intrahepatic cholestasis (PFIC), and bile acid synthesis defects may present in a similar clinical and histologic manner. However, in PFIC and bile acid synthesis defects the GGT levels are normal or low. Electron microscopy of the liver biopsy may help distinguish NPC and PFIC.

Intrauterine growth retardation, prematurity, poor feeding, emesis, poor growth, and partially or intermittently acholic stools are characteristic of intrahepatic cholestasis. Patients with neonatal lupus erythematosus may present with giant-cell hepatitis; however, thrombocytopenia, skin rash, or congenital heart block is usually also present.

In cases of suspected idiopathic neonatal hepatitis (diagnosed in the absence of infectious, metabolic, and toxic causes), patency of the biliary tree should be verified to exclude extrahepatic surgical disorders. DIDA scanning and ultrasonography may be helpful in this regard. Some clinicians have used the enteral string test during DIDA scanning to confirm bile duct patency. Liver biopsy findings are usually diagnostic after age 6–8 weeks (see Table 21–2) but may be misleading before age 6 weeks. Failure to detect patency of the biliary tree, nondiagnostic liver biopsy findings, or persisting complete cholestasis (acholic stools) are indications for minilaparotomy and intraoperative cholangiography performed by an experienced surgeon, ERCP, percutaneous cholecystography, or magnetic resonance cholangiopancreatography (MRCP). Occasionally, a small but patent (hypoplastic) extrahepatic biliary tree is demonstrated (as in Alagille syndrome) and is probably the result rather than the cause of diminished bile flow; surgical reconstruction of hypoplastic biliary trees should not be attempted.

Once a patent extrahepatic tree is confirmed, therapy should include choleretics, a special formula with medium-chain triglycerides (Pregestimil, Alimentum), and supplemental fat-soluble vitamins in water-miscible form (see Table 21–4). This therapy is continued as long as significant cholestasis remains (conjugated bilirubin > 1 mg/dL). Fat-soluble vitamin levels should be monitored while supplements are given and at least once after their discontinuation.

Eighty percent of patients recover without significant hepatic fibrosis. However, in 20% of cases with this presentation, the patient has PFIC and is likely to progress to cirrhosis. In general, failure to resolve the cholestatic picture by age 6–12 months is associated with progressive liver disease and evolving cirrhosis. This may occur with either normal or diminished numbers of interlobular bile ducts (paucity of interlobular ducts). Liver transplantation has been successful when signs of hepatic decompensation are noted (rising bilirubin, coagulopathy, intractable ascites).

Balistreri WF et al: Intrahepatic cholestasis: Summary of an American Association for the Study of Liver Diseases single-topic conference. Hepatology 2005;42:222 [PMID: 15898074].

Roberts EA: Neonatal hepatitis syndrome. Semin Neonatol 2003; 8:357 [PMID: 15001124].

Yerushalmi B et al: Niemann–Pick disease type C in neonatal cholestasis at a North American Center. J Pediatr Gastroenterol Nutr 2002;35(1):44 [PMID: 12142809].

4. Paucity of Interlobular Bile Ducts

Forms of intrahepatic cholestasis caused by decreased numbers of interlobular bile ducts (< 0.5 bile ducts per portal tract) may be classified according to whether they are associated with other malformations. Alagille syndrome (syndromic paucity or arteriohepatic dysplasia) is caused by mutations in the gene *Jagged 1*, located on chromosome 20p which codes for a ligand of the notch receptor. Alagille syndrome is sometimes recognized by identification of the characteristic facies, which becomes more obvious with age. The forehead is prominent, as is the nasal bridge. The eyes are set deep and sometimes widely apart (hypertelorism). The chin is small and slightly pointed and projects forward. The ears are prominent. The stool color varies with the severity of cholestasis. Pruritus begins by age 3–6 months. Firm, smooth hepatomegaly may be present. Cardiac murmurs are present in 95% of patients, and butterfly vertebrae (incomplete fusion of the vertebral body or anterior arch) are present in 50%. Xanthomas develop later in the disease as hypercholesterolemia becomes a problem. Occasionally, early cholestasis is mild and not recognized or the patient may present with complex congenital heart disease (eg, tetralogy of Fallot).

Conjugated hyperbilirubinemia may be mild to severe (2–15 mg/dL). Serum alkaline phosphatase, GGT, and cholesterol are markedly elevated, especially early in life. Serum bile acids are always elevated. Aminotransferases are mildly increased, but clotting factors and other liver proteins are usually normal.

The cardiovascular abnormalities include peripheral, branch pulmonary artery or pulmonary valvular stenoses (most common), atrial septal defect, coarctation of the aorta, and tetralogy of Fallot. Up to 10–15% of patients have intracranial vascular abnormalities and may develop intracranial hemorrhage early in childhood.

Eye abnormalities (posterior embryotoxon) and renal abnormalities (dysplastic kidneys, renal tubular ectasia, single kidney, hematuria) can also be present. Growth retardation with normal to increased levels of growth hormone (growth hormone resistance) is common. A variable portion of patients may have pancreatic insufficiency that may contribute to the fat malabsorption. Although variable, the intelligence quotient is frequently low. Hypogonadism with micropenis may be present. A weak, high-pitched voice may develop. Neurologic disorders resulting from vitamin E deficiency (areflexia, ataxia, ophthalmoplegia) eventually develop in many unsupplemented children.

In the nonsyndromic form, paucity of interlobular bile ducts occurs in the absence of the extrahepatic malformations. Paucity of interlobular bile ducts may also occur in α_1-antitrypsin deficiency, Zellweger syndrome, in association with lymphedema (Aagenaes syndrome), PFIC, cystic fibrosis, CMV or rubella infection, and inborn errors of bile acid metabolism.

High doses (250 mg/kg/d) of cholestyramine may control pruritus, lower cholesterol, and clear xanthomas. Ursodeoxycholic therapy (15–25 mg/kg/d) appears to be more effective and causes fewer side effects than cholestyramine. Nutritional therapy to prevent wasting and deficiencies of fat-soluble vitamins is of particular importance because of the severity of cholestasis (see Table 21–4).

Prognosis is more favorable in the syndromic than in the nonsyndromic varieties. In the former, only 30–40%

of patients have severe complications of disease, whereas over 70% of patients with nonsyndromic varieties progress to cirrhosis. Many of this latter group may have PFIC. In Alagille syndrome, cholestasis may improve by age 2–4 years, with minimal residual hepatic fibrosis. Survival into adulthood despite raised serum bile acids, aminotransferases, and alkaline phosphatase occurs in about 50% of cases. Several patients have developed hepatocellular carcinoma. Hypogonadism has been noted; however, fertility is not obviously affected in most cases. Cardiovascular anomalies may shorten life expectancy. Some patients have persistent, severe cholestasis, rendering their quality of life poor or recurrent bone fractures caused by metabolic bone disease; liver transplantation has been successfully performed under these circumstances.

Emerick KM et al: Intracranial vascular abnormalities in patients with Alagille syndrome. J Pediatr Gastroenterol Nutr 2005; 41:99 [PMID: 15990638].

Lykavieris P et al: Bleeding tendency in children with Alagille syndrome. Pediatrics 2003;111(1):167 [PMID: 12509572].

Piccoli DA, Spinner NB: Alagille syndrome and the Jagged 1 gene. Semin Liver Dis 2001;21:525 [PMID: 11745040].

PROGRESSIVE FAMILIAL INTRAHEPATIC CHOLESTASIS (Byler Disease)

PFIC is a group of disorders presenting as pruritus, diarrhea, jaundice, and failure to thrive in the first 6–12 months of life. PFIC type I (Byler disease), caused by mutations in the *FIC1* gene, is associated with low to normal serum levels of GGT and cholesterol and elevated levels of bilirubin, aminotransferases, and bile acids. Diarrhea is common. Liver biopsy results are similar to those found with giant-cell hepatitis but sometimes with a paucity of interlobular bile ducts and centrolobular fibrosis that progresses to cirrhosis. Electron microscopy shows diagnostic granular "Byler bile" in canaliculi.

Treatment includes administration of UDCA, partial biliary diversion if the condition is unresponsive to UDCA, and liver transplantation. With partial biliary diversion or ileal exclusion surgery, many patients show improved growth and liver histology, reduction in symptoms and, thus, avoidance of liver transplantation. PFIC type II is caused by mutations in the bile salt export pump (*BSEP*) gene, which codes for an adenosine triphosphate-dependent canalicular bile salt transport protein. These patients are clinically and biochemically similar to PFIC type I patients and have similar liver histology and treatment options. PFIC type III is caused by mutations in the *MDR₃* (multiple drug resistance protein type 3) gene, which encodes a canalicular protein that pumps phospholipid into bile. Serum GGT and bile acid levels are ele-

vated, bile duct proliferation and portal tract fibrosis are seen in liver biopsies, and bile phospholipid levels are low. Treatment is similar to that for other forms of PFIC. Bile acid synthesis defects are clinically similar to those in PFIC I and PFIC II, with low serum levels of GGT and cholesterol; however, the serum level of total bile acids is inappropriately normal or low and urine bile acid analysis may identify a synthesis defect. Treatment is with oral cholic acid and UDCA.

Carlton VE et al: Molecular basis of intrahepatic cholestasis. Ann Med 2004;36:606 [PMID: 15768832].

Kurbegov AC et al: Biliary diversion for progressive familial intrahepatic cholestasis: Improved liver morphology and bile acid profile. Gastroenterology 2003;125:1227 [PMID: 14517804].

Shneider BL: Progressive intrahepatic cholestasis: Mechanisms, diagnosis and therapy. Pediatr Transplant 2004;8:609[Review] [PMID: 15598335].

Wanty C et al: Fifteen years single center experience in the management of progressive familial intrahepatic cholestasis of infancy. Acta Gastroenterol Belg 2004;67:313 [PMID: 15727074].

EXTRAHEPATIC NEONATAL CHOLESTASIS

Extrahepatic neonatal cholestasis is characterized by complete and persistent cholestasis (acholic stools) in the first 3 months of life; lack of patency of the extrahepatic biliary tree proved by intraoperative, percutaneous, or endoscopic cholangiography; firm to hard hepatomegaly; and typical features on histologic examination of liver biopsy tissue (see Table 21–2). Causes include biliary atresia, choledochal cyst, spontaneous perforation of the extrahepatic ducts, and intrinsic obstruction of the common duct.

1. Biliary Atresia

Biliary atresia is the progressive fibroinflammatory obliteration of the lumen of all, or part of, the extrahepatic biliary tree presenting within the first 3 months of life. In European Americans, biliary atresia occurs in 1:10,000–1:18,000 births, and the incidence in both sexes is equal. In Asian Americans the incidence is higher and the disorder is twice as common in girls. The abnormality found most commonly is complete atresia of all extrahepatic biliary structures. There appear to be at least two types of biliary atresia: the perinatal form (80% of cases), in which a perinatal insult is believed to initiate inflammatory obstruction of the biliary tree, and the fetal–embryonic form (20% of cases), in which the extrahepatic biliary system did not develop normally. In the perinatal form, meconium and first-passed stools are usually normal in color, suggesting early patency of the ducts. Evidence obtained from surgically removed remnants of the extrahepatic biliary tree suggests an inflammatory or sclerosing cholangiopathy. Although an infectious cause seems reasonable, no agent has been consistently found in such cases. A role for reovirus type 3 and rotavirus group C has been suggested. Certain histocompatibility locus antigen types may predispose to biliary atresia. In the fetal–embryonic type, the bile duct presumably developed abnormally and is associated with other nonhepatic congenital anomalies. The association of biliary atresia with the polysplenia syndrome (heterotaxia, preduodenal portal vein, interruption of the inferior vena cava, polysplenia, and midline liver) supports an embryonic origin of biliary atresia in these cases.

Jaundice may be noted in the newborn period but is more often delayed until age 2–3 weeks. The urine stains the diaper; and the stools are often pale yellow, buff-colored, gray, or acholic. Seepage of bilirubin products across the intestinal mucosa may give some yellow coloration to the stools. Hepatomegaly is common, and the liver may feel firm to hard; splenomegaly develops later. Pruritus, digital clubbing, xanthomas, and a rachitic rosary may be noted in older patients. By age 2–6 months, the growth curves reveal poor weight gain. Late in the course, ascites, failure to thrive, and bleeding complications occur.

No single laboratory test will consistently differentiate biliary atresia from other causes of complete obstructive jaundice. A study of hepatic 2,6-dimethyliminodiacetic acid (HIDA) excretion performed early in the course of disease may help to distinguish intrahepatic from extrahepatic causes of cholestasis, although there is considerable overlap. MRCP shows guarded promise as an imaging study to define biliary atresia. Although biliary atresia is suggested by persistent elevation of serum GGT or alkaline phosphatase levels, high cholesterol levels, and prolonged prothrombin times, these findings have also been reported in severe neonatal hepatitis, α_1-antitrypsin deficiency, and bile duct paucity. Furthermore, these tests will not differentiate the location of the obstruction within the extrahepatic system. Generally, the aminotransferases are elevated only modestly in biliary atresia. Serum proteins and blood clotting factors are not affected early in the disease. Routine chest radiograph may reveal abnormalities suggestive of polysplenia syndrome. Ultrasonography of the biliary system should be performed to ascertain the presence of choledochal cyst and intra-abdominal anomalies. Liver biopsy specimens can differentiate intrahepatic causes of cholestasis from biliary atresia in over 90% of cases (see Table 21–2).

The major diagnostic dilemma is distinguishing between this entity and neonatal hepatitis, bile duct paucity, metabolic liver disease (particularly α_1-antitrypsin deficiency), choledochal cyst, or intrinsic bile duct obstruction (stones, bile plugs). Although spontaneous perforation of extrahepatic bile ducts leads to jaundice and acholic stools, the infants are usually quite ill with chemical peritonitis from biliary ascites, and hepatomegaly is not found.

If the diagnosis of biliary atresia cannot be excluded by the diagnostic evaluation before age 60 days, surgical exploration is necessary. Laparotomy must include liver biopsy and an operative cholangiogram if a gallbladder is present. The presence of yellow bile in the gallbladder implies patency of the proximal extrahepatic duct system. Radiographic visualization of cholangiographic contrast in the duodenum excludes obstruction to the distal extrahepatic ducts.

In the absence of surgical correction or transplantation, the following eventually develop: failure to thrive, marked pruritus, portal hypertension, hypersplenism, bleeding diathesis, rickets, ascites, and cyanosis. Eventually, hepatic failure and death occur, almost always by age 18–24 months.

Except for the occasional example of correctable biliary atresia, in which choledochojejunostomy is feasible, the standard procedure is hepatoportoenterostomy (Kasai procedure). Occasionally, portocholecystostomy (gallbladder Kasai procedure) may be performed if the gallbladder is present and the passage from it to the duodenum is patent. These procedures are best done in specialized centers where experienced surgical, pediatric, and nursing personnel are available. Surgery should be performed as early as possible (before 60 days of life); the Kasai procedure should generally not be undertaken in infants older than age 4 months, because the likelihood of bile drainage at this age is very low. Orthotopic liver transplantation is now indicated for patients who do not undergo the Kasai procedure, who fail to drain bile after the Kasai procedure, or who progress to end-stage biliary cirrhosis despite surgical treatment. The 3–5-year survival rate following liver transplantation is 80–90%.

Whether or not the Kasai procedure is performed, supportive medical treatment measures consist of vitamin and caloric support (vitamins A, D, K, and E and formulas containing medium-chain triglycerides [Pregestimil or Alimentum]) (see Table 21–4). Suspected bacterial infections (eg, ascending cholangitis) should be treated promptly with broad-spectrum antibiotics, and signs of bleeding tendency should be corrected with intramuscular vitamin K. Ascites can be managed initially with reduced sodium intake and spironolactone. Choleretics and bile acid-binding products (cholestyramine, aluminum hydroxide gel) are of little use. The value of UDCA remains to be determined.

When bile flow is sustained following portoenterostomy, the 10-year survival rate is 25–35%. Death is usually caused by liver failure, sepsis, acidosis, or respiratory failure secondary to intractable ascites. Esophageal variceal hemorrhage develops in 40% of patients. Surprisingly, terminal hemorrhage is unusual. Occasional long-term survivors develop hepatopulmonary syndrome (intrapulmonary right to left shunting of blood resulting in hypoxia) or portopulmonary hypertension (pulmonary arterial hypertension in patients with portal hypertension). Liver transplantation has dramatically changed the outlook for these patients.

Condino AA et al:. Portopulmonary hypertension in pediatric patients. J Pediatr 2005;147:3. [PMID: 16027687].

Mack CL, Sokol RJ: Unraveling the pathogenesis and etiology of biliary atresia. Pediatr Res 2005;57:87R [PMID: 15817506].

Meyers RL et al: High-dose steroids, ursodeoxycholic acid, and chronic intravenous antibiotics improve bile flow after Kasai procedure in infants with biliary atresia. J Pediatr Surg 2003;38(3):406 [PMID: 12632357].

Muraji T et al: Japanese Biliary Atresia Society: Postoperative corticosteroid therapy for bile drainage in biliary atresia—a nationwide survey. J Pediatr Surg 2004;39:1803 [PMID: 15616935].

Nio M et al: Japanese Biliary Atresia Registry: Five- and 10-year survival rates after surgery for biliary atresia: A report from the Japanese Biliary Atresia Registry. J Pediatr Surg 2003; 38(7):997 [PMID: 12861525].

Sokol RJ et al: Pathogenesis and outcome of biliary atresia: Current concepts. J Pediatr Gastroenterol Nutr 2003;37:4 [PMID: 12827000].

2. Choledochal Cyst

Choledochal cysts cause 2–5% of cases of extrahepatic neonatal cholestasis; the incidence is fourfold higher in girls and higher in patients of Asian descent. In most cases, the clinical manifestations, basic laboratory findings, and histopathologic features on liver biopsy are indistinguishable from those associated with biliary atresia. Neonatal symptomatic cysts are usually associated with atresia of the distal common duct—accounting for the diagnostic dilemma—and may simply be part of the spectrum of biliary atresia. Ultrasonography or MRI reveals the presence of a cyst. Immediate surgery is indicated once abnormalities in clotting factors have been corrected and bacterial cholangitis, if present, has been treated with intravenous antibiotics. In older children, choledochal cyst presents as recurrent episodes of right upper quadrant abdominal pain, vomiting, obstructive jaundice, or pancreatitis, or as a right abdominal mass.

Excision of the cyst and choledocho–Roux-en-Y jejunal anastomosis are recommended. In some cases, because of technical problems, only the mucosa of the cyst can be removed with jejunal anastomosis to the proximal bile duct. Anastomosis of cyst to jejunum or duodenum is not recommended.

The prognosis depends on the presence or absence of associated evidence of atresia and the appearance of the intrahepatic ducts. If atresia is found, the prognosis is similar to that described in the preceding section. If an isolated extrahepatic cyst is encountered, the outcome is generally excellent, with resolution of the jaundice and return to normal liver architecture. However,

bouts of ascending cholangitis, particularly if intrahepatic cysts are present, or obstruction of the anastomotic site may occur. The risk of biliary carcinoma developing within the cyst is about 5–15% at adulthood; therefore, cystectomy or excision of cyst mucosa should be undertaken whenever possible.

Bismuth H, Krissat J: Choledochal cyst malignancies. Ann Oncol 1999;10:94 [PMID: 10436795].

He X et al: Congenital choledochal cyst—Report of 56 cases. Chin Med Sci J 2000;15(1):52 [PMID: 12899402].

Miyano G et al: Cholecystectomy alone is inadequate for treating forme fruste choledochal cyst: Evidence from a rare but important case report. Pediatr Surg Int 2005;21:61 [PMID: 15316725].

Wong AM et al: Prenatal diagnosis of choledochal cyst using magnetic resonance imaging: A case report. World J Gastroenterol 2005;11:5082 [PMID: 16124073].

3. Spontaneous Perforation of the Extrahepatic Bile Ducts

The sudden appearance of obstructive jaundice, acholic stools, and abdominal enlargement with ascites in a sick newborn is suggestive of this condition. The liver is usually normal in size, and a yellow-green discoloration can often be discerned under the umbilicus or in the scrotum. In 24% of cases, stones or sludge obstructs the common bile duct. DIDA scan or ERCP shows leakage from the biliary tree, and ultrasonography confirms ascites or fluid around the bile duct.

Treatment is surgical. Simple drainage, without attempts at oversewing the perforation, is sufficient in primary perforations. A diversion anastomosis is constructed in cases associated with choledochal cyst or stenosis. The prognosis is generally good.

Chardot C et al: Spontaneous perforation of the biliary tract in infancy: A series of 11 cases. Eur J Pediatr Surg 1996;6:341 [PMID: 9007467].

Xanthakos SA et al: Spontaneous perforation of the bile duct in infancy: A rare but important cause of irritability and abdominal distension. J Pediatr Gastroenterol Nutr 2003;36(2):287 [PMID: 12548069].

OTHER NEONATAL HYPERBILIRUBINEMIC CONDITIONS (Noncholestatic Nonhemolytic)

This group of disorders associated with hyperbilirubinemia is of two types: (1) unconjugated hyperbilirubinemia, consisting of breast milk jaundice, Lucey–Driscoll syndrome, congenital hypothyroidism, upper intestinal obstruction, Gilbert disease, Crigler–Najjar syndrome, and drug-induced hyperbilirubinemia; and (2) conjugated noncholestatic hyperbilirubinemia, consisting of Dubin–Johnson syndrome and Rotor syndrome.

1. Unconjugated Hyperbilirubinemia

Breast Milk Jaundice

Persistent elevation of the indirect bilirubin fraction may occur in up to 36% of breast-fed infants. Enhanced β-glucuronidase activity in breast milk is one factor that increases absorption of unconjugated bilirubin. Substances (eg, L-aspartic acid) in casein hydrolysate formulas inhibits this enzyme. The increased enterohepatic shunting of unconjugated bilirubin exceeds the normal conjugating capacity in the liver of these infants. The mutation for Gilbert syndrome predisposes to breast milk jaundice and to more prolonged jaundice. Low volumes of ingested breast milk may also contribute to jaundice in the first week of life.

Hyperbilirubinemia does not usually exceed 20 mg/dL, with most cases in the range of 10–15 mg/dL. In patients whose bilirubin levels are above 4–5 mg/dL, the jaundice is noticeable by the fifth to seventh day of breast feeding. It may accentuate the underlying physiologic jaundice—especially early, when total fluid intake may be less than optimal. Except for jaundice, the physical examination is usually normal; urine does not stain the diaper, and the stools are golden yellow.

The jaundice peaks by the third week of life and clears before age 3 months in almost all infants, even when breast feedings are continued. All infants who remain jaundiced past age 2–3 weeks should have measurements of conjugated bilirubin to exclude hepatobiliary disease.

Kernicterus has rarely been reported in association with this condition. In special situations, breast feeding may be discontinued temporarily and replaced by formula feedings for 2–3 days until serum bilirubin decreases by 2–8 mg/dL. Cow's milk formulas inhibit the intestinal reabsorption of unconjugated bilirubin. When breast feeding is reinstituted, the serum bilirubin may increase slightly but not to the previous level. Phototherapy is not indicated in the healthy full-term infant with this condition unless bilirubin levels meet high-risk levels as defined by the American Academy of Pediatrics.

American Academy of Pediatrics. Subcommittee on Hyperbilirubinemia. Management of hyperbilirubinemia in the newborn infant 35 or more weeks of gestation. Pediatrics 2004;114:297 [PMID: 15231951].

Gourley GR: A controlled, randomized, double-blind trial of prophylaxis against jaundice among breastfed newborns. Pediatrics 2005;116:385 [PMID: 16061593].

Kreamer BL et al: A novel inhibitor of beta-glucuronidase: 1-Aspartic acid. Pediatr Res 2001;50(4):460 [PMID: 11568288].

Mauro Y et al: Prolonged unconjugated hyperbilirubinemia associated with breast milk and mutations of the bilirubin uridine diphosphate-glucuronosyl transferase gene. Pediatrics 2000;106:E59 [PMID: 11061796].

Monaghan G et al: Gilbert's syndrome is a contributory factor in prolonged unconjugated hyperbilirubinemia of the newborn. J Pediatr 1999;134:441 [PMID: 10190918].

Congenital Hypothyroidism

Although the differential diagnosis of indirect hyperbilirubinemia should always include congenital hypothyroidism, the diagnosis may be obvious from other clinical and physical clues or from the newborn screening results. The jaundice clears quickly with replacement thyroid hormone therapy, although the mechanism is unclear.

Tiker F: Congenital hypothyroidism and early severe hyperbilirubinemia. Clin Pediatr (Phila) 2003;42:365 [PMID: 12800733].

Upper Intestinal Obstruction

The association of indirect hyperbilirubinemia with high intestinal obstruction (eg, duodenal atresia, annular pancreas, pyloric stenosis) in the newborn has been observed repeatedly; the mechanism is unknown. Diminished levels of hepatic glucuronyl transferase have been found on liver biopsy in pyloric stenosis, and genetic studies suggest that this indirect hyperbilirubinemia is an early sign of Gilbert syndrome.

Treatment is that of the underlying obstructive condition (usually surgical). Jaundice disappears once adequate nutrition is achieved.

Trioche P et al: Jaundice with hypertrophic pyloric stenosis is an early manifestation of Gilbert's syndrome. Arch Dis Child 1999;81:301 [PMID: 10490432].

Gilbert Syndrome

Gilbert syndrome is a common form (3–7% of the population) of familial hyperbilirubinemia associated with a partial reduction of hepatic bilirubin uridine diphosphate-glucuronyl transferase activity and perhaps an abnormality in the function or amount of one or more hepatocyte membrane protein carriers. Accelerated jaundice of the newborn, breast milk jaundice, and jaundice with intestinal obstruction may be present in affected infants. During puberty and beyond, mild fluctuating jaundice, especially with illness, and vague constitutional symptoms are common. Shortened red blood cell survival time in some patients is thought to be caused by reduced activity of enzymes involved in heme biosynthesis (protoporphyrinogen oxidase). Subsidence of hyperbilirubinemia has been achieved in patients by administration of phenobarbital (5–8 mg/kg/d), although this therapy is not justified.

The disease is inherited as an abnormality of the promoter region of uridine diphosphate-glucuronyl transferase-1; however, another factor is necessary for disease expression. The homozygous (16%) and heterozygous states (40%) are common. Males are affected more often than females (4:1). Serum unconjugated bilirubin is generally less than 3–6 mg/dL, although unusual cases may exceed 8 mg/dL. The findings on liver biopsy and most other LFTs are normal except for prolonged indocyanine green and bromosulfophthalein retention. An increase of 1.4 mg/dL or more in the level of unconjugated bilirubin after a 2-day fast (300 kcal/d) is consistent with the diagnosis of Gilbert syndrome. Genetic testing is available but rarely needed. No treatment is necessary.

Bancroft JD et al: Gilbert syndrome accelerates development of neonatal jaundice. J Pediatr 1998;132:656 [PMID: 9580766].

Ulgenalp A et al: Analyses of polymorphism for UGT1*1 exon 1 promoter in neonates with pathologic and prolonged jaundice. Biol Neonate 2003;83(4):258 [PMID: 12743455].

Crigler–Najjar Syndrome

Infants with type 1 Crigler–Najjar syndrome usually develop rapid severe elevation of unconjugated bilirubin (> 30–40 mg/dL) with neurologic consequences (kernicterus). Consanguinity is often present. Prompt recognition of this entity and treatment with exchange transfusions are required, followed by phototherapy. Some patients have no neurologic signs until adolescence or early adulthood, at which time deterioration may occur suddenly. For diagnosis of this condition it is useful to obtain a duodenal bile specimen, which characteristically will be colorless and contain a predominance of unconjugated bilirubin, small amounts of monoconjugates, and only traces of diconjugated bilirubin. Phenobarbital administration in these patients does not significantly alter these findings, nor does it lower serum bilirubin levels. The deficiency in uridine diphosphate-glucuronyl transferase-1 is inherited in an autosomal recessive pattern. A combination of phototherapy and cholestyramine may keep bilirubin levels below 25 mg/dL. The use of tin protoporphyrin or tin mesoporphyrin remains experimental. Liver transplantation is curative and may prevent kernicterus if performed early. An auxiliary orthotopic transplantation also relieves the jaundice while the patient retains native liver. Hepatocyte transplantation is experimental.

A milder form (type 2) with both autosomal dominant and recessive inheritance is rarely associated with neurologic complications. Hyperbilirubinemia is less severe, and the bile is pigmented and contains bilirubin monoglucuronide and diglucuronide. Patients with this form respond to phenobarbital with lowering of serum bilirubin levels. An increased proportion of monoconjugated and diconjugated bilirubin in the bile follows phenobarbital treatment. Liver biopsy findings and LFTs are consistently normal in both types.

Ambrosino G et al: Isolated hepatocyte transplantation for Crigler-Najjar syndrome type 1. Cell Transplant 2005;14(2–3):151 [PMID: 15881424].

Kaplan M et al: Bilirubin genetics for the nongeneticist: Hereditary defects of neonatal bilirubin conjugation. Pediatrics 2003; 111:886 [PMID: 12671128].

Schauer R et al: Treatment of Crigler–Najjar type 1 disease: Relevance of early liver transplantation. J Pediatr Surg 2003;38(8):1227 [PMID: 12891498].

Drug-Induced Hyperbilirubinemia

Vitamin K_3 (menadiol) may elevate indirect bilirubin levels by causing hemolysis. Vitamin K_1 (phytonadione) can be used safely in neonates. Carbamazepine can cause conjugated hyperbilirubinemia in infancy. Rifampin and antiretroviral protease inhibitors may cause unconjugated hyperbilirubinemia. Other drugs (eg, ceftriaxone, sulfonamides) may displace bilirubin from albumin, potentially increasing the risk of kernicterus—especially in the sick premature infant.

2. Conjugated Noncholestatic Hyperbilirubinemia (Dubin–Johnson Syndrome & Rotor Syndrome)

These diagnoses are suspected when persistent or recurrent conjugated hyperbilirubinemia and jaundice occur and liver function tests are normal. The basic defect in Dubin–Johnson syndrome affects the multiple organic anion transport protein (MRP_2) of the bile canaliculus, causing impaired hepatocyte excretion of conjugated bilirubin into bile. A variable degree of impairment in uptake and conjugation complicates the clinical picture. Transmission is autosomal recessive, so a positive family history is occasionally obtained. In Rotor syndrome, the defect lies in hepatic uptake and storage of bilirubin. Bile acids are metabolized normally, so that cholestasis does not occur. Bilirubin values range from 2–5 mg/dL, and other LFTs are normal.

In Rotor syndrome, the liver is normal; in Dubin–Johnson syndrome, it is darkly pigmented on gross inspection and may be enlarged. Microscopic examination reveals numerous dark-brown pigment granules consisting of polymers of epinephrine metabolites, especially in the centrilobular regions. However, the amount of pigment varies within families, and some jaundiced family members may have no demonstrable pigmentation in the liver. Otherwise, the liver is histologically normal. Oral cholecystography fails to visualize the gallbladder in Dubin–Johnson syndrome but is normal in Rotor syndrome. Differences in the excretion patterns of bromosulfophthalein, in results of DIDA cholescintigraphy, in urinary coproporphyrin I and III levels, and in the serum pattern of monoglucuronide and diglucuronide conjugates of bilirubin can help distinguish between these two conditions.

Choleretic agents (eg, UDCA) may help reduce the cholestasis in infants with Dubin–Johnson syndrome.

Kaplan M et al: Bilirubin genetics for the nongeneticist: Hereditary defects of neonatal bilirubin conjugation. Pediatrics 2003; 111(4 Pt 1):886 [PMID: 12671128].

Regev RH et al: Treatment of severe cholestasis in neonatal Dubin–Johnson syndrome with ursodeoxycholic acid. J Perinat Med 2002;30(2):185 [PMID: 12012642].

HEPATITIS A

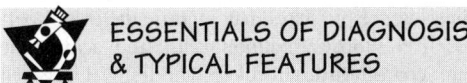

ESSENTIALS OF DIAGNOSIS & TYPICAL FEATURES

- *Gastrointestinal upset (anorexia, vomiting, diarrhea).*
- *Jaundice.*
- *Liver tenderness and enlargement.*
- *Abnormal LFTs.*
- *Local epidemic of the hepatitis A infection.*
- *Positive anti-hepatitis A virus (HAV) IgM antibody.*

General Considerations

Hepatitis A virus (HAV) infection occurs in both epidemic and sporadic fashion (Table 21–6). Trans-mission by the fecal–oral route explains epidemic outbreaks from contaminated food or water supplies, including by food handlers. Viral particles 27 nm in diameter have been found in stools during the acute phase of hepatitis A infection and are similar in appearance to the enteroviruses. Sporadic cases usually result from contact with an affected individual. Transmission through blood products obtained during the viremic phase is a rare event, although it has occurred in a newborn nursery. The overt form of the disease is easily recognized by the clinical manifestations. However, two-thirds of children are asymptomatic, and two-thirds of symptomatic children are anicteric. Therefore, most symptomatic children with HAV are believed to have a gastroenteritis. Lifelong immunity to HAV follows infection. In developing countries, most children are exposed to HAV by age 10 years, while only 20% are exposed by age 20 years in developed countries.

Antibody to HAV appears within 1–4 weeks of clinical symptoms. Although the great majority of children with infectious hepatitis are asymptomatic or have mild disease and recover completely, some will develop fulminant hepatitis leading to death or requiring liver transplantation.

Table 21–6. Hepatitis viruses.

	HAV	HBV	HCV	HDV	HEV
Type of virus	Enterovirus (RNA)	Hepadnavirus (DNA)	Flavivirus (RNA)	Incomplete (RNA)	Calicivirus (RNA)
Transmission routes	Fecal-oral	Parenteral, sexual, vertical	Parenteral, sexual, vertical	Parenteral, sexual	Fecal-oral
Incubation period (days)	15–40	50–150	30–150	20–90	14–65
Diagnostic test	Anti-HAV IgM	HBsAg, anti-HBc IgM	Anti-HCV, PCR-RNA test	Anti-HDV	Anti-HEV
Mortality rate (acute)	0.1–0.2%	0.5–2%	1–2%	2–20%	1–2% (in pregnant women, 20%)
Carrier state	No	Yes	Yes	Yes	No
Vaccine available	Yes	Yes	No	Yes (HBV)	No
Treatment	None	Interferon-α, nucleoside analogues (lamivudine, tenofovir, adefovir, entecovir)	Interferon-α (pegylated interferon in adults) plus ribavirin	Treatment for HBV	None

HAV, hepatitis A virus; HBc, hepatitis B core; HBsAg, hepatitis B surface antigen; HBV, hepatitis B virus; HDV, hepatitis D (delta) virus; PCR, polymerase chain reaction.

HEPATITIS VIRUS ABBREVIATIONS

HAV	Hepatitis A virus
Anti-HAV IgM	IgM antibody to HAV
HBV	Hepatitis B virus
HBsAg	HBV surface antigen
HBcAg	HBV core antigen
HBeAg	HBVe antigen
Anti-HBs	Antibody to HBsAg
Anti-HBc	Antibody to HBcAg
Anti-HBc IgM	IgM antibody to HBcAg
Anti-HBe	Antibody to HBeAg
HCV	Hepatitis C virus
Anti-HCV	Antibody to HCV
HDV	Hepatitis D (delta) virus
Anti-HDV	Antibody to HDV
HEV	Hepatitis E virus
Anti-HEV	Antibody to HEV
~~NANBNC~~	Non-A, non-B, non-C hepatitis virus

Clinical Findings

A. History

Features of the patient's history may elicit direct exposure to a previously jaundiced individual, consumption of seafood, contaminated water or imported fruits or vegetables, attendance in a day care center, or recent travel to an area of endemic infection. Following an incubation period of 15–40 days, the initial nonspecific symptoms usually precede the development of jaundice by 5–10 days.

B. Symptoms and Signs

Fever, anorexia, vomiting, headache, and abdominal pain are typical symptoms. Dark urine precedes jaundice, which peaks in 1–2 weeks and then begins to subside. The stools may become light or clay-colored during this time. Clinical improvement can occur as jaundice develops. Tender hepatomegaly and jaundice are typically present; splenomegaly is variable.

C. Laboratory Findings

Aminotransferases and conjugated and unconjugated bilirubin levels are elevated. The leukocyte count is normal to low; the sedimentation rate is elevated. Serum proteins are generally normal, but an elevation of the γ-globulin fraction (> 2.5 g/dL) can occur and indicates a worse prognosis. Hypoalbuminemia, hypoglycemia, and marked prolongation of prothrombin time (international normalized ratio [INR] > 2.0) are serious prognostic findings. Diagnosis is made by serology. A posi-

tive anti-HAV IgM indicates acute disease, whereas IgG anti-HAV persists after recovery.

Percutaneous liver biopsy is rarely indicated but may be performed safely in most children provided that the partial thromboplastin time and platelet count are normal and the prothrombin time is prolonged less than 4–5 seconds. The presence of ascites may increase the risk of percutaneous liver biopsy. "Balloon cells" and acidophilic bodies are characteristic histologic findings. Liver cell necrosis may be diffuse or focal, with accompanying infiltration of inflammatory cells containing polymorphonuclear leukocytes, lymphocytes, macrophages, and plasma cells, particularly in portal areas. Some bile duct proliferation may be seen in the perilobular portal areas alongside areas of bile stasis. Regenerative liver cells and proliferation of reticuloendothelial cells are present. Occasionally massive hepatocyte necrosis occurs, portending a bad prognosis.

Differential Diagnosis

Before jaundice appears, the symptoms are those of a nonspecific viral enteritis. Other diseases with somewhat similar onset include pancreatitis, infectious mononucleosis, leptospirosis, drug-induced hepatitis, Wilson disease, autoimmune hepatitis, and other hepatitis viruses. Acquired CMV disease may also mimic HAV, although lymphadenopathy is usually present in the former.

Prevention

Some attempt at isolation of the patient during initial phases of illness is indicated, although most patients with hepatitis A are noninfectious by the time the disease becomes overt. Stool, diapers, and other fecally stained clothing should be handled with care for 1 week after the appearance of jaundice.

Passive–active immunization of exposed susceptible persons can be achieved by giving standard immune globulin, 0.02–0.04 mL/kg intramuscularly. Illness is prevented in 80–90% of individuals if immune globulin is given within 1–2 weeks of exposure. Individuals traveling to endemic disease areas should receive HAV vaccine or 0.02–0.06 mL/kg of immune globulin as prophylaxis if there is insufficient time (< 2 weeks) for the initial dose of vaccine. All children older than age 2 years with chronic liver diseases should receive two doses of HAV vaccine 6 months apart. It is currently recommended that universal childhood immunization for HAV be implemented in U.S. states with 20 or more cases per 100,000 population per year, and in local areas with a high prevalence.

Treatment

No specific treatment measures are required. Sedatives and corticosteroids should be avoided. At the start of the illness, a light diet is preferable. During the icteric phase, lower-fat foods may diminish gastrointestinal symptoms but do not affect overall outcome. Drugs and elective surgery should be avoided.

Prognosis

Ninety-nine percent of children recover without sequelae. In rare cases of fulminant hepatitis, the patient may die in 5 days or may survive as long as 1–2 months without liver transplantation. The prognosis is poor if hepatic coma or ascites develop; orthotopic liver transplantation is indicated under these circumstances. Incomplete resolution can cause a prolonged hepatitis; however, resolution invariably occurs without long-term hepatic sequelae. Rare cases of aplastic anemia following acute infectious hepatitis have been reported. A benign relapse of symptoms may occur in 10–15% of cases after 6–10 weeks of apparent resolution.

Craig AS, Schaffner W: Prevention of hepatitis A with the hepatitis A vaccine. N Engl J Med 2004;350:476 [PMID: 14749456].

Demicheli V, Tiberti D: The effectiveness and safety of hepatitis A vaccine: A systematic review. Vaccine 2003;21(19–20):2242 [PMID: 12744850].

Jenson HB: The changing picture of hepatitis A in the United States. Curr Opin Pediatr 2004;16:89 [PMID: 14758121].

HEPATITIS B

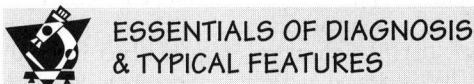

ESSENTIALS OF DIAGNOSIS & TYPICAL FEATURES

- *Gastrointestinal upset, anorexia, vomiting, diarrhea.*
- *Jaundice, tender hepatomegaly, abnormal LFTs.*
- *Serologic evidence of hepatitis B disease: HBsAg, HBeAg, anti-HBc IgM.*
- *History of parenteral, sexual, or household exposure or maternal HBsAg carriage.*

General Considerations

In contrast to hepatitis A, hepatitis B virus (HBV) infection has a longer incubation period of 21–135 days (see Table 21–5). The disease is caused by a DNA virus that is usually acquired perinatally from a carrier mother, or later in life from blood products, shared needles, needle sticks, skin piercing, or tattoos. It can also be sexually transmitted. Transmission via blood products has been almost eliminated by anti-HBc antibody donor-screening protocols. The complete HBV particle is composed of a core (28-nm particle) that is found in the nucleus of infected liver cells and a double outer shell (surface antigen). The surface antigen in blood is termed HBsAg. The antibody to it is anti-HBs. The core antigen is termed HBcAg and its antibody is anti-HBc. A specific anti-HBc IgM antibody occurs during primary viral replication.

Another important antigen–antibody system associated with HBV disease is the "e" antigen system. HBeAg, a truncated soluble form of HBcAg, appears in the serum of infected patients early and correlates with active virus replication. Persistence of HBeAg is a marker of infectivity, whereas the appearance of anti-HBe generally implies termination of viral replication. However, HBV mutant viruses (precore mutant) may replicate with negative HBeAg tests and positive tests for anti-HBe antibody. Other serologic markers indicating viral replication include the presence of DNA polymerase and circulating HBV DNA.

Clinical Findings

A. SYMPTOMS AND SIGNS

Symptoms include slight fever (which may be absent) and mild gastrointestinal upset. Visible jaundice is usually the first significant finding. It is accompanied by darkening of the urine and pale or clay-colored stools. Many patients, particularly infants, are asymptomatic. Hepatomegaly is frequently present. Occasionally a symptom complex (caused by antigen–antibody complexes) of macular rash, urticarial lesions, and arthritis antedates the appearance of icterus. Occasionally, HBV infection presents as a glomerulonephritis or nephrotic syndrome from immune complexes. When acquired vertically at birth, chronic disease is frequently completely asymptomatic despite ongoing liver injury.

B. LABORATORY FINDINGS

To diagnose acute HBV infection, the HBsAg and anti-HBc IgM are the only tests needed. To document recovery, immunity, or response to the HBV vaccine, the anti-HBs is useful. To document previous HBV infection, the anti-HBc is most useful. If HBsAg persists after 8 weeks in acute infections, it may signify a chronic infection, although chronic infection is defined as lasting 6 months or more. Vertical transmission to newborns is documented by positive HBsAg. LFT results are similar to those discussed earlier for hepatitis A. Liver histology is similar for HAV and HBV disease, although specific stains may detect HBcAg or HBsAg in the liver, and ground-glass appearance to hepatocytes may be present.

Renal involvement may be suspected on the basis of urinary findings suggesting glomerulonephritis or nephrotic syndrome.

Differential Diagnosis

The differentiation between HAV and HBV disease is made easier by a history of parenteral exposure, an HBsAg-positive parent, or an unusually long period of incubation. HBV and hepatitis C virus (HCV) infection or Epstein-Barr virus (EBV) infection are differentiated serologically. The history may suggest a drug-induced hepatitis, especially if a serum sickness prodrome is reported. Autoimmune hepatitis, Wilson disease, hemochromatosis, nonalcoholic steatohepatitis, and α_1-antitrypsin deficiency should also be considered.

Non-A non-B non-C (NANBNC) hepatitis is diagnosed when test results for the serologic markers of HAV, HBV, HCV, and EBV are negative; drug-induced hepatitis is diagnosed if there is a history of specific drug exposure; autoimmune hepatitis is diagnosed if autoimmune markers are present; Wilson disease is diagnosed if ceruloplasmin levels are abnormal; hemochromatosis is diagnosed if transferrin saturation is high; α_1-antitrypsin deficiency is diagnosed if serum concentration is decreased, and steatohepatitis is diagnosed if liver biopsy findings are suggestive.

Prevention

Control of hepatitis B in the population is based on screening of blood donors and pregnant women, use of properly sterilized needles and surgical equipment, avoidance of sexual contact with carriers, and vaccination of all infants and adolescents, as well as household contacts, sexual partners, medical personnel, and those at high risk. Universal immunization of all infants born in the United States and of adolescents is now recommended, as it is in most other countries. When acquired vertically at birth, chronic disease is frequently asymptomatic despite ongoing liver injury or a benign carrier state. The vaccine is highly effective for preexposure prophylaxis. (See Chapter 9.) For postexposure prophylaxis, administration of HBIG (0.06 mL/kg intramuscularly, given as soon as possible after exposure, up to 7 days) and initiation of vaccination are recommended.

Treatment

Supportive measures such as bed rest and a nutritious diet are used during the active symptomatic stage of disease. Corticosteroids are contraindicated. No other treatment is needed for acute HBV infection. For patients with progressive disease (chronic hepatitis with fibrosis), there are currently two treatment options. Treatment with α-interferon (5–6 million units/m^2 body surface area injected subcutaneously three times a week for 4–6 months) inhibits viral replication in 30–40% of patients, normalizes the ALT level, and leads to the disappearance of HBeAg and the appearance of anti-HBe. Side effects are common. Younger children may respond better than older children. Orally administered lamivudine therapy (3 mg/kg/day up to 100 mg per day for 12 months) leads to a successful response in 25% of treated children, with minimal side effects. However, resistant organisms can emerge. Pegylated interferon and adefovir are promising agents being tested in children. Asymptomatic HBsAg carriers (normal serum ALT, no hepatomegaly) do not respond to either therapy. Liver transplantation is successful in acute fulminant hepatitis B; however, reinfection is common following liver transplantation for chronic hepatitis B. Chronic HBIG therapy or lamivudine therapy reduces recurrence after transplantation.

Prognosis

The prognosis is good, although fulminant hepatitis or chronic hepatitis and cirrhosis may supervene in up to 10% of patients. The course of the acute disease is variable, but jaundice seldom persists for more than 2 weeks. HBsAg disappears in 95% of cases at the time of clinical recovery. Persistent asymptomatic infection may occur, particularly in children with vertical transmission, Down syndrome, or leukemia and in those undergoing chronic hemodialysis. Persistence of neonatally acquired HBsAg occurs in 70–90% of infants without immunoprophylaxis or vaccination, and the presence of e antigen in the HBsAg carrier indicates ongoing viral replication. However, 1–2% of children infected at birth will show spontaneous seroconversion of HBeAg each year. If HBV infection is acquired later in childhood, HBV is cleared and recovery occurs in 90–95% of patients. Chronic hepatitis B disease predisposes the patient to development of hepatocellular carcinoma. Once chronic HBV infection is established, surveillance for development of hepatocellular carcinoma with hepatic ultrasonography and serum α-fetoprotein is performed annually. Routine HBV vaccination of newborns in endemic countries has reduced the incidence of fulminant hepatic failure, chronic hepatitis, and hepatocellular carcinoma in children.

Broderick AL, Jonas MM: Hepatitis B in children. Semin Liver Dis 2003;23(1):59 [PMID: 12616451].

Dentinger CM et al: Persistence of antibody to hepatitis B and protection from disease among Alaska natives immunized at birth. Pediatr Infect Dis J 2005;24:786 [PMID: 16148845].

Ni YH et al: Lamivudine treatment in maternally transmitted chronic hepatitis B virus infection patients. Pediatr Int 2005;47:372 [PMID: 16091071].

Schwarz KB: Pediatric issues in new therapies for hepatitis B and C. Curr Gastroenterol Rep 2003;5(3):233 [PMID: 12734046].

Shepard CW et al: Epidemiology of hepatitis B and hepatitis B virus infection in United States children. Pediatr Infect Dis J 2005;24:755 [PMID: 16148839].

HEPATITIS C

General Considerations

Hepatitis C virus (HCV) virus is the most common cause of most non-B chronic hepatitis (90% of posttransfusion hepatitis cases) (see Table 21–6). Risk factors in adults and older children include illicit use of intravenous drugs (40%), occupational or sexual exposure (10%), and transfusions (10%); 30% of cases have no known risk factors. In children, most cases are associated with blood or blood product transfusions, transmission from an infected mother, or other household transmission. In the past, children with hemophilia or on chronic hemodialysis were at significant risk. The risk from transfused blood products has diminished greatly (from 1–2:100 to 1:100,000 units of blood) since the advent of blood testing for ALT and anti-HCV. HCV infection has also been caused by contaminated immune serum globulin preparations. Vertical transmission from HCV-infected mothers occurs more commonly with mothers who are HIV-positive (10–20%) compared with those who are HIV-negative (5–6%). About 0.4% of adolescents and 1.5% of adults in the United States have serologic evidence of infection. Vertically infected infants have elevated ALT levels, but do not appear ill; long-term outcome is unknown, however 20–30% of infants recover completely. Transmission of the virus from breast milk is probably rare. HCV rarely causes fulminant hepatitis in children or adults in Western countries, but different serotypes do so in Asia.

HCV is a single-stranded RNA virus in the flavivirus family. At least seven genotypes of HCV exist. Several well-defined HCV antigens are the basis for serologic antibody tests. The third-generation enzyme-linked immunosorbent assay (ELISA) test for anti-HCV is highly accurate. Anti-HCV is generally present when symptoms occur; however, test results may be negative in the first few months of infection. The presence of HCV RNA in serum, detected by polymerase chain reaction and branched-DNA test indicates active infection.

Clinical Findings

A. SYMPTOMS AND SIGNS

The incubation period is 1–5 months, with insidious onset of symptoms. Many childhood cases, especially those acquired vertically, are asymptomatic despite development of chronic hepatitis. Flulike prodromal symptoms and jaundice occur in less than 25% of cases. Hepatosplenomegaly may or may not be evident in chronic hepatitis. Ascites, clubbing, palmar erythema, or spider angiomas indicate progression to cirrhosis.

B. LABORATORY FINDINGS

Fluctuating mild to moderate elevations of aminotransferases over long periods are characteristic of chronic HCV infection. Diagnosis is established by the presence of anti-HCV (second-generation ELISA) confirmed by the radioimmunoblot assay or HCV RNA by polymerase chain reaction. Anti-HCV is acquired passively at birth from infected mothers and cannot be used to confirm disease in the neonate for the first 15 months. HCV RNA testing should be performed in suspected cases. Results of this test may be negative in the first month of life, but become positive by 4 months.

Percutaneous liver biopsy should be considered in chronic cases. Histologic examination shows portal triaditis with chronic inflammatory cells, occasional lymphocyte nodules in portal tracts, mild macrovesicular steatosis, and variable bridging necrosis, fibrosis, and cirrhosis. Cirrhosis in adults generally requires 10–30 years of chronic HCV infection, but it has occasionally developed sooner in children.

Differential Diagnosis

HCV hepatitis should be distinguished from HAV, HBV, and NANBNC hepatitis by serologic testing. Other causes of cirrhosis in children should be considered in cases of chronic illness, such as Wilson disease or α_1-antitrypsin deficiency. Chronic hepatitis may also be caused by drug reactions, autoimmune disease, or steatohepatitis.

Treatment

Treatment of acute HCV hepatitis is supportive. Indications for treatment of chronic infection will be determined by current clinical trials. Currently, infants with normal or minimally elevated ALT are not treated. Chronic hepatitis caused by HCV responds to interferon-α (3 million units/m^2 three times a week for 6–12 months) in 30–50% of cases. Relapses are common and appear to depend on genotype of the virus. Overall only 10–20% are sustained responders, and the response is poorer with infections with genotype 1a or 1b. Combined interferon plus ribavirin is more successful in adults and in children. Long-acting (pegylated) interferon (with or without ribavirin) is more effective in adults, with sustained response rates up to 60–70%. This is being tested in children. End-stage liver disease secondary to HCV responds well to liver transplantation, although reinfection is common and gradually progressive. Pre- and post-transplant antiviral therapy may reduce the risk of reinfection. There is no vaccine, and no benefit from using immune globulin in infants born to infected mothers. Elective C-section of HCV-infected pregnant women with a high titer of circulating virus may lessen the likelihood for vertical transmission.

Prognosis

In adults, 70–80% of HCV cases develop chronic hepatitis, and cirrhosis develops in 20% of those with chronic infection for 10–30 years. Alcohol intake, and concomitant obesity and fatty liver, increase this risk. HCV is now the leading indication for liver transplantation in adults. A strong association exists between chronic HCV disease and the development of hepatocellular carcinoma after as little as 15 years. The outcome in children is less well defined, although cirrhosis may develop rapidly in rare cases or after decades. About 50% of children infected by transfusion in the first few years of life develop chronic infection. Infants infected at birth often have concomitant HIV infection; their long-term outcome is unknown at present but appears benign for the first 10 years of life. In adults, chronic HCV infection has been associated with mixed cryoglobulinemia, polyarteritis nodosa, a sicca-like syndrome, and membranoproliferative glomerulonephritis.

Di Ciommo V et al: Interferon alpha in the treatment of chronic hepatitis C in children: A meta-analysis. J Viral Hepat 2003; 10(3):210 [PMID: 12753340].

England K et al: Growth in the first 5 years of life is unaffected in children with perinatally-acquired hepatitis C infection. J Pediatr 2005;147:227 [PMID: 16126055].

European Paediatric Hepatitis C Virus Network. Three broad modalities in the natural history of vertically acquired hepatitis C virus infection. Clin Infect Dis 2005;41:45 [PMID: 15937762].

European Paediatric Hepatitis C Virus Network: Effects of mode of delivery and infant feeding on the risk of mother-to-child transmission of hepatitis C virus. BJOG 2001;108:371 [PMID: 11305543].

Pembreya L et al; EPHN Collaborators. The management of HCV infected pregnant women and their children European Paediatric HCV Network. J Hepatol 2005;43:515 [PMID: 16144064].

Rumbo C. Hepatitis C: Current approaches in pediatrics. Pediatr Transplant 2005;9:662 [PMID: 16176427].

Syriopoulou V et al: Mother to child transmission of hepatitis C virus: Rate of infection and risk factors. Scand J Infect Dis 2005;37:350 [PMID: 16051571].

Tovo PA et al: Hepatitis B virus and hepatitis C virus infections in children. Curr Opin Infect Dis 2005;18(3):261 [PMID: 15864105].

HEPATITIS D (Delta Agent)

General Considerations

The hepatitis D virus (HDV) is a 35-nm defective virus that requires a coat of HBsAg to be infectious (see Table 21–6). Thus, HDV infection can occur only in the presence of HBV infection. In developing countries, transmission is by intimate contact; in Western countries, by parenteral exposure. HDV is rare in North America. HDV can infect simultaneously with HBV, causing acute hepatitis, or can superinfect a patient with chronic HBV infection, predisposing the individual to chronic hepatitis or fulminant hepatitis. In children, the association between chronic HDV coinfection with HBV and chronic hepatitis and cirrhosis is strong. Vertical HDV transmission is rare.

The diagnosis of HDV is made by anti-HDV IgM. Treatment is directed at therapy for HBV infection (eg, interferon-α) or for fulminant hepatic failure.

Dalekos GN et al: Interferon-alpha treatment of children with chronic hepatitis D virus infection: The Greek experience. Hepatogastroenterology 2001;47:1072.

Niro GA et al: .Treatment of hepatitis D. J Viral Hepat 2005;12:2 [PMID: 15655042].

HEPATITIS E

General Considerations

Hepatitis E virus (HEV) infection is a cause of enterically transmitted, epidemic non-A, non-B hepatitis (see Table 21–6). It is rare in the United States. HEV is a calicivirus-like agent that is transmitted via the fecal–oral route. It occurs predominantly in developing countries in association with water-borne epidemics, and has only a 3% secondary attack rate in household contacts. Areas reporting epidemics include Southeast Asia, China, the Indian subcontinent, the Middle East, northern and western Africa, Mexico, and Central America. Its clinical manifestations resemble HAV infection except that symptomatic disease is rare in children, more common in adolescents and adults, and is associated with a high mortality (10–20%) in pregnant women, particularly in the third trimester. Diagnosis is established by detecting anti-HEV antibody. The outcome in nonpregnant individuals is benign, with no chronic hepatitis or chronic carrier state reported. There is no effective treatment.

Piper-Jenks N et al: Risk of hepatitis E infection to travelers. J Travel Med 2000;7:1949 [PMID: 11003732].

Wang L et al: An overview and recent advances in vaccine research. World J Gastroenterol 2004;10(15):2157 [PMID: 15259057].

OTHER HEPATITIS VIRUSES

The hepatitis G virus (HGV), also called the GB virus, is relatively common and parenterally and vertically transmitted, but it has not been shown to produce acute or chronic liver disease. TT virus is also commonly transmitted, but is not a significant cause of hepatitis.

Other undiscovered NANBNC viruses may be the cause of cases of fulminant hepatitis in children. Infection with these uncharacterized agents is associated with the development of aplastic anemia in a small proportion of patients recovering from hepatitis and in 10–20% of those undergoing liver transplantation for indeterminate fulminant hepatitis. Parvovirus has been associated with fulminant hepatitis; the prognosis is relatively good in children. Infectious mononucleosis (EBV) is commonly associated with acute hepatitis. CMV, adenovirus, HIV, brucella, and leptospirosis are other infectious causes of acute hepatitis.

Polgreen PM et al: GB virus type C/hepatitis G virus: A non-pathogenic flavivirus associated with prolonged survival in HIV-infected individuals. Microbes Infect 2003;5:1255 [PMID: 14623022].

Sokal EM et al: Acute parvovirus B19 infection associated with fulminant hepatitis of favorable prognosis in young children. Lancet 1998;352:1739 [PMID: 9848349].

FULMINANT HEPATIC FAILURE
(Acute Massive Hepatic Necrosis, Acute Liver Failure)

ESSENTIALS OF DIAGNOSIS & TYPICAL FEATURES

- *Acute hepatitis with deepening jaundice.*
- *Extreme elevation of AST and ALT.*
- *Prolonged prothrombin time and INR.*
- *Encephalopathy and cerebral edema.*
- *Asterixis and fetor hepaticus.*

General Considerations

Fulminant hepatic failure (FHF) is defined as acute liver dysfunction resulting in hepatic coma and coagulopathy (INR > 2.0) within 6 weeks after onset. In young children, encephalopathy may be difficult to detect or not present. Mortality is 60–80% in children (without liver transplantation). An unusually virulent infectious agent or aggressive host immune response is postulated in many cases. In the first few weeks of life, FHF can be caused by herpes simplex, enteroviruses, adenovirus, galactosemia, fructose intolerance, tyrosinemia, neonatal iron storage disease, respiratory chain and fatty acid oxidation defects, familial erythrophagocytic histiocytosis, bile acid synthesis defects, and peroxisomal diseases. In older infants and children, HBV, NANBNC hepatitis, parvovirus, and HEV are sometimes causative. HAV rarely is responsible. Patients with immunologic deficiency diseases and those receiving immunosuppressive drugs are vulnerable to herpes viruses. In children with HIV infection, nucleoside reverse transcriptase inhibitors have triggered lactic acidosis and liver failure. In patients with underlying respiratory chain defects, valproic acid may trigger FHF. In older children, Wilson disease, acute fatty liver of pregnancy, Reye syndrome, autoimmune hepatitis, drugs (eg, acetaminophen, anesthetic agents, valproic acid) or toxins (eg, poisonous mushrooms, herbs, "ecstasy"), leukemia, and cardiac dysfunction must also be considered. Some 20–30% of cases in children are without identifiable cause and labeled indeterminate.

Clinical Findings

In some patients, the disease proceeds in a rapidly fulminant course with deepening jaundice, coagulopathy, hyperammonemia, ascites, a rapidly shrinking liver, and progressive coma. Terminally, AST and ALT, which were greatly elevated (2000–10,000 units/L), may improve at the time when the liver is getting smaller and undergoing massive necrosis and collapse. Some patients start with a course typical of benign hepatitis and then suddenly become severely ill during the second week of the disease. Fever, anorexia, vomiting, and abdominal pain may be noted, and worsening of LFTs parallels changes in sensorium or impending coma. Hyperreflexia and a positive extensor plantar response are seen. A characteristic breath odor (fetor hepaticus) is present. A severe coagulopathy precedes impairment of renal function, manifested by either oliguria or anuria, which is an ominous sign. Characteristic laboratory findings include elevated serum bilirubin levels (usually > 15–20 mg/dL), sustained very high AST and ALT (> 3000 units/L) that may decrease, terminally, low serum albumin, hypoglycemia, and prolonged prothrombin time/INR. Blood ammonia levels become elevated, whereas blood urea nitrogen is often very low. Hyperpnea is frequent, and mixed respiratory alkalosis and metabolic acidosis are present.

Differential Diagnosis

Infectious, metabolic, and drug/toxin causes are most common. Patients with Reye syndrome or urea cycle defects are typically anicteric. Wilson disease, autoimmune hepatitis, acute leukemia, cardiomyopathy, and Budd–Chiari syndrome should be considered. Acetaminophen overdose, herbal remedies, and other toxins (eg, "Ecstasy") need to be considered even if there is a negative history.

Complications

The development of renal failure and depth of hepatic coma determine the prognosis. Patients in grade 4 coma (unresponsiveness to verbal stimuli, decorticate or decerebrate posturing) rarely survive without transplantation, and may have residual central nervous system deficits. Cerebral edema, which usually accompanies coma, is frequently the cause of death. Extreme prolongation of prothrombin time or INR greater than 4 predicts poor recovery. Acetaminophen overdose is the exception. Sepsis, hemorrhage, renal failure, or cardiorespiratory arrest is a common terminal event. The rare survivor of advanced disease without transplantation may have residual fibrosis or even cirrhosis.

Treatment

The most effective therapy is excellent critical care. A number of therapies have failed to affect outcome, including exchange transfusion, plasmapheresis with plasma exchange, total body washout, charcoal hemoperfusion, and hemodialysis using a special high-permeability membrane. Hyperammonemia and bleeding should be controlled. Extracorporeal hepatic support devices are being developed to help bridge patients to liver transplant or allow for liver regeneration. Orthotopic liver transplantation is successful in 60–85% of cases; however, patients in grade 4 coma may not always recover cerebral function. Therefore, patients in FHF should be transferred prior to the development of hepatic coma to centers where liver transplantation can be performed. Criteria for deciding when to perform transplantation are not firmly established; however, serum bilirubin over 20 mg/dL, INR greater than 4, and factor V levels less than 20% indicate a poor prognosis. Living related donors may be required for transplantation in a timely fashion. The prognosis is better for acetaminophen ingestion, particularly when *N*-acetylcysteine treatment is given.

Corticosteroids may be harmful, except in autoimmune hepatitis for which steroids may reverse the FHF. Acyclovir is essential in herpes simplex disease. Sterilization of the colon with oral antibiotics such as metronidazole, neomycin, or gentamicin is recommended. An alternative is acidification of the colon with lactulose, 1–2 mL/kg three or four times daily, which reduces blood ammonia levels and traps ammonia in the colon. Some centers use *N*-acetylcysteine in all patients, although it is only of proven benefit in acetaminophen toxicity.

Close monitoring of fluid and electrolytes is mandatory and requires a central venous line. Ten percent dextrose solutions should be infused (6–8 mg/kg/min) to maintain normal blood glucose. Diuretics, sedatives, and tranquilizers are to be used sparingly. Early signs of cerebral edema are treated with infusions of mannitol (0.5–1.0 g/kg). Comatose patients are intubated, given mechanical ventilatory support, and monitored for signs of infection. Coagulopathy is treated with fresh-frozen plasma, other clotting factor concentrates, platelet infusions, or exchange transfusion. Plasmapheresis and hemodialysis may help stabilize a patient while awaiting liver transplantation. Epidural monitoring for increased intracranial pressure (hepatic coma stages 3 and 4) in patients awaiting liver transplantation is advocated. Artificial hepatic support devices are being developed. Continuous venous–venous dialysis may be helpful to maintain fluid balance. Prophylactic immune globulin, 0.02 mL/kg intramuscularly, should be given to close contacts of patients with HAV infection.

Prognosis

The overall prognosis remains poor without liver transplantation. Exchange transfusions or other modes of heroic therapy do not improve survival figures. The presence of nests of liver cells seen on liver biopsy amounting to more than 25% of the total cells and rising levels of clotting factors V and VII coupled with rising levels of serum α-fetoprotein may signify a more favorable prognosis for survival. The survival rate in patients who undergo liver transplantation (60–85%) exceeds that of those who do not (20–40%).

Dhawan A et al: Approaches to acute liver failure in children. Pediatr Transplant 2004;8:584 [PMID: 15598330].

Lee WS et al:. Etiology, outcome and prognostic indicators of childhood fulminant hepatic failure in the United kingdom. J Pediatr Gastroenterol Nutr 2005;40:575 [PMID: 15861019].

Liu E et al: Characterization of acute liver failure and development of a continuous risk of death staging system in children. J Hepatol 2006;44:134 [PMID: 16169116].

AUTOIMMUNE HEPATITIS

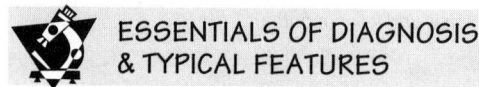

ESSENTIALS OF DIAGNOSIS & TYPICAL FEATURES

- *Acute or chronic hepatitis.*
- *Hypergammaglobulinemia.*
- *Positive ANA, ASMA, or anti-LKM.*

General Considerations

Autoimmune hepatitis (AIH) is most common in adolescent girls, although it occurs at all ages and in either sex. Rarely, AIH evolves from drug-induced hepatitis (eg, pemoline) or may develop in conjunction with such diseases as ulcerative colitis, Sjögren syndrome, or autoimmune hemolytic anemia. Wilson disease, α_1-antitrypsin deficiency, cystic fibrosis, and bile acid synthesis defects may present similarly as chronic hepatitis. A positive HBsAg test implicates HBV, and anti-HCV and anti-HDV suggest HCV and HDV, respectively. Positive antinuclear (ANA) antibodies, anti-smooth muscle antibodies (ASMA, type I AIH) or liver–kidney microsomal (LKM) antibodies (type II AIH), elevated serum IgG, and systemic manifestations (eg, arthralgia, weight loss, acne, and amenorrhea) are characteristic of AIH.

A genetic susceptibility to development of this entity is suggested by the increased incidence of the histocompatibility antigens HLA-A1 and HLA-B8. Increased autoimmune disease in families of patients and a high prevalence of seroimmunologic abnormalities have been noted in relatives. Occasionally patients have an "overlap syndrome" of AIH and primary sclerosing cholangitis.

Clinical Findings

Fever, malaise, recurrent or persistent jaundice, skin rash, arthritis, amenorrhea, gynecomastia, acne, pleurisy, pericarditis, or ulcerative colitis may be found in the history of these patients, or asymptomatic hepatomegaly or splenomegaly may be found on examination. Occasionally patients present in acute liver failure. Cutaneous signs of chronic liver disease may be noted (eg, spider angiomas, palmar erythema, and digital clubbing). Hepatosplenomegaly is frequently present.

LFTs reveal moderate elevations of serum bilirubin, AST, ALT, and serum alkaline phosphatase. Serum albumin may be low. Serum IgG levels are strikingly elevated (in the range of 2–6 g/dL). Low levels of C3 complement have been reported. Three subtypes have been described based on autoantibodies present: type 1: anti-smooth muscle (anti-actin); type 2: anti-LKM (anti-cytochrome P-450); and type 3: anti-soluble liver antigen.

Histologic examination of liver biopsy specimens shows loss of the lobular limiting plate, and interface hepatitis ("piecemeal" necrosis). Portal fibrosis, an inflammatory reaction of lymphocytes and plasma cells in the portal areas and perivascularly, and some bile duct and Kupffer cell proliferation and pseudolobule formation may be present. Cirrhosis may exist at diagnosis in up to 50% of patients.

Differential Diagnosis

Laboratory and histologic findings differentiate other types of chronic hepatitis (eg, HBV, HCV, and HDV infection; steatohepatitis; Wilson disease; α_1-antitrypsin deficiency; primary sclerosing cholangitis). Primary sclerosing cholangitis occasionally presents in a manner similar to AIH, including the presence of autoantibodies. Wilson disease and α_1-antitrypsin deficiency must be excluded if HBV and HCV studies are negative. Drug-induced (isoniazid, methyldopa, pemoline) chronic hepatitis should be ruled out.

Complications

Untreated disease that continues for months to years eventually results in postnecrotic cirrhosis, with complications of portal hypertension. Persistent malaise, fatigue, amenorrhea, and anorexia parallel disease activity. Bleeding from esophageal varices and development of ascites usually usher in hepatic failure.

Treatment

Corticosteroids (prednisone, 2 mg/kg/d) decrease the mortality rate during the early active phase of the disease. Azathioprine, 1–2 mg/kg/d, is of value in decreasing the side effects of long-term corticosteroid therapy but should not be used alone during the induction phase of treatment. Steroids are reduced over a 3- to 12-month period, and azathioprine is continued for 1–2 years if AST and ALT are normal. Liver biopsy is performed before stopping azathioprine therapy; if inflammation persists, then azathioprine is continued. Thiopurine methyltransferase activity should be assessed prior to starting azathioprine, to prevent extremely high blood levels and severe bone marrow toxicity. Relapses are treated similarly. Many patients require chronic azathioprine therapy. UCDA, cyclosporine, tacrolimus, or methotrexate may be helpful in poorly responsive cases. Use of mycophenolate mofetil instead of azathioprine is under study. Liver transplantation is indicated when disease progresses to decompensated cirrhosis despite therapy or in unresponsive cases presenting in acute liver failure. Steroid therapy may be life-saving in those presenting in acute liver failure.

Prognosis

The overall prognosis for AIH is improved significantly with early therapy. Some studies report cures (normal histologic findings) in 15–20% of patients. Relapses (seen clinically and histologically) occur in 40–50% of patients after cessation of therapy; remissions follow repeat treatment. Survival for 10 years is common despite residual cirrhosis. Of children with AIH, 20–50% eventually require liver transplantation. Complications of portal hypertension (bleeding varices, ascites, spontaneous bacterial peritonitis, and hepatopulmonary syndrome) require specific therapy. Liver transplantation is successful 70–90% of the time. Disease recurs after transplantation 10–50% of the time and is treated similarly to pretransplant disease.

Alvarez F: Treatment of autoimmune hepatitis: Current and future therapies. Curr Treat Options Gastroenterol 2004;7:413 [PMID: 15345212].

Czaja AJ: Autoimmune liver disease. Curr Opin Gastroenterol 2003;19:232 [PMID: 15703563].

Czaja AJ et al: Treatment challenges and investigational opportunities in autoimmune hepatitis. Hepatology 2005;41:207 [PMID: 15690485].

Mieli-Vergani G, Vergani D: Autoimmune liver disease in children. Ann Acad Med Singapore 2003;32(2):239 [PMID: 12772529].

NONALCOHOLIC FATTY LIVER DISEASE (NAFLD)

Patients with NAFLD present with asymptomatic soft hepatomegaly. If nonalcoholic steatohepatitis (NASH) is present, mild to moderately elevated aminotransferases (2–10 times the upper limit of normal) are also present. ALT is frequently higher than AST. Alkaline phosphatase and GGT may be mildly elevated, but bilirubin is normal. Liver biopsy shows micro- or macrovesicular steatosis in simple NAFLD, with the addition of portal tract inflammation, Mallory bodies, and variable degrees of portal fibrosis to cirrhosis in NASH. Ultrasonography or CT scanning indicates fat density in the liver. Most cases are associated with overweight state or type 2 diabetes mellitus. One to three percent of adolescents in the United States may have NASH, based on the observation that 15–25% of American adolescents are overweight or obese and that roughly 10% of these individuals will have NASH. Steatohepatitis is also associated with Wilson disease, hereditary fructose intolerance, tyrosinemia, HCV hepatitis, cystic fibrosis, fatty acid oxidation defects, kwashiorkor, Reye syndrome, respiratory chain defects, and toxic hepatopathy (ethanol and others). Treatment is weight reduction and exercise for obesity or treatment for the other causes. A pilot trial suggests that vitamin E may be helpful and is currently under study. In addition, improved control of insulin resistance with metformin or pioglitazone is also under study in NASH. Cirrhosis and liver failure have been described in adults with this disease.

Lavine JE, Schwimmer JB: Nonalcoholic fatty liver disease in the pediatric population. Clin Liver Dis 2004;8:549 [PMID: 15331063].

Molleston JP et al: Obese children with steatohepatitis can develop cirrhosis in childhood. Am J Gastroenterol 2002;97(9):2460 [PMID: 12358273].

Schwimmer JB et al: Obesity, insulin resistance, and other clinico-pathological correlates of pediatric nonalcoholic fatty liver disease. J Pediatr 2003;143:500 [PMID: 14571229].

Wieckowska A, Feldstein AE: Nonalcoholic fatty liver disease in the pediatric population: A review. Curr Opin Pediatr 2005; 17:636 [PMID: 16160540].

α_1-ANTITRYPSIN DEFICIENCY LIVER DISEASE

ESSENTIALS OF DIAGNOSIS & TYPICAL FEATURES

- Serum α_1-antitrypsin level less than 50–80 mg/dL.
- Identification of a specific protease inhibitor (Pi) phenotype (PiZZ, PiSZ).
- Detection of diastase-resistant glycoprotein deposits in periportal hepatocytes.
- Histologic evidence of liver disease.
- Family history of early-onset pulmonary disease or liver disease.

General Considerations

The disease is caused by a deficiency in α_1-antitrypsin, a protease inhibitor (Pi) system, predisposing patients to chronic liver disease and an early onset of pulmonary emphysema. It is most often associated with the Pi phenotypes *ZZ* and *SZ*. Heterozygotes may have a slightly higher incidence of liver disease. The exact relationship between low levels of serum α_1-antitrypsin and the development of liver disease is unclear. Emphysema develops because of a lack of inhibition of neutrophil elastase, which destroys pulmonary connective tissue. Although all patients with the *ZZ* genotype eventually have antitrypsin inclusions in hepatocytes, only about 20% develop significant liver disease. An associated abnormality in the microsomal disposal of accumulated aggregates may be necessary for the liver disease phenotype.

About 10–20% of affected individuals present with neonatal cholestasis. About 10% of individuals with α_1-antitrypsin deficiency have had clinically significant liver injury by age 18 years. Very few children have significant pulmonary involvement. Most affected children are completely asymptomatic, with no laboratory or clinical evidence of liver or lung disease.

Clinical Findings

A. SYMPTOMS AND SIGNS

α_1-Antitrypsin deficiency should be considered in all infants with neonatal cholestasis. Serum GGT is usually elevated. Jaundice, acholic stools, and malabsorption may also be present. Infants are often small for gestational age, and hepatosplenomegaly may be present. The family history may be positive for emphysema or cirrhosis.

In older children, hepatomegaly or physical findings suggestive of cirrhosis and portal hypertension, especially in the face of a negative history of liver disease, should always lead one to consider α_1-antitrypsin deficiency. Recurrent pulmonary disease (bronchitis, pneumonia) may be present in a few older children.

B. LABORATORY FINDINGS

Levels of the α_1-globulin fraction may be less than 0.2 mg/dL on serum protein electrophoresis. α_1-Antitrypsin levels are low (< 50–80 mg/dL) in homozygotes (*ZZ*). Specific Pi phenotyping should be done to confirm the diagnosis. Genotyping is rarely necessary. LFTs often reflect underlying hepatic pathologic changes. Hyperbilirubinemia (mixed) and elevated aminotransferases, alkaline phosphatase, and GGT are present early. Hyperbilirubinemia generally resolves, while aminotransferase and GGT elevation may persist. Signs of cirrhosis and hypersplenism may develop.

Liver biopsy after age 6 months shows diastase-resistant, periodic acid-Schiff staining intracellular granules, with hyaline masses, particularly in periportal zones. These may be absent prior to age 6 months, but when present are characteristic of α_1-antitrypsin deficiency.

Differential Diagnosis

In newborns, other specific causes of neonatal cholestasis need to be considered, including biliary atresia. In older children, other causes of insidious cirrhosis (eg, HBV or HCV infection, autoimmune hepatitis, Wilson disease, cystic fibrosis, hemochromatosis, and glycogen storage disease) should be considered.

Complications

Of all infants with PiZZ α_1-antitrypsin deficiency, only 20% develop liver disease in childhood. The complications of portal hypertension, cirrhosis, and chronic cholestasis predominate in affected children. Occasionally, children develop paucity of interlobular bile ducts.

Early-onset pulmonary emphysema occurs in young adults (age 30–40 years), particularly in smokers. An increased susceptibility to hepatocellular carcinoma has been noted in cirrhosis associated with α_1-antitrypsin deficiency.

Treatment

There is no specific treatment for the liver disease of this disorder. Replacement of the protein by transfusion therapy is successful in preventing pulmonary disease in affected adults. The neonatal cholestatic condition is treated with choleretics, medium-chain triglyceride-containing formula, and water-miscible vitamins (see Table 21–4). UCDA may reduce AST, ALT, and GGT, but its effect on outcome is unknown. Portal hypertension, esophageal bleeding, ascites, and other complications are treated as described elsewhere. Hepatitis A and B vaccines should be given to children with α_1-antitrypsin deficiency. Genetic counseling is indicated whenever the diagnosis is made. Diagnosis by prenatal screening is possible. Liver transplantation, performed for development of end-stage liver disease, cures the deficiency. Passive and active cigarette smoke exposure should be eliminated to help prevent pulmonary manifestations.

Prognosis

Of those patients presenting with neonatal cholestasis, approximately 10–25% will need liver transplantation in the first 5 years of life, 15–25% during childhood or adolescence, and 50–75% will survive into adulthood with variable degrees of liver fibrosis. A correlation between histologic patterns and clinical course has been documented in the infantile form of the disease. Liver failure can be expected 5–15 years after development of cirrhosis. Recurrence or persistence of hyperbilirubinemia along with worsening coagulation studies indicates the need for evaluation for possible liver transplantation. Decompensated cirrhosis caused by this disease is an excellent indication for liver transplanta-

tion; the survival rate should reach 80–90%. Pulmonary involvement is prevented by liver transplantation.

Rudnick DA, Perlmutter DH: Alpha-1-antitrypsin deficiency: A new paradigm for hepatocellular carcinoma in genetic liver disease. Hepatology 2005;42(3):514 [PMID: 16044402].

Schilsky ML, Oikonomou I: Inherited metabolic liver disease. Curr Opin Gastroenterol 2005;21:275 [PMID: 15818147].

Stoller JK, Aboussouan LS: Alpha1-antitrypsin deficiency. Lancet 2005;365:2225 [PMID: 15978931].

Sveger T, Eriksson S: The liver in adolescents with α_1-antitrypsin deficiency. Hepatology 1995;22:514 [PMID: 7635419].

WILSON DISEASE (Hepatolenticular Degeneration)

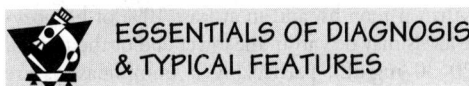

ESSENTIALS OF DIAGNOSIS & TYPICAL FEATURES

- *Acute or chronic liver disease.*
- *Deteriorating neurologic status.*
- *Kayser–Fleischer rings.*
- *Elevated liver copper.*
- *Abnormalities in levels of ceruloplasmin and serum and urine copper.*

General Considerations

Wilson disease is caused by a mutation in the gene on chromosome 13 coding for a specific P-type adenosine triphosphatase involved in copper transport. This results in impaired bile excretion of copper and incorporation of copper into ceruloplasmin by the liver. The accumulated hepatic copper causes oxidant (free-radical) damage to the liver. Subsequently, copper accumulates in the basal ganglia and other tissues. The disease should be considered in all children older than 4 years with evidence of liver disease (especially with hemolysis) or with suggestive neurologic signs. A family history is often present, and 25% of patients are identified by screening asymptomatic homozygous family members. The disease is autosomal recessive and occurs in 1:30,000 live births in all populations.

Clinical Findings

A. SYMPTOMS AND SIGNS

Hepatic involvement may be fulminant, present as an acute hepatitis, may masquerade as chronic liver disease, or may progress insidiously to postnecrotic cirrhosis. Findings include jaundice; hepatomegaly early in childhood; splenomegaly; Kayser–Fleischer rings; and later onset of neurologic manifestations such as tremor, dysarthria, and drooling beginning after age 10 years. Deterioration in school performance is often the earliest neurologic expression of disease. Psychiatric symptoms may also occur. The Kayser–Fleischer rings can sometimes be detected by unaided visual inspection as a brown band at the junction of the iris and cornea, but slitlamp examination is always necessary. Absence of Kayser–Fleischer rings does not exclude this diagnosis.

B. LABORATORY FINDINGS

The laboratory diagnosis is sometimes difficult. Serum ceruloplasmin levels (measured by the oxidase method) are usually less than 20 mg/dL. (Normal values are 23–43 mg/dL.) Low values, however, occur normally in infants younger than 3 months, and in at least 10% of homozygotes the levels may be within the lower end of the normal range (20–30 mg/dL), particularly if immunoassays are used to measure ceruloplasmin. Rare patients with higher ceruloplasmin levels have been reported. Serum copper levels are low, but the overlap with normal is too great for satisfactory discrimination. In acute fulminant Wilson disease serum copper levels are elevated markedly, owing to hepatic necrosis and release of copper. The presence of anemia, hemolysis, very high serum bilirubin levels (> 20–30 mg/dL), low alkaline phosphatase, and low uric acid are characteristic of acute Wilson disease. Urine copper excretion in children older than 3 years is normally less than 30 μg/d; in Wilson disease, it is generally greater than 150 μg/d. Finally, the tissue content of copper from a liver biopsy, normally less than 50 μg/g dry tissue, is greater than 250 μg/g in Wilson disease.

Glycosuria and aminoaciduria have been reported. Hemolysis and gallstones may be present; bone lesions simulating those of osteochondritis dissecans have also been found.

The coarse nodular cirrhosis, steatosis, and glycogenated nuclei seen on liver biopsy may distinguish Wilson disease from other types of cirrhosis. Early in the disease, vacuolation of liver cells, steatosis, and lipofuscin granules can be seen, as well as Mallory bodies. The presence of Mallory bodies in a child is strongly suggestive of Wilson disease. Stains for copper may sometimes be negative despite high copper content in the liver. Therefore, liver copper levels must be determined biochemically on biopsy specimens. Electron microscopy findings of abnormal mitochondria may be helpful.

Differential Diagnosis

During the icteric phase, acute viral hepatitis, α_1-antitrypsin deficiency, autoimmune hepatitis, Indian childhood cirrhosis, and drug-induced hepatitis are the usual diagnostic possibilities. Later, other causes of cirrhosis and portal

hypertension require consideration. Laboratory testing for serum ceruloplasmin, 24-hour urine copper excretion, liver copper concentration, and a slitlamp examination of the cornea will differentiate Wilson disease from the others. Urinary copper excretion during penicillamine challenge (500 mg twice a day in the older child or adult) may help differentiate Wilson disease from other causes. Genetic testing may be necessary in confusing cases. Other copper storage diseases that occur in early childhood include Indian childhood cirrhosis, Tyrolean childhood cirrhosis, and idiopathic copper toxicosis. However, ceruloplasmin concentrations are normal in these conditions.

Complications

Progressive liver disease, postnecrotic cirrhosis, hepatic coma, progressive neurologic degeneration, and death are the rule in the untreated patient. The complications of portal hypertension (variceal hemorrhage, ascites) are poorly tolerated by these patients. Progressive degenerating central nervous system disease and terminal aspiration pneumonia are common in untreated older people. Acute hemolytic disease may result in acute renal failure and profound jaundice as part of the presentation of fulminant hepatitis.

Treatment

Copper chelation with D-penicillamine or trientine hydrochloride, 1000–2000 mg/d orally, is the treatment of choice in all cases, whether or not the patient is symptomatic. It is best to begin with 250 mg/d and increase the dose weekly by 250 mg increments. The target dose for children is 20 mg/kg/d. Strict dietary restriction of copper intake is not practical. Supplementation with zinc acetate (25–50 mg orally, three times daily) may reduce copper absorption. Copper chelation is continued for life, although doses may be reduced transiently at the time of surgery or early in pregnancy. Vitamin B_6 (25 mg) is given daily while on penicillamine to prevent optic neuritis. In some countries, after a clinical response to penicillamine or trientine, zinc therapy is substituted and continued for life. Tetrathiomolybdate is being tested as an alternative therapy. Noncompliance with the drug regimen can lead to sudden fulminant liver failure and death.

Liver transplantation is indicated for all cases of acute fulminant disease with hemolysis and renal failure, progressive hepatic decompensation despite several months of penicillamine, and severe progressive hepatic insufficiency in patients who unadvisedly discontinue penicillamine, triene, or zinc therapy.

Prognosis

The prognosis of untreated Wilson disease is poor. Without liver transplantation, all patients with the fulminant presentation succumb. Copper chelation reduces hepatic copper content, reverses many of the liver lesions, and can stabilize the clinical course of established cirrhosis. Neurologic symptoms generally respond to therapy. All siblings should be immediately screened and homozygotes given treatment with copper chelation or zinc acetate therapy, even if asymptomatic. Genetic testing (haplotype analysis or genotyping) is available at a few centers for family members.

Dhawan A et al: et al Wilson's disease in children: 37-year experience and revised King's score for liver transplantation. Liver Transpl 2005;11:441 [PMID: 15776453].

Marcellini M et al: Treatment of Wilson's disease with zinc from the time of diagnosis in pediatric patients: A single-hospital, 10-year follow-up study. J Lab Clin Med 2005;145:139 [PMID: 15871305].

Roberts EA, Schilsky ML: A practice guideline on Wilson disease. Hepatology 2003;37(6):1475 [PMID: 12774027].

Wang XH et al: Living-related liver transplantation for Wilson's disease. Transpl Int 2005;18:651 [PMID: 15910288].

Wilson DC et al: Severe hepatic Wilson's disease in preschool-aged children. J Pediatr 2000;137:719 [PMID: 11060541].

REYE SYNDROME (Encephalopathy with Fatty Degeneration of the Viscera)

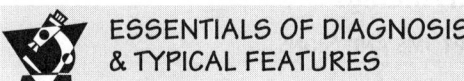 ESSENTIALS OF DIAGNOSIS & TYPICAL FEATURES

- *Prodromal upper respiratory tract infection, influenza A or B illness, or varicella.*
- *History of salicylate ingestion.*
- *Vomiting.*
- *Lethargy, drowsiness progressing to semicoma.*
- *Elevated AST, hyperammonemia, normal or slightly elevated bilirubin, prolonged prothrombin time.*
- *Microvesicular steatosis of the liver, kidneys, brain.*
- *Absence of other metabolic diseases.*

General Considerations

Reported cases of Reye syndrome have decreased dramatically, perhaps because of a decline in the use of salicylates among younger children, who seem to be at greater risk. In addition, many cases currently diagnosed as a variety of metabolic diseases (eg, fatty acid oxidation defects) were previously diagnosed as Reye syndrome. Infection with varicella, influenza A and B, echovirus 2,

coxsackievirus A, and EBV are associated, as is the use of salicylates.

The pathogenesis is thought to be damage to mitochondria caused by salicylate metabolites or some other toxin or chemical in the milieu of a viral infection or underlying polymorphism in mitochondrial function. Mitochondrial dysfunction leads to elevated short-chain fatty acids and hyperammonemia as well as directly to cerebral edema. The liver injury recovers despite the progression of cerebral edema in many cases.

Clinical Findings

A. SYMPTOMS AND SIGNS

Varicella, influenza, or minor upper respiratory tract illness precedes the development of vomiting, irrational and combative behavior, progressive stupor, and coma. Restlessness and convulsions may also occur. Striking physical findings are hyperpnea, irregular respirations, and dilated, sluggishly reacting pupils. Jaundice is minimal or absent. The liver may be normal or enlarged. Splenomegaly is absent. A positive Babinski sign, hyperreflexia, and decorticate and decerebrate posturing are consistent with increased intracranial pressure.

B. LABORATORY FINDINGS

CSF is acellular, and CSF glucose may be low in younger patients who have hypoglycemia. CSF pressure is increased. Moderate to severe elevations of AST, ALT, and lactate dehydrogenase and normal serum bilirubin and alkaline phosphatase values are characteristic. The prothrombin time/INR is usually mild to moderately prolonged, and the blood ammonia is elevated to varying degrees. A mixed respiratory alkalosis and metabolic acidosis is typical. Hyperaminoacidemia (glutamine, alanine, lysine) and hypocitrullinemia are present.

Histology of the liver shows diffuse microvesicular steatosis with minimal inflammatory changes. Glycogen is virtually absent from the hepatocytes in biopsy specimens taken before administration of hypertonic glucose. Mitochondria are large, pleomorphic, and have decreased matricial density on electron microscopy. The kidney changes include swelling and fatty degeneration of the proximal tubules.

C. ELECTROENCEPHALOGRAPHY

The electroencephalogram shows diffuse slow-wave activity.

Differential Diagnosis

Differentiation of Reye syndrome from encephalitis, acute toxic encephalopathy, hepatic coma, or fulminant hepatitis can be made on clinical and laboratory grounds. A negative history and urine screen for ingestion of poisons and drugs, absence of cells in the CSF, and absence of jaundice favor a diagnosis of Reye syndrome. The fatty acid oxidation defects (eg, medium-chain acyl-CoA dehydrogenase deficiency) and other metabolic disorders may resemble Reye syndrome; gas chromatographic analysis of urine and serum acyl-carnitine levels will help differentiate them. Liver biopsy and electron microscopy can be helpful and are indicated in atypical cases.

Treatment

Treatment in an intensive care unit is supportive. If cerebral edema can be minimized, the liver makes a full recovery. Mechanical ventilation may become necessary if the patient reaches grade 3 coma (agitated delirium, combativeness). Intracranial pressure should be monitored directly and kept below 15–20 mm Hg, and systemic blood pressure should be kept high enough to maintain cerebral perfusion pressure above 45–50 mm Hg. Hyperventilation, mannitol infusions (0.5–1.0 g/kg every 4 hours), barbiturates, or ventricular drainage is used to lower intracranial pressure. Maintenance fluids using 10% glucose should be given at a rate sufficient to produce a urine flow of 1.0–1.5 mL/kg/h. Vitamin K, 3–5 mg intramuscularly, should be administered. Hypothermia and pentobarbital coma have been used to decrease body (brain) metabolic needs during the period of uncontrolled intracranial pressure.

Prognosis

At least 70% of patients with Reye syndrome survive. The prognosis is related to the depth of coma and the peak ammonia level on admission. Because Reye syndrome is uncommon now, many patients are diagnosed only when in deep coma. All patients should be screened for fatty acid oxidation and other metabolic defects. Survivors should not be given aspirin.

Auret-Leca E et al: Incidence of Reye syndrome in France: A hospital-based survey. J Clin Epidemiol 2001;54:857 [PMID: 11470397].

Bhutta AT et al: Reye's syndrome: Down but not out. South Med J 2003;96:43 [PMID: 12602712].

Chow EL et al: Reassessing Reye syndrome. Arch Pediatr Adolesc Med 2003;157:1241 [PMID: 14662583].

CIRRHOSIS

Cirrhosis is a histologically defined condition of the liver characterized by diffuse hepatocyte injury and regeneration, an increase in connective tissue (bridging fibrosis), and disorganization of the lobular and vascular architecture (regenerative nodules). It may be micronodular or macronodular in appearance. It is the vasculature distortion that leads to increased resistance to blood flow, producing portal hypertension and its consequences.

Many liver diseases may progress to cirrhosis. In children, the two most common forms of cirrhosis are postnecrotic and biliary, with different causes, symptomatology, and treatment requirements. Both forms can eventually lead to liver failure and death.

In the pediatric population, postnecrotic cirrhosis is often a result of acute or chronic liver disease (eg, idiopathic neonatal giant-cell hepatitis; viral hepatitis [HBV, HCV, or NANBNC hepatitis]; autoimmune or drug-induced hepatitis); or certain inborn errors of metabolism (see Table 21–5). Cirrhosis is an exceptional outcome of HAV infection and only follows massive hepatic necrosis. The evolution to cirrhosis may be insidious, with no recognized icteric phase, as in some cases of HBV or HCV infection, Wilson disease, hemochromatosis, or α_1-antitrypsin deficiency. At the time of diagnosis of cirrhosis, the underlying liver disease may be active, with abnormal LFTs; or it may be quiescent, with normal LFTs. Most cases of biliary cirrhosis result from congenital abnormalities of the bile ducts (biliary atresia, choledochal cyst), tumors of the bile duct, Caroli disease, PFIC, primary sclerosing cholangitis, paucity of the intrahepatic bile ducts, and cystic fibrosis.

Occasionally, cirrhosis may follow a hypersensitivity reaction to certain drugs such as phenytoin. Parasites (*Opisthorchis sinensis, Fasciola,* and *Ascaris*) may be causative in children living in endemic areas.

Clinical Findings

A. SYMPTOMS AND SIGNS

General malaise, loss of appetite, failure to thrive, and nausea are frequent complaints, especially in anicteric varieties. Easy bruising may be reported. Jaundice may or may not be present. The first indication of underlying liver disease may be ascites, gastrointestinal hemorrhage, or hepatic encephalopathy. Variable hepatosplenomegaly, spider angiomas, warm skin, palmar erythema, or digital clubbing may be present. A small, shrunken liver may present. Most often, the liver is enlarged slightly, especially in the subxiphoid region, where it has a firm to hard quality and an irregular edge. Ascites may be detected as shifting dullness or a fluid wave. Gynecomastia may be noted in males. Digital clubbing occurs in 10–15% of cases. Pretibial edema often occurs, reflecting underlying hypoproteinemia. In adolescent girls, irregularities of menstruation and amenorrhea may be early complaints.

In biliary cirrhosis, patients often have jaundice, dark urine, pruritus, hepatomegaly, and sometimes xanthomas in addition to the previously mentioned clinical findings. Malnutrition and failure to thrive due to steatorrhea may be more apparent in this form of cirrhosis.

B. LABORATORY FINDINGS

Mild abnormalities of aminotransferases (AST, ALT) are often present, with a decreased level of albumin and a variable increase in the level of γ-globulins. Prothrombin time is prolonged and may be unresponsive to vitamin K administration. Burr and target red cells may be noted on the peripheral blood smear. Anemia, thrombocytopenia, and leukopenia are present if hypersplenism exists. However, cirrhosis may be present despite normal blood tests.

In biliary cirrhosis, elevated conjugated bilirubin, bile acids, GGT, alkaline phosphatase, and cholesterol are common.

C. IMAGING

Hepatic ultrasound or CT examination may demonstrate abnormal hepatic texture and nodules. In biliary cirrhosis, abnormalities of the biliary tree may be apparent by ultrasonography, CT, hepatobiliary scintigraphy, or cholangiography.

D. PATHOLOGIC FINDINGS

Liver biopsy findings of regenerating nodules and surrounding fibrosis are hallmarks of cirrhosis. Pathologic features of biliary cirrhosis also include canalicular and hepatocyte cholestasis, as well as plugging of bile ducts. The interlobular bile ducts may be increased or decreased, depending on the cause and the stage of the disease process.

Complications & Treatment

Major complications of cirrhosis in childhood include progressive nutritional disturbances, hormonal disturbances, and the evolution of portal hypertension and its complications. Hepatocellular carcinoma occurs with increased frequency in the cirrhotic liver, especially in patients with the chronic form of hereditary tyrosinemia or after long-standing HBV or HCV disease. At present, there is no proven medical treatment for cirrhosis, but whenever a treatable condition is identified (eg, Wilson disease, galactosemia, congenital fructose intolerance, autoimmune hepatitis) or an offending agent eliminated (HBV, HCV, drugs, toxins), disease progression can be altered; occasionally regression of fibrosis has been noted. Children with cirrhosis should receive the hepatitis A and B vaccines, and they should be monitored for the development of hepatocellular carcinoma with serial serum α-fetoprotein determination and abdominal ultrasound for hepatic nodules. Liver transplantation may be appropriate in patients with cirrhosis whose disease is continuing to progress, with evidence of worsening hepatic synthetic function, or in whom the complications of cirrhosis are no longer manageable.

Prognosis

Postnecrotic cirrhosis has an unpredictable course. Without transplantation, affected patients may die from liver failure within 10–15 years. Patients with a rising bilirubin, a vitamin K-resistant coagulopathy, or diuretic refractory ascites usually survive less than 1–2 years. The terminal event in some patients may be generalized hemorrhage, sepsis, or cardiorespiratory arrest. For patients with biliary cirrhosis, the prognosis is similar, except for those with surgically corrected lesions that result in regression or stabilization of the underlying liver condition. With liver transplantation, the long-term survival rate is 70–90%.

Bissell DM, Maher JJ: Hepatic fibrosis and cirrhosis. In: Zakim D, Boyer TD (eds): *Hepatology: A Textbook of Liver Disease.* Saunders, 2003.

Fattovich G et al: Hepatocellular carcinoma in cirrhosis: Incidence and risk factors. Gastroenterology 2004;127:S35 [PMID: 15508101].

Hardy SC, Kleinman RE: Cirrhosis and chronic liver failure. In: Suchy FJ, Sokol RJ, Balistreri WF (editors): *Liver Disease in Children.* Lippincott Williams & Wilkins, 2001.

PORTAL HYPERTENSION

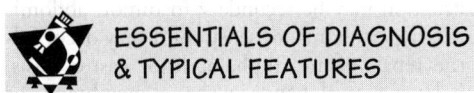

ESSENTIALS OF DIAGNOSIS & TYPICAL FEATURES

- *Splenomegaly.*
- *Recurrent ascites.*
- *Variceal hemorrhage.*
- *Hypersplenism.*

General Considerations

Portal hypertension is defined as an increase in the portal venous pressure to more than 5 mm Hg greater than the inferior vena caval pressure. Portal hypertension is most commonly a result of cirrhosis. However, portal hypertension without cirrhosis may be divided into prehepatic, suprahepatic, and intrahepatic causes. Although the specific lesions vary somewhat in their clinical signs and symptoms, the consequences of portal hypertension are common to all.

A. PREHEPATIC PORTAL HYPERTENSION

Prehepatic portal hypertension from acquired abnormalities of the portal and splenic veins accounts for 30–50% of cases of variceal hemorrhage in children. A history of neonatal omphalitis, sepsis, dehydration, or umbilical vein catheterization may be present. Causes in older children include local trauma, peritonitis (pyelophlebitis), hypercoagulable states, and pancreatitis. Symptoms may occur before age 1 year, but in most cases the diagnosis is not made until age 3–5 years. Patients with a positive neonatal history tend to be symptomatic earlier.

A variety of portal or splenic vein malformations, some of which may be congenital, have been described, including defects in valves and atretic segments. Cavernous transformation is probably the result of attempted collateralization around the thrombosed portal vein rather than a congenital malformation. The site of the venous obstruction may be anywhere from the hilum of the liver to the hilum of the spleen.

B. SUPRAHEPATIC VEIN OCCLUSION OR THROMBOSIS (BUDD–CHIARI SYNDROME)

In most instances, no cause can be demonstrated. Suggested causes include endothelial injury to hepatic veins by bacterial endotoxin, which has been demonstrated experimentally. The occasional association of hepatic vein thrombosis in inflammatory bowel disease favors the presence of endogenous toxins traversing the liver. Vasculitis leading to endophlebitis of the hepatic veins has been described occasionally. In addition, hepatic vein obstruction may be secondary to tumor, abdominal trauma, hyperthermia, or sepsis, or it may occur following the repair of an omphalocele or gastroschisis. Congenital vena caval bands, webs, a membrane, or stricture above the hepatic veins are sometimes causative. Hepatic vein thrombosis may be a complication of oral contraceptive medications. Underlying thrombotic conditions (deficiency of antithrombin III, protein C or protein S, factor V Leiden; antiphospholipid antibodies; or mutations of the prothrombin gene) should be evaluated.

C. INTRAHEPATIC PORTAL HYPERTENSION

1. Cirrhosis (see previous section).

2. Venoocclusive disease (acute stage)—This now occurs most frequently in bone marrow transplant patients. It may also develop after chemotherapy for acute leukemia, particularly with thioguanine. Additional causes include the ingestion of pyrrolizidine alkaloids ("bush tea") or other herbal teas and a familial form of the disease occurring in congenital immunodeficiency states.

The acute form of the disease generally occurs in the first month after bone marrow transplantation and is heralded by the triad of weight gain (ascites), tender hepatomegaly, and jaundice.

3. Congenital hepatic fibrosis—This is a rare autosomal recessive cause of intrahepatic presinusoidal portal hypertension (Table 21–7). Liver biopsy is generally diagnostic, demonstrating Meyenburg complexes. On angiography, the intrahepatic branches of the portal vein may be duplicated. Autosomal recessive polycystic

kidney disease is often associated with the hepatic lesion; therefore, renal ultrasonography and urography should be routinely performed.

4. Other rare causes—Hepatoportal sclerosis (idiopathic portal hypertension, noncirrhotic portal fibrosis), noncirrhotic nodular transformation of the liver, and schistosomal hepatic fibrosis are also rare causes of intrahepatic presinusoidal portal hypertension.

Clinical Findings

A. SYMPTOMS AND SIGNS

For prehepatic portal hypertension, splenomegaly in an otherwise well child is the most constant physical sign. Recurrent episodes of abdominal distention resulting from ascites may be noted. The usual presenting symptoms are hematemesis and melena.

The presence of prehepatic portal hypertension is suggested by the following: (1) an episode of severe infection in the newborn period or early infancy—especially omphalitis, sepsis, gastroenteritis, severe dehydration, or prolonged or difficult umbilical vein catheterizations; (2) no previous evidence of liver disease; (3) a history of well-being prior to onset or recognition of symptoms; and (4) normal liver size and tests with splenomegaly.

Most patients with suprahepatic portal hypertension present with abdominal pain, tender hepatomegaly of acute onset, and abdominal enlargement caused by ascites. Jaundice is present in only 25% of patients. Vomiting, hematemesis, and diarrhea are less common. Cutaneous signs of chronic liver disease are often absent, as the obstruction is usually acute. Distended superficial veins on the back and the anterior abdomen, along with dependent edema, are seen when inferior vena cava obstruction affects hepatic vein outflow. Absence of hepatojugular reflux (jugular distention when pressure is applied to the liver) is a helpful clinical sign.

The symptoms and signs of intrahepatic portal hypertension are generally those of cirrhosis (see section on Cirrhosis).

B. LABORATORY FINDINGS AND IMAGING

Most other common causes of splenomegaly or hepatosplenomegaly may be excluded by proper laboratory tests. Cultures, EBV titers, hepatitis serologies, blood smear examination, bone marrow studies, and LFTs may be necessary. In prehepatic portal hypertension, LFTs are generally normal. In Budd–Chiari syndrome and venoocclusive disease, mild to moderate hyperbilirubinemia with modest elevations of aminotransferases and prothrombin time are often present. Significant early increases in fibrinolytic parameters (especially plasminogen activator inhibitor 1) have been reported in venoocclusive disease. Hypersplenism with mild leu-

Table 21–7. Biliary tract diseases of childhood.

	Acute Hydrops Transient Dilatation of Gallbladder[a,b]	Choledochal Cyst[c] (See Figure 21–1.)	Acalculous Cholecystitis[d]	Caroli Disease[e] (Idiopathic Intrahepatic Bile Duct Dilation)	Congenital Hepatic Fibrosis[f]	Biliary Dyskinesia[g]
Predisposing or associated conditions	Premature infants with prolonged fasting or systemic illness. Hepatitis. Abnormalities of cystic duct. Kawasaki disease. Bacterial sepsis, EBV.	Congenital lesion. Female sex. Asians. Rarely with Caroli or congenital hepatic fibrosis.	Systemic illness, sepsis (*Streptococcus*, *Salmonella*, *Klebsiella*, etc), HIV infection. Gallbladder stasis, obstruction of cystic duct (stones, nodes, tumor).	Congenital lesion. Also found in congenital hepatic fibrosis or with choledochal cyst. Female sex. Autosomal-recessive polycystic kidney disease.	Familial (autosomal-recessive 25% with autosomal-recessive polycystic kidney disease. Choledochal cyst. Meckel-Gruber, Ivemark, or Jeune syndrome.	Adolescents.
Symptoms	Absent in premature infants. Vomiting, abdominal pain in older children.	Abdominal pain, vomiting, jaundice.	Acute severe abdominal pain, vomiting, fever.	Recurrent abdominal pain, vomiting. Fever, jaundice when cholangitis occurs.	Hematemesis, melena from bleeding esophageal varices.	Intermittant RUQ pain.
Signs	Right upper quadrant abdominal mass. Tenderness in some.	Icterus, acholic stools, dark urine in neonatal period. Right upper quadrant abdominal mass or tenderness in older children.	Tenderness in mid and right upper abdomen. Occasional palpable mass in right upper quadrant.	Icterus, hepatomegaly.	Hepatosplenomegaly.	Usually normal exam.
Laboratory abnormalities	Most are normal. Increased WBC count in sepsis (may be decreased in premature infants). Abnormal LFTs in hepatitis.	Conjugated hyperbilirubinemia, elevated GGT, slightly increased AST. Elevated pancreatic serum amylase common.	Elevated WBC count, normal or slight abnormality of LFTs.	Abnormal LFTs. Increased WBC count with cholangitis. Urine abnormalities if associated with congenital hepatic fibrosis.	Low platelet and WBC count (hypersplenism), slight elevation of AST, GGT. Inability to concentrate urine.	Usually normal.
Diagnostic studies most useful	Gallbladder ultrasonography.	Gallbladder ultrasonography hepatobiliary scintigraphy, MRCP, or ERCP.	Scintigraphy to confirm nonfunction of gallbladder. Ultrasonography or abdominal CT scan to rule out other neighboring disease.	Transhepatic cholangiography, MRCP, ERCP, scintigraphy, ultrasonography, intravenous pyelography.	Liver biopsy. Ultrasonography of the liver and kidneys. Upper endoscopy.	CCK stimulated scinitgraphy demonstrating reduced ejection fraction.

(continued)

Table 21-7. Biliary tract diseases of childhood. (continued)

	Acute Hydrops Transient Dilatation of Gallbladder[a,b]	Choledochal Cyst[c] (See Figure 21-1.)	Acalculous Cholecystitis[d]	Caroli Disease[e] (Idiopathic Intrahepatic Bile Duct Dilation)	Congenital Hepatic Fibrosis[f]	Biliary Dyskinesia[9]
Treatment	Treatment of associated condition. Needle or tube cystostomy rarely required. Cholecystectomy seldom indicated.	Surgical resection and choledochojejunostomy.	Broad-spectrum antibiotic coverage, then cholecystectomy.	Antibiotics and surgical or endoscopic drainage for cholangitis. Liver transplantation for some. Lobectomy for localized disease.	Treatment of portal hypertension. Liver/kidney transplantation for some.	Cholecystectomy in well selected cases.
Complications	Perforation with bile peritonitis rare.	Progressive biliary cirrhosis. Increased incidence of cholangiocarcinoma. Cholangitis in some.	Perforation and bile peritonitis, sepsis, abscess or fistula formation. Pancreatitis.	Sepsis with episodes of cholangitis, biliary cirrhosis, portal hypertension. Intraductal stones. Cholangiocarcinoma.	Bleeding from varices. Splenic rupture, severe thrombocytopenia. Progressive renal failure.	Continued pain after surgery.
Prognosis	Excellent with resolution of underlying condition. Consider cystic duct obstruction if disorder fails to resolve.	Depends on anatomic type of cyst, associated condition, and success of surgery. Liver transplantation required in some.	Good with early diagnosis and treatment.	Poor, with gradual deterioration of liver function. Multiple surgical drainage procedures expected. Liver transplantation should alter long-term prognosis.	Good in absence of serious renal involvement and with control of portal hypertension. Slightly increased risk of cholangiocarcinoma.	Good short-term outcome in well-selected patients.

Ultrasonography, liver and biliary tract scanning; scintigraphy, hepatobiliary scan using radiolabeled [99m]technetium; AST, aspartate aminotransferase (SGOT); CT, computed tomography; ERCP, endoscopic retrograde cholangiopancreatography; EBV, Epstein-Barr virus; GGT, γ-glutamyl transpeptidase; LFT, liver function tests; MRCP, magnetic resonance cholangiopancreatography; RUQ, right upper quadrant; WBC, white blood count.

[a]Crankson S et al: Acute hydrops of the gallbladder in childhood. Eur J Pediatr 1992;151:318 [PMID: 9788647].

[b]Zulian F et al: Acute surgical abdomen as presenting manifestation of Kawasaki disease. J Pediatr 2003;142:731 [PMID: 12838207].

[c]deVries JS et al: Choledochal cysts: Age of presentation, symptoms and late complications related to Todani's classification. J Pediatr Surg 2002;37:1568 [PMID: 12407541].

[d]Imamoglu M et al: Acute acalculous cholecystitis in children: Diagnosis and treatment. J Pediatr Surg 2002;37:36 [PMID: 11781983].

[e]Madjov R et al: Caroli's disease. Report of 5 cases and review of literature. Hepatogastroenterology 2005;52:606 [PMID: 15816487].

[f]Perisic VN: Long term studies on congenital hepatic fibrosis in children. Acta Paediatr 1995;85:695 [PMID: 7670259].

[9]Carney DE et al: Predictors of successful outcome after cholecystectomy for biliary dyskinesia. J Pediatr Surg 2004;39:813 [PMID: 15785202].

kopenia and thrombocytopenia is often present. Upper endoscopy may reveal varices in symptomatic patients.

Doppler-assisted ultrasound scanning of the liver, portal vein, splenic vein, inferior vena cava, and hepatic veins may assist in defining the vascular anatomy. In prehepatic portal hypertension, abnormalities of the portal or splenic vein may be apparent, whereas the hepatic veins are normal. When noncirrhotic portal hypertension is suspected, angiography often is diagnostic. Selective arteriography of the superior mesenteric artery or MRI is recommended prior to surgical shunting to determine the patency of the superior mesenteric vein.

For suprahepatic portal hypertension, an inferior venacavogram using catheters from above or below the suspected obstruction may reveal an intrinsic filling defect, an infiltrating tumor, or extrinsic compression of the inferior vena cava by an adjacent lesion. A large caudate lobe of the liver suggests Budd–Chiari syndrome. Care must be taken in interpreting extrinsic pressure defects of the subdiaphragmatic inferior vena cava if ascites is significant.

Simultaneous wedged hepatic vein pressure and hepatic venography are useful to demonstrate obstruction to major hepatic vein ostia and smaller vessels. In the absence of obstruction, reflux across the sinusoids into the portal vein branches can be accomplished. Pressures should also be taken from the right heart and supradiaphragmatic portion of the inferior vena cava to eliminate constrictive pericarditis and pulmonary hypertension from the differential diagnosis.

Differential Diagnosis

All causes of splenomegaly must be included in the differential diagnosis. The most common ones are infections, immune thrombocytopenic purpura, blood dyscrasias, lipidosis, reticuloendotheliosis, cirrhosis of the liver, and cysts or hemangiomas of the spleen. When hematemesis or melena occurs, other causes of gastrointestinal bleeding are possible, such as gastric or duodenal ulcers, tumors, duplications, and inflammatory bowel disease.

Because ascites is almost always present in suprahepatic portal hypertension, cirrhosis resulting from any cause must be excluded. Other suprahepatic (cardiac, pulmonary) causes of portal hypertension must also be ruled out. Although ascites may occur in prehepatic portal hypertension, it is uncommon.

Complications

The major manifestation and complication of portal hypertension is bleeding esophageal varices. Fatal exsanguination is uncommon, but hypovolemic shock or resulting anemia may require prompt treatment. Hyper-

splenism with leukopenia and thrombocytopenia occurs but seldom causes major symptoms. Rupture of the enlarged spleen secondary to trauma is always a threat. Retroperitoneal edema has been reported (Clatworthy sign).

Without treatment, complete and persistent hepatic vein obstruction leads to liver failure, coma, and death. A nonportal type of cirrhosis may develop in the chronic form of hepatic venoocclusive disease in which small- and medium-sized hepatic veins are affected. Death from renal failure may occur in rare cases of congenital hepatic fibrosis.

Treatment

Definitive treatment of noncirrhotic portal hypertension is generally lacking. Aggressive medical treatment of the complications of prehepatic portal hypertension is generally quite effective. The early experience with surgical portosystemic shunts was unfavorable. Recently, several centers have reported excellent results with either portosystemic shunt or the meso-rex (mesenterico-left portal bypass) shunt. When possible, the meso-rex shunt is the preferred technique. Venoocclusive disease may be prevented somewhat by the prophylactic use of UCDA or defibrotide prior to conditioning for bone marrow transplantation. Treatment with defibrotide and withdrawal of the suspected offending agent, if possible, may increase the chance of recovery. For suprahepatic portal hypertension, efforts should be directed at correcting the underlying cause, if possible. Either surgical or angiographic relief of obstruction should be attempted if a defined obstruction of the vessels is apparent. Liver transplantation, if not contraindicated, should be considered early in the course if direct correction is not possible. In most cases, management of portal hypertension is directed at management of the complications (Table 21–8).

Prognosis

For prehepatic portal hypertension, the prognosis depends on the site of the block, the effectiveness of variceal eradication, the availability of suitable vessels for shunting procedures, and the experience of the surgeon. In patients treated by medical means, bleeding episodes seem to diminish with adolescence.

The prognosis in patients treated by medical and supportive therapy may be better than in the surgically treated group, especially when surgery is performed at an early age, although no comparative study has been done. Portacaval encephalopathy is unusual after shunting except when protein intake is excessive, but neurologic outcome may be better in patients who receive a meso-rex shunt when compared with medical management alone.

Table 21–8. Treatment of complications of portal hypertension.

Complication	Diagnosis	Treatment
Bleeding esophageal varices	Endoscopic verification of variceal bleeding.	Endosclerosis or variceal band ligation. Octreotide, 30 μg/m²/h intravenous. Pediatric Sengstaken-Blakemore tube. Surgical variceal ligation, selective venous embolization, TIPS, OLT. Propranolol may be useful to prevent recurrent bleeding.
Ascites	Clinical examination (fluid wave, shifting dullness), abdominal ultrasonography.	Sodium restriction (1–2 mEq/kg/d), spironolactone (3–5 mg/kg/d), furosemide (1–2 mg/kg/d), intravenous albumin (0.5–1 g/kg per dose), paracentesis, peritoneovenous (LeVeen) shunt, TIPS, surgical portosystemic shunt, OLT.[a]
Hepatic encephalopathy	Abnormal neurologic examination, elevated plasma ammonia.	Protein restriction (0.5–1 g/kg/d), intravenous glucose (6–8 mg/kg/min), neomycin (2–4 g/m² BSA PO in 4 doses), lactulose (1 mL/kg per dose [up to 30 mL] every 4–6 h PO), plasmapheresis, hemodialysis, OLT.[a]
Hypersplenism	Low WBC count, platelets, and/or hemoglobin. Splenomegaly.	No intervention, partial splenic embolization, TIPS, surgical portosystemic shunt, OLT. Splenectomy may worsen variceal bleeding.

[a]In order of sequential management.
BSA, body surface area; OLT, orthotopic liver transplantation; TIPS, transjugular intrahepatic portosystemic shunt; WBC, white blood cell.

The mortality rate of hepatic vein obstruction is very high (95%). In venoocclusive disease, the prognosis is better, with complete recovery possible in 50% of acute forms and 5–10% of subacute forms.

Bogin V et al: Budd-Chiari syndrome: In evolution. Eur J Gastroenterol Hepatol 2005;17:33 [PMID 15647637].

Botha JF et al: Portosystemic shunts in children: A 15-year experience. J Am Coll Surg 2004;199:179 [PMID 15275870].

Broxson EG et al: Portal hypertension develops in a subset of children with standard risk acute lymphoblastic leukemia treated with oral 6-thioguanine during maintenance therapy. Pediatr Blood Cancer 2005;44:226 [PMID 15503293].

Chalandon Y et al: Prevention of veno-occlusive disease with defibrotide after allogeneic stem cell transplantation. Biol Blood Marrow Transplant 2004;10:347 [PMID 15111934].

Dhiman RK et al: Non-cirrhotic portal fibrosis (idiopathic portal hypertension): Experience with 151 patients and a review of the literature. J Gastroenterol Hepatol 2002;17:6 [PMID 11895549].

Fuchs J et al: Mesenterico-left portal vein bypass in children with congenital extrahepatic portal vein thrombosis: A unique curative approach. J Pediatr Gastroenterol Nutr 2003;36:213 [PMID 12548056].

McKiernan PJ: Treatment of variceal bleeding. Gastrointest Endosc Clin North Am 2001;11:789 [PMID 11689366].

Menon P et al: Extrahepatic portal hypertension: Quality of life and somatic growth after surgery. Eur J Pediatr Surg 2005;15:82 [PMID 15877255].

Price MR et al: Management of esophageal varices in children by endoscopic variceal ligation. J Pediatr Surg 1996;31:1056 [PMID: 8863233].

Sartori MT et al: Role of fibrinolytic and clotting parameters in the diagnosis of liver veno-occlusive disease after hematopoietic stem cell transplantation in a pediatric population. Thromb Haemost 2005;93:682 [PMID 15142875].

Vogelsang GB, Dalal J: Hepatic venoocclusive disease in blood and bone marrow transplantation in children: Incidence, risk factors and outcome. J Pediatr Hematol Oncol 2002;24:746 [PMID 12468908].

BILIARY TRACT DISEASE

1. Cholelithiasis

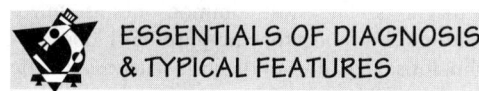 **ESSENTIALS OF DIAGNOSIS & TYPICAL FEATURES**

- *Episodic right upper quadrant abdominal pain.*
- *Elevated bilirubin, alkaline phosphatase, and GGT.*
- *Stones or sludge seen on abdominal ultrasound.*

General Considerations

Gallstones may develop at all ages in the pediatric population and in utero. Gallstones may be divided into cholesterol stones, which contain more than 50% cholesterol, and pigment, black (sterile bile) and brown (infected bile) stones. Pigment stones predominate in the first decade of life, while cholesterol stones account for up to 90% of gallstones in adolescence. For some patients, gallbladder dysfunction is associated with biliary sludge formation, which may evolve into "sludge balls" or tumefaction bile and then into gallstones. The process is reversible in many patients.

Clinical Findings

A. HISTORY

Most symptomatic gallstones are associated with acute or recurrent episodes of moderate to severe, sharp right upper quadrant or epigastric pain. The pain may radiate substernally or to the right shoulder. On rare occasions, the presentation may include a history of jaundice, back pain, or generalized abdominal discomfort, when it is associated with pancreatitis, suggesting stone impaction in the common duct or ampulla hepatopancreatica. Nausea and vomiting may occur during attacks. Pain episodes often occur postprandially, especially after ingestion of fatty foods. The groups at risk for gallstones include patients with known or suspected hemolytic disease; females; teenagers with prior pregnancy; obese individuals; individuals with rapid weight loss; children with portal vein thrombosis; certain racial or ethnic groups, particularly Native Americans (Pima Indians) and Hispanics; infants and children with ileal disease (Crohn disease) or prior ileal resection; patients with cystic fibrosis or Wilson disease; and infants on prolonged parenteral hyperalimentation. Other, less certain risk factors include a positive family history, use of birth control pills, and diabetes mellitus.

B. SYMPTOMS AND SIGNS

During acute episodes of pain, tenderness is present in the right upper quadrant or epigastrium, with a positive inspiratory arrest (Murphy sign), usually without peritoneal signs. While rarely present, scleral icterus is helpful. Evidence of underlying hemolytic disease in addition to icterus may include pallor (anemia), splenomegaly, tachycardia, and high-output cardiac murmur. Fever is unusual in uncomplicated cases.

C. LABORATORY FINDINGS

Laboratory tests are usually normal unless calculi have lodged in the extrahepatic biliary system, in which case the serum bilirubin and GGT (or alkaline phosphatase) may be elevated. Amylase and lipase levels may be increased if stone obstruction occurs at the ampulla hepatopancreatica.

D. IMAGING

Ultrasound evaluation is the best imaging technique, showing abnormal intraluminal contents (stones, sludge) as well as anatomic alterations of the gallbladder or dilation of the biliary ductal system. The presence of an anechoic acoustic shadow differentiates calculi from intraluminal sludge or sludge balls. Ceftriaxone may cause similar findings. Plain abdominal radiographs will show calculi with a high calcium content in the region of the gallbladder in up to 15% of patients. Lack of visualization of the gallbladder with hepatobiliary scintigraphy suggests chronic cholecystitis. In selected cases, ERCP, MRCP, or endoscopic ultrasound may be helpful in defining subtle abnormalities of the bile ducts and locating intraductal stones.

Differential Diagnosis

Other abnormal conditions of the biliary system with similar presentation are summarized in Table 21–7. Liver disease (hepatitis, abscess, or tumor) can cause similar symptoms or signs. Peptic disease, reflux esophagitis, paraesophageal hiatal hernia, cardiac disease, and pneumomediastinum must be considered when the pain is epigastric or substernal in location. Renal or pancreatic disease is a possible explanation if the pain is localized to the right flank or mid back. Subcapsular or supracapsular lesions of the liver (abscess, tumor, or hematoma) or right lower lobe infiltrate may also be a cause of nontraumatic right shoulder pain.

Complications

Major problems are related to stone impaction in either the cystic or common duct and lead to stricture formation or perforation. Acute distention and subsequent perforation of the gallbladder may occur when gallstones cause obstruction of the cystic duct. Stones impacted at the level of the ampulla hepatopancreatica often cause gallstone pancreatitis.

Treatment

Symptomatic cholelithiasis is treated by laparoscopic cholecystectomy or open cholecystectomy in selected cases. Intraoperative cholangiography via the cystic duct is recommended so that the physician can be certain the biliary system is free of retained stones. Calculi in the extrahepatic bile ducts may be removed at ERCP.

Gallstones developing in premature infants on total parenteral nutrition can be followed by ultrasound examination. Most of the infants are asymptomatic, and the stones will resolve in 3–36 months. Gallstone dissolution using cholelitholytics (UCDA) or mechanical means (lithotripsy) has not been approved for use in children. Asymptomatic gallstones do not usually require treatment, as less than 20% will eventually cause problems.

Prognosis

The prognosis is excellent in uncomplicated cases that come to standard cholecystectomy.

Burch Bruch SW et al: The management of nonpigmented gallstones in children. J Pediatr Surg 2000;35:729 [PMID: 10813336].

Jaffray B: Minimally invasive surgery. Arch Dis Child 2005;90:537 [PMID 15851444].

Lobe, TE: Cholelithiasis and cholecystitis in children. Semin Pediatr Surg 2000;9:170 [PMID: 11112834].

Mah D et al: Management of suspected common bile duct stones in children: Role of selective intraoperative cholangiogram and endoscopic retrograde cholangiopancreatography. J Pediatr Surg 2004;39:808 [PMID 15185201].

Miltenburg DM et al: Changing indications for pediatric cholecystectomy. Pediatrics 2000;105:1250 [PMID: 10835065].

2. Primary Sclerosing Cholangitis

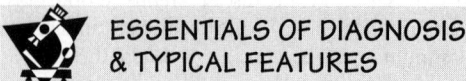

ESSENTIALS OF DIAGNOSIS & TYPICAL FEATURES

- *Pruritus and jaundice.*
- *Elevated GGT.*
- *Associated with inflammatory bowel disease.*
- *Abnormal ERCP or MRCP.*

General Considerations

Primary sclerosing cholangitis (PSC) is a progressive liver disease of unknown cause, characterized by chronic inflammation and fibrosis of the intra- and/or extrahepatic bile ducts, with eventual obliteration of peripheral bile ducts, cholangiographic evidence of strictures, and dilation of all or parts of the biliary tree. PSC is more common in males with inflammatory bowel disease, particularly ulcerative colitis. It can also be seen with histiocytosis X, sicca syndromes, congenital and acquired immunodeficiency syndromes, and cystic fibrosis.

Clinical Findings

A. SYMPTOMS AND SIGNS

PSC often has an insidious onset. Clinical symptoms may include abdominal pain, fatigue, pruritus, and jaundice. Acholic stools and steatorrhea can occur. Physical findings include hepatomegaly, splenomegaly, and jaundice.

B. LABORATORY FINDINGS

The earliest finding may be asymptomatic elevation of the GGT. Subsequent laboratory abnormalities include elevated levels of alkaline phosphatase and bile acids. Later, cholestatic jaundice and elevated AST and ALT may occur. Patients with associated inflammatory bowel disease often test positive for perinuclear antineutrophil cytoplasmic antibodies. Other markers of autoimmune liver disease (ANA and ASMA) are often found

but are not specific for PSC. Sclerosing cholangitis due to cryptosporidia is common in immunodeficiency syndromes.

C. RADIOLOGIC FINDINGS

Ultrasound may show dilated intrahepatic bile ducts behind strictures. MRCP is now the diagnostic study of choice, demonstrating irregularities of the biliary tree.

Differential Diagnosis

The differential diagnosis includes infectious hepatitis, secondary cholangitis, autoimmune hepatitis, metabolic liver disease, cystic fibrosis, choledochal cyst, or other anomalies of the biliary tree, including Caroli disease and congenital hepatic fibrosis.

Complications

Complications include secondary bacterial cholangitis, pancreatitis, biliary fibrosis, and cirrhosis. Progression to liver failure is common and the risk of cholangiocarcinoma is higher in PSC.

Treatment

No completely effective treatment is available. Patients with early disease may benefit from high-dose UCDA (25–30 mg/kg/d). Patients with autoimmune markers may benefit from treatment with corticosteroids and azathioprine. Antibiotic treatment of cholangitis and dilation and stenting of dominant bile duct strictures can reduce symptoms.

Prognosis

The majority of patients will eventually require liver transplantation and PSC is the fifth leading indication for liver transplantation in the United States. The median duration from the time of diagnosis to end-stage liver disease is 12–15 years.

Gregorio GV et al: Autoimmune hepatitis/sclerosing cholangitis overlap syndrome in childhood: A 16-year prospective study. Hepatology 2001;33:544 [PMID: 11230733].

Mieli-Vergani G, Vergani D: Sclerosing cholangitis in the paediatric patient. Best Pract Res Clin Gastroenterol 2001;15:681 [PMID: 11492976].

Talwalkar JA, Lindor KD: Primary sclerosing cholangitis. Inflamm Bowel Dis 2005;11:62 [PMID 15674115].

3. Other Biliary Tract Disorders

For a schematic representation of the various types of choledochal cysts, see Figure 21–1. For summary information on acute hydrops, choledochal cyst, acalculous

TYPE		FINDINGS
I	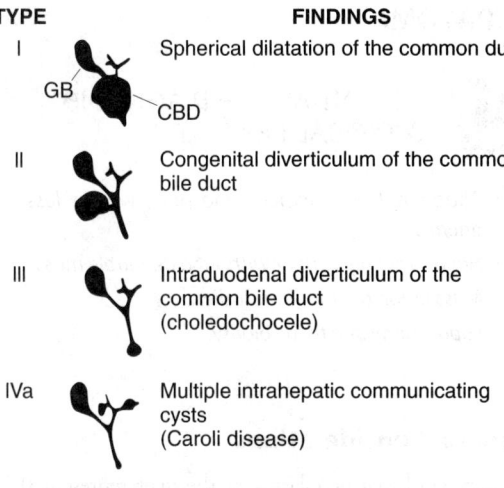	Spherical dilatation of the common duct
II		Congenital diverticulum of the common bile duct
III		Intraduodenal diverticulum of the common bile duct (choledochocele)
IVa		Multiple intrahepatic communicating cysts (Caroli disease)
IVb		Mixed extrahepatic and intrahepatic fusiform or cystic dilation (possibly variants of Caroli disease, congenital hepatic fibrosis)

Figure 21–1. Classification of cystic dilation of the bile ducts. Types I, II, and III are extrahepatic choledochal cysts. Type IVa is solely intrahepatic, and type IVb is both intrahepatic and extrahepatic. GB, gallbladder; CBD, common bile duct.

cholecystitis, Caroli disease, biliary dyskinesia, and congenital hepatic fibrosis, see Table 21–7.

PYOGENIC & AMEBIC LIVER ABSCESS

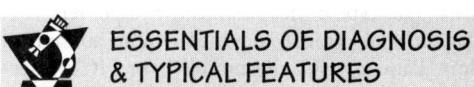

ESSENTIALS OF DIAGNOSIS & TYPICAL FEATURES

- *Fever and painful enlarged liver.*
- *Ultrasound of liver demonstrating an abscess.*
- *Positive serum ameba antigen titer or positive bacterial culture of abscess fluid.*

General Considerations

Pyogenic liver abscesses are often caused by intestinal bacteria seeded via the portal vein from infected viscera and occasionally from ascending cholangitis or gangrenous cholecystitis. Blood cultures are positive in up to 60% of patients. The resulting lesion tends to be solitary and located in the right hepatic lobe. Bacterial seeding may also occur from infected burns, pyodermas, and osteomyelitis. Unusual causes include ompha-

litis, subacute infective endocarditis, pyelonephritis, Crohn disease, and perinephric abscess. In immunocompromised patients, *S aureus,* gram-negative organisms, and fungi may seed the liver from the arterial system. Multiple pyogenic liver abscesses are associated with severe sepsis. Children receiving anti-inflammatory and immunosuppressive agents and children with defects in white blood cell function (chronic granulomatous disease) are prone to pyogenic hepatic abscesses, especially those caused by *S aureus.*

Amoebic liver abscess is rare in children. An increased risk is associated with travel through areas of endemic infection (Mexico, Southeast Asia) within 5 months of presentation. *Entamoeba histolytica* invasion occurs via the large bowel, although a history of diarrhea (colitis-like picture) is not always obtained.

Clinical Findings

With pyogenic liver abscess, nonspecific complaints of fever, chills, malaise, and abdominal pain are frequent. Weight loss is very common, especially in delayed diagnosis. A few patients have shaking chills and jaundice. The dominant complaint is a constant dull pain over an enlarged liver that is tender to palpation. An elevated hemidiaphragm with reduced or absent respiratory excursion may be demonstrated on physical examination and confirmed by fluoroscopy. Laboratory studies show leukocytosis and, at times, anemia. LFTs may be normal or reveal mild elevation of transaminases and alkaline phosphatase. Fever and abdominal pain are the two most common symptoms of amebic liver abscess. Abdominal tenderness and hepatomegaly are present in over 50%. Early in the course, LFTs may suggest mild hepatitis. An occasional prodrome may include cough, dyspnea, and shoulder pain as rupture of the abscess into the right chest occurs. Consolidation of the right lower lobe is common (10–30% of patients).

Ultrasound liver scan is the most useful diagnostic aid in evaluating pyogenic and amebic abscesses, detecting lesions as small as 1–2 cm. Nuclear scanning with gallium or technetium sulfur colloid or CT imaging may be useful in differentiating tumor or hydatid cyst.

The distinction between pyogenic and amebic abscesses is best made by indirect hemagglutination test (which is positive in more than 95% of patients with amebic liver disease) and the prompt response of the latter to antiamebic therapy (metronidazole). Examination of material obtained by needle aspiration of the abscess using ultrasound guidance is often diagnostic.

Differential Diagnosis

Hepatitis, hepatoma, hydatid cyst, gallbladder disease, or biliary tract infections can mimic liver abscess. Subphrenic abscesses, empyema, and pneumonia may give a similar picture. Inflammatory disease of the intestines or of the biliary system may be complicated by liver abscess.

Complications

Spontaneous rupture of the abscess may occur with extension of infection into the subphrenic space, thorax, peritoneal cavity, and, occasionally, the pericardium. Bronchopleural fistula with large sputum production and hemoptysis can develop in severe cases. Simultaneously, the amebic liver abscess may be secondarily infected with bacteria (in 10–20% of patients). Metastatic hematogenous spread to the lungs and the brain has been reported.

Treatment

Ultrasound- or CT-guided percutaneous needle aspiration for aerobic and anaerobic culture with simultaneous placement of a catheter for drainage, combined with appropriate antibiotic therapy, is the treatment of choice for solitary pyogenic liver abscess. Multiple liver abscesses may also be treated successfully by this method. Surgical intervention may be indicated if rupture occurs outside the capsule of the liver or if enterohepatic fistulae are suspected.

Amebic abscesses in uncomplicated cases should be treated promptly with oral metronidazole, 35–50 mg/kg/d, in 3 divided doses for 10 days. Intravenous metronidazole can be used for patients unable to take oral medication. Failure to improve after 72 hours of drug therapy suggests superimposed bacterial infection or an incorrect diagnosis. At this point, needle aspiration or surgical drainage is indicated. Once oral feedings can be tolerated, a luminal amebicide such as iodoquinol should be initiated. Resolution of the abscess cavity occurs over 3–6 months.

Prognosis

An unrecognized and untreated pyogenic liver abscess is universally fatal. With drainage and antibiotics, the cure rate is about 90%. Most amebic abscesses are cured with conservative medical management; the mortality rate is less than 3%. If extrahepatic complications occur (empyema, bronchopleural fistula, or pericardial complications), 10–15% of patients will succumb.

Kurland JE, Brann OS: Pyogenic and amebic liver abscesses. Curr Gastroenterol Rep 2004;6:273 [PMID 15245694].

Rajak CL et al: Percutaneous drainage of liver abscesses: Needle aspiration versus catheter drainage. AJR Am J Roentgenol 1998;170:1035 [PMID 9530055].

Wells CD, Arguedas M: Amebic liver abscess. South Med J 2004; 97:673 [PMID 15301125].

HEPATOMA

ESSENTIALS OF DIAGNOSIS & TYPICAL FEATURES

- *Abdominal enlargement and pain, weight loss, anemia.*
- *Hepatomegaly with or without a definable mass.*
- *Mass lesion on imaging studies.*
- *Laparotomy and tissue biopsy.*

General Considerations

Primary epithelial neoplasms of the liver represent 0.2–5.8% of all malignant conditions in children. After Wilms tumor and neuroblastoma, hepatomas are the third most common intra-abdominal cancer. The incidence is higher in Southeast Asia, where childhood cirrhosis is more common. There are two basic morphologic types with certain clinical and prognostic differences. Hepatoblastoma predominates in male infants and children and accounts for 79% of liver cancer in children, with most cases appearing before age 5 years. There is an increased risk of hepatoblastoma in Beckwith–Wiedemann syndrome, hemihypertrophy, familial adenomatosis polyposis coli, and in premature or low-birth-weight infants. Most lesions are found in the right lobe of the liver. Pathologic differentiation from hepatocarcinoma may be difficult. Hepatocarcinoma, the other major malignant tumor of the liver, occurs more frequently after age 3 years. This type of neoplasm carries a poorer prognosis than hepatoblastoma and causes more abdominal discomfort. Patients with chronic HBV or HCV infection, cirrhosis, glycogen storage disease type I, tyrosinemia, or α_1-antitrypsin deficiency have an increased risk for hepatocellular carcinoma. The late development of hepatoma in patients receiving androgens for treatment of Fanconi syndrome and aplastic anemia must also be kept in mind. The use of anabolic steroids by body-conscious adolescents poses a risk of hepatic neoplasia. An interesting aspect of primary epithelial neoplasms of the liver has been the increased incidence of associated anomalies and endocrine abnormalities. Virilization has been reported as a consequence of gonadotropin activity of the tumor. Feminization with bilateral gynecomastia may occur in association with high estradiol levels in the blood, the latter a consequence of increased aromatization of circulating androgens by the liver. Leydig cell hyperplasia without spermatogenesis is found on testicular biopsy. Hemihypertrophy, congenital absence of the kidney, macroglossia, and Meckel diverticulum have been found in association with hepatocarcinoma.

Clinical Findings

A noticeable increase in abdominal girth with or without pain is the most constant feature of the history. A parent may note a bulge in the upper abdomen or report feeling a hard mass. Constitutional symptoms (eg, anorexia, fatigue, fever, and chills) may be present. Teenage boys may complain of gynecomastia.

A. SYMPTOMS AND SIGNS

Weight loss, pallor, and abdominal pain associated with a large abdomen are common. Physical examination reveals hepatomegaly with or without a definite tumor mass, usually to the right of the midline. In the absence of cirrhosis, signs of chronic liver disease are usually absent. However, evidence of virilization or feminization in prepubertal children may be noted.

B. LABORATORY FINDINGS

Normal LFTs are the rule. Anemia frequently occurs, especially in cases of hepatoblastoma. Cystathioninuria has been reported. α-Fetoprotein levels are often elevated, especially in hepatoblastoma. Estradiol levels are sometimes elevated. Final tissue diagnosis is best obtained at laparotomy, although ultrasound- or CT-guided needle biopsy of the liver mass can be used.

C. IMAGING

Ultrasonography, CT, and MRI are useful for diagnosis, staging, and following tumor response to therapy. A scintigraphic study of bone and lung and selective angiography are generally part of the preoperative work-up to evaluate metastatic disease.

Differential Diagnosis

In the absence of a palpable mass, the differential diagnosis is that of hepatomegaly with or without anemia or jaundice. Hematologic and nutritional conditions should be ruled out, as well as HBV and HCV infection, α$_1$-antitrypsin deficiency disease, lipid storage diseases, histiocytosis X, glycogen storage disease, tyrosinemia, congenital hepatic fibrosis, cysts, adenoma, focal nodular hyperplasia, inflammatory pseudotumor, and hemangiomas. If fever is present, hepatic abscess (pyogenic or amebic) must be considered. Venoocclusive disease and hepatic vein thrombosis are rare possibilities. Tumors in the left lobe may be mistaken for pancreatic pseudocysts.

Complications

Progressive enlargement of the tumor, abdominal discomfort, ascites, respiratory difficulty, and widespread metastases (especially to the lungs and the abdominal lymph nodes) are the rule. Rupture of the neoplastic liver and intraperitoneal hemorrhage have been reported. Progressive anemia and emaciation predispose the patient to an early septic death.

Treatment

An aggressive surgical approach has resulted in the only long-term survivals. Complete resection of the lesion offers the only chance for cure. It appears that every isolated lung metastasis should also be surgically resected. Radiotherapy and chemotherapy have been disappointing in the treatment of primary liver neoplasms, although they may be used for initial cytoreduction of tumors found to be unresectable at the time of primary surgery. Second-look celiotomy has, in some cases, allowed resection of the tumor, resulting in a reduced mortality rate. Liver transplantation can be an option in hepatoblastoma with 85% 10-year survival in patients with unresectable disease limited to the liver. For hepatocellular carcinoma, the survival rate is poor due to the typically advanced stage at diagnosis. The survival rate may be better for those patients in whom the tumor is incidental to another disorder (tyrosinemia, biliary atresia, cirrhosis). In HBV-endemic areas, childhood HBV vaccination has reduced the incidence of hepatocellular carcinoma.

Prognosis

If the tumor is completely removed the survival rate is 90% for hepatoblastoma and 33% for hepatocellular carcinoma. If metastases are present, survival is reduced to 40% for hepatoblastoma.

Chang MH et al: Universal hepatitis B vaccination in Taiwan and the incidence of hepatocellular carcinoma in children. N Engl J Med 1997;336:1855 [PMID: 9197213].

Emre S, McKenna GJ: Liver tumors in children. Pediatr Transpl 2004;8:632 [PMID: 15598339].

Stringer MD: Liver tumors. Semin Pediatr Surg 2000;9:196 [PMID: 11112837].

Tiao GM et al: The current management of hepatoblastoma: A combination of chemotherapy, conventional resection, and liver transplantation. J Pediatr 2005;146:204 [PMID: 15689909].

LIVER TRANSPLANTATION

Orthotopic liver transplantation is indicated in children with end-stage liver disease, acute fulminant hepatic failure, or complications from metabolic liver disorders. Recent advances in immunosuppression (eg, cyclosporine and tacrolimus, use of monoclonal antibodies against T cells, introduction of mycophenolate mofetil and sirolimus), better candidate selection, improvements in surgical techniques, antiviral medications, and experience in postoperative management have contributed to improved results.

The major indications for childhood transplantation are

1. A failed Kasai operation or decompensated cirrhosis caused by biliary atresia.

2. α_1-Antitrypsin deficiency.

3. Posthepatitic (autoimmune chronic hepatitis, hepatitis B or C disease) cirrhosis.

4. Tyrosinemia.

5. Crigler–Najjar syndrome type 1.

6. Wilson disease.

7. Acute fulminant hepatic failure when recovery is unlikely.

8. Primary sclerosing cholangitis.

9. Hepatic-based malignancies.

10. Cases in which the consequences of chronic cholestasis severely impair the patient's quality of life (eg, Alagille syndrome).

Children should be referred early for evaluation because the limiting factor for success is the small donor pool. Pared-down adult livers, organs from living related donors, and split adult donor livers have expanded the donor pool, in addition to whole pediatric donor organs. Ten percent of recipients require retransplantation. In general, 80–90% of children survive at least 2–5 years after transplantation, with long-term survival expected to be comparable. Lifetime immunosuppression therapy using combinations of tacrolimus, cyclosporine, prednisone, azathioprine, mycophenolate mofetil, or sirolimus with its incumbent risks, is necessary to prevent rejection. The minimal amount of immunosuppression that will prevent allograft rejection is chosen. The overall quality of life for children with a transplanted liver appears to be excellent. The lifelong risk of EBV-induced lymphoproliferative disease is approximately 5% and is related to age and EBV exposure status at time of transplant and intensity of immunosuppression. Various protocols are being tested for prevention and treatment of lymphoproliferative disease.

Alonso EM et al: Functional outcomes of pediatric liver transplantation. J Pediatr Gastroenterol Nutr 2003;37:155 [PMID: 12883302].

Bucuvalas JC et al: A novel approach to managing variation: Outpatient therapeutic monitoring of calcineurin inhibitor blood levels in liver transplant recipients. J Pediatr 2005;146:744 [PMID: 15973310].

Heo JS et al: Posttransplantation lymphoproliferative disorder in pediatric liver transplantation. Transpl Proc 2004;36:2307 [PMID: 15561231].

Utterson EC et al; The Split Research Group: Biliary atresia: clinical profiles, risk factors, and outcomes of 755 patients listed for liver transplantation. J Pediatr 2005;147:180 [PMID: 16126046].

■ PANCREAS

ACUTE PANCREATITIS

ESSENTIALS OF DIAGNOSIS & TYPICAL FEATURES

- *Epigastric abdominal pain radiating to the back.*
- *Nausea and vomiting.*
- *Elevated serum amylase and lipase.*
- *Evidence of pancreatic inflammation by CT or ultrasound.*

General Considerations

Most cases of acute pancreatitis are the result of drugs, viral infections, systemic diseases, abdominal trauma, or obstruction of pancreatic flow. More than 20% are idiopathic. Causes of pancreatic obstruction include stones, choledochal cyst, tumors of the duodenum, pancreas divisum, and ascariasis. Acute pancreatitis has been seen following treatment with sulfasalazine, thiazides, valproic acid, azathioprine, mercaptopurine, asparaginase, antiretroviral drugs (especially ddI), high-dose corticosteroids, and other drugs. It may also occur in cystic fibrosis, systemic lupus erythematosus, α_1-antitrypsin deficiency, diabetes mellitus, Crohn disease, glycogen storage disease type I, hyperlipidemia types I and V, hyperparathyroidism, Henoch–Schönlein purpura, Reye syndrome, organic acidopathies, Kawasaki disease, or chronic renal failure; during rapid refeeding in cases of malnutrition; following spinal fusion surgery; and in familial cases. Alcohol-induced pancreatitis should be considered in the teenage patient.

Clinical Findings

A. SYMPTOMS AND SIGNS

An acute onset of persistent (hours to days), moderate to severe upper abdominal and midabdominal pain occasionally referred to the back, and vomiting, is the common presenting picture. The abdomen is tender but not rigid, and bowel sounds are diminished, suggesting peritoneal irritation. Abdominal distention is common in infants and younger children. Jaundice is unusual. Ascites may be noted, and a left-sided pleural effusion is present in some patients. Periumbilical and flank bruising indicate hemorrhagic pancreatitis.

B. Laboratory Findings

Leukocytosis and an elevated serum amylase(> 3 times normal) should be expected early, except in infants younger than 6 months who may have hypoamylasemia. Serum lipase is elevated and persists longer than serum amylase. The immunoreactive trypsinogen may also be elevated. Pancreatic amylase isoenzyme determination can help differentiate nonpancreatic causes (eg, salivary, intestinal, or tuboovarian) of serum amylase elevation. Hyperglycemia (serum glucose > 300 mg/dL), hypocalcemia, falling hematocrit, rising blood urea nitrogen, hypoxemia, and acidosis may all occur in severe cases and imply a poor prognosis.

C. Imaging

Plain radiographic films of the abdomen may show a localized ileus (sentinel loop). Ultrasonography shows decreased echodensity of the gland in comparison with the left lobe of the liver. Pseudocyst formation can occasionally be seen early in the course. CT scanning is better for detecting pancreatic phlegmon, or abscess formation. ERCP or MRCP may be useful in confirming patency of the main pancreatic duct in cases of abdominal trauma; in recurrent acute pancreatitis; or in revealing stones, ductal strictures, and pancreas divisum.

Differential Diagnosis

Other causes of acute upper abdominal pain include lesions of the stomach, duodenum, liver, and biliary system; acute gastroenteritis or atypical appendicitis; pneumonia; volvulus; intussusception; and nonaccidental trauma.

Complications

Complications early in the disease include shock, fluid and electrolyte disturbances, ileus, acute respiratory distress syndrome, and hypocalcemia. Hypervolemia is seen between the third and fifth days, at which time renal tubular necrosis may occur. The gastrointestinal, neurologic, musculoskeletal, hepatobiliary, dermatologic, and hematologic systems may also be involved.

Later, 5–20% of patients develop a pseudocyst heralded by recurrence of abdominal pain and rise in the serum amylase. Up to 60–70% of pseudocysts resolve spontaneously. Infection, hemorrhage, rupture, or fistulization may occur. Phlegmon formation is common and may extend from the gland into the retroperitoneum or into the lesser sac. Most regress, but some require drainage. Infection in this inflammatory mass may occur. Pancreatic abscess formation, which is rare (3–5%), develops 2–3 weeks after the initial insult. Fever, leukocytosis, and pain suggest this complication; diagnosis is made by ultrasound or CT scanning.

Chronic pancreatitis, exocrine or endocrine pancreatic insufficiency, and pancreatic lithiasis are rare sequelae of acute pancreatitis.

Treatment

Medical management includes careful attention to fluids, electrolytes. and respiratory status. Gastric decompression may be helpful if there is significant vomiting. Pain should be controlled with opioids. Acid suppression may be helpful. Nutrition is provided by the parenteral or enteral (jejunal) route. Broad-spectrum antibiotic coverage is useful only in necrotizing pancreatitis. Drugs known to produce acute pancreatitis should be discontinued. Surgical treatment is reserved for traumatic disruption of the gland, intraductal stone, other anatomic obstructive lesions, and unresolved or infected pseudocysts or abscesses. Early endoscopic decompression of the biliary system reduces the morbidity associated with pancreatitis caused by obstruction of the common bile duct.

Prognosis

In the pediatric age group, the prognosis is surprisingly good with conservative management. The mortality rate is 5–10% in patients treated surgically and 1% in those treated only with medication. The morbidity rate is high with surgery as a result of fistula formation.

Jackson WD: Pancreatitis: Etiology, diagnosis, and management. Curr Opin Pediatr 2001;13:447 [PMID: 11801891].

Lowe ME: Pancreatitis in childhood. Curr Gastroenterol Rep 2004;6:240 [PMID 15128492].

CHRONIC PANCREATITIS

Chronic pancreatitis is differentiated from acute pancreatitis in that the pancreas remains structurally or functionally abnormal after an attack.

The causes are multiple and can be divided into toxic-metabolic (eg, alcohol, chronic renal failure, hypercalcemia), idiopathic, genetic, autoimmune, recurrent and severe acute pancreatitis, and obstructive pancreatitis (eg, pancreas divisum, choledochal cyst).

Clinical Findings

The diagnosis often is delayed by the nonspecific symptoms and the lack of persistent laboratory abnormalities.

A. Symptoms and Signs

There is usually a prolonged history of recurrent upper abdominal pain of variable severity. Radiation of the pain into the back is a frequent complaint. Fever and vomiting are not common. Steatorrhea and symptoms of diabetes may develop later in the course, and malnutrition secondary to failure of pancreatic exocrine secretions may also occur.

B. LABORATORY FINDINGS

Serum amylase and lipase levels are usually elevated during early acute attacks but are often normal later. Pancreatic insufficiency and reduced volume and bicarbonate response may be found during pancreatic stimulation testing or by determination of fecal pancreatic elastase 1. Mutations of the cationic trypsinogen gene, the pancreatic secretory trypsin inhibitor, and the cystic fibrosis transmembrane conductance regulator gene (*CFTR*) are associated with recurrent acute and chronic pancreatitis. Elevated blood glucose and glycohemoglobin levels and glycosuria frequently occur in protracted disease. Sweat chloride should be checked for cystic fibrosis and serum calcium for hyperparathyroidism.

C. IMAGING

Radiographs of the abdomen may show pancreatic calcifications in up to 30% of patients. Ultrasound or CT examination demonstrates pancreatic enlargement, ductal dilation, and calculi in up to 80%. CT is the initial imaging procedure of choice. MRCP or ERCP can show ductal dilation, stones, strictures, or stenotic segments. Endoscopic ultrasound in the diagnosis and staging of chronic pancreatitis is being evaluated.

Differential Diagnosis

Other causes of recurrent abdominal pain must be considered. Specific causes of pancreatitis such as hyperparathyroidism; systemic lupus erythematosus; infectious disease; and ductal obstruction by tumors, stones, or helminths must be excluded by appropriate tests.

Complications

Disabling abdominal pain, steatorrhea, malnutrition, pancreatic pseudocysts, and diabetes are the most frequent long-term complications. Pancreatic carcinoma occurs more frequently in chronic pancreatitis, and in up to 40% of patients with hereditary pancreatitis by age 70.

Treatment

Medical management of acute attacks is indicated (see Acute Pancreatitis section). If ductal obstruction is strongly suspected, endoscopic therapy (balloon dilation, stenting, stone removal, or sphincterotomy) should be pursued. Relapses occur in most patients. Orally ingested nonenteric-coated pancreatic enzymes at mealtime may reduce pain episodes in some patients. Antioxidant therapy is being investigated. Pseudocysts may be marsupialized to

the surface or drained into the stomach or into a loop of jejunum if they fail to regress spontaneously. Experience in pediatric patients indicates that lateral pancreaticojejunostomy can reduce pain in patients with a dilated pancreatic duct and may prevent or delay progression of functional pancreatic impairment. Pancreatectomy and islet cell autotransplantation have been used in selected cases of chronic pancreatitis.

Prognosis

In the absence of a correctable lesion, the prognosis is not good. Disabling episodes of pain, pancreatic insufficiency, diabetes, and pancreatic cancer may ensue. Narcotic addiction and suicide are risks in teenagers with disabling disease.

Lowe ME: Pancreatitis in childhood. Curr Gastroenterol Rep 2004;6:240 [PMID: 15128492].

Witt H: Gene mutations in children with chronic pancreatitis. Pancreatology 2001;1:432 [PMID: 12120220].

GASTROINTESTINAL & HEPATOBILIARY MANIFESTATIONS OF CYSTIC FIBROSIS

Cystic fibrosis is a disease with protean manifestations. Although pulmonary and pancreatic involvement dominate the clinical picture for most patients (see Chapter 18), a variety of other organs can be involved. Table 21–9 lists the important gastrointestinal, pancreatic, and hepatobiliary conditions that may affect patients with cystic fibrosis along with their clinical findings, incidence, most useful diagnostic studies, and preferred treatment.

Baker SS et al: Pancreatic enzyme therapy and clinical outcomes in patients with cystic fibrosis. J Pediatr 2005;146:189 [PMID: 15689904].

Borowitz D et al: Gastrointestinal outcomes and confounders in cystic fibrosis. J Pediatr Gastroenterol Nutr 2005;41:273 [PMID: 16131979].

Borowitz D et al: Use of fecal elastase-1 to classify pancreatic status in patients with cystic fibrosis. J Pediatr 2004;145:322 [PMID: 15343184].

Corbett K et al: Cystic fibrosis-associated liver disease: A population-based study. J Pediatr 2004;145:327 [PMID: 15343185].

Lenaerts C et al: Surveillance for cystic fibrosis-associated hepatobiliary disease: Early ultrasound changes and predisposing factors. J Pediatr 2003;143:343 [PMID: 14517517].

Ratjen F, Doring G: Cystic fibrosis. Lancet 2003;361:681 [PMID 12606185].

SYNDROMES WITH PANCREATIC EXOCRINE INSUFFICIENCY

Several syndromes are associated with exocrine pancreatic insufficiency. Clinically, patients present

Table 21–9. Gastrointestinal and hepatobiliary manifestations of cystic fibrosis.

Organ	Condition	Symptoms	Age at Presentation	Incidence (%)	Diagnostic Evaluation	Management
Esophagus	Gastroesophageal reflux, esophagitis	Pyrosis, dysphagia, epigastric pain, hematemesis.	All ages	10–20	Endoscopy and biopsy, overnight pH study	H_2 blockers, antacids, carafate, PPIs, surgical antireflux procedure.
	Varices	Hematemesis, melena.	Childhood and adolescents	3–10	Endoscopy	Endosclerosis, band ligation, drugs (see text), TIPS, liver transplantation. (see Table 21–8).
Stomach	Gastritis	Upper abdominal pain, vomiting, hematemesis.	School age and older	10–25	Endoscopy and biopsy	H_2 blockers, antacids, carafate, PPIs.
	Hiatal hernia	Reflux symptoms (see above). epigastric pain.	School age and older	3–5	Endoscopy; UGI	As above. Surgery in some.
Intestine	Meconium ileus	Abdominal distention, bilious emesis.	Neonate	10–15	Radiologic studies, plain abdominal films; contrast enema shows microcolon	Dislodgement of obstruction with Gastrografin enema. Surgery if unsuccessful or if case complicated by atresia, perforation, or volvulus.
	Distal intestinal obstruction syndrome	Abdominal pain, acute and recurrent; distention; occasional vomiting.	Any age, usually school age through adolescence	10–15	Palpable mass in right lower quadrant, radiologic studies	Gastrografin enema, intestinal lavage solution, diet, bulk laxatives, adjustment of pancreatic enzyme intake.
	Fibrosing colonopathy	As above. History of high enzyme dosage.	≥3 years	< 1	Barium enema or UGI/SBFT, abdominal ultrasound, or CT	Reduce pancreatic enzyme dose to < 2000 units of lipase/kg per dose if indicated. Surgical resection may be necessary.
	Intussusception	Acute, intermittent abdominal pain; distention; emesis.	Infants through adolescence	1–3	X-ray studies, barium enema	Reduction by barium or air enema or surgery if needed. Diet. Bulk laxatives. Adjustment of pancreatic enzyme intake.
	Rectal prolapse	Anal discomfort, rectal bleeding.	Infants and children to age 4–5 years	15–25	Visual mass protruding from anus	Manual reduction, adjustment of pancreatic enzyme dosage, reassurance as problem resolves by age 3–5 years.

(continued)

679

Table 21-9. Gastrointestinal and hepatobiliary manifestations of cystic fibrosis. (continued)

Organ	Condition	Symptoms	Age at Presentation	Incidence (%)	Diagnostic Evaluation	Management
Intestine (cont'd)	Carbohydrate intolerance	Abdominal pain, flatulence, continued diarrhea with adequate replacement therapy.	Any age	10–25	Intestinal mucosal biopsy and disaccharidase analysis. Breath hydrogen after lactose load.	Reduce lactose intake; lactase; reduction of gastric hyperacidity if mucosa shows partial villous atrophy. Beware concurrent celiac disease or *Giardia* infection.
Pancreas	Total exocrine insufficiency	Diarrhea, steatorrhea, malnutrition, failure to thrive. Specific fat-soluble vitamin deficiency states.	Neonate through infancy	85–90	72-h fecal fat evaluation, fecal pancreatic elastase, direct pancreatic function tests	Pancreatic enzyme replacement, may need elemental formula, fat-soluble vitamin and vitamin E supplements.
	Pancreatic sufficiency (partial exocrine insufficiency)	Occasional diarrhea, mild growth delay.	Any age	10–15	72-hour fecal fat evaluation, direct pancreatic function tests, fecal pancreatic elastase	Pancreatic enzyme replacement in selected patients. Fat-soluble vitamin supplements as indicated by biochemical evaluation.
	Pancreatitis	Recurrent abdominal pain, vomiting.	Older children through adolescence. Primarily in patients with partial pancreatic sufficiency.	0.1	Increased serum lipase and amylase, pancreatic provocative test, MRCP, ERCP	Addition of pancreatic enzymes to feeds, endoscopic removal of sludge or stones if present, endoscopic papillotomy.
	Diabetes	Weight loss, polyuria, polydipsia.	Older children through adolescence	5–7	Glucose tolerance test and insulin levels	Diet, insulin, oral hypoglycemics.
Liver	Steatosis	Hepatomegaly.	Neonates and infants, but can be seen at all	20–60	Liver biopsy	Improved nutrition, replacement of pancreatic enzymes and vitamins.
	Focal biliary cirrhosis	Hepatomegaly.	Infants and older patients. Prevalence increases with age.	10–70	Liver biopsy	As above. Taurine supplements (still experimental), ursodeoxycholic acid.
	Multilobular biliary cirrhosis	Hepatosplenomegaly, hematemesis from esophageal varices; hypersplenism, jaundice, ascites late in course.	School age through adolescence	5–15	Liver biopsy, endoscopy	Improved nutrition, ursodeoxycholic acid, endosclerosis or band ligation of varices, or partial splenic embolization, liver transplantation.

Liver (cont'd)	Neonatal jaundice	Cholestatic jaundice hepatomegaly; often seen with meconium ileus.	Neonates	0.1–1	Sweat chloride test, liver biopsy	Nutritional support, special formula with medium-chain triglyceride–containing oil, pancreatic enzyme replacement, vitamin supplements.
Gallbladder	Microgallbladder	None.	Congenital—present at any age	30	Ultrasound or hepatobiliary scintigraphy	None needed.
	Cholelithiasis	Recurrent abdominal pain, rarely jaundice.	School age through adolescence	1–10	Ultrasound	Surgery if symptomatic and low risk, trial of cholelitholytics in others.
Extrahepatic bile ducts	Intraluminal obstruction (sludge, stones, tumor)	Jaundice, hepatomegaly, abdominal pain.	Neonates, then older children through adolescence	Rare in neonates (< 0.1)	Ultrasound and hepatobiliary scintigraphy, MRCP	Surgery in neonates; ERCP in older patients or surgery.
	Extraluminal obstruction (intrapancreatic compression, tumor)	As above.	Older children to adults	Rare (< 1)	As above	Surgical biliary drainage procedure or ERCP.

CT, computed tomography; ERCP, endoscopic retrograde cholangiopancreatography; MRCP, magnetic resonance cholangiopancreatography; PPI, proton pump inhibitor; TIPS, transjugular intrahepatic portosystemic shunt; UGI/SBFT, upper gastrointestinal/small bowel follow-through radiologic series.

with a history of failure to thrive, diarrhea, fatty stools, and an absence of respiratory symptoms. Laboratory findings include a normal sweat chloride; low fecal pancreatic elastase 1; and low to absent pancreatic lipase, amylase, and trypsin levels on duodenal intubation. Each disorder has several associated clinical features that aid in the differential diagnosis. In Shwachman syndrome, pancreatic exocrine hypoplasia with widespread fatty replacement of the glandular acinar tissue is associated with neutropenia because of maturational arrest of the granulocyte series. Metaphyseal dysostosis and an elevated fetal hemoglobin are common; immunoglobulin deficiency and hepatic dysfunction are also reported. CT examination of the pancreas demonstrates the widespread fatty replacement. Serum immunoreactive trypsinogen levels are extremely low.

Other associations of exocrine pancreatic insufficiency include (1) aplastic alae, aplasia cutis, deafness (Johanson–Blizzard syndrome); (2) sideroblastic anemia, developmental delay, seizures, and liver dysfunction (Pearson bone marrow pancreas syndrome); (3) duodenal atresia or stenosis; (4) malnutrition; and (5) pancreatic hypoplasia or agenesis.

The complications and sequelae of deficient pancreatic enzyme secretion are malnutrition, diarrhea, and growth failure. The degree of steatorrhea may lessen with age. Intragastric lipolysis primarily caused by lingual lipase may compensate in patients with low or absent pancreatic function. In Shwachman syndrome, the major sequela is short stature. Increased numbers of infections may result from chronic neutropenia. Neutrophil mobility is also impaired in many patients. In addition, an increased incidence of leukemia has been noted in these patients.

Pancreatic enzyme and fat-soluble vitamin replacement are required therapy in most patients. The prognosis appears to be good for those able to survive the increased number of bacterial infections early in life and those patients without severe associated defects.

Boocock GR et al: Mutations in SBDS are associated with Shwachman-Diamond syndrome. Nat Genet 2003;33:97 [PMID: 12496757].

Durie PR: Pancreatic aspects of cystic fibrosis and other inherited causes of pancreatic dysfunction. Med Clin North Am 2000; 84:609 [PMID: 10872418].

Rothbaum R et al: Shwachman–Diamond syndrome: Report from an international conference. J Pediatr 2002;141:266 [PMID: 12183725].

Sarles J et al: Pancreatic function and congenital duodenal abnormalities. J Pediatr Gastroenterol Nutr 1993;16:284 [PMID: 8492257].

Seneca S et al: Pearson marrow pancreas syndrome: A molecular study and clinical management. Clin Genet 1997;51:338 [PMID: 9212183].

Wright NM et al: Permanent neonatal diabetes mellitus and pancreatic exocrine insufficiency resulting from congenital pancreatic agenesis. Am J Dis Child 1993;147:607 [PMID: 8506821].

ISOLATED EXOCRINE PANCREATIC ENZYME DEFECT

Normal premature infants and most newborns produce little, if any, pancreatic amylase following meals or exogenous hormonal stimulation. This temporary physiologic insufficiency may persist for the first 3–6 months of life and be responsible for diarrhea when complex carbohydrates (cereals) are introduced into the diet.

Congenital pancreatic lipase deficiency and congenital colipase deficiency are extremely rare disorders, causing diarrhea and variable malnutrition with malabsorption of dietary fat and fat-soluble vitamins. The sweat chloride level is normal, and neutropenia is absent. Treatment is oral replacement of pancreatic enzymes and a low-fat diet or formula containing medium-chain triglycerides.

Exocrine pancreatic insufficiency of proteolytic enzymes (eg, trypsinogen, trypsin, chymotrypsin) is caused by enterokinase deficiency, a duodenal mucosal enzyme required for activation of the pancreatic proenzymes. These patients present with malnutrition associated with hypoproteinemia and edema but are free of respiratory symptoms and have a normal sweat test. They respond to pancreatic enzyme replacement therapy and feeding formulas that contain a casein hydrolysate (eg, Nutramigen, Pregestimil).

Durie PR: Pancreatic aspects of cystic fibrosis and other inherited causes of pancreatic dysfunction. Med Clin North Am 2000; 84:609 [PMID: 10872418].

Mann NS, Mann SK: Enterokinase. Proc Soc Exp Biol Med 1994;206:114 [PMID: 8208733].

McKenna LL: Pancreatic disorders in the newborn. Neonatal Netw 2000;19:13 [PMID: 11949098].

Stormon MO, Durie PR: Pathophysiologic basis of exocrine pancreatic dysfunction in childhood. J Pediatr Gastroenterol Nutr 2002;35:8 [PMID: 12142803].

PANCREATIC TUMORS

Pancreatic tumors, whether benign or malignant, are rare lesions. They most often arise from ductal or acinar epithelium (malignant adenocarcinoma) or from islet (endocrine) components within the gland, such as the benign insulinoma (adenoma) derived from β cells. Other pancreatic tumors also originate from these pluripotent endocrine cells (gastrinoma, VIPoma, glucagonoma). These malignant lesions produce diverse symptoms, because they release biologically active polypeptides from this ectopic

Table 21–10. Pancreatic tumors.

	Age	Major Findings	Diagnosis	Treatment	Associated Conditions
Insulinoma	Any age	Hypoglycemia, seizures; high serum insulin; weight gain; abdominal pain and mass infrequent	CT scan, MRI, EUS, SRS	Surgery, diazoxide, SSTA	
Adenocarcinoma	Any age	Epigastric pain, mass weight loss, anemia, biliary obstruction	Ultrasound, CT scan, MRI, EUS	Surgery	Chronic pancreatitis
Gastrinoma	Older than age 5–8 years	Male sex, gastric hypersecretion, peptic symptoms, multiple ulcers, gastrointestinal bleeding, anemia, diarrhea	Elevated fasting gastrin and postsecretin suppression test (> 300 pg/mL), CT scan, MRI, EUS, SRS, laparotomy	PPI, surgical resection, total gastrectomy, SSTA	Zollinger-Ellison syndrome, multiple endocrine neoplasia syndrome type I, neurofibromatosis
VIPoma	Any age	Secretory diarrhea, hypokalemia, hypochlorhydria, weight loss, flushing	Elevated VIP levels; sometimes, elevated serum gastrin and pancreatic polypeptide; SRS	Surgery, SSTA, IV fluids	
Glucagonoma	Older patients	Diabetes, necrolytic rash, diarrhea, anemia, thrombotic events, depression	Elevated glucagon, gastrin, VIP, MRI, SRS	Surgery, SSTA	

CT, computed tomography; EUS, endoscopic ultrasound; MRI, magnetic resonance imaging; PPI, proton pump inhibitor; SRS, somatostatin-receptor scintigraphy; SSTA, somatostatin analog; VIP, vasoactive intestinal polypeptide.

location. The clinical features of these tumors are summarized in Table 21–10. The differential diagnosis of these pancreatic tumors includes Wilms tumor, neuroblastoma, and malignant lymphoma. In older children, endoscopic ultrasonography can aid in localizing these tumors.

Jaksic T et al: A 20-year review of pediatric pancreatic tumors. J Pediatr Surg 1992;27:1315 [PMID: 1328584].

Johnson PRV, Spitz L: Cysts and tumors of the pancreas. Semin Pediatr Surg 2000;9:209 [PMID 11112838].

Vossen S et al: Therapeutic management of rare malignant pancreatic tumors in children. World J Surg 1998;22:879 [PMID: 9673563].

REFERENCES

Suchy FJ et al (editors): *Liver Disease in Children,* 2nd ed. Lippincott, Williams & Wilkins, 2001.

Walker WA et al (editors): *Pediatric Gastrointestinal Disease: Pathophysiology, Diagnosis, Management,* 4th ed. BC Decker, 2004.

Wyllie R, Hyams JS (editors): *Pediatric Gastrointestinal and Liver Disease,* 3rd ed. Elsevier, 2006.

Kidney & Urinary Tract

Gary M. Lum, MD

◼ EVALUATION OF THE KIDNEY & URINARY TRACT

HISTORY

When renal disease is suspected, the history should include

1. Family history of cystic disease, hereditary nephritis, deafness, dialysis, or renal transplantation.
2. Preceding acute or chronic illnesses (eg, urinary tract infection [UTI], pharyngitis, impetigo, or endocarditis).
3. Rashes or joint pains.
4. Growth delay or failure to thrive.
5. Polyuria, polydipsia, enuresis, urinary frequency, or dysuria.
6. Documentation of hematuria, proteinuria, or discolored urine.
7. Pain (abdominal, costovertebral angle, or flank) or trauma.
8. Sudden weight gain or edema.
9. Drug or toxin exposure.

For the newborn or small infant, the physician should obtain birth history and information regarding prenatal ultrasonographic studies, birth asphyxia, Apgar scores, oligohydramnios, dysmorphic features, abdominal masses, voiding patterns, anomalous development, and umbilical artery catheterization.

PHYSICAL EXAMINATION

Important aspects of the physical examination include the height, weight, skin lesions (café-au-lait or ash leaf spots), pallor, edema, or skeletal deformities. Anomalies of the ears, eyes, or external genitalia may be associated with renal disease. The blood pressure should be measured in a quiet setting. The cuff should cover two-thirds of the child's upper arm, and peripheral pulses should be noted. The abdomen should be palpated, with attention to the kidneys, abdominal masses, mus-

culature, and the presence of ascites. An ultrasonic device is useful for measurements in infants.

LABORATORY EVALUATION OF RENAL FUNCTION

Urinalysis

Commercially available dipsticks can be used to screen for the presence of red blood cells, hemoglobin, leukocytes, nitrites, and protein and to approximate pH. Positive results for blood should always be confirmed by microscopy, as should any suspicion of crystalluria. Significant proteinuria (> 150 mg/dL) detected by dipstick should be confirmed by quantitation either with a 24-hour collection or by the protein/creatinine ratio (see following section) of a random specimen.

Serum Analysis

The standard indicators of renal function are serum levels of urea nitrogen and creatinine; their ratio is normally about 10:1. This ratio may increase when renal perfusion or urine flow is decreased, as in urinary tract obstruction or dehydration. Because serum urea nitrogen levels are more affected by these and other factors (eg, nitrogen intake, catabolism, use of corticosteroids) than are creatinine levels, the most reliable single indicator of glomerular function is the serum level of creatinine. For example, serum creatinine increasing from 0.5 mg/dL to 1.0 mg/dL represents a 50% decrease in glomerular filtration rate. Small children should have serum creatinine levels well under 0.8 mg/dL, and only larger adolescents should have levels exceeding 1 mg/dL. Less precise but nonetheless important indicators of the possible presence of renal disease are abnormalities of serum electrolytes, pH, calcium, phosphorus, magnesium, albumin, or complement.

Measurement of Glomerular Filtration Rate

The endogenous creatinine clearance (C_{cr}) in milliliters per minute estimates the glomerular filtration rate (GFR). A 24-hour urine collection is usually obtained; however, in small children from whom collection is difficult, a 12-hour daytime specimen, collected when urine flow rate is greatest, is acceptable. The procedure for collecting a timed urine specimen should be explained carefully so that the parent or patient understands fully the rationale of (1) first emptying the bladder (discarding that urine) and noting the time; and (2) putting all urine subsequently voided into the collection receptacle, including the last void, 12 or 24 hours later. Reliability of the 24-hour collection can be checked by measuring the total 24-hour creatinine excretion in the specimen. Total daily creatinine excretion (creatinine index) should be in the range of 14–20 mg/kg. Creatinine indices on either side of this range suggest collections that were either inadequate or excessive. Calculation by the following formula requires measurements of plasma creatinine (P_{cr}) in mg/mL, urine creatinine (U_{cr}) in mg/mL, and urine volume (V) expressed as mL/min:

$$C_{Cr} = \frac{U_{Cr}\, V}{P_{Cr}}$$

Creatinine is a reflection of body muscle mass. Because accepted ranges of normal C_{cr} are based on adult parameters, correction for size is needed to determine normal ranges in children. Clearance is corrected to a standard body surface area of 1.73 m^2 in the formula:

$$\text{"Corrected" } C_{Cr} = \frac{\text{Patient's } C_{Cr} \times 1.73 \text{ m}^2}{\text{Patient's body surface area}}$$

Although 80–125 mL/min/1.73 m^2 is the normal range for C_{cr}, estimates at the lower end of this range may indicate problems.

A simple and tested formula for quick approximation of C_{cr} incorporates use of the plasma creatinine level and the child's length in centimeters:

$$C_{Cr}\ (\text{mL}/\text{min}/1.73\ \text{m}^2) = \frac{0.55 \times \text{Height in cm}}{P_{Cr} \text{ in mg}/\text{dL}}$$

Note: Because this formula takes into account the body surface area, further correction is not necessary. Use 0.45 × length in centimeters for newborns and for infants younger than age 1 year. This method of calculation is not meant to detract from the importance of clearance determinations, but is useful when a suspicious plasma creatinine needs to be checked.

Urine Concentrating Ability

Inability to concentrate urine is associated with polyuria, polydipsia, or enuresis and is often the first sign of chronic renal failure. The first morning void should be concen-

trated. Evaluation of other abnormalities of urinary concentration or dilution is discussed later in the sections on specific disease entities, such as diabetes insipidus.

Microhematuria or Isolated Proteinuria

In children with asymptomatic hematuria or proteinuria, the search for renal origins will yield the most results. Isolated proteinuria may reflect urologic abnormalities, benign excretion, or glomerular alterations. The presence of red cell casts suggests glomerulonephritis (GN), but the absence of casts does not rule out this disease. Anatomic abnormalities such as cystic disease may be a source of hematuria.

Benign hematuria, including benign familial hematuria, is diagnosed by exclusion. In this group are children whose hematuria is caused by asymptomatic hypercalciuria. Figure 22–1 suggests an approach to the renal work-up of hematuria. GN is discussed in more detail later in this chapter.

The association of proteinuria with hematuria is characteristic of more significant glomerular disease. Quantitation of the proteinuria is customarily accomplished by a time collection (eg, over a 24-hour period). However, an assessment of the degree of proteinuria may be made with the performance of the urine protein/creatinine ratio in a random urine sample. A protein-to-creatinine ratio of more than 0.2 is abnormal. A timed urine collection is performed as described previously for C_{cr}. In the evaluation of asymptomatic proteinuria, orthostatic or postural proteinuria should be ruled out. The protein present in urine voided on arising in the morning is compared with that in urine formed in the upright position during the rest of the day. This can be accomplished more simply by comparing the protein/creatinine ratios. If the quantitation is accomplished by separation of the "upright" and "supine" portions of a 24-hour collection, if the upright collection contains 80–100% of the entire 24-hour measured protein, and if there are no other markers of renal disease, the diagnosis of benign postural proteinuria is acceptable.

An approach to the work-up of isolated proteinuria is shown in Figure 22–2. Note that corticosteroid therapy is indicated in the algorithm because this may be initiated prior to referral. Other renal lesions with proteinuric manifestations are discussed later in this chapter.

Butani L, Kalia A: Idiopathic hypercalciuria in children—How valid are the existing diagnostic criteria? Pediatr Nephrol 2004;19:577 [PMID: 15054648].

Gordon C, Stapleton FB: Hematuria in adolescents. Adolesc Med Clin 2005;16:229 [PMID: 15844394].

Morgenstern BZ et al: Validity of protein-osmolality versus protein-creatinine ratios in the estimation of quantitative proteinuria from random samples of urine in children. Am J Kidney Dis 2003;41:760 [PMID:12666062].

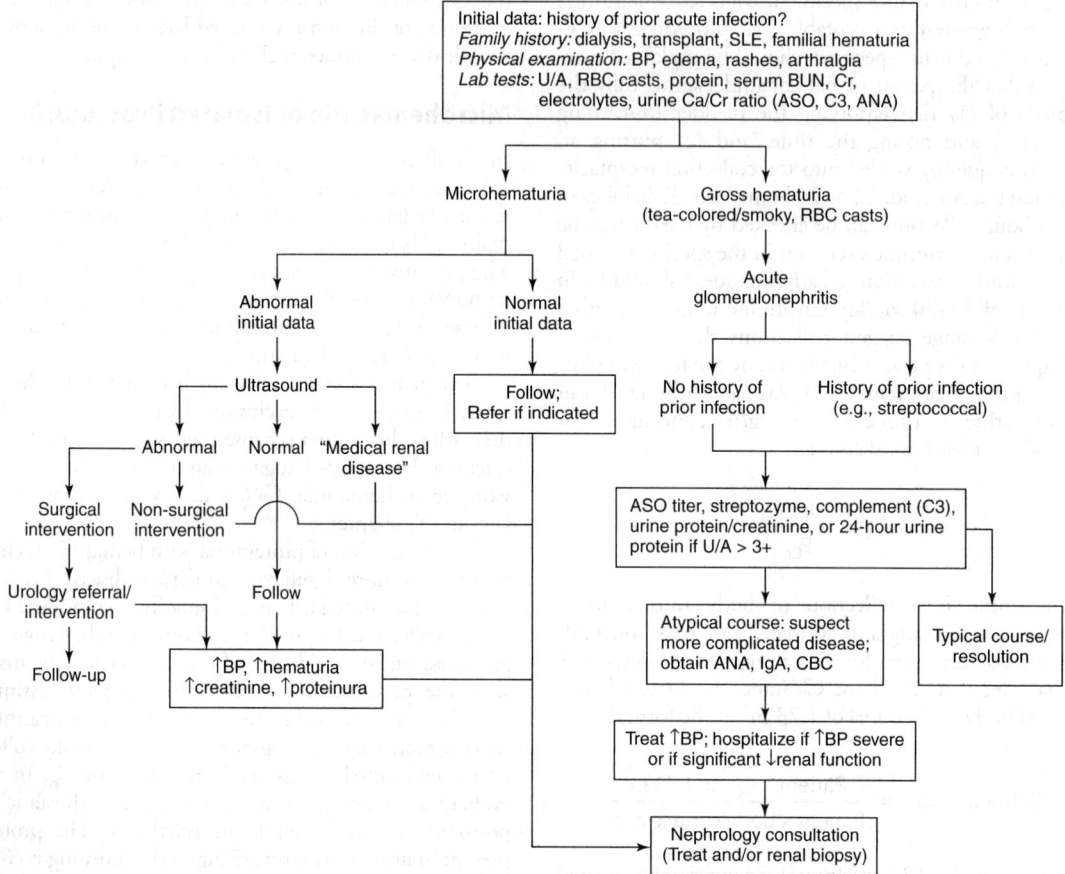

Figure 22–1. Approach to the renal work-up of hematuria. (Exclude UTI, lithiasis, trauma, bleeding disorders, sickle cell disease.) ANA, antinuclear antibody; ASO, antistreptolysin antibody; BP, blood pressure; BUN, blood urea nitrogen; C3, complement; Ca, calcium; Cr, creatinine; GN, glomerulonephritis; IgA, immunoglobulin A; PSGN, poststreptococcal glomerulonephritis; RBC, red blood cell; SLE, systemic lupus erythematosus; U/A, urinalysis.

Special Tests of Renal Function

Measurements of urinary sodium, creatinine, and osmolality are useful in differentiating prerenal from renal causes of renal insufficiency, such as acute tubular necrosis. The physiologic response to decreased renal perfusion is decreased urinary output, increased urine osmolality, increased urinary solutes (eg, creatinine), and decreased urinary sodium (usually < 20 mEq/L). Prolonged underperfusion results in varying increases in the serum creatinine and blood urea nitrogen (BUN) concentrations, prompting the need to differentiate between this state and acute tubular necrosis (see Acute Renal Failure section).

The presence of certain substances in urine may suggest tubular dysfunction. For example, urine glucose should be less than 5 mg/dL. Hyperphosphaturia occurs

with significant tubular abnormalities (eg, Fanconi syndrome). Measurement of the phosphate concentration of a 24-hour urine specimen and evaluation of tubular reabsorption of phosphorus (TRP) will help document renal tubular diseases as well as hyperparathyroid states. TRP (expressed as percentage of reabsorption) is calculated as follows:

$$TRP = 100 \left[1 - \frac{S_{Cr} \times U_{PO4}}{S_{PO_4} \times U_{Cr}} \right]$$

where S_{cr} = serum creatinine; U_{cr} = urine creatinine; S_{PO_4} = serum phosphate; and U_{PO_4} = urine phosphate. All values for creatinine and phosphate are expressed in milligrams per deciliter for purposes of calculation. A

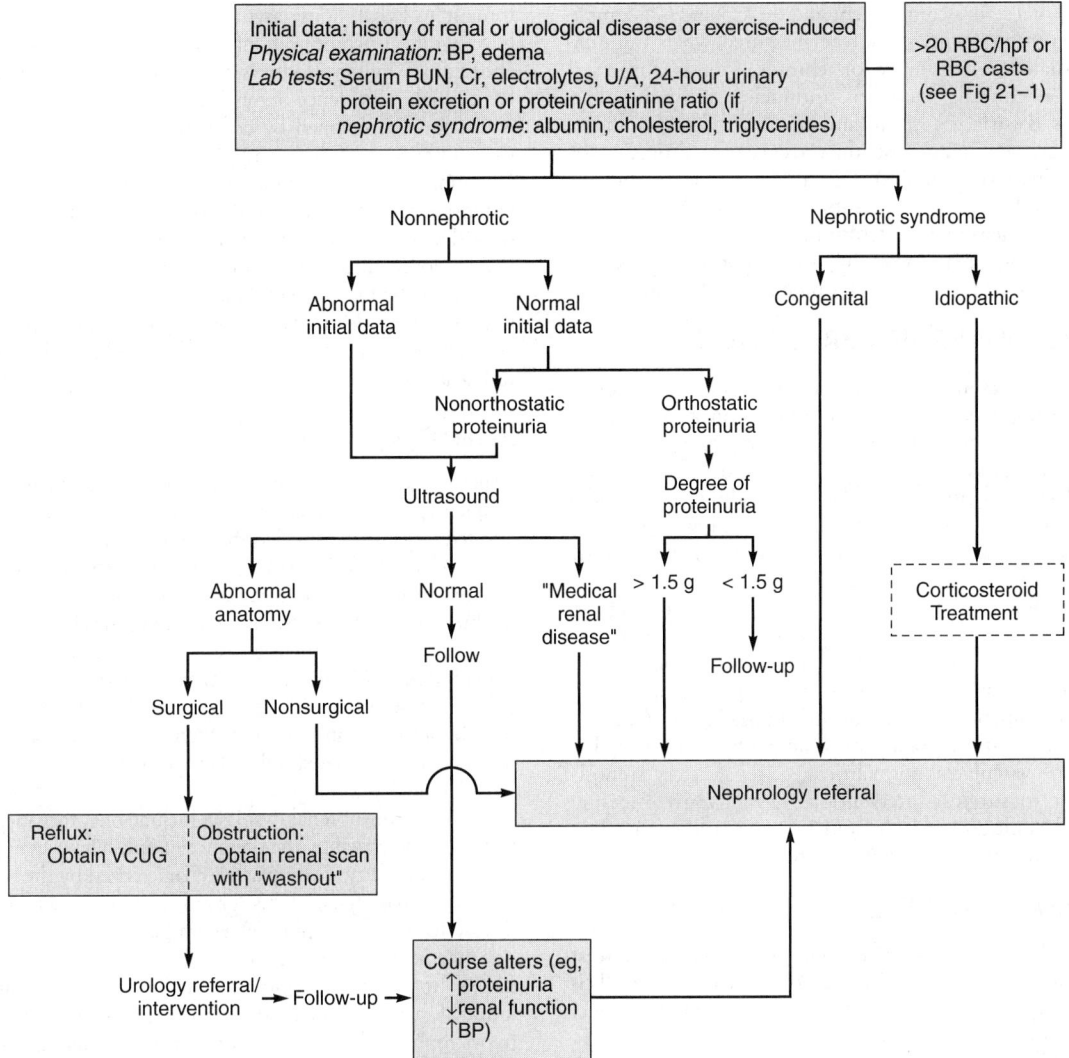

Figure 22–2. Approach to the work-up of isolated proteinuria. BP, blood pressure; Cr, creatinine; hpf, high-power field; RBC, red blood cell; U/A, urinalysis; VCUG, voiding cystourethrogram. *Complement is depressed in acute poststreptococcal glomerulonephritis, chronic glomerulonephritis, and lupus. Will normalize within a month in poststreptococcal glomerulonephritis.

TRP value of 80% or more is considered normal, although it depends somewhat on the value of S_{PO_4}.

The urinary excretion of amino acids in generalized tubular disease reflects a quantitative increase rather than a qualitative change. Diseases affecting proximal tubular reabsorption of bicarbonate—including isolated renal tubular acidosis (RTA), Fanconi syndrome (which occurs in diseases such as cystinosis), and chronic renal failure—are discussed later in the chapter.

LABORATORY EVALUATION OF IMMUNOLOGIC FUNCTION

Many parenchymal renal diseases are thought to have immune causation, although the mechanisms are largely unknown. Examples include (1) deposition of circulating antigen–antibody complexes that are directly injurious or incite injurious responses and (2) formation of antibody directed against the glomerular basement membrane (rare in children).

Total serum complement and the C3 and C4 complement components should be measured when immune-mediated renal injury or chronic GN is suspected. Where clinically indicated, antinuclear antibodies, hepatitis B surface antigen, and rheumatoid factor should be obtained. In rare cases the presence of cold-precipitable proteins (cryoglobulins), C3 "nephritic" factor, or anti-glomerular basement membrane (anti-GBM) antibody may be helpful in determining a specific diagnosis. At some point in the work-up, the diagnosis may be supported or confirmed by determining renal histology.

RADIOGRAPHIC EVALUATION

Renal ultrasonography is a useful noninvasive tool for evaluating renal parenchymal disease, urinary tract abnormalities, or renal blood flow. Excretory urography is used to assess the anatomy and function of the kidney, collecting system, and bladder. Radioisotope studies provide valuable information concerning renal anatomy, blood flow, and integrity and function of the glomerular, tubular, and collecting systems.

Evaluation of the lower urinary tract (voiding cystourethrography or cystoscopy) is indicated when vesicoureteral reflux or bladder outlet obstruction is suspected. Cystoscopy is rarely useful in the evaluation of asymptomatic hematuria or proteinuria in children.

Renal arteriography or venography is indicated to define vascular abnormalities (eg, renal artery stenosis) prior to surgical intervention. Less invasive measures such as ultrasonography and Doppler studies can demonstrate renal blood flow or thromboses.

RENAL BIOPSY

Histologic information is valuable for diagnosis, treatment, and prognosis. Satisfactory evaluation of renal tissue requires examination by light, immunofluorescence, and electron microscopy.

When a biopsy is anticipated, a pediatric nephrologist should be consulted. In children, percutaneous renal biopsy with a biopsy needle is an acceptable low-risk procedure—avoiding the risks of general anesthesia—when performed by an experienced physician. A surgeon should perform the biopsy procedure if operative exposure of the kidney is necessary, if an increased risk factor (eg, bleeding disorder) is present, or if a "wedge" biopsy is preferred.

■ CONGENITAL ANOMALIES OF THE URINARY TRACT

RENAL PARENCHYMAL ANOMALIES

About 10% of children have congenital anomalies of the genitourinary tract, which range in severity from asymp-

tomatic to lethal. Some asymptomatic abnormalities may have significant complications. For example, patients with "horseshoe" kidney (kidneys fused in their lower poles) have a higher incidence of renal calculi. Unilateral agenesis is usually accompanied by compensatory hypertrophy of the contralateral kidney and thus should be compatible with normal renal function. Supernumerary and ectopic kidneys are usually of no significance. Abnormal genitourinary development can result in varying degrees of renal maldevelopment and function, of which complete renal agenesis is the most severe. When the agenesis is bilateral, it causes early death. Severe oligohydramnios is present and can result in pulmonary hypoplasia and peculiar (Potter) facies.

Renal Dysgenesis

Renal dysgenesis represents a spectrum of anomalies. In simple hypoplasia, which may be unilateral or bilateral, the affected organs are smaller than normal. In the various forms of dysplasia, immature, undifferentiated renal tissue persists. In some of the dysplasias, the number of normal nephrons is insufficient to sustain life once the child reaches a critical body size. Such lack of renal tissue may not be readily discernible in the newborn period because the infant's urine production, though poor in concentration, may be adequate in volume. Often, the search for renal insufficiency is initiated only when growth fails or chronic renal failure develops.

Other forms of renal dysplasia include oligomeganephronia (characterized by the presence of only a few large glomeruli) and the cystic dysplasias (characterized by the presence of renal cysts). This group includes microcystic disease (congenital nephrosis). A simple cyst within a kidney may be clinically unimportant because it does not predispose to progressive polycystic development. An entire kidney lost to multicystic development with concomitant hypertrophy and normal function of the contralateral side may also be of little clinical consequence. Nonetheless, even a simple cyst could pose problems if it becomes a site for lithiasis, infection, or hematuria.

Polycystic Kidney Disease

Autosomal recessive polycystic kidney disease is increasingly diagnosed by prenatal ultrasound. In its most severe form the cystic kidneys are nonfunctional in utero, and, therefore, newborns can have Potter facies and other complications of oligohydramnios. In infancy and childhood, kidney enlargement by cysts may initially be recognized by abdominal palpation of the renal masses. Hypertension is an early problem. The rate of the progression of renal insufficiency varies, as does growth failure and other complications of chronic renal failure. Two genes (*ADPKD-1* and *ADPKD-2*) account for 80% and 10% of cases of the autosomal dominant polycystic kidney disease, respectively. Susceptibility of family members is detected by gene linkage studies. Renal ultrasound identifies cysts in about 80% of affected children by age 5 years. Children with this diagnosis need close monitoring for the development and treatment of hypertension, and their families should be offered genetic counseling. Management of end-stage renal failure is by dialysis or renal transplantation.

Gabow PA: Utility of ultrasonography in the diagnosis of autosomal dominant polycystic kidney disease in children. J Am Soc Nephrol 1997;8:105 [PMID: 9013454].

Guay-Woodford LM, Desmond RA: Autosomal recessive polycystic kidney disease: The clinical experience in North America. Pediatrics 2003;111:1072 [PMID: 12728091].

Medullary Cystic Disease (Juvenile Nephronophthisis)

Medullary cystic disease is characterized by varying sizes of cysts in the renal medulla and is associated with tubular and interstitial nephritis. Children present with renal failure and signs of tubular dysfunction (decreased concentrating ability, Fanconi syndrome). This lesion should not be confused with medullary sponge kidney (renal tubular ectasia), a frequently asymptomatic disease occurring in adults.

DISTAL URINARY TRACT ANOMALIES

Obstruction at the ureteropelvic junction may be the result of intrinsic muscle abnormalities, aberrant vessels, or fibrous bands. The lesion can cause hydronephrosis and usually presents as an abdominal mass in the newborn. Obstruction can occur in other parts of the ureter, especially at its entrance into the bladder, with resulting proximal hydroureter and hydronephrosis. Whether intrinsic or extrinsic, urinary tract obstruction should be relieved surgically as soon as possible to minimize damage to the kidneys.

Severe bladder malformations such as exstrophy are clinically obvious and provide a surgical challenge. More subtle—but urgent in terms of diagnosis—is obstruction of urine flow from vestigial posterior urethral valves. This anomaly, which occurs almost exclusively in males, usually presents as anuria or a poor voiding stream in the newborn period, with severe obstruction of urine flow. Ascites may occur, and the kidneys and bladder may be easily palpable. Surgical drainage of urine is urgently required to prevent irreversible damage.

Complex Anomalies

Prune belly syndrome is an association of urinary tract anomalies with cryptorchidism and absent abdominal musculature. Although complex anomalies, especially renal dysplasia, usually cause early death or the need for dialysis or transplantation, some patients have lived into the third decade with varying degrees of renal insufficiency. Timely urinary diversion is essential to sustain renal function.

Other complex malformations and external genital anomalies such as hypospadias are beyond the scope of this text. Overall, urologic abnormalities resulting in severe compromise and destruction of renal tissue provide therapeutic and management challenges aimed at preserving all remaining function and treating the complications of progressive chronic renal failure.

Chevalier RL: Perinatal obstructive nephropathy. Semin Perinatol 2004;28:124 [PMID: 15200251].

Mesrobian HG et al: Urologic problems of the neonate. Pediatr Clin North Am 2004;51:1051 [PMID: 15275988].

HEMATURIA & GLOMERULAR DISEASE

Children with painful hematuria should be investigated for urinary tract infection (UTI) or direct injury to the urinary tract. Dysuria commonly suggests cystitis or urethritis; back pain may support the presence of pyelonephritis; and colicky flank pain may mean the passage of a stone. Bright red blood or clots in the urine are associated with bleeding disorders, trauma, and arteriovenous malformations. Abdominal masses suggest the presence of urinary tract obstruction, cystic disease, or tumors involving the renal or perirenal structures.

Asymptomatic hematuria is a challenge because clinical and diagnostic data are required to decide whether to refer the child to a nephrologist. Figure 22–1 delineates the outpatient approach to renal hematuria. The concern regarding the differential diagnosis is the possible presence of glomerular disease.

GLOMERULONEPHRITIS

Poststreptococcal Glomerulonephritis

Acute poststreptococcal GN is the most common form of "postinfectious" GN. The epidemiologic relationship between certain strains of streptococci and GN is well recognized. Antigen–antibody complexes are formed in the bloodstream and deposited in the glomeruli where they incite glomerular inflammation and activate the complement system.

The diagnosis of poststreptococcal disease is supported by a recent history (7–14 days previously) of group A β-hemolytic streptococcal infection. If a positive culture is not available, recent infection may be supported by an elevated antistreptolysin O titer or by high titers of other antistreptococcal antibodies. Other infections can cause similar glomerular injury; thus, "postinfection GN" may be a better term for this type of acute GN. In most cases recovery is expected and usually complete within weeks. In cases when the diagnosis is in some question, or in patients whose renal function progressively deteriorates, a renal biopsy should be performed.

The clinical presentation of GN is usually gross hematuria (coffee-colored or tea-colored urine), with or without edema (eg, periorbital), which in mild cases occurs secondary to the alteration in glomerular function, resulting in sodium and water retention. Symptoms are usually nonspecific. In cases accompanied by hypertension (a common finding), headache may be present. Fever is uncommon. Severe glomerular injury (which usually occurs in severe, acute presentations of the more chronic or destructive forms of GN) may be accompanied by massive proteinuria (nephrotic syndrome), anasarca or ascites, and severe compromise of renal function.

Typical poststreptococcal GN has no specific treatment. Appropriate antibiotic therapy is indicated if an infection is still present. The disturbances in renal function and resulting hypertension may require close follow-up and management, with reduction in salt intake, treatment with diuretics, or antihypertensive drugs. In severe cases, with profound renal failure, hemodialysis or peritoneal dialysis may be necessary; corticosteroids may also be administered in an attempt to influence the course of the GN.

The acute abnormalities generally resolve in 2–3 weeks. Serum complement (C3) may be normal as early as 3 days or as late as 30 days after onset. The complement consuming glomerulonephritides also include membranoproliferative GN (chronic GN with persistent complement depression) and lupus GN. (See Chapter 26.) Although microscopic hematuria may persist for as long as a year, most children recover completely (85%). Persistent deterioration in renal function, urinary abnormalities beyond 18 months, persistent hypocomplementemia, and nephrotic syndrome are ominous signs. If any one of these is present, a renal biopsy is indicated.

IgA Nephropathy

When asymptomatic gross hematuria appears to accompany a minor acute febrile illness or other stressful occurrence, the diagnosis of IgA nephropathy may be entertained. In contrast to postinfection GN, with IgA nephropathy there is no evidence of prior infection, complement is not depressed, and serum immunoglobin A is elevated in 50% of all cases. Often there are no associated clinical factors. The gross hematuria resolves within days, and there are no serious sequelae in 85% of cases of IgA nephropathy. Treatment is not indi-

cated, and the prognosis is good in most cases. Prognosis is guarded, however, if severe proteinuria, hypertension, or renal insufficiency is present or ensues. In such instances, although no treatment is universally accepted, corticosteroids and other immunosuppressive drugs are used. Omega-3 fatty acids present in fish oils are thought to be helpful.

Donadio JV, Grande JP: The role of fish oil/omega-3 fatty acids in the treatment of IgA nephropathy. Semin Nephrol 2004;24: 225 [PMID: 15156528].

Yoshikawa N et al: Pathophysiology and treatment of IgA nephropathy in children. Pediatr Nephrol 2001;16:446 [PMID: 11405121].

Henoch–Schönlein Purpura

The diagnosis of Henoch–Schönlein purpura rests on the presence of a typical maculopapular rash found primarily, but not exclusively, on the dorsal surfaces of lower extremities and buttocks. Most children have abdominal pain and bloody diarrhea. Joint pain is common, and, depending on the extent of renal involvement, hypertension may be present. Joint and abdominal pain responds to treatment with corticosteroids. Renal involvement ranges from mild GN with microhematuria to severe GN and varying degrees of renal insufficiency. GN with massive proteinuria and renal insufficiency carries the worst prognosis. Twenty percent of such cases result in end-stage renal failure. There is no universally accepted treatment, but corticosteroids are often administered.

Delos Santos NM, Wyatt RJ. Pediatric IgA nephropathies: Clinical aspects and therapeutic approaches. Semin Nephrol 2004; 24:269 [PMID: 15156531].

Membranoproliferative Glomerulonephritis

The most common "chronic" form of GN occurring in children is membranoproliferative GN. The diagnosis is established from the histologic appearance of the glomeruli. The discussion of the various types of this form of GN is complex. Clinically, type II carries the worse prognosis, as end-stage renal failure develops in most cases. Type I more often responds to treatment with corticosteroids. C3 is depressed (in both types) and may be useful as a marker of response to treatment.

The various types of GN have similar manifestations. Table 22–1 lists the most commonly encountered entities in the differential diagnosis of GN in childhood and their clinical and histopathologic descriptions. Severe glomerular histopathologic and clinical entities, such as anti-GBM antibody disease (Goodpasture syndrome), Wegener granulomatosis, and idiopathic, rapidly pro-

Table 22–1. Glomerular diseases encountered in childhood.

Entity	Clinical Course	Prognosis
Postinfection glomerulonephritis. Onset occurs 10–14 days after acute illness, commonly streptococcal. Characteristics include acute onset, tea-colored urine, mild to severe renal insufficiency, and edema.	Acute phase is usually over in 2 wk. There is complete resolution in 95% of cases. Severity of renal failure and hypertension varies. Microhematuria may persist to 18 mo. Hypocomplementemia resolves in 1–30 d.	Excellent. Chronic disease is rare. Severe proteinuria, atypical presentation or course, or persistent hypocomplementemia suggest another entity.
Membranoproliferative glomerulonephritis. Presentation ranges from mild microhematuria to acute GN syndrome. Diagnosis is made by renal biopsy. Etiology is unknown. Type I and type II are most common. Lesion is chronic.	Course can be mild to severe (rapid deterioration in renal function); may mimic postinfection GN. Proteinuria can be severe. Complement depression is intermittent to persistent. Hypertension is usually significant.	Type I may respond to corticosteroids. Type II (dense deposit disease) is less treatable; function decrease varies from immediate to as long as 15 y in 30–50% of untreated cases.
IgA nephropathy. Classic presentation consists of asymptomatic gross hematuria during acute unrelated illness, with microhematuria between episodes. There are occasional instances of acute GN syndrome. Etiology is unknown. Diagnosis is made by biopsy.	90% of cases resolve in 1–5 y. Gross hematuric episodes resolve with recovery from acute illness. Severity of renal insufficiency and hypertension varies. Proteinuria occurs in more severe, atypical cases.	Generally good. Small percentage develop chronic renal failure. Proteinuria in the nephrotic range is a poor sign. There is no universally accepted medication. (Corticosteroids may be useful in severe cases.)
Henoch–Schönlein purpura glomerulonephritis. Degree of renal involvement varies. Asymptomatic microhematuria is most common, but GN syndrome can occur. Renal biopsy is recommended in severe cases; it can provide prognostic information.	Presentation varies with severity of renal lesion. In rare cases, may progress rapidly to serious renal failure. Hypertension varies. Proteinuria in the nephrotic range and severe decline in function can occur.	Overall, prognosis is good. Patients presenting with greater than 50% reduction in function or proteinuria exceeding 1 g/ 24 h may develop chronic renal failure. Severity of renal biopsy picture can best guide approach in such cases. There is no universally accepted medication.
Glomerulonephritis of systemic lupus erythematosus (SLE). Microhematuria and proteinuria are rarely first signs of this systemic disease. Renal involvement varies. GN often causes the most concern.	Renal involvement is mild to severe. Clinical complexity depends on degree of renal insufficiency and other systems involved. Hypertension is significant. Manifestations of the severity of the renal lesion guide therapeutic intervention.	Renal involvement accounts for most significant morbidity in SLE. Control of hypertension affects renal prognosis. Medication is guided by symptoms, serology, and renal lesion. End-stage renal failure can occur.
Hereditary glomerulonephritis (eg, Alport syndrome). Transmission is autosomal-dominant/X-linked, with family history marked by end-stage renal failure, especially in young males. Deafness and eye abnormalities are associated.	There is no acute syndrome. Females are generally less affected but are carriers. Hypertension and increasing proteinuria occur with advancing renal failure. There is no known treatment.	Progressive proteinuria and hypertension occur early, with gradual decline in renal function in those most severely affected. Disease progresses to end-stage renal failure in most males.

GN, glomerulonephritis.

gressive GN, may be considered in the differential diagnosis of acute GN. But these disorders are exceedingly rare in children.

ACUTE INTERSTITIAL NEPHRITIS

Acute interstitial nephritis is characterized by diffuse or focal inflammation and edema of the renal interstitium and secondary involvement of the tubules. It seems to be related most often to drugs (eg, β-lactam–containing antibiotics, such as methicillin).

Fever, rigor, abdominal or flank pain, and rashes may occur in drug-associated cases. Urinalysis should reveal leukocyturia and hematuria. Hansel staining of the urinary sediment often demonstrates eosinophils. The inflammation can cause significant deterioration of renal function. If the diagnosis is unclear because of the absence of drug or toxin exposure history or the absence of eosinophils in the urine, a renal biopsy may be performed to demonstrate the characteristic tubular and interstitial inflammation. Immediate identification and removal of the causative agent is imperative and may be all that is necessary. Treatment with corticosteroids is helpful in cases with progressive renal insufficiency or nephrotic syndrome. Severe renal failure requires supportive dialysis.

PROTEINURIA & RENAL DISEASE

Urine is rarely completely protein-free, but the average excretion is well below 150 mg/24 h. Small increases in urinary protein can accompany febrile illnesses or exertion and in some cases occur while in the upright posture (discussed earlier).

An algorithm for investigation of isolated proteinuria is presented in Figure 22–2. In idiopathic nephrotic syndrome without associated features of GN, treatment with corticosteroids may be initiated as described later in this chapter. Nephrologic advice or follow-up should be sought, especially in difficult or frequently relapsing cases.

CONGENITAL NEPHROSIS

Congenital nephrosis is a rare autosomal recessive disorder. The kidneys are pale and large and may show microcystic dilations (microcystic disease) of the proximal tubules and glomerular abnormalities. The latter consist of proliferation, crescent formation, and thickening of capillary walls. The pathogenesis is not well understood.

Infants with congenital nephrosis commonly have low birth weight, a large placenta, wide cranial sutures, and delayed ossification. Mild edema may be seen after the first few weeks of life. Anasarca follows, and the abdomen can become greatly distended by ascites. Massive proteinuria associated with typical-appearing nephrotic syndrome and hyperlipidemia is the rule. Hematuria is common. If the patient lives long enough, progressive renal failure occurs. Most affected infants succumb to infections at the age of a few months.

Treatment prior to dialysis and transplantation has little to offer other than nutritional support and management of the chronic renal failure.

IDIOPATHIC NEPHROTIC SYNDROME OF CHILDHOOD (Nil Disease, Lipoid Nephrosis, Minimal Change Disease)

Nephrotic syndrome is characterized by proteinuria, hypoproteinemia, edema, and hyperlipidemia. It may occur as a result of any form of glomerular disease and may rarely be associated with a variety of extrarenal conditions. In young children, the disease usually takes the form of idiopathic nephrotic syndrome of childhood (nil disease, lipoid nephrosis, minimal change disease), which has characteristic clinical and laboratory findings, but no well-understood cause.

Clinical Findings

Affected patients are generally younger than age 6 years at the time of their first episode. Often following an influenza-like syndrome, periorbital swelling and perhaps oliguria are noticed. Within a few days, increasing edema—even anasarca—becomes evident. Other than vague malaise and occasionally abdominal pain, complaints are few. With significant "third spacing" of plasma volume, however, some children may present with hypotension. With marked edema, dyspnea due to pleural effusions may also occur.

Despite heavy proteinuria, the urine sediment is usually normal, although microscopic hematuria may be present. Plasma albumin levels are low, and lipid levels are increased. When azotemia occurs, it is usually secondary to intravascular volume depletion.

Glomerular morphology is unremarkable except for fusion of foot processes of the glomerular basement membrane. This finding, however, is nonspecific and is associated with many proteinuric states.

Complications

Infections (eg, peritonitis) sometimes occur, and pneumococci are frequently the cause. Hypercoagulability may be present, and thromboembolic phenomena are commonly reported. In cases of minimal-change disease (no significant glomerular lesions are demonstrated), hypertension can still be noted, and renal insufficiency can result from decreased renal perfusion.

Treatment & Prognosis

As soon as the diagnosis of idiopathic nephrotic syndrome is made, corticosteroid treatment should be started. Prednisone, 2 mg/kg/d (maximum, 60 mg/d), is given for 6 weeks as a single daily dose. The same dose is then administered on an alternate-day schedule for 6 weeks; thereafter, the dose is tapered gradually and discontinued over the ensuing 2 months. In following this regimen, one assumes that proteinuria has ceased. If remission is not achieved during the initial phase of corticosteroid treatment additional nephrologic consultation should be obtained. If remission is achieved, only to be followed by relapse, the treatment course may be repeated. A renal biopsy is also often considered when there is little or no response to treatment. One should take into account that the histologic findings may not alter the treatment plan, which is designed to eliminate the nephrotic syndrome regardless of underlying renal histology.

Unless the edema is symptomatic (eg, respiratory compromise due to ascites), diuretics should be used with extreme care; patients may have decreased circulating volume and are also at risk for intravenous thrombosis. Careful restoration of compromised circulating volume with intravenous albumin infusion and administration of diuretics is helpful in mobilizing edema. Infections (eg, acute peritonitis) should be treated promptly to reduce morbidity. Immunization with pneumococcal vaccine is advised.

The initial, and all subsequent responses to corticosteroids suggest a good prognosis. Failure to respond or early relapse usually heralds a prolonged series of relapses. This not only may indicate the presence of more serious nephropathy, but presents a challenge in choosing future therapy. Chlorambucil or cyclophosphamide drug therapy is predictably successful only in children who respond to corticosteroids. Patients who do not respond to corticosteroids or who relapse frequently should be referred to a pediatric nephrologist. Intravenous Solu-Medrol in more refractory cases is helpful. In some cases, when the continued usage of corticosteroids raises concerns of toxicity, concomitant treatment with either ciclosporin A or tacrolimus appears to be helpful.

Filler G: Treatment of nephrotic syndrome in children and controlled trials. Nephrol Dial Transplant 2003;18:vi75 [PMID: 12953047].

Loeffler K et al: Tacrolimus therapy in pediatric patients with treatment-resistant nephrotic syndrome. Pediatr Nephrol 2004; 19:281 [PMID: 14758528].

FOCAL GLOMERULAR SCLEROSIS

Focal glomerular sclerosis is one cause of corticosteroid-resistant or frequent relapsing nephrotic syndrome. The cause is unknown. The diagnosis is made by renal biopsy, which shows normal-appearing glomeruli as well as some partially or completely sclerosed glomeruli. The lesion has serious prognostic implications because as many as 15–20% of cases can progress to end-stage renal failure. The clinical response to corticosteroid treatment is variable. In difficult cases, cyclosporin A or tacrolimus have been used in addition to corticosteroids.

Raafat RH et al: High-dose oral cyclosporin therapy for recurrent focal segmental glomerulosclerosis in children. Am J Kidney Dis 2004;44:50 [PMID: 15211437].

MESANGIAL NEPHROPATHY
(Mesangial Glomerulonephritis)

Mesangial nephropathy is another form of corticosteroid-resistant nephrotic syndrome. The renal biopsy shows a distinct increase in the mesangial matrix of the glomeruli. Very often the expanded mesangium contains deposits of IgM demonstrable on immunofluorescent staining. The cause is unknown. Corticosteroid therapy may induce remission, but relapses are common. Choices for treating this type of nephrotic syndrome are the same as noted earlier.

MEMBRANOUS NEPHROPATHY
(Membranous Glomerulonephritis)

Although largely idiopathic in nature, membranous nephropathy can be found in association with diseases such as hepatitis B antigenemia, systemic lupus erythematosus, congenital and secondary syphilis, and renal vein thrombosis; with immunologic disorders such as autoimmune thyroiditis; and with administration of drugs such as penicillamine. The pathogenesis is unknown, but the glomerular lesion is thought to be the result of prolonged deposition of circulating antigen–antibody complexes.

The onset of membranous nephropathy may be insidious or may resemble that of idiopathic nephrotic syndrome of childhood (see preceding section). It occurs more often in older children and adults. The proteinuria of membranous nephropathy responds poorly to corticosteroid therapy, although low-dose corticosteroid therapy may reduce or delay development of chronic renal insufficiency. The diagnosis is made by renal biopsy.

■ DISEASES OF THE RENAL VESSELS

RENAL VEIN THROMBOSIS

In the newborn period, renal vein thrombosis may complicate sepsis or dehydration. It may be observed in an infant of a diabetic mother; may be associated with umbilical vein catheterization; or may result from any condition that produces a hypercoagulable state (eg, clotting factor deficiency, systemic lupus erythematosus, or thrombocytosis). Renal vein thrombosis is less common in older children and adolescents. It may develop following trauma or without any apparent predisposing factors. Spontaneous renal vein thrombosis has been associated with membranous glomerulonephropathy. Nephrotic syndrome may either cause or result from renal vein thrombosis.

Clinical Findings

Renal vein thrombosis in newborns is generally characterized by the sudden development of an abdominal mass. If the thrombosis is bilateral, oliguria may be present; urine output may be normal with a unilateral thrombus. In older children, flank pain, sometimes with a palpable mass, is a common presentation.

No single laboratory test is diagnostic of renal vein thrombosis. Hematuria usually is present; proteinuria is less constant. In the newborn, thrombocytopenia may be found, but is rare in older children. The diagnosis is made by ultrasonography and Doppler flow studies.

Treatment

Anticoagulation with heparin is the treatment of choice both in newborns and in older children. In the newborn, a course of heparin combined with treatment of the underlying problem is usually all that is required. Management in other cases is less straightforward. The tendency for recurrence and embolization has led some to recommend long-term anticoagulation. If an underlying membranous GN is suspected, biopsy should be performed.

Course & Prognosis

The mortality rate in newborns from renal vein thrombosis depends on the underlying cause. With unilateral thromboses, the prognosis for adequate renal function is good. Renal vein thrombosis may rarely recur in the same kidney or occur in the other kidney years after the original episode of thrombus formation. Extension into the vena cava, with pulmonary emboli, is possible.

RENAL ARTERIAL DISEASE

Arterial disease (eg, fibromuscular hyperplasia and congenital stenosis) is a rare cause of hypertension in children. Although there are few clinical clues to underlying arterial lesions, this should be suspected in children whose hypertension is severe, with onset at or before age 10 years, or associated with delayed visualization with nuclear scan. The diagnosis is established by renal arteriography with selective renal vein renin measurements. Some of these lesions may be approached by transluminal angioplasty or surgery (see Hypertension section), but repair may be technically impossible in many small children. Although thrombosis of renal arteries is rare, it should be considered in a patient experiencing acute onset of hypertension and hematuria in an appropriate setting (eg, in association with hyperviscosity or umbilical artery catheterization). Early diagnosis and treatment (eg, heparin) provides the best chance of reestablishing renal blood flow.

HEMOLYTIC–UREMIC SYNDROME

Hemolytic–uremic syndrome is the most common glomerular vascular cause of acute renal failure in childhood. It is usually the result of infection with Shiga-toxin–producing (also called verotoxin-producing) strains of *Shigella* or *Escherichia coli*. Ingestion of undercooked ground beef or unpasteurized foods is a common source. There are many serotypes, but the most common pathogen in the United States is *E coli* 0157:H7. Bloody diarrhea is the usual presenting complaint, followed by hemolysis and renal failure. Circulating verotoxin causes endothelial damage, which leads to platelet deposition, microvascular occlusion with subsequent hemolysis, and thrombocytopenia. Similar microvascular endothelial activation may also be triggered by some drugs (eg, cyclosporin A); by viruses (human immunodeficiency virus); and by pneumococcal infections, in which bacterial neuraminidase exposes the Thomsen–Friedenreich antigen on red cells, platelets, and endothelial cells, thereby causing platelet aggregation, endothelial damage, and hemolysis. Rare cases are caused by predisposing genetic factors (eg, congenitally depressed C3 complement and factor H deficiency).

Clinical Findings

The epidemic form begins with a prodrome of abdominal pain, diarrhea, and vomiting. Oliguria, pallor, and bleeding manifestations, principally gastrointestinal, occur next. Hypertension and seizures develop in some children—especially those who develop severe renal failure and fluid overload. There may also be significant endothelial involvement in the central nervous system (CNS).

Anemia is profound, and red blood cell fragments are seen on blood smears. A high reticulocyte count confirms the hemolytic nature of the anemia, but may not be noted in the presence of renal failure. Thrombocytopenia is profound, but other coagulation abnormalities are less consistent. Serum fibrin split products are often present, but fulminant disseminated intravascular coagulation is rare. Hematuria and proteinuria are often present. The serum complement level is normal except in those cases related to congenital predisposition.

Complications

These usually result from renal failure. Neurologic problems, particularly seizures, may result from electrolyte abnormalities such as hyponatremia, hypertension, or from CNS vascular disease. Severe bleeding, transfusion requirements, and hospital-acquired infections must be anticipated.

Treatment

Meticulous attention to fluid and electrolyte status is crucial. The use of antimotility agents and antibiotics is believed to worsen the disease. Antibiotics may up-regulate and cause the release of large amounts of bacterial Shiga toxin. Timely dialysis improves the prognosis. Since prostacyclin-stimulating factor, a potent inhibitor of platelet aggregation, may be absent in some cases, plasma infusion or plasmapheresis has been advocated in severe cases (generally in those cases with severe CNS involvement). Platelet inhibitors have also been tried, but the results have not been impressive, especially late in the disease. Nonetheless, using a platelet inhibitor early in the disease in an attempt to halt platelet consumption and microvascular occlusion may obviate the need for platelet transfusions and reduce the progression of renal failure. Red cell and platelet transfusions may be necessary. Although the risk of volume overload is significant, this can be minimized by dialysis. Erythropoietin (epoetin alfa) treatment may reduce red cell transfusion needs. Although no therapy is universally accepted, strict control of hypertension and nutrition and the timely use of dialysis reduce morbidity and mortality. If renal failure is "nonoliguric," and output is sufficient to ensure against fluid overload and electrolyte abnormalities, management of renal failure without dialysis is possible.

Course & Prognosis

Most commonly, children recover from the acute episode within 2–3 weeks. Some residual renal disease (including hypertension) occurs in about 30%, and end-stage renal failure occurs in about 15%. Thus follow-up of children recovering from hemolytic–uremic syndrome should include serial determinations of renal function for 1–2 years and meticulous attention to blood pressure for 5 years. Mortality (about 3–5%) is most likely in the early phase, primarily resulting from CNS complications.

Ault BH: Factor H and the pathogenesis of renal diseases. Pediatr Nephrol 2000;14:1045 [PMID: 10975323].

Corrigan JJ Jr, Boineau FG: Hemolytic uremic syndrome. Pediatr Rev 2001;22:365 [PMID: 11691946].

▇ RENAL FAILURE

ACUTE RENAL FAILURE

Acute renal failure is the sudden inability to excrete urine of sufficient quantity or adequate composition to maintain body fluid homeostasis. The most common cause in children is dehydration. However, encountering signs of acute renal insufficiency in a hospitalized patient raises many other possibilities: impaired renal perfusion or renal ischemia, acute renal disease, renal vascular compromise,

acute tubular necrosis, or obstructive uropathy. Table 22–2 lists such prerenal, renal, and postrenal causes.

Clinical Findings

The hallmark of early renal failure is oliguria. Although an exact etiologic diagnosis may be unclear at the onset, classifying the oliguria as outlined in Table 22–2 is helpful in determining if any immediately reversible cause is present.

If the cause of elevation in serum BUN and creatinine or oliguria is unclear, entities that can be quickly addressed and corrected (eg, volume depletion) should be considered first. Once normal renal perfusion is ensured and no clinical evidence for de novo renal disease is present, a diagnosis of acute tubular necrosis (vasomotor nephropathy, ischemic injury) may be entertained.

A. PRERENAL CAUSES

The most common cause of decreased renal function in children is compromised renal perfusion. It is usually

Table 22–2. Classification of renal failure.

Prerenal
  Dehydration due to gastroenteritis, malnutrition, or diarrhea
  Hemorrhage, aortic or renal vessel injury, trauma, cardiac disease and/or surgery, renal arterial thrombosis
  Diabetic acidosis
  Hypovolemia associated with capillary leak or nephrotic syndrome
  Shock
  Heart failure
Renal
  Hemolytic-uremic syndrome
  Acute glomerulonephritis
  Prolonged renal hypoperfusion
  Nephrotoxins
  Acute tubular necrosis or vascular nephropathy
  Renal (cortical) necrosis
  Intravascular coagulation—septic shock, hemorrhage
  Diseases of renal vessels
  Iatrogenic disorders
  Severe infections
  Drowning, especially fresh water
  Crystalluria: sulfonamide or uric acid
  Hyperuricacidemia from cancer treatment
  Hepatic failure
Postrenal
  Obstruction due to tumor, hematoma, posterior urethral valves, ureteropelvic junction stricture, ureterovesical junction stricture, ureterocele
  Stones
  Trauma to a solitary kidney or collecting system
  Renal vein thrombosis

Table 22-3. Urine studies.

Prerenal Failure	Acute Tubular Necrosis
Urine osmolality 50 mOsm/kg greater than plasma osmolality	Urine osmolality equal to or less than plasma osmolality
Urine sodium < 10 mEq/L	Urinary sodium > 20 mEq/L
Ratio of urine creatinine to plasma creatinine > 14:1	Ratio of urine creatinine to plasma creatinine < 14:1
Specific gravity > 1.020	Specific gravity 1.012–1.018

secondary to dehydration, although abnormalities of renal vasculature and poor cardiac performance may also be considered. Table 22–3 lists the urinary indices helpful in distinguishing these "prerenal" conditions from true renal parenchymal insult, such as in acute tubular necrosis.

B. RENAL CAUSES

Causes of renal failure intrinsic to the kidney include acute glomerulonephritides, hemolytic–uremic syndrome, acute interstitial nephritis, and nephrotoxic injury. The diagnosis of acute tubular necrosis (vasomotor nephropathy)—which is reserved for those cases in which renal ischemic insult is believed to be the likely cause—should be considered when correction of prerenal or postrenal problems does not improve renal function and there is no evidence of de novo renal disease.

C. POSTRENAL CAUSES

Postrenal failure, usually found in newborns with urologic anatomic abnormalities, is accompanied by varying degrees of renal insufficiency. The approach to the problem in the very young is addressed earlier in the chapter, but one should always keep in mind the possibility of acute urinary tract obstruction in acute renal failure, especially in the setting of anuria of acute onset.

Complications

The clinical severity of the complications depends on the degree of renal functional impairment and oliguria. Common complications include (1) fluid overload (hypertension, congestive heart failure, pulmonary edema), (2) electrolyte disturbances (hyperkalemia), (3) metabolic acidosis, (4) hyperphosphatemia, and (5) uremia.

Treatment

An indwelling bladder catheter is inserted to ascertain urine output. If urine volume is insignificant and renal failure is established, the catheter should be removed to minimize infection risks. Prerenal or postrenal factors should be excluded or rectified, and normal circulating volume established and maintained with appropriate fluids. Strict measurements of input and output must be maintained, and input adjusted as reduction in output dictates. The patient's response is assessed by physical examination and measuring urinary output. Measurement of central venous pressure may be indicated. Increasing urine output with diuretics, such as furosemide (1–5 mg/kg, per dose, intravenously, maximum of 200 mg), can be attempted. The effective dose will depend on the amount of functional compromise (if < 50% function, initiate attempt at diuresis with maximum dose). If a response does not occur within 1 hour (ie, the urine output remains low [< 0.5 mL/kg/h]), the furosemide dose, if not already at maximum, should be increased up to 5 mg/kg. In some cases the addition of a long-acting thiazide diuretic, such as metolazone, may work. If no diuresis occurs with maximum dosing, further administration of diuretics should cease.

If these maneuvers stimulate some urine flow but biochemical evidence of acute renal failure persists, the resulting nonoliguric acute renal failure should be more manageable. Fluid overload and dialysis may be averted. However, if the medications and nutrients required exceed the urinary output, dialysis is indicated. Institution of dialysis before the early complications of acute renal failure develop is likely to improve clinical management and outcome. It is important to adjust medication dosage according to the degree of renal function.

Acute Dialysis

A. INDICATIONS FOR DIALYSIS

Immediate indications for dialysis are (1) severe hyperkalemia; (2) unrelenting metabolic acidosis (usually in a situation where fluid overload prevents sodium bicarbonate administration); (3) fluid overload with or without severe hypertension or congestive heart failure (a situation that would seriously compromise nutrition or drug administration); and (4) symptoms of uremia, usually manifested in children by CNS depression.

B. METHODS OF DIALYSIS

Peritoneal dialysis is generally preferred in children because of the ease of performance and patient tolerance. Although peritoneal dialysis is technically less efficient than hemodialysis, hemodynamic stability and metabolic control can be better sustained because this technique can be applied on a relatively continuous basis. Hemodialysis should be considered (1) if rapid removal of toxins is desired, (2) if the size of the patient makes hemodialysis less technically cumbersome and hemodynamically well tolerated, or (3) if impediments to efficient peritoneal dialysis are present (eg, ileus).

Furthermore, if vascular access and usage of anticoagulation are not impediments, a slow, continuous hemodialytic process (continuous renal replacement treatment) may be applied.

C. COMPLICATIONS OF DIALYSIS

Complications of peritoneal dialysis include peritonitis, volume depletion, and technical complications such as dialysate leakage and respiratory compromise from intra-abdominal dialysate fluid. Peritonitis can be avoided by strict observance of aseptic technique. Peritoneal fluid cultures are obtained as clinically indicated. Leakage is reduced by good catheter placement technique and appropriate intra-abdominal dialysate volumes. Dialysis is useful in maintaining electrolyte balance. Potassium (absent from standard dialysate solutions) can be added to the dialysate as required. Phosphate is also absent because hyperphosphatemia is an expected problem in renal failure. Nonetheless, if phosphate intake is inadequate, hypophosphatemia must be addressed. Correction of fluid overload is accomplished by using high osmolar dialysis fluids. Higher dextrose concentrations (maximum 4.25%) can correct fluid overload rapidly at the risk of causing hyperglycemia. Fluid removal may also be increased with more frequent exchanges of the dialysate, but rapid osmotic transfer of water may result in hypernatremia.

Even in small infants, hemodialysis can rapidly correct major metabolic and electrolyte disturbances, as well as volume overload. The process is highly efficient, but the speed of the changes can cause problems such as hemodynamic instability. Anticoagulation is usually required. Careful monitoring of the appropriate biochemical parameters is important. Note that during or immediately following the procedure, blood sampling will produce misleading results because equilibration between extravascular compartments and the blood will not have been achieved. Vascular access must be obtained and carefully monitored.

Course & Prognosis

Severe oliguria, if it occurs, usually lasts about 10 days. Oliguria lasting longer than 3 weeks, or anuria, makes the diagnosis of acute tubular necrosis very unlikely and favors vascular injury, severe ischemia (cortical necrosis), GN, or obstruction. The diuretic phase begins with an increase in urinary output to large volumes of isosthenuric urine containing sodium levels of 80–150 mEq/L. During the recovery phase, signs and symptoms subside rapidly, although polyuria may persist for several days or weeks. Urinary abnormalities usually disappear completely within a few months. If renal recovery does not ensue, arrangements are made for chronic dialysis and eventual renal transplantation.

Andreoli SP: Acute renal failure. Curr Opin Pediatr 2002;14:183 [PMID: 11981288].

Barletta GM, Bunchman TE: Acute renal failure in children and infants. Curr Opin Crit Care 2004;10:499 [PMID: 15616392].

CHRONIC RENAL FAILURE

Chronic renal failure in children most commonly results from developmental abnormalities of the kidneys or urinary tract. Infants with renal agenesis are not expected to survive. Depending on the degree of dysgenesis (including multicystic development) the resulting renal function will determine outcome. Abnormal development of the urinary tract may not permit normal renal development. Obstructive uropathy or severe vesicoureteral reflux nephropathy, without (or despite) surgical intervention, continues to cause a significant amount of progressive renal insufficiency in children. In older children, the chronic glomerulonephritides and nephropathies, irreversible nephrotoxic injury, or hemolytic–uremic syndrome may also result in chronic renal failure.

When chronic renal failure is congenital, the inability to concentrate urine results in polyuria. Affected patients often fail to thrive. Without medical care, children with long-standing chronic renal failure may present with complications such as rickets or anemia.

Chronic renal failure may follow acute GN or develop with chronic GN in the absence of an obvious acute episode. Growth failure depends on age at presentation and the rapidity of functional decline. Some of the chronic glomerulonephritides (eg, membranoproliferative GN) can progress unnoticed if subtle abnormalities of the urinary sediment are undetected or ignored. Any child with a history of chronic GN or significant renal injury needs close follow-up and monitoring of renal function and blood pressure.

Complications

Any remaining unaffected renal tissue can compensate for gradual loss of functioning nephrons in progressive chronic renal failure, but complications of renal insufficiency appear when compensatory ability is overwhelmed. In children who have developmentally reduced function and are unable to concentrate the urine, polyuria and dehydration is more likely to be a problem than fluid overload. Output may be expected to gradually diminish with time as renal failure progresses to end stage; however, some children can continue to produce generous quantities of urine (but not of good quality) even though they require dialysis. Moreover, a salt-wasting state can occur. In contrast, children who develop chronic renal failure due to the glomerular disease or renal injury will characteristically retain sodium and water and develop hypertension.

Metabolic acidosis and growth retardation occur early in chronic renal failure. Disturbances in calcium, phosphorus, and vitamin D metabolism leading to renal osteodystrophy require prompt attention. Although renal compensation and increased parathyroid hormone can maintain a normal serum phosphate level early in the course, this pathophysiologic response to hyperphosphatemia will be reflected by an increase in parathyroid hormone and alkaline phosphatase.

Uremic symptoms occur late in chronic renal failure, and include anorexia, nausea, and malaise. CNS features range from confusion, apathy, and lethargy to stupor and coma. Associated electrolyte abnormalities may precipitate seizures (more commonly, a result of untreated hypertension or the presence of hypocalcemia, especially with too rapid correction of acidosis). Anemia (normochromic and normocytic from decreased renal erythropoietin synthesis) is usual. Platelet dysfunction and other abnormalities of the coagulation system may be present. Bleeding—especially gastrointestinal bleeding—may be a problem. Uremic pericarditis, congestive heart failure, pulmonary edema, and hypertension may occur.

Treatment

Treatment of chronic renal failure is primarily aimed at controlling the associated complications. Hypertension, hyperkalemia, hyperphosphatemia, acidosis, and anemia are among the earlier problems. Acidosis may be treated with sodium citrate solutions, as long as the added sodium will not aggravate hypertension. Sodium restriction is advisable when hypertension is present. Hyperphosphatemia is controlled by dietary restriction and dietary phosphate binders (eg, calcium carbonate). Vitamin D should be given to maintain normal serum calcium. When the BUN level exceeds approximately 50 mg/dL, or if the child is lethargic or anorexic, dietary protein should be restricted. Potassium restriction will be necessary as the GFR falls to a level where urinary output decreases sharply. Diet must be maintained to provide the child's specific daily requirements.

Renal function must be monitored regularly (creatinine and BUN), and serum electrolytes, calcium, phosphorus, alkaline phosphatase, and hemoglobin and hematocrit levels monitored to guide changes in fluid and dietary management as well as dosages of phosphate binder, citrate buffer, vitamin D, blood pressure medications, and epoetin alfa. Growth failure may also be treated with human recombinant growth hormone. These treatment areas require careful monitoring to minimize symptoms while the need for chronic dialysis and transplantation continues to be assessed.

Care must be taken to avoid medications that aggravate hypertension; increase the body burden of sodium, potassium, or phosphate; or increase production of BUN. Successful management relies greatly on education of the patient and family.

Attention must also be directed toward the psychosocial needs of the patient and family as they adjust to chronic illness and the eventual need for dialysis and kidney transplantation.

Roth KS et al: Obstructive uropathy: An important cause of chronic renal failure in children. Clin Pediatr 2002;41:309 [PMID: 12086196].

Swinford RD, Portman RJ: Measurement and treatment of elevated blood pressure in the pediatric patient with chronic kidney disease. Adv Chronic Kidney Dis 2004;11:143 [PMID: 15216486].

Dialysis & Transplantation

At present there is a 1-year graft survival rate of living-related kidney transplants of 90%; 85% at 2 years; and 75% at 5 years. With cadaveric transplantation, percentages of graft survivals are 76%, 71%, and 62%, respectively. Overall, the mortality rate is 4% for recipients of living-related donors and 6.8% for recipients of cadaver organs. These percentages are affected by the increased mortality, reported to be as high as 75% in infants younger than age 1 year, primarily due to technical issues and complications of immunosuppression. A body weight of at least 15 kg is associated with a significantly improved survival rate. Adequate growth and well-being are directly related to acceptance of the graft, the degree of normal function, and the side effects of medications.

Chronic peritoneal dialysis (home-based) and hemodialysis provide life-saving treatment for those children awaiting renal transplantation. The best measure of the success of chronic dialysis in children is the level of physical and psychosocial rehabilitation achieved, such as continued participation in day-to-day activities and school attendance. Although catch-up growth rarely occurs, patients can grow at an acceptable rate even though they may remain in the lower percentiles. Use of epoetin alfa, growth hormone, and better control of renal osteodystrophy contribute to improved outcome.

Bartosh SM et al: Long-term outcomes in pediatric renal transplant recipients who survive into adulthood. Transplantation 2003; 76:1195 [PMID: 14578753].

Fine RN et al: Recombinant human growth hormone post-renal transplantation in children: A randomized controlled study of the NAPRTCS. Kidney Int 2002;62:688 [PMID: 12110034].

Neu AM et al: Chronic dialysis in children and adolescents. The 2001 NAPRTCS Annual Report. Pediatr Nephrol 2002;17: 656 [PMID: 12185477].

HYPERTENSION

Hypertension in children is commonly of renal origin. It is anticipated as a complication of known renal parenchymal disease, but it may be found on routine physical examination in an otherwise normal child. Increased understanding of the roles of water and salt retention and overactivity of the renin–angiotensin system has done much to guide therapy; nevertheless, not all forms of hypertension can be explained by these two mechanisms.

The causes of renal hypertension in the newborn period include (1) congenital anomalies of the kidneys or renal vasculature, (2) obstruction of the urinary tract, (3) thrombosis of renal vasculature or kidneys, and (4) volume overload. Some instances of apparent paradoxic elevations of blood pressure have been reported in clinical situations in which chronic diuretic therapy is used, such as in bronchopulmonary dysplasia. Hypertensive infants should also be examined for renal, vascular, or aortic abnormalities (eg, thrombosis, neurofibromatosis, coarctation) as well as some endocrine disorders, including, pheochromocytoma and glucocorticoid-remedial aldosteronism.

Diagnosis

A child is normotensive if the average recorded systolic and diastolic blood pressures are lower than the 90th percentile for age and sex. The 90th percentile in the newborn period is approximately 85–90/55–65 mm Hg for both sexes. In the first year of life, the acceptable levels are 90–100/60–67 mm Hg. Incremental increases with growth occur, gradually approaching young adult ranges of 100–120/65–75 mm Hg in the late teens. Careful measurement of blood pressure requires correct cuff size and reliable equipment. The cuff should be wide enough to cover two-thirds of the upper arm and should encircle the arm completely without an overlap in the inflatable bladder. Although an anxious child may have an elevation in blood pressure, abnormal readings must not be too hastily attributed to this cause. Repeat measurement is helpful, especially after the child has been consoled.

Routine laboratory studies include a complete blood count, urinalysis, and urine culture. Radiography and ultrasonography are used to study the anatomy of the urinary tract, the blood flow to the kidneys, and their function. A renal biopsy (which rarely reveals the cause of hypertension unless clinical evidence of renal disease is present) should always be undertaken with special care in the hypertensive patient and preferably after pressures have been controlled by therapy. Figure 22–3 presents a suggested approach to the outpatient work-up of hypertension.

Treatment

A. TREATMENT OF ACUTE EMERGENT HYPERTENSION

A hypertensive emergency exists when CNS signs of hypertension appear, such as papilledema or encephalopathy. Retinal hemorrhages or exudates indicate a need for prompt and effective control. In children, however, end-organ abnormalities secondary to hypertension commonly are not present. Treatment varies with the clinical presentation. The primary classes of useful antihyperten-

sive drugs are (1) diuretics, (2) α- and β-adrenergic blockers, (3) angiotensin-converting enzyme inhibitors, (4) calcium channel blockers, and (5) vasodilators.

Whatever method is used to control emergent hypertension, medications for sustained control should also be initiated so that the effect will be maintained when the emergent measures are discontinued (Table 22–4). Acute elevations of blood pressure not exceeding the 95th percentile for age may be treated with oral antihypertensives, aiming for progressive improvement and control within 48 hours.

1. Sublingual nifedipine—This calcium channel blocker is rapid acting, and, in appropriate doses, should not result in hypotensive blood pressure levels. The liquid from a 10-mg capsule can be drawn into a syringe and the dosage approximated. The exact dosage for children who weigh less than 10–30 kg is difficult to ascertain by this method, but 5 mg is a safe starting point. Because the treatment is given for rising blood pressure, it is unlikely that the effects will be greater than desired. Larger children with malignant hypertension require 10 mg. In such cases, the capsule may simply be pierced and the medication squeezed under the patient's tongue.

2. Intravenous hydralazine—This vasodilator is sometimes effective. Dosage varies according to the severity of the hypertension and should begin at about 0.15 mg/kg.

3. Sodium nitroprusside—In an intensive care setting, this powerful vasodilator is very effective for reducing severely elevated blood pressure. Intravenous administration of 0.5–10 mg/kg/min will reduce blood pressure in seconds; the dose must be monitored carefully. Metabolism of the drug results in thiocyanate; thus, with prolonged usage, levels of thiocyanate must be monitored, especially in renal insufficiency.

4. Furosemide—Administered at 1–5 mg/kg intravenously, this diuretic will reduce blood volume and enhance the effectiveness of antihypertensive drugs.

B. TREATMENT OF SUSTAINED HYPERTENSION

Several choices are available (Table 22–5). A single drug such as a β-blocker (unless contraindicated, eg, in reactive airway disease) may be adequate to treat mild hypertension. Diuretics are useful to treat renal insufficiency, but disadvantages of possible electrolyte imbalance must be considered. Single-drug therapy with an angiotensin-converting enzyme inhibitor is useful, especially because most hypertension in children is renal in origin. Calcium channel blockers are increasingly useful, and appear well tolerated in children. The use of the vasodilator type of antihypertensive drug requires concomitant administration of a diuretic to counter the effect of vasodilation on increasing renal sodium and water retention and a β-blocker to counter reflex tachycardia. Minoxidil, considered the most powerful of the orally administered vasodi-

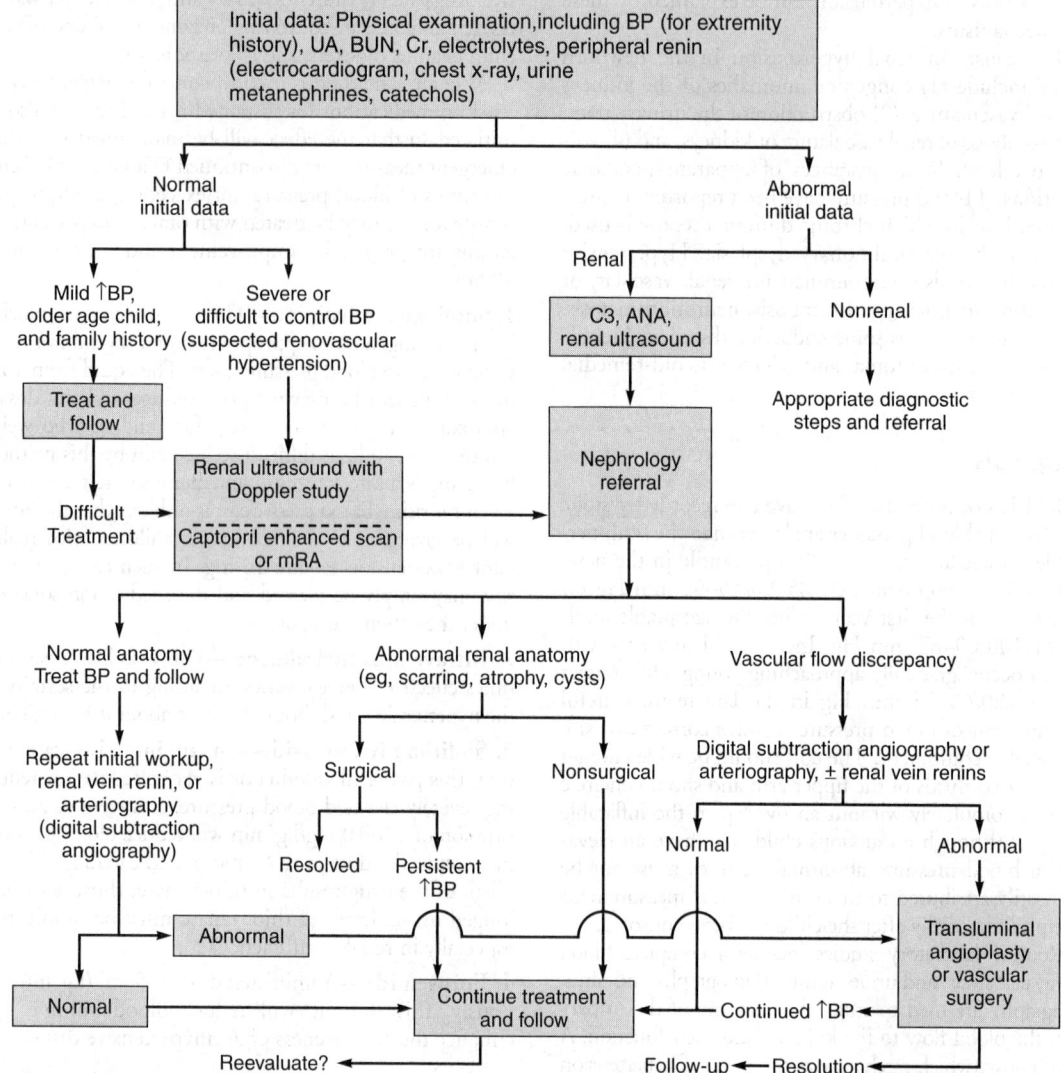

Figure 22–3. Approach to the outpatient work-up of hypertension. ANA, antinuclear antibody; BUN, blood urea nitrogen; Cr, creatinine.

lators, can be extremely efficacious in the treatment of severe, sustained hypertension, but its effect is greatly off-set by the other effects described. Hirsutism is a significant side effect. Hydralazine hydrochloride may still be the most common vasodilator in pediatric use—but, again, the necessity of using two additional drugs for maximum benefit relegates to severe situations calling for management with three or four drugs. The advice of a pediatric nephrologist should be sought.

Nehal US, Ingelfinger JR: Pediatric hypertension: Recent literature. Curr Opin Pediatr 2002;14:189 [PMID: 11981289].

INHERITED OR DEVELOPMENTAL DEFECTS OF THE URINARY TRACT

There are many developmental, hereditary, or metabolic defects of the kidneys and collecting system. The clinical consequences include metabolic abnormalities, failure to thrive, nephrolithiasis, renal glomerular or tubular dysfunction, and chronic renal failure. Table 22–6 lists some

Table 22–4. Antihypertensive drugs for emergent treatment.

Drug	Oral Dose	Major Side Effects[a]
Nifedipine	0.25–0.5 mg/kg/SL	Flushing, tachycardia
Labetalol	1–3 mg/kg/h IV	Secondary to β-blocking activity
Sodium nitroprusside	0.5–10 mg/kg/min IV drip	Cyanide toxicity, sodium and water retention
Furosemide	1–5 mg/kg IV	Secondary to severe volume contraction, hypokalemia
Diazoxide	2–10 mg/kg IV bolus	Hyperglycemia, hyperuricemia, sodium and water retention
Hydralazine	0.1–0.2 mg/kg IV	Sodium and water retention, tachycardia, flushing

[a]Many more side effects than those listed have been reported.

of the major entities; discussion of the rarer conditions is beyond the scope of this book.

DISORDERS OF THE RENAL TUBULES

Three subtypes of renal tubular acidosis (RTA) are well recognized: (1) the classic form, called type I or distal RTA; (2) the bicarbonate-wasting form, called type II or proximal RTA; and (3) type IV, or hyperkalemic RTA (rare in children), which is associated with hyporeninemic hypoaldosteronism. Type I and type II and their variants are encountered most frequently in children. Type III is a combination of types I and II.

Primary tubular disorders in childhood, such as glycinuria, hypouricemia, or renal glycosuria, may result from a defect in a single tubular transport pathway (see Table 22–6).

1. Distal Renal Tubular Acidosis (Type I)

The most common form of distal RTA in childhood is the hereditary form. The clinical presentation is one of failure to thrive, anorexia, vomiting, and dehydration. Hyperchloremic metabolic acidosis occurs, with hypokalemia and a urinary pH exceeding 6.5. The acidosis is more severe in the presence of a bicarbonate "leak." This variant of distal RTA with bicarbonate wasting has been called type III, but for clinical purposes need not be considered as

a distinct entity. Concomitant hypercalciuria may lead to rickets, nephrocalcinosis, nephrolithiasis, and renal failure.

Other situations that may be responsible for distal RTA are found in some of the entities listed in Table 22–6.

Distal RTA results from a defect in the distal nephron, in the tubular transport of hydrogen ion, or in the maintaining of a steep enough gradient for proper excretion of hydrogen ion. This defect can be accompanied by degrees of bicarbonate wasting.

The classic test for distal RTA is an acid load from NH_4Cl. The test is cumbersome and can produce severe acidosis. A clinical trial of alkali administration should be used to rule out proximal (type II) RTA. The dose of alkali required to achieve a normal plasma bicarbonate concentration in patients with distal RTA is low (seldom exceeding 2–3 mEq/kg/24 h)—in contrast to that required in proximal RTA (> 10 mEq/kg/24 h). Higher doses are needed, however, if distal RTA is accompanied

Table 22–5. Antihypertensive drugs for ambulatory treatment.

Drug	Oral Dose	Major Side Effects[a]
Hydrochlorothiazide	2–4 mg/kg/24 h as single dose or in 2 individual doses	Potassium depletion, hyperuricemia
Furosemide	1–5 mg/kg/dose, 2–3 doses per day	Potassium and volume depletion
Hydralazine	0.75 mg/kg/24 h in 4–6 divided doses	Lupus erythematosus, tachycardia, headache
Amlodipine	0.2–0.5 mg/kg/d in 2 divided doses	Fatigue, headache, facial flushing
Propranolol	0.2–5 mg/kg/dose, 2–3 doses per day	Syncope, cardiac failure, hypoglycemia
Minoxidil	0.15 mg/kg/dose, 2–3 doses per day	Tachycardia, angina, fluid retention, hirsutism
Captopril	0.3–2 mg/kg/dose, 2–3 doses per day	Rash, hyperkalemia, glomerulopathy
Enalapril	0.2–0.5 mg/kg/d in 2 divided doses	Proteinuria, cough, hyperkalemia
Nifedipine	0.5–1 mg/kg/d, 3 doses per day	Flushing, tachycardia
Verapamil	3–7 mg/kg/d in 2 or 3 divided doses	AV conduction disturbance

[a]Many more side effects than those listed have been reported. AV, atrioventricular.

Table 22–6. Inherited or developmental defects of the urinary tract.

Cystic diseases of genetic origin
Polycystic disease
  Autosomal-recessive form (infantile)
  Autosomal-dominant form (adult)
  Other syndromes that include either form
Cortical cysts
  Several syndromes are known to have various renal cystic manifestations, including "simple" cysts; may not have significant effect on renal functional status or be associated with progressive disease
Medullary cysts
  Medullary sponge kidney
  Medullary cystic disease (nephronophthisis)
Hereditary and familial cystic dysplasia
  Congenital nephrosis
  "Finnish" disease
Dysplastic renal diseases
Renal aplasia (unilateral, bilateral)
Renal hypoplasia (unilateral, bilateral, total, segmental)
Multicystic renal dysplasia (unilateral, bilateral, multilocular, postobstructive)
Familial and hereditary renal dysplasias
Oligomeganephronia
Hereditary diseases associated with nephritis
Hereditary nephritis with deafness and ocular defects (Alport syndrome)
Nail-patella syndrome
Familial hyperprolinemia
Hereditary nephrotic syndrome
Hereditary osteolysis with nephropathy
Hereditary nephritis with thoracic asphyxiant dystrophy syndrome
Hereditary diseases associated with intrarenal deposition of metabolites
Angiokeratoma corporis diffusum (Fabry disease)
Heredopathia atactica polyneuritiformis (Refsum disease)
Various storage diseases (eg, G_{M1} monosialogangliosido-

sis, Hurler syndrome, Niemann-Pick disease, familial metachromatic leukodystrophy, glycogenosis type I [von Gierke disease], glycogenosis type II [Pompe disease])
Hereditary amyloidosis (familial Mediterranean fever, heredofamilial urticaria with deafness and neuropathy, primary familial amyloidosis with polyneuropathy)
Hereditary renal diseases associated with tubular transport defects
Hartnup disease
Fanconi anemia
Oculocerebrorenal syndrome of Lowe
Cystinosis (infantile, adolescent, adult types)
Wilson disease
Galactosemia
Hereditary fructose intolerance
Renal tubular acidosis (many types)
Hereditary tyrosinemia
Renal glycosuria
Vitamin D–resistant rickets
Pseudohypoparathyroidism
Vasopressin-resistant diabetes insipidus
Hypouricemia
Hereditary diseases associated with lithiasis
Hyperoxaluria
L-Glyceric aciduria
Xanthinuria
Lesch-Nyhan syndrome and variants, gout
Nephropathy due to familial hyperparathyroidism
Cystinuria (types I, II, III)
Glycinuria
Miscellaneous
Hereditary intestinal vitamin B_{12} malabsorption
Total and partial lipodystrophy
Sickle cell anemia
Bartter syndrome

by bicarbonate wasting. Correction of acidosis can result in reduced complications and improved growth.

Distal RTA is usually permanent, although it sometimes occurs as a secondary complication. If the defect is not caused by a significant tubular disorder and renal damage is prevented, the prognosis is good.

2. Proximal Renal Tubular Acidosis (Type II)

Proximal RTA, the most common form of RTA in childhood, is characterized by an alkaline urine pH, loss of bicarbonate in the urine, and mildly reduced serum bicarbonate concentration. This occurs as a result of a lower than normal bicarbonate threshold, above which

bicarbonate appears in the urine. Thus, urinary acidification can occur when the concentration of serum bicarbonate drops below that threshold, and bicarbonate disappears from the urine; this ability to eventually acidify the urine thus reflects normal distal tubular function.

Proximal RTA is often an isolated defect, and in the newborn can be considered an aspect of renal immaturity. Onset in infants is accompanied by failure to thrive, hyperchloremic acidosis, hypokalemia, and, rarely, nephrocalcinosis. Secondary forms result from reflux or obstructive uropathy or occur in association with other tubular disorders (see Table 22–6). Proximal RTA requires greater than 3 mEq/kg of alkali per day to correct the acidosis. Serum bicarbonate should be monitored weekly until a level of at least 20 mEq/L is attained.

Citrate solutions (eg, Bicitra, Polycitra) are somewhat more easily tolerated than sodium bicarbonate. Bicitra contains 1 mEq of Na^+ and citrate per milliliter. Polycitra contains 2 mEq per milliliter of citrate and 1 mEq each of Na^+ and K^+. The required daily dosage is divided into three doses. Potassium supplementation may be required, because the added sodium load presented to the distal tubule may exaggerate potassium losses.

The prognosis is excellent in cases of isolated defects, especially when the problem is related to renal immaturity. Alkali therapy can usually be discontinued after several months to 2 years. Growth should be normal, and the gradual increase in the serum bicarbonate level to above 22 mEq/L heralds the presence of a raised bicarbonate threshold in the tubules. If the defect is part of a more complex tubular abnormality (Fanconi syndrome with attendant phosphaturia, glycosuria, and amino aciduria), the prognosis depends on the underlying disorder or syndrome.

Roth KS, Chan JC: Renal tubular acidosis: A new look at an old problem. Clin Pediatr (Phila) 2001;40:533 [PMID: 11681819].

OCULOCEREBRORENAL SYNDROME (Lowe Syndrome)

Lowe syndrome results from a range of mutations in the *ORCL1* gene that codes for a Golgi apparatus phosphatase. Affected males have anomalies involving the eyes, brain, and kidneys. The physical stigmas and the degree of mental retardation vary with the location of the mutation. In addition to congenital cataracts and buphthalmos, the typical facies includes prominent epicanthal folds, frontal prominence, and a tendency to scaphocephaly. Muscle hypotonia is a prominent finding. The renal abnormalities are of tubule function and include hypophosphatemic rickets with low serum phosphorus levels, low to normal serum calcium levels, elevated serum alkaline phosphatase levels, RTA, and aminoaciduria. Treatment includes alkali therapy, phosphate replacement, and vitamin D. Antenatal diagnosis is possible.

CONGENITAL HYPOKALEMIC ALKALOSIS (Bartter Syndrome and Gitelman Syndrome)

Bartter syndrome is characterized by severe hypokalemic, hypochloremic metabolic alkalosis, extremely high levels of circulating renin and aldosterone, and a paradoxic absence of hypertension. On renal biopsy, a striking juxtaglomerular hyperplasia is seen.

A neonatal form of Bartter syndrome is thought to result from mutations in two genes affecting either Na^+–K^+ or K^+ transport. These patients have life-threatening episodes of fever and dehydration with hypercalciuria and early-onset nephrocalcinosis. Classic Bartter syndrome presenting in infancy with polyuria and growth retardation (but not nephrocalcinosis) is thought to result from mutations in a chloride channel gene. Gitelman syndrome occurs in older children and features episodes of muscle weakness, tetany, hypokalemia, and hypomagnesemia. These children have hypocalciuria.

Treatment with prostaglandin inhibitors and potassium-conserving diuretics (eg, amiloride combined with magnesium supplements) and potassium may be beneficial. Although the prognosis is guarded, a few patients seem to have less severe forms of the disease that are compatible with long survival times.

CYSTINOSIS

Three types of cystinosis have been identified: adult, adolescent, and infantile. The adolescent type is characterized by cystine deposition, which if not treated with phosphocysteamine (Cystagon), is accompanied by the development of the renal Fanconi syndrome and varying degrees of renal failure. Growth is usually normal. The infantile type is the most common and the most severe. Characteristically, children present in the first or second year of life with Fanconi syndrome and, without the metabolic benefit of Cystagon treatment, progress to end-stage renal failure.

Cystinosis results from mutations in the *CTNS* gene that codes for a cystine transporter. About 50% of patients share an identical deletion. Inheritance is autosomal recessive. Cystine is stored in cellular lysosomes in virtually all tissues. Eventually, cystine accumulation results in cell damage and cell death, particularly in the renal tubules. Renal failure between ages 6 and 12 years is common.

Whenever the diagnosis of cystinosis is suspected, slit-lamp examination of the corneas by an ophthalmologist should be performed, because cystine crystal deposition causes an almost pathognomonic ground-glass "dazzle" appearance. Increased white cell cystine levels are diagnostic. Hypothyroidism is common.

Cystagon therapy is helpful in the treatment of cystinosis. Depending on the progression of chronic renal failure, management is directed toward all side effects of renal failure, with particular attention paid to the control of renal osteodystrophy. Dialysis and transplantation may be needed.

Gahl WA: Early oral cysteamine therapy for nephropathic cystinosis. Eur J Pediatr 2003;162:S38 [PMID: 14610675].

NEPHROGENIC DIABETES INSIPIDUS

The congenital X-linked recessive form of nephrogenic diabetes insipidus results from mutations in the vasopressin receptor, *AVPR2*. Autosomal (recessive and dominant) forms of nephrogenic diabetes insipidus are caused by mutations of the *AQP2* gene that codes for a water channel protein, aquaporin-2. Genetic counseling and mutation testing are available.

The symptoms are polyuria, polydipsia, and failure to thrive. In some children, particularly if the solute intake is unrestricted, adjustment to an elevated serum osmolality may develop. These children are particularly susceptible to episodes of dehydration, fever, vomiting, and convulsions.

Clinically, the diagnosis can be made on the basis of a history of polydipsia and polyuria that are not sensitive to the administration of vasopressin, desmopressin acetate, or lypressin. The diagnosis is confirmed by performing a vasopressin test. Carefully monitored water restriction does not increase the tubular reabsorption of water (TcH$_2$O) to above 3 mL/min/m^2. Urine osmolality will remain lower than 450 mOsm/kg, whereas serum osmolality rises and total body weight falls. Before weight reduction greater than 5% occurs or before serum osmolality exceeds 320 mOsm/kg, vasopressin should be administered. Urine concentrating ability is impaired in a number of conditions—sickle cell anemia, pyelonephritis, potassium depletion, hypercalcemia, cystinosis and other renal tubular disorders, and obstructive uropathy—and as a result of nephrotoxic drugs. Children receiving lithium treatment should be monitored for the development of nephrogenic diabetes insipidus.

In infants, it is usually best to allow water as demanded and to restrict salt. Serum sodium levels should be evaluated at intervals to avoid hyperosmolality from inadvertent water restriction. In later childhood, sodium intake should continue to be restricted to 2.0–2.5 mEq/kg/24 h.

Treatment with hydrochlorothiazide is helpful, and many patients show improvement with administration of prostaglandin inhibitors such as indomethacin or tolmetin.

Pattaragarn A, Alon US: Treatment of congenital nephrogenic diabetes insipidus by hydrochlorothiazide and cyclooxygenase-2 inhibitor. Pediatr Nephrol 2003;18:1073 [PMID: 12883974].

NEPHROLITHIASIS

Renal calculi in children may result from inborn errors of metabolism, such as cystine in cystinosis, glycine in hyperglycinuria, urates in Lesch–Nyhan syndrome, and oxalates in oxalosis. Stones may occur secondary to hypercalciuria in distal tubular acidosis, and large stones are quite often seen in children with spina bifida who have paralyzed lower limbs. Treatment is limited to that of the primary condition, if possible. Surgical removal of stones should be considered only for obstruction, intractable severe pain, and chronic infection.

Cystinuria

Cystinuria, like Hartnup disease and a number of other disorders, is primarily an abnormality of amino acid transport across both the enteric and proximal renal tubular epithelium. There are at least three biochemical types. In the first type, the bowel transport of basic amino acids and cystine is impaired, but transport of cysteine is not impaired. In the renal tubule, basic amino acids are again rejected by the tubule, but cystine absorption appears to be normal. The reason for cystinuria remains obscure. Heterozygous individuals have no aminoaciduria. The second type is similar to the first except that heterozygous individuals excrete excess cystine and lysine in the urine, and cystine transport in the bowel is normal. In the third type, only the nephron is involved. The only clinical manifestations are related to stone formation: ureteral colic, dysuria, hematuria, proteinuria, and secondary UTI. Urinary excretion of cystine, lysine, arginine, and ornithine is increased.

The most reliable way to prevent stone formation is to maintain a constantly high free-water clearance. This involves generous fluid intake. Alkalinization of the urine is helpful. If these measures do not prevent significant renal lithiasis, the use of tiopronin (Thiola) is recommended.

Primary Hyperoxaluria

Oxalate production in humans is derived from the oxidative deamination of glycine to glyoxylate, from the serine-glycolate pathway, and from ascorbic acid. At least two enzymatic blocks have been described. Type I is a deficiency of liver-specific peroxisomal alanine:glyoxylate aminotransferase. Type II is glyoxylate reductase deficiency.

Excess oxalate combines with calcium to form insoluble deposits in the kidneys, lungs, and other tissues, beginning during childhood. The joints are occasionally involved, but the main effect is on the kidneys, where progressive oxalate deposition leads to fibrosis and eventual renal failure.

Pyridoxine supplementation and a low-oxalate diet have been tried as therapy, but the overall prognosis is poor, and most patients succumb to uremia by early adulthood. Renal transplantation is not very successful because of destruction of the transplant kidney. However, encouraging results have been obtained with concomitant liver transplantation, correcting the metabolic defect.

Hyperoxaluria may also occur secondary to ileal disease or after ileal resection.

Bartosh SM: Medical management of pediatric stone disease. Urol Clin North Am 2004;31:575 [PMID: 15313066].

Langman CB: The molecular basis of kidney stones. Curr Opin Pediatr 2004;16:188 [PMID: 15021200].

Milliner DS: The primary hyperoxalurias: An algorithm for diagnosis. Am J Nephrol 2005;25:154 [PMID: 15855742].

Sterberg K et al: Pediatric stone disease: An evolving experience. J Urol 2005;174:1711 [PMID: 16148688].

URINARY TRACT INFECTIONS

It is estimated that 8% of girls and 2% of boys will acquire UTIs in childhood. Girls older than age 6 months have UTIs far more commonly than boys, whereas uncircumcised boys younger than 3 months of age have more UTIs than girls. Circumcision reduces the likelihood of UTI in boys. The density of distal urethral and periurethral bacterial colonization with uropathogenic bacteria correlates with the risk of UTI in children. Most UTIs are ascending infections. Specific adhesins present on the fimbria of uropathogenic bacteria allow colonization of the uroepithelium in the urethra and bladder and increase the likelihood of UTI.

Dysfunctional voiding, which is uncoordinated relaxation of the urethral sphincter during voiding leading to incomplete emptying of the bladder, and similarly, any condition that interferes with complete emptying of the bladder, such as constipation or a neurogenic bladder, is associated with an increased risk of UTI. Poor perineal hygiene, structural abnormalities of the urinary tract, catheterization, instrumentation of the urinary tract, and sexual activity increase the risk as well.

The inflammatory response to infection during pyelonephritis may result in renal parenchymal scars. Renal parenchymal scars in infancy and childhood may contribute to hypertension, renal disease, and renal failure later in life. The organisms most commonly responsible for UTI are normal fecal flora, most commonly *E coli* (> 85%), *Klebsiella, Proteus,* other gram-negative bacteria, and, less frequently, *Enterococcus* or coagulase-negative staphylococci.

A. SYMPTOMS AND SIGNS

Newborns and infants demonstrate nonspecific signs, including fever, hypothermia, jaundice, poor feeding, irritability, vomiting, failure to thrive, and sepsis. Strong, foul-smelling or cloudy urine may be noted. Preschool children may have abdominal or flank pain, vomiting, fever, urinary frequency, dysuria, urgency, or enuresis. School-age children commonly have classic signs of cystitis (frequency, dysuria, and urgency) or pyelonephritis (fever, vomiting, and flank pain). Costovertebral tenderness is unusual in young children, but may be demonstrated by school-age children. Physical examination should include attention to blood pressure determination, abdominal exam, and a genitourinary exam. Urethritis, poor perineal hygiene, herpes simplex virus, or other genitourinary infections may be apparent on examination.

B. LABORATORY TESTS

Collection of urine for urinalysis and culture is difficult in children due to frequent contamination of the sample. In toilet-trained, cooperative, older children, a midstream, clean-catch method is satisfactory. Although cleaning of the perineum does not improve specimen quality, straddling of the toilet to separate the labia in girls, retraction of the foreskin in boys, and collecting midstream urine significantly reduce contamination. In infants and young children, bladder catheterization or suprapubic collection is necessary in most cases to avoid contaminated samples. Bagged urine specimens are helpful only if negative.

Screening urinalysis indicates pyuria (> 5 WBC/hpf) in most children with UTI, but many children with pyuria do not have UTI. White cells from the urethra or vagina may be present in urine or may be in the urine because of a systemic infection. The leukocyte esterase test correlates well with the presence of pyuria, but has a similar false-positive rate. The detection of urinary nitrite by dipstick is highly correlated with enteric organisms being cultured from urine. Most young children (70%) with UTI have negative nitrite tests because they empty their bladder frequently, and it requires several hours for bacteria to convert ingested nitrates to nitrite in the bladder. The sensitivity of nitrite detection is highest on a first morning void. Gram stain of unspun urine correlates well with culture recovery of 10^5 cfu/mL or more, but is infrequently available outside of the hospital.

The gold standard for diagnosis remains the properly collected urine specimen. Specimens that are not immediately cultured should be refrigerated and kept cold during transport. Any growth is considered significant from a suprapubic culture. Quantitative recovery of 10^5 cfu/mL or more is considered significant on clean-catch specimens, and 10^4–10^5 is considered significant on catheterized specimens. Usually the recovery of multiple organisms indicates contamination, but some contaminated specimens will yield only a single species.

Asymptomatic bacteriuria is detected in 0.5–1.0% of children who are screened with urine culture. Asymptomatic bacteriuria is believed to represent colonization of the urinary tract with nonuropathogenic bacteria. Treatment may increase the risk of symptomatic UTI by eliminating nonpathogenic colonization. Screening urine cultures in nonsymptomatic children are, therefore, generally discouraged. Repeated urine cultures are often helpful in differentiating asymptomatic bacteriuria from contamination of the culture versus true UTI.

In children with pyelonephritis, a serum creatinine should be determined.

C. Treatment

Management of UTI is influenced by clinical assessment. Very young children (< 3 months) and children with dehydration, toxicity, or sepsis should be admitted to the hospital and treated with parenteral antimicrobials. Older infants and children who are not seriously ill can be treated as outpatients. Initial antimicrobial therapy is based on prior history of infection and antimicrobial use, as well as location of the infection in the urinary tract. Uncomplicated cystitis can be treated with amoxicillin, trimethoprim–sulfamethoxazole, or a first-generation cephalosporin. Each of these antimicrobials is concentrated in the lower urinary tract, and high cure rates are common. There are significant differences in the rates of antimicrobial resistance, so knowledge of the rates in the local community is important. More seriously ill children are initially treated parenterally with a third-generation cephalosporin or aminoglycoside. The initial antimicrobial choice is adjusted after culture and susceptibility are known. The recommended duration of antimicrobial therapy for uncomplicated cystitis is 7–10 days. For sexually mature teenagers, fluoroquinolones such as ciprofloxacin and levofloxacin given for 3 days for cystitis are usually cost-effective. Short-course therapy of cystitis is not recommended in children, because differentiating upper and lower tract disease may be difficult, and higher failure rates are reported in most studies of short-course therapy.

Acute pyelonephritis is usually treated for 10 days. The duration of parenteral therapy in uncomplicated pyelonephritis is not well defined, but most children can complete therapy orally once symptomatic improvement has occurred. A repeat urine culture 24–48 hours after beginning therapy is not needed if the child is improving and doing well.

D. Radiologic Evaluation

Because congenital urologic abnormalities increase the risk of UTI, radiologic evaluation of first UTI has been routinely recommended. These recommendations usually include routine ultrasound of the kidneys and voiding cystourethrogram (VCUG). Vesicoureteral reflux (VUR) is a congenital abnormality present in about 1% of the population. VUR is graded using the international scale (I—reflux into ureter; II—reflux to the kidney; III—reflux to kidney with dilation of ureter only; IV—reflux with dilation of ureter and mild blunting of renal calyces; V—reflux with dilation of ureter and blunting of renal calyces). Reflux is detected in 30–50% of children 1 year of age and younger. The natural history of reflux is to improve, and 80% of reflux of grades I, II, or III will resolve or significantly improve within 3 years following detection.

VCUG should be done selectively on children with first UTI. Children with suspected urologic abnormality due to weak stream, dribbling, or perineal abnormalities should be studied with VCUG. Boys with first UTI should be studied to detect posterior urethral valves, an important congenital abnormality that requires surgery. Children older than 3 years who are otherwise healthy and growing well usually can be followed clinically and do not need VCUG with first UTI. The yield in sexually active teenagers is also very low.

Ultrasonographic examination of kidneys should be done in children with acute pyelonephritis who have not improved after 3–5 days of antimicrobial treatment adjusted for the susceptibility of the organism. The examination is done to detect renal or perirenal abscesses or obstruction of the kidney.

E. Follow-Up

Children with UTI should be followed with screening urinalysis 1 and 2 months after resolution of UTI. Dipstick nitrate determination can be used at home by parents on first morning voided urine in children with frequently recurring UTI.

F. Prophylactic Antimicrobials

Selected children with frequently recurring UTI may benefit from prophylactic antimicrobials. In children with high-grade VUR, prophylactic antimicrobials may be beneficial in reducing UTI, as an alternative to surgical correction, or in the interval prior to surgical therapy. Many experts recommend surgical correction of higher-grade reflux, particularly grade V. Trimethoprim–sulfamethoxazole and nitrofurantoin are approved for prophylaxis. Use of broader-spectrum antimicrobials leads to colonization and infection with resistant strains.

Children with dysfunctional voiding generally do not benefit from prophylactic antimicrobials; rather, addressing the underlying dysfunctional voiding is most important.

Baker PC et al: The addition of ceftriaxone to oral therapy does not improve outcome in febrile children with urinary tract infections. Arch Pediatr Adolesc Med 2001;155(2):133 [PMID: 11177086].

Greenfield SP: Management of vesicoureteral reflux in children. Curr Urol Rep 2001;2:113.

Hoberman A et al: Imaging studies after a first febrile urinary tract infection in young children. N Engl J Med 2003;348(3):195 [PMID: 12529459].

Huicho L et al: Meta-analysis of urine screening tests for determining the risk of urinary tract infection in children. Pediatr Infect Dis J 2002;21(1):1 [PMID: 11791090].

Smellie JM et al: Outcome at 10 years of severe vesicoureteric reflux managed medically: Report of the international reflux study in children. J Pediatr 2001;139(5):656 [PMID: 11713442].

Subcommittee on Urinary Tract Infection, American Academy of Pediatrics: Practice parameter: The diagnosis, treatment, and evaluation of the initial urinary tract infection in febrile infants and young children. Pediatrics 1999;103(4):843 [PMID:10103321].

REFERENCES

Barratt TM et al: *Pediatric Nephrology,* 5th ed. Lippincott Williams & Wilkins, 2003.

Webb N, Postlethwaite R: *Clinical Paediatric Nephrology,* 3rd ed. Oxford University Press, 2003.

Neurologic & Muscular Disorders

Paul G. Moe, MD, Tim A. Benke, MD, PhD, & Tim J. Bernard, MD

◼ NEUROLOGIC ASSESSMENT & NEURODIAGNOSTIC PROCEDURES

NEUROLOGIC HISTORY & EXAMINATION

Despite recent advances in neurodiagnostic testing and neuroimaging, a thorough history remains the most important tool in accurately diagnosing neurologic disorders. The chief complaint(s) and present illness should clearly delineate the temporal profile and sequence of neurologic symptoms. From a detailed history, the clinician will determine if the neurologic symptoms are acute or chronic, static or progressive, recurrent or monophasic, periodic or randomly intermittent, short or prolonged. The patient's description of his or her symptoms will provide clues as to the anatomic localization of the disturbance and possible pathogenic mechanisms. The history should also include what precipitates, palliates, or changes the symptoms.

The history and review of systems provide essential background information about the patient and may provide evidence for a more generalized disorder or for associated or predisposing conditions. Similarly, the family history and social history frequently provide clues for underlying genetic, hereditary, environmental, or psychological conditions that are the basis of the patient's complaints. The social history also provides insight into how the symptoms affect the child's and family's day-to-day living, school performance, and quality of life. A developmental history may provide the earliest clues of a degenerative disorder. Some developmental milestones are summarized in Table 23–1.

The physical examination should include the child's height, weight, head circumference, blood pressure, pulse rate, general appearance, and level of alertness and attentiveness. It is important to observe the child's spontaneous activity, behavior, and responses to light, noise, and touch. Is the child abnormally irritable or demonstrating odd behavior for his or her age? Are there dysmorphic features of the face, head, ears, trunk, extremities, or digits? Are any discolored patches of skin such as hemangio-

mas, ash-leaf depigmented patches, or café au lait spots present? Is the fontanel open or closed, too big or too small? A more detailed mental status examination may be appropriate for school-age children (Table 23–2). The child should be observed for truncal sway or loss of balance (Romberg test). Testing for vibratory appreciation requires that the child be old enough to report whether he or she can feel the vibrations of a tuning fork applied to the digits or bony prominences. Muscle mass, consistency, tone, and strength should be assessed in all four limbs, across multiple joints, and in the neck and trunk. Muscle stretch reflexes can be elicited normally from infancy to adulthood at the biceps, triceps, knees, and ankles. The presence, absence, or asymmetry of automatic infantile movements and reflexes (automatisms) should be noted (see Table 23–1).

The examiner should then proceed with a systematic neurologic examination, including an assessment of cranial nerves II through XII, funduscopy, and testing of eye movements and pupillary light and near-vision reflexes. Cerebellar control of body and extremity posture, ambulation, and fine coordinated movements can usually be evaluated by watching the child walk, run, play with or reach for toys, sit, and stand still. Responses to light touch and mildly painful stimulation can be assessed by tickling or touching the child and lightly pinching toes or fingers and observing facial expression and withdrawal and avoidance movements. Position sensation can be assessed in older children by having them stand with eyes closed. The clinician should construct a differential diagnostic list of disorders that could account for the patient's symptoms and develop a systematic approach to neurodiagnostic testing and neuroimaging procedures.

LUMBAR PUNCTURE

Spinal fluid is usually obtained by inserting a small-gauge needle (eg, no. 22) through the L3–L4 intervertebral space into the thecal sac while the patient is lying on his or her side. After an opening pressure is measured, a small amount of fluid is removed most frequently to examine for evidence of infection or inflammation (Table 23–3). Fluid is sent for red and white cell counts, for determination of the concentrations of protein and glucose, and for viral and bacterial cultures. In some cases, additional information is obtained with

Table 23–1. Neurologic developmental milestones.

	Birth	3 Months	6 Months	9 Months	12–15 Months	24 Months
Motor	Flexor posture, lifts head prone, hands grasped	Sits: head forward, bobbing, lifts head supine, hands open, retains briefly	Rolls both ways, begins to sit alone, supports (erect), bounces	Creeps, pulls up standing, pincer grasp, sits well	Walks with one or both hands held, stands alone briefly, releases on command	Walks and runs well, walks downstairs, turns pages singly
Special senses	Regards (vision), may follow 45 degrees	Looks at hands, follows 90–180 degrees	Discriminates voices, localizes sounds	Picks up raisin, "bye-bye"	Localizes noises, localizes pain	Towers six or seven cubes, imitates scribble
Adaptive	Startles to sound, delayed nociceptive response	Smiles socially, vocalizes socially, follows vertically	Holds cube, palmar grasp, retrieves toy, transfers and rakes raisin	Bangs toys together, pat-a-cake	Assists in dressing, attempts spoon feeding, tries two-cube tower	Asks for toilet, pulls on garments, spoon-feeds well, parallel play
Language	Throaty noises	Coos, chuckles, vocal social response	Babbles (polysyllables), "mmm-mmm"	"Ma-ma, Da-da," one other "word"	Understands simple command, speaks one to three words	Speaks in phrases, names three to five pictures, pronouns: "I, me, you"
Reflex	Tonic neck, palmar grasp	Disappearing tonic neck, Moro reflex	Begins voluntary stepping	Parachute response		
Automatisms	Moro reflex, sucks, roots, stepping, supporting, traction: head lag	Landau response, traction: no head lag	Neck righting, blinks to threat			

special staining techniques for mycobacteria and fungus. Additional fluid may be sent for polymerase chain reaction (PCR) testing for specific viral agents, antibody titer determinations, cytopathologic study, lactate and pyruvate concentrations, and amino acid and neurotransmitter analysis. Lumbar puncture is imperative when bacterial meningitis is suspected. Caution must be exercised, however, when signs of increased intracranial pressure (eg, papilledema) or focal neurologic signs are present that might indicate a substantial risk of precipitating tentorial or tonsillar herniation.

ELECTROENCEPHALOGRAPHY

Electroencephalography (EEG), a widely used noninvasive electrophysiologic method for recording cerebral activity, has its greatest clinical applicability in the study of seizure disorders. Activation techniques to accentuate abnormalities or disclose latent abnormalities include photic stimulation, sustained hyperventila-

tion for 3 minutes, and sleep deprivation, the last of which is an excellent, though less widely used, activation method.

Table 23–2. Mental status examination for school-age children.

Orientation: Time, place, situation, name, date, year.
Memory: Recent and remote, eg, "What did you have for lunch?" "What did you do on your birthday?" Remember (for 10 min): "Red flag, Washington's birthday, Christmas presents."
Calculation: Depends on educational background. Example: Subtract serial sevens.
Proverbs: Interpret: "Too many cooks spoil the broth." "A rolling stone gathers no moss."
Situation: "What would you do if you saw a fire?"
Aphasia: "What's this?" (chalk). "Stick out your tongue." "Put your right finger on your left ear." Sample speech, reading, and writing.

Table **23–3.** Characteristics of cerebrospinal fluid in the normal child and in central nervous system infections and inflammatory conditions.

Condition	Initial Pressure (mm H_2O)	Appearance	Cells/μL	Protein (mg/dL)	Glucose (mg/dL)	Other Tests	Comments
Normal	< 160	Clear	0–5 lymphocytes; first 3 months, 1–3 PMNs; neonates, up to 30 lymphocytes, 20–50 RBCs	15–35 (lumbar), 5–15 (ventricular); up to 150 (lumbar) for short time after birth; to 6 months up to 65	50–80 (two-thirds of blood glucose); may be increased after seizure	CSF-IgG index[a] < 0.7[a]; LDH 2–27 U/L	CSF protein in first month may be up to 170 mg/dL in small-for-date or premature infants; no increase in WBCs due to seizure.
Bloody tap	Normal or low	Bloody (sometimes with clot)	One additional WBC/ 700 RBCs[b]; RBCs not crenated	One additional milligram per 800 RBCs[b]	Normal	RBC number should fall between first and third tubes; wait 5 min between tubes	Spin down fluid, supernatant will be clear and colorless.[c]
Bacterial meningitis, acute	200–750+	Opalescent to purulent	Up to thousands, mostly PMNs; early, few cells	Up to hundreds	Decreased; may be none	Smear and culture mandatory; LDH > 24 U/L; lactate, IL-8, TNF elevated, correlate with prognosis	Very early, glucose may be normal; PCR (meningo- and pneumococcus) plasma, CSF may aid diagnosis
Bacterial meningitis, partially treated	Usually increased	Clear or opalescent	Usually increased; PMNs usually predominate	Elevated	Normal or decreased	LDH usually > 24 U/L; PCR	Smear and culture may be negative if antibiotics have been in use.
Tuberculous meningitis	150–750+	Opalescent; fibrin web or pellicle	250–500, mostly lymphocytes; early, more PMNs.	45–500; parallels cell count; increases over time	Decreased; may be none	Smear for acid-fast organism:CSF culture and inoculation; PCR	Consider AIDS
Fungal meningitis	Increased	Variable; often clear	10–500; early, more PMNs; then mostly lymphocytes	Elevated and increasing	Decreased	India ink preparations, cryptococcal antigen, PCR, culture, inoculations, immunofluorescence tests	Often superimposed in patients who are debilitated or on immuno-suppressive therapy
Aseptic meningoencephalitis (viral meningitis, or parameningeal disease); encephalitis is similar	Normal or slightly increased	Clear unless cell count > 300/μL	None to a few hundred, mostly lymphocytes; PMNs predominate early	20–125	Normal; may be low in mumps, herpes, or other viral infections	CSF, stool, blood, throat washings for viral cultures; LDH < 28 U/L; PCR for HSV, CMV, EBV, enterovirus, etc	Acute and convalescent antibody titers for some viruses; in mumps, up to 1000 lymphocytes, serum amylase often elevated; rarely, a thousand cells present in enteroviral infection

Parainfectious encephalomyelitis (ADEM)	80–450, usually increased	Usually clear	0–50+, mostly lymphocytes	15–75	Normal	CSF-IgG index may be increased; oligoclonal bands variable	No organisms; fulminant cases resemble bacterial meningitis
Polyneuritis	Normal and occasionally increased	Early: normal; late: xanthochromic if protein high	Normal; occasionally slight increase	Early: normal; late: 45–1500	Normal	CSF-IgG index may be increased; oligoclonal bands variable	Try to find cause (viral infections, toxins, lupus, diabetes, etc)
Meningeal carcinomatosis	Often elevated	Clear to opalescent	Cytologic identification of tumor cells	Often mildly to moderately elevated	Often depressed	Cytology	Seen with leukemia, medulloblastoma, meningeal melanosis, histiocytosis X. **Notes:** May mimic infectious meningitis
Brain abscess	Normal or increased	Usually clear	5–500 in 80%; mostly PMNs	Usually slightly increased	Normal; occasionally decreased	Imaging study of brain (MRI)	Cell count related to proximity to meninges; findings as in purulent meningitis if abscess ruptures

[a]CSF-IgG index = CSF IgG/serum IgG ÷ CSF albumin/serum albumin.

[b]Many studies document pitfalls in using these ratios due to WBC lysis. Clinical judgment and repeat taps may be necessary to rule out meningitis in this situation.

[c]CSF WBC (predicted) = CSF RBC × (blood WBC/blood RBC). O:P ratio = observed CSF WBC ÷ predicted CSF WBC. Also, do WBC:RBC ratio. If O:P ratio ≤ 0.01, and WBC:RBC ratio ≤ 1:100, meningitis is absent.

ADEM, acute disseminated encephalomyelitis; AIDS, acquired immunodeficiency syndrome; CMV, cytomegalovirus; CSF, cerebrospinal fluid; EBV, Epstein–Barr virus; HSV, herpes simplex virus; IL-8, interleukin 8; LDH, lactate dehydrogenase; MRI, magnetic resonance imaging; PCR, polymerase chain reaction; PMN, polymorphonuclear neutrophil; RBC, red blood cell; TNF, tumor necrosis factor; WBC, white blood cell.

EEG is also used in the evaluation of tumors, cerebrovascular accidents, neurodegenerative diseases, and other neurologic disorders causing brain dysfunction. Recordings over a 24-hour period or all-night recordings are invaluable in the diagnosis of sleep disturbances and narcolepsy. EEG with telemetry or simultaneous monitoring of behavior on videotape has great usefulness in selected cases. The EEG can be helpful in determining a possible cause or mechanism of coma, whether subclinical seizures are contributing to the coma, and can help determine whether coma is irreversible and brain death has occurred.

The limitations of EEG are considerable. In most cases, the duration of the actual tracing is about 45 minutes and reflects only surface cortical function. Many drugs, especially barbiturates and benzodiazepines, may cause artifact on the tracing and may confuse interpretation. Moreover, about 15% of nonepileptic individuals, especially children, may have an abnormal EEG. EEG findings such as those occasionally seen in migraine, learning disabilities, or behavior disorders are often nonspecific and do not reflect permanent brain damage. A major usefulness of EEG is to show epileptiform activity in children with seizure disorders. Sometimes the findings are diagnostic, as in the hypsarrhythmia EEG of infantile spasms or the prolonged 3/s spike-wave of absence seizures.

Computed tomography (CT) scans, evoked potentials, positron emission tomography (PET), regional cerebral blood flow studies, single-photon emission computed tomography, and magnetic resonance imaging (MRI) supplement the EEG as a diagnostic and prognostic tool.

EVOKED POTENTIALS

Cortical visual, auditory, or somatosensory evoked potentials (evoked responses) may be recorded from the scalp surface over the temporal, occipital, or frontoparietal cortex after repetitive stimulation of the retina by light flashes, the cochlea by sounds, or a nerve by galvanic stimuli of varying frequency and intensity, respectively. Computer averaging is used to recognize and enhance these responses while subtracting or suppressing the asynchronous background EEG activity. The presence or absence of evoked potential waves and their latencies (time from stimulus to wave peak or time between peaks) figures in the clinical interpretation.

The reproducible and quantifiable results obtained from brainstem auditory, pattern-shift visual, and short-latency somatosensory evoked potentials (see section on short-latency somatosensory evoked potentials) indicate the level of function of the relevant sensory pathway or system and identify the site of anatomic disruption. Although results of these tests alone are usually not diagnostic, the tests are noninvasive, sensitive, objective, and relatively inexpensive extensions of the clinical neurologic examination. Because the auditory and somatosensory tests and one type of visual test are completely passive, requiring only that the patient remain still, they are particularly useful in the evaluation of neonates, young children, and patients unable to cooperate. Knowledge of normal values and experience in testing are mandatory.

Brainstem Auditory Evoked Potentials

A brief auditory stimulus (click) of varying intensity and frequency is delivered to the ear to activate the auditory nerve (nerve VIII) and sequentially activate the cochlear nucleus, tracts and nuclei of the lateral lemniscus, and inferior colliculus. Thus this technique assesses hearing and function of the brainstem auditory tracts.

Hearing in the neonate or uncooperative patient can be assessed objectively, making the technique particularly useful in high-risk infants and in mentally retarded or autistic patients. Brainstem auditory evoked potentials are used to judge brainstem dysfunction in sleep apnea, Arnold-Chiari malformation, and achondroplasia. Because high doses of anesthetic agents or barbiturates do not seriously affect results, the test is used to assess and monitor brainstem function of surgical patients (in the operating room) and those in hypoxic-ischemic coma or coma following head injury. Absence of evoked potential waves beyond the first wave from the auditory nerve usually signifies brain death. Brainstem auditory evoked potentials are also useful in the early evaluation of diseases affecting myelin such as the leukodystrophies and multiple sclerosis, although auditory evoked potentials are less valuable than visual evoked potentials in the evaluation of multiple sclerosis. Intrinsic brainstem gliomas can also be evaluated with auditory evoked potentials. They are sometimes useful in evaluation of hereditary ataxias, Wilson disease, and other degenerative disorders of the brainstem.

Pattern-Shift Visual Evoked Potentials

The preferred stimulus is a shift (reversal) of a checkerboard pattern, and the response is a single wave (called P-100) generated in the striate and parastriate visual cortex. The absolute latency of P-100 (time from stimulus to wave peak) and the difference in latency between the two eyes are sensitive indicators of disease. The amplitude of response is affected by any process resulting in poor fixation on the stimulus screen or affecting visual acuity. Ability to focus on a checkerboard pattern is necessary. An LED (light-emitting diode) in goggles, or bright flash stimulus can be used in younger and uncooperative children, but the norms are less standardized. This is a crude whole retina (rather than only macula) stimulation that can give normal results in a blind child.

Clinical applications of the test include detection and monitoring of strabismus (eg, in amblyopia ex anopsia), optic neuritis, and lesions near the optic nerve and chiasm such as optic gliomas and craniopharyngiomas. Degenerative and immunologic diseases that affect visual transmission may be detected early and followed by serial evaluations. Examples of such diseases include adrenoleukodystrophy, Pelizaeus-Merzbacher disease, some spinocerebellar degenerations, sarcoidosis, and even multiple sclerosis. Flash visual evoked potentials are used to monitor function during surgery on the eyes or optic nerve, to assess cortical or hysterical blindness, and to evaluate patients with photosensitive epilepsy, who may have exaggerated responses.

Short-Latency Somatosensory Evoked Potentials

Responses are commonly produced by electrical stimulation of peripheral sensory nerves, because this evokes potentials of greatest amplitude and clarity. Finger tapping and muscle stretching may also be used to stimulate somatosensory potentials. The function of this test is similar to that of the auditory test in closely correlating waveforms with function of the sensory pathways and permitting localization of conduction defects.

Short-latency somatosensory evoked potentials are used in the assessment of a wide variety of lesions of the peripheral nerve, root, spinal cord, and central nervous system (CNS) following trauma, neuropathies (eg, in diabetes mellitus or Guillain-Barré syndrome), myelodysplasias, cerebral palsy, and many other disorders. The procedure is often performed on an outpatient basis. One method is stimulation of the median nerve at the wrist with small (nonpainful) electrical shocks and recording of responses from the brachial plexus above the clavicle, the neck (cervical cord), and the opposite scalp area overlying the sensorimotor cortex. After stimulation from the knee (peroneal nerve) or ankle (tibial nerve), impulses are recorded from the lower lumbar spinal cord, cervical cord, and sensorimotor cortex. Such potentials are used to monitor spinal cord sensory functioning during surgery for scoliosis, myelodysplasias, tumors, and other lesions of the spinal cord or its blood vessels. The technique is also used in leukodystrophies involving peripheral nerves, in multiple sclerosis, and in the evaluation of hysteria and malingering (anesthetic limbs). In the diagnosis of coma and brain death, somatosensory evoked potentials supplement the results of auditory evoked potentials.

PEDIATRIC NEURORADIOLOGIC PROCEDURES

Sedation for Procedures

Oral chloral hydrate, 30–60 mg/kg/dose, is safest. Many radiology departments, however, use intravenously administered agents because of the risks of vomiting and aspiration. One favorite is pentobarbital, 6 mg/kg for children weighing less than 15 kg and 5 mg/kg for larger children (up to a maximum of 200 mg) given intramuscularly or rectally (at least 20 minutes before a procedure) or 2–4 mg/kg given intravenously. Equipment to support blood pressure and respiration must be available. This dosage usually achieves sedation for up to 2 hours. If, however, sedation is inadequate 30 minutes after injection, and if the child's condition permits a second dose of pentobarbital, 2 mg/kg is given. Midazolam 0.1 mg/kg IV or 0.2 mg/kg intranasally is gaining popularity for brief procedures (eg, Botox injection).

Computed Tomography

CT scanning consists of a series of cross-sectional (axial) roentgenograms. Radiation exposure is approximately the same as that from a skull radiographic series. The images can be viewed on a television screen as the scan is being done, and later examined on films. Both record variations in tissue density. CT scanning is of high sensitivity (88–96% of lesions larger than 1–2 cm can be seen) but low specificity (tumor, infection, or infarct may look the same).

The CT scan is often repeated after intravenous injection of iodized contrast for enhancement, which reflects the vascularity of a lesion or its surrounding tissues. Precautions should be taken to ensure that the patient is not sensitive to iodinated dyes and that allergic reactions can be managed promptly. Sufficient information is often obtained from a nonenhanced scan, thus reducing both cost and risk.

Magnetic Resonance Imaging

MRI is a noninvasive technique that uses the magnetic properties of certain nuclei to produce diagnostically useful signals. Currently the technique is based on detecting the response (resonance) of hydrogen proton nuclei to applied radiofrequency electromagnetic radiation. These nuclei are abundant in the body and more sensitive to MRI than other nuclei. The strength of MRI signals varies with the relationship of water to protein and the amount of lipid in the tissue. The MRI image displayed provides high-resolution contrast of soft tissues. MRI can provide information about the histologic, physiologic, and biochemical status of tissues in addition to gross anatomic data.

MRI has been used to delineate brain tumors, edema, ischemic and hemorrhagic lesions, hydrocephalus, vascular disorders, inflammatory and infectious lesions, and degenerative processes. MRI can be used to study myelination and demyelination, and through the demonstration of changes in relaxation time, metabolic disorders of the brain, muscles, and glands. Because bone causes no artifact in the images, the posterior fossa and its contents can be studied far better using MRI than with CT scans. Even blood vessels and the cranial nerves can be imaged. In contrast, the inability of MRI to detect calcification limits its usefulness in the investigation of calcified lesions such as craniopharyngioma and leptomeningeal angiomatosis.

Magnetic resonance angiography (MRA) is a noninvasive (no arterial or venous puncture or dye injection) technique to show large extra- and intracranial blood vessels. It often replaces the more hazardous intra-arterial injection angiogram.

Perfusion imaging using a paramagnetic contrast agent is used in stroke patients to evaluate brain ischemic penumbra. Similarly, diffusion imaging (measuring random motion of water molecules) may show reduced diffusion in areas of cytotoxic edema, and is useful in acute strokes and toxic or metabolic brain injuries. The area of involvement often exceeds the T1 hypodense or T2 hyperdense stroke area, and possibly reflects recoverable tissue injury as compared with totally infarcted tissue, cell death, or apoptosis (programmed cell death) in the center of the stroke.

Another new MRI technique, proton MR spectroscopy, measures signals of increased cellular activity and oxidative metabolism; neuronal acetyl aspartate, phosphocreatinine, and phosphomonoester are increased. Ratios are often calculated to choline and P_i (inorganic phosphate). Increased lactate (anaerobic metabolism), choline, and creatinine, reflecting increased cell surface area—as in gliosis or scarring—can be assessed in a chosen voxel or tiny area of interest. An epileptic focus in the medial temporal lobe is an example; an active seizure site might show increased metabolism. Sclerosis and gliosis ("scar") would show the converse.

Functional MRI can be performed at the same time as an ongoing regular MRI. Blood oxygenation changes in an area of interest (eg, an area of language acquisition) during rest and then during a verbal work paradigm can identify and lateralize the language cortex. A change in ratio of oxyhemoglobin to deoxyhemoglobin results in a detectable MRI signal.

Positron Emission Tomography

PET is an imaging technique that measures the metabolic rate at a given site by CT scanning. For measurement of local cerebral metabolism, the radiolabeled substrate most frequently used has been intravenously administered fluorodeoxyglucose. Gray matter and white matter are clearly distinguishable; the skull and air- or fluid-filled cavities are least active metabolically.

PET has been used to study the cerebral metabolism of neonates and brain activation by visual or auditory stimuli. Pathologic states that have been studied include epilepsy, brain infarcts, brain tumors, and dementias. This functional test of brain metabolism is useful in preoperative evaluation for epilepsy surgery. The epileptogenic zone will often be hypermetabolic during seizures and hypoactive during the time between seizures. The information from PET scan complements EEG and MRI findings to aid in the decision about tissue removal. In infants with infantile spasms, PET scan has occasionally detected focal lesions, thereby leading to successful surgical removal. Clinical application is limited by the cost of the procedure and the clinician's need for access to a nearby cyclotron for preparation of the radiopharmaceuticals.

Ultrasonography

Ultrasonography offers a pictorial display of the varying densities of tissues in a given anatomic region by recording the echoes of ultrasonic waves reflected from it. These waves, modulated by pulsations, are introduced into the tissue by means of a piezoelectric transducer. The many advantages of ultrasonography include the ability to assess a structure and its positioning quickly with easily portable equipment, without ionizing radiation, and at about one-fourth the cost of CT scanning. Sedation is usually not necessary, and the procedure can be repeated as often as needed without risk to the patient. In brain imaging, B-mode and real-time sector scanners are usually used, permitting excellent detail in the coronal and sagittal planes. Contiguous structures can be studied by a continuous sweep and reviewed on videotape.

Ultrasonography has been used for in utero diagnosis of hydrocephalus and other anomalies. In neonates, the thin skull and the open anterior fontanelle have facilitated imaging of the brain, and ultrasonography is used to screen and follow infants of less than 32 weeks' gestation or weighing less than 1500 g for intracranial hemorrhage. Other uses in neonates include detection of hydrocephalus, major brain and spine malformations, and calcifications from intrauterine infection with cytomegalovirus (CMV) or *Toxoplasma*.

Cerebral Angiography

Arteriography remains a useful procedure in the diagnosis of many cerebrovascular disorders, particularly in cerebrovascular accidents or in potentially operable vascular malformations. In some brain tumors, arteriography may be necessary to define the precise location or vascular bed, to differentiate among tumors, or to distinguish tumor from abscess or infarction. Noninvasive CTs, MRIs, and MRAs can diagnose many cases of static or flowing blood disorders (eg, sinus thromboses). If necessary, invasive arteriography is usually done via femoral artery-aorta catheterization.

Myelography

Radiographic examination of the spine may be indicated in cases of spinal cord tumors or various forms of spinal dysraphism and in the rare instance of herniated disks in children. MRI has largely replaced sonography and CT.

Aydin K et al: Utility of electroencephalography in the evaluation of common neurologic conditions in children. J Child Neurol 2003;18:394 [PMID: 128896973].

Bonsu BK, Harper MB: Accuracy and test characteristics of ancillary tests of cerebrospinal fluid for predicting acute bacterial meningitis in children with low white blood cell counts in cerebrospinal fluid. Acad Emerg Med 2005;12:303 [PMID: 15805320].

Davies NW et al: Factors influencing PCR detection of viruses in cerebrospinal fluid of patients with suspected CNS infections. J Neurol Neurosurg Psychiatry 2005;76:82 [PMID: 15608000].

Dooley JM et al: The utility of the physical examination and investigations in the pediatric neurology consultation. Pediatr Neurol 2003;28:96 [PMID: 12699858].

Halsted HJ, Jones BV: Pediatric neuroimaging for the pediatrician. Pediatr Ann 2002;31:661 [PMID: 12389370].

Kleine TO et al: New and old diagnostic markers of meningitis in cerebrospinal fluid (CSF). Brain Res Bull 2003;61:287 [PMID: 12909299].

Krishnamoorthy KS et al: Diffusion-weighted imaging in neonatal cerebral infarction: Clinical utility and follow-up. J Child Neurol 2000;15:592 [PMID: 11019790].

Mazor SS et al: Interpretation of traumatic lumbar punctures: Who can go home? Pediatrics 2003;111:525 [PMID: 12612231].

Straussberg R et al: Absolute neutrophil count in aseptic and bacterial meningitis related to time of lumbar puncture. Pediatr Neurol 2003;28:365 [PMID: 12878298].

DISORDERS AFFECTING THE NERVOUS SYSTEM IN INFANTS & CHILDREN

ALTERED STATES OF CONSCIOUSNESS

ESSENTIALS OF DIAGNOSIS & TYPICAL FEATURES

- *Reduction or alteration in cognitive and affective mental functioning and in arousability or attentiveness.*
- *Acute onset.*

General Considerations

Many terms are used to describe the continuum from full alertness to complete unresponsiveness and deep coma, including clouding, obtundation, somnolence or stupor, semicoma or light coma, and deep coma. Several scales have been used to grade the depth of unconsciousness (Table 23–4). The commonly used Glasgow Coma Scale is summarized in Table 11–5. Physicians should use one of these tables and provide further descriptions in case narratives. These descriptions help subsequent observers quantify unconsciousness and evaluate changes in the patient's condition.

The neurologic substrate for consciousness is the reticular activating system in the brainstem, up to and

Table 23–4. Gradation of coma.

	Deep Coma		Light Coma		
	Grade 4	Grade 3	Grade 2	Grade 1	Stupor
Response to pain	0	+	Avoidance	Avoidance	Arousal unsustained
Tone/posture	Flaccid	Decerebrate	Variable	Variable	Normal
Tendon reflexes	0	+/–	+	+	+
Pupil response	0	+	+	+	+
Response to verbal stimuli	0	0	0	0	+
Other corneal reflex	0	+	+	+	+
Gag reflex	0	+	+	+	+

including the thalamus and paraventricular hypothalamus. Large lesions of the cortex, especially of the left hemisphere, can also cause coma. The term "locked-in syndrome" describes patients who are conscious but have no access to motor or verbal expression because of massive loss of motor function of the brainstem. "Coma vigil" refers to patients who seem comatose but have some spontaneous motor behavior, such as eye opening or eye tracking, almost always at a reflex level. Persistent vegetative state denotes a chronic condition in which there is preservation of the sleep-wake cycle but no awareness and no recovery of mental function.

Emergency Measures

The clinician's first response is to ensure that the patient will survive. The ABCs of resuscitation are pertinent. The airway must be kept open with positioning or even endotracheal intubation. Breathing and adequate air exchange can be assessed by auscultation; hand bag respiratory assistance with oxygen may be needed. Circulation must be ensured by assessing pulse and blood pressure. An intravenous line is always necessary. Fluids, plasma, blood, or even a dopamine drip (1–20 μg/kg/min) may be required in cases of hypotension. An extremely hypothermic or febrile child may require vigorous cooling or warming to save life. The assessment of vital signs may signal the diagnosis. Slow, insufficient respirations suggest poisoning by hypnotic drugs; apnea may indicate diphenoxylate hydrochloride poisoning. Rapid, deep respirations suggest acidosis, possibly metabolic, as with diabetic coma; toxic, such as that due to aspirin; or neurogenic, as in Reye syndrome. Hyperthermia may indicate infection or heat stroke; hypothermia may indicate cold exposure, ethanol poisoning, or hypoglycemia (especially in infancy).

The signs of impending brain herniation are another priority of the initial assessment. Bradycardia, high blood pressure, irregular breathing, increased extensor tone, and third nerve palsy with the eye deviated outward and the pupil dilated are possible signs of impending temporal lobe or brainstem herniation. These signs suggest a need for slight hyperventilation, reducing cerebral edema, prompt neurosurgical consultation, and possibly, in an infant with a bulging fontanelle, subdural or ventricular tap (or both). Initial intravenous fluids should contain glucose until further assessment disproves hypoglycemia as a cause.

A history obtained from parents or witnesses is desirable. Sometimes the only history will be obtained from ambulance attendants. An important point is whether the child is known to have a chronic illness, such as diabetes, hemophilia, epilepsy, or cystic fibrosis. Recent acute illness raises the possibility of coma caused by viral or bacterial meningitis. Trauma is a common cause of coma. Lack of a history of trauma, especially in infants, does not rule it out. Nonaccidental trauma or a fall not witnessed by caregivers may have occurred. In coma of unknown cause, poisoning is always a possibility. Absence of a history of ingestion of a toxic substance or of medication in the home does not rule out poisoning as a cause.

Often the history is obtained concurrently with a brief pediatric and neurologic screening examination. After the assessment of vital signs, the general examination proceeds with a trauma assessment. Palpation of the head and fontanelle, inspection of the ears for infection or hemorrhage, and a careful examination for neck stiffness are indicated. If circumstances suggest head or neck trauma, the head and neck must be immobilized so that any fracture or dislocation will not be aggravated. The skin must be inspected for petechiae or purpura that might suggest bacteremia, infection, bleeding disorder, or traumatic bruising. Examination of the chest, abdomen, and limbs is important to exclude enclosed hemorrhage or traumatic fractures.

Neurologic examination quantifies the stimulus response and depth of coma, such as responsiveness to verbal or painful stimuli. Examination of the pupils, optic fundi, and eye movements is important. Are the eye movements spontaneous, or is it necessary to do the doll's-eye maneuver (rotating the head rapidly to see whether the eyes follow)? Motor and sensory examinations assess reflex asymmetries, Babinski sign, and evidence of spontaneous posturing or posturing induced by noxious stimuli (eg, decorticate or decerebrate posturing).

If the cause of the coma is not obvious, emergency laboratory tests must be obtained. Table 23–5 lists some of the causes of coma in children. An immediate blood glucose (or Dextrostix), complete blood count, urine obtained by catheterization if necessary, pH and electrolytes (including bicarbonate), serum urea nitrogen, and aspartate aminotransferase are initial screens. Urine, blood, and even gastric contents must be saved for toxin screen if the underlying cause is not obvious. Spinal tap is often necessary to rule out CNS infection. Papilledema is a relative contraindication to lumbar puncture. Occasionally, blood culture is obtained, antibiotics started, and imaging study of the brain done prior to a diagnostic spinal tap. If meningitis is suspected and a tap is believed to be hazardous, antibiotics should be started and the diagnostic spinal puncture done later. Tests that are helpful in obscure cases of coma include partial oxygen pressure, partial carbon dioxide pressure, ammonia levels, serum and urine osmolality, porphyrins, lead levels, and urine and serum amino acids and urine organic acids.

If head trauma or increased pressure is suspected, an emergency CT scan or MRI is necessary. Bone win-

Table 23–5. Some causes of coma in childhood.

Mechanism of Coma	Likely Cause	
	Newborn Infant	Older Child
Anoxia		
Asphyxia	Birth asphyxia	CO poisoning
Respiratory obstruction	Meconium aspiration, infection (especially respiratory syncytial virus)	Croup, epiglottitis
Severe anemia	Hydrops fetalis	Hemolysis, blood loss
Ischemia		
Cardiac	Shunting lesions, hypoplastic left heart	Shunting lesions, aortic stenosis, myocarditis
Shock	Asphyxia, sepsis	Blood loss, infection
Head trauma	Birth contusion, hemorrhage, nonaccidental trauma	Falls, auto accidents, athletic injuries
Infection	Gram-negative meningitis, herpes encephalitis, sepsis	Bacterial meningitis, viral encephalitis, postinfectious encephalitis
Vascular	Intraventricular hemorrhage, sinus thrombosis	Arterial or venous occlusion with congenital heart disease, idiopathic trauma
Neoplasm	Rare this age. Choroid plexus papilloma with severe hydrocephalus.	Brainstem glioma, increased pressure with posterior fossa tumors
Drugs	Maternal sedatives, injected analgesics	Overdose, many drugs
Epilepsy	Constant minor motor seizures; electrical seizure without motor manifestations	Constant minor motor seizures, absence status, postictal state; drugs given to stop seizures
Toxins	Maternal sedatives or injections	Arsenic, alcohol, drugs, pesticides
Hypoglycemia	Birth injury, diabetic progeny, toxemic progeny	Diabetes, "prediabetes," hypoglycemic agents
Increased intracranial pressure	Anoxic brain damage, hydrocephalus, metabolic disorders (urea cycle; amino-, organic acidurias)	Toxic encephalopathy, Reye syndrome, head trauma, tumor of posterior fossa
Hepatic causes	Hepatic failure, inborn metabolic errors in bilirubin conjugation	Hepatic failure
Renal causes	Hypoplastic kidneys	Nephritis, acute (AGN) and chronic
Hypertensive encephalopathy		AGN, vasculitis, hemolytic uremic syndrome (HUS), reversible posterior leukoencephalopathy
Hypercapnia	Congenital lung anomalies, bronchopulmonary dysplasia (BPD)	Cystic fibrosis (hypercapnia, anoxia)
Electrolyte abnormalities		
Hypernatremia	Iatrogenic ($NaHCO_3$ use), salt poisoning	Diarrhea, dehydration
Hyponatremia	Inappropriate antidiuretic hormone, adrenogenital syndrome, dialysis (iatrogenic)	Diarrhea, dehydration
Severe acidosis	Septicemia, cold injury, metabolic errors	Infection, diabetic coma, poisoning (eg, aspirin)
Hyperkalemia	Renal failure, adrenogenital syndrome	Poisoning (aspirin)
Purpuric	Disseminated intravascular coagulation	Disseminated intravascular coagulation, leukemia, thrombotic thrombocytopenic purpura (TTP)

Modified and reproduced, with permission, from Lewis J, Moe PG: The unconscious child. In: Conn H, Conn R (editors). *Current Diagnosis,* 5th ed. WB Saunders, 1977.

dows on the former study or skull radiographs can be done at the same sitting. The absence of skull fracture does not rule out coma caused by closed head trauma. Injury that results from shaking a child is one example. In a child with an open fontanelle, a real-time ultrasound may be substituted for the other, more definitive imaging studies if there is good local expertise.

Rarely, an emergency EEG aids in diagnosing the cause of coma. A nonconvulsive status epilepticus or focal finding seen with herpes encephalitis (periodic lateralized epileptiform discharges) and focal slowing as seen with stroke or cerebritis are cases in which the EEG might be helpful. The EEG also may correlate with the stage of coma and add prognostic information.

Treatment

A. GENERAL MEASURES

Vital signs must be monitored and maintained. Most emergency departments and intensive care units have flow sheets that provide space for repeated monitoring of the coma; one of the coma scales (described earlier) can be a useful tool for this purpose. The patient's response to vocal or painful stimuli and orientation to time, place, and situation are monitored. Posture and movements of the limbs, either spontaneously or in response to pain, are serially noted. Pupillary size, equality, and reaction to light, and movement of the eyes to the doll's-eye maneuver or ice-water caloric tests should be recorded. Intravenous fluids can be tailored to the situation, as for treatment of acidosis, shock, or hypovolemia. Nasogastric suction is initially important. The bladder should be catheterized for monitoring urine output and for urinalysis.

B. SEIZURES

An EEG should be ordered if seizures are suspected. If obvious motor seizures have occurred, treatment for status epilepticus is given with intravenous drugs (see section on seizure disorders). If brainstem herniation or increased pressure is possible, an intracranial monitor may be necessary. This procedure is described in more detail in Chapter 13. Initial treatment of impending herniation includes keeping the patient's head up (15–30 degrees) and providing slight hyperventilation. The use of mannitol, diuretics, corticosteroids, and drainage of cerebrospinal fluid (CSF) are more heroic measures covered in detail in Chapter 13.

Prognosis

About 50% of children with nontraumatic causes of coma have a good outcome. In studies of adults assessed on admission or within the first days after the onset of coma, an analysis of multiple variables was most helpful in assessing prognosis. Abnormal neuro-ophthalmologic signs (eg, the absence of pupillary reaction or of eye movement in response to the doll's-eye maneuver or ice water caloric testing and the absence of corneal responses) were unfavorable. Delay in the return of motor responses, tone, or eye opening was also unfavorable. In children, the assessment done on admission is about as predictive as one done in the succeeding days. Approximately two-thirds of outcomes can be successfully predicted at an early stage on the basis of coma severity, extraocular movements, pupillary reactions, motor patterns, blood pressure, temperature, and seizure type. Other characteristics, such as the need for assisted respiration, the presence of increased intracranial pressure, and the duration of coma, are not significantly predictive. Published reports suggest that an anoxic (in contrast to traumatic, metabolic, or toxic) coma, such as that caused by near drowning, has a much grimmer outlook.

BRAIN DEATH

Many medical and law associations have endorsed the following definition of death: An individual who has sustained either (1) irreversible cessation of circulatory and respiratory functions or (2) irreversible cessation of all functions of the entire brain, including the brainstem, is dead. A determination of death must be made in accordance with accepted medical standards. Representatives from several pediatric and neurologic associations have endorsed the Guidelines for the Determination of Brain Death in Children. The criteria in full-term infants (ie, those born at greater than 38 weeks' gestation) were applicable 1 week after the neurologic insult. Difficulties in assessing premature infants and full-term infants shortly after birth were acknowledged.

Prerequisites

In assessment of brain death, the history is important. The physician must determine proximate causes to make sure no remediable or reversible conditions are present. Examples of such causes are metabolic conditions, toxic agents, sedative-hypnotic drugs, surgically remediable conditions, hypothermia, and paralytic agents.

Physical Examination Criteria

(See also Chapter 13.)

The following criteria are those established by the Task Force on Brain Death in Children:

1. **Coexistence of coma and apnea:** The patient must exhibit complete loss of consciousness, vocalization, and volitional activity.
2. **Absence of brainstem function:** As defined by the following: (a) Midposition or fully dilated pupils that do not respond to light; drugs may influence and invalidate pupillary assessment. (b) Absence of sponta-

neous eye movements and those induced by side-to-side passive head movements (oculocephalic reflex) and ice water instillation in the external auditory canal (ice water caloric test; intact tympanic membranes must be documented). (c) Absence of movement of bulbar musculature, including facial and oropharyngeal muscles; the corneal, gag, cough, sucking, and rooting reflexes are absent. (d) Absence of respiratory movements when the patient is off the respirator; apnea testing using standardized methods can be performed but is done after other criteria are met.

3. **Temperature and blood pressure:** The patient must not be significantly hypothermic or hypotensive for age.

4. **Tone:** Tone is flaccid, and spontaneous or induced movements are absent, excluding spinal cord events such as reflex withdrawal or spinal myoclonus.

5. **General examination findings:** The examination should remain consistent with brain death throughout the observation and testing period.

Confirmation

Apnea testing should be carried out at a partial carbon dioxide pressure level greater than 60 mm Hg, and with normal oxygenation maintained throughout the test period. This level may be reached 3–15 minutes after taking the patient off the respirator. The recommended observation period to confirm brain death (repeated examinations) is 12–24 hours (longer in infants); reversible causes must be ruled out. If an irreversible cause is documented, laboratory testing is not essential. Helpful tests to support the clinical assertion of brain death include EEG and angiography. Electrocerebral silence on EEG should persist for 30 minutes, and drug concentrations must be insufficient to suppress EEG activity. Absence of intracerebral arterial blood flow can be confirmed by carotid angiography and cerebral radionuclide angiography. Persistence of dural sinus flow does not invalidate the diagnosis of brain death.

Cerebral evoked potentials, intracranial blood pulsations on ultrasound, and xenon-enhanced CT have not been sufficiently studied to be considered definitive in the diagnosis of brain death. In rare cases, preserved intracranial perfusion in the presence of EEG silence has been documented, and the converse has also been reported.

Claassen J et al: Detection of electrographic seizures with continuous EEG monitoring in critically ill patients. Neurology 2004;62:1743 [PMID: 15159471].

Hosain SA et al: Electroencephalographic patterns in unresponsive pediatric patients. Pediatr Neurol 2005;32:162 [PMID: 15730895].

Lazar NM et al: Bioethics for clinicians: 24. Brain death. CMAJ 2001;164:833 [PMID: 11276553].

Morenski JD et al: Determination of death by neurological criteria. J Intensive Care Med 2003;18:211 [PMID: 15035767].

Oropello JM: Determination of brain death: theme, variations, and preventable errors. Crit Care Med 2004;32:1417 [PMID: 15187532].

Ruiz-Garcia M et al: Brain death in children: Clinical, neurophysiological and radioisotopic angiography findings in 125 patients. Childs Nerv Syst 2000;16:40 [PMID: 10672428].

Shewmon DA: Coma prognosis in children. Part II: Clinical application. J Clin Neurophysiol 2000;17:467 [PMID: 11085550].

Wijdicks EFM: Brain death worldwide: Accepted fact but no global consensus in diagnostic criteria. Neurology 2002;58:20 [PMID: 11781400].

Worrall K: Use of the Glasgow coma scale in infants. Paediatr Nurs 2004;16:45 [PMID: 15160621].

SEIZURE DISORDERS (Epilepsies)

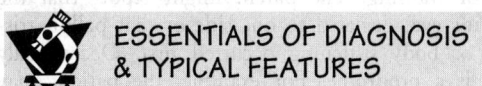
ESSENTIALS OF DIAGNOSIS & TYPICAL FEATURES

- *Recurrent nonfebrile seizures.*
- *Often, interictal electroencephalographic changes.*

General Considerations

A seizure is a sudden, transient disturbance of brain function, manifested by involuntary motor, sensory, autonomic, or psychic phenomena, alone or in any combination, often accompanied by alteration or loss of consciousness. A seizure may occur after a metabolic, traumatic, anoxic, or infectious insult to the brain.

Repeated seizures without evident cause justify the label of epilepsy. Seizures and epilepsy occur most commonly at the extremes of life. The incidence is highest in the newborn period and higher in childhood than in later life. Epilepsy in childhood often remits. Prevalence flattens out after age 10–15 years. The chance of having a second seizure after an initial unprovoked episode is 30%. The chance of remission from epilepsy in childhood is 50%. The recurrence rate after the withdrawal of drugs is about 30%. Factors adversely influencing recurrence include (1) difficulty in getting the seizures under control (ie, the number of seizures occurring before control is achieved), (2) neurologic dysfunction or mental retardation, (3) age at onset younger than 2 years, and (4) abnormal EEG at the time of discontinuing medication. The type of seizure also often determines prognosis.

Seizures are caused by any factor that disturbs brain function. Seizures and epilepsy are often classified as symptomatic (the cause is identified or presumed) or idiopathic (the cause is unknown or presumed to be genetic). The younger the infant or child, the more likely it is the cause can be identified. Idiopathic or genetic epilepsy most often appears between ages 4 and 16 years. A seizure disorder or epilepsy should not be considered idiopathic unless thorough history, examination, and laboratory tests have revealed no apparent cause.

Clinical Findings

A. SYMPTOMS AND SIGNS

The key to the diagnosis of epilepsy is the history. An aura sometimes precedes the seizure itself. The patient describes a feeling of fear, numbness or tingling in the fingers, or bright lights in one visual field. Sometimes the patient recalls nothing because there has been no aura or warning. The parent might report that the patient's eyes deviated to one side or that pallor, trismus, or body stiffening occurred first. Occasionally there is a prodrome. For example, the patient may experience a feeling of unwellness, a premonition that something is about to happen, or a recurrent thought for minutes or hours prior to the aura and seizure itself.

Minute details of the seizure can help determine the site of onset and aid in classification. Did the patient become extremely pale before falling? Was the patient able to respond to queries during the episode? Did the patient become completely unconscious? Did the patient fall stiffly or gradually slump to the floor? Was there an injury? How long did the stiffening or jerking last? Where in the body did the jerking take place? Events after the seizure can be helpful in diagnosis. Was there loss of speech? Was the patient able to respond accurately before going to sleep? All the events prior to, during, and after the seizure can help to classify the seizure, and indeed may help to determine if the event actually was an epileptic seizure or a pseudoseizure (a nonepileptic phenomenon mimicking a seizure). Classifying the seizure may aid in diagnosis or prognosis and may suggest appropriate laboratory tests and medications (Tables 23–6 and 23–7).

B. STATUS EPILEPTICUS

Status epilepticus is a clinical or electrical seizure lasting at least 30 minutes, or a series of seizures without complete recovery over the same period of time. After 30 minutes of seizure activity, hypoxia and acidosis occur, with depletion of energy stores, cerebral edema, and structural damage. Eventually, high fever, hypotension, respiratory depression, and even death may occur. Status epilepticus is a medical emergency.

Status epilepticus is classified as (1) convulsive (the common tonic-clonic, or grand mal, status epilepticus) or (2) nonconvulsive (characterized by altered mental status or behavior with subtle or absent motor compo-

nents). Absence status, or spike-wave stupor, and (very rare) partial complex status epilepticus are examples of the nonconvulsive type (Table 23–8). An EEG may be necessary to aid in diagnosing nonconvulsive status, because these patients sometimes appear merely stuporous and lack typical convulsive movements.

A child with status epilepticus may have a high fever with or without intracranial infection. Studies show that 25–75% of children with status epilepticus experience it as their initial seizure. Often it is a reflection of a remote insult (eg, anoxic or traumatic). Tumor, stroke, or head trauma, which are common causes of status epilepticus in adults, are uncommon causes in childhood. Fifty percent of cases are symptomatic of acute (25%) or chronic (25%) CNS disorders. Infection and metabolic disorders are the most common causes of status epilepticus in children. The cause is unknown in 50% of patients, but many of these patients will be febrile. Status epilepticus occurs most commonly in children age 5 years and younger (85%). The most common age is 1 year or younger (37%), and the distribution is even for each year thereafter (approximately 12% per year). For treatment options, see Table 23–9.

C. FEBRILE SEIZURES

Criteria for febrile seizures are (1) age 3 months to 5 years (most occur between ages 6 and 18 months), (2) fever of greater than 38.8 °C, and (3) non-CNS infection. More than 90% of febrile seizures are generalized, last less than 5 minutes, and occur early in the illness causing the fever. Febrile seizures occur in 2–3% of children. Acute respiratory illnesses are most commonly associated with febrile seizures. Gastroenteritis, especially when caused by *Shigella* or *Campylobacter,* and urinary tract infections are less common causes. Roseola infantum is a rare but classic cause. One study implicated viral causes in 86% of cases. Immunizations may be a cause.

Rarely status epilepticus may occur during a febrile seizure. Febrile seizures rarely (1–2.4%) lead to epilepsy or recurrent nonfebrile seizures in later childhood and adult life. The chance of later epilepsy is higher if the febrile seizures have complex features, such as a duration of longer 15 minutes, more than one seizure in the same day, or focal features. Other adverse factors are an abnormal neurologic status preceding the seizures (eg, cerebral palsy or mental retardation), early onset of febrile seizure (before age 1 year), and a family history of epilepsy. Even with adverse factors, the risk of epilepsy after febrile seizures is low, in the range of 15–20%. Recurrent febrile seizures occur in 30–50% of cases, but in general do not worsen the long-term outlook.

The child with a febrile seizure must be examined. Routine studies such as serum electrolytes, glucose, calcium, skull radiographs, or brain imaging studies are seldom helpful. A white count above 20,000/μL or an

Table 23–6. Seizures by age at onset, pattern, and preferred treatment.

Age Group and Seizure Type	Age at Onset	Clinical Manifestations	Causative Factors	Electroencephalographic Pattern	Other Diagnostic Studies	Treatment and Comments (Anticonvulsants by Order of Choice)
Neonatal seizures	Birth to 2 wk	Often atypical; sudden limpness or tonic posturing, brief apnea, and cyanosis; odd cry; eyes rolling up; blinking or mouthing or chewing movements; nystagmus, twitchiness or clonic movements—focal, multifocal, or generalized. Some seizures are nonepileptic: decerebrate, or other posturings, release from forebrain inhibition; poor response to drugs.	Neurologic insults (hypoxia/ischemia; intracranial hemorrhage) present more in first 3 d or after eighth day; metabolic disturbances alone between third and eighth days; hypoglycemia, hypocalcemia, hyper- and hyponatremia. Drug withdrawal. Pyridoxine dependency. CNS infections. Structural abnormalities.	May correlate poorly with clinical seizures. Focal spikes or slow rhythms; multifocal discharges. Electroclinical dissociation may occur: EEG-electrical seizure without clinical manifestations and vice versa.	Lumbar puncture; CSF PCR for herpes, enterovirus; serum Ca^{2+}, PO_4^{3-}, glucose, Mg^{2+}; BUN, amino acid screen, blood ammonia, organic acid screen, TORCHS[a] IgM. Ultrasound or CT/MRI for suspected intracranial hemorrhage and structural abnormalities	Phenobarbital, IV or IM; if seizures not controlled, add phenytoin IV (loading dose 20 mg/kg each). Diazepam 0.3 mg/kg. Treat underlying disorder. Seizures due to brain damage often resistant to anticonvulsants. When cause in doubt, stop protein feedings until enzyme deficiencies of urea cycle or amino acid metabolism ruled out.
West syndrome infantile spasms (See also Lennox–Gastaut syndrome, below.)	3–18 mos; occasionally up to 4 y	Sudden, usually symmetric adduction and flexion of limbs with concomitant flexion of head and trunk; also abduction and extensor movements like Moro reflex. Tendency for spasms to occur in clusters, on waking or falling asleep, or when fatigued, or may be noted particularly when the infant is being handled, is ill, or is otherwise irritable. Tendency for each patient to have own stereotyped pattern.	Pre- or perinatal brain damage or malformation in approximately one-third; biochemical, infectious, degenerative causes in approximately one-third; unknown in approximately one-third. With early onset, pyridoxine dependency, amino- or organic aciduria. Tuberous sclerosis in 5–10%. Chronic inflammatory disease, eg, TORCHS[a], homeobox gene mutations.	Hypsarrhythmia; chaotic high-voltage slow waves, random spikes, all leads (90%); other abnormalities in 10%. Rarely normal. EEG normalization early in course usually correlates with reduction of seizures; not helpful prognostically regarding mental development.	Funduscopic and skin examination, trial of pyridoxine. Amino and organic acid screen. Chronic inflammatory disease. TORCHS[a] screen, CT, or MRI scan should be done to (1) establish definite diagnosis, (2) aid in genetic counseling. SPECT or PET scan may identify focal lesion.	ACTH preferred (2–4 U/kg/d) IM corticotropin gel once daily, then slow withdrawal. Some prefer oral corticosteroids. Zonisamide, valproic acid, vigabatrin, B6 pyridoxine trial (Japan). In resistant cases, ketogenic or medium-chain triglyceride diet (see text). New drugs: topiramate, lamotrigine, off-label use. Retardation of varying degree in approximately 90% of cases. Occasionally, surgical extirpation of focal lesion may be curative.

(continued)

Table 23–6. Seizures by age at onset, pattern, and preferred treatment. (continued)

Age Group and Seizure Type	Age at Onset	Clinical Manifestations	Causative Factors	Electroencephalographic Pattern	Other Diagnostic Studies	Treatment and Comments (Anticonvulsants by Order of Choice)
Febrile convulsions	3 mos to 5 y (maximum 6–18 mos). Most common childhood seizure: incidence 2%	Usually generalized seizures, less than 15 mins; rarely focal in onset. May lead to status epilepticus. Latter usually benign. Recurrence risk of second febrile seizure 30%; 50% if under 1 y of age; recurrence risk is same after status epilepticus.	Nonneurologic febrile illness (temperature rises to 39°C or higher); positive family history, day care, slow development, prolonged neonatal hospitalization are other risk factors.	Normal interictal EEG, especially when obtained 8–10 d after seizure. In older infants, 3/s generalized spike waves often seen (suggests genetic epilepsy underpinnings).	Lumbar puncture in infants or whenever suspicion of meningitis exists.	Treat underlying illness, fever. Diazepam orally or rectally as needed, 0.3–0.5 mg/kg tid during illness or for prolonged (> 5–15 mins) seizure. Prophylaxis with phenobarbital or valproic acid rarely needed: maybe with neurologic deficits, prolonged seizures, family anxiety.
Myoclonic-astatic (akinetic, atonic) seizures, formerly atypical absence. When mental retardation is presented, this is called Lennox–Gastaut syndrome.	Any time in childhood; usually 2–7 y	Shock-like violent contractions of one or more muscle groups, singly or irregularly repetitive; may fling patient suddenly to side, forward, or backward. Usually no or only brief loss of consciousness. Half of patients or more also have generalized grand mal seizures.	Multiple causes, usually resulting in diffuse neuronal damage. History of West's syndrome; prenatal or perinatal brain damage; viral meningoencephalitides; CNS degenerative disorders; lead or other encephalopathies; structural cerebral abnormalities, eg, migrational abnormalities.	Atypical slow (1–2.5 Hz) spike-wave complexes and bursts of high-voltage generalized spikes, often with diffusely slow background frequencies. See text.	As dictated by index of suspicion. Nerve conduction studies. Skin or conjunctival biopsy for electron microscopy. MRI scan, WBC lysosomal enzymes if metabolic degenerative disease suspected.	Difficult to treat. Valproic acid, clonazepam, ethosuximide, felbamate, topiramate. Ketogenic or medium-chain triglyceride diet. ACTH or corticosteroids as in West syndrome. Perhaps off-label lamotrigine, levetiracetam, zonisomide. Protect head with helmet and chin padding.
Absence (petit mal). Also juvenile and myoclonic absence.	3–15 y	Lapses of consciousness or vacant stares, lasting about 3–10 s, often in clusters. Automatisms of face and hands; clonic activity in 30–45%. Often confused with complex partial seizures but no aura or postictal confusion.	Unknown. Genetic component; probably an autosomal dominant gene.	3/s bilaterally synchronous, symmetric, high-voltage spikes and waves. EEG normalization correlates closely with control of seizures.	Hyperventilation when patient on inadequate or no medication often provokes attacks. Imaging studies rarely of value.	Valproic acid, lamotrigine, or ethosuximide; with latter, switch to valproate if major motor seizures. In resistant cases, ketogenic diet, zonisamide, topiramate, levetiracetam, acetazolamide.

Simple partial or focal seizures (motor/sensory/jacksonian).	Any age	Seizure may involve any part of body; may spread in fixed pattern (jacksonian march), becoming generalized. In children, epileptogenic focus often "shifts," and epileptic manifestations may change concomitantly.	Focal spikes or slow waves in appropriate cortical region; sometimes diffusely abnormal or even normal. "Rolandic spikes" (centrotemporal spikes) are typical; ?genetic, often benign (nonlesional) pattern	If seizures are difficult to control or progressive deficits occur, neuroradiodiagnostic studies, particularly MRI brain scan, imperative (see text).	Carbamazepine. Also used: oxcabazepine, phenytoin, lamotrigine, gabapentin, topiramate, levetiracetam, and zonisamide. Valproic acid useful adjunct.
Complex partial seizures (psychomotor, temporal lobe, or limbic seizures are older terms).	Any age	Aura may be a sensation of fear, epigastric discomfort, odd smell or taste (usually unpleasant), visual or auditory hallucination. Aura and seizure stereotyped for each patient. Seizure may consist of vague stare; facial, tongue, or swallowing movements and throaty sounds; or various complex automatisms. Usually brief, 15–90 s, followed by confusion. History of aura and of automatisms involving more than face and hands establish diagnosis.	As above, but occurring in temporal lobe and its connections, eg, frontotemporal, temporoparietal, temporo-occipital regions.	MRI when structural lesions suspected. PCR of cerebrospinal fluid in acute febrile situation for herpes or enteroviral encephalitis. SPECT, PET scan, video EEG monitoring when epilepsy surgery considered.	Carbamazepine, phenytoin. More than one drug may be necessary. Valproic acid may be useful. In cases uncontrolled by drugs and where a primary epileptogenic focus is identifiable, excision of anterior third of temporal lobe. Oxcarbazepine, topiramate, lamotrigine, levetiracetam, and zonisamide.
Benign epilepsy of childhood (with centrotemporal or rolandic foci)	5–16 y	Partial motor or generalized seizures. Similar seizure patterns may be observed in patients with focal cortical lesions. Usually nocturnal simple partial seizures of face, tongue, hand.	Seizure history or abnormal EEG findings in relatives of 40% of affected probands and 18–20% of parents and siblings, suggesting transmission by a single autosomal-dominant gene, possibly with age-dependent penetrance.	Centrotemporal spikes or sharp waves ("rolandic discharges") appearing paroxysmally against a normal EEG background.	Seldom need CT or MRI scan.	Carbamazepine or other agent. (See simple complex partial seizures.) Often no medication is necessary, especially if seizure is exclusively nocturnal and infrequent. Lamotrigine, topiramate, levetiracetam, zonisamide.

(continued)

Table 23–6. Seizures by age at onset, pattern, and preferred treatment. (continued)

Age Group and Seizure Type	Age at Onset	Clinical Manifestations	Causative Factors	Electroencephalographic Pattern	Other Diagnostic Studies	Treatment and Comments (Anticonvulsants by Order of Choice)
Juvenile myo-clonic epilepsy (of Janz)	Late childhood and adolescence, peaking at 13 y	Mild myoclonic jerks of neck and shoulder flexor muscles after awakening. Intelligence usually normal. Often absence seizures, and generalized tonic-clonic seizures as well.	40% of relatives have myoclonias, especially in females; 15% have the abnormal EEG pattern with clinical attacks.	Interictal EEG shows variety of spike-and-wave sequences or 4- to 6-Hz multispike and wave complexes ("fast spikes")	If course is unfavorable, differentiate from progressive myoclonic syndromes by appropriate biopsies (muscles, liver, etc).	Valproic acid, lamotrigine, topiramate, ?levetiracetam, zonisamide.
Generalized tonic-clonic seizures (grand mal) (GTCS)	Any age	Loss of consciousness; tonic-clonic movements, often preceded by vague aura or cry. Incontinence in 15%. Postictal confusion; sleep. Often mixed with or masking other seizure patterns.	Often unknown. Genetic component. May be seen with metabolic disturbances, trauma, infection, intoxication, degnerative disorders, brain tumors.	Bilaterally synchronous, symmetrical multiple high-voltage spikes, spikes/waves (eg, 3/s). EEG often normal in those younger than age 4. Focal spikes may become "secondarily generalized."	As above	Phenobarbital in infants; carbamazepine or valproic acid; phenytoin; topiramate, lamotrigine. Combinations may be necessary.

aTORCHS is a mnemonic for toxoplasmosis, other infections, rubella, cytomegalovirus, herpes simplex, and syphilis.
ACTH, adrenocorticotropic hormone; BUN, blood urea nitrogen; CNS, central nervous system; CSF, cerebrospinal fluid; CT, computed tomography; EEG, electroencephalogram; IM, intramuscularly; IV, intravenously; MRI, magnetic resonance imaging; PCR, polymerase chain reaction; PET, positron emission tomography; SPECT, single photon emission computed tomography; WBC, white blood cell.

Table 23–7. Benign childhood epileptic syndromes.

Syndrome	Characteristics
Benign idiopathic neonatal convulsions (BINC)	6% of neonatal convulsions; 97% have onset on 3rd to 7th day of life (so-called 5th day fits); clonic; multifocal; usually brief; occasional status epilepticus
Benign familial neonatal convulsions (BFNC)	Autosomal-dominant; onset in 2–90 d; 20% have linkage to chromosome 20q13; clonic; 86% recover
Generalized tonic-clonic seizures (GTCS)	Age at onset, 3–11 y; may have family or personal history of febrile convulsions; 50% have 3/s spike-wave EEG; may have concurrent absence seizures
Childhood absence seizures	Incidence higher in girls than in boys; age at onset, 3–12 y (peak 6–7 years); 10–200 seizures per day; 3/s spike–wave EEG; 40% have GTCS; most remit at puberty
Juvenile absence seizures	Incidence higher in boys than in girls; age at onset, 10–12 y; uncommon; less frequent seizures; 3–4/s general spike-wave EEG; most have GTCS; some remit
Juvenile myoclonic epilepsy (Janz syndrome)	Age at onset, 12–18 y (average, 15 y); myoclonic jerks upper limbs, seldom fall; 4–6/s general spike-wave EEG; untreated, 90% have GTCS, mostly on waking; 20–30% have absence seizures; 25–40% are photosensitive; 10% remission rate (90% do not remit)
Benign epilepsy with centrotemporal spikes (BECTS); "rolandic epilepsy"	Autosomal-dominant; age at onset 3–13 y (most at 4–10 y); 80% have brief, 2–5 min sleep seizures only; usually simple partial seizures (face, tongue, cheek, hand) sensory or motor; occasionally have GTCS; bilateral spikes on EEG; may not need medication if seizures infrequent; remits at puberty

EEG, electroencephalogram.

Table 23–8. Status epilepticus: clinical types.

Generalized seizure (common)
  Convulsive (tonic, clonic, myoclonic); 90%
  Nonconvulsive (absence, atypical absence, atonic); 10%
Focal (partial) seizures (rare)
  Simple partial
  Complex partial
Neonatal
  Many clinical varieties
  May be electrical (ie, on electroencephalogram) status only with no visible clinical findings; called electroclinical dissociation

Table 23–9. Status epilepticus treatment.

1. ABCs
  a. Airway: Maintain oral airway; intubation may be necessary.
  b. Breathing: Oxygen.
  c. Circulation: Assess pulse, blood pressure; support with IV fluids, drugs. Monitor vital signs.
2. Start glucose-containing IV; evaluate serum glucose; electrolytes, HCO_3^-, CBC, BUN, anticonvulsant levels.
3. May need arterial blood gases, pH.
4. Give 50% glucose if Dextrostix low (1–2 mL/kg).
5. Begin IV drug therapy; goal is to control status epilepticus in 20–60 min.
  a. Diazepam 0.3–0.5 mg/kg over 1–5 min (20 mg maximum); may repeat in 5–20 min; or, lorazepam 0.05–0.2 mg/kg (less effective with repeated doses, longer-acting than diazepam). [a]Midazolam IV: 0.1–0.2 mg/kg; intranasally, 0.2 mg/kg.
  b. Phenytoin 10–20 mg/kg IV (not IM) over 5–20 min; 1000 mg maximum); monitor with blood pressure and ECG. Fosphenytoin may be given more rapidly in the same dosage; order 10–20 mg/kg of "phenytoin equivalent."
  c. Phenobarbital 5–20 mg/kg (sometimes higher in newborns or refractory status in intubated patients).
6. Correct metabolic perturbations (eg, low-sodium, acidosis).
7. Other drug approaches in refractory status:
  a. Repeat phenytoin, phenobarbital (10 mg/kg). Monitor blood levels. Support respiration, blood pressure as necessary.
  b. [a]Midazolam drip: 1–5 μg/kg/min (even to 20 kg/min). Valproate sodium, available as 100 mg/mL for IV use; give 15–30 mg/kg over 5–20 min.
  c. Pentobarb coma. Propofol. General anesthetic.
8. Consider underlying causes:
  a. Structural disorders or trauma. MRI or CT scan.
  b. Infection: Spinal tap, blood culture, antibiotics.
  c. Metabolic disorders: Consider lactic acidosis, toxins, uremia. May need to evaluate medication levels, toxin screen, judicious fluid administration.
9. Give maintenance drug (if diazepam only was sufficient to halt status epilepticus): phenytoin 10 mg/kg, phenobarbital 5 mg/kg, daily dose IV (or by mouth) divided every 12 hours.

[a]Much new supportive data.
BUN, blood urea nitrogen; CBC, complete blood count; CT, computed tomography; ECG, electrocardiogram; IM, intramuscularly; IV, intravenously; MRI, magnetic resonance imaging.

extreme left shift may correlate with bacteremia. Complete blood count and blood cultures may be appropriate studies. Serum sodium is often slightly low but not low enough to require treatment or to cause the seizure. Meningitis must be ruled out. Patients with bacterial meningitis can present with a fever and seizure. Signs of meningitis (eg, bulging fontanelle, stiff neck, stupor, and irritability) may all be absent, especially in a child younger than age 18 months.

After controlling the fever and stopping an ongoing seizure, the physician must decide whether to do a spinal tap. The fact that the child has had a previous febrile seizure does not rule out meningitis as the cause of the current episode. The younger the child, the more important the tap, because physical findings are less reliable in diagnosing meningitis. Although the yield is low, a tap should probably be done if the child is younger than age 18 months, if recovery is slow, if no other cause for the fever is found, or if close follow-up will not be possible. Occasionally observation in the emergency department for several hours obviates the need for a tap. A negative tap does not rule out the emergence of meningitis during the same febrile illness. Sometimes a second tap must be done.

Prophylactic anticonvulsants are not required after the uncomplicated febrile seizure. If febrile seizures are complicated or prolonged, or if medical reassurance fails to relieve family anxiety, anticonvulsant prophylaxis may be indicated and can reduce the incidence of recurrent febrile or nonfebrile seizures. One remedy is to use diazepam at the first onset of fever for the duration of the febrile illness (0.5 mg/kg two or three times per day orally or rectally). Diastat is an expensive rectal diazepam preparation. Phenobarbital, 3–5 mg/kg/d as a single bedtime dose, is an inexpensive long-term prophylaxis. Often, increasing the dosage gradually (eg, starting with 2 mg/kg/d the first week, increasing to 3 mg/kg/d the second week, and so on) decreases side effects and noncompliance. A plasma phenobarbital level in the range of 15-40 mg/mL is desirable. Valproate sodium is more hazardous. In infants, the commonly used liquid suspension has a short half-life and causes more gastrointestinal upset than do the sprinkle capsules. The dosage is 15–60 mg/kg/d in two (sprinkles) divided doses. Precautionary laboratory studies are necessary. Phenytoin and carbamazepine have not shown effectiveness in the prophylaxis of febrile seizures (see Table 23–9). Measures to control fever such as sponging or tepid baths, antipyretics, and the administration of antibiotics for proven bacterial illness are reasonable but unproven to prevent recurrent febrile seizures.

Simple febrile seizures do not have any long-term adverse consequences. An EEG should be performed if the febrile seizure is complicated or unusual. In uncomplicated febrile seizures, the EEG is usually normal. About 22% of patients will show slowing or epileptiform abnormalities. Ideally the EEG should be done at least a week after the illness to avoid transient changes due to fever or the seizure itself. In older children, 3/s spike-wave discharge, suggestive of a genetic propensity to epilepsy, may occur. In the young infant, EEG findings seldom aid in assessing the chance of recurrence of febrile seizures or in long-term prognosis.

D. LABORATORY FINDINGS AND IMAGING

Ordering of laboratory tests depends on the child's age, the severity and type of seizure, whether the child is ill or injured, and the clinician's suspicion about the underlying cause. Every case of afebrile suspected seizure disorder warrants an EEG. Other studies are used selectively. Seizures in early infancy are often symptomatic. Therefore, the younger the child, the more careful must be the laboratory assessment (Table 23–10).

Metabolic abnormalities are seldom found in the well child with seizures. Unless there is a high clinical suspicion

Table 23–10. Laboratory studies after first seizure (nonneonatal).

Well infant	EEG, calcium, BUN, or urinalysis, and perhaps CT or MRI. (Abnormal examination or focally abnormal EEG: do imaging study.) Rule out nonaccidental trauma.
Well older child	EEG; consider CT or MRI
Ill infant	Calcium, magnesium, CBC, BUN, glucose, electrolytes, blood culture, lumbar puncture, EEG, possibly CT or MRI
Ill older child	CBC, BUN, lumbar puncture, EEG, CT or MRI
Generalized tonic-clonic seizure	Practice parameter: EEG only. Circumstances may suggest need for: calcium, glucose, CBC, BUN, electrolytes, lumbar puncture (may omit if afebrile, looks well)
Generalized absence	EEG only
Atypical absence	EEG, MRI: Consider studies for mental retardation: serum and urine amino and organic acids and chromosomes, including fragile X. If there is progressive worsening, consider lysosomal enzymes, lumbar puncture, long-chain fatty acids, skin or conjunctival biopsies.
Infantile spasms	See Atypical absence
Myoclonic progressive seizure with mental retardation	See Atypical absence
Focal	EEG. In cases of mental retardation, positive neurologic examination, EEG focal slow wave, or poorly controlled seizures, do MRI. In refractory cases, consider surgical evaluation.

BUN, blood urea nitrogen; CBC, complete blood count; CT, computed tomography; EEG, electroencephalogram; MRI, magnetic resonance imaging.

of uremia, hyponatremia, or other serious conditions, laboratory tests are not necessary. Special studies may be necessary in unusual circumstances, for example, when hemolytic uremic syndrome or lead poisoning is a suspected cause. CT scans are overused in patients with seizures. The youngster with a routine febrile seizure, a nonfebrile generalized seizure with normal examination and normal EEG, or an absence seizure does not need a CT or MRI scan. The yield in a child with normal neurologic examination and EEG is less than 5%. Conversely, in children with symptomatic epileptic syndromes, the EEG will be abnormal in as many as 60–80% of patients. Examples include infantile spasms, Lennox-Gastaut syndrome, and progressive myoclonic epilepsy.

In focal seizures, children with benign rolandic epilepsy do not need a CT scan; it will invariably be normal. The yield with other focal seizures is 15–30%, with most of the findings unimportant in relation to diagnosis and prognosis (eg, a mildly dilated single ventricle or superficial atrophy). Nonetheless, an imaging study eases anxiety and rules out the remote possibility of tumor or vascular malformation. Other indications for MRI scan (the superior study) include difficulty in controlling seizures, progressive neurologic findings on serial examinations, worsening focal findings on the EEG, suspicion of increased pressure, and of course any case in which surgery is being considered. A previously normal scan does not rule out an emerging tumor; if the course is unsatisfactory, repeating the scan may be necessary. A neoplasm or other unexpected treatable lesion is found in a small number, perhaps 2–3%, of scans.

E. Electroencephalography

The limitations of EEG—even with epilepsy, for which it is most useful—are considerable. A seizure is a clinical phenomenon; an EEG showing epileptiform activity may confirm and even extend the clinical diagnosis, but it only occasionally is diagnostic (eg, in absence seizures).

The EEG need not be abnormal in the epileptic child. Normal EEGs are seen following a first generalized seizure in one-third of children younger than age 4 years. The initial EEG is normal in about 20% of older epileptic children and in about 10% of epileptic adults. These percentages are reduced when serial tracings are obtained. Focal spikes and generalized spike-wave discharges are seen in 30% of close nonepileptic relatives of patients with epilepsy.

1. Diagnostic value—The greatest value of the EEG in convulsive disorders is to help classify seizure types and select appropriate therapy (see Table 23–6). "Petit mal" absences and partial complex/"psychomotor seizures" are sometimes difficult to distinguish, especially when the physician must rely on the history and cannot observe the seizure. The differing EEG patterns of these seizures will then prove most helpful. Finding a mixed seizure EEG pattern in a child who clinically has only major motor sei-

zures or only focal seizures will help the clinician select anticonvulsants effective for both seizure types identified by the EEG. The EEG may help in diagnosing infant seizures with minimal or atypical clinical manifestations; it may show hypsarrhythmia (high-amplitude spikes and slow waves with a disorganized background) in infantile spasms or the 1–4/s slow spike-wave pattern of the Lennox-Gastaut syndrome. Both are expressions of diffuse brain dysfunction and generally of grave significance. The EEG may show focal slowing that, if constant, particularly when corresponding focal seizure manifestations and abnormal neurologic findings are present, will alert the physician to the presence of a structural lesion. In this case, brain imaging may establish the cause and help determine further investigation and treatment.

2. Prognostic value—A normal EEG following a first convulsion suggests (but does not guarantee) a favorable prognosis. Markedly abnormal EEGs may become normal with treatment (1) immediately following intravenous injection of 50 mg of vitamin B_6 in pyridoxine dependency or deficiency; (2) in infantile spasms and sometimes the Lennox-Gastaut syndrome (with the use of adrenocorticotropic hormone [ACTH] or corticosteroids); (3) in absence seizures (with appropriate anticonvulsants); and (4) in akinetic and other minor motor seizures, including the Lennox-Gastaut syndrome (ketogenic diet). If so, it is likely that seizure control will be achieved (although this may not correlate with the ultimate developmental status of the patient).

Electroencephalography should be repeated when the severity and frequency of seizures increase despite adequate anticonvulsant therapy, when the clinical seizure pattern changes significantly, or when progressive neurologic deficits develop. Emergence of new focal or diffuse slowing may indicate a progressive lesion. Conversely, a normalized tracing may help confirm remission of absence seizures.

The EEG may be helpful in determining when to discontinue anticonvulsant therapy. The presence or absence of epileptiform activity on the EEG prior to withdrawal of anticonvulsants after a seizure-free period of several years on the medications has been shown to be correlated with the degree of risk of recurrence of seizures.

Differential Diagnosis

It is extremely important to be accurate in the diagnosis of epilepsy and not to make the diagnosis without ample proof. To the layperson, epilepsy often has connotations of brain damage and limitation of activity. A person so diagnosed may be excluded from certain occupations in later life. It is often very difficult to change an inaccurate diagnosis of many years' standing. Some of the common nonepileptic events that mimic seizure disorder are listed in Table 23–11.

Table 23–11. Nonepileptic paroxysmal events.

Breath-holding attacks

Age 6 mo to 3 y. Always precipitated by trauma and fright. Cyanosis; sometimes stiffening, tonic (or jerking-clonic) convulsion (anoxic seizure). Patient may sleep following attack. Family history positive in 30%. Electroencephalogram (EEG) normal. Treatment is interpretation and reassurance.

Infantile syncope (pallid breath-holding)

No external precipitant (perhaps internal pain, cramp, or fear?). Pallor may be followed by seizure (anoxic-ischemic). Vagally (heart-slowing) mediated, like adult syncope. EEG normal; may see cardiac slowing with vagal stimulation (cold cloth on face) during EEG.

Tics or Tourette syndrome

Simple or complex stereotyped (the same time after time) jerks or movements, coughs, grunts, sniffs. Worse at repose or with stress. May be suppressed during physician visit. Family history often positive. EEG negative. Nonanticonvulsant drugs may benefit.

Night terrors, sleep talking, walking, "sit-ups"

Age 3–10. Usually occur in first sleep cycle (30–90 min after going to sleep), with crying, screaming, and autonomic discharge (pupils dilated, perspiring, etc). Lasts minutes. Child goes back to sleep and has no recall of event next day. Sleep studies (polysomnogram and EEG) are normal. Disappears with maturation. Sleep talking and walking and short "sit-ups" in bed are fragmentary arousals. If a spell is recorded, EEG shows arousal from deep sleep, but the behavior seems wakeful. The youngster needs to be protected from injury and gradually settled down and taken back to bed.

Nightmares

Nightmares or vivid dreams occur in subsequent cycles of sleep, often in the early morning hours, and generally are partially recalled the next day. The bizarre and frightening behavior may sometimes be confused with complex partial seizures. These occur during REM (rapid eye movement) sleep; epilepsy usually does not occur during that phase of sleep. In extreme or difficult cases, an all-night sleep EEG may help to differentiate seizures from nightmares.

Migraine

One variant of migraine can be associated with an acute confusional state. There may be the usual migraine prodrome with spots before the eyes, dizziness, visual field defects, and then agitated confusion. A history of other, more typical migraine with severe headache and vomiting but without confusion may aid in the diagnosis. The severe headache with vomiting as the youngster comes out of the spell may aid in distinguishing the attack from epilepsy. Other seizure manifestations are practically never seen, eg, tonic-clonic movements, falling, and complete loss of consciousness. The EEG in migraine is usually normal and seldom has epileptiform abnormalities often seen in patients with epilepsy. Lastly, migraine and epilepsy are sometimes linked: migraine-caused ischemia on the brain surface sometimes leads to later epilepsy. Are both channelopathies?

Benign nocturnal myoclonus

Common in infants and may last even up to school age. Focal or generalized jerks (the latter also called hypnic or sleep jerks) may persist from onset of sleep on and off all night. A video record for physician review can aid in diagnosis. EEG taken during jerks is normal, proving that these jerks are not epilepsy. Treatment is reassurance.

Shuddering

Shuddering or shivering attacks can occur in infancy and be a forerunner of essential tremor in later life. Often, the family history is positive for tremor. The shivering may be very frequent. EEG is normal. There is no clouding or loss of consciousness.

Gastroesophageal reflux

Seen more commonly in children with cerebral palsy or brain damage; reflux of acid gastric contents may cause pain that cannot be described by the child. At times, there may be unusual posturings (dystonic or other) of the head and neck or trunk, an apparent attempt to stretch the esophagus or close the opening. There is no loss of consciousness, but there may be eye rolling, apnea, and occasional vomiting that may simulate a seizure. An upper gastrointestinal series, cine of swallowing, sometimes even an EEG (normal during episode) may be necessary to distinguish this from seizures.

Masturbation

Rarely in infants, repetitive rocking or rubbing motions may simulate seizures. The youngster may look out of contact, be poorly responsive to the environment, and have autonomic expressions (eg, perspiration, dilated pupils) that may be confused with seizures. Observation by a skilled individual, sometimes even in a hospital situation, may be necessary to distinguish this from seizures. EEG is of course normal between or during attacks. Interpretation and reassurance are the only necessary treatment.

Conversion reaction/pseudoseizures

As many as 50% of patients with pseudoseizures have epilepsy. Episodes may be writhing, intercourse-like movements, tonic episodes, bizarre jerking and thrashing around, or even apparently sudden unresponsiveness. Often, there is ongoing psychological trauma. Often, but not invariably, the patients are developmentally delayed. The spells must often be seen or recorded on videotape in a controlled situation to distinguish them from epilepsy. A normal EEG during a spell is a key diagnostic feature. Often, the spells are so bizarre that they are easily distinguished. Sometimes, pseudoseizures can be precipitated by suggestion with injection of normal saline in a controlled situation. Combativeness is common; self-injury and incontinence rare.

Temper tantrums and rage attacks

These are sometimes confused with epilepsy. The youngster is often amnesic or at least claims amnesia for events during the spell. The attacks are usually precipitated by frustration or anger and are often directed either verbally or physically and subside with behavior modification and isolation. EEGs are generally normal but unfortunately seldom obtained during an attack. Anterior temporal leads may be helpful in ruling out temporal or lateral frontal abnormalities, the latter sometimes seen in partial complex seizures. Improvement of the attacks with psychotherapy, milieu therapy, or behavioral modification helps rule out epilepsy.

(continued)

Table 23–11. Nonepileptic paroxysmal events. (continued)

Benign paroxysmal vertigo	Staring spells
These are brief attacks of vertigo in which the youngster often appears frightened and pale and clutches the parent. The attacks last 5–30 s. Sometimes, nystagmus is identified. There is no loss of consciousness. Usually, the child is well and returns to play immediately afterward. The attacks may occur in clusters, then disappear for months. Attacks are usually seen in infants and preschoolers age 2–5. EEG is normal. If caloric tests can be obtained (often very difficult in this age group), abnormalities with hypofunction of one side are sometimes seen. Medications are usually not desirable or necessary.	Teachers often make referral for absence or petit mal seizures in youngsters who stare or seem preoccupied at school. Helpful in the history is the lack of these spells at home, eg, before breakfast, a common time for absence seizures. A lack of other epilepsy in the child or family history often is helpful. Sometimes, these children have difficulties with school and a cognitive or learning disability. The child can generally be brought out of this spell by a firm command. An EEG is sometimes necessary to confirm that absence seizures are not occurring. A 24-hour ambulatory EEG to record attacks during the child's everyday school activities is occasionally necessary.

Complications

Emotional disturbances—notably anxiety, depression, anger, and feelings of guilt and inadequacy—often occur not only in the patient but also in the parents of the child with seizures. The seizures, particularly the hallucinatory auras and psychomotor attacks, frequently set off in the prepubescent and adolescent patient fantasies (and sometimes obsessive ruminations) about dying and death that may become so strong that they lead to suicidal behavior. The limitations many school systems place on epileptic children add to the problem. Some children may react by acting out.

Pseudoretardation may occur in children with poorly controlled epilepsy because their seizures (or the subclinical paroxysms sustained) interfere with their learning ability. Anticonvulsants are less likely to cause such interference but may do so when given in toxic amounts. Phenobarbital is particularly implicated. Mental retardation may be part of the same pathologic process that causes the seizures but may occasionally be worsened when seizures are frequent, prolonged, and accompanied by hypoxia.

Physical injuries, especially lacerations of the forehead and chin, are frequent in astatic or akinetic seizures (so-called drop attacks), necessitating protective headgear. In all other seizure disorders in childhood, injuries as a direct result of an attack are rare.

Treatment

The ideal treatment of seizures is the correction of specific causes. However, even when a biochemical disorder, a tumor, meningitis, or another specific cause is being treated, anticonvulsant drugs are often still required.

A. PRECAUTIONARY MANAGEMENT OF INDIVIDUAL BRIEF SEIZURES

Caregivers should be instructed to protect the patient against self-injury and aspiration of vomitus; beyond that, no specific therapy is necessary. The less done to the patient during a brief seizure of less than 15 minutes, the better. Thrusting a spoon handle or tongue depressor into the clenched mouth of a convulsing patient or trying to restrain tonic-clonic movements may cause worse injuries than a bitten tongue or bruised limb. Mouth-to-mouth resuscitation is rarely necessary.

B. GENERAL MANAGEMENT OF THE YOUNG EPILEPTIC PATIENT

1. Education—The patient and parents must be helped to understand the problem of seizures and their management. Many children—some even as young as age 3 years—are capable of cooperating with the physician in problems of seizure control.

All bottles containing antiepileptic drugs should be labeled. The parents should know the names and dosage of the anticonvulsants being administered.

Materials on epilepsy—including pamphlets, monographs, films, and videotapes suitable for children and teenagers, parents, teachers, and medical professionals—may be purchased through the Epilepsy Foundation of America, Materials Service Center, 4351 Garden City Drive, Landover, MD 20785. The Foundation's local chapter and other community organizations are eager to provide guidance and other services. Support groups exist in many cities for older children and adolescents and for their parents and others concerned.

2. Privileges and precautions in daily life—Encourage normal living within reasonable bounds. Children should engage in physical activities appropriate to their age and social group. After seizure control is established, swimming is generally permissible with a buddy system or adequate lifeguard coverage. Scuba diving and high climbing should not be permitted. Physical training and sports are usually to be welcomed rather than restricted. Driving is discussed in the next section.

Loss of sleep should be avoided. Emotional disturbances may need to be treated. Alcohol intake should be avoided because it may precipitate seizures. Prompt attention should be given to infections. Further neurologic disturbances should be brought to the physician's attention promptly.

Although every effort should be made to control seizures, this must not interfere with a child's ability to function. Sometimes a child is better off having an occasional mild seizure than being so heavily sedated that function at home, in school, or at play is impaired. Therapy and medication adjustment often require much art and fortitude on the physician's part. Some patients with infrequent seizures, especially if only nocturnal partial seizures (eg, rolandic seizures) may not need anticonvulsant medications.

3. Driving—Driving becomes important to most young people at age 15 or 16 years. Restrictions vary from state to state. In most states, a learner's permit or driver's license will be issued to an epileptic individual if he or she has been under a physician's care and free of seizures for at least 1 year, provided that the treatment or basic neurologic problem does not interfere with the ability to drive. A guide to this and other legal matters pertaining to persons with epilepsy is published by the Epilepsy Foundation of America, whose legal department may be able to provide additional information (see reference at the end of this section).

4. Pregnancy—In the pregnant teenager with epilepsy, the possibility of teratogenic effects of anticonvulsants, such as facial clefts (two to three times increased risk), must be weighed against the risks from seizures. Such malformations occur in the infants of about 2.5% of mothers with untreated epilepsy. Some antiepileptic drugs (eg, valproate), are more teratogenic.

C. Principles of Anticonvulsant Therapy

1. Drug selection—Treat with the drug appropriate to the clinical situation, as outlined in Table 23–12.

2. Treatment strategy—Start with one drug in conventional dosage, and increase the dosage until seizures are controlled. If seizures are not controlled on the tolerated maximal dosage of one major anticonvulsant, gradually switch to another before using two-drug therapy. The dosages and usually effective blood levels are listed in Table 23–12. Individual variations must be expected. The therapeutic range may also vary somewhat with the method used to determine levels.

3. Counseling—Advise the parents and the patient that the prolonged use of anticonvulsant drugs will not produce significant or permanent mental slowing (although the underlying cause of the seizures might) and that prevention of seizures for 1–2 years substantially reduces the chances of recurrence. Advise them also that anticonvulsants are given to prevent further seizures and that they should be taken as prescribed. Changes in medications or dosages should not be made without the physician's knowledge. Unsupervised sudden withdrawal of anticonvulsant drugs may precipitate severe seizures or even status epilepticus. Anticonvulsants must be kept where they cannot be ingested by small children or suicidal patients.

4. Follow-up—Check the patient at intervals, depending on the underlying cause of the seizures, the degree of control, and the toxic properties of the anticonvulsant drug or drugs used. Blood counts and liver function tests must be obtained periodically in the case of some anticonvulsants, as indicated in Table 23–12. Periodic neurologic reevaluation is important. Repeat EEGs are not needed to achieve seizure control. Indications for repeat EEGs are discussed earlier.

5. Long-term management—Continue anticonvulsant treatment until the patient is free of seizures for at least 1–2 years, or in some cases until the patient reaches adolescence. In about 75% of patients, seizures may not recur. Variables such as younger age at onset, normal EEG, and ease of controlling seizures carry a favorable prognosis, whereas later onset, epileptiform spikes on EEG, difficulty in controlling the seizures, polytherapy, generalized tonic-clonic or myoclonic seizures, and an abnormal neurologic examination are associated with a higher risk of recurrence.

6. Withdrawal of treatment—In general, there is no need to withdraw anticonvulsants before taking an EEG. Discontinue anticonvulsants gradually. If it becomes necessary to withdraw anticonvulsants abruptly, the patient should be under close medical surveillance. If seizures recur during or after withdrawal, anticonvulsant therapy should be reinstituted and again maintained for at least 1–2 years.

D. Blood Levels of Antiepileptic Drugs

1. General comments—Most anticonvulsants take two or three times the length of their half-life to reach the steady-state levels indicated in Table 23–12. This must be considered when blood levels are assessed after anticonvulsants are started or dosages are changed. Individuals vary in their metabolism and their particular pharmacokinetic characteristics. These and external factors, including, for example, food intake or illness, also affect the blood level. Thus the level reached on a milligram per kilogram basis varies among patients. Experience and clinical research in the determination of antiepileptic blood levels have shown that there is some correlation between (1) drug dose and blood level, (2) blood level and therapeutic effect, and (3) blood level and some toxic effects.

2. Effective levels—The ranges given in Table 23–12 are those within which seizure control without toxicity will be achieved in most patients. The level for any given individual will vary not only with metabolic makeup (including biochemical defects) but also with the nature and

Table 23–12. Guide to pediatric anticonvulsant drug therapy.[a]

Drug	Average Total Dosage (mg/kg/d)	Steady State	Effective Blood Levels[b]	Side Effects and Precautions	Directions and Remarks
Primary anticonvulsant					
Carbamazepine (Tegretol) (Carbatrol, Tegretol XR are sustained-release formulations)	15–25 mg/kg/d in 2–4 divided doses	3–6 d	4–12 µg/mL (> 15)	Dizziness, ataxia, diplopia, drowsiness, nausea, rash. *Rare:* hepatotoxicity, bone marrow depression, dystonia, inappropriate ADH secretion, bizarre behaviors, tics.	Monitor CBC, platelet count, liver function tests periodically. Blood effects usually early and transient. *Drug interactions:* ↑ by fluoxetine, propoxyphene, erythromycin, cimetidine; ↓ by felbamate, phenobarbital, phenytoin.
Valproic acid (Depakene, Depakote) (Depacon Extended-Release)	15–60 mg/kg/d in 2–4 divided doses	2–4 d	50–120 µg/mL (> 140)	Weight gain, occasional gastric discomfort, constipation. Tremor, hair loss in 5%. *Rare:* hepatotoxicity, hyperammonemia, leukopenia, polycystic ovaries (more toxic in infants younger than 2 years)	For prophylaxis in febrile convulsions, see text. Monitor CBC, platelets, liver function tests closely in first 6 months, then periodically. Can be given rectally (suspension: 250 mg/5 mL). Depacon is an IV preparation, 100 mg/mL. *Drug interactions:* ↓ by phenobarbital, phenytoin, carbamazepine, ↑ by lamotrigine, felbamate.
Phenytoin (Dilantin)	5–10 mg/kg/d in 1 or 2 doses	5–10 d	5–20 µg/mL (> 25)	Gum hypertrophy, hirsutism, ataxia, nystagmus, diplopia, rash, anorexia, nausea, osteomalacia. *Rare:* macrocytic anemia, lymph node involvement, exfoliative dermatitis, peripheral neuropathy.	Good dental hygiene reduces gum hyperplasia. May aggravate absence and myoclonic seizures. Poorly absorbed by neonatal gut. Use 50 mg Infant tabs in infants (may be crushed to adjust dosage). Suspension not recommended. *Drug interactions:* ↑ by felbamate; ↓ by carbamazepine, phenobarbital, antacids.
Phenobarbital	3–5 mg/kg/d as single daily dose	10–21 d	15–40 µg/mL (> 45)	Irritability and overactivity in many children; sedative effects in others. Mild ataxia, depression, skin rash. May interfere with learning.	Overall, the safest drug. Bitter taste. Higher blood levels sometimes required and tolerated in severe chronic epileptics. Useful in neonatal seizures and status epilepticus. Valproate increases unbound phenobarbital levels.
Primidone (Mysoline)	10–25 mg/kg/d in 3 or 4 divided doses	1–5 d	4–12 µg/mL (> 15)	Drowsiness, ataxia, vertigo, anorexia, nausea, vomiting, rash. (Like phenobarbital.)	Start slowly with 25–35% of expected maintenance dose; useful in essential tremor.
Ethosuximide (Zarontin)	10–40 mg/kg/d in 1 or 2 doses	5–6 d	40–100 µg/mL (> 150)	Nausea, gastric discomfort, hiccups, blood dyscrasias.	May aggravate generalized seizures. Combine with valproic acid in refractory absence seizures.
Clonazepam (Klonopin)	0.01–0.1 mg/kg/dose	5–10 d	15–80 ng/mL (> 80)	Drowsiness (> 50%): soporific effects greatest drawback. Behavior problems in 25%. Slurred speech, ataxia, salivation.	Start slowly with 25% of expected maintenance dosage; increase every 2 or 3 d. Useful with refractory minor motor seizures (astatic, myoclonic, infantile spasms; absences). Tolerance may occur.

(continued)

Table 23–12. Guide to pediatric anticonvulsant drug therapy.[a] (continued)

Drug	Average Total Dosage (mg/kg/d)	Steady State	Effective Blood Levels[b]	Side Effects and Precautions	Directions and Remarks
Adjunctive or secondary drug					
Acetazolamide (Diamox)	5–20 mg/kg/d in 2 or 3 divided doses	1–2 d	10–14 µg/mL	Anorexia; numbness and tingling. Renal stones (rare).	Supplement to other medications, especially in absence and complex partial seizures. Catamenial seizures.
Levetiracetam (Keppra)	10–20 mg/kg/d to maximal 40–60 over 2–6 weeks	1–3 d	20–40 µg/mL	Personality change, irritability in 5–10%. Somnolence, dizziness, headache, asthenia.	Complex partial seizures, myoclonic. Little effect on other drugs.
Oxcarbazepine (Trileptal)	8–10 mg/kg/d initial, 20–50 mg/kg/d maint in 2 doses	1–3 d	MHD (breakdown product) 12–30 µg/mL	Dizziness, fatigue, somnolence, nausea, ataxia, headache, hyponatremia, rash	Partial seizures. Little effect on other drug levels. No need for lab (CBC, LFTs).
Felbamate (Felbatol)	15–45 mg/kg/d in 3 or 4 divided doses	5–7 d	22–137 µg/mL	Anorexia, vomiting, insomnia, headache, somnolence. Rash in 1%. Aplastic anemia and hepatic failure are significant hazards.	A dangerous drug. Used in children with Lennox-Gastaut syndrome and other refractory epilepsies. Obtain informed consent. *Drug interactions:* ↓ by phenytoin, carbamazepine.
Vigabatrin (Sabril)	20–100 mg/kg/d in 2–3 divided doses	Not known	Not known	Drowsiness, confusion, weight gain, retinal changes, visual loss	Infantile spasms, especially tuberous sclerosis. Add-on drug for partial seizures. Not licensed by FDA in United States as of 1999.
Gabapentin (Neurontin) > 12 years	30–60 mg/kg/d in 3 divided doses (900–4800 mg total per day)	1–2 d	12–25 µg/mL	Drowsiness, dizziness, ataxia.	Add-on drug for partial seizures; no effect on other anticonvulsant drug levels.
Topiramate (Topamax)	Start 0.5–1 mg/kg/d to 10 mg/kg/d) in 2 divided doses (maximum, 400 mg/d)	Not known	8–25 µg/mL	Somnolence, slowed mentation, dizziness, language problems, kidney stones, anorexia, weight loss (rarely, metabolic acidosis).	Slow dose titration advisable. Minimal effect on other drug levels. Lennox–Gastaut, West syndrome. Broad-spectrum drug.
Tiagabine (Gabitril)	0.1–1.5 mg/kg/d in 2 divided doses	1–2 d	20–70 µg/mL	Dizziness, tremor, abnormal thinking	Adjunctive drug for partial seizures.
Zonisamide (Zonegran)	1–2 mg/kg/d to maximum 8–12 mg/kg/d in 1 or 2 divided doses	5–7 d	20–30 µg/mL	Drowsiness, anorexia, GI symptoms, weight loss, behavior changes, renal stones (0.2–2%), hypohidrosis, rash.	Broad-spectrum drug. A sulfonamide (don't use if allergic to sulfa drugs). Hazard: oligohydrosis-fever syndrome. Widely used in Japan.

(continued)

Table 23–12. Guide to pediatric anticonvulsant drug therapy.[a] (continued)

Drug	Average Total Dosage (mg/kg/d)	Steady State	Effective Blood Levels[b]	Side Effects and Precautions	Directions and Remarks
Lamotrigine (Lamictal)	5–15 mg/kg/d in 2 divided doses (1–5 mg/ kg if taking valproic acid); 5– 400 mg/d total	8–15 d	10–20 μg/mL	Dizziness, headaches, diplopia, ataxia, nausea. Rash in 5–10%. 1% Stevens-Johnson usually in first 4–8 wk.	Complex partial seizures, Lennox–Gastaut syndrome, absence seizures. Valproate increases drug half-life. Increase dose slowly over 2 mos.
Treatment of status epilepticus[a]					
Diazepam (Valium)	0.3 mg/kg IV. Repeat dose: 0.1–0.3 mg/kg IV.			Administer slowly. Monitor pulse and blood pressure. May cause respiratory depression in presence of phenobarbital.	May need to be repeated every 3–4 h. Follow with phenytoin or phenobarbital for long-range control. ***Note:*** Intramuscular administration for status epilepticus ineffective.
Phenobarbital	5–20 mg/kg IV initially. Repeat dose: 5–10 mg/kg IV.			See above.	In infancy, rule out pyridoxine dependency; load with 15–20 mg/kg IV.
Phenytoin (Dilantin); (Fosphenytoin, safer)	10–20 mg/kg IV initially. Repeat dose: 5–10 mg/kg IV.			Administer IV over a 5-min period. Administer fosphenytoin IM only if no IV access.	Adjunct in neonatal seizures (20 mg/kg IV) if phenobarbital alone fails.
Lorazepam (Ativan)	0.05–0.2 mg/kg IV. May repeat.			Mild respiratory depression.	May be more effective than diazepam. Longer-acting.
Midazolam (Versed)	0.1–0.2 mg/kg IM or IV; 0.2 mg/kg as nasal spray. IV drip 1–5++μg/kg/min			See other benzodiapines.	Short-acting. Many new favorable reports.
Valproate sodium (depacon)	5–60 mg/kg IV (20 mg/min). Depacon rapid injection form (see Table 23–9)			Administer slowly. Dizziness, nausea, and injection-site pain.	Half-life 16 h. Useful when child can't take valproate orally, or for status epilepticus

[a]Treatment of infantile spasms: See text regarding use of corticotropin or corticosteroids. See also clonazepam or valproic acid, especially with recurrences.

[b]In parentheses are shown the levels at which clinical toxicity becomes manifest in monotherapy.

ADH, antidiuretic hormone; CBC, complete blood count; IM, intramuscularly; IV, intravenously; MHD, mono hydroxy metabolite; LFT, liver function tests.

severity of the seizures and their underlying cause, and with other medications being taken, among other factors. Seizure control may be achieved at lower levels in some patients, and higher levels may be reached without toxicity in others. When control is achieved at a lower level, the dosage should not be increased merely to get the level into the therapeutic range. Likewise, toxic side effects will be experienced at different levels even within the therapeutic range. Lowering the dosage usually resolves the problem, but sometimes the drug must be withdrawn or another added (or both). Some serious toxic effects, including aller-

gic reactions and bone marrow or liver toxicity, are independent of dosage.

3. Interaction of antiepileptic drugs—Blood levels of anticonvulsants may be affected by other drugs. Individual variations occur; adjustment of dosages may be required. (See Table 23–12.)

4. Indications for determination of blood levels—Drug blood levels should be measured after a new drug is introduced and seizure control without toxicity is achieved to determine the effective level for that patient.

Blood level monitoring is useful also when expected control on a usual dosage has not been achieved either with a single drug or after adding another, when seizures recur in a patient with previously well-controlled seizures, or when control is poor in a patient taking anticonvulsants who is being seen for the first time. A low level may indicate inadequate dosage, drug interaction, or noncompliance with the prescribed regimen. A high level may indicate slowed metabolism or excretion or drug interaction.

Blood levels are mandatory when signs and symptoms of toxicity are present, especially when more than one drug is being used or when the dosage of a single drug has been changed. Blood levels may be the only means of detecting intoxication in a comatose patient or very young child. Toxic levels also occur with drug abuse and liver or renal disease. Blood levels of anticonvulsants are unnecessary when the patient's seizure control is satisfactory and he or she is free of toxic signs or symptoms.

E. SIDE EFFECTS OF ANTIEPILEPTIC DRUGS

(See also Table 23–12.)

1. Allergic reactions—Serious allergic reactions usually necessitate discontinuance of a drug. However, not every rash in a child receiving an anticonvulsant is drug-related. If a useful antiepileptic drug is discontinued and the rash disappears, restarting the drug in a smaller dosage may be warranted to see if the rash recurs.

2. Drug toxicity—Signs of drug toxicity often disappear when the daily dosage is reduced by 25–30%.

3. Avoiding sedation—The sedative effect of many of the anticonvulsants may be avoided by slowly working up to the usual therapeutic dose—for example, over 3–4 weeks for phenobarbital or topiramate.

4. Avoiding side effects—Gingival hyperplasia secondary to phenytoin is best minimized through good dental hygiene but occasionally requires gingivectomy. This condition may recede within about 6 months after the drug is discontinued. The hypertrichosis associated with phenytoin does not regress when the drug is discontinued.

F. ADRENOCORTICOTROPIC HORMONE AND CORTICOSTEROIDS

1. Indications—These drugs are indicated for infantile spasms not due to causes amenable to specific therapy and in the Lennox-Gastaut syndrome, which cannot be controlled by anticonvulsant drugs. Duration of therapy is guided by cessation of clinical seizures and normalization of the EEG. ACTH or oral corticosteroids are usually continued in full doses for 2 weeks and then, if seizures have ceased, tapered over 1 week. Others use

a total treatment period of about 2 months. If seizures recur, the dosage is increased to the last effective level and repeated for 2–4 weeks, or switching to or from prednisone is tried. Some clinicians keep the patient at this dosage for up to 6 months before attempting withdrawal. There is no strong evidence, however, that longer courses of treatment are more beneficial.

2. Dosages—

a. ACTH gel—Start with 2–4 units/kg/d intramuscularly in a single morning dose. Parents can be taught to give injections.

b. Prednisone—Start with 2–4 mg/kg/d orally in two or three divided doses.

3. Precautions—Give additional potassium, guard against infections, follow for possible hypertension, and discuss the cushingoid appearance and its disappearance. Do not withdraw oral corticosteroids suddenly. Side effects in some series occur in up to 40% of patients, especially with higher dosages than those listed here (used by some authorities). With long-term use, prophylaxis against *Pneumocystis* infection may be required.

G. KETOGENIC OR MEDIUM-CHAIN TRIGLYCERIDES

1. Diet in Treatment of Epilepsy—A ketogenic diet should be recommended in astatic and myoclonic seizures and absence seizures not responsive to drug therapy. It is occasionally recommended for infantile spasms that do not respond to ACTH or corticosteroids. Ketosis is induced by a diet high in fats and very limited in carbohydrates with sufficient protein for body maintenance and growth. The ratio of fat calories to carbohydrate calories may range from 2.5:1 up to 4:1. Adding medium-chain triglycerides to the diet induces ketosis more readily than does a high level of dietary fats and thus requires less carbohydrate restriction. The mechanism for the anticonvulsant action of the ketogenic diet is not understood. It is, however, the ketosis, not the acidosis, that raises the seizure threshold. The diet is most effective in children younger than age 8 years.

The ketogenic diet is difficult and expensive, tends to be monotonous, and depends on the caregiver's ability to weigh out the foods as well as on absolute adherence to the diet prescribed. Whether the ketosis is achieved by high-fat meals or by adding medium-chain triglycerides to the diet is often a matter of the physician's, the dietitian's, or the patient's preference. The result may also depend on which form of the diet is better tolerated. Full cooperation of all family members is required, including the patient if old enough. However, when seizure control is achieved by this method, the child is alert, he or she often needs no (or only small amounts of) anticonvulsants, and parental and patient satisfaction is most gratifying.

H. SURGERY

In seizure disorders intractable to anticonvulsant therapy and primarily of focal origin, neurosurgery should be considered. Useful procedures, depending on the lesion, include corticectomy, hemispherectomy, anterior temporal lobectomy (for complex partial seizures), callosotomy (or commissurotomy), and stereotactic ablation. Vagal nerve stimulation with an implanted electrode is another new, expensive surgical approach for intractable epilepsy.

Arts WF et al: Course and prognosis of childhood epilepsy: 5-year follow-up of the Dutch study of epilepsy in childhood. Brain 2004;127:1774 [PMID: 15201192].

Benbadis SR et al: Idiopathic generalized epilepsy and choice of antiepileptic drugs. Neurology 2003;61:1793 [PMID: 14694051].

Berg AT et al: How long does it take for partial epilepsy to become intractable? Neurology 2003;60:186 [PMID: 12552028].

Berg AT et al: Longitudinal assessment of adaptive behavior in infants and young children with newly diagnosed epilepsy: Influences of etiology, syndrome, and seizure control. Pediatrics 2004;114:645 [PMID: 15342834].

Berg AT et al: Status epilepticus after the initial diagnosis of epilepsy in children. Neurology 2004;63:1027 [PMID: 15452294].

Bourgeois BFD: Chronic management of seizures in the syndromes of idiopathic generalized epilepsy. Epilepsia 2003;44:27 [PMID: 12752459].

Brevoord JC et al: Status epilepticus: clinical analysis of a treatment protocol based on midazolam and phenytoin. J Child Neurol 2005;20:476 [PMID: 15996395].

Buchhalter JR, Jarrar RG: Therapeutics in pediatric epilepsy, Part 2: Epilepsy surgery and vagus nerve stimulation. Mayo Clin Proc 2003;78:371 [PMID: 12630591].

Camfield P, Camfield C: Childhood epilepsy: What is the evidence for what we think and what we do? J Child Neurol 2003; 18:272 [PMID: 12760431].

Caplan R et al: Depression and anxiety disorders in pediatric epilepsy. Epilepsia 2005;46:720 [PMID: 15857439].

Capovilla G et al: Short-term nonhormonal and nonsteroid treatment in West syndrome. Epilepsia 2003;44:1085 [PMID: 12887441].

Ceulemans BP et al: Clinical correlations of mutations in the SCN1A gene: from febrile seizures to severe myoclonic epilepsy in infancy. Pediatr Neurol 2004;30:236 [PMID: 15087100].

Chin RF et al: Meningitis is a common cause of convulsive status epilepticus with fever. Arch Dis Child 2005;90:66 [PMID: 15613516].

Daulin M et al: Reduction of seizures with low-dose clonazepam in children with epilepsy. Pediatr Neurol 2003;28:48 [PMID: 12657920].

Dooley JM, Hayden JD: Benign febrile myoclonus in childhood. Can J Neurol Sci 2004;31:504 [PMID: 15595256].

Freeman JM: Less testing is needed in the emergency room after a first afebrile seizure. Pediatrics 2003;111:194 [PMID: 12509575].

French JA et al: Efficacy and tolerability of the new antiepileptic drugs I: treatment of new onset epilepsy. Neurology 2004;62:1252 [PMID: 15111659].

French JA et al: Efficacy and tolerability of the new antiepileptic drugs II: treatment of refractory epilepsy. Neurology 2004;62:1261 [PMID: 15111660].

Goh S et al: Infantile spasms and intellectual outcomes in children with tuberous sclerosis complex. Neurology 2005;65:235 [PMID: 16043792].

Harbord MG et al: Use of intranasal midazolam to treat acute seizures in paediatric community settings. J Paediatr Child Health 2004;40:556 [PMID: 15367152].

Hermann B, Sheth R: Cognitive consequences of antiepilepsy medications in children. Neurology 2004;62:841.

Hawash KY, Rosman P: Do partial seizures predict an increased risk of seizure recurrence after antiepilepsy drugs are withdrawn? J Child Neurol 2003;18:331 [PMID: 12822817].

Hirtz D et al: Practice parameter: Evaluating a first nonfebrile seizure in children. Neurology 2000;55:616 [PMID: 10980722].

Hirtz D et al: Practice parameter: Treatment of the child with a first unprovoked seizure. Neurology 2003;60:166 [PMID: 12552027].

Jarrar RG, Buchhalter JR: Therapeutics in pediatric epilepsy, Part 1: The new antiepileptic drugs and the ketogenic diet. Mayo Clin Proc 2003;78:359 [PMID: 12630590].

Kanazawa O: Shuddering attacks—Report of four children. Pediatr Neurol 2000;23:421 [PMID: 11118798].

Kang HC et al: Early- and late-onset complications of the ketogenic diet for intractable epilepsy. Epilepsia 2004;45:1116 [PMID: 15329077].

Kim HL et al: Clinical experience with zonisamide monotherapy and adjunctive therapy in children with epilepsy at a tertiary care referral center. J Child Neurol 2005;20:212 [PMID: 15832611].

Kivity S et al: Long-term cognitive outcomes of a cohort of children with cryptogenic infantile spasms treated with high-dose adrenocorticotropic hormone. Epilepsia 2004;45:255 [PMID: 15009227].

Knudsen JF et al: Oligohydrosis and fever in pediatric patients treated with zonisamide. Pediatr Neurol 2003;28:184 [PMID: 12770670].

Kothare SV et al: Efficacy and tolerability of zonisamide in juvenile myoclonic epilepsy. Epileptic Disord 2004;6:267 [PMID: 15634623].

Kwan P, Brodie MJ: Pheobarbital for the treatment of epilepsy in the 21st century: a critical review. Epilepsia 2004;45:114 [PMID: 15329080].

Lagae L et al: Clinical experience with levetiracetam in childhood epilepsy: an add-on and mono-therapy trial. Seizure 2005; 14:66 [PMID: 15642504].

Mackay MT et al: Practice parameter: Medical treatment of infantile spasms. Neurology 2004;62:1668 [PMID: 15159460].

Majorie JF et al: Vagus nerve stimulation in patients with catastrophic childhood epilepsy, a 2-year follow-up study. Seizure 2005;14:10 [PMID: 15642494].

Mulley JC et al: Channelopathies as a genetic cause of epilepsy. Curr Opin Neurol 2003;16:171 [PMID: 12644745].

Nadkarni S et al: Current treatments of epilepsy. Neurology 2005; 64:S2.

Narchi H: Benign afebrile cluster convulsions with gastroenteritis: an observational study. BMC Pediatr 2004;5:2 [PMID: 15005806].

Okumura A et al: Unconsciousness and delirious behavior in children with febrile seizures. Pediatr Neurol 2004;30:316 [PMID: 1516532].

Ozdemir D et al: Efficacy of continuous midazolam infusion and mortality in childhood refractory generalized convulsive status epilepticus. Seizure 2005;14:129 [PMID: 15694567].

Papavasiliou A et al: Psychogenic status epilepticus in children. Epilepsy Behav 2004;5:539 [PMID: 15256192].

Posner EB et al: A systematic review of treatment of typical absence seizures in children and adolescents with ethosuximide, sodium valproate or lamotrigine. Seizure 2005;14:117 [PMID: 15694565].

Prasad A et al: Evolving antiepileptic drug treatment in juvenile myoclonic epilepsy. Arch Neurol 2003;60:1100 [PMID: 12925366].

Riikonen R: The latest on infantile spasms. Curr Opin Neurol 2005;18:91 [PMID: 15791136].

Sankar R: Initial treatment of epilepsy with antiepileptic drugs: pediatric issues. Neurology 2004;63:S30 [PMID: 15557549].

Sahin M et al: Prolonged treatment for acute symptomatic refractory status epilepticus. Neurology 2003;61:398 [PMID: 12913208].

Schor N et al: Treatment with propofol. The new status quo for status epilepticus? Neurology 2005;65:506 [PMID: 16116104].

Shahar E et al: Primary generalized epilepsy during infancy and early childhood. J Child Neurol 2004;19:170 [PMID: 15119477].

Sinclair DB: Prednisone therapy in pediatric epilepsy. Pediatr Neurol 2003;28:194 [PMID: 12770672].

Sullivan JE, Dlugos DJ: Idiopathic generalized epilepsy. Curr Treat Options Neurol 2004;6:231 [PMID: 15043806].

Tan M, Appleton R: Attention deficit and hyperactivity disorder, methylphenidate, and epilepsy. Arch Dis Child 2005;90:57 [15613514].

Than KD et al: Can you predict an immediate, complete, and sustained response to the ketogenic diet? Epilepsia 205;46:580 [PMID: 15816955].

Tromp SC et al: Relative influence of epileptic seizures and of epilepsy syndrome on cognitive function. J Child Neurol 2003;18:407 [PMID: 12886976].

Uneri A, Turkdogan D: Evaluation of vestibular functions in children with vertigo attacks. Arch Dis Child 2003;88:510 [PMID: 12765917].

van Gestel JPJ: Propofol and thiopental for refractory status epilepticus in children. Neurology 2005;65:591 [PMID: 16116121].

Verotti A et al: Intermittent oral diazepam prophylaxis in febrile convulsions: its effectiveness for febrile seizure recurrence. Eur J Paediatr Neurol 2004;8:131 [PMID: 15120684].

Vigevano F: Levetiracetam in pediatrics. J Child Neurol 2005;20:87 [PMID: 15794171].

Waruiru C, Appleton R: Febrile seizures: an update. Arch Dis Child 2004;89:751 [PMID: 15269077].

Watemburg N et al: Clinical experience with open-label topiramate use in infants younger than 2 years of age. J Child Neurol 2003;18:258 [PMID: 12760428].

Wheless JW et al: Topiramate, carbamazepine, and valproate monotherapy: double-blind comparison in children with newly diagnosed epilepsy. J Child Neurol 2005;19:135 [PMID: 15072107].

Wheless JW et al: Rapid infusion with valproate sodium is well tolerated in patients with epilepsy. J Child Neurol 2004;63:1507 [PMID: 15505177].

Wilfong AA: Zonisamide monotherapy for epilepsy in children and young adults. Pediatr Neurol 2005;32:77 [PMID: 15664764].

Wirrell EC: Valproic acid-associated weight gain in older children and teens with epilepsy. Pediatr Neurol 2003;28:126 [PMID: 12699863].

Yanagaki S et al: Zonisamide for West syndrome: a comparison of clinical responses among different titration rate. Brain Dev 2005;27:286 [PMID: 15862192].

Zupane ML: Neonatal seizures. Pediatr Clin North Am 2004;51:961 [PMID: 15275983].

SYNCOPE & FAINTING

Fainting is transient loss of consciousness and postural tone due to cerebral ischemia or anoxia. Up to 20–50% of children (age birth–20 years) will faint at some time. There may be a prodrome of dizziness, lightheadedness, nausea, so-called gray-out, sweating, and pallor. After falling, many children stiffen or have jerking motions when unconscious, a tonic-clonic, anoxic-ischemic seizure mimicking epilepsy. Watching or undergoing a venipuncture is a common precipitant of fainting, as is prolonged standing, fatigue, illness, overheating and sweating, dehydration, hunger, and athleticism with slow baseline pulse. The family history is positive for similar episodes in 90% of patients.

Classification

Ninety-five percent of cases of syncope are of the vasovagal-vasodepressive or neurocardiogenic type (Table 23–13). Vasodilation, cardiac slowing, and hypotension cause transient (1–2 minutes) cerebral ischemia and result in the patient passing out. The patient arouses in 1–2 minutes, but full recovery may take an hour or more. Besides those already listed, rare precipitants include hair grooming, cough, micturition, neck stretching, and emotional stress. More ominous is cardiac syncope, which often occurs during exercise. Angina or palpitations may occur. An obstructive lesion such as aortic stenosis, cardiomyopathy, coronary disease, or dysrhythmia may be the cause. Other spells that may mimic syncope are listed in Table 23–13.

Table 23–13. Classification of syncope in childhood.

Vasovagal, neurocardiogenic (neurally mediated)
  Orthostatic
  Athleticism
  Pallid breath-holding
  Situational (stress, blood drawing)
Cardiac
  Obstructive
  Arrhythmia
  Prolonged QTc
  Hypercyanotic (eg, in tetralogy of Fallot)
Nonsyncope mimicker
  Migraine with confusion or stupor
  Seizure
  Hypoglycemia
  Hysteria
  Hyperventilation
  Vertigo

Clinical Findings

A. SYMPTOMS AND SIGNS

The work-up of fainting includes a personal and a detailed family history, and a physical examination with emphasis on blood pressure and cardiac and neurologic features. In the adolescent, a blood pressure drop of more than 30 mm Hg after standing for 5–10 minutes or a baseline systolic pressure of less than 80 mm Hg suggests orthostasis.

B. LABORATORY FINDINGS AND IMAGING

Hemoglobin should be checked if anemia is suggested by the history. Electrocardiography should be done. Consider cardiology referral, Holter monitoring, and echocardiography if cardiac causes seem likely. Tilt testing (though norms are vague) may have a role in frequent recurrent syncope to confirm a vasodepressor cause and avoid more expensive diagnostic investigations.

Treatment

Treatment consists mostly of giving advice about the benign nature of fainting and about avoiding precipitating situations. The patient should be cautioned to lie down if prodromal symptoms occur. Good hydration and reasonable salt intake are advisable. In some cases β-blockers and rarely fludrocortisone may have a role.

Allan WC, Gospe SM Jr: Seizures, syncope, or breath-holding presenting to the pediatric neurologist—when is the etiology a life-threatening arrhythmia? Semin Pediatr Neurol 2005;12:2 [PMID: 15929459].

Britton JW: Syncope and seizures—differential diagnosis and evaluation. Clin Auton Res 2004;14:148 [PMID: 15241643].

DiVasta AD, Alexander ME: Fainting freshmen and sinking sophomores: cardiovascular issues of the adolescent. Curr Opin Pediatr 2004;16:350 [PMID: 15273492].

Narchi H: The child who passes out. Pediatr Rev 2000;21:384 [PMID: 11077022].

Sateriades ES et al: Incidence and prognosis of syncope. N Engl J Med 2002;347:878 [PMID: 12239256].

HEADACHES

Headache is one of the most common complaints in pediatric neurology clinics, accounting for 25–30% of all referrals. Epidemiologic studies indicate that headache occurs in 37% of children by age 7 years and in 69% of children by age 14 years. Migraine headache occurs in 5% and 15%, respectively, of children at these ages. Successful treatment requires an accurate diagnosis and proper classification of headache. Based on the patient's history, a simplified initial categorization as summarized in Table 23–14 can be made. A more exhaustive classification scheme has been developed by the International Headache Society and modified for use in children. Muscle contraction tension headaches are common in older children and adolescents. They are frequently generalized over the head with a "hat band" pressure or squeezing quality. Although appetite may be diminished, nausea and vomiting are usually not present. Symptoms specifically referable to the CNS are absent. If this type of headache becomes very frequent (three or more days per week) consideration should be given to drug (analgesic) overuse or misuse, depression, or sleep disorder. The neurologic examination is normal, neuroimaging tests are generally not needed, and treatment is judicious use of ibuprofen with or without a limited trial of amitriptyline. If simple measures are not satisfactory, biofeedback may be useful.

Table 23–14. Differential features of headaches in children.

	Muscle Contraction (Tension/Psychogenic)	Vascular (Migraine)	Traction and Inflammatory (Increased Intracranial Pressure)
Time course	Chronic, recurrent	Acute, paroxysmal, recurrent	Chronic or intermittent but increasingly frequent; progressive severity
Prodromes	No	Yes (sometimes in children)	No
Description	Diffuse, band-like, tight	Intense, pulsatile, unilateral in older child (70%); usually forehead in or behind one or both eyes.	Diffuse; more occipital with infratentorial mass, more frontal with supratentorial mass
Characteristic findings	Feelings of inadequacy, depression, or anxiety	Neurologic symptoms and signs usually transient	Positive neurologic signs, especially papilledema
Predisposing factors	Problems at home or school or socially (sexually)	Positive family history (75%); trivial head trauma may precipitate	None

Between 65% and 75% of children referred to neurology clinics for consultation regarding headaches have migraine. Many of these children are referred after they have seen ophthalmologists for "eye strain" or otolaryngologists to rule out sinusitis. Approximately 30% of children are referred after already undergoing one or more neuroimaging tests, the vast majority of which are normal.

Clinical Findings

The diagnosis and proper classification of migraine depends primarily on a thorough and detailed history (Table 23–15). Migraine headaches are paroxysmal, recurrent events separated by symptom-free intervals in a child with normal growth and development and whose neurologic examination is normal. Migraine affects children of all ages but is difficult to diagnose before age 4 years. The family history is positive for vascular, migrainous headaches in 75% of patients. The headaches have a pulsatile quality and are located unilaterally or bilaterally in the frontal or temporal regions, or commonly in the retro-orbital and cheek regions. The headaches last from 2 to more than 24 hours. A nonspecific prodrome of decreased or increased appetite and change in mood and temperament may precede the headache by hours or days. Headaches may be triggered by specific foods, minor head injuries, sleep deprivation, or irregular eating patterns, but more often no precipitant can be identified. An aura such as visual scotomata is uncommon in children. The headache is frequently accompanied by nausea, vomiting, photophobia, sensitivity to sound, vertigo, lightheadedness, fatigue, and mood alterations. Occasionally children may have loss of speech, hemiparesis, ataxia, confusional states, and bizarre visual distortions (so-called Alice in Wonderland syndrome). Very young children may experience recurrent or cyclical vomiting, abdominal pain, or recurrent self-limited bouts of ataxia or vertigo as the early manifestations of migraine.

Occasionally the frequency of migraine may spontaneously increase and become almost daily, a condition referred to as transformed migraine. When this change in frequency happens, it should at least raise suspicion of medication overuse with development of rebound headache; successful treatment requires medication withdrawal for 6–12 weeks or longer.

In contrast to tension and migraine headaches, headaches caused by intracranial disorders or increased intracranial pressure rarely occur in children who are otherwise healthy and well and who have completely normal examinations.

Laboratory studies and neuroimaging tests are rarely needed if a thorough history has been taken and the neurologic examination is normal. If the progression of headache is atypical for migraine or tension-type headaches or if the neurologic examination is abnormal, an MRI scan should be considered. When papilledema is present but the MRI is normal, a lumbar puncture may be needed to diagnose pseudotumor cerebri.

Treatment

Successful treatment of migraine is usually achieved with the systematic use of simple analgesics such as ibuprofen. The key to successful results is to take enough early enough to do the job. As soon as possible after the headache starts, the child is given ibuprofen 10 mg/kg followed

Table 23–15. Proposed revised IHS classification.

Pediatric Migraine without Aura (Common)	Pediatric Migraine with Aura[a] (Rare)
Diagnostic Criteria	**Diagnostic Criteria**
A. At least five attacks fulfilling B-D	A. At least two attacks fulfilling B
B. Headache attack lasting 1-48 hours	B. At least three of the following:
C. Headache has at least two of the following:	1. One or more fully reversible aura aymptoms indicating focal cortical and/or brainstem dysfunction
1. Bilateral location (frontal/temporal) or unilateral location	2. At least one aura developing gradually over more than 4 minutes or 2 or more symptoms occurring in succession
2. Pulsating quality	3. No auras lasting more than 60 minutes
3. Moderate to severe intensity	4. Headache follows in less than 60 minutes
4. Aggravation by routine physical acitivity	
D. During headache, at least one of the following	
1. Nausea and/or vomiting	
2. Photophobia and/or phonophobia	

[a]Idiopathic recurring disorder; headache usually lasts 1–48 hours.
IHS, International Headache Society.
Adapted, with permission, from: Winner P et al: Classification of pediatric migraine: proposed revisions of the IHS criteria. Headache 1995;35:407.

in 45 minutes by 5 mg/kg if needed. Additional doses of analgesics rarely provide additional benefit. The addition of 40–65 mg of caffeine, caffeine-ergotamine combinations, or 65 mg of isometheptene (Midrin) to ibuprofen may provide more reliable relief for some patients. Nausea and vomiting can be treated with metoclopramide, taken 10–20 minutes before other medications. For frequently recurring migraine, prophylaxis with propranolol, amitriptyline, cyproheptadine, valproate, or calcium channel blockers should be considered. At this time experience with using triptan and dihydroergotamine (nasal spray) in young children is limited; in teens, studies show sumatriptan, rizatriptan, naratriptan, and dihydroergotamine to be effective. Biofeedback, relaxation therapy, and other non-pharmacologic approaches to managing headache may be useful in children, and they provide an alternative method of treatment that avoids medication-related side effects.

Allen KD: Using biofeedback to make childhood headaches less of a pain. Pediatr Ann 2004;33:241 [PMID: 15101230].

Andrasik F et al: Brief neurologist-administered behavioral treatment of pediatric episodic tension-type headache. Neurology 2003;60:1215 [PMID: 12682344].

Anttila P: Tension-type headache in children and adolescents. Curr Pain Headache Rep 2004;8:500 [PMID: 15509465].

Curran MP et al: Intranasal sumatriptan: in adolescents with migraine. CNS Drugs 2005;19:335 [PMID: 15813647].

Damen L et al: Symptomatic treatment of migraine in children: A systematic review of medication trials. Pediatrics 2005;116:e295 [PMID: 16061583].

Just U et al: Emotional and behavioral problems in children and adolescents with primary headache. Cephalalgia 2003;23:206 [PMID: 12662188].

Kondev L, Minster A: Headache and facial pain in children and adolescents. Otolaryngol Clin North Am 2003;36:1153 [PMID: 15025014].

Lewis D et al: Practice parameter: pharmacological treatment of migraine headache in children and adolescents. Neurology 2004; 28:2215 [PMID: 15623677].

Millichap JG, Yee MM: The diet factor in pediatric and adolescent migraine. Pediatr Neurol 2003;28:9 [PMID: 12657413].

Termine C et al: Alternative therapies in the treatment of headache in childhood, adolescence and adulthood. Funct Neurol 2005;20:9 [PMID: 15948561].

Victor S, Ryan SW: Drugs for preventing migraine headaches in children. Cochrane Database Syst Rev 2003;4:CD002761 [PMID: 14583952].

Virtanen R et al: Externalizing problem behaviors and headache: A follow-up study of adolescent Finnish twins. Pediatrics 2004p; 114:981 [PMID: 15466094].

SLEEP DISORDERS

1. Sleep Apnea Syndrome in Older Children

Sleep apnea syndrome should be considered if there is a history of restless sleep with snoring or respiratory noise during sleep and frequent awakenings in an older child who shows poor school performance associated with excessive daytime sleepiness or irritability and hyperactivity. Children with these problems frequently have hypertrophied tonsils or adenoids, causing partial airway obstruction. Sleep apnea may be associated with facial dysmorphism; neuromuscular disorders with poor pharyngeal muscle control; and conditions with swelling of soft tissue in the pharynx and neck such as myxedema, Hodgkin disease, and massive obesity (pickwickian syndrome). Evaluation includes soft tissue radiographs of the lateral neck; chest radiograph; electrocardiogram (ECG) to rule out cardiomegaly, sinus dysrhythmias, and right-sided heart failure; arterial blood gas determinations while awake and during sleep; and polysomnography. Therapy is generally surgical, ranging from tonsillectomy and adenoidectomy when appropriate, to tracheostomy when medical measures fail.

2. Narcolepsy

Narcolepsy, a primary disorder of sleep, is characterized by chronic, excessive daytime sleeping that occurs regardless of activity or surroundings and is not relieved by increased sleep at night. Onset occurs as early as age 3 years. Of children with narcolepsy, 18% are younger than age 10, and 60% are between puberty and their late teens. Narcolepsy usually interferes severely with normal living. Months to years after onset, there may also be cataplexy (transient partial or total loss of muscle tone, often triggered by laughter, anger, or other emotional upsurge), hypnagogic hallucinations (visual or auditory), and sensations of paralysis on falling asleep. Studies have shown that rapid eye movement (REM) sleep, with loss of muscle tone and an EEG low-amplitude mixed frequency pattern, occurs soon after sleep onset in patients with cataplexy, whereas normal subjects experience 80–100 minutes or longer of non-REM (NREM) sleep before the initial REM period.

Recent research suggests absence of a hypothalamic neuropeptide, hypocretin (genetic? or from autoimmune injury?), causes narcolepsy and cataplexy. Spinal fluid (but not plasma) levels of hypocretin-1 (also called orexin) are diagnostic (level will be zero). The condition persists throughout life.

Modafinil is a new effective treatment for narcolepsy or excessive daytime sleepiness. Other CNS stimulants may have a role. Amphetamine mixtures (Adderall) or long-acting methylphenidate are examples. Cataplexy responds to venlafaxine, fluoxetine, or clomipramine. Rarely, acute narcolepsy/cataplexy (autoimmune) responds to intravenous immune globulin (IVIg).

3. Somnambulism

Somnambulism is one of a group of sleep disturbances known as disorders of arousal. The onset is abrupt, usually early in the night. It is characterized by coordinated activity (eg, walking and sometimes moving objects seemingly without purpose) in a state of veiled consciousness. The episode is relatively brief and ceases spontaneously. There is poor recall of the event on waking in the morning. Somnambulism may be related to mental activities occurring in stages 3 and 4 of NREM sleep. Incidence has been estimated at only 2–3%, but up to 15% of cases are reported in children age 6–16 years. Boys are affected more often than girls, and many have recurrent episodes. Psychopathologic features are rarely demonstrated, but a strong association (30%) between childhood migraine and somnambulism has been noted. Episodes of somnambulism may be triggered in predisposed children by stresses, including febrile illnesses. No treatment of somnambulism is required, and it is not necessary to seek psychiatric consultation.

4. Night Terrors

Night terrors (pavor nocturnus) are a disorder of arousal from NREM sleep. Most cases occur in children age 3–8 years, and the disorder rarely occurs after adolescence. It is characterized by sudden (but only partial) waking, with the severely frightened child unable to be fully roused or comforted. Concomitant autonomic symptoms include rapid breathing, tachycardia, and perspiring. The child has no recall of any nightmare. Psychopathologic mechanisms are unclear, but falling asleep after watching scenes of violence on television or hearing frightening stories may play a role. Elimination of such causes and administration of a mild antianxiety agent such as chlordiazepoxide may be helpful. It is important to differentiate these episodes from complex partial (psychomotor) seizures. (See also Chapter 2.)

Arii J et al: DSF hypocretin-1 (orexin-A) levels in childhood narcolepsy and neurologic disorders. Neurology 2004;63:2440 [PMID: 15623725].

Dauvilliers Y et al: A narcolepsy susceptibility locus maps to a 5 Mb region of chromosome 21q. Ann Neurol 2004;56:382 [PMID: 15349865].

Dauvilliers Y et al: Successful management of cataplexy with intravenous immunoglobulins at narcolepsy onset. Ann Neurol 2004;56:905 [PMID: 15562415].

Ivanenko A et al: Modafinil in the treatment of excessive daytime sleepiness in children. Sleep Med 2003;4:579 [PMID: 14607353].

Kotagal S et al: A putative link between childhood narcolepsy and obesity. Sleep Med 2004;5:147 [PMID: 15033134].

Kotagal S: Sleep disorders in childhood. Neurol Clin 2003;21:961 [PMID: 14743660].

Lecendreux M et al: Clinical efficacy of high-dose intravenous immunoglobulins near the onset of narcolepsy in a 10-year-old boy. J Sleep Res 2003;12:347 [PMID: 14633248].

Macleod S et al: Symptoms of narcolepsy in children misinterpreted as epilepsy. Epileptic Disord 2005;7:13 [PMID: 15741135].

Scammell TE: The neurobiology, diagnosis, and treatment of narcolepsy. Ann Neurol 2003;53:154 [PMID: 12557281].

PSEUDOTUMOR CEREBRI

Pseudotumor cerebri is characterized by increased intracranial pressure in the absence of an identifiable intracranial mass or hydrocephalus. An obese teenage girl (or adult) is the typical phenotype. Symptoms are headache, tinnitus, and visual loss; signs are those of increased intracranial pressure as outlined in Table 23–16. The cause is usually unknown, but pseudotumor cerebri has been described in association with a variety of inflammatory, metabolic, toxic, and connective tissue disorders (Table 23–17). The diagnosis of pseudotumor cerebri is one of exclusion. MRI scan of the head is needed to exclude hydrocephalus and intracranial masses. This study demonstrates ventricles of small or normal size but no other structural abnormalities. Venous thrombosis, an underrecognized cause, must be ruled out by magnetic resonance venogram or even injected venograms of cerebral sinuses. Lumbar puncture should be performed to document elevated CSF pressure. Examination of CSF reveals normal findings except for elevated pressure. In some inflammatory and connective tissue diseases, however, the CSF protein concentration may be increased.

Treatment of pseudotumor cerebri is aimed at correcting the identifiable predisposing condition. In addition, some patients may benefit from the use of furosemide or acetazolamide to decrease the volume and pressure of CSF within the CNS. These drugs may be used in combination with repeated lumbar punctures to remove CSF. If a program of repeated CSF removal and medical management is not successful or if central

Table 23–16. Signs of increased intracranial pressure.

Acute, Subacute
Macrocephaly
Excessive rate of head growth
Altered behavior
Decreased level of consciousness
Vomiting
Blurred vision
Double vision
Optic disc swelling
Abducens nerve paresis
Chronic
Macrocephaly
Growth impairment
Developmental delay
Optic atrophy
Visual field loss

Table 23–17. Conditions associated with pseudotumor cerebri.

Metabolic-toxic disorders
  Hypervitaminosis A
  Hypovitaminosis A
  Prolonged steroid therapy
  Steroid withdrawal
  Tetracycline therapy
  Nalidixic acid therapy
  Iron deficiency
  Lead poisoning
  Hypocalcemia
  Hyperparathyroidism
  Adrenal insufficiency
  Systemic lupus erythematosus
  Chronic CO_2 retention
Infectious and parainfectious disorders
  Chronic otitis media
    (Lateral sinus thrombosis)
  Guillain-Barré syndrome
Dural sinus thrombosis
Minor head injury

---

vision or visual field loss is detected despite these measures, lumboperitoneal or ventriculoperitoneal shunt or optic nerve fenestration may be necessary to prevent irreparable visual loss and damage to the optic nerves.

Bynke G et al: Ventriculoperitoneal shunting for idiopathic intracranial hypertension. Neurology 2004;63:1314 [PMID: 15477563].

Lim M et al: Visual failure without headache in idiopathic intracranial hypertension. Arch Dis Child 2005;90:206 [PMID: 15665183].

Rajpal S et al: Transverse venous sinus stent placement as treatment for benign intracranial hypertension in a young male: case report and review of the literature. J Neurosurg 2005;102:342 [PMID: 15881764].

Said RR, Rosman NP: A negative cranial computed tomographic scan is not adequate to support a diagnosis of pseudotumor cerebri. J Child Neurol 2004;19:609 [PMID: 15605471].

Sylaja PN et al: Differential diagnosis of patients with intracranial sinus venous thrombosis related isolated intracranial hypertension from those with idiopathic intracranial hypertension. J Neurol Sci 2003;215:9 [PMID: 14568121].

Tabassi A et al: Serum and CSF vitamin A concentrations in idiopathic intracranial hypertension Neurology 2005;64:1893 [PMID: 15955940].

CEREBROVASCULAR DISEASE

Childhood stroke is emerging as a serious and increasingly recognized disorder, affecting two to eight out of every 100,000 children. There are numerous adverse outcomes which include death in 10%, neurologic deficits or seizures in 60–80%, and recurrent strokes in 20–35%.

The initial approach to the patient should recognize that childhood stroke represents a neurologic emergency, for which promptness in diagnosis can affect treatment considerations and outcome. Unfortunately, most pediatric stroke is not recognized until 24–36 hours after onset, when treatment considerations matter most. When possible, all children who present with stroke should be transferred to a tertiary care center that specializes in pediatric stroke management. The evaluation should include a thorough history of prior illnesses, especially those associated with varicella (even in the prior 1–2 years), *Mycoplasma*, human immunodeficiency virus (HIV), minor trauma to the head and neck, and familial clotting tendencies. A systematic search for evidence of cardiac, vascular, hematologic, or intracranial disorders should be undertaken (Table 23–18). Though many strokes are not associated with a single underlying systemic disorder, previously diagnosed congenital heart disease followed by hematologic and neoplastic disorders are the most common predisposing illnesses. In many instances the origin is multifactorial, necessitating a thorough investigation even when the cause may seem obvious. As a result, the cause of childhood stroke is increasingly determined, whereas in past studies up to 30% remained idiopathic. This is particularly important when considering that recurrence risk may be as high as 35%.

Clinical Findings

A. SYMPTOMS AND SIGNS

Manifestations of stroke in childhood vary according to the vascular distribution to the brain structure that is involved. Because many conditions leading to childhood stroke result in emboli, multifocal neurologic involvement is common. Children may present with acute hemiplegia similarly to stroke in adults. Symptoms of unilateral weakness, sensory disturbance, dysarthria, and dysphagia may develop over a period of minutes, but at times progressive worsening of symptoms may evolve over several hours. Bilateral hemispheric involvement may lead to a depressed level of consciousness. The patient may also demonstrate disturbances of mood and behavior and experience focal or multifocal seizures. Physical examination of the patient is aimed not only at identifying the specific deficits related to impaired cerebral blood flow, but also at seeking evidence for any predisposing disorder. Retinal hemorrhages, splinter hemorrhages in the nail beds, cardiac murmurs, rash, neurocutaneous stigmata, and signs of trauma are especially important findings.

B. LABORATORY FINDINGS AND ANCILLARY TESTING

In the acute phase, certain investigations should be carried out emergently with consideration of treatment options. This should include complete blood count, erythrocyte

Table 23–18. Etiologic risk factors for stroke in children.

Cardiac disorders
   Cyanotic heart disease
   Valvular disease
      Rheumatic
      Endocarditis
   Cardiomyopathy
   Cardiac dysrhythmia
Vascular occlusive disorders
   Arterial trauma (carotid dissections)
   Homocystinuria/homocysteinemia
   Vasculitis
      Meningitis
      Polyarteritis nodosa
      Systemic lupus erythematosus
      Drug abuse (amphetamines)
   Varicella
   Mycoplasma
   Human immunodeficiency virus
   Fibromuscular dysplasia
   Moyamoya disease
   Diabetes
   Nephrotic syndrome
   Systemic hypertension
   Dural sinus and cerebral venous thrombosis
   Cortical venous thrombosis
Hematologic disorders
   Iron deficiency anemia
   Polycythemia
   Thrombotic thrombocytopenia
   Thrombocytopenic purpura
   Hemoglobinopathies
      Sickle cell disease
   Coagulation defects
      Hemophilia
      Vitamin K deficiency
   Hypercoagulable states
      Prothrombin gene mutation
      Lipoprotein (a)
      Factor V Leiden
      Antiphospholipid antibodies
      Hypercholesterolemia
      Hypertriglyceridemia
      Factor VIII deficiency
      Pregnancy
      Systemic lupus erythematosus
      Use of oral contraceptives
      Antithrombin III deficiency
      Protein C and S deficiencies
   Leukemia
Intracranial vascular anomalies
   Arteriovenous malformation
   Arterial aneurysm
   Carotid-cavernous fistula

---

sedimentation rate, basic chemistries, blood urea nitrogen, creatinine, prothrombin time/partial thromboplastin time, chest radiograph, ECG, urine toxicology, and imaging (see following section). Subsequent studies can be carried out systemically, with particular attention paid to disorders involving the heart, blood vessels, platelets, red cells, hemoglobin, and coagulation proteins. Twenty to fifty percent of all pediatric stroke patients will have a prothrombotic state. Additional laboratory tests for systemic disorders such as vasculitis, mitochondrial disorders, and metabolic disorders are sometimes indicated. Neonatal infarctions require pathologic examination of the placenta.

Examination of CSF is indicated in patients with fever, nuchal rigidity, or obtundation when the diagnosis of intracranial infection requires exclusion. Lumbar puncture may be deferred until a neuroimaging scan (excluding brain abscess or a space-occupying lesion that might contraindicate lumbar puncture) has been obtained. In the absence of infection and frank intracranial subarachnoid hemorrhage, CSF examination is rarely helpful in defining the cause of the cerebrovascular disorder.

When seizures are prominent, an EEG may be used as an adjunct in the patient's evaluation. An EEG and sequential EEG monitoring may help in patients with severely depressed consciousness.

ECG and echocardiography are useful both in the diagnostic approach to the patient and in ongoing monitoring and management, particularly when hypotension or cardiac arrhythmias complicate the clinical course.

C. IMAGING

CT and MRI scans of the brain are often helpful in defining the extent of cerebral involvement with ischemia or hemorrhage. CT scans may be normal within the first 12–24 hours of an ischemic stroke and may need to be repeated several hours later. A CT scan early after the onset of neurologic deficits is valuable in excluding intracranial hemorrhage. This information may be helpful in the early stages of management and in the decision to treat with anticoagulants. State-of-the-art management of stroke in the adult population omits CT scanning but proceeds directly to urgent MRI, MRA, and diffusion-weighted imaging since these modalities are sensitive to acute stroke in the initial 3 hours, when intravenous thrombolytics might be indicated. In consideration of venous occlusion either CT scan with contrast or magnetic resonance venogram is indicated.

Except in cases in which trauma resulting in arterial dissection is suspected, cerebral angiography or MRA is usually not urgently needed but may be needed to diagnose disorders such as moya-moya disease, dissecting aneurysm, aneurysm, fibromuscular dysplasia, and cerebral arteritis. If vessel imaging is performed, all major vessels should be studied from the aortic arch. If evidence of fibromuscular dysplasia is present in the intracranial or extracranial vessels, renal arteriography is indicated. In studies in which both MRA or cerebral angiography have been used, nearly 80% of patients with ischemic stroke demonstrated a cerebrovascular abnormality.

Differential Diagnosis

Patients with an acute onset of neurologic deficits must be evaluated for other disorders that can cause focal neurologic deficits. Hypoglycemia, prolonged focal seizures, a prolonged postictal paresis (Todd paralysis), acute disseminated encephalomyelitis, meningitis, encephalitis, and brain abscess should all be considered. Migraine with focal neurologic deficits may be difficult to differentiate initially from ischemic stroke. Occasionally the onset of a neurodegenerative disorder (eg, adrenoleukodystrophy or mitochondrial disorder) may begin with the abrupt onset of seizures and focal neurologic deficits. The possibility of drug abuse (particularly cocaine) and other toxic exposures must be investigated diligently in any patient with acute mental status changes.

Treatment

The initial management of stroke in a child is aimed at providing support for pulmonary, cardiovascular, and renal function. Patients should be administered oxygen. Typically, maintenance fluids without added glucose are indicated to augment vascular volume. Specific treatment of stroke, including blood pressure management, fluid management, and anticoagulation measures, depends partly on the underlying pathogenesis. Sickle cell patients require specialists in hematology to perform urgent exchange transfusion. In most other cases of childhood stroke without hemorrhage, aspirin 2–5 mg/kg daily is indicated as soon as the diagnosis is made. Aspirin use appears safe and has not been associated with Reye syndrome in pediatric stroke patients. In some situations, emergent heparinization for arterial dissection, stuttering stroke, emboli, and consumptive coagulopathies is indicated. In adults with cerebrovascular thrombosis, thrombolytic agents (tissue plasminogen activator) used systemically or delivered directly to a vascular thrombotic lesion using interventional radiologic techniques has been shown to improve outcome; although case reports exist, studies in children have not been completed.

Long-term management requires intensive rehabilitation efforts and therapy aimed at improving the child's language, educational, and psychological performance. Length of treatment with various agents, such as low-molecular-weight heparin and aspirin, is still being studied and depends on the etiology. Multidisci-plinary stroke teams are the best resource for making these decisions.

Prognosis

The outcome of stroke in infants and children is variable. Roughly 40% may have minimal deficits, 30% are moderately affected, and 30% are severely affected. Underlying predisposing conditions and the vascular territory involved all play a role in dictating the outcome for an individual patient. When the stroke involves extremely large portions of one hemisphere or large portions of both hemispheres and cerebral edema develops, the patient's level of consciousness may deteriorate rapidly, and death may occur within the first few days. Some patients may achieve almost complete recovery of neurologic function within several days if the cerebral territory is small. Seizures, either focal or generalized, may occur in 30–50% of patients at some point in the course of their cerebrovascular disorder. Recurrence is 20–35%, and is more prominent in some conditions, such as protein C deficiency and lipoprotein (a) abnormalities. Chronic problems with learning, behavior, and activity are common. Long-term follow-up with a multidisciplinary stroke team is indicated.

Barnes C et al: Arterial ischaemic stroke in children. J Paediatr Child Health 2004;40:384 [PMID: 15228568].

Barnes C et al: Prothrombotic abnormalities in childhood ischaemic stroke. Thromb Res 2005;1 [PMID: 16039697].

deVeber G: Arterial ischemic strokes in infants and children: an overview of current approaches. Semin Thromb Hemost 2003;29: 567 [PMID: 14719173].

deVeber G: In pursuit of evidence-based treatments for paediatric stroke: the UK and Chest guidelines. Lancet Neurol 2005; 7:432 [PMID: 15963446].

Duran R et al: Factor V Leiden mutation and other thrombophilia markers in childhood ischemic stroke. Clinical and applied thrombosis/hemostasis. Clin Appl Thromb Hemost 2005;11:83 [PMID: 15678277].

Friefeld S et al: Health-related quality of life and its relationship to neurological outcome in child survivors of stroke. CNS Spectr 2004;6:465 [PMID: 15162094].

Gabis LV et al: Time lag to diagnosis of stroke in children. Pediatrics 2002;110:924 [PMID: 12415031].

Ganesan V et al: Clinical guidelines for the management of childhood stroke. Hosp Med 2005;1:4 [PMID: 15686158].

Ganesan V et al: Investigation of risk factors in children with arterial ischemic stroke. Ann Neurol 2003;53:167 [PMID: 12557282].

Gruber A et al: Intra-arterial thrombolysis for the treatment of perioperative childhood cardioembolic stroke. Neurology 2000;54: 1684 [PMID: 10762516].

Husson B et al: Magnetic resonance angiography in childhood arterial brain infarcts: A comparative study with contrast angiography. Stroke 2002;33:1280 [PMID: 11988604].

Monagle et al: Antithrombotic therapy in children: The seventh ACCP conference on antithrombotic and thrombolytic therapy. Chest 2004;126:645 [PMID: 15383489].

Zahuranec DB et al: Is it time for a large, collaborative study of pediatric stroke? Stroke 2005;36:1825 [PMID: 16100029].

CONGENITAL MALFORMATIONS OF THE NERVOUS SYSTEM

Malformations of the nervous system occur in 1–3% of living neonates and are present in 40% of infants who die. Developmental anomalies of the CNS may result from a variety of causes, including infectious, toxic, metabolic, and vascular insults that affect the fetus. The specific type of malformation that results from such insults, however, may depend more on the gestational period during which the insult occurs than on the specific cause. The period of induction, days 0–28 of gestation, is the period during which the neural plate appears and the neural tube forms and closes. Insults during this phase can result in a major absence of neural structures, such as anencephaly, or in a defect of neural tube closure, such as spina bifida, meningomyelocele, or encephalocele. Cellular proliferation and migration characterize neural development that occurs after 28 days' gestation. Lissencephaly, pachygyria, agyria, and agenesis of the corpus callosum may be the result of disruptions (genetic, toxic, infectious, or metabolic) that can occur during the period of cellular proliferation and migration.

1. Abnormalities of Neural Tube Closure

Defects of neural tube closure constitute some of the most common congenital malformations affecting the nervous system. Spina bifida with associated meningomyelocele or meningocele is commonly found in the lumbar region. Depending on the extent and severity of the involvement of the spinal cord and peripheral nerves, lower extremity weakness, bowel and bladder dysfunction, and hip dislocation may be present. Delivery via cesarean section followed by early surgical closure of meningoceles and meningomyeloceles is usually indicated. Additional treatment is necessary to manage chronic abnormalities of the urinary tract, orthopedic abnormalities such as kyphosis and scoliosis, and paresis of the lower extremities. Hydrocephalus associated with meningomyelocele usually requires ventriculoperitoneal shunting.

Arnold-Chiari Malformations

Arnold-Chiari malformation type I consists of elongation and displacement of the caudal end of the brainstem into the spinal canal with protrusion of the cerebellar tonsils through the foramen magnum. In association with this hindbrain malformation, minor to moderate abnormalities of the base of the skull often occur, including basilar impression (platybasia) and small foramen magnum. Arnold-Chiari malformation type I may remain asymptomatic for years, but in older children and young adults it may cause progressive ataxia, paresis of the lower cranial nerves, and progressive vertigo; rarely it may present with apnea or disordered breathing. Posterior cervical laminectomy may be necessary to provide relief from cervical cord compression. Ventriculoperitoneal shunting is required for hydrocephalus.

Arnold-Chiari malformation type II consists of the malformations found in Arnold-Chiari type I plus an associated lumbar meningomyelocele. Hydrocephalus develops in approximately 90% of children with Arnold-Chiari malformation type II. These patients may also have aqueductal stenosis, hydromyelia or syringomyelia, and cortical dysplasias. The clinical manifestations of Arnold-Chiari malformation type II are most commonly caused by the associated hydrocephalus and meningomyelocele. In addition, dysfunction of the lower cranial nerves may be present. Up to 25% may have epilepsy, likely secondary to the cortical dysplasias. With the advent of "aggressive-selective" therapy, mortality is 14%; of survivors 74% are ambulatory and 73% have a normal IQ.

Arnold-Chiari malformation type III is characterized by occipital encephalocele, a closure defect of the rostral end of the neural tube. Hydrocephalus is extremely common with this malformation.

In general, the diagnosis of neural tube defects is obvious at the time of birth. The diagnosis may be strongly suspected prenatally on the basis of ultrasonographic findings and the presence of elevated α-fetoprotein in the amniotic fluid. All women of childbearing age should take prophylactic folate, which can prevent these defects and decrease the risk of recurrence by 70%.

2. Disorders of Cellular Proliferation & Migration

Lissencephaly

Lissencephaly is a severe malformation of the brain characterized by an extremely smooth cortical surface with minimal sulcal and gyral development. Such a smooth surface is characteristic of fetal brain at the end of the first trimester. In addition, lissencephalic brains have a primitive cytoarchitectural construction with a four-layered cerebral mantle instead of the mature six-layered mantle. Pachygyria (thick gyri) and agyria (absence of gyri) may vary in an anterior to posterior gradient, which can be suggestive of the underlying genetic defect. Patients with lissencephaly usually have severe neurodevelopmental delay, microcephaly, and seizures (including infantile spasms); however, there is significant phenotypic heterogeneity, which can depend on the specific mutation. These disorders are autosomal recessive, except for the X-linked disorders. *LIS1* mutations on chromosome 17 are associated with dysmorphic features (Miller-Dieker syndrome). X-linked syndromes involving mutations in *DCX* (double cortin) and

ARX (associated with ambiguous genitalia) affect males with lissencephaly and females with band heterotopias or agenesis of the corpus callosum. Lissencephaly in association with hydrocephalus, cerebellar malformations, and muscular dystrophy may occur in Walker-Warburg syndrome (*POMT1* mutation), Fukuyama muscular dystrophy (*fukutin* mutation), and muscle-eye-brain disease (*POMGnT1* mutation). It is particularly important to identify these syndromes not only because clinical tests are available, but also because of their genetic implications. Lissencephaly may also be a component of Zellweger syndrome, a metabolic peroxisomal abnormality associated with the presence of elevated concentrations of very-long-chain fatty acids in plasma. No specific treatment for lissencephaly is available and seizures are often difficult to control with standard medications.

MRI scans have helped to define a number of presumed migrational defects that are similar to but anatomically more restricted than lissencephaly. A distinctive example is bilateral perisylvian cortical dysplasia. Patients with this disorder have pseudobulbar palsy, variable cognitive deficits, facial diplegia, dysarthria, developmental delay, and epilepsy. Seizures are often difficult to control with antiepileptic drugs; some patients have benefited from corpus callosotomy. The cause of this syndrome is as yet unknown, though intrauterine cerebral ischemic injury has been postulated. Therapy is aimed at improving speech and oromotor functions and controlling seizures.

Agenesis of the Corpus Callosum

Agenesis of the corpus callosum, once thought to be a rare cerebral malformation, is more frequently diagnosed with modern neuroimaging techniques. The cause of this malformation is unknown. Occasionally it appears to be inherited in either an autosomal dominant or recessive pattern. X-linked recessive patterns have also been described (*ARX* as mentioned earlier). Agenesis of the corpus callosum has been found in some patients with pyruvate dehydrogenase deficiency and in others with nonketotic hyperglycinemia. Most cases are sporadic. Maldevelopment of the corpus callosum may be partial or complete. No specific syndrome is typical of agenesis of the corpus callosum, although many patients have seizures, developmental delay, microcephaly, or mental retardation. Neurologic abnormalities may be related to microscopic cytoarchitectural abnormalities of the brain that occur in association with agenesis of the corpus callosum. The malformation may be found coincidentally by neuroimaging studies in otherwise normal patients and has been described as a coincidental finding at autopsy in neurologically normal individuals. A special form of agenesis of the corpus callosum occurs in Aicardi syndrome. In this X-linked disorder, agenesis of the corpus callosum is associated with other cystic intracerebral abnormalities, infantile spasms, mental retardation, lacunar chorioretinopathy, and vertebral body abnormalities.

Dandy-Walker Syndrome

Despite being described nearly a century ago, the exact definition of the Dandy-Walker syndrome is still debated. Classically, it is characterized by aplasia of the vermis, cystic enlargement of the fourth ventricle, rostral displacement of the tentorium, and absence or atresia of the foramina of Magendie and Luschka. Although hydrocephalus is usually not present congenitally, it develops within the first few months of life. Ninety percent of patients who develop hydrocephalus do so by age 1 year. Variants have cerebellar hypoplasia without dilation of the fourth ventricle and hydrocephalus and may suggest other subtle cortical abnormalities not classically present and could be confused with other disorders such as Joubert syndrome and its variants. On physical examination, a rounded protuberance or exaggeration of the cranial occiput often exists. In the absence of hydrocephalus and increased intracranial pressure, few physical findings may be present to suggest neurologic dysfunction. An ataxic syndrome occurs in fewer than 20% of patients and is usually late in appearing. Many long-term neurologic deficits result directly from hydrocephalus. Diagnosis of Dandy-Walker syndrome is confirmed by CT or MRI scanning of the head. Treatment is directed at the management of hydrocephalus.

3. Craniosynostosis

Craniosynostosis, or premature closure of cranial sutures, is usually sporadic and idiopathic. However, some patients have hereditary disorders, such as Apert syndrome and Crouzon disease, that are associated with abnormalities of the digits, extremities, and heart. Occasionally craniosynostosis may be associated with an underlying metabolic disturbance such as hyperthyroidism and hypophosphatasia. The most common form of craniosynostosis involves the sagittal suture and results in scaphocephaly, an elongation of the head in the anterior to posterior direction. Premature closure of the coronal sutures causes brachycephaly, an increase in cranial growth from left to right. Unless many or all cranial sutures close prematurely, intracranial volume will not be compromised, and the brain's growth will not be impaired. Closure of only one or a few sutures will not cause impaired brain growth or neurologic dysfunction. Management of craniosynostosis is directed at preserving normal skull shape and consists of excising the fused suture and applying material to the edge of the craniectomy to prevent reossification of the bone edges. The best cosmetic effect on the skull is achieved when surgery is done during the first 6 months of life.

4. Hydrocephalus

Hydrocephalus is characterized by an increased volume of CSF in association with progressive ventricular dilation. In communicating hydrocephalus, CSF circulates through the ventricular system and into the subarachnoid space without obstruction. In noncommunicating hydrocephalus, an obstruction blocks the flow of CSF within the ventricular system or blocks the egress of CSF from the ventricular system into the subarachnoid space. A wide variety of disorders, such as hemorrhage, infection, tumors, and congenital malformations, may play a causal role in the development of hydrocephalus. Attention to an X-linked inheritance pattern, the presence of radialized thumbs and aqueductal stenosis, is suggestive of X-linked hydrocephalus due to the clinically testable neural cell adhesion molecule-L1 deficiency.

Clinical features of hydrocephalus include macrocephaly, an excessive rate of head growth, irritability, vomiting, loss of appetite, impaired upgaze, impaired extraocular movements, hypertonia of the lower extremities, and generalized hyperreflexia. Without treatment, optic atrophy may occur. In infants, papilledema may not be present, whereas older children with closed cranial sutures can eventually develop swelling of the optic disk. Hydrocephalus can be diagnosed on the basis of the clinical course, findings on physical examination, and CT or MRI scan.

Treatment of hydrocephalus is directed at providing an alternative outlet for CSF from the intracranial compartment. The most common method is ventriculoperitoneal shunting. Other treatment should be directed, if possible, at the underlying cause of the hydrocephalus.

For genetic testing, see http://www.genetests.org

Barkovich AJ et al: Radiologic classification of malformations of cortical development. Curr Opin Neurobiol 2001;12:145 [PMID: 11262727].

Kato M, Dobyns WB: Lissencephaly and the molecular basis of neuronal migration. Hum Mol Gen 2003;12:R89 [PMID: 12668601].

Lekvoc GP, Bristol RE, Rekate, HL: Cognitive impact of craniosynostosis. Semin Pediatr Neurol 2004;11:305 [PMID: 158287151].

Leventer RJ et al: LIS1 missense mutations cause milder lissencephaly phenotypes including a child with normal IQ. Neurology 2001;57:416 [PMID: 11502906].

Patel S, Barkovich AJ: Analysis and classification of cerebellar malformations. AJNR Am J Neuroradiol 2002;23:1074 [PMID: 12169461].

ABNORMAL HEAD SIZE

Bone plates of the skull have almost no intrinsic capacity to enlarge or grow. Unlike long bones, they depend on extrinsic forces to stimulate new bone formation at the suture lines. Although gravity and traction on bone by muscle and scalp probably stimulate some growth, the single most important stimulus for head growth during infancy and childhood is brain growth. Therefore, accurate assessment of head growth is one of the most important aspects of the neurologic examination of young children. A head circumference that is two standard deviations above or below the mean for age requires investigation and explanation.

1. Plagiocephaly

An abnormal skull shape is plagiocephaly ("oblique head"). Flatness of the head (brachycephaly) is a common complaint, and nowadays is usually secondary to supine sleep position ("back to sleep"), not from occipital lambdoid suture craniosynostosis.

Repositioning the head during naps (eg, with a rolled towel under one shoulder), and "tummy time" when awake are remedies. Rarely is a skull film and/or consultation necessary to rule out craniosynostosis. Most positional non-synostotic plagiocephaly resolves by age 2 years.

2. Microcephaly

A head circumference more than two standard deviations below the mean for age and sex is by definition microcephaly. More important, however, than a single head circumference measurement is the rate or pattern of head growth over time. Head circumference measurements that progressively drop to lower percentiles with increasing age are indicative of a process or condition that has impaired the brain's capacity to grow. The causes of microcephaly are numerous. Some examples are listed in Table 23–19.

Clinical Findings

A. SYMPTOMS AND SIGNS

Microcephaly may be suspected in the full-term newborn and in infants up to age 6 months whose chest circumference exceeds the head circumference (unless the child is very obese). Microcephaly may be discovered when the child is examined because of delayed developmental milestones or neurologic problems, such as seizures or spasticity. There may be a marked backward slope of the forehead (as in familial microcephaly) with narrowing of the bitemporal diameter. The fontanelle may close earlier than expected, and sutures may be prominent.

B. LABORATORY FINDINGS

Laboratory findings vary with the cause. Abnormal dermatoglyphics may be present when the injury occurred before 19 weeks' gestation. In the newborn, IgM antibody titers for toxoplasmosis, rubella, CMV, herpes simplex virus, and syphilis may be assessed. Elevated specific IgM titer is indicative of congenital infection.

Table 23–19. Causes of microcephaly.

Causes	Examples
Chromosomal	Trisomy 13, 18, 21
Malformation	Lissencephaly, schizencephaly
Syndromes	Rubenstein-Taybi, Cornelia de Lange, Angelman
Toxins	Alcohol, anticonvulsants (?), maternal phenylketonuria (PKU)
Infections (intrauterine)	TORCHS[a]
Radiation	Maternal pelvis, first and second trimester
Placental insufficiency	Toxemia, infection, small for gestational age
Familial	Autosomal-dominant, autosomal-recessive
Perinatal hypoxia, trauma	Birth asphyxia, injury
Infections (perinatal)	Bacterial meningitis (especially group B streptococci) Viral encephalitis (enterovirus, herpes simplex)
Metabolic	Glut-1 deficiency, PKU, maple syrup urine disease
Degenerative disease	Tay–Sachs, Krabbe

[a]TORCHS is a mnemonic for toxoplasmosis, other infections, rubella, cytomegalovirus, herpes simplex, and syphilis.

The urine culture for CMV will be positive at birth when this virus is the cause of microcephaly. Eye, cardiac, and bone abnormalities may also be clues to congenital infection. The child's serum and urine amino and organic acid determinations are occasionally diagnostic. The mother may require screening for phenylketonuria. Karyotyping should be considered.

C. IMAGING

CT or MRI scans may aid in diagnosis and prognosis. These studies may demonstrate calcifications, malformations, or atrophic patterns that suggest specific congenital infections or genetic syndromes. Plain skull radiographs are of limited value. Genetic counseling should be offered to the family of any infant with significant microcephaly.

Differential Diagnosis

Congenital craniosynostosis involving multiple sutures is easily differentiated by inspection of the head, history, identification of syndromes, hereditary pattern, and some-

times signs and symptoms of increased intracranial pressure. Common forms of craniosynostosis involving sagittal, coronal, and lambdoidal sutures are associated with abnormally shaped heads but do not cause microcephaly. Recognizing treatable causes of undergrowth of the brain such as hypopituitarism/hypothyroidism, and severe protein-calorie undernutrition is critical so that therapy can be initiated as early as possible.

Treatment & Prognosis

Except for the treatable disorders already noted, treatment is usually supportive and directed at the multiple neurologic and sensory deficits, endocrine disturbances (eg, diabetes insipidus), and seizures. Many, but not all, children with microcephaly are developmentally delayed. The notable exceptions are found in cases of hypopituitarism (rare) or familial autosomal dominant microcephaly.

Bardin C et al: Outcome at 5 years of age of SGA and AGA infants born less than 28 weeks of gestation. Semin Perinatol 2004; 28:288 [PMID: 15565789].

Freeman JM, Carson BS: Management of infants with potentially misshapen heads. Pediatrics 2003;111:918.

Glass RB et al: The infant skull: a vault of information. Radiographics 2004;507:22 [PMID: 15026597].

Gnamey DK et al: Primary autosomal recessive microcephaly: a novel clinical phenotype. Genet Couns 2005;16:107 [PMID: 15844788].

Hutchison BL et al: Plagiocephaly and brachycephaly in the first two years of life: A prospective cohort study. Pediatrics 2004; 114:970.

Maugans TA: The misshapen head [commentary]. Pediatrics 2002; 100:166.

Sztriha L et al: Microcephaly associated with abnormal gyral pattern. Neuropediatrics 2004;35:346.

Wang D et al: Glut-1 deficiency syndrome: clinical, genetic, and therapeutic aspects. Ann Neurol 2005;57:111 [PMID: 15622525].

3. Macrocephaly

A head circumference more than two standard deviations above the mean for age and sex denotes macrocephaly. Rapid head growth rate suggests increased intracranial pressure, most likely caused by hydrocephalus, extra-axial fluid collections, or neoplasms. Macrocephaly with normal head growth rate suggests familial macrocephaly or true megalencephaly, as might occur in neurofibromatosis. Other causes and examples of macrocephaly are listed in Table 23–20.

Clinical Findings

Clinical and laboratory findings vary with the underlying process. In infants, transillumination of the skull with an intensely bright light in a completely darkened room may disclose subdural effusions, hydrocephalus, hydranenceph-

Table 23–20. Causes of macrocephaly.

Causes	Examples
Pseudomacrocephaly, pseudohydrocephalus, catch-up growth crossing percentiles	Growing premature infant; recovery from malnutrition, congenital heart disease, postsurgical correction
Increased intracranial pressure	
With dilated ventricles	Progressive hydrocephalus, subdural effusion
With other mass	Arachnoid cyst, porencephalic cyst, brain tumor
Benign familial macrocephaly (idiopathic external hydrocephalus)	External hydrocephalus, benign enlargement of the subarachnoid spaces (synonyms)
Megalencephaly (large brain)	
With neurocutaneous disorder	Neurofibromatosis, tuberous sclerosis, etc
With gigantism	Sotos syndrome
With dwarfism	Achondroplasia
Metabolic	Mucopolysaccharidoses
Lysosomal	Metachromatic leukodystrophy (late)
Other leukodystrophy	Canavan spongy degeneration
Thickened skull	Fibrous dysplasia (bone), hemolytic anemia (marrow), sicklemia, thalassemia

aly, and cystic defects. A surgically or medically treatable condition must be ruled out. Thus the first decision is whether and when to perform an imaging study.

A. IMAGING STUDY DEFERRED

1. Catch-up growth—Catch-up growth may be evident, as it is in the thriving, neurologically intact premature infant whose rapid head enlargement is most marked in the first weeks of life, or the infant in the early phase of recovery from deprivation dwarfism. As the expected normal size is reached, head growth slows and then resumes a normal growth pattern. If the fontanelle is open, cranial ultrasonography can assess ventricular size and diagnose or exclude hydrocephalus.

2. Familial macrocephaly—This condition may exist when another family member has an unusually large head with no signs or symptoms referable to such disorders as neurocutaneous dysplasias (especially neurofibromatosis) or cerebral gigantism (Sotos syndrome), or when there are no significant mental or neurologic abnormalities in the child.

B. IMAGING STUDY

CT or MRI scans (or ultrasonography, if the anterior fontanelle is open) are used to define any structural cause of macrocephaly and to identify an operable disorder. Even when the condition is untreatable (or does not require treatment), the information gained may permit more accurate diagnosis and prognosis, guide management and genetic counseling, and serve as a basis for comparison should future abnormal cranial growth or neurologic changes necessitate a repeat study. An imaging study is necessary if signs or symptoms of increased intracranial pressure are present (see Table 23–16).

Aquilina K et al: Choroid plexus adenoma: case report and review of the literature. Childs Nerv Syst 2005;21:410.

Cutting LE et al: Megalencephaly in NF1. Neurology 2002;59: 1388 [PMID: 12427889].

Dementieva YA et al: Accelerated head growth in early development of individuals with autism. Peditr Neurol 2005;32:102 [PMID: 15664769].

Ravid S, Maytal J: External hydrocephalus: A probable cause for subdural hematoma in infancy. Pediatr Neurol 2003;28:139 [PMID: 12699866].

Riel-Romero RM et al: Megalencephalic leukoencephalopathy with subcortical cysts in two siblings owing to two novel mutations: case reports and review of the literature. J Child Neurol 2005;20:230 [PMID: 1583614].

NEUROCUTANEOUS DYSPLASIAS

Neurocutaneous dysplasias are diseases of the neuroectoderm and sometimes involve endoderm and mesoderm. Birthmarks and skin growths appearing later often suggest a need to look for brain, spinal cord, and eye disease. Hamartomas (histologically normal tissue growing abnormally rapidly or in aberrant sites) are common. The most common dysplasias are dominantly inherited. Benign and even malignant tumors may develop.

Dahan D et al: Neurocutaneous syndromes. Adolesc Med 2002; 13:495 [PMID: 12270797].

Kandt RS: Tuberous sclerosis complex and neurofibromatosis type 1: the two most common neurocutaneous diseases. Neurol Clin 2003;21:983 [PMID: 14743661].

Korf BR: The phakomatoses. Clin Dermatol 2005;23:78 [PMID: 15708292].

1. Neurofibromatosis (von Recklinghausen Disease)

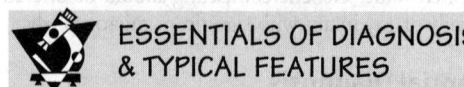

ESSENTIALS OF DIAGNOSIS & TYPICAL FEATURES

- *More than six café au lait spots 5 mm in greatest diameter in prepubertal individuals and over 15 mm in greatest diameter in postpubertal individuals.*

- *Two or more neurofibromas of any type or one plexiform neurofibroma.*
- *Freckling in the axillary or inguinal regions.*
- *Optic glioma.*
- *Two or more Lisch nodules (iris hamartomas).*
- *Distinctive osseous lesions, such as sphenoid dysplasia or thinning of long bone with or without pseudarthroses.*
- *First-degree relative (parent, sibling, offspring) with neurofibromatosis type 1 by above criteria.*

General Considerations

Neurofibromatosis is a multisystem disorder with a prevalence of 1:4000. Fifty percent of cases are due to new mutations in the *NF1* gene. Forty percent of patients will develop medical complications of the disorder in their lifetime.

Clinical Findings

A. SYMPTOMS AND SIGNS

The most common presenting symptoms are cognitive or psychomotor problems; 40% of patients have learning disabilities, and mental retardation occurs in 8%. The family history is important in identifying dominant gene manifestations in parents. Parents should be examined in detail. The history should focus on lumps or masses causing disfigurement, functional problems, or pain. The clinician should ask about visual problems. Strabismus or amblyopia dictates a search for optic glioma, a common tumor in neurofibromatosis. Any progressive neurologic deficit calls for studies to rule out tumor of the spinal cord or CNS. Tumors of cranial nerve VIII virtually never occur in neurofibromatosis type 1 but are the rule in neurofibromatosis type 2, a rare autosomal dominant disease.

The physician should check blood pressure and examine the spine for scoliosis and the limbs for pseudarthroses. Head measurement often shows macrocephaly. Hearing and vision need to be assessed. The eye examination should include a check for proptosis and iris Lisch nodules. The optic disk should be examined for atrophy or papilledema. Short stature and precocious puberty are occasional findings. An examination for neurologic manifestations of tumors (eg, asymmetrical reflexes or spasticity) is important.

B. LABORATORY FINDINGS

Laboratory tests are not likely to be of value in asymptomatic patients. Selected patients require brain MRI with special cuts through the optic nerves to rule out optic glioma.

Hypertension necessitates evaluation of renal arteries for dysplasia and stenosis. Cognitive and school achievement testing may be indicated. Scoliosis or limb abnormalities should be studied by appropriate roentgenograms such as an MRI scan of the spinal cord and roots.

Differential Diagnosis

Patients with McCune-Albright syndrome often have larger café au lait spots with precocious puberty, polyostotic fibrous dysplasia, and hyperfunctioning endocrinopathies. One or two café au lait spots are often seen in normal children. A large solitary café au lait spot is usually innocent, not neurofibromatosis type 1.

Treatment

Genetic counseling is important. The risk to siblings is up to 50%. The disease may be progressive, with serious complications occasionally seen. Patients sometimes worsen during puberty or pregnancy. Genetic screening of family members is required. Annual or semiannual visits are important in the early detection of school problems or bony or neurologic abnormalities.

Multidisciplinary clinics at medical centers around the U.S. are excellent resources. Prenatal diagnosis is probably on the horizon, but the variability of manifestations (trivial to severe) will make therapeutic abortion an unlikely option. Chromosomal linkage studies are under way (chromosome 17q11.2). Information for laypeople and physicians is available from the National Neurofibromatosis Foundation, Inc., 70 West 40th Street, New York, NY 10018.

Arun D, Gutmann DH: Recent advances in neurofibromatosis type 1. Curr Opin Neurol 2005;17:101 [PMID: 15021234].

Collins MT et al: Thyroid carcinoma in the McCune-Albright syndrome: contributory role of activating Gs alpha mutations. Clin Endocrinol Metab 2003;88:4413 [PMID: 12970318].

Han M, Criado E: Renal artery stenosis and aneurysms associated with neurofibromatosis. J Vasc Surg 2005;41:539 [PMID: 15838492].

Kanowitz SJ et al: Auditory brainstem implantation in patients with neurofibromatosis type 2. Laryngoscope 2004;114:3135 [PMID: 15564834].

Listernick R, Charrow J: Neurofibromatosis-1 in childhood. Adv Dermatol 2004;20:75 [PMID: 15544197].

Nguyen JT et al: Large solitary café au lait spots: a report of 5 cases and review of the literature. Cutis 2004;73:311, 316 [PMID: 15186045].

Rosser TL et al: Cerebrovascular abnormalities in a population of children with neurofibromatosis type 1. Neurology 2005;64:553 [PMID: 15699396].

Ruggieri M et al: Earliest clinical manifestations and natural history of neurofibromatosis type 2 (NF2) in childhood: a study of 24 patients. Neuropediatrics 2005;36:21 [PMID: 15776319].

Tekin M et al: Cafe au lait spots: The pediatrician's perspective. Pediatr Rev 2001;22:82 [PMID: 11230626].

Vivarelli R et al: Epilepsy in neurofibromatosis 1. J Child Neurol 2003;18:338 [PMID: 12822818].

Ward BA, Gutmann DH: Neurofibromatosis 1: from lab bench to clinic. Pediatr Neurol 2005;32:221 [PMID: 15797177].

2. Tuberous Sclerosis (Bourneville Disease)

ESSENTIALS OF DIAGNOSIS & TYPICAL FEATURES

- Facial angiofibromas or subungual fibromas.
- Often hypomelanotic macules, gingival fibromas.
- Retinal hamartomas.
- Cortical tubers or subependymal glial nodules, often calcified.
- Renal angiomyolipomas.

General Considerations

Tuberous sclerosis is a dominantly inherited disease. Almost all patients have deletions on chromosome 9 (*TSC1* gene) or 16 (*TSC2* gene). The gene products hamartin and tuberin have tumor-suppressing effects. A triad of seizures, mental retardation, and adenoma sebaceum occurs in only 33% of patients. The disease was earlier thought to have a high rate of mutation. As a result of more sophisticated techniques such as MRI, parents formerly thought not to harbor the gene are now being diagnosed as asymptomatic carriers.

Like neurofibromatosis, tuberous sclerosis is associated with a wide variety of symptoms. The patient may be asymptomatic except for skin findings or may be devastated by severe infantile spasms in early infancy, by continuing epilepsy, and by mental retardation. Seizures in early infancy correlate with later mental retardation.

Clinical Findings

A. SYMPTOMS AND SIGNS

1. Dermatologic features—Skin findings bring most patients to the physician's attention. Ninety-six percent of patients have one or more hypomelanotic macules, facial angiofibromas, ungual fibromas, or shagreen patches. Adenoma sebaceum, the facial skin hamartomas, may first appear in early childhood, often on the cheek, chin, and dry sites of the skin where acne is not usually seen. They often have a reddish hue. The off-white hypomelanotic macules are seen more easily in tanned or dark-skinned individuals than in those with lighter skin. The macules often are oval or "ash leaf" in shape and follow derma-tomes. A Wood lamp (ultraviolet light) shows the macules more clearly, a great help in the light-skinned patient. In the scalp, poliosis (whitened hair) is the equivalent. In infancy, the presence of these macules accompanied by seizures is virtually diagnostic of the disease. Subungual or periungual fibromas are more common in the toes. Leathery, orange peel–like shagreen patches support the diagnosis. Café au lait spots are occasionally seen. Fibrous or raised plaques may resemble coalescent angiofibromas.

2. Neurologic features—Seizures are the most common presenting symptom. Five percent of patients with infantile spasms (a serious epileptic syndrome) have tuberous sclerosis. Thus any patient presenting with infantile spasms (and the parents as well) should be evaluated for this disorder. An imaging study of the CNS, such as a CT scan, may show calcified subependymal nodules; MRI may show dysmyelinating white matter lesions or cortical tubers. Virtually any kind of symptomatic seizure (eg, atypical absence, partial complex, and generalized tonic-clonic seizures) may occur.

3. Mental retardation—Mental retardation occurs in up to 50% of patients referred to tertiary care centers; the incidence is probably much lower in randomly selected patients. Patients with seizures are more prone to mental retardation or learning disabilities.

4. Renal lesions—Renal cysts or angiomyolipomas may be asymptomatic. Hematuria or obstruction of urine flow sometimes occurs; the latter requires operation. Ultrasonography of the kidneys should be done in any patient suspected of tuberous sclerosis, both to aid in diagnosis if lesions are found and to rule out renal obstructive disease.

5. Cardiopulmonary involvement—Rarely cystic lung disease may occur. Rhabdomyomas of the heart may be asymptomatic but can lead to outflow obstruction, conduction difficulties, and death. Chest radiographs and echocardiograms can detect these rare manifestations. Cardiac rhabdomyoma may be detected on prenatal ultrasound examination.

6. Eye involvement—Retinal hamartomas are often near the disc.

7. Skeletal involvement—Findings sometimes helpful in diagnosis are cystic rarefactions of the bones of the fingers or toes.

B. DIAGNOSTIC STUDIES

Plain radiographs may detect areas of thickening within the skull, spine, and pelvis, and cystic lesions in the hands and feet. Chest radiographs may show lung honeycombing. More helpful is CT scanning, which can show the virtually pathognomonic subependymal nodular calcifications and sometimes widened gyri or tubers and brain tumors. Contrast material may show the often classically located tumors near the interventricular foramen.

Hypomyelinated lesions may be seen with MRI. EEG is helpful in delineating the presence of seizure discharges.

Treatment

Therapy is as indicated by underlying disease (eg, seizures and tumors of the brain, kidney, and heart). Skin lesions on the face may need dermabrasion or laser treatment. Genetic counseling emphasizes identification of the carrier. The risk of appearance in offspring if either parent is a carrier is 50%. The patient should be seen annually for counseling and reexamination in childhood. Identification of the chromosomes (9,16; *TSC1* and *TSC2* genes) may in the future make intrauterine diagnosis possible.

Au KS et al: Molecular genetic basis of tuberous sclerosis complex: from bench to bedside. J Child Neurol 2004;19:699 [PMID: 15563017].

Bader RS et al: Fetal rhabdomyoma: prenatal diagnosis, clinical outcome, and incidence of associated tuberous sclerosis complex. J Pediatr 2003;143:620 [PMID: 14615733].

DiMario FJ Jr: Brain abnormalities in tuberous sclerosis complex. J Child Neurol 2004;19:650 [PMID: 15563010].

Roach ES, Sparagana SP: Diagnosis of tuberous sclerosis complex. J Child Neurol 2004;19:643 [PMID: 15563009].

Thiele EA: Managing epilepsy in tuberous sclerosis complex. J Child Neurol 2004;19:680 [PMID: 15563014].

Wiznitzer M: Autism and tuberous sclerosis. J Child Neurol 2004;19:675 [PMID: 15563013].

3. Encephalofacial Angiomatosis (Sturge-Weber Disease)

Sturge-Weber disease consists of a facial port wine nevus involving the upper part of the face (in the first division of cranial nerve V), a venous angioma of the meninges in the occipitoparietal regions, and choroidal angioma. The syndrome has been described without the facial nevus (rare, type III, exclusive leptomeningeal angioma).

Clinical Findings

In infancy, the eye may show congenital glaucoma, or buphthalmos, with a cloudy, enlarged cornea. In early stages, the facial nevus may be the only indication, with no findings in the brain even on radiologic studies. The characteristic cortical atrophy, calcifications of the cortex, and meningeal angiomatosis may appear with time, solidifying the diagnosis.

Physical examination may show focal seizures or hemiparesis on the side opposite the cerebral lesion. The facial nevus may be much more extensive than the first division of cranial nerve V; it can involve the lower face, mouth, lip, neck, and even torso. Hemiatrophy of the opposite limbs may occur. Mental handicap may result from poorly controlled seizures. Late-appearing glaucoma and rarely CNS hemorrhage occur.

Radiologic studies may show calcification of the cortex; CT scanning may show this much earlier than plain radiographic studies. MRI often shows underlying brain involvement.

The EEG often shows depression of voltage over the involved area in early stages; later, epileptiform abnormalities may be present focally.

Treatment

Sturge-Weber disease is sporadic. Early control of seizures is important to avoid consequent developmental setback. If seizures do not occur, normal development can be anticipated. Careful examination of the newborn, with ophthalmologic assessment to detect early glaucoma, is indicated. Rarely, surgical removal of the involved meninges and the involved portion of the brain may be indicated, even hemispherectomy.

Comi AM et al: Encephalofacial angiomatosis sparing the occipital lobe and without facial nevus: On the spectrum of Sturge-Weber syndrome variants? J Child Neurol 2003;18:35 [PMID: 12661936].

Feller L, Lemmer J: Encephalotrigeminal angiomatosis. SADJ 2003;58:370 [PMID: 14964051] .

Kossoff EH et al: Outcomes of 32 hemispherectomies for Sturge-Weber syndrome worldwide. Neurology 2002;59:1735 [PMID: 12473761].

Menzel JF et al: Early diagnosis of cerebral involvement in Sturge-Weber syndrome using high-resolution BOLD MR venography. Pediatr Radiol 2005;35:85 [PMID: 15480615].

Miyama S, Goto T: Leptomeningeal angiomatosis with infantile spasms. Pediatr Neurol 2004;31:353 [PMID: 15519118].

Taddeucci G et al: Migraine-like attacks in a child with Sturge-Weber syndrome without facial nevus. Pediatr Neurol 2005;32:131 [PMID: 15664776].

4. von Hippel-Lindau Disease (Retinocerebellar Angiomatosis)

von Hippel-Lindau disease is a rare, dominantly inherited condition with retinal and cerebellar hemangioblastomas; cysts of the kidneys, pancreas, and epididymis; and sometimes renal cancers. The patient may present with ataxia, slurred speech, and nystagmus due to a hemangioblastoma of the cerebellum or with a medullary spinal cord cystic hemangioblastoma. Retinal detachment may occur from hemorrhage or exudate in the retinal vascular malformation. Rarely a pancreatic cyst or renal tumor may be the presenting symptom.

The diagnostic criteria for the disease are a retinal or cerebellar hemangioblastoma with or without a positive family history, intra-abdominal cyst, or renal cancer.

Fitz EW, Newman SA: Neuro-ophthalmology of von Hippel-Lindau. Curr Neurol Neurosci Rep 2004;4:384 [PMID: 15324605].

Maher ER: von Hippel-Lindau disease. Curr Mol Med 2004; 4:833 [PMID: 15579030].

Richard S et al: von Hippel-Lindau disease. Lancet 2004;363:1231 [PMID: 15081659].

CENTRAL NERVOUS SYSTEM DEGENERATIVE DISORDERS OF INFANCY & CHILDHOOD

The CNS degenerative disorders of infancy and childhood are characterized by arrest of psychomotor development and loss, usually progressive but at variable rates, of mental and motor functioning and often of vision as well. Seizures are common in some disorders. Symptoms and signs vary with age at onset and primary sites of involvement of specific types.

These disorders are fortunately rare. An early clinical pattern of decline often follows normal early development. Referral for sophisticated biochemical testing is usually necessary before a definitive diagnosis can be made (Tables 23–21 and 23–22).

Auvin S, Valee L: Neuronal lipofuscinosis. Lancet 2004;364:786 [PMID: 15337405].

Damen G et al: Gastrointestinal and other clinical manifestations in 17 children with congenital disorders of glycosylation type Ia, Ib, and Ic. J Pediatr Gastroenterol Nutr 2004;38:282 [PMID: 15076627].

Davidzon G et al: POLG mutations and Alpers syndrome. Ann Neurol 2005;56:921 [PMID: 15929042].

Dubey P et al: Adrenal insufficiency in asymptomatic adrenoleukodystrophy patients identified by very long-chain fatty acid screening. J Pediatr 2005;146:528 [PMID: 15812458].

Deusterhus P: Huntington disease: a case study of early onset presenting as depression. J Am Acad Child Adolesc Psychiatry 2004;43:1293 [PMID: 15381897].

Huntsman RJ et al: A typical presentation of Leigh syndrome: a case series and review. Pediatr Neurol 2005;32:335 [PMID: 15866434].

Mole SE: The genetic spectrum of human neuronal ceroid-lipofuscinoses. Brain Pathol 2004;14:70 [PMID: 14997939].

Moser H et al: Progress in X-linked adrenoleukodystrophy. Curr Opin Neurol 2004;17:263 [PMID: 15167059].

Moser HW et al: Follow-up of 89 asymptomatic patients with adrenoleukodystrophy treated with Lorenzo's oil. Arch Neurol 2005;62:1073 [PMID: 16009761].

Noetzel MJ: Diagnosing "undiagnosed" leukodystrophies: The role of molecular genetics. Neurology 2004;62:847 [PMID: 15037679].

Riel-Romero RM et al: Megalencephalic leukoencephalopathy with subcortical cysts in two siblings owing to two novel mutations: case reports and review of the literature. J Child Neurol 2005;20:230 [PMID: 15832614].

Schiffmann R, van der Knaap MS: The latest on leukodystrophies. Curr Opin Neurol 2004;17:187 [PMID: 15021247].

Seneca S et al: Early onset Huntington disease: a neuronal degeneration syndrome. Eur J Pediatr 2004;163:717 [PMID: 15338298].

Sinha S et al: Neuronal ceroid lipofuscinosis: a clinicopathological study. Seizure 2004;13:235 [PMID: 15121131].

Vanhanen SL et al: Neuroradiological findings (MRS, MRI, SPECT) in infantile neuronal ceroid-lipofuscinosis (infantile CLN1) at different stages of the disease. Neuropediatrics 2004;35:27 [PMID: 15002049].

Vargas AP: Unusual early-onset Huntington's disease. J Child Neurol 2003;18:429 [PMID: 12886981].

Vermeulen G et al: Fright is a provoking factor in vanishing white matter disease. Ann Neurol 2005;57:560 [PMID: 15786451].

Wilson CG et al: Vanishing white matter disease in a child presenting with ataxia. J Paediatr Child Health 2005;41:65 [PMID: 15670229].

ATAXIAS OF CHILDHOOD

1. Acute Cerebellar Ataxia

Acute cerebellar ataxia occurs most commonly in children age 2–6 years. The onset is abrupt, and the evolution of symptoms is rapid. In about 50% of patients, a prodromal illness occurs with fever, respiratory or gastrointestinal symptoms, or an exanthem within 3 weeks of onset. Associated viral infections include varicella, rubeola, mumps, rubella, echovirus infections, poliomyelitis, infectious mononucleosis, and influenza. Bacterial infections such as scarlet fever and salmonellosis have also been incriminated.

Clinical Findings

A. SYMPTOMS AND SIGNS

Ataxia of the trunk and extremities may be so severe that the child exhibits a staggering, reeling gait and inability to sit without support or to reach for objects; or he or she may show only mild unsteadiness. Hypotonia, tremor of the extremities, and horizontal nystagmus may be present. Speech may be slurred. The child is frequently irritable, and vomiting may occur.

There are no clinical signs of increased intracranial pressure. Sensory and reflex testing usually shows no abnormalities.

B. LABORATORY FINDINGS

CSF pressure and protein and glucose levels are normal; slight lymphocytosis ($\leq 30/mL$) may be present. Attempts should be made to identify the etiologic viral agent.

C. IMAGING

CT scans are normal; MRI may show cerebellar postinfectious demyelinating lesions. The EEG may be normal or may show nonspecific slowing.

Differential Diagnosis

Acute cerebellar ataxia must be differentiated from acute cerebellar syndromes due to phenytoin, phenobarbital, primidone, or lead intoxication. For phenytoin, the toxic level in serum is usually above 25 µg/mL; for phenobarbital, above 50 µg/mL; for primidone, above 14 µg/mL. (See section on seizure disorders.) Papilledema, anemia, basophilic stippling of erythrocytes, proteinuria, typical radiographs, and elevated CSF protein are clinical clues to lead intoxication, which is confirmed by serum, urine, or hair lead levels. Polymyoclonus-opsoclonus syndrome with an occult neuroblastoma (see following section) occasionally begins as acute cerebellar ataxia.

In rare cases, acute cerebellar ataxia may be the presenting sign of acute bacterial meningitis or may be mimicked by corticosteroid withdrawal, vasculitides such as in polyarteritis nodosa, trauma, the first attack of ataxia in a metabolic disorder such as Hartnup disease, or the onset of acute disseminated encephalomyelitis or of multiple sclerosis. The history and physical findings may differentiate these disturbances, but appropriate laboratory studies are often necessary. For ataxias with more chronic onset and course, see the sections on spinocerebellar degeneration and the other degenerative disorders.

Treatment & Prognosis

Treatment is supportive. Corticosteroids do not help; IVIg has been used. Between 80% and 90% of children with acute cerebellar ataxia not secondary to drug toxicity recover without sequelae within 6–8 weeks. In the remainder, neurologic disturbances, including disorders of behavior and of learning, ataxia, abnormal eye movements, and speech impairment, may persist for months or years, and recovery may remain incomplete.

Bodensteiner JB, Johnsen SD: Cerebellar injury in the extremely premature infant: newly recognized but relatively common outcome. J Child Neurol 2005;20:139 [PMID: 15794181].

De Bruecker Y et al: MRI findings in acute cerebellitis. Eur Radiol 2004;14:1478 [PMID: 14968261].

Dinolfo E: Evaluation of ataxia. Pediatr Rev 2001;22:177 [PMID: 11331741].

Go T: Intravenous immunoglobulin therapy for acute cerebellar ataxia. Acta Paediatr 2003;92:504 [PMID: 12801122].

Lamperti C et al: Cerebellar ataxia and coenzyme Q10 deficiency. Neurology 2003;60:1206 [PMID: 12682339].

Ryan MM, Engle EC: Acute ataxia I childhood. J Child Neurol 2003;18:309 [PMID: 12822814].

2. Polymyoclonus-Opsoclonus Syndrome of Childhood (Infantile Myoclonic Encephalopathy, "Dancing Eyes-Dancing Feet" Syndrome)

The symptoms and signs of this syndrome are at first similar to those of acute cerebellar ataxia. Often of sudden onset, polymyoclonus-opsoclonus syndrome is characterized by severe incoordination of the trunk and extremities with lightninglike jerking or flinging movements of a group of muscles, causing the child to be in constant motion while awake. Extraocular muscle involvement results in sudden irregular eye movements (opsoclonus). Irritability and vomiting are often present, but there is no depression of level of consciousness. This syndrome occurs in association with viral infections and tumors of neural crest origin among other disorders. Immunologic mechanisms have been postulated. Usually no signs of increased intracranial pressure are present. CSF may show normal or mildly increased protein levels. Special techniques show increased CSF levels of plasmacytes and abnormal immunoglobulins. The EEG may be slightly slow, but when performed together with EMG, it shows no evidence of association between cortical discharges and the muscle movements. An assiduous search must be made to rule out tumor of neural crest origin by chest radiographs and CT, MRI, or ultrasound of the adrenal area as well as by assays of urinary catecholamine metabolites (vanillylmandelic acid and others) and cystathionine.

The symptoms respond to variably to ACTH or to IVIg. Plasmapheresis has been successful. Usually the underlying neural crest tumor is benign (ganglioneuroblastoma); surgical excision may be the only oncologic therapy needed. Lifespan is determined by the biologic behavior of the tumor. The syndrome is usually self-limited but may be characterized by exacerbations and remissions, even after the removal of the neural crest tumor and without other evidence of its recurrence, symptoms may reappear. Mild mental retardation may be a sequela.

Gesundheit B et al: Ataxia and secretory diarrhea: two unusual paraneoplastic syndromes occurring concurrently in the same patient with ganglioneuroblastoma. J Pediatr Hematol Oncol 2004;26:549 [PMID: 15342979].

Glatz K et al: Parainfectious opsoclonus-myoclonus syndrome: high dose intravenous immunoglobulins are effective. J Neurol Neurosurg Psychiatry 2003;74:279 [PMID: 12531974].

Krolczyk S: Opsoclonus: An early sign of neonatal herpes encephalitis. J Child Neurol 2003;18:356 [PMID: 12822821].

Mutch LS, Johnston DL: Late presentation of opsoclonus-myoclonus-ataxia syndrome in a child with stage 4S neuroblastoma. J Pediatr Hematol Oncol 2005;27:341 [PMID: 15956891].

Pranzatelli MR et al: Evidence of cellular immune activation in children with opsoclonus-myoclonus: cerebrospinal fluid neopterin. J Child Neurol 2004;19:919 [PMID: 15704863].

Pranzatelli MR et al: Immunologic and clinical responses to rituximab in a child with opsoclonus-myoclonus syndrome. Pediatrics 2005;115:115 [PMID: 15601813].

Pranzatelli MR et al: Screening for autoantibodies in children with opsoclonus-myoclonus-ataxia. Pediatr Neurol 2002;27:384 [PMID: 12504207].

Tate ED et al: Neuroepidemiologic trends in 105 US cases of pediatric opsoclonus-myoclonus syndrome. J Pediatr Oncol Nurs 2005;22:8 [PMID: 15574722].

Table 23–21. Central nervous system degenerative disorders of infancy.

Disease	Enzyme Defect and Genetics	Onset	Early Manifestations	Vision and Hearing	Somatic Findings
WHITE MATTER					
Globoid (Krabbe) leukodystrophy	Recessive galactocerebroside b-galactosidase deficiency. Chromosome 14.	First 6 mos; late-onset form 2–6 y. Rare adolescent, adult form.	Feeding difficulties. Shrill cry. Irritability. Arching of back.	Optic atrophy, mid-course to late. Hyperacusis occasionally.	Head often small. Often underweight.
Metachromatic leukodystrophy	Recessive. Arylsulfatase A deficiency. 22q13.	Second year; less often, later childhood or adult	Incoordination, especially gait disturbance; then general regression. Reverse in juveniles.	Optic atrophy, usually late. Hearing normal.	Head enlarged late. No change in juvenile form.
Neuroaxonal dystrophy	Familial, (?) recessive. More common in girls than boys; defect unknown.	6 mo to 2 y	Arrest of development and dementia. Loss of motor functions. Occasionally hypesthesia over trunk and legs.	Nystagmus occasional; optic atrophy, blindness; abnormal VER.	Early, may lie in "frog position."
Hallervorden–Spatz syndrome or PKAN	Mutations in *PANK2* gene.	By age 10 y	Rigidity, dystonia, gait disturbance, tremor.	Abnormal ERG. Retinal degeneration.	Dystonia, gait disturbance.
Pelizaeus–Merzbacher disease	X-linked recessive; rare female. Proteolipid protein (myelin) decreased. Xq22	Birth (connatal) to 2 y	Eye rolling often shortly after birth. Head bobbing. Slow loss of intellect.	Slowly developing optic atrophy. Hearing normal. Nystagmus.	Head and body normal
DIFFUSE, BUT PRIMARILY GRAY MATTER					
Poliodystrophy (Alpers disease or syndrome)	Occasionally familial, recessive. Metabolic forms.	Infancy to adolescence	Variable: loss of intellect, seizures, incoordination. Vomiting, hepatic failure.	Cortical blindness and deafness.	Head normal initially; may fail to grow.
Tay-Sachs disease and G$_{M2}$ gangliosidosis variants: Sandhoff disease; juvenile; chronic-adult	Recessive. Hexosaminidase deficiencies. Tay-Sachs (93% East European Jewish), hexosaminidase A deficiency. Sandhoff-hexosaminidase A and B deficiency. Juvenile-partial hexosaminidase A	Tay-Sachs, and Sandhoff; 3–6 mos; others 2–6 y or later.	Variable: shrill cry, loss of vision, infantile spasms, arrest of development. In juvenile and chronic forms: motor difficulties; later, mental difficulties.	Cherry-red macula, early blindness. Hyperacusis early. Strabismus in juvenile form, blindness late.	Head enlarged late. Liver occasionally enlarged. None in juvenile chronic forms.
Niemann-Pick disease and variants	50% Jewish. Recessive. Sphingomyelinase deficiency in types A and C involving the CNS.	First 6 mos. In variants, later onset: often non-Jewish.	Slow development. Protruding belly.	Cherry-red macula in 35–50%. Blindness late. Deafness occasionally.	Head usually normal. Spleen enlarged more than liver. Occasional xanthomas of skin.
Infantile Gaucher disease (glucosylceramide lipidosis)	Recessive. Glucocerebrosidase deficiency.	First 6 mos; rarely, late infancy	Stridor or hoarse cry; retraction; feeding difficulties	Occasional cherry-red macula. Convergent squint. Deafness occasionally.	Head usually normal. Liver and spleen equally enlarged.

Motor System	Seizures	Laboratory and Tissue Studies	Course
WHITE MATTER			
Early spasticity, occasionally preceded by hypotonia. Prolonged nerve conduction.	Early. Myoclonic and generalized, decerebrate posturing	CSF protein elevated; usually normal in late-onset forms. Sural nerve; nonspecific myelin breakdown. Enzyme deficiency in leukocytes, cultured skin fibroblasts. Demyelination, gliosis with low-signal CT scan, high-signal T_2-weighted MRI.	Rapid. Death usually by $1\,^1/_2$–2 y. Late-onset cases may live 5–10 y.
Combined upper and lower motor neuron signs. Ataxia. Prolonged nerve conduction.	Infrequent, usually late and generalized	Metachromatic cells in urine: negative sulfatase A test. CSF protein elevated. Urine sulfatide increased. Sural nerve biopsy; metachromasia. Enzyme deficiency in leukocytes, cultured skin fibroblasts. Imaging: Same as globoid leukodystrophy.	Moderately slow. Death in infantile form by 3–8 y, in juvenile form by 10–15 y.
Combined upper and lower motor neuron lesions. Hypotonia, extrapyramidal manifestations.	Variable, but usually not a prominent feature	Denervation on EMG. Increased iron uptake in region of basal ganglia. Brain and sural nerve: axonal swellings or "spheroids" Cerebellar atrophy. Cause unknown. Conjunctival biopsy may yield nerves with "spheroids."	Progressive, with death early in second decade or earlier.
Extrapyramidal signs, dysarthria, increased deep tendon reflexes.	Variable, EEG may be abnormal	Axonal degeneration (spheroids). Iron deposits in basal ganglia on MRI: eye-of-the-tiger appearance.	Progressive mental/motor deterioration
Cerebellar signs early, hyperactive deep reflexes. Spasticity.	Usually only late	None specific. Brain biopsy: extensive demyelination with small perivascular islands of intact myelin. Exon abnormalities in proteolipid protein gene in 10–25%.	Very slow, often seemingly stationary.
DIFFUSE, BUT PRIMARILY GRAY MATTER			
Variable: incoordination, spasticity	Often initial manifestation: myoclinic, akinetic, and generalized	POLG1 mutation: multiple deletions, depletions of mitochondrial DNA. Neuronal loss in cortex: may occur very late. Variably increased serum pryuvate, lactate; liver steatosis, cirrhosis late.	Usually rapid, with death within 1–3 y after onset. Variants in older children, adults.
Initially floppy. Eventual decerebrate rigidity. In juvenile and chronic forms: dysarthria, ataxia, spasticity.	Frequent, in midcourse and late. Infantile spasms and generalized	Blood smears: vacuolated lymphocytes; basophillic hypergranulation. Enzyme deficiencies in serum, leukocytes, culture skin fibroblasts. High-density thalami on CT scan, low-density white matter.	Moderately rapid. Death usually by 2–5 y. In juvenile form, 5–15 y.
Initially floppy. Eventually spastic. Occasionally extrapyramidal signs. Ataxia, dystonia.	Rare and late	Blood: vacuolated lymphocytes; increased lipids. X-rays: "mottled" lungs, decalcified bones. "Foam cells" in bone marrow, spleen, lymph nodes. WBC, fibroblast enzyme studies are diagnostic.	Moderately slow. Death usually by 3–5 y.
Opisthotonos early, followed rapidly by decerebrate rigidity	Rare and late	Anemia. Increased acid phosphatase. X-rays: thinned cortex, trabeculation of bones. "Gaucher cells" in bone marrow, spleen. Enzyme deficiency in leukocytes or cultured skin fibroblasts.	Very rapid

(continued)

Table 23–21. Central nervous system degenerative disorders of infancy. (continued)

Disease	Enzyme Defect and Genetics	Onset	Early Manifestations	Vision and Hearing	Somatic Findings
DIFFUSE, BUT PRIMARILY GRAY MATTER					
Lipogranulomatosis (Farber disease)	Ceramidase deficiency.	Early in infancy	Hoarseness, irritability, restricted joint movements.	Usually normal.	Painful nodular swelling of joints; subcutaneous nodules.
Generalized gangliosidosis and juvenile type (G_{m1} gangliosidoses)	Recessive; b-galactosidase deficiency.	First year; less often, second year	Arrest of development. Protruding belly. Coarse facies in infantile (generalized) form.	50% "cherry-red spot." Hearing usually normal. In juvenile type. Occasionally retinitis pigmentosa.	Head enlarged early: liver enlarged more than spleen.
Subacute necrotizing encephalomyelopathy (Leigh disease)	Recessive or variable. May have deficiency of pyruvate carboxylase, pyruvate dehydrogenase, cytochrome enzymes.	Infancy to late childhood	Difficulties in feeding; feeble or absent cry; floppiness, apnea.	Optic atrophy, often early. Roving eye movements. Ophthalmoplegia.	Head usually normal, occasionally small; cardiac and renal tubular dysfunction occasionally.
Menkes disease (kinky hair disease)	X-linked recessive; defect in copper absorption.	Infancy	Peculiar facies; secondary hair white, twisted, split; hypothermia.	May show optic disc pallor and microcysts of pigment epithelium.	Normal to small.
Carbohydrate-deficient glycoprotein syndrome	Recessive glycoprotein abnormality; glycosolation faulty.	Infancy	Failure to thrive, retardation, protein-losing enteropathy.	Strabismus, retinopathy.	Dysmorphic facies. Prominent fat pads.
Abetalipoproteinemia (Bassen-Kornzweig disease)	Recessive; primary defect unknown.	Early childhood	Diarrhea in infancy.	Retinitis pigmentosa; late ophthalmoplegia.	None.

3. Spinocerebellar Degeneration Disorders

Spinocerebellar degeneration disorders may be hereditary or may occur in sporadic fashion. Hereditary disorders include Friedreich ataxia, dominant hereditary ataxia, and a group of miscellaneous diseases.

Friedreich Ataxia

This is a recessive disorder characterized by onset of gait ataxia or scoliosis before puberty that becomes progressively worse. Reflexes, light touch, and position sensation are reduced. Dysarthria becomes progressively more severe. Cardiomyopathy usually develops, and diabetes mellitus occurs in 40% of patients, half of whom require insulin. Pes cavus typically is found. The GAA trinucleotide repeats on chromosome 9 can be used for laboratory diagnosis.

Treatment includes surgery for scoliosis and intervention as needed for cardiac disease and diabetes. Antioxidants may slow cardiac deterioration. Patients are usually confined to a wheelchair after age 20 years. Death occurs, usually from heart failure or dysrhythmias, in the third or fourth decade; some patients survive longer.

Motor System	Seizures	Laboratory and Tissue Studies	Course
DIFFUSE, BUT PRIMARILY GRAY MATTER			
Psychomotor retardation and progressive paralysis	Usually none	Chest radiographs may show pulmonary infiltrates. Nodules: granulomatous lesions, resembling those in reticuloendotheliosis. Multiple infarcts on CNS imaging.	Rapid: death usually in 1–2 y.
Initially floppy, eventually spastic	Usually late	Blood: vacuolated lymphocytes. X-rays: dorsolumbar kyphosis, "beaking" of vertebrae. "Foam cells" similar to those in Niemann-Pick disease.	Very rapid. Death within a few years. Slower in juvenile type (to 10 y).
Flaccid and immobile; may become spastic. Spinocerebellar forms; ataxia, myelopathy.	Rare and late tonic seizures	Increased CSF and blood lactate and pyruvate. High-signal MRI T_2 foci in thalami; globus pallidus, putamen, subthalamic nuclei. May be considered a mitochondrial disorder. DNA, enzyme tests on muscle.	Usually rapid in infants, but may be slow with death after several years. Central hypoventilation a frequent cause of death.
Variable: floppy to spastic	Myoclonic infantile spasms, status epilepticus	Defective absorption of copper. Cerebral angiography shows elongated arteries. Hair shows pili torti, split shafts. Copper and ceruloplasmin low.	Moderately rapid. Death usually by 3–4 y.
Variable hypotonia, neuropathy	Rare	Normal transferrin decreased. Carbohydrate-deficient transferrin increased. Liver steatosis. Cerebellar hypoplasia.	Cardiomyopathy, thrombosis. Hepatic fibrosis.
Ataxia, late extrapyramidal movement disorder	None	Abetalipoproteinemia: acanthocytosis, low serum vitamin E; cerebellar atrophy on imaging.	Progression arrested with vitamin E.

CSF, cerebrospinal fluid; CNS, central nervous system; CT, computed tomography; EEG, electroencephalogram; EMG, electromyelogram; ERG, electroretinogram; MRI, magnetic resonance imaging; PKAN, pantothenate kinase associated neurodegeneration; VER, visual evoked response; WBC, white blood cell.

Dominant Ataxia

These diseases (in the past known as olivopontocerebellar atrophy, Holmes ataxia, Marie ataxia, and the like) occur with varying manifestations, even among members of the same family. Ataxia occurs at onset, and progression continues with ophthalmoplegias (in some patients), extrapyramidal syndromes, polyneuropathy, and dementia. Several types have been found to be caused by CAG trinucleotide repeats. Levodopa may ameliorate rigidity and bradykinesia, but no other therapy is available. Only 10% of patients experience onset in childhood, and the course in these patients is often more rapid.

Miscellaneous Hereditary Ataxias

Associated findings permit identification of these recessive disorders. These include ataxia-telangiectasia (telangiectasia and immune defects; see below); Wilson disease (Kayser-Fleischer rings); Refsum disease (ichthyosis, cardiomyopathy, retinitis pigmentosa, and large nerves); Rett syndrome (regression to autism at age 7–18 months in girls, loss of use of hands, and progressive failure of brain growth); and abetalipoproteinemia (infantile diarrhea, acanthocytosis, and retinitis pigmentosa). Gluten sensitivity may cause ataxia. Patients with juvenile and chronic gangliosidoses and some hemolytic anemias and long-term survivors of Chédiak-Higashi disease may develop spinocerebellar degeneration. Idiopathic familial ataxia is called Behr syndrome. Neuropathies such as Charcot-Marie-Tooth disease produce ataxia.

Alper G, Narayanan V: Friedreich's ataxia. Pediatr Neurol 2003; 28:335 [PMID: 12878293].

Hadjivassiliou M: Gluten ataxia I perspective: Epidemiology, genetic susceptibility and clinical characteristics. Brain 2003; 126:685 [PMID: 12566288].

Hart PE et al: Antioxidant treatment of patients with Friedreich ataxia: four-year follow-up. Arch Neurol 2005;62:621 [PMID: 15824263].

Table 23–22. Central nervous system degenerative disorders of childhood. [a]

Disease	Enzyme Defect and Genetics	Onset	Early Manifestations	Vision and Hearing	Motor System	Seizures	Laboratory and Tissue Studies	Course
Adrenoleukodystrophy and variants (peroxisomal disease)	X-linked recessive. Neonatal form recessive Xq28. Acyl-CoA synthetase deficiency.	5–10 years. May also present as newborn, adolescent or adult.	Impaired intellect; behavioral problems	Cortical blindness and deafness	Ataxia, spasticity; motor deficits may be asymmetrical or one-sided initially; adrenomyeloneuropathy in adults	Occasionally	Hyperpigmentation and adrenocortical insufficiency. ACTH elevated. Accumulation of very-long-chain fatty acids in plasma. ?Stem cell, marrow transplant early on.	Variable course, many mildly involved. Severe variant with death in 2–5 y.
Neuronal ceroid lipofuscinosis (NCL; cerebromacular degeneration); infantile NCL (INCL); late infantile (LINCL); juvenile NCL (JNCL; Batten disease)	Recessive; multiple gene mutations, polymorphisms.	6–24 months INCL; 2–4 y LINCL; 4–8 y JNCL	Ataxia; visual difficulties; arrested intellectual development. Seizures	Pigmentary degeneration of macula; optic atrophy; ERG, VER abnormal	Ataxia; spasticity progressing to decerebrate rigidity	Often early: myoclonus and later generalized; refractory	Blood: vacuolated lymphocytes. Biopsy, EM of skin, conjunctiva; WBC: "curvilinear bodies, fingerprint profiles." Molecular testing of *CLN1, CLN2, CLN3* genes. Protein gene product testing for CLN1 and CLN2.	Moderately slow. Death in 3–8 y.
Subacute sclerosing panencephalitis (Dawson disease)	None. Measles "slow virus" infection. Also reported as result of rubella.	3–22 years; rarely earlier or later	Impaired intellect; emotional lability; incoordination	Occasionally chorioretinitis or optic atrophy; hearing normal	Ataxia; slurred speech; occasionally involuntary movements; spasticity progressing to decerebrate rigidity	Myoclonic and akinetic seizures relatively early; later, focal and generalized	CSF protein normal to moderately elevated. High CSF IgG[b], oligoclonal bands. Elevated CSF (and serum) measles (or rubella) antibody titers. Characteristic EEG. Brain biopsy; inclusion (acidophilic) body encephalitis; culturing of measles virus, perhaps rubella virus.	Variable, death in months to years. Remissions occasional. Treatment: INF-α intrathecal?
Megalencephalic leucodystrophy with subcortical cysts (MLC)	*MLC-1* gene defect usually 22q	Infancy	Macrocephaly		Ataxia; spasticity; ?dystonia	Varied; epilepsy	Characteristic MRI dysmyelination.	Slowly progressive to adulthood.

Disease	Genetics	Age of onset	Early/clinical features	Ophthalmologic	Motor/neurologic signs	Seizures	Laboratory/imaging	Course/treatment
Vanishing white matter/childhood ataxia with CNS hypomyelination VWM/CACH	*eIF2B* 3q27 autosomal recessive	Fatal infancy variant; other (slower) variants	Episodic deterioration with fever, head trauma, fear		Ataxia, spasticity		MRI: dramatic disappearance of white matter.	Fatal infantile form. Slowly progressive form. Adult variant (autosomal dominant) with ovarian dysgenesis.
Alexander disease	*GFAP* gene mutation autosomal dominant	Infancy	Macrocephaly key finding		As above		Demyelination; Rosenthal fibers characteristic of biopsy.	Fatal infantile. Juvenile: bulbar signs, less retardation.
Multiple sclerosis	None. Diagnosis difficult in childhood.	Adolescent; rare in childhood	Highly variable: may strike one or more sites of CNS; paresthesias common	Optic neuritis; diplopia, nystagmus at some time; vestibulocochlear nerves occasionally affected	Motor weakness; spasticity; ataxia; sphincter disturbances; slurred speech; mental difficulties.	Rare: focal or generalized	CSF may show slight pleocytosis, elevation of protein and gamma globulin;[b] oligoclonal bands present. CT scan may show areas of demyelination. Auditory, visual, and somatosensory evoked responses often show lesions in respective pathways. Changes in T-cell subsets.	Variable: complete remission possible. Recurrent attacks and involvement of multiple sites are prerequisites for diagnosis.
Cerebrotendinous xanthomatosis	?Recessive. Abnormal accumulation of cholesterol.	Late childhood to adolescence	Xanthomas in tendons; mental deterioration	Cataracts; xanthelasma	Cerebellar defects; bulbar paralysis late	Myoclonus	Xanthomas may appear in lungs. Xanthomas in tendons (especially Achilles).	Very slowly progressive into middle life. Replace bile deficient bile acid.
Huntington disease	Dominant. Chromosome 4p CAG repeat.	10% childhood onset	Rigidity; dementia	Ophthalmoplegia late	Rigidity; chorea frequently absent in children	50% with major motor seizures	CT scan may show "butterfly" atrophy of caudate and putamen.	Moderately rapid with death in 15 y.
Refsum disease (peroxisomal disease)	Recessive. Phytanic acid oxidase deficiency.	5–10 y	Ataxia;ichthyosis; cardiomyopathy	Retinitis pigmentosa; nystagmus	Ataxia; neuropathy; tendon reflexes absent	None	Serum phytanic acid elevated. Slow nerve conduction velocity. Elevated CSF protein. Peroxisomal disease.	Treat with low phytanic acid diet.

[a]For late infantile metachromatic leukodystrophy, Pelizaeus-Merzbacher disease, poliodystrophy, Gaucher disease of later onset, and subacute necrotizing encephalomyelopathy, see Table 23–21.

[b]CSF gamma globulin (IgG) is considered elevated in children when IgG is > 9% of total protein (possibly even > 8.3%); definitively elevated when > 14%.

ACTH, adrenocorticotropic hormone; CLN, ceroid lipofuscinosis; CSF, cerebrospinal fluid; CT, computed tomography; EEG, electroencephalogram; EM, electron microscopy ERG, electroretinogram; IFN-α, interferon-α; VER, visual evoked response; WBC, white blood cell.

Koenig M: Rare forms of autosomal recessive neurodegenerative ataxia. Semin Pediatr Neurol 2003;10:183 [PMID: 14653406].

Macpherson J et al: Observation of an excess of fragile-X permutations in a population of males referred with spinocerebellar ataxia. Hum Genet 2003;112:619 [PMID: 12612802].

Mahajnah M et al: Familial cognitive impairment with ataxia with oculomotor apraxia. J Child Neurol 2005;20:523 [PMID: 15996403].

Morrison PJ: Hereditary ataxias and paediatric neurology: new movers and shakers enter the field. Eur J Paediatr Neurol 2003;7:217 [PMID: 14511625].

Parmeggiani A et al: Epilepsy, intelligence and psychiatric disorders in patients with cerebellar hypoplasia. J Child Neurol 2003;18:1 [PMID: 12661930].

Vedanarayanan VV: Mitochondrial disorders and ataxia. Semin Pediatr Neurol 2003;10:200 [PMID: 14653408].

Yapici Z, Eraksoy M: Non-progressive congenital ataxia with cerebellar hypoplasia in three families. Acta Paediatr 2005;94:248 [PMID: 15981765].

ATAXIA-TELANGIECTASIA (Louis-Bar Syndrome)

Ataxia-telangiectasia is a multisystem disorder inherited as an autosomal recessive trait. It is characterized by progressive ataxia; telangiectasia of the bulbar conjunctivae, external ears, nares, and (later) other body surfaces, appearing in the third to sixth year; and recurrent respiratory, sinus, and ear infections. Ocular dyspraxia, slurred speech, choreoathetosis, hypotonia and areflexia, and psychomotor and growth retardation may be present. Endocrinopathies are common. Nerve conduction velocities may be reduced. The entire nervous system may be affected in late stages of the disease. A spectrum of involvement may be seen in the same family. Immunodeficiencies of IgA and IgE are common (see Chapter 29), and the incidence of certain cancers is high. Elevated serum α-fetoprotein is a screen for this disease.

Cabana MD et al: Consequences of the delayed diagnosis of ataxia-telangiectasia. Pediatrics 1998;102:98 [PMID: 9651420].

Crawford TO: Ataxia-telangiectasia. Semin Pediatr Neurol 1998;5:287 [PMID: 9874856].

Nowak-Wegrzyn A et al: Immunodeficiency and infections in ataxia-telangiectasia. J Pediatr 2004;144:505 [PMID: 15069401].

Sandoval C, Swift M: Hodgkin disease in ataxia-telangiectasia patients with poor outcomes. Med Pediatr Oncol 2003;40:162 [PMID: 12518345].

Tavani F et al: Ataxia-telangiectasia: The pattern of cerebellar atrophy on MRI. Neuroradiology 2003;45:315 [PMID: 12740724].

EXTRAPYRAMIDAL DISORDERS

Extrapyramidal disorders are characterized by the presence in the waking state of one or more of the following features: dyskinesias, athetosis, ballismus, tremors, rigidity, and dystonias.

For the most part, the precise pathologic and anatomic localization of these disorders is not understood. Motor pathways synapsing in the striatum (putamen and caudate nucleus), globus pallidus, red nucleus, substantia nigra, and the body of Luys are involved; this system is modulated by pathways originating in the thalamus, cerebellum, and reticular formation.

1. Sydenham Postrheumatic Chorea

Sydenham chorea is characterized by an acute onset of choreiform movements and variable degrees of psychological disturbance. It is frequently associated with rheumatic endocarditis and arthritis. Although the disorder follows infections with group A β-hemolytic streptococci, the interval between infection and chorea may be greatly prolonged; throat cultures and antistreptolysin O titers may therefore be negative. Chorea has also been associated with hypocalcemia; with vascular lupus erythematosus; and with toxic, viral, infectious, parainfectious, and degenerative encephalopathies.

Clinical Findings

A. SYMPTOMS AND SIGNS

Chorea, or rapid involuntary movements of the limbs and face, is the hallmark physical finding. In addition to the jerky incoordinate movements, the following are noted: emotional lability, waxing and waning ("milkmaid's") grip, darting tongue, "spooning" of the extended hands and their tendency to pronate, and knee jerks slow to return from the extended to their prestimulus position ("hung up"). Seizures, while uncommon, may be masked by choreic jerks.

B. LABORATORY FINDINGS

Anemia, leukocytosis, and an increased erythrocyte sedimentation rate and C-reactive protein may be present. The antistreptolysin O and/or anti-DNA-ase titer may be elevated and C-reactive protein present. Throat culture is sometimes positive for group A-hemolytic streptococci.

ECG and echocardiography are often essential to detect cardiac involvement. Antineuronal antibodies are present in most patients but are not specific for this disease. Specialized radiologic procedures (MRI and single-photon emission computed tomography) may show basal ganglia abnormalities.

Differential Diagnosis

The diagnosis of Sydenham chorea is usually not difficult. Tics, drug-induced extrapyramidal syndromes, Huntington chorea, and hepatolenticular degeneration (Wilson disease), as well as other rare movement disorders, can usually be ruled out on historical and clinical grounds. Immunologic linkages among chorea, tics, and obsessive-compulsive disorder are being studied in pediatric patients. Other causes of chorea can be ruled out by laboratory tests, such as antinuclear antibody for lupus, thyroid screening tests, serum calcium for hypocalcemia, and immunologic tests for Epstein-Barr virus infection.

Treatment

There is no specific treatment. Dopaminergic blockers such as haloperidol, 0.5 mg to 3–6 mg/d, and pimozide, 2–10 mg/d, have been used. Parkinsonian side effects such as rigidity and masked facies, and with high doses tardive dyskinesia, rarely occur in childhood. A variety of other drugs have been used with success in individual cases, such as the anticonvulsant sodium valproate, 50–60 mg/kg/d in divided doses; or prednisone, 0.5–2 mg/kg/d in divided doses. IVIg has been successful in severe cases. Emotional lability and depression sometimes warrant administration of antidepressants. All patients should be given antistreptococcal rheumatic fever prophylaxis, possibly through childbearing age.

Prognosis

Sydenham chorea is a self-limited disease that may last from a few weeks to months. Relapse of chorea may occur with nonspecific stress or illness—or with breakthrough streptococcal infections (if penicillin prophylaxis is not done). Two-thirds of patients relapse one or more times, but the ultimate outcome does not appear to be worse in those with recurrences. In older studies, eventual valvular heart disease occurs in about one-third of patients, particularly if other rheumatic manifestations appear. Psychoneurotic disturbances occur in a significant percentage of patients.

Barash J et al: Corticosteroid treatment in patients with Sydenham's chorea. Pediatr Neurol 2005;32:205 [PMID: 15730904].

Citak EC et al: Functional brain imaging in Sydenham's chorea and streptococcal tic disorders. J Child Neurol 2004;19:387 [PMID: 15224712].

Garvey MA et al: Treatment of Sydenham's chorea with intravenous immunoglobulin, plasma exchange, or prednisone. J Child Neurol 2005;20:424 [PMID: 15968928].

Korn-Lubetzki I et al: Recurrence of Sydenham chorea: implications for pathogenesis. Arch Neurol 2004;61:1261 [PMID: 15313844].

Murphy ML, Pichichero ME: Prospective identification and treatment of children with pediatric autoimmune neuropsychiatric disorder associated with group A streptococcal infection (PANDAS). Arch Pediatr Adolesc Med 2002;156:356 [PMID: 11929370].

van Toorn et al: Distinguishing PANDAS from Sydenham's chorea: case report and review of the literature. Eur J Paediatr Neurol 2004;8:211 [PMID: 15261885].

2. Tics (Habit Spasms)

Clinical Findings

Tics, or habit spasms, are quick repetitive but irregular movements, often stereotyped, and briefly suppressible. Coordination and muscle tone are not affected. A psychogenic basis is seldom discernible. Transient tics of childhood (12–24% incidence in school-age children) last from 1 month to 1 year and seldom need treatment. Many children with tics have a history of encephalopathic past events, neurologic soft signs, and school problems. Facial tics such as grimaces, twitches, and blinking predominate, but the trunk and extremities are often involved and twisting or flinging movements may be present. Vocal tics are less common.

Tourette syndrome is characterized by multiple fluctuating motor and vocal tics with no obvious cause lasting more than 1 year. Tics evolve slowly, new ones being added to or replacing old ones. Coprolalia and echolalia are relatively infrequent. Partial forms are common. The usual age at onset is 2–15 years, and the familial incidence is 35–50%. The disorder occurs in all ethnic groups. Tourette syndrome may be triggered by stimulants such as methylphenidate and dextroamphetamine. An imbalance of or hypersensitivity to neurotransmitters, especially dopamine and serotonin, has been hypothesized.

In mild cases, tics are self-limited, and when disregarded disappear. When attention is paid to one tic, it may disappear only to be replaced by another that is often worse. If the tic and its underlying anxiety or compulsive neuroses are severe, psychiatric evaluation and treatment are needed.

Important comorbidities are attention-deficit/hyperactivity disorder and obsessive-compulsive disorder. Learning disabilities, sleep difficulties, anxiety states, and mood swings are also common. Medications such as methylphenidate and dextroamphetamine should be carefully titrated to treat attention-deficit/hyperactivity disorder and avoid worsening tics. Fluoxetine and clomipramine may be useful for obsessive-compulsive disorder and rage episodes in patients with tics.

Treatment

The most effective medications for treating Tourette syndrome are dopamine blockers; however, many pediatric patients can manage without drug treatment. Medications are generally reserved for patients with disabling symptoms; treatment may be relaxed or discontinued when the symptoms abate (Table 23–23). Nonpharmacologic treatment of Tourette syndrome includes education of patients, family members, and school personnel. In some cases, restructuring the school environment to prevent tension and teasing may be necessary. Supportive counseling, either at or outside school, should be provided. Medica-

Table 23–23. Medications for Tourette syndrome and tics.

Dopamine blockers (many are antipsychotics)[c]
   Haloperidol (Haldol)
   Pimozide (Orap)
   Aripiprazole (Abilify)[c]
   Olanzapine (Zyprexa)[c]
   Risperidone (Risperdal)
Serotonergic drugs[a]
   Fluoxetine (Prozac)
   Anafranil (Clomipromine)
Noradrenergic drugs[b]
   Clonidine (Catapres)
   Guanfacine (Tenex)
Other
   Clonazepam (Klonopin)
   Baclofen (Lioresal)
   Pergolide (Permax)

---

[a]Useful for obsessive-compulsive disorder.
[b]Useful for attention-deficit/hyperactivity disorder.
[c]Some off-label use.

tions usually do not eradicate the tics. The goal of treatment should be to reduce the tics to tolerable levels without inducing undesirable side effects. Medication dosage should be increased at weekly intervals until a satisfactory response is obtained. Often a single dose at bedtime is sufficient. The two neuroleptic agents used most often are pimozide and risperidone. Sleepiness and weight gain are the most common side effects; rare are prolonged QT interval (ECG), akathisia, and tardive dyskinesia. Clonidine, clonazepam, and calcium channel blockers have been used in individual patients with some success. Sometimes these agents are used in combination (eg, clonidine with pimozide). IVIg has been unsuccessful.

Sydenham chorea is a well-documented pediatric autoimmune disorder associated with streptococcal infections (pediatric autoimmune neuropsychiatric disorder associated with streptococcal infection; PANDAS). Patients with tic disorders occasionally have obsessive-compulsive disorder precipitated or exacerbated by streptococcal infections. Less definite (much less frequent) are tic flare-ups with streptococcal infection. Active prospective antibody (antineuronal and antistreptococcal) and clinical studies are in progress. Research centers have used experimental treatments (IVIG, plasmapheresis, and steroids) in severe cases. At present, most patients with a tic do not worsen with group A streptococcal infections; with rare exceptions, penicillin prophylaxis is not generally necessary for the majority of patients with tic disorders.

Cuker A et al: Candidate locus for Gilles de la Tourette syndrome/obsessive compulsive disorder/chronic tic disorder at 18q22. Am J Med Genet A 2004;130:37 [PMID: 15368493].

Hoekstra J et al: Lack of effect of intravenous immunoglobulins on tics: a double-blind placebo-controlled study. J Clin Psychiatry 2004;65:537 [PMID: 14119917].

Leckman JF: Tourette's syndrome. Lancet 2002;360:1577 [PMID: 12443611].

Loiselle CR et al: Antistreptococcal, neuronal, and nuclear antibodies in Tourette syndrome. Pediatr Neurol 2003;28:119 [PMID: 12699862].

March JS: Pediatric autoimmune neuropsychiatric disorders associated with streptococcal infection (PANDAS): implications for clinical practice. Arch Pediatr Adolesc Med 2004;158:926 [PMID: 15351762].

Murphy ML, Pichichero ME: Prospective identification and treatment of children with pediatric autoimmune neuropsychiatric disorder associated with a group A streptococcal infection (PANDAS). Arch Pediatr Adolesc Med 2002;156:356 [PMID: 11929370].

Perrin EM et al: Does group A beta-hemolytic streptococcal infection increase risk for behavioral and neuropsychiatric symptoms in children? Arch Pediatr Adolesc Med 2004;158:848 [PMID: 15351749].

Snider LA et al: Tics and problem behavior in school children: Prevalence, characterization, and associations. Pediatrics 2002;110:331 [PMID: 12165586].

Swedo SE, Grant PJ: Annotation: PANDAS: a model for human autoimmune disease. J Child Psychol Psychiatry 2005;46:227 [PMID: 15755299].

3. Paroxysmal Dyskinesias/ Chronic Dystonia

Sudden-onset, short-duration choreoathetosis or dystonia episodes occur in childhood. Most often these episodes are familial and genetic. Episodes may occur spontaneously or be set off by actions ("kinesiogenic," or movement-induced) such as rising from a chair, reaching for a glass, or walking. Sometimes only hard sustained exercise will induce the dyskinesia. (Nocturnal dyskinesia/dystonic episodes are currently thought to be frontal lobe seizures.)

The diagnosis is clinical. Onset is usually in childhood (1.5–14 years). The patient is alert and often disconcerted during an episode.

Episodes may last seconds to 5–20 minutes and occur several times daily or monthly. Laboratory work is normal. EEG is normal between or during an attack; brain imaging is normal. Inheritance is usually autosomal dominant. Anticonvulsants (eg, carbamazepine) usually prevent further attacks. Patients often grow out of this disease in one or two decades.

Nonkinesiogenic dyskinesia is often secondary to an identifiable brain lesion, less or not responsive to medications, and nongenetic.

Disorders of ion channels underlie many of the genetic cases; some cases are linked to epilepsy and hemiplegic migraine. Chromosome loci are known.

The diagnosis of chronic persistent dystonia (sometimes L-dopa–responsive) may be aided by spinal fluid neurotransmitter and genetic chromosome studies. Rarely, dyskinesia (eg, dystonia) may be precipitated by fever, and chorea (rarely) may be a benign lifelong genetic disease.

Anca MH et al: Natural history of Oppenheim's dystonia (DYT1) in Israel. J Child Neurol 2003;18:325 [PMID: 12822816].

Bruno MK et al: Clinical evaluation of idiopathic paroxysmal kinesigenic dyskinesia: new diagnostic criteria. Neurology 2004;63:2280 [PMID: 15623687].

Dooley JM et al: Fever-induced dystonia. Pediatr Neurol 2003;28:149 [PMID: 12699869].

Jan MM: Misdiagnoses in children with dopa-responsive dystonia. Pediatr Neurol 2004;31:298 [PMID: 15464646].

Kleiner-Fisman G et al: Benign hereditary chorea: Clinical, genetic and pathological findings. Ann Neurol 2003:54:244 [PMID: 12891678].

Li Z et al: Childhood paroxysmal kinesigenic dyskinesia: report of seven cases with onset at an early age. Epilepsy Behav 2005;6:435 [PMID: 15820356].

McGrath TM, Dure LS: Paroxysmal dyskinesias in children. Curr Treat Options Neurol 2003;5:275 [PMID: 12791193].

4. Tremor

The most common cause of persisting tremors in childhood is essential tremor. Of those with this lifelong malady, 4.6% have onset in childhood (2–16 years). A genetic dominant inheritance is probable; 20–80% afflicted report a relative with tremors. Tremor, a mild fine motor and cosmetic handicap is worsened by anxiety, fatigue, stress, physical activity, and caffeine, and transiently improved by alcohol. Comorbidities include attention-deficit/hyperactivity disorder, dystonia, and possibly Tourette syndrome. Hand/arm tremor is the major manifestation; voice and head tremors are rare. Sometimes, "shuddering attacks" in infancy are a forerunner.

Laboratory studies are normal. Progression is minimal. Helpful medications (rarely needed long-term) include propranolol or primidone.

Differential diagnosis include birth asphyxia, Wilson disease, hyperthyroidism, and hypocalcemia; history and laboratory tests rule out these rare possibilities.

Jankovic J et al: Essential tremor among children. Pediatrics 2004;114:1203 [PMID: 15520096].

Schlaggar BL, Mink JW: Movement disorders in children. Pediatr Rev 2003;24:39 [PMID: 15972843].

Zesiewicz TA et al: Practice Parameter: Therapies for essential tremor. Neurology 2005;64:2008 [PMID: 15972843].

▓ INFECTIONS & INFLAMMATORY DISORDERS OF THE CENTRAL NERVOUS SYSTEM

Infections of the CNS are among the most common neurologic disorders encountered by pediatricians. Although infections are among the CNS disorders most amenable to treatment, they also have a very high potential for causing catastrophic destruction of the nervous system. It is imperative for the clinician to recognize infections early in order to treat and prevent massive tissue destruction.

Clinical Findings

A. SYMPTOMS AND SIGNS

Patients with CNS infections, whether caused by bacteria, viruses, or other microorganisms, present with similar manifestations. Systemic signs of infection include fever; malaise; and impaired heart, lung, liver, or kidney function. General features suggesting CNS infection include headache, stiff neck, fever or hypothermia, changes in mental status (including hyperirritability evolving into lethargy and coma), seizures, and focal sensory and motor deficits. Meningeal irritation is manifested by the presence of Kernig and Brudzinski signs. In very young infants, signs of meningeal irritation may be absent, and temperature instability and hypothermia are often more prominent than fever. In young infants, a bulging fontanelle and an increased head circumference are common. Papilledema may eventually develop, particularly in older children and adolescents. Cranial nerve palsies may develop acutely or gradually during the course of neurologic infections. No specific clinical sign or symptom is reliable in distinguishing bacterial infections from infections caused by other microbes.

During the initial clinical assessment, conditions that predispose the patient to infection of the CNS should be sought. Infections involving the sinuses or other structures in the head and neck region can result in direct extension of infection into the intracranial compartment. Open head injuries, recent neurosurgical procedures, immunodeficiency, and the presence of a mechanical shunt may predispose to intracranial infection.

B. LABORATORY FINDINGS

When CNS infections are suspected, blood should be obtained for a complete blood count, general chemistry panel, and culture. Most important, however, is obtaining CSF. In the absence of focal neurologic deficits or signs of increased intracranial pressure, CSF should be obtained immediately from any patient in whom serious CNS infection is suspected. When papilledema or focal motor signs are present, a lumbar puncture may be delayed until a neuroimaging procedure has been done to exclude space-occupying lesion. Start treatment for bacterial meningitis. It is generally safe to obtain spinal fluid from infants with nonfocal neurologic examination even if the fontanelle is bulging. Spinal fluid should be examined for the presence of red and white blood cells, protein concentration, glucose concentration, bacteria, and other microorganisms; a sample should be cultured. In addition, serologic, immunologic, and nucleic acid detection (PCR) tests may be performed on the spinal fluid in an attempt to identify the specific organism. Spinal fluid that contains a high proportion of polymorphonuclear leukocytes, a high protein concentration, and a low glucose concentration strongly suggests bacterial infection (see Chapter 38). CSF containing predominantly lymphocytes, a high protein concentration, and a low glucose concentration suggests infection with mycobacteria, fungi, uncommon bacteria, and some viruses such as lymphocytic choriomeningitis virus, herpes simplex virus, mumps virus, and arboviruses (see Chapters 36 and 39). CSF that contains a high proportion of lymphocytes, normal or only slightly elevated protein concentration, and a normal glucose concentration is most suggestive of viral infections, although partially treated bacterial meningitis and parameningeal infections may also result in this type of CSF formula. Typical CSF findings in a variety of infectious and inflammatory disorders are shown in Table 23–3.

In some cases, brain biopsy may be needed to identify the presence of specific organisms and clarify the diagnosis. Herpes simplex virus infections can be confirmed using the PCR test to assay for herpes DNA in spinal fluid. This test has a 95% sensitivity and 99% specificity. Brain biopsy may be needed to detect the rare PCR-negative case of herpes simplex and various parasitic infections, brain tumors, and other structural abnormalities.

C. IMAGING

Neuroimaging with CT and MRI scans may be helpful in demonstrating the presence of brain abscess, meningeal inflammation, or secondary problems such as venous and arterial infarctions, hemorrhages, and subdural effusions when these are expected. In addition, these procedures may identify sinus or other focal infections in the head or neck region that are related to the CNS infection. CT bone windows may demonstrate bony abnormalities such as basilar fractures.

EEGs may be helpful in the assessment of patients who have had seizures at the time of presentation. The changes are often nonspecific and characterized by generalized slowing. In some instances, such as herpes simplex virus or focal enterovirus infection, lateralized epileptiform discharges may be seen early in the course and may be one of the earliest laboratory abnormalities to suggest the diagnosis. EEGs may also show focal slowing over regions of abscesses.

BACTERIAL MENINGITIS

Bacterial infections of the CNS may present acutely (symptoms evolving rapidly over 1–24 hours), subacutely (symptoms evolving over 1–7 days), or chronically (symptoms evolving over more than 1 week). Diffuse bacterial infections involve the leptomeninges, superficial cortical

structures, and blood vessels. Although the term "meningitis" is used to describe these infections, it should not be forgotten that the brain parenchyma is also inflamed and that blood vessel walls may be infiltrated by inflammatory cells that result in endothelial cell injury, vessel stenosis, and secondary ischemia and infarction. Overall characteristics of meningitis are outlined in Table 23–24.

Pathologically, the inflammatory process involves all intracranial structures to some degree. Acutely, this inflammatory process may result in cerebral edema or impaired CSF flow through and out of the ventricular system, resulting in hydrocephalus.

Treatment

A. SPECIFIC MEASURES

(See also Chapter 35 and the section on *Haemophilus influenzae* type B infections in Chapter 38.)

While awaiting the results of diagnostic tests, the physician should start broad-spectrum antibiotic coverage as noted in the following discussion. After specific organisms are identified, antibiotic therapy can be tailored based on antibiotic sensitivity patterns. Bacterial meningitis in children younger than age 3 months is treated initially with cefotaxime (or ceftriaxone if the child is older than age 1 month) and ampicillin; the latter agent is used to treat *Listeria* and enterococci infections, which rarely affect older children. Children older than age 3 months are given ceftriaxone, cefotaxime, or ampicillin plus gentamicin. If *Streptococcus pneumoniae* cannot be ruled out by the initial Gram stain, vancomy-

Table 23–24. Encephalitis.

Definition: Brain inflammation (usually acute)
  Clinical: (Fever, headache) Seizures, motor paralysis, impaired consciousness
  Laboratory: CSF cells, protein increased; culture/PCR; serology CSF/blood
  Radiographic: Swelling (?focal), dysmyelination, ?infarcts
  Pathologic: Perivascular cells, gray matter, even neuronophagia; edema, dysmyelination, gliosis
Infectious: (95%) Enteroviruses, herpes, EBV, other viral (rare bacteria, fungi, protozoa); (some causes mosquito- or tick-borne; seasonal)
Para/post-infectious (ADEM): (25%) During or after banal respiratory infection, exanthema; most often no etiologic agent is identified
Treatment: Supportive. Herpes: acyclovir. ADEM: ?steroids, intravenous immune globulin.

ADEM, acute disseminated encephalomyelitis; EBV, Epstein-Barr virus; PCR, polymerase chain reaction.
Reproduced from: Lewis P, Glaser CA: Encephalitis. Pediatr Rev 2005;26:347.

cin or rifampin is added until cultures are reported, because penicillin-resistant pneumococci are common in the United States. Therapy may be narrowed when organism sensitivity allows. Duration of therapy is 7 days for meningococcal infections, 10 days for *H influenzae* or pneumococcal infection, and 14–21 days for other organisms. Slow clinical response or the occurrence of complications may prolong the need for therapy. Although therapy for 7 days has proved successful in many children with *H influenzae* infection, it cannot be recommended without further study if steroids are also used (see following discussion).

B. GENERAL AND SUPPORTIVE MEASURES

Children with bacterial meningitis are often systemically ill. The following complications should be looked for and treated aggressively: hypovolemia, hypoglycemia, hyponatremia, acidosis, septic shock, increased intracranial pressure, seizures, disseminated intravascular coagulation, and metastatic infection (eg, pericarditis, arthritis, or pneumonia). Children should initially be monitored closely (cardiorespiratory monitor, strict fluid balance and frequent urine specific gravity assessment, daily weights, and neurologic assessment every few hours), not fed until neurologically very stable, isolated until the organism is known, rehydrated with isotonic solutions until euvolemic, and then given intravenous fluids containing dextrose and sodium at no more than maintenance rate (assuming no unusual losses occur).

Complications

Abnormalities of water and electrolyte balance result from either excessive or insufficient production of antidiuretic hormone and require careful monitoring and appropriate adjustments in fluid administration. Monitoring serum sodium every 8–12 hours during the first 1–2 days, and urine sodium if the inappropriate secretion of antidiuretic hormone is suspected, usually uncovers significant problems.

Seizures occur in up to 30% of children with bacterial meningitis. Seizures tend to be most common in neonates and less common in older children. Persistent focal seizures or focal seizures associated with focal neurologic deficits strongly suggest subdural effusion, abscess, or vascular lesions such as arterial infarct, cortical venous infarcts, or dural sinus thrombosis. Because generalized seizures in a metabolically compromised child may have severe sequelae, early recognition and therapy are critical; some practitioners prefer phenytoin for acute management because it is less sedating than phenobarbital.

Subdural effusions occur in as many as 50% of young children with *S pneumoniae* meningitis. Subdural effusions are often seen on CT scans of the head during the course of meningitis. They do not require treatment unless they

are producing increased intracranial pressure or progressive mass effect. Although subdural effusions may be detected in children who have persistent fever, such effusions do not usually have to be sampled or drained if the infecting organism is *H influenzae,* meningococcus, or pneumococcus. These are usually sterilized with the standard treatment duration, and slowly waning fever during an otherwise uncomplicated recovery may be followed clinically. Under any other circumstance, however, aspiration of the fluid for documentation of sterilization or for relief of pressure should be considered.

Cerebral edema can participate in the production of increased intracranial pressure, requiring treatment with dexamethasone, osmotic agents, diuretics, or hyperventilation; continuous pressure monitoring may be needed.

Long-term sequelae of meningitis result from direct inflammatory destruction of brain cells, vascular injuries, or secondary gliosis. Focal motor and sensory deficits, visual impairment, hearing loss, seizures, hydrocephalus, and a variety of cranial nerve deficits can result from meningitis. Sensorineural hearing loss in *H influenzae* meningitis occurs in approximately 5–10% of patients during long-term follow-up. Recent studies have suggested that early addition of dexamethasone to the antibiotic regimen may modestly decrease the risk of hearing loss in some children with *bacterial* meningitis (see Chapter 38).

In addition to the variety of disorders mentioned earlier in this section, some patients with meningitis have mental retardation and severe behavioral disorders that limit their function at school and later performance in life.

BRAIN ABSCESS

Clinical Findings

Patients with brain abscess often appear to have systemic illness similar to patients with bacterial meningitis, but in addition they show signs of focal neurologic deficits, papilledema, and other evidence of increased intracranial pressure or a mass lesion. Symptoms may be present for a week or more; children with bacterial meningitis usually present within a few days. Conditions predisposing to development of brain abscess include penetrating head trauma; chronic infection of the middle ear, mastoid, or sinuses (especially the frontal sinus); chronic dental or pulmonary infection; cardiovascular lesions allowing right-to-left shunting of blood (including arteriovenous malformations); and endocarditis.

When brain abscess is strongly suspected, a neuroimaging procedure such as CT or MRI scans should be done prior to lumbar puncture. If a brain abscess is identified, lumbar puncture may be dangerous and rarely alters the choice of antibiotic or clinical management since the CSF abnormalities usually reflect only parameningeal inflammation. With spread from contagious septic foci, streptococci and anaerobic bacteria are most common. Staphylococci most often enter from trauma or from infections. Enteric organisms may form an abscess from chronic otitis. Unfortunately, cultures from a large number of brain abscesses remain negative.

The diagnosis of brain abscess is based primarily on a strong clinical suspicion and confirmed by a neuroimaging procedure. EEG changes are nonspecific but frequently demonstrate focal slowing in the region of brain abscess.

Treatment

Initial therapy for infection from presumed contagious foci uses penicillin and metronidazole. Cefotaxime is a good alternative to penicillin, especially if enteric organisms are suspected. Enteric organisms are also often susceptible to trimethoprim-sulfamethoxazole. Suspicion of infection by staphylococci, or their recovery from an aspirate, should be treated with nafcillin or vancomycin. Treatment may include neurologic consultation and anticonvulsant and edema therapy if necessary. In their early stages, brain abscesses are areas of focal cerebritis and can be "cured" with antibiotic treatment alone. Well-developed abscesses require surgical drainage.

Differential Diagnosis

Differential diagnosis of brain abscess includes any condition that produces focal neurologic deficits and increased intracranial pressure, such as neoplasms, subdural effusions, cerebral infarctions, and certain infections (herpes simplex, cysticercosis, and toxocariasis).

Prognosis

The surgical mortality rate in the treatment of brain abscess is lower than 5%. Untreated cerebral abscesses lead to irreversible tissue destruction and may rupture into the ventricle, producing catastrophic deterioration in neurologic function and death. Because brain abscesses are often associated with systemic illness and systemic infections, the death rate is frequently high in these patients.

VIRAL INFECTIONS

Viral infections of the CNS can involve primarily meninges (meningitis) (see Chapter 36) or cerebral parenchyma (encephalitis). All patients, however, have some degree of involvement of both the meninges and cerebral parenchyma (meningoencephalitis). Many viral infections are generalized and diffuse, but some viruses, notably herpes simplex and some enteroviruses, characteristically cause prominent focal disease. Focal cerebral involvement is clearly evident on neuroimaging procedures. Some viruses have an affinity for specific CNS cell populations. Poliovirus and other enteroviruses can selectively infect anterior horn cells (poliomyelitis) and some intracranial motor neurons.

Although most viral infections of the nervous system have an acute or subacute course in childhood, chronic infections can occur. Subacute sclerosing panencephalitis, for example, represents a chronic indolent infection caused by measles virus and is characterized clinically by progressive neurodegeneration and seizures.

Inflammatory reactions within the nervous system may occur during the convalescent stage of systemic viral infections. Parainfectious or postinfectious inflammation of the CNS results in several well-recognized disorders: acute disseminated encephalomyelitis (25% of encephalitis), transverse myelitis, optic neuritis, polyneuritis, and Guillain-Barré syndrome.

Congenital viral infections can also affect the CNS. CMV, herpes simplex virus, and rubella virus are the most notable causes of viral brain injury in utero.

Treatment of CNS viral infections is usually limited to symptomatic and supportive measures, except for herpes simplex virus. Acyclovir is the treatment in suspected or proved cases of herpes simplex virus encephalitis. Acyclovir is also useful in some patients with varicella-zoster virus infections of the CNS. West Nile virus, new in the United States, is an arthropod-borne flavivirus. It is found in mosquitoes, birds, and horses, and accounts for 27% of hospitalized patients in New York (1991) with encephalitis and muscle weakness. Fourteen percent had encephalitis alone, and 6% had aseptic meningitis. CSF antibody studies and PCR (57% positive for viral RNA) were diagnostic aids. The infection is now endemic as far as the western United States, particularly now in California. Recent studies have suggested spread of the infection to mosquitoes further south along the Atlantic seaboard.

Encephalopathy of Human Immunodeficiency Virus Infection

Neurologic syndromes associated directly with HIV infection include subacute encephalitis, meningitis, myelopathy, polyneuropathy, and myositis. In addition, secondary opportunistic infections of the CNS occur in patients with HIV-induced immunosuppression. *Toxoplasma* and CMV infections are particularly common. Progressive multifocal leukoencephalopathy, a secondary papillomavirus infection, and herpes simplex and varicella-zoster infections also occur frequently in patients with HIV infection. A variety of fungal (especially cryptococcal), mycobacterial, and bacterial infections have been described.

Neurologic abnormalities in these patients can also be the result of noninfectious neoplastic disorders. Primary CNS lymphoma and metastatic lymphoma to the nervous system are the most frequent neoplasms of the nervous system in these patients. See Chapters 29, 35, and 37 for diagnosis and management of HIV infection.

OTHER INFECTIONS

A wide variety of other microorganisms, including *Toxoplasma,* mycobacteria, spirochetes, rickettsiae, amoebae, and mycoplasmas, can cause CNS infections. CNS involvement in these infections is usually secondary to systemic infection or other predisposing factors. Appropriate cultures and serologic testing are required to confirm infections by these organisms. Parenteral antimicrobial treatment for these infections is discussed in Chapter 35.

NONINFECTIOUS INFLAMMATORY DISORDERS OF THE CENTRAL NERVOUS SYSTEM

The differential diagnosis of bacterial, viral, and other microbial infections of the CNS includes disorders that cause inflammation but for which no specific causal organism has been identified. Sarcoidosis, Behçet disease, systemic lupus erythematosus, other collagen-vascular disorders, and Kawasaki disease are examples. In these disorders, CNS inflammation usually occurs in association with characteristic systemic manifestations that allow proper diagnosis. Management of CNS involvement in these disorders is the same as the treatment of the systemic illness.

OTHER PARAINFECTIOUS ENCEPHALOPATHIES

In association with systemic infections or other illnesses, CNS dysfunction may occur in the absence of direct CNS inflammation or infection. Reye syndrome is a prominent example of this type of encephalopathy that often occurs in association with varicella virus or other respiratory or systemic viral infections. In Reye syndrome, cerebral edema and cerebral dysfunction occur, but there is no evidence of any direct involvement of the nervous system by the associated microorganism or inflammation. Cerebral edema in Reye syndrome is accompanied by liver dysfunction and fatty infiltration of the liver. As a result of efforts to discourage use of aspirin in childhood febrile illnesses, the number of patients with Reye syndrome has markedly decreased. The precise relationship, however, between aspirin and Reye syndrome is unclear.

Abzug MJ: Presentation, diagnosis, and management of enterovirus infections in neonates. Paediatr Drugs 2004;6:1 [PMID: 14969566].

Chaudhuri A: Adjunctive dexamethasone treatment in acute bacterial meningitis. Lancet Neurol 2004;3:54 [PMID: 14693112].

Chavez-Bueno S, McCracken GH Jr: Bacterial meningitis in children. Pediatr Clin North Am 2005;52:795 [PMID: 15925663].

Feigin RD: Use of corticosteroids in bacterial meningitis. Pediatr Infect Dis J 2004;23:355 [PMID: 15071293].

Grose C: The puzzling picture of acute necrotizing encephalopathy after influenza A and B virus infection in young children. Pediatr Infect Dis J 2004;23:253 [PMID: 15014302].

Hayes EG, O'Leary DR: West Nile virus infection: a pediatric perspective. Pediatrics 2004;113:1375 [PMID: 15121956].

Hunson JL et al: Clinical and neuroradiologic features of acute disseminated encephalomyelitis in children. Neurology 2001; 56:1308 [PMID: 11376179].

Kennedy PG: Neurological infection. Lancet Neurol 2004;3:13 [PMID: 14693102].

Khurana DS et al: Acute disseminated encephalomyelitis in children: Discordant neurologic and neuroimaging abnormalities and response to plasmapheresis. Pediatrics 2004;116:431 [PMID: 16061599].

Lewis P, Glaser CA: Encephalitis. Pediatr Rev 2005;26:353 [PMID: 16199589].

Nolan MA et al: Survival after pulmonary edema due to enterovirus 71 encephalitis. Neurology 2003;60:1651 [PMID: 12771257].

Sazgar M et al: Influenza B acute necrotizing encephalopathy: A case report and literature review. Pediatr Neurol 2003;28:396 [PMID: 12878304].

Sejvar JJ et al: Neurologic manifestations and outcome of West Nile virus infection. JAMA 2003;290:511 [PMID: 12876094].

Silvia MT, Licht DJ: Pediatric central nervous system infections and inflammatory white matter disease. Pediatr Clin North Am 2005;52:1107 [PMID: 16009259].

Studahl M: Influenza virus and CNS manifestations. J Clin Virol 2003;28:225 [PMID: 14522059].

Toth C et al: Neonatal herpes encephalitis: A case series and review of clinical presentations. Can J Neurol Sci 2003;30:36 [PMID: 12619782].

Tyler KL: West Nile Virus Infection in the United States. Arch Neurol 2004;61:1190 [PMID: 15313835].

Whitley RJ, Kimberlin DW: Herpes simplex encephalitis: children and adolescents. Semin Pediatr Infect Dis 2005;16:17 [PMID: 15685145].

Yim R et al: Spectrum of clinical manifestations of West Nile Virus infection in children. Pediatrics 2004;114:1674 [PMID: 15574633].

SYNDROMES PRESENTING AS ACUTE FLACCID PARALYSIS

Flaccid paralysis evolving over hours or a few days suggests involvement of the lower motor neuron complex (see section on floppy infant syndrome). Anterior horn cells (spinal cord) may be involved by viral infection (paralytic poliomyelitis) or by paraviral or postviral immunologically mediated disease (acute transverse myelitis). The nerve trunks (polyneuritis) may be diseased as in Guillain-Barré syndrome or affected by toxins (diphtheria or porphyria). The neuromuscular junction may be blocked by tick toxin or botulinum toxin. The paralysis rarely will be due to metabolic (periodic paralysis) or inflammatory muscle disease (myositis). A lesion compressing the spinal cord must be ruled out.

Clinical Findings

A. SYMPTOMS AND SIGNS

Features assisting diagnosis are age, a history of preceding or waning illness, the presence (at time of paralysis) of fever, rapidity of progression, cranial nerve findings, and sensory findings (Table 23–25). The examination may show long tract findings (pyramidal tract), causing increased reflexes and a positive Babinski sign. The spinothalamic tract may be interrupted, causing loss of pain and temperature. Back pain, even tenderness to percussion, may occur, as well as bowel and bladder incontinence. Often the paralysis is ascending, symmetric, and painful (muscle tenderness or myalgia). Laboratory findings occasionally are diagnostic.

B. LABORATORY FINDINGS (SEE TABLE 23–25.)

Examination of CSF is helpful. Imaging studies of the spinal column (plain radiographs) and spinal cord (MRI) are occasionally essential. Viral cultures (CSF, throat, and stool) and titers aid in diagnosing poliomyelitis. A high sedimentation rate may suggest tumor or abscess; the presence of antinuclear antibody may suggest lupus arteritis.

EMG and nerve conduction velocity can be helpful in diagnosing polyneuropathy. Nerve conduction is usually slowed after 7–10 days. Findings in botulism and tick-bite paralysis can be specific and diagnostic. Rarely, elevation of muscle enzymes or even myoglobinuria may aid in diagnosis of myopathic paralysis. Porphyrin urine studies and heavy-metal assays (arsenic, thallium, and lead) can reveal those rare toxic causes of polyneuropathic paralysis.

Differential Diagnosis

The child who has been well and becomes paralyzed often has polyneuritis. Acute transverse myelitis sometimes occurs in an afebrile child. The child who is ill and febrile at the time of paralysis often has acute transverse myelitis or poliomyelitis. Acute epidural spinal cord abscess (or other compressive lesion) must be ruled out. Poliomyelitis is very rare in our immunized population. Enterovirus 71 and West Nile disease are two new causes. Paralysis due to tick bites occurs seasonally (spring and summer). The tick is usually found in the occipital hair. Removal is curative.

Paralysis due to botulinum toxin occurs most commonly in those younger than age 1 year (see Chapter 38). Intravenous drug abuse can lead to myelitis and paralysis. Furthermore, chronic myelopathy occurs with two human immunodeficiency virus infections: HTLV-I and HTLV-III (now called HIV-1).

Complications

A. RESPIRATORY PARALYSIS

Early and careful attention to oxygenation is essential. Administration of oxygen, intubation, mechanical respiratory assistance, and careful suctioning of secretions may be required. Increasing anxiety and a rise in diastolic and systolic blood pressures are early signs of hypoxia. Cyanosis is a late sign. Deteriorating spirometric findings (forced expiratory volume in 1 second and total vital capacity) may indicate the need for controlled intubation and respiratory support. Blood gases (usually late changes with increased CO_2 and decreased O_2) can aid decisions.

B. INFECTIONS

Pneumonia is common, especially in patients with respiratory paralysis. Antibiotic therapy is best guided by results of cultures. Bladder infections occur when an indwelling catheter is required because of bladder paralysis. Recovery from myelitis may be delayed by urinary tract infection.

C. AUTONOMIC CRISIS

This may be a cause of death in Guillain-Barré syndrome. Strict attention to vital signs to detect and treat hypotension or hypertension and cardiac arrhythmias in an intensive care setting is advisable, at least early in the course and in severely ill patients.

Treatment

Most of these syndromes have no specific treatment. Ticks causing paralysis must be removed. Other therapies include the use of erythromycin in *Mycoplasma* infections and botulism immune globulin in infant botulism. Recognized associated disorders (eg, endocrine, neoplastic, or toxic) should be treated by appropriate means. Supportive care also involves pulmonary toilet, adequate fluids and nutrition, bladder and bowel care, prevention of decubitus ulcers, and in many cases, psychiatric support.

A. CORTICOSTEROIDS

These agents are believed by most to be of no benefit in Guillain-Barré syndrome. Autonomic symptoms (eg, hypertension) in polyneuritis may require treatment.

B. PLASMAPHERESIS, INTRAVENOUS IMMUNOGLOBULIN

Plasma exchange or intravenous IgG has been beneficial in moderate or severe cases of Guillain-Barré syndrome. Some clinicians use inability to ambulate as a criterion to use IVIg.

C. PHYSICAL THERAPY

Rehabilitative measures are best instituted when acute symptoms have subsided and the patient is stable.

D. ANTIBIOTICS

Appropriate antibiotics and drainage are required for epidural abscess.

Table 23–25. Acute flaccid paralysis in children.

	Poliomyelitis (Paralytic, Spinal, and Bulbar), With or Without Encephalitis	Landry-Guillain-Barré Syndrome ("Acute Idiopathic Polyneuritis")	Botulism	Tick-Bite Paralysis	Transverse Myelitis and Neuromyelitis Optica
Etiology	Poliovirus types I, II, and III; other enteroviruses, eg, EV71; vaccine strain polio virus (rare); West Nile virus: epidemic in birds. Mosquitoes infect horses, humans	Likely delayed hypersensitivity—with T-cell–mediated antiganglioside antibodies. Mycoplasmal and viral infections (EBV, CMV), *Campylobacter jejuni*, Hepatitis B.	*Clostridium botulinum* toxin. Block at neuromuscular junction. Under age 1, toxin synthesized in bowel by organisms in ingested dust or honey. At older ages toxin ingested in food. Rarely from wound infection.	Probable interference with transmission of nerve impulse caused by toxin in tick saliva.	Usually unknown; multiple viruses (herpes, EBV, varicella, hepatitis A) often postviral (see Guillain–Barré syndrome).
History	None, or inadequate polio immunization. Upper respiratory or gastrointestinal symptoms followed by brief respite. Bulbar paralysis more frequent after tonsillectomy. Often in epidemics, in summer and early fall.	Nonspecific respiratory or gastrointestinal symptoms in preceding 5–14 d common. Any season, though slightly lower incidence in summer.	Infancy: dusty environment (eg, construction area), honey. Older: food poisoning. Multiple cases hours to days after ingesting contaminated food.	Exposure to ticks (dog tick in eastern United States; wood ticks). Irritability 12–24 h before onset of a rapidly progressive ascending paralysis.	Rarely symptoms compatible with multiple sclerosis or optic neuritis. Progression from onset to paraplegia often rapid, usually without a history of bacterial infection.
Presenting complaints	Febrile at time of paralysis. Meningeal signs, muscle tenderness, and spasm. Asymmetrical weakness widespread or segmental (cervical, thoracic, lumbar). Bulbar symptoms early or before extremity weakness; anxiety; delirium.	Symmetrical weakness of lower extremities, which may ascend rapidly to arms, trunk, and face. Verbal child may complain of paresthesias. Fever uncommon. Facial weakness early. Miller-Fisher variant presents as ataxia and ophthalmoplegia (rare).	Infancy: constipation, poor suck and cry. "Floppy." Apnea. Lethargy. Choking (cause of SIDS?). Older: blurred vision, diplopia, ptosis, choking, weakness.	Rapid onset and progression of ascending flaccid paralysis; often accompanied by pain and paresthesias. Paralysis of upper extremities second day after onset. Sometimes acute ataxia presentation.	Root and back pain in about one-third to one-half of cases. Sensory loss below level of lesion accompanying rapidly developing paralysis. Sphincter difficulties common. Fever (58%).
Findings	Flaccid weakness, usually asymmetrical. Cord level: Lumbar: legs, lower abdomen. Cervical: shoulder, arm, neck, diaphragm. Bulbar: respiratory, lower cranial nerves. Encephalopathy accompanies paralysis in West Nile.	Flaccid weakness, symmetric, usually greater proximally, but may be more distal or equal in distribution. Rarely cranial nerves IX–XI, III–VI. Miller-Fisher variant: ophthalmoplegia, ataxia. Bulbar involvement may occur. Slight distal impairment of position, vibration, touch; difficult to assess in young children.	Infants: Flaccid weakness. Alert. Eye, pupil, facial weakness. Deep tendon reflexes decreased. Absent suck, gag. Constipation. Older: paralysis accommodation, eye movements. Weak swallow. Respiratory paralysis.	Flaccid, symmetric paralysis. Cranial nerve and bulbar (respiratory) paralysis, ataxia, sphincter disturbances, and sensory deficits may occur. Some fever. Diagnosis rests on finding tick, which is especially likely to be on occipital scalp.	Paraplegia with areflexia below level of lesion early; later, may have hyperreflexia. Sensory loss below and hyperesthesia or normal sensation above level of lesion. Paralysis of bladder and rectum. Optic neuritis rarely may be present.

(continued)

Table 23–25. Acute flaccid paralysis in children. (continued)

	Poliomyelitis (Paralytic, Spinal, and Bulbar), With or Without Encephalitis	Landry-Guillain-Barré Syndrome ("Acute Idiopathic Polyneuritis")	Botulism	Tick-Bite Paralysis	Transverse Myelitis and Neuromyelitis Optica
CSF	Pleocytosis (20–500+ cells) with PMN predominance in first few days, later monocytic preponderance. Protein frequently elevated (50–150 mg/dL). CSF IgM + in West Nile.	Cytoalbuminologic dissociation; ten or fewer mononuclear cells with high protein after first week. Normal glucose. IgG may be elevated. West Nile will have cells; nerves can be involved in a myeloradiculitis.	Normal.	Normal.	Usually no manometric block; CSF may show increased protein, pleocytosis with predominantly mononuclear cells, increased IgG.
Electromyogram (EMG)	Denervation after 10–21 days. Nerve conduction normal. Amplitude reduced in West Nile.	Nerve conduction velocities markedly decreased; may be normal early, or if axon only damage.	EMG distinctive: BSAP (brief small abundant potentials).	Nerve conduction slowed; returns rapidly to normal after removal of tick.	Normal early. Denervation at level of lesion after 10–21 d.
Other studies	Virus in stool and throat. Serial serologic titers IgG, IgM in West Nile. Hyponatremia 30% in West Nile.	Search for specific cause such as infection, intoxication, autoimmune disease. Antiganglioside antibodies to GM$_1$ (GQ1b in Miller-Fisher)	Infancy: stool culture, toxin. Rare serum toxin positive. Older: serum (or wound) toxin.	Leukocytosis, often with moderate eosinophilia	Normal spine x-rays do not exclude spinal epidural abscess. MRI to ruleout cord-compressive lesions. Cord may be swollen in myelitis.
Course and prognosis	Paralysis usually maximal 3–5 d after onset. Transient bladder paralysis may occur. Outlook varies with extent and severity of involvement. **Note:** Mortality greatest from respiratory failure and superinfection. West Nile paralysis may be permanent.	Course progressive over a few days to about 2 weeks. **Note:** Threat greatest from respiratory failure (10%), autonomic crises (eg, widely variable blood pressure, arrhythmia), and superinfection. Majority recover completely. Plasmapheresis may have a role. Intravenous IgG. Relapses occasionally occur.	Infancy: supportive. Penicillin. Botulism immune globulin intravenous (BIG-IV). Respiratory support, gavage feeding. Avoid aminoglycosides. Older: penicillin, antitoxin, prolonged respiratory support. Prognosis: excellent. Fatality 3%.	Total removal of tick is followed by rapid improvement and recovery. Otherwise, mortality rate due to respiratory paralysis is very high.	Large degree of functional recovery possible. Corticosteroids are of controversial benefit in shortening duration of acute attack or altering the overall course. Plasmapheresis, IVIg: anecdotal benefit.

CMV, cytomegalovirus; CSF, cerebrospinal fluid; EBV, Ebstein–Barr virus; IVIg, intravenous immune globulin; MRI, magnetic resonance imaging; PMN, polymorphonuclear neutrophil; SIDS, sudden infant death syndrome.

Bakker J, Metz L: Devic's neuromyelitis optica treated with intravenous gamma globulin (IVIG). Can J Neurol Sci 2004;31:265 [PMID: 15198456].

Dalakas MC: Intravenous immunoglobulin in autoimmune neuromuscular diseases. JAMA 2004;291:2367 [PMID: 15150209].

Defresne P et al: Acute transverse myelitis in children: Clinical course and prognostic factors. J Child Neurol 2003;18:401 [PMID: 12886975].

Dimario FJ Jr: Intravenous immunoglobulin in the treatment of childhood Guillain-Barré syndrome: A randomized trial. Pediatrics 2005;116:226 [PMID: 15995056].

Fox CK et al: Recent advances in infant botulism. Pediatr Neurol 2005;32:149 [PMID: 15730893].

Hughes RA et al: Practice parameter: immunotherapy for Guillain-Barré syndrome. Neurology 2003;61:736 [PMID: 14504313].

Jeha LE et al: West Nile virus infection: A new acute paralytic illness. Neurology 2003;61:55 [PMID: 12847156].

Korinthenberg R et al: Intravenously administered immunoglobulin in the treatment of childhood Guillain-Barré syndrome: A randomized trial. Pediatrics 2004;116:8 [PMID: 15995024].

Krishnan C et al: Transverse myelitis: pathogenesis, diagnosis and treatment. Front Biosci 2004;9:1483 [PMID: 14977560].

Li Z, Turner RP: Pediatric tick paralysis: discussion of two cases and literature review. Pediatr Neurol 2004;31:304 [PMID: 15464647].

Miyazawa R et al: Determinants of prognosis of acute transverse myelitis in children. Pediatr Int 2003;45:512 [PMID: 14521523].

Sejvar JJ et al: West Nile virus-associated flaccid paralysis. Emerg Infect Dis 2005;11:1021 [PMID: 16022775].

Shaharao V et al: Recurrent acute transverse myelopathy: association with antiphospholipid antibody syndrome. Indian J Pediatr 2004;71:559 [PMID: 15226572].

Soloman T, Willison H: Infectious causes of acute flaccid paralysis. Curr Opin Infect Dis 2003;16:375 [PMID: 14501988].

Tekgul H et al: Outcome of axonal and demyelinating forms of Guillain-Barre syndrome in children. Pediatr Neurol 2003;28:295 [PMID: 12849884].

Thompson JA et al: Infant botulism in the age of botulism immune globulin. Neurology 2005;64:2029 [PMID: 15917401].

Vedanarayanan VV et al: Tick paralysis in children: Electrophysiology and possibility of misdiagnosis. Neurology 2002;59:1088 [PMID: 12370471].

Yim R et al: Spectrum of clinical manifestations of West Nile virus infection in children. Pediatrics 2004;114:1673 [PMID: 15574633].

■ DISORDERS OF CHILDHOOD AFFECTING MUSCLES (Table 23–26)

DIAGNOSTIC STUDIES

Serum Enzymes

Creatine kinase reflects muscle damage or "leaks" from muscle into plasma. Blood should be drawn before EMG or muscle biopsy, which may lead to release of the enzyme. Corticosteroids may suppress levels despite very active muscle disease, for example, as in polymyositis.

Electromyography

EMG is often helpful in grossly differentiating myopathic from neurogenic processes. Fibrillations occur in both. In the myopathies, very low spikes are more typical, and the motor unit action potentials seen during contraction characteristically are of short duration, are polyphasic, and are increased in number for the strength of the contraction (increased interference pattern). Neurogenic findings include decreased numbers of motor units, which may be polyphasic, larger than normal, or both. The interference pattern is decreased. In myotonic dystrophy, the EMG is characterized by prolonged discharge of electrical activity on movement of the probing needle (so-called "dive-bomber" sound).

Muscle Biopsy

Properly executed (by open biopsy or by using the Bergstrom muscle biopsy needle), this procedure is usually helpful. Histochemical techniques, histogram analysis of muscle fiber types and sizes, and electron microscopy are offering new classifications of the myopathies. Findings common to the muscular dystrophies include variation in the size and shape of muscle fibers, increase in connective tissue, interstitial infiltration of fatty tissue, degenerative changes in muscle fibers, and central location of nuclei.

Dystrophin is a normal intracellular plasma membrane protein in muscle, the gene product missing in Duchenne and Becker muscular dystrophies. Staining the muscle for dystrophin aids in differentiating Duchenne and Becker muscular dystrophies; dystrophin is absent in Duchenne muscular dystrophy and reduced in Becker muscular dystrophy. Electrophoresis can confirm whether the dystrophin is absent or present in small amounts and whether there is a qualitative difference from normal dystrophin, the latter two patterns being characteristic of Becker muscular dystrophy.

Genetic Testing & Carrier Detection

Previously, detection of carriers for Duchenne muscular dystrophy (mothers and sisters of affected boys) rested on creatine kinase elevations (two-thirds of patients will have this finding); physical findings of mild dystrophy (large calves and muscle weakness); abnormal muscle EMGs; or biopsy results. All are unreliable for diagnostic purposes.

DNA probes are now available for carrier detection and prenatal diagnosis of Duchenne and Becker muscular dystrophies. Deletions are often (60%) found on the short arm of the X chromosome; it is postulated that all

Table 23–26. Muscular dystrophies and myotonias of childhood.

Disease	Genetic Pattern	Age at Onset	Early Manifestations	Involved Muscles	Reflexes
Muscular dystrophies Duchenne muscular dystrophy (pseudohypertrophic infantile)	X-linked recessive; autosomal-recessive unusual. 30–50% have no family history.	2–6 y; rarely in infancy	Clumsiness, easy fatigability on walking, running, and climbing stairs. Walking on toes; waddling gait. Lordosis. (Climbing up on legs rising from supine position—Gower maneuver.)	Axial and proximal before distal. Pelvic girdle; pseudohypertrophy of gastrocnemius (90%), triceps brachii, and vastus lateralis. Shoulder girdle usually later, also articulation difficulties. Eventually cardiomyopathy (50%).	Knee jerks ± or 0; ankle jerks + to ++
Becker muscular dystrophy (late onset)	X-linked recessive. (Allele at Xp21.)	Childhood (usually later than in Duchenne)	Similar to Duchenne.	Similar to Duchenne.	Similar to Duchenne.
Limb-girdle muscular dystrophy A. Pelvifemoral (Leyden-Möbius) B. Scapulohumeral (Erb juvenile)	Autosomal-recessive in 60%; high sporadic incidence. A. Relatively common B. Rare	Variable; early childhood to adulthood	Weakness, with distribution according to type. Waddling gait, difficulty climbing stairs. Lordosis.	A. Pelvic girdle usually involved first and to greater extent. B. Shoulder girdle often asymmetric. Quadriceps and hamstrings may be weakest.	Usually present
Facioscapulohumeral muscular dystrophy (Landouzy-Déjérine) Scapuloperoneal variant (rare)	Autosomal-dominant; sporadic cases not uncommon: Linkage to 4q35; variable number of (decreased) D4Z4 repeats	Usually late in childhood and adolescence; rare in infancy; not uncommon in 20s	Diminished facial movements with inability to close eyes, smile, or whistle. Face may be flat; unlined. Difficulty in raising arms over head. Lordosis. Tripping in scapuloperoneal type.	Facial muscles followed by shoulder girdle, with occasional spread to hips or distal legs (scapuloperoneal variant). (Face may be *un*involved.)	Present
Spinal muscular atrophy (SMA) Infantile SMA (Werdnig-Hoffman disease)	Autosomal-recessive	0–2 y	Floppy infant.	Pelvic and shoulder girdle. Tongue. Intercostals. Fingers and toes spared.	0 or nearly so
Juvenile SMA (Kugelburg-Welander disease)	Autosomal-recessive	Onset after age 2 usually (age 5–15 typical)	Weakness. "Fasciculations" 50%. Rarely a cause of floppy infant.	Same	Same
Metabolic myopathies Carnitine deficiency (lipid storage myopathy) Primary (rare) Secondary: multiple forms	Genetics variable, often recessive	Infancy to adolescence	Fasting hypoglycemia and coma; less ketosis than expected. Myopathy. Cardiomyopathy. Fatty liver. Don't confuse with Reye, SIDS.	Weakness variable; may be precipitated by exercise (with resultant myoglobulinuria) or fasting	Normal to decreased

Muscle Biopsy Findings	Other Diagnostic Tests	Treatment	Prognosis
Degeneration and variation in fiber size; proliferation of connective tissue. Basophilia, phagocytosis. Poor differentiation of fiber types on ATPase reaction; deficiency of type IIB fibers. Dystrophin absent.	EMG myopathic. CK (4000–5000 IU) very high with decrease toward normal over the years. 60% have C-terminal Xp21 deletion on blood, amniotic fluid or chorionic villi. Positive test obviates need for muscle biopsy	Physical therapy, braces, wheelchair eventually, weight control. Prednisone, deflazacort improve motor function temporarily. Creatine, some benefit. Gene transfer minidystrophin by viral vectors. Utrophin.	Ten percent show nonprogressive mental retardation. Osteoporosis, scoliosis common. Death from cardiac or respiratory failure 10–15 y after diagnosis with 75% of patients dead by age 20.
Similar to above, except type IIB fibers present. Reduced or abnormal size dystrophin.	Similar to above, although muscle enzymes may not be as elevated	As above. Wheelchair in late childhood or early adult life.	Slower progression than Duchenne's, with death usually in adulthood.
Dystrophic muscle changes (see Duchenne). Dystrophin normal. Special stains for sarcoglycan (dystrophin associated glycoprotein [DAG] deficiency).	EMG myopathic. CK variable; many severe cases have sarcoglycan deficiency (severe autosomal recessive type). Must exclude dystrophinopathy and SMA.	Physical therapy, weight control	Mildly progressive: spread from lower to upper limbs may take 15–20 y. Life expectancy mid to late adulthood.
Predominantly large fibers with scattered tiny atrophic fibers, "moth-eaten" and whorled fibers. Inflammatory response. Little or no fiber splitting, fibrosis, or type 1 fiber predominance.	EMG myopathic. Muscle enzymes usually normal. 4q35ter deletion. If blood test positive, biopsy unnecessary.	Physical therapy where indicated. Wheelchair in 20%. Forty percent of biopsies show inflammation; steroids ineffective, however.	Very slowly progressive, often with plateaus, except in infantile form where there may be difficulties in walking by adolescence. Usually normal life span.
Small, group atrophy. Twin peak fiber size. Fiber type grouping. Minimal fibrosis.	EMG neuropathic. Nerve conduction, CSF, muscle enzymes normal. 90–95% have deletions or abnormalities in *SMN* (survival motor neuron) or other genes at band 5q13. Carrier detection available.	Supportive: respiratory care, positioning, secretion management. Genetic counseling.	80–95% of patients 0–4 y die of pneumonia and respiratory failure.
Same.		Physical therapy, wheelchair positioning to avoid scoliosis. May walk, usually later lose this.	Fairly normal life expectancy. 4–40+ y.
Lipid droplets ± or ragged red fibers may be present.	Muscle biochemistry (carnitine, CPT enzyme). Urine organic acids (at time of illness). Plasma carnitine: deficiency may be in blood alone or blood and muscle.	Avoid fasting and mitochondrial toxins, eg, ASA, valproic acid. Carbohydrate. Treat acidosis. Carnitine orally.	Variable: occasionally fatal in infants. Progressive weakness, developmental delay, cardiomyopathy may occur.

(continued)

Table 23–26. Muscular dystrophies and myotonias of childhood. (continued)

Disease	Genetic Pattern	Age at Onset	Early Manifestations	Involved Muscles	Reflexes
"Oculocraniosomatic syndrome" (ophthalmoplegia and "ragged reds"; progressive external ophthalmoplegia) Kearns-Sayre	Mitochondrial DNA deletion; other hereditary neurologic disorders may be found in patient or family.	Variable; from infancy to adult life; most at about 10 y of age	Ptosis and limitation of eye movements; hearing and visual loss (retinitis pigmentosa); intellectual loss; cerebellar disturbance (ataxia).	Extraocular muscles, often asymmetric. Variable involvement of axial muscles; cardiac muscles, with conduction defect.	Depressed to ± or 0
Myasthenia gravis Transient neonatal	Variable.	At birth	Difficulty sucking, swallowing; trouble with secretions.	Somatic and cranial muscles.	Normal to decreased
Persistent neonatal	Variable.	Variable: birth, neonatal, infancy	Same as transient form.	Same as transient form.	Same as transient form.
Congenital myopathies Myotonic dystrophy (Neonatal onset)	Autosomal-dominant.	At birth	Same as myasthenia. Ptosis. Facial diplegia. Arthrogyposis, club feet, thin ribs.	Cranial and somatic, pharyngeal.	Decreased to 0
"Other" myopathies Central core Nemaline (rod body) Myotubular (centronuclear)	Dominant or rarely autosomal-recessive x-linked recessive in neonatal form.	Severe variants present at birth; milder variants (more common) infancy, childhood	Severe variant, newborns with severe hypotonia and respiratory failure is rare. Later presentation—facial weakness, mild to moderate weakness, even "toe walking" only.	Similar to myotonic dystrophy.	Decreased to 0
Congenital muscular dystrophy (Fukayama) (FCMD)	Genetic; recessive; chromosome 9q31–33. fuKutin mutations.	Birth to 9 mo	Hypotonia, joint contractures, mental retardation.	Heterogenous. Facial (cranial) and somatic. Contracture common.	Variable
Congenital muscular dystrophy (occidental)	Unknown; usually not familial; merosin-deficient variant 6q2. Many variants (8).	Birth (or early infancy)	As above. Normal IQ.	Same (merosin negative may involve heart, nerves, and brain).	Same
Benign congenital hypotonia (Oppenheim)	Variable.	Variable	Hypotonia only. Deep tendon reflexes positive. Laboratory tests, biopsy normal.	Somatic muscles (respiratory muscles spared).	Normal to decreased
Myotonias Myotonia congenita (Thomsen)	Autosomal-dominant (autosomal-recessive cases reported).	Early infancy to late childhood	Difficulty in relaxing muscles after contracting them, especially after sleep; aggravated by cold, excitement.	Hands especially; muscles may be diffusely enlarged, giving patient herculean appearance.	Normal

Muscle Biopsy Findings	Other Diagnostic Tests	Treatment	Prognosis
Mitochondrial abnormalities. "Ragged red" fibers. Changes in fiber size, usually due to type 2 fiber atrophy.	CK usually normal. ECG with conduction block. CSF protein elevated. Nerve conduction slowed. MRI of brain and brainstem auditory evoked response may be abnormal. Mitochondrial deletions.	Plastic retraction of eyelids. Cardiac support. Anticipate diabetes mellitus. Coenzyme Q?	Dysphagia may develop (50%) as well as generalized muscle weakness. Prognosis poor. In severe cases, spongy vacuolization of brain and brainstem.
Unnecessary.	Edrophonium or neostigmine tests. Acetylcholine receptor (AChR) antibodies. Repetitive nerve stimulation, EMG.	Supportive. Anticholinergic drugs.	Usually transient (< 2 months).
Sophisticated end plate, nerve terminal ultrastructural studies may be necessary.	May be similar to above. AChR antibodies negative.	May not respond to ACh-ase drugs, steroids, or immunosuppressants.	Variable, may have long-term severe course.
Generalized fiber hypertrophy, delay in maturation. Type I atrophy. Internal nuclei.	EMG myotonic in some (waning amplitude and pitch). Test mother. CK often normal. DNA testing (chromosome 19) for GCT repeat.	Supportive, even respiratory support. Genetic counseling.	Severely involved infant may improve dramatically over months; expect mental retardation in this same variant.
Distinctive diagnostic histochemistry, eg, "central cores,""nemaline rods," myotubes type II–I fibers of unequal size.	Myopathic EMG.	Supportive. Genetic counseling.	Variable. May shorten life. Death in infancy or severe handicap in severe neonatal form. Scoliosis prominent.
"Dystrophic" changes. Fibrosis. Necrotic fibers. Internal nuclei. ?Regenerative fibers.	Myopathic EMG. CK increased. Positive CT, MRI scans: white matter low density, etc.	Supportive.	Physical and mental handicap lifelong. Virtually all are of Japanese ancestry.
Same. Evaluate for merosin (a-laminen-2 deficiency).	Brain imaging normal in pure form. Merosin-deficient form may have white matter abnormalities.	Supportive.	May improve, walk. Scoliosis.
Normal with sophisticated studies (histochemistry, electron microscopy, even metabolic studies).	Use of this diagnosis is shrinking with increasingly sophisticated biochemical (eg, cytochrome oxidase) studies.	Supportive.	Good (by definition). (Few documented long-term studies.)
Nonspecific and minor changes; type IIB fibers may be absent.	EMG myotonic.	Usually none. Phenytoin, especially in cold weather, may improve muscle functioning.	Normal life expectancy, with only mild disability.

(continued)

Table 23–26. Muscular dystrophies and myotonias of childhood. (continued)

Disease	Genetic Pattern	Age at Onset	Early Manifestations	Involved Muscles	Reflexes
Myotonic dystrophy I (Steinert) (childhood and adult form) Myotonic dystrophy II [Proximal myotonic myopathy (PROMM)]	Autosomal-dominant.	Late childhood to adolescence; neonatal and infantile forms increasingly recognized (see above)	Myotonia of grasp, tongue; worsened by cold, emotions. "Hatchet-face." Nasal voice. Weakness and easy fatigability. Mild to moderate mental retardation noted.	Wasting, weakness of facial muscles, (mastication); sternocleidomastoids, hands. Myotonic phenomena: "bunching up" of muscles of tongue, thenar eminance, finger extensors after tapping with percussion hammer.	In infantile form, marked hyporeflexia

patients and most mothers will show deletions when sufficient probes are developed to search the whole Duchenne genome (perhaps 4000 kb in length).

Amplification of DNA by the PCR test can detect the deletion. Moreover, this technique plus Southern blot analysis can detect abnormal DNA base repeats. For example, in myotonic dystrophy, a GCT triplet excess is currently the most sensitive test for that disease. The tests can be used for intrauterine diagnosis and prediction of whether the triplet is within the normal or mutant range. Thus, in many cases, the greater the number of repeats, the more severely involved the fetus or patient.

Mutations (especially deletions) of survivor motor neuron and neuronal apoptosis inhibitory protein genes on chromosome 5q13 are present in 95% of patients with spinal muscular atrophy.

Finally, Kearns-Sayre progressive external ophthalmoplegia with retinopathy is inherited via maternal cytoplasmic mitochondria. Assay of mutations and deletions from blood or muscle samples are now commercially available.

Therapy for Duchenne muscular dystrophy continues to be frustrating. Prednisone in low doses has increased muscle strength and prolonged ambulation. Research emphasis is on gene therapy, but there is great difficulty in finding viral vectors able to carry the very large dystrophin gene into muscle cells.

Aslan M et al: Merosin-negative congenital muscular dystrophy: magnetic resonance spectroscopy findings. Brain Dev 2005;27:308 [PMID: 15862197].

Berven S, Bradford DS: Neuromuscular scoliosis: Causes of deformity and principles for evaluation and management. Semin Neurol 2002;22:167 [PMID: 12524562].

Bianchi ML et al: Bone mineral density and bone metabolism in Duchenne muscular dystrophy. Osteporos Int 2003;12:761 [PMID: 12897980].

Dubowitz V: Prednisone for Duchenne muscular dystrophy. Lancet Neurol 2005;4:264 [PMID: 15847833].

Escolar DM et al: CINRG randomized controlled trial of creatine and glutamine in Duchenne muscular dystrophy. Ann Neurol 2005;58:151 [PMID: 15984021].

Felice KJ et al: Fascioscapulohumeral dystrophy presenting as infantile facial diplegia and late-onset limb-girdle myopathy in members of the same family. Muscle Nerve 2005;32:368 [PMID: 15880682].

Grewal PK, Hewitt JE: Glycosylation defects: A new mechanism for muscular dystrophy? Hum Mol Genet 2003;12(Spec No 2):R259 [PMID: 12925572].

Kapsa R et al: Novel therapies for Duchenne muscular dystrophy. Lancet Neurol 2003;2:299 [PMID: 12849184].

Kesari A et al: SMNI dosage analysis in spinal muscular atrophy from India. BMC Med Genet 2005;6:22 [PMID: 15910686].

Kirschner J, Bonnemann CG: The congenital and limb-girdle muscular dystrophies: sharpening the focus, blurring the boundaries. Arch Neurol 2004;61:189 [PMID: 14967765].

Komura K et al: Effectiveness of creatine monohydrate in mitochondrial encephalomyopathies. Pediatr Neurol 2003;28:53 [PMID: 12657421].

Lois M et al: Beneficial effects of creatine supplementation in dystrophic patients. Muscle Nerve 2003;27:604 [PMID: 12707981].

Mathrew KD, Moore SA: Limb-girdle muscular dystrophy. Curr Neurol Neurosci Rep 2003;3:78 [PMID: 12507416].

Mendell JR: Congenital muscular dystrophy (editorial). Neurology 2001;56:993 [PMID: 11320168].

Mercuri E et al: Phenotypic spectrum associated with mutations in the fukutin-related protein gene. Ann Neurol 2003;53:537 [PMID: 12666124].

Moxley RT 3rd et al: Practice parameter: corticosteroid treatment of Duchenne dystrophy. Neurology 2005;64:13 [PMID: 15642897].

Muntoni F: Cardiac complications of childhood myopathies. J Child Neurol 2003;18:191 [PMID: 12731645].

Muntoni F et al: Defective glycosylation in muscular dystrophy. Lancet 2002;360:1419 [PMID: 12424008].

Riggs JE et al: Congenital myopathies/dystrophies. Neurol Clin 2003;21:779 [PMID: 14743649].

Muscle Biopsy Findings	Other Diagnostic Tests	Treatment	Prognosis
Type I fiber atrophy, type II hypertrophy, sarcoplasmic masses, internal nuclei, phagocytosis, fibrosis, and cellular reaction.	EMG markedly myotonic. Glucose tolerance test, thyroid tests. ECG. Chest radiograph and pulmonary function tests. Immunoglobulins. PCR amplification of GCT repeat on chromosome 19q13 to distinguish normal from mutant alleles. CCTG repeat in zinc finger protein gene.	Procainamide, 250 mg tid orally, increased to tolerance; phenytoin 5–7 mg/kg/d orally. (Drugs usually have little role.)	Frontal baldness, cataracts (85%), gonadal atrophy (85% of males), thyroid dysfunction, diabetes mellitus (20%). Cardiac conduction defects; impaired pulmonary function. Low IgG. Life expectancy decreased. Type II—slowly progressive weakening; good outlook.

ASA, acetylsalicyclic acid; CK, creatine kinase; CPT, carnitine palmityl transferase; CSF, cerebrospinal fluid; CT, computed tomography; ECG, electrocardiogram; EMG, electromyogram; MRI, magnetic resonance imaging; PCR, polymerase chain reaction; SIDS, sudden infant death syndrome.

Zatz M et al: The 10 autosomal recessive limb-girdle muscular dystrophies. Neuromuscul Disord 2003;13:532 [PMID: 12921790].

Zhang W et al: Enzymatic diagnostic test for muscle-eye-brain type congenital muscular dystrophy using commercially available reagents. Clin Biochem 2003;36:339 [PMID: 12849864].

BENIGN ACUTE CHILDHOOD MYOSITIS

Benign acute childhood myositis (myalgia cruris epidemica) is characterized by transient severe muscle pain and weakness affecting mainly the calves and occurring 1–2 days following an upper respiratory tract infection. Although symptoms involve mainly the gastrocnemius muscles, all skeletal muscles appear to be invaded directly by virus; recurrent episodes are due to different viral types. By seroconversion or isolation of the virus, acute myositis has been shown to be largely due to influenza types B and A and occasionally due to parainfluenza and adenovirus.

Agyeman P et al: Influenza-associated myositis in children. Infection 2004;32:199 [PMID: 15293074].

MYASTHENIA GRAVIS

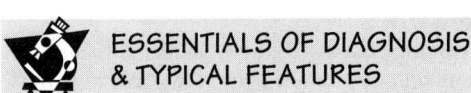

ESSENTIALS OF DIAGNOSIS & TYPICAL FEATURES

- *Weakness, chiefly of muscles innervated by the brainstem, usually coming on or increasing with use (fatigue).*
- *Positive response to neostigmine and edrophonium.*
- *Acetylcholine receptor antibodies in serum (except in congenital form).*

General Considerations

Myasthenia gravis is characterized by easy fatigability of muscles, particularly the extraocular muscles and those of mastication, swallowing, and respiration. In the neonatal period, however, or in early infancy, the weakness may be so constant and general that an affected infant may present nonspecifically as a "floppy infant." Girls are affected more frequently than boys. The age at onset is older than 10 years in 75% of patients, often shortly after menarche. If diagnosed before age 10 years, congenital myasthenia should be considered in retrospect. Thyrotoxicosis is found in almost 10% of affected female patients. The essential abnormality is a circulating antibody that binds to the acetylcholine receptor protein and thus reduces the number of motor end plates for binding by acetylcholine.

Clinical Findings

A. SYMPTOMS AND SIGNS

1. Neonatal (transient) myasthenia gravis—This disorder occurs in 12% of infants born to myasthenic mothers. The condition is due to maternal acetylcholine receptor antibody transferred across the placenta; a thymic factor in the infant may also be involved.

2. Congenital (persistent) myasthenia gravis—In this form of the disease, the mothers of the affected infants rarely have myasthenia gravis, but other relatives may. Sex distribution is equal. Symptoms are often subtle and not recognized initially. Differential diagnosis includes many other causes of the "floppy infant" syndrome, such as infant botulism, ocular myopathy, congenital ptosis, and Möbius syndrome (facial nuclear aplasia and other anomalies). Congenital myasthenia gravis is not caused by receptor antibodies and often responds poorly to therapy. It may result from a genetic abnormality of the acetylcholine receptor protein, postsynaptic membrane structure, or other myoneural transmission defects.

3. Juvenile myasthenia gravis—In this autoimmune form, the symptoms and signs are similar to those in adults. Receptor antibodies are usually present. The patient may be first seen by an ophthalmologist or psychiatrist. The more prominent signs are difficulty in chewing, dysphagia, a nasal voice, ptosis, and ophthalmoplegia. Pathologic fatigability of limbs, chiefly involving the proximal limb and neck muscles, may be more prominent than the bulbar signs and may lead to an initial diagnosis of conversion hysteria, muscular dystrophy, or polymyositis. Weakness may be limited to ocular muscles only. Associated disorders include autoimmune conditions, especially thyroid disease.

An acute fulminant form of myasthenia gravis has been reported in children age 2–10 years, who present with rapidly progressive respiratory difficulties. Bulbar paralysis may evolve within 24 hours. The differential diagnosis includes Guillain-Barré syndrome and bulbar poliomyelitis. Administration of anticholinesterase agents establishes the diagnosis and is life-saving. Rarely, myasthenia can be postinfectious, and slowly resolve to normal.

B. LABORATORY FINDINGS

1. Neostigmine test—In newborns and very young infants, the neostigmine test may be preferable to the edrophonium (Tensilon) test because the longer duration of its response permits better observation, especially of sucking and swallowing movements. The test dose of neostigmine is 0.02 mg/kg subcutaneously, usually given with atropine, 0.01 mg/kg subcutaneously. There is a delay of about 10 minutes before the effect may be manifest. The physician should be prepared to suction secretions.

2. Edrophonium test—Testing with edrophonium is used in older children who are capable of cooperating in certain tasks, such as raising and lowering their eyelids and squeezing a sphygmomanometer bulb or the examiner's hands. Ophthalmologic tests of ocular motility with edrophonium are often positive in patients able to cooperate. The test dose is 0.1–1 mL intravenously, depending on the size of the child. Maximum improvement occurs within 2 minutes.

3. Other laboratory tests—Serum acetylcholine receptor antibodies or muscle-specific receptor tyrosine kinase

are often found in the neonatal and juvenile forms. In juveniles, thyroid studies are appropriate.

C. ELECTRICAL STUDIES OF MUSCLE

Repetitive stimulation of a motor nerve at slow rates (3/s) with recording over the appropriate muscle reveals a progressive fall in amplitude of the muscle potential in myasthenic patients. A maximal stimulus must be given. At higher rates of stimulation (50/s), there may be a transient repair of this defect before the progressive decline is seen. If this study is negative, single-fiber EMG may be helpful diagnostically.

D. IMAGING

Chest radiograph and CT scanning in older children may disclose benign thymus enlargement. Thymus tumors are rare in children.

Treatment

A. GENERAL AND SUPPORTIVE CARE

In the newborn or in a child in myasthenic or cholinergic crisis (see item 5 in the following section), suctioning of secretions is essential. Respiratory assistance may be required. Treatment should be conducted by physicians with experience in this disorder.

B. ANTICHOLINESTERASE DRUG THERAPY

1. Pyridostigmine bromide—The dosage must be adjusted for each patient. A frequent starting dosage is 15–30 mg orally every 6 hours.

2. Neostigmine—Fifteen milligrams of neostigmine are roughly equivalent to 60 mg of pyridostigmine bromide. Neostigmine often causes gastric hypermotility with diarrhea, but it is the drug of choice in newborns, in whom prompt treatment may be life-saving. It may be given parenterally.

3. Atropine—Atropine may be added on a maintenance basis to control mild cholinergic side effects such as hypersecretion, abdominal cramps, and nausea and vomiting.

4. Immunologic intervention—Such intervention is achieved primarily with prednisone and recently with mycophenolate mofetil. Plasmapheresis is effective in removing acetylcholine receptor antibody in severely affected patients. More potent immunomodulators are occasionally necessary.

5. Myasthenic crisis—Relatively sudden difficulties in swallowing and respiration may be observed in myasthenic patients. Edrophonium results in dramatic but brief improvement; this may make evaluation of the condition of the small child difficult. Suctioning, tracheostomy, respiratory assistance, and fluid and electrolyte maintenance may be required.

6. Cholinergic crisis—Cholinergic crisis may result from overdosage of anticholinesterase drugs. The resulting weakness may be similar to that of myasthenia, and the muscarinic effects (diarrhea, sweating, lacrimation, miosis, bradycardia, and hypotension) are often absent or difficult to evaluate. The edrophonium test may help to determine whether the patient is receiving too little of the drug or is manifesting toxic symptoms due to overdosage. Improvement after the drugs are withdrawn suggests cholinergic crisis. A respirator should be available. The patient may require atropine and tracheostomy.

C. Surgical Measures

Early video thoracoscopic thymectomy is beneficial in many patients whose disease is not confined to ocular symptoms; the effects may be delayed. Experienced surgical and postsurgical care are prerequisites.

Prognosis

Neonatal (transient) myasthenia presents a great threat to life, primarily because of secretion aspiration. With proper treatment, the symptoms usually begin to disappear within a few days to 2–3 weeks, after which the child usually requires no further treatment. In the congenital (persistent) form, the symptoms may initially be as acute as in the transient variety. More commonly, however, they are relatively benign and constant, with gradual worsening as the child grows older. Fatal cases occur. In the juvenile form, patients may become resistant or unresponsive to anticholinesterase compounds and require corticosteroids or treatment in a hospital where respiratory assistance can be given. The overall prognosis for survival, for remission, and for improvement after therapy with prednisone and thymectomy is favorable. Death in myasthenic or cholinergic crisis may occur unless prompt treatment is given.

Andrews PI: Autoimmune myasthenia gravis in childhood. Semin Neurol 2004;24:101 [PMID: 15229797].

Felice KJ et al: Postinfectious myasthenia gravis: report of two children. J Child Neurol 2005;20:441 [PMID: 15968930].

Juel VC, Massey JM: Autoimmune myasthenia gravis: Recommendations for treatment and immunologic modulation. Curr Treat Opt Neurol 2005;7:3 [PMID: 15610702].

Meriggioli MN et al: Mycophenolate mofetil for myasthenia gravis: an analysis of efficacy, safety, and tolerability. Neurology 2003;61:1438 [PMID: 14638974].

Skelly CL et al: Thoracoscopic thymectomy in children with myasthenia gravis. Am Surg 2003;69:1087 [PMID: 14700296].

PERIPHERAL NERVE PALSIES

1. Facial Weakness

Facial asymmetry may be present at birth or may develop later, either suddenly or gradually, unilaterally or bilaterally. Nuclear or peripheral involvement of the facial nerves results in sagging or drooping of the mouth and inability to close one or both eyes, particularly when newborns and infants cry. Inability to wrinkle the forehead may be demonstrated in infants and young children by getting them to follow a light moved vertically above the forehead. Loss of taste of the anterior two-thirds of the tongue on the involved side may be demonstrated in cooperative children by age 4 or 5 years. Playing with a younger child and the judicious use of a tongue blade may enable the physician to note whether the child's face puckers up when something sour (eg, lemon juice) is applied with a swab to the anterior tongue. Ability to wrinkle the forehead is preserved, owing to bilateral innervation, in supranuclear facial paralysis.

Injuries to the facial nerve at birth occur in 0.25–6.5% of consecutive live births. Forceps delivery is the cause in some cases; in others, the side of the face affected may have abutted in utero against the sacral prominence. Often, no cause can be established.

Acquired peripheral facial weakness (Bell's palsy) of sudden onset and unknown cause is common in children. It often follows a viral illness (postinfectious) or physical trauma (eg, cold). It may be a presenting sign of Lyme disease, infectious mononucleosis, herpes simplex, or Guillain-Barré syndrome and is usually diagnosable by the history, physical examination, and appropriate laboratory tests. Chronic VII nerve palsy may be a sign of brainstem tumor.

Bilateral facial weakness in early life may be due to agenesis of the facial nerve nuclei or muscles (part of Möbius syndrome) or may even be familial. Myasthenia gravis, polyneuritis (Miller-Fisher syndrome), and myotonic dystrophy or other congenital myopathies must be considered.

Asymmetrical crying facies, in which one side of the lower lip depresses with crying (this is the normal side) and the other does not, is usually an innocent form of autosomal dominant inherited congenital malformation. The defect in the parent (the asymmetry often improves with age) may be almost inapparent. EMG suggests congenital absence of the depressor anguli oris muscle of the lower lip. Forceps pressure is often erroneously incriminated as a cause of this innocent congenital anomaly. Occasionally other major (eg, cardiac septal defects) congenital defects accompany the palsy. Authorities vary in the incidence of major anomalies (10%) and extent of investigations; chromosome 22q11 deletion, careful cardiac evaluation, and serum calcium may be pertinent.

In the vast majority of cases of isolated peripheral facial palsy—both those present at birth and those acquired later—improvement begins within 1–2 weeks, and near or total recovery of function is observed within

2 months. Methylcellulose drops, 1%, should be instilled into the eyes to protect the cornea during the day; at night the lid should be taped down with cellophane tape. Upward massage of the face for 5–10 minutes three or four times a day may help maintain muscle tone. Prednisone therapy (2–4 mg/kg PO for 5–7 days) likely does not aid recovery. In the older child, acyclovir (herpes antiviral agent) therapy or antibiotics (Lyme disease) may have a role in Bell palsy.

In the few children with permanent and cosmetically disfiguring facial weakness, plastic surgical intervention at age 6 years or older may be of benefit. New procedures, such as attachment of facial muscles to the temporal muscle and transplantation of cranial nerve XI, are being developed.

Akcakus M et al: Asymmetric crying facies associated with congenital hypoparathyroidism and 22q11 deletion. Turk J Pediatr 2004;46:191 [PMID: 15214756].

Ashtekar CS et al: Best evidence topic report. Do we need to give steroids in children with Bell's palsy? Emerg Med J 2005; 22:505 [PMID: 15983089].

Couch RB: Nasal vaccination, *Escherichia coli* enterotoxin, and Bell's palsy. N Engl J Med 2004;350:860 [PMID: 14985482].

Gilden DH: Clinical practice. Bell's palsy: N Engl J Med 2004; 351:1323 [PMID: 15385659].

Salinas RA et al: Corticosteroids for Bell's palsy (idiopathic facial paralysis). Cochrane Database Syst Rev 2004;(4):CD001942 [PMID: 15495021].

Sapin SO et al: Neonatal asymmetric crying facies: a new look at an old problem. Clin Pediatr (Phila) 2005;44:109 [PMID: 15735828].

Singhi P, Jain V: Bell's palsy in children. Semin Pediatr Neurol 2003;10:289 [PMID: 14992461].

Terada K et al: Bilateral facial nerve palsy associated with Epstein-Barr virus infection with a review of the literature. Scand J Infect Dis 2004;36:75 [PMID: 15000569].

Vorstman JA, Kuiper H: Peripheral facial palsy in children: test for Lyme borreliosis only in the presence of other clinical signs. Ned Tijdschr Geneeskd 2004;148:655 [PMID: 15106315].

CHRONIC POLYNEUROPATHY

Polyneuropathy, usually insidious in onset and slowly progressive, occurs in children of any age. The presenting complaints are chiefly disturbances of gait and easy fatigability in walking or running, and slightly less often, weakness or clumsiness of the hands. Pain, tenderness, or paresthesias are mentioned less frequently. Neurologic examination discloses muscular weakness, greatest in the distal portions of the extremities, with steppage gait and depressed or absent deep tendon reflexes. Cranial nerves are sometimes affected. Sensory deficits occur in a stocking-and-glove distribution. The muscles may be tender, and trophic changes such as glassy or parchment skin and absent sweating may occur. Thickening of the ulnar and peroneal nerves may

be felt. Pure sensory neuropathies show up as chronic trauma. That is, the patient does not feel minor trauma or burns, and thus allows trauma to occur.

Known causes include (1) toxins (lead, arsenic, mercurials, vincristine, and benzene); (2) systemic disorders (diabetes mellitus, chronic uremia, recurrent hypoglycemia, porphyria, polyarteritis nodosa, and lupus erythematosus); (3) inflammatory states (chronic or recurrent Guillain-Barré syndrome and neuritis associated with mumps or diphtheria); (4) hereditary, often degenerative conditions, which in some classifications include certain storage diseases, leukodystrophies, spinocerebellar degenerations with neurogenic components, and Bassen-Kornzweig syndrome; and (5) hereditary sensory or combined motor and sensory neuropathies (Table 23–27). Polyneuropathies associated with malignancies, beriberi, or other vitamin deficiencies, or excessive vitamin B_6 intake are not reported or are exceedingly rare in children.

The most common chronic neuropathy of insidious onset often has no identifiable cause. This chronic inflammatory demyelinating neuropathy (CIDP) is assumed to be immunologically mediated and may have a relapsing course. Sometimes facial weakness occurs. CSF protein levels are elevated. Nerve conduction is slowed, and nerve biopsies are abnormal. Immunologic abnormalities are seldom demonstrated, although nerve biopsies may show round cell infiltration. Corticosteroids and other immunosuppressants may give long-term benefit.

Of the four defined hereditary sensory neuropathies, one rarer variant is familial dysautonomia, also called Riley-Day syndrome. Transmitted as an autosomal recessive trait and occurring mostly in Jewish children, this disorder has its onset in infancy. It is characterized by vomiting and difficulties in feeding that are due to abnormal esophageal motility, pulmonary infections, decreased or absent tearing, indifference to pain, diminished or absent tendon reflexes, absence of fungiform papillae of the tongue, emotional lability, abnormal temperature control with excessive sweating, labile blood pressure, abnormal intradermal histamine responses, and other evidence of autonomic dysfunction.

Rarely, a careful genetic history (pedigree) and examination and electrical testing (motor and sensory nerve conduction and EMG) of relatives are keys to diagnosis of hereditary neuropathy. This is the most common cause of chronic neuropathy in children. Other hereditary neuropathies may have ataxia as a prominent finding often overshadowing the neuropathy. Examples are Friedreich ataxia, dominant cerebellar ataxia, and Marinesco-Sjögren syndrome. Finally, some hereditary neuropathies are associated with identifiable and occasionally treatable metabolic errors (see Table 23–22). These disorders are described in more detail in Chapter 32 (see also Table 23–21).

Table 23–27. Hereditary motor and sensory neuropathies; metabolic error unknown.

Name	Prototype	Inheritance	Clinical Features	Nerve Biopsy
Sensory and autonomic neuropathy	Familial dysautonomia	Autosomal-recessive	See text.	Decreased unmyelinated fibers posterior column and cord
HMSN I (if tremor is present, Roussy-Lévy syndrome) (60–90% of HMSN are type I) (CMT I)	"Classic" Charcot-Marie-Tooth (CMT) type I (1) CMT 1A (2) CMT 1B (3) CMT 1C (4) X-linked (5) Type 4	Autosomal-dominant 17p11.2 1q22 Connexin 32	Onset 0–15 y. Weakness, atrophy of feet, calves (pes cavus, "stork legs"), hands. Sensory loss 0 or variable. Deep tendon reflexes 0. Motor nerve conduction velocities slowed. 10% have hypertrophic (palpable) nerves. Type 1B is linked to Duffy blood group.	Segmental demyelination
HMSN II (10–30% of cases) (CMT 2)	Neuronal, axonal type 2	Autosomal-dominant. Multiple gene sites	Less severe; onset 10–30y. Leg cramps, numbness, motor nerve conduction velocities normal or slightly slow. CSF protein often normal.	Axonal loss, secondary demyelination
HMSN III (CMT 3)	Hypertrophic CMT disease; Déjérine-Sottas disease	Autosomal-recessive (or autosomal-dominant, sporadic)	Onset in infancy. Severe. CSF protein increased. Very slow MNCV. Slowly progressive.	Hypertrophic ("onion bulb") interstitial changes
HMSN IV (CMT 4)	Refsum disease	Autosomal-recessive demyelinating, or axonal	Severe sensory, mild motor. Thick nerves. CSF protein elevated. Ichthyosis, retinitis pigmentosa, ataxia, deafness. Urine phytanic acid.	See HMSN III
HMSN V	CMT disease with spastic paraparesis		Abnormal pyramidal tract findings. Rule out adrenomyelopathy (blood test).	Defined in pedigrees. Rule out adrenomyelopathy with long-chain fatty acids
HNPP	Hereditary neuropathy with liability to pressure palsies	Autosomal-dominant *PMP22* 17p11.2 deletion	Adolescent onset. Episodic numbness, peroneal palsy, carpal tunnel syndrome.	Occasional "tomaculous sausage" nerve formations

CSF, cerebrospinal fluid; HMSN, hereditary motor and sensory neuropathy; MNCV, motor nerve conduction velocity; PMP, peripheral myelin protein.

Laboratory diagnosis of chronic polyneuropathy is made by measurement of motor and sensory nerve conduction velocities. EMG may show a neurogenic polyphasic pattern. CSF protein levels are often elevated, sometimes with an increased IgG index. Nerve biopsy, with teasing of the fibers and staining for metachromasia, may demonstrate loss of myelin, and to a lesser degree, loss of axons and increased connective tissue or concentric lamellas (so-called onion-skin appearance) around the nerve fiber. Muscle biopsy may show the pattern associated with denervation. Other laboratory studies directed toward specific causes mentioned above include screening for heavy metals and for metabolic, renal, or vascular disorders.

Therapy is directed at specific disorders whenever possible. Occasionally the weakness is profound and involves bulbar nerves, in which case tracheostomy and respiratory assistance are required. Corticosteroid therapy may be of considerable benefit in cases where the cause is unknown or neuropathy is considered to be due to chronic inflammation (this is not the case in acute Guillain-Barré syndrome or acute inflammatory demyelinating neuropathy). Prednisone is recommended, 1–2.5 mg/kg/d orally, with tapering to the lowest effective dose; it should be discontinued if the process seems to be arresting and reinstituted when symptoms recur. Prednisone should probably not be used for treatment of hereditary neuropathy. In all cases considered for corticosteroid therapy, the risks and benefits should be carefully weighed. When treatment is appropriate, symptoms regress and may disappear altogether over a period of months. Immunotherapy may be safer or "steroid-sparing"; IVIg, plasmapheresis, mycophenolate mofetil, and rituximab are choices.

The long-term prognosis varies with the cause and the ability to offer specific therapy. In the corticosteroid-dependent group, residual deficits and even deaths within a few years are more frequent.

Burns TM et al: Current therapeutic strategies for patients with polyneuropathies secondary to inherited metabolic disorders. Mayo Clin Proc 2003;78:858 [PMID: 12839082].

Donofrio PD: Immunotherapy of idiopathic inflammatory neuropathies. Muscle Nerve 2003;28:273 [PMID: 12929187].

Finsterer J: Treatment of immune-mediated, dysimmune neuropathies. Acta Neurol Scand 2005;112:115 [PMID: 16008538].

Gorson KC et al: Efficacy of mycophenolate mofetil in patients with chronic immune demyelinating polyneuropathy. Neurology 2004;63:715 [PMID: 15326250].

Hughes R et al: Randomized controlled trial of intravenous immunoglobulin versus oral prednisone in chronic inflammatory demyelinating polyradiculoneuropathy. Ann Neurol 2001; 50:195 [PMID: 11506402].

Pareyson D: Differential diagnosis of Charcot-Marie-Tooth disease and related neuropathies. Neurol Sci 2004;25:72. [PMID: 15221625].

Pleasure DE, Chance PF: Neurotrophin-3 therapy for Charcot-Marie-Tooth disease type 1A. Neurology 2005;65:681 [PMID: 16157894].

Ropper AH: Current treatments for CIDP. Neurology 2003; 60(Suppl 3):S16 [PMID: 12707418].

Ruts L et al: Distinguishing acute-onset DIDP from Guillain-Barré syndrome with treatment related fluctuations: Neurology 2005;65:138 [PMID: 16009902].

Sander HW, Hedley-Whyte ET: Case records of the Massachusetts General Hospital. Weekly clinicopathological exercises: Case 6-2003: A nine-year-old girl with progressive weakness and areflexia. N Engl J Med 2003;348:735 [PMID: 12594319].

van Doorn PA: Treatment of Guillain-Barré syndrome and CIDP. J Peripher Nerv Syst 2005;10:113 [PMID: 15958124].

■ MISCELLANEOUS NEUROMUSCULAR DISORDERS

FLOPPY INFANT SYNDROME

ESSENTIALS OF DIAGNOSIS & TYPICAL FEATURES

- *In early infancy, decreased muscular activity, both spontaneous and in response to postural reflex testing and to passive motion.*
- *In young infants, "frog posture" or other unusual positions at rest.*
- *In older infants, delay in motor milestones.*

General Considerations

In the young infant, ventral suspension (ie, supporting the infant with a hand under the chest) normally results in the infant's holding its head slightly up (45 degrees or less), the back straight or nearly so, the arms flexed at the elbows and slightly abducted, and the knees partly flexed. The "floppy" infant droops over the hand like an inverted U. The normal newborn attempts to keep the head in the same plane as the body when pulled up from supine to sitting by the hands (traction response). Marked head lag is characteristic of the floppy infant. Hyperextensibility of the joints is not a dependable criterion.

The usual reasons for seeking medical evaluation in older infants are delays in walking, running, or climbing stairs or motor difficulties and lack of endurance. Hypotonia or decreased motor activity is a frequent presenting complaint in neuromuscular disorders but may also accompany a variety of systemic conditions or may be due to certain disorders of connective tissue.

1. Paralytic Group

The hypotonic infant who is weak (appearing paralyzed) usually has a lesion of the lower motor neuron complex (Table 23–28). The child has significant lack of movement against gravity (eg, fails to kick the legs, hold up the arms, or attempt to stand when held) or in response to stimuli such as tickling or slight pain. Infantile progressive spinal muscular atrophy (Werdnig-Hoffman disease) is the most common cause. Neuropathy is rare. Botulism and myasthenia gravis (rare) are neuromuscular junction causes. Myotonic dystrophy

Table 23–28. Floppy infant: paralytic causes.

Disease	Genetic	Early Manifestations
IPSMA (Infantile progressive spinal muscular atrophy) "Malignant" form	AR; diagnose by SMN deletion exon 7,8 (98% of cases)	In utero movements decreased in one-third. Gradual weakness, delay in gross motor milestones. Weak cry. Abdominal breathing. Poor limb motion ("no kicking"). No deep tendon reflexes. Fasciculations of tongue. Normal personal-social behavior.
"Intermediate" form	AR; same as above. EMG helpful.	Onset under age 1 year usual. *Progression slower:* may be impossible to predict early course of IPSMA. Hand tremors common.
Infantile botulism	Acquired younger than age 1 y (mostly under 6 mo); botulism spore in stool makes toxin	Poor feeding. Constipation. Weak cry. Failure to thrive. Lethargy. Facial weakness, ptosis, ocular muscle palsy. Inability to suck, swallow. Apnea. Source: soil dust (outdoor construction workers or family gardeners may bring it home on clothes), honey. EMG helpful, RMNS.
Myasthenia gravis Neonatal transient	12% of infants born from a myasthenia mother	Floppiness. Poor sucking and feeding; choking. Respiratory distress. Weak cry. Autoimmune antibodies from mother.
Congenital persistent	Mother normal. Rare AR (AD)	As above; may improve and later exacerbate. Multiple syndromes (rare).
Myotonic dystrophy	AD 99%—mother transmits gene. DNA testing 98% accurate.	Polyhydramnios; failure of suck, respirations. Facial diplegia. Ptosis. Arthrogryposis. Thin ribs. Later, developmental delay. Examine mother for myotonia, physiognomy. EMG variable in infant.
Neonatal "rare myopathy," severe variant Nemaline, central core, "minimal change," etc	AR, AD	Virtually all of the rare myopathies may have a severe (even fatal) neonatal or early infant form. Clinical features similar in infancy to infantile myotonic dystrophy. Muscle biopsy for definitive diagnosis.
Congenital muscular dystrophy Fukayama (FCMD)	Genetic	Early onset. Facial weakness. Joint contractures. Severe mental retardation. Seizures. Brain structural abnormalities; MRI helpful.
Other		Severe or benign. No mental retardation (see text).
Infantile neuropathy Hypomyelinating (rare)	HSMN most common cause	Demyelinating or axonal; a rare cause. Rule out mimicking IPSMA (deletion study). EMG, NCV are key studies. Nerve biopsy.
Benign congenital hypotonia	Unknown cause	Diagnosis of exclusion. Family history variable. Mild to moderate hypotonia with weakness. (This term being used less with increasing genetic, microscopy advances.) Improves with time.

AD, autosomal dominant; AR, autosomal recessive; EMG, electromyogram; HSMN, hereditary sensory motor neuropathy; MRI, magnetic resonance imaging; NCV, nerve conduction velocity; RMNS, repetitive motor nerve stimulation; SMN, survival motor neuron.

and rare myopathies (eg, central core myopathy) are muscle disease entities.

In anterior horn cell or muscle disease, weakness is proximal (ie, in shoulders and hips); finger movement is preserved. Tendon reflexes are absent or depressed; strength (to noxious stimuli) is decreased (paralytic). Intelligence is preserved. Fine motor, language, and personal and social milestones are normal, as measured, for example, on a Denver Developmental Screening Test (DDST, or Denver II) (see Chapter 2).

Myopathies

The congenital, relatively nonprogressive myopathies, muscular dystrophy, myotonic dystrophy, polymyositis, and periodic paralysis were discussed earlier in this chapter. Most cases of congenital or early infantile muscular dystrophy reported in the past probably represented congenital myopathies (see Table 23–28). Congenital muscular dystrophy, diagnosed by muscle biopsy, occurs in two forms: (1) a benign form, with gradual improvement in strength; and (2) a severe form, in which either weakness progresses rapidly and death occurs in the first months or year of life or severe disability is present with little or no progression but lifelong marked limitation of activity.

Glycogenosis with Muscle Involvement

Glycogen storage diseases are described in Chapter 32. Patients with type II disease (Pompe disease, due to a deficiency of acid maltase) are most likely to present as floppy infants. Muscle cramps on exertion or easy fatigability, rather than floppiness in infancy, is the presenting complaint in type V disease (McArdle phosphorylase deficiency) or in the glycogenosis due to phosphofructokinase deficiency or phosphohexose isomerase inhibition.

Myasthenia Gravis

Neonatal transient and congenital persistent myasthenia gravis, with patients presenting as paralytic floppy infants, is described earlier in this chapter.

Arthrogryposis Multiplex (Congenital Deformities About Multiple Joints)

This symptom complex, sometimes associated with hypotonia, may be of neurogenic or myopathic origin (or both) and may be associated with a variety of other anomalies. Orthopedic aspects are discussed in Chapter 24.

Spinal Cord Lesions

Severe limpness in newborns following breech extraction with stretching or actual tearing of the lower cervical to upper thoracic spinal cord is rarely seen today, owing to improved obstetric delivery. Klumpke lower brachial plexus paralysis may be present; the abdomen is usually exceedingly soft, and the lower extremities are flaccid. Urinary retention is present initially; later, the bladder may function autonomously. MRI spinal scanning may define the lesion. After a few weeks, spasticity of the lower limbs becomes obvious. Treatment is symptomatic and consists of bladder and skin care and eventual mobilization on crutches or in a wheelchair.

2. Nonparalytic Group

The nonparalytic hypotonic infant often has a damaged brain (Table 23–29). Rarely, tendon reflexes may be depressed or absent; usually, brisk reflexes (with hypotonia) point to "suprasegmental" or cerebral dysfunction. Intrauterine or perinatal insults to brain or spinal cord, while sometimes difficult to document, are major causes. (Occasionally, severe congenital myopathies presenting in the newborn period simulate nonparalytic hypotonia.) Persisting severe hypotonia is ominous. Tone will often vary. Spasticity and other forms of cere-

bral palsy may emerge; hypertonia and hypotonia may occur at varying times in the same infant. Choreoathetoid or ataxic movements and developmental delay can clarify the diagnosis. Tendon reflexes are usually increased; pathologic infant reflexes (Babinski and tonic neck) may persist or worsen.

The creatine kinase level and the EMG are usually normal. Prolonged nerve conduction velocities (rare in this situation) point to polyneuritis or leukodystrophy. Muscle biopsies, using special stains and histographic analysis, often show a remarkable reduction in size of type II fibers associated with decreased voluntary motor activity.

Limpness in the neonatal period and early infancy and subsequent delay in achieving motor milestones are the presenting features in a large number of children with a variety of CNS disorders, including mental retardation, as in trisomy 21. In many such cases, no specific diagnosis can be made. Close observation and scoring of motor patterns and adaptive behavior, as by the DDST, are helpful.

Anagnostou E et al: Type I spinal muscular atrophy can mimic sensory-motor axonal neuropathy. J Child Neurol 2005;20:147 [PMID: 15794183].

Barash JR et al: First case of infant botulism caused by *Clostridium baratii* type F in California. J Clin Microbiol 2005;43:4280 [PMID: 16082001].

Castrodale V: The hypotonic infant: Case study of central core disease. Neonatal Netw 2003;22:53 [PMID: 12597091].

Darras BT, Jones HR Jr: Neuromuscular problems of the critically ill neonate and child. Semin Pediatr Neurol 2004;11:147 [PMID: 15259868].

Johnston HM: The floppy weak infant revisited. Brain Dev 2003; 25:155 [PMID: 12689691].

Kim CT et al: Neuromuscular rehabilitation and electrodiagnosis. 4. Pediatric issues. Arch Phys Med Rehabil 2005:86(3 Suppl 1):S28 [PMID: 15761797].

Kroksmark AK et al: Myotonic dystrophy: muscle involvement in relation to disease type and size of expanded CTG-repeat sequence. Dev Med Child Neurol 2005;47:478 [PMID: 15991869].

Paro-Panjan D, Neubauer D: Congenital hypotonia: Is there an algorithm? J Child Neurol 2005;19:439 [PMID: 15446393].

Premasiri MK, Lee YS: The myopathology of floppy and hypotonic infants in Singapore. Pathology 2003;35:409 [PMID: 14555385].

Richer LP et al: Diagnostic profile of neonatal hypotonia: An 11-year study. Pediatr Neurol 2001;25:32 [PMID: 11483393].

Thompson JA et al: Infant botulism in the age of botulism immune globulin. Neurology 2005;64:2029 [PMID: 15917401].

Vasta I et al: Can clinical signs identify newborns with neuromuscular disorders? J Pediatr 2005;146:73 [PMID: 15644826].

Wilmshurst JM et al: Peripheral neuropathies of infancy. Dev Med Child Neurol 2003;45:408 [PMID: 12785442].

CEREBRAL PALSY

The term "cerebral palsy" is a nonspecific term used to describe a chronic, static impairment of muscle tone,

Table 23–29. Floppy infant: nonparalytic causes.

	Causes	Manifestations
Central nervous system disorders		
Atonic diplegia (prespastic diplegia)	Intrauterine, perinatal asphyxia, cord injury	Limpness, stupor; poor suck, cry, Moro reflex, grasp; later, irritability, increased tone and reflexes
Choreoathetosis	As above; kernicterus	Hypotonic early; movement disorder emerges later (6–18 mo)
Ataxic cerebral palsy	Same as choreoathetosis	Same as choreoathetosis
Syndromes with hypotonia (CNS origin)		
Trisomy 21	Genetic	All have hypotonia early
Prader-Willi syndrome	Genetic deletion 15q11	Hypotonia, hypomentia, hypogonadism, obesity ("H_3O")
Marfan syndrome	Autosomal-dominant	Arachnodactyly
Dysautonomia	Autosomal-recessive	Respiratory infections, corneal anesthesia
Turner syndrome	45X, or mosaic	Somatic stigmata (see Chapter 32: Inborn Errors of Metabolism)
Degenerative disorders		
Tay-Sachs disease	Autosomal-recessive	Cherry-red spot on macula
Metachromatic leukodystrophy	Autosomal-recessive	Deep tendon reflexes increased early, polyneuropathy late; mental retardation
Systemic diseases[a] Malnutrition	Deprivation, cystic fibrosis, celiac disease	
Chronic illness	Congenital heart disease; chronic pulmonary disease (eg, bronchopulmonary dysplasia); uremia, renal acidosis	
Metabolic disease	Hypercalcemia, Lowe disease, Pompe disease, Leigh disease	
Endocrinopathy	Hypothyroid	

[a]See elsewhere in text for manifestations.
CNS, central nervous system.

strength, coordination, or movements. The term implies that the condition is nonprogressive and originated from some type of cerebral insult or injury before birth, during delivery, or in the perinatal period. Other neurologic deficits or disorders (eg, blindness, deafness, or epilepsy) often coexist. Some form of cerebral palsy occurs in about 0.2% of neonatal survivors. The fundamental course, severity, precise manifestations, and prognosis vary widely.

The most common forms of cerebral palsy (75% of cases) involve spasticity of the limbs. A variety of terms denote the specific limb or combination of limbs affected: monoplegia (one limb); hemiplegia (arm and leg on same side of body, but arm more affected than leg); paraplegia (both legs affected with arms unaffected); quadriplegia (all four limbs affected equally).

Ataxia is the second most common form of cerebral palsy, accounting for about 15% of cases. The ataxia frequently affects fine coordinated movements of the upper extremities, but may also involve lower extremities and trunk. An involuntary movement disorder usually in the form of choreoathetosis accounts for 5% of cases and persistent hypotonia without spasticity 1%.

Depending on the type and severity of the motor deficits, associated neurologic deficits or disorders may occur: seizures in up to 50%, mild mental retardation in 26%, and severe retardation in up to 27%. Disorders of language, speech, vision, hearing, and sensory perception are found in varying degrees and combinations.

The findings on physical examination are variable and are predominantly those of spasticity, hyperreflexia, ataxia, and involuntary movements. Microcephaly is frequently present. In patients with hemiplegia, the affected arm and leg may be smaller and shorter than the unaffected limbs. Cataracts, retinopathy, and congenital heart defects may be indicative of congenital infections such as CMV and rubella.

Appropriate laboratory studies depend on the history and physical findings. MRI scans may be helpful in understanding the full extent of cerebral injury, and occasionally neuroimaging results suggest specific etiologies (eg, periventricular calcifications in congenital CMV infections). Other diagnostic tests that may be considered include genetic studies based on history or MRI findings; urine amino acids and organic acids; and blood amino acids, lactate, pyruvate, and ammonia concentrations.

The determination that a child has cerebral palsy is based in part on excluding other neurologic disorders and following the child for a sufficient amount of time to ascertain the static, nonprogressive nature of the disorder.

Treatment and management are directed at assisting the child to attain maximal physical functioning and potential physical, occupational, and speech therapy; orthopedic monitoring and intervention and special educational assistance may all contribute to an improved outcome. Medications and injections (eg, botulinum toxin) for spasticity and seizures are needed in many children. Also important is the general support of the parents and family with counseling, educational programs, and support groups.

The prognosis for patients with cerebral palsy depends greatly on the severity of the motor deficits and the degree of incapacity the patients ultimately experience. In severe cases, lifespan is greatly shortened to 10 years or less. Aspiration, pneumonia, or other intercurrent infections are the most common causes of death.

In contrast, patients with mild cerebral palsy may improve with age. Some patients experience resolution of their motor deficits by age 7 years. Many children with normal intellect have normal lifespans and are able to lead productive, satisfying lives.

The cause is often obscure or multifactorial. No definite etiologic diagnosis is possible in 25% of cases. The incidence is high among infants small for gestational age. Intrauterine hypoxia is a frequent cause. Other known causes are intrauterine bleeding, infections, toxins, congenital malformations, obstetric complications (including birth hypoxia), neonatal infections, kernicterus, neonatal hypoglycemia, metabolic disorders, and a small number of genetic syndromes.

Awaad V et al: Functional assessment following intrathecal baclofen therapy in children with spastic cerebral palsy. J Child Neurol 2003;18:26 [PMID: 12661935].

Cooley WD: Providing a primary care medical home for children and youth with cerebral palsy. Pediatrics 2004;114:1106 [PMID: 15466117].

Gibson CS et al: Antenatal causes of cerebral palsy: Associations between inherited thrombophilias, viral and bacterial infection, and inherited susceptibility to infection. Obstet Gynecol Surv 2003;58:209 [PMID: 12612461].

Koman LA et al: Cerebral palsy. Lancet 2004;363:1619 [PMID: 15145637].

Oskoui M, Shevell MI: Profile of pediatric hemiparesis. J Child Neurol 2005;20:471 [PMID: 15996394].

Pidcock FS: The emerging role of therapeutic botulinum toxin in the treatment of cerebral palsy. J Pediatr 2004;145(2 Suppl): S33 [PMID: 15292885].

Russman BS, Ashwal S: Evaluation of the child with cerebral palsy. Semin Pediatr Neurol 2004;11:47 [PMID: 15132253].

Shevell MI et al: Etiologic yield of cerebral palsy: A contemporary case series. Pediatr Neurol 2003;28:352 [PMID: 12878296].

Singhi P et al: Epilepsy in children with cerebral palsy. J Child Neurol 2003;18:174 [PMID: 12731642].

Wu YW et al: Prognosis for Ambulation in Cerebral Palsy: A Population-Based Study. Pediatrics 2004;14:1264 [PMID: 15520106].

REFERENCES

Internet References

Child Neurology Society

http://www.childneurologysociety.org

This site contains information about new developments and research and has practice parameters.

Child Neurology Foundation

http://www.childneurologyfoundation.org/index.html

Describes sites, resources, and tests related to child neurology.

E-Medicine

http://www.emedicine.com/neuro/PEDIATRIC_NEUROLOGY.htm

This contains a list of various topics within pediatric neurology.

American Association of Child and Adolescent Psychiatry

http://www.aacp.org

Contains practice parameters and other information.

National Institute of Neurological Disorders and Stroke

http://www.ninds.nih.gov

Brief descriptions of neurological disorders.

Gene Tests

http://www.genetests.org

Lengthy descriptions of many of the genetic disorders.

Epilepsy Foundation of America

http://www.epilepsyfoundation.org

Describes epilepsy research and some basics about epilepsy.

American Epilepsy Society

http://www.aesnet.org

Gives information about the society and general in formation about epilepsy. A good section on drugs is given.

Neurofibromatosis Foundation

http://www.nf.org

Neurofibromatosis information.

Tuberous Sclerosis Association

http://www.tsalliance.org

Orthopedics

Robert E. Eilert, MD

Orthopedics is the medical discipline that deals with disorders of the neuromuscular and skeletal systems. Patients with orthopedic problems present with one or more of the following complaints: pain, loss of function, or deformity. Although review of the history reveals the patient's expectation, physical examination is the most important feature of orthopedic diagnosis.

■ DISTURBANCES OF PRENATAL ORIGIN

CONGENITAL AMPUTATIONS & LIMB DEFICIENCIES

Congenital amputations may be due to teratogens (eg, drugs or viruses), amniotic bands, or metabolic diseases (eg, diabetes in the mother).

Children with congenital limb deficiencies, such as absence of the femur, tibia, or fibula, also have a high incidence of associated congenital anomalies, including genitourinary and cardiac defects and cleft palate. A limb deficiency usually consists of partial absence of structures in the extremity along one side or the other. For example, in radial club hand, the entire radius is absent, but the thumb may be either hypoplastic or completely absent; that is, the effect on structures distal to the amputation varies. Complex tissue defects are nearly always associated with longitudinal bone deficiency in that the associated nerves and muscles are not completely represented when a bone is absent.

Terminal amputations are treated by prosthesis, for example, to compensate for shortness of one leg. For certain types of severe anomalies, operative treatment is indicated to remove a portion of the malformed extremity (eg, foot) so that a prosthesis can be fitted early. An extension prosthesis fitted over the foot to equalize limb length is a reasonable nonsurgical alternative.

Lower extremity prostheses are best fitted between ages 12 and 15 months, when walking starts. They are consistently well accepted, because they are necessary for balancing and walking. For a unilateral upper extremity amputation, fitting the child with a dummy-type prosthesis as early as age 6 months has the advantage of instilling an accustomed pattern of proper length and bimanual manipulation. Although myoelectric prostheses have a technologic appeal, the majority of patients use the simplest construct in the long run.

Children quickly learn how to function with their prostheses and can lead active lives, even participating in sports with peers.

Kant P et al: Treatment of longitudinal deficiency affecting the femur: Comparing patient mobility and satisfaction outcomes of Syme amputation against extension prosthesis. J Pediatr Orthop 2003;23:236 [PMID: 12604957].

Congenital Limb Deficiency: http://www.reach.org.uk/content/files/standards.pdf

DEFORMITIES OF THE EXTREMITIES

1. Metatarsus Varus

Metatarsus varus is a common congenital foot deformity characterized by inward deviation of the forefoot. A vertical crease in the arch occurs when the deformity is more rigid. The angulation is at the level of the base of the fifth metatarsal, and this bone will be prominent. Most flexible deformities are secondary to intrauterine posture and usually resolve spontaneously. Several investigators have noticed that 10–15% of children with metatarsus varus have hip dysplasia; therefore, a careful hip examination is necessary. If the deformity is rigid and cannot be manipulated past the midline, it is worthwhile to use a cast changed at intervals of 2 weeks to correct the deformity. So-called corrective shoes do not live up to their name, although they can be used to maintain correction obtained by casting.

Lincoln TL, Suen PW: Common rotational variations in children. J Am Acad Orthop Surg 2003;11:312 [PMID: 14565753].

2. Club Foot (Talipes Equinovarus)

The diagnosis of classic talipes equinovarus, or club foot, requires three features: (1) plantar flexion of the foot at the ankle joint (equinus), (2) inversion deformity of the heel (varus), and (3) medial deviation of the forefoot (varus). The incidence of club foot is approximately 1:1000 live births. There are three major categories of club foot: (1) idiopathic, (2) neurogenic, and (3) those associated with syndromes such as arthrogryposis and Larsen syndrome. Any infant with a club foot should be examined carefully for associated anomalies, especially of the spine. Idiopathic club feet may be hereditary.

Treatment consists of manipulation of the foot to stretch the contracted tissues on the medial and posterior aspects, followed by splinting to hold the correction. When this treatment is instituted shortly after birth, correction is rapid. When treatment is delayed, the foot tends to become more rigid within a matter of days. After full correction is obtained, a night brace is necessary for long-term maintenance of correction. Treatment by means of casting requires patience and experience, but fewer patients require surgery when attention is paid to details of the Ponsetti technique. If the foot is rigid and resistant to cast treatment, surgical release and correction are appropriate. Fifteen to fifty percent require a surgical release.

Colburn M, Williams M: Evaluation of the treatment of idiopathic clubfoot by using the Ponsetti method. J Foot Ankle Surg 2003;42:259 [PMID: 14566717].

Clubfoot: http://www.marchofdimes.com/professionals/681_1211.asp

3. Infantile Dysplasia of the Hip Joint

The definition of dysplasia is abnormal growth or development. Dysplasia of the hip encompasses a spectrum of conditions in which an abnormal relationship exists between the proximal femur and the acetabulum. In the most severe condition, the femoral head is not in contact with the acetabulum and is classified as a dislocated hip. A dislocatable hip is one in which the hip is within the acetabulum but can be dislocated with a provocative maneuver. A subluxatable hip is one in which the femoral head comes partially out of the joint with a provocative maneuver. Acetabular dysplasia is the term used to denote insufficient acetabular development on radiograph.

Congenital dislocation of the hip occurs in approximately 1:1000 live births. At birth, both the acetabulum and femur are underdeveloped. The dysplasia is progressive with growth unless the dislocation is corrected. If the dislocation is corrected in the first few days or weeks of life, the dysplasia is completely reversible and a normal hip will develop. As the child becomes older and the dislocation or subluxation persists, the deformity will worsen to the point at which it will not be completely reversible, especially after the walking age. For this reason, it is important to diagnose the deformity early.

Clinical Findings

The diagnosis of hip dislocation in the newborn depends on demonstrating instability of the joint by placing the infant on its back and obtaining complete relaxation by feeding with a bottle if necessary. The examiner's long finger is then placed over the greater trochanter and the thumb over the inner side of the thigh. Both hips are flexed 90 degrees and then slowly abducted from the midline, one hip at a time. With gentle pressure, an attempt is made to lift the greater trochanter forward. A feeling of slipping as the head relocates is a sign of instability (Ortolani sign). When the joint is more stable, the deformity must be provoked by applying slight pressure with the thumb on the medial side of the thigh as the thigh is adducted, thus slipping the hip posteriorly and eliciting a jerk as the hip dislocates (Barlow sign). The signs of instability are more reliable than a radiograph for diagnosing congenital dislocation of the hip in the newborn. Ultrasonography can be used but tends to result in overdiagnosis in the newborn. Asymmetrical skinfolds are present in about 40% of newborns and therefore are not particularly helpful.

After the first month of life, the signs of instability become less evident. Contractures begin to develop about the hip joint, limiting abduction to less than 90 degrees. It is important to hold the pelvis level to detect asymmetry of abduction. If the knees are at unequal heights when the hips and knees are flexed, the dislocated hip will be on the side with the lower knee. After the first 6 weeks of life, radiologic examination becomes more valuable, with lateral displacement of the femoral head being the most reliable sign. In mild cases, the only abnormality may be increased steepness of acetabular alignment, so that the acetabular angle is greater than 35 degrees.

If dysplasia of the hip has not been diagnosed during the first year of life and the child begins to walk, there will be a painless limp and a lurch to the affected side. When the child stands on the affected leg, a dip of the pelvis will be evident on the opposite side, owing to weakness of the gluteus medius muscle. This is called the Trendelenburg sign and accounts for the unusual swaying gait. In children with bilateral dislocations, the loss of abduction is almost symmetrical and may be deceiving. A radiograph of the pelvis is indicated in children with incomplete abduction in the first few months of life. As a child with bilateral dislocation of the hips begins to walk, the gait is waddling. The perineum is widened as a result of lateral displacement of the hips, and there is flexion contracture as a result of posterior displacement of the hips. This flexion contracture contributes to marked lumbar lordosis, and the greater trochanters are easily palpable in their elevated position. Treatment is still possible in the first 2 years of life, but the results are not nearly as effective as in children receiving treatment in the nursery.

Treatment

Dislocation or dysplasia diagnosed in the first few weeks or months of life can easily be treated by splinting, with the hip maintained in flexion and abduction. Forced abduction is contraindicated, because this can lead to avascular necrosis of the femoral head. The use of double or triple diapers is never indicated because diapers are not adequate to obtain proper positioning of the hip. An orthopedic surgeon with experience managing the problem is best to supervise treatment of children requiring splints.

In the first 4 months of life, reduction can be obtained by simply flexing and abducting the hip; no other manipulation is usually necessary. In late cases, preoperative traction for 2–3 weeks relaxes soft tissues about the hip. Following traction in which the femur is brought down opposite the acetabulum, reduction can be easily achieved without force under general anesthesia. After reduction a hip spica is used for 6 months. If the reduction is not stable within a reasonable range of motion after closed reduction, open reduction is indicated. If reduction is done at an older age, operations to correct the deformities of the acetabulum and femur may be necessary as well as open reduction.

Weinstein SL, Mubarak SJ, Wenger DR: Developmental hip dysplasia and dislocation: Part I. Instr Course Lect 2004;53:523 (Review) [PMID: 15116641].

Weinstein SL, Mubarak SJ, Wenger DR: Developmental hip dysplasia and dislocation: Part II. Instr Course Lect 2004;53:531 (Review) [PMID: 15116642].

4. Torticollis

Wryneck deformities in infancy may be due either to injury to the sternocleidomastoid muscle during delivery or to disease affecting the cervical spine. When contracture of the sternocleidomastoid muscle causes torticollis, the chin is rotated to the side opposite to the affected muscle, and the head is tilted toward the side of the contracture. A mass felt in the midportion of the sternocleidomastoid muscle is not a true tumor but rather fibrous transformation within the muscle.

In most cases, passive stretching is effective. If the deformity has not been corrected by passive stretching within the first year of life, surgical release of the muscle origin and insertion will correct it. Excising the "tumor" of the sternocleidomastoid muscle creates an unsightly scar and is unnecessary. If the deformity is left untreated, a striking facial asymmetry will persist.

Torticollis is occasionally associated with congenital deformities of the cervical spine, and radiographs of the spine are indicated in all cases. In addition, there is a 20% incidence of hip dysplasia.

Acute torticollis may follow upper respiratory infection or mild trauma in children. Rotatory subluxation of the upper cervical spine requires computed tomography for accurate imaging. Traction or a cervical collar usually results in resolution of the symptoms within 1 or 2 days. Other causes of torticollis include spinal cord or cerebellar tumors, syringomyelia, and rheumatoid arthritis.

Fernandez Cornejo VJ et al: Inflammatory atlanto-axial subluxation (Grisel's syndrome) in children: Clinical diagnosis and management. Childs Nerv Syst 2003;19:342 [PMID: 12783261].

GENERALIZED DISORDERS OF SKELETAL OR MESODERMAL TISSUES

1. Arthrogryposis Multiplex Congenita (Amyoplasia Congenita)

Arthrogryposis multiplex congenita consists of incomplete fibrous ankylosis (usually bilateral) of many or all joints of the body. Upper extremity contractures usually consist of adduction of the shoulders; extension of the elbows; flexion of the wrists; and stiff, straight fingers with poor muscle control of the thumbs. In the lower extremities, common deformities are dislocation of the hips, extension contractures of the knees, and severe club feet. The joints are fusiform and the joint capsules decreased in volume due to lack of movement during fetal development. Various investigations have attributed the basic defect to an abnormality of muscle or the lower motor neurons. Muscle development is poor, and muscles may be represented only by fibrous bands. Passive mobilization of joints is the early treatment. Prolonged casting for correction of deformities is contraindicated in these children because further stiffness results. Use of removable splints combined with vigorous therapy is the most effective conservative treatment. Surgical release of the affected joints is often necessary. The club foot associated with arthrogryposis is very stiff and nearly always requires an operation. Surgery about the knees, including capsulotomy, osteotomy, and tendon lengthening, is used to correct deformity. In the young child, a dislocated hip may be reduced operatively by the medial approach. Multiple operative procedures about the hip are contraindicated because further stiffness may be produced with consequent impairment of motion. Affected children are often able to walk if the dislocations and contractures are reduced surgically. The long-term prognosis for physical and vocational independence is guarded. These patients have normal intelligence, but they have such severe physical restrictions that gainful employment is hard to find.

must be sought. Secondary curvature will resolve as the primary problem is treated.

Clinical Findings

A. Symptoms and Signs

Scoliosis in adolescents does not cause significant pain. If a patient has significant pain, seek the underlying cause because the scoliosis is usually secondary to some other disorder such as a bone or spinal cord tumor. Deformity of the rib cage and asymmetry of the waistline are evident with curvatures of 30 degrees or more. A lesser curvature may be detected by the forward bending test described in the preceding section, which is designed to detect early abnormalities of rotation that may not be apparent when the patient is standing erect.

B. Imaging

The most valuable radiographs are those taken of the entire spine in the standing position in both the antero-posterior and lateral planes. Usually one primary curvature is evident with a compensatory curvature that develops to balance the body. At times two primary curvatures may be seen, usually in the right thoracic and left lumbar regions. Any left thoracic curvature should be suspected of being secondary to neurologic disease, prompting a more meticulous neurologic examination. If the curvatures of the spine are balanced (compensated), the head is centered over the center of the pelvis and the patient is "in balance." If the spinal alignment is uncompensated, the head will be displaced to one side, which produces an unsightly deformity. Rotation of the spine may be measured by scoliometer. This rotation is associated with a marked rib hump as the lateral curvature increases in severity. Deformity of the rib cage causes long-term problems when lung volumes are reduced.

Treatment

Treatment of scoliosis depends on curve magnitude, skeletal maturity, and risk of progression. Curvatures of less than 20 degrees usually do not require treatment unless they show progression. Bracing is indicated for curvature of 20–40 degrees in a skeletally immature child. Treatment is indicated for any curvature that demonstrates progression on serial radiologic examination. Curvatures greater than 40 degrees are resistant to treatment by bracing. Thoracic curvatures greater than 60 degrees have been correlated with poor pulmonary function in adult life. Curvatures of such severity are an indication for surgical correction and posterior spinal fusion to maintain the correction. Curvatures of 40–60 degrees may also require spinal fusion if they are progressive, are causing decompensation of the spine, or cause unacceptable deformity.

Surgical fusion involves decortication of the bone over the laminas and spinous processes, with the addition of bone graft. Rods, hooks, or pedicle screws maintain postoperative correction, with activity restriction for several months until the bone fusion is solid. Treatment requires a team approach and is best done in centers with full support facilities.

Prognosis

Compensated small curves that do not progress may be well tolerated throughout life, with minor deformity. Counsel the patients regarding the genetic transmission of scoliosis and caution that their children's backs should be examined as part of routine physicals. Early detection allows for simple brace treatment. Severe scoliosis may require correction by spinal arthrodesis, although fusionless techniques are being developed.

Braun JT, Akyuz E, Ogilvie JW: The use of animal models in fusionless scoliosis investigations. Spine 2005;30(17 Suppl):S35 [PMID: 16138065].

Danielsson AJ, Nachemson AL: Back pain and function 22 years after brace treatment for adolescent idiopathic scoliosis: A case-control study—part I. Spine 2003;28:2078 [PMID: 14501917].

SLIPPED CAPITAL FEMORAL EPIPHYSIS

Slipped capital femoral epiphysis is a condition caused by displacement of the proximal femoral epiphysis due to disruption of the growth plate. The head of the femur is usually displaced medially and posteriorly relative to the femoral neck. The condition occurs in adolescence and is most common in obese males. The cause is unclear, although some authorities have shown experimentally that the strength of the perichondrial ring stabilizing the epiphysial area is sufficiently weakened by hormonal changes during adolescence such that the overload of excessive body weight can produce a pathologic fracture through the growth plate. Hormonal studies in these children are usually normal, although slipped capital femoral epiphysis is associated with hypothyroidism.

The condition occasionally occurs acutely following a fall or direct trauma to the hip. More commonly, vague symptoms occur over a protracted period in an otherwise healthy child who presents with pain and limp. The pain can be referred into the thigh or the medial side of the knee. Examine the hip joint in any obese child complaining of knee pain. The consistent finding on physical examination is limitation of internal rotation of the hip. The diagnosis may be clearly apparent only in the lateral radiographic view.

Treatment is based on the same principles that govern treatment of any fracture of the femoral neck in that the head of the femur is internally fixed to the neck of the femur and the fracture line allowed to heal. Unfortunately, the severe complication of avascular necrosis occurs in 30% of these patients. There is a positive correlation between forceful reduction of the slip and avascular necrosis. In cases of acute slip, as evidenced by the absence of any callus formation about the growth plate, it may be possible to reduce the hip by gentle traction. In more chronic cases, a more expeditious procedure is to pin the slip as it lies. Remodeling of the fracture site often improves the position of the hip without further surgery.

The long-term prognosis is guarded because most of these patients continue to be overweight and overstress their hip joints. Follow-up studies have shown a high incidence of premature degenerative arthritis in this disease, even in those who do not develop avascular necrosis. The development of avascular necrosis almost guarantees a poor prognosis, because new bone does not readily replace the dead bone at this late stage of skeletal development. About 30% of patients have bilateral involvement, which may occur as late as 1 or 2 years after the primary episode.

Slipped capital femoral epiphysis: http://www.emedicine.com/sports/topic122.htm

GENU VARUM & GENU VALGUM

Genu varum (bowleg) is normal from infancy through age 2 years. The alignment then changes to genu valgum (knock-knee) until about age 8 years, at which time adult alignment is attained. Criteria for referral to an orthopedist include persistent bowing beyond age 2 years, bowing that is increasing rather than decreasing, bowing of one leg only, and knock-knee associated with short stature.

Bracing may be appropriate. Rarely an osteotomy is necessary for a severe problem such as Blount disease (proximal tibial epiphysial dysplasia).

Bowen RE, Dorey FJ, Moseley CF: Relative tibial and femoral varus as a predictor of progression of varus deformities of the lower limbs in young children. J Pediatr Orthop 2002;22: 105 [PMID: 11744864].

TIBIAL TORSION

"Toeing in" in small children is a common parental concern. Tibial torsion is rotation of the leg between the knee and the ankle. Internal rotation amounts to about 20 degrees at birth but decreases to neutral rotation by age 16 months. The deformity is sometimes accentuated by laxity of the knee ligaments, allowing excessive internal rotation of the leg in small children. In children who have a persistent internal rotation of the tibia beyond age 16–18 months, the condition is often due to sleeping with feet turned in and can be reversed with an external rotation splint worn only at night.

FEMORAL ANTEVERSION

Toeing in beyond age 2 or 3 years is usually secondary to femoral anteversion, which is characterized by more internal rotation of the hip compared with external rotation. This femoral alignment follows a natural history of progressive decrease toward neutral during growth. Studies comparing the results of treatment with shoes or braces to the natural history have shown that little is gained by active treatment. Active external rotation exercises, such as skating or bicycle riding, can be encouraged. Osteotomy for rotational correction is rarely required. Children who have no external rotation of hip in extension are candidates for orthopedic consultation.

Lincoln TL, Suen PW: Common rotational variations in children. J Am Acad Orthop Surg 2003;11:312.

COMMON FOOT PROBLEMS

When a child begins to stand and walk, the long arch of the foot is flat with a medial bulge over the inner border of the foot. The forefeet are mildly pronated or rotated inward, with a slight valgus alignment of the knees. As the child grows and joint laxity decreases, the long arch is better supported and more normal relationships occur in the lower extremities. (See also sections on metatarsus varus and talipes equinovarus.)

1. Flatfoot

Flatfoot is a normal condition in infants. If the heel cord is of normal length, full dorsiflexion is possible with the heel in the neutral position. As long as the heel cord is of normal length and a longitudinal arch is noted when the child is sitting in a non–weight-bearing position, the parents can be assured that a normal arch will probably develop. There is usually a familial incidence of relaxed flatfeet in children who have no apparent arch. In any child with a shortened heel cord or stiffness of the foot, other causes of flatfoot such as tarsal coalition or vertical talus should be ruled out by a complete orthopedic examination and radiograph.

In the child with an ordinary relaxed flatfoot, no active treatment is indicated unless calf or leg pain is present. In children who have leg pains attributable to flatfoot, a supportive shoe with scaphoid pad, such as a good-quality sports shoe, is useful. An orthotic that holds the heel in neutral and supports the arch may relieve discomfort if more support is needed. An arch insert should not be prescribed unless passive correction of the arch is easily accomplished; otherwise, the skin over the medial side of the foot will be irritated.

2. Talipes Calcaneovalgus

Talipes calcaneovalgus is characterized by excessive dorsiflexion at the ankle and eversion of the foot. It is often present at birth and is due to intrauterine position. Treatment consists of passive exercises, stretching the foot into plantar flexion. In rare instances, it may be necessary to use plaster casts to help with manipulation and positioning. Complete correction is the rule.

Gore AI, Spencer JP: The newborn foot. Am Fam Physician 2004;69:865 (Review) [PMID: 14989573].

3. Cavus Foot

This deformity consists of an unusually high longitudinal arch of the foot. It may be hereditary or associated with neurologic conditions such as poliomyelitis, Charcot-Marie-Tooth disease, Friedreich ataxia, and diastematomyelia. There is usually an associated contracture of the toe extensor, producing a claw toe deformity in which the metatarsal phalangeal joints are hyperextended and the interphalangeal joints acutely flexed. Any child presenting with cavus feet should receive a careful neurologic examination and radiographs of the spine.

Conservative therapy is ineffective. In symptomatic cases, surgery may be necessary to lengthen the contracted extensor and flexor tendons and to release the plantar fascia and other tight plantar structures. The associated varus heel deformity causes more problems than the high arch.

Statler TK, Tullis BL: Pes cavus. J Am Podiatr Med Assoc 2005; 95:42 (Review) [PMID: 15659413].

4. Bunions (Hallux Valgus)

Adolescents may present with lateral deviation of the great toe associated with a prominence over the head of the first metatarsal. This deformity is painful only with shoe wear and almost always can be relieved by fitting shoes that are wide enough in the toe. Surgery should be avoided in the adolescent, because further growth tends to cause recurrence of the deformity.

Talab YA: Hallux valgus in children: A 5–14-year follow-up study of 30 feet treated with a modified Mitchell osteotomy. Acta Orthop Scand 2002;73:195.

■ DEGENERATIVE PROBLEMS (ARTHRITIS, BURSITIS, & TENOSYNOVITIS)

Degenerative arthritis may follow childhood skeletal problems, such as infection, slipped capital femoral epiphysis, avascular necrosis, or trauma, or it may occur in association with hemophilia. Early effective treatment of these disorders can prevent arthritis. Degenerative changes in the soft tissues around joints may occur as a result of overuse syndrome in adolescent athletes. Young boys throwing excessive numbers of pitches, especially curve balls, may develop "little leaguer" elbow, consisting of degenerative changes around the humeral condyles associated with pain, swelling, and limitation of motion (see Chapter 25). In order to enforce the rest necessary for healing, a plaster cast may be necessary. A more reasonable preventive measure is to limit the number of pitches thrown by children.

Acute bursitis is uncommon in childhood, and other causes should be ruled out before this diagnosis is accepted.

Tenosynovitis is most common in the region of the knees and feet. Children taking dancing lessons, particularly toe dancing, may have pain around the flexor tendon sheaths in the toes or ankles. Rest is effective treatment. At the knee level, the patellar ligament may be irritated, with associated swelling in the infrapatellar fat pad. Synovitis in this area is usually due to overuse and is treated by rest and nonsteroidal anti-inflammatory drugs. Corticosteroid injections are contraindicated.

■ TRAUMA

SOFT TISSUE TRAUMA (Sprains, Strains, & Contusions)

A sprain is the stretching of a ligament, and a strain is a stretch of a muscle or tendon. Contusions are generally due to tissue compression, with damage to blood vessels within the tissue and the formation of hematoma.

A severe sprain is one in which the ligament is completely disrupted, resulting in instability of the joint. A mild or moderate sprain is one in which incomplete tearing of the ligament occurs but in which local pain and swelling results.

Mild or moderate sprains are treated by rest of the affected joint, with ice and elevation to prevent prolonged symptoms. By definition, mild or moderate sprain is not associated with instability of the joint.

If more severe trauma occurs, resulting in tearing of a ligament, instability of the joint may be demonstrated by gross examination or by stress testing with radiographic documentation. Such deformity of the joint may cause persistent instability resulting from inaccurate apposition of the ligament ends during healing. If instability is evident, surgical repair of the torn ligament may be indicated. If a muscle is torn at its tendinous insertion, it should be repaired.

The initial treatment of any sprain consists of ice, compression, and elevation. Splinting of the affected joint protects against further injury and relieves swelling and pain. Ibuprofen and other nonsteroidal anti-inflammatory drugs are useful for pain.

1. Ankle Sprains

The history will indicate that the injury was by either forceful inversion or eversion. The more common inversion injury results in tearing or injury to the lateral ligaments, whereas an eversion injury will injure the medial ligaments of the ankle. The injured ligaments may be identified by means of careful palpation for point tenderness around the ankle. The joint should be supported or immobilized at a right angle, which is the functional position. Adhesive taping may be effective but should be changed frequently to prevent blisters. Use of a posterior plaster splint or air splint produces joint rest, and the extremity can be protected by using crutches. Prolonged use of a plaster cast is usually not necessary, but the sprained ankle should be rested sufficiently to allow complete healing, which may take 3–6 weeks. Rehabilitation to include strengthening and restitution of kinesthetic sensation can prevent long-term disability.

Lord J, Winell JJ: Overuse injuries in pediatric athletes. Curr Opin Pediatr 2004;16:47 (Review) [PMID: 14758113].

2. Knee Sprains

Sprains of the collateral and cruciate ligaments are uncommon in children. These ligaments are so strong that it is more common to injure the epiphysial growth plates, which are the weakest structures in the region of the knees of children. In adolescence, however, the physes have started to close, and the knee joint is more like that of an adult, so that rupture of the anterior cruciate ligament can result from a hyperextension injury. If the injury produces avulsion of the tibial spine, open anatomic reduction is often required.

Effusion of the knee after trauma deserves referral to an orthopedic specialist. The differential diagnosis includes torn ligament, torn meniscus, and osteochondral fracture. Nontraumatic effusion should be evaluated for inflammatory conditions (eg, juvenile rheumatoid arthritis) or patellar malalignment.

Vaquero J, Vidal C, Cubillo A: Intra-articular traumatic disorders of the knee in children and adolescents. Clin Orthop Relat Res 2005;432:97 (Review) [PMID: 15738809].

3. Internal Derangements of the Knee

Meniscal injuries are uncommon in children younger than age 12 years. Clicking or locking of the knee may occur in young children as a result of a discoid lateral meniscus, which is a rare congenital anomaly. As the child approaches adolescence, internal damage to the knee from a torsion weight-bearing injury may result in locking of the knee if tearing and displacement of a meniscus occurs. Osteochondral fractures secondary to osteochondritis dissecans may also present as internal derangements of the knee in adolescence. Posttraumatic synovitis may mimic a meniscal lesion. In any severe injury to the knee, epiphysial injury should be suspected; stress films will sometimes demonstrate separation of the distal femoral epiphysis in such cases. Epiphysial injury should be suspected whenever tenderness is present on both sides of the metaphysis of the femur after injury.

Smith AD: The skeletally immature knee: What's new in overuse injuries. Instr Course Lect 2003;52:691.

4. Back Sprains

Sprains of the ligaments and muscles of the back are unusual in children but may occur as a result of violent trauma from automobile accidents or athletic injuries. Back pain in a child may be the only symptom of significant disease and warrants clinical investigation. Inflammation, infection, renal disease, or tumors can cause back pain in children, and sprain should not be accepted as a routine diagnosis.

Balague F et al: Low-back pain in children. Lancet 2003;361:1403.

Wall EJ et al: Backpacks and back pain: Where's the epidemic? J Pediatr Orthop 2003;23:437.

5. Contusions

Contusion of muscle with hematoma formation produces the familiar "charley horse" injury. Treatment of such injuries is by application of ice, compression, and rest. Exercise should be avoided for 5–7 days. Local heat may hasten healing once the acute phase of tenderness and swelling is past.

6. Myositis Ossificans

Ossification within muscle occurs when there is sufficient trauma to cause a hematoma that later heals in the manner of a fracture. The injury is usually a contusion and occurs most commonly in the quadriceps of the thigh or the triceps of the arm. When a severe injury with hematoma is recognized, it is important to splint the extremity and avoid activity. If further trauma causes recurrent injury, ossification may reach spectacular proportions and resemble an osteosarcoma.

Disability is great, with local swelling and heat and extreme pain on the slightest motion of the adjacent joint. The limb should be rested, with the knee in extension or the elbow in 90 degrees of flexion, until the local reaction has subsided. After local heat and tenderness have decreased, gentle active exercises may be initiated. Passive stretching exercises are not indicated, because they may stimulate the ossification reaction. If surgery is necessary, it should not be attempted before 9 months to 1 year after injury, because it may restart the process and lead to an even more severe reaction.

TRAUMATIC SUBLUXATIONS & DISLOCATIONS

Dislocation of a joint is always associated with severe damage to the ligaments and joint capsule. In contrast to fracture reduction, which may be safely postponed, dislocations must be reduced immediately. Dislocations can usually be reduced by gentle sustained traction. It often happens that no anesthetic is necessary for several hours after the injury, because of the protective anesthesia produced by the injury. Following reduction, the joint should be splinted for transportation of the patient.

The dislocated joint should be treated by immobilization for at least 3 weeks, followed by graduated active exercises through a full range of motion. Vigorous passive manipulation of the joint by a therapist may be harmful.

1. Subluxation of the Radial Head (Nursemaid Elbow)

Infants may sustain subluxation of the radial head as a result of being lifted or pulled by the hand. The child appears with the elbow fully pronated and painful. The usual complaint is that the child's elbow will not bend. Radiographic findings are normal, but there is point tenderness over the radial head. When the elbow is placed in full supination and slowly moved from full flexion to full extension, a click may be palpated at the level of the radial head. The relief of pain is remarkable, as the child usually stops crying immediately. The elbow may be immobilized in a sling for comfort for a day. Occasionally, symptoms last for several days, requiring more prolonged immobilization.

Pulled elbow may be a clue to battering. This should be considered during examination, especially if the problem is recurrent.

2. Recurrent Dislocation of the Patella

Recurrent dislocation of the patella is more common in loose-jointed individuals, especially adolescent girls. If the patella completely dislocates, it nearly always goes laterally. Pain is severe, and the patient is brought to the doctor with the knee slightly flexed and an obvious bony mass lateral to the knee joint associated with a flat area over the anterior knee. Radiologic examination confirms the diagnosis. The patella may be reduced by extending the knee and placing slight pressure on the patella while gentle traction is exerted

on the leg. In subluxation of the patella, the symptoms may be more subtle, and the patient will complain that the knee "gives out" or "jumps out of place."

In the case of complete dislocation, the knee should be immobilized for 3–4 weeks, followed by a physical therapy program for strengthening the quadriceps muscle. Operation may be necessary to tighten the knee joint capsule if dislocation or subluxation is recurrent. In such instances, if the patella is not stabilized, repeated dislocation produces damage to the articular cartilage of the patellofemoral joint and premature degenerative arthritis.

Buchner M, Baudendistel B, Sabo D, Schmitt H: Acute traumatic primary patellar dislocation: long-term results comparing conservative and surgical treatment. Clin J Sport Med 2005; 15:62 [PMID: 15782048].

FRACTURES

1. Epiphysial Separations

In children, epiphysial separations and fractures are more common than ligamentous injuries. This finding is based on the fact that the ligaments of the joints are generally stronger than the associated growth plates. In instances in which dislocation is suspected, a radiograph should be taken in order to rule out epiphysial fracture. Radiographs of the opposite extremity, especially for injuries around the elbow, may be valuable for comparison. Reduction of a fractured epiphysis should be done under anesthesia to align the growth plate with the least amount of force. Fractures across the growth plate may produce bony bridges that will cause premature cessation of growth or angular deformities of the extremity. Epiphysial fractures around the shoulder, wrist, and fingers can usually be treated by closed reduction, but fractures of the epiphyses around the elbow often require open reduction. In the lower extremity, accurate reduction of the epiphysial plate is necessary to prevent joint deformity if a joint surface is involved. If angular deformities result, corrective osteotomy may be necessary.

Mehlman CT: Growth plate fractures. http://www.emedicine.com/orthoped/topic627.htm

2. Torus Fractures

Torus fractures consist of "buckling" of the cortex due to compression of the bone. They usually occur in the distal radius or ulna. Alignment is usually satisfactory, and simple immobilization for 3 weeks is sufficient.

3. Greenstick Fractures

Greenstick fractures involve frank disruption of the cortex on one side of the bone but no discernible cleavage plane on the opposite side. These fractures are angulated but not displaced, because the bone ends are not separated. Reduction is achieved by straightening the arm into normal alignment, and reduction is maintained by a snugly fitting plaster cast. It is necessary to get a radiograph of greenstick fractures again in a week to 10 days to make certain that the reduction has been maintained in the cast. A slight angular deformity can be corrected by remodeling of the bone. The farther the fracture is from the growing end of the bone, the longer the time required for remodeling. The fracture can be considered healed when no tenderness or local heat is present and when adequate bony callus is seen on radiograph.

4. Fracture of the Clavicle

Clavicular fractures are very common injuries in infants and children. The patient can be immobilized in a sling for comfort. The healing callus will be apparent when the fracture has consolidated, but this unsightly lump will generally resolve over a period of months to a year.

5. Supracondylar Fractures of the Humerus

Supracondylar fractures tend to occur in children age 3–6 years and are potentially dangerous because of the proximity to the brachial artery in the distal arm. They are usually associated with a significant amount of trauma, so that swelling may be severe. Most often, these fractures are treated by closed reduction and percutaneous pinning. Complications associated with supracondylar fractures include Volkmann ischemic contracture of the forearm due to vascular compromise and cubitus varus (decreased carrying angle) secondary to poor reduction. The so-called gunstock deformity of the elbow may be somewhat unsightly but does not usually interfere with joint function.

Gosens T, Bongers KJ: Neurovascular complications and functional outcome in displaced supracondylar fractures of the humerus in children. Injury 2003;34:267 [PMID: 12667778].

6. General Comments on Other Fractures in Children

Reduction of fractures in children is usually accomplished by simple traction and manipulation; open reduction is indicated if a satisfactory alignment is not obtained. Remodeling of the fracture callus usually produces an almost normal appearance of the bone over a matter of months. The younger the child, the more remodeling is possible. Angular deformities remodel reliably. Rotatory malalignment does not remodel.

The physician should be suspicious of child abuse whenever the age of a fracture does not match the history given or when the severity of the injury is more than the alleged accident would have produced. In suspected cases of battering in which no fracture is present on the initial radiograph, a repeat radiograph 10 days later is in order. Bleeding beneath the periosteum will be calcified by 7–10 days, and the radiographic appearance is almost diagnostic of severe closed trauma characteristic of a battered child.

■ INFECTIONS OF THE BONES & JOINTS

OSTEOMYELITIS

Osteomyelitis is an infectious process that usually starts in the spongy or medullary bone and then extends to involve compact or cortical bone. The lower extremities are most often affected, and there is commonly a history of trauma. Osteomyelitis may occur as a result of direct invasion from the outside through a penetrating wound (nail) or open fracture, but hematogenous spread of infection (eg, pyoderma or upper respiratory tract infection) from other infected areas is much more common. The most common infecting organism is *Staphylococcus aureus,* which has a tendency to infect the metaphyses of growing bones. Anatomically, circulation in the long bones is such that the arterial supply to the metaphysis just below the growth plate is close to end arteries, which turn sharply to end in venous sinusoids, causing a relative stasis. In the infant younger than age 1 year, there is direct vascular communication with the epiphysis across the growth plate, so that direct spread may occur from the metaphysis to the epiphysis and subsequently into the joint. In the older child, the growth plate provides an effective barrier, the epiphysis is usually not involved, and the infection spreads retrograde from the metaphysis into the diaphysis, and by rupture through the cortical bone, down along the diaphysis beneath the periosteum.

1. Exogenous Osteomyelitis

To avoid osteomyelitis by direct extension, all wounds must be carefully examined and cleansed. Osteomyelitis is a common occurrence from pressure sores in anesthetic areas, such as in patients with spina bifida. Cultures of the wound made at the time of exploration and debridement may be useful if signs of infection develop subsequently. Copious irrigation is necessary, and all nonviable skin, subcutaneous tissue, fascia, and muscle must be excised. In extensive or contaminated wounds, antibiotic coverage is indicated. Contaminated lacerations should be left open and secondary closure performed 3–5 days later. If at the time of delayed closure further necrotic tissue is present, it should be excised. Leaving the wound open allows the infection to stay at the surface rather than extend inward to the bone. Puncture wounds are especially liable to lead to osteomyelitis and should be carefully debrided.

Initially, broad-spectrum antibiotics should be administered, but the final choice of antibiotics is directed by culture results. A tetanus toxoid booster may be indicated. Gas gangrene is best prevented by adequate debridement.

After exogenous osteomyelitis has become established, treatment becomes more complicated, requiring extensive surgical debridement and intravenous antibiotics.

2. Hematogenous Osteomyelitis

Hematogenous osteomyelitis is usually caused by pyogenic bacteria; 85% of cases are due to staphylococci. Streptococci are a less common cause of osteomyelitis. *Pseudomonas* organisms are common in cases of nail puncture wounds. Children with sickle cell anemia are especially prone to osteomyelitis caused by *Salmonella* spp.

Clinical Findings

A. SYMPTOMS AND SIGNS

In infants, the manifestations of osteomyelitis may be subtle, presenting as irritability, diarrhea, or failure to feed properly; the temperature may be normal or slightly low; and the white blood cell count may be normal or only slightly elevated. There may be pseudoparalysis of the involved limb. In older children, the manifestations are more striking, with severe local tenderness and pain, often high fever, rapid pulse, and elevated white blood cell count and erythrocyte sedimentation rate (ESR). Osteomyelitis of a lower extremity often occurs around the knee joint in children age 7–10 years. Tenderness is most marked over the metaphysis of the bone where the process has its origin. For a child who refuses to bear weight, osteomyelitis is high in the differential diagnosis.

B. LABORATORY FINDINGS

Blood cultures are often positive early. The most significant test in infancy is the aspiration of pus. It is useful to needle the bone in the area of suspected infection and aspirate any fluid present. This fluid should be stained for organisms and cultured. Even edema fluid may be useful for determining the causative organism. Elevation of the ESR above 50 mm/h is typical for osteomyelitis. C-reactive protein is elevated earlier than the ESR.

C. IMAGING

Nonspecific local swelling is the first radiographic finding. This is followed by elevation of the periosteum, with formation of new bone from the cambium layer of the periosteum occurring after 3–6 days. As the infection becomes chronic, areas of cortical bone are isolated by pus spreading down the medullary canal, causing rarefaction and demineralization of the bone. Such isolated pieces of cortex become ischemic and form sequestra (dead bone fragments). These radiographic findings are late but specific. Osteomyelitis should be diagnosed clinically before significant radiographic findings are present. Bone scan is sensitive but nonspecific and should be interpreted in the clinical context before radiographic findings become positive. Magnetic resonance imaging can demonstrate edema early or soft-tissue thickening later.

Treatment

A. SPECIFIC MEASURES

Antibiotics should be started intravenously as soon as the diagnosis of osteomyelitis is made. Oral antibiotics are begun when tenderness, fever, the white cell count, and the ESR are all decreasing and the culture is positive. Agents that cover *S aureus* and *Streptococcus pyogenes* (eg, oxacillin, nafcillin, cefazolin, and clindamycin) are appropriate for most cases. For specific recommendations and for possible *Pseudomonas* infection, see Chapter 38.

Chronic infections are treated for months. Following surgical debridement, *Pseudomonas* foot infections usually respond to 1–2 weeks of antibiotic treatment.

B. GENERAL MEASURES

Splinting of the limb minimizes pain and decreases spread of the infection by lymphatic channels through the soft tissue. The splint should be removed periodically to allow active use of adjacent joints and prevent stiffening and muscle atrophy. In chronic osteomyelitis, splinting may be necessary to guard against fracture of the weakened bone.

C. SURGICAL MEASURES

Aspiration of the metaphysis for culture and Gram stain is the most useful diagnostic measure in any case of suspected osteomyelitis. In the first 24–72 hours, it may be possible to treat osteomyelitis with antibiotics alone. If frank pus is aspirated from the bone, however, surgical drainage is indicated. If the infection has not shown a dramatic response within 24 hours, surgical drainage is also indicated. It is important that all devitalized soft tissue be removed and adequate exposure of the bone obtained to permit free drainage. Excessive amounts of bone should not be removed when draining acute osteomyelitis, because it will not be completely replaced by the normal healing process. Bone damage is limited by surgical drainage, whereas failure to evacuate pus in acute cases may lead to widespread damage.

Prognosis

When osteomyelitis is diagnosed in the early clinical stages and prompt antibiotic therapy is begun, the prognosis is excellent. If the process has been unattended for a week to 10 days, there is almost always some permanent loss of bone structure, as well as the possibility of growth abnormality.

Moumile K et al: Bacterial aetiology of acute osteoarticular infections in children. Acta Paediatr 2005;94:419 [PMID: 16092454].

PYOGENIC ARTHRITIS

The source of pyogenic arthritis varies according to the child's age. In the infant, pyogenic arthritis often develops by spread from adjacent osteomyelitis. In the older child, it presents as an isolated infection, usually without bony involvement. In teenagers with pyogenic arthritis, an underlying systemic disease or an organism (eg, gonococcus) that has an affinity for joints is usually the cause.

The infecting organism varies with age: group B streptococcus and *S aureus* in those younger than age 4 months; *Haemophilus influenzae* and *S aureus* in those age 4 months to 4 years; and *S aureus* and *S pyogenes* in older children and adolescents. *H influenzae* is now uncommon because of effective immunization. *Kingella kingae* is a gram-negative bacterium that occasionally causes pyarthrosis.

The initial effusion of the joint rapidly becomes purulent. An effusion of the joint may accompany osteomyelitis in the adjacent bone. A white cell count exceeding 100,000/µL in the joint fluid indicates a definite purulent infection. Generally, spread of infection is from the bone into the joint, but unattended pyogenic arthritis may also affect adjacent bone. The ESR is often above 50 mm/h.

Clinical Findings

A. SYMPTOMS AND SIGNS

In older children, the signs may be striking, with fever, malaise, vomiting, and restriction of motion. In infants, paralysis of the limb due to inflammatory neuritis may be evident. Infection of the hip joint in infants should be suspected if decreased abduction of the hip is present in an infant who is irritable or feeding poorly. A history of umbilical catheter treatment in the newborn nursery should alert the physician to the possibility of pyogenic arthritis of the hip.

B. IMAGING

Early distention of the joint capsule is nonspecific and difficult to measure by radiograph. In the infant with unrecognized pyogenic arthritis, dislocation of the joint may follow within a few days as a result of distention of the capsule by pus. Later changes include destruction of the joint space, resorption of epiphysial cartilage, and erosion of the adjacent bone of the metaphysis. The bone scan shows increased flow and increased uptake about the joint.

Treatment

Aspiration of the joint is the key to diagnosis. In the hip joint, pyogenic arthritis is most easily treated by surgical drainage because the joint is deep and difficult to aspirate and is also inaccessible to thorough cleaning through needle aspiration. Arthroscopic irrigation and debridement have been successful in treating pyogenic arthritis of the knee. If fever and clinical symptoms do not subside within 24 hours after treatment is begun, open surgical drainage is indicated. Antibiotics can be selected based on the child's age, results of the Gram stain, and culture of the aspirated pus. Reasonable empiric therapy in infants is nafcillin or oxacillin plus a third-generation cephalosporin. An antistaphylococcal agent alone is usually adequate for children older than age 5 years. For staphylococcal infections, 3 weeks of therapy is recommended; for other organisms, 2 weeks is usually sufficient. Oral therapy may be begun when clinical signs have improved markedly. It is not necessary to give intra-articular antibiotics, because good levels are achieved in the synovial fluid with parenteral administration.

Prognosis

The prognosis for the patient with pyogenic arthritis is excellent if the joint is drained early, before damage to the articular cartilage has occurred. If infection is present for more than 24 hours, dissolution of the proteoglycans in the articular cartilage takes place, with subsequent arthrosis and fibrosis of the joint. Damage to the growth plate may also occur, especially within the hip joint, where the epiphyseal plate is intracapsular.

Frank G, Mahoney HM, Eppes SC: Musculoskeletal infections in children. Pediatr Clin North Am 2005;52:1083 (Review) [PMID: 16009258].

TUBERCULOUS ARTHRITIS

Tuberculous arthritis is now a rare disease in the United States. Children in poor social circumstances, however, such as homeless families, are prone to tuberculous arthritis. Generally the infection may be ruled out by negative skin testing. The joints most commonly affected in children are the intervertebral discs, resulting in gibbus or dorsal angular deformity at the site of involvement.

Treatment is by local drainage of the abscess, followed by antituberculous therapy. Prolonged immobilization in a plaster cast or prolonged bed rest is necessary to promote healing. Spinal fusion may be required to preserve stability of the vertebral column.

Mkandawire NC, Kaunda E: Bone and joint TB at Queen Elizabeth Central Hospital 1986 to 2002. Trop Doct 2005;35:14 [PMID: 15712533].

DISKITIS

Diskitis is pyogenic infectious spondylitis in children; supportive treatment and intravenous antibiotics are likely to lead to rapid relief of symptoms and signs without recurrence.

McCarthy JJ et al: Musculoskeletal infections in children: basic treatment principles and recent advancements. Instr Course Lect 2005;54:515-28 (Review) [PMID: 15948476].

TRANSIENT SYNOVITIS OF THE HIP

The most common cause of limping and pain in the hip in children in the United States is transitory synovitis, an acute inflammatory reaction that often follows an upper respiratory infection and is generally self-limited. In questionable cases, aspiration of the hip yields only yellowish fluid, ruling out pyogenic arthritis. Generally, however, toxic synovitis of the hip is not associated with elevation of the ESR, white blood cell count, or temperature above 38.3 °C. It classically affects children age 3–10 years and is more common in boys than girls. There is limitation of motion of the hip joint, particularly internal rotation, and radiographic changes are nonspecific, with some swelling apparent in the soft tissues around the joint.

Treatment consists of bed rest and the use of traction with slight flexion of the hip. Nonsteroidal antiinflammatory drugs shorten the course of the disease, although even with no treatment, the disease usually runs its course in days. It is important to maintain radiographic follow-up because toxic synovitis may be the precursor of avascular necrosis of the femoral head (described in the next section) in a small percentage of patients. Radiographs can be obtained at 6 weeks, or earlier if either a persistent limp or pain is present.

Yagupsky P: Differentiation between septic arthritis and transient synovitis of the hip in children. J Bone Joint Surg Am 2005;87:459; author reply 459 (no abstract available) [PMID: 15687174].

■ VASCULAR LESIONS & AVASCULAR NECROSIS (Osteochondroses)

Osteochondrosis due to vascular lesions may affect various growth centers. Table 24–1 indicates the common sites and the typical ages at presentation.

Table 24–1. The osteochondroses.

Ossification Center	Eponym	Typical Age (years)
Capital femoral	Legg-Calvé-Perthes disease	4–8
Tarsal navicular	Köhler bone disease	6
Second metatarsal head	Freiberg disease	12–14
Vertebral ring	Scheuermann disease	13–16
Capitellum	Panner disease	9–11
Tibial tubercle	Osgood-Schlatter disease	11–13
Calcaneus	Sever disease	8–9

In contrast to other body tissues that undergo infarction, bone removes necrotic tissue and replaces it with living bone in a process called creeping substitution. This replacement of necrotic bone may be so complete and so perfect that a completely normal bone results. Adequacy of replacement depends on the patient's age, the presence or absence of associated infection, the congruity of the involved joint, and other physiologic and mechanical factors.

Because of their rapid growth in relation to their blood supply, the secondary ossification centers in the epiphyses are subject to avascular necrosis. Despite the number of different names referring to avascular necrosis of the epiphyses, the process is identical, necrosis of bone followed by replacement (see Table 24–1).

Even though the pathologic and radiographic features of avascular necrosis of the epiphyses are well known, the cause is not generally agreed upon. Necrosis may follow known causes such as trauma or infection, but idiopathic lesions usually develop during periods of rapid growth of the epiphyses.

AVASCULAR NECROSIS OF THE PROXIMAL FEMUR (Legg-Calvé-Perthes Disease)

The vascular supply of the proximal femur is precarious, and when it is interrupted, necrosis results.

Clinical Findings

A. SYMPTOMS AND SIGNS

The highest incidence of Legg-Calvé-Perthes disease is between ages 4 and 8 years. Persistent pain is the most common symptom, and the patient may present with limp or limitation of motion.

B. LABORATORY FINDINGS

Laboratory findings, including studies of joint aspirates, are normal.

C. IMAGING

Radiographic findings correlate with the progression of the process and the extent of necrosis. The early finding is effusion of the joint associated with slight widening of the joint space and periarticular swelling. Decreased bone density in and around the joint is apparent after a few weeks. The necrotic ossification center appears more dense than the surrounding viable structures, and the femoral head is collapsed or narrowed.

As replacement of the necrotic ossification center occurs, rarefaction of the bone occurs in a patchwork fashion, producing alternating areas of rarefaction and relative density, referred to as "fragmentation" of the epiphysis.

In the hip, widening of the femoral head may occur associated with flattening, or coxa plana. If infarction has extended across the growth plate, a radiolucent lesion will be evident within the metaphysis. If the growth center of the femoral head has been damaged so that normal growth is arrested, shortening of the femoral neck results.

Eventually, complete replacement of the epiphysis develops as living bone replaces necrotic bone by creeping substitution. The final shape of the head depends on the extent of the necrosis and collapse of weakened bone.

Differential Diagnosis

Differential diagnosis must include inflammation and infection and dysplasia. Transient synovitis of the hip may be distinguished from Legg-Calvé-Perthes disease by serial radiographs.

Treatment

The principle of treatment is protection of the joint. If the joint is deeply seated within the acetabulum and normal joint motion is maintained, a reasonably good hip can result. Little benefit has been shown from bracing.

Prognosis

The prognosis for complete replacement of the necrotic femoral head in a child is excellent, but the functional result depends on the amount of deformity that develops during the time the softened structure exists. In Legg-Calvé-Perthes disease, the prognosis depends on the completeness of involvement of the epiphysial center. In general, patients with metaphysial defects, those in whom the disease develops late in childhood, and those who have more complete involvement of the femoral head have a poorer prognosis.

Hesse B, Kohler G: Does it always have to be Perthes' disease? What is epiphyseal dysplasia? Clin Orthop 2003;414:219 [PMID: 12966296].

Joseph B et al: Natural evolution of Perthes disease: A study of 610 children under 12 years of age at disease onset. J Pediatr Orthop 2003;23:590 [PMID: 12960621].

OSTEOCHONDRITIS DISSECANS

In osteochondritis dissecans, a wedge-shaped necrotic area of bone and cartilage develops adjacent to the articular surface. The fragment of bone may be broken off from the host bone and displaced into the joint as a loose body. If it remains attached, the necrotic fragment may be completely replaced by creeping substitution.

The pathologic process is the same as that described previously for avascular necrosing lesions of ossification centers. Because these lesions are adjacent to articular cartilage, however, joint damage may occur.

The most common sites of these lesions are the knee (medial femoral condyle), the elbow joint (capitellum), and the talus (superior lateral dome). Joint pain is the usual presenting complaint. However, local swelling or locking may be present, particularly if a fragment is free in the joint. Laboratory studies are normal.

Treatment consists of protection of the involved area from mechanical damage. If a fragment is free within the joint as a loose body, it must be removed. For some marginal lesions, it may be worthwhile to drill the necrotic fragment to encourage more rapid vascular ingrowth and replacement. If large areas of a weight-bearing joint are involved, secondary degenerative arthritis may result.

Wall E, Von Stein D: Juvenile osteochondritis dissecans. Orthop Clin North Am 2003;34:341 [PMID: 12974484].

■ NEUROLOGIC DISORDERS INVOLVING THE MUSCULOSKELETAL SYSTEM

ORTHOPEDIC ASPECTS OF CEREBRAL PALSY

Early physical therapy to encourage completion of the normal developmental patterns may benefit patients with cerebral palsy. The greatest gains from this therapy are obtained during the first few years of life, and therapy should not be continued when no improvement is apparent.

Bracing and splinting are of questionable benefit, although night splints may be useful in preventing equinus deformity of the feet or adduction contractures of the hips. Orthopedic surgery is useful for treating joint contractures that interfere with function. In general, muscle transfers are unpredictable in cerebral palsy, and most orthopedic procedures are directed at tendon lengthening or bony stabilization by osteotomy or arthrodesis.

Flexion and adduction of the hip due to hyperactivity of the adductors and flexors may produce a progressive paralytic dislocation of the hip, which can lead to pain and dysfunction. Treatment of this dislocation is difficult and unsatisfactory. The principal preventive measure is abduction bracing, but this must often be supplemented by release of the adductors and hip flexors in order to prevent dislocation. In severe cases, osteotomy of the femur may also be necessary to correct the bony deformities of femoral anteversion and coxa valga that are invariably present. Patients with a predominantly athetotic pattern are poor candidates for any surgical procedure or bracing.

Because it is difficult to predict the outcome of surgical procedures in cerebral palsy, the surgeon must examine patients on several occasions before any operative procedure is undertaken. Follow-up care by a physical therapist to maximize the anticipated long-term gains should be arranged before the operation.

Sussman MD, Aiona MD: Treatment of spastic diplegia in patients with cerebral palsy. J Pediatr Orthop B 2004;13:S1 (Review) [PMID: 15076595].

Aiona MD, Sussman MD: Treatment of spastic diplegia in patients with cerebral palsy: Part II. J Pediatr Orthop B 2004;13:S13 (Review) [PMID: 15083127].

ORTHOPEDIC ASPECTS OF MYELODYSPLASIA

Patients born with spina bifida cystica (aperta) should be examined early by an orthopedic surgeon. The level of neurologic involvement determines the muscle imbalance that will be present and apt to produce deformity with growth. The involvement is often asymmetrical and tends to change during the first 12–18 months of life. Early closure of the sac is the rule, although there has been some hesitancy to provide treatment to all of these patients because of the extremely poor prognosis associated with congenital hydrocephalus, high levels of paralysis, and associated congenital anomalies. A high percentage of these children have hydrocephalus, which may be evident at birth or shortly thereafter, requiring shunting. Associated musculoskeletal problems may include club foot, congenital dislocation of the hip, arthrogryposis-type changes of the lower extremities, and congenital scoliosis. The most common lesions are at the level of L3–4

and tend to affect the hip joint, with progressive dislocation occurring during growth. Foot deformities may be in any direction and are complicated by the fact that sensation is generally absent. Spinal deformities develop in a high percentage of these children, with scoliosis present in approximately 40%. Ambulation may require long leg braces. Careful urologic follow-up must be obtained to prevent complications from bladder dysfunction.

In children who have a reasonable likelihood of walking, operative treatment consists of reduction of the hip and alignment of the feet in the weight-bearing position as well as stabilization of the scoliosis. In children who lack active quadriceps function and extensor power of the knee, the likelihood of ambulation is greatly decreased. In such patients, aggressive surgery in the hip region may result in stiffening of the joints, thus preventing sitting. Multiple foot operations are also contraindicated in these children.

The overall treatment of the child with spina bifida should be coordinated in a multidisciplinary clinic where various medical specialists work with therapists, social workers, and teachers to provide the best possible care.

Mazur JM, Kyle S: Efficacy of bracing the lower limbs and ambulation training in children with myelomeningocele. Dev Med Child Neurol 2004;46:352 (Review) (no abstract available) [PMID: 15132267].

NEOPLASIA OF THE MUSCULOSKELETAL SYSTEM

Neoplastic diseases of the musculoskeletal system are a serious problem because of the poor prognosis of malignant tumors arising in bone or other tissues derived from mesoderm. Fortunately, few of the benign lesions undergo malignant transformation. Accurate diagnosis depends on correlation of the clinical, radiographic, and microscopic findings. Complaints about the knee should be investigated for tumor, although the usual causes of knee pain are traumatic, infectious, or developmental in origin.

Lewis VO: Limb salvage in the skeletally immature patient. Curr Oncol Rep 2005;7:285 (Review) [PMID: 15946588].

Osteochondroma

Osteochondroma is the most common bone tumor in children. It usually presents as a pain-free mass. When present, pain is caused by adventitious bursitis or tendinitis due to irritation by the tumor. The lesion may be single or multiple. Pathologically, the lesion is a bone mass capped with cartilage. These masses tend to grow during childhood and adolescence in proportion to the child's growth.

On radiograph the tumors tend to be in the metaphysial region of long bones and may be pedunculated or sessile. The cortex of the underlying bone "flows" into the base of the tumor.

An osteochondroma should be excised if it interferes with function, is frequently traumatized, or is large enough to be deforming. The prognosis is excellent. Malignant transformation is very rare.

Bottner F et al: Surgical treatment of symptomatic osteochondroma: A three- to eight-year follow-up study. J Bone Joint Surg Br 2003;85:1161 [PMID: 14653600].

Osteoid Osteoma

Osteoid osteoma classically produces night pain that can be relieved by aspirin. On physical examination there usually is tenderness over the lesion. An osteoid osteoma in the upper femur may cause pain referred to the knee.

On radiograph the lesion is a radiolucent nidus surrounded by dense osteosclerosis that may obscure the nidus. Bone scan shows intense uptake in the lesion.

Surgical incision of the nidus is curative and may be done using computed tomography imaging and minimally invasive technique. The prognosis is excellent, with no known cases of malignant transformation, although the lesion has a tendency to recur.

Enchondroma

Enchondroma is usually a silent lesion unless it produces a pathologic fracture. On radiograph it is radiolucent, usually in a long bone. A speckled calcification may be present. The classic lesion looks as though someone dragged his or her fingernails through clay, making streaks in the bones. Enchondroma is treated by surgical curettage and bone grafting. The prognosis is excellent. Malignant transformation may occur but is very rare in childhood.

Chondroblastoma

In chondroblastoma, the presenting complaint is pain around a joint. This neoplasm may produce a pathologic fracture. On radiograph the lesion is radiolucent and can perforate the epiphysial cartilage. Calcification is unusual, with little or no reactive bone. The lesion is treated by surgical curettage and bone grafting. The prognosis is excellent if complete curettage is performed. There is no known malignant transformation.

Masui F et al: Chondroblastoma: A study of 11 cases. Eur J Surg Oncol 2002;28:869 [PMID: 12477480].

Nonossifying Fibroma

Nonossifying fibroma is also called benign cortical defect and is nearly always an incidental finding on radiograph.

The most frequent sites are the distal femur and proximal tibia. Nonossifying fibroma is a radiolucent lesion eccentrically located in the bone. Usually a thin sclerotic border is evident. Multiple lesions may be present. No treatment is needed because these lesions heal as they ossify with maturation of the bone and growth.

Osteosarcoma

In osteosarcoma, the presenting complaint is usually pain in a long bone, although functional loss, the mass of the tumor, or limp may be the complaint. Pathologic fracture is common. The malignant osseous tumor produces a destructive expanding and invasive lesion. A triangle may be adjacent to the tumor produced by elevated periosteum and subsequent tumor ossification. The lesion may contain calcification and violates the cortex of the bone. Femur, tibia, humerus, and other long bones are the sites usually affected.

Surgical excision (limb salvage) or amputation is indicated based on the extent of the tumor. The lesion is radioresistant and does not respond to chemotherapy. Adjuvant chemotherapy is routinely used prior to surgical excision. The prognosis is improving, with 30% 5-year survival rates being reported in modern series. Death usually occurs as a result of lung metastasis.

Kuhelj D, Jereb B: Pediatric osteosarcoma: a 35-year experience in Slovenia. Pediatr Hematol Oncol 2005;22:335 [PMID: 1602012].

Ewing Sarcoma

In Ewing sarcoma, the presenting complaint is usually pain and tenderness. Fever and leukocytosis may also be present, which makes osteomyelitis the main differential diagnosis. The lesion may be multicentric. Ewing sarcoma is radiolucent and destroys the cortex, frequently in the diaphysial region. Reactive bone formation may occur about the lesion, seen as successive layers of so-called onion skin layering.

Treatment is with multiagent chemotherapy, radiation, and surgical resection. The prognosis is poor with large tumor size, pelvic lesions, and poor response to chemotherapy.

MISCELLANEOUS DISEASES OF BONE

FIBROUS DYSPLASIA

Dysplastic fibrous tissue replacement of the medullary canal is accompanied by the formation of metaplastic bone in fibrous dysplasia. Three forms of the disease are recognized: monostotic, polyostotic, and polyostotic with endocrine disturbances (precocious puberty in females, hyperthyroidism, and hyperadrenalism [Albright syndrome]).

Clinical Findings

A. SYMPTOMS AND SIGNS

The lesion or lesions may be asymptomatic. Pain, if present, is probably due to pathologic fractures. In females, endocrine disturbances may be present in the polyostotic variety and associated with café au lait spots.

B. LABORATORY FINDINGS

Laboratory findings are normal unless endocrine disturbances are present, in which case secretion of gonadotropic, thyroid, or adrenal hormones may be increased.

C. IMAGING

The lesion begins centrally within the medullary canal, usually of a long bone, and expands slowly. Pathologic fracture may occur. If metaplastic bone predominates, the contents of the lesion will be of the density of bone. The disease is often asymmetrical, and limb length disturbances may occur as a result of stimulation of epiphysial cartilage growth. Marked deformity of the bone may result, and a shepherd's crook deformity of the upper femur is a classic feature of the disease.

Differential Diagnosis

The differential diagnosis includes other fibrous lesions of bone as well as destructive lesions such as unicameral bone cyst, eosinophilic granuloma, aneurysmal bone cyst, nonossifying fibroma, enchondroma, and chondromyxoid fibroma.

Treatment

If the lesion is small and asymptomatic, no treatment is needed. If the lesion is large and produces or threatens pathologic fracture, curettage and bone grafting are indicated.

Prognosis

Unless the lesions impair epiphysial growth, the prognosis for patients with fibrous dysplasia is good. Lesions tend to enlarge during the growth period but are stable during adult life. Malignant transformation is rare.

UNICAMERAL BONE CYST

Unicameral bone cyst occurs in the metaphysis of a long bone, usually in the femur or humerus. It begins within the medullary canal adjacent to the epiphysial cartilage. It probably results from some fault in enchondral ossification. The cyst is considered active as long as it abuts onto the metaphysial side of the epiphysial cartilage, and there is a risk of growth arrest with or without treatment.

When a border of normal bone exists between the cyst and the epiphysial cartilage, the cyst is inactive. The lesion is usually identified when a pathologic fracture occurs, producing pain. Laboratory findings are normal. On radiograph, the cyst is identified centrally within the medullary canal, producing expansion of the cortex and thinning over the widest portion of the cyst.

Treatment consists of curettage and bone grafting. The cyst may heal after a fracture.

Dormans JP, Pill SG: Fractures through bone cysts: unicameral bone cysts, aneurysmal bone cysts, fibrous cortical defects, and nonossifying fibromas. Instr Course Lect 2002;51:457 (Review) (no abstract available) [PMID: 12064135].

ANEURYSMAL BONE CYST

Aneurysmal bone cyst is similar to unicameral bone cyst, but it contains blood rather than clear fluid. It usually occurs in a slightly eccentric position in the long bone, expanding the cortex of the bone but not breaking the cortex. Involvement of the flat bones of the pelvis is less common. On radiographs, the lesion appears somewhat larger than the width of the epiphysial cartilage. This feature distinguishes it from unicameral bone cyst.

Chromosomal abnormalities have been associated with aneurysmal bone cyst. The lesion may appear aggressive histologically, and it is important to differentiate it from osteosarcoma or hemangioma. Treatment is by curettage and bone grafting. The prognosis is good.

INFANTILE CORTICAL HYPEROSTOSIS (Caffey Syndrome)

Infantile cortical hyperostosis is a benign disease of unknown cause that has its onset before age 6 months and is characterized by irritability; fever; and nonsuppurating, tender, painful swellings. Swellings may involve almost any bone of the body and are frequently widespread. Classically, swellings of the mandible and clavicle occur in 50% of patients; swellings of the ulna, humerus, and ribs also occur. The disease is limited to the shafts of bones and does not involve subcutaneous tissues or joints. It is self-limited but may persist for weeks or months. Anemia, leukocytosis, an increased ESR, and elevation of the serum alkaline phosphatase concentration are usually present. Cortical hyperostosis is demonstrable by a typical radiographic appearance and may be diagnosed on physical examination by an experienced pediatrician.

Fortunately the disease appears to be decreasing in frequency. Indomethacin may be useful for treatment. The prognosis is good, and the disease usually terminates without deformity.

GANGLION

A ganglion is a smooth, small cystic mass connected by a pedicle to the joint capsule, usually on the dorsum of the wrist. It may also occur in the tendon sheath over the flexor surfaces of the fingers. These ganglia can be excised if they interfere with function or cause persistent pain.

BAKER CYST

A Baker cyst is a herniation of the synovium in the knee joint into the popliteal region. In children, the diagnosis may be made by aspiration of mucinous fluid, but the cyst nearly always disappears with time. Whereas Baker cysts may be indicative of intra-articular disease in the adult, they occur without internal derangement in children and rarely require excision.

Kocher MS, Klingele K, Rassman SO: Meniscal disorders: normal, discoid, and cysts. Orthop Clin North Am 2003;34:329 (Review) [PMID: 12974483].

Rehabilitation & Sports Medicine

25

Pamela E. Wilson, MD, & Dennis J. Matthews, MD

The development of sports medicine as a unique discipline has grown since the 1980s in response to the expanding body of knowledge in the areas of exercise physiology, biomechanics, and musculoskeletal medicine. The boom in physical fitness and physical activity has generated a need for specialty training in these areas. As more and more children become involved in recreational and competitive activities an understanding of sports medicine and developmental issues will be of major importance to health care providers in today's modern pediatric practice.

■ BASIC PRINCIPLES

The basic unit of the musculoskeletal system is the muscle fiber which can be classified as either slow twitch, fast twitch, or of intermediate type. Slow twitch, or type 1, fibers have a tendency to be smaller, are recruited in muscle contractions first, and are innervated by smaller motor neurons. Fast twitch, or type 2, fibers make up white muscle and have a tendency to be larger. They are recruited when the body needs to produce rapid muscle tension. In general they produce more lactic acid than type 1 fibers. An intermediate type 2a fiber also exists and is called fast oxidative glycolytic, or FOG. Untrained individuals have a 50:50 proportion of type 1 to type 2 fibers. Elite long-distance runners can have up to 90% type 1 fibers. This apparent adaptation raises the interesting question as to whether an athlete is genetically programmed or can develop adaptations to be successful in sports.

Exercise generates specific effects on the cardiorespiratory system that include increased VO_2 max (maximum amount of oxygen that can be consumed), increased cardiac output, reduced resting heart rate, and improved blood pressure responses.

Biomechanics, the study of movement and how the forces generated by the neuromuscular system translate into these movements, integrates principles of biology and physics. Through biomechanics we can understand the intricacies of movement and how these movements affect athletic performance and result in injuries.

Types of Muscle Contraction Associated with Exercise

Muscle contractions can be divided into three types: isometric, isotonic, and isokinetic. An isometric exercise is exercise against a fixed load in which no movement is achieved. Isometric exercise can improve strength at a given angle, but does not impact endurance. These exercises are beneficial in therapy prescriptions during the acute phase of an injury in which certain muscles or groups of muscles need strengthening. Isometric exercise can cause an increase in blood pressure and heart rate and should be used cautiously when a cardiac condition is present. Isokinetic exercise uses the concept of constant velocity and can provide maximal muscle contractions through full range of motion. This type of exercise generally requires special equipment. Lastly, isotonic exercise uses the principle of constant load and muscle length changes to strengthen muscles. It is the most common type of exercise and can be sport-specific. Isotonic exercises can be further classified as below:

A. CONCENTRIC

In concentric exercises the force of a muscle contraction overcomes an external resistance, which results in shortening of the muscle. These muscles accelerate a distal segment in the kinetic chain and are therefore referred to as open kinetic chain movements. An example of such an exercise is a biceps curl, during which the biceps is actively contracting or shortening to lift the weight.

B. ECCENTRIC

In eccentric exercises, contractions increase muscle tension associated with lengthening of the muscle and are used to decelerate a distal segment in the kinetic chain. This type of exercise is exemplified by the squatting motion, in which the quadriceps lengthens under tension to control downward motion. If the terminal segment in the chain is fixed, this type of movement is called closed kinetic chain movement.

De Ste Croix M et al: Assessment and interpretation of isokinetic muscle strength during growth and maturation. Sports Med 2003;33:727 [PMID: 12895130].

806

Strength Training

Strength is defined as the peak force that can be generated during a maximal single contraction. Strength training is therefore the use of progressive resistance to improve an athlete's ability to resist or exert force. This can be achieved by a variety of techniques including body weight, free weight, or machine resistance. The benefits of weight-training programs are improved performance, endurance, and muscular strength. These programs can be started in prepubescent athletes and if designed appropriately can be done safely with minimal risk for injury. Tanner staging (see Chapter 30) helps to define readiness for progression into more strenuous programs. Power lifting and weight lifting should be restricted to those athletes who have reached or passed Tanner stage V. Individuals at Tanner stage IV or less can safely participate in a strength training program that is specifically and carefully designed for younger athletes. These programs incorporate submaximal resistance with multiple repetitions. They can be generalized or sport-specific. Care should be taken to prevent injuries while using weight training equipment at home. Children and adults with disabilities can benefit from the same type of programs modified to meet their specific needs.

Benjamin HJ, Glow KM: Strength training for children and adolescents: What physicians can recommend. Phys Sportsmed 2003;31:9.

Faigenbaum AD: Strength training for children and adolescents. Clin Sports Med 2000:19;4:593 [PMID: 11019731].

Guy JA, Micheli LJ: Strength training for children and adolescence. J Am Acad Orthop Surg 2001;9:29 [PMID: 11174161].

PREPARTICIPATION HISTORY & PHYSICAL EXAMINATION

The preparticipation medical examination is designed to evaluate children and screen for potential medical problems that could occur during athletic participation. The objectives of this evaluation are to establish baseline medical information, detect any medical condition that may limit athletic participation, evaluate the athlete for preventable injuries, meet the legal or insurance requirements of most states, assess the athlete's maturity, and make recommendations for necessary protective equipment. The ideal timing of this examination is in preseason, at least 4–6 weeks before training starts. This allows time for any needed interventions by the physician.

Preparticipation History

The history is the most important part of the encounter. Many key elements need to be explored with the athlete. There are many standardized history forms available both on the Internet and in monographs. Figure 25–1A is one example of the essential questions contained in a preparticipation history. The history must include the following areas:

A. CARDIOVASCULAR HISTORY

The physician should note any history of cardiac murmurs, chest pain at rest or with exertion, syncopal episodes or sudden fatigue, shortness of breath, or recent illnesses with chest pain. The family history should specifically ask about underlying cardiac diseases including hypertrophic cardiomyopathy, prolonged QT syndrome, Marfan syndrome, arrhythmias, and sudden death in family members. These questions are necessary to identify potentially life-threatening cardiac lesions. The most common causes of sudden death in young athletes on the playing field are hypertrophic cardiomyopathy and congenital heart lesions.

B. HISTORY OF HYPERTENSION

Any history of hypertension requires further investigation. The current guidelines for the diagnosis of hypertension are blood pressure over 130/75 mm Hg in a child under age 10 years or blood pressure over 140/85 mm Hg in a child 10 years of age or older.

C. HISTORY OF CHRONIC DISEASES

Diseases such as reactive airway disease or exercise-induced asthma, diabetes, renal disease, liver disease, chronic infections, neurologic disorders, or hematologic diseases should be noted.

D. MUSCULOSKELETAL LIMITATIONS AND PRIOR INJURIES

The physician should explore limited range of motion and muscle weakness along with prior injuries that may affect future performance. Chronic pain or soreness long after activity may reflect overuse syndromes and should also be evaluated.

E. MENSTRUAL HISTORY IN FEMALES

The physician should pay particular attention to the so-called female athletic triad: amenorrhea, eating disorders, and osteoporosis.

F. NUTRITIONAL ISSUES

The physician should record methods the athlete uses to maintain, gain, or lose weight.

G. MEDICATION HISTORY

This information will provide data on current medications whose side effects may suggest activity modifications. Also, documenting drug use may provide the opportunity to explore with the patient any benefits or drawbacks of using performance-enhancing compounds such as anabolic steroids, creatine, stimulants, and narcotics.

PREPARTICIPATION HISTORY

Name_____ DOB_____ Age_____ Sex (M or F)

Primary Physician_____Sports _____

Allergies (medications, latex, foods, bees, etc) _____

Medications (include prescription, nonprescription, supplements and vitamins) _____
_____

Answer questions by checking yes (Y)/no (N)/don't know (?)

	Y	N	?
General Health			
1. Have you had any injuries or illnesses?			
2. Have you ever been hospitalized?			
3. Do you think you are too thin or overweight?			
4. Have you ever used anything to gain or lose weight?			
5. Any problems exercising in the heat: heat cramps, heat exhaustion or heat stroke?			
6. Ever had frostbite?			
7. Any vision problems?			
8. Do you wear glasses, contact lens, or eye protection?			
9. Any dental appliances?			
10. Have you had any surgeries?			
11. Any organs missing?			
12. Immunizations (tetanus/ hepatitis B) are they current?			
13. Any concerns about participating in sports?			
Cardiac/Respiratory History			
1. Has any family member died suddenly, had heart disease before age 50 or other heart problems?			
2. Do you have any dizziness, chest pain, a racing heart, or shortness of breath with exercise?			
3. Have you ever passed out?			
4. Do you have a heart murmur, high blood pressure, or any heart condition?			
5. Can you exercise as much as your friends?			
6. Any history of asthma, problems breathing, coughing with exercise?			
Neurologic History			
1. Any history of a head injury/concussion: being knocked out, dazed, or having memory loss?			
2. Have you ever had a seizure or convulsion?			
3. Any nerve problems: stingers, burners, pinched nerves or numbness?			
4. Any problems with headaches?			
Musculoskeletal History			
1. Do you have a history of sprains, strains or fractures?			
2. Any hip, knee or ankle injuries?			
3. Any shoulder, elbow, wrist, hand or finger injuries?			
4. Any back or neck problems?			
5. Ever have to be in a splint, cast or use crutches?			
6. Do you use any special equipment when competing (braces, orthotics, pads etc)			
Females Only			
1. Any problems with menstruation: cramps, irregularity, etc.			
2. When was your last period? _____			

COMMENT ON YES ANSWERS

_____
_____
_____
_____
_____
_____

Figure 25–1. **A:** Preparticipation history.

PREPARTICIPATION PHYSICAL EXAM

Name_____

Date of birth/age_____

Height_____Weight_____BP_____

Pulse R wrist_____L wrist_____other_____

Vision R 20/_____L 20/_____ (was it corrected Y or N)

GENERAL EXAM *(circle normal or abnormal and record results on the form)*

APPEARANCE	normal	
	abnormal	_____
HEENT	normal	
	abnormal	_____
LUNGS	normal	
	abnormal	_____
HEART	normal	
& PULSES	abnormal	_____
ABDOMEN	normal	
	abnormal	_____
GU	normal	
	abnormal	_____
SKIN &	normal	
LYMPH NODES	abnormal	_____
NEURO	normal	
	abnormal	_____

MUSCULOSKELETAL EXAM *(record ROM or instabilities if abnormal)*

NECK	normal	
	abnormal	_____
BACK	normal	
	abnormal	_____
SHOULDERS	normal	
	abnormal	_____
ELBOW &	normal	
WRIST	abnormal	_____
HANDS &	normal	
FINGERS	abnormal	_____
HIP	normal	
	abnormal	_____
KNEE	normal	
	abnormal	_____
ANKLE &	normal	
FOOT	abnormal	_____

Cleared for sports: **YES or NO**   If not cleared for sport **WHY?**_____

Further evaluation/rehab or/secondary clearance: _____

Signature examinee:_____   **Date**_____

Figure 25–1. **B:** Preparticipation exam.

Armsey TD, Hosey RG: Medical aspects of sports: Epidemiology of injuries, preparticipation examination, and drugs in sports. Clin Sports Med 2004;23:255 [PMID: 15183571].

Kutscher EC et al: Anabolic steroids: A review for the clinician. Sports Med 2002;32:285 [PMID: 11929356].

Sabatini S: The female athlete triad. Am J Med Sci 2001;322:193.

Physical Examination

The physical examination should be focused on the needs of the athlete. It may be the only time that an athlete has contact with medical personnel, and can be used to promote wellness along with screening for physical activity. Figure 25–1B includes a preparticipation physical exam form. The examination should include routine vital signs including blood pressure measurements obtained in the upper extremity. The cardiovascular examination should include palpation of pulses, auscultation for murmurs in both sitting and standing, and evaluation of the effects of exercise on the individual. The musculoskeletal examination is used to determine strength, range of motion, flexibility, and previous injuries. Included is a quick guide that can be used to screen for abnormalities in this area (Table 25–1). The remainder of the examination should emphasize the following areas:

A. SKIN

Are there any contagious lesions such as herpes or impetigo?

B. VISUAL

Are there any visual problems? Is there any evidence of retinal problems? Are both eyes intact?

C. ABDOMINAL

Is there any evidence of hepatosplenomegaly?

D. GENITOURINARY

Are any testicular abnormalities or hernias present?

E. NEUROLOGIC

Are there any problems with coordination, gait, or mental processing?

F. SEXUAL MATURITY

What Tanner stage is this individual?

Recommendations for Participation

After completing the medical examination (history and physical) the physician can make recommendations to the athlete on sports clearance. The options are unrestricted participation, limited participation, or no participation. Table 25–2 is a composite of recommendations for sports participation organized by body system. In addition, recommendations for sports participation based

Table 25–1. The screening sports exam.[a]

General evaluation	Have person stand in front of the examiner and evaluate both front and back along with posture
	Look at general body habitus
	Look for asymmetry in muscle bulk, scars, or unusual postures
	Watch how the patient moves when instructed
Neck evaluation	Evaluate range of motion (ROM) by having person bend head forward (chin to chest), rotate from side to side, and laterally bend (ear to shoulder)
	Observe for asymmetry, lack of motion, or pain with movement
Shoulder and upper extremity evaluation	Observe clavicles, shoulder position, scapular position, elbow position, and fingers
	ROM screening
	Fully abduct arms with palms in jumping jack position
	Internally and externally rotate shoulder
	Flex and extend wrist, pronate and supinate wrist, flex and extend fingers
	Do the following manual muscle testing:
	Have person shrug shoulders (testing trapezius)
	Abduct to 90 degrees (testing deltoid)
	Flex elbow (testing biceps)
	Extend elbow over head (testing triceps)
	Test wrist flexion and extension
	Have person grasp fingers
Back evaluation	General inspection to look for scoliosis or kyphosis
	ROM screening
	Bend forward touching toes with knees straight (spine flexion and hamstring range)
	Rotation, side bending, and spine extension
Gait and lower extremity evaluation	General observation while walking
	Walk short distance normally (look at symmetry, heel-toe gait pattern, look at all joints involved in gait and leg lengths, any evidence of joint effusions or pain)
	Have person toe-walk and heel-walk for short distance and check tandem walking (balance beam walking)

[a]If any abnormalities are found, then a more focused evaluation is required.

Table 25–2. Recommendations and considerations for participation in sports.

Disorders	Considerations and Recommendations	References
Cardiac		
Anticoagulation treatment	Need to avoid all contact sports	

Aortic stenosis	Individualize treatment based on disease and systolic gradient
	  Mild: < 20 mm Hg, all sports if asymptomatic.
	  Moderate: limited sports.
	  Severe: no competitive sports.	

Arrhythmias	Consult with cardiologist as WPW and long QT syndrome can have serious consequences.	
Congestive heart failure (CHF)	Screen patient with LVEF < 30% for ischemia. Use AHA risk stratification criteria to define exercise capacity.	Braith, 2002
Heart implants	No jumping, swimming, or contact sports.	
Hypertrophic cardiomyopathy	Single most common cause of cardiac death in young athletes. Athletes should not participate in sports except possibly low-intensity forms (eg, golf, bowling). Consult with cardiologist.	Maron, 2002a,b
Marfan syndrome	Aortic root dilation is associated with mitral valve prolapse and regurgitation. Participate in sports with minimal physical demands.	Salim et al, 2001
Mitral valve prolapse	Fairly common condition. No restrictions unless there is a history of syncope, positive family history of sudden death, arrhythmias with exercise, or moderate regurgitation.	
Syncope	Unexplained syncopal episodes during exercise must be evaluated by ECG, echocardiograph, Holter, and tilt test prior to resumption of any activities.	Firoozi, 2002
Endocrine		

Diabetes type I	No restrictions to activity, however:
	  Short-term exercise = no insulin changes.
	  Vigorous exercise = 25% reduction in insulin with 15–30 g of carbohydrates before and every 30 min during exercise.
	  Strenuous exercise = may require up to an 80% reduction in insulin with extra carbohydrates.
	  Generally monitor blood glucose closely.
		Birrer et al, 2003;
		Draznin, 2000

Eye		
Detached retina	Do not participate in strenuous sports regardless of contact risk.	Moeller, 1996
One eye	Consider avoiding contact sports although if patient does participate use of eye protection is a must.	Vinger, 2000
Gentiourinary		
One testicle	Need to wear protective cups in collision/contact sports.	
Solitary kidney	Advise not to participate in collision/contact sports.	Terrell, 1997
Hematologic		
Hemophilia	Avoid contact/collision sports.	
Sickle cell trait	No restrictions if disorder well under control. Athletes should avoid dehydration and acclimate to altitude. There is however a known association between exercise and sudden death.	

(continued)

Vinger PF: A practical guide for sports eye protection. Phys Sportsmed 2000;28:49.

Winell J, Burke SW: Sports participation of children with Down syndrome. Orthop Clin North Am 2003;34:439.

REHABILITATION OF SPORTS INJURIES

Participation in sports can have tremendous benefits for the individual. It provides physical activity, acquisition of motor skills, and social opportunities. All sports participation, however, carries an inherent risk of injuries. These injuries are classified as either acute or chronic. Chronic injuries occur over time and are related to repetitive stress. These injuries develop in response to overuse, repeated microtrauma, and inadequate repair of injured tissue. Acute injuries, or macrotrauma, are one-time events that can cause alterations in biomechanics and physiology. In response to an acute injury the body responds in a predictable fashion. The first week is characterized by an acute inflammatory response. During this time initial vasoconstriction is followed by vasodilatation. Chemical mediators of inflammation are released and result in the classical physical findings of local swelling, warmth, pain, and loss of function. This phase is essential in healing of the injury. The proliferative phase occurs over 2–4 weeks and involves repair and clean-up. Fibroblasts infiltrate and lay down new collagen. Lastly, the maturation phase allows for repair and regeneration of the damaged tissues.

The management of acute sports injuries is geared toward optimizing healing and restoring function. The goals of immediate care are to minimize the effects of the injury by reducing pain and swelling, to educate the athlete about the nature of the injury and how to take care of it, and to maintain the health of the rest of the body. The treatment for an acute injury is captured in the acronym **PRICE:**

- **P**rotect the injury from further damage (taping, splints, braces)
- **R**est the area
- **I**ce
- **C**ompression of the injury
- **E**levation immediately

The use of nonsteroidal anti-inflammatory agents reduces the inflammatory response and reduces discomfort. These medications may be used immediately after the injury. Glucocorticoids should be administered judiciously. If administered inappropriately they may prolong the acute phase of recovery. Therapeutic use of physical modalities, including early cold and later heat, hydrotherapy, massage, electrical stimulation, iontophoresis, and ultrasound, can enhance recovery in the acute phase.

The recovery phase can be lengthy and requires athlete participation. Initial treatment is focused on joint range of motion and flexibility. Range-of-motion exercises should follow a logical progression of starting with passive motion, then moving to active assistive, and finally to active movement. Active range of motion is initiated once normal joint range has been reestablished. Flexibility is sport-specific and aimed at reducing tight musculature. Strength training can begin early in this phase of rehabilitation. Initially only isometric exercises are encouraged. As recovery progresses and flexibility increases, isotonic and isokinetic exercises can be added to the program. These should be done at least three times per week. As the athlete approaches near-normal strength and is pain-free, the final maintenance phase can be introduced. During this phase the athlete will continue to build strength and work on endurance. The biomechanics of sport-specific activity needs to be analyzed and retraining incorporated into the exercise program. Generalized cardiovascular conditioning should continue during the entire rehabilitation treatment.

■ COMMON SPORTS MEDICINE ISSUES AND INJURIES

INFECTIOUS DISEASES

Infectious diseases are common in both recreational and competitive athletes. These illnesses have an effect on basic physiologic function and athletic performance. Given this knowledge, physicians, parents, and coaches can adopt the common-sense guidelines listed in Table 25–3.

Table 25–3. Sports participation guidelines: infectious diseases.

Athletes with temperatures higher than 100 °F should not participate in sporting activities.

Athletes who have had recent infectious mononucleosis can return to noncontact training at 3 wk as long as there is no splenic enlargement. They may return to contact sports after 4 wk and a normal abdominal examination.

Athletes with a streptococcal pharyngitis can resume activity once treatment has been initiated and they are afebrile.

If a localized herpes gladiatorum or impetigo lesion is present, no contact sports are allowed until the lesions have resolved. Athletes with herpes zoster have the same restrictions. There are no restrictions for athletes with common warts. Athletes with molluscum contagiosum can compete if the affected areas are covered. Athletes with furuncles cannot be involved in contact sports or swimming until the lesions are healed.

Athletes with HIV infection may compete in all types of sports. Universal precautions should be used with all athletes who have sustained injuries.

Rihn JA et al: Community-acquired methicillin-resistant *Staphylococcus aureus*: An emerging problem in the athletic population. Am J Sports Med 2005;33:1924 [PMID: 16314668].

HEAD & NECK INJURIES

Head and neck injuries occur most commonly in contact and individual sports. The sports with the highest incidence of brain injury are football, bicycling, baseball, horseback riding, and golf. The treatment of these is controversial with multiple guidelines being developed. Injuries in young children should err on the conservative side as they have developing central nervous systems.

Concussion is a temporary and immediate impairment of neurologic function and may or may not have an unconscious period associated. Classically it has been defined by length of unconsciousness (LOC), post-traumatic amnesia (PTA), and confusion. Concussions have been categorized as grade 1 (mild), grade 2 (moderate), or grade 3 (severe). Return-to-play guidelines have been developed by several resources and are compiled in Table 25–4. Recently, other tools for assessment have gained popularity including the Standardized Assessment of Concussion (SAC) used for on-field evaluation, Balance Error Scoring System (BESS), computerized testing, and symptoms checklist. Athletes should never be allowed to return to play if any symptoms are present or if there is an abnormal neurologic exam. Once symptoms have resolved a recommended six-step progression is outlined for return to play: (1) assess at rest; once asymptomatic progress to (2) light aerobic exercise, followed by (3) sport-specific exercise, then begin (4) noncontact drills followed by (5) contact drills, and finally (6) release to game play. If any symptoms present the athlete should be not move to the next step. Neuropsychology testing is advocated for athletes with persistent symptoms.

Second impact syndrome is a rare but potentially deadly complication of head injuries. Athletes who have had a prior brain injury that has not healed and have a second injury are at risk for a loss of vascular autoregulation and subsequent malignant cerebral edema.

Cervical spine injuries are fairly common but potentially serious. They can cause fractures, ligamentous injuries, and associated spinal cord injuries. The most frequent neck injury is a cervical strain. Return to play for cervical strain is allowed when neck range of motion is full and pain-free, strength is normal, vertebral column is stable, and there is a normal neurologic exam.

Atlantoaxial instability is common in children with Down syndrome because of underlying ligamentous laxity, including the annular ligament of C1, and hypotonia. Cervical neck films including flexion, extension, and neutral position evaluate the atlanto-dens interval (ADI). ADI is normally less than 2.5 mm, but up to 4.5 mm is acceptable in this population. Children with greater than 4.5 mm should be limited from contact and collision activities.

Table 25–4. Return-to-competition guidelines following concussion.

Grade 1 or mild concussion
No loss of consciousness (LOC)
PTA or confusion lasting less than 15 min
First Injury
- Remove from game
- Return to play in 15 minutes if exam is normal
Second Injury
- Return to play if asymptomatic after 1 wk

Grade 2 or moderate concussion
No LOC
PTA or confusion lasting longer than 15 minutes
First Injury
- Remove from game
- Hospital evaluation if symptoms persist for more than 1 hour
- Return to play if asymptomatic after 1 wk
- CT or MRI if symptoms persist for more than 1 wk
Second Injury
- Return to play if asymptomatic after 2 wks
Third Injury
- Out for season

Grade 3 or severe concussion
Any LOC
First Injury
- Transport to hospital for evaluation
- With a brief LOC (seconds), return to play if asymptomatic after 1 wk
- With a longer LOC (minutes), return to play if asymptomatic after 2 wk
Second Injury
- No play for at least 1 mo following absence of symptoms; consider ending season

PTA, post-traumatic amnesia; CT, computed tomography; MRI, magnetic resonance imaging.

American Academy of Neurology: Practice parameter: The management of concussion in sports (Summary statement). Report of the Quality standards subcommittee. Neurology 1997;48:581 [PMID: 9065530].

Cantu RC: Guidelines for return to contact sports after a cerebral concussion. Phys Sportsmed 1986;14:75.

Cole AJ et al: Cervical spine athletic injuries: A pain in the neck. Phys Med Rehabil Clin N Am 1994;5:37.

Colorado Medical Society: *Report of the Sports Medicine Committee: Guidelines for the Management of Concussion in Sports* (revised). Colorado Medical Society, 1991.

Dimberg EL: Management of common neurologic conditions in sports. Clin Sports Med 2005;24:637 [PMID: 16004923].

Patel DR: The pediatric athlete with disabilities. Pediatr Clin North Am 2002;49:803 [PMID: 12296534].

Winell J: Sports participation of children with Down syndrome. Orthop Clin North Am 2003;34:439 [PMID: 12974493].

Burners and stingers are common injuries in contact sports, especially football. These types of cervical radiculopathies or brachial plexopathies occur when the head is laterally bent and the shoulder depressed. Symptoms include immediate burning pain and paresthesias down one arm generally lasting only minutes. Weakness in the muscles of the upper trunk—supraspinatus, deltoid, and biceps—can persist for weeks. Workup includes a thorough neurologic assessment. If symptoms persist, then a diagnostic evaluation should include cervical spine x-rays, magnetic resonance imaging (MRI) scans, and electromyography. The athlete can return to play once symptoms have resolved, neck and shoulder range of motion is pain-free, reflexes and strength are normal, and the Spurling test is negative. Preventative strategies include always wearing protective gear, proper blocking and tackling techniques, and maintaining neck and shoulder strength.

Feinberg JH: Burners and stingers. Phys Med Rehabil Clin N Am 2000;11:771 [PMID: 11092018].

SPINE INJURIES

Injuries to the spine are fairly common even in the pediatric population. As children have become more competitive in sports, the number of reported injuries has increased. Sports with a fairly high incidence of back injuries include golf, gymnastics, football, dance, wrestling, and weightlifting. Pain lasting more than 2 weeks indicates a possible structural problem and needs to be investigated.

Herniated discs account for a small percentage of back injuries in children. These injuries are almost unheard of in preadolescence. Most injuries occur at the L4-L5 and L5-S1 vertebrae. Symptoms include back and leg pain. Pain may be increased with activities such as bending, sitting, and coughing. Pain often radiates down the lower extremity in a radicular pattern. Evaluation includes physical and neurologic exam including straight leg testing, sensory testing, and checking reflexes. If symptoms persist then the evaluation includes electromyography, CT, and MRI scans. Treatment generally is conservative as most back injuries improve spontaneously. The athlete can rest the back for a short period and then begin on a structured exercise program of extension and isometrics followed by flexion exercises. If symptoms persist, then a short course of steroids may be indicated. Surgery is recommended only if neurologic compromise persists.

Spondylolysis is an injury to the pars interarticularis. Pars defects are present in 4–6% of the population. Repetitive stress to this area results in fractures. The injury is common in gymnasts, dancers, and football players. Spondylolysis occurs at L5 in 85% of cases. Pain usually develops during an adolescent growth spurt. Back pain may radiate into the buttock or thigh area. Extension of the spine increases pain. Evaluation includes an oblique x-ray view of the spine in order to look for the so-called "Scottie dog sign." Treatment includes rest from sporting activities, stretching of the hamstrings, stabilization exercises, lumbosacral bracing, and occasionally surgery.

If a bilateral pars injury occurs, then slippage of one vertebra over another (**spondylolisthesis**) can occur. These injuries are graded on a scale of 1 to 4 based on the percentage of slippage: grade 1 (0–25%); grade 2 (25–49%); grade 3 (50–74%); and grade 4 (75–100%). Diagnosis is based on lateral x-rays although further studies may be indicated, and treatment is often symptomatic. Asymptomatic athletes with less than 30% slippage have no restrictions and are followed up on a routine basis. Slippage of 50% requires interventions of stretching hip flexors and hamstrings, along with bracing or surgery.

Eddy D et al: A review of spine injuries and return to play. Clin J Sport Med 2005;15:453 [PMID: 16278551].

Herman MJ: Spondylolysis and spondylolisthesis in the child and adolescent athlete. Orthop Clin North Am 2003;34:461 [PMID: 12974495].

SHOULDER INJURIES

In evaluating shoulder injuries it is necessary to look at both macro- and microtrauma. Fractures and dislocations account for most macrotrauma. The balance of other injuries are related to repetitive overuse and tissue failure. **Rotator cuff injuries** are common in sports that require repetitive overhead motions. Muscle imbalances and injury cause the position of the humeral head to be abnormal which may cause impingement of the supraspinatous tendon under the acromial arch. Pain is usually reported in the anterior and lateral shoulder and is increased with overhead activities. Diagnostic workup includes plain x-rays and an outlet view to look for anatomic variability. The rehabilitation of this injury is geared toward reduction of inflammation, improved flexibility, and strengthening of the scapular stabilizers and rotator cuff muscles. This is achieved by a progression of isometric exercise followed by isotonic or isokinetic exercises. A biomechanics evaluation can assist in the recovery process by building sport-specific skills and eliminating substitution patterns.

Tythweleigh-Strong G et al: Rotator cuff disease. Curr Opin Rheumatol 2001:13:135 [PMID: 11224738].

Wasserlauf BF: Shoulder disorders in the skeletally immature throwing athlete. Orthop Clin North Am 2003;34:427 [PMID: 12974492].

ELBOW & FOREARM INJURIES

Injuries in the forearm are quite common with both chronic and acute etiologies (eg, the chronic overuse "Little League elbow" and the frequent childhood fracture typical of falls on an outstretched arm). When evaluating the elbow consider dividing the exam into specific anatomic areas as discussed below.

Table 25–5. Guidelines for pitching limits in youth baseball.

Age (years)	Pitches/game[a]
8–10	52 ± 15
11–12	68 ± 18
13–14	76 ± 16
15–16	91 ± 16
16–17	106 ± 16

[a]Based on 2 games/week.

Medial Elbow Pain

Medial elbow pain can have multiple etiologies, but one of the most common is **medial epicondylitis,** an overuse injury caused by valgus stress at the elbow. **Little League elbow** consists of a group of abnormalities that develop in young baseball pitchers. These abnormalities are secondary to the biomechanical forces generated around the elbow during throwing. These forces can result in shearing, inflammation, traction, and abnormal bone development. Pitching can be divided into six phases: windup, early cocking, late cocking, acceleration, deceleration, and follow-through. The acceleration phase is where most forces are generated. The symptoms are primarily swelling, pain, performance difficulties, and weakness. The pain localizes to the medial epicondyle, which may be tender to palpation. Wrist flexion and pronation increase symptoms. The different phases of throwing should be analyzed to isolate when the pain appears. If pain is present in all phases this may indicate a severe injury. Workup includes a series of elbow x-rays, including stress films and comparison films, to look for widening of the epiphyseal lines and MRI studies. Treatment of the acute injury includes rest. It is not uncommon for a player to be benched for up to 6 weeks. Competition can be resumed once the player is asymptomatic.

The key to treating this injury is prevention. Children should be properly conditioned and coached in correct throwing biomechanics. There are guidelines for pitching limits in youth baseball. Little League limits 10- to 12-year-old children to 6 innings/week and 13- to 15-year-old children to 9 innings/week. Limiting pitches per game is outlined in Table 25–5.

Other causes of medial elbow pain include ulnar collateral ligament injury, ulnar neuritis, apophysitis, and fractures.

Lateral Elbow Pain

Lateral elbow pain can be the result of a few unique problems in growing athletes. **Panner disease** is also caused by valgus stress at the elbow. It is a focal process in the capitellum and occurs in players between 5 and 12 years of age. The child presents with dull aching in the lateral elbow that generally worsens when the child throws something. Swelling and reduced elbow extension are usually present. X-rays show an abnormal capitellum with fragmentation and areas of sclerosis. Treatment is conservative, using rest, ice, and splinting. The child can return to play after the x-rays normalize.

The same type of pain in a 13- to 15-year-old athlete is usually **osteochondritis dissecans.** This injury is basically avascular necrosis of the capitellum which can result in the formation of loose bodies. X-rays are needed in the diagnosis and help to classify the injury into one of three categories. Treatment is based on this classification and can be either conservative or surgical in nature. The child should be seen by an orthopedic specialist.

Lateral epicondylitis is common in racquet sports, particularly tennis. It is an overuse of the extensor muscle in the forearm and causes pain in the lateral elbow. Pain is increased by wrist extension. Initial treatment is aimed at inflammation control. Stretching and strengthening of forearm muscles are the primary interventions during the subsequent phases. Stroke mechanics may need to be altered and a forearm brace used to decrease the forces in the extensor muscles.

Posterior Elbow Pain

Posterior elbow pain is not very common. Etiologies include dislocations, fractures, triceps avulsions, and olecranon bursitis.

Axe M: Recommendation for protecting youth baseball pitches. Sports Med and Arthroscopy Rev 2001;9.

Gerbino PG: Elbow disorders in throwing athletes. Orthop Clin North Am 2003;34:417 [PMID: 12974491].

Hang DW et al: A clinical and roentgenographic study of Little League elbow. Am J Sports Med 2004;32:79 [PMID: 14754727].

Johnson EW: Tennis elbow. Misconceptions and widespread mythology. Am J Phys Med Rehabil 2000;79:2:113 [PMID: 10744183].

HAND & WRIST INJURIES

All hand and wrist injuries have the potential for long-term, often serious disability and deserve a thorough evaluation.

1. Hand Injuries

Distal Phalanx Injuries

Tuft injury requires splinting for 6 weeks or until the patient is pain-free. If there is significant displacement, then a K-wire can be used for reduction. **Nail bed injury** often requires splinting and drainage of subungual hematomas.

Distal Interphalangeal Injuries

Mallet finger or **extensor tendon avulsion** occurs in ball-handling sports. The mechanism of injury is a force applied to an extended finger. Treatment is splinting in extension for 6 weeks for fractures and 8 weeks for tendon rupture.

Thumb Injuries

Gamekeeper's thumb is an injury to the ulnar collateral ligament from forced abduction of the metacarpal phalangeal joint. It is a common skiing injury. If a radiograph shows an avulsed fragment is displaced less than 2 mm, a thumb spica cast can be used. If there is no fragment and less than 35 degrees of lateral joint space opening, a spica cast for 6 weeks is indicated. Surgery is required for more serious injuries.

Fractures

Boxer's fracture is a neck fracture of the fifth digit. These fractures can be treated by closed reduction and casting for 3 weeks. A displaced fracture requires open reduction and internal fixation.

2. Wrist Injuries

Most swollen wrists without evidence of instability can be splinted for several weeks. Radial and ulnar fractures must be ruled out because these are fairly common in children.

Scaphoid fractures are caused by a force applied to a hyperextended wrist. If evidence of snuffbox tenderness and swelling is present, the wrist must be immobilized for 10 days and then reassessed, even if x-rays are normal. A nondisplaced fracture requires at least 6 weeks of immobilization in a thumb spica cast.

Brook S et al: The management of scaphoid fractures. J Sci Med Sports 2005;8:181.

Geissler WB: Carpal fractures in athletes. Clin Sports Med 2001; 20:167 [PMID: 11227704].

Wang QC, Johnson BA: Fingertip injuries. Am Fam Physician 2001; 63:1961 [PMID: 11388710].

HIP INJURIES

Because the pelvis and hip articulate with both the lower extremities and the spine, this is an area rich in ligaments, muscle attachments, and nerves. Injuries in young children are rare, but sprains and strains are common.

Groin pull, or **adductor strain,** is generally caused by forced abduction as in running, falling, twisting, or tackling. The associated pain is in the adductor muscle. There may be pain with adduction or hip flexion and tenderness over the adductor tubercle. Treatment includes rest, ice, protection, and strengthening of the muscle when it heals.

Quadriceps contusion is caused by a direct macroinjury to the muscle, resulting in bruising, swelling, and pain. The anterior and lateral thigh regions are most commonly injured. Treatment is rest, ice, and protection for the first 24 hours. The knee should be kept in a fully flexed position. Two to three days after the injury, range-of-motion exercises may begin in both flexion and extension. Once 120 degrees of motion has been established and movement does not cause pain, the athlete may return to competitive activity. If the muscle remains firm on examination after 2 weeks, then x-rays of the thigh should be done to rule out myositis ossificans. **Myositis ossificans** is an abnormal deposition of calcium in the muscle that may be induced by aggressive stretching of the muscle too early in the clinical course.

Hamstring strain is very common in multiple sports. The mechanism of injury is forced extension of the knee. Examination reveals pain on palpation of the muscle. Pain also occurs with knee flexion against resistance. Treatment is rest, ice, and compression. The athlete can walk as soon as he or she can tolerate the activity. It is particularly important to stretch the hamstring because, as a two-joint muscle, it is more susceptible to injury than other types of muscle.

The bursa is a structure that allows for improved motion by reducing friction. When a bursa becomes inflamed, movement is painful and may be limited. Areas susceptible to bursa inflammation are the shoulder, elbow, patella, and hip. **Trochanteric bursitis,** causing pain when the hip is flexed, often results from reduced flexibility of the iliotibial band and gluteus medius tendons. It is best evaluated in a side-lying position, and pain is reproduced when the hip is actively flexed from a fully extended hip. Initial treatment is to alter the offending activity and then start a stretching program geared at the iliotibial band and hip abductors. Corticosteroid injections may be used after conservative treatment has failed.

Most **hip dislocations** are in the posterior direction. Athletes with this injury classically present with hip flexion, adduction, and internal rotation.

Hip dislocations in skeletally mature athletes are almost always associated with acetabular and femoral neck fracture. The preadolescent, skeletally immature competitor may have an isolated injury. This is a true on-field emergency, and the athlete should be transported to the nearest facility that has an orthopedic surgeon available. Severe bleeding, avascular necrosis, and nerve damage can result. Once reduction has been established in a noncomplicated case, protected weight bearing on crutches for 6 weeks is recommended followed by another 6 weeks of range-of-motion and strengthening exercises. An athlete may return gradually to competition after 3 months when strength and motion are normal.

Femoral neck fractures (**stress fractures**) are generally the result of repetitive microtrauma. They commonly occur in track athletes who have increased their mileage.

Athletes with this type of injury present with persistent pain in the groin and pain with internal and external rotation. Range of motion may be limited in hip flexion and internal rotation. If plain x-rays are negative, then a bone scan is indicated. Treatment is based on the type of fracture. A **transverse fracture** generally requires internal fixation to prevent femoral displacement from occurring and potentially causing avascular necrosis. A **compression fracture** is less likely to be displaced; treatment is conservative and involves resting the hip until it heals. Cardiovascular conditioning can be maintained easily through nonimpact exercises and activity.

Cooper DE: Severe quadriceps muscle contusions in athletes. Am J Sports Med 2004;32:820 [PMID: 15090402].

Maffulli N: Lower limb injuries in children in sports. Clin Sports Med 2000;19:637 [PMID: 11019733].

KNEE INJURIES

Knee injuries are one of the most common problems evaluated by any practitioner. The function of the knee is for mobility and stability. Knee movements include flexion, extension, rotation, rolling, and gliding. The knee is stabilized through a variety of ligaments, tendons, and the meniscus.

Anterior Knee Pain

The most common knee complaint is anterior knee pain. This complaint can have multiple etiologies but should always include hip pathology as a possible source. Patellofemoral etiology is a common cause of anterior knee pain. The differential diagnosis is quite extensive and requires a thorough examination.

Patellofemoral overuse syndrome occurs in runners and in athletes participating in sports with repetitive stress in the lower extremity. Classically, pain is located over the medial surface and under surface of the patella. It is associated with swelling and crepitus of the knee joint. The Q-angle often is increased. The Q-angle is measured by drawing a line from the anterosuperior iliac spine down to the center of the patella and then through the tibial tubercle. The intersecting angle is the Q-angle. Normal is 14 degrees for males and 17 degrees for females. Q-angles greater than 20 degrees tend to track the patella laterally changing the knee biomechanics.

Plicae alares are normal synovial folds in the knee joint. If they become thickened or fibrosed they can become entrapped. This happens with direct macrotrauma or repetitive microtrauma. The athlete complains of snapping or popping in the knee. The knee pain is worse with knee flexion and activity intensifies symptoms. On examination the hamstrings may be tight. Physical findings include localized tenderness and occasionally popping palpable at 30–60 degrees of knee flexion.

Tendonitis of the patellar tendon is caused by overuse. The mechanism is repetitive loading of the quadriceps during running or jumping. **Osgood-Schlatter disease** occurs in the preteen and adolescent years. It is most common in boys between 12 and 15 years and in girls between 11 and 13 years. Pain usually is present at the tibial tubercle, and activities using eccentric quadriceps muscle movement aggravate the pain. The pain can become so extensive that routine activity must be curtailed. X-rays may or may not show abnormalities. Type 1 disease has no findings, whereas type 2 has evidence of fragmentation of the tibial tubercle. Many other conditions can cause anterior knee pain and need to be ruled out, including arthritis, complex regional pain syndrome, infections, and neoplasm. Finally, **chondromalacia patellae** is an arthroscopic diagnosis and should not be used as a clinical diagnosis.

Treatment of Anterior Knee Pain

As with any acute injury, control of inflammation is essential. This begins with rest and ice. Alignment problems should be corrected with stretching and strengthening. Orthotics may need to be used for correction of foot deformities. Quadriceps strengthening begins with isometric exercises that progress to a concentric program. These include short arc vastus medialis contractions, which are the last 10 degrees of knee extension. In the last part of the therapy program eccentric loading of the quadriceps can be incorporated. During this time the athlete should be working on endurance and cardiovascular conditioning. Knee bracing is controversial, and the major benefits are proprioceptive feedback and patellar tracking.

Lateral Knee Pain

Lateral knee pain is most commonly associated with a tight iliotibial band, which can lead to **tendonitis** and **bursitis.** Pain over the lateral femoral condyle is present along with a positive Ober test. The Ober test is done with the athlete in a side-lying position. The knee and hip are flexed to 90 degrees then the hip is maximally abducted and extended. From this position the leg is allowed to drop by gravity while the knee is still controlled. It will not relax if the iliotibial band is tight. Treatment involves rest and stretching. Athletics should not be resumed until the patient is pain-free. This may take up to 6 weeks. Other sources of lateral knee pain are popliteus tendonitis and biceps tendonitis.

Posterior Knee Pain

Posterior knee pain usually results from an injury to the gastrocnemius-soleus complex caused by overuse. It can also include a Baker cyst, tibial stress fracture, or tendonitis of the hamstring. Treatment is rest, ice, and strengthening exercises after symptoms have improved.

Meniscal Injuries

The meniscus of the knee cushions forces in the knee joint, increases nutrient supply to the cartilage, and stabilizes the knee. Most injuries are related to directional changes on a weight-bearing extremity. **Medial meniscus injuries** have a history of tibial rotation in a weight-bearing position. This happens frequently in ball-handling sports. **Lateral meniscus injuries** occur with tibial rotation with a flexed knee. These injuries are uncommon in children under age 10 years. The athlete with such an injury has a history of knee pain, swelling, snapping, or locking or may report a feeling of the knee giving way. Physical examination reveals joint line tenderness and a positive McMurray hyperflexion/rotation test. The diagnostic test of choice is MRI of the knee, although standard knee x-rays should be included. Arthrograms are still used by some practitioners. Treatment may be symptomatic for isolated injuries of the meniscus and no ligamentous involvement or mechanical blocks. If surgery is needed the athlete should not bear weight on the knee for 3 weeks. During this time, range-of-motion and strengthening exercises can be done.

Medial & Lateral Collateral Ligament Injuries

The medial and lateral collateral ligaments are positioned along either side of the knee and act to stabilize it. They help to control varus and valgus stress applied to the knee joint. Excessive varus or valgus stress causes stretching of the ligament, producing tears. Medial injuries occur with a blow to the lateral aspect of the knee, as seen in a football tackle. The athlete may feel a pop or lose sensation along the medial aspect of the knee. The examination reveals an effusion and tenderness medially. A valgus stress test done in full extension and 20–30 degrees of flexion will reproduce pain. Diagnosis is made by routine and stress x-rays of the knee.

Treatment is almost always conservative. Initial injuries should be iced and elevated. A protective brace needs to be worn, and full knee motion in the brace can be done after 7 days. Weight bearing is allowed, and a strengthening program can be started. The athlete should use the brace until he or she is pain-free and has full range of motion. The use of a functional brace is often required when a player returns to competition. This is only temporary until the ligaments heal properly.

Anterior Cruciate Ligament Injuries

The anterior cruciate ligament (ACL) has three bands and prevents anterior subluxation of the tibia. The ACL is injured by deceleration, twisting, and cutting motions. The mechanism of the injury involves force applied to the knee during hyperextension, with excessive valgus stress and forced external rotation of the femur on a fixed tibia. Evaluation of the knee begins with examining the non-injured knee. The Lachman test will provide information on knee stability in relation to the ACL. All other structures of the knee need to be examined to rule out concomitant injuries. Imaging of the knee includes plain x-rays along with MRI scan.

Treatment options include both conservative and surgical procedures. Conservative treatment includes bracing, strengthening, and restricting physical activity. Braces enhance proprioception and control terminal extension. Surgical repair is quite popular, and a patellar tendon graft is used frequently. Rehabilitation of the knee starts immediately after surgery. A continuous passive range of motion machine is used postoperatively. Partial weight bearing is allowed in a brace that is set in full extension as the quadriceps strengthen. After 2 weeks, partial weight bearing and walking are started. The goals of the subsequent program are continued strength, muscle reeducation, endurance, agility, and coordination.

Posterior Cruciate Ligament Injuries

The posterior cruciate ligament (PCL) runs from the medial femoral condyle to the posterior tibial plateau and has two parts. Its main function is to prevent posterior tibial subluxation. This is an extremely rare injury and occurs when the individual falls on a flexed knee with the ankle in plantarflexion or with forced hyperflexion of the knee. The examination begins with the non-injured knee and proceeds to the injured side. Confirmatory testing includes the posterior drawer test done in supine with the knee flexed to 90 degrees and the foot stabilized. Grading is based on the amount of translation. Grade 1 (mild) is up to 5 mm, grade 2 (moderate) is 5–10 mm, and grade 3 (severe) is greater than 10 mm. Diagnostic imaging includes plain x-rays and MRI scan.

Treatment can be determined as soon as the exact injury has been isolated. Treatment is controversial with respect to surgical versus nonsurgical management. The use of braces and a progressive rehabilitation program have been used successfully in athletes with grade 1 and 2 injuries. Grade 3 injuries generally require surgery.

Andrish JT: Anterior cruciate ligament injuries in the skeletally immature patient. Am J Orthop 2001;30:103 [PMID: 11234936].

Evans NA et al: The natural history and tailored treatment of ACL injury. Phys Sportsmed 2001;29:19.

Kyist J: Rehabilitation following anterior cruciate ligament injury: Current recommendations for sports participation. Sports Med 2004;34:269 [PMID: 15049718].

FOOT & ANKLE INJURIES

Injuries in the lower leg, ankle, and foot are quite common in pediatric athletes. The types of injuries sustained tend to depend on the age group. Young children tend to have diaphyseal injuries, in contrast to older children in rapid growth, who tend to have epiphyseal and apophyseal injuries. Perhaps the most common injury evaluated is the **ankle sprain.** When a ligament is overloaded tearing occurs. These injuries are graded on a scale of 1 to 3. A grade 1 injury is a stretch without instability, grade 2 is a partial tear with some instability, and grade 3 is a total disruption of the ligament with instability of the joint. The ankle has three lateral ligaments (anterior talofibular, calcaneofibular, and posterior talofibular) and a medial deltoid ligament. Inversion of the foot generally damages the anterior talofibular ligament, whereas eversion injures the deltoid ligament. Physical examination often reveals swelling, bruising, and pain. The anterior drawer test is easy to perform and reliably tests the anterior talofibular ligament. Other maneuvers include the talar tilt and valgus stress test. Diagnostic testing should be done when a bony injury is suspected. The adult Ottawa criteria do not pertain to those younger than 18 years of age. Tenderness over the malleoli, tenderness beyond ligament attachments, and excessive swelling are reasons to obtain radiographs.

Treatment of ankle injuries is imperative to ensure full recovery and should begin immediately after the injury. Phase 1 care involves immediate compressive wrapping and icing to control swelling and inflammation. Protected weight bearing is allowed in the early phase of rehabilitation. The second phase begins when the athlete can ambulate without pain. During this time ankle range of motion is emphasized, along with isometric contractions of the ankle dorsiflexors. Once 90% of strength has returned, active isotonic (eccentric and concentric exercises) and isokinetic exercises can be added. Phase 3 is designed to increase strength, improve proprioception, and add ballistic activity. The "foot alphabet" and "tilt board" are excellent methods to improve ankle proprioception. This program may take up to 6 weeks before an athlete can return to full activity. The athlete should wear a protective brace for 3 to 4 months and continue to ice after exercising.

Plantar fascitis is a common problem that manifests itself as heel pain. It happens in runners who log more than 30 miles per week and in athletes who have tight Achilles tendons or poorly fitting shoes. It is common in people with cavus feet and in individuals who are overweight. The pain is worse upon first standing up in the morning and taking a few steps. A bone spur is often found on examination. Treatment involves local massage, stretching of the gastrocsoleus, nonsteroidal anti-inflammatory drugs, arch supports, and local steroid injections. Runners may need to cut back on their weekly mileage until these measures eliminate pain.

Hockenbury RT, Sammarco J: Evaluation and treatment of ankle sprains: Clinical recommendations for a positive outcome. Phys Sportsmed 2001;29:57.

Osborne MD, Rizzo Jr TD: Prevention and treatment of ankle sprains in athletes. Sports Med 2003;33:1145 [PMID: 14719982].

Verhagen E et al: The effects of a proprioceptive balance board training program for the prevention of ankle sprains: A proprioceptive controlled trial. Am J Sports Med 2004;32:1385 [PMID: 15310562].

PREVENTION

As in all activities most sports-related injuries can be prevented by the use of protective equipment, common sense, and proper training. Protective equipment should be properly fitted and maintained by an individual with training and instruction. Helmets should be used in football, baseball, hockey, bicycling, skiing, in-line skating, skateboarding, or any sport with risk for head injury. Eye protection should be used in sports that have a high incidence of eye injuries. Proper protective padding should be identified and used including chest pads for catchers; shin guards in soccer; shoulder, arm, chest, and leg padding in hockey; and wrist and elbow protectors in skating. A few common-sense concepts should be addressed by coaches, parents, and physicians in order to ensure the safety of children participating in sports. These include inspecting playing fields for potential hazards, adapting rules to the developmental level of the participants, and matching opponents equally.

The use of the preparticipation history and physical examination can identify potential problems and allow for prevention and early intervention. Proper training techniques reduce injuries by encouraging flexibility, promoting endurance, and teaching correct biomechanics. Sports education reinforces the concepts of fitness and a healthy lifestyle along with sport-specific training. Early identification of an injury allows the athlete to modify techniques and avoid micro- and macrotrauma. Once an injury has occurred it needs to be identified properly and appropriate measures used to minimize inflammation. Rehabilitation of the injury starts as soon as it has been identified. Early and appropriate care offers the athlete an optimal chance for full recovery and return to full participation.

Rheumatic Diseases

26

J. Roger Hollister, MD

JUVENILE RHEUMATOID ARTHRITIS
(Juvenile Chronic Arthritis)

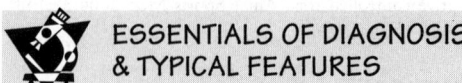

ESSENTIALS OF DIAGNOSIS & TYPICAL FEATURES

- *Nonmigratory monarticular or polyarticular arthropathy, with a tendency to involve large joints or proximal interphalangeal joints and lasting more than 3 months.*
- *Systemic manifestations with fever, erythematous rashes, nodules, leukocytosis, and, occasionally, iridocyclitis, pleuritis, pericarditis, anemia, fatigue, and growth failure.*

General Considerations

Patients with juvenile rheumatoid arthritis (JRA) have different immunogenetic traits than those with adult rheumatoid arthritis. In JRA, HLA-DR5 is associated with iritis and the production of antinuclear antibodies (ANA), whereas HLA-DR4 is found in seropositive, polyarticular disease. These traits may be important in the formation of antisuppressor cell antibodies, immune complex generation, and consequent chronic inflammatory disease. Genomics by microarray analysis shows great promise in understanding the genetic predisposition to JRA. Tumor necrosis factor may be the final common cytokine that perpetuates the inflammation.

Clinical Findings

A. SYMPTOMS AND SIGNS

Three major patterns of presentation in JRA provide clues to the prognosis and possible sequelae of the disease. In the acute febrile form, an evanescent salmon-pink macular rash, arthritis, hepatosplenomegaly, leukocytosis, and polyserositis characterize the constellation described by George Still. Patients with this form have episodic illness, and remission of the systemic features can be expected within 1 year. They do not develop iridocyclitis.

The polyarticular pattern resembles the adult disease, with chronic pain and swelling of many joints in a symmetric fashion. Both large and small joints are usually involved. Systemic features are less prominent, although low-grade fever, fatigue, rheumatoid nodules, and anemia may be present. Patients with this form tend to have long-standing arthritis, although the disease may wax and wane. Iridocyclitis occurs occasionally in this group. Older children may have a positive rheumatoid factor test.

The third pattern consists of pauciarticular disease, characterized by chronic arthritis of a few joints—often the large weight-bearing joints—in an asymmetric distribution. The synovitis is usually mild and may be painless. Systemic features are uncommon, but there is severe extra-articular involvement with inflammation in the eye. Up to 30% of children with pauciarticular JRA develop insidious, asymptomatic iridocyclitis, which may cause blindness if untreated. The activity of the eye disease does not correlate with that of the arthritis. Therefore, routine ophthalmologic screening with slit-lamp examination must be performed at 3-month intervals if the ANA test is positive and at 6-month intervals if the ANA test is negative for 4 years after the onset of arthritis.

B. LABORATORY FINDINGS

There is no diagnostic test for JRA. Rheumatoid factor is positive in about 15% of patients, usually when onset of polyarticular disease occurs after age 8 years. ANA are most often present in pauciarticular disease with iridocyclitis and may serve as an indication of this complication; they are also fairly common in the late-onset rheumatoid factor-positive group. A normal erythrocyte sedimentation rate (ESR) does not exclude the diagnosis.

Table 26–1 lists the general characteristics of joint fluid in various conditions. A positive Gram stain or culture is the only definitive test for infection. A leukocyte count over 2000/µL suggests inflammation; this may be due to infection, any of the collagen-vascular diseases, leukemia, or reactive arthritis. A very low glucose concentration (< 40 mg/dL) or very high polymorphonuclear leukocyte count (> 60,000/µL) is highly suggestive of bacterial arthritis in a child. Chemical

Table 26–1. Joint fluid analysis.

Disorder	Cells/μL	Glucose[a]
Trauma	More red cells than white cells; usually < 2000 white cells	Normal
Reactive arthritis	3000–10,000 white cells, mostly mono-nuclears	Normal
Juvenile rheuma-toid arthritis and other inflamma-tory arthritides	5000–60,000 white cells, mostly neutro-phils	Usually normal or slightly low
Septic arthritis	> 60,000 white cells, > 90% neutrophils	Low to normal

[a]Normal value is 75% or more of serum glucose value.

analysis of synovial fluid is otherwise of little diagnostic benefit.

C. IMAGING

In the early stages of the disease, only soft-tissue swelling and regional osteoporosis are seen. Magnetic resonance imaging (MRI) of involved joints may show joint damage earlier in the course of the disease than other imaging modalities.

Differential Diagnosis

Table 26–2 lists the most common causes of limb pain in childhood. A few points of information may indicate the most likely diagnosis. For instance, orthopedic causes are due to increased physical activity, not major trauma. Reactive arthritides are suggested by a preceding viral infection, strep throat, or purpuric rash, and their course is waxing and waning over several days.

Monarticular arthritis is the most important differential disorder to establish. Pain in the hip or lower extremity is a frequent symptom of childhood cancer, especially leukemia, neuroblastoma, and rhabdomyosarcoma. Infiltration of bone by tumor and actual joint effusion may be seen. X-rays of the affected site and a careful examination of the blood smear for unusual cells and thrombocytopenia are necessary. A normal lactate dehydrogenase value is helpful in the exclusion of neoplastic disease. In doubtful cases, bone marrow examination is indicated.

Bacterial arthritis is usually acute and monarticular except for arthritis associated with *Haemophilus influenzae* infection and gonorrhea, both of which may be associated with a migratory pattern. Fever, leukocytosis,

and increased ESR with an acute process in a single joint, demand synovial fluid examination and culture to identify the pathogen.

The arthritis of rheumatic fever is migratory, transient, and often more painful than that of JRA. Rheumatic fever is very rare in children under age 5 years. Evidence of rheumatic carditis should be sought. Evidence of recent streptococcal infection is essential to the diagnosis. The fever pattern in rheumatic fever is low grade and persistent compared with the spiking fever in the systemic form of JRA. Lyme arthritis resembles

Table 26–2. Differential diagnosis of limb pain in children.

Orthopedic
 Stress fracture
 Overuse syndrome
 Chondromalacia patellae
 Osgood-Schlatter disease
 Slipped capital femoral epiphysis
 Legg-Calvé-Perthes disease
 Hypermobility syndrome
Reactive arthritis
 Henoch-Schonlein purpura
 Reactive arthritis following diarrhea
 Toxic synovitis of the hip
 Transient synovitis following viral infection
 Rheumatic fever
Infections
 Bacterial
  Lyme arthritis
  Osteomyelitis
  Septic arthritis
  Discitis
 Viral
  Parvovirus (in adolescents)
  Rubella
  Hepatitis B arthritis
Collagen-vascular
 Juvenile rheumatoid arthritis
 Spondyloarthropathy
 Systemic lupus erythematosus
 Dermatomyositis
Neoplastic
 Leukemia
 Lymphoma
 Neuroblastoma
 Reticuloendotheliosis
 Osteoid osteoma
 Bone tumors (benign or malignant)
Syndromes of psychoorganic origin
 Growing pains
 Fibromyalgia
 Reflex neurovascular dystrophy

pauciarticular JRA, but the former occurs as discrete, recurrent episodes of arthritis lasting 2–6 weeks. A negative test for antibodies to *Borrelia burgdorferi* argues strongly against this diagnosis.

Treatment

The objectives of therapy are to restore function, relieve pain, and maintain joint motion. In recent years, other nonsteroidal anti-inflammatory drugs (NSAIDs) have replaced salicylates in the medical treatment of JRA. Although their anti-inflammatory potency is not different from that of aspirin, their liquid form, decreased frequency of dosing, and diminished side effects appear to enhance compliance, cause fewer side effects, and justify their increased cost. Naproxen, 7.5 mg/kg twice daily; ibuprofen, 10 mg/kg four times daily; or diclofenac 1 mg/kg, given twice daily, may be used. If benefit occurs in the first 2 days, there will be continued improvement, with the maximum effect at 6 weeks. Celecoxib, a new NSAID that is a selective cyclooxygenase-2 inhibitor, shows promise in relieving the gastrointestinal irritation seen with previous NSAIDs. Dosages for children are under investigation. Range-of-motion and muscle-strengthening exercises should be taught and supervised by a therapist, and a home program should be instituted. Bed rest is to be avoided except in the most acute stages. Joint casting is almost never indicated.

Patients with JRA that fails to respond to aspirin or NSAIDs have a number of alternatives. Methotrexate is the second-line medication of choice. Symptomatic response usually occurs within 3–4 weeks. The low dosages used (5–10 mg/m^2/wk as a single dose) have been associated with few side effects. Stomatitis usually resolves with continued administration. Nausea may be prevented by splitting the dose. Hepatotoxicity, including fibrosis, is a concern. A complete blood count and liver function tests should be obtained at 2-month intervals. Liver biopsy may be performed if there are recurrent elevations of aminotransferases. Two new second-line agents are available for patients with progressive disease. Leflunomide is an antipyrimidine medication shown to be as effective as methotrexate. Side effects may include diarrhea and alopecia. Etanercept is a tumor necrosis factor receptor construct that must be administered subcutaneously twice a week (0.4 mg/kg/dose). Infliximab, an anti-tumor necrosis factor antibody, administered in combination with methotrexate, is another second-line treatment. Combination trials with second-line agents are in progress.

Iridocyclitis should be treated by an ophthalmologist, and methotrexate may be used in difficult cases. Local corticosteroid injections into joints, synovectomy, or joint replacement may be indicated in selected patients.

Prognosis

In the primarily articular forms of JRA, disease activity diminishes progressively with age and ceases by puberty in about 85% of patients. In a few instances, the disorder will persist into adult life. Problems after puberty relate primarily to residual joint damage. Presentation in the teen years usually presages adult disease. The children most likely to be handicapped permanently are those with unremitting synovitis, hip involvement, or positive rheumatoid factor tests.

Anthony KK, Schanberg LE: Pain in children with arthritis: A review of the current literature. Arthritis Rheum 2003;49:272 [PMID: 12687523].

Bowyer SL et al: Health status of patients with juvenile rheumatoid arthritis at 1 and 5 years after diagnosis. J Rheumatol 2003;30:394 [PMID: 12563701].

Flato B et al: Prognostic factors in juvenile rheumatoid arthritis: A case-control study revealing early predictors and outcomes after 14.9 years. J Rheumatol 2003;30:386 [PMID: 12563700].

Franco CA et al: Factors related to severe uveitis at diagnosis in children with juvenile idiopathic arthritis in a screening program. Am J Ophthalmol 2003;135:757 [PMID: 12788113].

Hashkes PJ, Laxer RM: Medical treatment of juvenile idiopathic arthritis. JAMA 2005;294:1671 [PMID: 16204667].

Selvaag AM et al: Early disease course and predictors of disability in juvenile rheumatoid arthritis and juvenile spondyloarthropathy: a 3 year prospective study. J Rheumatol 2005;32:1122 [PMID: 15940778].

Shaw KL et al: Growing up and moving on in rheumatology: a multicentre cohort of adolescents with juvenile idiopathic arthritis. Rheumatology (Oxford) 2005;44:806 [PMID: 15769786].

Weiss JE, Ilowite NT: Juvenile idiopathic arthritis. Pediatr Clin N Am 2005;52:413 [PMID: 15820374].

SPONDYLOARTHROPATHY

Lower extremity arthritis, particularly in males over age 10 years, suggests a form of spondyloarthropathy. Inflammation of tendinous insertions (enthesopathy) such as the tibial tubercle or the heel occurs in these diseases and not in JRA. Low back pain and sacroiliitis are quite specific for this form of arthritis. Carriage of HLA-B27 antigen occurs in 80% of patients with this disorder. No autoantibodies are found, but inflammatory indicators such as an elevated ESR or C-reactive protein are usually present. The episodes are usually intermittent, in contrast to the more chronic symptoms of JRA. Acute, not chronic, uveitis may occur.

The NSAIDs, particularly indomethacin (2–4 mg/kg/d) and naproxen (15 mg/kg/d), are more effective than salicylates in treating the spondyloarthropathies. Refractory cases may respond to methotrexate, etanercept, or infliximab. Local corticosteroid injections are contraindicated in Achilles tendinitis.

Unlike in adults, the disorder does not frequently progress to joint destruction or ankylosis in children.

Briot K et al: Body weight, body composition, and bone turnover changes in patients with spondyloarthropathy receiving anti-tumor necrosis factor α treatment. Ann Rheum Dis 2005; 64:1137 [PMID: 15642695].

ENTEROPATHIC ARTHRITIS

Enteropathic arthritis includes several syndromes such as Reiter syndrome, reactive arthritis, and the arthritis of inflammatory bowel disease and celiac disease. The unifying feature of these arthritides is the association of lower extremity arthritis with preceding or concurrent gastrointestinal symptoms. Reactive arthritis that follows diarrhea caused by *Salmonella, Shigella, Yersinia,* or *Chlamydia* infection occurs in individuals who are HLA-B27 positive. The human gene product shares a six–amino acid homology with the cell wall of the provocative organism. Transvection experiments with human HLA-B27 genes inserted into rats and mice have strongly supported the central role of the genetic predisposition in this form of arthritis. However, animals raised in a germ-free environment have less disease, emphasizing the role of enteric organisms in these spondyloarthropathies. In an analogous manner, the arthritis associated with Crohn disease and ulcerative colitis usually begins after or concurrent with active bowel disease. Other extraintestinal manifestations such as uveitis, stomatitis, hepatitis, and erythema nodosum may occur in these individuals.

Treatment for the musculoskeletal manifestations of inflammatory bowel disease, in addition to controlling the bowel disease, is primarily NSAIDs, similar to those detailed for ankylosing spondylitis.

Demetter P et al: Colon mucosa of patients both with spondyloarthritis and Crohn's disease is enriched with macrophages expressing the scavenger receptor CD163. Ann Rheum Dis 2005;64:321 [PMID: 15166002].

SYSTEMIC LUPUS ERYTHEMATOSUS

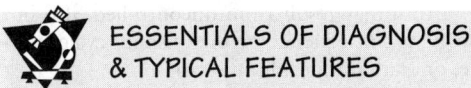

ESSENTIALS OF DIAGNOSIS & TYPICAL FEATURES

- *Multisystem inflammatory disease of joints, serous linings, skin, kidneys, and the central nervous system (CNS).*
- *ANA must be present in active, untreated disease.*

GENERAL CONSIDERATIONS

Systemic lupus erythematosus (SLE) is the prototype of immune complex diseases; its pathogenesis is related to deposition in the tissue of soluble immune complexes existing in the circulation. The spectrum of symptoms appears to be due not to tissue-specific autoantibodies but rather to damage to the tissue by lymphocytes, neutrophils, and complement evoked by the deposition of antigen-antibody complexes. Many such antigen-antibody systems are present in this disorder, but the best correlation exists between DNA/anti-DNA complexes and the activity of the disease. Laboratory tests of these antibodies and complement components give an objective assessment of disease pathogenesis and response to therapy. Autoreactive T lymphocytes that have escaped clonal deletion and unregulated B lymphocyte production of autoantibodies may initiate the disease. A genetic predisposition to lupus appears critical to causation of the disease.

Clinical Findings

A. SYMPTOMS AND SIGNS

The onset of SLE is most common in girls (8:1) between ages 9 and 15 years. The symptoms depend on the organ involved with immune complex deposition.

1. Joint symptoms—Joint symptoms are the most common presenting feature. Nondeforming arthritis may involve any joint, often in a symmetric manner. Myositis may also occur and is more painful than the inflammation in dermatomyositis.

2. Systemic manifestations—These include weakness, anorexia, fever, fatigue, and weight loss.

3. Skin lesions—Lesions include butterfly erythema and induration, small ulcerations in skin and mucous membranes, purpura, alopecia, and Raynaud phenomenon. The sun sensitivity of the dermal lesions may be striking.

4. Polyserositis—Polyserositis may include pleurisy with effusions, peritonitis, and pericarditis. Libman-Sacks endocarditis may occur in patients with antiphospholipid antibodies.

5. Gastrointestinal findings—Hepatosplenomegaly and lymphadenopathy may occur. Gastrointestinal presentations of SLE are unusual, with the exception of acute pancreatitis.

6. Renal manifestations—Renal SLE produces few symptoms at onset but is often progressive and is the leading cause of death among patients with SLE. Renal biopsy is indicated in patients who do not respond to corticosteroids or who cannot have corticosteroids tapered to a less toxic alternate-day regimen. The histologic pattern of diffuse proliferative nephritis requires the most aggressive treatment. Late complications are nephrosis and uremia. Control of hypertension is critical to maintain renal function.

7. Central nervous system (CNS)— CNS involvement produces a variety of symptoms such as seizures, coma, hemiplegia, focal neuropathies, chorea, and behavior disturbances, including psychosis.

B. LABORATORY FINDINGS

Leukopenia and anemia are frequently found with a low incidence of Coombs positivity. Thrombocytopenia and purpura may be early manifestations even in the absence of other organ involvement. The ESR is elevated, and hypergammaglobulinemia is often present. Renal involvement is indicated by the presence in the urine of red cells, white cells, red cell casts, and proteinuria.

The ANA test is invariably positive in patients with active untreated SLE, and a negative ANA test effectively excludes the diagnosis. For patients with a positive ANA test, a profile identifying individual disease-specific antibodies should be ordered. Anticardiolipin antibody and the lupus anticoagulant are two autoantibodies that identify patients with lupus at risk for thrombotic events.

In managing the disease, elevated titers of anti-DNA antibody and depressed levels of serum complement (C3) accurately reflect active disease, especially renal, CNS, and skin disease. A computed tomography (CT) or MRI scan may identify pathologic conditions of the brain in lupus cerebritis, such as infarction, vasculitis, or atrophy.

Differential Diagnosis

SLE may simulate many inflammatory diseases such as rheumatic fever, rheumatoid arthritis, and viral infections. It is essential to review all organ systems carefully to establish a clinical pattern. Renal and CNS involvement is unique to SLE. A negative ANA test excludes the diagnosis of SLE. Tests yielding false-positive results are usually of low titer (1:320).

An overlap syndrome known as mixed connective tissue disease, with features of several collagen-vascular diseases, occurs in adults and children. The symptom complex is diverse and does not readily fit previous classifications. Arthritis, fever, skin tightening, Raynaud phenomenon, muscle weakness, and rashes are most commonly present. Important factors in recognition of this disease entity are the relative infrequency of renal disease, which implies a better prognosis than SLE, and the corticosteroid responsiveness of symptoms, which distinguishes mixed connective tissue disease from scleroderma. The definition of the disease includes the presence of serum antibody to a ribonuclear protein. The initial ANA test is positive in very high titers. The ANA profile demonstrates the antibody to ribonuclear protein. Pulmonary disease in childhood produces major morbidity.

Treatment

The treatment of SLE should be tailored to the organ system involved so that toxicities may be minimized.

Prednisone, 0.5–1 mg/kg/d orally, has significantly lowered the mortality rate in SLE and should be used in all patients with renal, cardiac, or CNS involvement. The dosage should be varied using clinical and laboratory parameters of disease activity, and the minimum amount of corticosteroid to control the disease should be used. Alternate-day regimens of corticosteroid are frequently possible. Skin manifestations, arthritis, and fatigue may frequently be treated with antimalarials such as hydroxychloroquine, 5–7 mg/kg/d orally. Pleuritic pain or arthritis can often be managed with NSAIDs.

If disease control is inadequate with prednisone or if the dose required produces intolerable side effects, an immunosuppressant should be added. Either azathioprine, 2–3 mg/kg/d orally, or cyclophosphamide, 0.5–1 g/m², administered intravenously once a month, has been most widely used. Recent studies indicate that mycophenolate mofetil may used in place of intravenous cyclophosphamide to induce remission or sustain remission after intravenous cyclophosphamide therapy. These drugs are ineffective during acute crises such as seizures. Thrombotic events due to clotting antibodies require long-term anticoagulation.

The toxicities of the regimens must be carefully considered. Growth failure, osteoporosis, Cushing syndrome, adrenal suppression, and aseptic necrosis are serious side effects of chronic use of prednisone. When high doses of corticosteroids are used (> 2 mg/kg/d), the risk of sepsis is very real. Cyclophosphamide causes bladder epithelial dysplasia, hemorrhagic cystitis, and sterility. Azathioprine has been associated with liver damage and bone marrow suppression. Immunosuppressant treatment should be withheld if the total white count falls below 3000/µL or the neutrophil count below 1000/µL. Retinal damage from chloroquine derivatives has not been observed with recommended dosages. Intravenous pulse steroid therapy and plasmapheresis are treatments that may be useful in selected cases.

Amenorrhea may result from uncontrolled SLE but may also be a consequence of prednisone, cyclophosphamide, or azathioprine administration.

Course & Prognosis

The prognosis in SLE relates to the presence of renal involvement or infectious complications of treatment. With improved diagnosis, milder cases are now identified. Nonetheless, the survival rate has improved from 51% at 5 years in 1954 to 90% today. The disease has a natural waxing and waning cycle, and periods of complete remission are not unusual.

Arbuckle MR et al: Development of autoantibodies before the clinical onset of systemic lupus erythematosus. N Engl J Med 2003;349:1526 [PMID: 14561795].

Bijl M et al: Mycophenolate mofetil prevents a clinical relapse in patients with systemic lupus erythematosus at risk. Ann Rheum Dis 2003;62:534 [PMID: 12759290].

Ginzler EM, Dvorkina O: Newer therapeutic approaches for systemic lupus erythematosus. Rheum Dis Clin N Am 2005;31:315 [PMID: 15922148].

Lilleby V et al: Frequency of osteopenia in children and young adults with childhood-onset systemic lupus erythematosus. Arthritis Rheum 2005;52:2051 [PMID: 15986346].

McGhee JL et al: Clinical utility of antinuclear antibody tests in children. BMC Pediatr 2004;4:13 [PMID: 15245579].

Urowitz MB et al: Prolonged remission in systemic lupus erythematosus. J Rheumatol 2005;32:1467 [PMID: 16078321].

DERMATOMYOSITIS (Polymyositis)

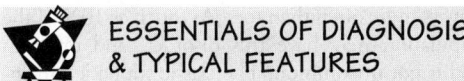

ESSENTIALS OF DIAGNOSIS & TYPICAL FEATURES

- *Pathognomonic skin rash.*
- *Weakness of proximal muscles and occasionally of pharyngeal and laryngeal groups.*
- *Pathogenesis related to vasculitis.*

General Considerations

Dermatomyositis, a rare inflammatory disease of muscle and skin in childhood, is uniquely responsive to corticosteroid treatment. The vasculitis observed in childhood dermatomyositis differs pathologically from the adult disease. Small arteries and veins are involved, with an exudate of neutrophils, lymphocytes, plasma cells, and histiocytes. The lesion progresses to intimal proliferation and thrombus formation. These vascular changes are found in the skin, muscle, kidney, retina, and gastrointestinal tract. Postinflammatory calcinosis is frequent.

The autoimmune pathogenesis of dermatomyositis has been difficult to unravel. Recent studies have shown that both cellular and humoral mechanisms may be involved. Lymphocytes from patients are stimulated to undergo blastogenesis in the presence of muscle tissue and will release lymphotoxin, which destroys cultured fetal muscle cells. Biopsies studied with immunofluorescence techniques demonstrate immunoglobulin and complement in perivascular distribution. The putative antigen has not been identified, and results of viral studies have been negative.

Clinical Findings

A. SYMPTOMS AND SIGNS

The predominant symptom is muscular weakness in proximal distribution affecting pelvic and shoulder girdles. Tenderness, stiffness, and swelling may be found but are not striking. Neurologic findings such as absence of tendon reflexes are not seen until late in the disease. Pharyngeal and respiratory involvement can be life-threatening. Flexion contractures and muscle atrophy produce significant residual deformities. Calcinosis may follow the inflammation in muscle and skin.

The rash of dermatomyositis is very helpful in the diagnosis of unknown muscle disease. Characteristically, the rash involves the upper eyelids and extensor surfaces of the knuckles, elbows, and knees with a distinctive heliotrope color that progresses to a scaling and atrophic appearance. Periorbital edema is not uncommon. Nail-fold capillary abnormalities may identify patients with a poorer prognosis. None of the rashes associated with other childhood rheumatic diseases have these features of distribution. The activity of the rash frequently does not parallel the muscle disease.

B. LABORATORY FINDINGS

Determination of muscle enzyme levels is the most helpful tool in diagnosis and treatment. All enzymes, including serum aldolase, should be screened to detect an abnormality that reflects activity of the disease. In later years of the illness, MRI of weak muscles may show disease activity when the enzymes are normal. The ANA test may be positive. Electromyography is useful to distinguish myopathic from neuropathic causes of muscle weakness. Muscle biopsy is indicated in doubtful cases of myositis without the pathognomonic rash.

Treatment

Prednisone in high dosages (1–2 mg/kg/d orally) has been shown to speed recovery. The dosage should be maintained or increased until muscle enzymes have returned to normal. Functional recovery will lag somewhat behind laboratory improvement. With improvement, the dosage may be cut to that level which maintains disease control and normal muscle enzymes. Treatment must be continued for an average of 2 years. Methotrexate, 1 mg/kg/wk, is an effective, steroid-sparing treatment. Intravenous immune globulin or cyclosporine therapy may be tried in refractory cases. Physical therapy is critical to prevent or allay contractures.

Course & Prognosis

Most children will recover and discontinue medications in 1–3 years. Relapses may occur. Functional ability is very good in most patients. Myositis in childhood is not associated with an increased risk of cancer.

Compeyrot-Lacassagne S, Feldman BM: Inflammatory myopathies in children. Ped Clin N Am 2005;52:493 [PMID: 15820377].

Pachman LM et al: History of infection before the onset of juvenile dermatomyositis: results from the National Institute of Arthritis and Musculoskeletal and Skin Diseases Research Registry. Arthritis Rheum 2005;53:166 [PMID: 15818654].

Smith RL et al: Skin involvement in juvenile dermatomyositis is associated with loss of end row nailfold capillary loops. J Rheumatol 2004;31:1644 [PMID: 15290747].

Rennebohm R: Juvenile dermatomyositis. Pediatr Ann 2002;31:426 [PMID: 12149796].

Takken T et al: The reliability of an aerobic and an anaerobic exercise tolerance test in patients with juvenile onset dermatomyositis. J Rheumatol 2005;32:734 [PMID: 15801033].

POLYARTERITIS NODOSA

Polyarteritis nodosa is a rare disease, but a significant number of cases have been reported in childhood and infancy. No single cause has been found, but evidence of a streptococcal trigger and poorly controlled parvovirus infection has been found in some series.

Pathologically, the disease is a vasculitis of medium-sized arteries with fibrinoid degeneration in the media extending to the intima and adventitia. Neutrophils and eosinophils comprise the inflammatory reaction. Aneurysms may be palpated or seen radiographically. Thrombosis of diseased arteries may cause infarction in many organs. Fibrosis of vessels and surrounding tissues accompanies the healing stages.

Symptomatology involves many tissues, and diagnosis is difficult. Unexplained fever, conjunctivitis, CNS involvement, and cardiac disease are more prominent in children than in adults. Many cases appear as acute myocarditis, and the peripheral neuropathy so common in adults with the disease is unusual in children. Diagnosis depends on biopsy-proved vasculitis or characteristic aneurysms on angiography.

The mortality rate is high, especially with cardiac involvement. Treatment consists of prednisone, 1–1.5 mg/kg/d orally, immunosuppressants, and intravenous immune globulin, but controlled studies of the efficacy of therapy of this rare disease are not yet available.

Ozen S et al. Juvenile polyarteritis: results of a multicenter survey of 110 children. J Pediatrics 2004;145:517 [PMID: 15480378].

Frankel SK et al: Vasculitis: Wegener granulomatosis, Churg-Strauss, microscopic polyangiitis, polyarteritis, Takayasu arteritis. Crit Care Clin 2002;18:855 [PMID: 12418444].

SCLERODERMA

Fortunately, the most common forms of scleroderma in childhood are linear scleroderma and morphea, not the systemic disease. The skin disease begins as indurated and depigmented patches (morphea) or streaks of skin on an extremity (linear scleroderma). As the linear form progresses over a 2- or 3-year period, subcutaneous tissue becomes atrophied and contractures develop in affected joints. Physical therapy and treatment with methotrexate or vitamin D analogues may limit extension of the lesions but not reverse previous

damage. It is rare for the limited form to progress to systemic sclerosis.

In systemic sclerosis, the dermal process is generalized. Raynaud phenomenon is almost invariably present. Arthralgias, esophageal dysfunction, and renal disease indicate systemic disease. Involvement of the lungs and kidneys may lead to rapid demise. Because the pathogenesis of systemic scleroderma is unknown, there are no effective therapies.

Zulian F et al: Localized scleroderma in childhood is not just a skin disease. Arthritis Rheum 2005;52:2873 [PMID: 16142730].

RAYNAUD PHENOMENON

Raynaud phenomenon is an intermittent vasospastic disorder of fingers more often than toes. As much as 10% of the adult population may have this disorder, and onset in childhood is not uncommon. The classic triphasic presentation is cold-induced pallor and cyanosis, followed by hyperemia, but incomplete forms are frequent. In adults over age 35 years who are ANA-positive, Raynaud phenomenon may be a harbinger of rheumatic disease. This progression is rarely seen in childhood. Evaluation should include a detailed history with review of systems relevant to rheumatic disease and examination for nail-fold capillary abnormalities. In the absence of positive findings, Raynaud phenomenon is likely to be idiopathic.

Treatment involves education about hand warming (eg, using mittens not gloves); the role of stress, which may be a precipitant; and in very symptomatic patients, treatment with calcium channel blockers such as nifedipine during winter months.

Nigrovic PA et al: Raynaud's phenomenon in children: A retrospective review of 123 patients. Pediatrics 2003;111:715 [PMID: 12671102].

■ NONRHEUMATIC PAIN SYNDROMES

1. Reflex Sympathetic Dystrophy

Reflex sympathetic dystrophy is a painful condition that is frequently confused with arthritis. There appears to be an increasing prevalence and increasing recognition of the condition. Severe extremity pain leading to nearly complete loss of function is the hallmark of the condition. Evidence of autonomic dysfunction is demonstrated by color changes, temperature differences, and dyshidrosis in the affected extremity. Foot involvement is more common than hand involvement. A puffy swelling of the entire hand or foot is common. On examination, there is marked cutaneous hyperesthesia to even the slightest touch. Results of laboratory tests are negative. X-ray findings are normal except for late development of osteoporosis. Bone scans are very helpful and demonstrate either increased or decreased blood supply to the painful extremity.

The cause of this condition remains elusive. Unlike adults with the disorder, children only occasionally have a history of significant physical trauma at onset. How the autonomic dysfunction causes severe somatic pain is not known, but the feedback cycle does provide the basis for treatment. In mild cases, a program of rehabilitative physical therapy in combination with desensitization techniques will restore function and relieve pain. Patients with treatment-refractory reflex sympathetic dystrophy need family counseling and may respond to steroids or ganglionic blocks by local anesthesia. Long-term prognosis is good if recovery is rapid; recurrent episodes imply a less favorable prognosis.

Maillard SM et al: Reflex sympathetic dystrophy: a multidisciplinary approach. Arthritis Rheum 2004;51:284 [PMID: 15077274].

2. Fibromyalgia

Fibromyalgia is a diffuse pain syndrome in which patients experience pain all over their bodies without objective swelling. Weather changes and fatigue exacerbate symptoms. A sleep disturbance, such as insomnia or prolonged waking periods in the night, is an almost universal symptom; therefore, patients should be carefully questioned in this regard. On examination, patients appear normal except for characteristic trigger points at the insertion of muscles, especially along the neck, spine, and pelvis.

Treatment consists of physical therapy and relieving the sleep disorder. Low-dose antidepressant medication (amitriptyline, 25 mg) taken before sleep may produce remarkable benefit in reduction of pain. Physical therapy should emphasize a graded rehabilitative approach to stretching and exercise. Analgesic medications provide poor pain relief and should be avoided because their use leads to escalation of medication, including narcotics.

The prognosis for young patients is not clear, and long-term strategies may be necessary to enable them to cope with the condition.

Conte PM et al: Termperament and stress response in children with juvenile primary fibromyalgia syndrome. Arthritis Rheum 2003;48:2923 [PMID: 14558099].

Worrel LM et al: Treating fibromyalgia with a brief interdisciplinary program: initial outcomes and predictors of response. Mayo Clin Proc 2001;76:384 [PMID: 11322354].

3. Chronic Fatigue Syndrome

Since 1985, chronic fatigue syndrome has become an increasingly common diagnosis. The distinction between this apparent organic fatigue and emotional causes of fatigue is not easily made. Criteria have been developed by the National Institutes of Health to assist in classification. The fatigue should have a defined date of onset, and there is a long list of excludable diagnoses. Other clinical manifestations include low-grade fevers, sore throat, painful lymph nodes, and neuropsychiatric problems. Epstein-Barr virus infection does not account for all the patients described. Treatment is symptomatic and somewhat unsatisfactory.

Moss-Morris R et al: A randomized controlled graded exercise trial for chronic fatigue syndrome: outcomes and mechanisms of change. J Health Psych 2005;10:245 [PMID: 15723894].

Solomon L, Reeves WC: Factors influencing the diagnosis of chronic fatigue syndrome. Arch Int Med 2004;164:2241 [PMID: 15534161].

HYPERMOBILITY SYNDROME

Ligamentous laxity, which previously was thought to occur only in Ehlers-Danlos syndrome or Down syndrome, is now recognized as a common cause of joint pain in our physically competitive society.

Children are now participating in a wide range of physically demanding sports and activities. Patients with hypermobility present with episodic joint pain and occasionally with swelling that lasts a few days after increased physical activity. Depending on the activity, almost any joint may be affected.

Physical examination may reveal joint swelling and tenderness, but the key to diagnosis is the demonstration of ligamentous laxity. Five criteria have been established: (1) passive opposition of the thumb to the flexor surface of the forearm; (2) passive hyperextension of the fingers so that they are parallel to the extensor surface of the forearm; (3) hyperextension of the elbow; (4) hyperextension of the knee (genu recurvatum); and (5) palms on floor with knees extended. Results of laboratory tests are normal. The pain associated with the syndrome is produced by improper joint alignment caused by the laxity during exercise.

Treatment consists of a graded conditioning program designed to provide muscular support of the joints to compensate for the loose ligaments. The prognosis is good provided conditioning before activities is adequate.

Seckin U et al: The prevalence of joint hypermobility among high school students. Rheumatology Int 2005;25:260 [PMID: 14745505].

REFERENCES

Cassidy JT et al: *Textbook of Pediatric Rheumatology,* 5th ed. Elsevier Saunders, 2005.

Hematologic Disorders

27

Daniel R. Ambruso, MD, Taru Hays, MD, & Neil Goldenberg, MD

NORMAL HEMATOLOGIC VALUES

The normal ranges for peripheral blood counts vary significantly with age. Normal neonates show a relative polycythemia with a hematocrit of 45–65%. The reticulocyte count at birth is relatively high at 2–8%. Within the first few days of life, erythrocyte production decreases, and the levels of hemoglobin and hematocrit fall to a nadir at about 6–8 weeks. During this period, known as physiologic anemia of infancy, normal infants have hemoglobins as low as 10 g/dL and hematocrits as low as 30%. Thereafter, the normal values for hemoglobin and hematocrit gradually increase until adult values are reached after puberty. Premature infants can reach a nadir hemoglobin level of 7–8 g/dL at 8–10 weeks.

Newborns have larger red cells than children and adults, with a mean corpuscular volume (MCV) at birth of more than 94 fL. The MCV subsequently falls to a nadir of 70–84 fL at about age 6 months. Thereafter, the normal MCV increases gradually until it reaches adult values after puberty.

The normal number of white blood cells is higher in infancy and early childhood than later in life. Neutrophils predominate in the differential white count at birth and in the older child. Lymphocytes predominate (up to 80%) between about ages 1 month and 6 years.

Normal values for the platelet count are 150,000–400,000/μL and vary little with age.

BONE MARROW FAILURE

Failure of the marrow to produce adequate numbers of circulating blood cells may be congenital or acquired and may cause pancytopenia (aplastic anemia) or involve only one cell line (single cytopenia). Constitutional and acquired aplastic anemias are discussed in this section and the more common single cytopenias in later sections. Bone marrow failure caused by malignancy or other infiltrative disease is discussed in Chapter 28. It is important to remember that many drugs and toxins may affect the marrow and cause single or multiple cytopenias.

Suspicion of bone marrow failure is warranted in children with pancytopenia and in children with single cytopenias who lack evidence of peripheral red cell, white cell, or platelet destruction. Macrocytosis often accompanies bone marrow failure. Many of the constitutional bone marrow disorders are associated with a variety of congenital anomalies.

Young NS: The pathophysiology of acquired aplastic anemia. N Engl J Med 1997;336:1365 [PMID: 9134878].

CONSTITUTIONAL APLASTIC ANEMIA (Fanconi Anemia)

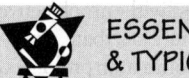

ESSENTIALS OF DIAGNOSIS & TYPICAL FEATURES

- *Progressive pancytopenia.*
- *Macrocytosis.*
- *Multiple congenital anomalies.*
- *Increased chromosome breakage in peripheral blood lymphocytes.*

General Considerations

Fanconi anemia is a syndrome characterized by defective DNA repair that is caused by a variety of genetic mutations. Inheritance is autosomal recessive, and the disease occurs in all ethnic groups. Hematologic manifestations usually begin with thrombocytopenia or neutropenia and subsequently progress over the course of months or years to pancytopenia. Typically the diagnosis is made between ages 2 and 10 years.

Clinical Findings

A. SYMPTOMS AND SIGNS

Symptoms are determined principally by the degree of hematologic abnormality. Thrombocytopenia may cause purpura, petechiae, and bleeding; neutropenia may cause severe or recurrent infections; and anemia may cause weakness, fatigue, and pallor. Congenital anomalies are present in at least 50% of patients. The most common include abnormal pigmentation of the skin (generalized hyperpigmentation, café-au-lait or hypopigmented spots), short stature with delicate features, and skeletal malformations (hypoplasia, anomalies, or absence of the thumb and radius). More subtle anomalies are hypoplasia of the thenar eminence or a weak or absent radial pulse. Associated renal anomalies include aplasia, "horseshoe" kidney, and duplication of the collecting system. Other anomalies are microcephaly, microphthalmia, strabismus, ear anomalies, and hypogenitalism.

B. LABORATORY FINDINGS

Thrombocytopenia or leukopenia typically occurs first, followed over the course of months to years by anemia and progression to severe aplastic anemia. Macrocytosis is virtually always present, is usually associated with anisocytosis and an elevation in fetal hemoglobin levels, and is an important diagnostic clue. The bone marrow reveals hypoplasia or aplasia. The diagnosis is confirmed by the demonstration of an increased number of chromosome breaks and rearrangements in peripheral blood lymphocytes. The use of diepoxybutane to stimulate these breaks and rearrangements provides for a sensitive assay that is virtually always positive in children with Fanconi anemia, even before the onset of hematologic abnormalities.

Specific molecular markers/genes called Fanc-A, B, C, and others are found in different ethnic populations. These markers are identified in research laboratories and are not available as routine clinical tests.

Differential Diagnosis

Because patients with Fanconi anemia frequently present with thrombocytopenia, the disorder must be differentiated from idiopathic thrombocytopenic purpura (ITP) and other more common causes of decreased platelets. In contrast to patients with ITP, those with Fanconi anemia usually exhibit a gradual fall in the platelet count, and counts less than $20,000/\mu L$ are often accompanied by neutropenia or anemia, along with phenotypical features. Fanconi anemia may also be manifested initially by pancytopenia, and must be differentiated from acquired aplastic anemia and other disorders such as acute leukemia. Examination of the bone marrow and chromosome studies of peripheral blood lymphocytes will usually distinguish between these disorders.

Complications

The most important complications of Fanconi anemia are those related to thrombocytopenia and neutrope-

nia. Endogenous endocrine dysfunction may include growth hormone deficiency, hypothyroidism, or impaired glucose metabolism. In addition, persons with Fanconi anemia have a significantly increased risk of developing malignancies, especially acute nonlymphocytic leukemia, solid tumors, and myelodysplastic syndromes. Death is usually the result of thrombocytopenic hemorrhage, overwhelming infection, or malignancy.

Treatment

Attentive supportive care is a critical feature of management. Patients with neutropenia who develop fever require prompt evaluation and parenteral broad-spectrum antibiotics. Transfusions are important, but should be used judiciously, especially in the management of thrombocytopenia, which frequently becomes refractory to platelet transfusions as a consequence of alloimmunization. Transfusions from family members should be discouraged because of the negative effect on the outcome of bone marrow transplantation. At least 50% of patients with Fanconi anemia respond, albeit incompletely, to oxymetholone, and many recommend institution of androgen therapy before transfusions are needed. However, oxymetholone is associated with hepatotoxicity, hepatic adenomas, and masculinization, and is particularly troublesome for female patients.

Successful bone marrow transplantation cures the aplastic anemia and is an important treatment option for children with Fanconi anemia who have a human leukocyte antigen (HLA)-identical sibling donor. Before transplantation the prospective donor must be screened for Fanconi anemia by testing his or her lymphocytes for chromosome breakage.

Prognosis

Many patients succumb to bleeding, infection, or malignancy in adolescence or early adulthood. The long-term outlook for those undergoing successful bone marrow transplantation is uncertain, particularly with regard to the risk of subsequently developing malignancies.

Alter BP: Fanconi's anemia and malignancies. Am J Hematol 1996;3:99 [PMID: 8892734].

Butturini A: Hematologic abnormalities in Fanconi anemia: An international Fanconi anemia registry study. Blood 1994;84:1650 [PMID: 8068955].

Dufour C: Stem cell transplantation from HLA-matched related donor for Fanconi's anaemia: A retrospective review of the multicentric Italian experience on behalf of AIEOP-GITMO. Br J Haematol 2001;112:796 [PMID: 11260086].

Joenje H: The emerging genetic and molecular basis of Fanconi anemia. Nat Rev Genet 2001;2:446 [PMID: 11389461].

ACQUIRED APLASTIC ANEMIA

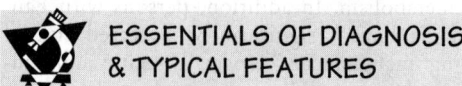

ESSENTIALS OF DIAGNOSIS & TYPICAL FEATURES

- *Weakness and pallor.*
- *Petechiae, purpura, and bleeding.*
- *Frequent or severe infections.*
- *Pancytopenia with hypocellular bone marrow.*

General Considerations

Acquired aplastic anemia is characterized by peripheral pancytopenia with a hypocellular bone marrow. Approximately 50% of the cases in childhood are idiopathic. Other cases are secondary to idiosyncratic reactions to drugs such as phenylbutazone, sulfonamides, nonsteroidal anti-inflammatories, and anticonvulsants. Toxic causes include exposure to benzene, insecticides, and heavy metals. Infectious causes include viral hepatitis (usually non-A, non-B, non-C), infectious mononucleosis, and human immunodeficiency virus (HIV). In immunocompromised children, aplastic anemia has been associated with human parvovirus B19. Immune mechanisms of marrow suppression are suspected in most cases.

Clinical Findings

A. SYMPTOMS AND SIGNS

Weakness, fatigue, and pallor result from anemia; petechiae, purpura, and bleeding occur because of thrombocytopenia; and fevers due to generalized or localized infections are associated with neutropenia. Hepatosplenomegaly and significant lymphadenopathy are unusual.

B. LABORATORY FINDINGS

Anemia is usually normocytic, with a low reticulocyte count. The white blood cell count is low, with a marked neutropenia. The platelet count is typically below 50,000/μL and frequently below 20,000/μL. Bone marrow aspiration and biopsy show hypocellularity, often marked.

Differential Diagnosis

Examination of the bone marrow usually excludes pancytopenia caused by peripheral destruction of blood cells or by infiltrative processes such as acute leukemia, storage diseases, and myelofibrosis. Many of these other conditions are associated with hepatosplenomegaly. Preleukemic conditions also may present with pancytopenia and hypocellular bone marrows. Cytogenetic analysis of the marrow is helpful, because a clonal abnormality may predict the subsequent development of leukemia. Since some children with Fanconi anemia may not have congenital anomalies appreciated, patients with newly diagnosed aplastic anemia should be studied for chromosome breaks and rearrangements in peripheral blood lymphocytes.

Complications

Acquired aplastic anemia is characteristically complicated by infection and hemorrhage, which are the leading causes of death. Other complications are those associated with therapy.

Treatment

Comprehensive supportive care is most important in the management of acute acquired aplastic anemia. Febrile illnesses require prompt evaluation and usually parenteral antibiotics. Red blood cell transfusions alleviate symptoms of anemia. Platelet transfusions may be lifesaving, but they should be used sparingly because many patients eventually develop platelet alloantibodies and become refractory to platelet transfusions.

Bone marrow transplantation is generally considered the treatment of choice for severe aplastic anemia when an HLA-compatible sibling donor is available. Because the likelihood of success with transplantation is influenced adversely by multiple transfusions, HLA typing of family members should be undertaken as soon as the diagnosis of aplastic anemia is made. An increasing number of patients who lack HLA-matched siblings are able to find matched donors through cord blood banks or the National Bone Marrow Registry.

An alternative to bone marrow transplantation from an HLA-matched sibling donor is immunomodulation, usually with antithymocyte globulin and cyclosporine. Responses are very good. Most patients show hematologic improvement and become transfusion-independent.

Prognosis

Children receiving early bone marrow transplantation from an HLA-identical sibling have a long-term survival rate of greater than 80%. Sustained, complete remissions may be seen in 65–80% of patients receiving immunosuppressive therapy. However, both therapies are associated with an increased risk of myelodysplastic syndromes, acute leukemia, and other malignancies in long-term survivors.

Brodsky R: Acquired severe aplastic anemia in children: Is there a standard of care? Pediatr Blood Cancer 2004;43:711 [PMID: 15503299].

Fouladi M: Improved survival in severe acquired aplastic anemia of childhood. Bone Marrow Transplant 2000;26:1149 [PMID: 11149724].

Goldenberg NA: Successful treatment of severe aplastic anemia in children using standardized immunosuppressive therapy with antithymocyte globulin and cyclosporine A. Pediatr Blood Cancer 2004;43:718 [PMID: 15390303].

Ohara A: Myelodysplastic syndrome and acute myelogenous leukemia as a late clonal complication in children with aplastic anemia. Blood 1997;90:1009 [PMID: 9242530].

Rosenfeld S: Antithymocyte globulin and cyclosporine for severe aplastic anemia: Association between hematologic response and long-term outcome. JAMA 2003;289:1130 [PMID: 12622583].

■ ANEMIAS

APPROACH TO THE CHILD WITH ANEMIA

Anemia is a relatively common finding, and identifying the cause is important. Even though anemia in childhood has many causes, the correct diagnosis can usually be established with relatively little laboratory cost.

Frequently the cause is identified with a careful history. The possibility of nutritional causes should be addressed by inquiry about dietary intake; growth and development; and symptoms of chronic disease, malabsorption, or blood loss. Hemolytic disease may be associated with a history of jaundice (including neonatal jaundice) or by a family history of anemia, jaundice, gallbladder disease, splenomegaly, or splenectomy. The child's ethnic background may suggest the possibility of certain hemoglobinopathies or of deficiencies of red cell enzymes such as glucose-6-phosphate dehydrogenase (G6PD). The review of systems may reveal clues to a previously unsuspected systemic disease associated with anemia. The patient's age is important because some causes of anemia are age-related. For example, patients with iron-deficiency anemia and β-globin disorders present more commonly at ages 6–36 months than at other times in life.

The physical examination may also reveal clues to the cause of anemia. Poor growth may suggest chronic disease or hypothyroidism. Congenital anomalies may be associated with constitutional aplastic anemia (Fanconi anemia) or with congenital hypoplastic anemia (Diamond–Blackfan anemia). Other disorders may be suggested by the findings of petechiae or purpura (leukemia, aplastic anemia, hemolytic–uremic syndrome), jaundice (hemolysis or liver disease), generalized lymphadenopathy (leukemia, juvenile rheumatoid arthritis, HIV infection), splenomegaly (leukemia, sickle hemoglobinopathy syndromes, hereditary spherocytosis, liver disease, hypersplenism), or evidence of chronic or recurrent infections.

The initial laboratory evaluation of the anemic child consists of a complete blood count (CBC) with differential and platelet count, review of the peripheral blood smear, and a reticulocyte count. The algorithm in Figure 27–1 uses limited laboratory information, together with the history and physical examination, to reach a specific diagnosis or to focus additional laboratory investigations on a limited diagnostic category (eg, microcytic anemia, bone marrow failure, pure red cell aplasia, or hemolytic disease). This diagnostic scheme depends principally on the MCV to determine whether the anemia is microcytic, normocytic, or macrocytic, according to the percentile curves of Dallman and Siimes (Figure 27–2).

Although the incidence of iron deficiency in the United States has decreased significantly with improvements in infant nutrition, it remains an important cause of microcytic anemia, especially at ages 6–24 months. A trial of therapeutic iron is appropriate in such children, provided the dietary history is compatible with iron deficiency and the physical examination or CBC count does not suggest an alternative cause for the anemia. If this is not the case or if a trial of therapeutic iron fails to correct the anemia and microcytosis, further laboratory evaluation is warranted.

Another key element of Figure 27–1 is the use of both the reticulocyte count and the peripheral blood smear to determine whether a normocytic or macrocytic anemia is due to hemolysis. Typically hemolytic disease is associated with an elevated reticulocyte count, but some children with chronic hemolysis initially present during a period of virus-induced aplasia when the reticulocyte count is not elevated. Thus, review of the peripheral blood smear for evidence of hemolysis (eg, spherocytes, red cell fragmentation, sickle forms) is important in the evaluation of children with normocytic anemias and low reticulocyte counts. When hemolysis is suggested, the correct diagnosis may be suspected by specific abnormalities of red cell morphology or by clues from the history or physical examination. Autoimmune hemolysis is usually excluded by direct antiglobulin testing. Review of blood counts and the peripheral blood smears of the mother and father may suggest genetic disorders such as hereditary spherocytosis. Children with normocytic or macrocytic anemias, with relatively low reticulocyte counts and no evidence of hemolysis on the blood smear, usually have anemias caused by inadequate erythropoiesis in the bone marrow. The presence of neutropenia or thrombocytopenia in such children suggests the possibility of aplastic anemia, malignancy, or severe folate/vitamin B_{12} deficiency, and usually dictates examination of the bone marrow.

Pure red cell aplasia may be congenital (Diamond–Blackfan anemia), acquired and transient (transient

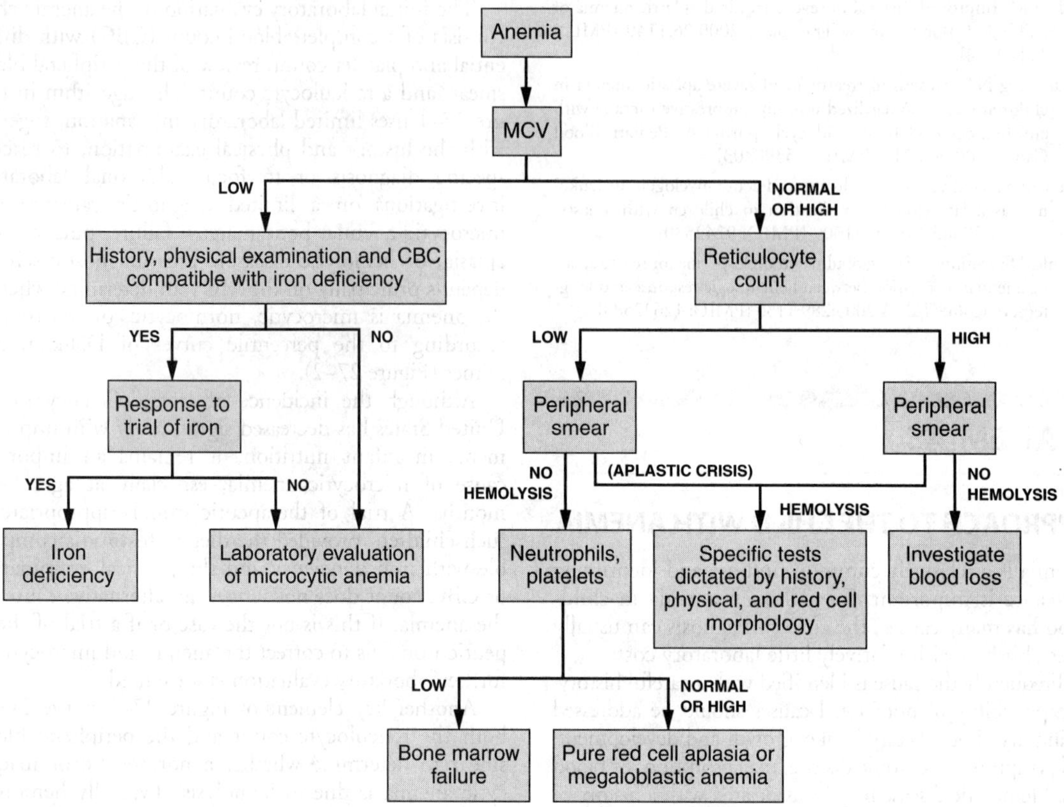

```
                              ┌──────────┐
                              │  Anemia  │
                              └────┬─────┘
                                   │
                              ┌────▼─────┐
                              │   MCV    │
                              └──┬────┬──┘
                  LOW           │    │         NORMAL
                  ┌─────────────┘    └──────────OR HIGH
```

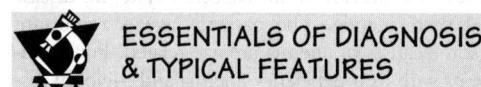

Figure 27–1. Investigation of anemia.

erythroblastopenia of childhood), a manifestation of a systemic disease such as renal disease or hypothyroidism, or due to malnutrition or mild deficiencies of folate or vitamin B_{12}.

Hermiston ML: A practical approach to the evaluation of the anemic child. Pediatr Clin North Am 2002;49:877 [PMID: 12430617].

PURE RED CELL APLASIA

Infants and children with normocytic or macrocytic anemia, a low reticulocyte count, and normal or elevated numbers of neutrophils and platelets should be suspected of having pure red cell aplasia. Examination of the peripheral blood smear in such cases is important because signs of hemolytic disease suggest chronic hemolysis complicated by an aplastic crisis due to parvovirus infection. Appreciation of this phenomenon is important because chronic hemolytic disease may not be diagnosed until the anemia is exacerbated by an episode of red cell aplasia and subsequent rapidly falling hemoglobin level. In such cases, cardiovascular compromise and congestive heart failure may develop quickly.

1. Congenital Hypoplastic Anemia (Diamond–Blackfan Anemia)

ESSENTIALS OF DIAGNOSIS & TYPICAL FEATURES

- *Age: birth to 1 year.*
- *Macrocytic anemia with reticulocytopenia.*
- *Bone marrow with erythroid hypoplasia.*
- *Short stature or congenital anomalies in one-third of patients.*

GENERAL CONSIDERATIONS

Diamond–Blackfan anemia is a relatively rare cause of anemia that usually presents in infancy or early childhood. Early diagnosis is important because treatment with corticosteroids results in increased erythropoiesis

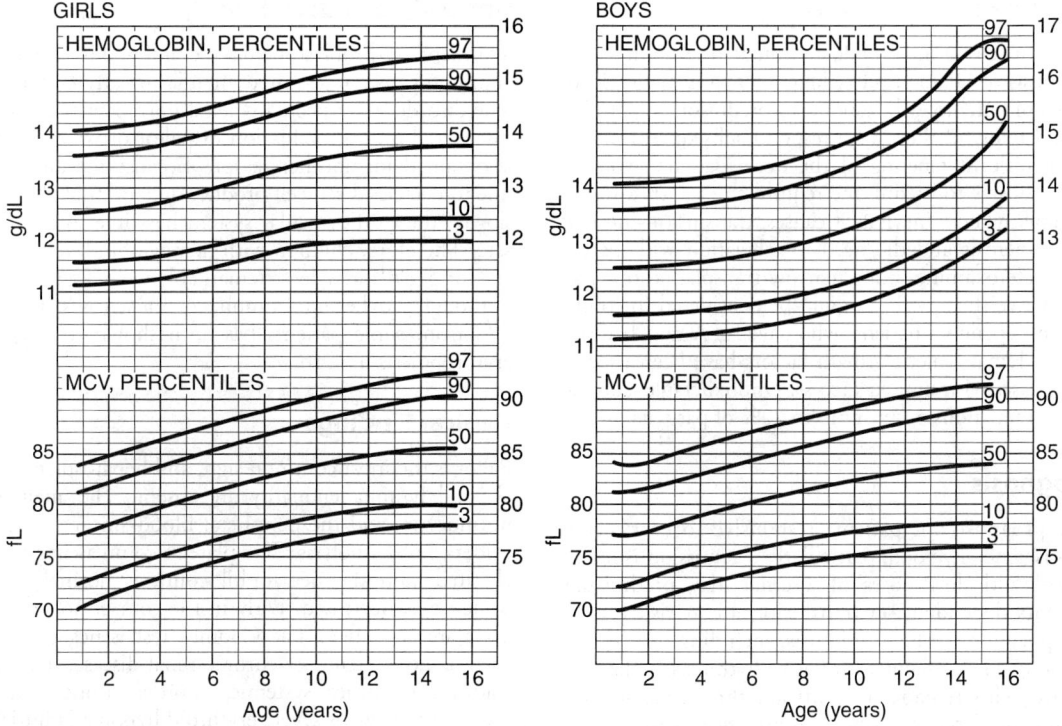

Figure 27–2. Hemoglobin and red cell volume in infancy and childhood. (Reproduced, with permission, from Dallman PR, Siimes MA: Percentile curves for hemoglobin and red cell volume in infancy and childhood. J Pediatr 1979;94:26.)

in about two-thirds of patients, thus avoiding the difficulties and complications of long-term chronic transfusion therapy. The cause is unclear; both autosomal dominant and autosomal recessive modes of inheritance occur.

Clinical Findings

A. SYMPTOMS AND SIGNS

Signs and symptoms are generally those of chronic anemia, such as pallor; congestive heart failure sometimes follows. Jaundice, splenomegaly, or other evidence of hemolysis is usually absent. Short stature or other congenital anomalies are present in one-third of patients. A wide variety of anomalies have been described; those affecting the head, face, and thumbs are the most common.

B. LABORATORY FINDINGS

Diamond–Blackfan anemia is characterized by severe macrocytic anemia and marked reticulocytopenia. The neutrophil count is usually normal or slightly decreased, and the platelet count is normal or elevated. The bone

marrow usually shows a marked decrease in erythroid precursors but is otherwise normal. In older children, fetal hemoglobin levels are usually increased and there is evidence of persistent fetal erythropoiesis, such as the presence of the i antigen on erythrocytes. In addition, the level of adenosine deaminase in erythrocytes is elevated.

Differential Diagnosis

The principal differential diagnosis is transient erythroblastopenia of childhood. Children with Diamond–Blackfan anemia generally present at an earlier age, often have macrocytosis, and have evidence of fetal erythropoiesis and an elevated level of red cell adenosine deaminase. In addition, short stature and congenital anomalies, are not associated with transient erythroblastopenia. Lastly, transient erythroblastopenia of childhood usually resolves within 6–8 weeks of diagnosis, whereas Diamond–Blackfan anemia is a lifelong affliction. Other disorders associated with decreased red cell production such as renal failure, hypothyroidism, and the anemia of chronic disease need to be considered.

Treatment

Oral corticosteroids should be initiated as soon as the diagnosis of Diamond–Blackfan anemia is made. Two-thirds of patients will respond to prednisone, 2 mg/kg/d, and many of those who respond subsequently tolerate significant tapering of the dose. Patients who are unresponsive to prednisone require chronic transfusion therapy, which inevitably causes transfusion-induced hemosiderosis and the need for chelation with parenteral deferoxamine. Bone marrow transplantation is an alternative therapy that should be considered for transfusion-dependent patients who have HLA-matched siblings. Hematopoietic growth factors have been used in some cases with limited success. Unpredictable, spontaneous remissions occur in up to 20% of patients.

Prognosis

The prognosis for patients responsive to corticosteroids is generally good, particularly if remission is maintained with low doses of alternate-day prednisone. Patients dependent on transfusion are at risk for the complications of hemosiderosis, including death from congestive heart failure, cardiac arrhythmias, or hepatic failure. This remains a significant threat, particularly during adolescence, when compliance with nightly subcutaneous infusions of deferoxamine is often difficult to ensure.

Berndt A: Successful transplantation of CD34+ selected peripheral blood stem cells from an unrelated donor in an adult patient with Diamond-Blackfan anemia and secondary hemochromatosis. Bone Marrow Transplant 2005;35:99 [PMID: 15516941].

Vlachos A: Hematopoietic stem cell transplantation for Diamond–Blackfan anemia: A report from the Diamond–Blackfan Anemia Registry. Bone Marrow Transplant 2001;27:381 [PMID: 11313667].

2. Transient Erythroblastopenia of Childhood

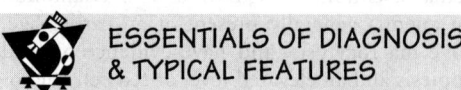

ESSENTIALS OF DIAGNOSIS & TYPICAL FEATURES

- Age: 6 months to 4 years.
- Normocytic anemia with reticulocytopenia.
- Absence of hepatosplenomegaly or lymphadenopathy.
- Erythroid precursors initially absent from bone marrow.

General Considerations

Transient erythroblastopenia of childhood is a relatively common cause of acquired anemia in early childhood. The disorder is suspected when a normocytic anemia is discovered during evaluation of pallor or when a CBC is obtained for another reason. Because the anemia is due to decreased red cell production, and thus develops slowly, the cardiovascular system has time to compensate. Therefore, children with hemoglobin levels as low as 4 or 5 g/dL may look remarkably well. The disorder is thought to be autoimmune in most cases, because IgG from some patients has been shown to suppress erythropoiesis in vitro.

Clinical Findings

Pallor is the most common sign, and hepatosplenomegaly and lymphadenopathy are absent. The anemia is normocytic, and the peripheral blood smear shows no evidence of hemolysis. The platelet count is normal or elevated, and the neutrophil count is normal or, in some cases, decreased. Early in the course, no reticulocytes are identified. The Coombs test is negative, and there is no evidence of chronic renal disease, hypothyroidism, or other systemic disorder. Bone marrow examination shows severe erythroid hypoplasia initially; subsequently, erythroid hyperplasia develops along with reticulocytosis, and the anemia resolves.

Differential Diagnosis

Transient erythroblastopenia of childhood must be differentiated from Diamond–Blackfan anemia, particularly in infants younger than age 1 year. In contrast to Diamond–Blackfan anemia, transient erythroblastopenia is not associated with macrocytosis, short stature, or congenital anomalies, or with evidence of fetal erythropoiesis prior to the phase of recovery. Also in contrast to Diamond–Blackfan anemia, transient erythroblastopenia is associated with normal levels of red cell adenosine deaminase. Transient erythroblastopenia of childhood must also be differentiated from chronic disorders associated with decreased red cell production, such as renal failure, hypothyroidism, and other chronic states of infection or inflammation. As with other single cytopenias, the possibility of malignancy (ie, leukemia) should always be considered, particularly if fever, bone pain, hepatosplenomegaly, or lymphadenopathy is present. In such cases, examination of the bone marrow is generally diagnostic. Confusion may sometimes arise when the anemia of transient erythroblastopenia is first identified during the early phase of recovery when the reticulocyte count is high. In such cases, the disorder may be confused with the anemia of acute blood loss or with hemolytic disease. In contrast to hemolytic disorders, transient erythroblastopenia of childhood is not associated with jaundice or peripheral destruction of red cells.

Treatment & Prognosis

By definition, this is a transient disorder. Some children require red cell transfusions if cardiovascular compromise is present. Resolution of the anemia is heralded by an increase in the reticulocyte count, which generally occurs within 4–8 weeks of diagnosis. In contrast to other autoimmune disorders of childhood (eg, ITP, autoimmune hemolytic anemia), transient erythroblastopenia of childhood is not treated with corticosteroids because of its short course.

Cherrick I: Transient erythroblastopenia of childhood: Prospective study of fifty patients. Am J Pediatr Hematol Oncol 1994;16:320 [PMID: 7978049].

Miller R: Transient erythroblastopenia of childhood in infants < 6 months of age. Am J Pediatr Hematol Oncol 1994;16:246 [PMID: 8037344].

NUTRITIONAL ANEMIAS

1. Iron-Deficiency Anemia

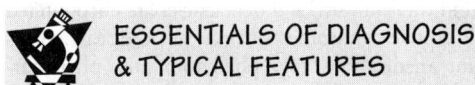

ESSENTIALS OF DIAGNOSIS & TYPICAL FEATURES

- *Pallor and fatigue.*
- *Poor dietary intake of iron (ages 6–24 months).*
- *Chronic blood loss (age > 2 years).*
- *Microcytic hypochromic anemia.*

General Considerations

Long considered the most common cause of anemia in pediatrics, the incidence of iron deficiency has decreased substantially due to improved nutrition and the increased availability of iron-fortified infant formulas and cereals. Thus, the current approach to anemia in childhood must take into consideration a relatively greater likelihood of other causes.

Normal-term infants are born with sufficient iron stores to prevent iron deficiency for the first 4–5 months of life. Thereafter, enough iron needs to be absorbed to support the needs of rapid growth. For this reason, nutritional iron deficiency is most common between 6 and 24 months of life. A deficiency earlier than age 6 months may occur if iron stores at birth are reduced by prematurity, small birth weight, neonatal

anemia, or perinatal blood loss or if there is subsequent iron loss due to hemorrhage. Iron-deficient children older than age 24 months should be evaluated for blood loss. Iron deficiency, in addition to causing anemia, has adverse effects on multiple organ systems. Thus, the importance of identifying and treating iron deficiency extends past the resolution of any symptoms directly attributable to a decreased hemoglobin concentration.

Clinical Findings

A. SYMPTOMS AND SIGNS

Symptoms and signs vary with the severity of the deficiency. Mild iron deficiency is usually asymptomatic. In infants with more severe iron deficiency, pallor, fatigue, irritability, and delayed motor development are common. Children whose iron deficiency is due in part to ingestion of unfortified cow's milk may be fat, with poor muscle tone. A history of pica is common.

B. LABORATORY FINDINGS

The severity of anemia depends on the degree of iron deficiency, and the hemoglobin level may be as low as 3–4 g/dL in severe cases. Red cells are microcytic and hypochromic, with a low MCV and low mean corpuscular hemoglobin. The red blood cell distribution width is typically elevated, even with mild iron deficiency. The reticulocyte count is usually normal or slightly elevated, but the reticulocyte index or absolute reticulocyte count is decreased. Iron studies show a decreased serum ferritin and a low serum iron, elevated total iron-binding capacity, and decreased transferrin saturation. These laboratory abnormalities are usually present with moderate to severe iron deficiency, but mild cases may be associated with variable laboratory results. The peripheral blood smear shows microcytic, hypochromic red blood cells with anisocytosis, and occasional target, teardrop, elliptical, and fragmented red cells. Leukocytes are normal, and very often platelet count is increased with normal morphology.

The bone marrow examination is not helpful in the diagnosis of iron deficiency in infants and small children because little or no iron is stored as marrow hemosiderin at these ages.

Differential Diagnosis

The differential diagnosis is that of microcytic, hypochromic anemia. The possibility of thalassemia (α-thalassemia, β-thalassemia, and hemoglobin E disorders) should be considered, especially in infants of African, Mediterranean, or Asian ethnic background. In contrast to infants with iron deficiency, those with thalassemia generally have an elevated number of erythrocytes (the index of the MCV divided by the red cell number is usually less than 13) and are less likely, in mild cases, to have an elevated red blood cell distribution width. Thalassemias are associated with normal or increased levels of serum iron and ferritin and with normal iron-binding capacity. The hemoglobin electrophoresis in β-thalassemia minor typically shows an elevation of hemoglobin A_2 levels, but coexistent iron deficiency may lower the percentage of hemoglobin A_2 into the normal range. Hemoglobin electrophoresis will also identify children with hemoglobin E, a cause of microcytosis common in Southeast Asians. In contrast, the hemoglobin electrophoresis in α-thalassemia trait is normal. Lead poisoning has also been associated with microcytic anemia, but anemia with lead levels less than 40 mg/dL is often due to coexistent iron deficiency.

The anemia of chronic inflammation or infection is normocytic but in late stages may be microcytic. This anemia is usually suspected because of the presence of a chronic systemic disorder. The level of serum iron is low, but the iron-binding capacity is normal, and the serum ferritin level is normal or elevated. Relatively mild infections, particularly during infancy, may cause transient anemia. As a result, caution should be exercised when the diagnosis of mild iron deficiency is entertained in infants and young children who have had recent viral or bacterial infections. Ideally, screening tests for anemia should not be obtained within 3–4 weeks of such infections.

Treatment

The recommended oral dose of elemental iron is 6 mg/kg/d in three divided daily doses. Mild cases may be treated with 2 mg/kg/d given once daily before breakfast. Parenteral administration of iron is rarely necessary. Iron therapy results in an increased reticulocyte count within 3–5 days, which is maximal between 5 and 7 days. The hemoglobin level begins to increase thereafter. The rate of hemoglobin rise is inversely related to the hemoglobin level at diagnosis. In moderate to severe cases, an elevated reticulocyte count 1 week after initiation of therapy confirms the diagnosis and documents compliance and response to therapy. When iron deficiency is the only cause of anemia, adequate treatment usually results in a resolution of the anemia within 4–6 weeks. Treatment is generally continued for a few additional months to replenish iron stores.

Hermiston ML: A practical approach to the evaluation of the anemic child. Pediatr Clin North Am 2002;49:877 [PMID: 12430617].

2. Megaloblastic Anemias

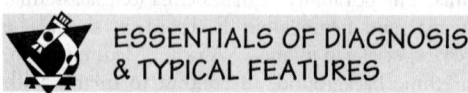

ESSENTIALS OF DIAGNOSIS & TYPICAL FEATURES

- *Pallor and fatigue.*
- *Nutritional deficiency or intestinal malabsorption.*

- *Macrocytic anemia.*
- *Megaloblastic bone marrow changes.*

General Considerations

Megaloblastic anemia is a macrocytic anemia caused by deficiency of cobalamin (vitamin B_{12}), folic acid, or both. Cobalamin deficiency due to dietary insufficiency may occur in infants who are breast-fed by mothers who are strict vegetarians or who have pernicious anemia. Intestinal malabsorption is the usual cause of cobalamin deficiency in pediatrics and occurs with Crohn disease, chronic pancreatitis, bacterial overgrowth of the small bowel, infection with the fish tapeworm (*Diphyllobothrium latum*), or after surgical resection of the terminal ileum. Deficiencies due to inborn errors of metabolism (transcobalamin II deficiency and methylmalonic aciduria) have also been described. Malabsorption of cobalamin due to deficiency of intrinsic factor (pernicious anemia) is rare in childhood.

Folic acid deficiency may be caused by inadequate dietary intake, malabsorption, increased folate requirements, or some combination of the three. Folate deficiency due to dietary deficiency alone is rare but occurs in severely malnourished infants and has been reported in infants fed goat's milk not fortified with folic acid. Folic acid is absorbed in the jejunum, and deficiencies are encountered in malabsorptive syndromes such as celiac disease. Anticonvulsant medications (eg, phenytoin and phenobarbital) and cytotoxic drugs (eg, methotrexate) have also been associated with folate deficiency, caused by interference with folate absorption or metabolism. Finally, folic acid deficiency is more likely to develop in infants and children with increased requirements. This occurs during infancy because of rapid growth and also in children with chronic hemolytic anemia. Premature infants are particularly susceptible to the development of the deficiency because of low body stores of folate.

Clinical Findings

A. SYMPTOMS AND SIGNS

Infants with megaloblastic anemia may show pallor and mild jaundice as a result of ineffective erythropoiesis. Classically, the tongue is smooth and beefy red. Infants with cobalamin deficiency may be irritable and may be poor feeders. Older children with cobalamin deficiency may complain of paresthesias, weakness, or an unsteady gait and may show decreased vibratory sensation and proprioception on neurologic examination.

B. LABORATORY FINDINGS

The laboratory findings of megaloblastic anemia include an elevated MCV and mean corpuscular hemoglobin. The peripheral blood smear shows numerous macro-ovalocytes with anisocytosis and poikilocytosis. Neutrophils are large and have hypersegmented nuclei. The white cell and platelet counts are normal with mild deficiencies, but may be decreased in more severe cases. Examination of the bone marrow typically shows erythroid hyperplasia with large erythroid and myeloid precursors. Nuclear maturation is delayed compared with cytoplasmic maturation, and erythropoiesis is ineffective. The serum indirect bilirubin concentration may be slightly elevated.

Children with cobalamin deficiency have a low serum vitamin B_{12} level, but decreased levels of serum vitamin B_{12} may also be found in about 30% of patients with folic acid deficiency. The level of red cell folate is a better reflection of folate stores than is the serum folic acid level. Serum levels of metabolic intermediates, methylmalonic acid, and homocysteine may help establish the correct diagnosis. Elevated methylmalonic acid levels are consistent with cobalamin deficiency, whereas elevated levels of homocysteine occur with both cobalamin and folate deficiency.

Differential Diagnosis

Most macrocytic anemias in pediatrics are not megaloblastic. Other causes of an increased MCV include drug therapy (eg, anticonvulsants, anti-HIV nucleoside analogues), Down syndrome, an elevated reticulocyte count (hemolytic anemias), bone marrow failure syndromes (Fanconi anemia, Diamond–Blackfan anemia), liver disease, and hypothyroidism.

Treatment

Treatment of cobalamin deficiency due to inadequate dietary intake is readily accomplished with oral supplementation. Most cases, however, are due to intestinal malabsorption and require parenteral treatment. In severe cases, parenteral therapy may induce life-threatening hypokalemia and require supplemental potassium. Folic acid deficiency is treated effectively with oral folic acid in most cases. Children at risk for the development of folic acid deficiencies, such as premature infants and those with chronic hemolysis, are often given folic acid prophylactically.

Rosenblatt DS: Cobalamin and folate deficiency: Acquired and hereditary disorders in children. Semin Hematol 1999;36:19 [PMID: 9930566].

ANEMIA OF CHRONIC DISORDERS

Anemia is a common manifestation of many chronic illnesses in children. In some instances, causes may be mixed. For example, children with chronic disorders involving intestinal malabsorption or blood loss may have anemia of chronic inflammation in combination with nutritional deficiencies of iron, folate, or cobalamin. In other settings, the anemia is due to dysfunction of a single organ (eg, renal failure, hypothyroidism), and correction of the underlying abnormality resolves the anemia.

1. Anemia of Chronic Inflammation

Anemia is frequently associated with chronic infections or inflammatory diseases. The anemia is usually mild to moderate in severity, with a hemoglobin level of 8–12 g/dL. In general, the severity of the anemia corresponds to the severity of the underlying disorder, and there may be microcytosis but not hypochromia. The reticulocyte count is low. The anemia is thought to be due to inflammatory cytokines that inhibit erythropoiesis, and shunting of iron into and impaired iron release from reticuloendothelial cells. Levels of erythropoietin are relatively low for the severity of the anemia. The serum iron concentration is low, but in contrast to iron deficiency, anemia of chronic inflammation is not associated with elevated iron-binding capacity and is associated with an elevated serum ferritin level. Treatment consists of correction of the underlying disorder, which, if controlled, generally results in improvement in hemoglobin level.

Hagar W: Diseases of iron metabolism. Pediatr Clin North Am 2002;49:893 [PMID: 12430618].

2. Anemia of Chronic Renal Failure

Severe normocytic anemia occurs in most forms of renal disease that have progressed to renal insufficiency. Although white cell and platelet production remain normal, the bone marrow shows significant hypoplasia of the erythroid series and the reticulocyte count is low. The principal mechanism is deficiency of erythropoietin, a hormone produced in the kidney, but other factors may contribute to the anemia. In the presence of significant uremia, a component of hemolysis may also be present. In the past, treatment of the anemia of chronic renal failure depended on transfusions of packed red blood cells. However, recombinant human erythropoietin (epoetin alfa) corrects the anemia, and its use has largely eliminated the need for transfusions.

Seeherunvong W: Identification of poor responders to erythropoietin among children undergoing hemodialysis. J Pediatr 2001;138: 710 [PMID: 11343048].

Yorgin PD: The clinical efficacy of higher hematocrit levels in children with chronic renal insufficiency and those undergoing dialysis. Semin Nephrol 2001;21:451 [PMID: 11559886].

3. Anemia of Hypothyroidism

Some patients with hypothyroidism develop significant anemia. Occasionally, anemia is detected before the diagnosis of the underlying disorder. A decreased growth velocity in an anemic child suggests hypothyroidism. The anemia is usually normocytic or macrocytic, but it is not megaloblastic and, hence not due to deficiencies of cobalamin or folate. Replacement therapy with thyroid hormone is usually effective in correcting the anemia.

CONGENITAL HEMOLYTIC ANEMIAS: RED CELL MEMBRANE DEFECTS

The congenital hemolytic anemias are usually divided into three categories: defects of the red cell membrane, hemoglobinopathies, and disorders of red cell metabolism. Hereditary spherocytosis and elliptocytosis are the most common red cell membrane disorders. The diagnosis is suggested by the peripheral blood smear, which shows characteristic red cell morphology (eg, spherocytes, elliptocytes). These disorders usually have an autosomal dominant inheritance, and the diagnosis may be suggested by a family history. The hemolysis is due to the deleterious effect of the membrane abnormality on red cell deformability. Decreased cell deformability leads to entrapment of the abnormally shaped red cells in the spleen. Many patients have splenomegaly, and splenectomy usually alleviates the hemolysis.

1. Hereditary Spherocytosis

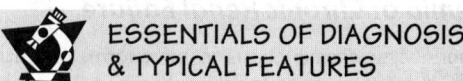

ESSENTIALS OF DIAGNOSIS & TYPICAL FEATURES

- Anemia and jaundice.
- Splenomegaly.
- Positive family history of anemia, jaundice, or gallstones.
- Spherocytosis with increased reticulocytes.
- Increased osmotic fragility.
- Negative direct antiglobulin test (DAT).

General Considerations

Hereditary spherocytosis is a relatively common inherited hemolytic anemia that occurs in all ethnic groups but is most common in persons of Northern European ancestry, in whom the incidence is about 1:5000. The disorder is a heterogeneous one, marked by variable degrees of anemia, jaundice, and splenomegaly. In some persons, the disorder is mild and there is no anemia because erythroid hyperplasia fully compensates for hemolysis. Severe cases are transfusion-dependent prior

to splenectomy. The hallmark of hereditary spherocytosis is the presence of microspherocytes in the peripheral blood. The disease is inherited in an autosomal dominant fashion in about 75% of cases; the remainder is thought to be autosomal recessive or to be caused by new mutations.

Hereditary spherocytosis is usually the result of a partial deficiency of spectrin, an important structural protein of the red cell membrane skeleton. Spectrin deficiency weakens the attachment of the cell membrane to the underlying membrane skeleton and causes the red cell to lose membrane surface area. This process creates spherocytes that are poorly deformable and have a shortened life span because they are trapped in the microcirculation of the spleen and engulfed by splenic macrophages. The extreme heterogeneity of hereditary spherocytosis is related directly to variable degrees of spectrin deficiency. In general, children who inherit spherocytosis in an autosomal dominant fashion have less spectrin deficiency and mild or moderate hemolysis. In contrast, those with nondominant forms of spherocytosis tend to have greater deficiency of spectrin and more severe anemia.

Clinical Findings

A. SYMPTOMS AND SIGNS

Hemolysis causes significant neonatal hyperbilirubinemia in 50% of affected children. Splenomegaly subsequently develops in the majority and is often present by age 5 years. Jaundice is variably present and in many patients may be noted only during infection. Patients with significant chronic anemia may complain of pallor, fatigue, or malaise. Intermittent exacerbations of the anemia are caused by increased hemolysis or by aplastic crises and may be associated with severe weakness, fatigue, fever, abdominal pain, or even congestive heart failure.

B. LABORATORY FINDINGS

Most patients have mild chronic hemolysis with hemoglobin levels of 9–12 g/dL. In some cases, the hemolysis is fully compensated and the hemoglobin level is in the normal range. Rare cases of severe disease require frequent transfusions. The anemia is usually normocytic and hyperchromic, and many patients have an elevated mean corpuscular hemoglobin concentration. The peripheral blood smear shows numerous microspherocytes and polychromasia. The reticulocyte count is elevated, often higher than might be expected for the degree of anemia. White blood cell and platelet counts are usually normal. The osmotic fragility is increased, particularly after incubation at 37 °C for 24 hours. Serum bilirubin usually shows an elevation in the unconjugated fraction. DAT is negative.

Differential Diagnosis

Spherocytes are frequently present in persons with immune hemolysis. Thus, in the newborn, hereditary spherocytosis must be distinguished from hemolytic disease caused by ABO or other blood type incompatibilities. Older patients with autoimmune hemolytic anemia frequently present with jaundice and splenomegaly and with spherocytes on the peripheral blood smear. The DAT is positive in most cases of immune hemolysis and negative in hereditary spherocytosis. Occasionally, the diagnosis is confused in patients with splenomegaly from other causes, especially when hypersplenism increases red cell destruction and when some spherocytes are noted on the blood smear. In such cases, the true cause of the splenomegaly may be suggested by signs or symptoms of portal hypertension or by laboratory evidence of chronic liver disease. In contrast to children with hereditary spherocytosis, those with hypersplenism typically have some degree of thrombocytopenia or neutropenia.

Complications

Severe jaundice may occur in the neonatal period and, if not controlled by phototherapy, may occasionally require exchange transfusion. Splenectomy is associated with an increased risk of overwhelming bacterial infections, particularly with pneumococci. Gallstones occur in 60–70% of adults who have not undergone splenectomy and may form as early as age 5–10 years.

Treatment

Supportive measures include the administration of folic acid to prevent the development of red cell hypoplasia due to folate deficiency. Acute exacerbations of anemia, due to increased rates of hemolysis or to aplastic crises due to infection with human parvovirus, may be severe enough to require red cell transfusions. Splenectomy is performed in many cases and always results in significant improvement. The procedure increases the survival of the spherocytic red cells and leads to complete correction of the anemia in most cases. Patients with more severe disease may show some degree of hemolysis after splenectomy. Except in unusually severe cases, the procedure should be postponed until the child is at least age 5 years because of the greater risk of postsplenectomy sepsis prior to this age. All patients scheduled for splenectomy should be immunized with pneumococcal, *Haemophilus influenzae* b, and meningococcal vaccines prior to the procedure, and some clinicians recommend penicillin prophylaxis afterward. The need for splenectomy in mild cases is controversial. Splenectomy in the middle childhood years prevents the subsequent development of cholelithiasis and eliminates the need for the activity restrictions recommended for children with splenomegaly. However, these benefits must be weighed against the risks of the surgical procedure and the subsequent lifelong risk of postsplenectomy sepsis.

Prognosis

Splenectomy eliminates signs and symptoms in all but the most severe cases and reduces the risk of cholelithiasis. The abnormal red cell morphology and increased osmotic fragility persist without clinical consequence.

Delhommeau F: Natural history of hereditary spherocytosis during the first year of life. Blood 2000;95:393 [PMID: 10627440].

2. Hereditary Elliptocytosis

Hereditary elliptocytosis is a heterogeneous disorder that ranges in severity from an asymptomatic state with an almost normal red cell morphology to severe hemolytic anemia. Most affected persons have numerous elliptocytes on the peripheral blood smear but mild or no hemolysis. Those with hemolysis have an elevated reticulocyte count and may have jaundice and splenomegaly. These disorders are caused by mutations of red cell membrane skeletal proteins, and most have an autosomal dominant inheritance. Because most patients are asymptomatic, no treatment is indicated. Patients with significant degrees of hemolytic anemia may benefit from folate supplementation or from splenectomy.

Some infants with hereditary elliptocytosis present in the neonatal period with moderate to marked hemolysis and significant hyperbilirubinemia. This disorder has been termed "transient infantile poikilocytosis" because such infants exhibit bizarre erythrocyte morphology with elliptocytes, budding red cells, and small misshapen cells that defy description. The MCV is low, and the anemia may be severe enough to require red cell transfusions. Typically, one parent has hereditary elliptocytosis, usually mild or asymptomatic. The infant's hemolysis gradually abates during the first year of life, and the erythrocyte morphology subsequently becomes more typical of hereditary elliptocytosis.

Mentzer WC: Modulation of erythrocyte membrane mechanical stability by 2,3-diphosphoglycerate in the neonatal poikilocytosis/elliptocytosis syndrome. J Clin Invest 1987;79:943 [PMID: 3818955].

Palek J: Mutations of the red cell membrane proteins: From clinical evaluation to detection of the underlying genetic defect. Blood 1992;8:308 [PMID: 1627793].

CONGENITAL HEMOLYTIC ANEMIAS: HEMOGLOBINOPATHIES

The hemoglobinopathies are an extremely heterogeneous group of congenital disorders that occur in many different ethnic groups. The relatively high frequency of these

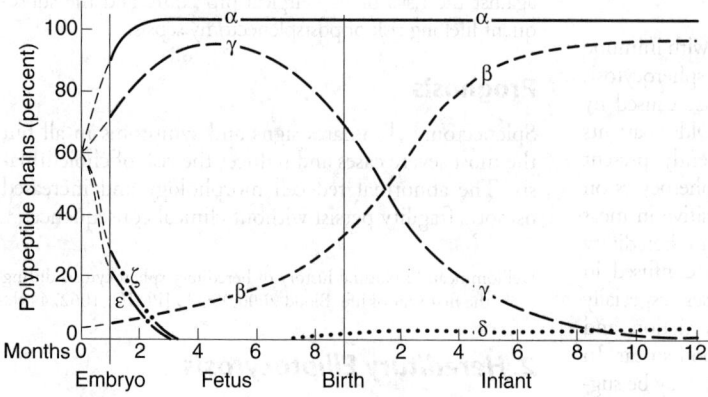

Figure 27-3. Changes in hemoglobin polypeptide chains during human development. (Reproduced, with permission, from Miller DR, Baehner RL: *Blood Diseases of Infancy and Childhood*, 6th ed. Mosby, 1989.)

genetic variants is related to the malaria protection afforded to heterozygous individuals. The hemoglobinopathies are generally classified into two major groups. The first, the thalassemias, are caused by quantitative deficiencies in the production of globin chains. These quantitative defects in globin synthesis cause microcytic and hypochromic anemias. The second group of hemoglobinopathies consists of those caused by structural abnormalities of globin chains. The most important of these, hemoglobins S, C, and E, are all the result of point mutations and single amino acid substitutions in β-globin. Many, but not all, infants with hemoglobinopathies are identified by routine neonatal screening.

Figure 27-3 shows the normal developmental changes that occur in globin-chain production during gestation and the first year of life. At birth, the predominant hemoglobin is fetal hemoglobin (hemoglobin F), which is composed of two α-globin chains and two γ-globin chains. Subsequently, the production of γ-globin decreases and the production of β-globin increases so that adult hemoglobin (two α chains and two β chains) predominates after 2–4 months. Because α-globin chains are present in both fetal and adult hemoglobin, disorders of α-globin synthesis (α-thalassemia) are clinically manifest in the newborn as well as later in life. In contrast, patients with β-globin disorders such as β-thalassemia and sickle cell disease are generally asymptomatic during the first 3–4 months of age and present clinically after γ-chain production—and therefore fetal hemoglobin levels—have decreased substantially.

1. α-Thalassemia

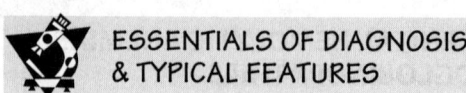

ESSENTIALS OF DIAGNOSIS & TYPICAL FEATURES

- *African, Mediterranean, Middle Eastern, Chinese, or Southeast Asian ancestry.*

- *Microcytic, hypochromic anemia of variable severity.*
- *Bart's hemoglobin detected by neonatal screening.*

General Considerations

Most of the α-thalassemia syndromes are the result of deletions of one or more of the α-globin genes on chromosome 16. Normal diploid cells have four α-globin genes; thus the variable severity of the α-thalassemia syndromes is related to the number of gene deletions (Table 27–1). The severity of the α-thalassemia syndromes varies among affected ethnic groups, depending on the genetic abnormalities prevalent in the population. In persons of African ancestry, α-thalassemia is usually caused by the deletion of only one of the two α-globin genes on each chromosome. Thus, in the African population, heterozygous individuals are silent carriers and homozygous individuals have α-thalassemia trait. In Asians, deletions of one or of both α-globin genes on the same chromosome are common; heterozygous individuals are either silent carriers or have α-thalassemia trait, and homozygous individuals or compound heterozygous individuals have α-thalassemia trait, hemoglobin H disease, or hydrops fetalis. Thus, the presence of α-thalassemia in a child of Asian ancestry may have important implications for genetic counseling, whereas this is not usually the case in families of African ancestry.

Clinical Findings

The clinical findings depend on the number of α-globin genes deleted. Table 27–1 summarizes the α-thalassemia syndromes.

Persons with three α-globin genes (one-gene deletion) are asymptomatic and have no hematologic abnormalities. Hemoglobin levels and MCV are normal. Hemoglo-

Table 27–1. The α-thalassemias.

Usual Genotypes[a]	α Gene Number	Clinical Features	Hemoglobin Electrophoresis[b]	
			Birth	> 6 mos
αα/αα	4	Normal	N	N
-α/αα	3	Silent carrier	0–3% Hb Bart's	N
--/αα or -α/-α	2	α-thal trait	2–10% Hb Bart's	N
--/-α	1	Hb H disease	15–30% Hb Bart's	Hb; H present
--/--	0	Fetal hydrops	> 75% Hb Bart's	-

[a]α indicates presence of α-globin gene, – indicates deletion of α-globin gene.
[b]N = normal results, Hb = hemoglobin, Hb Bart's $= \gamma_4$, Hb H $= \beta_4$.

bin electrophoresis in the neonatal period shows 0–3% Bart's hemoglobin, a variant hemoglobin composed of four γ-globin chains. Hemoglobin electrophoresis after the first few months of life is normal. Thus, this condition is usually suspected only in the context of family studies or when a small amount of Bart's hemoglobin is detected by neonatal screening for hemoglobinopathies.

Persons with two α-globin genes (two-gene deletion) are typically asymptomatic. The MCV is usually less than 100 fL at birth. Hematologic studies in older infants and children show a normal or slightly decreased hemoglobin level with a low MCV and a slightly hypochromic blood smear with some target cells. The hemoglobin electrophoresis typically shows 2–10% Bart's hemoglobin in the neonatal period but is normal in older children and adults.

Persons with one α-globin gene (three-gene deletion) have a mild to moderately severe microcytic hemolytic anemia (hemoglobin level of 7–10 g/dL), which may be accompanied by hepatosplenomegaly and some bony abnormalities caused by the expanded medullary space. The reticulocyte count is elevated, and the red cells show marked hypochromia and microcytosis with significant poikilocytosis and some basophilic stippling. Hemoglobin electrophoresis in the neonatal period typically shows 15–30% Bart's hemoglobin. Later in life, hemoglobin H (composed of four β-globin chains) is present. Incubation of red cells with brilliant cresyl blue (hemoglobin H preparation) shows inclusion bodies formed by denatured hemoglobin H.

The deletion of all four α-globin genes causes severe intrauterine anemia and asphyxia and results in hydrops fetalis and fetal demise or neonatal death shortly after delivery. Extreme pallor and massive hepatosplenomegaly are present. Hemoglobin electrophoresis reveals a predominance of Bart's hemoglobin with a complete absence of normal fetal or adult hemoglobin.

Differential Diagnosis

α-Thalassemia trait (two-gene deletion) must be differentiated from other mild microcytic anemias, including iron deficiency and β-thalassemia minor. In contrast to children with iron deficiency, children with α-thalassemia trait show normal or increased levels of ferritin and serum iron. In contrast to children with β-thalassemia minor, children with α-thalassemia trait have a normal hemoglobin electrophoresis after age 4–6 months. Finally, the history of a low MCV (96 fL) at birth or the presence of Bart's hemoglobin on the neonatal hemoglobinopathy screening test suggests α-thalassemia.

Children with hemoglobin H disease may have jaundice and splenomegaly, and the disorder must be differentiated from other hemolytic anemias. The key to the diagnosis is the decreased MCV and the marked hypochromia on the blood smear. With the exception of β-thalassemia, most other significant hemolytic disorders have a normal or elevated MCV and are not hypochromic. Infants with hydrops fetalis due to severe α-thalassemia must be distinguished from those with hydrops due to other causes of anemia such as alloimmunization.

Complications

The principal complication of α-thalassemia trait is the needless administration of iron, given in the belief that a mild microcytic anemia is due to iron deficiency. Persons with hemoglobin H disease may have intermittent exacerbations of their anemia, which occasionally require blood transfusions. Splenomegaly may exacerbate the anemia and may require splenectomy. Women pregnant with hydropic α-thalassemia fetuses are subject to increased complications of pregnancy, particularly toxemia and postpartum hemorrhage.

Treatment

Persons with α-thalassemia trait require no treatment. Those with hemoglobin H disease should receive supplemental folic acid and avoid the same oxidant drugs that cause hemolysis in persons with G6PD deficiency, because exposure to these drugs may exacerbate their anemia. The anemia may also be exacerbated during periods of infection, and transfusions may be required. Hypersplenism may develop later in childhood and require surgical splenectomy. Genetic counseling and prenatal diagnosis should be offered to families at risk for hydropic fetuses.

Chui DH: Hydrops fetalis caused by α-thalassemia: An emerging health care problem. Blood 1998;91:2213 [PMID: 9516118].

Clarke GM: Laboratory investigation of hemoglobinopathies and thalassemias: Review and update. Clin Chem 2000;46:1284 [PMID: 10926923].

Miller ST: A fast hemoglobin variant on newborn screening is associated with α-thalassemia trait. Clin Pediatr 1997;36:75 [PMID: 9118593].

2. β-Thalassemia

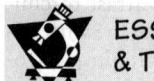

ESSENTIALS OF DIAGNOSIS & TYPICAL FEATURES

β-Thalassemia minor:
- Normal neonatal screening test.
- African, Mediterranean, Middle Eastern, or Asian ancestry.
- Mild microcytic, hypochromic anemia.
- No response to iron therapy.
- Elevated level of hemoglobin A₂.

β-Thalassemia major:
- Neonatal screening shows hemoglobin F only.
- Mediterranean, Middle Eastern, or Asian ancestry.
- Severe microcytic, hypochromic anemia with marked hepatosplenomegaly.

General Considerations

In contrast to the four α-globin genes, only two β-globin genes are present in diploid cells, one on each chromosome 11. Some β-thalassemia genes produce no β-globin chains and are termed β^0-thalassemia. Other β-globin genes produce some β-globin but in diminished quantities and are termed β^+-thalassemia. Persons affected by β-thalassemia may be heterozygous or homozygous. Individuals heterozygous for most β-thalassemia genes have β-thalassemia minor. Homozygous individuals have β-thalassemia major (Cooley anemia), a severe transfusion-dependent anemia, or a condition known as thalassemia intermedia, which is more severe than thalassemia minor but is not generally transfusion-dependent. β-Thalassemia major is the most common worldwide cause of transfusion-dependent anemia in childhood. In addition, β-thalassemia genes interact with genes for structural β-globin variants such as hemoglobin S and hemoglobin E to cause serious disease in compound heterozygous individuals. These disorders are discussed further in the sections dealing with sickle cell disease and with hemoglobin E disorders.

Clinical Findings

A. SYMPTOMS AND SIGNS

Persons with β-thalassemia minor are usually asymptomatic with a normal physical examination. Those with β-thalassemia major are normal at birth but develop significant anemia during the first year of life. If the disorder is not identified and treated with blood transfusions, such children grow poorly and develop massive hepatosplenomegaly and enlargement of the medullary space with thinning of the bony cortex. The skeletal changes cause characteristic facial deformities (prominent forehead and maxilla) and predispose the child to pathologic fractures.

B. LABORATORY FINDINGS

Children with β-thalassemia minor have normal neonatal screening results but subsequently develop a decreased MCV with or without mild anemia. The peripheral blood smear typically shows hypochromia, target cells, and sometimes basophilic stippling. Hemoglobin electrophoresis performed after 6–12 months of age is usually diagnostic when levels of hemoglobin A₂, hemoglobin F, or both are elevated. β-Thalassemia major is often initially suspected when hemoglobin A is absent on neonatal screening. Such infants are hematologically normal at birth but develop severe anemia after the first few months of life. The peripheral blood smear typically shows a severe hypochromic, microcytic anemia with marked anisocytosis and poikilocytosis. Target cells are prominent, and nucleated red blood cells often exceed the number of circulating white blood cells. The hemoglobin level usually falls to 5–6 g/dL or less, and the reticulocyte count is elevated but the reticulocyte index is normal to decreased. Platelet and white blood cell counts may be increased, and the serum bilirubin level is elevated. The bone marrow shows marked erythroid hyperplasia but is rarely needed for diagnosis. Hemoglobin electrophoresis shows only fetal hemoglobin and hemoglobin A₂ in children with homozygous β^0-thalassemia.

globin level may be normal or only slightly decreased because the rate of hemolysis is much less than in sickle cell anemia.

Most infants with sickle hemoglobinopathies born in the United States are now identified by neonatal screening. Results indicative of possible sickle cell disease require prompt confirmation with hemoglobin electrophoresis. Children with sickle cell anemia and with sickle β^0-thalassemia have only hemoglobins S and F. Persons with sickle β^+-thalassemia have a preponderance of hemoglobin S with a lesser amount of hemoglobin A. Persons with sickle hemoglobin C disease have equal amounts of hemoglobins S and C. The use of solubility tests to screen for the presence of sickle hemoglobin should be avoided because a negative result is frequently encountered in infants with sickle cell disease, and because a positive result in an older child does not differentiate sickle cell trait from sickle cell disease. Thus, hemoglobin electrophoresis is always necessary to accurately identify a sickle disorder.

Differential Diagnosis

Hemoglobin electrophoresis and sometimes hematologic studies of the parents are usually sufficient to confirm the correct diagnosis of a sickle cell disorder. Infants whose neonatal screening test shows only hemoglobins F and S occasionally have disorders other than sickle cell anemia or sickle β^0-thalassemia. The most important of these disorders is a compound heterozygous condition of sickle hemoglobin and pancellular hereditary persistence of fetal hemoglobin. Such children, when older, typically have 30% fetal hemoglobin and 70% hemoglobin S, but they do not have significant anemia nor are they subject to vasoocclusive episodes.

Complications

Repeated tissue ischemia and infarction causes damage to virtually every organ system. Table 27–2 lists the most important complications. Patients who require multiple transfusions are at risk for transfusional hemosiderosis and the development of red cell alloantibodies.

Treatment

The cornerstone of treatment is enrollment in a program involving patient and family education, comprehensive outpatient care, and appropriate treatment of acute complications. Important to the success of such a program are psychosocial services, blood bank services, and the ready availability of baseline patient information in the setting in which acute illnesses are evaluated and treated. Management of sickle cell anemia and sickle β^0-thalassemia includes prophylactic penicillin, which should be initiated by age 2 months and continued at least until age 5 years.

The routine use of penicillin prophylaxis in sickle hemoglobin C disease and sickle β^+-thalassemia is controversial. Pneumococcal conjugate and polysaccharide vaccine should be administered to all children who have sickle cell disease. Other routine immunizations, including yearly vaccination against influenza, should be provided. All illnesses associated with fever greater than 38.5 °C should be evaluated promptly, bacterial cultures performed, parenteral broad-spectrum antibiotics administered, and careful inpatient or outpatient observation conducted.

Treatment of painful vasoocclusive episodes includes the maintenance of adequate hydration (with avoidance of overhydration), correction of acidosis if present, administration of adequate analgesia, maintenance of normal oxygen saturation, and the treatment of any associated infections.

Red cell transfusions play an important role in management. Transfusions are indicated to improve oxygen-carrying capacity during acute severe exacerbations of anemia, as occurs during episodes of splenic sequestration or aplastic crisis. Red cell transfusions are not indicated for the treatment of chronic steady-state anemia, which is usually well tolerated, or for uncomplicated episodes of vasoocclusive pain. Simple or partial exchange transfusion to reduce the percentage of circulating sickle cells is indicated for some severe acute vasoocclusive events and may be lifesaving. These events include stroke, moderate to severe acute chest syndrome, and acute life-threatening failure of other organs. Transfusions may also be used prior to high-risk procedures such as surgery with general anesthesia and arteriograms with ionic contrast materials. Some patients who develop severe vasoocclusive complications may benefit from chronic transfusion therapy. The most common indication for this type of transfusion is stroke. Without transfusions, children with stroke have a 70–80% chance of recurrent stroke within a 2-year period. This risk of recurrent neurologic events is reduced markedly by the transfusion therapy.

Successful stem cell transplantation cures sickle cell disease, but to date its use has been limited because of the risks associated with the procedure, the inability to predict in young children the severity of future complications, and the paucity of HLA-identical sibling donors. Daily administration of oral hydroxyurea increases levels of fetal hemoglobin, decreases hemolysis, and reduces by 50% episodes of pain in severely affected adults with sickle cell anemia. The hematologic effects and short-term toxicity of hydroxyurea in children are similar to those in adults. Thus hydroxyurea is being used increasingly for selected children and adolescents who have frequent, severe complications.

Prognosis

Early identification by neonatal screening of infants with sickle cell disease, combined with comprehensive care that includes prophylactic penicillin, has markedly reduced mortality in childhood. Most patients now live well into adulthood, but eventually succumb to complications.

Academy of Pediatrics, Section on Hematology/Oncology and Committee on Genetics: Health supervision for children with sickle cell disease. Pediatrics 2002;109:526 [PMID: 11875155].

Kinney TR: Safety of hydroxyurea in children with sickle cell anemia: Results of the HUG-KIDS study, a phase I/II trial. Blood 1999;94:1550 [PMID: 10477679].

Raphael RI: Pathophysiology and treatment of sickle cell disease. Clin Adv Hematol Oncol 2005;3:492 [PMID: 16167028].

Vichinsky EP: Causes and outcomes of the acute chest syndrome in sickle cell disease. N Engl J Med 2000;342:1855 [PMID: 10861320].

Walters MC: Bone marrow transplantation for sickle cell disease. N Engl J Med 1996;335:369 [PMID: 8663884].

4. Sickle Cell Trait

Individuals who are heterozygous for the sickle gene are said to have sickle cell trait. This genetic carrier state occurs in 8% of African Americans and is more common in some areas of Africa and the Middle East. Infants with sickle cell trait are identified by neonatal screening results that show hemoglobin FAS. Accurate identification of older persons with sickle cell trait depends on hemoglobin electrophoresis, which typically shows about 60% hemoglobin A and about 40% hemoglobin S. No anemia or hemolysis is present, and the physical examination is normal. Persons with sickle cell trait are generally healthy, and experience no illness attributable to the presence of sickle hemoglobin in their red cells. Life expectancy is normal.

Sickle trait erythrocytes are capable of sickling, particularly under conditions of significant hypoxemia, and a number of clinical abnormalities have been linked to this genetic carrier state. Exposure to environmental hypoxia (altitude > 3100 m [10,000 ft] above sea level) may precipitate splenic infarction. However, most persons with sickle cell trait who choose to visit such altitudes for skiing, hiking, or climbing do so without difficulty. Many develop some degree of hyposthenuria, and about 4% experience painless hematuria, usually microscopic but occasionally macroscopic. For the most part, these renal abnormalities are subclinical and do not progress to significant renal dysfunction. The incidence of bacteriuria and pyelonephritis may be increased during pregnancy, but overall rates of maternal and infant morbidity and mortality are not affected by the presence of sickle cell trait in the pregnant woman.

An epidemiologic study of army recruits in military basic training found a higher risk of sudden unexplained death following strenuous exertion in recruits with sickle cell trait than in those with normal hemoglobin. This study has raised concerns about exercise and exertion for persons with the trait. However, considerable evidence suggests that exercise is generally safe and that athletic performance is not adversely affected by sickle cell trait. Exercise tolerance is normal, and the incidence of sickle cell trait in black professional football players is similar to that of the general African American population, suggesting no barrier to achievement in such a physically demanding profession. Thus, restrictions on athletic competition for children with sickle cell trait are not warranted. Sickle cell trait is most significant for its genetic implications.

Nuss R: Cardiopulmonary function in men with sickle cell disease who reside at moderately high altitude. J Lab Clin Med 1993;122:382 [PMID: 8228552].

5. Hemoglobin C Disorders

Hemoglobin C is detected by neonatal screening. Two percent of African Americans are heterozygous for hemoglobin C and are said to have hemoglobin C trait. Such individuals have no symptoms, anemia, or hemolysis, but the peripheral blood smear may show some target cells. Identification of persons with hemoglobin C trait is important for genetic counseling, particularly with regard to the possibility of sickle hemoglobin C disease in offspring.

Persons with homozygous hemoglobin C have a mild microcytic hemolytic anemia and may develop splenomegaly. The peripheral blood smear shows prominent target cells. As with other hemolytic anemias, complications of homozygous hemoglobin C include gallstones and aplastic crises.

Olson JF: Hemoglobin C disease in infancy and childhood. J Pediatr 1994;125:745 [PMID: 7965426].

6. Hemoglobin E Disorders

Hemoglobin E is the second most common hemoglobin variant worldwide, with a gene frequency greater than 10% in some areas of Thailand and Cambodia. In Southeast Asia, an estimated 30 million people have hemoglobin E trait. Persons heterozygous for hemoglobin E show hemoglobin FAE by neonatal screening and are asymptomatic and usually not anemic, but they may develop mild microcytosis. Persons homozygous for hemoglobin E are also asymptomatic but may have mild anemia; the peripheral blood smear shows microcytosis and some target cells.

Hemoglobin E is most important because of its interaction with β-thalassemia. Compound heterozygotes for hemoglobin E and β⁰-thalassemia are normal at birth and, like infants with homozygous E, show hemoglobin FE on neonatal screening. Unlike homozygotes, they subsequently develop mild to severe microcytic hypochromic anemia. Such children may exhibit jaundice, hepatosplenomegaly, and poor growth if the disorder is not recognized and treated appropriately. In some cases, the anemia becomes severe enough to require lifelong transfusion therapy. In certain areas of the United States, hemoglobin E/β⁰-thalassemia has become a more common cause of transfusion-dependent anemia than homozygous β-thalassemia.

Krishnamurti L: Coinheritance of α-thalassemia-1 and hemoglobin E/β⁰-thalassemia: Practical implications for neonatal screening and genetic counseling. J Pediatr 1998;132:863 [PMID: 9602201].

Weatherall DJ: Hemoglobin E–β⁰-thalassemia: An increasingly common disease with some diagnostic pitfalls. J Pediatr 1998;132:765 [PMID: 9602183].

7. Other Hemoglobinopathies

Hundreds of other human globin-chain variants have been identified and described. Some, such as hemoglobins D and G, are relatively common. Heterozygous individuals, who are frequently identified during the course of neonatal screening programs for hemoglobinopathies, are generally asymptomatic and usually have no anemia or hemolysis. The principal significance of most hemoglobin variants is the potential for disease in compound heterozygous individuals who also inherit a gene for β-thalassemia or sickle hemoglobin. For example, children who are compound heterozygous for hemoglobins S and D_{Punjab} ($D_{Los\ Angeles}$) have sickle cell disease.

CONGENITAL HEMOLYTIC ANEMIAS: DISORDERS OF RED CELL METABOLISM

Erythrocytes depend on the anaerobic metabolism of glucose for the maintenance of adenosine triphosphate levels sufficient for homeostasis. Glycolysis also produces the 2,3-diphosphoglycerate levels needed to modulate the oxygen affinity of hemoglobin. Glucose metabolism via the hexosemonophosphate shunt is necessary to generate sufficient reduced nicotinamide adenine dinucleotide phosphate and reduced glutathione to protect red cells against oxidant damage. Congenital deficiencies of many glycolytic pathway enzymes have been associated with hemolytic anemias. In general, the morphologic abnormalities present on the peripheral blood smear are nonspecific, and the inheritance of these disorders is autosomal recessive or X-linked. Thus, the possibility of a red cell enzyme defect should be considered during the evaluation of a patient with a congenital hemolytic anemia when the peripheral blood smear does not show red cell morphology typical of membrane or hemoglobin defects (eg, spherocytes, sickle forms, target cells), when hemoglobin disorders

are excluded by hemoglobin electrophoresis and by isopropanol precipitation tests, and when family studies do not suggest an autosomal dominant disorder. The diagnosis is confirmed by finding a low level of the deficient enzyme.

The two most common disorders of erythrocyte metabolism are G6PD deficiency and pyruvate kinase deficiency.

1. Glucose-6-Phosphate Dehydrogenase (G6PD) Deficiency

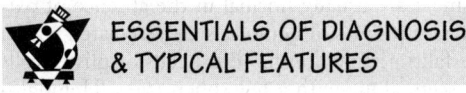

ESSENTIALS OF DIAGNOSIS & TYPICAL FEATURES

- *African, Mediterranean, or Asian ancestry.*
- *Neonatal hyperbilirubinemia.*
- *Sporadic hemolysis associated with infection or with ingestion of oxidant drugs or fava beans.*
- *X-linked inheritance.*

General Considerations

Deficiency of G6PD is the most common red cell enzyme defect that causes hemolytic anemia. The disorder has X-linked recessive inheritance and occurs with high frequency among persons of African, Mediterranean, and Asian ancestry. Hundreds of different G6PD variants have been characterized. In most instances, the deficiency is due to enzyme instability; thus, older red cells are more deficient than younger ones, and are unable to generate sufficient nicotinamide adenine dinucleotide phosphate to maintain the levels of reduced glutathione necessary to protect the red cells against oxidant stress. Thus, most persons with G6PD deficiency do not have a chronic hemolytic anemia but have episodic hemolysis at times of exposure to the oxidant stress of infection or of certain drugs or food substances. The severity of the disorder varies among ethnic groups; G6PD deficiency in persons of African ancestry usually is less severe than in other ethnic groups.

Clinical Findings

A. SYMPTOMS AND SIGNS

Infants with G6PD deficiency may have significant hyperbilirubinemia and require phototherapy or exchange transfusion to prevent kernicterus. The deficiency is an important cause of neonatal hyperbilirubinemia in infants of Mediterranean or Asian ancestry but less so in infants of African ancestry. Older children with G6PD deficiency are asymptomatic and appear normal between episodes of hemolysis. Hemolytic episodes are often triggered by infection or by the ingestion of oxidant drugs such as antimalarial compounds and sulfonamide antibiotics (Table 27–3). Ingestion of fava beans may trigger hemolysis in children of Mediterranean or Asian ancestry but usually not in children of African ancestry. Episodes of hemolysis are associated with pallor, jaundice, hemoglobinuria, and sometimes cardiovascular compromise.

B. LABORATORY FINDINGS

The hemoglobin, reticulocyte count, and peripheral blood smear are usually normal in the absence of oxidant stress. Episodes of hemolysis are associated with a variable fall in hemoglobin. "Bite" cells or blister cells may be seen, along with a few spherocytes. Hemoglobinuria is common, and the reticulocyte count increases within a few days. Heinz bodies may be demonstrated with appropriate stains. The diagnosis is confirmed by the finding of reduced levels of G6PD in erythrocytes. Because this enzyme is present in increased quantities in reticulocytes, the test is best performed at a time when the reticulocyte count is normal or near normal.

Complications

Kernicterus is a risk for infants with significant neonatal hyperbilirubinemia. Episodes of acute hemolysis in older children may be life-threatening. Rare G6PD variants are associated with chronic hemolytic anemia; the clinical course of patients with such variants may be complicated by splenomegaly and by the formation of gallstones.

Treatment

The most important treatment issue is avoidance of drugs known to be associated with hemolysis (see Table 27–3). For some patients of Mediterranean, Middle Eastern, or Asian ancestry, the consumption of fava beans must also be avoided. Infections should be treated promptly and

Table 27–3. Some common drugs and chemicals that can induce hemolytic anemia in persons with G6PD deficiency.

Acetanilide	Niridazole
Doxorubicin	Nitrofurantoin
Furazolidone	Phenazopyridine
Methylene blue	Primaquine
Nalidixic acid	Sulfamethoxazole

Reproduced, with permission, from Beutler E: Glucose-6-phosphate dehydrogenase deficiency. N Engl J Med 1991;324:171.

antibiotics given when appropriate. Most episodes of hemolysis are self-limiting, but red cell transfusions may be lifesaving when signs and symptoms indicate cardiovascular compromise.

Beutler E: G6PD deficiency. Blood 1994;84:3613 [PMID: 7949118].

Kaplan M: Conjugated bilirubin in neonates with glucose-6-phosphate dehydrogenase deficiency. J Pediatr 1996;128:695 [PMID: 8627445].

2. Pyruvate Kinase Deficiency

Pyruvate kinase deficiency is an autosomal recessive disorder observed in all ethnic groups but is most common in northern Europeans. The deficiency is associated with a chronic hemolytic anemia of varying severity. Approximately one-third of those affected present in the neonatal period with jaundice and hemolysis that require phototherapy or exchange transfusion. Occasionally, the disorder causes hydrops fetalis and neonatal death. In older children, the hemolysis may require red cell transfusions or be mild enough to go unnoticed for many years. Jaundice and splenomegaly frequently occur in the more severe cases. The diagnosis of pyruvate kinase deficiency is occasionally suggested by the presence of echinocytes on the peripheral blood smear, but these findings may be absent prior to splenectomy. The diagnosis depends on the demonstration of low levels of pyruvate kinase activity in red cells.

Treatment of pyruvate kinase depends on the severity of the hemolysis. Blood transfusions may be required for significant anemia, and splenectomy may be beneficial. The procedure does not cure the disorder but ameliorates the anemia and its symptoms. Characteristically, the reticulocyte count increases and echinocytes become more prevalent after splenectomy, despite the decreased hemolysis and increased hemoglobin level.

Gilsanz F: Fetal anaemia due to pyruvate kinase deficiency. Arch Dis Child 1993;69:523 [PMID: 8285758].

ACQUIRED HEMOLYTIC ANEMIA

1. Autoimmune Hemolytic Anemia

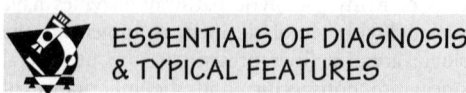

ESSENTIALS OF DIAGNOSIS & TYPICAL FEATURES

- *Pallor, fatigue, jaundice, and dark urine.*
- *Splenomegaly common.*
- *Positive DAT.*
- *Reticulocytosis and spherocytosis.*

General Considerations

Acquired autoimmune hemolytic anemia is rare during the first 4 months of life but is one of the more common causes of acute anemia after the first year. It may arise as an isolated problem or may complicate an infection (hepatitis, upper respiratory tract infections, mononucleosis, or cytomegalovirus infection); systemic lupus erythematosus and other autoimmune syndromes; immunodeficiency states; or, rarely, malignancies.

Clinical Findings

A. SYMPTOMS AND SIGNS

The disease usually has an acute onset manifested by weakness, pallor, dark urine, and fatigue. Jaundice is a prominent finding, and splenomegaly is often present. Some cases have a more chronic, insidious onset. Clinical evidence of an underlying disease may be present.

B. LABORATORY FINDINGS

The anemia is normochromic and normocytic and may vary from mild to severe (hemoglobin concentration < 5 g/dL). The reticulocyte count and index are usually increased but occasionally are normal or low. Spherocytes and nucleated red cells may be seen on the peripheral blood smear. Although leukocytosis and elevated platelet counts are a common finding, thrombocytopenia occasionally occurs. Other laboratory data consistent with hemolysis are present, such as increased indirect and total bilirubin, lactic dehydrogenase, aspartate aminotransferase, and urinary urobilinogen. Intravascular hemolysis is indicated by hemoglobinemia or hemoglobinuria. Examination of bone marrow shows marked erythroid hyperplasia and hemophagocytosis, but is seldom required.

Serologic studies are helpful in defining pathophysiology, planning therapeutic strategies, and assessing prognosis (Table 27–4). In almost all cases, the direct and indirect antiglobulin (DAT and IAT) tests are positive. Further evaluation allows distinction into one of three syndromes. The presence of IgG on the patient's red blood cells, maximal in vitro antibody activity at 37 °C, and either no antigen specificity or an Rh-like specificity constitute warm autoimmune hemolytic anemia with extravascular destruction by the reticuloendothelial system. In contrast, the detection of complement alone on red blood cells, optimal reactivity in vitro at 4 °C, and I

Table 27–4. Classification of autoimmune hemolytic anemia (AIHA) in children.

Syndrome	Warm AIHA	Cold AIHA	Paroxysmal Cold Hemoglobinuria
Specific antiglobulin test IgG Complement	Strongly positive Negative or mildly positive	Negative Strongly positive	Negative Strongly positive
Temperature at maximal reactivity (in vitro)	37 °C	4 °C	4 °C
Antigen specificity	May be panagglutinin or may have an Rh-like specificity	I or i	P
Other	...	...	Positive biphasic hemolysin test
Pathophysiology	Extravascular hemolysis, destruction by the RES (eg, spleen)	Intravascular hemolysis (may have extravascular component)	Intravascular hemolysis (may have extravascular component)
Prognosis	May be more chronic (> 3 months) with significant morbidity and mortality. May be associated with a primary disorder (lupus, immunodeficiency, etc).	Generally acute (< 3 months). Good prognosis: often associated with infection.	Acute, self-limited. Associated with infection.
Therapy	Respond to RES blockade, including steroids (prednisone, 2 mg/kg/d), IVIG (1 g/kg/d for 2 days), or splenectomy	May not respond to RES blockade. Severe cases may benefit from plasmapheresis.	Usually self-limited. Symptomatic management.

RES, reticuloendothelial system; IVIG , intravenous immune globulin.

or i antigen specificity are diagnostic of cold autoimmune hemolytic anemia with intravascular hemolysis. Although cold agglutinins are relatively common (~ 10%) in normal individuals, clinically significant cold antibodies exhibit in vitro reactivity at 30 °C or above.

Paroxysmal cold hemoglobinuria usually has a different cause. The laboratory evaluation is identical to cold autoimmune hemolytic anemia except for antigen specificity (P) and the exhibition of in vitro hemolysis. Paroxysmal cold hemoglobinuria is almost always associated with significant infections, such as *Mycoplasma*, Epstein–Barr virus (EBV), and cytomegalovirus (CMV). Warm IgM antibodies are rare.

Differential Diagnosis

Autoimmune hemolytic anemia must be differentiated from other forms of congenital or acquired hemolytic anemias. The DAT discriminates antibody-mediated hemolysis from other causes, such as hereditary spherocytosis.

Complications

The anemia may be very severe and result in cardiovascular collapse, requiring emergency management. The complications of the underlying disease such as disseminated lupus erythematosus or an immunodeficiency state may be present.

Treatment

Medical management of the underlying disease is important in symptomatic cases. Defining the clinical syndrome provides a useful guide to treatment. Most patients with warm autoimmune hemolytic anemia (in which hemolysis is mostly extravascular) respond to prednisone (2–4 mg/kg/d). After the initial treatment, the dose of corticosteroids may be decreased slowly. Patients may respond to 1 g of intravenous immune globulin (IVIG) per kilogram per day for 2 days, but fewer patients respond to IVIG than to prednisone. Although the rate of remission with splenectomy may be as high as 50%, particularly in warm autoimmune hemolytic anemia, this should be carefully considered in younger patients and withheld until other treatments have been tried. In severe cases unresponsive to more conventional therapy, immunosuppressive agents such as cyclophosphamide, azathioprine, busulfan, and cyclosporine may be tried alone or in combination with corticosteroids. In refractory cases, recent studies have documented responses to rituximab. Bone marrow transplantation has been used in a small number of cases.

Patients with cold autoimmune hemolytic anemia and paroxysmal cold hemoglobinuria are less likely to respond to corticosteroids or IVIG. Because these syndromes are most apt to be associated with infections and have an acute, self-limited course, supportive care may be all that is required. Plasma exchange may be effective in severe cold autoimmune (IgM) hemolytic anemia because the offending antibody has an intravascular distribution.

Supportive therapy is crucial. Patients with cold-reacting antibodies, particularly paroxysmal cold hemoglobinuria, should be kept in a warm environment. Transfusion may be necessary because of the complications of severe anemia but should be used only when there is no alternative. In most patients, cross-match–compatible blood will not be found, and the least incompatible unit should be identified. Transfusion must be conducted carefully, beginning with a test dose (see Transfusion Medicine section). Identification of the patient's phenotype for minor red cell alloantigens may be helpful in avoiding alloimmunization or in providing appropriate transfusions if alloantibodies arise after initial transfusions. Patients with severe intravascular hemolysis may have associated disseminated intravascular coagulation (DIC), and heparin therapy should be considered in such cases.

Prognosis

The outlook for autoimmune hemolytic anemia in childhood is usually good unless associated diseases are present (eg, congenital immunodeficiency, acquired immunodeficiency syndrome [AIDS], lupus erythematosus), in which case the hemolysis is likely to run a chronic course. In general, children with warm autoimmune hemolytic anemia are at greater risk for more severe and chronic disease with higher morbidity and mortality rates. Hemolysis and positive antiglobulin tests may continue for months or years. Patients with cold autoimmune hemolytic anemia or paroxysmal cold hemoglobinuria are more likely to have acute, self-limited disease (< 3 months). Paroxysmal cold hemoglobinuria is almost always associated with infection (eg, *Mycoplasma* infection, CMV, and EBV).

Petz LD: Unusual problems regarding autoimmune hemolytic anemias. In: *Acquired Immune Hemolytic Anemias.* Churchill Livingstone, 2004:341–344.

Shirey RS: Prophylactic antigen-matched donor blood for patients with warm autoantibodies: An algorithm for transfusion management. Transfusion 2002;42:1435 [PMID: 12421216].

Zecca M: Rituximab for the treatment of refractory autoimmune hemolytic anemia in children. Blood 2003;101:3857 [PMID: 12531800].

2. Nonimmune Acquired Hemolytic Anemia

Hepatic disease may alter the lipid composition of the red cell membrane. This usually results in the formation of target cells and is not associated with significant hemolysis.

Occasionally, hepatocellular damage is associated with the formation of spur cells and brisk hemolytic anemia. Renal disease may also be associated with significant hemolysis; hemolytic–uremic syndrome is one example. In this disorder, hemolysis is associated with the presence, on the peripheral blood smear, of echinocytes, helmet cells, fragmented red cells, and spherocytes.

A microangiopathic hemolytic anemia with fragmented red cells and some spherocytes may be observed in a number of conditions associated with intravascular coagulation and fibrin deposition within vessels. This occurs with DIC such as may complicate severe infection, but it may also occur when the intravascular coagulation is localized, as with giant cavernous hemangiomas (Kasabach–Merritt syndrome). Fragmented red cells may also be seen with mechanical damage (eg, associated with artificial heart valves).

POLYCYTHEMIA & METHEMOGLOBINEMIA

CONGENITAL ERYTHROCYTOSIS (Familial Polycythemia)

In pediatrics, polycythemia is usually secondary to chronic hypoxemia. However, a number of families with congenital erythrocytosis have been described. The disorder differs from polycythemia vera in that only red blood cells are affected; the white blood cell and platelet counts are normal. It occurs as an autosomal dominant or recessive disorder. There are usually no physical findings except for plethora and splenomegaly. The hemoglobin level may be as high as 27 g/dL. Patients usually have no symptoms other than headache and lethargy. Studies in a number of families have revealed (1) an abnormal hemoglobin with altered oxygen affinity, (2) reduced red cell diphosphoglycerate, (3) autonomous increase in erythropoietin production, or (4) hypersensitivity of erythroid precursors to erythropoietin.

Treatment is not indicated unless symptoms are marked. Phlebotomy is the treatment of choice.

SECONDARY POLYCYTHEMIA

Secondary polycythemia occurs in response to hypoxemia. The most common cause of secondary polycythemia in children is cyanotic congenital heart disease. It also occurs in chronic pulmonary disease such as cystic fibrosis. Persons living at extremely high altitudes, as well as some with methemoglobinemia, develop polycythemia. It has on rare occasions been described without hypoxemia in association with renal tumors, brain tumors, Cushing disease, or hydronephrosis.

Polycythemia may occur in the neonatal period; it is particularly exaggerated in infants who are preterm or small for gestational age. In these infants, polycythemia is sometimes associated with other symptoms. It may occur in infants of diabetic mothers, in Down syndrome, and as a complication of congenital adrenal hyperplasia.

Iron deficiency may complicate polycythemia and aggravate the associated hyperviscosity. This complication should always be suspected when the MCV falls below the normal range. Coagulation and bleeding abnormalities, including thrombocytopenia, mild consumption coagulopathy, and elevated fibrinolytic activity, have also been described in severely polycythemic cardiac patients. Bleeding at surgery may be severe.

The ideal treatment of secondary polycythemia is correction of the underlying disorder. When this cannot be done, phlebotomy may be necessary to control symptoms. Iron sufficiency should be maintained. Adequate hydration of the patient and phlebotomy with plasma replacement may be indicated prior to major surgical procedures; these measures prevent the complications of thrombosis and hemorrhage. Isovolumetric exchange transfusion is the treatment of choice in severe cases.

METHEMOGLOBINEMIA

Methemoglobin is continuously formed at a slow rate by the oxidation of heme iron to the ferric state. Normally, it is enzymatically reduced back to hemoglobin. Methemoglobin is unable to transport oxygen and causes a shift in the dissociation curve of the residual oxyhemoglobin. Cyanosis is produced with methemoglobin levels of approximately 15% or greater. Levels of methemoglobin increase by several mechanisms.

1. Hemoglobin M

The designation M is given to several abnormal hemoglobins associated with methemoglobinemia. Affected individuals are heterozygous for the gene, which is transmitted as an autosomal dominant disorder. The different types of hemoglobin M result from different amino acid substitutions in α-globin or β-globin. Hemoglobin electrophoresis at the usual pH will not always demonstrate the abnormal hemoglobin, and isoelectric focusing may be needed. The patient has cyanosis but is otherwise usually asymptomatic. Exercise tolerance may be normal, and life expectancy is not affected. This type of methemoglobinemia does not respond to any form of therapy.

2. Congenital Methemoglobinemia Due to Enzyme Deficiencies

Congenital methemoglobinemia is caused most frequently by congenital deficiency of the reducing enzyme diaphorase I (coenzyme factor I). It is transmitted as an autosomal recessive trait. Affected patients may have as much as 40% methemoglobin but usually have no symptoms, although a mild compensatory polycythemia may be present. Patients with methemoglobinemia associated with a deficiency of diaphorase I respond readily to treatment with ascorbic acid and methylene blue (see following section), but treatment is not usually indicated.

3. Acquired Methemoglobinemia

A number of compounds activate the oxidation of hemoglobin from the ferrous to the ferric state, forming methemoglobin. These include the nitrites and nitrates (contaminated water), chlorates, and quinones. Drugs in this group are the aniline dyes, sulfonamides, acetanilid, phenacetin, bismuth subnitrate, and potassium chlorate. Poisoning with a drug or chemical containing one of these substances should be suspected in any infant or child who presents with sudden cyanosis. Methemoglobin levels in such cases may be extremely high and can produce anoxia, dyspnea, unconsciousness, circulatory failure, and death. Young infants and newborns are more susceptible to acquired methemoglobinemia because their red cells have difficulty reducing hemoglobin, probably because their NADH methemoglobin reductase is transiently deficient. Infants with metabolic acidosis from diarrhea and dehydration or other causes may also develop methemoglobinemia.

Patients with the acquired form of methemoglobinemia respond dramatically to methylene blue in a dose of 1–2 mg/kg intravenously. For infants and young children, a smaller dose (1–1.5 mg/kg) is recommended. Ascorbic acid administered orally or intravenously also reduces methemoglobin, but the response is slower.

Mansouri A: Concise review: Methemoglobinemia. Am J Hematol 1993;42:7 [PMID: 8416301].

Osterhoudt KC: Rebound severe methemoglobinemia from ingestion of a nitroethane artificial-fingernail remover. J Pediatr 1995;126:819 [PMID: 7752015].

Sager S: Methemoglobinemia associated with acidosis of probable renal origin. J Pediatr 1995;126:59 [PMID: 7815226].

■ DISORDERS OF LEUKOCYTES

NEUTROPENIA

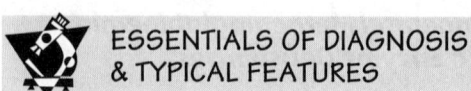

ESSENTIALS OF DIAGNOSIS & TYPICAL FEATURES

- *Increased frequency of infections.*

- *Ulceration of oral mucosa and gingivitis.*
- *Normal numbers of red cells and platelets.*

General Considerations

Neutropenia is an absolute neutrophil (granulocyte) count of less than 1500/μL in childhood, or below 1000/μL between ages 1 week and 2 years. During the first few days of life, an absolute neutrophil count of less than 3500 cells/μL may be considered neutropenia. Neutropenia results from absent or defective granulocyte stem cells, ineffective or suppressed myeloid maturation, decreased production of hematopoietic cytokines (eg, granulocyte colony-stimulating factor [G-CSF] or granulocyte-macrophage colony-stimulating factor [GM-CSF]), decreased marrow release, increased neutrophil destruction or consumption, or, in pseudoneutropenia, from an increased neutrophil marginating pool (Table 27–5).

The most severe types of congenital neutropenia include reticular dysgenesis (congenital aleukocytosis), Kostmann syndrome (severe neutropenia with maturation defect in the marrow progenitor cells), Shwachman syndrome (neutropenia with pancreatic insufficiency), neutropenia with immune deficiency states, cyclic neutropenia, and myelokathexis or dysgranulopoiesis. Genetic mutations for Chédiak–Higashi syndrome and Shwachman syndrome have recently been identified. Neutropenia may also be associated with storage and metabolic diseases and immunodeficiency states. The most common causes of neutropenia are viral infection or drugs resulting in decreased production in the marrow or increased destruction or both. Severe bacterial infections may be associated with neutropenia. Although rare, neonatal alloimmune neutropenia can be severe and associated with increased risk for infection. Autoimmune neutropenia in the mother can result in passive transfer of antibody to the fetus and neutropenia in the neonate. Malignancies, osteopetrosis, marrow failure syndromes, and hypersplenism are not usually associated with isolated neutropenia.

Clinical Findings

A. SYMPTOMS AND SIGNS

Acute severe bacterial or fungal infection is the most significant complication of neutropenia. Although the risk is increased when the absolute neutrophil count is less than 500/μL, the actual susceptibility is variable and depends on the cause of neutropenia, marrow reserves, and other factors. The most common types of infection include septicemia, cellulitis, skin abscesses, pneumonia, and perirectal abscesses. Sinusitis, aphthous ulcers, gingivitis, and periodontal disease also

Table 27–5. Classification of neutropenia of childhood.

Congenital neutropenia with stem cell abnormalities
    Reticular dysgenesis
    Cyclic neutropenia
Congenital neutropenia with abnormalities of committed myeloid progenitor cells
    Neutropenia with immunodeficiency disorders (T cells and B cells)
    Severe congenital neutropenia (Kostmann syndrome)
    Chronic idiopathic neutropenia of childhood
    Myelocathexis with dysmyelopoiesis
    Chédiak-Higashi syndrome
    Shwachman syndrome
    Cartilage-hair hypoplasia
    Dyskeratosis congenita
    Fanconi anemia
    Organic acidemias (eg, propionic, methylmalonic)
    Glycogenosis Ib
    Osteopetrosis
Acquired neutropenias affecting stem cells
    Malignancies (leukemia, lymphoma) and preleukemic disorders
    Drugs or toxic substances
    Ionizing radiation
    Aplastic anemia
Acquired neutropenias affecting committed myeloid progenitors and/or survival of mature neutrophils
    Ineffective granulopoiesis (vitamin B_{12}, folate, and copper deficiency)
    Infection
    Immune (neonatal alloimmune or autoimmune; autoimmune or chronic benign neutropenia of childhood)
    Hypersplenism

---

cause significant problems for these patients. In addition to local signs and symptoms, patients may have chills, fever, and malaise. In most cases, the spleen and liver are not enlarged. *Staphylococcus aureus* and gram-negative bacteria are the most common pathogens.

B. LABORATORY FINDINGS

Neutrophils are absent or markedly reduced in the peripheral blood smear. In most forms of neutropenia or agranulocytosis, the monocytes and lymphocytes are normal and the red cells and platelets are not affected. The bone marrow usually shows a normal erythroid series, with adequate megakaryocytes but a marked reduction in the myeloid cells or a significant delay in maturation of this series. Total cellularity may be decreased.

In the evaluation of neutropenia (eg, persistent, intermittent, cyclic), careful attention should be paid to the duration and pattern of neutropenia, the types of infections and their frequency, and phenotypic abnormalities on physical examination. A careful family history and blood counts from the parents are useful. If an acquired cause, such as viral infection or drug, is not obvious and no other primary disease is present, white blood cell counts, white cell differential, and platelet and reticulocyte counts should be completed once or twice weekly for 4–6 weeks to determine the possibility of cyclic neutropenia. Bone marrow aspiration and biopsy are most important to characterize the morphologic features of myelopoiesis. Measuring the neutrophil counts in response to steroid infusion will document the marrow reserves. Tests for specific causes of neutropenia include measurement of neutrophil antibodies, immunoglobulin levels, antinuclear antibodies, and lymphocyte phenotyping to detect immunodeficiency states. Cultures of bone marrow are important for defining the numbers of stem cells and progenitors committed to the myeloid series or the presence of cytotoxic lymphocytes or humoral inhibitory factors. Cytokine levels in plasma or mononuclear cells can be measured directly. Some neutropenia disorders have abnormal neutrophil function. Recent studies have documented abnormalities in the elastase gene in severe congenital and cyclic neutropenias. Increased apoptosis in marrow precursors or circulating neutrophils has been described in several congenital disorders.

Treatment

Identifiable toxic agents should be eliminated or associated diseases (eg, infections) treated. Prophylactic antimicrobial therapy is not indicated for afebrile, asymptomatic patients. Recombinant G-CSF and GM-CSF will increase neutrophil counts in most patients. Patients may be started on 3–5 μg/kg/d of G-CSF (filgrastim) given subcutaneously or intravenously once a day. Depending on the counts, the dose may be increased or decreased. For patients with congenital neutropenia, the dose should be regulated to keep the absolute neutrophil count less than 10,000/μL. Some patients maintain adequate counts with G-CSF given 2–3 times/week.

Prognosis

The prognosis varies greatly with the cause and severity of the neutropenia. In severe cases with persistent agranulocytosis, the prognosis is poor in spite of antibiotic therapy; in mild or cyclic forms of neutropenia, symptoms may be minimal and the prognosis for normal life expectancy excellent. Up to 50% of patients with Shwachman syndrome may develop aplastic anemia, myelodysplasia, or leukemia during their lifetime. Patients with Kostmann syndrome also have a potential for leukemia. Recombinant hematopoietic hormones (ie, G-CSF) increase peripheral counts and decrease infectious complications.

Ancliff PJ: Long-term follow-up of granulocyte colony-stimulating factor receptor mutations in patients with severe congenital neutropenia: Implications for leukaemogenesis and therapy. Br J Haematol 2003;120:685 [PMID: 12588357].

Bellanne-Chantelot C: Mutations in the ELA2 gene correlate with more severe expression of neutropenia: A study of 81 patients from the French Neutropenia Register. Blood 2004;103:4119 [PMID: 14962902].

Berliner N: Congenital and acquired neutropenia. Hematology 2004;63 [PMID: 15561677].

Dror Y: Update on childhood neutropenia: Molecular and clinical advances. Hematol Oncol Clin North Am 2004;18:1439 [PMID: 15511624].

Federman N: The genetic basis of bone marrow failure syndromes in children. Mol Genet Metab 2005;86:100 [PMID: 16125992].

Sera Y: A comparison of the defective granulopoiesis in childhood cyclic neutropenia and in severe congenital neutropenia. Haematologica 2005;90:1032 [PMID: 16079102].

NEUTROPHILIA

Neutrophilia is an increase in the absolute neutrophil count in the peripheral blood to greater than 7500–8500 cells/μL for infants, children, and adults. To support the increased peripheral count, neutrophils may be mobilized from bone marrow storage or peripheral marginating pools. Neutrophilia occurs acutely in association with bacterial or viral infections, inflammatory diseases (eg, juvenile rheumatoid arthritis, inflammatory bowel disease, Kawasaki disease), surgical or functional asplenia, liver failure, diabetic ketoacidosis, azotemia, congenital disorders of neutrophil function

(eg, chronic granulomatous disease, leukocyte adherence deficiency), and hemolysis. Drugs such as corticosteroids, lithium, and epinephrine increase the blood neutrophil count. Corticosteroids cause release of neutrophils from the marrow pool and inhibit egress from capillary beds and postpone apoptotic cell death. Epinephrine causes release of the marginating pool. Acute neutrophilia has been reported after stress such as from electric shock, trauma, burns, surgery, and emotional upset. Tumors involving the bone marrow, such as lymphomas, neuroblastomas, and rhabdomyosarcoma, may be associated with leukocytosis and the presence of immature myeloid cells in the peripheral blood. Infants with Down syndrome have defective regulation of proliferation and maturation of the myeloid series and may develop neutrophilia. At times this process may affect other cell lines and mimic myeloproliferative disorders or acute leukemia.

The neutrophilias must be distinguished from myeloproliferative disorders such as chronic myelogenous leukemia and juvenile chronic myelogenous leukemia. In general, abnormalities involving other cell lines, the appearance of immature cells on the blood smear, and the presence of hepatosplenomegaly are important differentiating characteristics.

DISORDERS OF NEUTROPHIL FUNCTION

Neutrophils play a key role in host defenses. Circulating in capillary beds, they adhere to the vascular endothelium adjacent to sites of infection and inflammation. Moving between endothelial cells, the neutrophil migrates toward the offending agent. Contact with a microbe that is properly opsonized with complement or antibodies triggers ingestion, a process in which cytoplasmic streaming results in the formation of pseudopods that fuse around the invader, encasing it in a phagosome. During the ingestion phase, the oxidase enzyme system assembles and is activated, taking oxygen from the surrounding medium and reducing it to form toxic oxygen metabolites critical to microbicidal activity. Concurrently, granules from the two main classes (azurophil and specific) fuse and release their contents into the phagolysosome. The concentration of toxic oxygen metabolites (eg, hydrogen peroxide, hypochlorous acid, hydroxyl radical) and other compounds (eg, proteases, cationic proteins, cathepsins, defensins) increases dramatically, resulting in the death and dissolution of the microbe. Complex physiologic and biochemical processes support and control these functions. Defects in any of these processes may lead to inadequate cell function and an increased risk of infection.

Classification

Table 27–6 summarizes congenital neutrophil function defects. Recently described is a syndrome of severe neu-

Table 27–6. Classification of congenital neutrophil function deficits.

Disorder	Clinical Manifestations	Functional Defect	Biochemical Defect	Inheritance
Chédiak-Higashi syndrome	Oculocutaneous albinism, photophobia, nystagmus, ataxia. Recurrent infections of skin, respiratory tract, and mucous membranes with gram-positive and gram-negative organisms. Many die during lymphoproliferative phase with hepatomegaly, fever. This may be a viral-associated hemophagocytic syndrome secondary to Epstein-Barr virus infection. Older patients may develop degenerative CNS disease.	Neutropenia. Neutrophils, monocytes, lymphocytes, platelets, and all granule-containing cells have giant granules. Most significant defect is in chemotaxis. Also milder defects in microbicidal activity and degranulation.	Gene deficit identified. Alterations in membrane fusion with formation of giant granules. Other biochemical abnormalities in cAMP and cGMP, microtubule assembly.	Autosomal recessive
Leukocyte adherence deficiency I	Recurrent soft-tissue infections, including gingivitis, otitis, mucositis, periodontitis, skin infections. Delayed separation of the cord in newborn and problems with wound healing.	Neutrophilia. Diminished adherence to surfaces, leading to decreased chemotaxis.	Absence or partial deficiency of CD11/CD18 cell surface adhesive glycoproteins.	Autosomal recessive
Leukocyte adherence deficiency II	Recurrent infections, mental retardation, craniofacial abnormalities, short stature.	Neutrophilia. Deficient "rolling" interaction with endothelial cells. Red cells have Bombay phenotype.	Deficient fucosyl transferase results in deficient sialyl Lewis X antigen, which interacts with P selectin on endothelial cell to establish neutrophil rolling, a prerequisite for adherence and diapedesis.	Autosomal recessive
Chronic granulomatous disease	Recurrent purulent infections with catalase-positive bacteria and fungi. May involve skin, mucous membranes. Also develop deep infections (lymph nodes, lung, liver, bones) and sepsis.	Neutrophilia. Neutrophils demonstrate deficient bactericidal activity but normal chemotaxis and ingestion. Defect in the oxidase enzyme system, resulting in absence or diminished production of oxygen metabolites toxic to microbes.	A number of molecular defects in oxidase components. Absent cytochrome b558 with decreased expression of either (1) or (2): (1) gp91-phox (2) p22-phox Absent p47-phox or p67-phox (cytosolic components).	(1) X-linked (60–65% of cases). (2) Autosomal recessive (< 5% of cases). Autosomal recessive (30% of cases).
Myeloperoxidase deficiency	Generally healthy. Fungal infections when deficiency associated with systemic diseases (eg, diabetes).	Diminished capacity to enhance hydrogen peroxide–mediated microbicidal activity.	Diminished or absent myeloperoxidase; post-translational defect in processing protein.	Autosomal recessive
Specific granule deficiency	Recurrent skin and deep tissue infections.	Decreased chemotaxis and bactericidal activity.	Failure to produce specific granules or their contents during myelopoiesis.	Autosomal recessive

CNS, central nervous system; cAMP, cyclic adenosine monophosphate; cGMP, cyclic guanosine monophosphate.

trophil dysfunction and severe infections associated with a mutation in a GTPase signaling molecule, Rac2. Other congenital or acquired causes of mild to moderate neutrophil dysfunction include metabolic defects (eg, glycogen storage disease, diabetes mellitus, renal disease, hypophosphatemia), viral infections, and certain drugs. Neutrophils from newborn infants have abnormal adherence, chemotaxis, and bactericidal activity. Cells from patients with thermal injury, trauma, and overwhelming infection have defects in cell motility and bactericidal activity similar to those seen in neonates.

Clinical Findings

Recurrent bacterial or fungal infections are the hallmark of neutrophil dysfunction. Although many patients will have infection-free periods, episodes of pneumonia, sinusitis, cellulitis, cutaneous and mucosal infections (including perianal or peritonsillar abscesses), and lymphadenitis are frequent. As with neutropenia, aphthous ulcers of mucous membranes, severe gingivitis, and periodontal disease are also major complications. In general, *S aureus,* along with gram-negative organisms, is commonly isolated from infected sites; other organisms may be specifically associated with a defined neutrophil function defect. In some disorders, fungi account for an increasing number of infections. Deep or generalized infections such as osteomyelitis, liver abscesses, sepsis, meningitis, and necrotic or even gangrenous soft-tissue lesions occur in specific syndromes (eg, leukocyte adherence deficiency or chronic granulomatous disease). Patients with severe neutrophil dysfunction may die in childhood from severe infections or associated complications. Table 27–6 summarizes pertinent laboratory findings.

Treatment

The mainstays of management of these disorders are anticipation of infections and aggressive attempts to identify the foci and the causative agents. Surgical procedures to achieve these goals may be both diagnostic and therapeutic. Broad-spectrum antibiotics covering the range of possible organisms should be initiated without delay, switching to specific antimicrobial agents when the microbiologic diagnosis is made. When infections are unresponsive or they recur, granulocyte transfusions may be helpful.

Chronic management includes prophylactic antibiotics. Trimethoprim–sulfamethoxazole and other antibiotic compounds enhance the bactericidal activity of neutrophils from patients with chronic granulomatous disease. Some patients with Chédiak–Higashi syndrome improve clinically when given ascorbic acid. Recombinant γ-interferon decreases the number and severity of infections in patients with chronic granulomatous dis-

ease. Demonstration of this activity with one patient group raises the possibility that cytokines, growth factors, and other biologic response modifiers may be helpful in other conditions in preventing recurrent infections. Bone marrow transplantation has been attempted in most major congenital neutrophil dysfunction syndromes, and reconstitution with normal cells and cell function has been documented. Combining genetic engineering with autologous bone marrow transplantation may provide a future strategy for curing these disorders.

Prognosis

For mild to moderate defects, anticipation and conservative medical management ensure a reasonable outlook. For severe defects, excessive morbidity and significant mortality exist. In some diseases, the development of noninfectious complications, such as the lymphoproliferative phase of Chédiak–Higashi syndrome or inflammatory syndromes in chronic granulomatous disease, may influence prognosis.

Ambruso DR: Human neutrophil immunodeficiency syndrome is associated with an inhibitory Rac2 mutation. Proc Natl Acad Sci U S A 2000;97:4654 [PMID: 10758162].

Hidalgo A: Insights into leukocyte adhesion deficiency type 2 from a novel mutation in the GDP-fucose transporter gene. Blood 2003;101:1705 [PMID: 12406889].

Kyono W: A practical approach to neutrophil disorders. Pediatr Clin North Am 2002;49:929 [PMID: 12430620].

LYMPHOCYTOSIS

From the first week up to the fifth year of life, lymphocytes are the most numerous leukocytes in human blood. The ratio then reverses gradually to reach the adult pattern of neutrophil predominance. An absolute lymphocytosis in childhood is associated with acute or chronic viral infections, pertussis, syphilis, tuberculosis, and hyperthyroidism. Other noninfectious conditions, drugs, and hypersensitivity and serum sickness-like reactions cause lymphocytosis.

Fever, upper respiratory symptoms, gastrointestinal complaints, and rashes are clues in distinguishing infectious from noninfectious causes. The presence of enlarged liver, spleen, or lymph nodes is crucial to the differential diagnosis, which includes acute leukemia and lymphoma. Most cases of infectious mononucleosis are associated with hepatosplenomegaly or adenopathy. The absence of anemia and thrombocytopenia helps to differentiate these disorders. Evaluation of the morphology of lymphocytes on peripheral blood smear is crucial. Infectious causes, particularly infectious mononucleosis, are associated with atypical features in the lymphocytes such as basophilic cytoplasm, vacuoles, finer and less-dense chromatin, and an indented nucleus. These features are distinct from the characteristic morphology associated with lymphoblastic leukemia. Lymphocytosis in childhood is most commonly associated with infections and resolves with recovery from the primary disease.

EOSINOPHILIA

Eosinophilia in infants and children is an absolute eosinophil count greater than 300/μL. Marrow eosinophil production is stimulated by the cytokine interleukin-5. Allergies, particularly eczema, are the most common primary causes of eosinophilia in children. Eosinophilia also occurs in drug reactions, with tumors (Hodgkin and non-Hodgkin lymphomas and brain tumors), and with immunodeficiency and histiocytosis syndromes. Increased eosinophil counts are a prominent feature of many invasive parasitic infections. Gastrointestinal disorders such as chronic hepatitis, ulcerative colitis, Crohn disease, and milk precipitin disease may be associated with eosinophilia. Increased blood eosinophil counts have been identified in several families without association with any specific illness. Rare causes of eosinophilia include the hypereosinophilic syndrome, characterized by counts greater than 1500/μL and organ involvement and damage (hepatosplenomegaly, cardiomyopathy, pulmonary fibrosis, and central nervous system injury). This is a disorder of middle-aged adults and is rare in children. Eosinophilic leukemia has been described, but its existence as a distinct entity is controversial.

Eosinophils are sometimes the last type of mature myeloid cell to disappear after marrow ablative chemotherapy. Increased eosinophil counts are associated with graft-versus-host disease after bone marrow transplantation, and elevations are sometimes documented during rejection episodes in patients who have solid organ grafts.

BLEEDING DISORDERS

Bleeding disorders may occur as a result of (1) quantitative or qualitative abnormalities of platelets, (2) quantitative or qualitative abnormalities in plasma procoagulant factors, (3) vascular abnormalities, or (4) accelerated fibrinolysis. The coagulation cascade and fibrinolytic system are shown in Figures 27–4 and 27–5.

The most critical aspect in evaluating the bleeding patient is obtaining detailed personal and family bleeding histories including manifestation of bleeding complications associated with dental interventions, surgeries, suture placement and removal, and trauma. Excessive mucosal bleeding is suggestive of a platelet disorder, von Willebrand disease, dysfibrinogenemia, or vasculitis. Bleeding into muscles and joints may be associated with a plasma procoagulant factor abnormality. In either sce-

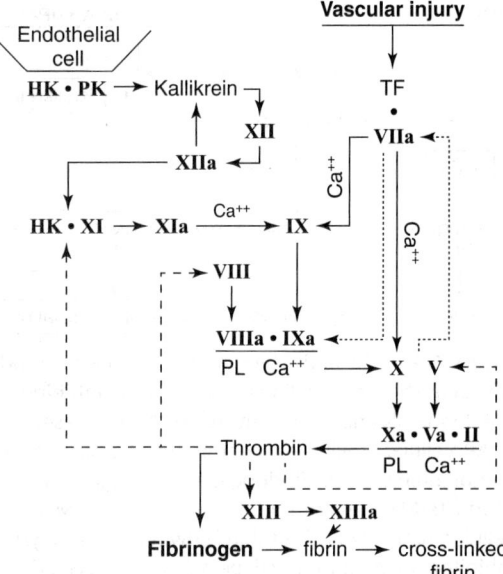

Figure 27–4. The procoagulant system and formation of a fibrin clot. Vascular injury initiates the coagulation process by exposure of tissue factor (TF); the dashed lines indicate thrombin actions in addition to clotting of fibrinogen. The finely dotted lines indicate the feedback activation of the VII-TF complex by Xa and IXa. HK, high molecular weight kininogen; PK, prekallikrein; Ca^{2+}, calcium; PL, phospholipid. (Reproduced, with permission, from Goodnight SH, Hathaway WE, editors: *Disorders of Hemostatis & Thrombosis: A Clinical Guide*, 2nd ed. McGraw-Hill, 2001.)

nario, the abnormality may be congenital or acquired. A thorough physical examination should be performed with special attention to the skin, oro- and nasopharynx, liver, spleen, and joints. Screening/diagnostic evaluation in patients with suspected bleeding disorders should initially include the following laboratory testing:

1. Prothrombin time (PT) to assess clotting function of factors VII, X, V, II, and fibrinogen.
2. Activated partial thromboplastin time (aPTT) to assess clotting function of high molecular weight kininogen, prekallikrein, XII, XI, IX, VIII, X, V, II, and fibrinogen.
3. Platelet count and size determined as part of a CBC.
4. Platelet functional assessment by platelet function analyzer-100 (PFA-100), or template bleeding time.

The following laboratory tests may also be useful:

1. Fibrinogen concentration.
2. Thrombin time to measure the generation of fibrin from fibrinogen following conversion of prothrom-

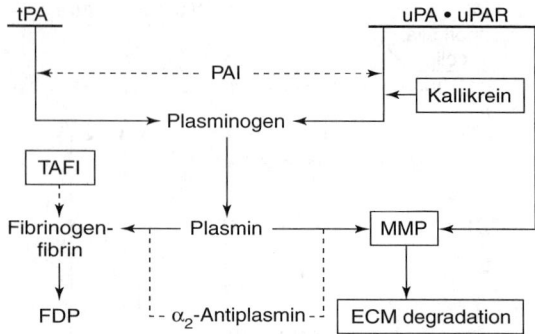

Figure 27–5. The fibrinolytic system. Solid arrows indicate activation; dotted line arrows indicate inhibition. tPA, tissue plasminogen activator; uPA, urokinase; uPAR, cellular urokinase receptor; PAI, plasminogen activator inhibitor; FDP, fibrinogen–fibrin degradation products; MMP, matrix metalloproteinases; ECM, extracellular matrix; TAFI, thrombin activatable fibrinolysis inhibitor. (Reproduced, with permission, from Goodnight SH, Hathaway WE, editors: *Disorders of Hemostatis & Thrombosis: A Clinical Guide,* 2nd ed. McGraw-Hill, 2001.)

bin to thrombin, as well as the antithrombin effects of fibrin-split products and heparin. The thrombin time may be prolonged in the setting of a normal fibrinogen concentration if the fibrinogen is dysfunctional (ie, dysfibrinogenemia).

3. Euglobulin lysis time (ELT), if available, to evaluate for accelerated fibrinolysis if the preceding work-up is nonrevealing despite documented history of pathological bleeding. If the ELT is shortened, assessment of plasminogen activator inhibitor-1 is warranted, as congenital deficiency in this fibrinolytic inhibitor may cause hyperfibrinolysis. In ill patients, measurement of fibrin degradation products may assist in the diagnosis of DIC.

Goodnight SH, Hathaway WE, eds: *Disorders of Hemostasis & Thrombosis: A Clinical Guide,* 2nd ed. New York: McGraw-Hill, 2001:41–51.

ABNORMALITIES OF PLATELET NUMBER OR FUNCTION

Thrombocytopenia in the pediatric age range is often immune-mediated (eg, idiopathic thrombocytopenic purpura, neonatal auto- or alloimmune thrombocytopenia, heparin-induced thrombocytopenia), but is also observed in consumptive coagulopathy (eg, DIC, Kasabach-Merrit syndrome), acute leukemias, rare disorders such as Wiskott-Aldrich syndrome and type IIb von Willebrand disease, and artifactually in automated cytometers (eg, Bernard–Soulier

syndrome), where giant forms may not be enumerated as platelets by automated cell counters.

1. Idiopathic Thrombocytopenic Purpura

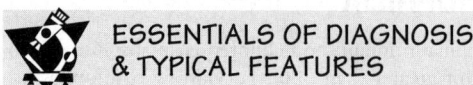

ESSENTIALS OF DIAGNOSIS & TYPICAL FEATURES

- *Otherwise healthy child.*
- *Decreased platelet count.*
- *Petechiae, ecchymoses.*

General Considerations

Acute idiopathic thrombocytopenic purpura (ITP) is the most common bleeding disorder of childhood. It occurs most frequently in children age 2–5 years and often follows infection with viruses such as rubella, varicella, measles, parvovirus, influenza, or EBV. Most patients recover spontaneously within a few months. Chronic ITP (> 6 months' duration) occurs in 10–20% of affected patients. The thrombocytopenia results from clearance of circulating IgM- or IgG-coated platelets by the reticuloendothelial system. The spleen plays a predominant role in the disease by forming the platelet cross-reactive antibodies and sequestering the antibody-bound platelets.

Clinical Findings

A. SYMPTOMS AND SIGNS

Onset of ITP is usually acute, with the appearance of multiple petechiae and ecchymoses. Epistaxis is also common at presentation. No other physical findings are usually present. Rarely, concurrent infection with EBV or CMV may cause hepatosplenomegaly or lymphadenopathy, simulating acute leukemia.

B. LABORATORY FINDINGS

1. Blood—The platelet count is markedly reduced (usually < 50,000/μL and often < 10,000/μL), and platelets frequently are of larger size on peripheral blood smear, suggesting accelerated production of new platelets. The white blood count and differential are normal, and the hemoglobin concentration is preserved unless hemorrhage has been significant.

2. Bone marrow—The number of megakaryocytes (which may be larger than normal) is increased. Erythroid and myeloid cellularity is normal.

3. Other laboratory tests—Platelet-associated IgG and/or IgM may be demonstrated on the patient's platelets or in the serum. PT and aPTT are normal.

Table 27–7. Common causes of thrombocytopenia.

Destruction			Decreased Production	
Antibody-Mediated	**Coagulopathy**	**Other**	**Congenital**	**Acquired**
Idiopathic thrombocytic purpura Infection Immunologic diseases	Disseminated intravascular coagulopathy Sepsis Necrotizing enterocolitis Thrombosis Cavernous hemangioma	Hemolytic-uremic syndrome Thrombotic thrombocytopenic purpura Hypersplenism Respiratory distress syndrome Wiskott-Aldrich syndrome	Fanconi anemia Wiskott-Aldrich syndrome Thrombocytopenia with absent radii Metabolic disorders Osteopetrosis	Aplastic anemia Leukemia and other malignancies Vitamin B_{12} and folate deficiencies

Differential Diagnosis

Table 27–7 lists common causes of thrombocytopenia. ITP is a diagnosis of exclusion. Family history or the finding of predominantly giant platelets on the peripheral blood smear is helpful in determining whether thrombocytopenia is hereditary. Bone marrow examination should be performed if the history is atypical (ie, the child is not otherwise healthy, or if there is a family history of bleeding), if abnormalities other than purpura and petechiae are present on physical examination, or if other cell lines are affected on the CBC. The importance of performing a bone marrow examination prior to using corticosteroids in the treatment for ITP is controversial.

Complications

Severe hemorrhage and bleeding into vital organs are the feared complications of ITP. Intracranial hemorrhage is the most serious but rarely seen complication, occurring in less than 1% of affected children. The most important risk factors for hemorrhage are a platelet count less than 10,000/μL and mean platelet volume less than 8 fL.

Treatment

A. General Measures

Most children require no therapy. Treatment should be given for bleeding, rather than for platelet count per se. Aspirin and other medications that compromise platelet function should be avoided. Bleeding precautions (eg, restriction from physical contact activities, use of helmets, etc) should be observed. Platelet transfusion should be avoided except in circumstances of life-threatening bleeding (wherein emergent splenectomy is to be pursued) or emergent surgery in the setting of severe thrombocytopenia.

B. Corticosteroids

Patients with clinically significant but non–life-threatening bleeding (ie, epistaxis, hematuria, and hematochezia) and those with a platelet count of less than 10,000/μL may benefit from prednisone at 2–4 mg/kg orally per day for 3–5 days, decreasing to 1–2 mg/kg/d for a total of 14 days. The dosage is then tapered and stopped. No further prednisone is given regardless of the platelet count unless significant bleeding recurs, at which time prednisone is administered in the smallest dose that achieves resolution of bleeding episodes (usually 2.5–5 mg twice daily). Follow-up continues until the steroid can again be discontinued, spontaneous remission occurs or other therapeutic measures are instituted.

C. Intravenous Immunoglobulin (IVIG)

IVIG is the treatment of choice for severe, life-threatening bleeding, and may also be used as an alternative or adjunct to corticosteroid treatment in both acute and chronic ITP of childhood. IVIG may be effective even when the patient is resistant to corticosteroids; responses are prompt and may last for several weeks. Most patients receive 1 g/kg/d for 1–3 days. Infusion time is typically 4–6 hours. Platelets may be given simultaneously during life-threatening hemorrhage, but are rapidly destroyed. Adverse effects of IVIG are common, including transient neurologic complications (eg, headache, nausea, and aseptic meningitis) in one-third of patients. These symptoms may mimic those of intracranial hemorrhage and necessitate radiologic evaluation of the brain. A transient decrease in neutrophil number may also be seen.

D. Anti-Rho(D) Immunoglobulin

This polyclonal immunoglobulin binds to the D antigen on red blood cells. The splenic clearance of anti-D-coated red cells interferes with removal of antibody-coated platelets, resulting in improvement in thrombocytopenia. This approach is effective only in Rh(+) patients with a functional spleen. The time required for platelet increase is slightly longer than with IVIG. However, approximately 80% of Rh(+) children with acute or chronic ITP respond well. Significant hemolysis may occur transiently with an average hemoglobin concentration decrease of 0.8 g/dL. However, severe hemolysis does occur in 5% of treated children, and clinical and laboratory evaluation approximately 5 days following administration is warranted in all patients. Although less expensive and time consuming to infuse than IVIG, Rho(D) immunoglobulin is more expensive than corticosteroids.

E. SPLENECTOMY

Most children with chronic ITP have platelet counts greater than 30,000/μL. Up to 70% of such children spontaneously recover with a platelet count greater than 100,000/μL within 1 year. For those who do not do so, corticosteroids, IVIG, and anti-D immunoglobulin are typically effective treatment for acute bleeding. Splenectomy produces a response in 70–90% but should be considered only after persistence of significant thrombocytopenia for at least 1 year. Preoperative treatment with corticosteroids, IVIG, or anti-D immunoglobulin is usually indicated. Postoperatively, the platelet count may rise to 1 million/μL, but is not often associated with thrombotic complications in the pediatric age group. The risk of overwhelming infection (predominantly with encapsulated organisms) is increased after splenectomy, particularly in the young child. Therefore, the procedure should be postponed, if possible, until the age of 5 years. Administration of pneumococcal and *Haemophilus influenzae* b vaccines at least 2 weeks prior to splenectomy is recommended. Meningococcal vaccine, although controversial, may be considered. Penicillin prophylaxis should be started postoperatively and continued for 1–3 years.

Prognosis

Ninety percent of children with ITP will have a spontaneous remission. Features associated with the development of chronic ITP include female gender, age greater than 10 years at presentation, insidious onset of bruising, and the presence of other autoantibodies. Older child- and adolescent-onset ITP is associated with an increased risk of chronic autoimmune diseases; appropriate screening by history and laboratory studies (eg, antinuclear antibody) is warranted.

Kaplan RN: Differential diagnosis and management of thrombocytopenia in childhood. Pediatr Clin North Am 2004;51:1109 [PMID: 15275991].

Tarantino MD: The pros and cons of drug therapy for immune thrombocytopenic purpura in children. Hematol Oncol Clin North Am 2004;18:1301 [PMID: 15511617].

2. Thrombocytopenia in the Newborn

Thrombocytopenia is one of the most common causes of neonatal hemorrhage and should be considered and investigated in any newborn with petechiae, purpura, or other significant bleeding. Defined as a platelet count less than 150,000/μL, thrombocytopenia occurs in approximately 0.9% of unselected neonates. A number of specific entities may be responsible (see Table 27–7); however, one-half of such neonates have alloimmune thrombocytopenia. Infection and DIC are the most common causes of thrombocytopenia in ill full-term newborns and in preterm newborns. In the healthy neonate, antibody-mediated thrombocytopenia (alloimmune or maternal autoimmune), viral syndromes, hyperviscosity, and major-vessel thrombosis are frequent causes of thrombocytopenia. Management is directed toward the underlying etiology.

Thrombocytopenia Associated with Platelet Alloantibodies (Neonatal *Allo*immune Thrombocytopenia)

Platelet alloimmunization occurs in 1 in approximately 350 pregnancies. Unlike in Rh incompatibility, 30–40% of affected neonates are first-born. Thrombocytopenia is progressive over the course of gestation and worse with each subsequent pregnancy. Alloimmunization occurs when a platelet antigen of the infant differs from that of the mother and the mother is sensitized by fetal platelets that cross the placenta into the maternal circulation. In Caucasians, alloimmune thrombocytopenia is most often due to HPA-1a incompatibility. Sensitization of a mother homozygous for human platelet antigen 1b to paternally acquired fetal HPA-1a antigen results in severe fetal thrombocytopenia in 1 in 1200 fetuses. Only 1 in 20 HPA-1a–positive fetuses of HPA-1a–negative mothers develop alloimmunization. The presence of antenatal maternal platelet antibodies on more than one occasion and persisting in the third trimester is predictive of severe neonatal thrombocytopenia; a weak or undetectable antibody does not exclude thrombocytopenia. Severe intracranial hemorrhage occurs in 10–30% of affected neonates as early as 20 weeks gestation. Petechiae or other bleeding manifestations are usually present shortly after birth. The disease is self-limited, and the platelet count normalizes within 4 weeks.

If alloimmunization is associated with clinically significant bleeding, transfusion of platelet concentrates harvested from the mother is more effective than random donor platelets in increasing the platelet count. Transfusion with HPA-matched platelets from unrelated donors or treatment with IVIG or methylprednisolone has also been successful in raising the platelet count and achieving hemostasis. If thrombocytopenia is not severe and bleeding is absent, observation alone is often appropriate.

Intracranial hemorrhage in a previous child secondary to alloimmune thrombocytopenia is the strongest risk factor for severe fetal thrombocytopenia and hemorrhage in a subsequent pregnancy. Amniocentesis or chorionic villus sampling to obtain fetal DNA for platelet antigen typing is sometimes performed if the father is heterozygous for HPA-1a. If alloimmunization has occurred with a previous pregnancy, irrespective of history of intracranial hemorrhage, screening cranial ultrasound for hemorrhage should begin at 20 weeks gestation and be repeated regularly. In addition, cordocentesis should be performed at approximately 20 weeks gestation, with prophylactic transfusion of irradiated, filtered, maternal platelet concentrates. If the fetal platelet count is less than 100,000/µL, the mother should be treated with weekly IVIG. Delivery by elective cesarean section is recommended if the fetal platelet count is less than 50,000/µL, to minimize the risk of intracranial hemorrhage associated with birth trauma.

Thrombocytopenia Associated with Idiopathic Thrombocytopenic Purpura in the Mother (Neonatal *Auto*immune Thrombocytopenia)

Infants born to mothers with ITP or other autoimmune diseases (eg, antiphospholipid antibody syndrome or systemic lupus erythematosus) may develop thrombocytopenia as a result of transfer of antiplatelet IgG from the mother to the infant. Unfortunately, maternal and fetal platelet counts and maternal antiplatelet antibody levels are unreliable predictors of bleeding risk. Antenatal corticosteroid administration to the mother is generally instituted once maternal platelet count falls below 50,000/µL, with or without a concomitant course of IVIG.

Most neonates with neonatal autoimmune thrombocytopenia do not develop clinically significant bleeding, and thus treatment for thrombocytopenia is not often required. The risk of intracranial hemorrhage is 0.2–2%. If diffuse petechiae or minor bleeding are evident, a 1- to 2-week course of oral prednisone, 2 mg/kg/d, may be administered. If the platelet count remains consistently less than 20,000/µL or if severe hemorrhage develops, IVIG should be given (1 g/kg daily for 1–3 days). Platelet transfusions are only indicated for life-threatening bleeding, and may only be effective after removal of antibody by exchange transfusion. The platelet nadir is typically between the 4th to 6th day of life, improves significantly by 1 month, and full recovery may take 2–4 months. Platelet recovery may be delayed in breast-fed infants because of transfer of IgG to the milk.

Neonatal Thrombocytopenia Associated with Infections

Thrombocytopenia is commonly associated with severe generalized infections during the newborn period. Between 50% and 75% of neonates with bacterial sepsis are thrombocytopenic. Intrauterine infections such as rubella, syphilis, toxoplasmosis, CMV, herpes simplex, enteroviruses, and parvovirus are often associated with thrombocytopenia. In addition to specific treatment for the underlying disease, platelet transfusions may be indicated in severe cases.

Thrombocytopenia Associated with Kaposiform Hemangioendotheliomas (Kasabach–Merritt Syndrome)

A rare but important cause of thrombocytopenia in the newborn is kaposiform hemangioendotheliomas, a benign neoplasm with distinct histopathology from that of classic infantile hemangiomas. Intense platelet sequestration in the lesion results in peripheral thrombocytopenia and may rarely be associated with a DIC-like picture and hemolytic anemia. The bone marrow typically shows megakaryocytic hyperplasia in response to the thrombocytopenia. Treatment with corticosteroids, α-interferon, and vincristine have all been shown to be useful to reduce the size of the lesion and are indicated if significant coagulopathy is present, the lesion compresses a vital structure, or the lesion is cosmetically unacceptable. If consumptive coagulopathy is present heparin or aminocaproic acid may be useful. Depending on the site, embolization may be tried. Surgery is often a last resort, due to the high risk of hemorrhage.

Hall GW: Kasabach–Merritt syndrome: Pathogenesis and management. Br J Haematol 2001;112:851 [PMID: 11298580].

Kaplan RN: Differential diagnosis and management of thrombocytopenia in childhood. Pediatr Clin North Am 2004;51:1109 [PMID: 15275991].

3. Disorders of Platelet Function

Individuals with platelet function defects typically develop skin and mucosal bleeding similar to that occurring in persons with thrombocytopenia. Historically, platelet function has been screened by measurement of the bleeding time. If the bleeding time is prolonged, in vitro platelet aggregation is then studied using agonists such as adenosine diphosphate, collagen, arachidonic acid, and ristocetin, with simultaneous comparison to a normal control subject. While labor-intensive, platelet aggregometry remains important in selected clinical situations. The PFA-100 has become available for evaluation of platelet dysfunction and von Willebrand disease, and has largely replaced the template bleeding time in many clinical laboratories. Unfortunately, none of these tests of platelet function is uniformly predictive of clinical bleeding severity.

Platelet dysfunction may be inherited or acquired, with the latter being more common. Acquired disorders of platelet function may occur secondary to uremia, cirrhosis, sepsis, myeloproliferative disorders, congenital heart disease, and viral infections. Many pharmacologic agents decrease platelet function. The most common offending agents in the pediatric population are aspirin and other nonsteroidal anti-inflammatory drugs (NSAIDs), synthetic penicillins, and valproic acid. In acquired platelet dysfunction, the PFA-100 closure time is typically prolonged with collagen-epinephrine but normal with collagen-ADP.

The inherited disorders are due to defects in platelet–vessel interaction, platelet–platelet interaction, platelet granule content or release (the latter including defects of signal transduction), thromboxane and arachidonic acid pathway, and platelet-procoagulant protein interaction. Individuals with hereditary platelet dysfunction generally have a prolonged bleeding time with normal platelet number and morphology by light microscopy. PFA-100 closure time, in contrast to that in acquired dysfunction, is typically prolonged with collagen-ADP in addition to collagen-epinephrine.

Congenital causes of defective platelet–vessel wall interaction include Bernard–Soulier syndrome. This condition is characterized by increased platelet size and decreased platelet number. The molecular defect in this autosomal recessive disorder is a deficiency or dysfunction of glycoprotein Ib-V-IX complex on the platelet surface resulting in impaired von Willebrand factor (vWF) binding, and hence, impaired platelet adhesion to the vascular endothelium.

Glanzmann thrombasthenia is an example of platelet-platelet dysfunction. In this autosomal recessive disorder, glycoprotein IIb–IIIa is deficient or dysfunctional. Platelets do not bind fibrinogen effectively and exhibit impaired aggregation. As in Bernard-Soulier syndrome, acute bleeding is treated by platelet transfusion.

Disorders involving platelet granule content include storage pool disease and Quebec platelet disorder. In individuals with storage pool disease, platelet-dense granules lack adenosine dinucleotide phosphate and adenosine trinucleotide phosphate and are often found to be low in number by electron microscopy. These granules are also deficient in Hermansky–Pudlak, Chédiak–Higashi, and Wiskott–Aldrich syndromes. Whereas deficiency of α-granules results in the gray platelet syndrome, Quebec platelet disorder is characterized by a normal platelet α-granule number, but with abnormal proteolysis of α-granule proteins and deficiency of platelet α-granule multimerin. Epinephrine-induced platelet aggregation is markedly impaired.

Platelet dysfunction has also been observed in other congenital syndromes, such as Down and Noonan syndromes, without a clear understanding of the molecular platelet defect.

Treatment

Acute bleeding in many individuals with acquired or selected congenital platelet function defects responds to therapy with desmopressin acetate, likely due to an induced release of vWF from endothelial stores. If this therapy is ineffective, or in the case of Bernard-Soulier and Glanzmann syndromes, the mainstay of treatment for bleeding episodes is platelet transfusion. Recombinant VIIa has variable efficacy and is not preferable to platelet transfusion.

Drachman JG: Inherited thrombocytopenia: When a low platelet count does not mean ITP. Blood 2004;103:390 [PMID: 14505084].

Sohal AS: Uremic bleeding: Pathophysiology and clinical risk factors. Thromb Res 2005;June 30 [Epub ahead of print] [PMID: 15993929].

INHERITED BLEEDING DISORDERS

Table 27–8 lists normal values for coagulation factors. The more common factor deficiencies are discussed in this section. Individuals with bleeding disorders should avoid exposure to medications that inhibit platelet function. Participation in contact sports such as football and ice hockey should be considered in the context of the severity of the bleeding disorder.

1. Factor VIII Deficiency (Hemophilia A, Classic Hemophilia)

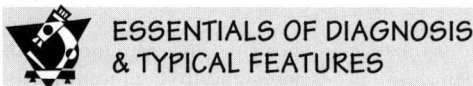

ESSENTIALS OF DIAGNOSIS & TYPICAL FEATURES

- Bruising, soft-tissue bleeding, hemarthrosis.
- Prolonged activated partial thromboplastin time (aPTT).
- Reduced factor VIII activity.

General Considerations

Factor VIII activity is reported in units per milliliter, with 1 unit/mL equal to 100% of the factor activity found in 1 mL of normal plasma. The normal range for factor VIII activity is 0.5–1.5 U/mL (50–150%). Hemophilia A occurs predominantly in males as an X-

Table 27–8. Physiologic alterations in measurements of the hemostatic system.

Measurement	Normal Adults	Fetus (20 wk)	Preterm (25–32 wk)	Term Infant	Infant (6 mo)	Pregnancy (term)	Exercise (acute)	Aging (70–80 y)
Platelets								
Count μL/10³	250	107–297	293	332	—	260	↑18–40%	225
Size (fL)	9.0	8.9	8.5	9.1	—	9.6	↑	—
Aggregation ADP	N	+	↓	↓	—	↑	↓15%	—
Collagen	N	↓	↓	↓	—	N	↓60%	N
Ristocetin	N	—	↑	↑	—	—	↓10%	—
BT (min)	2–9	—	3.6±2	3.4±1.8	—	9.0±1.4	—	5.6
Procoagulant System								
PTT*	1	4.0	3	1.3	1.1	1.1	↓15%	↓
PT*	1.00	2.3	1.3	1.1	1	0.95	N	—
TCT*	1	2.4	1.3	1.1	1	0.92	N	—
Fibrinogen mg/dL	278 (0.61)	96 (50)	250 (100)	240 (150)	251 (160)	450 (100)	↓25%	↑15%
II, U/mL	1 (0.7)	0.16 (0.10)	0.32 (0.18)	0.52 (0.25)	0.88 (0.6)	1.15 (0.68–1.9)	—	N
V, U/mL	1.0 (0.6)	0.32 (0.21)	0.80 (0.43)	1.00 (0.54)	0.91 (0.55)	0.85 (0.40–1.9)	—	N
VII, U/mL	1.0 (0.6)	0.27 (0.17)	0.37 (0.24)	0.57 (0.35)	0.87 (0.50)	1.17 (0.87–3.3)	↑200%	↑25%
VIIIc, U/mL	1.0 (0.6)	0.50 (0.23)	0.75 (0.40)	1.50 (0.55)	0.90 (0.50)	2.12 (0.8–6.0)	↑250%	1.50
vWF, U/mL	1.0 (0.6)	0.65 (0.40)	1.50 (0.90)	1.60 (0.84)	1.07 (0.60)	1.7	↑75–200%	↑
IX, U/mL	1.0 (0.5)	0.10 (0.05)	0.22 (0.17)	0.35 (0.15)	0.86 (0.36)	0.81–2.15	↑25%	1.0–1.40
X, U/mL	1.0 (0.6)	0.19 (0.15)	0.38 (0.20)	0.45 (0.3)	0.78 (0.38)	1.30	—	N
XI, U/mL	1.0 (0.6)	0.13 (0.08)	0.2 (0.12)	0.42 (0.20)	0.86 (0.38)	0.7	—	N
XII, U/mL	1.0 (0.6)	0.15 (0.08)	0.22 (0.09)	0.44 (0.16)	0.77 (0.39)	1.3 (0.82)	—	↑16%
XIII, U/mL	1.04 (0.55)	0.30	0.4	0.61 (0.36)	1.04 (0.50)	0.96	—	—
PreK, U/mL	1.12 (0.06)	0.13 (0.08)	0.26 (0.14)	0.35 (0.16)	0.86 (0.56)	1.18	—	↑27%
HK, U/mL	0.92 (0.48)	0.15 (0.10)	0.28 (0.20)	0.64 (0.50)	0.82 (0.36)	1.6	—	↑32%
Anticoagulant System								
AT-U/mL	1.0	0.23	0.35	0.56	1.04	1.02	↑14%	N
α₂MG, U/mL	1.05 (0.79)	0.18 (0.10)	—	1.39 (0.95)	1.91 (1.49)	1.53 (0.85)	—	—
C1IN, U/mL	1.01	—	—	0.72	1.41	—	—	—
PC, U/mL	1.0	0.10	0.29	0.50	0.59	0.99	N	N
Total PS, U/mL	1.0 (0.6)	0.15 (0.11)	0.17 (0.14)	0.24 (0.1)	0.87 (0.55)	0.89	—	N
Free, PS, U/mL	1.0 (0.5)	0.22 (0.13)	0.28 (0.19)	0.49 (0.33)	—	0.25	—	—
Heparin	1.01	0.10 (0.06)	0.25 (0.10)	0.49 (0.33)	0.97 (0.59)	—	—	↓15%
Cofactor II, U/mL	(0.73)							
TFPI, ng/mL	73	21	20.6	38	—	—	—	—
Fibrinolytic System								
Plasminogen U/mL	1.0	0.20	0.35 (0.20)	0.37 (0.18)	0.90	1.39	↓10%	N
t-PA, ng/mL	4.9	—	8.48	9.6	2.8	4.9	↑300%	N
α₂-AP, U/mL	1.0	1.0	0.74 (0.5)	0.83 (0.65)	1.11 (0.83)	0.95	N	N
PAI-1, U/mL	1.0	—	1.5	1.0	1.07	4.0	↓5%	N
Overall fibrinolysis	N	↑	↑	↑	—	↓	↑	↓

Except as otherwise indicated values are mean ±2 SD or values in () are lower limits (–2SD or lower range); +, positive or present; ↓, decreased; ↑, increased; N, normal or no change; *, values as ratio or subject/mean of reference range; ADP, adenosine diphosphate; BT, bleeding time; PTT, partial thromboplastin time; PT, prothrombin time; TCT, thrombin clotting time; vWF, von Willebrand factor; PreK, prekallikrein; HK, high molecular weight kininogen; AT, antithrombin; α₂-MG, α₂-macroglobulin; C1IN, C1 esterase inhibitor; PC, protein C; PS, protein S; TFPI, tissue factor pathway inhibitor; t-PA, tissue plasminogen activator; α₂-AP, α₂-antiplasmin; PAI, plasminogen activator inhibitor. Overall fibrinolysis is measured by euglobulin lysis time.
Adapted, with permission, from Goodnight SH, Hathaway WE (editors): *Disorders of Hemostasis & Thrombosis: A Clinical Guide.* McGraw-Hill, 2001.

linked disorder. One-third of cases are due to a new mutation. The incidence of factor VIII deficiency is 1:5000 male births.

Clinical Findings

A. SYMPTOMS AND SIGNS

Patients with severe hemophilia A (< 1% plasma factor VIII activity) have frequent spontaneous bleeding episodes involving skin, mucous membranes, joints, muscles, and viscera. In contrast, patients with mild hemophilia A (5–40% factor VIII activity) bleed only at times of trauma or surgery. Those with moderate hemophilia A (1– < 5% factor VIII activity) typically have intermediate bleeding manifestations. The most crippling aspect of factor VIII deficiency is the tendency to develop recurrent hemarthroses that incite joint destruction.

B. LABORATORY FINDINGS

Individuals with hemophilia A have a prolonged aPTT, except in some cases of mild deficiency. The prothrombin time (PT) is normal. The diagnosis is confirmed by finding decreased factor VIII activity with normal vWF activity. In two-thirds of families of hemophilic patients, the females are carriers and some are mildly symptomatic. Carriers of hemophilia can be detected by determination of the ratio of factor VIII activity to vWF antigen and by molecular genetic techniques. In a male fetus or newborn with a family history of hemophilia A, cord blood sampling for factor VIII activity is accurate and important in subsequent care.

Complications

Intracranial hemorrhage is the leading disease-related cause of death among patients with hemophilia. Up to 80% of intracranial hemorrhages are spontaneous (ie, not associated with trauma). Hemarthroses begin early in childhood and, if recurrent, result in joint destruction (ie, hemophilic arthropathy). Large intramuscular hematomas can lead to a compartment syndrome with resultant muscle and nerve death. Although these complications are most common in severe hemophiliacs, they may be experienced by individuals with moderate or mild disease. A serious complication of hemophilia is the development of an acquired circulating antibody to factor VIII after treatment with factor VIII concentrate. Such factor VIII inhibitors develop in 15–25% of patients with severe hemophilia A, and may be amenable to desensitization and immunosuppressive therapy. In recent years, recombinant factor VIIa has become a therapy of choice for treatment of acute hemorrhage in patients with hemophilia A and a high-titer inhibitor.

In prior decades, therapy-related complications in hemophilia A have included infection with the human immunodeficiency virus (HIV), hepatitis B virus (HBV), and hepatitis C virus (HCV). Through more stringent donor selection, the implementation of sensitive screening assays, the use of heat- or chemical viral inactivation methods, and the development of recombinant products, the risks of these infections have been eliminated. Inactivation methods do not eradicate viruses lacking a lipid envelope, however, so that transmission of parvovirus and hepatitis A remains a concern with the use of plasma-derived products. Immunization with hepatitis A and hepatitis B vaccines is recommended for all hemophilia patients.

Treatment

The general aim of management is to correct the factor VIII activity to within normal limits in order to prevent or stop bleeding. Some patients with mild factor VIII deficiency may respond to desmopressin via release of endothelial stores of factor VIII and vWF into plasma; however, most patients require administration of exogenous factor VIII to achieve hemostasis. The in vivo half-life of factor VIII is generally 8–12 hours, but may exhibit considerable variation among individuals depending on comorbid conditions. Non–life-threatening, non–limb-threatening hemorrhage is typically treated initially with 20–30 units of factor VIII per kilogram of body weight, to achieve a rise in plasma factor VIII activity to 40–60%. Large joint hemarthrosis and life- or limb-threatening hemorrhage is treated initially with approximately 50 U/kg factor VIII, targeting a rise to 100% factor VIII activity. Subsequent doses are determined according to the site and extent of bleeding and the clinical response and doses are rounded to the nearest whole vial size with excess factor VIII infused, not discarded. In circumstances of suboptimal clinical response, recent change in bleeding frequency, or comorbid illness, monitoring the plasma factor VIII activity response may be warranted. For most instances of non–life-threatening hemorrhage in experienced patients with moderate or severe hemophilia A, treatment can be administered at home, provided adequate intravenous access exists and close contact is maintained with the hemophilia clinician team.

Prophylactic factor VIII infusions (eg, two or three times weekly) may prevent the development of arthropathy in severe hemophiliacs, and is becoming more common in pediatric hemophilia care.

Prognosis

The development of safe and effective therapies for hemophilia A has resulted in improved long-term survival in recent decades. In addition, more aggressive management and the coordination of comprehensive care through hemophilia centers has the prospect of a greatly improved quality of life and level of function.

DiMichele D: Inhibitors in haemophilia: Clinical aspects. Haemophilia 2004;10(Suppl 4):140 [PMID: 15479387].

Dunn AL: Recent advances in the management of the child who has hemophilia. Hematol Oncol Clin North Am 2004;24:83 [PMID: 12612185].

2. Factor IX Deficiency (Hemophilia B, Christmas Disease)

The mode of inheritance and clinical manifestations of factor IX deficiency are the same as those of factor VIII deficiency. Hemophilia B is 15–20% as prevalent as hemophilia A. As in factor VIII deficiency, factor IX deficiency is associated with a prolonged aPTT, but the PT and thrombin time are normal. However, the aPTT is slightly less sensitive to factor IX deficiency than factor VIII deficiency. Diagnosis of hemophilia B is made by assaying factor IX activity, and severity is determined similarly to factor VIII deficiency. In general, clinical bleeding severity appears to correlate less well with factor activity in hemophilia B than hemophilia A.

The mainstay of treatment in hemophilia B is exogenous factor IX. Unlike factor VIII, about 50% of the administered dose of factor IX diffuses into the extravascular space. Therefore, one unit of plasma-derived factor IX concentrate or recombinant factor IX per kilogram is expected to increase plasma factor IX activity by approximately 1%. Factor IX typically has a half-life of 20–22 hours in vivo, but due to variability, therapeutic monitoring may be warranted. Similarly, as for factor VIII products, viral inactivation techniques for plasma-derived factor IX concentrates appear effective in eradicating HIV, HBV, and HCV. Only 1–3% of persons with factor IX deficiency develop an inhibitor to factor IX, but may be at risk for anaphylaxis when receiving exogenous factor IX. The prognosis for persons with factor IX deficiency is comparable to those with factor VIII deficiency. Gene therapy research efforts are ongoing for both hemophilias.

Shapiro AD: Hemophilia B (factor IX deficiency). In: Goodnight SH, Hathaway WE, editors. *Disorders of Hemostasis & Thrombosis: A Clinical Guide,* 2nd ed. New York: McGraw-Hill, 2001:140–148.

Shapiro AD: The safety and efficacy of recombinant human blood coagulation factor IX in previously untreated patients with severe or moderately severe hemophilia B. Blood 2005;105:518 [PMID: 15383463].

3. Factor XI Deficiency (Hemophilia C)

Factor XI deficiency is a genetic, autosomally transmitted coagulopathy typically of mild to moderate clinical severity. Cases of factor XI deficiency account for less than 5% of all hemophilia patients. Homozygotes generally bleed at surgery or following severe trauma but do not commonly have spontaneous hemarthroses. In contrast to factor VIII and IX deficiencies, factor XI activity is least predictive of bleeding risk. Although typically mild, pathologic bleeding may

be seen in heterozygous individuals with factor XI activity as high as 60%. The aPTT is often considerably prolonged. In individuals with deficiency of both plasma and platelet-associated factor XI, the PFA-100 may also be prolonged. Management typically consists of perioperative prophylaxis and episodic therapy for acute hemorrhage. Treatment includes infusion of fresh frozen plasma (FFP); platelet transfusion may also be useful for acute hemorrhage in patients with deficiency of platelet-associated factor XI. Desmopressin has been used in some cases. The prognosis for an average life span in patients with factor XI deficiency is excellent.

Salomon O: New observations on factor XI deficiency. Haemophilia 2004;10(Suppl 4):184 [PMID: 15479396].

4. Other Inherited Bleeding Disorders

Other hereditary single clotting factor deficiencies are rare. Transmission is generally autosomal. Homozygous individuals with a deficiency or structural abnormality of prothrombin, factor V, factor VII, or factor X may have excessive bleeding.

Persons with dysfibrinogenemia (ie, structurally and/or functionally abnormal fibrinogen) are usually asymptomatic but may develop recurrent venous thromboembolic episodes or bleeding. Immunologic assay of fibrinogen are normal, but the thrombin time is prolonged, as may also be the PT and aPTT. Cryoprecipitate, which is rich in fibrinogen, is the treatment of choice, given the present lack of availability of a plasma-derived or recombinant fibrinogen product in the United States.

Afibrinogenemia resembles hemophilia clinically but has an autosomal recessive inheritance. Affected patients can experience a variety of bleeding manifestations, including mucosal bleeding, ecchymoses, hematomas, hemarthroses, and intracranial hemorrhage, especially following trauma. Fatal umbilical cord hemorrhage has been reported in neonates. The PT, aPTT, and thrombin time are all prolonged. A severely reduced fibrinogen concentration in an otherwise well child is confirmatory of the diagnosis. As in dysfibrinogenemia, cryoprecipitate infusion is used for surgical prophylaxis and treatment for acute hemorrhage.

Bolton-Maggs PH: The rare coagulation disorders—Review with guidelines for management from the United Kingdom Haemophila Centre Doctors' Organisation. Haemophilia 2004;10:593 [PMID: 15357789].

VON WILLEBRAND DISEASE

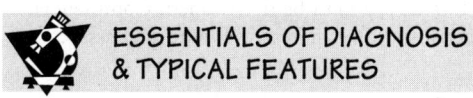

ESSENTIALS OF DIAGNOSIS & TYPICAL FEATURES

- *Easy bruising and epistaxis from early childhood.*
- *Menorrhagia.*

- *Prolonged PFA-100 (or bleeding time); normal platelet count; the absence of acquired platelet dysfunction.*
- *Reduced activity or abnormal structure of vWF.*

General Considerations

von Willebrand disease (vWD) is the most common inherited bleeding disorder among Caucasians, with a prevalence of 1%. It is caused by a quantitative or qualitative deficiency of vWF. vWF is a protein present as a multimeric complex in plasma, which binds factor VIII and also is a cofactor for platelet adhesion to the endothelium. Seventy to eighty percent of all patients with vWD have classic vWD (type 1). vWD type 1 is caused by a partial quantitative deficiency of vWF, type 2 involves a qualitative deficiency of (ie, dysfunctional) vWF, and type 3 is characterized by a nearly complete deficiency of vWF. The majority (> 90%) of individuals with type 1 disease are asymptomatic. vWD is most often transmitted as an autosomal dominant trait, but can be autosomal recessive. The disease can also be acquired, developing in association with hypothyroidism, Wilms tumor, cardiac disease, renal disease, or systemic lupus erythematosus and in individuals receiving valproic acid. Acquired vWD is most often caused by the development of an antibody to vWF.

Clinical Findings

A. SYMPTOMS AND SIGNS

A history of increased bruising and excessive epistaxis is often present. Prolonged bleeding also occurs with trauma or at surgery. Menorrhagia is often a presenting finding in females.

B. LABORATORY FINDINGS

The PT is normal, and the aPTT is sometimes prolonged. A prolongation of the PFA-100 or bleeding is usually present since vWF plays a role in platelet adherence to endothelium. Platelet number may be decreased in types 2 and 3. Factor VIII and vWF antigen are decreased in types 1 and 3, but may be normal in type 2 vWD. vWF activity (eg, ristocetin cofactor activity) is decreased in all types. Since normal vWF antigen levels vary by blood type (with type O normally having lower levels), blood type must be determined. Complete laboratory classification requires vWF multimer assay.

Treatment

The treatment to prevent or halt bleeding for most patients with vWD types 1 and 2 is desmopressin acetate,

which causes release of vWF from endothelial stores. Desmopressin may be administered intravenously at a dose of 0.3 µg/kg diluted in at least 20–30 mL of normal saline and given over 20–30 minutes. This dose typically elicits a three- to fivefold rise in plasma vWF. A high-concentration desmopressin nasal spray (150 µg/spray), different than the preparation used for enuresis, may alternatively be used. Because vWF response is variable among patients, factor VIII and vWF activities are typically measured before and 60 minutes after infusion, if no recent response has been measured. Desmopressin may cause fluid shifts, hyponatremia, and seizures in children under 2 years of age. Because stored vWF release is limited, tachyphylaxis often occurs with desmopressin. If further therapy is indicated, vWF-replacement therapy (eg, plasma-derived concentrate) is recommended; such therapy is also used in patients with type 1 or 2a vWD who exhibit suboptimal laboratory response to desmopressin, and for all individuals with type 2b or 3 vWD. Antifibrinolytic agents (eg, ε-aminocaproic acid) may be useful for control of mucosal bleeding. Topical thrombin and fibrin glue may also be of benefit. Estrogen-containing contraceptive therapy may be helpful for menorrhagia.

Prognosis

With the availability of effective treatment and prophylaxis for bleeding, life expectancy in vWD is normal.

Cox Gill J: Diagnosis and treatment of von Willebrand disease. Hematol Oncol Clin North Am 2004;18:1277 [PMID: 15511616].

Mannucci PM: Treatment of von Willebrand's disease. N Engl J Med 2004;351:683 [PMID: 15306670].

ACQUIRED BLEEDING DISORDERS

1. Disseminated Intravascular Coagulation (DIC)

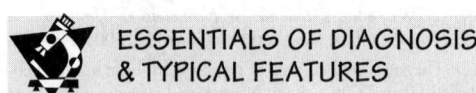 ESSENTIALS OF DIAGNOSIS & TYPICAL FEATURES

- *Presence of disorder known to trigger DIC.*
- *Evidence for consumptive coagulopathy (prolonged aPTT, PT, and/or thrombin time; increase in FSP (fibrin-fibrinogen split products); decreased fibrinogen or platelets).*

General Considerations

DIC is an acquired pathologic process characterized by tissue factor-mediated diffuse coagulation activation in the host. DIC involves dysregulated, excessive thrombin generation, with consequent intravascular fibrin deposition and consumption of platelets and procoagulant factors. Microthrombi, composed of fibrin and platelets, may produce tissue ischemia and end-organ damage. The fibrinolytic system is frequently activated in DIC, leading to plasmin-mediated destruction of fibrin and fibrinogen; this results in fibrin-fibrinogen degradation products (FDPs) which exhibit anticoagulant and platelet-inhibitory functions. DIC commonly accompanies severe infection and other critical illnesses in infants and children. Conditions known to trigger DIC include endothelial damage (eg, endotoxin, virus), tissue necrosis (eg, burns), diffuse ischemic injury (eg, shock, hypoxia acidosis), and systemic release of tissue procoagulants (eg, certain cancers, placental disorders).

Clinical Findings

A. SYMPTOMS AND SIGNS

Signs of DIC may include: (1) signs of shock, often including end-organ dysfunction; (2) diffuse bleeding tendency (eg, hematuria, melena, purpura, petechiae, persistent oozing from needle punctures or other invasive procedures); and (3) evidence of thrombotic lesions (eg, major vessel thrombosis, purpura fulminans).

B. LABORATORY FINDINGS

Tests that are most sensitive, easiest to perform, most useful for monitoring, and best reflect the hemostatic capacity of the patient are the PT, aPTT, platelet count, fibrinogen, and fibrin–fibrinogen split products. The PT and aPTT are typically prolonged and the platelet count and fibrinogen concentration may be decreased. However, in children, the fibrinogen level may be normal until late in the course. Levels of fibrin–fibrinogen split products are increased, and elevated levels of D-dimer, a cross-linked fibrin degradation byproduct, may be helpful in monitoring the degree of activation of both coagulation and fibrinolysis. However, D-dimer is nonspecific and may be elevated in the context of a triggering event (eg, severe infection) without concomitant DIC. Often, physiologic inhibitors of coagulation, especially antithrombin III and protein C, are consumed, predisposing to thrombosis. The specific laboratory abnormalities in DIC may vary with the triggering event and the course of illness.

Differential Diagnosis

DIC can be difficult to distinguish from coagulopathy of liver disease (ie, hepatic synthetic dysfunction), especially when the latter is associated with thrombocytopenia secondary to portal hypertension and hypersplenism. Generally, factor VII activity is decreased markedly in liver disease (due to deficient synthesis of this protein, which has the

shortest half-life among the procoagulant factors) but only mildly to moderately decreased in DIC (due to consumption). Factor VIII activity is often normal or even increased in liver disease, but decreased in DIC.

Treatment

A. THERAPY FOR UNDERLYING DISORDER

The most important aspect of therapy in DIC is the identification and treatment of the triggering event. If the pathogenic process underlying DIC is reversed, often no other therapy is needed for the coagulopathy.

B. REPLACEMENT THERAPY FOR CONSUMPTIVE COAGULOPATHY

Replacement of consumed procoagulant factors with FFP and of platelets via platelet transfusion is warranted in the setting of DIC with hemorrhagic complications, or as periprocedural bleeding prophylaxis. Infusion of 10–15 mL/kg FFP typically raises procoagulant factor activities by approximately 10–15%. Cryoprecipitate can also be given as a rich source of fibrinogen; one bag of cryoprecipitate per 3 kg in infants or one bag of cryoprecipitate per 6 kg in older children typically raises plasma fibrinogen concentration by 75–100 mg/dL.

C. ANTICOAGULANT THERAPY FOR COAGULATION ACTIVATION

Continuous intravenous infusion of unfractionated heparin is sometimes given in order to attenuate coagulation activation and consequent consumptive coagulopathy. The rationale for heparin therapy is to maximize the efficacy of, and minimize the need for, replacement of procoagulants and platelets; however, clinical evidence demonstrating benefit of heparin in DIC is lacking. Heparin dosing is provided in the section on thrombosis treatment.

D. SPECIFIC FACTOR CONCENTRATES

A nonrandomized pilot study of antithrombin concentrate in children with DIC and associated acquired antithrombin deficiency demonstrated favorable outcomes, suggesting that replacement of this consumed procoagulant may be of benefit. Protein C concentrate has also shown promise in two small pilot studies of meningococcal-associated DIC with purpura fulminans. Activated protein C has reduced mortality in septic adults in a large randomized multicenter trial; an international pediatric trial is ongoing.

2. Liver Disease

The liver is the major synthetic site of prothrombin, fibrinogen, high molecular weight kininogen, and factors V, VII, IX, X, XI, XII, and XIII. In addition, plasminogen and the physiologic anticoagulants (antithrombin III, protein C, and protein S) are hepatically synthesized. α_2-Antiplasmin, a regulator of fibrinolysis, is also produced in the liver. Deficiency of factor V and the vitamin K–dependent factors (II, VII, IX, and X) is most often a result of decreased hepatic synthesis and is manifested by a prolonged PT and often a prolonged aPTT. Extravascular loss and increased consumption of clotting factors may contribute to PT and aPTT prolongation. Fibrinogen production is often decreased, and/or an abnormal fibrinogen (dysfibrinogen) containing excess sialic acid residues may be synthesized. Hypo/dysfibrinogenemia is associated with prolongation of thrombin time and reptilase time. FDPs and D-dimers may be present because of increased fibrinolysis, particularly in the setting of chronic hepatitis/cirrhosis. Thrombocytopenia secondary to hypersplenism may occur. Distinction between DIC and coagulopathy of liver disease may also mimic vitamin K deficiency; the latter may be distinguished by normal factor V activity. Treatment of acute bleeding in the setting of coagulopathy of liver disease consists of replacement with FFP and platelets. Desmopressin may shorten the bleeding time and aPTT in patients with chronic liver disease, but its safety has not been well established. Recombinant VIIa also has been shown to be efficacious for life-threatening hemorrhage.

3. Vitamin K Deficiency

The newborn period is characterized by physiologically depressed activity of the vitamin K–dependent factors (II, VII, IX, and X). If vitamin K is not administered at birth, a bleeding diathesis previously called hemorrhagic disease of the newborn, now termed *vitamin K deficiency bleeding (VKDB)*, may develop. Outside of the newborn period, vitamin K deficiency may occur as a consequence of inadequate intake, excess loss, inadequate formation of active metabolites, or competitive antagonism.

One of three patterns is seen in the neonatal period:

1. Early VKDB of the newborn occurs within 24 hours of birth and is most often manifested by cephalohematoma, intracranial hemorrhage, or intra-abdominal bleeding. Although occasionally idiopathic, it is most often associated with maternal ingestion of drugs that interfere with vitamin K metabolism (eg, warfarin, phenytoin, isoniazid, and rifampin). Early VKDB occurs in 6–12% of neonates born to mothers taking these medications but not receiving vitamin K supplementation. The disorder is often life-threatening.

2. Classic VKDB of the newborn occurs at 24 hours to 7 days of age and usually is manifested as gastrointestinal, skin, or mucosal bleeding. Bleeding after circumcision may occur. Although occasionally associated with maternal drug usage, it most often occurs in well babies who do not receive vitamin K at birth and are solely breast-fed.

3. Late neonatal VKDB occurs on or after day 8. Manifestations include intracranial, gastrointestinal, or skin bleeding. This disorder is often associated with fat malabsorption (eg, in chronic diarrhea) or alterations in intestinal flora (eg, with prolonged antibiotic therapy). Like classic VKDB, late VKDB occurs almost exclusively in breast-fed infants.

The diagnosis of vitamin K deficiency is suspected based on the history, physical examination, and laboratory results. The PT is prolonged out of proportion to the aPTT (also prolonged). The thrombin time becomes prolonged late in the course. The platelet count is normal. This laboratory profile is similar to the coagulopathy of acute liver disease, but with normal fibrinogen level and absence of hepatic transaminase elevation. The diagnosis of vitamin K deficiency is confirmed by a demonstration of noncarboxylated proteins in vitamin K's absence in the plasma and by clinical and laboratory responses to vitamin K. Intravenous or subcutaneous treatment with vitamin K should be given immediately and not withheld awaiting test results. In the setting of severe bleeding, additional acute treatment with FFP or recombinant factor VIIa may be indicated.

4. Uremia

Uremia is frequently associated with acquired platelet dysfunction. Bleeding occurs in approximately 50% of patients with chronic renal failure. The bleeding risk conferred by platelet dysfunction associated with metabolic imbalance may be compounded by decreased vWF activity and procoagulant deficiencies (eg, factor II, XII, XI, IX) due to increased urinary losses of these proteins in some settings of renal insufficiency. In accordance with platelet dysfunction, uremic bleeding is typically characterized by purpura, epistaxis, menorrhagia, or gastrointestinal hemorrhage. Acute bleeding may be managed with infusion of desmopressin acetate, factor VIII concentrates containing vWF, or cryoprecipitate with or without coadministration of FFP. Red cell transfusion may be required. Prophylactic administration of erythropoietin before the development of severe anemia appears to decrease the bleeding risk. Recombinant VIIa may be useful in refractory bleeding.

Goldenberg NA: Pediatric hemostasis and use of plasma components. Best Pract Res Clin Haematol 2006;19:143 [PMID: 16377547].

Hey E: Vitamin K—What, why, and when. Arch Dis Child Fetal Neonatal Ed 2003;88:F80 [PMID: 12598491].

VASCULAR ABNORMALITIES ASSOCIATED WITH BLEEDING

1. Henoch–Schönlein Purpura (See Chapter 22) (Anaphylactoid Purpura)

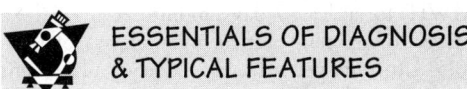

ESSENTIALS OF DIAGNOSIS & TYPICAL FEATURES

- *Purpuric cutaneous rash.*
- *Migratory polyarthritis or polyarthralgias.*
- *Intermittent abdominal pain.*
- *Nephritis.*

General Considerations

Henoch–Schönlein purpura (HSP), the most common type of small vessel vasculitis in children, primarily affects boys 2–7 years of age. Occurrence is highest in the spring and fall, and upper respiratory infection precedes the diagnosis in two-thirds of children.

Leukocytoclastic vasculitis in HSP principally involves the small vessels of the skin, gastrointestinal tract, and kidneys, with deposition of IgA immune complexes. The most common and earliest symptom is palpable purpura, which results from extravasation of erythrocytes into the tissue surrounding the involved venules. Antigens from group A β-hemolytic streptococci and other bacteria, viruses, drugs, foods, and insect bites have been proposed as inciting agents.

Clinical Findings

A. SYMPTOMS AND SIGNS

Skin involvement may be urticarial initially, progresses to a maculopapular appearance, and coalesces to a symmetrical, palpable purpuric rash distributed on the legs, buttocks, and elbows. New lesions may continue to appear for 2–4 weeks, and may extend to involve the entire body. Two-thirds of patients develop migratory polyarthralgias or polyarthritis, primarily of the ankles and knees. Intermittent, sharp abdominal pain occurs in approximately 50% of patients, and hemorrhage and edema of the small intestine can often be demonstrated. Intussusception may develop. Twenty-five to fifty percent of those affected develop renal involvement in the 2nd or 3rd week of illness with either a nephritic or, less commonly, nephrotic picture. Hypertension may accompany the renal involvement. In males, testicular torsion may also occur, and neurologic symptoms are possible due to small vessel vasculitis.

B. LABORATORY FINDINGS

The platelet count is normal or elevated, and other screening tests of hemostasis and platelet function are typically normal. Urinalysis frequently reveals hematuria, and sometimes proteinuria. Stool may be positive for occult blood. The antistreptolysin O (ASO) titer is often elevated and the throat culture positive for group A β-hemolytic streptococci. Serum IgA may be elevated.

Differential Diagnosis

The rash of septicemia (especially meningococcemia) may be similar to skin involvement in HSP, although the distribution tends to be more generalized. The possibility of trauma should be considered in any child presenting with purpura. Other vasculitides should also be considered. The lesions of thrombotic, thrombocytopenic purpura are not palpable.

Treatment

Generally, treatment is supportive. NSAIDs may useful for the arthritis. Corticosteroid therapy may provide symptomatic relief for severe gastrointestinal or joint manifestations but does not alter skin or renal manifestations. If culture for group A β-hemolytic streptococci is positive or if the ASO titer is elevated, a therapeutic course of penicillin is warranted.

Prognosis

The prognosis for recovery is generally good, although symptoms frequently (25–50%) recur over a period of several months. In patients who develop renal manifestations, microscopic hematuria may persist for years. Progressive renal failure occurs in less than 5% of patients with HSP, with an overall fatality rate of 3%.

Cuttica RJ: Vasculitis in children: A diagnostic challenge. Curr Probl Pediatr 1997;27:309 [PMID: 9399074].

2. Collagen Disorders

Mild to life-threatening bleeding occurs with some types of Ehlers–Danlos syndrome, the most common inherited collagen disorder. (See Chapter 33.) Ehlers–Danlos syndrome is characterized by joint hypermobility, skin extensibility, and easy bruising. Coagulation abnormalities may sometimes be present, including platelet dysfunction and deficiencies of coagulation factors VIII, IX, XI, and XIII. However, bleeding and easy bruising, in most instances, relates to fragility of capillaries and compromised vascular integrity. Individuals with Ehlers–Danlos syndrome types 4 and 6 are at risk for aortic dissection and spontaneous rupture of aortic aneurysms. Surgery should be avoided for patients with

Ehlers-Danlos syndrome, as should medications that induce platelet dysfunction.

De Paepe A: Bleeding and bruising in patients with Ehlers-Danlos syndrome and other collagen vascular disorders. Br J Haematol 2004;127:491 [PMID: 15566352].

THROMBOTIC DISORDERS

Although uncommon in children, thrombotic disorders are being recognized with increasing frequency, particularly with heightened physician awareness, and improved survival in pediatric intensive care settings. Clinical risk factors are present in more than 90% of children with acute venous thromboembolic events (VTE). These conditions include the presence of an indwelling vascular catheter, cardiac disease, malignancy, infection, trauma, surgery, immobilization, collagen vascular/chronic inflammatory disease, renal disease, and sickle cell anemia.

Initial evaluation of the child who has thrombosis includes an assessment for potential triggering factors, as well as a family history of thrombosis and early cardiovascular or neurovascular disease. Appropriate radiologic imaging is essential to objectively document the thrombus and to delineate the type (venous versus arterial), possible vasoocclusion, and extent of thrombosis. A comprehensive laboratory investigation for thrombophilia (ie, hypercoagulability) is recommended in order to disclose possible underlying congenital or acquired abnormalities that may affect acute or long-term management. Testing for intrinsic anticoagulant deficiencies (proteins C and S and antithrombin III), procoagulant factor excesses or activators (eg, factor VIII and antiphospholipid antibodies), genetic mutations mediating enhanced procoagulant activity or reduced sensitivity to inactivation (factor V Leiden and prothrombin 20210 polymorphisms), biochemical mediators of endothelial damage (homocysteine and antiphospholipid antibodies), and markers or regulators of fibrinolysis (eg, D-dimer, plasminogen activator inhibitor-1, and lipoprotein[a]) should be completed. Interpretation of procoagulant factor and intrinsic anticoagulant levels should take into account the age dependence of normal values for these proteins. Recent evidence suggests that elevated plasma levels of factor VIII and D-dimer may be predictive of long-term post-thrombotic outcomes in children. Such outcomes include recurrent VTE and the development of the post-thrombotic syndrome, a condition of venous insufficiency and valvular damage characterized by chronic skin changes, edema, and/or pain, and sometimes functional limitation.

Current guidelines for the treatment of first-episode VTE in children have been largely based upon adult experience, and include therapeutic anticoagulation for at least 3 months. During the period of anticoagulation, bleeding precautions should be followed as previously described for bleeding disorders. Initial therapy is with continuous intravenous unfractionated heparin or twice-daily subcutaneous low molecular weight heparin (LMWH) for at least 7 days, monitored by anti-Xa activity level to maintain anticoagulant levels of 0.3–0.7, or 0.5–1.0 units per mL, respectively. Subsequent extended anticoagulant therapy is given with LMWH or daily warfarin, an oral agent monitored by the PT to maintain an international normalized ratio (INR) of 2.0–3.0 (2.5–3.5 in the presence of an antiphospholipid antibody). During warfarin treatment, the INR should be within the therapeutic range for two consecutive days before discontinuation of heparin. Warfarin pharmacokinetics are affected by acute illness, numerous medications, and changes in diet, and require frequent monitoring. LMWH offers the advantage of only infrequent need for monitoring, but is far more expensive than warfarin. In cases of limb- or life-threatening VTE, including major proximal pulmonary embolus, and in cases of progressive VTE despite therapeutic anticoagulation, thrombolytic therapy (eg, tissue-type plasminogen activator) is often warranted.

Goldenberg NA: Long-term outcomes of venous thrombosis in children. Curr Opin Hematol 2005;12:370 [PMID: 16093782].

Monagle P: Antithrombotic therapy in children: The Seventh ACCP Conference on Antithrombotic and Thrombolytic Therapy. Chest 2004;126(3 Suppl):645S [PMID: 15383489].

INHERITED DISORDERS

1. Protein C Deficiency

Protein C is a vitamin K–dependent protein that is normally activated by thrombin bound to thrombomodulin and inactivates activated factors V and VIII. In addition, activated protein C promotes fibrinolysis. Two phenotypes of hereditary protein C deficiency exist. Heterozygous individuals with autosomal dominant protein C deficiency often present with VTE as young adults, but the disorder may manifest during childhood or in later adulthood. Following a second event, lifelong anticoagulation therapy should be instituted. Homozygous or compound heterozygous protein C deficiency is rare but phenotypically severe. Affected children generally present within the first 12 hours of life with purpura fulminans and/or VTE. Retinal thrombosis may result in blindness. Prompt protein C replacement by infusion of FFP every 6–12 hours, or of protein C concentrate (if available), along with therapeutic heparin administration is recommended. Subsequent management requires chronic anticoagulation with warfarin or protein C concentrate. Recurrent VTE is common, especially during periods of subtherapeutic anticoagulation.

2. Protein S Deficiency

Protein S is a cofactor for protein C. Neonates with homozygous protein S deficiency have a course similar to those with homozygous or compound heterozygous protein C deficiency. Lifelong warfarin therapy is indicated in severe deficiency, or in heterozygous individuals who have experienced recurrent VTE.

3. Antithrombin III (ATIII) Deficiency

ATIII is the most important physiologic inhibitor of thrombin and inhibits activated factors IX, X, XI, and XII. ATIII deficiency is transmitted in an autosomal dominant pattern and is associated with VTE, typically with onset in adolescence or young adulthood. Therapy for acute VTE involves replacement with antithrombin concentrate (if available) and therapeutic anticoagulation. The efficiency of heparin may be significantly diminished in the setting of severe ATIII deficiency and anticoagulation with warfarin required. Patients with recurrent VTE are maintained on lifelong warfarin.

4. Factor V Leiden Mutation

An amino acid substitution in the gene coding for factor V results in factor V Leiden, a factor V polymorphism that is resistant to inactivation by activated protein C. The most common cause of activated protein C resistance in Caucasians, factor V Leiden is present in approximately 5% of the Caucasian population, 20% of Caucasian adults with deep vein thrombosis, and 40–60% of those with a family history of VTE. VTE occurs in both heterozygous and homozygous individuals. In the former case, thrombosis is typically triggered by a clinical risk factor (or else develops in association with additional thrombophilia traits), whereas in the latter case, it is often spontaneous. Population studies suggest that the risk of VTE is increased 7-fold in the setting of heterozygous factor V Leiden, 35-fold among heterozygous individuals taking the oral contraceptives, and 80-fold in those homozygous for factor V Leiden.

5. Prothrombin Mutation

The 20210 glutamine to alanine mutation in the prothrombin gene is a relatively common polymorphism in Caucasians that enhances its activation to thrombin. In heterozygous form, prothrombin 20210 has been associated with a 3-fold increased risk for VTE.

6. Other Inherited Disorders

Qualitative abnormalities of fibrinogen (dysfibrinogenemias) are usually inherited in an autosomal dominant

manner. Most individuals with dysfibrinogenemia are asymptomatic. Some patients experience bleeding, while others develop venous or arterial thrombosis. The diagnosis is suggested by a prolonged thrombin time with a normal fibrinogen concentration. Hyperhomocysteinemia can be an inherited or an acquired condition and is associated with an increased risk for both arterial and venous thromboses. In children, it may also serve as a risk factor for ischemic arterial stroke. However, hyperhomocysteinemia is quite uncommon in the setting of dietary folate supplementation (as in the United States), and is observed almost uniquely in cases of metabolic disease (eg, homocystinuria). Furthermore, methylene tetrahydrofolate reductase receptor mutations do not appear to constitute a risk factor for thrombosis in U.S. children, except in rare circumstances in which homocysteine is elevated.

Lipoprotein(a) is a lipoprotein with homology to plasminogen. In vitro studies suggest that lipoprotein(a) may both promote atherothrombosis and inhibit fibrinolysis. Case-control studies suggest that elevated plasma concentrations of lipoprotein(a) are associated with an increased odds of VTE and ischemic arterial stroke in children.

Increased factor VIII may be demonstrated in patients with acute VTE. This increase has been implicated as a risk factor for both VTE in adults and may be familial.

ACQUIRED DISORDERS

1. Antiphospholipid Antibodies

The development of antiphospholipid antibodies is the most common form of acquired thrombophilia in children. Antiphospholipid antibodies include the lupus anticoagulant, anticardiolipin antibodies, and β_2-glycoprotein-1 antibodies and have become increasingly implicated in VTE. The lupus anticoagulant may be demonstrated in vitro via its inhibition of phospholipid-dependent coagulation assays (eg, aPTT) and dilute Russell viper venom time, whereas immunologic techniques (eg, enzyme-linked immunosorbent assays) are often used to detect anticardiolipin and β_2-glycoprotein-1 antibodies. Although common in persons with autoimmune diseases such as systemic lupus erythematosus, antiphospholipid antibodies may also develop following certain drug exposures, infection, acute inflammation, and lymphoproliferative diseases. Sometimes VTE and antiphospholipid antibodies may predate other signs of lupus for long periods of time. Viral illness is a common precipitant in children, and in many cases, the inciting infection may be asymptomatic.

If an antiphospholipid antibody persists for 6–12 weeks following the acute thrombotic event, anticoagulation should be continued at least until the antiphospholipid antibody becomes undetectable. In addition, consideration should be given to long-term anticoagulation.

2. Deficiencies of Intrinsic Anticoagulants

Acquired deficiencies of proteins C and S and ATIII may occur in the clinical context of excessive consumption, including sepsis, DIC, major-vessel or extensive VTE, and post–bone marrow transplant sinusoidal obstruction syndrome (formerly termed hepatic venoocclusive disease). Pilot studies in children have suggested a possible therapeutic role for antithrombin or protein C concentrates in sepsis associated DIC and severe post-transplant sinusoidal obstruction syndrome.

3. Acute Phase Reactants

As part of the acute phase response, plasma fibrinogen concentration, plasma factor VIII and elevations in platelet count activity may occur, all of which may contribute to an acquired prothrombotic state.

Reactive thrombocytosis is rarely associated with VTE in children when the platelet count is less than 1 million/μL.

Manco-Johnson MJ: Laboratory testing for thrombophilia in pediatric patients. On behalf of the Subcommittee for Perinatal and Pediatric Thrombosis of the Scientific and Standardization Committee of the International Society on Thrombosis and Haemostasis (ISTH). Thromb Haemost 2002;88:155 [PMID: 12152657].

Nowak-Göttl U: Thromboembolism in children. Curr Opin Hematol 2002;9:448 [PMID: 12172465].

■ SPLENIC ABNORMALITIES

SPLENOMEGALY & HYPERSPLENISM

The differential diagnosis of splenomegaly includes the general categories of congestive splenomegaly, chronic infections, leukemia and lymphomas, hemolytic anemias, reticuloendothelioses, and storage diseases (Table 27–9).

Splenomegaly due to any cause may be associated with hypersplenism and the excessive destruction of circulating red cells, white cells, and platelets. The degree of cytopenia is variable and, when mild, requires no specific therapy. In other cases, the thrombocytopenia may cause life-threatening bleeding, particularly when the splenomegaly is secondary to portal hypertension and associated with esophageal varices or the consequence of a storage disease. In such cases, treatment with surgical splenectomy or with splenic embolization may be warranted. Although more commonly associated with acute enlargement, rupture of an enlarged spleen can be seen in more chronic conditions such as Gaucher disease.

Stone DL: Life threatening splenic hemorrhage in two patients with Gaucher's disease. Am J Hematol 2000;64:140 [PMID: 10814997].

ASPLENIA & SPLENECTOMY

Children who lack normal splenic function are at risk for sepsis, meningitis, and pneumonia due to encapsulated bacteria such as pneumococci and *H influenzae*. Such infections are often fulminant and fatal because of inadequate antibody production and impaired phagocytosis of circulating bacteria.

Congenital asplenia is usually suspected when an infant is born with abnormalities of abdominal viscera and complex cyanotic congenital heart disease. Howell–Jolly bodies are usually present on the peripheral blood smear, and the absence of splenic tissue is confirmed by technetium radionuclide scanning. The prognosis depends on the underlying cardiac lesions, and many children die during the first few months. Prophylactic antibiotics, usually penicillin, and pneumococcal conjugate and polysaccharide vaccines are recommended.

The risk of overwhelming sepsis following surgical splenectomy is related to the child's age and to the underlying disorder. Because the risk is highest when the procedure is performed earlier in life, splenectomy is usually postponed until after age 5 years. The risk of postsplenectomy sepsis is also greater in children with malignancies, thalassemias, and reticuloendothelioses than in children whose splenectomy is performed for ITP, hereditary spherocytosis, or trauma. Prior to splenectomy, children should be immunized against *Pneumococcus, H influenzae,* and *Neisseria meningitidis.* Additional management should include penicillin prophylaxis and prompt evaluation for fever 38.8 °C or above or signs of severe infection.

Children with sickle cell anemia develop functional asplenia during the first year of life, and overwhelming sepsis is the leading cause of early deaths in this disease. Prophylactic penicillin has been shown to reduce the incidence of sepsis by 84%.

Pickering L: American Academy of Pediatrics: Immunization in special circumstances. Red Book 2000;25:66.

■ TRANSFUSION MEDICINE

DONOR SCREENING & BLOOD PROCESSING: RISK MANAGEMENT

Minimizing the risks of transfusion begins by asking the donor questions that will protect the recipient from transmission of infectious agents as well as other risks of transfusions. In addition, information defining high-

Table 27–9. Causes of chronic splenomegaly in children.

Cause	Associated Clinical Findings	Diagnostic Investigation
Congestive splenomegaly	History of umbilical vein catheter or neo-natal omphalitis; signs of portal hyper-tension (varices, hemorrhoids, dilated abdominal wall veins); pancytopenia, his-tory of hepatitis or jaundice	Complete blood count, platelet count, liver function tests, ultrasonography
Chronic infections	History of exposure to tuberculosis, his-toplasmosis, coccidioidomycosis, other fungal disease; chronic sepsis (foreign body in bloodstream; subacute infective endocarditis)	Appropriate cultures and skin tests, ie, blood cultures; PPD, fungal serology and antigen tests; chest film; HIV serology
Infectious mononucleosis	Fever, fatigue, pharyngitis, rash, adenop-athy, hepatomegaly	EBV antibody titers
Leukemia, lymphoma, Hodgkin disease	Evidence of systemic involvement with fe-ver, bleeding tendencies, hepatomegaly, and lymphadenopathy; pancytopenia	Blood smear, bone marrow examination, chest film, gallium scan, LDH, uric acid
Hemolytic anemias	Anemia, jaundice; family history of ane-mia, jaundice, and gallbladder disease in young adults	Reticulocyte count, Coombs test, blood smear, osmotic fragility test, hemoglobin electrophoresis
Reticuloendothelioses (histiocytosis X)	Chronic otitis media, seborrheic or pete-chial skin rashes, anemia, infections, lym-phadenopathy, hepatomegaly, bone le-sions	Skeletal x-rays for bone lesions; biopsy of bone, liver, bone marrow, or lymph node
Storage diseases	Family history of similar disorders, neu-rologic involvement, evidence of macu-lar degeneration, hepatomegaly	Biopsy of liver or bone marrow in search for storage cells
Splenic cyst	Evidence of other infections (postinfec-tious cyst) or congenital anomalies; pe-culiar shape of spleen	Radionuclide scan, ultrasonography
Splenic hemangioma	Other hemangiomas, consumptive co-agulopathy	Radionuclide scan, arteriography, platelet count, coagulation screen

PPD , purified protein derivative; HIV, human immunodeficiency virus; EBV, Epstein-Barr virus; LDH, lactic dehydrogenase.

risk groups whose behavior increases the possible trans-mission of HIV, hepatitis, and other diseases is pro-vided, with the request that persons in these groups not donate blood.

Before blood components can be released for transfu-sion, donor blood is screened for hepatitis B surface anti-gen; antibodies to hepatitis B, hepatitis C, HIV-1 and HIV-2, and human T-cell lymphotropic virus (HTLV) I and II; and a serologic test for syphilis (Table 27–10). Screening donor blood for viral genome (nucleic acid amplification testing) was mandated for HIV and HCV early in 2003 and for West Nile Virus later that year. HIV p24 antigen may not be required depending on HIV nucleic acid amplification testing used. Detection of other viral genomes may be added. Positive tests are repeated.

Upon their confirmation, the unit in question is destroyed; and the donor placed in a deferral category. Many of the screening tests used are very sensitive and have a high rate of false-positive results. As a result, confirmatory tests have been developed to check the initial screening results and separate the false-positives from the true-positives. Recently, bacterial culture of platelet concentrates was added to the screening paradigm.

With these techniques, the risk of an infectious compli-cation from blood components has been minimized (see Table 27–10), with the greatest risk being post-transfusion hepatitis (see sections on hepatitis C virus and non-A, non-B, non-C hepatitis in Chapter 21). Autologous donation is recognized by some centers as a safe alternative to homolo-gous blood. Issues of donor size make the techniques of

Table 27–10. Transmission risks of infectious agents for which screening of blood products is routinely performed.

Disease Entity	Transmission	Screening and Processing Procedures	Approximate Risk of Transmission
Syphilis	Low risk that fresh blood drawn during spirochetemia can transmit infection. Organism not able to survive beyond 72 hours during storage at 4 °C.	Donor history. RPR or VDRL.	< 1:100,000
Hepatitis A	Units drawn during prodrome could transmit virus. Because of brief viremia during acute phase, absence of asymptomatic carrier phase, and failure to detect transmission in multiple transfused individuals, infection by this agent is unlikely.	Donor history.	1:1,000,000
Hepatitis B	Prolonged viremia during various phases of the disease and asymptomatic carrier state make HBV infection a significant risk of transfusion. Incidence has markedly decreased with screening strategies.	Donor history, education, and self-exclusion. Hepatitis B surface antigen (HBsAg). Surrogate tests for non-A, non-B hepatitis and screen for hepatitis C and retroviruses have helped screen out population at risk for transmitting HBV.	1:250,000–1:30,000
Hepatitis C	Over two-thirds of cases of non-A, non-B post-transfusion hepatitis may be due to this agent. The virus has characteristics similar to those of HBV which are responsible for the risk from transfusion. Infection may lead to a significant incidence of cirrhosis and end-stage liver disease.	Donor history. Surrogate tests: ALT and hepatitis B core antibody (anti-HBc), anti-HCV. Nucleic acid testing for viral genome required.	1:1,600,000
Non-A, non-B, non-C hepatitis	Not a specific cause but a classification of agents other than HAV, HBV, HCV, Epstein-Barr virus, and cytomegalovirus, which can cause post-transfusion hepatitis.	Donor history. Surrogate tests: anti-HBc.	Undefined
Human immunodeficiency virus (HIV-1, HIV-2) infection	Cytotoxic retrovirus spread by sexual contact, parenteral (including transfusion) and vertical routes. Resultant destruction of CD4-positive cells leads to clinical manifestations of AIDS.	Donor history, education, and self-exclusion. Anti-HIV by EIA screening test. Western blot confirmatory. P^{24} antigen testing. Nucleic acid testing for viral genome required.	1:2,000,000–1:1,500,000
Human T-cell lymphotropic virus I and II (HTLV-I and -II) infection	Retroviruses spread by sexual contact, parenteral (including transfusion) and vertical modes. Over years to decades, infection with HTLV-I may cause lymphoid malignancies or myelopathy.	Donor history. Anti-HTLV-I and -II by enzyme immunoassay screening test. Western blot confirmatory.	1:600,000

RPR, rapid plasma reagin; VDRL, syphilis test; HAV, HBV, HCV, hepatitis A virus, hepatitis B virus, hepatitis C virus; ALT, alanine transaminase; AIDS, acquired immunodeficiency syndrome; EIA, enzyme-linked immunosorbent assay; HTLV, human T-cell lymphotropic virus.

autologous donation difficult to apply to the pediatric population.

Primary CMV infections are significant complications of blood transfusion in transplant recipients, neonates, and immunodeficient individuals. Transmission of CMV can be avoided by using seronegative donors, apheresis platelet concentrates collected by techniques ensuring low numbers of residual white cells, or red cell or platelet products leukocyte-depleted by filtering (white blood cell counts less than 5 million per packed red cell unit or apheresis platelet concentrate equivalent).

STORAGE & PRESERVATION OF BLOOD & BLOOD COMPONENTS

Whole blood is routinely fractionated into packed red cells, platelets, and FFP or cryoprecipitate for most efficient use of all blood components. The storage conditions and biologic characteristics of the fractions are summarized in Table 27–11. The conditions provide the optimal environment to maintain appropriate recovery, survival, and function and are different for each blood component. For example, red cells undergo dramatic metabolic changes during their 35–42-day storage, with a decrease in 2,3-DPG during the second week of storage, a decrease in adenosine triphosphate, and a gradual loss of intracellular potassium. Fortunately, these changes are reversed readily within hours to days after the red cells are transfused. However, in certain clinical conditions, these effects may define the type of components used. For example, blood less than 7–10 days old would be preferred for exchange transfusion in neonates or replacement of red cells in persons with cardiopulmonary disease to ensure adequate oxygen-carrying capacity. Storage time is not an issue when administering transfusions to those with chronic anemia.

Under certain conditions in which excessive potassium load is a problem, one has the option of using blood less than 10 days old, making packed cells out of an older unit of whole blood, or washing blood stored as packed cells. Regardless of the blood's age, over 70% of the red cells will circulate after transfusion and approximate normal survival in the circulation.

Platelets are stored at 22 °C for a maximum of 5 days; criteria for 7-day storage are being developed. At the extremes of storage, there should be at least a 60% recovery, a survival time that approximates turnover of fresh autologous platelets, and normalization of the bleeding time or PFA-100 in proportion to the peak platelet count. Frozen components, red cells, FFP, and cryoprecipitate are outdated at 3 years, 1 year, and 1 year, respectively. Frozen red cells out to 10 years retain the same biochemical and functional characteristics as the day they were frozen. FFP contains 80% or more of all of the clotting factors of fresh plasma. Factors VIII and XIII and fibrinogen are concentrated in cryoprecipitate.

PRETRANSFUSION TESTING

Both the donated blood and the recipient are tested for ABO and Rh(D) antigens and for auto- or alloantibodies in the serum. The cross-match is required on any component that contains red cells. In the major cross-match, washed donor red cells are incubated with the serum from the patient, and agglutination is detected and graded. The antiglobulin phase of the test is then performed; Coombs reagent, which will detect the presence of IgG or complement on the surface of the red cells, is added to the mixture, and any possible reaction is evaluated. In the presence of a negative antibody screen in the recipient, a negative immediate spin cross-match test confirms the compatibility of the blood and antiglobulin phase is not required. Further testing is required if the antibody screen or the cross-match is positive, and blood should not be given until the nature of the reactivity is delineated. An incompatible cross-match is evaluated first with a DAT or Coombs test to detect IgG or complement on the surfaces of the recipient's red cells. The indirect antiglobulin test is also used to determine the presence of antibodies that will coat or activate complement on the surfaces of normal red cells.

TRANSFUSION PRACTICE

General Rules

Several rules should be observed in administering any blood component:

1. In final preparation of the component, no solutions should be added to the bag or tubing set except for normal saline (0.9% sodium chloride for injection, USP), ABO-compatible plasma, or other specifically approved expanders. Hypotonic solutions cause hemolysis of red cells, and, if these are transfused, a severe reaction will occur.

2. Transfusion products should be protected from contact with any calcium-containing solution (eg, lactated Ringer's); recalcification and reversal of the citrate effect will cause clotting of the blood component.

3. Blood components should not be warmed to a temperature greater than 37 °C. If a component is incubated in a water bath, it should be enclosed in a watertight bag to prevent bacterial contamination of entry ports.

4. Whenever a blood bag is entered, the sterile integrity of the system is violated, and that unit should be discarded within 4 hours if left at room temperature or within 24 hours if the temperature is between 1 °C and 4 °C.

5. Transfusions of products containing red cells should not exceed 4 hours. Blood components in excess of what can be infused during this time period should be stored in the blood bank until needed.

Table 27–11. Characteristics of blood and blood components.

Component	Storage Conditions	Composition and Transfusion Characteristics	Indications	Risks and Precautions	Administration
Whole blood	4 °C for 35-day RBC characteristics: **Survival:** Recovery decreases during storage but is always > 70%. Cells that circulate approximate normal survival. **Function:** 2,3-DPG levels fall to undetectable after second week of storage. This defect repaired within 24 h of transfusion. **Electrolytes:** With storage, potassium increases in plasma. This rises to high levels after 2 wk of storage.	Contains RBCs and many plasma compounds of whole blood. Leukocytes and platelets lose activity or viability after a few days under these conditions. Procoagulant clotting factors (particularly VIII and V) deteriorate rapidly during storage. Each unit has about 500 mL volume and Hct 36–40%.	Oxygen carrying capacity (anemia). Volume replacement for blood loss (> 15–20%) or severe shock.	Must be ABO-identical and cross-match-compatible. Infectious diseases. Febrile or hemolytic transfusion reactions. Alloimmunization to red cell, white cell, or platelet antigens.	During acute blood loss, as rapidly as tolerated. In other settings, 2–4 h. 10 mL/kg will raise Hct by 5% and support volume.
Packed red cells	Same as for whole blood. Special rejuvenating solutions allow storage for 42 d.	Contains RBCs; plasma removed in preparation. Status of leukocytes, clotting factors, and platelets same as for whole blood. Hct about 70%, volume 200–250 mL. May request tighter pack to give Hct 80–90%.	Oxygen carrying capacity. Acute trauma or bleeding or situations requiring intensive cardiopulmonary support (Hct < 25–30%). Chronic anemia (Hct < 20%).	Same as for whole blood.	May be given as patient will tolerate based on cardiovascular status over 2–4 h. Dose of 3 mL packed RBC/kg will raise the Hct by 3%. If cardiovascular status stable, give 10 mL/kg over 2–4 h. If unstable, use smaller volume or do packed RBC exchange.

Washed or filtered red cells	When cells are washed, there is a 24-h outdate. Up to that time, they have the same characteristics as for packed red cells.	Same as for packed red cells.	Same as packed red cells. Depending on technique used and extent of reduction of white blood cells, washed red cells may achieve the following: • Avoid febrile reactions. • Decrease the transmission of CMV. • Decrease the incidence of allo-immunization to white cell antigens.	Same as whole blood. Removal of white cells diminishes the risk of febrile reactions. Filtration with high-efficiency white cell filters may decrease rate of alloimmunization to white cell antigens and transmission of CMV.	Same as for packed red cells.
Frozen red cells	Packed red cells frozen in 40% glycerol solution at less than −65 °C. Stored 10 years. Retain the same biochemical characteristics, function, and capacity for survival as the day in storage they were frozen; when thawed, 24-h outdate.	Same as for packed red cells.	Same as packed red cells. Useful for avoiding febrile reactions, decreasing transmission of CMV, autologous blood donation, and developing an inventory of rare red cell blood groups.	Same as for whole blood. Risk of CMV transmission is at same level as using seronegative components.	Same as for packed red cells.
Fresh frozen plasma	Plasma from whole blood stored at under −18 °C for up to 1 y.	Contains > 80% of all procoagulant and anticoagulant plasma proteins.	Replacement of plasma procoagulant and anticoagulant plasma proteins. May provide "other" factors, eg, treatment of TTP.	Need not be cross-matched; should be type-compatible. Volume overload, infectious diseases, allergic reactions. Solvent detergent–treated plasma or donor-retested plasma units have decreased risk for viral transmission.	As rapidly as tolerated by patient but not > 4 h. Dose: 10–15 mL/kg will increase level of all clotting factors by 10–20%.
Cryoprecipitate	Produced by freezing fresh plasma to under −65 °C, then allowing to thaw 18 h at 4 °C. After centrifugation, cryoprecipitable proteins are separated. May be stored at under −18 °C for up to 1 y.	Contains factor VIII, fibrinogen, and fibronectin at concentrations greater than those of plasma. Also contains factor XIII. VIII > 80 IU/pack, fibrinogen 100–350 mg/pack.	Treatment of acquired or congenital deficiencies of VIII, von Willebrand factor, and fibrinogen. Useful in making biologic glues that contain fibrinogen. Commercial clotting factor concentrates are the treatment of choice for factor VIII deficiency and von Willebrand disease because sterilization procedures further reduce the risk of viral transmission.	Same as for fresh frozen plasma. ABO agglutinogens may also be concentrated and can give positive direct agglutination test if not type-specific.	Cryoprecipitate can be given as a rapid infusion. Dose: 1/2 pack per kg body weight will increase factor VIII level by 80–100% and fibrinogen by 200–250 mg/dL.

(continued)

Table 27–11. Characteristics of blood and blood components. (continued)

Component	Storage Conditions	Composition and Transfusion Characteristics	Indications	Risks and Precautions	Administration
Platelet concentrates from whole blood donation	Separated from platelet-rich plasma and stored with gentle agitation at 22 °C for 3–5 d. Containers currently in use are plastic and allow for gas exchange, diffusion of CO_2 helps keep pH > 6, a major factor in keeping platelets viable and functional.	Each unit contains about 5×10^{10} platelets. Survival: Although there may be some loss with storage, 60–70% recovery should be achieved, with stored platelets correcting the bleeding time in proportion to the peak counts reached.	Treatment of thrombocytopenia or platelet function defects.	No cross-match necessary. Should be ABO type-specific. Other risks as for whole blood.	Can be given as rapid transfusion or as defined by cardiovascular status, not more than 4 h. Dose: 10 mL/kg should increase platelet count by at least 50,000/μL.
Platelet concentrates by apheresis techniques	Same as random donor units.	Platelet content is equivalent to 6–10 units of random donor concentrates. Depending on technique used, these may be relatively free of leukocytes, a product useful in avoiding alloimmunization.	As above, particularly useful in treating patients who have insufficient production in whom alloisoimmunization is a potential problem.	Same as above.	As above.
Granulocytes	Although they may be stored stationary at 20–24 °C, transfuse as soon as possible after collection.	Contains at least 1×10^{10} granulocytes but also platelets and red cells. When donors given 10 μg/kg G-CSF subcutaneously and 8 mg decadron orally 12–15 h before collection increases to $> 5 \times 10^{10}$ granulocytes.	Severely neutropenic individuals (< 500/μL) with poor marrow reserves and suspected bacterial or fungal infections not responding to 48–72 h of parenteral antibiotics. Also in patients with neutrophil dysfunction.	Same as for platelets. Pulmonary leukostasis reactions. Severe febrile reactions.	Given in an infusion over 2–4 h. Dose: 1 unit daily for newborns and infants, 1×10^9 granulocytes per kg.

CMV, cytomegalovirus; G-CSF, granulocyte colony-stimulating factor; Hct, hematocrit; RBC, red blood cell; TTP, thrombotic thrombocytopenic purpura.

6. Before transfusion, the blood component should be inspected visually for any unusual characteristics, such as the presence of flocculent material, hemolysis, or clumping of cells, and mixed thoroughly.

7. The unit and the recipient should be identified properly.

8. The administration set includes a standard 170–260 micron filter. Under certain clinical circumstances, an additional microaggregate filter may be used to eliminate small aggregates of fibrin, white cells, and platelets that will not be removed by the standard filter.

9. The patient should be observed during the entire transfusion but especially during the first 15 minutes. Any adverse symptoms or signs should be evaluated immediately and reactions to the transfusion reported promptly to the transfusion service.

10. When cross-match–incompatible red cells or whole blood unit(s) must be given to the patient (as with autoimmune hemolytic anemia), a test dose of 10% of the total volume (not to exceed 50 mL) should be administered over 15–20 minutes; the transfusion is then stopped and the patient evaluated for reaction. If no adverse effects are noted, the remainder of the volume can be infused carefully.

11. Blood for exchange transfusion in the newborn period may be cross-matched with either the infant's or the mother's serum. If the exchange is for hemolysis, 500 mL of whole blood stored for less than 7 days will be adequate. If replacement of clotting factors is a key issue, packed red cells (7 days old) reconstituted with FFP may be considered. Based on posttransfusion platelet counts, platelet transfusion may be considered. Other problems to be anticipated are acid–base derangements, hyponatremia, hyperkalemia, hypocalcemia, hypoglycemia, hypothermia, and hypervolemia or hypovolemia.

Choice of Blood Component

Several principles should be considered when deciding on the need for blood transfusion. Indications for blood or blood components must be well defined, and the patient's medical condition, not just the laboratory results, should be the basis for the decision. Specific deficiencies exhibited by the patient (eg, oxygen-carrying capacity, thrombocytopenia) should be treated with appropriate blood components and the use of whole blood minimized. Information about specific blood components is summarized in Table 27–11.

A. WHOLE BLOOD

Whole blood may be used in patients who require replacement of oxygen-carrying capacity and volume. More specifically, it should be considered when more than 15% of blood volume is lost. Doses vary depending on volume considerations (see Table 27–11). In acute situations, the transfusion may be completed rapidly to support blood volume.

B. PACKED RED CELLS

Packed red cells (which include leukocyte-poor, filtered, or frozen deglycerolized products) prepared from whole blood by centrifugal techniques are the appropriate choice for almost all patients with deficient oxygen-carrying capacity. Exact indications will be defined by the clinical setting, the severity of the anemia, the acuity of the condition, and any other factors affecting oxygen transport.

C. PLATELETS

The decision to transfuse platelets depends on the patient's clinical condition, the status of plasma phase coagulation, the platelet count, the cause of the thrombocytopenia, and the functional capacity of the patient's own platelets. With platelet counts less than 10,000–20,000/μL, the risk of severe, spontaneous bleeding is increased markedly, and—in the absence of antibody-mediated thrombocytopenia—transfusion should be considered. Under certain circumstances, especially with platelet dysfunction or treatment that inhibits the procoagulant system, transfusions at higher platelet counts may be necessary.

Transfused platelets are sequestered temporarily in the lungs and spleen before reaching their peak concentrations, 45–60 minutes after transfusion. A significant proportion of the transfused platelets never circulate but remain sequestered in the spleen. This phenomenon results in reduced recovery; only 60–70% of the transfused platelets are accounted for when peripheral platelet count increments are used as a measure of response.

In addition to cessation of bleeding, two variables indicate the effectiveness of platelet transfusions. The first is platelet recovery, as measured by the maximum number of platelets circulating in response to transfusion. The practical measure is the platelet count at 1 hour after transfusion. In the absence of immune or drastic nonimmune factors that markedly decrease platelet recovery, one would expect a 7000/μL increment for each random donor unit and a 40,000–70,000/μL increment for each single-donor apheresis unit in a large child or adolescent. For infants and small children, 10 mL/kg of platelets will increase the platelet count by at least 50,000/μL. The second variable is the survival of transfused platelets. Normally, if the recovery is great enough, transfused platelets have a half-life of 3–5 days. In the presence of increased platelet destruction, the life span may be shortened to a few days or a few hours. Frequent platelet transfusions may be required to maintain adequate hemostasis.

A particularly troublesome outcome in patients receiving long-term platelet transfusions is the develop-

Table 27–12. Adverse events following transfusions.

Event	Pathophysiology	Signs and Symptoms	Management
Acute hemolytic transfusion reaction	Preformed alloantibodies (most commonly to ABO) and occasionally autoantibodies cause rapid intravascular hemolysis of transfused cells with activation of clotting (DIC), activation of inflammatory mediators, and acute renal failure.	Fever, chills, nausea, chest pain, back pain, pain at transfusion site, hypotension, dyspnea, oliguria, dark urine.	The risk of this type of reaction overall is low (1:30,000), but the mortality rate is high (up to 40%). Stop the transfusion; maintain renal output with intravenous fluids and diuretics (furosemide or mannitol); treat DIC with heparin; and institute other appropriate supportive measures.
Delayed hemolytic transfusion reaction	Formation of alloantibodies after transfusion and resultant destruction of transfused red cells, usually by extravascular hemolysis.	Fever, jaundice, anemia. A small percentage may develop chronic hemolysis.	Detection, definition, and documentation (for future transfusions). Supportive care. Risk, 1:2500.
Febrile reactions	Usually caused by leukoagglutinins in recipient cytokines or other biologically active compounds.	Fever. May also involve chills.	Supportive. Consider leukocyte-poor products for future. Risk per transfusion, 1:200.
Allergic reactions	Most causes not identified. In IgA-deficient individuals, reaction occurs as a result of antibodies to IgA.	Itching, hives, occasionally chills and fever. In severe reactions, may see signs of anaphylaxis: dyspnea, pulmonary edema.	Mild to moderate reactions: diphenhydramine. More severe reactions: epinephrine subcutaneously and steroids intravenously. Risk for mild to moderate allergic reactions, 1:1000; severe anaphylactic reactions, 1:150,000.
Transfusion-related acute lung injury	Acute lung injury occurring within 6 h after transfusion. Two sets of factors interact to produce the syndrome. Patient factors: infection, surgery, cytokine therapy. Blood component factors: lipids, antibodies, cytokines. Two groups of factors interact during transfusion to result in lung injury indistinguishable from ARDS.	Tachypnea, dyspnea, hypoxia. Diffuse interstitial markings. Cardiac evaluation normal.	May consider younger products: packed red blood cells ≤ 2 weeks, platelets ≤ 3 days, washing components to prevent syndrome. Management: supportive care. Risk, 1:2000–1:3000 per transfusion.
Dilutional coagulopathy	Massive blood loss and transfusion with replacement with fluids or blood components and deficient clotting factors.	Bleeding.	Replacement of clotting factors or platelets with appropriate blood components.
Bacterial contamination	Contamination of units results in growth of bacteria or production of clinically significant levels of endotoxin.	Chills, high fever, hypotension, other symptoms of sepsis or endotoxemia.	Stop transfusion; make aggressive attempts to identify organism; provide vigorous supportive medical care including antibiotics.
Graft-versus-host disease	Lymphocytes from donor transfused in an immunoincompetent host.	Syndrome can involve a variety of organs, usually skin, liver, gastrointestinal tract, and bone marrow.	Preventive management: irradiation (> 1500 cGy) of cellular blood components transfused to individuals with congenital or acquired immunodeficiency syndromes, intrauterine transfusion, very premature infants, and when donors are relatives of the recipient.

(continued)

Table 27–12. Adverse events following transfusions. (continued)

Event	Pathophysiology	Signs and Symptoms	Management
Iron overload	There is no physiologic mechanism to excrete excess iron. Target organs include liver, heart, and endocrine organs. In patients receiving red cell transfusions over long periods of time, there is an increase in iron burden.	Signs and symptoms of dysfunctional organs affected by the iron.	Chronic administration of iron chelator such as deferoxamine.

ARDS, adult respiratory distress syndrome; DIC, disseminated intravascular coagulation.

ment of a refractory state characterized by poor (< 30%) recovery or no response to platelet transfusion (as measured at 1 hour). Most (70–90%) of these refractory states result from the development of alloantibodies directed against HLA antigens on the platelet. Platelets have class I HLA antigens, and the antibodies are primarily against HLA A or B determinants. A smaller proportion of these alloantibodies (< 10%) may be directed against platelet-specific alloantigens. The most effective approach to prevent HLA sensitization is to use leukocyte-depleted components (< 5 million leukocytes per unit of packed red cells or per apheresis or 6–10 random donor unit concentrates). For the alloimmunized, refractory patient, the best approach is to provide HLA-matched platelets for transfusion. Reports have suggested that platelet cross-matching procedures using HLA-matched or unmatched donors may be helpful in identifying platelet concentrates most likely to provide an adequate response.

D. FRESH FROZEN PLASMA

The indication for FFP is replacement of plasma coagulation factors in clinical situations in which a deficiency of one or more clotting factors exists and associated bleeding manifestations are present. In some hereditary factor deficiencies such as factor VIII deficiency or vWD, commercially prepared concentrates contain these factors in higher concentrations and, because of viral inactivation, impose less infectious risk and are more appropriate than plasma.

E. CRYOPRECIPITATE

This component may be used for acquired or congenital disorders of hypofibrinogenemia or afibrinogenemia. Although cryoprecipitate is a rich source for factor VIII or vWF, commercial concentrates that contain these factors are more appropriate (see preceding section). The dose given depends on the protein to be replaced. Cryoprecipitate can be given in a rapid transfusion over 30–60 minutes.

F. GRANULOCYTES

With better supportive care over the past 10 years, the need for granulocytes in neutropenic patients with severe bacterial infections has decreased. Indications still remain for severe bacterial infections unresponsive to vigorous medical therapy in either newborns or older children with bone marrow failure, or patients with neutrophil dysfunction. Newer mobilization schemes using G-CSF and steroids in donors result in granulocyte collections with at least 5×10^{10} neutrophils. This may provide a better product for patients requiring granulocyte support.

G. APHERESIS PRODUCTS AND PROCEDURES

Apheresis equipment allows one or more blood components to be collected from a donor while the rest are returned. Apheresis platelet concentrates, which have as many platelets as 6–10 units of platelet concentrates from whole blood donations, are one example; granulocytes another. Apheresis techniques can also be used to collect hematopoietic stem cells that have been mobilized into the blood by cytokines (G-CSF or GM-CSF) given alone or after chemotherapy. These stem cells are used for allogeneic or autologous bone marrow transplantation. Blood cell separators can be used for the collection of single-source plasma or removal of a blood component that is causing disease. Examples include red cell exchange in sickle cell disease and plasmapheresis in Goodpasture syndrome or in Guillain-Barré.

Adverse Effects

The noninfectious complications of blood transfusions are outlined in Table 27–12. Most complications present a small but significant risk to the recipient.

Busch MP: Current and emerging infectious risks of blood transfusions. JAMA 2003;289:959 [PMID: 12597733].

Goodnough LT: Transfusion medicine. First of two parts—Blood transfusion. N Engl J Med 1999;340:438 [PMID: 9971869].

Goodnough LT: Transfusion medicine. Second of two parts—Blood conservation. N Engl J Med 1999;340:525 [PMID: 10021474].

National Institutes of Health Consensus Conference: Fresh frozen plasma: Indications and risks. JAMA 1985;253:551 [PMID: 3968788].

National Institutes of Health Consensus Conference: Platelet transfusion therapy. JAMA 1987;257:1777 [PMID: 3820494].

Silliman CC: Transfusion-related acute lung injury: Epidemiology and a prospective analysis of etiologic factors. Blood 2003; 101:454 [PMID: 12393667].

Smith JW: Therapeutic apheresis: A summary of current indication categories endorsed by the AABB and the American Society for Apheresis. Transfusion 2003;43:820 [PMID: 12757535].

REFERENCES

Goodnight SH, Hathaway WE: *Disorders of Hemostasis and Thrombosis: A Clinical Guide.* McGraw-Hill, 2001.

Petz LD, Garratty G: *Acquired Immune Hemolytic Anemias,* 2nd ed. Churchill Livingstone, 2004.

Simon TL et al, (editors): *Rossi's Principles of Transfusion Medicine.* Lippincott Williams & Wilkins, 2002.

Vichinsky E, Walters U, Feusner J (editors): Pediatric hematology/oncology, part I. Pediatr Clin North Am 2002.

Neoplastic Disease

Kelley Maloney, MD, Brian S. Greffe, MD, Nicholas K. Foreman, MD, Christopher C. Porter, MD, Doug K. Graham, MD, Kelly Sawczyn, MD, Roger H. Giller, MD, Ralph R. Quinones, MD, & Amy K. Keating, MD

Each year approximately 150 out of every 1 million children younger than 20 years of age are diagnosed with cancer. For children between the ages of 1 and 20 years, cancer is the fourth leading cause of death, behind unintentional injuries, homicides, and suicides. However, combined-modality therapy, including surgery, chemotherapy, and radiation therapy, has improved survival dramatically, such that the overall 5-year survival rate of pediatric malignancies is now greater than 75%. It is estimated that by the year 2020, one in 600 adults will be a survivor of childhood cancer.

Because pediatric malignancies are rare, cooperative clinical trials have become the mainstay of treatment planning and therapeutic advances. The Children's Oncology Group (COG), representing the amalgamation of four prior pediatric cooperative groups (Children's Cancer Group, Pediatric Oncology Group, Intergroup Rhabdomyosarcoma Study Group, and the National Wilms Tumor Study Group), offers the most current therapeutic options and protocols and strives to answer important treatment questions in a timely manner. A child or adolescent newly diagnosed with cancer should be enrolled in a cooperative clinical trial whenever possible. Because many protocols are associated with significant toxicities, morbidity, and potential mortality, treatment of children with cancer should be supervised by a pediatric oncologist familiar with the hazards of treatment, preferably at a multidisciplinary pediatric cancer center.

Advances in molecular genetics, cell biology, and tumor immunology have contributed and are crucial to the continued understanding of pediatric malignancies and their treatment. Continued research in the biology of tumors will lead to the identification of targeted therapy for specific tumor types with hopefully fewer systemic effects.

Research in supportive care areas, such as prevention and management of infection, pain, and emesis, has improved the survival and quality of life for children undergoing cancer treatment. Long-term studies of childhood cancer survivors are yielding information that provides a rationale for modifying future treatment regimens to decrease morbidity. A guide for caring for childhood cancer survivors is now available to medical providers as well as families and details suggested exams and late effects by type of chemotherapy received.

Cure Search. Children's Oncology Group. http://www.survivorshipguidelines.org

Ries LAG et al: SEER Cancer Statistics Review, 1975–2000. http://seer.cancer.gov/csr/1975_2000

■ MAJOR PEDIATRIC NEOPLASTIC DISEASES

ACUTE LYMPHOBLASTIC LEUKEMIA

ESSENTIALS OF DIAGNOSIS & TYPICAL FEATURES

- Bone marrow aspirate or biopsy specimen shows more than 25% lymphoblasts.
- Pallor, petechiae, purpura (50%), bone pain (25%).
- Hepatosplenomegaly (60%), lymphadenopathy (50%).
- Single or multiple cytopenias: neutropenia, thrombocytopenia, anemia (99%).
- Leukopenia (15%) or leukocytosis (50%), often with lymphoblasts identifiable on blood smear.
- Diagnosis confirmed by bone marrow examination.

General Considerations

Acute lymphoblastic leukemia (ALL) is the most common malignancy of childhood, accounting for about 25% of all cancer diagnoses in patients younger than age 15 years. The worldwide incidence of ALL is about 1:25,000 children per year, including 3000 children per year in the United States. The peak age at onset is 4 years; 85% of patients are diagnosed between ages 2 and 10 years. Children with Down syndrome have a 14-fold increase in the overall rate of leukemia. Before the advent of chemotherapy, this disease was fatal, usually within 3–4 months, with virtually no survivors 1 year after diagnosis.

ALL results from uncontrolled proliferation of immature lymphocytes. Its cause is unknown, and genetic factors may play a role. Leukemia is defined by the presence of more than 25% malignant hematopoietic cells (blasts) on bone marrow aspirate. Leukemic blasts from the majority of cases of childhood ALL have an antigen on the cell surface called the common ALL antigen (CALLA). These blasts derive from B-cell precursors early in their development, called B-precursor ALL. Less commonly, lymphoblasts are of T-cell origin or of mature B-cell origin. Over 70% of children receiving aggressive combination chemotherapy and early presymptomatic treatment to the central nervous system (CNS) are now cured of ALL.

Clinical Findings

A. SYMPTOMS AND SIGNS

Presenting complaints of patients with ALL include those related to decreased bone marrow production of red blood cells (RBCs), white blood cells (WBCs), or platelets and to leukemic infiltration of extramedullary (outside bone marrow) sites. Intermittent fevers are common, as a result of either cytokines induced by the leukemia itself or infections secondary to leukopenia. Many patients present due to bruising or pallor. About 25% of patients experience bone pain, especially in the pelvis, vertebral bodies, and legs. Physical examination at diagnosis ranges from virtually normal to highly abnormal. Signs related to bone marrow infiltration by leukemia include pallor, petechiae, and purpura. Hepatomegaly or splenomegaly occurs in over 60% of patients. Lymphadenopathy is common, either localized or generalized to cervical, axillary, and inguinal regions. The testes may occasionally be unilaterally or bilaterally enlarged secondary to leukemic infiltration. Superior vena cava syndrome is caused by mediastinal adenopathy compressing the superior vena cava. A prominent venous pattern develops over the upper chest from collateral vein enlargement. The neck may feel full from venous engorgement. The face may appear plethoric, and the periorbital area may be edematous.

A mediastinal mass can cause tachypnea, orthopnea, and respiratory distress. Leukemic infiltration of cranial nerves may cause cranial nerve palsies with mild nuchal rigidity. The optic fundi may show exudates of leukemic infiltration and hemorrhage from thrombocytopenia. Anemia can cause a flow murmur, tachycardia, and, rarely, congestive heart failure.

B. LABORATORY FINDINGS

A complete blood count (CBC) with differential is the most useful initial test because 95% of patients with ALL have a decrease in at least one cell type (single cytopenia): neutropenia, thrombocytopenia, or anemia. Most patients have decreases in at least two blood cell lines. The WBC count is low or normal (= 10,000/μL) in 50% of patients, but the differential shows neutropenia (absolute neutrophil count < 1000/μL) along with a small percentage of blasts amid normal lymphocytes. In 30% of patients the WBC count is between 10,000 and 50,000/μL; in 20% of patients it is over 50,000/μL, occasionally higher than 300,000/μL. Blasts are usually readily identifiable on peripheral blood smears from patients with elevated WBC counts. Peripheral blood smears also show abnormalities in RBCs, such as teardrops. Most patients with ALL have decreased platelet counts (< 150,000/μL) and decreased hemoglobin (< 11 g/dL) at diagnosis. Fewer than 1% of patients diagnosed with ALL have entirely normal CBCs and peripheral blood smears but have bone pain that leads to bone marrow examination. Serum chemistries, particularly uric acid and lactate dehydrogenase (LDH), are often elevated at diagnosis as a result of cell breakdown.

The diagnosis of ALL is made by bone marrow examination, which shows a homogeneous infiltration of leukemic blasts replacing normal marrow elements. The morphology of blasts on bone marrow aspirate can usually distinguish ALL from acute myeloid leukemia (AML). Lymphoblasts are typically small, with cell diameters of approximately two erythrocytes. Lymphoblasts have scant cytoplasm, usually without granules. The nucleus typically contains no nucleoli or one small, indistinct nucleolus. Immunophenotyping of ALL blasts by flow cytometry helps distinguish precursor B-cell ALL from T-cell ALL or AML. Histochemical stains specific for myeloblastic and monoblastic leukemias (myeloperoxidase and nonspecific esterase) distinguish ALL from AML. About 5% of patients present with CNS leukemia, which is defined as a cerebrospinal fluid (CSF) WBC count greater than 5/μL with blasts present on cytocentrifuged specimen.

C. IMAGING

Chest radiograph may show mediastinal widening or an anterior mediastinal mass and tracheal compression secondary to lymphadenopathy or thymic infiltration, especially in T-cell ALL. Abdominal ultrasound may show kidney enlargement from leukemic infiltration or uric acid nephropathy as well as intra-abdominal adenopathy. Plain radiographs of the long bones and spine may show demineralization, periosteal elevation, growth arrest lines, or compression of vertebral bodies.

Differential Diagnosis

The differential diagnosis, based on the history and physical examination, includes chronic infections by Epstein–Barr virus (EBV) and cytomegalovirus (CMV), causing lymphadenopathy, hepatosplenomegaly, fevers, and anemia. Prominent petechiae and purpura suggest a diagnosis of immune thrombocytopenic purpura. Significant pallor could be caused by transient erythroblastopenia of childhood, autoimmune hemolytic anemias, or aplastic anemia. Fevers and joint pains, with or without hepatosplenomegaly and lymphadenopathy, suggest juvenile rheumatoid arthritis (JRA). The diagnosis of leukemia usually becomes straightforward once the CBC reveals multiple cytopenias and leukemic blasts. Serum LDH levels may help distinguish JRA from leukemia. LDH is usually normal in JRA but often elevated in ALL patients presenting with bone pain. An elevated WBC count with lymphocytosis is typical of pertussis; however, in pertussis the lymphocytes are mature, and neutropenia is rarely associated.

Treatment

A. SPECIFIC THERAPY

Intensity of treatment is determined by specific prognostic features present at diagnosis, the patient's response to therapy, and specific biologic features of the leukemia cells. The majority of patients with ALL are enrolled in clinical trials designed by clinical groups and approved by the National Cancer Institute; the largest group is the COG. The first month of therapy consists of induction, at the end of which over 95% of patients exhibit remission on bone marrow aspirates. The drugs most commonly used in induction include oral prednisone or dexamethasone, intravenous vincristine and daunorubicin, intramuscular asparaginase, and intrathecal methotrexate. For T-cell ALL, intravenous cyclophosphamide may be added during induction.

Consolidation is the second phase of treatment, during which intrathecal chemotherapy along with continued systemic therapy and sometimes cranial radiation therapy are given to kill lymphoblasts "hiding" in the meninges. Several months of intensive chemotherapy follows consolidation. This intensification has led to improved survival in pediatric ALL.

Maintenance therapy includes daily oral mercaptopurine, weekly oral methotrexate, and, often, monthly pulses of intravenous vincristine and oral prednisone or dexamethasone. Intrathecal chemotherapy, either with methotrexate alone or combined with cytarabine and hydrocortisone, is usually given every 2–3 months.

These drugs have significant potential side effects. Patients need to be monitored closely to prevent drug toxicities and to ensure early treatment of complications. The duration of treatment ranges between 2.2 years for girls and 3.2 years for boys. Treatment for ALL is tailored to prognostic, or risk, groups. A child age 1–9 years with a WBC count under 50,000/μL at diagnosis and without poor biologic features t(9;22) or t(4;11) is considered to be at "standard risk" and receives less intensive therapy than a "high-risk" patient who has a WBC count at diagnosis over 50,000/μL or is older than age 10 years. Also impor-

tant is the patient's response to treatment determined by minimal residual disease (MRD) monitoring. This risk-adapted treatment approach has significantly increased the cure rate among patients with less favorable prognostic features while minimizing treatment-related toxicities in those with favorable features. Bone marrow relapse is usually heralded by an abnormal CBC, either during treatment or for a few years thereafter.

The CNS and testes are sanctuary sites of extramedullary leukemia. Currently, about a third of all ALL relapses are isolated to these sanctuary sites. Systemic chemotherapy does not penetrate these tissues as well as it penetrates other organs. Thus, presymptomatic intrathecal chemotherapy is a critical part of ALL treatment, without which many more relapses would occur in the CNS, with or without bone marrow relapse. The majority of isolated CNS relapses are diagnosed in an asymptomatic child at the time of routine intrathecal injection, when CSF cell count and differential shows an elevated WBC with leukemic blasts. Occasionally, symptoms of CNS relapse develop: headache, nausea and vomiting, irritability, nuchal rigidity, photophobia, and cranial nerve palsies. Currently, testicular relapse occurs in less than 5% of boys. The presentation of testicular relapse is usually unilateral painless testicular enlargement, without a distinct mass. Routine follow-up of boys both on and off treatment includes physical examination of the testes.

Bone marrow transplantation, now called hematopoietic stem cell transplantation (HSCT), is rarely used as initial treatment for ALL, because most patients are cured with chemotherapy alone. Patients whose blasts contain certain chromosomal abnormalities, such as t(9;22) or hypodiploidy (< 44 chromosomes), and patients with a very slow response to therapy may have a better cure rate with early HSCT from an HLA-DR–matched sibling donor, or perhaps a matched unrelated donor, than with intensive chemotherapy alone. HSCT cures about 50% of patients who relapse, provided that a second remission is achieved with chemotherapy before transplant. Children who relapse more than 1 year after completion of chemotherapy (late relapse) may be cured with intensive chemotherapy without HSCT. A number of new biologic agents, including tyrosine kinase inhibitors and immunotoxins, are currently in various stages of research and development. Some of these therapies may prove relevant for future treatment of poor risk or relapsed ALL.

B. SUPPORTIVE CARE

Tumor lysis syndrome should be anticipated when treatment is started. Alkalinization of urine with intravenous sodium bicarbonate, maintaining brisk urine output, and treating with oral allopurinol are appropriate steps in managing tumor lysis syndrome. Serum levels of potassium, phosphorus, and uric acid should be monitored. If superior vena caval or superior mediastinal syndrome is present, general anesthesia is contraindicated temporarily. If hyperleukocytosis (WBC count > 100,000/μL) is accompanied by hyperviscosity and mental status changes, leukophoresis may be indicated to rapidly reduce the number of circulating blasts and minimize the potential thrombotic or hemorrhagic CNS complications. Throughout the course of treatment, all transfused blood and platelet products should be irradiated to prevent graft-versus-host disease from the transfused lymphocytes. Whenever possible, blood products should be leukodepleted to minimize CMV transmission, transfusion reactions, and sensitization to platelets.

Due to the immunocompromised state of the patient with ALL, bacterial, fungal, and viral infections are serious and can be life-threatening or fatal. During the course of treatment, fever (temperature = 38.3 °C) and neutropenia (absolute neutrophil count < 500/μL) require prompt assessment, blood cultures from each lumen of a central line, and prompt treatment with empiric broad-spectrum antibiotics. Patients receiving ALL treatment must receive prophylaxis against *Pneumocystis jiroveci* (formerly *Pneumocystis carinii*). Trimethoprim–sulfamethoxazole given twice each day on 2 or 3 consecutive days per week is the drug of choice. Patients nonimmune to varicella are at risk for very serious—even fatal—infection. Such patients should receive varicella-zoster immune globulin (VZIG) within 72 hours after exposure and treatment with intravenous acyclovir for active infection.

The treatment of a patient on chemotherapy for ALL is complex because of the infectious complications and potential toxicities of chemotherapy.

Prognosis

Cure rates depend on specific prognostic features present at diagnosis, biologic features of the leukemic blast, and the response to therapy. Two of the most important features are WBC count and age. Children age 1–9 years whose diagnostic WBC count is less than 50,000/μL have a higher rate of cure than other patients (~85% EFS [event free survival] for these children). The rapidity of response to induction treatment has prognostic significance as well, reflecting leukemic blast sensitivity to chemotherapy. Patients are categorized as rapid early responders (RER) or slow early responders (SER) based on the percentage of blasts present in bone marrow aspirates within 7–14 days after induction begins. More intensive treatment regimens are given to SERs than RERs to increase their chance of cure. Certain chromosomal abnormalities present in the leukemic blasts at diagnosis influence prognosis. Patients with t(9;22) generally have a very poor chance of cure even with intensive chemotherapy. Likewise, infants less than 6 months of age with t(4;11) have a poor chance of cure with conventional chemotherapy. In contrast, 15% of

patients whose blasts are hyperdiploid (containing over 50 chromosomes instead of the normal 46) with trisomies of chromosomes 4, 10, and 17, and 25% of patients whose blasts have a t(12;21) and TEL-AML1 rearrangement have a greater chance of cure than do children without these characteristics, approaching 90% survival. Techniques based on leukemic blast immunophenotyping or immunoglobulin rearrangements have been developed to detect residual lymphoblasts in bone marrow, called minimal residual disease (MRD), at the end of induction and during remission. Many groups have shown that even low levels of MRD predict an inferior outcome. In the current COG clinical trials, patients with levels of MRD above 0.1% at the end of remission induction will receive intensified therapy, in an attempt to improve their outcome.

Bostrom BC: Dexamethasone versus prednisone and daily oral versus weekly intravenous mercaptopurine for patients with standard-risk acute lymphoblastic leukemia: A report from the Children's Cancer Group. Blood 2003:101:3809 [PMID: 12531809].

Pearce JM et al: Childhood leukemia. Pediatr Rev 2005:26(3);96 [PMID: 15741325].

Peters C et al: Allogeneic haematopoitic stem cell transplantation in children with acute lymphoblastic leukaemia: The BFM/IBFM/EBMT concepts. Bone Marrow Transplant 2005:35:S9 [PMID: 15812540].

ACUTE MYELOID LEUKEMIA

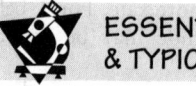 **ESSENTIALS OF DIAGNOSIS & TYPICAL FEATURES**

- Bone marrow aspirate or biopsy shows 20% or more leukemic blasts.
- Fatigue, bleeding, or infection.
- Adenopathy, hepatosplenomegaly, skin nodules (M4 and M5 subtypes).
- Cytopenias: neutropenia (69%), anemia (44%), thrombocytopenia (33%).

General Considerations

Approximately 500 new cases of acute myeloid leukemia (AML) occur per year in children and adolescents in the United States. Although AML accounts for only 25% of all leukemias in this age group, it is responsible for at least one-third of deaths from leukemia in children and teenagers. Congenital conditions associated with an increased risk of AML include Diamond–Blackfan anemia, neurofibromatosis, Down syndrome, Wiskott–Aldrich, Kostmann and Li–Fraumeni syndromes, as well as chromosomal instability syndromes such as Fanconi anemia. Acquired risk factors include exposure to ionizing radiation, cytotoxic chemo-

Table 28-1. FAB subtypes of acute myeloid leukemia.

FAB Classification	Common Name	Distribution in Childhood (Age)		Cytogenetic Associations	Clinical Features
		< 2 Years	> 2 Years		
M0	Acute myeloid leukemia, minimally differentiated		1%	inv (3q26), t(3;3)	
M1	Acute myeloblastic leukemia without maturation	17%	23%		
M2	Acute myeloblastic leukemia with maturation		26%	t(8;21) t(6;9); rare	Myeloblastomas or chloromas
M3	Acute promyelocytic leukemia		4%	t(15;17); rarely, t(11;17) or (5;17)	Disseminated intravascular coagulation
M4	Acute myelomonoblastic leukemia	30%	24%	11q23, inv 3, t(3;3), t(6;9)	Hyperleukocytosis, CNS involvement, skin and gum infiltration
M4Eo	Acute myelomonoblastic leukemia with abnormal eosinophils			inv16, t(16;16)	
M5	Acute monoblastic leukemia	46%	15%	11q23, t(9;11), t(8;16)	Hyperleukocytosis, CNS involvement, skin and gum infiltration
M6	Erythroleukemia		2%		
M7	Acute megakaryoblastic leukemia	7%	5%	t(1;22)	Down syndrome frequent (< 2 years of age)

FAB, French-American-British classification; CNS, central nervous system.

therapeutic agents, and benzenes. However, the vast majority of patients have no identifiable risk factors. Historically, the diagnosis of AML was based almost exclusively on morphology and immunohistochemical staining of the leukemic cells. AML has eight subtypes (M0–M7) according to the French–American–British (FAB) classification (Table 28–1). Immunophenotypic, cytogenetic, and molecular analyses are increasingly important in confirming the diagnosis of AML and subclassifying it into biologically distinct subtypes that have therapeutic and prognostic implications. Cytogenetic clonal abnormalities occur in 80% of patients with AML and are often predictive of outcome.

Aggressive induction therapy currently results in a 75–85% complete remission rate. However, long-term survival has improved only modestly to approximately 50%, despite the availability of a number of effective agents, improvements in supportive care, and increasingly intensive therapies.

Clinical and Laboratory Findings

The clinical manifestations of AML commonly include anemia (44%), thrombocytopenia (33%), and neutrope-

nia (69%). Symptoms may be few and innocuous or may be life-threatening. The median hemoglobin value at diagnosis is 7 g/dL, and platelets usually number fewer than 50,000/μL. Frequently the absolute neutrophil count is under 1000/μL, although the total WBC count is over 100,000/μL in 25% of patients at diagnosis.

Hyperleukocytosis may be associated with life-threatening complications. Venous stasis and sludging of blasts in small vessels cause hypoxia, hemorrhage, and infarction, most notably in the lung and CNS. This clinical picture is a medical emergency requiring rapid intervention, such as leukophoresis, to decrease the leukocyte count. CNS leukemia is present in 5–15% of patients at diagnosis, a higher rate of initial involvement than in ALL. Certain subtypes, such as M4 and M5, have a higher likelihood of meningeal infiltration than do other subtypes. Additionally, clinically significant coagulopathy may be present at diagnosis in patients with M3, M4, or M5 subtypes. This problem manifests as bleeding or an abnormal disseminated intravascular coagulation screen and should be at least partially corrected prior to initiation of treatment, which may transiently exacerbate the coagulopathy.

Treatment

A. SPECIFIC THERAPY

AML is less responsive to treatment than ALL and requires more intensive chemotherapy. Toxicities from therapy are common and likely to be life-threatening; therefore, treatment should be undertaken only at a tertiary pediatric oncology center.

Current AML protocols rely on intensive administration of anthracyclines, cytarabine, and etoposide for induction of remission. After remission is obtained those patients who have a matched sibling donor undergo allogeneic HSCT while those patients without an appropriate related donor are treated with additional cycles of aggressive chemotherapy for a total of 6–9 months.

The biologic heterogeneity of AML is becoming increasingly important therapeutically. The M3 subtype, associated with t(15;17) demonstrated either cytogenetically or molecularly, is currently treated with all *trans*-retinoic acid in addition to chemotherapy with high-dose cytarabine and daunorubicin. All *trans*-retinoic acid leads to differentiation of promyelocytic leukemia cells and can induce remission, but cure requires conventional chemotherapy as well. The use of arsenic trioxide has also been investigated in the treatment of this subtype of AML with favorable results.

Another biologically distinct subtype of AML occurs in children with Down syndrome, M7, or megakaryocytic AML. Using less intensive treatment, remission induction rate and overall survival of these children are dramatically superior to non-Down syndrome children with AML. It is important that children with Down syndrome receive appropriate treatment specifically designed to be less intensive.

Biologic agents are increasingly being studied in the treatment of AML. The development and early success of antibody-targeted cytotoxic agents such as gemtuzumab ozogamicin (Mylotarg, a humanized anti-CD33 monoclonal antibody conjugated with calicheamicin) are encouraging in the quest for therapeutic agents that result in higher survival rates. This agent is now being trialed with intensive chemotherapy for treatment of AML.

B. SUPPORTIVE CARE

Tumor lysis syndrome rarely occurs during induction treatment of AML. Nevertheless, when the diagnostic WBC cell count is greater than 100,000 or significant adenopathy or organomegaly is present, one should alkalinize urine with intravenous sodium bicarbonate, maintain brisk urine output, and follow potassium, uric acid, and phosphorous lab values closely. Hyperleukocytosis (WBC > 100,000/μL) is a medical emergency and, in a symptomatic patient, requires rapid intervention such as leukophoresis to rapidly decrease the number of circulating blasts and thereby decrease hyperviscosity. Delaying transfusion of packed RBCs until the WBC can be decreased to below 100,000/μL avoids exacerbating hyperviscosity. It is also important to correct the coagulopathy commonly associated with M3, M4, or M5 subtypes prior to beginning induction chemotherapy. As with the treatment of ALL, all blood products should be irradiated and leukodepleted; pneumocystis prophylaxis must be administered during treatment and for several weeks afterward; and patients not immune to varicella must receive VZIG within 72 hours of exposure and prompt treatment with intravenous acyclovir for active infection.

Onset of fever (temperature ≥ 38.3 °C) or chills associated with neutropenia requires prompt assessment, blood cultures from each lumen of a central venous line, other cultures such as throat or urine as appropriate, and prompt initiation of broad-spectrum intravenous antibiotics. Infections in this population of patients can rapidly become life-threatening. Because of the high incidence of invasive fungal infections, there should be a low threshold for initiating antifungal therapy. Filgrastim (granulocyte colony-stimulating factor) may be used to stimulate granulocyte recovery during the treatment of AML and results in shorter periods of neutropenia and hospitalization. It must be stressed that the supportive care for this group of patients is as important as the leukemia-directed therapy and that this treatment should be carried out only at a tertiary pediatric cancer center.

Prognosis

Published results from various centers show a 50–60% survival rate at 5 years following first remission for those patients that do not have matched sibling hematopoietic stem cell donors. Patients with matched sibling donors fare slightly better, with 5-year survival rates of 60–70% after allogeneic HSCT.

As treatment becomes more sophisticated, outcome is increasingly related to the subtype of AML. Currently, AML with t(8;21), t(15;17), inv 16, or in children with Down syndrome has the most favorable prognosis, with 65–75% long-term survival using modern treatments. The least favorable outcome occurs in AML with monosomy 7 or 5, 7q, 5q–, or 11q23 cytogenetic abnormalities.

Alonzo TA et al: Postremission therapy for children with acute myeloid leukemia: The children's cancer group experience in the transplant era. Leukemia 2005;19(6);965 [PMID: 15830007].

Neudorf S et al: Allogeneic bone marrow transplantation for children with acute myelocytic leukemia in first remission demonstrates a role for graft versus leukemia in the maintenance of disease-free survival. Blood 2004:103(10);3655 [PMID: 14751924].

Tallman MS et al: Drug therapy for acute myeloid leukemia. Blood 2005:106(4);1154 [PMID: 15870183].

MYELOPROLIFERATIVE DISEASES

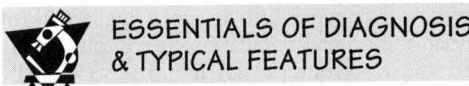

ESSENTIALS OF DIAGNOSIS & TYPICAL FEATURES

- *Leukocytosis with predominance of immature cells.*
- *Often indolent course.*
- *Fever, bone pain, respiratory symptoms.*
- *Hepatosplenomegaly.*

Myeloproliferative diseases in children are relatively rare. They are characterized by ineffective hematopoiesis that results in excessive peripheral blood counts. The three most important types are chronic myelogenous leukemia (CML), which accounts for less than 5% of the childhood leukemias, transient myeloproliferative disorder in children with Down syndrome, and juvenile myelomonocytic leukemia (Table 28–2).

1. Chronic Myelogenous Leukemia

General Considerations

CML with translocation of chromosomes 9 and 22 (the Philadelphia chromosome, Ph+) is identical to adult Ph+ CML. Translocation 9;22 results in the fusion of the *BCR* gene on chromosome 22 and the *ABL* gene on chromosome 9. The resulting fusion protein is a constitutively active tyrosine kinase that interacts with a variety of effector proteins and allows for deregulated cellular proliferation, decreased adherence of cells to the bone marrow extracellular matrix, and resistance to apoptosis. The disease usually progresses within 3 years to an accelerated phase and then to a blast crisis. It is generally accepted that Ph+ cells have an increased susceptibility to the acquisition of additional molecular changes that lead to the accelerated and blast phases of disease.

Clinical and Laboratory Findings

Patients with CML may present with nonspecific complaints similar to those of acute leukemia, including bone pain, fever, night sweats, and fatigue. However, patients can also be asymptomatic. Those patients with a total WBC count of more than 100,000/μL may have symptoms of leukostasis, such as dyspnea, priapism, or neurologic abnormalities. Physical findings may include fever, pallor, ecchymoses, and hepatosplenomegaly. Anemia, thrombocytosis, and leukocytosis are frequent

Table 28–2. Comparison of JMML, CML, and TMD.

	JMML	CML	TMD
Age at onset	< 2 years old	> 3 years old	< 3 months old
Clinical presentation	Abrupt onset; eczematoid skin rash, marked lymphadenopathy, bleeding tendency, moderate hepatosplenomegaly, fever	Nonspecific constitutional complaints, massive splenomegaly, variable hepatomegaly	DS features, often no or few symptoms; or hepatosplenomegaly, respiratory symptoms
Chromosomal alterations	Monosomy or del (7q) in 20% of patients	t(9;22)	Constitutional trisomy 21, but usually no other abnormality
Laboratory features	Moderate leukocytosis (> 10,000/μL), thrombocytopenia, monocytosis (> 1000/μL), elevated fetal hemoglobin, normal to diminished leukocyte alkaline phosphatase, elevated muramidase	Marked leukocytosis (> 100,000/μL), normal to elevated platelet count, decreased to absent leukocyte alkaline phosphatase, usually normal muramidase	Variable leukocytosis, normal to high platelet count, large platelets, myeloblasts

JMML, juvenile myelomonocytic leukemia; CML, chronic myelogenous leukemia; TMD, transient myeloproliferative disorder; DS, Down syndrome.

laboratory findings. The peripheral smear is usually diagnostic with a characteristic predominance of myeloid cells in all stages of maturation and relatively few blasts.

Treatment and Prognosis

Historically, hydroxyurea or busulfan has been used to reduce or eliminate Ph+ cells. However, HSCT is the only consistently curative intervention. Reported survival rates for patients younger than age 20 years transplanted in the chronic phase from matched related donors are 70–80%. Unrelated stem cell transplants result in survival rates of 50–65%.

The understanding of the molecular mechanisms involved in the pathogenesis of CML has led to the rational design of molecularly targeted therapy. Imatinib mesylate (Gleevec) is a tyrosine kinase inhibitor that has had dramatic success in the treatment of CML, with most adults and children achieving cytogenetic remission. The durability of the remission for children is unclear but is now the accepted upfront therapy. However, some patients are resistant to imatinib, and its role in the long-term management of children with CML awaits further studies.

2. Transient Myeloproliferative Disorder

General Considerations

Transient myeloproliferative disorder is unique to patients with trisomy 21 or mosaicism for trisomy 21. It is characterized by uncontrolled proliferation of blasts, usually of megakaryocytic origin, during early infancy and spontaneous resolution. The pathogenesis of this process is not well understood, although mutations in the *GATA1* gene have recently been implicated as initial events.

Although the true incidence is unknown, it is estimated to occur in up to 10% of patients with Down syndrome. Despite the fact that the process usually resolves by 3 months of age, organ infiltration may cause significant morbidity and mortality.

Clinical Findings, Treatment, and Prognosis

Patients can present with hydrops fetalis, pericardial or pleural effusions, or hepatic fibrosis. More frequently, they are asymptomatic or only minimally ill. Therefore, treatment is primarily supportive. Patients without symptoms are not treated, and those with organ dysfunction receive low doses of chemotherapy or leukophoresis (or both) to reduce peripheral blood blast counts. Although patients with transient myeloproliferative disorder have apparent resolution of the process, approximately 30% go on to

develop acute megakaryoblastic leukemia (AML M7) within 3 years.

3. Juvenile Myelomonocytic Leukemia

Clinical and Laboratory Findings

Juvenile myelomonocytic leukemia (JMML), accounts for approximately one-third of the myelodysplastic and myeloproliferative disorders in childhood. Patients with neurofibromatosis type 1 (NF-1) are at higher risk of JMML than the general population. It typically occurs in infants and very young children and is occasionally associated with monosomy 7 or a deletion of the long arm of chromosome 7.

Clinical Findings, Treatment, and Prognosis

Patients with JMML present similarly to those with other hematopoietic malignancies, with lymphadenopathy, hepatosplenomegaly, skin rash, or respiratory symptoms. Patients may have stigmata of NF-1 with neurofibromas or café au lait spots. Laboratory findings include anemia, thrombocytopenia, leukocytosis with monocytosis, and elevated fetal hemoglobin.

The results of chemotherapy for children with JMML have been disappointing, with estimated survival rates of less than 30%. Approximately 40–45% of patients are projected to survive long term using HSCT, although optimizing conditioning regimens and donor selection may improve these results.

Crispino JD: GATA1 mutations in Down syndrome: Implications for biology and diagnosis of children with transient myeloproliferative disorder and acute megakaryoblastic leukemia. Pediatr Blood Cancer 2005:44;40 [PMID: 15390312].

Cwynarski K et al: Stem cell transplantation for chronic myeloid leukemia in children. Blood 2003;102:1224 [PMID: 12714525].

Goldman JM, Melo JV: Chronic myeloid leukemia—Advances in biology and new approaches to treatment. N Engl J Med 2003;349:1451 [PMID: 14534339].

Mundschau G et al: Mutagenesis of GATA1 is an initiating event in Down syndrome leukemogenesis. Blood 2003;101:4298 [PMID: 12560215].

Passmore SJ et al: Paediatric myelodysplastic syndromes and juvenile myelomonocytic leukaemia in the UK: A population-based study of incidence and survival. Br J Haematol 2003;121;758 [PMID: 12780790].

Pulsipher MA: Treatment of CML in pediatric patients: Should imatinib mesylate (STI-571, Gleevec) or allogeneic hematopoietic cell transplant be front-line therapy? Pediatr Blood Cancer 2004:43(5);523 [PMID: 15382266].

Thornley I et al: Treating children with chronic myeloid leukemia in the imatinib era: A therapeutic dilemma? Med Pediatr Oncol 2003;41:115 [PMID: 12825214].

Woods WG et al: Prospective study of 90 children requiring treatment for juvenile myelomonocytic leukemia or myelodysplastic syndrome: A report from the Children's Cancer Group. J Clin Oncol 2002;20:434 [PMID: 11786571].

BRAIN TUMORS

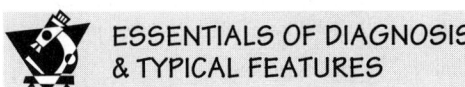

ESSENTIALS OF DIAGNOSIS & TYPICAL FEATURES

- *Classic triad: morning headache, vomiting, and papilledema.*
- *Increasing head circumference, cranial nerve palsies, dysarthria, ataxia, hemiplegia, papilledema, hyperreflexia, macrocephaly, cracked pot sign.*
- *Seizures, personality change, blurred vision, diplopia, weakness, decreased coordination, precocious puberty.*

General Considerations

The classic triad of morning headache, vomiting, and papilledema is present in less than 30% of children at presentation. School failure and personality changes are common in older children. Irritability, failure to thrive, and delayed development are common in very young children with brain tumors. Recent-onset head tilt can result from a posterior fossa tumor.

Brain tumors are the most common solid tumors of childhood, accounting for 1500–2000 new malignancies in children each year in the United States and for 25–30% of all childhood cancers. In general, children with brain tumors have a better prognosis than do adults. Favorable outcome occurs most commonly with low-grade and fully resectable tumors. Unfortunately, cranial irradiation in young children can have significant neuropsychological, intellectual, and endocrinologic sequelae.

Brain tumors in childhood are biologically and histologically heterogeneous, ranging from low-grade localized lesions to high-grade tumors with neuraxis dissemination. High-dose systemic chemotherapy is used frequently, especially in young children with high-grade tumors, in an effort to delay, decrease, or completely avoid cranial irradiation. Such intensive treatment may be accompanied by autologous HSCT or peripheral stem cell reconstitution.

The causes of pediatric brain tumors are unknown. The risk of developing astrocytomas is increased in children with neurofibromatosis or tuberous sclerosis. Several studies show that some childhood brain tumors occur in families with increased genetic susceptibility to childhood cancers in general, brain tumors, or leukemia and lymphoma. An excess of seizures has been observed in relatives of children with astrocytoma. Certain pediat-

ric brain tumors such as ependymoma have been linked to polyomavirus, but the exact relationship is unknown. The risk of developing a brain tumor is increased in children who received cranial irradiation for treatment of meningeal leukemia.

Because pediatric brain tumors are rare, they are often misdiagnosed or diagnosed late; most pediatricians see no more than two children with brain tumors during their careers.

Clinical Findings

A. SYMPTOMS AND SIGNS

Clinical findings at presentation vary depending on the child's age and the tumor's location. Children younger than age 2 years more commonly have infratentorial tumors. Children with such tumors usually present with nonspecific symptoms such as vomiting, unsteadiness, lethargy, and irritability. Signs may be surprisingly few or may include macrocephaly, ataxia, hyperreflexia, and cranial nerve palsies. Because the head can expand in young children, papilledema is often absent. Measuring head circumference and observing gait are essential in evaluating a child for possible brain tumor. Eye findings and apparent visual disturbances such as difficulty tracking can occur in association with optic pathway tumors such as optic glioma. Optic glioma occurring in a young child is often associated with neurofibromatosis.

Older children more commonly have supratentorial tumors, which are associated with headache, visual symptoms, seizures, and focal neurologic deficits. Initial presenting features are often nonspecific. School failure and personality changes are common. Vaguely described visual disturbance is often present, but the child must be directly asked. Headaches are common, but they often will not be predominantly in the morning. The headaches may be confused with migraine.

Older children with infratentorial tumors characteristically present with symptoms and signs of hydrocephalus, which include progressively worsening morning headache and vomiting, gait unsteadiness, double vision, and papilledema. Cerebellar astrocytomas enlarge slowly, and symptoms may worsen over several months. Morning vomiting may be the only symptom of posterior fossa ependymomas, which originate in the floor of the fourth ventricle near the vomiting center. Children with brainstem tumors may present with facial and extraocular muscle palsies, ataxia, and hemiparesis; hydrocephalus occurs in approximately 25% of these patients at diagnosis.

B. IMAGING AND STAGING

In addition to the tumor biopsy, neuraxis imaging studies are obtained to determine whether dissemination has occurred. It is unusual for brain tumors in children and adolescents to disseminate outside of the CNS.

Magnetic resonance imaging (MRI) has become the preferred diagnostic study for pediatric brain tumors. MRI provides better definition of the tumor and delineates indolent gliomas that may not be seen on computed tomography (CT) scan. In contrast, a CT scan can be done in less than 10 minutes—as opposed to the 30 minutes required for an MRI scan—and is still useful if an urgent diagnostic study is necessary or to detect calcification of a tumor. Both scans are generally done with and without contrast enhancement. Contrast enhances regions where the blood–brain barrier is disrupted. Postoperative scans to document the extent of tumor resection should be obtained within 48 hours after surgery to avoid postsurgical enhancement.

Imaging of the entire neuraxis and CSF cytologic examination should be part of the diagnostic evaluation for patients with tumors such as medulloblastoma, ependymoma, and pineal region tumors. Diagnosis of neuraxis drop metastases (tumor spread along the neuraxis) can be accomplished by gadolinium-enhanced MRI incorporating sagittal and axial views. MRI of the spine should be obtained preoperatively in all children with midline tumors of the fourth ventricle or cerebellum. A CSF sample should be obtained during the diagnostic surgery. Lumbar CSF is preferred over ventricular CSF for cytologic examination. Levels of biomarkers in the blood and CSF, such as human chorionic gonadotropin and α-fetoprotein, may be helpful at diagnosis and in follow-up. Both human chorionic gonadotropin and α-fetoprotein should be obtained from the blood preoperatively for all pineal and suprasellar tumors.

Table 28–3. Location and frequency of common pediatric brain tumors.

Location	Frequency of Occurrence (%)
Hemispheric	**37**
Low-grade astrocytoma	23
High-grade astrocytoma	11
Other	3
Posterior fossa	**49**
Medulloblastoma	15
Cerebellar astrocytoma	15
Brainstem glioma	15
Ependymoma	4
Midline	**14**
Craniopharyngioma	8
Chiasmal glioma	4
Pineal region tumor	2

Table 28–4. Prognostic factors in children with medulloblastoma.

Factor	Favorable	Unfavorable
Extent of disease	Nondisseminated	Disseminated
Size of primary tumor after surgery	≤ 3 cm (completely resected)	> 3 cm
Histologic features	Undifferentiated	Foci of glial, ependymal, or neuronal differentiation
Age	≥ 4 years	< 4 years

The neurosurgeon should discuss staging and sample collection with an oncologist before surgery in a child newly presenting with a scan suggestive of brain tumor.

C. CLASSIFICATION

About 50% of the common pediatric brain tumors occur above the tentorium and 50% in the posterior fossa. In the very young child, posterior fossa tumors are more common. Most childhood brain tumors can be divided into two categories according to the cell of origin: (1) glial tumors such as astrocytomas and ependymomas or (2) nonglial tumors such as medulloblastoma and other primitive neuroectodermal tumors. Some tumors contain both glial and neural elements (eg, ganglioglioma). A group of less common CNS tumors do not fit into either category (ie, craniopharyngiomas, germ cell tumors, choroid plexus tumors, and meningiomas). Low-grade and high-grade tumors are found in most categories. Table 28–3 lists the locations and frequencies of the common pediatric brain tumors.

Astrocytoma is the most common brain tumor of childhood. Most are juvenile pilocytic astrocytoma (WHO grade I) found in the posterior fossa with a bland cellular morphology and few or no mitotic figures. Low-grade astrocytomas are in many cases curable by complete surgical excision alone. Chemotherapy is effective in low-grade astrocytomas.

Medulloblastoma and related primitive neuroectodermal tumors are the most common high-grade brain tumors in children. These tumors usually occur in the first decade of life, with a peak incidence between ages 5 and 10 years and a female-to-male ratio of 2.1:1.3. These tumors typically arise in the midline cerebellar vermis, with variable extension into the fourth ventricle. Reports of neuraxis dissemination at diagnosis range from 10–46% of patients. Prognostic factors are outlined in Table 28–4.

Brainstem tumors are third in frequency of occurrence in children. They are frequently of astrocytic origin and often are high-grade. Children with tumors that diffusely infiltrate the brainstem and involve primarily the pons have a long-term survival rate of less than 15%. Brainstem tumors that occur above or below the pons and grow in an eccentric or cystic manner have a somewhat better outcome. Exophytic tumors in this location may be amenable to surgery. Generally, brainstem tumors are treated without a tissue diagnosis.

Other brain tumors such as ependymomas, germ cell tumors, choroid plexus tumors, and craniopharyngiomas are less common, and each is associated with unique diagnostic and therapeutic challenges.

Treatment

A. SUPPORTIVE CARE

Dexamethasone should be started prior to initial surgery (0.5–1.0 mg/kg initially, then 0.25–0.5 mg/kg/d in four divided doses). Anticonvulsants (usually phenytoin, 4–8 mg/kg/d) should be started if the child has had a seizure or if the surgical approach is likely to induce seizures. Because postoperative treatment of young children with high-grade brain tumors incorporates increasingly more intensive systemic chemotherapy, consideration should also be given to the use of prophylaxis for prevention of oral candidiasis and *Pneumocystis* infection. Dexamethasone and phenytoin potentially reduce the effectiveness of chemotherapy and should be discontinued as soon after surgery as possible.

Optimum care for the pediatric patient with a brain tumor requires a multidisciplinary team including subspecialists in pediatric neurosurgery, neurooncology, neurology, endocrinology, neuropsychology, radiation therapy, and rehabilitation medicine, as well as highly specialized nurses, social workers, and staff in physical therapy, occupational therapy, and speech and language science.

B. SPECIFIC THERAPY

The goal of treatment is to eradicate the tumor with the least short- and long-term morbidity. Long-term neuropsychological morbidity becomes an especially important issue related to deficits caused by the tumor itself and the sequelae of treatment. Meticulous surgical removal of as much tumor as possible is generally the preferred initial approach. Technologic advances in the operating microscope, the ultrasonic tissue aspirator, and the CO_2 laser (which is less commonly used in pediatric brain tumor surgery); the accuracy of computerized stereotactic resection; and the availability of intraoperative monitoring techniques such as evoked potentials and electrocorticography have increased the feasibility and safety of surgical resection of many pediatric brain tumors. Second-look surgery after chemo-

therapy is increasingly being used when tumors are incompletely resected at initial surgery.

Radiation therapy for pediatric brain tumors is in a state of evolution. For tumors with a high probability of neuraxis dissemination (eg, medulloblastoma), craniospinal radiation is still standard therapy in children older than age 3 years. In others (eg, ependymoma), craniospinal radiation has been abandoned because neuraxis dissemination at first relapse is rare. Approaches to the delivery of radiation to minimize the adverse effects on normal brain tissue are being explored and include stereotactic radiation and the use of three-dimensional treatment planning.

Chemotherapy is effective in treating low-grade and malignant astrocytomas and medulloblastomas. A series of brain tumor protocols for children younger than age 3 years involved administering intensive chemotherapy after tumor resection and delaying or omitting radiation therapy. The results of these trials have generally been disappointing but have taught valuable lessons regarding the varying responses to chemotherapy of different tumor types. Future trials may give shorter courses of more intense chemotherapy followed by conformal radiotherapy. Conformal techniques allow the delivery of radiation to strictly defined fields and may limit side effects.

In older children with malignant glioma, the current approach would be surgical resection of the tumor and combined-modality treatment with irradiation and intensive chemotherapy. In patients with glioblastoma, the use of high-dose chemotherapy and autologous bone marrow or peripheral stem cell reconstitution is being studied. Initial results are mixed, but the toxicity of such therapy remains a concern. Surgery is not indicated for diffuse brainstem gliomas. Traditional treatment of these tumors has been local irradiation. Hyperfractionation to increase the dose from the conventional 54 Gy to 72–78 Gy showed no apparent benefit in a recent Children's Cancer Group (CCG) study. New approaches are needed for this prognostically poor tumor.

The treatment of low-grade astrocytomas is evolving. Increasing numbers of young children are receiving antitumor chemotherapeutic agents such as carboplatin and vincristine after incomplete resection of these tumors. The role of irradiation after subtotal resection even in older children is being questioned.

Prognosis

Despite improvements in surgery and radiation therapy, the outlook for cure remains poor for children with high-grade glial tumors. For children with high-grade gliomas, an early CCG study showed a 45% progression-free survival rate for children who received radiation therapy and chemotherapy. A follow-up CCG study in which all patients had chemotherapy and radiation therapy showed a 5-year progression-free survival rate of 36%. There is a possibility of effective salvage therapy with high-dose chemotherapy for children who relapse. In addition, the extent of resection appeared to correlate positively with prognosis, with a 3-year progression-free survival rate of 17% for patients receiving biopsy only, 29–32% for patients receiving partial or subtotal resections, and 54% for those receiving 90% resections. Biologic factors that may affect survival are being increasingly recognized. The prognosis for diffuse pontine gliomas remains very poor, with no benefit from high-dose chemotherapy plus radiation versus radiation alone.

The 5- and even 10-year survival rate for low-grade astrocytomas of childhood is 60–90%. However, prognosis depends on both site and grade. A child with a pilocytic astrocytoma of the cerebellum has a considerably better prognosis than a child with a fibrillary astrocytoma of the cerebral cortex. Recently, a new entity of low-grade tumor of childhood, the pilomyxoid astrocytoma has been recognized. Pilomyxoid astrocytomas seem to have a poorer prognosis than juvenile pilocytic astrocytomas. For recurrent or progressive low-grade astrocytoma of childhood, relatively moderate chemotherapy may improve the likelihood of survival.

Conventional craniospinal irradiation for children with low-stage medulloblastoma results in survival rates of 60–90%. Ten-year survival rates are lower (40–60%). Chemotherapy allows a reduction in the craniospinal radiation dose while preserving survival rates for average-risk patients. However, even reduced-dose craniospinal radiation has an adverse effect on intellect, especially in children younger than 7 years of age. Five-year survival rates for high-risk medulloblastoma have been 25–40%, but recent trials suggest a dramatically improved prognosis for patients receiving intensive chemotherapy and radiation. Children with supratentorial primitive neuroectodermal tumors also benefit from the addition of chemotherapy to craniospinal radiation.

Major challenges remain in treating brain tumors in children younger than age 3 years and in treating brainstem gliomas and malignant gliomas. The increasing emphasis is on the quality of life of survivors, not just the survival rate.

Duffner PK et al: The treatment of malignant brain tumors in infants and very young children: An update of the pediatric oncology group experience. Neuro-oncol 1999;1:152 [PMID: 11554387].

Foreman NK et al: A study of sequential high dose cyclophosphamide and high dose carboplatin with peripheral stem cell rescue in resistant or recurrent pediatric brain tumors. J Neurooncol 2005;71:181 [PMID: 15690136].

Komotar RJ et al: Pilomyxoid astrocytoma: A review. MedGenMed 2004;6(4):42 [PMID: 15775869].

Packer RJ et al: Long-term neurologic and neurosensory sequelae in adult survivors of a childhood brain tumor: Childhood cancer survivor study. J Clin Oncol 2003;21:3255 [PMID: 12947060].

Pollack IF et al: Association between chromosome 1p and 19q loss and outcome in pediatric malignant gliomas: Results from the CCG-945 cohort. Pediatr Neurosurg 2003;39:114 [PMID: 12876389].

LYMPHOMAS AND LYMPHOPROLIFERATIVE DISORDERS

The term "lymphoma" refers to a malignant proliferation of lymphoid cells, usually in association with and arising from lymphoid tissues (ie, lymph nodes, thymus, spleen). In contrast, the term "leukemia" refers to a malignancy arising from the bone marrow, which may include lymphoid cells. Because lymphomas can involve the bone marrow, the distinction between the two can be confusing. The diagnosis of lymphoma is a common one among childhood cancers, accounting for 10–15% of all malignancies. The most common form is Hodgkin disease, which represents nearly half of all cases. The remaining subtypes, referred to collectively as non-Hodgkin lymphoma, are divided into four main groups: lymphoblastic, small non–cleaved-cell, large B-cell, and anaplastic large cell lymphomas.

In contrast to lymphomas, lymphoproliferative disorders (LPDs) are quite rare in the general population. Most are polyclonal, nonmalignant (though often life-threatening) accumulations of lymphocytes that occur when the immune system fails to control virally transformed lymphocytes. However, a malignant monoclonal proliferation can also arise. The post-transplant LPDs occur in patients who are immunosuppressed to prevent solid organ or bone marrow transplant rejection, particularly liver and heart transplant patients. Spontaneous LPDs occur in immunodeficient individuals and, less commonly, in immunocompetent persons.

1. Hodgkin Disease

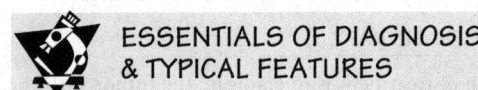

ESSENTIALS OF DIAGNOSIS & TYPICAL FEATURES

- *Painless cervical (70–80%) or supraclavicular (25%) adenopathy; mediastinal mass (50%).*
- *Fatigue, anorexia, weight loss, fever, night sweats, pruritus, cough.*

General Considerations

Children with Hodgkin disease have a better response to treatment than do adults, with a 75% overall survival rate at more than 20 years following diagnosis. Although adult therapies are applicable, the management of Hodgkin disease in children younger than age 18 years frequently differs. Because excellent disease control can result from several different therapeutic approaches, selection of staging procedures [radiographic, surgical, or other procedures to determine additional location(s) of disease] and treatment are often based on the potential long-term toxicity associated with the intervention.

Although Hodgkin disease represents 50% of the lymphomas of childhood, only 15% of all cases occur in children age 16 years or younger. Children younger than age 5 years account for 3% of childhood cases. There is a 4:1 male predominance in the first decade. Notably, in underdeveloped countries the age distribution is quite different, with a peak incidence in younger children.

Hodgkin disease is subdivided into four histologic groups, and the distribution in children parallels that of adults: lymphocyte-predominant (10–20%); nodular sclerosing (40–60%) (increases with age); mixed cellularity (20–40%); and lymphocyte-depleted (5–10%). Prognosis is independent of subclassification, with appropriate therapy based on stage (see Staging section).

Clinical Findings

A. SYMPTOMS AND SIGNS

Children with Hodgkin disease usually present with painless cervical adenopathy. The lymph nodes often feel firmer than inflammatory nodes and have a rubbery texture. They may be discrete or matted together and are not fixed to surrounding tissue. The growth rate is variable, and involved nodes may wax and wane in size over weeks to months.

As Hodgkin disease nearly always arises in lymph nodes and spreads to contiguous nodal groups, a detailed examination of all nodal sites is mandatory. Lymphadenopathy is common in children, so the decision to perform biopsy is often difficult or delayed for a prolonged period. Indications for consideration of early lymph node biopsy include lack of identifiable infection in the region drained by the enlarged node, a node greater than 2 cm in size, supraclavicular adenopathy or abnormal chest radiograph, and lymphadenopathy increasing in size after 2 weeks or failing to resolve within 4–8 weeks.

Constitutional symptoms occur in about one-third of children at presentation. Symptoms of fever greater than 38 °C, weight loss of 10%, and drenching night sweats are defined by the Ann Arbor staging criteria as B symptoms. The A designation refers to the absence of these symptoms. B symptoms are of prognostic value, and more aggressive therapy is usually required for cure. Generalized pruritus and pain with alcohol ingestion may also occur.

Half of patients have asymptomatic mediastinal disease (adenopathy or anterior mediastinal mass), although symptoms due to compression of vital structures in the thorax may occur. A chest radiograph should be obtained when lymphoma is being considered. The mediastinum must be evaluated thoroughly before any surgical procedure is undertaken to avoid airway obstruction or cardiovascular collapse during anesthesia and possible death. Splenomegaly or hepatomegaly is generally associated with advanced disease.

B. LABORATORY FINDINGS

The CBC is usually normal, although anemia, neutrophilia, eosinophilia, and thrombocytosis may be present. The erythrocyte sedimentation rate and other acute-phase reactants are often elevated and can serve as markers of disease activity. Immunologic abnormalities occur, particularly in cell-mediated immunity, and anergy is common in advanced-stage disease at diagnosis. Autoantibody phenomena such as hemolytic anemia and an idiopathic thrombocytopenic purpura-like picture have been reported.

C. STAGING

Staging of Hodgkin disease determines treatment and prognosis. The most common staging system is the Ann Arbor classification that describes extent of disease by I–IV and symptoms by an A or a B suffix (eg, stage IIIB). A systematic search for disease includes chest radiography, CT scan of the chest, abdomen and pelvis, and bilateral bone marrow aspirates and biopsies. Technetium bone scanning may show bony involvement and is usually reserved for patients with bone pain, as bone involvement is rare. Gallium scanning defines gallium-avid tumors and is most useful in evaluating residual mediastinal disease at the completion of treatment. Positron emission tomography is increasingly used in the staging and follow-up of patients with Hodgkin disease, often replacing gallium scanning.

The staging laparotomy in pediatrics is rarely performed because almost all patients are given systemic chemotherapy rather than radiation. This shift in favored therapy is due to the toxicities of high-dose, extended-field radiation in children and the complications of laparotomy, including postsplenectomy sepsis.

D. PATHOLOGY

The diagnosis of Hodgkin disease requires the histologic presence of the Reed–Sternberg cell or its variants in tissue. Reed–Sternberg cells are germinal-center B cells that have undergone malignant transformation. Nearly 20% of these tumors in developed countries are positive for EBV and there is growing evidence to implicate EBV in the development of Hodgkin disease.

Treatment & Prognosis

To achieve long-term disease-free survival while minimizing treatment toxicity, Hodgkin disease is increasingly treated by chemotherapy alone—and less often by radiation therapy.

Several combinations of chemotherapeutic agents are effective, but the most commonly used are COPP (cyclophosphamide, Oncovin [vincristine], procarbazine, and prednisone) and ABVD (Adriamycin [doxorubicin], bleomycin, vinblastine, and dacarbazine). When these schedules are alternated, exposure to an individual drug is decreased, and the toxicities associated with cumulative doses are minimized. The combination of dexamethasone, cisplatin, cytarabine, and etoposide is also being used increasingly.

Although risk-adapted chemotherapy alone is very effective in achieving cure, radiation continues to play a role in the treatment of childhood Hodgkin disease, because combined-modality therapy may increase the cure rate in advanced disease. The use of radiation therapy at the end of risk-adapted chemotherapy when no residual disease is present appears to improve short-term, event-free survival, but its benefit for long-term survival remains to be demonstrated. Current COG studies are evaluating the risks and benefits of radiation therapy in intermediate risk disease.

Current treatment gives children with stage I and stage II Hodgkin disease at least a 90% disease-free likelihood of survival 5 years after diagnosis, which generally equates with cure. Two-thirds of all relapses occur within 2 years after diagnosis and relapse rarely occurs beyond 4 years. In more advanced disease (stage III and stage IV), 5-year event-free survival rates range from over 60–90%. With more patients being long-term survivors of Hodgkin disease, the risk of secondary malignancies, both leukemias and solid tumors, is becoming more apparent and is higher in patients receiving radiation therapy. Therefore, elucidating the optimal treatment strategy that minimizes such risk should be the goal of future studies.

Patients with relapsed Hodgkin disease are often salvageable using chemotherapy and radiation therapy. An increasingly popular alternative is autologous HSCT, which may improve survival rates. Allogeneic HSCT is also used, but carries increased risks of complications and may not offer added survival benefit.

Lin HM: Second malignancy after treatment of pediatric Hodgkin disease. J Pediatr Hematol Oncol 2005;27:28 [PMID: 15654275].

O'Connor O: Developing new drugs for the treatment of lymphoma. Eur J Haematol 2005;[Suppl]66:150 [PMID: 16007885].

Schwartz CL: The management of Hodgkin disease in the young child. Curr Opin Pediatr 2003;15:10 [PMID: 12544266].

Velez MC: Consultation with the specialist: Lymphomas. Pediatr Rev 2003;24:380 [PMID: 14595035].

2. Non-Hodgkin Lymphoma

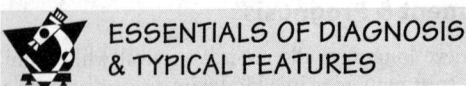

ESSENTIALS OF DIAGNOSIS & TYPICAL FEATURES

- Cough, dyspnea, orthopnea, swelling of the face, lymphadenopathy, mediastinal mass, pleural effusion.

- Abdominal pain, abdominal distention, vomiting, constipation, abdominal mass, ascites, hepatosplenomegaly.

- Adenopathy, fevers, neurologic deficit, skin lesions.

General Considerations

Non-Hodgkin lymphomas (NHLs) are a diverse group of cancers accounting for 5–10% of malignancies in children younger than age 15 years. About 500 new cases arise per year in the United States. The incidence of NHLs increases with age. Children age 15 years or younger account for only 3% of all cases of NHLs; it is uncommon before age 5 years. There is a male predominance of approximately 3:1. In equatorial Africa, NHLs cause almost 50% of pediatric malignancies.

Most children who develop NHL are immunologically normal. However, children with congenital or acquired immune deficiencies (eg, Wiskott–Aldrich syndrome, severe combined immunodeficiency syndrome, X-linked lymphoproliferative syndrome, HIV infection, or immunosuppressive therapy following solid organ or marrow transplantation) have an increased risk of developing NHLs. It has been estimated that their risk is 100–10,000 times that of age-matched control subjects.

Animal models suggest a viral contribution to the pathogenesis of NHL, and there is evidence of viral involvement in human NHL as well. In equatorial Africa, 95% of Burkitt lymphomas contain DNA from EBV. But in North America, less than 20% of Burkitt tumors contain the EBV genome. The role of other viruses, such as human herpes viruses 6 and 8, disturbances in host immunologic defenses, chronic immunostimulation, and specific chromosomal rearrangements, is under investigation as potential triggers in the development of NHL.

Unlike adult NHL, virtually all childhood NHLs are rapidly proliferating, high-grade, diffuse malignancies. These tumors exhibit aggressive behavior but are usually very responsive to treatment. Nearly all pediatric NHLs are histologically classified into four main groups: lymphoblastic lymphoma (LL), small non–cleaved-cell lymphoma (Burkitt lymphoma [BL] and Burkitt-like lymphoma [BLL]), large B-cell lymphoma (LBCL), and anaplastic large cell lymphoma (ALCL). Immunophenotyping and cytogenetic features, in addition to clinical presentation, are increasingly important in the classification, pathogenesis, and treatment of NHLs. Comparisons of pediatric NHLs are summarized in Table 28–5.

Clinical Findings

A. SYMPTOMS AND SIGNS

Childhood NHLs can arise in any site of lymphoid tissue, including lymph nodes, thymus, liver, and spleen. Common extralymphatic sites include bone, bone mar-

Table 28–5. Comparison of pediatric non-Hodgkin lymphomas.

	Lymphoblastic Lymphoma	Small Noncleaved Cell Lymphoma (BL and BLL)	Large B-Cell Lymphoma	Anaplastic Large Cell Lymphoma
Incidence (%)	30–40	35–50	10–15	10–15
Histopathologic features	Indistinguishable from ALL lymphoblasts	Large nucleus with prominent nucleoli surrounded by very basophilic cytoplasm that contains lipid vacuoles	Large cells with cleaved or non-cleaved nuclei	Large pleomorphic cells
Immunophenotype	Immature T cell	B cell	B cell	T cell or null cell
Cytogenetic markers	Translocations involving chromosome 14q11 and chromosome 7; interstitial deletions of chromosome 1	t(8;14), t(8;22), t(2;8)	Many	t(2;5)
Clinical presentation	Intrathoracic tumor, mediastinal mass (50–70%), lymphadenopathy above diaphragm (50–80%)	Intra-abdominal tumor (90%), jaw involvement (10–20% sporadic BL, 70% endemic BL), bone marrow involvement	Abdominal tumor most common; unusual sites: lung, face, brain, bone, testes, muscle	Lymphadenopathy, fever, weight loss, night sweats, extranodal sites including viscera and skin
Treatment	Similar to ALL therapy; 24 mos duration	Intensive administration of alkylating agents and methotrexate; CNS prophylaxis; 3–9 mos duration	Similar to therapy for BL/BLL	Similar to therapy for lymphoblastic lymphoma or BL/BLL

ALL, acute lymphoblastic leukemia; BL, Burkitt lymphoma; BLL, Burkitt-like lymphoma; CNS, central nervous system.

row, CNS, skin, and testes. Signs and symptoms at presentation are determined by the location of lesions and the degree of dissemination. Because NHL usually progresses very rapidly, the duration of symptoms is quite brief, from days to a few weeks. Nevertheless, children present with a limited number of syndromes, most of which correlate with cell type.

Children with LL often present with symptoms of airway compression (cough, dyspnea, orthopnea) or superior vena cava obstruction (facial edema, chemosis, plethora, venous engorgement), which are a result of mediastinal disease. *These symptoms are a true emergency necessitating rapid diagnosis and treatment.* Pleural or pericardial effusions may further compromise the patient's respiratory and cardiovascular status. CNS and bone marrow involvement are not common at diagnosis. When bone marrow contains more than 25% lymphoblasts, patients are diagnosed with ALL.

Most patients with BL and BLL present with abdominal disease. Abdominal pain, distention, a right lower quadrant mass, or intussusception in a child older than age 5 years suggests the diagnosis of BL. Bone marrow involvement is common (~ 65% of patients). BL is the most rapidly proliferating tumor known and

has a high rate of spontaneous cell death as it outgrows its blood supply. Consequently, children presenting with massive abdominal disease frequently have tumor lysis syndrome (hyperuricemia, hyperphosphatemia, and hyperkalemia). These abnormalities can be aggravated by tumor infiltration of the kidney or urinary obstruction by tumor. Although similar histologically, numerous differences exist between cases of BL occurring in endemic areas of equatorial Africa and the sporadic cases of North America (Table 28–6).

Large cell lymphomas are similar clinically to the small non–cleaved-cell lymphomas, although unusual sites of involvement are quite common, particularly with ALCL. Skin lesions, focal neurologic deficits, and pleural or peritoneal effusions without an obvious associated mass are frequently seen.

B. DIAGNOSTIC EVALUATION

Diagnosis is made by biopsy of involved tissue with histology, immunophenotyping, and cytogenetic studies. If mediastinal disease is present, general anesthesia must be avoided if the airway or vena cava is compromised by tumor. In these cases samples of pleural or ascitic fluid, bone marrow, or peripheral nodes obtained under local

Table 28–6. Comparison of endemic and sporadic Burkitt lymphoma.

	Endemic	Sporadic
Incidence	10 per 100,000	0.9 per 100,000
Cytogenetics	Chromosome 8 breakpoint upstream of c-*myc* locus	Chromosome 8 breakpoint within c-*myc* locus
EBV association	≥ 95%	≤ 20%
Disease sites at presentation	Jaw (58%), abdomen (58%), CNS (19%), orbit (11%), marrow (7%)	Jaw (7%), abdomen (91%), CNS (14%), orbit (1%), marrow (20%)

EBV, Epstein-Barr virus; CNS, central nervous system.

anesthesia may confirm the diagnosis. Major abdominal surgery and intestinal resection should be avoided in patients with an abdominal mass that is likely to be BL, as the tumor will regress rapidly with the initiation of chemotherapy. The rapid growth of these tumors and the associated life-threatening complications demand that further studies be done expeditiously so that specific therapy is not delayed.

After a thorough physical examination, a CBC, liver function tests, and a biochemical profile (electrolytes, calcium, phosphorus, uric acid, renal function) should be obtained. An elevated LDH reflects tumor burden and can serve as a marker of disease activity. Imaging studies should include a chest radiograph and chest CT scan, an abdominal ultrasound or CT scan, and possibly a gallium or positron emission tomography scan. Bone marrow and CSF examinations are also essential.

Treatment

A. SUPPORTIVE CARE

The management of life-threatening problems at presentation is critical. The most common complications are superior mediastinal syndrome and acute tumor lysis syndrome. Patients with airway compromise require prompt initiation of specific therapy. Because of the risk of general anesthesia in these patients, it is occasionally necessary to initiate steroids or low-dose emergency radiation until the mass is small enough for a biopsy to be undertaken safely. Response to steroids and radiation is usually prompt (12–24 hours).

Tumor lysis syndrome should be anticipated in all patients who have NHL with a large tumor burden. Maintaining a brisk urine output (> 5 mL/kg/h) with intravenous fluids and diuretics is the key to management. Allo-

purinol will reduce serum uric acid, and alkalinization of urine will increase its solubility. Rasburicase is an intravenous alternative to allopurinol. Because phosphate precipitates in alkaline urine, alkali administration should be discontinued if hyperphosphatemia occurs. Renal dialysis is occasionally necessary to control metabolic abnormalities. Every attempt should be made to correct or minimize metabolic abnormalities before initiating chemotherapy; however, this period of stabilization should not exceed 24–48 hours.

B. SPECIFIC THERAPY

Systemic chemotherapy is the mainstay of therapy for NHLs. Nearly all patients with NHL require intensive intrathecal chemotherapy for CNS prophylaxis. Surgical resection is not indicated unless the entire tumor can be resected safely, which is rare. Partial resection or debulking surgery has no role. Radiation therapy does not improve outcome, so its use is confined to exceptional circumstances.

Therapy for LL is generally based on treatment protocols designed for ALL and involves dose-intensive, multiagent chemotherapy. The duration of therapy is 2 years. Treatment of BL and BLL using alkylating agents and intermediate- to high-dose methotrexate administered intensively but for a relatively short time produce the highest cure rates. LBCL is treated similarly, whereas ALCL has been treated with both BL and LL protocols.

Monoclonal antibodies such as rituximab (anti-CD20) allow for more targeted therapy of lymphomas and have been successful in improving outcomes in adults. Clinical studies employing this type of therapy in children are underway in those with newly diagnosed as well as relapsed or refractory B-cell NHL.

Prognosis

A major predictor of outcome in NHL is the extent of disease at diagnosis. Ninety percent of patients with localized disease can expect long-term, disease-free survival. Patients with extensive disease on both sides of the diaphragm, CNS involvement, or bone marrow involvement in addition to a primary site have a 70–80% failure-free survival rate. Relapses occur early in NHL; patients with LL rarely have recurrences after 30 months from diagnosis, whereas patients with BL and BLL very rarely have recurrences beyond 1 year. Patients who experience relapse may have a chance for cure by autologous or allogeneic HSCT.

Cairo MS et al: Childhood and adolescent large-cell lymphoma (LCL): A review of the Children's Cancer Group experience. Am J Hematol 2003;72:53 [PMID: 12508269].

Cairo MS et al: Childhood and adolescent non-Hodgkin lymphoma: New insights in biology and critical challenges for the future. Pediatr Blood Cancer 2005;45:753 [PMID: 15929129].

Davidson MB et al: Pathophysiology, clinical consequences, and treatment of tumor lysis syndrome. Am J Med 2004;116:546 [PMID: 15063817].

Raetz E et al: B large-cell lymphoma in children and adolescents. Cancer Treat Rev 2003;29:91 [PMID 12670451].

Thorley-Lawson DA, Gross A: Persistence of the Epstein-Barr virus and the origins of associated lymphomas. N Engl J Med 2004;350:1328 [PMID: 15044644].

3. Lymphoproliferative Disorders

LPDs can be thought of as a part of a continuum with lymphomas. Whereas LPDs represent inappropriate, often polyclonal proliferations of nonmalignant lymphocytes, lymphomas represent the development of malignant clones, sometimes arising from recognized LPDs.

Post-Transplantation Lymphoproliferative Disorders

Post-transplantation lymphoproliferative disorders (PTLDs) arise in patient populations that have received substantial immunosuppressive medications for solid organ or bone marrow transplantation. In these patients, reactivation of latent EBV infection in B cells drives a polyclonal proliferation of these cells that is fatal if not halted. Occasionally a true lymphoma develops, often bearing a chromosomal translocation.

LPDs are an increasingly common and significant complication of transplantation. The incidence of PTLD ranges from approximately 2–15% of transplant recipients, depending on the organ transplanted and the immunosuppressive regimen.

Treatment of these disorders is a challenge for transplant physicians and oncologists. The initial treatment is reduction in immunosuppression, which allows the patient's own immune cells to destroy the virally transformed lymphocytes. However, this is only effective in approximately half of patients. For those patients who do not respond to reduced immune suppression, chemotherapy of various regimens may succeed. The use of anti–B-cell antibodies, such as rituximab (anti-CD20), for the treatment of PTLDs has been promising in early trials.

Spontaneous Lymphoproliferative Disease

Immunodeficiencies in which LPDs occur include Bloom syndrome, Chédiak–Higashi syndrome, ataxia–telangiectasia, Wiskott–Aldrich syndrome, X-linked lymphoproliferative syndrome, congenital T-cell immunodeficiencies, and HIV infection. Treatment depends on the circumstances, but unlike PTLD, few therapeutic options are often available. Castleman disease is an LPD occurring in pediatric patients without any apparent immunodeficiency. The autoimmune lymphoproliferative syndrome is characterized by widespread lymphadenopathy with hepatosplenomegaly, and autoimmune phenomena. Autoimmune lymphoproliferative syndrome results from muta-

tions in the Fas ligand pathway that is critical in regulation of apoptosis.

Gottschalk S et al: Post-transplant lymphoproliferative disorders. Annu Rev Med 2005;56:29 [PMID: 15660500].

Green M, Webber S: Posttransplantation lymphoproliferative disorders. Pediatr Clin North Am 2003;50:1471 [PMID: 14710788].

Pescovitz MD: The use of rituximab, anti-CD20 monoclonal antibody, in pediatric transplantation. Pediatr Transplant 2004;8:9 [PMID: 15009836].

Shroff R, Rees L: The post-transplant lymphoproliferative disorder—A literature review. Pediatr Nephrol 2004;19:369 [PMID: 14986084].

NEUROBLASTOMA

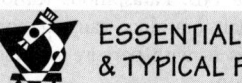

ESSENTIALS OF DIAGNOSIS & TYPICAL FEATURES

- *Bone pain, abdominal pain, anorexia, weight loss, fatigue, fever, irritability.*
- *Abdominal mass (65%), adenopathy, proptosis, periorbital ecchymosis, skull masses, subcutaneous nodules, hepatomegaly, spinal cord compression.*

General Considerations

Neuroblastoma (NB) arises from neural crest tissue of the sympathetic ganglia or adrenal medulla. It is composed of small, fairly uniform cells with little cytoplasm and hyperchromatic nuclei that may form rosette patterns. Pathologic diagnosis is not always easy, and NB must be differentiated from the other "small, round, blue cell" malignancies of childhood (Ewing sarcoma, rhabdomyosarcoma, peripheral neuroectodermal tumor, and lymphoma).

NB accounts for 7–10% of pediatric malignancies and is the most common solid neoplasm outside the CNS. Fifty percent of NBs are diagnosed before age 2 years and 90% before age 5 years.

NB is a biologically diverse disease with varied clinical behavior ranging from spontaneous regression to progression through very aggressive therapy. Unfortunately, despite significant advances in our understanding of this tumor at the cellular and molecular level, the overall survival rate in advanced disease has changed little in 20 years, with 3-year event-free survival being less than 15%.

Clinical Findings

A. SYMPTOMS AND SIGNS

Clinical manifestations vary with the primary site of malignant disease and the neuroendocrine function of the tumor. Many children present with constitutional symptoms such as fever, weight loss, and irritability. Bone pain suggests metastatic disease, which is present in 60% of children older than 1 year of age at diagnosis. Physical examination may reveal a firm, fixed, irregularly shaped mass that extends beyond the midline. The margins are often poorly defined. Although most children have an abdominal primary tumor (40% adrenal gland, 25% paraspinal ganglion), NB can arise wherever there is sympathetic tissue. In the posterior mediastinum, the tumor is usually asymptomatic and discovered on a chest radiograph obtained for other reasons. Patients with cervical NB present with a neck mass, which is often misdiagnosed as infection. Horner syndrome (unilateral ptosis, myosis, and anhydrosis) or heterochromia iridis (differently colored irises) may accompany cervical NB. Paraspinous tumors can extend through the spinal foramina, causing cord compression. Patients may present with paresis, paralysis, and bowel or bladder dysfunction.

The most common sites of metastases are bone, bone marrow, lymph nodes (regional as well as disseminated), liver, and subcutaneous tissue. NB has a predilection for metastasis to the skull, in particular the sphenoid bone and retrobulbar tissue. This causes periorbital ecchymosis and proptosis. Liver metastasis, particularly in the newborn, can be massive. Subcutaneous nodules are bluish in color and associated with an erythematous flush followed by blanching when compressed, probably secondary to catecholamine release.

NB may also be associated with unusual paraneoplastic manifestations. Perhaps the most striking example is opsoclonus-myoclonus, also called dancing eyes/dancing feet syndrome. This phenomenon is characterized by the acute onset of rapid and chaotic eye movements, myoclonic jerking of the limbs and trunk, ataxia, and behavioral disturbances. This process, which often persists after therapy is complete, is thought to be secondary to cross-reacting antineural antibodies. Intractable, chronic watery diarrhea is associated with tumor secretion of vasoactive intestinal peptides. Both of these paraneoplastic syndromes are associated with favorable outcomes.

B. Laboratory Findings

Anemia is present in 60% of children with NB and can be due to chronic disease or marrow infiltration. Occasionally, thrombocytopenia is present, but thrombocytosis is a more common finding, even with metastatic disease in the marrow. Urinary catecholamines (vanillylmandelic acid and homovanillic acid) are elevated in at least 90% of patients at diagnosis and should be measured prior to surgery.

C. Imaging

Plain radiographs of the primary tumor may show stippled calcifications. Metastases to bone appear irregular and lytic. Periosteal reaction and pathologic fractures may also be seen. CT scanning provides more information, including the extent of the primary tumor, its effects on surrounding structures, and the presence of liver and lymph node metastases. Classically, in tumors originating from the adrenal, the kidney is displaced inferolaterally, which helps to differentiate NB from Wilms tumor. MRI is useful in determining the presence of spinal cord involvement in tumors that appear to invade neural foramina.

Technetium bone scanning is obtained for the evaluation of bone metastases, because the tumor usually takes up technetium Metaiodobenzyl-guanidine (MIBG) scanning is also performed to detect metastatic disease.

D. Staging

Staging of NB is performed according to the International Neuroblastoma Staging System (INSS) (Table 28–7). A biopsy of the tumor is performed to deter-

Table 28–7. International Neuroblastoma Staging System.

Stage	Description
1	Localized tumor with complete gross excision, with or without microscopic residual disease; representative ipsilateral lymph nodes negative for tumor microscopically.
2A	Localized tumor with incomplete gross excision; representative ipsilateral non-adherent lymph nodes negative for tumor microscopically.
2B	Localized tumor with or without complete gross excision, with ipsilateral non-adherent lymph nodes positive for tumor. Enlarged lymph nodes must be negative microscopically.
3	Unresectable unilateral tumor infiltrating across the midline, with or without regional lymph node involvement; or localized unilateral tumor with contralateral regional lymph node involvement; or midline tumor with bilateral extension by infiltration (unresectable) or by lymph node involvement. The midline is defined as the vertebral column. Tumors originating on one side and crossing the midline must infiltrate to or beyond the opposite side of the vertebral column.
4	Any primary tumor with dissemination to distant lymph nodes, bone, bone marrow, liver, skin, and/or other organs, except as defined for stage 4S.
4S	Localized primary tumor, as defined for stage 1, 2A, or 2B, with dissemination limited to skin, liver, and/or bone marrow, and limited to infants younger than 1 year. Marrow involvement should be less than 10% of nucleated cells.

mine the biologic characteristics of the tumor. In addition, bilateral bone marrow aspirates and biopsies must be performed to evaluate marrow involvement.

Tumors are classified as favorable or unfavorable based on histologic characteristics. Amplification of the *MYCN* protooncogene is a reliable marker of aggressive clinical behavior with rapid disease progression. Tumor cell DNA content is also predictive of outcome. Hyperdiploidy is a favorable finding, whereas diploid DNA content is associated with a poorer outcome.

Treatment & Prognosis

Patients are treated based on a risk stratification system adopted by the COG based on INSS stage, age, *MYCN* status, histology, and DNA index. The mainstay of NB therapy is surgical resection coupled with chemotherapy. The usually massive size of the tumor often makes primary resection impossible. Under these circumstances, only a biopsy is performed. Following chemotherapy, a second surgical procedure may allow for resection of the primary tumor. Radiation is sometimes also necessary. Effective chemotherapeutic agents in the treatment of NB include cyclophosphamide, doxorubicin, etoposide, cisplatin, vincristine, and topotecan. About 80% of patients achieve complete or partial remission, although in advanced disease, remission is seldom durable.

For low-risk disease (stage I and II), surgical resection alone may be sufficient to affect a cure. Infants younger than 1 year with stage IV disease may need little if any therapy, although chemotherapy may be initiated because of bulky disease causing mechanical complications. In intermediate-risk NB (subsets of patients with stage III and IV disease) the primary treatment approach is surgical combined with chemotherapy. High-risk patients (the majority with stage III and IV disease) require multimodal therapy, including surgery, radiation, chemotherapy, and autologous HSCT. The administration of *cis* retinoic acid, a differentiating agent, can prolong disease-free survival in advanced-stage NB when administered in the setting of minimal residual disease after HSCT.

Cooperative clinical trials are underway in high-risk patients using ch14.18 (a monoclonal antibody specific for the predominant antigen on NB cells) and cytokines to eradicate minimal residual disease. A phase II study is underway using fenretinide, a synthetic retinoid, and radiolabeled MIBG is also being investigated.

For children with stage I, II, or IV-S disease, the 5-year survival rate is 70–90%. Infants younger than 460 days old have a greater than 80% likelihood of long-term survival. Children older than age 1 year with stage III disease have an intermediate prognosis (approximately 40–70%). Older patients with stage IV disease have a poor prognosis (5–50% survival 5 years from diagnosis), although patients 12–18 months old with hyperdiploidy and nonamplified *MYCN* have an excellent prognosis.

George RE et al: Hyperdiploidy plus nonamplified *MYCN* confers a favorable prognosis in children 12–18 months old with disseminated neuroblastoma: A Pediatric Oncology Group Study. J Clin Oncol 2005;23:6466 [PMID: 16116152].

London WB et al: Evidence for an age cutoff greater than 365 days for neuroblastoma risk group stratification in the children's oncology group. J Clin Oncol 2005;23:6459 [PMID: 16116153].

Matthay KK et al: Opsoclonus myoclonus syndrome in neuroblastoma a report from a workshop on the dancing eyes syndrome at the advances in neuroblastoma meeting in Genoa, Italy, 2004. Cancer Lett 2005;228:275 [PMID: 15922508].

National Cancer Institute. www.cancer.gov/cancertopics/types/neuroblastoma

Schmidt ML et al: Favorable prognosis for patients 12–18 months of age with stage 4 nonamplified *MYCN* neuroblastoma: A Children's Cancer Group Study. J Clin Oncol 2005;23:6474 [PMID: 16116154].

WILMS TUMOR (Nephroblastoma)

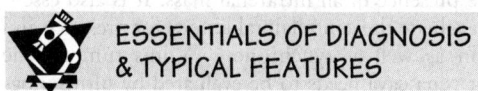

ESSENTIALS OF DIAGNOSIS & TYPICAL FEATURES

- *Asymptomatic abdominal mass or swelling (83%).*
- *Fever (23%), hematuria (21%).*
- *Hypertension (25%), genitourinary malformations (6%), aniridia, hemihypertrophy.*

General Considerations

Approximately 460 new cases of Wilms tumor occur annually in the United States, representing 5–6% of cancers in children younger than age 15 years. After neuroblastoma (NB), this is the second most common abdominal tumor in children. The majority of Wilms tumors are of sporadic occurrence. However, in a few children, Wilms tumor occurs in the setting of associated malformations or syndromes, including aniridia, hemihypertrophy, genitourinary malformations (eg, cryptorchidism, hypospadias, gonadal dysgenesis, pseudohermaphroditism, and horseshoe kidney), Beckwith–Wiedemann syndrome, Denys–Drash syndrome, and WAGR syndrome (Wilms tumor, aniridia, ambiguous genitalia, mental retardation).

The median age at diagnosis is related both to gender and laterality, with bilateral tumors presenting at a younger age than unilateral tumors, and males being diagnosed earlier than females. Wilms tumor occurs most commonly between ages 2 and 5 years; it is unusual after age 6 years. The mean age at diagnosis is 4 years.

Clinical Findings

A. SYMPTOMS AND SIGNS

Most children with Wilms tumor present with increasing size of the abdomen or an asymptomatic abdominal mass incidentally discovered by a parent. The mass is usually smooth and firm, well demarcated, and rarely crosses the midline, though it can extend inferiorly into the pelvis. About 25% of patients will be hypertensive at presentation. Gross hematuria is an uncommon presentation, although microscopic hematuria occurs in approximately 25% of patients.

B. LABORATORY FINDINGS

The CBC is usually normal, but some patients have anemia secondary to hemorrhage into the tumor. Blood urea nitrogen and serum creatinine are usually normal. Urinalysis may show some blood or leukocytes.

C. IMAGING AND STAGING

Ultrasonography or CT of the abdomen should establish the presence of an intrarenal mass. It is also essential to evaluate the contralateral kidney for presence and function as well as synchronous Wilms tumor. The inferior vena cava needs to be evaluated by ultrasonography for the presence and extent of tumor propagation. The liver should be imaged for the presence of metastatic disease. A plain chest radiograph (four views) or chest CT scans (or both) should be obtained to determine whether pulmonary metastases are present. Approximately 10% of patients will have metastatic disease at diagnosis. Of these, 80% will have pulmonary disease and 15% liver metastases. Bone and brain metastases are extremely uncommon and usually associated with different, more aggressive renal tumors, such as clear cell sarcoma or rhabdoid tumor; hence, bone scans and brain imaging are not routinely performed. The clinical stage is ultimately decided at surgery and confirmed by the pathologist.

Treatment & Prognosis

In the United States, treatment of Wilms tumor begins with surgical exploration of the abdomen via an anterior surgical approach to allow for inspection and palpation of the contralateral kidney. The liver and lymph nodes are inspected and suspicious areas biopsied or excised. En bloc resection of tumor is performed. Every attempt is made to avoid tumor spillage at surgery as this may change staging and treatment. Because therapy is tailored to tumor stage, it is imperative that a surgeon familiar with the staging requirements perform the operation.

In addition to the staging, the histologic type has implications for therapy and prognosis. Favorable histology (FH; see later discussion) refers to the classic triphasic

Table 28–8. Treatment of Wilms tumor.

Stage/Histologic Subtype	Treatment
I–II FH and I UH	18 wk (dactinomycin and vincristine)
III–IV FH and II–IV focal anaplasia	24 wk (dactinomycin, vincristine, and doxorubicin) with radiation
II–IV UH (diffuse anaplasia)	24 wks (vincristine, doxorubicin, etoposide, and cyclophosphamide with radiation

FH, favorable histology; UH, unfavorable histology.

Wilms tumor and its variants. Unfavorable histology (UH) refers to the presence of diffuse anaplasia (extreme nuclear atypia) and is present in 5% of Wilms tumors. Only a few small foci of anaplasia in a Wilms tumor give a worse prognosis to patients with stage II, III, or IV tumors. Loss of heterozygosity of chromosomes 1p and 16q are adverse prognostic factors in those with favorable histology. Following excision and pathologic examination, the patient is assigned a stage that defines further therapy.

Improvement in the treatment of Wilms tumor has resulted in an overall cure rate of approximately 90%. The National Wilms Tumor Study Group's fourth study (NWTS-4) demonstrated that survival rates were improved by intensifying therapy during the initial treatment phase while shortening overall treatment duration (24 weeks vs 60 weeks of treatment).

Table 28–8 provides an overview of the current treatment recommendations in NWTS-5. Patients with stage III or IV Wilms tumor require radiation therapy to the tumor bed and to sites of metastatic disease. Chemotherapy is optimally begun within 5 days after surgery, whereas radiation therapy should be started within 10 days. Stage V (bilateral Wilms tumor) disease dictates a different approach, consisting of bilateral renal biopsies followed by chemotherapy and second-look renal-sparing surgery. Radiation may also be necessary.

Using these approaches, 4-year overall survival rates through NWTS-4 are as follows: stage I FH, 96%; stage II–IV FH, 82–92%; stage I–III UH (diffuse anaplasia), 56–70%; stage IV UH, 17%. Patients with recurrent Wilms tumor have approximately a 50% salvage rate with surgery, radiation therapy, and chemotherapy (singly or in combination). HSCT is also being explored as a way to improve the chances of survival after relapse.

Future Considerations

Although progress in the treatment of Wilms tumor has been extraordinary, important questions remain to be answered. Questions have been raised regarding the role of pre-nephrectomy chemotherapy in the treatment of Wilms tumor. Presurgical chemotherapy seems to decrease tumor rupture at resection but may unfavorably affect outcome by changing staging. Future studies will be directed at minimizing acute and long-term toxicities for those with low-risk disease and improving outcomes for those with high-risk and recurrent disease.

Grundy PE et al: Loss of heterozygosity for chromosomes 1p and 16q is an adverse prognostic factor in favorable-histology Wilms tumor: A report from the National Wilms Tumor Study Group. J Clin Oncol 2005;23:7312 [PMID: 16129848].

Kalapurakal JA et al: Management of Wilms' tumour: Current practice and future goals. Lancet Oncol 2004;5:37 [PMID: 14700607].

National Cancer Institute. www.cancer.gov/cancertopics/types/wilms

Rivera MN, Haber DA: Wilms' tumour: Connecting tumorigenesis and organ development in the kidney. Natl Rev Cancer 2005;5:699 [PMID: 16110318].

BONE TUMORS

Primary malignant bone tumors are uncommon in childhood with only 650–700 new cases per year. Osteosarcoma accounts for 60% of cases and occurs mostly in adolescents and young adults. Ewing sarcoma is the second most common malignant tumor of bony origin and occurs from toddlers to young adults. Both tumors have a male predominance.

The cardinal signs of bone tumor are pain at the site of involvement, often following slight trauma, mass formation, and fracture through an area of cortical bone destruction.

1. Osteosarcoma

General Considerations

Although osteosarcoma is the sixth most common malignancy in childhood, it ranks third among adolescents and young adults. This peak occurrence during the adolescent growth spurt suggests a causal relationship between rapid bone growth and malignant transformation. Further evidence for this relationship is found in epidemiologic data showing patients with osteosarcoma to be taller than their peers, osteosarcoma occurring most frequently at sites where the greatest increase in length and size of bone occurs, and osteosarcoma occurring at an earlier age in girls than boys, corresponding to their earlier growth spurt. The metaphyses of long tubular bones are primarily affected. The distal femur accounts for more than 40% of cases, with the proximal tibia, proximal humerus, and mid and proximal femur following in frequency.

Clinical Findings

A. SYMPTOMS AND SIGNS

Pain over the involved area is the usual presenting symptom with or without an associated soft tissue mass. Patients generally have symptoms for several months prior to diagnosis. Systemic symptoms (fever, weight loss) are rare. Laboratory evaluation may reveal elevated serum alkaline phosphatase or LDH levels.

B. IMAGING AND STAGING

Radiographic findings show permeative destruction of the normal bony trabecular pattern with indistinct margins. In addition, periosteal new bone formation and lifting of the bony cortex may create a Codman triangle. A soft tissue mass plus calcifications in a radial or sunburst pattern are frequently noted. MRI is more sensitive in defining the extent of the primary tumor and in many centers has replaced CT scanning. The most common sites of metastases are the lung (≤ 20% of newly diagnosed cases) and the bone (10%). A CT scan of the chest and a bone scan are essential for detecting metastatic disease. Bone marrow aspirates and biopsies are not indicated.

Despite the rather characteristic radiographic appearance, a tissue sample is needed to confirm the diagnosis. Placement of the incision for biopsy is of critical importance. A misplaced incision could preclude a limb salvage procedure and necessitate amputation. The surgeon who will carry out the definitive surgical procedure should perform the biopsy. A staging system for osteosarcoma based on local tumor extent and presence or absence of distant metastasis has been proposed, but it has not been validated.

Treatment and Prognosis

Historical studies showed that over 50% of patients receiving surgery alone developed pulmonary metastases within 6 months after surgery. This suggests the presence of micrometastatic disease at diagnosis. Adjuvant chemotherapy trials showed improved disease-free survival rates of 55–85% after 3–10 years of follow-up.

Osteosarcomas are highly radioresistant lesions; for this reason, radiation therapy has no role in its primary management. Chemotherapy is often administered prior to definitive surgery (neoadjuvant chemotherapy). This permits an early attack on micrometastatic disease and may also shrink the tumor, facilitating a limb salvage procedure. Preoperative chemotherapy also makes detailed histologic evaluation of tumor response to the chemotherapy agents possible. If the histologic response is poor (> 10% viable tumor tissue), postoperative chemotherapy can be changed accordingly. Chemotherapy may be administered intra-arterially or intravenously, although the benefits of intra-arterial chemotherapy are disputed. Agents having efficacy in the treatment of osteosarcoma include doxorubicin, cisplatin, high-dose methotrexate, and ifosfamide.

Definitive cure requires en bloc surgical resection of the tumor with a margin of uninvolved tissue. Amputation and limb salvage are equally effective in achieving local control of osteosarcoma. Contraindications to limb-sparing surgery include major involvement of the neurovascular bundle by tumor; immature skeletal age, particularly for lower extremity tumors; infection in the region of the tumor; inappropriate biopsy site; and extensive muscle involvement that would result in a poor functional outcome.

Postsurgical chemotherapy is generally continued until the patient has received 1 year of treatment. Relapses are unusual beyond 3 years, but late relapses do occur. Histologic response to neoadjuvant chemotherapy is an excellent predictor of outcome. Patients with localized disease having 90% tumor necrosis have a 70–85% long-term, disease-free survival rate. Other favorable prognostic factors include distal skeletal lesions, longer duration of symptoms, age older than 20, female gender, and near-diploid tumor DNA index. Patients with metastatic disease at diagnosis or multifocal bone lesions do not fair well, despite advances in chemotherapy and surgical techniques.

2. Ewing Sarcoma

General Considerations

Ewing sarcoma accounts for only 10% of primary malignant bone tumors; fewer than 200 new cases occur each year in the United States. It is a disease primarily of white males, almost never affects blacks, and occurs mostly in the second decade of life. Ewing sarcoma is considered a "small, round, blue cell" malignancy. The differential diagnosis includes rhabdomyosarcoma, lymphoma, and NB. Although most commonly a tumor of bone, it may also occur in soft tissue (extraosseous Ewing sarcoma or peripheral neuroectodermal tumor [PNET]).

Clinical Findings

A. SYMPTOMS AND SIGNS

Pain at the site of the primary tumor is the most common presenting sign, with or without swelling and erythema. No specific laboratory findings are characteristic of Ewing sarcoma, but an elevated LDH may be present and is of prognostic significance.

B. IMAGING AND STAGING

The radiographic appearance of Ewing sarcoma overlaps with osteosarcoma, although Ewing sarcoma usually involves the diaphyses of long bones. The central axial skeleton gives rise to 40% of Ewing tumors. Evaluation of a patient diagnosed as having Ewing sarcoma should include CT scan or MRI (or both) of the primary lesion to define the extent of local disease as precisely as possible. This is imperative for planning future surgical procedures or radiation therapy. Metastatic disease is present in 25% of patients at diagnosis. The lung (38%), bone (particularly the spine) (31%), and the bone marrow (11%) are the most common sites for metastasis. CT scan of the chest, bone scanning, and bilateral bone marrow aspirates and biopsies are all essential to the staging work-up.

A biopsy is essential in establishing the diagnosis. Histologically, Ewing sarcoma consists of sheets of undifferentiated cells with hyperchromatic nuclei, well-defined cell borders, and scanty cytoplasm. Necrosis is common. Electron microscopy, immunocytochemistry, and cytogenetics may be necessary to confirm the diagnosis. A generous tissue biopsy specimen is often necessary for diagnosis but should not delay starting chemotherapy.

A consistent cytogenetic abnormality, t(11;22), has been identified in Ewing sarcoma and PNET and is present in 85–90% of tumors. These tumors also express the protooncogene c-*myc*, which may be helpful in differentiating Ewing sarcoma from NB, where it is not expressed.

Therapy usually commences with the administration of chemotherapy after biopsy and is followed by local control measures. Depending on many factors, including the primary site of the tumor and the response to chemotherapy, local control could be achieved by surgery, radiation therapy, or a combination of these methods. Following local control, chemotherapy continues for approximately 1 year. Effective treatment for Ewing sarcoma uses combinations of dactinomycin, vincristine, doxorubicin, cyclophosphamide, etoposide, and ifosfamide. Patients with small localized primary tumors have a 50–70% long-term, disease-free survival rate. For patients with metastatic disease and large pelvic primary tumors, survival is poor. Autologous HSCT is being investigated for the treatment of these high-risk patients.

Burdach S et al: High-dose therapy for patients with primary multifocal and early relapsed Ewing's tumors: Results of two consecutive regimens assessing the role of total-body irradiation. J Clin Oncol 2003;21:3072 [PMID: 12915596].

Goorin AM et al: Presurgical chemotherapy compared with immediate surgery and adjuvant chemotherapy for nonmetastatic osteosarcoma: Pediatric Oncology Group Study POG-8651. J Clin Oncol 2003;15:1574 [PMID: 12697883].

Goyal S et al: Symptom interval in young people with bone cancer. Eur J Cancer 2004;40;2280 [PMID: 15454254].

Grimer RJ et al: Surgical options for children with osteosarcoma. Lancet Oncol 2005;6(2);85 [PMID: 15683817].

Marec-Berard P, Philip T: Ewing sarcoma: The pediatrician's point of view. Pediatr Blood Cancer 2004:42(5);477 [PMID: 15049024].

Marina N et al: Biology and therapeutic advances for pediatric osteosarcoma. Oncologist 2004;19:422 [PMID: 15266096].

Rodriguez-Galindo C et al: Treatment of Ewing sarcoma family of tumors: Current status and outlook for the future. Med Pediatr Oncol 2003;40:276 [PMID: 12652615].

RHABDOMYOSARCOMA

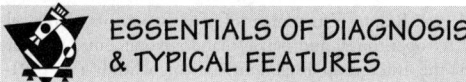

ESSENTIALS OF DIAGNOSIS & TYPICAL FEATURES

- *Painless, progressively enlarging mass; proptosis; chronic drainage (nasal, aural, sinus, vaginal); cranial nerve palsies.*
- *Urinary obstruction, constipation, hematuria.*

General Considerations

Rhabdomyosarcoma is the most common soft tissue sarcoma occurring in childhood and accounts for 10% of solid tumors in childhood. The peak incidence is at age 2–5 years; 70% of children are diagnosed before age 10 years. A second smaller peak is seen in adolescents with extremity tumors. Males are affected more commonly than females.

Rhabdomyosarcoma can occur anywhere in the body. When rhabdomyosarcoma imitates striated muscle and cross-striations are seen by light microscopy, the diagnosis is straightforward. Immunohistochemistry, electron microscopy, or chromosomal analysis is sometimes necessary to make the diagnosis. Rhabdomyosarcoma is further classified into subtypes based on pathologic features: embryonal (60–80%), of which botryoid is a variant; alveolar (about 15–20%); undifferentiated sarcoma (8%); pleomorphic, which is seen in adults (1%); and other (11%). These subtypes occur in characteristic locations and have different metastatic potentials and outcomes.

Although the pathogenesis of rhabdomyosarcoma is unknown, in rare cases a genetic predisposition has been determined. Li–Fraumeni syndrome is an inherited mutation of the *p53* tumor suppressor gene that results in a high risk of bone and soft tissue sarcomas in childhood plus breast cancer and other malignant neoplasms before age 45 years. Two characteristic chromosomal translocations [t(2;13) and t(1;13)] have been described in alveolar rhabdomyosarcoma. The t(1;13) translocation appears to be a favorable prognostic feature in patients with metastatic alveolar rhabdomyosarcoma, while the t(2;13) is associated with poor outcomes.

Clinical Findings

A. SYMPTOMS AND SIGNS

The presenting symptoms and signs of rhabdomyosarcoma result from disturbances of normal body function due to tumor growth (see Table 28–9). For example, patients with orbital rhabdomyosarcoma present with

Table 28–9. Characteristics of rhabdomyosarcoma.

Primary Site	Frequency (%)	Symptoms and Signs	Predominant Pathologic Subtype
Head and neck	35		Embryonal
Orbit	9	Proptosis	
Parameningeal	16	Cranial nerve palsies; aural or sinus obstruction with or without drainage	
Other	10	Painless, progressively enlarging mass	
Genitourinary	22		Embryonal (botryoid variant in bladder and vagina)
Bladder and prostate	13	Hematuria, urinary obstruction	
Vagina and uterus	2	Pelvic mass, vaginal discharge	
Paratesticular	7	Painless mass	
Extremities	18	Adolescents, swelling of affected body part	Alveolar (50%), undifferentiated
Other	25	Mass	Alveolar, undifferentiated

proptosis, whereas patients with rhabdomyosarcoma of the bladder can present with hematuria, urinary obstruction, or a pelvic mass.

B. IMAGING

A plain radiograph and a CT or MRI scan should be obtained to determine the extent of the primary tumor and to assess regional lymph nodes. A lung CT scan is obtained to rule out pulmonary metastasis, the most common site of metastatic disease at diagnosis. A skeletal survey and a bone scan are obtained to determine whether bony metastases are present. Bilateral bone marrow biopsies and aspirates are obtained to rule out bone marrow infiltration. Additional studies may be warranted in certain sites. For example, in parameningeal primaries, a lumbar puncture is performed to evaluate CSF for tumor cells.

Treatment

Optimal management and treatment of rhabdomyosarcoma is complex and requires combined modality therapy. When feasible, the tumor should be excised, but this is not always possible because of the site of origin and size of tumor. When only partial tumor resection is feasible, the operative procedure is usually limited to biopsy and sampling of lymph nodes. Debulking of unresectable tumor may improve outcomes. Chemotherapy can often convert an inoperable tumor to a resectable one. A second-look procedure to remove residual disease and confirm the clinical response to chemotherapy and radiation therapy is generally performed at about week 20 of therapy.

Radiation therapy is an effective method of local tumor control for both microscopic and gross residual disease. It is generally administered to all patients, the only exception being those with a localized tumor that has been completely resected. All patients with rhabdomyosarcoma receive chemotherapy, even when the tumor is fully resected at diagnosis. The exact regimen and duration of chemotherapy are determined by primary site, group, and tumor node metastasis (TNM) classification. Vincristine, dactinomycin, and cyclophosphamide have shown the greatest efficacy in the treatment of rhabdomyosarcoma.

Prognosis

The age of the patient, the extent of tumor at diagnosis, the primary site, the pathologic subtype, and the response to treatment all influence the long-term, disease-free survival rate from the time of diagnosis. Children with localized disease at diagnosis have a 70–75% 3-year disease-free survival rate, whereas children with metastatic disease at presentation have a poorer outcome (39% 3-year disease-free survival).

Newer treatment strategies for high-risk patients include different drug combinations and dosing schedules with hematopoietic growth factor support, hyperfractionated radiation therapy, and autologous HSCT.

Joshi D et al: Age is an independent prognostic factor in rhabdomyosarcoma: A report from the Soft Tissue Sarcoma Committee of the Children's Oncology Group. Pediatr Blood Cancer 2004;42:64 [PMID: 14752797].

National Cancer Institute. www.cancer.gov/cancertopics/types/childrhabdomyosarcoma

Raney RB et al: Results of treatment of fifty-six patients with localized retroperitoneal and pelvic rhabdomyosarcoma: A report from the Intergroup Rhabdomyosarcoma Study-IV, 1991–1997 [PMID: 15127417].

Stevens MCG: Treatment for childhood rhabdomyosarcoma: The cost of cure. Lancet Oncol 2005;6:77 [PMID: 15683816].

RETINOBLASTOMA

General Considerations

Retinoblastoma is a neuroectodermal malignancy arising from embryonic retinal cells that accounts for 3% of malignant disease in children younger than age 15 years. It is the most common intraocular tumor in pediatric patients and causes 5% of cases of childhood blindness. In the United States, 200 to 300 new cases occur per year. This is a malignancy of early childhood, with 90% of the tumors diagnosed before age 5 years. Bilateral involvement occurs in 20–30% of children and typically is diagnosed at a younger age (median age 14 months) than unilateral disease (median age 23 months).

Retinoblastoma is the prototype of hereditary cancers due to a mutation in the retinoblastoma gene (*RB1*), which is located on the long arm of chromosome 13 (13q14). This gene is a tumor-suppressor gene that normally controls cellular growth. When the gene is inactivated, as in retinoblastoma, cellular growth is uncontrolled. Uncontrolled cell growth leads to tumor formation. Inactivation of both *RB1* alleles within the same cell is required for tumor formation.

Retinoblastoma is known to arise in heritable and nonheritable forms. Based on the different clinical characteristics of the two forms, Knudson proposed a "two-hit" hypothesis for retinoblastoma tumor development. He postulated that two independent events were necessary for a cell to acquire tumor potential. Mutations at the *RB1* locus can be inherited or arise spontaneously. In heritable cases, the first mutation arises during gametogenesis, either spontaneously (90%) or through transmission from a parent (10%). This mutation is present in every retinal cell and in all other somatic and germ cells. Ninety percent of persons who carry this germline mutation will develop retinoblastoma. For tumor formation, the loss of the second *RB1* allele within a cell must occur; loss of only one allele is insufficient for tumor formation. The second mutation occurs in a somatic (retinal) cell. In nonheritable cases (60%), both mutations arise in a somatic cell after gametogenesis has taken place.

Clinical Findings

A. SYMPTOMS AND SIGNS

Children with retinoblastoma generally come to medical attention while the tumor is still confined to the globe. Although present at birth, retinoblastoma is not usually detected until it has grown to a considerable size. Leukocoria (white pupillary reflex) is the most common sign (found in 60% of patients). Parents may note an unusual appearance of the eye or asymmetry of the eyes in a photograph. The differential diagnosis of leukocoria includes *Toxocara canis* granuloma, astrocytic hamartoma, retinopathy of prematurity, Coats disease, and persistent hyperplastic primary vitreous. Strabismus (in 20% of patients) is seen when the tumor involves the macula and central vision is lost. Rarely (in 7% of patients), a painful red eye with glaucoma, a hyphema, or proptosis is the initial manifestation. A single focus or multiple foci of tumor may be seen in one or both eyes at diagnosis. Bilateral involvement occurs in 20–30% of children.

B. EVALUATION

Suspected retinoblastoma requires a detailed ophthalmologic examination under general anesthesia. An ophthalmologist makes the diagnosis of retinoblastoma by the appearance of the tumor within the eye without pathologic confirmation. A white to creamy pink mass protruding into the vitreous matter suggests the diagnosis; intraocular calcifications and vitreous seeding are virtually pathognomonic of retinoblastoma. A CT scan of the orbits detects intraocular calcification, evaluates the optic nerve for tumor infiltration, and detects extraocular extension of tumor. A single focus or multiple foci of tumor may be seen in one or both eyes at diagnosis. Metastatic disease of the marrow and meninges can be ruled out with bilateral bone marrow aspirates and biopsies plus CSF cytology.

Treatment

Each eye is treated according to the potential for useful vision, and every attempt is made to preserve vision. The choice of therapy depends on the size, location, and number of intraocular lesions. Absolute indications for enucleation include no vision, neovascular glaucoma, inability to examine the treated eye, and inability to control tumor growth with conservative treatment. External beam irradiation has been the mainstay of therapy. A total dose of 35–45 Gy is administered. However, many centers are investigating the role of systemic chemotherapy for the treatment of retinoblastoma confined to the globe and the elimination of external beam radiotherapy is now accepted. Cryotherapy, photocoagulation, and radioactive plaques can be used for local tumor control. Patients with metastatic disease receive chemotherapy.

Children with retinoblastoma confined to the retina (whether unilateral or bilateral) have an excellent prognosis, with 5-year survival rates greater than 90%. Mortality is correlated directly with extent of optic nerve involvement, orbital extension of tumor, and massive choroid invasion. Patients who have disease in the optic nerve beyond the lamina cribrosa have only a 40% 5-year survival rate. Patients with meningeal or metastatic spread rarely survive, although intensive chemotherapy and autologous HSCT have produced long-term survivors.

Patients with the germline mutation (heritable form) have a significant risk of developing second primary tumors. Osteosarcomas account for 40% of such tumors. Second malignant neoplasms occur both in patients who have and those who have not received radiation therapy. The 30-year cumulative incidence for a second neoplasm is 35% in patients who received radiation therapy and 6% in those who did not receive radiation therapy. The risk continues to increase over time. Although radiation contributes to the risk, it is the presence of the retinoblastoma gene itself that is responsible for the development of nonocular tumors in these patients.

Abramson DH, Sxhefler AC: Update on retinoblastoma. Retina 2004:24(6);828 [PMID: 15579980].

Antoneli CB et al: Extraocular retinoblastoma: A 13-year experience. Cancer 2003;15:1292 [PMID: 12973854].

Brichard B et al: Combined chemotherapy and local treatment in the management of intraocular retinoblastoma. Med Pediatr Oncol 2002;38:411 [PMID: 11984802].

Deegan WF: Emerging strategies for the treatment of retinoblastoma. Curr Opin Ophthalmol 2003;14(5);291 [PMID: 14502057].

Nahum MP et al: Long-term follow-up of children with retinoblastoma. Pediatr Hematol Oncol 2001;18:173 [PMID: 11293284].

Rodriguez-Galindo C et al: Treatment of intraocular retinoblastoma with vincristine and carboplatin. J Clin Oncol 2003; 15:2019 [PMID: 12743157].

Shields C et al: Continuing challenges in the management of retinoblastoma with chemotherapy. Retina 2004:24(6);849 [PMID: 15579981].

HEPATIC TUMORS

Two-thirds of liver masses found in childhood are malignant. Ninety percent of hepatic malignancies are either hepatoblastoma or hepatocellular carcinoma. Hepatoblastomas are somewhat more frequent than hepatocellular carcinomas (51% vs 39%). A comparison of the features of these hepatic malignancies is presented in Table 28–10. Of

Table 28–10. Comparison of hepatoblastoma and hepatocellular carcinoma in childhood.

	Hepatoblastoma	Hepatocellular Carcinoma
Median age at presentation	1 y (0–3 y)	12 y (5–18 y)
Male-to-female ratio	1.7:1	1.4:1
Associated conditions	Hemihypertrophy, Beckwith-Wiedemann syndrome, prematurity, Gardner syndrome	Hepatitis B virus infection, hereditary tyrosinemia, biliary cirrhosis, a_1-antitrypsin deficiency
Pathologic features	Fetal or embryonal cells; mesenchymal component (30%)	Large pleomorphic tumor cells and tumor giant cells
Solitary hepatic lesion	80%	20–50%
Unique features at diagnosis	Osteopenia (20–30%), isosexual precocity (3%)	Hemoperitoneum, polycythemia
Laboratory features		
Hyperbilirubinemia	5%	25%
Elevated AFP	> 90%	50%
Abnormal liver function tests	15–30%	30–50%

AFP, α-fetoprotein.

the benign tumors, 60% are hamartomas or vascular tumors such as hemangiomas.

Children with hepatic tumors usually come to medical attention because of an enlarging abdomen. Approximately 10% of hepatoblastomas are first discovered on routine examination. Anorexia, weight loss, vomiting, and abdominal pain are associated more commonly with hepatocellular carcinoma. Serum α-fetoprotein is often elevated and is an excellent marker for response to treatment.

Imaging studies should include abdominal ultrasound, CT scan, or MRI. Malignant tumors have a diffuse hyperechoic pattern on ultrasonography, whereas benign tumors are usually poorly echoic. Vascular lesions contain areas with varying degrees of echogenicity. Ultrasound is also useful for imaging the hepatic veins, portal veins, and inferior vena cava. CT scanning and, in particular, MRI are important for defining the extent of tumor within the liver. CT scanning of the chest and bone scan should be obtained to evaluate for metastatic spread.

Because bone marrow involvement is extremely rare, bone marrow aspirates and biopsies are not indicated. The prognosis for children with hepatic malignancies depends on the tumor type and the resectability of the tumor. Complete resectability is essential for survival. Chemotherapy can decrease the size of most hepatoblastomas. Following biopsy of the lesion, neoadjuvant chemotherapy is administered prior to attempting complete surgical resection. Chemotherapy can often convert an inoperable tumor to a completely resectable one and can also eradicate metastatic disease. Approximately 50–60% of hepatoblastomas are fully resectable, whereas only one-third of hepatocellular carcinomas

can be completely removed. Even with complete resection, only one-third of patients with hepatocellular carcinoma are long-term survivors. A recent CCG/Pediatric Oncology Group (POG) trial has shown cisplatin, fluorouracil, and vincristine to be as effective as but less toxic than cisplatin and doxorubicin in treating hepatoblastoma. Other drugs that have demonstrated benefit include fluorouracil and cyclophosphamide. Etoposide, carboplatin, and ifosfamide are under investigation. Radiation as well as liver transplantation is being investigated for patients whose tumors cannot be completely resected following chemotherapy.

Feusner J, Plaschkes J: Hepatoblastoma and low birth weight: A trend or chance observation? Med Pediatr Oncol 2002;39: 508 [PMID: 12228908].

Katzenstein HM et al: Hepatocellular carcinoma in children and adolescents: Results from the Pediatric Oncology Group and the Children's Cancer Group intergroup study. J Clin Oncol 2002;12:2789 [PMID: 12065555].

Katzenstein HM et al: Treatment of unresectable and metastatic hepatoblastoma: A Pediatric Oncology Group Phase II study. J Clin Oncol 2002;20:3438 [PMID: 12177104].

Malogolowkin MH et al: Feasibility and toxicity of chemoembolization for children with liver tumors. J Clin Oncol 2000; 18:1279 [PMID: 10715298].

Stocker JT: Hepatic tumors in children. Clin Liver Dis 2001; 5: 259 [PMID: 11218918].

LANGERHANS CELL HISTIOCYTOSIS

Langerhans cell histiocytosis (LCH; formerly called histiocytosis X) is a rare and poorly understood spectrum of disorders. It can occur as an isolated lesion or as widespread systemic disease involving virtually any body site. Eosinophilic granuloma, Hand–Schüller–Christian disease, and Letterer–Siwe disease are all syndromes encompassed by this disorder. LCH is not a true malignancy, but is a clonal, reactive proliferation of normal histiocytic cells, perhaps resulting from an immunoregulatory defect.

The distinctive pathologic feature is proliferation of histiocytic cells beyond what would be seen in a normal inflammatory process. Langerhans histiocytes have typical features: on light microscopy, the nuclei are deeply indented (coffee bean-shaped) and elongated, and the cytoplasm is pale, distinct, and abundant. Additional diagnostic characteristics include Birbeck granules on electron microscopy, expression of CD1 on the cell surface, and positive immunostaining for S-100 protein.

Clinical Findings

Because LCH encompasses a broad spectrum of diseases, its presentation can be variable, from a single asymptomatic lesion to widely disseminated disease.

Patients with localized disease present primarily with lesions limited to bone. Occasionally found incidentally on radiographs obtained for other reasons, these lesions are well-demarcated and frequently found in the skull, clavicles, ribs, and vertebrae. These lesions can be painful. Patients can also present with localized disease of the skin, often as a diaper rash that does not resolve.

Bony lesions, fever, weight loss, otitis media, exophthalmos, and diabetes insipidus occur in a small number of children with the disease. Formerly called Hand–Schüller-Christian disease, this multifocal disease commonly presents with generalized symptoms and organ dysfunction.

Children with disseminated LCH (formerly called Letterer–Siwe disease) typically present before age 2 years with a seborrheic skin rash, fever, weight loss, lymphadenopathy, hepatosplenomegaly, and hematologic abnormalities.

Diagnosis is made with biopsy of the involved organ. The work-up should include a CBC, liver and kidney function tests, a skeletal survey or technetium bone scan, and a urinalysis with specific gravity to rule out diabetes insipidus.

Treatment & Prognosis

The outcome of LCH is extremely variable, but the process usually resolves spontaneously. Isolated lesions may need no therapy at all. Intralesional corticosteroids, curettage, and low-dose radiation therapy are useful local treatment measures for symptomatic focal lesions. Patients with localized disease have an excellent prognosis.

Multifocal disease is often treated with systemic chemotherapy. Prednisone with vinblastine or etoposide can be given repeatedly or continuously until lesions heal; the drugs can then be reduced and finally stopped.

Multifocal disease is less predictable, but most cases resolve without sequelae. Age, degree of organ involvement, and response to therapy are the most important prognostic factors. Infants with disseminated disease tend to do poorly, with mortality rates approaching 50%. New treatment approaches for patients who do not respond to conventional chemotherapy have been evaluated in small studies. 2-Chlorodeoxyadenosine (2-CDA) has been used with some success. Therapeutic strategies targeting the dysregulated immune response using interferon-α or etanercept (antitumor necrosis factor-α) have also been reported.

Bernstrand C: Long-term follow-up of Langerhans cell histiocytosis: 39 years' experience at a single centre. Acta Paediatr 2005:94(8);1073 [PMID: 16188852].

Henter JI et al: Successful treatment of Langerhan's cell histiocytosis with etanercept. N Engl J Med 2001;345:1577 [PMID: 11794238].

Jubran RF et al: Predictors of outcome in children with Langerhans cell histiocytosis. Pediatr Blood Cancer 2005:45;37 [PMID: 15768381].

Kilborn TN et al: Paediatric manifestations of Langerhans cell histiocytosis: A review of the clinical and radiological findings. Clin Radiol 2003:58(4);269 [PMID: 12662947].

Kiss C et al: Interferon-alpha therapy in children with malignant diseases: Clinical experience in twenty-four patients treated in a single pediatric oncology unit. Med Pediatr Oncol 2002;39:115 [PMID: 12116059].

Rodriquez-Galindo C et al: Treatment of children with Langerhans cell histiocytosis with 2-chlorodeoxyadenosine. Am J Hematol 2002;69:179 [PMID: 11891804].

■ HEMATOPOIETIC STEM CELL TRANSPLANTATION

Amy K. Keating, MD, Roger H. Giller, MD, & Ralph R. Quinones, MD

Hematopoietic stem cell transplantation (HSCT), often referred to as bone marrow transplantation, involves the intravenous infusion of hematopoietic stem cells to reestablish normal hematopoiesis following marrow ablative or subablative chemotherapy or radiation therapy. The first successful human HSCTs were performed in the 1960s in ALL patients who received supralethal total body irradiation (TBI). The technology associated with HSCT subsequently has been expanded to include transplants that are either autologous (infusion of the patient's own hematopoietic stem cells) or allogeneic (infusion of another individual's hematopoietic stem cells). Different hematopoietic stem cell sources for transplantation include bone marrow, peripheral blood, and umbilical cord blood.

Advantages of peripheral and umbilical cord blood have led to increased use of these stem cell sources in recent years. Peripheral blood progenitor cells offer more rapid hematologic recovery and less supportive care needs after transplantation; however, they produce a higher risk of graft-versus-host disease (GVHD) than other stem cell sources. Umbilical cord blood provides an easily accessible, rich supply of hematopoietic stem cell precursors, but its use can be restricted due to limited cell doses available for larger adolescent and adult patients. Registries of bone marrow and umbilical cord blood from unrelated individuals catalogue several million potential donors worldwide for patients who lack suitably matched allogeneic family member donors.

HSCT is now considered standard therapy for a variety of malignancies, hematopoietic disorders (aplastic anemia, hemoglobinopathies), storage diseases, and severe immunodeficiencies. In many of these instances, transplantation is recommended only in high-risk situations or when conventional treatment fails. For example, HSCT has been used in sickle cell patients with a history of stroke, recurrent acute chest syndrome, or recurrent painful crises. Leukemia patients who have high-risk cytogenetic features such as monosomy 7 or the Philadelphia chromosome, t(9;22), may be candidates for transplantation in first clinical remission. In illnesses such as JMML, HSCT is used as primary therapy since no other curative treatment exists.

The rationale for HSCT in oncologic disorders is that much higher-dose chemotherapy, often in combination with myeloablative TBI, may overcome cancer cell resistance and achieve optimal tumor cell kill. This strategy is feasible because marrow toxicity from high-dose chemotherapy is circumvented by hematopoietic rescue. In allogeneic HSCT, graft-versus-tumor (GVT) effect may provide an immunologic supplement to the cytotoxic transplant preparative therapy. In GVT, donor lymphoid cells attack noncompatible antigens on malignant cells of the recipient. In patients with nonmalignant hematopoietic disorders or immunodeficiencies, HSCTs allow for replacement of absent or defective hematopoietic or lymphoid elements. In patients with storage disorders, such as Hurler disease, HSCT provides enzyme-making donor macrophages which populate host tissues.

A major challenge in performing allogeneic transplants is finding a closely HLA-matched sibling or unrelated donor. Also, sufficient host immunosuppression must be achieved to prevent allograft rejection and post-engraftment GVHD. The primary obstacle in autologous transplantation is collecting sufficient hematopoietic progenitor cells that are not contaminated by tumor cells. Purging of tumor cells (negative selection) can be achieved by several methods, including drug exposure, monoclonal antibodies, or cell culture techniques. Despite these advances, relapse of the original disease has been the greatest obstacle in autologous transplantation.

The selection of the most suitable donor for allogeneic transplant is critical since degree of compatibility is directly correlated with risk for graft rejection and GVHD. The principal genes known to encode for allogeneic recognition reside within the major histocompatibility complex (MHC) located on chromosome 6. The MHC class I antigens include HLA-A, HLA-B, and HLA-C. The important class II antigens include HLA-DR and HLA-DQ. Both class I and II antigens can mediate graft rejection or GVHD. Each child expresses one set of paternal and one set of maternal HLA antigens. Thus, the probability of one child inheriting any specific combination is 25%. Therefore, the chance of an individual sibling being a match for an allogeneic transplant is 1 in 4. Transplantation has four major treatment phases: preparative therapy, lymphohematopoietic rescue, supportive care, and long-term follow-up. The preparative phase is designed to be both myeloablative and anti-neoplastic. In the allogeneic transplant recipient, the preparative treatment also provides the necessary immunosuppression for successful donor engraftment. Preparative regimens use one or more chemotherapy drugs, often in combination with TBI.

Lymphohematopoietic rescue is accomplished by the intravenous infusion of bone marrow, peripheral blood progenitor cells, or umbilical cord blood. Graft failure after allogeneic transplant is rare in patients receiving stem cells from genotypically identical related donors but may be as high as 5–15% if the donor and patient are mismatched or unrelated. In allogeneic transplant, marrow processing prior to infusion may include removal of contaminating RBCs for ABO incompatibility or T-cell depletion to reduce the risk of GVHD. In autologous transplant, tumor purging or stem cell enrichment procedures can be performed for selected indications.

Supportive care in the initial months after transplant includes transfusions, infection prophylaxis and treatment, and nutritional support. GVHD prophylaxis is necessary in allogeneic transplants. All blood products should be leukocyte-depleted to reduce the risk of CMV transmission. Some institutions also use CMV seronegative blood to help prevent CMV transmission in selected patients. In addition, blood products must be irradiated to prevent GVHD from contaminating lymphocytes that remain in blood products.

Successful engraftment usually occurs 10–28 days following transplant. Peripheral blood stem cell transplant patients usually recover neutrophil counts earlier than patients receiving bone marrow or cord blood transplants. Platelet recovery generally occurs 6 or more weeks after HSCT. Hematopoietic growth factors such as granulocyte colony-stimulating factor or granulocyte/macrophage colony-stimulating factor may be used to hasten myeloid recovery.

The post-transplantation period can be complicated by bacterial, viral, fungal, and protozoal infections. Certain infections are typically seen at different time intervals after the transplant. During the early phase (0–1 month after transplant), when profound neutropenia and mucosal disruption occur, bacteria from the patient's aerodigestive tract are common culprits in bacteremia. Empiric antibiotic coverage and intravenous γ-globulin decrease the risk of bacterial sepsis immediately following transplant. The presence of central venous catheters makes antibiotic coverage against gram-positive bacteria an important consideration in infection management. Reactivation of herpes simplex virus may occur in as many as 70% of seropositive patients due to mucosal disruption and profound lymphopenia; thus, acyclovir prophylaxis is commonly employed. Fungal infections, particularly with *Candida* and *Aspergillus,* have made antifungal prophylaxis routine. In the intermediate post-HSCT phase (1–6 months after transplant), the patient often has reduced T-lymphocyte numbers and function and thus is susceptible to viral pathogens, including CMV, adenovirus, and respiratory syncytial virus. Prophylactic administration of acyclovir or ganciclovir helps limit CMV and other herpesvirus (herpes simplex virus, varicella-zoster virus) infections. Protozoan infections such as *Pneumocystis jiroveci* pneumonia are also a risk in this intermediate phase. HSCT patients receive trimethoprim–sulfamethoxazole, dapsone, or pentamidine as prophylaxis against *Pneumocystis.* The late phase (6–12 months after transplant), is characterized by infections from encapsulated bacteria such as *Pneumococcus* due to dysfunction of the reticuloendothelial system. Reactivation of varicella-zoster virus as shingles is also common. Patients on prolonged immunosuppressive treatment for chronic GVHD have increased and protracted risk of infections.

Despite the use of immunosuppressive agents, anti–T-cell antibodies, and T-cell depletion of the donor graft, approximately 20–70% of allogeneic HSCT patients experience some degree of acute GVHD. Factors influencing GVHD risk include the degree of HLA match, stem cell source, patient age, and donor gender. Acute GVHD occurs within the first 100 days after transplant. The first manifestation typically is a maculopapular skin rash. Skin biopsies may be done to confirm the diagnosis. Intestinal involvement results in secretory diarrhea, and hepatic involvement leads to cholestatic jaundice. Chronic GVHD occurs after day 100 and may involve multiple organ systems. Sclerotic skin, malabsorption, progressive weight loss, keratoconjunctivitis sicca, oral mucositis, chronic lung disease, and cholestatic jaundice are common manifestations. Treatment for GVHD consists of further use of immunosuppressive agents.

Long-term follow-up of HSCT patients is essential. Patients are at risk for numerous complications, including pulmonary disease, cataracts, endocrine dysfunction affecting growth and fertility, cardiac dysfunction, avascular necrosis of bone, developmental delay, and secondary malignancies. Although HSCT has many challenges, it represents an important advance in curative treatment for a variety of serious pediatric illnesses.

Bollard CEM et al: Hematopoietic stem cell transplantation in pediatric oncology. In Pizzo PA, Poplack DG (editors): *Principles and practice of pediatric oncology.* Lippincott Williams and Wilkins, 2006.

Guinan EC, et al: Principles of bone marrow and stem cell transplantation. In: Nathan DG, Orkin SH (editors): *Nathan and Oski's hematology of infancy and childhood,* 6th edition. WB Saunders, 2003.

Hahn T, et al: The role of cytotoxic therapy with hematopoietic stem cell transplantation in the therapy of acute lymphoblastic leukemia in children: an evidence-based review. Biol Blood Marrow Transplant 2005;11:823 [PMID: 16275588].

Rocha V, Sanz G, Gluckman E, et al: Umbilical cord blood transplantation. Curr Opin Hematol 2004;11:375 [PMID: 15548991].

LATE EFFECTS OF PEDIATRIC CANCER THERAPY

Late effects of treatment by surgery, radiation, and chemotherapy have been identified in survivors of pediatric cancer. Current estimates are that 1 in every 900 adults younger than age 45 years is a pediatric cancer survivor. In some studies, up to 60% of survivors of pediatric cancer will have some disability secondary to treatment. Virtually any organ system can demonstrate sequelae related to previous cancer therapy. This has necessitated the creation of specialized oncology clinics whose function it is to identify and provide treatment to these patients.

The Childhood Cancer Survivor Study, a pediatric multi-institutional collaborative project, was designed to investigate the various aspects of late effects of pediatric cancer therapy in a cohort of over 14,000 survivors of childhood cancer.

GROWTH COMPLICATIONS

Children who have received cranial irradiation are at highest risk of developing growth complications. Growth complications of cancer therapy in the pediatric survivor are generally secondary to direct damage to the pituitary gland, resulting in growth hormone deficiency. However, new evidence in children treated for ALL suggests that chemotherapy alone may result in an attenuation of linear growth without evidence of catch-up growth once therapy is discontinued. Up to 90% of patients who receive greater than 30 Gy of radiation to the CNS will show evidence of growth hormone deficiency within 2 years. Approximately 50% of children receiving 24 Gy will have growth hormone problems. The effects of cranial radiation appear to be age-related, with children younger than age 5 years at the time of therapy being particularly vulnerable. These patients usually benefit from growth hormone therapy. Currently, there is no evidence that such therapy causes a recurrence of cancer.

Spinal radiation inhibits vertebral body growth. In 30% of such individuals, standing heights may be less than the fifth percentile. Asymmetrical exposure of the spine to radiation may result in scoliosis.

Growth should be monitored closely, particularly in young survivors of childhood cancer. Follow-up studies should include height, weight, growth velocity, scoliosis examination, and, when indicated, growth hormone testing.

ENDOCRINE COMPLICATIONS

Thyroid dysfunction, manifesting as hypothyroidism, is common in children who received TBI, cranial radiation, or local radiation therapy to the neck. Particularly at risk are children with brain tumors who received more than 3000 cGy and those who received more than 4000 cGy to the neck region. The average time to develop thyroid dysfunction is 12 months after exposure, but the range is wide. Therefore, individuals at risk should be monitored yearly for at least 7 years from the completion of therapy. Although signs and symptoms of hypothyroidism may be present, most patients will have a normal thyroxine level with an elevated thyroid-stimulating hormone level. These individuals should be given thyroid hormone replacement because persistent stimulation of the thyroid from an elevated thyroid-stimulating hormone level may predispose to thyroid nodules and carcinomas. In a recent report from the Childhood Cancer Survivor Study, thyroid cancer occurred at 18 times the expected rate for the general population in pediatric cancer survivors who received radiation to the neck region. Hyperthyroidism, although rare, also occurs in patients who have received neck irradiation.

Precocious puberty, delayed puberty, and infertility are all potential consequences of cancer therapy. Precocious puberty, more common in girls, is usually a result of cranial irradiation causing premature activation of the hypothalamic–pituitary axis. This results in premature closure of the epiphysis and decreased adult height. Luteinizing hormone analogue and growth hormone are used to halt early puberty and facilitate continued growth.

Gonadal dysfunction in males is usually the result of radiation to the testes. Patients who receive testicular radiation as part of their therapy for ALL, abdominal radiation for Hodgkin disease, or TBI for HSCT are at highest risk. Radiation damages both the germinal epithelium, producing azoospermia, and Leydig cells, causing low testosterone levels and delayed puberty. Alkylating agents such as ifosfamide and cyclophosphamide can also interfere with male gonadal function, resulting in oligo- or azoospermia, low testosterone levels, and abnormal follicle-stimulating hormone (FSH) and luteinizing hormone (LH) levels. Determination of testicular size, semen analysis, and measurement of testosterone, FSH, and LH levels will help identify abnormalities in patients at risk. When therapy is expected to result in gonadal dysfunction, pretherapy sperm banking should be offered to adolescent males.

Exposure of the ovaries to abdominal radiation may result in delayed puberty with a resultant increase in FSH and LH and a decrease in estrogen. Girls receiving TBI as preparation for HSCT and those receiving craniospinal radiation are at particularly high risk for delayed puberty as well as premature menopause. In patients at high risk for development of gonadal complications, a detailed menstrual history should be obtained, and LH, FSH, and estrogen levels should be monitored if indicated.

No studies to date have confirmed an increased risk of spontaneous abortions, stillbirths, premature births, congenital malformations, or genetic diseases in the offspring of childhood cancer survivors. Women who have received abdominal radiation may develop uterine vascular insufficiency or fibrosis of the abdominal and pelvic musculature or uterus, and their pregnancies should be considered high-risk.

CARDIOPULMONARY COMPLICATIONS

Pulmonary dysfunction generally manifests as pulmonary fibrosis. Therapy-related factors known to cause pulmonary toxicities include certain chemotherapeutic agents, such as bleomycin, the nitrosoureas, and busulfan, as well as lung radiation or TBI. Pulmonary toxicity due to chemotherapy is related to the total cumulative dose received. Pulmonary function tests in patients with therapy-induced toxicity show restrictive lung disease, with decreased carbon monoxide diffusion and small lung volumes. Individuals exposed to these risk factors should be counseled to refrain from smoking and to give proper notification of the treatment history if they should require general anesthesia.

Cardiac complications usually result from exposure to anthracyclines (daunorubicin, doxorubicin, and mitoxantrone), which destroy myocytes and lead to inadequate myocardial growth as the child ages and eventually result in congestive heart failure. The incidence of anthracycline cardiomyopathy increases in a dose-dependent fashion. At least 5% of patients who have received a cumulative dose of more than 550 mg/m^2 of anthracyclines experience cardiac dysfunction. In a recent study, complications from these agents appeared 6–19 years following administration of the drugs. Pregnant women who have received anthracyclines should be followed up closely for signs and symptoms of congestive heart failure, as peripartum cardiomyopathy has been reported.

Radiation therapy to the mediastinal region, which is common as part of therapy for Hodgkin disease, has been linked to an increased risk of coronary artery disease; chronic restrictive pericarditis may also occur in these patients.

Current recommendations include an exercise echocardiogram and electrocardiogram every 1–5 years, depending on the age at therapy, total cumulative dose received, and presence or absence of mediastinal irradiation. Selective monitoring with various modalities is indicated for those who were treated with anthracyclines when they were younger than age 4 years or received more than 500 mg/m^2 of these drugs. Measurement of serum levels of cardiac troponin-T or atrial natriuretic peptide may be useful in assessing early cardiotoxicity of anthracyclines.

RENAL COMPLICATIONS

Long-term renal side effects stem from therapy with cisplatin, alkylating agents (ifosfamide and cyclophosphamide), or pelvic radiation. Patients who have received cisplatin may develop abnormal creatinine clearance, which may or may not be accompanied by abnormal serum creatinine levels, as well as persistent tubular dysfunction with hypomagnesemia. Alkylating agents can cause hemorrhagic cystitis, which may continue after chemotherapy has been terminated and has been associated with the development of bladder carcinoma. Ifosfamide can also cause Fanconi syndrome, which may result in clinical rickets if adequate phosphate replacement is not provided. Pelvic radiation may result in abnormal bladder function with dribbling, frequency, and enuresis.

Patients seen in long-term follow-up who have received nephrotoxic agents should be monitored with urinalysis, appropriate electrolyte profiles, and blood pressure. Urine collection for creatinine clearance or renal ultrasound may be indicated in individuals with suspected renal toxicity.

NEUROPSYCHOLOGICAL COMPLICATIONS

Pediatric cancer survivors who have received cranial radiation for ALL or brain tumors appear to be at greatest risk for neuropsychological sequelae. The severity of cranial radiation effects varies among individual patients and depends on the dose and dose schedule,

the size and location of the radiation field, the amount of time elapsed after treatment, the child's age at therapy, and the child's gender. Girls may be more susceptible than boys to CNS toxicity because of more rapid brain growth and development during childhood.

The main effects of CNS radiation appear to be related to attention capacities, ability with nonverbal tasks and mathematics, and short-term memory. Recent studies support the association between high-dose systemic methotrexate, triple intrathecal chemotherapy, and more recently, dexamethasone with more significant cognitive impairment.

Additionally, pediatric cancer patients have been reported as having more behavior problems and as being less socially competent than a sibling control group. Adolescent survivors of cancer demonstrate an increased sense of physical fragility and vulnerability manifested as hypochondriasis or phobic behaviors.

Finally, childhood cancer survivors are more likely to report symptoms of depression and somatic distress in adulthood. Pediatric cancer survivors may require ongoing counseling or other psychological interventions once they have completed therapy.

SECOND MALIGNANCIES

Approximately 3–12% of children receiving cancer treatment will develop a new cancer within 20 years of their first diagnosis. This is a tenfold increased incidence when compared with age-matched control subjects. Particular risk factors include exposure to alkylating agents, epipodophyllotoxins (VP-16), and radiation therapy, primary diagnosis of retinoblastoma or Hodgkin disease, or the presence of an inherited genetic susceptibility syndrome (Li-Fraumeni syndrome or NF). In a recent report, the cumulative estimated incidence of second malignant neoplasms for the cohort of the Childhood Cancer Survivor Study was 3.2% at 20 years from diagnosis.

Second hematopoietic malignances (acute myelogenous leukemia) occur as a result of therapy with epipodophyllotoxins or alkylating agents. It is unclear whether the schedule of drug administration and the total dose are related to the development of this secondary leukemia.

Children receiving radiation therapy are at risk for developing second malignancies, such as sarcomas, carcinomas, or brain tumors, in the field of radiation. A recent report examining the incidence of second neoplasms in a cohort of pediatric Hodgkin disease patients showed the cumulative risk of a second neoplasm to be as high as 8% at 15 years from diagnosis. The most common solid tumor was breast cancer (the majority located within the radiation field) followed by thyroid cancer. Girls age 10–16 years when they received radiation were at highest risk and had an actuarial incidence that approached 35% by age 40 years.

Friedman DL, Meadows AT: Late effects of childhood cancer therapy. Pediatr Clin North Am 2002;49:1083 [PMID: 12430627].

Hudson MM et al: Health status of adult long-term survivors of childhood cancer: A report from the Childhood Cancer Survivor Study. JAMA 2003;290:1583 [PMID: 14506117].

Kimball-Dalton V et al: Height and weight in children treated for acute lymphoblastic leukemia: Relationship to CNS treatment. J Clin Oncol 2003;21:2953 [PMID: 12885815].

Neglia IP et al: Second malignant neoplasms in five-year survivors of childhood cancer: Childhood Cancer Survivor Study. J Natl Cancer Inst 2001;93:618 [PMID: 11309438].

Poutanen T et al: Long-term prospective follow-up of cardiac function after cardiotoxic therapy for malignancy in children. J Clin Oncol 2003;21:2349 [PMID: 12805337].

Reiter-Purtill J et al: A controlled longitudinal study of the social functioning of children who completed treatment of cancer. J Pediatr Hematol Oncol 2003;25:467 [PMID: 12794525].

Zebrack BJ et al: Psychological outcomes in long-term survivors of childhood leukemia, Hodgkin's disease, and non-Hodgkin's lymphoma: A report from the Childhood Cancer Survivor Study. Pediatr 2002;110:42 [PMID: 12093945].

Immunodeficiency

29

Andrew H. Liu, MD, Lora J. Stewart, MD, & Richard Johnston, MD

Primary immunodeficiency (PID) commonly presents with recurrent or severe infections, but most children with frequent minor infections (eg, otitis media or sinusitis) do not have an underlying immune disorder. Immunodeficiency should be considered when infections are particularly severe, persistent, resistant to standard treatment, or caused by opportunistic organisms. Certain clinical patterns and recurring infections with certain types of microbes are indicative of specific immune deficiencies. Because delay in the diagnosis of PIDs is common, heightened diagnostic suspicion is warranted. Host immunity can be divided into four main groups for the purpose of categorizing PIDs: antibody immunity (B lymphocytes), combined immunity (T and B lymphocytes), phagocytic immunity (neutrophil or mononuclear cells), and complement (bactericidal proteins also involved in opsonization). Understanding the role each category plays in host defense allows critical evaluation for possible immunodeficiency as the etiology for recurrent infections.

Bonilla F et al: Primary immunodeficiency diseases. J Allergy Clin Immunol 2003;111:S571 [PMID: 12592303].

IMMUNODEFICIENCY EVALUATION: PRIMARY CONSIDERATIONS

Before evaluating for a defined primary immunodeficiency, consider conditions that increase susceptibility to infection, such as allergic rhinitis (causing sinusitis), cystic fibrosis (causing failure to thrive, pneumonia, and sinus disease), asthma (causing chronic cough and pneumonia), foreign bodies, and conditions that interfere with skin integrity. Also exclude common causes of secondary immunodeficiency such as human immunodeficiency virus infection, malnutrition, drugs, and protein loss via gastroenteropathy or kidney disease. If a single site is involved, exclude anatomic defects and foreign bodies. Figure 29–1 outlines the approach to considering PIDs.

Key clinical patterns can indicate the likelihood of a PID, the category of immune impairment (Table 29–1), and sometimes the specific PID. The frequency and severity of infections can be helpful when considering a PID. The Modell Foundation developed warning signs

for PID found in Figure 29–2. Children who meet two or more of these signs should be screened for PID. Age at the onset of infections can be a helpful clue, as defects in different arms of the immune system will present at typical ages. For instance, defects of phagocytes and cellular immunity typically present during the first months of life, whereas maternal antibody protects infants with antibody deficiency for 3–6 months. The type of infections should guide initial investigation, as antibody, complement, and phagocyte defects predispose mainly to bacterial infections; but diarrhea, superficial candidiasis, opportunistic infections, and severe herpes virus infections are more characteristic of T-lymphocyte immunodeficiency. Combined immunodeficiency syndromes will present with a combination of infections typical for B-lymphocyte and T-lymphocyte deficiencies. Table 29–1 classifies PID into four main host immunity categories based on differences in these revealing clinical parameters of age of onset, specific pathogens, affected organs, and other special features. Finally, male gender increases the likelihood of an X-linked PID, while consanguinity increases the likelihood of an autosomal recessive form of PID.

The level of laboratory investigation should be based on the clinical presentation and the suspected category of host immunity impairment. A complete blood count and quantitative immunoglobulin measurement will identify the majority of those with PID, as antibody deficiencies account for at least 50% of PIDs (Figure 29–3). Table 29–2 summarizes the approach to laboratory evaluation of PID.

Cunningham-Rundles C: Immune deficiency: Office evaluation and treatment. Allergy Asthma Proc 2003;24:409 [PMID: 14763242].

Woroniecka M, Ballow M: Primary immune deficiencies: Presentation, diagnosis, and management. Pediatr Clin 2000;47:1211 [PMID: 11130993].

Antibodies & Immunoglobulins

The initial screen for antibody deficiency is to measure serum immunoglobulins (IgG, IgM and IgA, but not IgD). The normal ranges of IgG, IgM, and IgA vary by age as their production by B lymphocytes matures (see Table 29–3 for normal ranges). Some patients may have normal

917

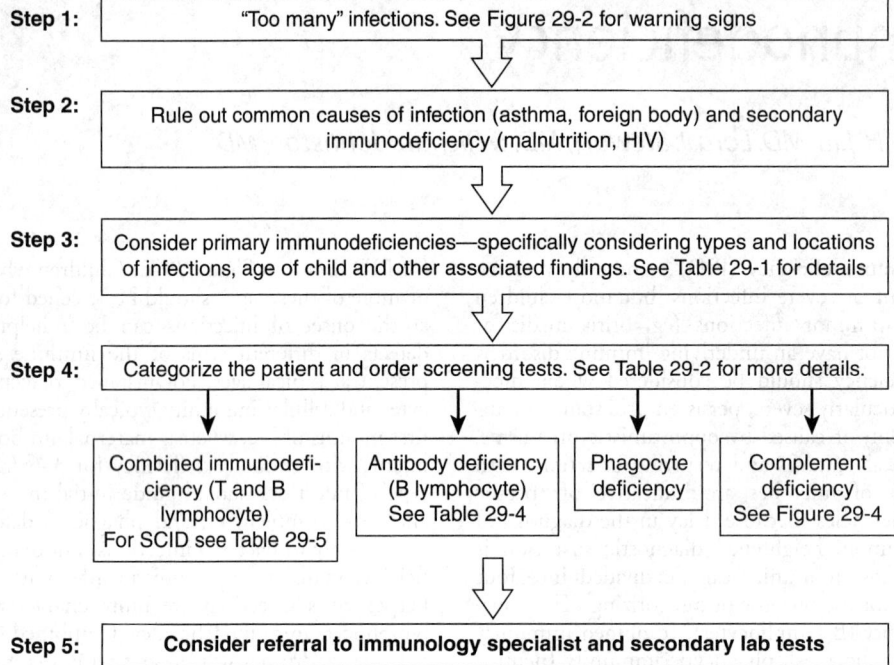

Step 1:   "Too many" infections. See Figure 29-2 for warning signs

Step 2:   Rule out common causes of infection (asthma, foreign body) and secondary immunodeficiency (malnutrition, HIV)

Step 3:   Consider primary immunodeficiencies—specifically considering types and locations of infections, age of child and other associated findings. See Table 29-1 for details

Step 4:   Categorize the patient and order screening tests. See Table 29-2 for more details.

Combined immunodeficiency (T and B lymphocyte) For SCID see Table 29-5

Antibody deficiency (B lymphocyte) See Table 29-4

Phagocyte deficiency

Complement deficiency See Figure 29-4

Step 5:   **Consider referral to immunology specialist and secondary lab tests**

Figure 29–1. General approach to primary immunodeficiencies.

immunoglobulin levels but do not make protective specific antibodies; other patients have abnormal immunoglobulin levels but make protective specific antibodies. When interpreting immunoglobulin concentrations, remember that infants have lower normal values compared to adults. Evaluation of specific antibodies includes isohemagglutinins, which are naturally occurring antibodies (except in patients with blood group AB) and are detectable by 6 months of age. Additional testing options include tetanus, diphtheria, *Haemophilus,* rubella, and mumps antibody levels following immunization. Assessing antibody response to pneumococcal polysaccharide can be helpful in the face of repeated pneumococcal infections, but as a screening tool it is often difficult to interpret, as the normal immune response to unconjugated polysaccharide vaccines may be weak or difficult to measure. The gold standard is pre- and post-immunization titers with at least a threefold increase in titers 3 weeks postimmunization. Obtaining T- and B-lymphocyte counts is recommended if an initial screen revealed very low immunoglobulin concentrations for all classes, as certain hypogammaglobulinemic syndromes have low or absent B lymphocytes (such as X-linked Bruton agammaglobulinemia). Protein electrophoresis can help identify the monoclonal increases seen in the oligoclonal gammopathy of Epstein-Barr virus (EBV) infections in X-linked lymphoproliferative syndrome, and in

heavy-chain diseases. Serum albumin should be measured in patients with hypogammaglobulinemia to exclude secondary deficiencies due to protein loss through bowel or kidneys. IgG or IgA subclass measurements may be abnormal in patients with varied immunodeficiency syndromes, but they are rarely helpful in an initial evaluation.

Ballow M: Primary immunodeficiency disorders: Antibody deficiency. J Allergy Clin Immunol 2002;109:581 [PMID: 11941303].

T Lymphocytes

The initial screen for T lymphocytes includes a complete blood cell count with differential to evaluate for a decreased absolute lymphocyte count (< 1000 K/µL). Delayed hypersensitivity skin tests (such as *Candida,* tetanus, or mumps) give good evidence for antigen-specific T-lymphocyte immunity, but a negative or anergic result is not helpful, as it may be due to young age, chronic illness, or poor test technique. Even T-lymphocyte deficiencies will often not manifest anergy until the impairment is severe (eg, acquired immunodeficiency syndrome). When T-lymphocyte abnormalities are suspected, it is important to check for specific antibody production and absolute numbers of T and B lymphocytes and their subsets (including CD3, CD4, CD8, CD19/CD20, and CD16/

Table 29–1. Categorical clinical features of primary immunodeficiencies.

Characteristic	Combined Deficiency (T- and B-Lymphocyte Defect)	Antibody Deficiency (B-Lymphocyte Defect)	Phagocyte Defect	Complement Defect
Age at onset of infections	Early onset, usually before 6 mo	Onset after maternal antibodies decline, usually after 3–6 mo; some later childhood or adult	Early onset	Any age
Specific pathogens	**Bacteria:** *Streptococcus pneumonia, Campylobacter fetus, Staphylococcus aureus, Haemophilus influenzae, Pseudomonas aeruginosa, Mycoplasma hominis, Ureaplasma urealyticum, Listeria monocytogenes, Salmonella typhi,* enteric flora, atypical mycobacteria, and BCG **Viruses:** CMV, EBV, varicella, RSV, enterovirus, rotavirus **Fungi/protozoa:** *Candida albicans, Aspergillus fumigatus* **Opportunistic:** *Pneumocystis carinii,* cryptosporidium, *Toxoplasma gondii*	**Bacteria:** *S pneumonia, C fetus, H influenzae, P aeruginosa, U urealyticum, S aureus, M hominis* **Viruses:** Enteroviruses **Fungi/protozoa:** *Giardia lamblia* **Opportunistic:** None	**Bacteria:** *S aureus,* enteric flora, *P aeruginosa, S typhi, Serratia* spp, *Nocardia asteroides, Klebsiella* spp, atypical mycobacteria, and BCG **Viruses:** None **Fungi/protozoa:** *C albicans, A fumigatus* **Opportunistic:** None	**Bacteria:** esp *Neisseria* spp, *S pneumoniae, S aureus, P aeruginosa, H influenzae, U urealyticum* **Viruses:** None **Fungi/protozoa:** None **Opportunistic:** None
Affected organs	**General:** Failure to thrive **Infectious:** Severe infection (meningitis, septicemia, sinopulmonary), recurrent candidiasis, protracted diarrhea	**Infections:** Recurrent sinopulmonary, pneumonia, meningitis **GI:** Chronic malabsorption and IBD-like symptoms **Other:** Arthritis	**Skin:** Dermatitis, impetigo, cellulitis **Lymph nodes:** Suppurative adenitis **Oral cavity:** Periodontitis, ulcers **Lungs:** Pneumonia, pneumatoceles **Other:** Abscesses, osteomyelitis	**Infections:** Meningitis, arthritis, septicemia, recurrent sinopulmonary
Special features	GVHD: Maternal T cells or blood product transfusion Postvaccination: Disseminated BCG or polio Absent lymphoid tissue Absent thymic shadow on chest x-ray	Autoimmunity Lymphoreticular malignancy Postvaccination paralytic polio Chronic enteroviral encephalitis	Poor wound healing; "cold" abscesses	Autoimmune disorders: SLE, vasculitis, dermatomyositis, scleroderma, glomerulonephritis, angioedema

BCG, bacille Calmette-Guérin; CMV, cytomegalovirus; EBV, Epstein-Barr virus; GVHD, graft-versus-host disease; IBD, inflammatory bowel disease; RSV, respiratory syncytial virus; SLE, systemic lupus erythematosus.
Adapted, with permission, from Woroniecka M, Ballow M: Primary immune deficiencies: presentation, diagnosis, and management. Pediatr Clin North Am 2000;47:1211.

10 Warning Signs of Primary Immunodeficiency

Primary Immunodeficiency (PI) causes children and young adults to have infections that come back frequently or are unusually hard to cure. In America alone, up to 1/2 million people suffer from one of the 100 known primary immunodeficiency diseases. If you or someone you know are affected by two or more of the following warning signs, speak to a physician about the possible presence of an underlying primary immunodeficiency.

1	Eight or more new ear infections in one year.	**6**	Recurrent, deep skin or organ abscesses.
2	Two or more serious sinus infections within 1 year.	**7**	Persistent thrush in mouth or elsewhere on skin, after age 1.
3	Two or more months on antibiotics with little effect.	**8**	Need for intravenous antibiotics to clear infections.
4	Two or more pneumonias within 1 year.	**9**	Two or more deap-seated infections.
5	Failure of an infant to gain weight or grow normally.	**10**	A family history of primary immunodeficiency.

Figure 29–2. Warning signs of primary immunodeficiency. (Adapted, with permission, from Jeffrey Modell Foundation.)

CD56). Because proper B-lymphocyte function and antibody production is dependent on T-lymphocyte function, most T-lymphocyte deficiencies manifest as combined impairments. Tests of T-lymphocyte proliferation and cytokine production can be supportive for characterizing immunodeficiency detected by initial tests, but they are not useful screening tests for children with chronic illness, recurrent infections, or young age; additionally, borderline function is often interpreted based on clinical correlation.

Phagocytic Immunity

Initial screening should include an evaluation for neutropenia with a complete blood count and differential. A blood smear can be done to exclude Howell-Jolly bodies of asplenia and to look for normal lysosomal granules in neutrophils. The respiratory burst and generation of bactericidal factors can be tested by nitroblue tetrazolium reduction, but this test has generally been replaced by assessing reduced nicotinamide adenine dinucleotide phosphate (NADPH) oxidase activity by flow cytometry (dihydrorhodamine flow cytometry assay). Leukocyte adhesion molecules are also screened by flow cytometry methods, although the difference in symptoms of suspected phagocyte defects should dictate which tests are used. Quantification of bacterial ingestion and microbicidal activity may be available.

Rosenzweig SD, Holland SM: Phagocyte immunodeficiencies and their infections. J Allergy Clin Immunol 2004;113:620 [PMID: 15100664].

Complement Pathways (Figure 29–4)

Deficiency of classic complement pathway components can be excluded by a normal hemolytic complement titer (CH50), for which the patient's serum must be separated and frozen to –70 °C within 30 minutes of collection to prevent auto-degradation of complement components. Alternative complement pathway deficiencies are similarly identified by AH50. Measuring individual complement component levels is not necessary if both CH50

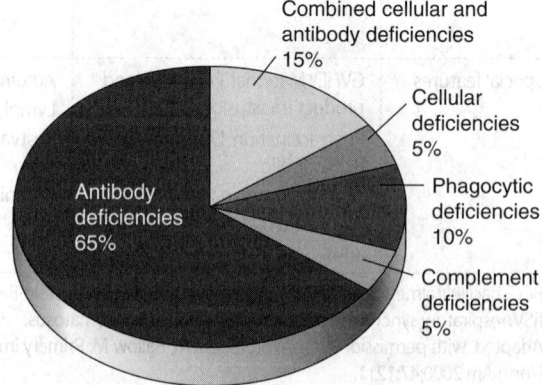

Figure 29–3. Relative frequencies of primary immunodeficiencies. (Adapted, with permission, from Stiehm ER, et al. *Immunologic disorders of infants and children*, 5th edition. Philadelphia: Elsevier, 2004.)

Table 29–2. Laboratory evaluation for primary immunodeficiency.

Suspected Defect	Screening Evaluation	Secondary Evaluation	Advanced Evaluation
B-lymphocyte defect	Quantitative immunoglobulins (IgG, IgM, and IgA)	B-lymphocyte enumeration panel (CD19/20) Antibody response to prior and/or repeat immunizations (tetanus, diphtheria, Hib) Isohemaglutinins	Screen for specific genetic mutations Screen for memory B cells (IgM-IgD-CD27+)
Combined T- and B-lymphocyte defect	Absolute lymphocyte count HIV testing	T- and B-lymphocyte enumeration panel (T = CD3, CD4 and CD8; B = CD19/20) Lymphocyte proliferation assay to mitogens and antigens Delayed-type hypersensitivity	DNA analysis for specific genetic mutations ADA or PNP levels of RBC Cytotoxicity studies
Phagocyte defect	WBC count with differential IgE level	Dihydrorodamine flow cytometry Nitroblue tetrazolium reduction assay	Bacteriocidal assays Chemotaxis assay
Complement defect	CH50	AH50	Individual complement levels and function.

ADA, adenosine deaminase; HIV, human immunodeficiency virus; PNP, purine nucleoside phosphorylase; RBC, red blood cell; WBC, white blood cell.
Adapted, with permission, from Cunningham-Rundles C: Immune deficiency: Office evaluation and treatment. Allergy Asthma Proc 2000;24:409.

Table 29–3. Normal values for immunoglobulins by age.

Age	IgG (mg/dL)	IgM (mg/dL)	IgA (mg/dL)
Newborn	1031 ± 200	11 ± 17	2 ± 3
1–3 months	430 ± 119	30 ± 11	21 ± 13
4–6 months	427 ± 186	43 ± 17	28 ± 18
7–12 months	661 ± 219	55 ± 23	37 ± 18
13–24 months	762 ± 209	58 ± 23	50 ± 24
25–36 months	892 ± 183	61 ± 19	71 ± 34
3–5 years	929 ± 228	56 ± 18	93 ± 27
6–8 years	923 ± 256	65 ± 25	124 ± 45
9–11 years	1124 ± 235	79 ± 33	131 ± 60
12–16 years	946 ± 124	59 ± 20	148 ± 63
Adults	1158 ± 305	99 ± 27	200 ± 61

Adapted, with permission, from Stiehm ER, et al. *Immunologic disorders of infants and children*, 5th edition. Philadelphia: Elsevier, 2004.

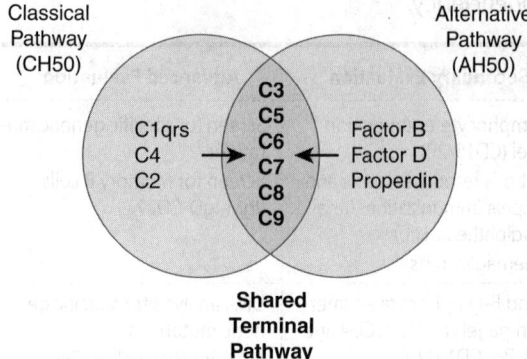

Figure 29–4. Complement proteins and laboratory test pathways.

and AH50 are normal. If the CH50 and AH50 are both low, the deficiency must be in their shared terminal pathway (C3, C5, C6, C7, C8, or C9). If CH50 is low, but AH50 is normal, the deficiency must be C1, C4, or C2; if AH50 is low and CH50 is normal, the deficiency must be factor D or B or properdin.

Wen L et al: Clinical and laboratory evaluation of complement deficiency. J Allergy Clin Immunol 2004;113:585 [PMID: 15100659].

ANTIBODY DEFICIENCY SYNDROMES

Antibody deficiencies include both congenital and acquired forms that result in low (hypogammaglobulinemia) or very low (agammaglobulinemia) levels of immunoglobulins (IgM, IgG, and IgA). Deficiencies result in recurrent bacterial infections, specifically with encapsulated bacteria, including pneumonia, otitis, sinusitis, meningitis, cellulitis, and sepsis. As a group, antibody deficiencies represent nearly half of all primary immunodeficiencies. Table 29–4 presents primary antibody deficiency syndromes, laboratory findings, and genetic inheritance. Patients who are unable to make specific antibody to vaccinations or infections are candidates for replacement gamma globulin therapy (ie, intravenous immune globulin [IVIG]). In contrast, those with secondary or transient hypogammaglobulinemia (ie, low total serum IgG level) but are able to make specific antibodies, generally do not need or benefit from replacement IVIG.

Ballow M: Primary immunodeficiency disorders: Antibody deficiency. J Allergy Clin Immunol 2002;109:581 [PMID: 11941303].

Bonilla FA, Geha RS: Primary immunodeficiency diseases. J Allergy Clin Immunol 2003;111:S571 [PMID: 12592303].

1. X-Linked Agammaglobulinemia (XLA)

X-linked agammaglobulinemia (XLA) typically presents with infections after 4 months of age, when maternally derived IgG levels have declined. Infections are usually due to *Haemophilus influenzae* and *Streptococcus pneumoniae,* but deep tissue infections and arthritis due to *Ureaplasma* species are seen as well. Antibody-deficient patients are also at risk for severe enterovirus infections with vaccine strains of poliovirus resulting in paralysis, and echoviruses causing chronic encephalitis. At presentation, male infants will have scant or absent lymphoid tissue including tonsils, adenoids, and lymph nodes. A small proportion will also have a history of poor growth. Most patients have low or absent immunoglobulins (IgM, IgG, and IgA) and, despite a normal leukocyte count, have low or absent B lymphocytes. XLA accounts for 85% of congenital hypogammaglobulinemia and occurs in about 1:200,000 male births. It results from mutations in the gene for the B lymphocyte tyrosine kinase (*btk*), which is important for B-lymphocyte maturation. A *btk* mutation by molecular analysis confirms the diagnosis of XLA. Current therapy is with lifelong replacement IgG. In addition to preventing infections, IVIG replacement usually results in resolution of inflammatory arthritis and improves growth. Because the severity of infections varies and antibiotics are widely used, diagnosis is often delayed for years, but XLA must be considered in males with recurrent infections regardless of severity.

Ballow M: Primary immunodeficiency disorders: Antibody deficiency. J Allergy Clin Immunol 2002;109:581 [PMID: 11941303].

2. Autosomal Recessive Congenital Agammaglobulinemia

Autosomal recessive congenital agammaglobulinemia is rare, accounting for less than 15% of all congenital hypogammaglobulinemia. The most common form results from defects of the μ heavy-chain gene, and these patients tend to have an earlier onset of infections than *btk*-deficient boys. Mutations in the μ heavy chain result in abnormal or absent IgM. Additional forms of autosomal recessive congenital antibody deficiency result from mutations in the Igα molecule, the BLNK adaptor protein, and the λ5 surrogate light chain. All of these mutations result in abnormal B-lymphocyte maturation with low B-cell numbers and poor specific antibody. Treatment and prognosis are similar to that of XLA.

Ballow M: Primary immunodeficiency disorders: Antibody deficiency. J Allergy Clin Immunol 2002;109:581 [PMID: 11941303].

3. Common Variable Immunodeficiency (CVID)

Common variable immunodeficiency (CVID) is a diagnosis of exclusion after other causes of hypogammaglobulinemia have been eliminated. Decreased levels of IgG and

Table 29–4. Predominantly antibody deficiency disorders.

Disease	Serum Ig	Circulating B Cells	Genetic Mutation	Mode of Inheritance
XLA	All isotypes absent	Less than 2%	Mutations in *BTK*	X linked
Autosomal recessive congenital				
Hypogammaglobulinemia				
Igα defect	All isotypes absent	Less than 2%	Defect in Igα molecule	AR
Surrogate light chain	All isotypes absent	Less than 2%	Mutations in λ5/14.1	AR
BLNK defect	All isotypes absent	Less than 2%	Mutations BLNK	?
μ heavy chain	All isotypes absent	Less than 2%	Mutations in μ heavy chain	AR
Common variable immunodeficiency	Variable, some or all isotypes decreased	Normal or decreased	Unknown, likely not a single gene, autosomal recessive form is ICOS	Variable
Autosomal recessive forms of hyper IgM syndrome	Normal or increased IgM, other isotypes decreased	IgM-bearing B cells only	Mutations in AID gene or UNG gene	AR
Transient hypogammaglobulinemia of infancy	IgG and IgA decreased, but IgM usually normal	Normal	Defect unknown	?
IgA deficiency	Very low or absent IgA	Normal	Defect unknown	Variable
IgG subclass deficiency	IgG subclasses decreased	Normal	Defect unknown	?

ICOS, inducible co-stimulatory molecule.
Adapted, with permission, from Ballow M: Primary immunodeficiency disorders: Antibody deficiency. J Allergy Clin Immunol 2002;109:581.

IgA, poor specific antibody to vaccine antigens, low or absent isohemagglutinins, and a history of recurrent infections characterize CVID. Sinopulmonary infections predominate, but additional chronic GI tract infections with *Giardia lamblia* and *Campylobacter jejuni* occur. Patients with CVID are at risk for developing bronchiectasis, autoimmune diseases (idiopathic thrombocytopenic purpura, autoimmune hemolytic anemia, rheumatoid arthritis, and inflammatory bowel disease), and malignancies (especially gastric carcinoma and lymphoma). Onset occurs at any age, and the incidence approaches 1:30,000. Many cases are sporadic, but a small percentage has autosomal dominant or recessive inheritance and some cases are associated with certain HL-DR/DQ alleles. Mutations in the gene for the inducible co-stimulatory molecule (ICOS) and its ligand are an example of autosomal recessive CVID. ICOS interactions with its ligand are important for developing memory B-lymphocyte function. Lab-oratory examination for CVID is variable but typically reveals low levels of IgG and IgA, normal numbers of B lymphocytes, low numbers of memory B lymphocytes (evaluated by flow cytometry) and abnormal specific antibodies. Some patients have evidence of T-lymphocyte abnormalities as well. Treatment includes lifelong replacement therapy with intravenous IgG and routine assessment for bronchiectasis, autoimmune disorders, and malignancies. Prognosis depends on time to diagnosis and implementation of IgG replacement, but can be good. Other complications include B-cell hyperplasia in the gut that may be severe enough to resemble Crohn's disease, and gastric atrophy with achlorhydria, sometimes followed by pernicious anemia. Lymphoreticular proliferation can occur after EBV infection and is not always malignant.

Abonia JP et al: Common variable immunodeficiency. Allergy Asthma Proc 2002;23:53 [PMID: 11894736].

Kokron CM et al: Clinical and laboratory aspects of common variable immunodeficiency. Ann Braz Acad Sci 2004;76:707 [PMID: 15558152].

Salzer U et al: ICOS deficiency in patients with common variable immunodeficiency. Clin Immunol 2004;113:234 [PMID: 15507837].

4. Autosomal Recessive Hyper-IgM Immunodeficiency

Autosomal recessive forms of hyper-IgM immunodeficiency differ from the X-linked form (see section on combined immunodeficiency), as affected patients have normal expression and function of CD40 ligand. Patients have mutations in activation-induced cytidine deaminase (AID) or uracil glycosylase (UNG). AID is required for B lymphocytes to switch from producing IgM to production of IgG, IgA, or IgE. UNG is also important for isotype class switching. The clinical presentation of AID- and UNG-deficient patients is less severe than that of X-linked hyper-IgM syndrome and also lacks opportunistic infections. Affected patients often have associated lymphoid hyperplasia compared to the paucity of lymphoid tissue seen with X-linked hyper-IgM syndrome. Treatment with IVIG replacement decreases infections and often normalizes IgM levels.

Etzioni A, Ochs HD: The hyper-IgM syndrome—An evolving story. Pediatr Res 2004;56:519 [PMID: 15319456].

5. Acquired Hypogammaglobulinemia

Acquired forms of hypogammaglobulinemia are common and may develop at any age. Causes of secondary hypogammaglobulinemia (nephrotic syndrome and protein-losing enteropathy) should be excluded by measuring serum albumin. Generally, we do not treat acquired forms with IVIG. Morphologic disorders or associated syndromes may point to a specific diagnosis.

Conley ME: Early defects in B cell development. Curr Opin Allergy Clin Immunol 2002;2:517 [PMID: 14752335].

6. Transient Hypogammaglobulinemia

Serum IgG levels normally decrease during an infant's first 4–5 months of life, as maternal IgG is lost. Transient hypogammaglobulinemia represents a delay in the onset of immunoglobulin synthesis that results in a prolonged nadir. Symptomatic patients present with recurrent infections, including upper respiratory tract infections, otitis, and sinusitis. Diagnosis is suspected in infants with low levels of IgG and IgA (usually two standard deviations below normal for age), but normal levels of IgM and normal numbers of circulating B lymphocytes. Importantly, infants have normal specific antibody responses and T-lymphocyte function. Apart from appropriate antibiotics, no treatment is required. Infants with severe infection and hypogammaglobulinemia could be given IVIG replacement, but benefits and risk must be considered and this is rarely necessary. Recovery occurs between 18 and 30 months of age and the prognosis for affected infants is excellent provided infections are treated promptly and appropriately.

Ballow M: Primary immunodeficiency disorders: Antibody deficiency. J Allergy Clin Immunol 2002;109:581 [PMID: 11941303].

7. Selective Immunoglobulin Deficiencies

Selective IgA deficiency is the most common immune abnormality, found in ~ 1:700 persons. It is defined by a serum IgA less than 7 mg/dL. Serum IgM, IgG, specific antibodies, and B- and T-lymphocyte numbers and function are normal. The majority of people with low serum IgA are without symptoms, but when symptoms are present, they include upper respiratory tract infections and/or diarrhea. Associations also exist with inflammatory bowel disease, allergic disease, asthma, and autoimmune disorders (thyroiditis, arthritis, vitiligo, thrombocytopenia, and diabetes). Because IgA has a short half-life in serum and it is primarily effective in its secreted form on mucosal surfaces, replacement is not feasible. For the majority of symptomatic IgA-deficient patients, antibiotics and appropriate autoimmune therapies are sufficient, but some patients have been treated with IVIG replacement. Caution must be exercised, as IgA-deficient patients are at risk for developing anti-IgA antibodies with blood product exposure, and the administration of blood products can result in anaphylaxis. Therefore when blood products are needed, washed packed red blood cells and volume expanders without blood products are recommended.

The possibility that deficiency of an IgG subclass (ie, abnormally low serum IgG2, IgG3, and/or IgG4) might predispose to recurrent upper respiratory tract infections in patients with normal total serum immunoglobulin levels is not well established. Normally, IgG1 comprises over 60% of total IgG and IgG2 over 10%. IgG3 accounts for about 5%, and IgG4 may be undetectable in up to 20% of healthy persons and serum levels are age-related. It has been difficult to establish a link between IgG subclass deficiencies and any consistent pattern of infections. IgG replacement should be reserved for patients with defects in specific antibody production, which is rarely seen in patients with selective IgA or IgG subclass deficiencies.

Ballow M: Primary immunodeficiency disorders: Antibody deficiency. J Allergy Clin Immunol 2002;109:581 [PMID: 11941303].

Bonilla FA, Geha RS: Primary immunodeficiency diseases. J Allergy Clin Immunol 2003;111:S571 [PMID: 12592303].

Treatment of Hypogammaglobulinemia

The mainstay of therapy for hypogammaglobulinemia is replacement IgG, but management of infections is also important. Additional treatment modalities have included the use of cytokine therapy such as interleukin (IL)-2, hormone replacement, and vitamin supplementation. Curative therapy with bone marrow transplantation (BMT) has been successful in patients with XLA, and gene therapy is not yet available outside a research setting. IgG is usually given by intravenous infusions at a dose of 400–600 mg/kg every 3–4 weeks to maintain a trough serum IgG of > 500–800 mg/dL (a higher trough level is important for patients with established pulmonary disease). Subcutaneous replacement is available but requires more frequent injections and may limit maximum dosing. The aim of treatment is to prevent future infections and minimize any progression of chronic lung disease (bronchitis or bronchiectasis). Despite the passive immunity provided by replacement IgG, infection remains a persistent risk and prognosis additionally depends on timely and appropriate antibiotics. Typical organisms include encapsulated bacteria, but *Ureaplasma* and *Mycoplasma* species must be considered. Infusions are generally well tolerated, with most reactions being mild including headache, back and limb pain, anxiety, and tightness of the chest. Rare systemic reactions can occur, including tachycardia, shivering, fever, and in severe cases, anaphylactoid shock. For patients with congenital hypogammaglobulinemia, replacement therapy is currently lifelong.

Durandy A et al: Immunoglobulin replacement therapy in primary antibody deficiency diseases—maximizing success. Int Arch Allergy Immunol 2005;136:217 [PMID: 15713984].

SEVERE COMBINED IMMUNODEFICIENCY DISEASES

Combined T- and B-lymphocyte diseases include severe combined immunodeficiency diseases (SCID) that encompass congenital diseases caused by different genetic mutations that result in severe deficiency of T and B lymphocytes. Despite differences in underlying mutations, affected patients present similarly, with recurrent infections caused by bacteria, viruses, fungi, and opportunistic pathogens. Additionally, patients often suffer from chronic diarrhea and failure to thrive. Without treatment, all patients with SCID typically die within the first years of life. SCID must be considered in the differential diagnosis in any infant with diarrhea and hypogammaglobulinemia. Additionally, common presentations include persistent cough, tachypnea or hypoxia secondary to underlying *Pneumocystis carinii* infection, or persistent oral or diaper candidiasis.

Physical examination is notable for a lack of lymphoid tissue including tonsils and lymph nodes. A chest x-ray usually demonstrates an absent thymic shadow. Laboratory evaluation often reveals lymphopenia and some degree of hypogammaglobulinemia. Occasionally, an infant with SCID will present with normal numbers of lymphocytes resulting from transfusion-related engraftment or maternal T-lymphocyte engraftment via peripartum transfusion. Natural killer (NK) cells and B-lymphocyte numbers may be decreased, normal, or elevated. Additionally, in vitro lymphocyte assays show poor response to mitogens, and specific antibodies are absent. Antenatal diagnosis is possible. Once SCID is suspected, *Pneumocystis* prophylaxis with trimethoprim-sulfamethoxazole and replacement IgG therapy should be initiated. Patients with suspected SCID should only be transfused with irradiated blood products and should not receive any live vaccines. Confirmation of the diagnosis usually employs a specialist and should include screening for SCID subtypes listed in Table 29–5. BMT offers the best possibility of cure, with use of a human leukocyte antigen (HLA)-matched sibling offering the highest chance of success. In affected patients without HLA-identical donors, T-lymphocyte–depleted HLA haplo-identical grafts or umbilical cord stem cells are used. For most patients, myeloablation is not necessary, as the patient is without T lymphocytes. Additionally, most patients do not require graft-versus-host disease (GVHD) prophylaxis unless the donor is unrelated. T-lymphocyte reconstitution takes approximately 4 months, but only ~ 50% of patients regain B-lymphocyte function, with the majority requiring long-term IVIG replacement. For months posttransplant, patients are susceptible to many serious infections and prophylaxis is usually continued. Additionally, any signs or symptoms of infection must be promptly investigated and aggressively treated. The highest rate of success is in the youngest patients prior to developing infections (> 95% survival), but overall rates of survival range from 50–100% depending on the underlying mutation. X-linked SCID has been treated with autologous bone marrow in which normal function was transduced to lymphocytes by retroviral gene transfer. Unfortunately, two patients developed leukemia due to insertion of the retroviral vector near an oncogene. At this time, safer vectors are still being sought.

There are currently nine described genes with mutations that result in SCID. Clinical presentation and treatment is generally similar. The variants of SCID can be organized by the presence or absence of specific lymphocytes, including T, B, and NK cells (Table 29–5).

Buckley RH: Molecular defects in human severe combined immunodeficiency and approaches to immune reconstitution. Annu Rev Immunol 2004;22:625 [PMID: 15032591].

Chinen J, Puck JM: Success and risks of gene therapy in primary immunodeficiencies. J Allergy Clin Immunol 2004;113:595 [PMID: 15100660].

Table 29–5. Severe combined immunodeficiency (SCID) variants.

Gene	Locus	Gene Product and Function	Presence of			Inheritance
			T Cell	B Cell	NK Cell	
IL2RG	xq13.1	Common γ chain of IL-2, 4, 7, 9, 15 cytokine receptors; necessary to activate JAK3 for intracellular signaling	—	+	—	XLR
ADA	20q13.11	Part of the purine salvage pathway; necessary for removal of toxic metabolites that inhibit all lymphoid cells	—	—	—	AR
JAK3	19p13.1	A tyrosine kinase important for differentiation of lymphoid cells	—	+	—	AR
IL7R	5p13	IL-7 receptor is necessary for T-cell development and activates *JAK3*	—	+	+	AR
RAG1/RAG2	11p13	DNA recombinases which mediate DNA recombination during B- and T-cell development	—	—	+	AR
CD3δ	11q23	Essential for T-cell development	—	+	+	AR
CD45	1q31-q32	Tyrosine kinase important for regulation of other kinases in T- and B-cell antigen receptor development	—	+	+	AR
AREMIS	20q13.11	Involved in repairing DNA ds breaks that occur during recombination	—	—	+	AR

AR, autosomal recessive; XLR, X-linked recessive; NK, natural killer.
Adapted, with permission, from Kalman et al: Mutations in genes for T-cell development: IL7R, CD45, IL2RG, JAK3, RAG1, RAG2, ARTEMIS, and ADA and severe combined immunodeficiency: HuGE review. Genet Med 2004;6:16.

1. X-Linked Severe Combined Immunodeficiency

X-linked SCID is the most common form (40%) of SCID resulting from mutations in the gene *IL2RG* (IL-2 receptor gene) that encodes the common γ chain. The γ-chain protein is shared by multiple cell surface receptors for cytokines that are essential for T lymphocyte maturation, including IL-2, IL-4, IL-7, IL-9, IL-15, and IL-21. Within the first 3 months of life, male infants present with diarrhea, cough, and rash. Laboratory examination reveals low T-lymphocyte numbers, normal numbers of B lymphocytes (which do not produce functional antibody), and absent NK cells.

2. Adenosine Deaminase Deficiency

Adenosine deaminase deficiency (ADA) is an autosomal recessive form of SCID due to absence of adenosine deaminase, which is important for removal of toxic metabolites, including adenosine, 2' deoxyadenosine, and 2'-O-methyladenosine. Increased levels of these metabolites result in T-

lymphocyte death. Subsequently, affected patients have complete absence of T-lymphocyte function. ADA SCID is distinguished from other variants of SCID by the following: the most profound lymphopenia (< 500/mm³), skeletal abnormalities including chondro-osseous dysplasia (flared costochondral junctions and bone-in-bone anomalies in vertebrae), and deficiency of all types of lymphocytes. Diagnosis is suspected in patients with profound lymphopenia and recurrent infections. The diagnosis is confirmed with a red blood cell assay for ADA activity. The genetic mutation is on chromosome 20q13.2–13.11. In addition to BMT, restoration of immune competence can occur in some patients with weekly infusions of polyethylene glycol–stabilized ADA enzyme conjugate. Gene therapy of stem cells with a retroviral vector has been successful, but the development of safer vectors is yet to come.

3. Janus Kinase 3 Deficiency

Another form of autosomal recessive SCID is due to mutations in the gene encoding janus kinase 3, which is important for intracellular signaling through the common γ chain. The clinical presentation and lymphocyte phenotype most closely resembles X-linked SCID, with low T and NK lymphocytes, and elevated, nonfunctional B lymphocytes.

4. IL-7-Receptor-Alpha-Chain Deficiency

IL-7-receptor-alpha-chain (IL-7Rα) deficiency SCID is transmitted by autosomal recessive inheritance. The IL-7 receptor is important for T-lymphocyte maturation and mutations result in low T-lymphocyte numbers, but normal numbers of dysfunctional B lymphocytes and NK cells.

5. Recombinase-Activating Gene Deficiencies

Another form of autosomal recessive SCID is due to mutations in recombinase activating genes (*RAG1* and *RAG2*), which encode proteins critical for assembling antigen receptor genes for both T and B lymphocytes. Several mutations have been described in both genes. The clinical presentation is similar to that of other forms of SCID, but the lymphocyte phenotype differs, as patients with SCID due to *RAG1* or *RAG2* mutations lack both T and B lymphocytes, but maintain normal or elevated numbers of NK cells.

Omenn syndrome is an autosomal recessive syndrome with severe combined immunodeficiency, but also eczematoid rash, hepatosplenomegaly, lymphadenopathy, and alopecia. The disease is due to mutations in *RAG1* or *RAG2* or Artemis (see below). Laboratory evaluation reveals absent B lymphocytes, normal to elevated T-lymphocyte numbers with restricted function, and normal functional NK cells. Additionally, affected patients often have eosinophilia and elevated levels of IgE. The syndrome is typically fatal, although BMT has been used.

Ege M et al: Ommen syndrome due to ARTEMIS mutations. Blood 2005;105:4179 [PMID: 15731174].

6. CD3-Delta-Chain Deficiency

CD3-delta-chain (CD3δ) deficiency is a rare form of autosomal recessive SCID. Homozygous defects in the CD3δ chain halt T-lymphocyte maturation. Clinical presentation and lymphocyte phenotype are similar to IL-7Rα deficiency, but CD3δ-chain deficiency differs from other forms of SCID in that these patients have a normal appearing thymic silhouette on chest radiograph.

Dadi H et al: Effect of CD3δ deficiency on maturation of alpha/beta and gamma/delta T-cell lineages in severe combined immunodeficiency. N Engl J Med 2003;349:1821 [PMID: 14602880].

7. CD45 Deficiency

Another rare form of autosomal recessive SCID is due to mutations in the gene for CD45. CD45 is a tyrosine phosphatase important for regulating signal transduction. Affected patients have similar presentation to other forms of SCID and a lymphocyte phenotype with low to absent T and NK cells, but elevated B lymphocytes.

8. Artemis Deficiency

Artemis is a DNA repair factor important for repairing cuts in the double-stranded DNA essential for the assembly of antigen receptors for T and B lymphocytes. Inheritance is autosomal recessive, and clinical presentation and lymphocyte phenotype are similar to *RAG1* and *RAG2* deficiencies.

9. ZAP-70 Deficiency

Deficiency of zeta-chain-associated protein (ZAP)-70 results in a rare form of autosomal recessive combined immunodeficiency. ZAP-70 is a tyrosine kinase critical for T-lymphocyte signaling and activation. Clinical presentation is similar to that of other forms of SCID, but most affected patients have palpable lymph nodes and visible thymic silhouette. Lymphocyte evaluation reveals absence of CD8+ T lymphocytes, normal but nonfunctional CD4+ T lymphocytes, normal numbers of poorly-functioning B lymphocytes, and normal numbers and function of NK cells.

Elder M: SCID due to ZAP-70 deficiency. Pediatr Hematol Oncol 1997;19:546 [PMID: 9407944].

OTHER COMBINED IMMUNODEFICIENCY DISORDERS

Combined immune deficiencies include defects that directly impair both T and B lymphocytes, as well as T-lymphocyte–specific defects, because proper B-lymphocyte function and antibody production is dependent on T-lymphocyte function. Therefore, most T-lymphocyte deficiencies manifest as combined impairments.

1. Wiskott-Aldrich Syndrome

Wiskott-Aldrich syndrome (WAS) is an X-linked recessive disease characterized by immune deficiency, microplatelet thrombocytopenia, and eczema. The syndrome results from mutations of the *WASP* gene at X11p. *WASP* is a protein involved in the rearrangement of actin and is important in interactions between T lymphocytes and antigen-presenting cells. Common presenting symptoms include bloody diarrhea, cerebral hemorrhage, and severe infections with polysaccharide-encapsulated bacteria, but clinical presentation can vary from classic severe WAS to mild thrombocytopenia without immune deficiency, or X-linked thrombocytopenia (XLT), depending on the mutation. A scoring system has been developed to help the clinician distinguish between WAS and XLT. Early deaths are due to bleeding and infections, but increased malignancies and autoimmune syndromes are seen over time. Survival through the teens is rare in patients not receiving treatment, although XLT is sometimes diagnosed in adults. Laboratory findings that suggest the diagnosis are a low platelet count, low or absent isohemagglutinins, and reduced antibody responses to polysaccharide antigens (*S pneumonae* and *H influenzae*). IgM may be low; IgA and IgE are often high. Treatment includes prophylaxis with antibiotics (including trimethoprim-sulfamethoxazole for *Pneumocystis carinii* pneumonia) and IVIG for patients with deficient antibody responses. Splenectomy has been helpful in patients with XLT, but must be followed by antibiotic prophylaxis because of the increased risk of septicemia and sudden death. Platelet transfusions should be avoided unless severe bleeding has occurred (such as central nervous system hemorrhage). Finally, BMT using the best-matched donor offers the possibility of a definitive cure, but is associated with potential morbidity and mortality.

Dupuis Girod S et al: Autoimmunity in Wiskott-Aldrich syndrome: Risk factors, clinical features, and outcome in a single-center cohort of 55 patients. Pediatrics 2003;111:e622 [PMID: 12728121].

Ochs HD, Notarangelo LD: X-linked immunodeficiencies. Curr Allergy Asthma Rep 2004;4:339 [PMID: 15283872].

2. 22q11.2 Deletion Syndrome (Digeorge Syndrome)

DiGeorge syndrome or 22q11.2 deletion syndrome is an autosomal dominant syndrome with defective development of the third and fourth pharyngeal pouches. Clinical characteristics include congenital heart defects, hypocalcemia due to hypoparathyroidism, distinctive craniofacial features, renal anomalies, and thymic hypoplasia. Presentation usually results from cardiac failure, or after 24–48 hours from hypocalcemia, and the diagnosis is sometimes made during the course of cardiac surgery, when no thymus is found in the mediastinum. Additional important clinical issues include delayed speech and behavioral problems. There is considerable variability in phenotype based on the location and extent of microdeletion. Overlapping syndromes include velocardiofacial syndrome and Shprintzen syndrome. The incidence is about 1 per 4000 births, and the abnormal chromosome is usually inherited from the mother. The associated immunodeficiency is secondary to the aplastic or hypoplastic thymus, where T-lymphocyte maturation occurs. Surprisingly, most patients have no or only mild immune defects. The term "partial DiGeorge syndrome" is commonly applied to these patients with impaired rather than absent thymus function. Typical laboratory examination reveals normal to decreased numbers of T lymphocytes with preserved T-lymphocyte function and normal B lymphocyte function, but in the rare patient with absent or dysfunctional T lymphocytes, B-lymphocyte function and antibody production may be abnormal as well. Over time, T-lymphocyte numbers normalize in the majority of patients who had low numbers of T lymphocytes at presentation. Diagnosis is confirmed via fluorescent in-situ hybridization chromosomal analysis for the microdeletion on chromosome 22. Treatment of the 22q11.2 deletion syndrome may require surgery for the cardiac defects and vitamin D, calcium, and/or parathyroid hormone replacement to correct hypocalcemia. Transfusion products should be irradiated. Both thymic grafts and bone marrow transplant have been successful in patients with absent T-lymphocyte immunity.

Sediva A et al: Early development of immunity in DiGeorge syndrome. Med Sci Monit 2005;11:CR182 [PMID: 15795698].

3. Ataxia-Telangiectasia

Ataxia-telangiectasia (A-T) is an autosomal recessive disorder characterized by progressive cerebellar ataxia (due to degeneration of Purkinje cells), telangiectasia, and variable immunodeficiency. The ataxia develops by age 5 years, followed by the appearance of telangiectasias of the conjunctivae and exposed areas (ie, nose, ears, and shoulders). The A-T mutated protein kinase is encoded on chromosome 11 and is required for cell-cycle regulation and DNA repair. The Nijmegen breakage syndrome is probably a variant of A-T with more severe clinical features, including microcephaly and birdlike facies. Abnormal findings in A-T include elevated serum α-fetoprotein levels (useful diagnostically), thymic hypoplasia and lymphopenia, immunoglobulin deficiencies including low levels of IgA, IgE, and/or IgG, and defective ability to repair radiation-induced DNA fragmentation. Clinically, the most important symptom is progressive loss of motor coordination, followed by weakness. Respiratory tract infections and many types of malignancy (including carcinomas and lymphomas) are the major causes of death. There is no definitive treatment, although IVIG and aggressive antibiotics have been used with limited success. Heterozygotes may have a small increased risk for breast cancer.

Nowak-Wegrzyn A et al: Immunodeficiency and infections in ataxia-telangiectasia. J Pediatr 2004;144:505 [PMID: 15069401].

Perlman S et al: Ataxia-telangiectasia: Diagnosis and treatment. Semin Pediatr Neurol 2003;10:173 [PMID: 14653405].

4. X-Linked Hyper-IgM Syndrome

X-linked hyper-IgM or CD40 ligand deficiency is the most common form of hyper-IgM and involves a defect in CD40 ligand (CD154) on T lymphocytes. Unlike the autosomal recessive forms of hyper-IgM, the mutation results in both antibody and cell-mediated deficiencies, as the interaction between CD40L (on T cells) and CD40 (on antigen-presenting cells) is important for antibody production and for T-cell activation. Affected males have low levels of IgG and IgA, but normal or elevated levels of IgM and normal numbers of B lymphocytes. Typically, male infants present with recurrent bacterial and opportunistic infections such as *Pneumocystis carinii* pneumonia or cryptosporidium diarrhea. Additionally, affected males have a high frequency of sclerosing cholangitis, increased liver and biliary tract carcinomas, neutropenia, and autoimmune syndromes including thrombocytopenia, arthritis, and inflammatory bowel disease. Conservative treatment includes IVIG and antibiotic prophylaxis, but because prognosis is still quite poor, BMT has been used with preliminary success.

Etzioni A, Ochs HD: The hyper-IgM syndrome—An evolving story. Pediatr Res 2004;56:519 [PMID: 15319456].

Jacobsohn DA et al: Nonmyeloablative hematopoietic stem cell transplant for X-linked hyper-immunoglobulin M syndrome with cholangiopathy. Pediatrics 2004;113:e122 [PMID: 14754981].

5. Immunodeficiency Due to Mutations of Nuclear Factor-κB–Essential Modulator

Immunodeficiency due to mutations in the gene for nuclear factor-κB–essential modulator (NEMO) is an X-linked syndrome in which male patients are characterized by ectodermal dysplasia (abnormal teeth, fine sparse hair, and abnormal or lacking sweat glands) and defects of T- and B-lymphocytes. Many mutations are fatal in utero for male patients. Female carriers may have incontinentia pigmenti. The mutation results in abnormal immunoreceptor signaling. Surviving males present with early serious infections, including opportunistic infections such as *Pneumocysitis* and atypical mycobacteria. Laboratory evaluation reveals hypogammaglobulinemia and poor specific antibody but normal numbers of T and B lymphocytes. Functional evaluation of lymphocytes demonstrates variable response. Because patients with confirmed NEMO mutations are quite rare, the best treatment course is unknown, but aggressive antibiotic therapy in combination with IVIG as well as BMT has been used. Prognosis is dependent on the severity of immunodeficiency, with most deaths due to infection.

Orange JS et al: The presentation and natural history of immunodeficiency caused by nuclear factor kappaB essential modulator mutation. J Allergy Clin Immunol 2004;113:725 [PMID: 15100680].

6. Combined Immunodeficiency with Defective Expression of Major Histocompatibility Complex Types I and II

Major histocompatibility complex class I (MHC I) deficiency or bare lymphocyte syndrome type I is an autosomal recessive combined immunodeficiency. Affected patients have abnormal TAP proteins important for intracellular transport and expression of MHC I on cell surfaces. Patients with bare lymphocyte syndrome type I present with recurrent sinopulmonary and skin infections. The diagnosis is confirmed by demonstrating an absence of MHC I expression.

Major histocompatibility complex class II (MHC II) deficiency or bare lymphocyte syndrome type II is a rare autosomal recessive combined immunodeficiency in which cells lack MHC II expression. Clinical presentation includes recurrent viral, bacterial, and fungal infections. Patients with bare lymphocyte syndrome type II have normal numbers of T and B lymphocytes, but low CD4+ lymphocytes, abnormal lymphocyte function, and hypogammaglobulinemia. They also have a high incidence of sclerosing cholangitis. When this diagnosis is suspected, demonstration of absent HLA class II molecules confirms the disorder. Severe cases are fatal without BMT, but milder phenotypes may be managed with IVIG replacement and aggressive use of antibiotics.

Nekrep N et al: When the lymphocyte loses its clothes. Immunity 2003:18;453 [PMID: 12705848].

Stiehm ER, et al. *Immunologic Disorders of Infants and Children*, 5th edition. Philadelphia: Elsevier, 2004.

7. Diseases Due to Defective Interferon Gamma & Interleukin 12 Pathways

The interferon-γ and interleukin 12 pathways are critical for macrophage, T-lymphocyte, and NK cell immunity towards mycobacterial infections. Multiple defects have been described both in the receptors for these cytokines and receptors for signal transducer and activator of transcription molecules, with affected patients variably susceptible to atypical mycobacterium or infection after bacille Calmette-Guérin vaccination. Age of onset is variable and can occur in early adulthood. Treatment with supplemental interferon-γ is effective for some patients in combination with appropriate antibiotics. Most patients should also receive long-term mycobacterial prophylaxis.

Fieschi C, Casanova J-L: The role of interleukin-12 in human infectious diseases: Only a faint signature. Eur J Immunol 2003; 33:1461 [PMID: 2778462].

Rosenzweig SD, Holland SM: Phagocyte immunodeficiencies and their infections. J Allergy Clin Immunol 2004;113:620 [PMID: 15100664].

8. Purine Nucleoside Phosphorylase Deficiency

Purine nucleoside phosphorylase (PNP) deficiency is an immunodeficiency due to defects in the gene encoding PNP, which is important in the purine salvage pathway. Deficiency of PNP causes toxic metabolites that results in T-lymphocyte death, but in many patients B lymphocytes are spared. This autosomal recessive disease not only has recurrent and serious infections, but affected patients have concomitant neurologic (developmental delay, ataxia, and spasticity) and autoimmune disorders. Infections present at variable ages. Laboratory evaluation reveals low or absent T lymphocytes and a variable B-lymphocyte deficiency, the disease is fatal due to infection or malignancy without BMT.

Dror Y et al: Purine nucleoside phosphorylase deficiency associated with a dysplastic marrow morphology. Pediatr Res 2004;55: 472 [PMID: 14711904].

Myers LA et al: Purine nucleoside phosphorylase deficiency presenting with lymphopenia and developmental delay: Successful correction with umbilical cord blood transplantation. J Pediatr 2004;145:710 [PMID: 15520787].

PHAGOCYTIC DEFECTS

Phagocytic defects include abnormalities of both numbers (neutropenia) and function of polymorphonuclear leukocytes (neutrophils, eosinophils, and basophils). Functional defects consist of impairments in adhesion, chemotaxis, or bacterial killing.

Rosenzweig SD, Holland SM: Phagocyte immunodeficiencies and their infections. J Allergy Clin Immunol 2004;113:620 [PMID: 15100664].

1. Neutropenia

Evaluation for the presence of neutropenia should be included when considering recurrent infections. The diagnosis and treatment is discussed in Chapter 27 (hematology). Additionally, some primary immunodeficiency syndromes have associated neutropenia (eg, XLA).

Dror Y, Sung L: Update on childhood neutropenia: molecular and clinical advances. Hematol Oncol Clin North Am 2004;18: 1439 [PMID: 15511624].

2. Chronic Granulomatous Disease

Chronic granulomatous disease is a rare immunodeficiency due to defective superoxide generation. Specifically, defects are seen in reduced nicotinamide adenine dinucleotide phosphate (NADPH) oxidase and most (65%) are inherited as X-linked recessive diseases, but autosomal recessive forms also exist. Clinical presenta-

tion is characterized by recurrent and serious infections of skin, lungs, and liver with catalase-positive bacteria, fungi, and subsequent granuloma formation. The five most common infecting species include *Staphylococcus aureus, Burkholderia cepacia, Serratia marcescens, Nocardia* species, and *Aspergillus* species. Diagnosis is performed by demonstrating lack of superoxide production via dihydrorhodamine flow cytometry. This test, unlike the nitroblue tetrazolium test, allows differentiation between X-linked and autosomal recessive forms and also demonstrates carrier status of X-linked disease. Treatment includes prophylactic and symptomatic use of antibiotics and antifungals in combination with interferon-γ. Additionally, BMT has been successful.

Jurkowska M et al: Genetic and biochemical background of chronic granulomatous disease. Arch Immunol Ther Exp (Warsz) 2004; 52:113 [PMID: 15179325].

Rosenzweig SD, Holland SM: Phagocyte immunodeficiencies and their infections. J Allergy Clin Immunol 2004;113:620 [PMID: 15100664].

3. Leukocyte Adhesion Deficiencies Types I & II

The ability of white blood cells to travel to distant sites of infections is critical for effectiveness of phagocytic immunity. In leukocyte adhesion deficiency (LAD), defects in molecules required for leukocyte adherence and migration prevent these cells from arriving at the sites of infections. LAD I is an autosomal recessive disease due to mutations in the common chain of the β2 integrin family (CD18) located on chromosome 21q22.3. These mutations result in impaired neutrophil migration in addition to poor adherence, phagocytosis, and antibody-dependent immunity. Clinically, patients present with variable phenotypes including recurrent serious infections, lack of pus formation, poor wound healing, and gingival and periodontal disease. The hallmark feature is little inflammation and absent neutrophils on histopathology (ie, cold abscesses) especially when concurrent with peripheral blood neutrophilia. The most severe phenotype presents with infections in the neonatal period, including delayed separation of the umbilical cord with associated omphalitis. Laboratory evaluation often demonstrates a striking leukocytosis. Diagnosis of suspected cases is confirmed by flow cytometry analysis for CD18. Treatment includes aggressive antibiotic therapy.

LAD II is a rare autosomal recessive disease due to inborn error in fucose metabolism that results in abnormal expression of sialyl-Lewis X (CD15s) that functions as a selectin ligand. The resulting phenotype is similar to LAD I, characterized by recurrent infections, lack of pus formation, poor wound healing, and periodontal disease, but additionally patients have developmental delays, short stature, dysmorphic facies, and the Bombay (hh) blood group. Diagnosis is confirmed by flow cytometry analysis for CD15s and treatment is usually limited to antibiotics, although fucose supplementation has been reported with some success.

Rosenzweig SD, Holland SM: Phagocyte immunodeficiencies and their infections. J Allergy Clin Immunol 2004;113:620 [PMID: 15100664].

4. Glucose-6-Phosphate Dehydrogenase Deficiency

Severe forms of X-linked glucose-6-phosphate dehydrogenase deficiency result in recurrent infections and increased risk of severe malarial infection due to abnormal neutrophil respiratory burst. Glucose-6-phosphate dehydrogenase–associated immunodeficiency is much less common than the associated hemolytic anemia.

Stiehm ER et al: *Immunologic Disorders in Infants and Children,* 5th ed. Elsevier Saunders, 2004.

5. Myeloperoxidase Deficiency

Leukocyte myeloperoxidase is important for intracellular destruction of *Candida albicans.* Although deficiency is quite common, few patients present with recurrent or chronic candidal infections. Diagnosis can be confirmed with assays measuring myeloperoxidase levels in leukocytes. Symptomatic and prophylactic antifungal therapy is often necessary in patients with recurrent infections. The myeloperoxidase gene has been localized to chromosome 17.

Stiehm ER et al: *Immunologic Disorders in Infants and Children,* 5th ed. Elsevier Saunders, 2004.

COMPLEMENT DEFECTS

As a component of the innate immune system, complement works through opsonization, lysis of target cells, and recruitment of phagocytic cells, and facilitates antibody-mediated immunity. The complement system includes three pathways of enzymatic reactions: classical, alternative, and lectin. All three pathways share C3 cleavage and result in promoting inflammation, eliminating pathogens, and enhancing the response of the immune system. Activation of the complement system occurs through bacterial proteins and surface-bound IgG and IgM antibodies.

1. Complement Factor Deficiencies

Rare deficiencies of individual complement factors (C1–C9) are inherited by autosomal recessive transmission. Deficiencies of factors C1, C4, and C2 do not predispose to increased infections, but are associated with autoimmune disorders such as systemic lupus erythematosus.

Primary C3 deficiency presents with severe pyogenic infections, as C3 is critical for opsonization in both the classical and alternative pathways. There are also acquired forms of C3 deficiency that predispose patients to similar infectious risks. Terminal complement factor deficiency (C5, C6, C7, C8, and C9) or properdin (an alternative pathway factor) deficiency results in recurrent infections with *Neisseria* species. Survivors of meningococcal meningitis and patients with recurrent neisserial infections should be screened for such a deficiency.

Deficiency of mannose binding lectin has been linked to increased risk of infections but recent studies have been unable to confirm deficiency as a risk factor.

Dahl M et al: A population-based study of morbidity and mortality in mannose-binding lectin deficiency. J Exp Med 2004;199:1391 [PMID: 15148337].

Wen L et al: Clinical and laboratory evaluation of complement deficiency. J Allergy Clin Immunol 2004;113:585 [PMID: 15100659].

2. Hereditary Angioedema Due to C1 Esterase Inhibitor Deficiency

Hereditary angioedema is a rare autosomal dominant disorder due to C1 esterase inhibitor (C1-INH) deficiency in which susceptibility to infection is not increased. There is also an acquired form associated with angiotensin-converting enzyme inhibitor medication use or some B-lymphocyte malignancies. Affected patients can experience edema of skin and bowel and potentially life-threatening edema of the airway. Trauma is a risk factor for the induction of edema, accidental or intentional (eg, due to surgery, childbirth, or dental work). The edema is usually nonpainful (unless it involves the bowel) and lasts 48–72 hours. There is no associated urticaria (ie, redness) or pruritus. Age at onset is quite variable and there is often a positive family history. Initial screening tests for complement that show decreased CH50 or low levels of C4 suggest the diagnosis. Confirmation comes from demonstration of low or absent levels of C1-INH or poor or absent C1-INH function. The synthetic androgen danazol (50–200 mg/d) prevents attacks by increasing C1-INH levels. Additionally, C1-inhibitor replacement is useful for the emergency treatment of acute edema, and during pregnancy when androgen therapy is contraindicated.

Bowen T et al: Canadian 2003 international consensus algorithm for the diagnosis, therapy and management of hereditary angioedema. J Allergy Clin Immunol 2004;114:629 [PMID: 15356569].

3. Paroxysmal Nocturnal Hemoglobinuria

Paroxysmal nocturnal hemoglobinuria is a rare X-linked disorder with variable disease expression in which affected patients have intravascular hemolysis, bone marrow failure, and thrombosis, but no associated immune defect. Paroxysmal nocturnal hemoglobinuria is due to a mutation in phosphatidylinositol-glycan complementation class A, which is critical for certain erythrocyte surface proteins. Without these surface proteins, erythrocytes are highly susceptible to complement-mediated lysis. Thrombotic events, particularly intra-abdominal, are the major cause of death. Additional morbidity and mortality is due to bone marrow failure and associated bone marrow malignancies.

Meletis J, Terpos E: Recent insights into the pathophysiology of paroxysmal nocturnal hemoglobinuria. Med Sci Monit 2003;9: RA161 [PMID: 12883466].

OTHER WELL-DEFINED IMMUNODEFICIENCY SYNDROMES

1. Hyper-IgE Syndrome

Hyper-IgE syndrome (HIES), also known as Job syndrome, is a rare primary immunodeficiency characterized by elevated levels of IgE (> 2000 IU/mL), neonatal eczematoid rash, recurrent infections with *Staphylococcus aureus,* recurrent pneumonia with pneumatocele formation, and typical facies. Inheritance appears to be sporadic, although autosomal dominant and recessive cases have been reported. Additional clinical findings include retained primary teeth, scoliosis, hyperextensibility, high palate, and osteoporosis. In addition to staphylococcal infections, affected patients also have increased incidence of infections due to *Streptococcus* species, *Pseudomonas* species, *Candida albicans,* and even opportunistic infections with *Pneumocystis carinii.* Laboratory evaluation reveals normal to profoundly elevated levels of IgE and occasionally an associated eosinophilia. However, elevated IgE levels themselves are not a risk factor for HIES, as atopic dermatitis and parasite infection are much more common causes of elevated IgE. Diagnosis is often difficult due to variable presentation, which may become progressively severe with increasing age. Subsequently, diagnosis is often only made over time and evolving syndrome characteristics. The underlying cause of HIES is unknown. The mainstay of treatment is prophylactic and symptomatic antibiotic use in combination with good skin care. IVIG has been used with some success to decrease infections and possibly modify IgE levels.

Grimbacher B et al: Hyper-IgE syndromes. Immunol Rev 2005;203: 244 [PMID: 15661034].

2. Immune Dysregulation, Polyendocrinopathy, Enteropathy, X-Linked Syndrome

Immune dysregulation, polyendocrinopathy, enteropathy, X-linked (IPEX) syndrome is a rare disease that usually presents with severe diarrhea and insulin-dependent diabetes mellitus within the first months of life. Affected males also have severe eczema, food allergy, autoimmune cytopenias, lymphadenopathy, splenomegaly, and recurrent infections. Most die before age 2 years due to malnutrition or sepsis. Immune dysregulation, polyendocrinopathy, enteropathy, X-linked syndrome results from mutations in the *FOXP3* gene that encodes a protein essential for developing regulatory T lymphocytes. Leukocyte counts and immunoglobulin levels are generally normal. Immunosuppression and nutritional supplementation has provided temporary improvements, but the prognosis is poor with most cases resulting in early death. Bone marrow transplantation has been attempted with variable success.

Chatila TA et al: JM2, encoding a fork head-related protein, is mutated in X-linked autoimmunity-allergic dysregulation syndrome. J Clin Invest 2000;106:R75 [PMID: 11120765].

Nieves DS et al: Dermatologic and immunologic findings in the immune dysregulation, polyendocrinopathy, enteropathy, X-linked syndrome. Arch Dermatol 2004;140:466 [PMID: 15096376].

3. X-Linked Lymphoproliferative Syndrome

X-linked lymphoproliferative syndrome is an immunodeficiency that develops following EBV infection. Affected males develop fulminant infectious mononucleosis with hemophagocytic syndrome, multiple organ system failure, and bone marrow aplasia. The mutated gene encodes a signaling protein used by T lymphocytes and NK cells called SLAM-adapter protein. Affected boys are immunologically normal prior to EBV infection, and during acute infection they produce antibody to EBV. In most instances, infection with EBV is fatal. Patients who survive the initial episode or who are never infected with EBV in childhood develop lymphomas, vasculitis, hypogammaglobulinemias (with elevated IgM) or common variable immunodeficiency in later life. Antenatal diagnosis is possible.

Latour S, Veilette A: Molecular and immunological basis of X-linked lymphoproliferative disease. Immunol Rev 2003;192: 221 [PMID: 12670406].

4. Chronic Mucocutaneous Candidasis

There are two forms of chronic mucocutaneous candidiasis (CMC). The first type is an autosomal dominant disorder, characterized by isolated candidal infections of the skin, nails, and mucous membranes, which is not due to other causes. Systemic disease is not characteristic, but case reports of intracranial mycotic aneurysms exist. Primary CMC most commonly occurs as an isolated syndrome, but can be associated with endocrine or autoimmune processes. The underlying defect is unknown, but the prognosis is quite good with antifungal therapy.

An autosomal recessive form of CMC with associated autoimmunity, also known as autoimmune polyendocrinopathy candidiasis ectodermal dysplasia (APECED) syndrome, is characterized by recurrent candidal infections, abnormal T-lymphocyte response to *Candida,* autoimmune endocrinopathies, and ectodermal dystrophies. APECED is due to mutations in the gene for an important transcription regulator protein called autoimmune regulator that is critical for normal thymocyte development. Treatment includes antifungal therapy in combination with therapy for associated endocrinopathies.

Lawrence T et al: Autosomal-dominant primary immunodeficiencies. Cur Opin Hematol 2004;12:22 [PMID: 15604887].

Soderbergh A et al: Prevalence and clinical associations of 10 defined autoantibodies in autoimmune polyendocrine syndrome type 1. J Clin Endocrinol Metab 2004;89:557 [PMID: 14764761].

5. Autoimmune Lymphoproliferative Syndrome

Autoimmune lymphoproliferative syndrome (ALPS) results from mutations of genes important for regulating programmed lymphocyte death (apoptosis). Most commonly the defect is in Fas (CD95) or Fas ligand, but other defects in the Fas pathway have also been described (eg, caspase 10). Clinical presentation includes lymphadenopathy, splenomegaly, and autoimmune disorders (autoimmune hemolytic anemia, neutropenia, thrombocytopenia, and sometimes arthritis). Occasionally, patients have frequent infections. The diagnosis is suspected when T-lymphocyte subsets by flow cytometry demonstrates elevated numbers of CD3+CD4⁻CD8⁻ (double negative) T lymphocytes. There are several different types of ALPS that are distinguished by the response of lymphocytes to Fas-induced apoptosis. Patients are often heterozygous, and inheritance is mostly dominant. Treatment with prednisone often controls the lymphadenopathy. Infections should be treated appropriately, and in some cases BMT has been curative. Affected patients are also at risk for lymphoma. Mutations affecting an apoptosis-related protein, caspase 8, cause an ALPS variant syndrome in which the susceptibility to infection by herpes simplex virus also increases.

Bleesing JJH: Autoimmune lymphoproliferative syndrome: A genetic disorder of abnormal lymphocyte apoptosis. Immunol Allergy Clin North Am 2002;22:339 [PMID: 11269222].

Rieux-Laucat F et al: Cell-death signaling and human disease. Curr Opin Immunol 2003;15:325 [PMID: 12787759].

GENETIC SYNDROMES ASSOCIATED WITH IMMUNODEFICIENCY

Several described genetic syndromes have associated immunodeficiency that is often identified after the syndrome has been diagnosed. Usually, the immune defect is not the major clinical problem.

Ming JE et al: Genetic syndromes associated with immunodeficiency. Immunol Allergy Clin North Am 2002;22:261.

Ming JE, Stiehm ER: Humoral immunodeficiencies: Syndromic immunodeficiencies with humoral defects. Immunol Allergy Clin North Am 2001;21:91 [PMID: 14708957].

1. Bloom Syndrome

Characteristics of Bloom syndrome include growth retardation, sun sensitivity, and telangiectasias of the face. The syndrome results from mutations in a DNA helicase which leads to excess sister chromatid exchanges. Affected patients have increased risk of malignancy and life-threatening infections. Serum IgA and IgM are variably low, and T-lymphocyte function is abnormal.

2. Transcobalamin 2 Deficiency

Transcobalamin 2 deficiency is due to defective cellular transport of cobalamin and results in megaloblastic anemia, diarrhea, and poor growth. Affected patients have hypogammaglobulinemia and poor specific antibody.

3. Immunodeficiency, Centromeric Instability, Facial Anomalies Syndrome

Immunodeficiency, centromeric instability, facial anomalies (ICF) syndrome is a rare condition due to abnormal DNA methyltransferase. Unlike other chromosome instability syndromes, immunodeficiency, centromeric instability, facial anomalies syndrome does not have an associated hypersensitivity to sunlight. Affected patients have severe respiratory, gastrointestinal, and skin infections due to low or absent immunoglobulins and abnormal T-lymphocyte numbers and function.

4. Trisomy 21

Patients with trisomy 21 or Down syndrome have increased susceptibility to respiratory infection. Immunodeficiency is variable with reported cases of abnormal T- and B-lymphocyte numbers and function. Additionally, patients have an increased incidence of autoimmune diseases.

5. Turner Syndrome

Turner syndrome is associated with increased risk of otitis media, respiratory infections, and malignancies. Immune defects are variable but may include abnormal T-lymphocyte numbers and function and hypogammaglobulinemia.

6. Chédiak-Higashi Syndrome

Chédiak-Higashi syndrome is a rare autosomal recessive disease caused by mutations of a lysosomal trafficking gene. The neutrophils of affected individuals have giant lysosomes, impaired chemotaxis, neutropenia, and abnormal NK-cell cytotoxicity. Patients present with recurrent infections (particularly periodontitis), partial oculocutaneous albinism, and neuropathy. Most patient progress to generalized lymphohistiocytic infiltration syndrome, which is a common cause of death. Treatment strategies address infections and neuropathy and the use of immunosuppression attempts to slow lymphoproliferative progression.

Stiehm ER et al: *Immunologic Disorders in Infants and Children,* 5th ed. Elsevier Saunders, 2004.

7. Griscelli Syndrome

Characterized by partial albinism, neutropenia, thrombocytopenia, and lymphohistiocytosis, Griscelli syndrome is a rare autosomal recessive syndrome due to mutations in the myosin VA gene. Affected patients have recurrent and serious infections caused by fungi, viruses, and bacteria. Immunologic evaluation demonstrates variable immunoglobulin levels and antibody function with impaired T-lymphocyte function. Bone marrow transplantation can correct the immunodeficiency. Griscelli syndrome is distinguished from Chédiak-Higashi syndrome by the lack of granules in white blood cells.

8. Netherton Syndrome

Patients with the autosomal recessive Netherton syndrome present with trichorrhexis (brittle hair), ichthyosiform rash, and allergic diseases. A subset of patients suffer recurrent infections. Immune function is variable but may include hypo- or hypergammaglobulinemia, abnormal T-lymphocyte function, or abnormal phagocyte function. The disease is due to mutations in a serine protease inhibitor encoded on the *SPINK5* gene.

Stiehm R et al: *Immunologic Disorders of Infants and Children,* 5th ed. Elsevier Saunders, 2004.

9. Cartilage-Hair Hypoplasia

Cartilage-hair hypoplasia is an autosomal recessive form of chondrodysplasia with short-limbed short stature, hypoplastic hair, defective immunity, and poor erythrogenesis. The immune defect is characterized by mild to moderate lymphopenia and abnormal lymphocyte function, but normal antibody function. Affected patients have increased susceptibility to infections and increased risk of lymphoma. The disorder results from mutation in the *RMRP* gene that encodes the RNA component of an RNase MRP complex. BMT can restore cell-mediated immunity but does not correct the cartilage abnormality.

Ridanpaa M et al: The major mutation in the *RMRP* gene causing CHH among the Amish is the same as that found in most Finnish cases. Am J Med Genet C Semin Med Genet 2003;121:81 [PMID: 12888988].

GRAFT-VERSUS-HOST DISEASE

Graft-versus-host disease (GVHD) occurs when immunologically competent donor T lymphocytes are grafted into a host who is unable to reject them. The immunocompetent donor T lymphocytes recognize the host as foreign, leading to significant morbidity and potentially death. In addition to BMT-associated disease, GVHD can also occur in immunodeficient patients who receive nonirradiated blood products or engraftment of maternally derived T lymphocytes during birth. A progressive skin rash followed by diarrhea, hepatitis, nephritis, pulmonary infiltrates, fever, and marrow damage characterize GVHD. Laboratory evaluation reveals eosinophilia and leukocytosis, and diagnosis is confirmed by biopsy. Prevention is the most successful approach to GVHD and is accomplished with prophylactic immunosuppressant regimens including methotrexate, cyclosporine, and mycophenolate mofetil. Treatment of GVHD includes similar regimens in addition to antithymocyte serum, corticosteroids, and monoclonal antibodies directed against T lymphocytes.

Jaksh M, Mattsson J: The pathophysiology of acute graft-versus-host disease. Scand J Immunol 2005;61:398.

Stiehm ER et al: *Immunologic Disorders in Infants and Children,* 5th ed. Elsevier Saunders, 2004.

Endocrine Disorders

30

Philip S. Zeitler, MD, PhD, Sharon H. Travers, MD, Francis Hoe, MD, Kristen Nadeau, MD, & Michael S. Kappy, MD, PhD

■ GENERAL CONCEPTS

One of the major functions of the endocrine system is to regulate enzymatic and other metabolic processes (eg, molecular transport) responsible for maintaining the equilibrium (homeostasis) of the internal environment to ensure survival of the individual. Other critical roles for the endocrine system are regulation of growth (in utero and postnatal), pubertal development and reproduction, energy production, blood pressure, and to a lesser extent, behavior.

The classic concept that endocrine effects are the result of hormones secreted into the blood to reach a target cell has been updated to account for other ways in which hormonal effects occur. Specifically, some hormone systems involve the stimulation or inhibition (or both) of metabolic processes in neighboring (as opposed to distant) cells (eg, within the pancreatic islets or cartilage). This phenomenon is termed *paracrine*. Other hormone effects reflect the action of particular hormones on the same cells that produced them. This action is termed *autocrine*. The discoveries of local production of insulin, glucagon, somatostatin, cholecystokinin, and many other hormones in the brain and gut support the concept of paracrine and autocrine processes in these tissues.

Another significant discovery in endocrine physiology was an appreciation of the role of specific hormone receptors in target tissues, without which the hormonal effects could not occur. In the complete androgen insensitivity (resistance) syndrome, androgen receptors are defective, and the 46,XY individual develops varying degrees of female external genitalia despite the presence of testes (usually intra-abdominal) and adequate testosterone production. Similarly, in nephrogenic diabetes insipidus or Albright hereditary osteodystrophy (pseudohypoparathyroidism), affected children have abnormal antidiuretic hormone or parathyroid hormone (PTH) receptor function and show the metabolic effects of diabetes insipidus or hypoparathyroidism (low serum calcium and high serum phosphate concentrations), despite more-than-adequate hormone secretion. Alternatively, abnormal activation of a hormone receptor leads to the effects of the hormone without its abnormal secretion. Examples of this phenomenon include McCune-Albright syndrome (precocious puberty and hyperthyroidism) and testotoxicosis (familial male precocious puberty).

HORMONE TYPES

Three main structural types of hormones exist: peptides and proteins, steroids, and amines. The peptide hormones include the releasing factors secreted by the hypothalamus, the hormones of the anterior and posterior pituitary gland, pancreatic islet cells, and parathyroid glands, insulin-like growth factor 1 (IGF-1) from the liver and other tissues, angiotensin II, atrial natriuretic hormone, and many local growth factors. Steroid hormones are secreted primarily by the adrenal cortex, the gonads, and the liver and kidney (active vitamin D). The amine hormones are secreted by the adrenal medulla (epinephrine) and the thyroid gland (triiodothyronine [T_3] and thyroxine [T_4]).

As a rule, the peptide hormones and epinephrine act more rapidly than the others and bind to specific receptors on the surface of their target cell. The metabolic effects of these hormones are usually stimulation or inhibition of the activity of preexisting enzymes or transport proteins (posttranslational effects). The steroid hormones, thyroid hormone, and active vitamin D, in contrast, act more slowly and bind to specific cytoplasmic receptors within the target cell and subsequently to specific regions (genes) on nuclear DNA, where they direct a read-out of specific protein(s). Their metabolic effects are generally caused by stimulating or inhibiting the synthesis of new enzymes or transport proteins (transcriptional effects), thereby increasing or decreasing the amount rather than the activity of these proteins in the target cell.

Metabolic processes that must be regulated rapidly (eg, blood glucose or calcium homeostasis) are usually under the control of the peptide hormones and epinephrine, whereas those processes that may be regulated more slowly (eg, pubertal development and metabolic rate) are under the control of the steroid hormones and thyroid hormone (Table 30–1). The control of electrolyte

Table 30–1. Hormonal regulation of metabolic processes.

First Level (Most Direct)			
Metabolite or Other Parameter	**Abnormality**	**Endocrine Gland**	**Hormone**
Glucose	Hyperglycemia	Pancreatic beta cell	Insulin
Glucose	Hypoglycemia	Pancreatic alpha cell	Glucagon
Glucose	Hypoglycemia	Adrenal medulla	Epinephrine
Calcium	Hypercalcemia	Thyroid C cell	Calcitonin (?)
Calcium	Hypocalcemia	Parathyroid	PTH
Sodium/plasma osmolality	Hypernatremia/hyperosmolality	Hypothalamus (posterior pituitary gland)	ADH
Plasma volume	Hypervolemia	Heart	ANH

Second Level: Sodium and Potassium Balance			
Metabolite or Other Parameter	**Abnormality**	**Endocrine Gland**	**Hormone**
Sodium/potassium	Hyponatremia	Kidney	Renin (an enzyme)
	Hyperkalemia	Liver and others	Angiotensin I
	Hypovolemia	Lung	Angiotensin II
		Adrenal cortex	Aldosterone

Third Level (Most Complex)			
Releasing Hormone	**Tropic Hormone**	**Endocrine Gland**	**Endocrine Gland Hormone**
CRH	ACTH	Adrenal cortex	Cortisol
GHRH	GH	Liver	IGF-1
GnRH	LH	Testis	Testosterone
GnRH	FSH/LH	Ovary	Estradiol/progesterone
TRH	TSH	Thyroid gland	T_4 (some T_3)

ACTH, corticotropin; ADH, antidiuretic hormone; ANH, antinaturietic hormone; CRH, corticotropin-releasing hormone; FSH, follicle-stimulating hormone; GH, growth hormone; GHRH, growth hormone-releasing hormone; GnRH, gonadotropin-releasing hormone; IGF, insulin-like growth factor; LH, luteinizing hormone; PTH, parathyroid hormone; T_3, triiodothyronine; T_4, thyroxine; TRH, thyrotropin-releasing hormone; TSH, thyroid-stimulating hormone.

homeostasis is intermediate and is regulated by a combination of peptide and steroid hormones (Table 30–1).

FEEDBACK CONTROL OF HORMONE SECRETION

Hormone secretion is regulated, for the most part, by feedback in response to changes in the internal environment as postulated by Claude Bernard in the nineteenth century (Table 30–1). When the metabolic imbalance is corrected, stimulation of the hormone's secretion ceases and may even be inhibited. Overcorrection of the imbalance stimulates secretion of a counterbalancing hormone or hormones, so that the circulating concentrations of all metabolites and plasma osmolality are kept within relatively narrow limits.

Hypothalamic-pituitary control of hormonal secretion is also regulated by feedback, so that end-organ failure (endocrine gland insufficiency) leading to decreased circulating concentrations of endocrine gland hormones results in increased secretion of their respective hypothalamic releasing and pituitary hormones (Table 30–1 and Figure 30–1). If restoration of normal circulating concentrations of hormones occurs, feedback inhibition at the pituitary and hypothalamus results in cessation of the previously stimulated secretion of releasing and pituitary hormones and restoration of their circulating concentrations to normal.

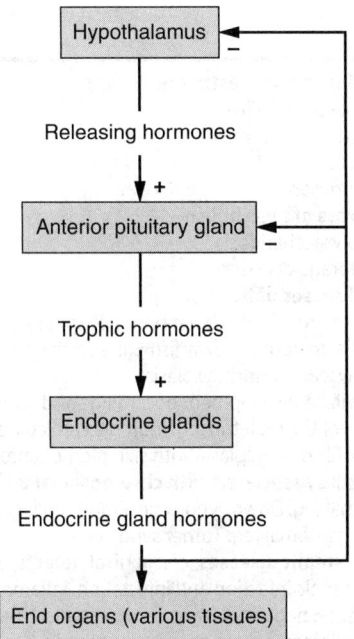

Figure 30–1. General scheme of the hypothalamus-pituitary-endocrine gland axis. Releasing hormones synthesized in the hypothalamus are secreted into the hypophysial portal circulation. Trophic hormones are secreted by the pituitary gland in response, and they in turn act on specific endocrine glands to stimulate the secretion of their respective hormones. The endocrine gland hormones exert their respective effects on various target tissues (end organs) and exert a negative feedback (feedback inhibition) on their own secretion by acting at the level of the pituitary and hypothalamus. This system is characteristic of those hormones listed in Table 30–1 (third level).

Similarly, if autonomous endocrine gland hyperfunction is present (eg, McCune-Albright syndrome, Graves disease, or adrenal tumor), the specific hypothalamic releasing and pituitary hormones are suppressed (Figure 30–1). An understanding of the basic phenomenon of feedback control of hormonal secretion is fundamental to the understanding of endocrine disorders and their evaluation in children.

■ DISTURBANCES OF GROWTH

Disturbances of growth and development are the most common presenting complaints in the pediatric endocrine clinic. It is critical to distinguish between normal and abnormal growth patterns, because deviation from a normal growth pattern can be the first or only manifestation of a wide variety of diseases. Determination of height velocity is the single most critical factor in evaluating the growth of a child, and a persistent increase or decrease in height percentiles between age 2 years and the onset of puberty should warrant further evaluation. It is a little more difficult to distinguish normal from abnormal growth in the first 2 years of life, as infants will show catch-up or catch-down growth during this period. It is also important to evaluate a child's growth in the context of normal standards. The National Center for Health Statistics provides standard growth charts derived from growth data of North American children (see Chapter 1). Height and weight measurements should be plotted on these charts. Growth charts are also available for children with specific growth disturbances, such as Turner syndrome and Down syndrome.

TARGET HEIGHT & SKELETAL MATURATION

The growth and height potential of a child is determined largely by genetic factors. The target (midparental) height of a child can be determined by calculating the mean parental height and adding or subtracting 6.5 cm for boys and girls, respectively. Most children will achieve an adult height that is within 8 cm of their target height; consequently, this calculation is very helpful in evaluating a child's genetic growth potential. Another important parameter in determining growth potential is bone age, which is a measure of skeletal maturation. Beyond the neonatal period, a radiograph of the left hand and wrist is obtained and compared with the published standards of Greulich and Pyle. The extent of skeletal maturation can be used to predict a child's ultimate height potential because growth ceases when epiphyseal fusion is complete. A delayed bone age is not diagnostic of a specific disease but indicates that there is residual growth potential.

SHORT STATURE

Short stature has many causes, and it is important to distinguish between normal variants of growth (familial short stature and constitutional growth delay) and pathologic conditions (Table 30–2). Pathologic short stature should be suspected in children who have an abnormal growth velocity (crossing major height percentiles on the growth curve) or in children who are significantly short for their family. Children with chronic illness or nutritional deficiencies may have poor linear growth, but this is typically associated with inadequate weight gain. In contrast, endocrine causes of short stat-

Table 30–2. Causes of short stature.

A. Genetic-familial short stature
B. Constitutional growth delay
C. Endocrine disturbances
 1. Growth hormone deficiency
  a. Hereditary—gene deletion
  b. Idiopathic—deficiency of growth hormone or growth hormone-releasing hormone (or both) with and without associated abnormalities of midline structures of the central nervous system
  c. Acquired
   Transient—eg, psychosocial short stature
   Organic—tumor, irradiation of the central nervous system, infection, or trauma
 2. Hypothyroidism
 3. Excess cortisol—Cushing disease and Cushing syndrome (including iatrogenic causes)
 4. Precocious puberty
 5. Diabetes mellitus (poorly controlled)
 6. Pseudohypoparathyroidism
 7. Rickets
D. Intrauterine growth restriction
 1. Intrinsic fetal abnormalities—chromosomal disorders
 2. Syndromes (eg, Russell-Silver, Noonan, Bloom, de Lange, Cockayne)
 3. Congenital infections
 4. Placental abnormalities
	D. Intrauterine growth restriction (*cont.*)
	 5. Maternal abnormalities
	  a. Hypertension/toxemia
	  b. Drug use
	  c. Malnutrition
	E. Inborn errors of metabolism
	 1. Mucopolysaccharidosis
	 2. Other storage diseases
	F. Intrinsic diseases of bone
	 1. Defects of growth of tubular bones or spine (eg, achondroplasia, metatropic dwarfism, diastrophic dwarfism, metaphyseal chondrodysplasia)
	 2. Disorganized development of cartilage and fibrous components of the skeleton (eg, multiple cartilaginous exostoses, fibrous dysplasia with skin pigmentation)
	G. Short stature associated with chromosomal defects
	 1. Autosomal (eg, Down syndrome, Prader-Willi syndrome)
	 2. Sex chromosomal (eg, Turner syndrome-XO)
	H. Chronic systemic diseases, congenital defects, and cancers (eg, chronic infection and infestation, inflammatory bowel disease, hepatic disease, cardiovascular disease, hematologic disease, central nervous system disease, pulmonary disease, renal disease, malnutrition, cancers, collagen vascular disease)
	I. Psychosocial short stature (deprivation dwarfism)

ure are usually associated with normal or excessive weight gain.

Familial Short Stature & Constitutional Growth Delay

Children with familial short stature are typically born with normal weight and length. In the first 2 years of life, however, they will have a deceleration in linear growth to reach their target percentile, which is determined largely by genetic factors. Once this target percentile is obtained, the child will have normal linear growth parallel to the growth curve. Skeletal maturation and the timing of puberty are consistent with chronologic age. Consequently, the height percentile the child has been following is maintained, and final height is short but appropriate for the family (Figure 30–2). For example, an infant boy of a mother who is 5'0" and father who is 5'5" may have a birth length at the fiftieth percentile. However, this child's length will probably change percentiles downward within the first 2 years of life to reach the fifth percentile. The calculated midparental height of this child is 5'5", which is at the fifth percentile for a full grown male. Consequently, the fifth percentile is an appropriate growth trajectory for this child.

Children with constitutional growth delay do not necessarily have short parents but have a growth pattern similar to those with familial short stature. The difference is that children with constitutional growth delay will have a delay in skeletal maturation and a delay in the onset of puberty. In these children, growth continues beyond the time the average child has stopped growing, and final height is appropriate for target height (Figure 30–3). There is often a history of other family members being so-called "late bloomers."

Growth Hormone Deficiency

Human growth hormone (GH) is produced by the anterior pituitary gland under the stimulation of growth hormone-releasing hormone (GHRH) and the inhibition of somatostatin. GH is secreted in a pulsatile pattern in response to sleep, exercise, and hypoglycemia and has direct growth-promoting and metabolic effects (Figure 30–4). GH also promotes growth indirectly by stimulating the production of insulin-like growth factors, primarily IGF-1.

Growth hormone deficiency (GHD) is characterized by decreased growth velocity, delay in skeletal maturation, absence of other explanations for poor growth, and laboratory tests indicating subnormal GH secretion. GHD may be isolated or may occur with other pituitary hormone deficiencies. Identifiable causes of GHD may be congeni-

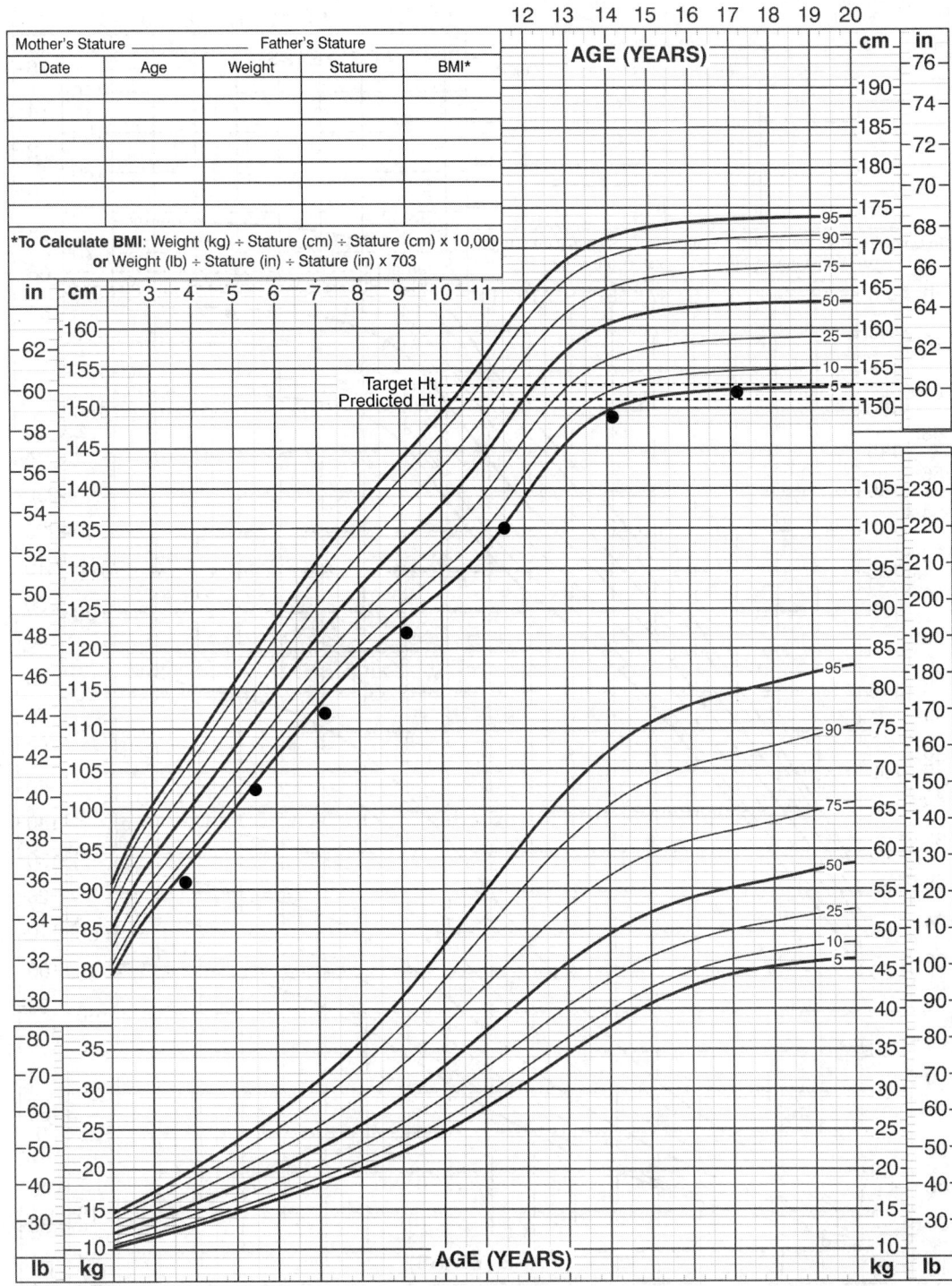

Figure 30–2. Typical pattern of growth in a child with familial short stature. After attaining an appropriate percentile during the first 2 years of life, the child will have normal linear growth parallel to the growth curve. Skeletal maturation and the timing of puberty are consistent with chronologic age. The height percentile the child has been following is maintained, and final height is short but appropriate for the family.

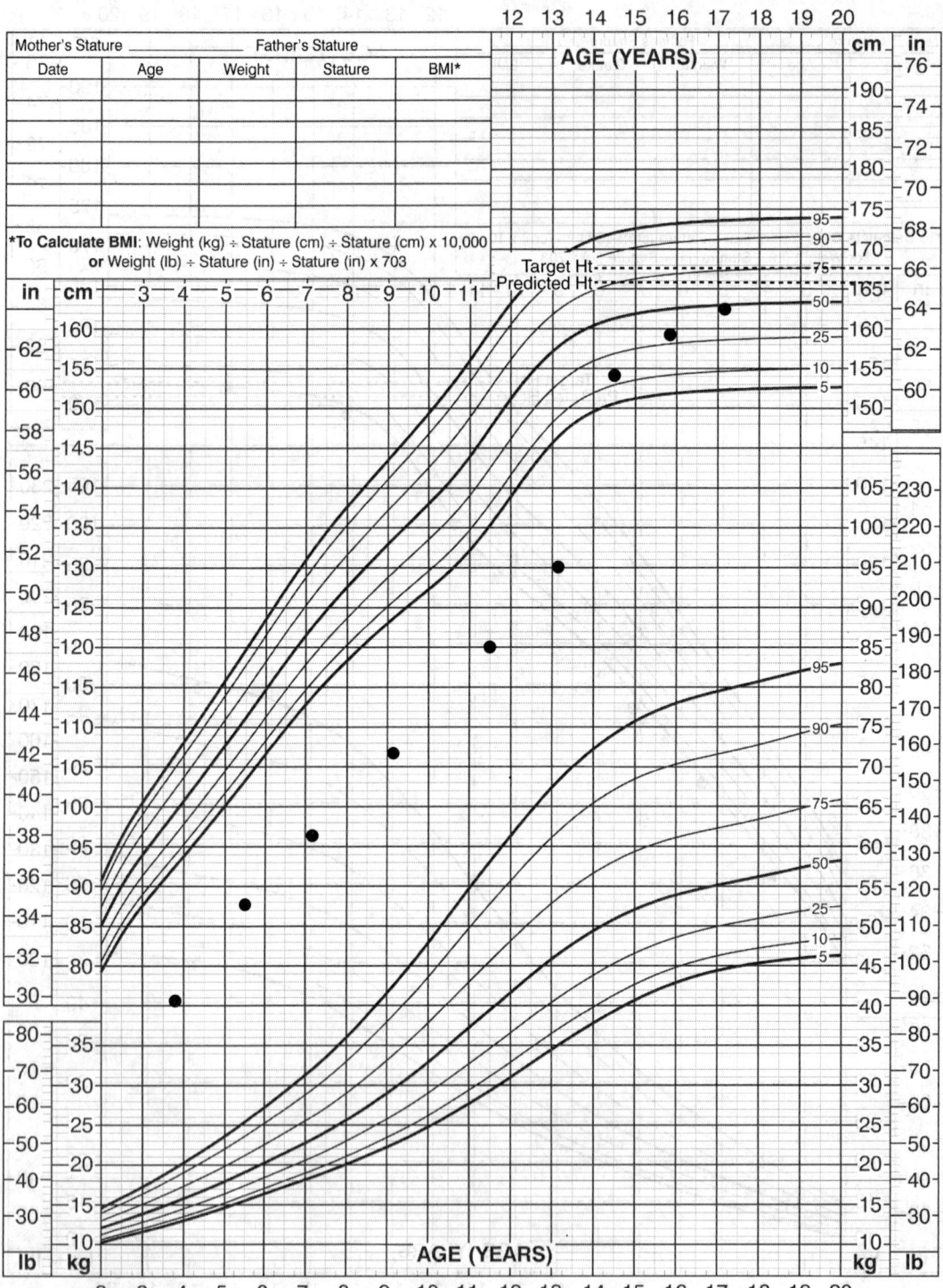

Figure 30–3. Typical pattern of growth in a child with constitutional growth delay. Growth slows during the first 2 years of life, similarly to children with familial short stature. Subsequently the child will have normal linear growth parallel to the growth curve. However, skeletal maturation and the onset of puberty are delayed. Growth continues beyond the time the average child has stopped growing, and final height is appropriate for target height.

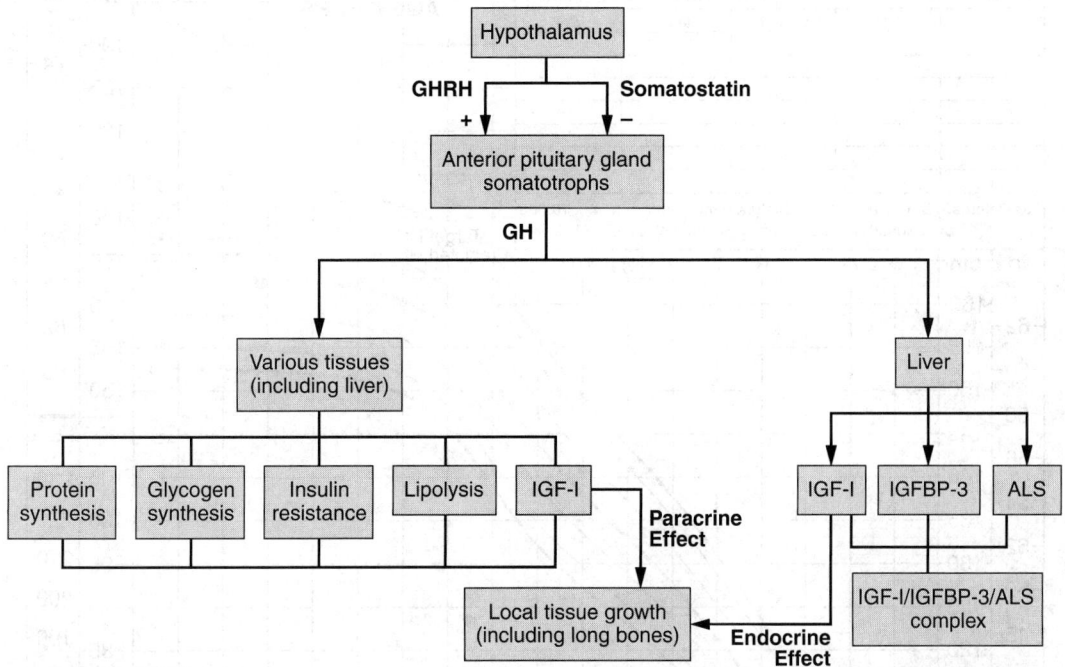

Figure 30–4. The GHRH/GH/IGF-1 system. The effects of growth hormone (GH) on growth are partly due to its direct anabolic effects in muscle, liver, and bone. In addition, GH stimulates many tissues to produce insulin-like growth factor 1 (IGF-1) locally, which stimulates the growth of the tissue itself (paracrine effect of IGF-1). The action of GH on the liver results in the secretion of IGF-1 (circulating IGF-1), which stimulates growth in other tissues (endocrine effect of IGF-1). The action of growth hormone on the liver also enhances the secretion of IGF-binding protein-3 (IGFBP-3) and acid-labile subunit (ALS), which form a high-molecular-weight complex with IGF-1. The function of this complex is to transport IGF-1 to its target tissues, but the complex also serves as a reservoir and possible inhibitor of IGF-1 action. In various chronic illnesses, the direct metabolic effects of growth hormone are inhibited; the secretion of IGF-1 in response to GH is blunted, and in some cases IGFBP-3 synthesis is enhanced, resulting in marked inhibition in the growth of the child. GHRH, growth hormone-releasing hormone.

tal (septo-optic dysplasia or empty-sella syndrome), genetic (GH or GHRH gene mutation), or acquired (craniopharyngioma, germinoma, histiocytosis, or cranial irradiation). Idiopathic GHD, however, occurs more commonly than any of these recognized causes, with an incidence of approximately 1:4000 children. The GH insensitivity syndrome (Laron dwarfism) is caused by a mutation in the GH receptor. These children present in a manner similar to those with GHD, but children with Laron dwarfism may have a distinctive facial appearance.

Infants with GHD are of normal birth weight; birth length may be reduced slightly, suggesting that GH is not a major contributor to intrauterine growth. Classic GH-deficient infants may present initially with hypoglycemia or evidence of other pituitary deficiencies such as central hypothyroidism or adrenal insufficiency. Gonadotropin and GH deficiency may be suspected in the newborn male who has a micropenis. Growth retardation may begin in

infancy or may be delayed until later childhood. In children with acquired or idiopathic GHD, the primary manifestation is a subnormal growth velocity (Figure 30–5). Because GH promotes lipolysis, many GH-deficient children will also have truncal adiposity.

Laboratory tests to assess GH status may be difficult to interpret. Children with normal and short stature have a broad range of GH secretion patterns, and significant overlap exists between test results of normal and GH-deficient children. Traditionally, provocative studies are performed using such agents as insulin-induced hypoglycemia, arginine, levodopa, clonidine, or glucagon. Serum concentrations of IGF-1 and IGF-binding protein 3 may give reasonable estimations of GH secretion in the adequately nourished child (see Figure 30–4). When results of GH tests are equivocal, a trial of GH treatment may be useful in determining whether an abnormally short child will benefit from

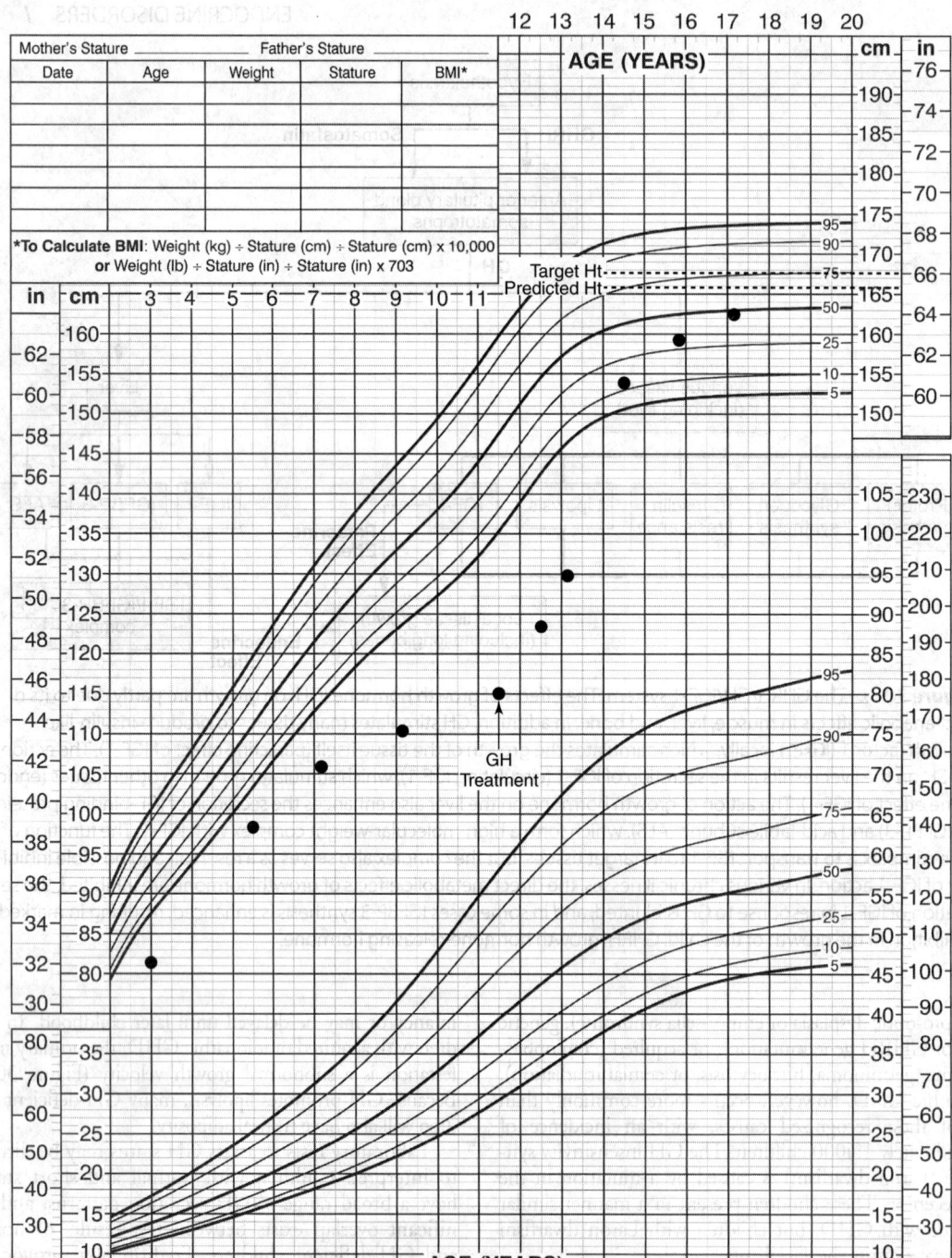

Mother's Stature		Father's Stature		
Date	Age	Weight	Stature	BMI*

*To Calculate BMI: Weight (kg) ÷ Stature (cm) ÷ Stature (cm) x 10,000
or Weight (lb) ÷ Stature (in) ÷ Stature (in) x 703

AGE (YEARS)

Target Ht
Predicted Ht

GH
Treatment

AGE (YEARS)

Figure 30–5. Typical pattern of growth in a child with acquired growth hormone deficiency. Children with acquired growth hormone deficiency have an abnormal growth velocity and fail to maintain height percentile during childhood. Other phenotypic features (central adiposity and immaturity of facies) may be present. Children with congenital growth hormone deficiency will cross percentiles during the first 2 years of life, similarly to the pattern seen in familial short stature and constitutional delay, but will fail to attain a steady height percentile subsequently.

GH. Currently the treatment of choice for GHD is recombinant GH in a dose of 0.15–0.3 mg/kg/wk administered subcutaneously divided into six or seven equal once-daily doses.

GH therapy is FDA-approved for children with GHD and growth restriction associated with chronic renal failure, for girls with Turner syndrome, children with Prader-Willi syndrome, and children born small for gestational age (SGA) who fail to demonstrate catch-up growth by age 4. GH therapy has been recently approved for children with idiopathic short stature whose current height is more than 2.25 standard deviations below the norm for age. Final height improvement may be 5–7 cm in this population. This indication has generated much controversy, and the role of GH in these children remains unclear. GH therapy is expensive, and indications other than these remain controversial. Reported side effects of recombinant GH therapy are uncommon but include benign intracranial hypertension and slipped capital femoral epiphysis. With early diagnosis and treatment, children with GHD reach normal or nearly normal adult height.

Small for Gestational Age/Intrauterine Growth Restriction

Small-for-gestational-age (SGA) infants are those who have birth weights less than the tenth percentile for the population's birth weight/gestational age relationship. SGA infants include those who are constitutionally small and growing at their potential, as well as those with intrauterine growth restriction (IUGR). IUGR refers to a heterogeneous group of patients who fail to grow at a normal rate in utero. SGA/IUGR occurs secondary to poor maternal environment, intrinsic fetal abnormalities, congenital infections, or other forms of fetal malnutrition. Conditions secondary to intrinsic fetal abnormalities are often referred to as primordial short stature and include the Russell–Silver, Seckel, Noonan, Bloom, and Cockayne syndromes, and progeria. Many children with milder degrees of SGA/IUGR (except those with intrinsic fetal abnormalities) exhibit catch-up growth during their first 3 years of life. However, 15–20% will remain short throughout life, particularly those whose growth restriction in utero occurred over several months rather than just the last 2 or 3 months of gestation, as well as those born preterm with subsequent inadequate postnatal nutrition. Those children who do not show catch-up growth will have a normal growth velocity, although they will follow a lower height percentile than expected for the family. In most instances, skeletal maturation corresponds to chronologic age or is delayed only mildly—in contrast to the delay occurring in children with constitutional growth delay. GH therapy has been evaluated in SGA children, and short-term studies have shown increases in growth velocity. Consequently, growth hormone has recently been approved for treatment in these children.

Disproportionate Short Stature

Skeletal dysplasias are disorders that result in disproportionate short stature. More than 200 different types of skeletal dysplasias may occur, either sporadically or genetically. Measurements of arm span and upper-to-lower body segment ratio are helpful in determining whether a child has normal body proportions. If disproportionate short stature is found, a skeletal survey may be useful because specific radiographic features characterize certain disorders. Because skeletal dysplasias are individually rare, the effect of GH on most types is largely unknown.

Short Stature Associated with Syndromes

Short stature is associated with many syndromes, including Turner, Down, and Prader-Willi. Girls with Turner syndrome typically have such other typical features as micrognathia, webbed neck, low posterior hairline, edema of hands and feet, multiple pigmented nevi, and an increased carrying angle. In some girls with Turner syndrome, however, short stature is the only clinical manifestation. Consequently, any girl with unexplained short stature should have a chromosomal evaluation. Although girls with Turner syndrome are not classically GH-deficient, GH therapy has been shown to improve final height by an average of 6.0 cm. The duration of GH therapy is a significant predictor of long-term height gain; consequently, it is important that Turner syndrome be diagnosed early and GH started as soon as possible.

GH is also approved for growth failure associated with Prader-Willi syndrome, a syndrome in which many individuals are GH-deficient. GH improves growth as well as body composition and physical activity in these patients. A few fatalities have been reported in Prader-Willi children treated with GH. All of these children were severely obese or had a history of respiratory impairment, sleep apnea, or an unidentified respiratory infection. The role of GH, if any, in contributing to these deaths is unknown. As a precaution, it is recommended that all Prader-Willi patients be evaluated for upper airway obstruction and sleep apnea prior to initiation of GH therapy.

Children with Down syndrome should be evaluated for GHD only if their linear growth is abnormal compared with the Down syndrome growth chart.

Psychosocial Short Stature (Psychosocial Dwarfism)

Psychosocial short stature is characterized by growth retardation in association with emotional deprivation. Undernutrition contributes to the growth retardation of some affected children. In addition to impaired growth, bizarre eating and drinking habits, bowel and bladder incontinence, social withdrawal, and delayed speech may occur. GH secretion in children with psychosocial short stature is diminished, but GH therapy is usually not beneficial. Foster home placement or a change in the psychological environment at home usually results in improved growth and normalization of GH secretion, personality, and eating behaviors.

Diagnostic Approach to Short Stature

Laboratory investigation should be guided by information gained from the history and physical examination. Initial considerations should include size at birth, presence of dysmorphology, pattern of growth since birth, family pattern of growth, pubertal stage, body segment proportion, and psychological problems. In a child who has poor weight gain as the primary disturbance, history of chronic illness and nutritional assessment are indicated. The following laboratory tests may be useful:

1. Radiograph of left hand and wrist for bone age
2. Complete blood count (to detect chronic anemia or infection)
3. Erythrocyte sedimentation rate (often elevated in collagen-vascular disease, cancer, chronic infection, and inflammatory bowel disease)
4. Urinalysis, blood urea nitrogen, and serum creatinine (occult renal disease)
5. Serum electrolytes, calcium, and phosphorus (renal tubular disease and metabolic bone disease)
6. Stool examination for fat, serum endomysial antibody (malabsorption or celiac disease)
7. Karyotype (in girls)
8. Thyroid function tests: free thyroxine (FT_4) and thyroid-stimulating hormone (TSH)
9. IGF-1 and IGF-binding protein 3

Carrel AL et al: Benefits of long-term GH therapy in Prader-Willi syndrome: A 4-year study. J Clin Endocrinol Metab 2002; 87:1581 [PMID: 11932286].

Kemp SF et al: Efficacy and safety results of long-term growth hormone treatment of idiopathic short stature. J Clin Endocrnol Metab 2005;90:5247 [PMID: 15998780].

Lee PA, Kendig JW, Kerrigan JR: Persistent short stature, other potential outcomes, and the effect of growth hormone treatment in children who are born small for gestational age. Pediatrics 2003;112:150 [PMID: 12837881].

TALL STATURE

Although we typically think of growth disturbances in relation to short stature, potentially serious pathologic conditions may be associated with tall stature and exces-

Table 30–3. Causes of tall stature.

A. Constitutional (familial)
B. Endocrine causes
   1. Growth hormone excess (pituitary gigantism)
   2. Precocious puberty
   3. Hypogonadism
C. Nonendocrine causes
   1. Klinefelter syndrome
   2. XYY males
   3. Marfan syndrome
   4. Cerebral gigantism (Soto syndrome)
   5. Homocystinuria

sive growth (Table 30–3). Excessive GH secretion is rare in children and is generally associated with a functioning pituitary adenoma. GH excess leads to gigantism if the epiphyses are open and to acromegaly if the epiphyses are closed. Affected children present with an accelerated growth velocity. The diagnosis is confirmed by demonstrating elevated GH and IGF-1 levels and failure of GH to suppress during a standard oral glucose tolerance test.

Constitutional tall stature may be a concern to adolescent girls. However, the upper limit of acceptable height in both sexes is increasing, and concerns about excessive growth for girls are becoming less frequent. When such concerns arise, the family history, growth curve, pubertal stage, and assessment of skeletal maturation allow assessment of predicted final adult height. Reassurance, counseling, and education may alleviate the family's concerns. In extremely rare instances in which the predicted height appears to be excessive and unacceptable, estrogen therapy may accelerate bone maturation and shorten the growth period.

Iughetti L, Bergomi A, Bernasconi S: Diagnostic approach and therapy of overgrowth and tall stature in childhood. Minerva Pediatr 2003;55:563 [PMID: 14676728].

■ THE POSTERIOR PITUITARY GLAND

The posterior pituitary (neurohypophysis) is an extension of the ventral hypothalamus. The two principal hormones of the posterior pituitary, oxytocin and arginine vasopressin, are synthesized in the supraoptic and paraventricular nuclei of the ventral hypothalamus. After synthesis, these peptide hormones are packaged in granules with specific neurophysins and transported via the axons to their storage site in the posterior pituitary. Vasopressin is essential for water balance; its primary action is on the kidney to promote reabsorption of water from urine. Oxytocin is primarily important during parturition and breast feeding and is not discussed further here.

Arginine Vasopressin (Antidiuretic Hormone)

The release of vasopressin is primarily influenced by serum osmolality and intravascular volume. Minor increases in plasma osmolality (detected by osmoreceptors in the anterolateral hypothalamus) and large decreases in intravascular volume (detected by baroreceptors in the cardiac atria) stimulate vasopressin release. Disorders of vasopressin release and action include (1) central (neurogenic) diabetes insipidus (discussed in the following section), (2) nephrogenic diabetes insipidus (see Chapter 22), and (3) the syndrome of inappropriate secretion of antidiuretic hormone (see Chapter 41).

CENTRAL DIABETES INSIPIDUS

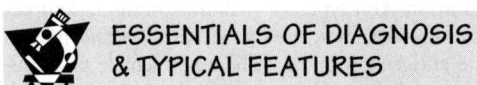

ESSENTIALS OF DIAGNOSIS & TYPICAL FEATURES

- *Polydipsia, polyuria (> 2 L/m²/d), and nocturia.*
- *Inability to concentrate urine after fluid restriction (urine specific gravity < 1.010; osmolality < 300 mOsm/kg).*
- *Hypernatremia and dehydration*
- *Plasma osmolality > 300 mOsm/kg with urine osmolality < 600 mOsm/kg.*
- *Subnormal plasma vasopressin concentration.*
- *Antidiuretic response to vasopressin administration.*

General Considerations

Central diabetes insipidus (DI) is caused by an inability to synthesize and release vasopressin. Without vasopressin, the kidneys are unable to concentrate the urine, resulting in excessive urinary water loss. Genetic causes of central DI are rare and include inherited mutations in the vasopressin gene (most are in the neurophysin portion of the vasopressin precursor), and the *WFS1* gene that causes Wolfram syndrome, also known as DID-MOAD (DI, diabetes mellitus, optic atrophy, and deafness). Midline brain abnormalities, such as septo-optic dysplasia and holoprosencephaly may also be associated with central DI. Traumatic brain injury or neurosurgery in or near the hypothalamus or pituitary can cause transient or permanent DI. In these cases, a triple phase

response is often seen. In the initial phase, transient DI occurs due to edema in the hypothalamus and/or pituitary area. This is followed in 2–5 days by the syndrome of inappropriate secretion of antidiuretic hormone, caused by unregulated release of vasopressin from dying neurons. The third phase of permanent DI results if a significant number of vasopressin neurons are destroyed.

Tumors and infiltrative diseases of the hypothalamus and pituitary are found in a significant number of children with DI. In children with craniopharyngiomas, DI usually develops after neurosurgical intervention. This is in contrast to germinomas in which DI is often the presenting symptom. Germinomas may be undetectable for several years; consequently, children with unexplained DI should have regularly repeated MRI. Infiltrative diseases such as histiocytosis and lymphocytic hypophysitis also can cause DI in children. In these conditions, as well as germinomas, MRI scans characteristically show thickening of the pituitary stalk. Infections involving the base of the brain can also cause transient DI.

Clinical Findings

Diabetes insipidus is often abrupt and is characterized by polyuria, nocturia, enuresis, and intense thirst. Children with DI typically crave cold. Hypernatremia, hyperosmolality, and dehydration may occur if fluid intake is not sufficient to keep up with urinary losses, either due to lack of access to fluids or an impaired thirst mechanism. In infants, symptoms may also include failure to thrive, vomiting, constipation, and unexplained fevers. Some infants may present with severe dehydration, circulatory collapse, and seizures. Vasopressin deficiency may be masked in patients with panhypopituitarism due to the impaired excretion of free water associated with adrenal insufficiency. Treating these patients with glucocorticoids may unmask their DI.

Diagnosis

The diagnosis of DI is confirmed when serum hyperosmolality is associated with hypo-osmolality. If the history reveals that the child can go through the night comfortably without drinking, screening tests can be obtained as an outpatient. Oral intake of fluid is prohibited after midnight. A first morning void is obtained to determine urine osmolality, sodium concentration, and specific gravity. If urine specific gravity is greater than 1.015, DI is excluded. If urine is not concentrated, a blood sample should be obtained within a few minutes of the urine collection and analyzed for osmolality and sodium, potassium, creatinine, and calcium levels. If screening results are unclear or if symptoms preclude safely withholding fluids at home, a water deprivation test performed in the hospital is indicated. During the water deprivation test, fluid is withheld and the child is closely monitored. A serum osmolality of greater than 290 mOsm/kg associated with an inappropriately dilute urine (osmolality < 300 mOsm/kg) is diagnostic for DI. Low serum vasopressin concentration and an antidiuretic response to vasopressin administration at the end of the test distinguishes central from nephrogenic DI. Children diagnosed with central DI should have a head magnetic resonance imaging (MRI) scan with contrast to look for tumors or infiltrative processes. The posterior pituitary "bright spot" on MRI is often absent in DI.

Decreased ability to concentrate urine may also occur with hypokalemia (eg, hyperaldosteronism), hypercalcemia, and with renal tubular abnormalities (eg, Fanconi syndrome). Children with primary polydipsia must be distinguished from those with diabetes insipidus. Children with primary polydipsia tend to have lower serum sodium levels and usually are able to appropriately concentrate their urine with overnight fluid deprivation. Some may have secondary nephrogenic diabetes insipidus due to dilution of the renal medullary interstitium and decreased renal concentrating ability, but this will resolve with restriction of intake.

Treatment

A. MEDICAL TREATMENT

The treatment of choice for central DI is desmopressin acetate (DDAVP) administered orally or intranasally. The aim of therapy is to provide the child with adequate antidiuresis allowing for uninterrupted sleep during the night and approximately 1 hour of diuresis before the next DDAVP dose. Children hospitalized with acute onset of diabetes insipidus, such as after neurosurgery, can be managed with intravenous vasopressin. Due to the amount of antidiuresis, intravenous fluids will need to be restricted to two-thirds the maintenance rate and electrolytes closely monitored to avoid water intoxication. Infants with diabetes insipidus should not be treated with DDAVP. Treatment with DDAVP in association with the volume of formula or breast milk needed to ensure adequate caloric intake would result in water intoxication. For this reason, infants are treated with extra free water, rather than DDAVP, to maintain normal hydration. Chlorothiazides may also be helpful in infants with central DI.

B. OTHER THERAPY

Therapy is directed toward the causative. Radiation therapy, chemotherapy, or surgery may be indicated for germinomas, histiocytosis, and craniopharyngiomas.

Cheetham T, Baylis PH: Diabetes insipidus in children: Pathophysiology, diagnosis and management. Paediatr Drugs 2002;4:785 [PMID: 12431131].

Wise-Faberowski L et al: Perioperative management of diabetes insipidus in children. J Neurosurg Anesthesiol 2004;16:14 [PMID: 14676564].

AUTOIMMUNE POLYGLANDULAR SYNDROMES

Autoimmune polyglandular syndrome (APS) types 1 and 2 are characterized by multiple autoimmune diseases that involve endocrine and nonendocrine tissues. APS type 1, also known as autoimmune polyendocrinopathy-candidiasis-ectodermal dystrophy (APECED) is a rare autosomal recessive disorder caused by mutations in the autoimmune regulator gene. In APS type 1, autoreactive T cells to organ-specific antigens in the thymus fail to be deleted, resulting in loss of self-tolerance and autoimmunity to multiple tissues and organs. APS type 1 usually presents in early childhood, typically with persistent mucocutaneous candidiasis. It is diagnosed clinically by the presence of at least two of the following three conditions: mucocutaneous candidiasis, hypoparathyroidism, and/or primary adrenal failure. Ectodermal dysplasia is often present. Other autoimmune diseases may also develop, including gonadal failure, alopecia, vitiligo, keratitis, hepatitis, intestinal dysfunction, atrophic gastritis, pernicious anemia, type 1 diabetes mellitus, and autoimmune thyroid disease.

In contrast, APS type 2 is a more common, complex polygenic disorder. It is associated with specific human leukocyte antigen genotypes. There is a female predominance. It is defined by primary adrenal failure with autoimmune thyroid disease and/or type 1 diabetes mellitus. Other autoimmune diseases such as vitiligo, alopecia, gonadal failure, celiac disease, atrophic gastritis, and pernicious anemia can also occur. Treatment is specific for each disease that develops. Long-term follow-up is needed to monitor for the early development of additional associated autoimmune diseases.

Dittmar M, Kahaly GJ: Polyglandular autoimmune syndromes: immunogenetics and long-term follow-up. J Clin Endocrinol Metab 2003;88:2983 [PMID: 12843130].

Eisenbarth GS, Gottlieb PA: Autoimmune polyendocrine syndromes. N Engl J Med 2004;350:2068 [PMID: 15141045].

Liston A et al: AIRE regulates negative selection of organ-specific T cells. Nat Immunol 2003;4:303 [PMID: 12612579].

Schatz DA, Winter WE: Autoimmune polyglandular syndrome II: Clinical syndrome and treatment. Endocrinol Metab Clin North Am 2002;31:339 [PMID: 12092454].

■ THE THYROID GLAND

FETAL DEVELOPMENT OF THE THYROID

The thyroid is capable of hormone synthesis in the fourteenth week of gestation, when TSH is detected in the fetal serum and pituitary gland. TSH does not normally cross the placenta, but T_4 and T_3 cross in limited amounts. The fetal pituitary-thyroid axis functions largely independently of the maternal pituitary-thyroid axis. Antithyroid drugs, including propylthiouracil (PTU) and methimazole, freely cross the placenta, and goitrous hypothyroid newborns may be born to hyperthyroid mothers who undergo treatment during pregnancy.

Graves disease is associated with thyroid-stimulating immunoglobulins (TSIs) and thyroid-binding inhibitory immunoglobulins (TBIIs). Mothers with TSIs can transmit these antibodies transplacentally, causing thyrotoxicosis in newborns. As TSI may still be present in the serum of previously hyperthyroid mothers, despite surgical or radioiodine-induced removal of their thyroid glands, transmission of TSI should be considered in all mothers with a history of hyperthyroidism. In addition, TBIIs can cross the placenta, causing hypothyroidism. Both maternal TSI and TBII usually disappear from the infant's circulation by 6–8 weeks.

Physiology

Pituitary TSH stimulates the thyroid gland to take up iodine and synthesize active thyroid hormones (ie, T_3 and T_4). Active hormone produced in excess of physiologic needs is stored within the thyroid follicles as thyroglobulin. The release of active thyroid hormones into the circulation is regulated by a negative feedback mechanism involving pituitary TSH and free thyroid hormone (see Figure 30–1).

Most T_3 and T_4 circulates bound to thyroid (hormone) binding globulin (TBG), albumin, and prealbumin, thus less than 1% of T_3 and T_4 is in the free form (FT_3 and FT_4). T_4 is deiodinated in the tissues to either T_3 or reverse T_3 (inactive). Receptors for T_3 are present on the cell surface, in the nucleus, in the cytosol, and on mitochondria.

At birth, the newborn's T_4 approximates that of the mother, but levels increase rapidly during the first 5 days of life in response to a TSH surge immediately following birth. TSH levels subsequently decrease to childhood levels by age 2–4 weeks. This physiologic neonatal TSH surge can cause falsely positive neonatal screens for hypothyroidism (ie, high TSH), if blood specimens for screening are collected on the first day of life.

The T_4 level is low in hypothyroidism and may also be reduced in premature infants (particularly those with sepsis or respiratory distress), hypopituitarism, malnutrition, and following therapy with T_3. In premature infants with low T_4, it is unclear whether treatment is beneficial, and may vary by gestational age. T_4 may also be low due to decreased TSH secretion with prolonged administration of adrenocorticoids, dopamine, or somatostatin. T_4 is also low in situations that affect TBG, namely decreased TBG (nephrosis, cirrhosis, hypoproteinemia, and familial TBG deficiency; following the administration of glucocorticoids, androgens, or anabolic steroids), abnormal TBG cleavage (sepsis), and abnormal

binding to TBG (heparin, furosemide, salicylates, and phenytoin). However, since these effects are primarily on TBG levels, and not on thyroid function per se, TSH and FT_4 levels remain in the normal range.

T_3 and T_4 levels are high in hyperthyroidism and may be elevated in acute forms of thyroiditis and hepatitis; in some types of inborn errors of thyroid hormone synthesis, release, or binding; following the administration of estrogens or clofibrate or during pregnancy; and following the administration of various iodine-containing globulins.

TBG levels are increased by pregnancy, estrogen therapy (including oral contraceptives), phenytoin or phenothiazines, occasionally as a genetic variation, in certain hepatic disorders, or for unknown causes. Because of the many "nonthyroidal" effects on T_4, FT_4 may provide additional information in certain settings.

HYPOTHYROIDISM (Congenital & Acquired Hypothyroidism)

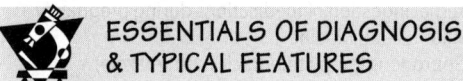

ESSENTIALS OF DIAGNOSIS & TYPICAL FEATURES

- *Growth retardation, diminished physical activity, impaired tissue perfusion, constipation, thick tongue, poor muscle tone, hoarseness, anemia, and intellectual retardation. (These findings can arise in the first 2 months of life, but are absent in 75% of newborns with documented hypothyroidism.)*
- *Thyroid hormone concentrations low (T_4, FT_4, and T_3 resin uptake [T_3RU]); TSH levels are elevated in primary hypothyroidism.*

Note: Most newborns with congenital hypothyroidism appear normal at birth and gain weight normally, even if not receiving treatment, for the first 3–4 months of life. Because congenital hypothyroidism must be treated as early as possible to avoid intellectual impairment, the diagnosis should be based on the newborn screening test and not on abnormal physical findings.

General Considerations

Thyroid hormone deficiency may be either congenital or acquired (juvenile hypothyroidism). Congenital hypothyroidism is the most common neonatal metabolic disorder and results in severe neurodevelopmental impairment if untreated. Although hypothyroidism in the newborn has many causes (Table 30–4), most cases are a result of hypoplasia or aplasia of the thyroid gland or failure of the gland to migrate into its normal anatomic location (ie, lingual or sublingual thyroid glands), with up to 2% of thyroid

Table 30–4. Causes of hypothyroidism.

A. Congenital	B. Acquired (juvenile hypothyroidism)

1. Aplasia, hypoplasia, or associated with maldescent of thyroid
   a. Embryonic defect of development
2. Familial iodine-induced goiter secondary to metabolic inborn errors
   a. Iodide transport defect (defect 1)
   b. Organification defect (defect 2)
     (1) Lack of iodine peroxidase
     (2) Lack of iodine transferase: Pendred syndrome, associated with congenital nerve deafness
   c. Coupling defect (defect 3)
   d. Iodotyrosine deiodinase defect (defect 4)
   e. Abnormal iodinated polypeptide (defects 5a and 5b)
     (1) Resulting from defect in intrathyroidal proteolysis of thyroglobulin
     (2) Abnormal plasma binding preventing use of T_4 by peripheral cells
   f. Inability of tissues to convert T_4 to T_3
3. Maternal ingestion of medications during pregnancy
   a. Maternal radioiodine
   b. Goitrogens (propylthiouracil, methimazole)
   c. Iodides
4. Iodide deficiency (endemic cretinism)
5. Idiopathic
	1. Autoimmune disease (lymphocytic thyroiditis)
	2. Thyroidectomy or radioiodine therapy for
	   a. Thyrotoxicosis
	   b. Cancer
	   c. Lingual thyroid
	   d. Isolated midline thyroid
	3. Destruction by x-ray
	4. Thyrotropin deficiency
	   a. Isolated
	   b. Associated with other pituitary tropic hormone deficiencies
	5. TRH deficiency due to hypothalamic injury or disease
	6. Chronic infections
	7. Medications
	   a. Iodides
	     (1) Prolonged, excessive ingestion
	     (2) Deficiency
	   b. Cobalt
	8. Idiopathic

T_3, triiodothyronine; T_4, thyroxine; TRH, thyrotropin-releasing hormone.

dysgenesis being familial. Another cause of congenital hypothyroidism is dyshormonogenesis. In children with enzymatic defects, thyroid enlargement is usually not present at birth, but occurs within the first two decades of life.

Cabbage, soybeans, aminosalicylic acid, thiourea derivatives, resorcinol, phenylbutazone, cobalt, and excessive iodine intake have been reported to cause goiter and hypothyroidism during pregnancy. Because many of these agents cross the placenta freely, they should be used with great caution during pregnancy. Iodine deficiency also causes hypothyroidism. Iodine deficiency leads to normal or slightly elevated T_3 at the expense of T_4, and as a consequence of the former, normal TSH. In the case of severe maternal iodine deficiency, both the fetus and the mother are T_4-deficient, both before and after onset of fetal thyroid function. This leads to irreversible, abnormal corticogenesis in the fetus.

Juvenile hypothyroidism, particularly if goiter is present, usually results from chronic lymphocytic (Hashimoto) thyroiditis (see later discussion).

Several hundred patients with clinical and laboratory features of resistance to thyroid hormone have been described. These syndromes are generally familial and are classified on the basis of the site of the resistance (eg, generalized; pituitary or peripheral tissue).

Clinical Findings

The severity of the findings in patients with thyroid deficiency depends on the age at onset and the degree of deficiency.

A. SYMPTOMS AND SIGNS

Note: Even with congenital absence of the thyroid gland, most newborns appear normal at birth and gain weight normally for the first 3–4 months of life, even without treatment. As congenital hypothyroidism must be treated as early as possible to prevent intellectual impairment, the diagnosis should be based on the newborn screening test and not on abnormal physical findings.

Findings may include physical and mental sluggishness; pale, gray, cool, or mottled skin; nonpitting myxedema; constipation; large tongue; poor muscle tone giving rise to a protuberant abdomen, umbilical hernia, and lumbar lordosis; hypothermia; bradycardia; diminished sweating (variable); decreased pulse pressure; hoarse voice or cry; transient deafness; and a slow relaxation component of deep tendon reflexes (best appreciated in the ankles). Nasal obstruction and discharge and persistent jaundice may be present in the neonatal period.

The skin may be dry, thick, scaly, and coarse, with a yellowish tinge due to excessive deposition of carotene. The hair may be dry, coarse, brittle, and excessive. Lateral thinning of the eyebrows may occur. The axillary and supraclavicular fat pads may be prominent in infants. Muscular hypertrophy (Kocher-Debré-Sémélaigne syndrome) is an unusual association with congenital hypothyroidism.

Growth changes include short stature; infantile skeletal proportions (relatively short extremities); infantile naso-orbital configuration (bridge of nose flat, broad, and underdeveloped; eyes seem to be widely spaced); delayed epiphyseal development; delayed closure of fontanelles; and retarded dental eruption. Metromenorrhagia may occur in older girls, and galactorrhea resulting from the stimulation of prolactin secretion or elevated thyrotropin-releasing hormone has been reported.

In hypothyroidism resulting from enzymatic defects, ingestion of goitrogens, or chronic lymphocytic thyroiditis, the thyroid gland may be enlarged. Thyroid enlargement in children is usually symmetrical, and the gland is moderately firm and without nodularity. In chronic lymphocytic thyroiditis, however, the thyroid frequently has a cobblestone surface; size and shape are readily apparent on inspection in children. Slowing of mental responsiveness and retardation of development of the brain may occur in neonates and infants, and a coincidental congenital malformation of the brain is present in some patients.

B. LABORATORY FINDINGS

T_4 and FT_4 levels are decreased. Radioiodine uptake is below 10% (normal: 10–30%). The binding of T_3 by erythrocytes or resin in vitro (T_3 resin uptake or T_3RU test) is lowered. With primary hypothyroidism, the serum TSH concentration is elevated. Normocytic anemia is common, but microcytic or macrocytic anemia may occur as a result of decreased iron, folate, and cobalamin absorption. Serum cholesterol and carotene are usually elevated in childhood but may be low or normal in infants. Cessation of therapy in previously treated hypothyroidism produces a marked rise in serum cholesterol levels in 6–8 weeks. Urinary creatinine excretion is decreased, and urinary hydroxyproline is low. Circulating autoantibodies to thyroid constituents may be present. Serum GH may be decreased, with subnormal GH response to stimulation in children with severe primary hypothyroidism, as well as low IGF-1 or IGF binding protein 3 (or both).

C. IMAGING

Thyroid imaging, while helpful in establishing the cause of congenital hypothyroidism, is not usually obtained, as it does not affect the treatment plan.

Skeletal maturation (bone age) is delayed. Centers of ossification, especially of the hip, may show multiple small centers or a single stippled, porous, or fragmented

center (epiphyseal dysgenesis). Vertebrae may show anterior beaking. Coxa vara and coxa plana may occur. Cardiomegaly is common.

Screening Programs for Neonatal Hypothyroidism

Congenital hypothyroidism should by diagnosed by neonatal screening within 10 days of birth. It may be recognized clinically during the first month of life or may be so mild that it is unrecognized clinically for months. Adequate treatment started as soon as possible improves the prognosis for intellectual performance later in life.

Differential Diagnosis

The causes of primary hypothyroidism due to intrinsic defects of the thyroid gland must be differentiated from pituitary and hypothalamic failure with secondary thyroid insufficiency. TSH and T_4 levels in combination are the most useful tests. When central hypothyroidism is diagnosed, screening for other pituitary abnormalities and MRI assessment are required.

Treatment

Levothyroxine is the drug of choice in a dosage of 75–100 µg/m²/d as a single dose. In newborns and infants, the dose is 10–12 µg/kg. The hypothyroid patient may be very responsive to thyroid and may be sensitive to slight excesses of thyroid hormone. A dose of 37.5 µg/day of levothyroxine is often recommended initially in neonates, although studies using 50 µg for the first 1–2 weeks suggest improved cognitive outcomes. Serum T_4 or FT_4 concentrations should be used to monitor the adequacy of therapy initially, because the elevated TSH may not fall into the normal range for several days to weeks. Subsequently, T_4 and TSH are used in combination, as elevations of serum TSH are sensitive early indicators of the need for increased medication (or increased compliance).

In the treatment of neonatal goiter with or without hypothyroidism resulting from drugs and goitrogens taken by the pregnant woman, temporary use of levothyroxine may be helpful in decreasing the size of the goiter.

Briet JM et al: Neonatal thyroxine supplementation in very preterm children. Pediatrics 2001;107:712 [PMID: 11335749].

Mitchell ML, Klein RZ: The sequelae of untreated maternal hypothyroidism. Eur J Endocrinol 2004;151(Suppl 3):U45 [PMID: 15554886].

Obregon MJ, Del Rey FE, de Escobar GM: The effects of iodine deficiency on thyroid hormone deiodination. Thyroid 2005;15:917 [PMID: 16131334].

Park SM, Chatterjee VK: Genetics of congenital hypothyroidism. J Med Genet 2005;42:379 [PMID: 15863666].

Rovet JF: Children with congenital hypothyroidism and their siblings: do they really differ? Pediatrics 2005;115:e52 [PMID: 15629966].

Simoneau-Roy J: Cognition and behavior at school entry in children with congenital hypothyroidism treated early with high-dose levothyroxine. J Pediatr 2004;144:747 [PMID: 15192621].

Van Vliet G: Treatment of congenital hypothyroidism. Lancet 2001; 358:86 [PMID: 11463405].

THYROIDITIS

Chronic lymphocytic (Hashimoto) thyroiditis is perhaps the most common pediatric endocrinopathy, particularly in adolescent girls. Acute and subacute thyroiditis are rare in all age groups.

1. Acute Suppurative Thyroiditis

Acute thyroiditis is rare. Oropharyngeal organisms are thought to reach the thyroid via a patent foramen cecum and thyroglossal duct tract. The most common pathogens are group A streptococci, pneumococci, *Staphylococcus aureus,* and anaerobes. The patient is invariably toxic, and the thyroid gland is exquisitely tender. Pain may radiate to adjacent areas of the neck or to the ear or chest. Thyroid tests are typically normal. Specific antibiotic therapy should be administered.

2. Subacute Nonsuppurative Thyroiditis

Subacute thyroiditis (de Quervain thyroiditis) is rare in the United States. In most cases, the cause is a virus (mumps, influenza, echovirus, coxsackievirus, Epstein-Barr virus, or adenovirus). Presenting features are similar to those of acute thyroiditis: fever, malaise, sore throat, dysphagia, and pain in the thyroid gland that may radiate to the ears. In contrast to acute thyroiditis, the onset of the subacute form is generally insidious and serum thyroid hormone concentrations may be elevated. The thyroid gland is firm, and the enlargement may be confined to one lobe. Radioiodine uptake is usually reduced. The differentiation from bacterial thyroiditis may be difficult, and antibiotic therapy is often recommended.

3. Chronic Lymphocytic Thyroiditis (Chronic Autoimmune Thyroiditis, Hashimoto Thyroiditis)

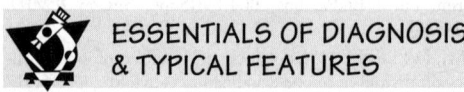

ESSENTIALS OF DIAGNOSIS & TYPICAL FEATURES

- Firm, freely movable, nontender, and diffusely enlarged goiter.

- Serum FT_4 concentrations are generally normal but may be elevated or decreased depending on the stage of the disease.

General Considerations

Chronic lymphocytic thyroiditis is occurring with increasing frequency in all age groups and currently is the most common cause of goiter and hypothyroidism in childhood. In children and adolescents, the incidence peaks between 8 and 15 years of age and occurs most commonly in females (4:1). The disease is the result of an autoimmune attack on the thyroid. Susceptibility to thyroid autoimmunity (and other endocrine autoimmune disorders) is associated with inheritance of certain histocompatibility alleles in APS type 2 (described earlier in this chapter).

Clinical Findings

A. SYMPTOMS AND SIGNS

The goiter is characteristically firm, freely movable, nontender, and symmetrical, with a pebbly consistency. Onset is usually insidious, and except for painless goiter, clinical manifestations are unusual. Occasionally a sensation of tracheal compression or fullness, hoarseness, and dysphagia are described by the patient. No local signs of inflammation or evidence of systemic infection are present.

B. LABORATORY FINDINGS

Laboratory findings vary. Serum concentrations of T_4, FT_4, and T_3RU are usually normal but may be elevated (hashitoxicosis) or depressed. Thyroid antibodies (antithyroglobulin, antithyroid peroxidase) are usually present, though titers are frequently low. A variety of abnormalities in radioactive iodide uptake studies have been described; thyroid scans usually show a diffuse or patchy pattern, and cold (nonfunctioning) nodules have been reported. Thyroid scans and uptake studies add little to the diagnosis. Surgical or needle biopsy is diagnostic but seldom indicated.

Treatment

The treatment of chronic lymphocytic thyroiditis is controversial. Full therapeutic doses of thyroid hormone (levothyroxine, 75–100 $\mu g/m^2/d$) may decrease the size of the goiter within 3 months, but in controlled trials the efficacy of thyroid hormone therapy is unsupported in the euthyroid child. Hypothyroidism is believed to be a common end result of autoimmune thyroiditis in the second to third decades of life; consequently, patients with adolescent goiter require lifelong surveillance, and children with documented hypothyroidism should receive levothyroxine in full replacement doses.

HYPERTHYROIDISM

> ### ESSENTIALS OF DIAGNOSIS & TYPICAL FEATURES
>
> - *Nervousness, emotional lability, fatigue, tremor, palpitations, excessive appetite, weight loss; increased perspiration, heat intolerance, and smooth, moist, warm skin.*
> - *Goiter, exophthalmos, tachycardia, widened pulse pressure (systolic hypertension), and weakness.*
> - *Thyroid hormone concentrations elevated (eg, T_4, FT_4, T_3, T_3RU); TSH concentration suppressed.*

General Considerations

Hyperthyroidism is caused by excess thyroid hormone. In children, most cases of hyperthyroidism are due to Graves disease, caused by antibodies directed at the TSH receptor that stimulate thyroid hormone production. Hyperthyroidism may also be due to acute, subacute, or chronic thyroiditis; autonomous functioning thyroid nodules, tumors producing TSH or TSH-like substances; or McCune-Albright syndrome, exogenous thyroid hormone excess and acute iodine exposure. Transient congenital hyperthyroidism (neonatal Graves disease) due to transplacental passage of maternal TSH receptor antibodies occurs in approximately 1% of babies born to mothers with Graves disease.

Clinical Findings

A. SYMPTOMS AND SIGNS

Hyperthyroidism is more common in females than in males. In children, the disease most frequently occurs during adolescence. The course of hyperthyroidism tends to be cyclic, with spontaneous remissions and exacerbations. Symptoms of hyperthyroidism include worsening school performance, fatigue, hyperactivity, emotional lability, nervousness, personality disturbances, insomnia, weight loss (despite increased appetite), palpitations, heat intolerance, increased perspiration, diarrhea, and irregular menses. Signs of hyperthyroidism include tachycardia, systolic hypertension with increased pulse pressure, exophthalmos, tremor, proximal muscle weakness, and moist, warm, skin. Accelerated growth and development may also occur. A diffuse firm goiter is present in almost all cases. A thyroid bruit and thrill may be present. In neonatal Graves disease, irritability, flushing, jaundice, hepatosplenomegaly, and thrombocytopenia are occasionally seen. Severe cases may result in arrhythmia, cardiac failure, and death.

B. LABORATORY FINDINGS

TSH is suppressed. T_4, FT_4, T_3, FT_3, and T_3RU are elevated except in rare cases in which only the serum T_3 is elevated (T_3 thyrotoxicosis). The presence of TSH-receptor autoantibodies (TSIs) and TSH-binding-inhibiting immunoglobulin (TBII) confirms the diagnosis of Graves' disease.

C. IMAGING

In Graves disease, radioactive iodine uptake by the thyroid is increased, whereas in subacute and chronic thyroiditis it is decreased. Autonomous hyperfunctioning nodules take up iodine while the surrounding tissue has decreased uptake. In children with hyperthyroidism, skeletal maturation assessed radiographically may be advanced. In infants, accelerated skeletal maturation may be associated with premature fusion of the cranial sutures. Long-standing hyperthyroidism is associated with osteoporosis.

Differential Diagnosis

Hypermetabolic states (severe anemia, chronic infections, pheochromocytoma, and muscle-wasting disease) may resemble hyperthyroidism clinically but differ in thyroid function studies.

Treatment

A. GENERAL MEASURES

In untreated hyperthyroidism, strenuous physical activity should be avoided. Bed rest may be required in severe cases.

B. MEDICAL TREATMENT

1. β-Adrenergic blocking agents—These agents serve as adjunct specific antithyroid therapies. They can rapidly ameliorate the symptoms of hyperthyroidism (nervousness, tremor, and palpitations) and are indicated in severe disease with cardiovascular abnormalities (tachycardia and hypertension). β_1-Specific agents such as atenolol are preferred because they are more cardioselective.

2. Antithyroid agents (propylthiouracil [PTU] and methimazole)—These drugs interfere with thyroid hormone synthesis, and in large doses PTU also inhibits the peripheral conversion of T_4 to T_3. Antithyroid agents are frequently used in the initial treatment of hyperthyroidism in children. It takes a few weeks to see a clinical response, adequate control may take 2–3 months, and treatment usually must be continued for at least 18–24 months. If medical therapy is unsuccessful in providing a sustained remission after this time, more definitive therapy, such as radioablation of the thyroid or thyroidectomy, should be considered.

a. Initial dosage—Methimazole is initiated at a dose of 10–60 mg/d, depending on severity of hyperthyroidism. It can be given once a day. PTU dosing is 10 times that for methimazole (150–600 mg/d) in three divided doses. Initial dosing is continued until FT_4 or T_4 have normalized and signs and symptoms have subsided.

b. Maintenance—The optimal dose of antithyroid agent for maintenance treatment remains somewhat unclear. Recent studies suggest that 10–15 mg/d of methimazole or 100–150 mg/d of PTU provide adequate long-term control in most patients with a minimum of side effects. If the TSH becomes elevated, many providers decrease the dose of the antithyroid agent. Some providers continue the same dose of antithyroid agent and add exogenous thyroid hormone replacement in this situation.

c. Toxicity—Rash, arthralgia, granulocytopenia, and hepatitis may occur. The drug must be discontinued, and antibiotics and a short course of corticosteroids should be prescribed if indicated.

3. Iodide—Iodide, in large doses, usually produces a rapid but short-lived blockade of thyroid hormone synthesis and release. It is generally recommended only for acute management of severely thyrotoxic patients.

C. RADIATION THERAPY

In radioactive iodine therapy, (^{131}I) is administered orally and concentrates in the thyroid, resulting in ablation of the gland. Radioablation is usually reserved for children with Graves disease associated with poor response to antithyroid agents, the development of adverse effects from the antithyroid agents, the lack of remission after several years of medical therapy, or poor medication adherence. However, some pediatric endocrinologists advocate radioablation as first-line therapy for children with Graves disease. Antithyroid agents should be discontinued 4–7 days prior to radioablation to allow radioiodine uptake by the thyroid. In the first 2 weeks following radioablation, hyperthyroidism may worsen as thyroid tissue is destroyed and thyroid hormone is released. Therapy with a β-adrenergic antagonist may be necessary for up to 4 months until FT_4 and T_4 fall into the normal range. In most cases, hypothyroidism develops and thyroid hormone replacement is needed. Long-term follow-up studies have not shown any increased incidence of thyroid cancer, leukemia, infertility, or birth defects when ablative doses of ^{131}I were used.

D. SURGICAL TREATMENT

Subtotal and total thyroidectomy are infrequently used to treat Graves disease in children. They are usually reserved for cases in whom definite therapy is indicated but the goiter is very large or associated with a suspicious nodule, the patient is very young or pregnant, or the family refuses radioiodine ablation. A β-adrenergic blocking agent should

be given to ameliorate the symptoms, and antithyroid agents should be given for several weeks prior to surgery to minimize the surgical risk from hyperthyroidism. In addition, iodide (eg, Lugol's solution 1 drop every 8 hours or saturated solution of potassium iodide 1–2 drops daily) should be given for 1–2 weeks prior to surgery in order to reduce thyroid vascularity and inhibit the release of thyroid hormone. Complications from surgery include hypoparathyroidism, recurrent laryngeal nerve damage, and death. It is crucial to have an experienced thyroid surgeon to minimize these complications. After thyroidectomy, the majority of children become hypothyroid and need thyroid hormone replacement.

Course & Prognosis

In children with Graves disease, improvement rarely occurs without therapy, but partial remissions and exacerbations may continue for several years. Treatment with an antithyroid agent results in prolonged remissions in one-third to two-thirds of children.

Cooper DS: Antithyroid drugs in the management of patients with Graves' disease: An evidence-based approach to therapeutic controversies. J Clin Endocrinol Metab 2003;88:3474 [PMID: 12915620].

Cooper DS: Hyperthyroidism. Lancet 2003;362:459 [PMID: 12927435].

Dotsch J et al: Graves disease in childhood: a review of the options for diagnosis and treatment. Paediatr Drugs 2003;5:95 [PMID: 12529162].

Read CH et al: A 36-year retrospective analysis of the efficacy and safety of radioactive iodine in treating young Graves' patients. J Clin Endocrinol Metab 2004;89:4229 [PMID: 15356012].

Management of Neonatal Graves Disease

Hyperthyroidism may develop several days after birth, especially if the mother was treated with PTU, which crosses the placenta. As a result, thyroid studies should be obtained at birth and repeated within the first week. Immediate management should focus on the cardiac manifestations. Temporary treatment may be necessary with iodide, antithyroid agents, β-adrenergic antagonists, and/or steroids. The hyperthyroidism gradually resolves over 1–3 months as maternal antibodies decline.

Polak M et al: Fetal and neonatal thyroid function in relation to maternal Graves' disease. Best Pract Res Clin Endocrinol Metab 2004;18:289 [PMID: 15157841].

Radetti G et al: Fetal and neonatal thyroid disorders. Minerva Pediatr 2002;54:383 [PMID: 12244277].

THYROID CANCER

Thyroid cancer is rare in childhood. Children usually present with a thyroid nodule or an asymptomatic asymmetrical neck mass. Dysphagia, hoarseness, and respiratory difficulty are unusual but may occur. Thyroid function tests are usually normal. A "cold" nodule is often seen on a technetium or radioiodine scan of the thyroid. Fine-needle aspirate or biopsy of the nodule may assist in the diagnosis.

The most common form of thyroid cancer is papillary thyroid carcinoma, a well-differentiated carcinoma that derives from the thyroid follicular cell. Children frequently present with local metastases to the cervical lymph nodes and occasionally with pulmonary metastasis. Despite its aggressive presentation, papillary thyroid carcinoma in children is associated with a relatively good prognosis, with a 20-year survival rate over 90%. Treatment consists of total or near-total thyroidectomy and removal of all involved lymph nodes. This is usually followed by radioiodine ablation to destroy the residual thyroid remnant and any metastatic tissue left behind after surgery. Thyroid hormone replacement is then started to suppress TSH and prevent stimulation of residual thyroid tissue. Since papillary thyroid carcinoma in children is associated with a high rate of recurrence, regular interval follow-up with serum thyroglobulin levels (a tumor marker) and radioiodine whole body scans are required.

Less common malignant tumors of the thyroid include follicular thyroid carcinoma, medullary thyroid carcinoma, anaplastic carcinoma, lymphoma, and sarcoma. Medullary thyroid carcinoma, due to autosomal dominant mutations in the RET proto-oncogene, arises from the C cells of the thyroid gland which secrete calcitonin and is associated with elevated serum calcitonin. It can occur sporadically or can be inherited in multiple endocrine neoplasia (MEN) type 2 and familial medullary thyroid carcinoma. In affected kindreds, all members should be screened for the mutation, and those identified with the mutation should be treated with prophylactic thyroidectomy in early childhood.

Bentley AA et al: Evaluation and management of a solitary thyroid nodule in a child. Otolaryngol Clin North Am 2003;36:117 [PMID: 12803013].

Hung W, Sarlis NJ: Current controversies in the management of pediatric patients with well-differentiated nonmedullary thyroid cancer: A review. Thyroid 2002;12:683 [PMID: 12225637].

Leboulleux S et al: Follicular cell-derived thyroid cancer in children. Horm Res 2005;63:145 [PMID: 15802922].

■ DISORDERS OF CALCIUM HOMEOSTASIS

Serum calcium concentration is tightly regulated by the coordinated actions of the parathyroid glands, kidney,

liver, and small intestine. Low serum calcium levels stimulate parathyroid hormone (PTH) release from the parathyroid glands. PTH in turn promotes release of calcium and phosphorus from bone, resorption of calcium from urinary filtrate, and excretion of phosphorus in the urine. PTH also activates the 1-hydroxylation of 25-hydroxylated vitamin D (made in the liver from dietary or endogenous vitamin D) to $1,25\text{-}(OH)_2$ vitamin D. The primary effect of $1,25\text{-}(OH)_2$ vitamin D is to promote the absorption of calcium from the intestines, though it also facilitates urinary and bone calcium and phosphorus handling in concert with PTH. Deficiencies or excesses of these agents, as well as abnormalities in their receptors or of vitamin D metabolism, lead to clinical disturbances described in the following section. Though calcitonin can reduce serum calcium concentration, it is not clinically relevant and is not discussed further.

HYPOCALCEMIC DISORDERS

A normal serum calcium concentration is 8.9–10.1 mg/dL or an ionized level of 1.2–1.4 mg/dL. Levels in newborns are slightly lower, whereas premature infants may have levels as low as 7 mg/dL. Because 50–60% of calcium in the serum is protein-bound, direct determination of ionized calcium level may be helpful in conditions with low serum protein or abnormal protein binding, such as acidosis.

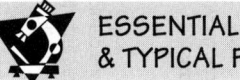

ESSENTIALS OF DIAGNOSIS & TYPICAL FEATURES

- *Tetany with facial and extremity numbness, tingling, cramps, spontaneous muscle contractures, carpopedal spasm, positive Trousseau and Chvostek signs, loss of consciousness, convulsions.*

- *Diarrhea, prolongation of electrical systole (QT interval), and laryngospasm.*

- *In hypoparathyroidism or pseudohypoparathyroidism: defective nails and teeth, cataracts, and ectopic calcification in the subcutaneous tissues and basal ganglia.*

General Considerations

Hypocalcemia is a consistent feature of conditions such as hypoparathyroidism, pseudohypoparathyroidism, transient tetany of the newborn, and severe vitamin D–deficiency rickets and may be present in rare disorders of vitamin D action. Hypocalcemia may also occur in malabsorption, chronic renal disease, tumor lysis syndrome, or rhabdomyolysis (Table 30–5).

Table 30–5. Hypocalcemia associated with rickets and other disorders.

Condition	Pathogenesis	Disease States/ Inheritance	Clinical Features	Biochemical Findings			
				Serum Calcium	Serum Phosphorus	Serum Alkaline Phosphatase	Other
Malabsorption	Impairment in intestinal absorption in any or all of the following: calcium, vitamin D, and magnesium	Cystic fibrosis, celiac disease, sprue, Shwachman syndrome	Failure to thrive, poor weight gain, steatorrhea, superimposed vitamin D–deficiency rickets.	Low or normal	Low or normal	Variable, may be low with concomitant zinc deficiency	Potentially low magnesium levels, potentially low 25-OH vitamin D
Chronic renal insufficiency	Decreased renal phosphate excretion, decreased 1-hydroxylase activity	Obstruction, glomerulonephritis, dysplastic kidneys	Uremia, growth failure, acidosis	Low or normal	Elevated	Elevated or normal	Elevated PTH levels in longstanding cases, low 1,25-OH vitamin D
Rhabdomyolysis	Muscle damage with liberation of large amounts of intracellular phosphate	Crush injuries of muscles, Pompe disease, carnitine deficiency	Hypocalcemic tetany, cardiac arrhythmia, risk of renal failure	Low	Elevated	Normal	Myoglobinuria
Tumor lysis syndrome	Release of intracellular phosphate and potassium	Initiation of chemotherapy for ALL, Burkitt lymphoma, or other malignancies	Hypocalcemic tetany, cardiac arrhythmia, risk of renal failure	Low	Elevated	Normal	Hyperkalemia, elevated uric acid
Vitamin D–deficiency rickets	Deficient dietary vitamin D intake, vitamin D malabsorption, other risk factors include dark skin and lack of sunlight exposure	May cluster in families due to various risk factors	Characteristic skeletal changes appear early, poor growth, symptomatic hypocalcemia is a late finding	Normal until late in course	Low or normal	Elevated	Elevated PTH levels, low 25-OH vitamin D
Vitamin D–refractory rickets–type I	Mutation in 1-hydroxylase enzyme required for synthesis of fully active 1,25-OH vitamin D	Autosomal recessive inheritance	Skeletal changes of rickets, symptomatic hypocalcemia	Low	Low or normal	Elevated	Elevated PTH, low 1,25-OH vitamin D
Vitamin D–refractory rickets–type II	Mutation in 1,25-OH vitamin D receptor	Autosomal recessive inheritance	Severe skeletal changes of rickets, total alopecia, symptomatic hypocalcemia	Low	Low or normal	Elevated	Elevated PTH, elevated 1,25-OH vitamin D
Hypophosphatemic rickets	Excessive loss of phosphate in the urine, ? abnormal humoral factor	X-linked dominant	Skeletal changes primarily in the lower extremities—genu varum or valgus, short stature	Normal or low	Very low	Usually normal	Normal PTH levels, abnormally high urinary phosphate excretion

PTH, parathyroid hormone; ALL, acute lymphoblastic leukemia.

Hypoparathyroidism may be idiopathic or may result from autoimmunity. Table 30–6 summarizes the findings in various disorders of parathyroid hormone secretion or action. Autoimmune parathyroid destruction with subsequent hypoparathyroidism may be isolated, or associated with other autoimmune disorders in the APECED syndrome (autoimmune polyendocrinopathy-candidiasis-ectodermal dystrophy, or APS-1). Hypoparathyroidism may also result from congenital absence of the parathyroid glands, as in DiGeorge syndrome. Other features of this disorder include congenital absence of the thymus (with resultant thymus-dependent immunologic deficiency) and cardiovascular anomalies.

Autosomal dominant hypocalcemia is associated with a gain-of-function mutation in the calcium receptor, resulting in low serum PTH despite hypocalcemia, and excessive urinary loss of calcium. A family history of hypocalcemia may provide a clue to differentiate this condition from other forms of hypoparathyroidism.

Hypoparathyroidism may develop following thyroidectomy, with either acute or insidious onset, and may be transient or permanent. Parathyroid deficiency following irradiation of the neck or the administration of therapeutic doses of radioactive iodine for carcinoma of the thyroid has also been reported.

Transient neonatal hypoparathyroidism, also known as transient tetany of the newborn, is caused by a relative deficiency of PTH or hormone action (see Table 30–6). There are two forms of this condition. The early form occurs within the first 2 weeks of life in newborns with a history of birth asphyxia or in those born to mothers with diabetes mellitus or hyperparathyroidism. Hypomagnesemia may occur in the early form and augments the severity of hypocalcemia. The late form occurs after 2 weeks and has been associated with infant formulas high in phosphate.

Both tumor lysis syndrome and rhabdomyolysis involve cellular destruction with liberation of large amounts of intracellular phosphate that subsequently complex with serum calcium.

Malabsorption states result in hypocalcemia by impairing absorption of calcium, vitamin D, and magnesium (see Table 30–6). Hypomagnesemia, due to losses from the gastrointestinal tract or kidney, may cause or augment the severity of hypocalcemia by impairing the release of PTH.

Rickets describes a characteristic radiographic appearance, including metaphyseal cupping and irregularity. Vitamin D deficiency caused by lack of sunlight exposure or dietary deficiency is the most common cause of rickets. It is classically described in dark-skinned, breast-fed infants born in the winter months. However, occult vitamin D deficiency may be more common than initially recognized. This concern forms the basis for the recommendation by the American Association of Pediatrics that breast-fed infants receive vitamin D supplementation of 200 IU/d. Rickets can also be caused by several defects in the metabo-

lism of vitamin D (see Table 30–6), including liver disease (with impaired 25-hydroxylation of vitamin D), kidney disease [with impaired 1-hydroxylation of 25-(OH) vitamin D], an inherited deficiency of 1α-hydroxylase (vitamin D–dependent rickets type 1), or end-organ resistance to vitamin D (vitamin D–dependent rickets type 2).

Familial hypophosphatemic rickets (vitamin D–resistant rickets) has skeletal findings similar to those of vitamin D–related rickets; however, the basic defect in this condition is abnormal renal phosphate loss. Dietary deficiency of calcium may also be an important cause of rickets.

Gartner LM, Greer FR: Prevention of rickets and vitamin D deficiency: New guidelines for vitamin D intake. Pediatrics 2003; 111:908 [PMID: 12671133].

Jan de Beur SM, Levine MA: Molecular pathogenesis of hypophosphatemic rickets. J Clin Endocrinol Metab 2002;87:2467 [PMID: 12050201].

Ladhani S et al: Presentation of vitamin D deficiency. Arch Dis Child 2004;89:781 [PMID 15269083].

Umpaichitra V, Bastian W, Castells S: Hypocalcemia in children: pathogenesis and management. Clin Pediatr (Phila) 2001;40:305 [PMID 11824172].

Clinical Findings

A. Symptoms and Signs

Prolonged hypocalcemia causes tetany, photophobia, blepharospasm, and diarrhea. The symptoms of tetany include numbness, cramps, and twitching of the extremities; carpopedal spasm and laryngospasm; a positive Chvostek sign (tapping of the face in front of the ear produces spasm of the facial muscles); unexplained bizarre behavior; irritability; loss of consciousness; convulsions; and retarded physical and mental development. Headache, vomiting, increased intracranial pressure, and papilledema may occur. In early infancy, respiratory distress may be the presenting finding.

B. Laboratory Findings

Calcium levels may be low or normal (see Tables 30–5 and 30–6). Phosphate levels may be low, normal, or high depending on the cause of the hypocalcemia. Magnesium levels may also be low. PTH levels are elevated in the hypocalcemic conditions, with the notable exception of hypoparathyroidism. Markedly elevated serum PTH may be associated with pseudohypoparathyroidism (see following discussion). Measurement of urinary excretion of calcium and phosphate can assist in diagnosis and monitoring of therapy.

C. Imaging

Soft tissue and basal ganglia calcification may occur in idiopathic hypoparathyroidism and pseudohypoparathyroidism. A variety of skeletal changes are associated

Table 30-6. Disorders of parathyroid hormone secretion or action.

Condition	Pathogenesis	Inheritance Pattern	Clinical Features	Biochemical Findings			
				Serum Calcium	Serum Phosphorus	Serum Alkaline Phosphatase	Serum PTH
Isolated hypoparathyroidism	Trauma, surgical destruction, isolated autoimmune destruction, rare familial forms	None; reports in familial forms of inheritance as X-linked recessive, autosomal recessive, or autosomal dominant	Symptoms of hypocalcemia	Low	High	Normal/Low	Low
DiGeorge syndrome	Deletion in chromosome 22	Majority represent new mutations	Symptoms of hypocalcemia, cardiac anomalies, immune disorder	Low	High	Normal/Low	Low
APS type I	Autoimmune destruction	Autosomal recessive	Mucocutaneous candidasis, Addison disease, potential for autoimmune destruction in other endocrine glands	Low	High	Normal/Low	Low
PHP type IA	Mutation in stimulatory G protein; resistance to PTH action	Autosomal dominant	AHO phenotype, variable hypocalcemia, may have resistance to other hormones using G protein signaling	Low or normal	Elevated or normal	Variable	Elevated
PPHP	Mutation in stimulatory G protein	Autosomal dominant—frequently found within same families with PHP type IA	AHO phenotype, biochemical parameters are normal	Normal	Normal	Normal	Normal
Transient tetany of the newborn—early onset	Defiency in PTH secretion and/or action	Sporadic—associated with difficult deliveries, infants of diabetic mothers, or maternal hyperparathyroidism	Onset of symptoms of hypocalcemia within 2 wk of birth	Low	Normal or low	Normal or low	Normal or low
Transient tetany of the newborn—late onset	Defiency in PTH secretion and/or action	Sporadic—associated with infant formulas that had a high phosphate content	Onset of symptoms of hypocalcemia after 2 wk of age	Low	Normal or low	Normal or low	Normal or low
Autosomal dominant hypocalcemia	Gain of function mutation of calcium receptor	Autosomal dominant	Symptoms of hypocalcemia family history	Low	High	Normal/Low	Low

PTH, parathyroid hormone; APS, autoimmune polyglandular syndrome; PHP, pseudohypoparathyroidism; PPHP, pseudopseudohypoparathyroidism; AHO, Albright hereditary osteodystrophy.

with rickets, including cupped and irregular appearance at the metaphysis of the long bones. Torsional deformities can result in genu varum (bowleg). Accentuation of the costochondral junction gives the rachitic rosary appearance seen on the chest wall.

Differential Diagnosis

Tables 30–5 and 30–6 outline the features of disorders associated with hypocalcemia. An artifactually low total serum calcium level may be seen with low serum albumin, and measurement of ionized calcium is advised in these cases.

Treatment

A. Acute or Severe Tetany

The objective of treatment is to correct hypocalcemia immediately by the administration of intravenous calcium. Calcium gluconate and calcium chloride 10 mg/kg are generally used for acute treatment. To avoid cardiac arrhythmia, intravenous calcium infusions should not exceed 50 mg/min. Cardiac monitoring should be performed during the infusion.

B. Maintenance Management of Hypoparathyroidism or Chronic Hypocalcemia

The objective of treatment is to maintain the serum calcium and serum phosphate at approximately normal levels without excessive urinary calcium excretion.

1. Diet—In addition to a diet high in calcium, calcium supplements are generally required. A starting dosage of 50–75 mg of elemental calcium per kilogram of body weight per day divided in three to four doses is used as initial management and should be titrated based on serum calcium levels and urinary calcium excretion. Therapy should be monitored to prevent hypercalcemia and its complications (see section on monitoring). Often, supplemental calcium can be decreased or discontinued after vitamin D therapy has stabilized.

2. Vitamin D supplementation—A variety of vitamin D preparations are available for treatment. Ergocalciferol (vitamin D_2) and calcitriol (1,25-dihydroxyvitamin D_3) are used in the majority of cases. Ergocalciferol is the preferred agent for the treatment of vitamin D deficiency. However, impaired metabolism of vitamin D to its active end product 1,25-$(OH)_2$ vitamin D, or impaired function of PTH requires supplementation with calcitriol. Selection and dosage of a vitamin D supplement vary with the condition to be treated and the patient's response to therapy. As with calcium supplementation, monitoring of therapy is essential to avoid toxicity.

3. Monitoring—Dosages of calcium and vitamin D must be tailored for each patient. Monitoring serum calcium, urine calcium, and serum alkaline phosphatase levels at 1- to 3-month intervals is necessary to ensure adequacy of therapy and to prevent hypercalcemia and nephrocalcinosis.

Basic goals in monitoring therapy include the following: (1) maintenance of serum calcium and phosphorus concentrations within normal ranges; (2) normalization of alkaline phosphatase concentrations for age; (3) regression of skeletal changes, if present; and (4) maintenance of spot urine calcium:creatinine ratio between 0.1 and 0.3 (0.05–0.15 if calcium is measured in milliequivalents per liter).

Hypophosphatemic rickets is an exception, since the monitoring goals are somewhat different. Serum calcium and alkaline phosphatase should be maintained within normal limits; however, phosphorus levels should be corrected only to the low normal range. Monitoring of serum PTH level is necessary to ensure that secondary hyperparathyroidism does not develop from excessive phosphate treatment or inadequate calcitriol replacement.

PSEUDOHYPOPARATHYROIDISM (Resistance to Parathyroid Hormone Action)

In pseudohypoparathyroidism (PHP), PTH production is adequate; however, target organs (renal tubule, bone, or both) fail to respond. This receptor resistance to PTH action is due to a heterozygous inactivating mutation in the stimulatory G protein subunit associated with the PTH receptor, which leads to impaired signaling. Resistance to other G protein–dependent hormones may also be present.

Several types of PHP have been identified, with variable biochemical and phenotypic features (see Table 30–6). PHP has biochemical abnormalities similar to hypoparathyroidism with hypocalcemia and hyperphosphatemia. However, PTH levels are elevated. It may be accompanied by a characteristic phenotype known as Albright hereditary osteodystrophy, which includes short stature; round, full facies; irregularly shortened fourth metacarpal; a short, thick-set body; delayed and defective dentition; and mild mental retardation. Corneal and lenticular opacities and ectopic calcification of the basal ganglia and subcutaneous tissues may occur with or without abnormal serum calcium levels. Treatment is the same as that for hypoparathyroidism.

Pseudopseudohypoparathyroidism (PPHP) describes individuals with the Albright hereditary osteodystrophy phenotype, but normal calcium homeostasis. PHP and PPHP can occur in the same cohort. Genomic imprinting is thought to be responsible for the differential phenotypic expression of disease, with heterozygous loss of maternal allele associated with PHP and heterozygous loss of paternal allele associated with PPHP.

Weinstein LS et al: Minireview: GNAS: normal and abnormal functions. Endocrinology 2004;145:5459 [PMID: 15331575].

HYPERCALCEMIC STATES

Hypercalcemia is defined as a serum level greater than 11 mg/dL. Severe hypercalcemia is defined as a level above 13.5 mg/dL.

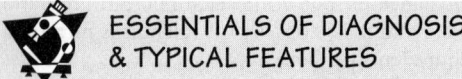

ESSENTIALS OF DIAGNOSIS & TYPICAL FEATURES

- *Abdominal pain, polyuria, polydipsia, hypertension, nephrocalcinosis, failure to thrive, renal stones, intractable peptic ulcer, constipation, uremia, and pancreatitis.*
- *Bone pain or pathologic fractures. Subperiosteal resorption on radiograph, renal parenchymal calcification or stones, and osteitis fibrosa cystica (brown tumors).*
- *Impaired concentration, altered mental status, mood swings, coma.*
- *Hypercalcemia and mild hyperparathyroidism noted as incidental findings in routine laboratory screening.*

General Considerations

More than 80% of hypercalcemic children or adolescents have either hyperparathyroidism or a malignant tumor as the underlying cause. Table 30–7 summarizes the differential diagnosis of childhood hypercalcemia.

Hyperparathyroidism is rare in childhood and may be primary or secondary. The most common cause of primary hyperparathyroidism is a parathyroid adenoma. Diffuse parathyroid hyperplasia or multiple adenomas have also been described in families. Familial hyperparathyroidism may be an isolated disease, or it may be associated with multiple endocrine neoplasia, usually type 1, and rarely type 2A. Hypercalcemia of malignancy can be associated with either solid or hematologic malignancies and is due to local destruction of bone by tumor infiltration or ectopic secretion of PTH-related protein. When ectopic PTH-related protein is present, calcium is elevated, serum PTH is suppressed, and serum PTH-related protein is elevated. Chronic renal disease with impaired phosphate excretion is the most common secondary cause of hyperparathyroidism.

Kollars J et al: Primary hyperparathyroidism in pediatric patients. Pediatrics 2005;115:974 [PMID: 15805373].

Table 30–7. Hypercalcemic states.

A. Primary hyperparathyroidism
 1. Parathyroid hyperplasia
 2. Parathyroid adenoma
 3. Familial, including MEN types 1 and 2
 4. Ectopic PTH secretion
B. Hypercalcemic states other than primary hyperparathyroidism associated with increased intestinal or renal absorption of calcium
 1. Hypervitaminosis D (including idiopathic hypercalcemia of infancy)
 2. Familial hypocalciuric hypercalcemia
 3. Lithium therapy
 4. Sarcoidosis
 5. Phosphate depletion
 6. Aluminum intoxication
C. Hypercalcemic states other than hyperparathyroidism associated with increased mobilization of bone minerals
 1. Hyperthyroidism
 2. Immobilization
 3. Thiazides
 4. Vitamin A intoxication
 5. Malignant neoplasms
   a. Ectopic PTH secretion or PTH-related protein
   b. Prostaglandin-secreting tumor and perhaps prostaglandin release from subcutaneous fat necrosis
   c. Tumors metastatic to bone
   d. Myeloma

MEN, multiple endocrine neoplasia; PTH, parathyroid hormone.

Clinical Findings

A. SYMPTOMS AND SIGNS

1. Due to hypercalcemia—Hypotonicity and weakness of muscles; apathy, mood swings, and bizarre behavior; nausea, vomiting, abdominal pain, constipation, and weight loss; hyperextensibility of joints; and hypertension, cardiac irregularities, bradycardia, and shortening of the QT interval. Coma occurs rarely. Calcium deposits in the cornea or conjunctiva (band keratopathy) may occur and are detected by slitlamp examination of the eye. Intractable peptic ulcer and pancreatitis occur in adults but rarely in children.

2. Due to increased calcium and phosphate excretion—Loss of renal concentrating ability with polyuria, polydipsia, precipitation of calcium phosphate in the renal parenchyma or as urinary calculi, and progressive renal damage.

3. Due to changes in the skeleton—Bone pain, osteitis fibrosa cystica, subperiosteal absorption of the distal clavicles and phalanges, absence of lamina dura around the teeth, spontaneous fractures, and a moth-eaten appearance of the skull on radiograph. Later, there is generalized demineralization with a predilection for subperiosteal cortical bone.

B. IMAGING

Bone changes may be subtle in children. Technetium sestamibi scintigraphy is preferred over conventional procedures such as ultrasonography, computed tomography (CT), and MRI for localizing parathyroid tumors.

Treatment

A. SYMPTOMATIC

Initial management consists of vigorous hydration with normal saline and forced calcium diuresis using a loop diuretic such as furosemide (1 mg/kg given every 6 hours). In cases of inadequate response to initial intervention, treatment with glucocorticoids or calcitonin may be helpful. Bisphosphonates, standard agents for the management of acute hypercalcemia in adults, are being used with increasing frequency for cases of refractory pediatric hypercalcemia.

B. CHRONIC

Treatment options vary depending on the condition. Removal of a parathyroid adenoma or subtotal removal of hyperplastic parathyroid glands is the preferred treatment. Postoperatively, hypocalcemia due to the rapid remineralization of chronically calcium-deprived bones may occur. A diet high in calcium and vitamin D is recommended immediately postoperatively and is continued until serum calcium concentrations are normal and stable. Treatment of secondary hyperparathyroidism from chronic renal disease is primarily directed at controlling serum phosphorus levels with phosphate binders. Pharmacologic doses of calcitriol are used to suppress PTH secretion.

Long-term therapy for hypercalcemia of malignancy is the treatment of the underlying disorder.

Course & Prognosis

The prognosis following removal of a single adenoma is excellent. The prognosis following subtotal parathyroidectomy for diffuse hyperplasia or removal of multiple adenomas is usually good and depends on correction of the underlying defect. In patients with multiple sites of parathyroid adenoma or hyperplasia, MEN is likely, and other family members may be at risk. Genetic counseling and DNA analysis to determine the specific gene defect are indicated.

FAMILIAL HYPOCALCIURIC HYPERCALCEMIA (Familial Benign Hypercalcemia)

Familial hypocalciuric hypercalcemia is distinguished by low to normal urinary calcium excretion as a result of high renal reabsorption of calcium. PTH is normal or slightly elevated.

In most cases, the gene defect has been identified as a mutation in the membrane-bound calcium-sensing receptor expressed on parathyroid and renal tubule cells. It is inherited as an autosomal dominant trait with high penetrance. There is a low rate of new mutations. The majority of patients are asymptomatic, and treatment is unnecessary. A severe form of symptomatic neonatal hyperparathyroidism may occur in infants homozygous for the receptor mutation.

Hypervitaminosis D

Vitamin D intoxication is almost always the result of ingestion of excessive amounts of vitamin D, some forms of which may be stored for months in adipose tissue.

Signs, symptoms, and treatment of vitamin D–induced hypercalcemia are the same as those in other hypercalcemic conditions.

Treatment depends on the stage of hypercalcemia. Severe hypercalcemia requires hospitalization and aggressive intervention. Due to the storage of vitamin D in the adipose tissue, several months of a low-calcium, low–vitamin D diet may be required.

IDIOPATHIC HYPERCALCEMIA OF INFANCY (Williams Syndrome)

Williams syndrome is an uncommon disorder of infancy characterized in its classic form by elfin-appearing facies and hypercalcemia in infancy. Other features include failure to thrive, mental and motor retardation, cardiovascular abnormalities (primarily supravalvular aortic stenosis), irritability, purposeless movements, constipation, hypotonia, polyuria, polydipsia, and hypertension. A gregarious and affectionate personality is the rule in older children with the syndrome. Hypercalcemia may not appear until several months after birth. Treatment consists of rigid restriction of dietary calcium and vitamin D, and in severe cases, moderate doses of glucocorticoids.

A defect in the metabolism of, or responsiveness to, vitamin D is postulated as the cause of Williams syndrome. Elastin deletions localized to chromosome 7 have been identified in over 90% of patients; thus, fluorescent in-situ hybridization analysis may be the best initial diagnostic tool. The risk of hypercalcemia generally resolves by age 4, and dietary restrictions can be relaxed.

Morris CA, Mervis CB: Williams syndrome and related disorders. Annu Rev Genomics Hum Genet 2000;1:461 [PMID: 11701637].

IMMOBILIZATION HYPERCALCEMIA

Abrupt immobilization, particularly in a rapidly growing adolescent, is a risk factor for hypercalcemia. Hypercalcemia and hypercalciuria often appear 1–3 weeks after immobilization. Medical or dietary intervention may be required in severe cases.

HYPOPHOSPHATASIA

Hypophosphatasia is an uncommon autosomal recessive condition characterized by a deficiency of alkaline phosphatase activity in serum, bone, and tissues. The deficiency of this enzyme leads to inadequate skeletal mineralization with clinical and radiographic features similar to rickets. Six different clinical forms have been identified. The perinatal form is characterized by severe skeletal deformity and death that occurs within a few days. The infantile form includes failure to thrive, hypotonia, and craniosynostosis. The childhood form has variable skeletal findings, reduced bone mineral density, and is associated with premature loss of deciduous teeth. Serum calcium levels may be elevated. The diagnosis of hypophosphatasia is made by demonstrating elevated levels of urinary phosphoethanolamine associated with low serum alkaline phosphatase.

Therapy is generally supportive. Children who survive the neonatal period may experience an improvement in severity of disease. Calcitonin may be of value for the temporary treatment of hypercalcemia.

◼ THE GONADS (Ovaries & Testes)

DEVELOPMENT & PHYSIOLOGY

The fetal gonads develop from bipotential anlagen in the genital ridge. In addition to gonadal tissue, both müllerian and wolffian structures are present and have the potential to differentiate into components of the internal reproductive structures. Table 30–8 summarizes the male and female structures arising from müllerian and wolffian ducts. The Y chromosome, specifically the *SRY* gene region of the chromosome, promotes testicular differentiation of the bipotential gonads. Once testicular differentiation has been determined, the fetal testis produces two substances critical for further male differentiation. Antimüllerian hormone promotes the regression of müllerian structures, and the rising concentrations of testosterone

Table 30–8. Sexual differentiation in the female and male.

Internal duct derivatives

Müllerian duct derivatives	Wolffian duct derivatives[a]
Fallopian tubes (oviducts) and fimbriae	Epididymis
	Vas deferens
Uterus	Seminal vesicles
Cervix	Ejaculatory duct
Vagina (posterior two thirds)	Prostatic urethra

External genitalia homologues

Primitive structure	Female genitalia	Male genitalia[b]
Undifferentiated gonad	Ovary	Testis
Genital tubercle	Clitoris	Glans penis
Genital swelling	Labia majora	Scrotum
Genital/urethral fold	Labia minora	Penile urethra/corpora

[a]Normal wolffian duct development is dependent on the local production of testosterone by Leydig cells of the adjacent testis and on testosterone's diffusion into the surrounding embryonic tissues. Thus females with congenital adrenal hyperplasia who are virilized as the result of circulating androgens do not have wolffian duct development. Normal male development is also dependent on regression of müllerian duct derivatives through the local action of müllerian inhibiting factor elaborated by the Sertoli cells of the adjacent testis.

[b]The normal development of male external genitalia is dependent on an adequate circulating concentration of testosterone, which is then further converted to dihydrotestosterone in the target tissues through the action of the enzyme 5α-reductase. Significantly elevated circulating concentrations of other (adrenal) androgens, as in females with congenital adrenal hyperplasia, can virilize the genital tubercle, and cause genital swelling and genital/urethral folds along the lines of their male homologues, resulting in varying degrees of female pseudohermaphroditism (ambiguity) (see text).

stimulate growth of wolffian derivatives into male internal structures. Dihydrotestosterone (DHT), formed by 1α-reductase action on testosterone, is primarily responsible for virilization of the external genitalia. In the absence of both antimüllerian hormone and testosterone, differentiation into female internal and external genitalia occurs.

AMBIGUOUS GENITALIA IN THE NEWBORN

A variety of abnormalities in chromosomal allocation, gonadal differentiation, gonadal function, testosterone synthesis and action, or adrenal function can lead to aberrant development of internal and external genital structures. These abnormalities can be divided into four categories.

Abnormalities in Normal Gonadal Differentiation

These abnormalities usually result from an abnormality in the number of sex chromosomes. Klinefelter syndrome (see Chapter 32), with a 47,XXY karyotype, is associated with a male phenotype but with poorly functioning testes. Turner syndrome, with a 45,XO karyotype (see Chapter 32), is associated with a female phenotype but with streak ovaries (gonadal dysgenesis) or premature ovarian failure. The phenotype is less severe if mosaicism or only partial absence of an X chromosome occurs. Mosaic forms of gonadal dysgenesis that contain a Y-bearing cell line have variable ambiguous internal and external phenotypes. Idiopathic testicular failure prior to completion of sexual differentiation results in ambiguous genitalia (incomplete virilization). True hermaphroditism, with the presence of both testicular and ovarian tissue, is rare and associated with external genitalia that range from fully masculine to almost completely feminine.

Abnormalities in Testosterone Synthesis or Action

These disorders generally present as micropenis, genital ambiguity, or complete absence of male external genitalia in an XY individual (Figure 30–6). Testicular tissue is present and produces antimüllerian hormone; therefore, internal structures are wolffian. Disorders in this category include enzymatic defects in testosterone synthesis (such as 12-ketoreductase deficiency) or defects in conversion of testosterone to DHT (5α-reductase deficiency). If the enzyme defect is incomplete, the external genitalia may masculinize at puberty when testosterone production increases. Since the gonads and adrenal gland share common enzymes of steroid hormone production, some of the enzymatic defects associated with male genital ambiguity may also affect production of cortisol and aldosterone, leading to cortisol deficiency and salt wasting. Defects in testosterone action result from absent or defective androgen receptors (androgen insensitivity) and, depending on the resultant degree of defect in androgen binding, the genital phenotype can range from relatively mild male ambiguity to complete female external development.

Disorders of Adrenal Androgen Production

These disorders can cause genital ambiguity in both XY and XX individuals. Excessive adrenal androgen production secondary to an enzyme defect in cortisol synthesis (ie, congenital adrenal hyperplasia, described in a later section) is the cause of 95% of inappropriate virilization in 46,XX newborns. An enzyme defect in adrenal androgen, cortisol, and aldosterone production (3β-hydroxysteroid dehydrogenase deficiency) is a rare cause of genital ambiguity in XY individuals.

Miscellaneous Syndromes

Various syndromes, such as VATER (vertebral defects, anal atresia, tracheoesophageal fistula with esophageal atresia, and radial and renal anomalies), WAGR (Wilms tumor, aniridia, genitourinary malformations, and mental retardation), Denys-Drash, and Smith-Lemli-Opitz, have a wide variety of congenital anomalies, including genital ambiguity. Maternal exposure to androgens or androgen antagonists is a rare cause of genital ambiguity in newborns.

Brown J, Warne G: Practical management of the intersex infant. J Pediatr Endocrinol Metab 2005;18:3 [PMID: 15679065].

MacLaughlin DR, Donahoe PK: Sex determination and differentiation. N Engl J Med 2004;350:367 [PMID: 14736929].

MacGillivray MH, Mazur T: Intersex. Adv Pediatr 2005;52:295 [PMID: 16124345].

ABNORMALITIES IN FEMALE PUBERTAL DEVELOPMENT & OVARIAN FUNCTION

1. Precocious Puberty in Girls

Precocious puberty is defined as pubertal development occurring below the limits of age set for normal onset of puberty. Puberty is considered precocious in girls if the onset of secondary sexual characteristics occurs before 8 years of age. Precocious puberty is more common in girls than in boys. This disparity is explained by the large number of girls with central idiopathic precocity, a condition that is unusual in boys. Girls between 6 and 8 years of age may also show signs of puberty but it can be a benign, slowly progressing form that requires no intervention. The age of pubertal onset may also be advanced by obesity.

Central (gonadotropin-releasing hormone [GnRH]-dependent) precocious puberty involves activation of the hypothalamic GnRH pulse generator, an increase in gonadotropin secretion, and a resultant increase in the production of sex steroids (Table 30–9). Consequently, the sequence of hormonal and physical events in central precocious puberty is identical to the progression of normal puberty. Central precocious puberty in girls is generally idiopathic but may be secondary to a demonstrable central nervous system (CNS) abnormality that disrupts the prepubertal restraint on the GnRH pulse generator. Such CNS abnormalities may include, but are not limited to, hypothalamic hamartomas, CNS tumors, cranial irradiation, hydrocephalus, and trauma. Peripheral precocious puberty (GnRH-independent) occurs independent of gonadotropin secretion. In girls, peripheral precocious puberty can be caused by ovarian or adrenal tumors, ovarian cysts, congenital adrenal hyperplasia, McCune-Albright syndrome, or exogenous

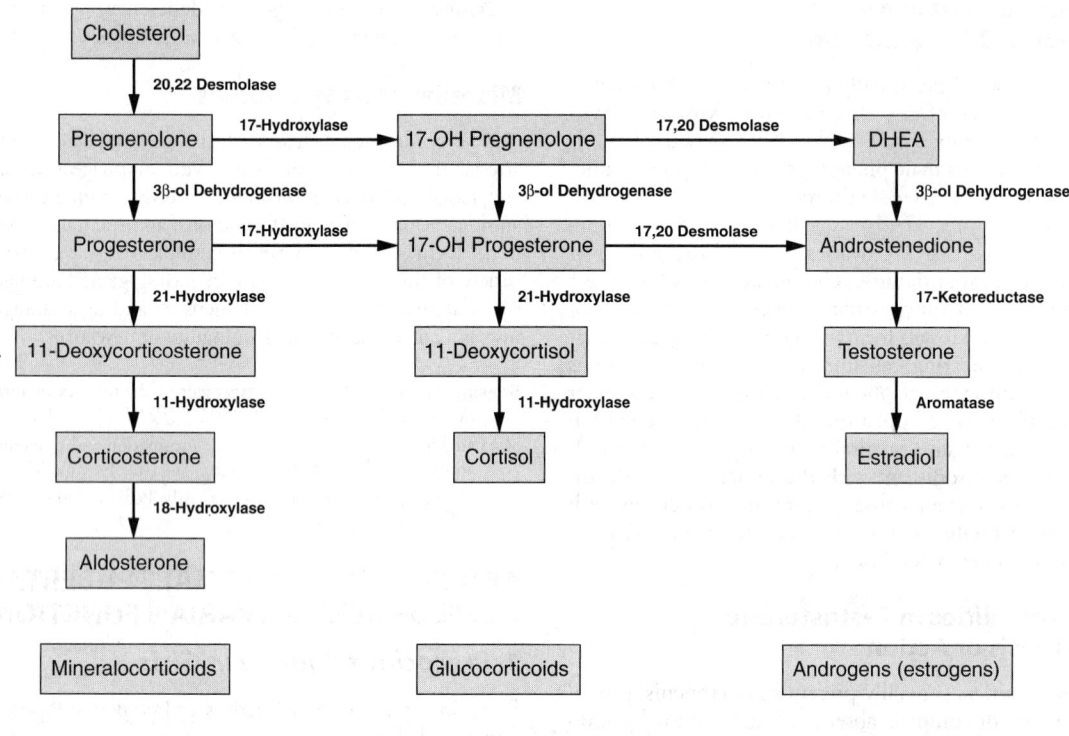

Figure 30–6. The corticosteroid hormone synthetic pathway. The pathways illustrated are present in differing amounts in the steroid-producing tissues: adrenal glands, ovaries, and testes. In the adrenal glands, mineralo-corticoids from the zona glomerulosa, glucocorticoids from the zona fasciculata, and androgens (and estro-gens) from the zona reticularis are produced. The major adrenal androgen is androstenedione, because the ac-tivity of 17-ketoreductase is relatively low. The adrenal gland does secrete some testosterone and estrogen, however. The pathways leading to the synthesis of mineralocorticoids and glucocorticoids are not present to any significant degree in the gonads; however, the testes and ovaries each produce both androgens and es-trogens. Further metabolism of testosterone to dihydrotestosterone occurs in target tissues of the action of the enzyme 5α-reductase. DHEA, dehydroepiandrosterone.

estrogen. McCune-Albright syndrome is a triad consisting of irregular café-au-lait lesions, polyostotic fibrous dysplasia, and GnRH-independent precocious puberty. It is caused by an activating mutation in the gene that encodes the α-subunit of G_s, the G-protein that stimulates adenyl cyclase. Consequently, endocrine cells with this mutation have autonomous hyperfunction and secrete excess amounts of their respective hormones.

Clinical Findings

A. Symptoms and Signs

Normal sexual development and precocity in girls usually starts with breast development, followed by pubic hair growth and menarche, but the order may vary. The inter-val between breast development and menarche can range from 1–6 years but is usually about 2 years. Girls with ovarian cysts or tumors will generally have signs of estrogen excess such as breast development and possibly vaginal bleeding. Adrenal tumors or congenital adrenal hyperplasia will present with signs of adrenarche (ie, pubic hair, axillary hair, acne, and/or increased body odor). Children with pre-cocious puberty usually have accelerated growth and may appear tall during childhood. However, because skeletal maturation (bone age) advances at a more rapid rate than linear growth, final adult stature may be compromised.

B. Laboratory Findings

One of the first steps in evaluating a child with early pubertal development is obtaining a radiograph of the left

Table 30–9. Causes of precocious pubertal development.

A. Central (GnRH-dependent) precocious puberty
  1. Constitutional (idiopathic)
  2. Hypothalamic lesions (hamartomas, tumors, congenital malformations)
  3. Dysgerminomas
  4. Hydrocephalus
  5. CNS infections
  6. CNS trauma, irradiation
  7. Pineal tumors (rare)
  8. Neurofibromatosis with CNS involvement
  9. Tuberous sclerosis
B. Peripheral (GnRH-independent) precocious puberty
  1. Congenital adrenal hyperplasia
  2. Adrenal tumors
  3. McCune-Albright syndrome (polyostotic fibrous dysplasia)
  4. Familial Leydig cell hyperplasia (testotoxicosis)—males
  5. Gonadal tumors
  6. Exogenous estrogen—oral (contraceptive pills) or topical
  7. Ovarian cysts (females)
  8. HCG-secreting tumors (eg, hepatoblastomas, choriocarcinomas) (males)

CAH, congenital adrenal hyperplasia; CNS, central nervous system; GnRH, gonadotropin-releasing hormone; HCG, human chorionic gonadotropin.

hand and wrist to determine skeletal maturity (bone age). If the bone age is advanced, further evaluation is typically warranted. In central precocious puberty, the basal serum concentrations of FSH and LH may still be in the prepubertal range. Thus documentation of the maturity of the hypothalamic-pituitary axis depends on demonstrating a pubertal LH response after stimulation with a GnRH agonist. In peripheral precocious puberty, basal serum FSH and LH are low, and the LH response to GnRH stimulation is suppressed as a result of feedback inhibition of the hypothalamic-pituitary axis by the autonomously secreted gonadal steroids (see Figure 30–1). In girls who have an ovarian cyst or tumor, estradiol levels will be markedly elevated. In girls who present with signs of adrenarche and an advanced bone age, androgen levels and possible adrenal intermediate metabolites (such as 17-hydroxyprogesterone) should be measured.

C. IMAGING

Once the diagnosis of central precocious puberty is made, an MRI of the brain should be done to evaluate for CNS lesions. It is unlikely that an abnormality will be found in girls between 6 and 8 years of age, so the need for an MRI in this age group should be individually assessed. In girls whose labs suggest peripheral precocious puberty, an ultrasound of the ovaries and/or adrenal gland should be considered.

Benign Variants of Precocious Puberty

Premature thelarche (benign early breast development) occurs most commonly between ages 12 and 36 months. It is often bilateral but may begin or remain as unilateral breast enlargement. In the absence of other signs of pubertal development (eg, accelerated growth rate or skeletal maturation, pubic hair, or vaginal mucosal maturation), no laboratory evaluation is necessary. Treatment consists of reassurance regarding the self-limited nature of this condition, but observation of the child at regular intervals (eg, twice a year) is also useful. Onset of thelarche after age 3 or in association with other signs of puberty requires more evaluation.

Premature adrenarche (benign early adrenal maturation) is manifested by gradual increase in pubic hair and body odor, and less commonly, axillary hair and acne. The average age at onset is 5–6 years. No increase in growth rate or skeletal maturation occurs, and no abnormal virilization (eg, clitoromegaly) is present. No treatment is required, though girls with premature adrenarche are at risk for developing polycystic ovarian syndrome later on during puberty.

Treatment

Girls with central precocious puberty can be treated with GnRH analogs, such as leuprolide. GnRH analogs downregulate pituitary GnRH receptors and thus decrease gonadotropin secretion. With treatment, physical changes of puberty regress or cease to progress, and linear growth slows down to a prepubertal rate. Projected final heights often increase as a result of slowing of skeletal maturation. Usually, GnRH analogs are given as a monthly depot intramuscular injection, and side effects are rare. After discontinuation of therapy, pubertal progression resumes, and in girls ovulation and pregnancy have been documented. Therapy is considered for both psychosocial and final height considerations. Treatment for peripheral precocious puberty is dependent on the underlying cause. In a girl who has an ovarian cyst, intervention is generally not necessary, as the cyst usually regresses spontaneously. For congenital adrenal hyperplasia, treatment with glucocorticoids would be initiated. Surgical resection is indicated for the rare adrenal or ovarian tumor.

In McCune-Albright syndrome, analogs of GnRH are not initially helpful. Therapy with antiestrogens (eg, tamoxifen) or agents that block estrogen synthesis (eg, ketoconazole or testolactone), or both, may be effective. Regardless of the cause of precocious puberty or the medical therapy selected, attention to the psychological needs of the patient and family is essential.

de Sanctis C et al: Pubertal development in patients with McCune-Albright syndrome or pseudohypoparathyroidism. J Pediatr Endocrinol Metab 2003;16(Suppl 2):293 [PMID: 12729407].

Gillis D, Schenker J: The evolving story of female puberty. Gynecol Endocrinol 2002;16:163 [PMID: 12012628].

Partsch CJ et al: Management and outcome of central precocious puberty. Clin Endocrinol (Oxf) 2002;56:129 [PMID: 11874402].

2. Delayed Puberty

Delayed puberty in girls should be evaluated if there are no pubertal signs by age 13 years or menarche by 15.5–16 years. Also, lack of completion of pubertal development to Tanner stage V within 4 years is considered delay. Primary amenorrhea refers to the absence of menarche and secondary amenorrhea refers to the cessation of established menses for at least 6 months.

Differential Diagnosis

The most common cause of delayed puberty is constitutional growth delay (Table 30–10). This growth pattern is reviewed earlier and characterized by short stature, normal growth velocity, and a delay in skeletal maturation. In this growth pattern, the timing of puberty is commensurate with bone age, not chronologic age. Girls may also have delayed puberty from any condition that delays growth and skeletal maturation, such as hypothyroidism, and growth hormonedeficiency.

Table 30–10. Cause of delayed puberty/amenorrhea.

A. Constitutional growth delay

B. Hypogonadism
1. Primary ovarian insufficiency
   a. Gonadal dysgenesis (Turner syndrome, true gonadal dysgenesis)
   b. Premature ovarian failure
      (1) Autoimmune disease
      (2) Surgery, radiation, chemotherapy
   c. Galactosemia
2. Central hypogonadism
   a. Hypothalamic or pituitary tumor, infection, irradiation
   b. Congenital hypopituitarism
   c. Kallmann syndrome
   d. Functional (chronic illness, undernutrition, exercise, hyperprolactinemia

C. Anatomic
1. Müllerian agenesis (Mayer-Rokitansky-Küster-Hauser syndrome)
2. Complete androgen resistance

Primary hypogonadism in girls refers to a primary abnormality of the ovaries. The most common diagnosis in this category is Turner syndrome, in which the lack of or an abnormal X chromosome leads to early loss of oocytes and accelerated stromal fibrosis. Other types of primary ovarian insufficiency are less common and include 46,XY gonadal dysgenesis, 46,XX gonadal dysgenesis, galactosemia, and autoimmune ovarian failure. Radiation and chemotherapy can also cause primary ovarian insufficiency.

Central hypogonadism refers to a hypothalamic or pituitary deficiency of GnRH or FSH/LH, respectively. Central hypogonadism can be functional, or reversible, and due to stress, undernutrition, prolactinemia, exercise, or chronic illness. Permanent central hypogonadism is typically associated with conditions that cause multiple pituitary hormone deficiencies such as congenital hypopituitarism, CNS tumors, or cranial irradiation. Isolated gonadotropin deficiency is rare but may occur in Kallman syndrome, which may be associated with anosmia. In either primary or central hypogonadism, signs of adrenarche are generally present.

Delayed menarche or secondary amenorrhea may result from lack of gonadotropin or ovarian failure, or may be the consequence of hyperandrogenism, anatomic obstruction precluding menstrual outflow, or müllerian agenesis. This latter disorder is called Mayer-Rokitansky-Küster-Hauser syndrome and is characterized by an absent vagina and various uterine abnormalities, with or without renal and skeletal anomalies.

Complete androgen insensitivity syndrome (androgen receptor defect) may be manifested as primary amenorrhea because the affected individual (46,XY) has functioning testes that produce müllerian-inhibiting hormone during fetal life. Thus no müllerian duct (oviduct or uterus) development occurs, but external sexual characteristics appear female because of the aromatization of testosterone to estrogen. Girls with this disorder develop breasts at the appropriate age but have amenorrhea and lack of sexual hair.

Evaluation

The history should include whether and when puberty commenced, level of exercise, nutritional intake, presence of stressors, sense of smell, symptoms of chronic illness, and family history of delayed puberty. Growth patterns should be assessed to determine if growth velocity and weight gain have been appropriate. Physical examination should focus on body proportions, breast and genital development, and stigmata of Turner syndrome. A pelvic exam or pelvic ultrasound should be considered, especially in a girl presenting with primary amenorrhea.

Prior to any laboratory testing, a bone age radiograph should be obtained. If the patient has not attained a bone age consistent with pubertal onset (ie, > 12 years in girls), further evaluation should focus on determining the cause of the bone age delay. If there is short stature and normal growth velocity, growth rate is normal and constitutional growth delay is likely. If growth rate is abnormal, laboratory studies may include a complete blood count, erythrocyte sedimentation rate, chemistry panel, and renal and liver function tests to screen for undiagnosed chronic medical illness. Evaluation for hypothyroidism and growth hormone deficiency may also be indicated. Measurement of FSH and LH will not be helpful in this setting since prepubertal levels are normally low. Determination of a karyotype should be considered if there is short stature, or any stigmata of Turner syndrome.

If the patient has attained a bone age consistent with onset of puberty and there are minimal or no signs of puberty on physical exam, determination of FSH and LH will distinguish between primary ovarian failure and central hypogonadism. Primary ovarian failure is also referred to as hypergonadotropic hypogonadism, as there is lack of estrogen feedback to the brain, resulting in elevations of FSH and consequently, if gonadotropins are elevated, a karyotype is the next step in the evaluation process, as Turner syndrome is the most common cause of hypergonadotropic hypogonadism in girls. Central hypogonadism is characterized by low gonadotropin levels and subsequent evaluation is geared toward determining if the hypogonadism is functional or permanent. In this setting, laboratory tests to evaluate for chronic disease and hyperprolactinemia and a cranial MRI may be helpful.

In a girl who presents with adequate breast development and amenorrhea, a progesterone challenge may be helpful to determine if sufficient estrogen is being produced. Girls who are producing estrogen will have a withdrawal bleed after 5–10 days of oral progesterone, whereas those who are estrogen deficient have no or very little bleeding. The exception is for girls with an absent uterus (androgen insensitivity or Mayer-Rokitansky-Küster-Hauser syndrome), as they have sufficient estrogen but will not have a withdrawal bleed. The most common cause of amenorrhea in girls who are making sufficient estrogen is polycystic ovarian syndrome. Girls who are estrogen deficient should be evaluated similarly to those who have delayed puberty.

Treatment

Replacement therapy in hypogonadal girls is begun with estrogen alone at the lowest available dosage. Cyclic estrogen-progesterone therapy is started 12–18 months later, and this can be given as a low-dose birth control pill. Progesterone therapy is needed to counteract the effects of estrogen on the uterus, as unopposed estrogen can promote endometrial hyperplasia. Estrogen is also necessary for normal bone mineralization and to prevent osteoporosis.

Hoffman B, Bradshaw KD: Delayed puberty and amenorrhea. Semin Reprod Med 2003;21:353 [PMID: 14724768].

Kaplowitz P: Precocious puberty: update on secular trends, definitions, diagnosis, and treatment. Adv Pediatr 2004;51:37 [PMID: 15366770].

Sybert VP, McCauley E: Turner's syndrome. N Engl J Med 2004; 351:1227 [PMID: 15371580].

Secondary Amenorrhea

See Chapter 3, on adolescence.

OVARIAN TUMORS

Ovarian tumors are not rare in children. They may occur at any age and are usually large, benign, and unilateral, and they may be producing estrogen. Ovarian tumors account for about 1% of cases of female sexual precocity. The most common estrogen-producing tumor is the granulosa cell tumor. Other tumors causing sexual precocity include thecomas, luteomas, mixed types, theca-lutein and follicular cysts, and ovarian tumors (teratomas, choriocarcinomas, and dysgerminomas). Ovarian tumors are usually palpated on rectal examination and are seen readily by ovarian ultrasonography. Treatment is surgical removal. Recurrences are uncommon.

ABNORMALITIES IN MALE PUBERTAL DEVELOPMENT & TESTICULAR FUNCTION

1. Precocious Puberty in Boys

Puberty is considered precocious in boys if secondary sexual characteristics appear before age 9 years. Precocious puberty appears to be much less common in boys than in girls. In boys presenting with sexual precocity, pseudoprecocious (peripheral, GnRH-independent) puberty is as common as true (central, GnRH-dependent) precocious puberty. In addition, boys with true precocious puberty are more likely to have an identifiable pathologic process (eg, CNS abnormality) than are girls. Early studies that documented this, however, included large numbers of girls aged 6–8 years of age in whom only minimal signs of breast development and a slowly-progressive pubertal course were seen. In retrospect, these girls were probably normal variants. In general, the younger the child presents with precocious puberty, the more likely a CNS abnormality can be detected.

Two primary GnRH-independent forms of precocious puberty have been described in boys: McCune-Albright syndrome (described previously) and familial Leydig cell hyperplasia, or testotoxicosis, a condition in which a mutated LH receptor on the Leydig cell is autonomously activated, resulting in testicular production of testosterone despite prepubertal LH concentrations.

Clinical Findings

A. Symptoms and Signs

In precocious development, increases in growth rate and growth of pubic hair are the most common presenting signs. Testicular size may differentiate true precocity, in which the testes enlarge, from pseudoprecocity (most commonly due to a virilizing form of congenital adrenal hyperplasia [CAH], such as 21- or 11-hydroxylase deficiency), in which the testes usually remain small. Some exceptions do occur—for example, testicular enlargement may occur in pseudoprecocity of long-standing due to secondary activation of central precocity from prolonged elevation of androgen levels, as in poorly controlled CAH. Tumors of the testis are associated with asymmetrical testicular enlargement.

B. Laboratory Findings

Basal serum LH and FSH concentrations are usually not in the pubertal range in boys with true sexual precocity, but the LH response to GnRH stimulation testing is pubertal (> 8 IU/L). Sexual precocity caused by CAH is usually associated with abnormal plasma concentrations of dehydroepiandrosterone, androstenedione, 17-hydroxyprogesterone (in CAH due to 21-hydroxylase deficiency), 11-deoxycortisol (in CAH due to 11-hydroxylase deficiency), or a combination of these steroids (see section on the adrenal cortex). Serum β-human chorionic gonadotropin (β-HCG) concentrations can identify the presence of an HCG-producing tumor (eg, CNS dysgerminoma or hepatoma) in boys who present with apparent true isosexual precocity (ie, accompanied by testicular enlargement) but suppressed gonadotropins following GnRH testing.

C. Imaging

Diagnostic studies are similar to those used to evaluate sexual precocity in girls. Ultrasonography may be useful in detecting hepatic, presacral, and testicular tumors.

Differential Diagnosis

The causes of isosexual precocity are outlined in Table 30–9. It is particularly important to differentiate pseudoprecocity from true sexual precocity. Seventy percent of boys with pseudoprecocious puberty have an adrenal enzyme abnormality (virilizing CAH). Of boys with true precocious puberty, 70% have benign CNS mass lesions. Premature adrenarche (described earlier) may occur in males as well as females.

Treatment

Treatment of idiopathic true precocious puberty in boys is similar to that in girls (see previous discussion). Treatment of McCune-Albright syndrome or familial Leydig cell hyperplasia with agents that block steroid synthesis (eg, ketoconazole), with an antiandrogen (eg, spironolactone), or a combination of both has been successful. Estrogen antagonists (eg, tamoxifen) or aromatase inhibitors (eg, anastrazole or letrazole) have been used to delay skeletal maturation and early epiphyseal closure.

2. Delayed Puberty

Lack of development of secondary sexual characteristics after age 14 years suggests abnormal testicular maturation. Although delay of puberty until age 14 years may be physiologically normal, boys generally become concerned if pubertal changes do not occur by then, and evaluation should be initiated at that time. Hypogonadism may be difficult to differentiate from constitutionally delayed puberty. Although the latter may be associated with a delay in testicular function, normal puberty occurs at a later date.

Testicular failure or insufficiency may be primary, resulting from the absence, malfunction, or destruction of testicular tissue, or secondary (central), due to pituitary or hypothalamic insufficiency. Primary testicular failure may be due to anorchia, Klinefelter syndrome or other sex chromosome abnormalities, enzymatic defects in testosterone synthesis, or inflammation and destruction of the testes following infection (eg, mumps), autoimmune disorders, radiation (in the treatment of leukemia), trauma, or tumor.

Secondary testicular failure may accompany panhypopituitarism, empty-sella syndrome, Kallmann syndrome (GnRH deficiency accompanied by anosmia), or isolated LH or FSH deficiencies. Destructive lesions in or near the anterior pituitary, especially craniopharyngiomas, gliomas, or infection, may also result in hypothalamic or pituitary dysfunction. Prader-Willi syndrome and Laurence-Moon syndrome (Bardet-Biedl syndrome) are frequently associated with LH and FSH deficiency secondary to GnRH deficiency. Miscellaneous causes of secondary testicular failure include chronic debilitating disease and hypothyroidism.

Clinical Findings

A. Symptoms and Signs

Physical examination may not be helpful in differentiating primary from secondary testicular insufficiency. Whereas cryptorchidism suggests primary testicular failure, hypothalamic or pituitary insufficiency as well as anatomic abnormalities may also lead to failure of testicular descent.

B. LABORATORY FINDINGS

In primary testicular failure, the plasma testosterone concentration is low, whereas LH and FSH values are elevated into the castrate range in children who have attained a pubertal skeletal age. In secondary testicular failure, circulating concentrations of all three hormones are below normal for age. To establish the presence of the testes and their ability to respond to stimulation, 1500 units of HCG may be given intramuscularly on days 1, 3, and 5. The plasma testosterone concentration should rise to > 200 mg/dL 24 hours after the final dose. A karyotype should be determined in primary testicular failure of unknown cause.

C. IMAGING

Skeletal maturation is usually delayed. A cranial CT scan or MRI should be performed in cases of secondary testicular failure.

TREATMENT

Specific therapy is indicated when the cause of testicular failure is known. Boys with simple constitutional delay may be offered a short (4–6 months) course of low-dose depot testosterone (75–100 mg/month) to stimulate their pubertal appearance and "jump-start" their endogenous development. In adolescents with permanent hypogonadism, treatment with depot testosterone, beginning with 75–100 mg intramuscularly each month, may be used until growth is complete. Thereafter, more adult dosing (150–200 mg every 2–3 weeks) may be used. A recent alternative to intramuscular injections is testosterone in gel, either as individual packets or in a pump that dispenses a preset dose of gel. This must be applied daily, usually after showering. Specific therapy for GnRH deficiency (eg, pulsatile subcutaneous delivery of GnRH) may result in fertility in patients with hypothalamic-pituitary insufficiency. However, the inconvenience and need for ongoing use to be effective has limited usefulness in pediatrics.

3. Cryptorchidism

Cryptorchidism (undescended testis) is a common disorder in children. It may be unilateral or bilateral and may be classified as ectopic or true cryptorchidism. Approximately 3% of full-term male newborns have an undescended testis at birth, with a higher proportion among premature infants. In over 50% of these patients, the cryptorchid testis descends by the third month; by age 1 year, 80% of all undescended testes are in the scrotum. Further descent may occur through puberty, the latter perhaps stimulated by endogenous gonadotropins.

Infertility and testicular malignancy risk must be considered in cases of cryptorchidism. The exact incidence of impairment in fertility is unknown and incidence figures vary in reported studies. However, histologic changes clearly occur as early as age 6 months in children with undescended testes. The reported malignancy rate in the cryptorchid testis is 48.9 per 100,000, which is 22 times higher than that seen in the general population. In addition, 25% of tumors develop in the contralateral testis, indicating that abnormality of testicular development (dysgenesis) may be bilateral in unilateral cryptorchidism. Ectopic testes are presumed to develop normally but are diverted as they descend through the inguinal canal. In most cases, true cryptorchidism is thought to be the result of testicular dysgenesis. Cryptorchid testes frequently have a short spermatic artery, poor blood supply, or both. Although early scrotal positioning of these testes (orchidopexy) will obviate further damage related to intra-abdominal location, the testes generally remain abnormal, spermatogenesis is rare, and the risk of malignant neoplasm is increased. These testes should probably be removed if spermatogenesis does not occur after a reasonable period of observation.

Cryptorchidism can occur in an isolated fashion or may be associated with other findings. Abnormalities in the hypothalamic-pituitary-gonadal axis predispose to cryptorchidism. Androgen biosynthesis or receptor defects may also predispose to cryptorchidism and undervirilization.

The diagnosis of bilateral cryptorchidism in an apparently male newborn should never be made until ruling out the possibility that the child is actually a fully virilized female with potentially fatal salt-losing CAH (see section on the adrenal cortex).

Clinical Findings

Plasma testosterone concentrations may be obtained after HCG stimulation to confirm the presence or absence of abdominal testes (see preceding section).

Differential Diagnosis

In palpating the testis, the cremasteric reflex may be elicited, causing the testis to be retracted into the inguinal canal or abdomen (pseudocryptorchidism). To prevent retraction, the fingers first should be placed across the abdominal ring and the upper portion of the inguinal canal, obstructing ascent. Examination while the child is in the squatting position or in a warm bath is also helpful. No treatment for retractile testes is necessary, and the prognosis for testicular descent and competence is excellent.

Treatment

A. SURGICAL TREATMENT

The current recommendation for treatment of cryptorchidism is that surgical orchidopexy be performed by an experienced surgeon if no descent has occurred by 1 year of age.

B. HORMONAL TREATMENT

Various treatment regimens have been used, ranging from 250–1000 IU HCG given twice weekly for 5 weeks. Such therapy will generally cause descent of retractile testes, but is generally not successful in treating cryptorchidism. Androgen treatment (eg, depot testosterone) is indicated as replacement therapy in the male child who lacks functional testes beyond the normal age of puberty.

4. Gynecomastia

Adolescent gynecomastia is a common, self-limited finding in boys that may occur in up to 75% of normal boys during puberty. Adolescent gynecomastia typically resolves within 2 years, but may not totally resolve if the degree of gynecomastia is extreme. Gynecomastia may sometimes occur as part of Klinefelter syndrome, or it may occur in boys who are taking drugs such as antidepressants or marijuana. Therapy, either medical (antiestrogens or aromatase inhibitors) or surgical, should be considered in cases that are prolonged or severe. This topic is discussed in more detail in Chapter 3.

TESTICULAR TUMORS

The major malignant tumors of the testis are seminomas and teratomas. Seminomas are rare in childhood; they may be hormone-producing. The major hormone-producing tumor of the testis is the Leydig cell tumor. It is frequently associated with sexual precocity. Other testicular tumors (choriocarcinomas and dysgerminomas) have been reported in association with sexual precocity.

Treatment of testicular tumors is surgical removal; chemotherapy and radiation therapy are not used in childhood unless a high-grade malignancy or metastasis is present. The prognosis in patients with Leydig cell tumors is generally good.

Grumbach MM: The neuroendocrinology of human puberty revisited. Horm Res 2002;57(Suppl 2):2 [PMID: 12065920].

Kaplowitz P: Precocious puberty: update on secular trends, definitions, diagnosis, and treatment. Adv Pediatr 2004;51:37 [PMID: 15366770].

Leung AK, Robson WL: Current status of cryptorchidism. Adv Pediatr 2004;51:351 [PMID: 15366780].

■ ADRENAL CORTEX

The adult adrenal cortex displays relative regional specificity of terminal steroid production. The outermost zona glomerulosa is the predominant source of aldosterone, ~reas the zona fasciculata makes cortisol, the major glu-

cocorticoid, as well as small amounts of mineralocorticoids. The innermost zona reticularis produces mainly androgens and estrogens. During fetal life, a fetal zone, or provisional cortex, predominates. This fetal zone produces glucocorticoids, mineralocorticoids, androgens, and estrogens, but is relatively deficient in 3β-ol dehydrogenase (see Figure 30–6). Therefore, placentally-produced progesterone serves as the major precursor for the fetal adrenal production of cortisol and aldosterone.

The adrenal cortex produces cortisol under the control of pituitary corticotropin (adrenocorticotropic hormone; ACTH) (see Figure 30–1 and Table 30–1), which is in turn regulated by corticotropin-releasing hormone (CRH), a hypothalamic peptide. The complex interaction of CNS influences on CRH secretion coupled with negative feedback of serum cortisol leads to a distinct diurnal pattern of ACTH and cortisol release. ACTH concentrations are greatest during the early morning hours, display a smaller peak in the late afternoon, and are lowest during the night. The pattern of serum cortisol concentration closely follows with a lag of a few hours. In the absence of cortisol feedback, both CRH and ACTH display dramatic hypersecretion.

Glucocorticoids are critical for normal gene expression in a wide variety of cells. In excess, glucocorticoids are both catabolic and antianabolic; that is, they promote the release of amino acids from muscle and increase gluconeogenesis while decreasing incorporation of amino acids into muscle protein. They also antagonize insulin action and facilitate lipolysis. Glucocorticoids help maintain blood pressure through their supportive effect on peripheral vascular tone and by promoting sodium and water retention.

Mineralocorticoids (primarily aldosterone in humans) promote sodium retention and stimulate potassium excretion in the distal tubule. Although ACTH can stimulate aldosterone production, the predominant regulator of aldosterone secretion is the volume- and sodium-sensitive renin-angiotensin-aldosterone system. Elevations of serum potassium concentrations also directly influence aldosterone release from the cortex.

Androgen (dehydroepiandrosterone and androstenedione) production by the zona reticularis is insignificant in prepubertal children. At the onset of puberty, androgen production increases and may be an important factor in the dynamics of puberty in both sexes. The adrenal gland is a major source of androgen in the pubertal and adult female.

ADRENOCORTICAL INSUFFICIENCY (Adrenal Crisis, Addison Disease)

The leading causes of adrenal insufficiency today are hereditary enzymatic defects (congenital adrenal hyperplasia), autoimmune destruction of the glands (Addison disease), and central adrenal insufficiency following an intracranial neoplasm or its treatment, or congenital midline defects in association with optic nerve hypoplasia (septooptic dysplasia). A rare form of familial adrenal insufficiency can occur in association with cerebral sclerosis and spastic paraplegia (adrenoleukodystrophy). Addison disease may be familial and has been described in association with hypoparathyroidism, candidiasis, hypothyroidism, pernicious anemia, hypogonadism, and diabetes mellitus as one of the polyglandular autoimmune syndromes. Less commonly, the gland is destroyed by tumor, calcification, or hemorrhage (Waterhouse-Friderichsen syndrome). Adrenal disease secondary to opportunistic infections (fungal or tuberculous) is again being reported in adults who have acquired immunodeficiency syndrome. A similar relationship is likely in children. In children, central adrenal insufficiency due to a primary anterior pituitary tumor is rare. A temporary salt-losing disorder due to partial mineralocorticoid deficiency or renal underresponsiveness (pseudohypoaldosteronism) may occur during infancy or with pyelonephritis.

Any acute illness, surgery, trauma, or exposure to excessive heat may precipitate an adrenal crisis in patients with adrenal insufficiency. Patients with primary adrenal insufficiency are generally at greater risk for life-threatening crisis than patients with central ACTH deficiency. This is a consequence of intact mineralocorticoid secretion and low-level autonomous cortisol secretion in central ACTH deficiency.

Clinical Findings

A. SYMPTOMS AND SIGNS

1. Acute form (adrenal crisis)—Manifestations include nausea and vomiting, diarrhea, abdominal pain, dehydration, fever (which may be followed by hypothermia), weakness, hypotension, circulatory collapse, and confusion or coma. Increased pigmentation may be associated with primary adrenal insufficiency as a result of the melanocyte-stimulating activity of the hypersecreted parent molecule of ACTH.

2. Chronic form—Manifestations include fatigue, hypotension, weakness, failure to gain or loss of weight, increased appetite for salt (primary insufficiency), vomiting (which may become forceful and sometimes projectile), and dehydration. Diffuse tanning with increased pigmentation over pressure points, scars, and mucous membranes may be present in primary adrenal insufficiency. A small heart may be seen on chest radiograph.

B. LABORATORY FINDINGS

1. Suggestive of adrenocortical insufficiency—In primary adrenal insufficiency, serum sodium and bicarbonate levels, arterial partial pressure of carbon dioxide, blood pH, and blood volume are decreased. Serum potassium and urea nitrogen levels are increased. Urinary sodium levels and the ratio of sodium to potassium are inappropriate for the degree of hyponatremia. In central adrenal insufficiency, serum sodium levels may be mildly decreased as a result of impaired water excretion. Eosinophilia and moderate lymphopenia may be present in either form of insufficiency.

2. Confirmatory tests—
a. The ACTH (cosyntropin) stimulation test—In primary adrenal insufficiency (ie, originating in the gland itself), plasma cortisol and aldosterone concentrations fail to increase significantly over baseline 60 minutes after an intravenous dose of ACTH (250 μg). To diagnose central adrenal insufficiency, a low dose of ACTH is given (1 μg).

b. Baseline serum ACTH concentrations—These are elevated in primary adrenal failure and are low in central adrenal insufficiency.

c. Urinary free cortisol and 17-hydroxycorticosteroid excretion—These values are decreased.

d. The CRH test—This test can be used to assess responsiveness of the entire hypothalamic-pituitary-adrenal axis. After administration of ovine CRH, serum concentrations of ACTH and cortisol are measured over a period of 2 hours. Verification of the presence of an intact axis or localization of the site of impairment is possible with careful interpretation of these results.

Differential Diagnosis

Acute adrenal insufficiency must be differentiated from severe acute infections, diabetic coma, various disturbances of the CNS, and acute poisoning. In the neonatal period, adrenal insufficiency may be clinically indistinguishable from respiratory distress, intracranial hemorrhage, or sepsis.

Chronic adrenocortical insufficiency must be differentiated from anorexia nervosa, certain muscular disorders (eg, myasthenia gravis), salt-losing nephritis, and chronic debilitating infections (eg, tuberculosis), and must be considered in cases of recurrent spontaneous hypoglycemia.

Treatment

A. ACUTE (ADRENAL CRISIS)

1. Hydrocortisone sodium succinate—Hydrocortisone sodium succinate, initially 50 mg/m^2 intravenously over 2–5 minutes or intramuscularly; thereafter, it is given intravenously, 12.5 mg/m^2, every 4–6 hours until stabilization is achieved and oral therapy can be tolerated.

2. Fluids and electrolytes—In primary adrenal insufficiency, 5–10% glucose in normal saline, 10–20 mL/kg intravenously, is given over the first hour and repeated if necessary to reestablish vascular volume. Normal saline is continued thereafter at one and one-half to two times the maintenance fluid requirements. In addition, intravenous boluses of glucose (10% glucose, 2 mL/kg) may be needed every 4–6 hours for hypoglycemia. In central adrenal insufficiency, routine fluid management is generally adequate following reinstatement of vascular volume and institution of cortisol replacement.

3. Fludrocortisone—When oral intake is tolerated, fludrocortisone, 0.05–0.15 mg daily, is started and continued as necessary every 12–24 hours for primary adrenal insufficiency.

4. Inotropic agents—Rarely, inotropic agents such as dopamine and dobutamine are needed. However, adequate cortisol replacement is critical because pressor agents may be ineffective in adrenal insufficiency.

5. Waterhouse-Friderichsen syndrome with fulminant infections—The use of adrenocorticosteroids and norepinephrine in the treatment or prophylaxis of fulminant infections remains controversial; corticosteroids may augment the generalized Shwartzman reaction in fatal cases of meningococcemia. However, corticosteroids should be considered in the presence of possible adrenal insufficiency, particularly with hypotension and circulatory collapse.

B. Maintenance Therapy

Following initial stabilization, the most effective substitution therapy is hydrocortisone, combined with fludrocortisone in primary adrenal insufficiency. Overtreatment should be avoided because it may result in obesity, growth retardation, and other cushingoid features. Additional hydrocortisone, fludrocortisone, or sodium chloride, singly or in combination, may be necessary with acute illness, surgery, trauma, or other stress reactions.

Supportive adrenocortical therapy should be given whenever surgical operations are performed in patients who have at some time received prolonged therapy with adrenocorticosteroids (see below).

1. Glucocorticoids—A maintenance dosage of 6–10 mg/m^2/d of hydrocortisone (or equivalent) is given orally in two or three divided doses. The dosage of all glucocorticoids is increased to 30–50 mg/m^2/d during intercurrent illnesses or other times of stress.

2. Mineralocorticoids—In primary adrenal insufficiency, give fludrocortisone, 0.05–0.15 mg orally daily as a single dose or in two divided doses. Periodic monitoring of blood pressure is recommended to avoid overdosing.

3. Salt—The child should be given ready access to table salt. Frequent blood pressure determinations in the recumbent position should be made to ensure that hypertension is avoided. In the infant, supplementation of 3–5 mEq Na$^+$/kg/d by adding the injectable solution (4 mg/mL) to formula or breast milk is generally required until table foods are introduced.

C. Corticosteroids in Patients with Adrenocortical Insufficiency Who Undergo Surgery

1. Before operation—Hydrocortisone sodium succinate, 30–50 mg/m^2/d intravenously, is given 1 hour before surgery.

2. During operation—Hydrocortisone sodium succinate, 25–100 mg intravenously, is administered with 5–10% glucose in saline throughout surgery.

3. During recovery—Hydrocortisone sodium succinate, 12.5 mg/m^2 intravenously, is given every 4–6 hours until oral doses are tolerated. The oral dose of three to five times the maintenance dose is continued until the acute stress is over, at which time the patient can be returned to the maintenance dose.

Course & Prognosis

A. Acute Adrenal Insufficiency

The course of acute adrenal insufficiency is rapid, and death may occur within a few hours, particularly in infants, unless adequate treatment is given. Spontaneous recovery is unlikely. Patients who have received long-term treatment with adrenocorticosteroids may exhibit adrenal collapse if they undergo surgery or other acute stress. Pharmacologic doses of glucocorticoids during these episodes may be needed throughout life.

In all forms of acute adrenal insufficiency, the patient should be observed carefully once the crisis has passed and evaluated with laboratory tests to assess the degree of permanent adrenal insufficiency.

B. Chronic Adrenal Insufficiency

Adequately treated, chronic adrenocortical insufficiency is consistent with a normal life.

Eisenbarth GS, Gottlieb PA: Autoimmune polyendocrine syndromes. N Engl J Med 2004;350:2068 [PMID: 15141045].

CONGENITAL ADRENAL HYPERPLASIAS

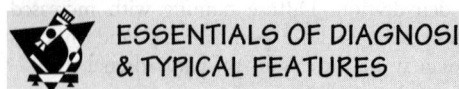

ESSENTIALS OF DIAGNOSIS & TYPICAL FEATURES

- Genital virilization in females, with labial fusion, urogenital sinus, enlargement of the clitoris, or other evidence of androgen action.
- Salt-losing crisis in infant males or isosexual precocity in older males with infantile testes.

- *Increased linear growth; advancement of skeletal maturation.*
- *Elevation of plasma 17-hydroxyprogesterone concentrations in the most common form; may be associated with electrolyte and water disturbances (hyponatremia, hyperkalemia, and metabolic acidosis), particularly in the newborn period.*

General Considerations

Autosomal recessive mutations in enzymes involved in adrenal steroidogenesis lead to impairment in cortisol biosynthesis with resultant increased ACTH secretion during fetal life. ACTH excess subsequently results in adrenal hyperplasia with increased production of various adrenal hormone precursors, including androgens. Increased pigmentation, especially of the scrotum, labia majora, and nipples, frequently results from excessive ACTH secretion. Congenital adrenal hyperplasia (CAH) is most commonly (in > 80% of patients) the result of homozygous 21-hydroxylase (cytochrome P-450 C21) deficiency (see Figure 30–6). In its severe form, excess adrenal androgen production beginning in the first trimester of fetal development results in virilization of the female infant and life-threatening hypovolemic, hyponatremic shock (adrenal crisis) in the newborn. Other enzyme defects that less commonly result in congenital adrenal hyperplasia include 11-hydroxylase, 3β-ol dehydrogenase, 20,22-desmolase, 18-hydroxylase-17, and 22-desmolase deficiencies. The clinical syndromes associated with each of these defects can be predicted from Figure 30–6 and Table 30–11.

Studies of patients with 21-hydroxylase deficiency indicate that the clinical type (salt-wasting versus non–salt-wasting) is usually consistent within a family and that a close genetic linkage exists between the 21-hydroxylase gene and the human leukocyte antigen complex on chromosome 6. The latter finding has allowed more precise heterozygote detection and prenatal diagnosis. Population studies indicate that the defective gene is present in 1:250–1:100 people and that the incidence of the disorder is 1:15,000–1:5000. Mass screening for this enzyme defect, using a microfilter paper technique to measure serum 17-hydroxyprogesterone, has been established in some U.S. states.

Nonclassic presentations of 21-hydroxylase deficiency have been reported with increasing frequency.

Table 30–11. Clinical and laboratory findings in adrenal enzyme defects resulting in congenital adrenal hyperplasia.

Enzyme Deficiency[a]	Urinary 17-Ketosteroids	Elevated Plasma Metabolite	Plasma Androgens	Aldosterone	Hypertension/ Salt Loss	External Genitalia
20,22-Desmolase	↓↓↓	—	↓↓↓	↓↓↓	–/+	Males: ambiguous Females: normal
3β-ol Dehydrogenase	↑↑ (DHEA)	17-OH pregnenolone (DHEA)	↑ (DHEA)	↓↓↓	–/+	Males: ambiguous Females: possibly virilized
17-Hydroxylase	↓↓↓	Progesterone	↓↓	Normal to ↑	+/–	Males: ambiguous Females: normal
21-Hydroxylase[a]	↑↑↑	17-OHP	↑↑	↓↓	–/+	Males: normal Females: virilized
11-Hydroxylase	↑↑	11-Deoxycortisol	↑↑	↓↓ (↑ Deoxycorticosterone)	+/–	Males: normal Females: virilized
17,20-Desmolase	↓↓↓	17-Hydroxysteroids (?)	↓↓	Normal	–/–	Males: ambiguous Females: normal

[a]Children with "simple virilizing (non–salt-wasting)" forms of 21-hydroxylase deficiency congenital adrenal hyperplasia (CAH) may have normal aldosterone production and serum electrolytes, but some children have normal aldosterone production and serum electrolytes at the expense of elevated plasma renin activity and are, by definition, compensated salt-wasters. These children usually receive mineralocorticoid as well as glucocorticoid treatment. Children with 21-hydroxylase deficiency CAH should therefore have documented normal plasma renin activity in addition to normal serum electrolytes before they are considered non–salt-wasters.
DHEA, dehydroepiandrosterone; 17-OHP, 17- hydroxyprogestrone.

Affected persons have a normal phenotype at birth but develop evidence of virilization during later childhood, adolescence, or early adulthood. In these cases, previously referred to as late-onset or acquired enzyme deficiency, results of hormonal studies are characteristic of 21-hydroxylase deficiency. An asymptomatic form has also been identified in which individuals have none of the phenotypic features of the disorder, but have hormonal study results identical to those of patients with nonclassic 21-hydroxylase deficiency. The nonclassic form appears to be less severe than the classic form. Because members of the same family may have classic, nonclassic, and asymptomatic forms, the disorders may be due to allelic variations of the same enzyme.

Clinical Findings

A. SYMPTOMS AND SIGNS

1. In females—The abnormality of the external genitalia may vary from mild enlargement of the clitoris to complete fusion of the labioscrotal folds, forming a scrotum, a penile urethra, a penile shaft, and enlargement of the clitoris to form a normal-sized glans (see Table 30–8). Signs of adrenal insufficiency (salt loss) may be present during the first days of life (typically in the first or second week). In rare cases, adrenal insufficiency does not occur for months or years. When the enzyme defect is milder, salt loss may not occur, and virilization predominates (simple virilizing form). In untreated, non–salt-losing 21-hydroxylase or 11-hydroxylase deficiency, growth rate and skeletal maturation are accelerated, and patients may become muscular. Pubic hair appears early (often before the second birthday), acne may be excessive, and the voice may deepen. Excessive pigmentation may develop. Final adult height is often compromised.

2. In males—The male infant usually appears normal at birth but may present with a salt-losing crisis in the first 2–4 weeks of life. In milder forms, salt-losing crises may not occur. In this circumstance, enlargement of the penis and increased pigmentation may be noted during the first few months. Other symptoms and signs are similar to those seen in females. The testes are not enlarged except in the rare male in whom aberrant adrenal cells (adrenal rests) are present in the testes and produce unilateral or bilateral enlargement, often asymmetrical. In the rare isolated defect of 17,20-desmolase activity, ambiguous genitalia may be present because of impaired androgen production (see Figure 30–6).

B. LABORATORY FINDINGS

1. Blood—Hormonal studies are essential for accurate diagnosis. Findings characteristic of the enzyme deficiencies are shown in Table 30–11.

2. Genetic studies—Rapid chromosomal diagnosis should be obtained in any newborn with ambiguous genitalia.

C. IMAGING

Adrenal ultrasonography, CT scanning, and MRI may be useful in defining pelvic anatomy or enlarged adrenals or in localizing an adrenal tumor. Vaginograms using contrast material and pelvic ultrasonography may be helpful in delineating the internal anatomy in a newborn with ambiguous genitalia.

Treatment

A. MEDICAL TREATMENT

Treatment goals in congenital adrenal hyperplasia consist of normalizing growth velocity and skeletal maturation using the smallest dose of glucocorticoid that will suppress adrenal function. The use of excessive amounts of glucocorticoids results in the undesirable side effects of Cushing syndrome. Mineralocorticoid replacement helps to sustain normal electrolyte homeostasis, although excessive mineralocorticoid dosing results in hypertension.

1. Glucocorticoids—Initially hydrocortisone given in a dosage of 30–50 mg/m^2/d parenterally or orally suppresses abnormal adrenal steroidogenesis within 2 weeks. When adrenal suppression has been accomplished, as evidenced by normalization of serum 17-hydroxyprogesterone, the patients are placed on maintenance doses of 15–20 mg/m^2/d in two or three divided doses. Between 50% and 60% of the daily dose should be given in the late evening to suppress the early morning ACTH rise. Dosage is adjusted to maintain normal growth rate and skeletal maturation. A variety of serum and urine androgens have been used to monitor adequacy of therapy, including 17-hydroxyprogesterone, androstenedione, and urinary pregnanetriol. However, none of these has been universally accepted. In adolescent females, normal menses are a sensitive index of the adequacy of therapy. Therapy should be continued throughout life in both males and females because of the possibility of malignant degeneration of the hyperplastic adrenal gland. In pregnant females who have congenital adrenal hyperplasia, adequate suppression of adrenal androgen secretion is critical to avoid virilization of the fetus, particularly a female fetus.

2. Mineralocorticoids—Fludrocortisone in a dose of 0.05–0.15 mg is given orally once a day or in two divided doses. Periodic monitoring of blood pressure and plasma renin is recommended to adjust dosing.

B. SURGICAL TREATMENT

Consultation with a urologist experienced with female genital reconstruction is indicated in affected females as soon as possible during infancy.

Course & Prognosis

When therapy is initiated in early infancy, abnormal metabolic effects and progression of masculinization can be avoided. Treatment with glucocorticoids permits normal growth, development, and sexual maturation. However, if not adequately controlled, congenital adrenal hyperplasia results in sexual precocity and masculinization throughout childhood. Affected individuals will be tall as children but short as adults because the rate of skeletal maturation is rapid with resultant premature closure of the epiphyses. If treatment is delayed or inadequate until somatic development is over, 12–14 years as determined by skeletal maturation (bone age), true central sexual precocity may occur in males and females.

Patient education stressing lifelong therapy is important to ensure compliance in adolescence and later life.

Virilization and multiple surgical genital reconstructions are associated with a high risk of psychosexual disturbances in female patients. Ongoing psychological evaluation and support is a critical component of care.

Merke DP, Bornstein SR: Congenital adrenal hyperplasia. Lancet 2005;365:2135 [PMID: 15964450].

Speiser PW, White PC: Congenital adrenal hyperplasia. N Engl J Med 2003;349:776 [PMID: 12930931].

ADRENOCORTICAL HYPERFUNCTION
(Cushing Disease, Cushing Syndrome)

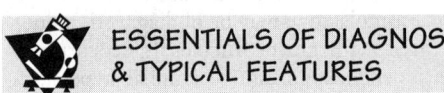

ESSENTIALS OF DIAGNOSIS & TYPICAL FEATURES

- Truncal adiposity with thin extremities, moon facies, muscle wasting, weakness, plethora, easy bruising, purplish striae, decreased growth rate, delayed skeletal maturation.
- Hypertension, osteoporosis, glycosuria.
- Elevated serum corticosteroids; low serum potassium levels; eosinopenia, lymphopenia.

General Considerations

Cushing syndrome may result from excessive secretion of adrenal steroids autonomously (adenoma or carcinoma), from excessive ACTH secretion from the pituitary (Cushing disease) or ectopic sources, or from chronic exposure to pharmacologic doses of exogenous glucocorticoids.

In children younger than 12 years, Cushing syndrome is usually iatrogenic (secondary to pharmacologic doses of ACTH or one of the glucocorticoids). It may rarely be due to an adrenal tumor, adrenal hyperplasia, an adenoma of the pituitary gland, or even more rarely, an extrapituitary (ectopic) ACTH-producing tumor.

Clinical Findings

A. SYMPTOMS AND SIGNS

1. Excess glucocorticoid—Adiposity, most marked on the face, neck, and trunk (a fat pad in the interscapular area is characteristic); fatigue; plethoric facies; purplish striae; easy bruising; osteoporosis; hypertension; glucose intolerance; back pain; muscle wasting and weakness; and marked retardation of growth and skeletal maturation.

2. Excess mineralocorticoid—Hypokalemia, mild hypernatremia with water retention, increased blood volume, edema, and hypertension.

3. Excess androgen—Hirsutism, acne, and varying degrees of virilization. Menstrual irregularities in older girls.

B. LABORATORY FINDINGS

1. Blood—

   a. Plasma cortisol concentrations—These are elevated, with loss of the normal diurnal variation in cortisol secretion. Determination of cortisol level between midnight and 2 AM may be a sensitive indicator of loss of variation.

   b. Serum chloride and potassium concentrations—These values may be lowered. Serum sodium and bicarbonate concentrations may be elevated (metabolic alkalosis).

   c. Serum ACTH concentrations—ACTH concentrations are decreased in cases of adrenal tumor, and increased with ACTH-producing pituitary or extrapituitary tumors.

   d. The leukocyte count—This measurement shows polymorphonuclear leukocytosis with lymphopenia, and the eosinophil count is low. The erythrocyte count may be elevated.

2. Saliva—

   a. Salivary cortisol—This value is elevated and is a less invasive means by which to measure several samples (may be performed at home). A salivary cortisol obtained at midnight is a highly specific and sensitive test for hypercortisolism.

3. 24-Hour urinary free cortisol excretion—This value is elevated. This is currently considered the most useful initial diagnostic test to document hypercortisolism, though midnight salivary cortisol is considered a reasonable, and more practical, alternative.

4. Response to dexamethasone suppression testing—The suppression of adrenal function by a small dose (0.5 mg) of dexamethasone is reduced in adrenal hyperfunction; larger doses (4–16 mg/d in four divided doses) of dexamethasone cause suppression of adrenal activity when the disease is due to ACTH hypersecretion, while hypercortisolism due to adenomas and adrenal carcinomas are rarely suppressed.

5. CRH test—The CRH stimulation test, in conjunction with petrosal sinus sampling, is effective at distinguishing pituitary and ectopic sources of ACTH excess and for lateralization of pituitary sources prior to surgery.

C. IMAGING

Pituitary imaging may demonstrate a pituitary adenoma. Adrenal imaging (eg, CT scan) may demonstrate adenoma or bilateral hyperplasia. Radionuclide studies of the adrenals may be useful in complex cases. Osteoporosis (evident first in the spine and pelvis) with compression fractures may occur in advanced cases, and skeletal maturation is usually delayed.

Differential Diagnosis

Children with exogenous obesity, particularly when accompanied by striae and hypertension, are frequently suspected of having Cushing syndrome. The child's height, growth rate, and skeletal maturation are helpful in differentiating the two, since children with Cushing syndrome have a poor growth rate, relatively short stature, and delayed skeletal maturation, whereas those with exogenous obesity usually have a normal or slightly increased growth rate, normal to tall stature, and advanced skeletal maturation. In addition, the color of the striae (purplish in Cushing syndrome, pink in obesity) and the distribution of the obesity assist in the differentiation. The urinary free cortisol excretion (in milligrams per gram of creatinine) may be mildly elevated in obesity, but midnight salivary cortisol is normal.

Treatment

In all cases of primary adrenal hyperfunction due to tumor, surgical removal, if possible, is indicated. Glucocorticoids should be administered parenterally in pharmacologic doses during and after surgery until the patient is stable. Supplemental oral glucocorticoids, potassium, salt, and mineralocorticoids may be necessary until the suppressed contralateral adrenal gland has recovered, sometimes over a period of several months.

The use of mitotane, a DDT derivative that is toxic to the adrenal cortex, and aminoglutethimide, an inhibitor of steroid synthesis, has been suggested, but the efficacy of these agents in children with adrenal tumors has not been determined.

Pituitary microadenomas may respond to pituitary surgery or irradiation.

Prognosis

If the tumor is malignant, the prognosis is poor if it cannot be completely removed. If it is benign, cure is to be expected following proper preparation and surgery.

Raff H, Findling JW: A physiologic approach to diagnosis of the Cushing syndrome. Ann Intern Med 2003;138:980 [PMID: 12809455].

Yehuda R et al: Relationship between 24-hour urinary-free cortisol excretion and salivary cortisol levels sampled from awakening to bedtime in healthy subjects. Life Sci 2003;73:349 [PMID: 12757842].

PRIMARY HYPERALDOSTERONISM

Primary hyperaldosteronism may be caused by an adrenal adenoma or by adrenal hyperplasia. It is characterized by paresthesias, tetany, weakness, nocturnal enuresis, periodic paralysis, low serum potassium and elevated serum sodium levels, hypertension, metabolic alkalosis, and production of a large volume of alkaline urine with a low specific gravity; the latter does not respond to vasopressin. The glucose tolerance test is frequently abnormal. Plasma and urinary aldosterone are elevated. In contrast to renal disease or Bartter syndrome, plasma renin activity is suppressed, creating a high aldosterone:renin ratio. In patients with adrenal tumor, the administration of ACTH may further increase the excretion of aldosterone. Marked improvement after the administration of an aldosterone antagonist such as spironolactone may be of diagnostic value.

Treatment is with glucocorticoids (glucocorticoid-remediable hyperaldosteronism or familial hyperaldosteronism type 1), spironolactone (familial hyperaldosteronism type 2), or subtotal or total adrenalectomy for hyperplasia, and surgical removal if a tumor is present.

Hood S et al: Prevalence of primary hyperaldosteronism assessed by aldosterone/renin ratio and spironolactone testing. Clin Med 2005;5:55 [PMID: 15745200].

Mulatero P et al: Diagnosis of primary aldosteronism: from screening to subtype differentiation. Trends Endocrinol Metab 2005;16:114 [PMID: 15808809].

Young WF Jr: Minireview: Primary aldosteronism—Changing concepts in diagnosis and treatment. Endocrinology 2003; 144:2208 [PMID: 12746276].

USES OF GLUCOCORTICOIDS & ADRENOCORTICOTROPIC HORMONE IN TREATMENT OF NONENDOCRINE DISEASES

Glucocorticoids are used for their anti-inflammatory and immunosuppressive properties in a variety of conditions in childhood. Pharmacologic doses are necessary to achieve these effects, and side effects are common.

Table 30–12. Potency equivalents for adrenocorticosteroids.

Adrenocorticosteroid	Trade Names	Potency/mg Compared with Cortisol (Glucocorticoid Effect)	Potency/mg Compared with Cortisol (Sodium-Retaining Effect)
Glucocorticoids			
Hydrocortisone (cortisol)	Cortef	1	1
Cortisone	Cortone Acetate	0.8	1
Prednisone	Meticorten, others	4–5	0.4
Methylprednisolone	Medrol, Meprolone	5–6	Minimal
Triamcinolone	Aristocort, Kenalog Kenacort, Atolone	5–6	Minimal
Dexamethasone	Decadron, others	25–40	Minimal
Betamethasone	Celestone	25	Minimal
Mineralocorticoid			
Fludrocortisone	Florinef	15–20	300–400

Numerous synthetic preparations possessing variable ratios of glucocorticoid to mineralocorticoid activity are available (Table 30–12).

Actions

Glucocorticoids exert a direct or permissive effect on virtually every tissue of the body; major known effects include the following:

1. Gluconeogenesis in the liver
2. Stimulation of fat breakdown (lipolysis) and redistribution of body fat
3. Catabolism of protein with an increase in nitrogen and phosphorus excretion
4. Decrease in lymphoid and thymic tissue and a decreased cellular response to inflammation and hypersensitivity
5. Alteration of CNS excitation
6. Retardation of connective tissue mitosis and migration, decreased wound healing
7. Improved capillary tone and increased vascular compartment volume and pressure

Side Effects of Therapy

When prolonged use of pharmacologic doses of glucocorticoids is necessary, clinical manifestations of Cushing syndrome are common. Side effects may occur with the use of synthetic exogenous agents by any route, including inhalation and topical administration, or with the use of ACTH. Use of a larger dose of glucocorticoids given once every 48 hours (alternate-day therapy) lessens the incidence and severity of some of the side effects (Table 30–13).

Tapering of Pharmacologic Doses of Steroids

Prolonged use of pharmacologic doses of glucocorticoids results in suppression of ACTH secretion and consequent adrenal atrophy. Thus the abrupt discontinuation of glucocorticoids may result in adrenal insufficiency. Furthermore, ACTH secretion generally does not restart until the administered steroid has been given in subphysiologic doses (< 6 mg/m^2/d orally) for several weeks.

If pharmacologic glucocorticoid therapy has been given for less than 10–14 days, the drug can be discontinued abruptly (if the condition for which it was prescribed allows) because adrenal suppression will be short-lived. However, it is advisable to educate the patient and family about the signs and symptoms of adrenal insufficiency in case problems arise.

If tapering is necessary in treating the condition for which the glucocorticoid is prescribed, a reduction of 25–50% every 2–7 days is sufficiently rapid to permit observation of clinical symptomatology. Moreover, the use of an alternate-day schedule (ie, a single dose given every 48 hours) will allow for a 50% decrease in the total 2 days' dosage while providing the desired pharmacologic effect. If tapering is not necessary for the underlying disease, the dosage can be decreased safely to the physiologic range. However, although a rapid decrease in dose to the physiologic range will not lead to frank adrenal insufficiency (because adequate exogenous cortisol is being provided), some patients may

Table 30–13. Side effects of glucocorticoid use.

A. Endocrine and metabolic effects
1. Hyperglycemia and glycosuria (chemical diabetes)
2. Cushing syndrome
3. Persistent suppression of pituitary-adrenal responsiveness to stress with resultant hypoadrenocorticism

B. Effects on electrolytes and minerals
1. Marked retention of sodium and water, producing edema, increased blood volume, and hypertension (more common in endogenous hyperadrenal states)
2. Potassium loss with symptoms of hypokalemia
3. Hypocalcemia, tetany

C. Effects on protein metabolism and skeletal maturation
1. Negative nitrogen balance, with loss of body protein and bone protein, resulting in osteoporosis, pathologic fractures, and aseptic bone necrosis
2. Suppression of growth, retarded skeletal maturation
3. Muscular weakness and wasting
4. Osteoporosis

D. Effects on the gastrointestinal tract
1. Excessive appetite and intake of food
2. Activation or production of peptic ulcer
3. Gastrointestinal bleeding from ulceration or from unknown cause (particularly in children with hepatic disease)
4. Fatty liver with embolism, pancreatitis, nodular panniculitis

E. Lowering of resistance to infectious agents; silent infection; decreased inflammatory reaction
1. Susceptibility to fungal infections; intestinal parasitic infections
2. Activation of tuberculosis; false-negative tuberculin reaction
3. Stimulation of activity of herpes simplex virus

F. Neuropsychiatric effects
1. Euphoria, excitability, psychotic behavior, and status epilepticus with electroencephalographic changes
2. Increased intracranial pressure with pseudotumor cerebri syndrome

G. Hematologic and vascular effects
1. Bleeding into the skin as a result of increased capillary fragility
2. Thrombosis, thrombophlebitis, cerebral hemorrhage

H. Miscellaneous effects
1. Myocarditis, pleuritis, and arteritis following abrupt cessation of therapy
2. Cardiomegaly
3. Nephrosclerosis, proteinuria
4. Acne (in older children), hirsutism, amenorrhea, irregular menses
5. Posterior subcapsular cataracts; glaucoma

experience a steroid withdrawal syndrome, characterized by malaise, fatigue, and loss of appetite. These symptoms may necessitate a two- or three-step decrease in dose to the physiologic range.

Once a physiologic equivalent dose (8–10 mg/m^2/d hydrocortisone or equivalent) is achieved and the patient's underlying disease is stable, the dose can be decreased to 4–5 mg/m^2/d given only in the morning. This will allow the adrenal axis to recover. After this dose has been given for 4–6 weeks, assessment of endogenous adrenal activity can be estimated by obtaining fasting plasma cortisol concentrations between 7 and 8 AM prior to the morning steroid dose or by a low-dose ACTH stimulation test (1 μg cosyntropin with cortisol measured after 45–60 minutes). When an alternate-day schedule is followed, plasma cortisol is measured the morning prior to treatment. A plasma cortisol concentration within the physiologic range (> 10 mg/dL) demonstrates return of basal physiologic adrenal rhythm. Exogenous steroids may then be discontinued safely, although it is advisable to continue to give the patient stress doses of glucocorticoids when appropriate until recovery of the response to stress has been documented.

After basal physiologic adrenal function returns, the adrenal reserve or capacity to respond to stress and infection can be estimated by the low-dose ACTH stimulation test, in which 1 μg of synthetic ACTH (cosyntropin) is administered intravenously. Plasma cortisol is measured prior to (zero time) and at 45–60 minutes after the infusion. A plasma cortisol concentration of > 18 mg/dL at 60 minutes indicates a satisfactory adrenal reserve.

Even if the results of testing are normal, patients who have received prolonged treatment with glucocorticoids may exhibit signs and symptoms of adrenal insufficiency during acute stress, infection, or surgery for months to years after treatment has been stopped. Careful monitoring, and when necessary the use of stress doses of glucocorticoids, should be considered during severe illnesses and surgery.

Allen DB: Inhaled steroids for children: effects on growth, bone, and adrenal function. Endocrinol Metab Clin North Am 2005;34:555 [PMID: 16085159].

Gulliver T, Eid N: Effects of glucocorticoids on the hypothalamic-pituitary-adrenal axis in children and adults. Immunol Allergy Clin North Am 2005;25:541 [PMID: 16054542].

National Asthma Education and Prevention Program: Long-term management of asthma in children: Safety of inhaled corticosteroids. J Allergy Clin Immunol 2002;110(5 Suppl):S160 [PMID: 12542074].

ADRENAL MEDULLA
PHEOCHROMOCYTOMA

Pheochromocytoma is an uncommon tumor in childhood. Only 10% of the reported cases occur in pediatric patients. The tumor may be located wherever chromaffin tissue (eg, adrenal medulla, sympathetic ganglia, or carotid body) is present, possibly from decreased apoptosis of neural crest cells during development. It may be multiple, recurrent, and sometimes malignant. Familial forms include pheochromocytomas associated with the dominantly inherited neurofibromatosis type 1, MEN type 2 (described earlier), and von Hippel-Lindau syndromes, as well as mutations of the succinate dehydrogenase genes. Neuroblastomas, ganglioneuromas, and other neural tumors, as well as carcinoid tumors may also secrete pressor amines and mimic a pheochromocytoma.

The symptoms of pheochromocytoma are generally caused by excessive secretion of epinephrine or norepinephrine and most commonly include headaches, sweating, tachycardia, and hypertension. Other symptoms include anxiety, hypertension, dizziness, weakness, nausea and vomiting, diarrhea, dilated pupils with blurring of vision, abdominal and precordial pain, and vasomotor instability (flushing and postural hypotension). Sustained symptoms may lead to cardiac, renal, optic, or cerebral damage.

Laboratory diagnosis is possible in over 90% of cases. Serum and urine catecholamines are elevated, particularly while the patient is symptomatic, but may be limited to the period of a paroxysm. Testing of plasma free metanephrine levels (while off of phenoxybenzamine, tricyclic antidepressants, and β-adrenoreceptor blockers, which can create false-positive results) is the most sensitive test and the gold standard for diagnosis, with negative levels, or levels three times above the normal range being diagnostic. Intermediate values may require additional testing with urinary vanillylmandelic acid and urinary total metanephrines providing the highest specificity. Provocative tests using histamine, tyramine, or glucagon and the phentolamine tests may be abnormal but are dangerous and are rarely necessary for diagnosis. After demonstrating a tumor biochemically, imaging methods including CT or MRI are then used to localize the tumor. When available, functional ligands such as (123)I-MIBG, [^{18}F]DA positron emission tomography scanning and somatostatin receptor scintigraphy (with either [^{123}I]Tyr3-octreotide or [^{111}In]DTPA-octreotide) are of utility in further diagnostic work-up of pheochromocytoma.

Laparoscopic tumor removal is the treatment of choice; however, the procedure must be undertaken with great caution and with the patient properly stabilized. Oral phenoxybenzamine or intravenous phentolamine are used preoperatively. Profound hypotension may occur as the tumor is removed but may be controlled with an infusion of norepinephrine, which may have to be continued for 1–2 days.

Unless irreversible secondary vascular changes have occurred, complete relief of symptoms is to be expected after recovery from removal of a benign tumor. However, prognosis is poor in patients with metastases, which occur more commonly with large, extra-adrenal pheochromocytomas.

Ilias I, Pacak K: Current approaches and recommended algorithm for the diagnostic localization of pheochromocytoma. J Clin Endocrinol Metab 2004;89:479 [PMID: 14764749].

Kinney MA et al: Perioperative management of pheochromocytoma. J Cardiothorac Vasc Anesth 2002;16:359 [PMID: 12073213].

Lenders JW et al: Phaeochromocytoma. Lancet 2005;366:665. [PMID: 16112304].

Maxwell PH: A common pathway for genetic events leading to pheochromocytoma. Cancer Cell 2005;8:91 [PMID: 16098460].

Newman KD, Ponsky T: The diagnosis and management of endocrine tumors causing hypertension in children. Ann N Y Acad Sci 2002;970:155 [PMID: 12381550].

Pozo J et al: Sporadic phaeochromocytoma in childhood: clinical and molecular variability. J Pediatr Endocrinol Metab 2005;18:527 [PMID: 16042317].

Sawka AM et al: Systematic review of the literature examining the diagnostic efficacy of measurement of fractionated plasma free metanephrines in the biochemical diagnosis of pheochromocytoma. BMC Endocr Disord 2004;29:2 [PMID: 15225350].

Diabetes Mellitus

31

H. Peter Chase, MD, & George S. Eisenbarth, MD, PhD

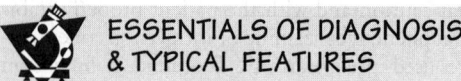

ESSENTIALS OF DIAGNOSIS & TYPICAL FEATURES

- *Polyuria, polydipsia, and weight loss.*
- *Hyperglycemia and glucosuria with or without ketonuria.*

General Considerations

Type 1 diabetes or immune-mediated diabetes (previously called juvenile diabetes or insulin-dependent diabetes mellitus [IDDM]) is the most common type of diabetes in people younger than age 40 years. It is associated with islet cell antibodies (immunologic markers), diminished insulin production, and being ketosis-prone.

Type 2 diabetes (non–insulin-dependent diabetes mellitus [NIDDM], non–immune-mediated) is the most common type in persons older than age 40 years; it is associated with being overweight, insensitivity to insulin, and not being prone to ketosis. Type 2 diabetes is increasing in frequency in children and is found in up to half of black and Hispanic children and in over two-thirds of American Indian children who develop diabetes. It occurs most frequently in overweight teenagers.

Maturity-onset diabetes of youth (MODY) is much less common and comprises several forms of diabetes in non-obese children with identified genetic mutations (eg, mutations of glucokinase or hepatic nuclear factor 1 or 2 genes). It presents as a nonketotic form of diabetes without islet cell antibodies and often is associated with a family history in several generations.

Etiology

A. TYPE 1 DIABETES

Type 1 diabetes results from immunologic damage to the insulin-producing β-cells of the pancreatic islets. This damage occurs gradually—over months or years in most people—and symptoms do not appear until about 90% of the pancreatic islets have been destroyed. The immunologic damage requires a genetic predisposition and is probably influenced by environmental factors.

The importance of genetics is shown by the fact that 35–50% of second identical twins develop diabetes after the first twin develops the disease. About 6% of siblings or offspring of persons with type 1 diabetes also develop diabetes (compared with a prevalence in the general population of 0.2–0.3%). The condition is more common in white children but occurs in all racial groups. There is an association with human leukocyte antigen (HLA)-DR3 and HLA-DR4, and about 95% of white diabetic children have at least one of these HLA types. Forty percent have both HLA-DR3 and HLA-DR4 (one from each parent), compared with only 3% of the general population.

The importance of environmental factors is suggested because not all second identical twins develop diabetes. Important environmental factors may be viral infections or factors in the diet.

The immunologic basis of diabetes is demonstrated by the ability of cyclosporine, a potent immunosuppressive agent, to preserve islet tissue for 1–2 years when given to newly diagnosed patients. However, renal damage from cyclosporine precludes its use. White blood cells are found in the islets of newly diagnosed patients and may release toxic products (free radicals, interleukin-1, and tumor necrosis factor) that injure the islets. Antibodies to islet cells, insulin, glutamic acid decarboxylase, ICA512 (IA-2), and other antibodies are present for months to years prior to diagnosis in the serum of over 90% of patients who will develop type 1 diabetes. These antibodies are probably the effect and not the cause of islet β-cell destruction.

B. TYPE 2 DIABETES

Type 2 diabetes has a strong genetic component, although the inherited defects vary in different families. Obesity (particularly central) and lack of exercise are often major environmental contributing factors. Insulin insensitivity results from all of the above-mentioned circumstances. The prevalence is increased among females, which may be related to the association with polycystic ovary syndrome. Acanthosis nigricans, a thickening and darkening of the skin over the posterior neck, armpits, or elbows, may aid in the diagnosis of type 2 diabetes.

Prevention

A. TYPE 1 DIABETES

Free antibody screening is now available for families having a relative with type 1 diabetes (1-800-425-8361). Intervention trials on antibody-positive first-degree relatives have begun in an effort to try to prevent type 1 diabetes.

B. TYPE 2 DIABETES

The prevention of type 2 diabetes was evaluated in a large study, the Diabetes Prevention Program. The study found that 30 minutes of exercise per day (5 days/week) and a low-fat diet reduced the risk for diabetes by 58%. Taking metformin also reduced the risk for type 2 diabetes by 31%.

Diagnosis

The classic symptoms of polyuria, polydipsia, and weight loss are now so well recognized that friends or family members often suspect the diagnosis of type 1 diabetes in affected individuals. Other cases may be detected by finding glucosuria on routine office urinalysis. Up to 50% of new cases of diabetes used to be diagnosed in patients presenting in coma, but most are now diagnosed before the individuals develop severe ketonuria, ketonemia, and secondary acidosis. Children often have a preceding minor illness, such as a flulike episode. The check of a blood or urine glucose can be done in a few seconds and could be life-saving. No disease other than diabetes (mellitus or insipidus) presents with continued frequent urination in spite of a dry tongue. An oral glucose tolerance test is rarely necessary in children. A random blood glucose level above 300 mg/dL (16.6 mmol/L) or a fasting blood glucose above 200 mg/dL (11 mmol/L) is sufficient to make the diagnosis of diabetes. The 1997 revised guidelines for the diagnosis of diabetes (see references) are a fasting plasma glucose level over 126 mg/dL (7 mmol/L) or a plasma glucose level above 200 mg/dL (11.1 mmol/L) taken randomly (with symptoms of diabetes) or 2 hours after an oral glucose load (1.75 g glucose/kg up to a maximum of 75 g). Confirmation of such abnormalities on more than one occasion is recommended as transient hyperglycemia can occur, particularly with illness. Impaired (not yet diabetic) fasting glucose values are 100–125 mg/dL (5.5–6.9 mmol/L) and impaired 2-hour values are 140–200 mg/dL (7.8–11.1 mmol/L). If the presentation is mild, hospitalization is usually not necessary.

Education about diabetes for all family members is essential for the home management of diabetes. The use of an educational book (see *Understanding Diabetes* in the references) can be very helpful to the family. All caregivers need to learn about diabetes, how to give insulin injections, perform home blood glucose monitoring, and handle acute complications. The stress imposed on the family around the time of initial diagnosis may lead to feelings of shock, denial, sadness, anger, fear, and guilt. Meeting with a counselor to express these feelings at the time of diagnosis helps with long-term adaptation.

Treatment

Most children have type 1 diabetes. The five major variables in treatment are (1) insulin type and dosage, (2) diet, (3) exercise, (4) stress management, and (5) blood glucose and ketone monitoring. All must be considered to obtain safe and effective metabolic control. Although teenagers can be taught to perform many of the tasks of diabetes management, they do better when supportive—not overbearing—parents continue to be involved in management of their disease. Children younger than age 10 or 11 years cannot reliably administer insulin without adult supervision because they lack fine motor control and may not understand the importance of accurate dosage.

A. INSULIN

Insulin functions (1) to allow glucose to pass into the cell, (2) to decrease the physiologic production of glucose, particularly in the liver, and (3) to turn off ketone production.

1. Treatment of new-onset diabetes—The greater the acidemia and ketone production, the greater the amount of insulin needed. If ketonemia is significant, the venous blood pH low (< 7.30), and the patient dehydrated, intravenous insulin and fluid therapy should be given (see section on ketonuria, ketonemia, and ketoacidosis). If the child is adequately hydrated and has a normal venous blood pH, one or two intramuscular or subcutaneous injections of 0.1–0.2 U/kg of regular insulin—or preferably of insulin lispro (Humalog, [H]) or insulin aspart (NovoLog, [NL])—1 hour apart will help shut down ketone production. If ketone production is insignificant or absent, this regimen is not necessary, and routine subcutaneous injections can be started.

When ketones are not present, the child is usually more responsive to insulin, and a total daily dosage of 0.25–0.5 U/kg/24 h (by subcutaneous injection) can be used. If ketones are or were present, the child usually does not produce as much insulin and will require 0.5–1 U/kg of total insulin per 24 hours.

Children usually receive mixtures of a short-acting insulin (to cover food intake or high blood sugars) and a longer-acting insulin (to suppress endogenous hepatic glucose production). This is achieved by combining insulins of different formulations with the desired properties (Table 31–1). The dosages are adjusted with each injection during the first week. In the past, most physicians began newly diagnosed children with two injections per day of an intermediate-acting insulin (eg, NPH) and a short-acting insulin such as Humalog or NovoLog (H or NL). About two-thirds of the total dosage is usually given before breakfast and the remainder before dinner. If human regular insulin is used, the injections are given 30–60 minutes before meals; when

Table 31–1. Kinetics of insulin action.

Type of Insulin	Begins Working	Main Effect	All Gone
Short-acting			
Regular	$1/2$ h	2–4 h	6–9 h
Humalog or NovoLog	10–15 min	30–80 min	4 h
Intermediate-acting			
NPH	2–4 h	6–8 h	12–15 h
Long-acting			
Lantus	1–2 h	2–23 h	24–26 h
Premixed			
NPH/Regular	$1/2$ h	Variable[a]	12–18 h
NPH/75/25[b]	$1/4$ h	1–8 h	12–15 h

[a]Available in various combinations to fit individual needs.
[b]A mixture of 75% NPH and 25% Humalog.
NPH, neutral protamine Hagedorn insulin.

using H or NL as the short-acting insulin, the injections are given just before eating. In young children who eat irregular amounts of food, it is often helpful to wait until after the meal to give the injection and decide on the appropriate dose of H or NL. Children younger than age 4 years usually need 1 or 2 units of rapid-acting insulin to cover meals, and the remainder of the dosage is NPH insulin. Children age 4–10 years may require up to 4 units of rapid-acting insulin to cover breakfast and dinner, whereas proportionately higher doses (usually 4–10 units) of H or NL or regular insulin are used for older children.

A 24-hour basal insulin, insulin glargine (Lantus), is now available, and many physicians now initiate therapy with this insulin. It has an acidic pH and must be given alone in the syringe. It is given once daily in the morning, or at dinner, or at bedtime depending on patient and family wishes. The Lantus dose is adjusted up or down depending on the morning fasting glucose levels. The most physiologic insulin regimen is then to add H/NL prior to each meal/snack. Children who are unable to consistently get H or NL at lunch or with snacks can receive H/NL with NPH at breakfast. The main advantage of Lantus over two injections of NPH daily is that severe hypoglycemic episodes (particularly at night) are greatly reduced with its use.

2. Continuing insulin dosage—The total daily insulin dosage may need to be increased gradually to 1 U/kg (especially if ketones are present at onset). When gluconeogenesis and glycolysis are suppressed by insulin, a honeymoon or grace period is a common phenomenon.

This often occurs 1–4 weeks after diagnosis in over 50% of children and tends to last longer in older children.

In helping families with day-to-day dosing of regular insulin or H or NL, some physicians initially use sliding scales, more recently referred to as "thinking" scales, to emphasize that the family must always be thinking about food recently eaten, or to be eaten, and recent or forthcoming exercise in addition to the blood glucose level. Examples of thinking scales are given in *Understanding Diabetes* (see references).

After the appropriate dosage of intermediate (eg, NPH) or long-acting (Lantus) insulin is achieved, daily adjustments usually are not needed. However, small decreases may be made for heavy activity (eg, afternoon sports or overnight events). Many families gradually learn to make small (0.5–1 unit) weekly adjustments in insulin dosage based on home blood glucose testing. Understanding the onset, peak, and duration of insulin activity is essential (see Table 31–1).

As noted earlier, when the more physiologic (closer to human insulin output) basal insulin, Lantus, is used, it must be given alone in the syringe or pen. When changing a patient from two shots/day of NPH insulin to Lantus, the total 24-hour dose of NPH is divided in half to use as the initial dose of Lantus. The Lantus dose is then increased or decreased 1 or 2 units every few days based on the fasting morning blood sugars. Common glucose level goals are 70–180 mg/dL (3.9–10 mmol/L) for preteens and 70–150 mg/dL (3.9–8.3 mmol/L) for teens. A short-acting insulin (H or NL) is then given prior to meals/snacks or a mixture of H or NL and NPH is given in the morning and H or NL at dinner. The dosages of H or NL may initially be based on a "thinking" scale (see previous discussion), and may later be based on carbohydrate-counting as the family becomes more knowledgeable (see section on diet).

Continuous subcutaneous insulin (insulin pump) therapy is being used more often in children, particularly for emotionally mature teens who are willing to do frequent blood glucose monitoring and to count carbohydrates. Basal insulin doses (usually H/NL) to use are chosen by the physician, with bolus doses prior to meals selected by the patient (or an appropriate adult) depending on the carbohydrate content of the food to be eaten. Insulin pump therapy is discussed in depth in Chapter 26 of *Understanding Diabetes*.

The following constitutes intensive diabetes management: (1) three or more insulin injections per day, or insulin pump therapy; (2) four or more blood glucose determinations per day; (3) careful attention to dietary intake; and (4) frequent contact with the health care provider. This was shown in the Diabetes Control and Complications Trial (DCCT; see section on diet) to result in improved glucose control and to reduce the risk for retinal, renal, cardiovascular, and neurologic complications of diabetes. All teenagers with suboptimal glucose control who are willing to comply should be considered for intensive diabetes management.

3. Treatment of type 2 diabetes—The treatment of type 2 diabetes in children varies with the severity of the disease. If the glycosylated hemoglobin (HbA_{1c}) is still normal (or near normal) and ketone levels are not moderately or significantly increased, modification of lifestyle (preferably for the entire family) is the first line of therapy. This must include reducing caloric intake and increasing exercise. If the HbA_{1c} is mildly elevated (6.2–9.0%) and ketone levels are not moderately or significantly increased, an oral hypoglycemia agent can be tried. Metformin is usually tried along with modification of lifestyle, starting with a dose of 250–500 mg once daily. If needed, and if gastrointestinal adaptation has occurred, the dose can be gradually increased to 1 g bid. If the presentation is more severe, with moderately or significantly increased urine ketone levels, or blood β-hydroxybutyrate is > 1.0 mmol/L, the initial treatment is similar to that of type 1 diabetes (including intravenous or subcutaneous insulin). Oral hypoglycemic agents may be tried at a later date, particularly if weight loss has been successful.

B. DIET

The mainstays of dietary treatment are discussed in detail in *Understanding Diabetes* (see references). The American Diabetes Association no longer recommends any one diabetic diet or its own diet. Instead, nutrition therapy for diabetics should be individualized, with consideration given to the patient's customary cultural eating habits and other lifestyle circumstances. Some families and children (particularly those with weight problems) find exchange diets helpful initially while they are learning food categories. Most centers now just use exchanges of carbohydrates, referred to below as carbohydrate-counting or "carb-counting."

The DCCT found that four nutrition factors contributed to better sugar control (lower HbA_{1c} levels). These factors are (1) adherence to a meal plan, (2) avoidance of extra snacks, (3) avoidance of overtreatment of low blood sugars (hypoglycemia), and (4) prompt treatment of high blood sugars. Two other nutritional factors include adjusting insulin levels for meals and maintaining a consistent schedule of nighttime snacks. The DCCT popularized the carb-counting dietary plan in which the dosage of H/NL or regular insulin is altered with each injection to adjust for the amount of carbohydrate to be eaten and the amount of exercise contemplated. One carbohydrate choice is 15 g of glucose in the United States (10 g in Canada and the United Kingdom). A common formula is to use 1 unit of H/NL for each 15 g of carbohydrate eaten, although this ratio must be adjusted (using blood glucose levels 2 hours after meals) for each person.

C. EXERCISE

Regular aerobic exercise—at least 30 minutes a day—is important for children with diabetes. Exercise fosters a sense of well-being; helps increase insulin sensitivity; and helps maintain proper weight, blood pressure, and blood fat levels. Exercise may also help maintain normal peripheral circulation in later years. It is particularly important for children with type 2 diabetes.

Hypoglycemia during exercise or in the 2–8 hours after exercise (delayed hypoglycemia) can be prevented by careful monitoring of blood sugar before, during, and after exercise; sometimes by reducing the dosage of the insulin active at the time of (or after) the exercise; and by providing extra snacks. Children using insulin pumps should reduce preexercise bolus insulin dosages as well as the basal dosages during (and sometimes after) the exercise. In general, the longer and more vigorous the activity, the greater the reduction in insulin dose. Extra snacks should also be eaten. Fifteen grams of glucose usually covers about 30 minutes of exercise. The use of drinks containing 5–10% dextrose, such as Gatorade, during the period of exercise is often beneficial.

D. STRESS MANAGEMENT

Management of stress is important on a short-term basis because stress hormones increase blood glucose levels. Chronic emotional upsets may lead to missed injections or other compliance problems. When this happens, counseling for the family and child becomes an important part of diabetes management.

E. BLOOD GLUCOSE MEASUREMENTS

All families must be able to monitor blood glucose levels three or four times daily—and more frequently in small infants and patients who have glucose control problems or intercurrent illnesses. Blood glucose levels can be monitored using any of the available meters, which generally have an accuracy of 90% or better. Target levels when no food has been eaten for 2 or more hours vary according to age (Table 31–2).

Blood glucose results should be recorded even if the meter has a memory feature. This allows the family to look for patterns and make changes in insulin dosage. If more than 50% of the values are above the desired range for age or more than 14% below the desired range, the insulin dosage usually needs to be adjusted. Some families are able to make these changes independently (particularly after the first year), whereas others need help from the health care provider. Children with diabetes should have clinic visits every 3 months. This provides an opportunity to adjust insulin dosages according to changes in growth and blood glucose levels as well as to check for changes noted on physical examination (eg, eyes and thyroid). Continuous subcutaneous glucose monitoring using the Guardian

Table 31–2. Ideal glucose levels after 2 or more hours of fasting.[a]

Age (years)	Glucose Level
≤ 4	80–200 mg/dL (4.6–11 mmol/L)
5–11	70–180 mg/dL (3.9–10 mmol/L)
≥ 12	70–150 mg/dL (3.9–8.3 mmol/L)

[a]At least half of the values must be below the upper limit to have a good HbA_{1c} value. The values should also be below the upper limits for age when tested 2 h after a meal.

Continuous Glucose Monitoring System by Medtronic/MiniMed or the Navigator by Abbott may also be helpful in monitoring glucose levels and trends.

Laboratory Evaluations

In addition to home measurements of blood glucose and blood or urine ketone levels, HbA_{1c} should be measured every 3 months. This test reflects the frequency of elevated blood glucose levels over the previous 3 months. Normal values vary among laboratories but are usually below 6.2% HbA_{1c}. The desired ranges are based on age. For the HbA_{1c} method, these ranges are as follows: 12–19 years, less than 7.5%; 6–11 years, less than 8.0%; and younger than 5 years, 7.5–8.5%. Higher levels are allowed in younger children to reduce the risk of hypoglycemia because their brains are still developing and they may not relate symptoms of hypoglycemia to a need for treatment. Low HbA_{1c} values are generally associated with a greater risk for hypoglycemia (see following section). Using either method, researchers found that longitudinal averages more than 33% above the upper limit of normal are associated with a higher risk for later renal and retinal complications. In the intensive treatment group of the DCCT, the lower HbA_{1c} values resulted in greater than 50% reductions in the retinal, renal, cardiovascular, and neurologic complications of diabetes.

Since atherosclerosis is the major cause of death in older patients with diabetes it is important to measure serum cholesterol, low-density lipoprotein cholesterol, and high-density lipoprotein cholesterol levels once yearly. Cholesterol levels should be below 200 mg/dL and low-density lipoprotein cholesterol levels below 100 mg/dL in postpubertal people with diabetes.

When puberty is reached and the individual has had diabetes for 3 years or longer, the urinary excretion of albumin should be measured (as microalbumin) in two separate urine samples once yearly (see section on chronic complications). This can be done using timed overnight urine collections or first-morning voids (expressed per milligram of creatinine). Normal values differ with the methodology

of the laboratory but are generally below 20 µg/min (or 30 µg/mg creatinine). People with type 2 diabetes should have this test done soon after diagnosis and then annually.

If the thyroid is enlarged (about 20% of patients with type 1 diabetes), the thyroid-stimulating hormone level should be measured yearly. This is usually the first test to become abnormal in the autoimmune thyroiditis commonly associated with type 1 diabetes.

In recent years antiendomysial and transglutaminase antibodies, reliable predictors of celiac disease, have been shown to be more common in children with diabetes as well as in their siblings. Risk of celiac disease is associated with HLA-DR3 and is more frequent in children with diabetes (celiac disease occurring in about 5%). The celiac antibodies should be checked in diabetic children with poor growth (especially when not related to poor glucose control) or those who present with gastrointestinal symptoms. The 21-hydroxylase autoantibody, a marker of increased risk of Addison disease, is present in approximately 1.3% of patients with type 1 diabetes, although Addison disease is found in only 1 in 200.

Type 2 diabetes is not an autoimmune disease, and the islet antibody tests are negative. An elevated insulin or C-peptide level is also helpful, indicating that insulin production is normal or elevated.

A checklist of the physician's contributions to good diabetes care is presented in Table 31–3.

Table 31–3. Physician's checklist of good diabetes management.

Variable	Frequency of Measurement	Tests and Values
Blood sugars	3–4 times daily	See age-appropriate values
Hemoglobin A_{1c}	Every 3 mo	See age-appropriate values
Urine microalbumin	Annually after 3 y of diabetes (pubertal patients)	< 20 µg/min
Ophthalmology referral	Annually after 3 y of diabetes (10 y old or greater)	Retinal photographs
Signs of other endocrinopathy	Evaluate at least annually (eg, thyroid enlargement)	(eg: TSH: 0.5–5.0 IU/mL)
Blood lipid panel	Annually	Cholesterol < 200 mg/dL; LDL < 100

TSH, thyroid-stimulating hormone.

Acute Complications

A. HYPOGLYCEMIA

Hypoglycemia (or insulin reaction) is defined as a blood glucose level below 60 mg/dL (or 3.3 mmol/L). For preschool children, values below 70 mg/dL (3.9 mmol/L) should be cause for concern. The common symptoms of hypoglycemia are hunger, weakness, shakiness, sweating, drowsiness (at an unusual time), headache, and behavioral changes. Children learn to recognize hypoglycemia at different ages but can often report "feeling funny" as young as age 4–5 years. If low blood sugar is not treated immediately with simple sugar, the hypoglycemia may result in loss of consciousness or convulsions. If hypoglycemia is left untreated for several hours, brain damage or death can occur.

Consistency in daily routine, correct insulin dosage, regular blood glucose monitoring, controlled snacking, compliance of patients and parents, and good education are all important in preventing severe hypoglycemia. In addition, insulin should not be injected prior to getting into a hot tub, bath, or shower. The heat will increase circulation to the skin and cause more rapid insulin uptake. The use of H/NL insulin and of Lantus insulin has also helped to reduce the occurrence of hypoglycemia.

The treatment of mild hypoglycemia involves giving 4 oz of juice, a sugar-containing soda drink, or milk, and waiting 10 minutes. If the blood glucose level is still below 60 mg/dL (3.3 mmol/L), the liquids are repeated. If the glucose level is above 60 mg/dL, solid foods are given. Moderate hypoglycemia, in which the person is conscious but incoherent, is treated by squeezing one-half tube of concentrated glucose (eg, Insta-Glucose or cake frosting) between the gums and lips and stroking the throat to encourage swallowing.

In the DCCT study, 10% of patients with standard management and 25% of those with intensive insulin management—insulin pumps or three or more insulin shots per day—had one or more severe hypoglycemic reactions each year. Families are advised to have glucagon in the home and to treat hypoglycemia by giving subcutaneous or intramuscular injections of 0.3 mL (30 units in an insulin syringe) for children younger than age 5 years and 0.5 mL (50 units) to those older than age 5 years. Some patients (usually those who have had diabetes for more than 10 years) fail to recognize the symptoms of low blood sugar (hypoglycemic unawareness). For these individuals, glucose control must be liberalized to prevent severe hypoglycemic reactions. School personnel, sports coaches, and baby-sitters must be trained to recognize and treat hypoglycemia.

B. KETONURIA, KETONEMIA, AND KETOACIDOSIS

Families must be educated to check blood or urine ketone levels during any illness (including vomiting even once) or any time a fasting blood glucose level is above 240 mg/dL (13.3 mmol/L), or a randomly measured glucose level is above 300 mg/dL (16.6 mmol/L). If moderate or significant ketonuria is detected, or the blood ketone (β-hydroxy-butyrate—using the Precision Xtra meter) is above 1.0 mmol/L, the health care provider must be called. Usually 10–20% of the total daily insulin dosage is given subcutaneously as H or NL (or regular) insulin every 2–3 hours until the elevated ketones are gone. This prevents ketonuria/ketonemia from progressing to ketoacidosis and allows most patients to receive treatment at home by telephone management. Juices and other fluids to help wash out the ketones and to prevent dehydration are encouraged, and suppositories of promethazine to prevent vomiting may be indicated. If deep breathing (Kussmaul respirations) or excessive weakness occurs, the patient should be evaluated promptly by a physician.

Acidosis (venous blood pH < 7.30) is now present in fewer than 25% of newly diagnosed children. Acidosis may also occur in those with known diabetes who do not check blood or urine ketone levels or fail to call the health care provider when ketones levels are elevated. Repeated episodes of ketoacidosis usually result from missed insulin injections and signify that counseling may be indicated, and that a responsible adult must take over the diabetes management. If for any reason this is not possible, a change in the child's living situation may be necessary.

Treatment of diabetic ketoacidosis (DKA) is based on four physiologic principles: (1) restoration of fluid volume, (2) inhibition of lipolysis and return to glucose utilization, (3) replacement of body salts, and (4) correction of acidosis. Laboratory tests at the start of treatment should include venous blood pH, blood glucose, and an electrolyte panel. Mild DKA is defined as a venous blood pH of 7.2–7.3; moderate DKA, a pH of 7.10–7.19; and severe DKA, a pH below 7.10. Patients with severe DKA should be hospitalized in a pediatric intensive care unit, if available in the area. More severe cases may benefit from determination of osmolality, calcium and phosphorus, and blood urea nitrogen levels. Severe and moderate episodes of DKA generally require hourly determinations of serum glucose, electrolytes, and venous pH levels, whereas these parameters can be measured every 2 hours if the pH level is 7.20–7.30.

1. Restoration of fluid volume—Dehydration is judged by (1) acute loss of body weight (if a recent weight is known), (2) dryness of oral mucous membranes, (3) low blood pressure, and (4) tachycardia. Initial treatment is with physiologic saline (0.9%), 10–20 mL/kg during the first hour. If indicated by continued signs of dehydration, this is repeated during the second hour. The total volume of fluid in the first 4 hours of treatment should not exceed 40 mL/kg because of the danger of cerebral edema (see section on management of cerebral edema). Human albumin,

10 mL/kg of 5% solution, can be given over 30 minutes if the patient is in shock. After initial reexpansion, half-physiologic (0.45%) saline usually is given at 1.5 times maintenance. Maintenance fluids are as shown in Chapter 41.

2. Inhibition of lipolysis and return to glucose utilization—Insulin turns off fat breakdown and ketone formation. Regular insulin is usually given intravenously at a rate of 0.1 U/kg/h. The insulin solution should be administered by pump and can be made by diluting 30 units of regular insulin in 150 mL of 0.9% saline (1 U/5 mL). If the glucose level falls below 250 mg/dL (13.9 mmol/L), 5% dextrose is added to the intravenous fluids. If the glucose level continues to decrease below 120 mg/dL (6.6 mmol/L), 10% dextrose can be added. If necessary, the insulin dosage can be reduced to 0.05 U/kg/h, but it should not be discontinued before the venous blood pH reaches 7.30. The half-life of intravenous insulin when discontinued is 6 minutes, whereas subcutaneous H or NL insulin takes 10–15 minutes, and regular insulin takes 30–60 minutes, to begin activity. Thus it is often better to continue intravenous insulin until subcutaneous insulin can begin acting.

3. Replacement of body salts—In patients with DKA, both sodium and potassium pass into the urine with the ketones and are depleted. Serum sodium concentrations may be falsely lowered by hyperglycemia, causing water to be drawn into the intravenous space, and by hyperlipidemia if fat replaces some of the water in the serum used for electrolyte analysis. Sodium is usually replaced adequately by the use of physiologic and half-physiologic saline in the rehydration fluids as discussed earlier.

Serum potassium levels may be elevated initially because of inability of potassium to stay in the cell in the presence of acidosis (even though total body potassium is low). Potassium should not be given until the serum potassium level is known to be low or normal and the pH is above 7.10. It is then usually given at a concentration of 40 mEq/L, with one-half of the potassium (20 mEq/L) either as potassium acetate or potassium chloride and the other half as potassium phosphate (20 mEq/L). Hypocalcemia can occur if all of the potassium is given as the phosphate salt; hypophosphatemia occurs if none of the potassium is of the phosphate salt.

4. Correction of acidosis—Acidosis is corrected as the fluid volume and aerobic glycolysis are restored and as insulin is administered to inhibit ketogenesis. As noted earlier, measurement of the venous blood pH (identical to arterial blood pH) reveals the severity of acidosis. Bicarbonate is usually not given, even with severe DKA.

5. Management of cerebral edema—Some degree of cerebral edema has been shown by computed tomography scan to be common in DKA. Associated clinical symptoms are rare, unpredictable, and often associated with demise. Cerebral edema may be related to overhydration with hypotonic fluids, although the cause is not well understood. It is now recommended that no more than 40 mL/kg of fluids be given in the first 4 hours of treatment. Cerebral edema is more common with a pH lower than 7.1, a arterial partial carbon dioxide pressure lower than 20 mm Hg, or when the serum sodium is noted to be falling rather than rising. Early neurologic signs may include headache, excessive drowsiness, and dilated pupils. Prompt initiation of therapy should include elevation of the head of the bed, hyperventilation, mannitol (1 g/kg over 30 minutes), and fluid restriction. If the cerebral edema is not recognized and treated early, over 50% of patients will die or have permanent brain damage.

Chronic Complications

In the past, about 30–40% of persons with type 1 diabetes eventually developed renal failure or loss of vision. Factors that greatly reduce this likelihood are longitudinal HbA_{1c} levels in a good range, maintenance of blood pressure below the 90th percentile for age, and abstinence from smoking or chewing tobacco. Annual retinal examinations and urine microalbumin measurements are important for children age 10 years or older who have had diabetes for 3 years or longer (see section on laboratory evaluations). Data now show that the use of angiotensin-converting enzyme inhibitors may reverse or delay kidney damage when it is detected in the microalbuminuria stage (20–300 µg/min). Similarly, laser treatment to coagulate proliferating capillaries prevents bleeding and leakage of blood into the vitreous fluid or behind the retina. This treatment helps to prevent retinal detachment and to preserve useful vision for many people with proliferative diabetic retinopathy.

REFERENCES

American Diabetes Association: Standards of medical care for patients with diabetes mellitus. Diabetes Care 2005;28(Suppl 1):S4 [PMID: 15618112].

American Diabetes Association: Type 2 diabetes in children and adolescents. Diabetes Care 2000;23:381 [PMID: 10868870].

Chase HP et al: Continuous subcutaneous glucose monitoring in children with type 1 diabetes. Pediatrics 2001;107:222 [PMID: 11158450].

Chase HP et al: The impact of the diabetes control and complications trial and humalog insulin on glycohemoglobin levels and severe hypoglycemia in type 1 diabetes. Diabetes Care 2001;24:430 [PMID: 11289463].

Chase HP: *Understanding Diabetes*, 11th ed. SFI, 2006. Available from Children's Diabetes Foundation, 777 Grant Street, Suite 302, Denver, CO 80203 for $18.00 (phone: 1-800-695-2873 or at the website www.barbaradaviscenter.org).

Diabetes Control and Complications Trial Research Group: The effect of intensive treatment of diabetes on the development and progression of long-term complications in insulin-dependent diabetes mellitus. N Engl J Med 1993;329:977 [PMID: 8366922].

Diabetes Prevention Program Research Group: Reduction in the incidence of type 2 diabetes with lifestyle intervention or metformin. N Engl J Med 2002;346:393 [PMID: 11832527].

Glaser N et al: Risk factors for cerebral edema in children with diabetic ketoacidosis. The Pediatric Emergency Medicine Collaborative Research Committee of the American Academy of Pediatrics. N Engl J Med 2001;344:264 [PMID: 11172153].

Maniatis AK et al: Continuous subcutaneous insulin infusion therapy for children and adolescents: an option for routine diabetes care. Pediatrics 2001;107:351 [PMID: 11158469].

Report of the Expert Committee on the Diagnosis and Classification of Diabetes Mellitus. Diabetes Care 1997;20:1183 [PMID: 9203460].

Roberts MD et al: Diabetic ketoacidosis with intracerebral complications. Pediatr Diabetes 2001;2:109 [PMID: 15016193].

Inborn Errors of Metabolism

Janet A. Thomas, MD, & Johan L.K. Van Hove, MD

Disorders in which single gene defects cause clinically significant blocks in metabolic pathways are called inborn errors of metabolism. For many years after Garrod first described them in 1908, these conditions were considered rare. Because the number of recognized inborn errors has increased, they are now acknowledged to be important causes of disease in children (estimated incidence 1:1500 children). Many of these disorders can now be treated effectively. Even when treatment is not available, correct diagnosis permits parents to make informed decisions about future offspring.

The pathology is almost always due either to accumulation of enzyme substrate behind a metabolic block or to deficiency of the reaction product. In some cases, the accumulated enzyme substrate is diffusible and has adverse effects on distant organs; in other cases, as in lysosomal storage diseases, the substrate primarily accumulates locally.

The clinical manifestations of inborn errors vary widely with both mild and severe forms of virtually every disorder. Many patients do not match the classic phenotype because mutations are not identical in different patients, even though they are in the same gene.

A first treatment strategy is to enhance the reduced enzyme activity. Gene replacement is a long-term goal, but problems of gene delivery to target organs and control of gene action make this an unrealistic option at present. Enzyme replacement therapy using intravenously administered recombinant enzyme has been developed as an effective strategy in lysosomal storage disorders. Organ transplantation (liver or bone marrow) can provide a source of enzyme for some conditions. Pharmacologic doses of a cofactor such as a vitamin can sometimes be effective. Alternatively, some strategies are designed to cope with the consequences of enzyme deficiency. Strategies used to avoid substrate accumulation include restriction of precursor in the diet (eg, low-phenylalanine diet for phenylketonuria), avoidance of catabolism, inhibition of an enzyme in the synthesis of the precursor (eg, NTBC in tyrosinemia type I), or removal of accumulated substrate pharmacologically (eg, glycine therapy for isovaleric acidemia) or by dialysis. An inadequately produced metabolite can also be supplemented (eg, glucose administration for glycogen storage disease type I).

Inborn errors can manifest at any time, can affect any organ system, and can mimic many common pediatric problems. This chapter focuses on when to consider metabolic disorder in the differential diagnosis of common pediatric problems. A few of the more important disorders are then discussed in detail.

DIAGNOSIS

SUSPECTING INBORN ERRORS

Inborn errors must be considered in the differential diagnosis of critically ill newborns, children with seizures, neurodegeneration, mental retardation, developmental delay, recurrent vomiting, Reye-like syndrome, parenchymal liver disease, cardiomyopathy, unexplained acidosis, hyperammonemia, and hypoglycemia. Inborn errors should be suspected when (1) symptoms accompany changes in diet, (2) the child's development regresses, (3) the child shows specific food preferences or aversions, or (4) the family has a history of parental consanguinity or problems suggestive of inborn error such as retardation or unexplained deaths in first- and second-degree relatives.

Physical findings associated with inborn errors include alopecia or abnormal hair, retinal cherry-red spot or retinitis pigmentosa, cataracts or corneal opacity, hepatomegaly or splenomegaly, coarse features, skeletal changes (including gibbus), neurologic regression, and intermittent or progressive ataxia or dystonia. Other features that may be important in the context of a suspicious history include failure to thrive, microcephaly, rash, jaundice, hypotonia, and hypertonia.

Finding an immediate cause of symptoms does not rule out an underlying inborn error. For example, renal tubular acidosis and cirrhosis may be due to an underlying inborn error. Acute crises may be brought on by intercurrent infections in some inborn errors. Some inborn errors suggest a diagnosis of nonaccidental trauma (eg, glutaric acidemia type I) or poisoning (eg, methylmalonic acidemia). In addition, children with inborn errors may be at higher risk for child abuse or neglect because of their frustrating irritability.

LABORATORY STUDIES

Table 32–1 lists common clinical and laboratory features of different groups of inborn errors. Table 32–2

Table 32–1. Presenting clinical and laboratory features of inborn errors.[a]

	Defects of Carbohydrate Metabolism	Defects of Amino Acid Metabolism[b]	Organic Acid Disorders[c]	Defects of Fatty Acid Oxidation	Defects of Purine Metabolism	Lysosomal Storage Diseases	Disorders of Peroxisomes
Neurodevelopmental							
Mental/developmental retardation	+++	+++	+++	+	++	+++	+++
Developmental regression	–	–	+	–	–	+++	+++
Acute encephalopathy	+++	+++	+++	+++	–	–	–
Seizures	++	+++	+++	+	–	+++	++
Ataxia/movement disorder	–	+	++	–	+++	–	–
Hypotonia	++	++	++	+++	–	+	+++
Hypertonia	–	++	+++	–	++	+	–
Abnormal behavior	–	++	++	–	++	+++	–
Growth							
Failure to thrive	+++	+++	+++	+	–	+	–
Short stature	++	–	+	–	–	++	–
Macrocephaly	–	–	+	–	–	+++	++
Microcephaly	+	++	+++	–	–	+	–
General							
Vomiting/anorexia	++	+++	+++	+++	–	–	++
Food aversion or craving	++	+++	+++	+++	–	–	–
Odor	–	++	++	–	–	–	–
Dysmorphic features	–	+	+	–	–	++	++
Congenital malformations	–	++	++	–	–	–	++
Organ-specific							
Hepatomegaly	+++	–	++	+++	–	+++	+++
Liver disease/cirrhosis	++	+	–	+	–	–	+
Splenomegaly	–	–	–	–	–	++	+
Skeletal dysplasia	–	–	–	–	–	++	++
Cardiomyopathy	++	–	+	+++	–	++	–
Tachypnea/hyperpnea	++	++	++	++	–	–	–
Rash	–	++	++	–	–	–	–
Alopecia or abnormal hair	–	+	++	–	–	–	+
Cataracts or corneal opacity	++	–	–	–	–	++	–
Retinal abnormality	–	+	+	+	–	++	++
Frequent infections	++	–	++	–	++	–	–
Deafness	–	–	+	–	–	++	–

(continued)

Table 32–1. Presenting clinical and laboratory features of inborn errors.[a] (continued)

	Defects of Carbohydrate Metabolism	Defects of Amino Acid Metabolism[b]	Organic Acid Disorders[c]	Defects of Fatty Acid Oxidation	Defects of Purine Metabolism	Lysosomal Storage Diseases	Disorders of Peroxisomes
Laboratory							
Hypoglycemia	+++	+	++	++	–	–	–
Hyperammonemia	–	++	++	++	–	–	–
Metabolic acidosis	++	++	+++	+++	–	–	–
Respiratory alkalosis	–	++	–	–	–	–	–
Elevated lactate/pyruvate	++	–	+++	++	–	–	–
Elevated liver enzymes	++	++	++	+++	–	+	+
Neutropenia or thrombocytopenia	+	–	+		++	+	–
Ketosis	+++	++	+++	–	–	–	–
Hypoketosis	–	–	+	+++	–	–	–

[a]+++, most conditions in group; ++, some; +, one or few; –, not found.
[b]Includes disorders of the urea cycle but not maple syrup urine disease.
[c]Includes maple syrup urine disease and disorders of pyruvate oxidation.

lists the most common laboratory tests used to diagnose these diseases and offers suggestions about their use.

Laboratory studies are almost always needed for the diagnosis of inborn errors. Serum electrolytes and pH should be used to estimate anion gap and acid-base status. Serum lactate, pyruvate, and ammonia levels are available in most hospitals but care is needed in obtaining samples appropriately. Amino acid and organic acid studies must be performed at specialized facilities to ensure accurate analysis and interpretation. An increasing number of inborn errors are diagnosed with DNA probes, but this method may require that the precise mutation in the family be known.

The physician should know what conditions a test can detect and when it can detect them. For example, urine organic acids may be normal in patients with medium-chain acyl-CoA dehydrogenase deficiency or biotinidase deficiency; glycine may be elevated only in cerebrospinal fluid (CSF) in patients with glycine encephalopathy. A result that is normal in one physiologic state may be abnormal in another. For instance, the urine of a child who becomes hypoglycemic upon prolonged fasting should be positive for ketones. In such a child, the absence of ketones in the urine suggests a defect in fatty acid oxidation.

Samples used to diagnose metabolic disease may be obtained at autopsy. Samples must be obtained in a timely fashion and may be analyzed directly or stored frozen until a particular analysis is justified by the results of postmortem examination, new clinical information, or developments in the field. Studies of other family members may help establish the diagnosis of a deceased patient. It may be possible to demonstrate that parents are heterozygous carriers of a particular disorder or that a sibling has the condition.

COMMON CLINICAL SITUATIONS

Mental Retardation

Some inborn errors can cause mental retardation without other distinguishing characteristics. Measurements of serum amino acids, urine organic acids, and serum uric acid should be obtained in every patient with nonspecific mental retardation. Urine screens for mucopolysaccharides and succinylpurines, and serum testing for carbohydrate-deficient glycoproteins are useful because these disorders do not always have specific physical findings. Absent speech can point to disorders of creatine. Abnormalities of the brain detected by MRI can suggest specific groups of disorders (eg, cortical migrational abnormalities in peroxisomal biogenesis disorders).

Acute Presentation in the Neonate

Acute metabolic disease in the neonate is most often a result of disorders of protein or carbohydrate metabolism and may be clinically indistinguishable from sepsis. Prominent symptoms include poor feeding, vomiting, altered mental status or muscle tone, jitteriness, seizures, and jaun-

Table 32–2. Obtaining and handling samples to diagnose inborn errors.

Test	Comments
Acid-base status	Accurate estimation of anion gap must be possible. Samples for blood gases should be kept on ice and analyzed immediately.
Blood ammonia	Sample should be collected without a tourniquet, kept on ice, and analyzed immediately.
Blood lactic acid and pyruvic acid	Sample should be collected without a tourniquet, kept on ice, and analyzed immediately. Reduction of pyruvic acid to lactic acid must be prevented. Normal literature values are for the fasting, rested state.
Amino acids	Blood and urine should be examined. CSF glycine should be measured if nonketotic hyperglycinemia is to be ruled out. Normal literature values are for the fasting state. Growth of bacteria in urine should be prevented. At autopsy: liver, kidney, or aqueous humor may be analyzed if urine is not available.
Organic acids	Urine preferred for analysis. At autopsy: liver, kidney, or aqueous humor may be analyzed if urine is not available.
Carnitine and acylcarnitine profile	Blood (plasma) may be analyzed for total, free, and esterified carnitine; normal values are for the healthy, nonfasted state. Acylcarnitine profile in blood may identify compounds esterified to carnitine, and urine and tissue studies may be needed for certain conditions.
Urine mucopoly-saccharides	Variations in urine concentration may cause errors in screening tests. Diagnosis requires knowing which mucopolysaccharides are increased. Some patients with Morquio disease do not have abnormal mucopolysacchariduria.
Enzyme assays	Specific assays must be requested. Exposure to heat may cause loss of enzyme activity. Enzyme activity in whole blood may become normal after transfusion or vitamin therapy. Leukocyte or fibroblast pellets should be kept frozen prior to assays. Fibroblasts may be grown from skin biopsies taken up to 72 h after death. Tissues such as liver and kidney should be taken as soon as possible after death, frozen immediately, and kept at –70 °C until assayed.

CSF, cerebrospinal fluid.

dice. Acidosis or altered mental status out of proportion to systemic symptoms should increase suspicion of a metabolic disorder. Laboratory measurements should include: electrolytes, ammonia, lactate, glucose, blood pH, and urine ketones and reducing substances. Glycine in CSF should be measured if glycine encephalopathy is suspected. Serum and urine amino acid, urine organic acid, and serum acylcarnitine analysis should be performed on samples collected before oral intake is discontinued and sent later for analysis if indicated by the results of initial studies. Neonatal cardiomyopathy or ventricular arrhythmias should be investigated with serum acylcarnitine analysis.

Vomiting & Encephalopathy in the Infant or Older Child

Electrolytes, ammonia, glucose, urine pH, urine reducing substances, and urine ketones should be measured in all patients with vomiting and encephalopathy before any treatment affects the results. Samples for serum amino acids, serum acylcarnitine profile, and urine organic acid analysis should be obtained early and frozen pending the results of initial studies. In the presentation of a Reye-like syndrome (ie, vomiting, encephalopathy, and hepatomegaly), amino acids, acylcarnitines, carnitine levels, and organic acids should be assessed immediately. Hypoglycemia with inappropriately low urine or serum ketones suggests the diagnosis of fatty acid oxidation defects.

Hypoglycemia

Duration of fasting, presence or absence of hepatomegaly, and Kussmaul breathing provide clues to the differential diagnosis of hypoglycemia. Serum insulin, cortisol, and growth hormone should be obtained on presentation. Urine ketones, urine organic acids, plasma lactate, serum acylcarnitine profile, carnitine levels, ammonia, and uric acid should be measured. Ketone body production is usually not efficient in the neonate, and ketonuria in a hypoglycemic or acidotic neonate suggests an inborn error. In the older child, inappropriately low urine ketone levels suggest an inborn error of fatty acid oxidation.

Hyperammonemia

Symptoms of hyperammonemia may appear and progress rapidly or insidiously. Decreased appetite, irritability, and behavioral changes appear first with vomiting, ataxia, lethargy, seizures, and coma appearing as ammonia levels increase. Tachypnea is also characteristic and is due to a direct effect on respiratory drive. Physical examination cannot exclude the presence of hyperammonemia, and serum ammonia should be measured whenever hyperammonemia is possible.

Severe hyperammonemia may be due to urea cycle disorders, organic acidemias, or fatty acid oxidation disorders (such as carnitine-acylcarnitine translocase deficiency) or, in the premature infant, transient hyperammonemia of the newborn. The cause can usually be ascertained by measuring quantitative serum amino acids (eg, citrulline), plasma carnitine and acylcarnitine esters, and urine organic acids and orotic acid. Respiratory alkalosis is usually present in urea cycle defects and transient hyperammonemia of the newborn, while acidosis is characteristic of hyperammonemia due to organic acidemias.

Acidosis

Inborn errors may cause chronic or acute acidosis at any age, with or without an increased anion gap. Inborn errors should be considered when acidosis occurs with recurrent vomiting or hyperammonemia and when acidosis is out of proportion to the clinical status. Acidosis due to an inborn error can be difficult to correct. The main causes of anion gap metabolic acidosis are lactic acidosis, ketoacidosis (including abnormal ketone body production such as in β-ketothiolase deficiency), methylmalonic acidemia or other organic acidurias, intoxication (ethanol, methanol, ethylene glycol, and salicylate), and uremia. Causes of non–anion gap metabolic acidosis includes loss of base in diarrhea or renal tubular acidosis (isolated renal tubular acidosis or renal Fanconi syndrome). Inborn errors associated with renal tubular acidosis or renal Fanconi syndrome include cystinosis, tyrosinemia type I, carnitine palmitoyltransferase I and mitochondrial diseases. Serum glucose and ammonia levels and urinary pH and ketones should be examined. Samples for amino acids and organic acids should be obtained at once and may be evaluated immediately or frozen for later analysis, depending on how strongly an inborn error is suspected. It is useful to test blood lactate and pyruvate levels in the chronically acidotic patient even if urine organic acid levels are normal. Lactate and pyruvate levels are difficult to interpret in the acutely ill patient, but in the absence of shock, high levels of lactic acid suggest primary lactic acidosis.

■ MANAGEMENT OF METABOLIC EMERGENCIES

Patients with severe acidosis, hypoglycemia, and hyperammonemia may be very ill; initially mild symptoms may worsen quickly, and coma and death may ensue within hours. With prompt and vigorous treatment, however, patients can recover completely, even from deep coma. All oral intake should be stopped. Sufficient glucose should be given intravenously to avoid or minimize catabolism in a patient with a known inborn error

who is at risk for crisis. Most conditions respond favorably to glucose administration, and few (eg, primary lactic acidosis due to pyruvate dehydrogenase deficiency) do not. After exclusion of fatty acid oxidation disorders, institution of intravenous fat emulsions (eg, intralipid) can provide crucial caloric input. Severe or increasing hyperammonemia should be treated pharmacologically or with dialysis, and severe acidosis should be treated with bicarbonate. More specific measures can be instituted when a diagnosis is established.

■ NEWBORN SCREENING

Criteria for screening newborns for a disorder include its frequency, its consequences if untreated, the ability of therapy to mitigate consequences, the cost of testing and the cost of treatment. All states in the U.S. screen newborns for phenylketonuria and hypothyroidism. In most states newborns are screened for galactosemia. Other metabolic disorders for which newborns are frequently screened include maple syrup urine disease, homocystinuria due to cystathionine β-synthase deficiency, and biotinidase deficiency. Expanded newborn screening using tandem mass spectrometry detects several disorders of amino acid, organic acid, and fatty acid metabolism.

Some screening tests measure a metabolite (eg, phenylalanine) that becomes abnormal with time and exposure to diet. In such instances the disease cannot be detected reliably until intake of the enzyme substrate is established. Other tests (eg, for biotinidase deficiency) measure an enzyme activity and can be performed at any time. Transfusions may cause false-negative results in this instance, and exposure of the sample to heat may cause false-positive results. Technologic advances have extended the power of newborn screening but have brought additional challenges. For example, although tandem mass spectrometry can detect many more disorders in the newborn period, consensus on diagnosis and treatment for some conditions is still under development.

Screening tests are not diagnostic, and diagnostic tests must be undertaken when an abnormal screening result is obtained. Further, because false-negative results occur, a normal newborn screening test does not rule out a condition.

The timing of newborn screening recommended by the American Academy of Pediatrics is appropriate for the detection of phenylketonuria, but hypothyroidism, for instance, can be missed when screening is carried out at the same time. Early discharge of neonates causes significant problems in newborn screening, with both false-negative and false-positive results. Nevertheless, all babies should be screened before discharge from the hospital.

The appropriate response to an abnormal screening test depends on the condition in question and the predictive value of the test. For example, when screening for galactosemia by enzyme assay, complete absence of enzyme activity is highly predictive of classic galactosemia. Failure to treat may rapidly lead to death. In this case, treatment must be initiated immediately while diagnostic studies are pending. In phenylketonuria, however, a diet restricted in phenylalanine is harmful to the baby whose screening test is a false-positive, while diet therapy produces an excellent outcome in the truly affected baby if treatment is established within the first weeks of life. Therefore, initiation of treatment for phenylketonuria is contraindicated until the diagnosis is confirmed. Physicians should combine current American Academy of Pediatrics recommendations, state laws and regulations, and consultation with their local metabolic center to arrive at appropriate strategies for each hospital and practice.

Bryant KG et al: A primer on newborn screening. Adv Neonatal Care 2004;4:306 [PMID: 15517524].

Buist NR et al: Metabolic evaluation of infantile epilepsy: Summary recommendations of the Amalfi Group. J Child Neurol 2002;17(Suppl 3):3S98 [PMID: 12597059].

Carpenter KH, Wiley V: Application of tandem mass spectrometry to biochemical genetics and newborn screening. Clin Chim Acta 2002;322:1 [PMID: 12104075].

Carreiro-Lewandowski E: Newborn screening: an overview. Clin Lab Sci 2002;15:229 [PMID: 12776783].

Chace DH, Kalas TA: A biochemical perspective on the use of tandem mass spectrometry for newborn screening and clinical testing. Clin Biochem 2005;38:296 [PMID: 15766731].

Christodoulou J: Clinical evaluation and emergency management of inborn errors of metabolism presenting in the newborn. Southeast Asian J Trop Med Public Health 2003;34(Suppl 3):189 [PMID: 15906734].

Claudius I et al: The emergency department approach to newborn and childhood metabolic crisis. Emerg Med Clin North Am 2005;23:843 [PMID: 15982549].

Clayton PT: Inborn errors presenting with liver dysfunction. Semin Neonatol 2002;7:49 [PMID: 12069538].

de Lonlay P et al: Neonatal hypoglycaemia: aetiologies. Semin Neonatol 2004;9:49 [PMID: 15013475].

Ellaway CJ et al: Clinical approach to inborn errors of metabolism presenting in the newborn period. J Paediatr Child Health 2002;38:511 [PMID: 12354271].

Gilbert-Barness E: Review: Metabolic cardiomyopathy and conduction system defects in children. Ann Clin Lab Sci 2004;34:15 [PMID: 15038665].

Hardelid P, Dezateux C: Neonatal screening for inborn errors of metabolism. Lancet 2005;365:2176 [PMID: 15978919].

Horster F et al: Disorders of intermediary metabolism: toxic leukoencephalopathies. J Inherit Metab Dis 2005;28:345 [PMID: 15868467].

Jones PM, Bennett MJ: The changing face of newborn screening: Diagnosis of inborn errors of metabolism by tandem mass spectrometry. Clin Chim Acta 2002;324:121 [PMID: 12204433].

Kahler SG, Fahey MC: Metabolic disorders and mental retardation. Am J Med Genet C Semin Med Genet 2003;117:31 [PMID: 12561056].

Marsden D: Expanded newborn screening by tandem mass spectrometry: the Massachusetts and New England experience. Southeast Asian J Trop Med Public Health 2003;34(Suppl 3): 111 [PMID: 15906712].

Ogier de Baulny H: Management and emergency treatments of neonates with a suspicion of inborn errors of metabolism. Semin Neonatol 2002;7:17 [PMID: 12069535].

Olpin SE: The metabolic investigation of sudden infant death. Ann Clin Biochem 2004;41(Pt 4):282 [PMID: 15298740].

Saudubray JM et al: Clinical approach to inherited metabolic disorders in neonates: An overview. Semin Neonatol 2002;7:3 [PMID: 12069534].

Schulze A et al: Expanded newborn screening for inborn errors of metabolism by electrospray ionization-tandem mass spectrometry: Results, outcome, and implications. Pediatrics 2003:111:1399 [PMID: 12777559].

Schweitzer-Krantz S: Early diagnosis of inherited metabolic disorders towards improving outcome: the controversial issue of galactosaemia. Eur J Pediatr 2003;162(Suppl 1):S50 [PMID: 14614623].

Walter JH: Arguments for early screening: a clinician's perspective. Eur J Pediatr 2003;162(Suppl 1):S2 [PMID: 14648212].

Wilcken B et al: Screening newborns for inborn errors of metabolism by tandem mass spectrometry. N Engl J Med 2003;348:2304 [PMID: 12788994].

■ DISORDERS OF CARBOHYDRATE METABOLISM

GLYCOGEN STORAGE DISEASES

Glycogen is a highly branched polymer of glucose that is stored in liver and muscle. Different enzyme defects affect its biosynthesis and degradation. The hepatic forms of the glycogenoses cause growth failure, hepatomegaly, and severe fasting hypoglycemia. They include glucose-6-phosphatase deficiency (type I; von Gierke disease), debrancher enzyme deficiency (type III), hepatic phosphorylase deficiency (type VI), and phosphorylase kinase deficiency (type IX), which normally regulates hepatic phosphorylase activity. There are two forms of glucose-6-phosphatase deficiency: in type Ia, the catalytic glucose-6-phosphatase is deficient, and in type Ib, the glucose-6-phosphate transporter is deficient. The latter form also has neutropenia. Glycogenosis type IV, brancher enzyme deficiency, usually presents with progressive liver cirrhosis.

The myopathic forms of glycogenosis affect skeletal muscle. Skeletal myopathy with weakness or rhabdomyolysis may be seen in muscle phosphorylase deficiency (type V), phosphofructokinase deficiency (type VII), and acid maltase deficiency (type II; Pompe disease). The infantile form of Pompe disease also has hypertrophic cardiomyopathy and macroglossia. The gluconeogenetic disorder fructose-1,6-bisphosphatase deficiency presents with major lactic acidosis and delayed hypoglycemia on fasting.

Diagnosis

Initial tests include glucose, lactate, triglycerides, cholesterol, uric acid, transaminases, and creatine kinase. Functional testing includes responsiveness of blood glucose to fasting and glucagon, or at times, an ischemic exercise test is helpful. Diagnostic confirmation requires enzyme assays on leukocytes, liver, or muscle. Disorders diagnosable on red or white blood cells include deficiency of debrancher enzyme (type III) and phosphorylase kinase (type IX). Pompe disease can usually be diagnosed by assaying acid maltase in fibroblasts. Glycogenosis type I can sometimes be diagnosed by molecular analysis.

Treatment

Treatment is designed to prevent hypoglycemia and avoid secondary metabolite accumulations such as elevated lactate in glycogenosis type I. In the most severe hepatic forms, the special diet must be strictly monitored with restriction of free sugars and measured amounts of uncooked cornstarch which slowly releases glucose and small glucose polymers in the intestinal lumen. Good results have been reported following continuous nighttime carbohydrate feeding or uncooked cornstarch therapy. Late complications even after years of treatment include focal segmental glomerulosclerosis, hepatic adenoma or carcinoma, and gout. Early trials of enzyme replacement therapy in Pompe disease have been promising.

Bruno C et al: Clinical and genetic heterogeneity of branching enzyme deficiency (glycogenosis type IV). Neurology 2004;63: 1053 [PMID: 15452297].

Chou JY et al: Type I glycogen storage diseases: disorders of the glucose-6-phosphatase complex. Curr Mol Med 2002;2:121 [PMID: 11949931].

Hagemans ML et al: Clinical manifestation and natural course of late-onset Pompe's disease in 54 Dutch patients. Brain 2005;128:671 [PMID: 15659425].

Kannourakis G: Glycogen storage disease. Semin Hematol 2002; 39:103 [PMID: 11957192].

Kishnani PS, Howell RR: Pompe disease in infants and children. J Pediatr 2004;144(5 Suppl):S35 [PMID: 15126982].

Moses SW: Historical highlights and unsolved problems in glycogen storage disease type 1. Eur J Pediatr 2002;161(Suppl 1): S2 [PMID: 12373565].

Ollivier K et al: Exercise tolerance and daily life in McArdle's disease. Muscle Nerve 2005;31:637 [PMID: 15614801].

Rake JP et al: Guidelines for management of glycogen storage disease type I—European Study on Glycogen Storage Disease Type I (ESGSD I). Eur J Pediatr 2002;161(Suppl 1):S112 [PMID: 12373584].

Visser G et al: Consensus guidelines for management of glycogen storage disease type 1b—European Study on Glycogen Storage Disease Type 1. Eur J Pediatr 2002;161(Suppl 1):S120 [PMID: 12373585].

Winkel LP et al: Enzyme replacement therapy in late-onset Pompe's disease: a three-year follow-up. Ann Neurol 2004; 55:495 [PMID: 15048888].

GALACTOSEMIA

Classic galactosemia is caused by almost total deficiency of galactose-1-phosphate uridyltransferase. Accumulation of galactose-1-phosphate in liver and renal tubules causes hepatic parenchymal disease and renal Fanconi syndrome. Onset of the severe disease is marked in the neonate by vomiting, jaundice (both direct and indirect), hepatomegaly, and rapid onset of liver insufficiency after initiation of milk feeding. Hepatic cirrhosis is progressive. Without treatment, death frequently occurs within a month, often from *Escherichia coli* sepsis. Cataracts, caused by accumulation of galactitol in the lens, usually develop within 2 months in untreated cases, but usually reverse with treatment. With prompt institution of a galactose-free diet, the prognosis for survival without liver disease is excellent. Even when dietary restriction is instituted early, patients with galactosemia are at increased risk for speech and language deficits and ovarian failure. Some patients develop progressive mental retardation, tremor, and ataxia. Milder variants of galactosemia with better prognosis exist in all populations.

The disorder is autosomal recessive with an incidence of approximately 1:40,000 live births. Because disease in infancy may be severe, newborn screening is common. Screening is accomplished by demonstrating enzyme deficiency in red cells with the Beutler test or by demonstrating increased serum galactose.

Diagnosis

In infants receiving foods containing galactose, laboratory findings include galactosuria and hypergalactosemia together with proteinuria and aminoaciduria. Absence of urine-reducing substances does not exclude the diagnosis. Galactose-1-phosphate is elevated in red blood cells. When the diagnosis is suspected, galactose-1-phosphate uridyltransferase should be assayed in erythrocytes. Blood transfusions give false-negative results and sample deterioration false-positive results.

Treatment

A galactose-free diet should be instituted as soon as the diagnosis is made. Compliance with the diet must be monitored by following galactose-1-phosphate levels in red blood cells. Appropriate diet management requires not only the exclusion of milk but an understanding of the galactose content of foods. Avoidance of galactose should be lifelong with appropriate calcium replacement.

Antshel KM et al: Cognitive strengths and weaknesses in children and adolescents homozygous for the galactosemia Q188R mutation: a descriptive study. Neuropsychology 2004;18:658 [PMID: 15506833].

Bosch AM et al: Clinical features of galactokinase deficiency: a review of the literature. J Inherit Metab Dis 2002;25:629 [PMID: 12705493].

Bosch AM et al: Living with classical galactosemia: health-related quality of life consequences. Pediatrics 2004;113:e423 [PMID: 15121984].

Lambert C, Boneh A: The impact of galactosemia on quality of life—a pilot study. J Inherit Metab Dis 2004;27:601 [PMID: 15669675].

Leslie ND: Insights into the pathogenesis of galactosemia. Annu Rev Nutr 2003;23:59 [PMID: 12704219].

Panis B et al: Bone metabolism in galactosemia. Bone 2004;35:982 [PMID: 15454106].

Ridel KR et al: An updated review of the long-term neurological effects of galactosemia. Pediatr Neurol 2005;33:153 [PMID: 16087312].

Webb AL et al: Verbal dyspraxia and galactosemia. Pediatr Res 2003;53:396 [PMID: 12595586].

Zaffanello M et al: Neonatal screening, clinical features and genetic testing for galactosemia. Genet Med 2005;7:211 [PMID: 15775761].

A patient/parent support group website with useful information for families: www.galactosemia.org

HEREDITARY FRUCTOSE INTOLERANCE

Hereditary fructose intolerance is an autosomal recessive disorder in which deficient activity of fructose-1-phosphate aldolase causes hypoglycemia and tissue accumulation of fructose-1-phosphate on fructose ingestion. Other abnormalities include failure to thrive, vomiting, jaundice, hepatomegaly, proteinuria, and generalized aminoaciduria. The untreated condition can progress to death from liver failure.

Diagnosis

The diagnosis is suggested by finding fructosuria or abnormal transferrin glycoform in the untreated patient. The appearance of hypoglycemia and hypophosphatemia after a closely monitored intravenous fructose loading test (200 mg/kg) is diagnostic. The diagnosis is confirmed by finding reduced enzyme activity of fructose-1-phosphate aldolase in the liver. Some patients may be diagnosed by identification of one of the common mutations on DNA analysis, but their absence does not exclude the diagnosis.

Treatment

Treatment consists of strict dietary avoidance of fructose. Vitamin supplementation is usually needed. Management is complicated by the fact that many drugs and

vitamins are dispensed in a sucrose base. Treatment monitoring can be done with transferrin glycoform analysis. If diet compliance is poor, physical growth retardation may occur. Growth will resume when more stringent dietary restrictions are reinstituted. If the disorder is recognized early, the prospects for normal development are good. As affected individuals grow up, they may recognize the association of nausea and vomiting with ingestion of fructose-containing foods and selectively avoid them.

Choi YK et al: Fructose intolerance: an under-recognized problem. Am J Gastroenterol 2003;98:1348 [PMID: 12818280].

Wong D: Hereditary fructose intolerance. Mol Genet Metab 2005; 85:165 [PMID: 16086449].

■ DISORDERS OF ENERGY METABOLISM

The most common disorders of central mitochondrial energy metabolism are pyruvate dehydrogenase deficiency and deficiencies of respiratory chain components. In many but not all patients, lactate is elevated in either blood or CSF. In pyruvate dehydrogenase deficiency, the lactate:pyruvate ratio is normal, whereas in respiratory chain disorders, the ratio is increased. Care must be taken to distinguish an elevated lactate that is due to these conditions (called primary lactic acidoses) from elevated lactate that is a consequence of hypoxia, ischemia, or sampling problems. Table 32–3 lists some causes of primary lactic acidosis.

Patients with a defect in the pyruvate dehydrogenase complex often have agenesis of the corpus callosum or Leigh syndrome (lesions in the globus pallidus, the dentate nucleus, and the periaqueductal gray matter). They can have mild facial dysmorphism. Recurrent altered mental status, recurrent ataxia, and recurrent acidosis are typical of many disturbances of pyruvate metabolism. The most common genetic defect is in the X-linked E_1 component, with males carrying milder mutations and females carrying severe mutations leading to cystic brain lesions.

The respiratory chain disorders are frequent (1:5000), and involve a heterogenous group of genetic defects that produce a variety of clinical syndromes (now > 50) of varying severity and presentation. The disorders can affect multiple organs. The following set of symptoms can indicate a respiratory chain disorder: brain: progressive neurodegeneration, Leigh syndrome, myoclonic seizures, brain atrophy, and subcortical leukodystrophy; eye: optic neuropathy, retinitis pigmentosa, and progressive external ophthalmoplegia; ears: nerve deafness; general: failure to

Table 32–3. Causes of primary lactic acidosis in childhood.

Defects of the pyruvate dehydrogenase complex
 E$_1$ (pyruvate decarboxylase) deficiency
 E$_2$ (dihydrolipoyl transacetylase) deficiency
 E$_3$ (lipoamide dehydrogenase) deficiency
 Pyruvate decarboxylase phosphate phosphatase deficiency
Abnormalities of gluconeogenesis
 Pyruvate carboxylase deficiency
  Isolated
  Biotinidase deficiency
  Holocarboxylase synthetase deficiency
 Fructose-1,6-diphosphatase deficiency
 Glucose-6-phosphatase deficiency (von Gierke disease)
Defects in the mitochondrial respiratory chain
 Complex I deficiency
 Complex IV deficiency (cytochrome C oxidase deficiency; frequent cause of Leigh disease)
 ATPase deficiency (frequent cause of Leigh disease)
 Other respiratory chain disorders

---

thrive; muscle: myopathy with decreased endurance; kidney: renal Fanconi syndrome; endocrine: diabetes mellitus and hypoparathyroidism; intestinal: pancreatic or liver insufficiency, or pseudo-obstruction; skin: areas of hypopigmentation; and heart: cardiomyopathy, conduction defects, and arrhythmias. Respiratory chain disorders are among the more common causes of static, progressive, or self-limited neurodevelopmental problems in children. Patients may present with nonspecific findings such as hypotonia, failure to thrive, or renal tubular acidosis, or with more specific features such as ophthalmoplegia or cardiomyopathy. Symptoms are often combined in recognizable clinical syndromes with ties to specific genetic causes. Ragged red fibers and mitochondrial abnormalities may be noted on histologic examination of muscle. Thirteen of the more than 100 genes that control activity of the respiratory chain are part of the mitochondrial genome. Therefore inheritance of defects in the respiratory chain may be mendelian or maternal.

Diagnosis

Pyruvate dehydrogenase deficiency is diagnosed by enzyme assay in leukocytes or fibroblasts. Confirmation can be obtained by molecular analysis. Diagnosis of respiratory chain disorders is based on a convergence of clinical, biochemical, morphologic, enzymatic, and molecular data. Classic pathologic features of mitochondrial disorders are the accumulation of mitochondria which produce ragged red fibers in skeletal muscle biopsy, and abnormal shapes and inclusions on electron microscopy. Unfortunately these findings are only present in 5% of children. Enzyme analysis on skeletal muscle or liver tissue is complicated by an overlap between normal and affected range. Mitochondrial DNA analysis in blood or tissue may identify a diagnostic mutation. A rapidly increasing number of nuclear genes causing respiratory chain defects are being recognized. Although diagnostic criteria have been published, the cause of lactic acidemia still cannot be defined in many patients. In some instances, the genetics and prognosis may be clear, but in many cases neither prognosis nor genetic risk can be predicted.

Treatment

A ketogenic diet is useful in some cases of pyruvate dehydrogenase deficiency. In rare patients with primary coenzyme Q deficiency, coenzyme Q treatment is very effective. Other treatments are of theoretical value, with little data on efficacy. Thiamine and lipoic acid have been tried in patients with pyruvate dehydrogenase complex deficiencies, and coenzyme Q and riboflavin have been helpful in some patients with respiratory chain defects. Dichloroacetic acid has been tried in pyruvate dehydrogenase complex deficiencies and in respiratory chain disorders, with variable clinical response and adverse effects.

Bernier FP et al. Diagnostic criteria for respiratory chain disorders in adults and children. Neurology 2002;59:1406 [PMID: 12427892].

Borchert A et al: Current concepts of mitochondrial disorders in childhood. Semin Pediatr Neurol 2002;9:151 [PMID: 12138999].

Brown GK: Congenital brain malformations in mitochondrial disease. J Inherit Metab Dis 2005;28:393 [PMID: 15868471].

Chaturvedi S et al: Mitochondrial encephalomyopathies: advances in understanding. Med Sci Monit 2005;11:RA238 [PMID: 15990701].

De Meirleir L: Defects of pyruvate metabolism and the Krebs cycle. J Child Neurol 2002;17(Suppl 3):3S26; discussion 3S33 [PMID: 12597053].

DiMauro S et al: Mitochondrial encephalomyopathies: diagnostic approach. Ann N Y Acad Sci 2004;1011:217 [PMID: 15126299].

DiMauro S et al: Mitochondrial encephalomyopathies: therapeutic approach. Ann N Y Acad Sci 2004;1011:232 [PMID: 15126300].

DiMauro S, Hirano M: Mitochondrial encephalomyopathies: an update. Neuromuscul Disord 2005;15:276 [PMID: 15792866].

Gillis L, Kaye E: Diagnosis and management of mitochondrial diseases. Pediatr Clin North Am 2002;49:203 [PMID: 11826805].

Huntsman RJ et al: Atypical presentations of Leigh syndrome: a case series and review. Pediatr Neurol 2005;32:334 [PMID: 15866434].

Lerman-Sagie T et al: White matter involvement in mitochondrial diseases. Mol Genet Metab 2005;84:127 [PMID: 15670718].

Scaglia F et al: Clinical spectrum, morbidity, and mortality in 113 pediatric patients with mitochondrial disease. Pediatrics 2004;114:925 [PMID: 15466086].

Schmiedel J et al: Mitochondrial cytopathies. J Neurol 2003;250:267 [PMID: 12638015].

Skladal D et al: The clinical spectrum of mitochondrial disease in 75 pediatric patients. Clin Pediatr (Phila) 2003;42:703 [PMID: 14601919].

Taylor RW, Turnbull DM: Mitochondrial DNA mutations in human disease. Nat Rev Genet 2005;6:389 [PMID: 15861210].

Thorburn DR et al: Biochemical and molecular diagnosis of mitochondrial respiratory chain disorders. Biochim Biophys Acta 2004;1659:121 [PMID: 15576043].

Vallance H: Biochemical approach to the investigation of pediatric mitochondrial disease. Pediatr Dev Pathol 2004;7:633 [PMID: 15630534].

Wong LJ: Comprehensive molecular diagnosis of mitochondrial disorders: qualitative and quantitative approach. Ann N Y Acad Sci 2004;1011:246 [PMID: 15126301].

Zeviani M, Di Donato S: Mitochondrial disorders. Brain 2004;127(Pt 10):2153 [PMID: 15358637].

A patient/parent support group website with useful information for families: www.umdf.org

DISORDERS OF AMINO ACID METABOLISM

DISORDERS OF THE UREA CYCLE

Ammonia is mostly derived from the catabolism of amino acids and is converted to an amino group in urea by enzymes of the urea cycle. Patients with severe defects (often those enzymes early in the urea cycle) usually present in infancy with severe hyperammonemia, vomiting, and encephalopathy, which is rapidly fatal. In patients with milder genetic defects, the course may be milder with vomiting and encephalopathy after protein ingestion or infection. Although defects in argininosuccinic acid synthetase (citrullinemia) and argininosuccinic acid lyase (argininosuccinic acidemia) may cause severe hyperammonemia in infancy, the usual clinical course is chronic with mental retardation. Ornithine transcarbamylase deficiency is X-linked. The rest of the urea cycle disorders are autosomal recessive. Age at onset of symptoms varies with residual enzyme activity, protein intake, growth, and stresses such as infection. Even within a family, males with ornithine transcarbamylase deficiency may differ by decades in the age of symptom onset. Many female carriers of ornithine transcarbamylase deficiency have protein intolerance. Some develop migrainelike symptoms after protein loads, and others develop potentially fatal episodes of vomiting and encephalopathy after protein ingestion, infections, or during labor and delivery. Trichorrhexis nodosa is common in patients with the chronic form of argininosuccinic acidemia.

Diagnosis

Blood ammonia should be measured in any acutely ill newborn in whom a cause is not obvious. In urea cycle defects, early hyperammonemia is associated with respiratory alkalosis. Serum citrulline is low or undetectable in carbamoyl phosphate synthetase and ornithine transcarbamylase deficiency, high in argininosuccinic acidemia, and very high in citrullinemia. Large amounts of argininosuccinic acid are found in the urine of patients with argininosuccinic acidemia. Urine orotic acid is increased in infants with ornithine transcarbamylase deficiency. Citrullinemia and argininosuccinic acidemia can be diagnosed in utero by appropriate enzyme assays, but carbamoyl phosphate synthetase and ornithine transcarbamylase deficiency can be diagnosed in utero only by using specific gene probes, and then only in certain families.

Treatment

During treatment of acute hyperammonemic crisis, protein intake should be stopped, and glucose and lipids should be given to reduce endogenous protein breakdown from catabolism. Arginine should be given intravenously, both because it is an essential amino acid for patients with urea cycle defects and because it increases the excretion of waste nitrogen in patients with citrullinemia and argininosuccinic acidemia. Sodium benzoate, either alone or with sodium phenylacetate, can be given intravenously to treat hyperammonemic coma. Additionally, hemodialysis is indicated for severe or persistent hyperammonemia, as is usually the case in the newborn. Peritoneal dialysis and double-volume exchange transfusion are insufficiently effective in this setting.

Long-term treatment includes oral administration of arginine (or citrulline), adherence to a low-protein diet, and administration of sodium benzoate and sodium phenylacetate or its prodrug, sodium phenylbutyrate, to increase excretion of nitrogen as hippuric acid and phenylacetylglutamine. Symptomatic heterozygous female carriers of ornithine transcarbamylase deficiency should also receive such treatment. Liver transplantation may be curative and is indicated for severe disorders.

The outcome of argininosuccinic acidemia and citrullinemia is better than that of ornithine transcarbamylase and carbamoyl phosphate synthetase deficiency. Most patients with urea cycle defects, no matter what the enzyme defect, develop permanent neurologic and intellectual impairments, with cortical atrophy and ventricular dilation seen on computed tomographic scan. Rapid identification and treatment of the initial hyperammonemic episode improves outcome.

Bachmann C: Long-term outcome of patients with urea cycle disorders and the question of neonatal screening. Eur J Pediatr 2003;162(Suppl 1):S29 [PMID: 14634803].

Bachmann C: Outcome and survival of 88 patients with urea cycle disorders: a retrospective evaluation. Eur J Pediatr 2003;162:410 [PMID: 12684900].

Cohn RM, Roth KS: Hyperammonemia, bane of the brain. Clin Pediatr (Phila) 2004;43:683 [PMID: 15494874].

Endo F et al: Clinical manifestations of inborn errors of the urea cycle and related metabolic disorders during childhood. J Nutr 2004;134(6 Suppl):1605S [PMID: 15173438].

Gropman AL, Batshaw ML: Cognitive outcome in urea cycle disorders. Mol Genet Metab 2004;81(Suppl 1):S58 [PMID: 15050975].

Gyato K et al: Metabolic and neuropsychological phenotype in women heterozygous for ornithine transcarbamylase deficiency. Ann Neurol 2004;55:80 [PMID: 14705115].

Leonard JV, McKiernan PJ: The role of liver transplantation in urea cycle disorders. Mol Genet Metab 2004;81(Suppl 1):S74 [PMID: 15050978].

Leonard JV, Morris AA: Urea cycle disorders. Semin Neonatol 2002;7:27 [PMID: 12069536].

Nassogne MC et al: Urea cycle defects: management and outcome. J Inherit Metab Dis 2005;28:407 [PMID: 15868473].

Nicolaides P et al: Neurological outcome in patients with ornithine carbamoyltransferase deficiency. Arch Dis Child 2002;86:54 [PMID: 11806886].

Scaglia F et al: Effect of alternative pathway therapy on branched chain amino acid metabolism in urea cycle disorder patients. Mol Genet Metab 2004;81(Suppl 1):S79 [PMID: 15050979].

Wilcken B: Problems in the management of urea cycle disorders. Mol Genet Metab 2004;81(Suppl 1):S86 [PMID: 15050980].

A patient/parent support group website with useful information for families: www.nucdf.org

PHENYLKETONURIA & THE HYPERPHENYLALANINEMIAS

Probably the best-known disorder of amino acid metabolism is the classic form of phenylketonuria caused by decreased activity of phenylalanine hydroxylase, the enzyme that converts phenylalanine to tyrosine. In classic phenylketonuria, there is little or no phenylalanine hydroxylase activity. In the less severe hyperphenylalaninemias there may be significant residual activity. Rare variants can be due to deficiency of dihydropteridine reductase or defects in biopterin synthesis.

Phenylketonuria is an autosomal recessive trait, with an incidence in Caucasians of approximately 1:10,000 live births. On a normal neonatal diet, affected patients develop hyperphenylalaninemia. Patients with untreated phenylketonuria exhibit severe mental retardation, hyperactivity, seizures, a light complexion, and eczema. The patient's urine has a "mouse-like" odor.

Success in preventing severe mental retardation in phenylketonuric children by restricting phenylalanine starting in early infancy led to screening programs to detect the disease early. Because the outcome is best when treatment is begun in the first month of life, infants should be screened during the first few days. A second test is necessary when newborn screening is done before 24 hours of age. In such cases the second test should be completed by the third week of life.

Diagnosis & Treatment

The diagnosis of phenylketonuria in a severely mentally retarded older child with typical biochemical and physical characteristics is straightforward, but in the newborn period, especially when there is no family history, the condition must be differentiated from other forms of hyperphenylalaninemia. This is usually done by determining serum phenylalanine and tyrosine levels on a normal diet and by examining pterins in blood and urine.

Prenatal diagnosis of phenylketonuria is possible using DNA probes. Molecular approaches are replacing serum measurements of phenylalanine and tyrosine to determine carrier status. Prenatal diagnosis of defects in pterin metabolism can often be made.

A. CLASSIC PHENYLKETONURIA

Findings include persistently elevated serum levels of phenylalanine (> 20 mg/dL or 1200 µM on a regular diet), normal or low serum levels of tyrosine, and normal pterins. Poor phenylalanine tolerance persists throughout life. Restriction of dietary phenylalanine intake (see section on treatment) is indicated, and a favorable outcome is the rule.

B. PERSISTENT HYPERPHENYLALANINEMIA

In infants receiving a normal protein intake, serum phenylalanine levels are usually 4–20 mg/dL, and pterins are normal. Phenylalanine restriction is indicated if phenylalanine levels consistently exceed 10 mg/dL (600 µM).

C. TRANSIENT HYPERPHENYLALANINEMIA

Serum phenylalanine levels are elevated early but progressively decline toward normal. Dietary restriction is only temporary, if required at all.

D. DIHYDROPTERIDINE REDUCTASE DEFICIENCY

Serum phenylalanine levels vary. The pattern of pterin metabolites is abnormal. Seizures and psychomotor regression occur even with diet therapy, probably because the enzyme defect also causes neuronal deficiency of serotonin and dopamine. These deficiencies require treatment with levodopa, carbidopa, 5-hydroxytryptophan, and folinic acid.

E. DEFECTS IN BIOPTERIN BIOSYNTHESIS

Serum phenylalanine levels vary. Total pterins are low, and their pattern may suggest the specific defect, which can be at one of several steps in the biosynthetic pathway. Clinical findings include myoclonus, tetraplegia, dystonia, oculogyric crises, and other movement disorders. Treatment is the same as for dihydropteridine reductase deficiency. Tetrahydrobiopterin may be added.

F. TYROSINEMIA OF THE NEWBORN

Serum phenylalanine levels are lower than those associated with phenylketonuria and are accompanied by marked hypertyrosinemia. Tyrosinemia of the newborn usually occurs in premature infants and is due to immaturity of 4-hydroxyphenylpyruvic acid oxidase. The condition resolves spontaneously within 3 months, almost always without sequelae.

G. MATERNAL PHENYLKETONURIA

Offspring of phenylketonuric mothers may have transient hyperphenylalaninemia at birth. Elevated maternal phenylalanine causes mental retardation, microcephaly, growth retardation, and often congenital heart disease or other malformations in the offspring. The risk to the fetus is lessened considerably by maternal phenylalanine restriction with maintenance of phenylalanine levels below 6 mg/dL (360 µM) before conception and throughout pregnancy.

Treatment of Classic Phenylketonuria

Treatment of classic phenylketonuria is to limit dietary phenylalanine intake to amounts that permit normal growth and development. Dietary goals usually aim for a phenylalanine level less than 6 mg/dL (360 µM). Metabolic formulas deficient in phenylalanine are available but must be supplemented with normal milk and other foods to supply enough phenylalanine to permit normal growth and development. Serum phenylalanine concentrations must be monitored frequently while ensuring that growth, development, and nutrition are adequate. This monitoring is best done in clinics experienced in dealing with such problems. Although dietary treatment is most effective when initiated during the first months of life, it may also be of benefit in reversing behaviors such as hyperactivity, irritability, and distractibility when started later in life.

Phenylalanine restriction should continue throughout life, both because of subtle changes in intellect and behavior in persons receiving treatment early who later stop the diet, and because of the risk of late development of potentially irreversible neurologic damage after stopping the diet. Counseling should be given during adolescence, and the woman's diet should be monitored closely prior to conception and throughout pregnancy.

Children with classic phenylketonuria who receive treatment promptly after birth and achieve phenylalanine and tyrosine homeostasis will develop well physically and can be expected to have normal or near-normal intellectual development.

Blau N, Erlandsen H: The metabolic and molecular bases of tetrahydrobiopterin-responsive phenylalanine hydroxylase deficiency. Mol Genet Metab 2004;82:101 [PMID: 15171997].

Blau N, Scriver CR: New approaches to treat PKU: how far are we? Mol Genet Metab 2004;81:1 [PMID: 14728984].

Brumm VL et al: Neuropsychological outcome of subjects participating in the PKU adult collaborative study: a preliminary review. J Inherit Metab Dis 2004;27:549 [PMID: 15669671].

Cederbaum S: Phenylketonuria: An update. Curr Opin Pediatr 2002;14:702 [PMID: 12436039].

Channon S et al: Executive functioning, memory, and learning in phenylketonuria. Neuropsychology 2004;18:613 [PMID: 15506828].

Feillet F et al: Maternal phenylketonuria: the French survey. Eur J Pediatr 2004;163:540 [PMID: 15241684].

Gassio R et al: Cognitive functions in classic phenylketonuria and mild hyperphenylalaninaemia: experience in a paediatric population. Dev Med Child Neurol 2005;47:443 [PMID: 15991863].

Hanley WB et al: Maternal Phenylketonuria Collaborative Study (MPKUCS)—the 'outliers'. J Inherit Metab Dis 2004;27:711 [PMID: 15505376].

Kim W et al: Trends in enzyme therapy for phenylketonuria. Mol Ther 2004;10:220 [PMID: 15294168].

Koch R: Maternal phenylketonuria: the importance of early control during pregnancy. Arch Dis Child 2005;90:114 [PMID: 15665159].

Lee PJ et al: Maternal phenylketonuria: report from the United Kingdom Registry 1978-97. Arch Dis Child 2005;90:143 [PMID: 15665165].

Leuzzi V et al: Executive function impairment in early-treated PKU subjects with normal mental development. J Inherit Metab Dis 2004;27:115 [PMID: 15159642].

Lucke T et al: BH4-sensitive hyperphenylalaninemia: New case and review of literature. Pediatr Neurol 2003;28:228 [PMID: 12770680].

Macdonald A et al: Protein substitutes for PKU: what's new? J Inherit Metab Dis 2004;27:363 [PMID: 15190194].

Matalon R et al: Biopterin responsive phenylalanine hydroxylase deficiency. Genet Med 2004;6:27 [PMID: 14726806].

Moats RA et al: Brain phenylalanine concentrations in phenylketonuria: research and treatment of adults. Pediatrics 2003;112(6 Pt 2):1575 [PMID: 14654668].

Perez-Duenas B et al: Tetrahydrobiopterin responsiveness in patients with phenylketonuria. Clin Biochem 2004;37:1083 [PMID: 15589814].

Pey AL et al: Mechanisms underlying responsiveness to tetrahydrobiopterin in mild phenylketonuria mutations. Hum Mutat 2004;24:388 [PMID: 15459954].

Spaapen LJ, Rubio-Gozalbo ME: Tetrahydrobiopterin-responsive phenylalanine hydroxylase deficiency, state of the art. Mol Genet Metab 2003;78:93 [PMID: 12618080].

Steinfeld R et al: Efficiency of long-term tetrahydrobiopterin monotherapy in phenylketonuria. J Inherit Metab Dis 2004; 27:449 [PMID: 15303001].

Patient/parent support group websites with useful information for families: www.pkunews.org and www.pkunetwork.org

HEREDITARY TYROSINEMIA

Type 1 hereditary tyrosinemia is caused by deficiency of fumarylacetoacetase. It presents with acute or progressive hepatic parenchymal damage, renal tubular dystrophy with generalized aminoaciduria, hypophosphatemic rickets, or neuropathic crises. Tyrosine and methionine are increased in blood and tyrosine metabolites and aminolevulinic acid in urine. The key diagnostic metabolite is elevated succinylacetone in urine. Liver failure may be rapidly fatal in infancy or somewhat more chronic, with liver cell carcinoma almost invariable in long-term survivors. The condition is autosomal recessive and is especially common in Scandinavia and in the Chicoutimi–Lac St. Jean region of Quebec. Prenatal diagnosis is possible.

Diagnosis

Similar clinical and biochemical findings may occur in other liver diseases such as galactosemia and hereditary fructose intolerance. Increased succinylacetone occurs only in fumarylacetoacetase deficiency, and is diagnostic. Enzyme assay in liver biopsy or mutation analysis can provide further diagnostic confirmation.

Treatment

A diet low in phenylalanine and tyrosine is indicated and can ameliorate liver disease, but does not prevent carcinoma development. Pharmacologic therapy to inhibit 4-hydroxyphenylpyruvate dehydrogenase using 2-(2-nitro-4-trifluoromethylbenzoyl)-1,3-cyclohexanedione (NTBC) decreases the production of toxic metabolites, maleylacetoacetate and fumarylacetoacetate. It improves the liver disease and renal disease, prevents acute neuronopathic attacks, and greatly reduces the risk of hepatocellular carcinoma. Liver transplantation is effective therapy for these children.

Joshi SN, Venugopalan P: Experience with NTBC therapy in hereditary tyrosinaemia type I: an alternative to liver transplantation. Ann Trop Paediatr 2004;24:259 [PMID: 15479577].

MAPLE SYRUP URINE DISEASE (Branched-Chain Ketoaciduria)

Maple syrup urine disease is due to deficiency of the enzyme catalyzing oxidative decarboxylation of the branched-chain keto acid derivatives of leucine, isoleucine, and valine. Accumulated keto acids of leucine and isoleucine cause the characteristic odor. Only leucine and its corresponding keto acid have been implicated in causing central nervous system dysfunction. Many variants of this disorder have been described, including mild, intermittent, and thiamin-dependent forms. All are autosomal recessive traits.

Patients with classic maple syrup urine disease are normal at birth but after about 1 week develop feeding difficulties, coma, and seizures. Unless diagnosis is made and dietary restriction of branched-chain amino acids is begun, most will die in the first month of life. Nearly normal growth and development may be achieved if treatment is begun before about age 10 days.

Diagnosis

Amino acid analysis shows marked elevations of branched-chain amino acids including alloisoleucine in serum and urine. Alloisoleucine, a transamination product of the keto acid of isoleucine, is almost pathognomonic. Urine organic acids demonstrate the characteristic keto acids. The magnitude and consistency of amino acid and organic acid changes are altered in mild and intermittent forms of the disease. Prenatal diagnosis is possible.

Treatment

Metabolic formulas deficient in branched-chain amino acids are available but must be supplemented with normal milk and other foods to supply enough branched-chain amino acids to permit normal growth and development. Serum levels of branched-chain amino acids must be monitored frequently in the first months of life to deal with changing protein requirements. Acute episodes must be aggressively treated to prevent catabolism and negative nitrogen balance.

Heldt K et al: Diagnosis of MSUD by newborn screening allows early intervention without extraneous detoxification. Mol Genet Metab 2005;84:313 [PMID: 15781191].

Morton DH et al: Diagnosis and treatment of maple syrup disease: A study of 36 patients. Pediatrics 2002;109:999 [PMID: 12042535].

Schonberger S et al: Dysmyelination in the brain of adolescents and young adults with maple syrup urine disease. Mol Genet Metab 2004;82:69 [PMID: 15110325].

Strauss KA, Morton DH: Branched-chain ketoacyl dehydrogenase deficiency: maple syrup disease. Curr Treat Options Neurol 2003;5:329 [PMID: 12791200].

HOMOCYSTINURIA

Homocystinuria is most often due to deficiency of cystathionine β-synthase, but may also be due to deficiency of methylenetetrahydrofolate reductase (MTHR) or to defects in the biosynthesis of methyl-B_{12}, the coenzyme for N^5-methyltetrahydrofolate methyltransferase. All known inherited forms of homocystinuria are transmitted as autosomal recessive traits and can be diagnosed in the fetus.

About 50% of patients with untreated cystathionine β-synthase deficiency are mentally retarded, and most have arachnodactyly, osteoporosis, and a tendency to develop dislocated lenses and thromboembolic phenomena. Milder elevations of homocystine are increasingly recognized as a factor in the etiology of vascular disease leading to myocardial infarction and stroke. These mild elevations are often caused by mutations leading to heat-sensitive defects in MTHR. Patients with remethylation defects usually exhibit failure to thrive and a variety of neurologic symptoms, including brain atrophy, microcephaly, and seizures in infancy and early childhood.

Diagnosis

Diagnosis is made by demonstrating homocystinuria in a patient who is not severely deficient in vitamin B_{12}. Serum methionine levels are usually high in patients with cystathionine β-synthase deficiency and often low in patients with remethylation defects. When the remethylation defect is due to deficiency of methyl-B_{12}, megaloblastic anemia or hemolytic uremic syndrome may be present, and an associated deficiency of adenosyl-B_{12} may cause methylmalonic aciduria. Studies of cultured fibroblasts may be necessary to make a specific diagnosis.

Treatment

About 50% of patients with cystathionine β-synthase deficiency respond to large oral doses of pyridoxine. Early treatment of pyridoxine nonresponders is by dietary methionine restriction. Oral administration of betaine will increase methylation of homocystine to methionine in patients with remethylation defects and may also improve neurologic function. Early treatment prevents mental retardation, lens dislocation, and thromboembolic manifestations, which justifies the screening of newborn infants. Large doses of vitamin B_{12} (eg, 1–5 mg hydroxycobalamin administered daily intramuscularly or subcutaneously) are indicated in some patients with defects in cobalamin metabolism.

Kelly PJ et al: Stroke in young patients with hyperhomocysteinemia to cystathionine beta-synthase deficiency. Neurology 2003; 60:275 [PMID: 12552044].

Moat SJ et al: The molecular basis of cystathionine beta-synthase (CBS) deficiency in UK and US patients with homocystinuria. Hum Mutat 2004;23:206 [PMID: 14722927].

Orendac M et al: Homocystinuria due to cystathionine beta-synthase deficiency: novel biochemical findings and treatment efficacy. J Inherit Metab Dis 2003;26:761 [PMID: 14739681].

Refsum H et al: Birth prevalence of homocystinuria. J Pediatr 2004;144:830 [PMID: 15192637].

Sakamoto A, Sakura N: Limited effectiveness of betaine therapy for cystathionine beta synthase deficiency. Pediatr Int 2003;45:333 [PMID: 12828591].

Singh RH et al: Cystathionine beta-synthase deficiency: effects of betaine supplementation after methionine restriction in B6-nonresponsive homocystinuria. Genet Med 2004;6:90 [PMID: 15017331].

Smith DL, Bodamer OA: Practical management of combined methylmalonicaciduria and homocystinuria. J Child Neurol 2002;17:353 [PMID: 12150582].

Yap S: Classical homocystinuria: vascular risk and its prevention. J Inherit Metab Dis 2003;26(2-3):259 [PMID: 12889665].

NONKETOTIC HYPERGLYCINEMIA

Inherited deficiency of various subunits of the glycine cleavage enzyme causes nonketotic hyperglycinemia. Glycine accumulation in the brain disturbs neurotransmission of the glycinergic receptors and the N-methyl-D-aspartate receptor. In its most severe form, also termed glycine encephalopathy, the condition presents in the newborn as hypotonia, lethargy proceeding to coma, myoclonic seizures, and hiccups, with a burst suppression pattern on electroencephalography. Apnea spells may develop requiring ventilator assistance in the first 2 weeks. The majority of patients develop severe mental retardation and seizures. Some patients have agenesis of the corpus callosum or posterior fossa malformations. Some patients present with seizures later in infancy or with developmental delay in childhood. All forms of the condition are autosomal recessive.

Diagnosis

Nonketotic hyperglycinemia should be suspected in any neonate or infant with seizures and is confirmed by demonstrating a large increase in glycine in nonbloody CSF with the ratio of CSF glycine to serum glycine being abnormally high. Enzyme analysis in a liver sample can confirm the diagnosis and can distinguish between defects in the T-protein or the P- and H-proteins. Molecular analysis is diagnostic in many cases. Prenatal diagnosis is possible only by assaying the enzyme in uncultured chorionic villus samples or by molecular analysis if both mutations are known in advance.

Treatment

Treatment of mild patients with sodium benzoate aimed at normalizing serum glycine levels and with dextromethorphan or ketamine to block N-methyl-D-aspartate receptors controls seizures and improves outcome. Treatment of severely affected patients is generally unsuccessful. High-dose benzoate therapy can aid in seizure control, but does not prevent severe mental retardation.

Aliefendioglu D et al: Transient nonketotic hyperglycinemia: Two case reports and literature review. Pediatr Neurol 2003;28:151 [PMID: 12699870].

Applegarth DA, Toone JR: Glycine encephalopathy (nonketotic hyperglycinaemia): review and update. J Inherit Metab Dis 2004;27:417 [PMID: 15272469].

Chien YH et al: Poor outcome for neonatal-type nonketotic hyperglycinemia treated with high-dose sodium benzoate and dextromethorphan. J Child Neurol 2004;19:39 [PMID: 15032382].

Hoover-Fong JE et al: Natural history of nonketotic hyperglycinemia in 65 patients. Neurology 2004;63:1847 [PMID: 15557500].

■ ORGANIC ACIDEMIAS

Organic acidemias are disorders of amino and fatty acid metabolism in which non-amino organic acids accumulate in serum and urine. These conditions are usually diagnosed by examining organic acids in urine, a complex procedure that requires considerable interpretive expertise and is usually performed only in specialized laboratories. Table 32–4 lists the clinical features of organic acidemias, together with the urine organic acid patterns typical of each. Additional details about some of the more important organic acidemias are provided in the sections that follow.

PROPIONIC & METHYLMALONIC ACIDEMIA (Ketotic Hyperglycinemias)

Idiopathic hyperglycinemia was first reported in 1961 as a syndrome of mental retardation and episodic ketoacidosis, neutropenia, thrombocytopenia, osteoporosis, and hyperglycinemia induced by protein intake or infection. It was then renamed ketotic hyperglycinemia to distinguish it from nonketotic hyperglycinemia, described in the preceding section. It is now known that the syndrome is almost always due to propionic or methylmalonic acidemia.

The oxidation of threonine, valine, methionine, and isoleucine results in propionyl-CoA, which propionyl-CoA carboxylase converts into L-methylmalonyl-CoA, which is metabolized through methylmalonyl-CoA mutase to succinyl-CoA. Gut bacteria and the breakdown of odd-chain-length fatty acids also substantially contribute to propionyl-CoA production. Propionic acidemia is due to a defect in the biotin-containing enzyme propionyl-CoA carboxylase, and methylmalonic acidemia is due to a defect in methylmalonyl-CoA mutase. In most cases the latter is due to a defect in the mutase apoenzyme, but in others it is due to a defect in the biosynthesis of its adenosyl-B_{12} coenzyme. In some of these defects, only the synthesis of adenosyl-B_{12} is blocked; in others, the synthesis of methyl-B_{12} is also blocked.

Clinical symptoms in propionic and methylmalonic acidemia vary according to the location and severity of the enzyme block. Children with severe blocks present with acute, life-threatening metabolic acidosis, hyperammonemia, and bone marrow depression early in infancy or with metabolic acidosis, vomiting, and failure to thrive during the first few months of life. Most patients with severe disease have mild or moderate mental retardation. Late complications include pancreatitis, cardiomyopathy, and basal ganglia stroke, and in methylmalonic aciduria, interstitial nephritis.

All known forms of propionic and methylmalonic acidemia are transmitted as autosomal recessive traits and can be diagnosed in utero.

Diagnosis

Laboratory findings consist of increases in urinary organic acids derived from propionyl-CoA or methylmalonic acid (see Table 32–4). Hyperglycinemia can be present. In some forms of abnormal B_{12} metabolism homocysteine can be elevated.

Treatment

Patients with enzyme blocks in B_{12} metabolism usually respond to massive doses of vitamin B_{12} given intramuscularly. Vitamin B_{12} non-responsive methylmalonic acidemia and propionic acidemia require amino acid restriction, strict prevention of catabolism, and carnitine supplementation to enhance propionylcarnitine excretion. Intermittent metronidazole can help reduce the propionate load from the gut. In the acute setting, hemodialysis may be needed. Combined liver-renal transplantation is an option for patients with renal insufficiency.

Andersson HC et al: Long-term outcome in treated combined methylmalonic acidemia and homocystinemia. Genet Med 1999; 1:146 [PMID: 11258350].

Ogier de Baulny H, Saudubray JM: Branched-chain organic acidurias. Semin Neonatol 2002;7:65 [PMID: 12069539].

Sass JO et al: Propionic acidemia revisited: a workshop report. Clin Pediatr (Phila) 2004;43:837 [PMID: 15583780].

Tanpaiboon P: Methylmalonic acidemia (MMA). Mol Genet Metab 2005;85:2 [PMID: 15959932].

Patient/parent support group website with useful information for families: www.oaanews.org

ISOVALERIC ACIDEMIA

Isovaleric acidemia, due to deficiency of isovaleryl-CoA dehydrogenase in the leucine oxidative pathway, was the first organic acidemia to be described in humans. Patients with this disorder usually present with poor feeding, metabolic acidosis, seizures, and an odor of sweaty feet during the first few days of life, with coma and death occurring if the condition is not recognized and treated. Other patients have a more chronic course, with episodes of vomiting and lethargy, hair loss, and pancreatitis precipitated by intercurrent infections or increased protein intake. The condition is autosomal recessive and can be diagnosed in utero.

Diagnosis

Isovalerylglycine is consistently detected in the urine by organic acid chromatography.

Treatment

Providing a low-protein diet or a diet low in leucine is effective. Conjugation with either glycine or carnitine helps in maintaining metabolic stability. Outcome is usually good.

CARBOXYLASE DEFICIENCY

Isolated pyruvate carboxylase deficiency presents with lactic acidosis and hyperammonemia in early infancy. Even if

Table 32–4. Clinical and laboratory features of organic acidemias.

Disorder	Enzyme Defect	Clinical and Laboratory Features
Isovaleric acidemia	Isovaleryl-CoA dehydrogenase	Acidosis and odor of sweaty feet in infancy, or growth retardation and episodes of vomiting, lethargy, acidosis, and odor. Isovalerylglycine always present in urine, with 3-hydroxyisovaleric acid during acute episodes.
3-Methylcrotonyl-CoA carboxylase deficiency	3-Methylcrotonyl-CoA carboxylase	Acidosis and feeding problems in infancy, or Reye-like episodes in older child. 3-Methylcrotonylglycine in urine, usually with 3-hydroxyisovaleric acid.
Combined carboxylase deficiency	Holocarboxylase synthetase	Hypotonia and lactic acidosis in infancy. 3-Hydroxyisovaleric acid in urine, often with small amounts of 3-hydroxypropionic and methylcitric acids. Often biotin-responsive.
	Biotinidase	Alopecia, seborrheic rash, and ataxia in infancy or childhood. Urine organic acids as above. Usually biotin-responsive.
3-Hydroxy-3-methylglutaric acidemia	Hydroxymethylglutaryl-CoA lyase	Hypoglycemia and acidosis in infancy; Reye-like episodes with non-ketotic hypoglycemia in older children. 3-Hydroxy-3-methylglutaric, 3-methylglutaconic, and 3-hydroxyisovaleric acids in urine.
3-Ketothiolase deficiency	3-Ketothiolase	Ketotic hyperglycinemia syndrome in infancy, or developmental and growth retardation with episodes of vomiting, acidosis, and encephalopathy. 2-Methyl-3-hydroxybutyric and 2-methylacetoacetic acids and tiglylglycine in urine, especially after isoleucine load.
Propionic acidemia	Propionyl-CoA carboxylase	Hyperammonemia and metabolic acidosis in infancy; ketotic hyperglycinemia syndrome later. 3-Hydroxypropionic and methylcitric acids in urine, with 3-hydroxy- and 3-ketovaleric acids during ketotic episodes.
Methylmalonic acidemia	Methylmalonyl-CoA mutase	Clinical features same as in propionic acidemia. Methylmalonic acid in urine, often with 3-hydroxypropionic and methylcitric acids.
	Defects in B_{12} biosynthesis	Clinical features same as above when only adenosyl-B_{12} synthesis is decreased: early neurologic features prominent when accompanied by decreased synthesis of methyl-B_{12}. In latter instance, hypomethioninemia and homocystinuria accompany methylmalonic aciduria.
Pyroglutamic acidemia	Glutathione synthetase	Acidosis and hemolytic anemia in infancy; chronic acidosis later. Pyroglutamic acid in urine.
Glutaric acidemia type I	Glutaryl-CoA dehydrogenase	Progressive extrapyramidal movement disorder in childhood, with episodes of acidosis, vomiting, and encephalopathy. Glutaric acid in urine, usually with 3-hydroxyglutaric acid.
Glutaric acidemia type II	Electron transfer flavoprotein (ETF) ETF:ubiquinone oxidoreductase (ETF dehydrogenase)	Hypoglycemia, acidosis, hyperammonemia, and odor of sweaty feet in infancy, often with polycystic and dysplastic kidneys. Later onset may be with episodes of hypoketotic hypoglycemia or slowly progressive skeletal myopathy. Glutaric, ethylmalonic, 3-hydroxyisovaleric, isovalerylglycine, and 2-hydroxyglutaric acids in urine, often with sarcosine in serum and urine.
4-Hydroxybutyric acidemia	Succinic semialdehyde dehydrogenase	Seizures and developmental retardation. 4-Hydroxybutyric acid in urine.

CoA, coenzyme A.

biochemically stabilized, the neurologic outcome is dismal. Isolated 3-methylcrotonyl-CoA carboxylase deficiency is frequently recognized on newborn screening using tandem mass spectrometric analysis of acylcarnitines. It is usually a benign condition that only rarely causes symptoms of acidosis and neurologic depression. All carboxylases require biotin as a cofactor. Holocarboxylase synthetase and biotinidase are two enzymes of biotin metabolism in mammals. Holocarboxylase synthetase covalently binds biotin to the apocarboxylases for pyruvate, 3-methylcrotonyl-CoA, and propionyl-CoA; and biotinidase releases biotin from these proteins and from proteins in the diet. Recessively inherited deficiency of either enzyme causes deficiency of all three carboxylases (ie, multiple carboxylase deficiency). Patients with holocarboxylase synthetase deficiency usually present as neonates with hypotonia, skin problems, and massive acidosis. Those with biotinidase deficiency more often present somewhat later with a syndrome of ataxia, seizures, seborrhea, and alopecia. Newborn screening for the condition is justified because many patients with biotinidase deficiency do not have typical symptoms, but do develop preventable neurologic sequelae.

Diagnosis

This diagnosis should be considered in patients with typical symptoms or in those with primary lactic acidosis. Urine organic acids are usually but not always abnormal (see Table 32–4). Diagnosis is made by enzyme assay. Biotinidase can be assayed in serum, and holocarboxylase synthetase in leukocytes or fibroblasts.

Treatment

Oral administration of biotin in large doses often reverses the organic aciduria within days and the clinical symptoms within days to weeks. Hearing loss can occur in patients with biotinidase deficiency despite treatment.

Grunewald S et al: Biotinidase deficiency: a treatable leukoencephalopathy. Neuropediatrics 2004;35:211 [PMID: 15328559].

Morrone A et al: Clinical findings and biochemical and molecular analysis of four patients with holocarboxylase synthetase deficiency. Am J Med Genet 2002;111:10 [PMID: 12124727].

Moslinger D et al: Molecular characterisation and neuropsychological outcome of 21 patients with profound biotinidase deficiency detected by newborn screening and family studies. Eur J Pediatr 2003;162(Suppl 1):S46 [PMID: 14628140].

Pacheco-Alvarez D et al: Biotin in metabolism and its relationship to human disease. Arch Med Res 2002;33:439 [PMID: 12459313].

Santer R et al: Partial response to biotin therapy in a patient with holocarboxylase synthetase deficiency: clinical, biochemical, and molecular genetic aspects. Mol Genet Metab 2003;79:160 [PMID: 12855220].

Seymons K et al: Dermatologic signs of biotin deficiency leading to the diagnosis of multiple carboxylase deficiency. Pediatr Dermatol 2004;21:231 [PMID: 15165201].

Weber P et al: Outcome in patients with profound biotinidase deficiency: relevance of newborn screening. Dev Med Child Neurol 2004;46:481 [PMID: 15230462].

Wiznitzer M, Bangert BA: Biotinidase deficiency: clinical and MRI findings consistent with myelopathy. Pediatr Neurol 2003;29:56 [PMID: 13679123].

Wolf B: Biotinidase deficiency: new directions and practical concerns. Curr Treat Options Neurol 2003;5:321 [PMID: 12791199].

GLUTARIC ACIDEMIA TYPE I

Glutaric acidemia type I is due to deficiency of glutaryl-CoA dehydrogenase. Patients have frontotemporal atrophy with enlarged sylvian fissures and macrocephaly. Sudden or chronic neurodegeneration secondary to neuronal degeneration in the caudate and putamen causes a progressive extrapyramidal movement disorder in childhood with dystonia and athetosis. Children with glutaric acidemia type I may present with retinal hemorrhages and intracranial bleeding and may thus be considered victims of child abuse. Severely debilitated children often die in the first decade, but several reported patients have had only mild neurologic abnormalities. Most patients develop symptoms in the first four years of life. The condition is autosomal recessive and prenatal diagnosis is possible.

Diagnosis

Glutaric acidemia type I should be suspected in patients with acute or progressive dystonia in the first four years of life. The MRI of the brain is highly suggestive. The diagnosis is supported by finding glutaric and 3-hydroxyglutaric acids in urine or glutarylcarnitine in serum. Demonstration of deficiency of glutaryl-CoA dehydrogenase in fibroblasts, leukocytes, or a mutation in the GCDH gene confirms the diagnosis. Prenatal diagnosis is by enzyme assay, quantitative metabolite analysis of amniotic fluid, or mutation analysis.

Treatment

Aggressive management of catabolism during intercurrent illness and supplementation with large amounts of carnitine may prevent degeneration of the basal ganglia. Dietary lysine and tryptophan are frequently restricted in young patients. Neurologic symptoms, once present, do not resolve. Symptomatic treatment of severe dystonia is important for affected patients.

Funk CB et al: Neuropathological, biochemical and molecular findings in a glutaric acidemia type 1 cohort. Brain 2005;128(Pt 4):711 [PMID: 15689364].

Strauss KA et al: Type I glutaric aciduria, part 1: Natural history of 77 patients. Am J Med Genet 2003;121C:38 [PMID: 12888985].

Strauss KA, Morton DH: Type I glutaric aciduria, part 2: A model of acute striatal necrosis. Am J Med Genet 2003;121C:53 [PMID: 12888986].

■ DISORDERS OF FATTY ACID OXIDATION & CARNITINE

FATTY ACID OXIDATION DISORDERS

Deficiency of very-long-chain and medium-chain acyl-CoA dehydrogenase (VLCAD, MCAD) and long-chain 3-hydroxyacyl-CoA dehydrogenase (LCHAD), three enzymes of fatty acid β-oxidation, usually causes Reye-like episodes of hypoketotic hypoglycemia, mild hyperammonemia, hepatomegaly, and encephalopathy. Sudden death in infancy is a less common presentation. The long-chain defects, which also include carnitine palmitoyltransferase deficiency I and II and carnitine acylcarnitine translocase deficiency, often cause skeletal myopathy with hypotonia and cardiomyopathy, and ventricular arrhythmias. Less severe defects present with recurrent episodes of rhabdomyolysis. LCHAD deficiency may produce progressive liver cirrhosis, peripheral neuropathy, and retinitis pigmentosa. Mothers of affected infants can have acute fatty liver of pregnancy or HELLP syndrome (hemolysis, elevated liver enzymes, and low platelets). Carnitine palmitoyltransferase II deficiency may cause renal tubular acidosis. MCAD deficiency is common, occurring in perhaps 1:9000 live births. Reye-like episodes may be fatal or cause residual neurologic damage. Episodes tend to become less frequent and severe with time. After the diagnosis is made and treatment instituted, morbidity decreases and mortality is avoided in MCAD deficiency.

Short-chain acyl-CoA dehydrogenase (SCAD) deficiency is characterized by the presence of ethylmalonic acid in the urine, and although some patients have symptoms similar to those in MCAD deficiency, many are asymptomatic. Glutaric acidemia type II results from defects in the transfer of electrons from fatty acid oxidation and some amino acid oxidation into the respiratory chain. Some patients with glutaric acidemia type II have a clinical presentation resembling MCAD deficiency. Patients with a severe neonatal presentation also have renal cystic disease and dysmorphic features. The least affected patients can present with late-onset myopathy and be riboflavin responsive. These conditions are autosomal recessive.

Diagnosis

The hypoglycemic presentation of the Reye episode is associated with a lack of an appropriate ketone response to fasting. Patients with MCAD deficiency may excrete hexanoylglycine, suberylglycine, and phenylpropionylglycine in the urine organic acids. Urine and blood findings in glutaric acidemia type II and SCAD deficiency are often diag-

nostic. The finding of normal urine organic acids does not exclude these conditions, because excretion of dicarboxylic acids and other products of microsomal and peroxisomal oxidation of fatty acids can be intermittent.

The analysis of acylcarnitine esters is currently the first-line diagnostic test and shows diagnostic metabolites regardless of clinical status. MCAD deficiency is characterized by elevated octanoylcarnitine. A similar typical pattern can be recognized in deficiencies of VLCAD, LCHAD, carnitine acylcarnitine translocase, and severe carnitine palmitoyltransferase. This is used in neonatal screening. Further confirmation can be obtained from analysis of fatty acid oxidation in fibroblasts. A common mutation in MCAD and in LCHAD deficiency is useful in confirming the diagnosis. Enzyme assays for each enzyme can be done in fibroblasts in specialized laboratories, and molecular analysis can confirm the mutations.

Treatment

Acutely, management involves prevention of hypoglycemia by avoiding prolonged fasting (> 8–12 hours). Chronic therapy includes providing carbohydrate snacks before bedtime and vigorous treatment of intercurrent infections. Because fatty acid oxidation can be compromised by associated carnitine deficiency, patients with MCAD deficiency usually receive oral carnitine. Carnitine use in VLCAD and LCHAD deficiency is less clear. Restriction of dietary long-chain fats is controversial in MCAD deficiency, but is required for VLCAD and LCHAD deficiencies. Medium-chain triglycerides are contraindicated in MCAD deficiency, but are an essential energy source for patients with VLCAD and LCHAD deficiencies or carnitine acylcarnitine translocase deficiency. Riboflavin may be beneficial in some patients with glutaric acidemia type II. Outcome in MCAD deficiency is excellent, but is more guarded in patients with the other disorders.

Alonso EM: Acute liver failure in children: the role of defects in fatty acid oxidation. Hepatology 2005;41:696 [PMID: 15789368].

Bartlett K, Pourfarzam M: Defects of beta-oxidation including carnitine deficiency. Int Rev Neurobiol 2002;53:469 [PMID: 12512350].

Deschauer M et al: Muscle carnitine palmitoyltransferase II deficiency: clinical and molecular genetic features and diagnostic aspects. Arch Neurol 2005;62:37 [PMID: 15642848].

Jamerson PA: The association between acute fatty liver of pregnancy and fatty acid oxidation disorders. J Obstet Gynecol Neonatal Nurs 2005;34:87 [PMID: 15673650].

Kilfoyle D et al: Recurrent myoglobinuria due to carnitine palmitoyltransferase II deficiency: clinical, biochemical, and genetic features of adult-onset cases. N Z Med J 2005;118:U1320 [PMID: 15776096].

Rakheja D et al: Long-chain L-3-hydroxyacyl-coenzyme A dehydrogenase deficiency: A molecular and biochemical review. Lab Invest 2002;82:815 [PMID: 12118083].

Rinaldo P et al: Fatty acid oxidation disorders. Annu Rev Physiol 2002;64:477 [PMID: 11826276].

Rubio-Gozalbo ME et al: Carnitine-acylcarnitine translocase deficiency: Case report and review of the literature. Acta Paediatr 2003;92:501 [PMID: 12801121].

Shekhawat PS et al: Fetal fatty acid oxidation disorders, their effect on maternal health and neonatal outcome: impact of expanded newborn screening on their diagnosis and management. Pediatr Res 2005;57(5 Pt 2):78R [PMID: 15817498].

Sigauke E et al: Carnitine palmitoyltransferase II deficiency: a clinical, biochemical, and molecular review. Lab Invest 2003;83:1543 [PMID: 14615409].

Sim KG et al: Strategies for the diagnosis of mitochondrial fatty acid beta-oxidation disorders. Clin Chim Acta 2002;323:37 [PMID: 12135806].

Treem WR: Mitochondrial fatty acid oxidation and acute fatty liver of pregnancy. Semin Gastrointest Dis 2002;13:55 [PMID: 11944635].

Vockley J, Whiteman DA: Defects of mitochondrial beta-oxidation: A growing group of disorders. Neuromuscul Disord 2002;12:235 [PMID: 11801395].

Wieser T et al: Carnitine palmitoyltransferase II deficiency: molecular and biochemical analysis of 32 patients. Neurology 2003;60:1351 [PMID: 12707442].

Patient/parent support group website with useful information for families: www.fodsupport.org

CARNITINE

Carnitine is an essential nutrient found in highest concentration in red meat. Its primary function is to transport long-chain fatty acids into mitochondria for oxidation. Primary defects of carnitine transport may manifest as Reye syndrome, cardiomyopathy, or skeletal myopathy with hypotonia. These disorders are rare compared with secondary carnitine deficiency, which may be due to diet (especially intravenous alimentation or ketogenic diet), renal losses, drug therapy (especially valproic acid), and other metabolic disorders (especially disorders of fatty acid oxidation and organic acidemias). The prognosis depends on the cause of the carnitine abnormality.

Free and esterified carnitine can be measured in blood. Muscle carnitine may be low despite normal blood levels, particularly in respiratory chain disorders. If carnitine insufficiency is suspected, the patient should be evaluated to rule out disorders that might cause secondary carnitine deficiency.

Oral or intravenous L-carnitine is used in carnitine deficiency or insufficiency in doses of 25–100 mg/kg/d or higher. Treatment is aimed at maintaining normal carnitine levels. Carnitine supplementation in patients with some disorders of fatty acid oxidation and organic acidosis may also augment excretion of accumulated metabolites. Supplementation may not prevent metabolic crises in such patients.

Evangeliou A, Vlassopoulos D: Carnitine metabolism and deficit— When supplementation is necessary? Curr Pharm Biotechnol 2003;4:211 [PMID: 12769764].

Foster DW: The role of the carnitine system in human metabolism. Ann N Y Acad Sci 2004;1033:1 [PMID: 15590999].

Hoppel C: The role of carnitine in normal and altered fatty acid metabolism. Am J Kidney Dis 2003;41(4 Suppl 4):S4 [PMID: 12751049].

Stanley CA: Carnitine deficiency disorders in children. Ann N Y Acad Sci 2004;1033:42 [PMID: 15591002].

Tein I: Carnitine transport: pathophysiology and metabolism of known molecular defects. J Inherit Metab Dis 2003;26:147 [PMID: 12889657].

HYPOXANTHINE-GUANINE PHOSPHORIBOSYLTRANSFERASE DEFICIENCY (Lesch-Nyhan Syndrome)

Hypoxanthine-guanine phosphoribosyltransferase is an enzyme converting the purine bases hypoxanthine and guanine to inosine monophosphate and guanosine monophosphate, respectively. The X-linked recessive disorder with complete deficiency is characterized by central nervous system dysfunction and purine overproduction with hyperuricemia and hyperuricuria. Depending on the residual activity of the mutant enzyme, male hemizygous individuals may be severely disabled by choreoathetosis, spasticity, and compulsive, mutilating lip and finger biting, or they may have only gouty arthritis and urate ureterolithiasis. Enzyme deficiency can be measured in erythrocytes, fibroblasts, and cultured amniotic cells; this disorder can thus be diagnosed in utero.

Diagnosis

Diagnosis is made by demonstrating an elevated uric acid:creatinine ratio in urine, followed by demonstration of enzyme deficiency in red blood cells or fibroblasts.

Treatment

Hyperhydration and alkalinization are essential to prevent kidney stones and urate nephropathy. Allopurinol and probenecid may be given to reduce hyperuricemia and prevent gout, but do not affect the neurologic status. Physical restraints are often more effective than neurologic medications for automutilation.

Deutsch SI et al: Hypothesized deficiency of guanine-based purines may contribute to abnormalities of neurodevelopment, neuromodulation, and neurotransmission in Lesch-Nyhan syndrome. Clin Neuropharmacol 2005;28:28 [PMID: 15711436].

Nyhan WL: Inherited hyperuricemic disorders. Contrib Nephrol 2005;147:22 [PMID: 15604603].

Nyhan WL: Lesch-Nyhan disease. J Hist Neurosci 2005;14:1 [PMID: 15804753].

■ LYSOSOMAL DISEASES

Lysosomes are cellular organelles in which complex macromolecules are degraded by specific acid hydrolases. Deficiency of a lysosomal enzyme causes its substrate to accumulate in the lysosomes of tissues that degrade it and a characteristic clinical picture develops. These storage disorders are classified as mucopolysaccharidoses, lipidoses, or mucolipidoses, depending on the nature of the stored material. Two additional disorders, cystinosis and Salla disease, are caused by defects in lysosomal proteins that normally transport material from the lysosome to the cytoplasm. Table 32–5 lists clinical and laboratory features of these conditions. Most are inherited as autosomal recessive traits, and all can be diagnosed in utero.

Diagnosis

The diagnosis of mucopolysaccharidosis is suggested by certain clinical and radiologic findings (dysostosis multiplex). Urine screening tests can detect increased mucopolysaccharides and further identify which specific mucopolysaccharides are present. Diagnosis must be confirmed by enzyme assays of leukocytes or cultured fibroblasts. Analysis of urinary oligosaccharides indicates a specific disorder prior to enzymatic testing. Lipidoses present with visceral symptoms or neurodegeneration. Diagnosis is made by appropriate enzyme assays of peripheral leukocytes or cultured skin fibroblasts.

Treatment

Most conditions cannot be treated effectively, but new avenues have given hope in many conditions. Hematopoietic stem cell transplantation can greatly improve the course of some lysosomal diseases, and is first-line treatment in some such as infantile Hurler syndrome. Several disorders are treated with infusions of recombinant modified enzyme. Treatment of Gaucher disease is very effective and long-term data suggest excellent outcome. Similar treatments have been developed for Fabry disease, several mucopolysaccharidoses, and Pompe disease. Substantial improvements in these conditions have been reported but with limitations. New avenues for treatment under development are offered through substrate inhibition and chaperone therapy. Treatment of cystinosis with cysteamine results in depletion of stored cystine and prevention of complications including renal disease.

Barker PB, Horska A: Neuroimaging in leukodystrophies. J Child Neurol 2004;19:559 [PMID: 15605464].

Brady RO: Gaucher and Fabry diseases: from understanding pathophysiology to rational therapies. Acta Paediatr Suppl 2003;92:19 [PMID: 14989461].

Brady RO, Schiffmann R: Enzyme-replacement therapy for metabolic storage disorders. Lancet Neurol 2004;3:752 [PMID: 15556808].

Burin MG et al: Investigation of lysosomal storage disease in non-immune hydrops fetalis. Prenat Diagn 2004;24:653 [PMID: 15305357].

Cox TM: Substrate reduction therapy for lysosomal storage disease. Acta Paediatr Suppl 2005;94:69 [PMID: 15895716].

Desnick RJ: Enzyme replacement and enhancement therapies for lysosomal diseases. J Inherit Metab Dis 2004;27:385 [PMID: 15190196].

Desnick RJ et al: Fabry disease, an under-recognized multisystemic disorder: Expert recommendations for diagnosis, management, and enzyme replacement therapy. Ann Intern Med 2003;138:338 [PMID: 12585833].

Elstein D et al: Gaucher disease: Pediatric concerns. Paediatr Drugs 2002;4:417 [PMID: 12083970].

Eto Y et al: Treatment of lysosomal storage disorders: cell therapy and gene therapy. J Inherit Metab Dis 2004;27:411 [PMID: 15190197].

Germain DP: Gaucher's disease: a paradigm for interventional genetics. Clin Genet 2004;65:77 [PMID: 14984463].

Ginzburg L et al: The pathogenesis of glycosphingolipid storage disorders. Semin Cell Dev Biol 2004;15:417 [PMID: 15207832].

Krivit W: Stem cell bone marrow transplantation in patients with metabolic storage diseases. Adv Pediatr 2002;49:359 [PMID: 12214779].

Masson C et al: Fabry disease: a review. Joint Bone Spine 2004; 71:381 [PMID: 15474388].

Meikle PJ et al: Newborn screening for lysosomal storage disorders: clinical evaluation of a two-tier strategy. Pediatrics 2004; 114:909 [PMID: 15466084].

Millington DS: Newborn screening for lysosomal storage disorders. Clin Chem 2005;51:808 [PMID: 15855665].

Ozkara HA: Recent advances in the biochemistry and genetics of sphingolipidoses. Brain Dev 2004;26:497 [PMID: 15533650].

Sauer M et al: Hematopoietic stem cell transplantation for mucopolysaccharidoses and leukodystrophies. Klin Padiatr 2004; 216:163 [PMID: 15175961].

Vellodi A: Lysosomal storage disorders. Br J Haematol 2005; 128:413 [PMID: 15686451].

Wenger DA et al: Insights into the diagnosis and treatment of lysosomal storage diseases. Arch Neurol 2003;60:322 [PMID: 12633142].

Wilcox WR: Lysosomal storage disorders: the need for better pediatric recognition and comprehensive care. J Pediatr 2004; 144(5 Suppl):S3 [PMID: 15126978].

Wraith JE: Lysosomal disorders. Semin Neonatol 2002;7:75 [PMID: 12069540].

Wraith JE: The clinical presentation of lysosomal storage disorders. Acta Neurol Taiwan 2004;13:101 [PMID: 15508935].

Patient/parent support group websites with useful information for families: www.mpssociety.org and www.ulf.org

■ PEROXISOMAL DISEASES

Peroxisomes are intracellular organelles that contain a large number of enzymes, many of which are oxidases linked to catalase. Among the enzyme systems in peroxisomes is one for β-oxidation of unusual very-long-chain fatty acids, phytanic acid, and bile acids, and one for plasmalogen biosynthesis. In addition, peroxisomes contain oxidases for D- and L-amino acids, pipecolic acid, and phytanic acid, and an enzyme (alanine-glyox-

Table 32–5. Clinical and laboratory features of lysosomal storage diseases.

Disorder	Enzyme Defect	Clinical and Laboratory Features
I. Mucopolysaccharidoses		
Hurler syndrome	α-Iduronidase	Autosomal recessive. Mental retardation, hepatosplenomegaly, umbilical hernia, coarse facies, corneal clouding, dorsolumbar gibbus, severe heart disease. Heparan sulfate and dermatan sulfate in urine.
Scheie syndrome	α-Iduronidase (incomplete)	Autosomal recessive. Corneal clouding, stiff joints, normal intellect. Clinical types intermediate between Hurler and Scheie common. Heparan sulfate and dermatan sulfate in urine.
Hunter syndrome	Sulfoiduronate sulfatase	X-linked recessive. Coarse facies, hepatosplenomegaly, mental retardation variable. Corneal clouding and gibbus not present. Heparan sulfate and dermatan sulfate in urine.
Sanfilippo syndrome: Type A Type B Type C Type D	 Sulfamidase α-N-Acetylglucosaminidase Acetyl-CoA: α-glucosaminide-N-acetyltransferase α-N-acetylglucosamine-6-sulfatase	Autosomal recessive. Severe mental retardation with comparatively mild skeletal changes, visceromegaly, and facial coarseness. Types cannot be differentiated clinically. Heparan sulfate in urine.
Morquio syndrome	N-Acetylgalactosamine-6-sulfatase	Autosomal recessive. Severe skeletal changes, platyspondylisis, corneal clouding. Keratan sulfate in urine.
Maroteaux-Lamy syndrome	N-Acetylgalactosamine-4-sulfatase	Autosomal recessive. Coarse facies, growth retardation, dorsolumbar gibbus, corneal clouding, hepatosplenomegaly, normal intellect. Dermatan sulfate in urine.
β-Glucuronidase deficiency	β-Glucuronidase	Autosomal recessive. Varies from mental retardation, dorsolumbar gibbus, corneal clouding, and hepatosplenomegaly to mild facial coarseness, retardation, and loose joints. Hearing loss common. Dermatan sulfate or heparan sulfate in urine.
II. Mucolipidoses		
Mannosidosis	α-Mannosidase	Autosomal recessive. Varies from severe mental retardation, coarse facies, short stature, skeletal changes, and hepatosplenomegaly to mild facial coarseness and loose joints. Hearing loss common. Abnormal oligosaccharides in urine.
Fucosidosis	α-Fucosidase	Autosomal recessive. Variable: coarse facies, skeletal changes, hepatosplenomegaly, occasional angiokeratoma corporis diffusum. Abnormal oligosaccharides in urine.
I-cell disease (mucolipidosis II)	N-Acetylglucosaminylphosphotransferase	Autosomal recessive; severe and mild forms known. Very short stature, mental retardation, early facial coarsening, clear cornea, stiffness of joints. Increased lysosomal enzymes in serum. Abnormal sialyl oligosaccharides in urine.
Sialidosis	N-Acetylineuraminidase (sialidase)	Autosomal recessive. Mental retardation, coarse facies, skeletal dysplasia, myoclonic seizures, macular cherry-red spot. Abnormal sialyl oligosaccharides in urine.

(continued)

Table 32–5. Clinical and laboratory features of lysosomal storage diseases. (continued)

Disorder	Enzyme Defect	Clinical and Laboratory Features
III. Lipidoses		
Niemann-Pick disease	Sphingomyelinase	Autosomal recessive. Acute and chronic forms known. Acute neuronopathic form common in eastern European Jews. Accumulation of sphingomyelin in lysosomes of RE system and CNS. Hepatosplenomegaly, developmental retardation, macular cherry-red spot. Death by 1–4 y.
Metachromatic leukodystrophy	Arylsulfatase A	Autosomal recessive. Late infantile form, with onset at 1–4 y, most common. Accumulation of sulfatide in white matter. Gait disturbances (ataxia), motor incoordination, and dementia. Death usually in first decade.
Krabbe disease (globoid cell leukodystrophy)	Galactocerebroside β-galactosidase	Autosomal recessive. Globoid cells in white matter. Onset at 3–6 mo with seizures, irritability, and retardation. Death by 1–2 y. Juvenile and adult forms are rare.
Fabry disease	α-Galactosidase A	X-linked recessive. Storage of trihexosylceramide in endothelial cells. Pain in extremities, angiokeratoma corporis diffusum and (later) poor vision, hypertension, and renal failure.
Farber disease	Ceramidase	Autosomal recessive. Storage of ceramide in tissues. Subcutaneous nodules, arthropathy with deformed and painful joints, and poor growth and development. Death within first year.
Gaucher disease	Glucocerebroside β-glucosidase	Autosomal recessive. Acute neuronopathic form: Accumulation of glucocerebroside in lysosomes of RE system and CNS. Retardation, hepatosplenomegaly, macular cherry-red spot, and Gaucher cells in bone marrow. Death by 1–2 y. Chronic form common in eastern European Jews. Accumulation of spingomyelin in lysosomes of RE system. Hepatosplenomegaly and flask-shaped osteolytic bone lesions. Consistent with normal life expectancy.
G_{M1} gangliosidosis	G_{M1} ganglioside β-galactosidase	Autosomal recessive. Accumulation of G_{M1} ganglioside in lysosomes of RE system and CNS. Infantile form: Abnormalities at birth with dysostosis multiplex, hepatosplenomegaly, macular cherry-red spot, and death by 2 years. Juvenile form: Normal development to 1 year of age, then ataxia, weakness, dementia, and death by 4–5 y. Occasional inferior beaking of vertebral bodies of L1 and L2.
G_{M2} gangliosidoses Tay-Sachs disease Sandhoff disease	β-N-Acetylhexos aminidase A β-N-Acetylhexos aminidase A & B	Autosomal recessive. Tay-Sachs disease common in eastern European Jews; Sandhoff disease is panethnic. Clinical phenotypes are identical, with accumulation of G_{M2} ganglioside in lysosomes of CNS. Onset at age 3–6 months, with hypotonia, hyperacusis, retardation, and macular cherry-red spot. Death by 2–3 years. Juvenile and adult onset forms of Tay-Sachs disease are rare.
Wolman disease	Acid lipase	Autosomal recessive. Accumulation of cholesterol esters and triglycerides in lysosomes of reticuloendothelial system. Onset in infancy with gastrointestinal symptoms and hepatosplenomegaly, and death by 3–6 mo. Adrenals commonly enlarged and calcified.

CNS, central nervous system; RE, reticuloendothelial.

ylate aminotransferase) that effects transamination of glyoxylate to glycine.

In some peroxisomal diseases, many enzymes are deficient. Zellweger (cerebrohepatorenal) syndrome, the best known among these, is caused by several defects in organelle assembly. Patients present in infancy with seizures, hypotonia, characteristic facies with a large forehead, and cholestatic hepatopathy. At autopsy renal cysts and absent peroxisomes are seen. Patients with a similar but milder biochemical and clinical phenotype have neonatal adrenoleukodystrophy or neonatal Refsum disease. They often have detectable peroxisomes.

In other peroxisomal diseases, only a single enzyme is deficient. Primary hyperoxaluria (alanine-glyoxylate aminotransferase deficiency) causes renal stones and nephropathy. Mutations in the X-linked very-long-chain fatty acid transporter gene, *ABCD1*, cause either a rapid leukodystrophy with loss of function (adrenoleukodystrophy), slow progressive spasticity and neuropathy (adrenomyeloneuropathy), or adrenal insufficiency. Defective phytanic acid oxidation in adult Refsum disease causes ataxia, leukodystrophy, cardiomyopathy, neuropathy, and cataracts. Other isolated enzyme deficiencies can mimic Zellweger syndrome.

Abnormalities of plasmalogen synthesis are clinically associated with rhizomelic chondrodysplasia punctata. Except for adrenoleukodystrophy, all peroxisomal diseases are autosomal recessive and can be diagnosed in utero.

Diagnosis

The best screening test for Zellweger syndrome and other biogenesis disorders is determination of very-long-chain fatty acids in serum or plasma. Urine bile acids are abnormal in other peroxisomal disorders. Phytanic acid and plasmalogens can also be measured. Together, these studies identify most peroxisomal diseases. Tissue biopsy and appropriate enzyme assays are needed for confirmation, especially when the parents plan further pregnancies.

Treatment

Bone marrow transplantation may be an effective treatment at the early stages of adrenoleukodystrophy. Lorenzo's oil, in combination with a very-low-fat diet and essential fatty acid supplementation, is ineffective in patients with established symptoms, but shows promise in prevention of neurologic symptoms in presymptomatic males with adrenoleukodystrophy. Dietary treatment is used for adult Refsum disease. Liver transplantation protects the kidneys in severe primary hyperoxaluria.

Baumgartner MR, Saudubray JM: Peroxisomal disorders. Semin Neonatol 2002;7:85 [PMID: 12069541].

Faust PL et al: Peroxisome biogenesis disorders; the role of peroxisomes and metabolic dysfunction in developing brain. J Inherit Metab Dis 2005;28:369 [PMID: 15868469].

Ferri R, Chance PF: Lorenzo's oil: advances in the treatment of neurometabolic disorders. Arch Neurol 2005;62:1045 [PMID: 16009756].

Moser H et al: Progress in X-linked adrenoleukodystrophy. Curr Opin Neurol 2004;17:263 [PMID: 15167059].

Moser HW et al: Follow-up of 89 asymptomatic patients with adrenoleukodystrophy treated with Lorenzo's oil. Arch Neurol 2005;62:1073 [PMID: 16009761].

Oglesbee D: An overview of peroxisomal biogenesis disorders. Mol Genet Metab 2005;84:299 [PMID: 15875330].

Peters C et al: Cerebral X-linked adrenoleukodystrophy: the international hematopoietic cell transplantation experience from 1982 to 1999. Blood 2004;104:881 [PMID: 15073029].

Poll-The BT et al: Peroxisome biogenesis disorders with prolonged survival: phenotypic expression in a cohort of 31 patients. Am J Med Genet A 2004;126:333 [PMID: 15098231].

Shimozawa N et al: Molecular and neurologic findings of peroxisome biogenesis disorders. J Child Neurol 2005;20:326 [PMID: 15921234].

Steinberg S et al: The PEX Gene Screen: molecular diagnosis of peroxisome biogenesis disorders in the Zellweger syndrome spectrum. Mol Genet Metab 2004;83:252 [PMID: 15542397].

Wander RJ: Metabolic and molecular basis of peroxisomal disorders: a review. Am J Med Genet A 2004;126:355 [PMID: 15098234].

Wanders RJ: Peroxisomes, lipid metabolism, and peroxisomal disorders. Mol Genet Metab 2004;83:16 [PMID: 15464416].

Wanders RJ, Waterham HR: Peroxisomal disorders I: biochemistry and genetics of peroxisome biogenesis disorders. Clin Genet 2005;67:107 [PMID: 15679822].

■ CONGENITAL DISORDERS OF GLYCOSYLATION

Many proteins, including many enzymes, require glycosylation with carbohydrate moieties for normal function. The carbohydrate-deficient glycoprotein syndromes are a family of disorders that result from failure of glycosylation. Children with type Ia disease usually present with prenatal growth disturbance, often with abnormal fat distribution, cerebellar hypoplasia, typical facial dysmorphic features, and mental retardation. The typical course includes chronic liver disease, peripheral neuropathy, endocrinopathies, retinopathy, and in some patients, acute life-threatening events. Patients with type Ib disease have a variable combination of liver fibrosis, protein-losing enteropathy, and hypoglycemia. More than a dozen other forms are characterized with additional key symptoms including coloboma, cutis laxa, severe epilepsy, ichthyosis, and Dandy-Walker malformation. Biochemical differences and variations in clinical course (eg, the absence of peripheral neuropathy) characterize the other types. Pathophysiology probably relates to defects of those biochemical pathways that require glycosylated proteins. The syndromes appear so far to be inherited in an autosomal recessive manner, and frequency was initially estimated to be as high as 1:20,000 in northern Europe.

Diagnosis

Diagnosis is supported by finding altered levels of glycosylated enzymes or other proteins such as transferrin, thyroxine-binding globulin, lysosomal enzymes, and clotting factors. Unfortunately these levels may be normal in carbohydrate-deficient glycoprotein syndromes or abnormal in other conditions. Diagnosis is confirmed by finding typical patterns of altered isoelectric focusing of selected proteins. Most diagnostic laboratories examine serum transferrin. Follow-up diagnosis is by assaying enzyme activity, analysis of lipid-linked oligosaccharides in fibroblasts, and mutation analysis.

Treatment

Treatment is supportive, with opportunity to monitor and provide early treatment for expected clinical features. Mannose supplementation has been beneficial in the treatment of patients with type 1b deficiency.

Damen G et al: Gastrointestinal and other clinical manifestations in 17 children with congenital disorders of glycosylation type Ia, Ib, and Ic. J Pediatr Gastroenterol Nutr 2004;38:282 [PMID: 15076627].

Grunewald S et al: Congenital disorders of glycosylation: A review. Pediatr Res 2002;52:618 [PMID: 12409504].

Jaeken J: Congenital disorders of glycosylation (CDG): update and new developments. J Inherit Metab Dis 2004;27:423 [PMID: 15272470].

Jaeken J, Carchon H: Congenital disorders of glycosylation: a booming chapter in pediatrics. Curr Opin Pediatr 2004;16:434 [PMID: 15273506].

Marquardt T, Denecke J: Congenital disorders of glycosylation: review of their molecular bases, clinical presentations, and specific therapies. Eur J Pediatr 2003;162:359 [PMID: 12756558].

■ SMITH-LEMLI-OPITZ SYNDROME & DISORDERS OF CHOLESTEROL SYNTHESIS

Several defects of cholesterol synthesis are associated with malformations and neurodevelopmental disability. Smith-Lemli-Opitz (SLO) syndrome is an autosomal recessive disorder caused by a deficiency of the enzyme 7-dehydrocholesterol δ^7-reductase. It is characterized by microcephaly, poor growth, mental retardation, typical dysmorphic features of face and extremities (particularly 2–3 toe syndactyly), and often malformations of the heart and genitourinary system. Severity ranges from moderate to severe mental retardation to early death. Although deficient synthesis of cholesterol leads directly to deficiency of some hormones and bile acids, the pathophysiology of the malformations is unclear. Frequency is estimated to be between 1:40,000 and 1:20,000. Other cholesterol synthetic defects are seen in Conradi

Hünnermann syndrome with chondrodysplasia punctata and atrophic skin. Cholestanolosis (cerebrotendinous xanthomatosis) presents with progressive ataxia and cataracts.

Diagnosis

In SLO, elevated 7- and 8-dehydrocholesterol in serum or other tissues, including amniotic fluid, is diagnostic. Serum cholesterol levels may be low, but may be in the normal range. Enzymes of cholesterol synthesis may be assayed in cultured fibroblasts or amniocytes and mutation analysis is possible.

Treatment

Although postnatal treatment does not resolve prenatal injury, supplementation with cholesterol in SLO improves growth and behavior. The role of supplemental bile acids is controversial.

Hennekam RC: Congenital brain anomalies in distal cholesterol biosynthesis defects. J Inherit Metab Dis 2005;28:385 [PMID: 15868470].

Herman GE: Disorders of cholesterol biosynthesis: prototypic metabolic malformation syndromes. Hum Mol Genet 2003;12(Spec No 1):R75 [PMID: 12668600].

Jira PE et al: Smith-Lemli-Opitz syndrome and the DHCR7 gene. Ann Hum Genet 2003;67(Pt 3):269 [PMID: 12914579].

Nowaczyk MJ et al: Incidence of Smith-Lemli-Opitz syndrome in Canada: results of three-year population surveillance. J Pediatr 2004;145:530 [PMID: 15480380].

Porter FD: Human malformation syndromes due to inborn errors of cholesterol synthesis. Curr Opin Pediatr 2003;15:607 [PMID: 14631207].

Porter FD: Malformation syndromes due to inborn errors of cholesterol synthesis. J Clin Invest 2002;110:715 [PMID: 12235098].

Rossi M et al: Characterization of liver involvement in defects of cholesterol biosynthesis: long-term follow-up and review. Am J Med Genet A 2005;132:144 [PMID: 15580635].

Sikora DM et al: Cholesterol supplementation does not improve developmental progress in Smith-Lemli-Opitz syndrome. J Pediatr 2004;144:783 [PMID: 15192627].

Starck L et al: Cholesterol treatment forever? The first Scandinavian trial of cholesterol supplementation in the cholesterol-synthesis defect Smith–Lemli–Opitz syndrome. J Intern Med 2002;252:314 [PMID: 12366604].

■ DISORDERS OF NEUROTRANSMITTER METABOLISM

Abnormalities of neurotransmitter metabolism are increasingly recognized as causes of significant neurodevelopmental disabilities. Affected patients may present with movement disorders (especially dystonia and oculogyric crises), seizures, abnormal tone, ataxia, or mental retardation.

Patients may be mildly affected (eg, dopa-responsive dystonia with diurnal variation) or severely affected (eg, intractable seizures with profound mental retardation). Deficient serine synthesis leads to congenital microcephaly, infantile seizures, and failure of myelination.

Diagnosis

Although some disorders can be diagnosed by examining serum amino acids or urine organic acids (eg, 4-hydroxybutyric aciduria), in most cases, diagnosis requires analysis of CSF. Spinal fluid samples for neurotransmitter analysis require special collection and handling, as the neurotransmitter levels are graduated along the axis of the central nervous system and are highly unstable once the sample is collected.

Treatment

For some conditions, such as pyridoxine-responsive seizures, pyridoxal-phosphate responsive encephalopathy, or dopa-responsive dystonia, response to treatment can be dramatic. For others, response to therapy is less satisfactory in part because of poor penetration of the blood-brain barrier. Supplementation with serine and glycine can substantially improve outcome in serine deficiency.

Baxter P: Pyridoxine-dependent seizures: A clinical and biochemical conundrum. Biochim Biophys Acta 2003;1647:36 [PMID: 12686105].

de Koning TJ et al: L-serine in disease and development. Biochem J 2003;371:653 [PMID: 12534373].

de Koning TJ, Klomp LW: Serine-deficiency syndromes. Curr Opin Neurol 2004;17:197 [PMID: 15021249].

Fiumara A et al: Aromatic L-amino acid decarboxylase deficiency with hyperdopaminuria: Clinical and laboratory findings in response to different therapies. Neuropediatrics 2002;33:203 [PMID: 12368991].

Hyland K, Arnold LA: Value of lumbar puncture in the diagnosis of infantile epilepsy and folinic acid-responsive seizures. J Child Neurol 2002;17(Suppl 3):3S48; discussion 3S56 [PMID: 12597055].

Jaeken J: Genetic disorders of gamma-aminobutyric acid, glycine, and serine as causes of epilepsy. J Child Neurol 2002;17(Suppl 3):3S84; discussion 3S88 [PMID: 12597057].

Ramaekers VT, Blau N: Cerebral folate deficiency. Dev Med Child Neurol 2004;46:843 [PMID: 15581159].

Swoboda KJ, Hyland K: Diagnosis and treatment of neurotransmitter-related disorders. Neurol Clin 2002;20:1143 [PMID: 12616685].

CREATINE SYNTHESIS DISORDERS

Creatine and creatine phosphate are essential for storage and transmission of phosphate-bound energy in muscle and brain. They are catabolized to creatinine. Three disorders of creatine synthesis are now known: arginine:glycine amidinotransferase (AGAT) deficiency, guanidinoacetate methyltransferase (GAMT) deficiency, and creatine transporter (CrT1) deficiency. GAMT and AGAT deficiencies are autosomal-recessive disorders, whereas CrT1 deficiency is X-linked. All patients demonstrate developmental delay, mental retardation, autistic behavior, seizures, and severe expressive language disturbance. Patients may also show developmental regression and brain atrophy. Patients with GAMT deficiency have more severe seizures and an extrapyramidal movement disorder. The seizure disorder is milder in CrT1-deficient patients. Some female heterozygotes of CrT1 deficiency may also show developmental delay or learning disabilities.

Diagnosis

The common feature of all creatine synthesis defects is a severe depletion of creatine/phosphocreatine in the brain demonstratable by reduction to absence of signal on magnetic resonance spectroscopy. In GAMT deficiency, guanidinoacetate accumulates, whereas in AGAT deficiency, guanidinoacetate is decreased, particularly in urine. Guanidinoacetate seems to be responsible for the severe seizures and movement disorder found in GAMT deficiency. Blood, urine, and CSF creatine levels are decreased in GAMT deficiency, but normal in AGAT deficiency. Urine excretion of creatine/creatinine is elevated in CrT1 deficiency. Enzyme and molecular analyses are available for diagnostic confirmation.

Treatment

Treatment with oral creatine supplementation is in part successful in GAMT and AGAT deficiencies. It is not beneficial in CrT1 deficiency. Treatment by combined arginine restriction and ornithine substitution in GAMT deficiency can decrease guanidinoacetate concentrations and improve the clinical course.

Schulze A: Creatine deficiency syndromes. Mol Cell Biochem 2003;244:143 [PMID: 12701824].

Stromberger C et al: Clinical characteristics and diagnostic clues in inborn errors of creatine metabolism. J Inherit Metab Dis 2003;26:299 [PMID: 12889668].

Sykut-Cegielska J et al: Biochemical and clinical characteristics of creatine deficiency syndromes. Acta Biochim Pol 2004;51:875 [PMID: 15625559].

Genetics & Dysmorphology

Ellen R. Elias, MD, Anne Chun-Hui Tsai, MD, MSc, & David K. Manchester, MD

Genetics is an exciting and rapidly developing field, the knowledge of which is critical to the understanding of human embryology, physiology, and disease processes. Tremendous advances in molecular biology and biochemistry are allowing more comprehensive understanding of mechanisms inherent in genetic disorders, as well as improved diagnostic tests and management options. However, some of the newer technologies and terms may be unfamiliar to the clinician in practice. To best cover this complex and varied subject, this chapter contains two major parts. The first part serves as an introduction and review of the basic principles of genetics, including basic knowledge of cytogenetics and molecular biology. The principles of inherited human disorders are reviewed, including different causes of genetic disorders, with a discussion of dysmorphology and teratology. The second part introduces common clinical disorders including descriptions of the diseases, with a discussion of their pathogenesis, diagnosis, and management.

PART I
Principles of Genetics

■ FOUNDATIONS OF GENETIC DIAGNOSIS

CYTOGENETICS

Cytogenetics is the study of genetics at the chromosome level. Chromosomal anomalies occur in 0.4% of all live births and are a prevalent cause of mental retardation and congenital anomalies. The prevalence of chromosomal anomalies is much higher among spontaneous abortions and stillbirths.

Chromosomes

Human chromosomes consist of DNA (the blueprint of genetic material), specific proteins forming the backbone of the chromosome (called histones), and other chromatin structural and interactive proteins. Chromosomes contain most of the genetic information necessary for growth and differentiation. The nuclei of all normal human cells, with the exception of gametes, contain 46 chromosomes, consisting of 23 pairs (Figure 33–1). Of these, 22 pairs are called autosomes. They are numbered according to their size; chromosome 1 is the largest and chromosome 22 the smallest. In addition, there are two sex chromosomes: two X chromosomes in females and one X and one Y chromosome in males. The two members of a chromosome pair are called homologous chromosomes. One homolog of each chromosome pair is maternal in origin (from the egg); the second is paternal (from the sperm). The egg and sperm each contain 23 chromosomes (haploid cells). During formation of the zygote, they fuse into a cell with 46 chromosomes (diploid cell).

Cell Division

Cells undergo cycles of growth and division that are controlled according to their needs and functions.

Mitosis is a kind of cell division, occurring in stages, during which DNA replication takes place and two daughter cells, genetically identical to the original parent cells, are formed. This cell division is typical for all somatic cells (cells other than the sperm or egg, which are called germline cells). There are four phases of mitosis: interphase, prophase, metaphase, and anaphase (Figure 33–2). In interphase, chromosomes are long, thin, and nonvisible. At this time, the genetic material is replicated. In prophase, the chromosomes are more condensed. During metaphase (the phase following DNA replication but preceding cell division), individual chromosomes can be visualized. Each arm consists of two identical parts, called chromatids. Chromatids of the same chromosome are called sister chromatids. In anaphase, the genetic material is separated into two cells.

Meiosis (Figure 33–3), during which eggs and sperm are formed, is cell division limited to gametes. During meiosis, three unique processes take place:

1. Crossing over of genetic material between two homologous chromosomes. This is preceded by the pairing of both members of each chromosome pair, which facilitates the physical exchange of homologous genetic material.

2. Random assortment of maternally and paternally derived homologous chromosomes into the daughter

Normal Male

Normal Female

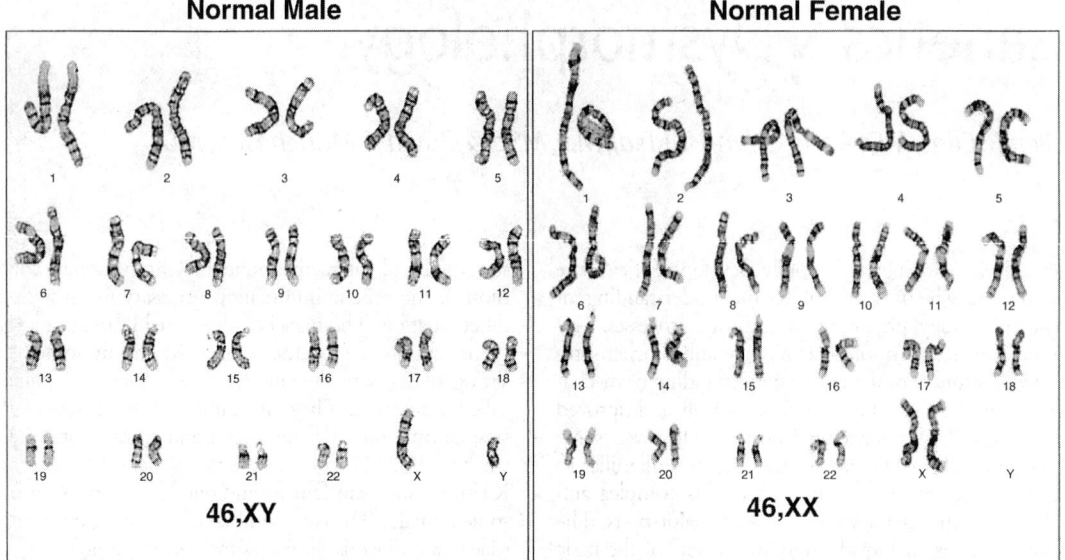

46,XY

46,XX

Figure 33–1. Normal male and female human karyotype. (Courtesy of Billie Carstens at CGL.)

cells. The distribution of maternal or paternal chromosomes to a particular daughter cell occurs independently in each cell.

3. Two cell divisions, the first of which is a reduction division—that is, separation between the homologous chromosomes. The second meiotic division is like mitosis, separating two sister chromatids into two genetically identical daughter cells.

Chromosome Preparation & Analysis

Chromosome structure is visible only during mitosis, most often achieved in the laboratory by stimulating a

blood lymphocyte culture with a mitogen for 3 days. Other tissues used for this purpose include skin, products of conception, cartilage, and bone marrow. Chorionic villi or amniocytes are used for prenatal diagnosis. Spontaneously dividing cells without a mitogen are present in bone marrow, and historically, bone marrow biopsy was done when immediate identification of a patient's chro-

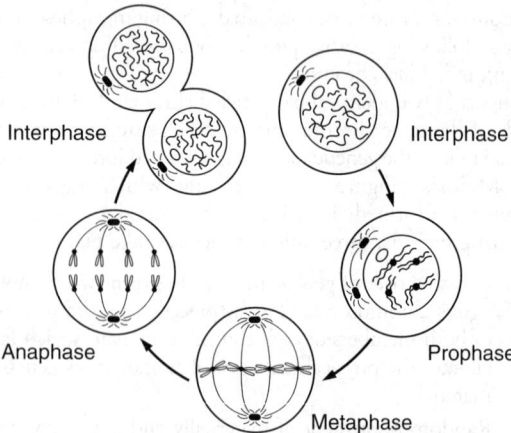

Figure 33–2. Stages of mitotic division.

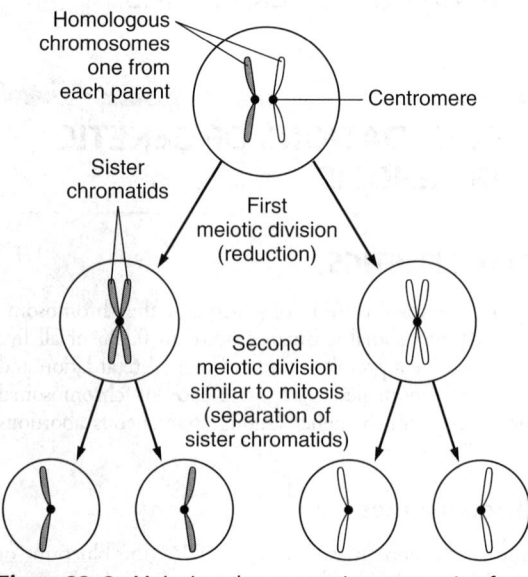

Figure 33–3. Meiosis—demonstrating conversion from the diploid somatic cell to the haploid gamete.

mosome constitution was necessary for appropriate management (eg, to rule out trisomy 13 in a newborn with a complex congenital heart disease). However, this invasive test has been replaced by the availability of the FISH technique (see following discussion).

Cells processed for routine chromosome analysis are stained on glass slides to yield a light-and-dark band pattern across the arms of the chromosomes (see Figure 33–1). This band pattern is characteristic and reproducible for each chromosome, allowing the chromosomes to be identified. Using different staining techniques, different banding patterns result: G, Q, and R banding. The most commonly used is G banding. The layout of chromosomes on a sheet of paper in a predetermined order is called a karyotype. High-resolution chromosome analysis is the study of more elongated chromosomes in prometaphase. In such an analysis, the bands can be visualized in greater detail, allowing detection of smaller, more subtle chromosomal rearrangements.

Fluorescent in situ hybridization (FISH) is a powerful technique that labels a known chromosome sequence with DNA probes attached to fluorescent dyes, thus enabling visualization of specific regions of chromosomes by fluorescent microscopy. There are many different kinds of probes, including paint probes (a mixture of sequences throughout one chromosome), sequence-specific probes, centromere probes, and telomere probes. A cocktail of differently colored probes, one color for each chromosome, called multicolor FISH, or M-FISH, can detect complex rearrangements between chromosomes. FISH can detect submicroscopic structural rearrangements undetectable by classic cytogenetic techniques and can identify marker chromosomes. For pictures of FISH studies, go to www.kumc.edu/gec/prof/cytogene.html

FISH also allows interphase cells (lymphocytes, amniocytes) to be screened for numerical abnormalities such as trisomy 13, 18, or 21, and sex chromosome anomalies. However, because of the possible background or contamination of the signal, the abnormality must be confirmed by conventional chromosome analysis.

Comparative Genomic Hybridization

Advances in computer chip technology have led to the development of new genetic testing using comparative genomic hybridization with microarray technique. This technique allows detection of very small genetic imbalances anywhere in the genome. Its usefulness has been well documented in cancer research and more recently in assessing small chromosomal rearrangements. In particular it has been used to detect interstitial and subtelomeric submicroscopic imbalances, to characterize their size at the molecular level, and to define the breakpoints of translocations.

Bejjani BA et al: Array-based comparative genomic hybridization in clinical diagnosis. Exp Rev Mol Diagn 2005;5(3):421 [PMID: 15934818].

Chromosome Nomenclature

Visible under the microscope is a constriction site on the chromosome called the centromere, which separates the chromosome into two arms: p, for petite, refers to the short arm, and q, the letter following p, refers to the long arm. Each arm is further subdivided into numbered bands visible using different staining techniques. Centromeres are positioned at different sites on different chromosomes and are used to differentiate the chromosome structures seen during mitosis as **metacentric** (p arm and q arm of almost equal size), **submetacentric** (p arm shorter than q arm), and **acrocentric** (almost no p arm). The use of named chromosome arms and bands provides a universal method of chromosome description. Common symbols include *del* (deletion), *dup* (duplication), *inv* (inversion), *ish* (in situ hybridization), *i* (isochromosome), *pat* (paternal origin), *mat* (maternal origin), and *r* (ring chromosome). These terms are further defined under Chromosomal Abnormalities, below.

Chromosomal Abnormalities

There are two types of chromosomal anomalies: numerical and structural.

A. ABNORMALITIES OF CHROMOSOMAL NUMBER

When a human cell has 23 chromosomes, such as human ova or sperm, it is in the haploid state (n). After conception, in cells other than the reproductive cells, 46 chromosomes are present in the diploid state (2n). Any number that is an exact multiple of the haploid number [eg, 46(2n), 69(3n), or 92(4n)] is referred to as euploid. Polyploid cells are those that contain any number other than the usual diploid number of chromosomes. Polyploid conceptions are usually not viable except in a "mosaic state," with the presence of more than one cell line in the body (see later text for details).

Cells deviating from the multiple of the haploid number are called aneuploid, meaning not euploid, indicating an abnormal number of chromosomes. Trisomy, an example of aneuploidy, is the presence of three of a particular chromosome rather than two. It results from unequal division, called nondisjunction, of chromosomes into daughter cells. Trisomies are the most common numerical chromosomal anomalies found in humans (eg, trisomy 21 [Down syndrome], trisomy 18, and trisomy 13). Monosomies, the presence of only one member of a chromosome pair, may be complete or partial. Complete monosomies may result from nondisjunction or anaphase lag. All complete autosomal monosomies appear to be lethal early in development and only survive in mosaic forms. Sex chromosome monosomy, however, can be viable.

B. ABNORMALITIES OF CHROMOSOMAL STRUCTURE

Many different types of structural chromosomal anomalies exist. Figure 33–4 displays the formal

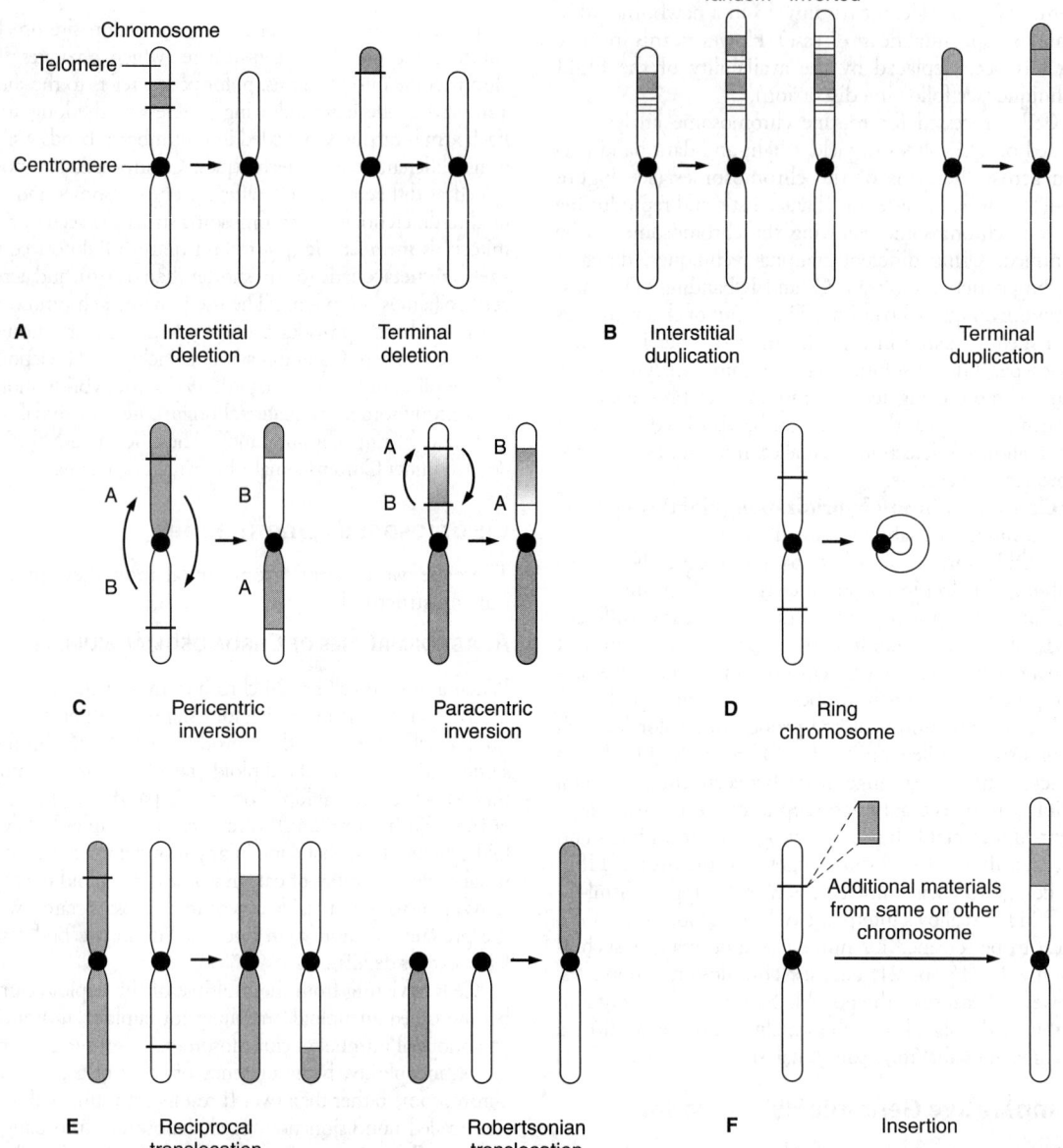

Figure 33–4. Examples of structural chromosomal abnormalities: deletion, duplication, inversion, ring chromosome, translocation, and insertion.

nomenclature as well as the ideogram demonstrating chromosomal anomalies. In clinical context, the sign (+) or (–) *preceding* the chromosome number indicates increased or decreased number, respectively, of that particular whole chromosome in a cell. For example, 47,XY+21 designates a male with three copies of chromosome 21. The sign (+) or (–) *after* the chromosome number signifies extra material or missing material, respectively, on one of the arms of the chromosome. For example, 46,XX,8q– denotes a deletion on the long arm of chromosome 8. Detailed nomenclature, such as 8q11, is required to further demonstrate a specific missing region so that genetic counseling can be provided.

1. Deletion (del) (see Figure 33–4A)—This refers to an absence of normal chromosomal material. It may be terminal (at the end of a chromosome) or interstitial (within a chromosome). The missing part is described using the code "del," followed by the number of the chromosome involved in parentheses, and a description of the missing region of that chromosome, also in parentheses, for example, 46,XX,del(1)(p36.3). This chromosome nomenclature describes the loss of genetic material from band 36.3 of the short arm of chromosome 1, which results in 1p36.3 deletion syndrome. Some more common deletions result in clinically recognizable conditions associated with mental handicaps and characteristic facial features. (See Part II of this chapter for descriptions of common genetic disorders caused by chromosomal deletions.)

2. Duplication (dup) (see Figure 33–4B)—An extra copy of a chromosomal segment can be tandem (genetic material present in the original direction) or inverted (genetic material present in the opposite direction). A well-described duplication of chromosome 22q11 causes cat eye syndrome, resulting in iris coloboma and anal or ear anomalies.

3. Inversion (inv) (see Figure 33–4C)—In this aberration, a rearranged section of a chromosome is inverted. It can be paracentric (not involving the centromere) or pericentric (involving the centromere).

4. Ring chromosome (r) (see Figure 33–4D)—Deletion of the normal telomeres (and possibly other subtelomeric sequences) leads to subsequent fusion of both ends to form a circular chromosome. Ring chromosomal anomalies often cause growth retardation and mental handicap.

5. Translocation (trans) (see Figure 33–4E)—This describes the interchromosomal rearrangement of genetic material. These may be balanced (the cell has a normal content of genetic material arranged in a structurally abnormal way) or unbalanced (the cell has gained or lost genetic material as a result of chromosomal interchange). Balanced translocations may further be described as reciprocal, the exchange of genetic material between two nonhomologous chromosomes, or robertsonian, the fusion of two acrocentric chromosomes.

6. Insertion (ins) (see Figure 33–4F)—Breakage within a chromosome at two points and incorporation of another piece of chromosomal material is called insertion. This requires three breakpoints and may occur between two chromosomes or within the same chromosome. The clinical presentation or phenotype depends on the origin of the inserted materials.

C. SEX CHROMOSOMAL ANOMALIES

Abnormalities involving sex chromosomes, including aneuploidy and mosaicism, are relatively common in the general population. The most common sex chromosome anomalies include 45,X (Turner syndrome), 47,XXX, 47,XXY (Klinefelter syndrome), 47,XYY, and different mosaic states. (Please see later text for clinical discussion.)

D. MOSAICISM

Mosaicism is the presence of two or more different chromosome constitutions in different cells of the same individual. For example, a patient may have some cells with 47 chromosomes and others with 46 chromosomes (46,XX/47,XX,+21 indicates mosaicism for trisomy 21; similarly, 45,X/46,XX/47,XXX indicates mosaicism for a monosomy and a trisomy X). Mosaicism should be suspected if clinical symptoms are milder than expected in a nonmosaic patient with the same chromosomal abnormality, or if the patient's skin shows unusual pigmentation. The prognosis is frequently better for a patient with mosaicism than for one with a corresponding chromosomal abnormality without mosaicism. In general, the smaller the proportion of the abnormal cell line, the better the prognosis. In the same patient, however, the proportion of normal and abnormal cells in various tissues, such as skin, brain, internal organs and peripheral blood, may be significantly different. Therefore, the prognosis for a patient with chromosomal mosaicism can seldom be assessed reliably based on the karyotype in peripheral blood alone.

E. UNIPARENTAL DISOMY

Under normal circumstances, one member of each homologous pair of chromosomes is of maternal origin from the egg and the other is of paternal origin from the sperm (Figure 33–5A). In uniparental disomy (UPD), both copies of a particular chromosome pair originate from the same parent. If UPD is caused by an error in the first meiotic division, both homologous chromosomes of that parent will be present in the gamete—a phenomenon called heterodisomy (see Figure 33–5B). If the disomy is caused by an error in the second meiotic division, two copies of the same chromosome will be present through the mechanism of rescue, duplication, and complementation (see Figure 33–5C–E)—a phenomenon called isodisomy. Isodisomy may also occur as a postfertilization error (see Figure 33–5F).

A chromosomal analysis would not reveal an abnormality, but DNA analysis would reveal that the child inherited two copies of DNA of a particular chromosome from one parent without the contribution from the other parent. Possible mechanisms for the adverse effects of UPD include homozygosity for deleterious recessive genes and the consequences of imprinting (see discussion in the Imprinting section). It is suspected that UPD of some chromosomes is lethal.

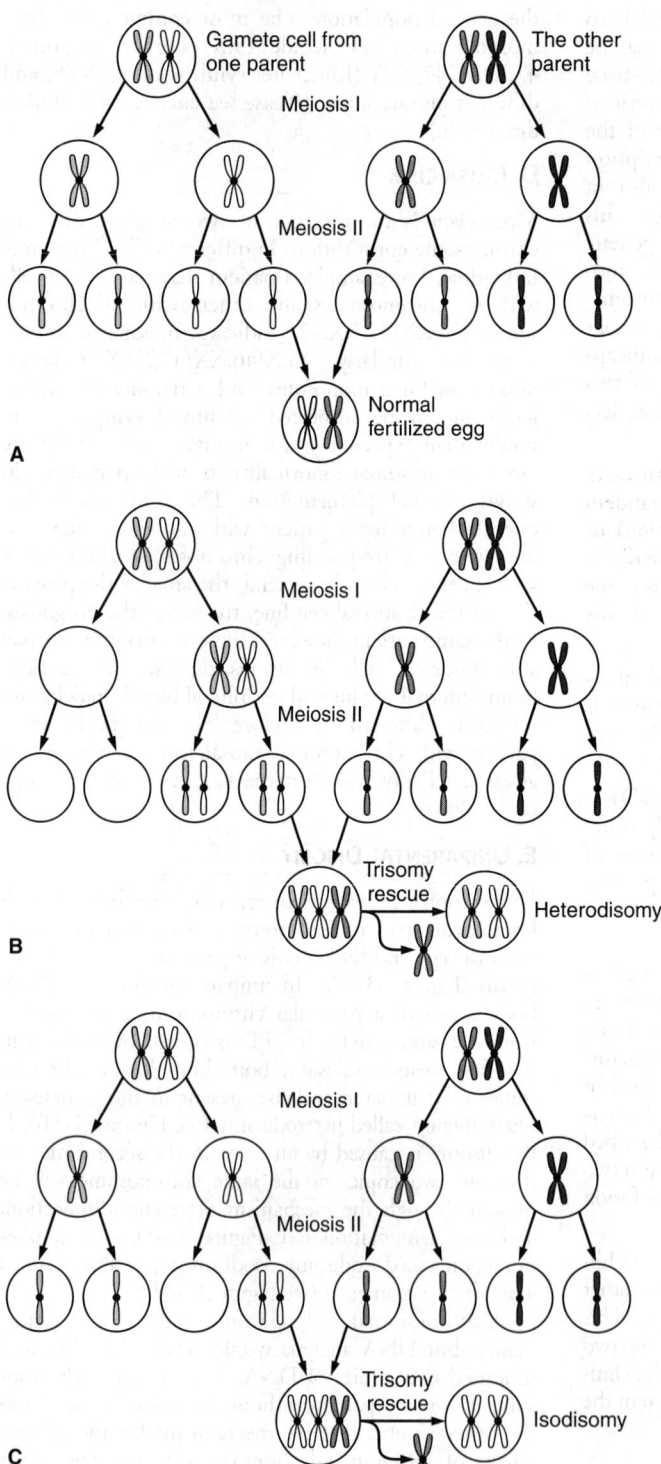

Figure 33–5. The assortment of homologous chromosomes during normal gametogenesis and uniparental disomy. **A:** Fertilization of normal gametes. **B:** Heterodisomy by trisomy rescue. **C:** Isodisomy by trisomy rescue.

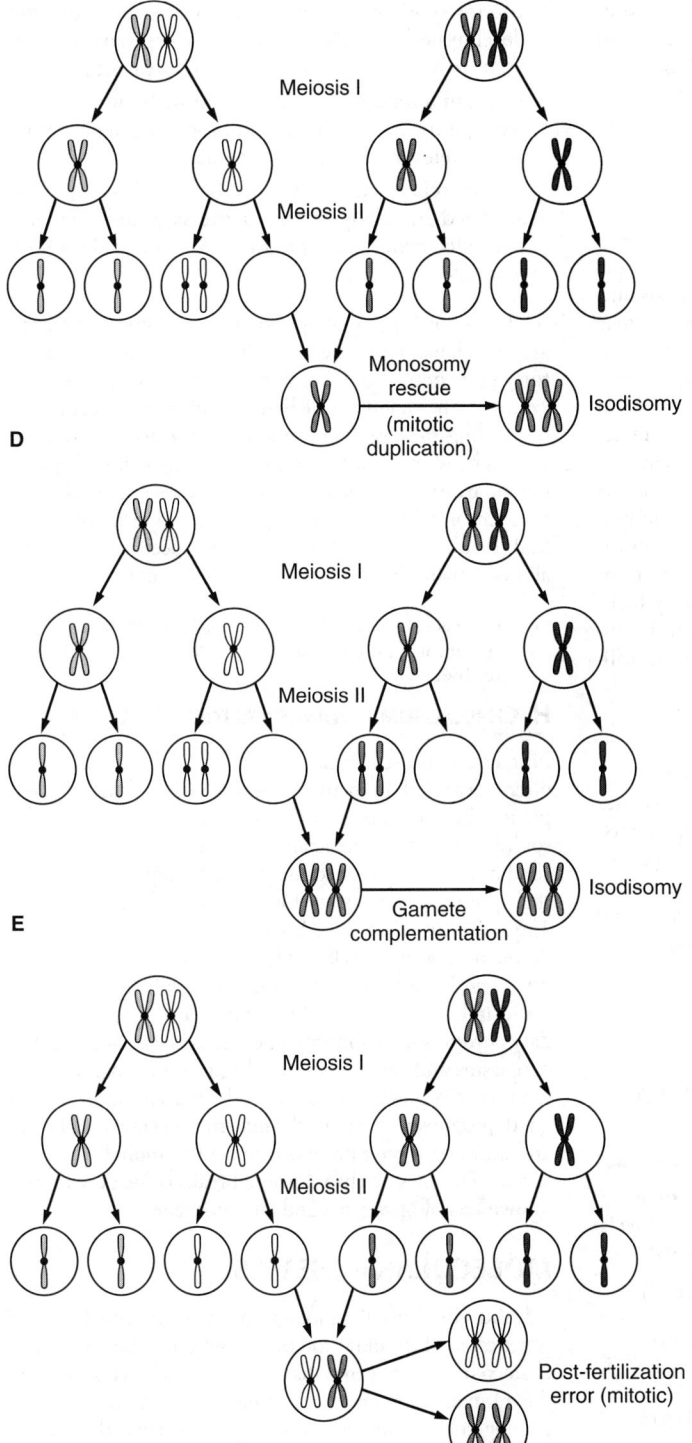

Figure 33–5. (continued) **D:** Isodisomy by monosomy rescue (mitotic duplication). **E:** Gamete complementation. **F:** Postfertilization error.

UPD has been documented for certain human chromosomes, including chromosomes 7, 11, 15, and X, and has been found in patients with Prader–Willi, Angelman, and Beckwith–Wiedemann syndromes. In addition, cystic fibrosis with only one carrier parent (caused by maternal isodisomy) has been reported. UPD may cause severe prenatal and postnatal growth retardation.

F. Contiguous Gene Syndromes

Contiguous gene syndromes result when a deletion causes the loss of genes adjacent to each other on a chromosome. Although many genes may be missing, the deletion may still be too small to be detected by routine karyotype. Therefore, contiguous gene syndromes are sometimes called "microdeletion syndromes." The genes involved in these syndromes are related only through their linear placement on the same chromosome segments and may not influence each other's functions directly. Table 33–1 lists examples of some currently known contiguous gene syndromes and their associated chromosomal abnormalities. These deletions may be familial (passed on by a parent), or occur de novo. The deletions may be diagnosed by high-resolution chromosome analysis in some affected individuals, or may be submicroscopic and detectable only with FISH or DNA analysis.

G. Chromosome Fragility

It is well known that environmental factors such as exposure to radiation, certain chemicals, and viruses contribute to chromosome breaks and rearrangements. There are also several well-defined autosomal recessive syndromes with DNA repair defects, associated with a greatly increased risk of chromosome aberrations. These are called chromosome instability or breakage syndromes. Examples are:

- **Bloom syndrome,** characterized by small stature and development of telangiectasias on exposure to sunlight. It is caused by a defect in a DNA helicase
- **Fanconi anemia,** often associated with radial ray defect, pigmentary changes, mild mental retardation, and development of pancytopenia.
- **Ataxia–telangiectasia** (Louis–Bar syndrome), characterized by telangiectasia of the skin and eyes, immunodeficiency, and progressive ataxia; a DNA repair defect.

The knowledge that specific chromosome aberrations are associated with these syndromes is often the basis for cytogenetic confirmation of their diagnosis. For example, the diagnosis of Fanconi anemia, is confirmed by finding increased chromosomal breakage and translocations between nonhomologous quadriradii after diepoxybutane treatment. Assessment of chromosome breaks and sister chromatid exchanges requires special techniques that lead to enhancement of the breaks, or special staining that allows visualization of the exchanged chromatids.

Levran O et al: The BRCA 1-interacting helicase BRIP1 is deficient in Fanconi anemia. Nat Genet 2005:37(9):931 [PMID: 16116424].

H. Chromosomal Abnormalities in Cancer

Numerical and structural chromosomal abnormalities are often identified in hematopoietic and solid-tumor neoplasms in individuals with otherwise normal chromosomes. These cytogenetic abnormalities have been categorized as primary and secondary. In primary abnormalities, their presence is necessary for initiation of the cancer (eg, 13q– in retinoblastoma). Secondary abnormalities appear de novo in somatic cells, only after the cancer has developed [eg, Philadelphia chromosome, t(9;22)(q34;q11), in acute and chronic myeloid leukemia]. Primary and secondary chromosomal abnormalities are specific for particular neoplasms and can be used for diagnosis or prognosis. For example, the presence of the Philadelphia chromosome is a good prognostic sign in chronic myelogenous leukemia and indicates a poor prognosis in acute lymphoblastic leukemia. The sites of chromosome breaks coincide with the known loci of oncogenes and antioncogenes.

MOLECULAR GENETICS

Advances in molecular biology have revolutionized human genetics, as they allow for the localization, isolation, and characterization of genes that encode protein sequences. As the Human Genome Project has moved into the post-cloning era, the function of gene products and their interaction with one another has become the main theme of molecular genetics. Molecular genetics can help explain the complex underlying biology involved in many human diseases.

Table 33–1. Examples of common contiguous gene syndromes.

Syndrome	Abnormal Chromosome Segment
Prader-Willi/Angelman syndrome	del 15q11
Shprintzen/DiGeorge spectrum	del 22q11
Miller-Dieker syndrome	del 17p13
Wilms tumor with aniridia, genitourinary malformations, and mental retardation	del 11p13
Williams syndrome	del 7q11
Smith-Magenis	del 17p11

Recombinant DNA Technology

Recombinant DNA technology was developed using restriction endonucleases, which cleave DNA at specific nucleotide sequences. A difference in DNA sequence caused by a normal variation of DNA or by a gene mutation either produces or eliminates an endonuclease recognition site, resulting in a DNA fragment of different size. Thus, the number and arrangement of restriction sites (called a restriction map) are characteristic of a given DNA sequence.

Before a DNA fragment of interest can be analyzed, multiple copies of it must be produced. This can be achieved by incorporating the human DNA fragment into a vector (ie, a DNA segment containing the means of replication and selection in bacteria). The vector-containing human DNA insert is replicated, thus producing multiple copies of the segment of interest. The source of inserts can be genomic DNA, obtained directly from cleaving of the target organism, or complementary DNA (cDNA), obtained by copying messenger RNA (mRNA) into DNA by reverse transcription.

A genomic library can be assembled by fragmenting human genomic DNA with restriction enzymes and then inserting the fragments into a vector. Such a library contains large numbers of different DNA sequences. Some of these specific DNA fragments are used to manufacture human proteins (eg, insulin, growth hormone, interferon, and blood clotting factors) for pharmacologic applications; others are used as probes (DNA segment-specific, radioactively labeled reagents for mapping and diagnosis).

Southern blot analysis is the molecular genetic technique used to look for changes in genomic DNA. A similar technique called Northern blot analysis is used to look for RNA abnormalities. Southern blot analysis relies on the use of restriction endonucleases to cleave human genomic DNA at specific nucleotide sequences and to produce DNA fragments of different lengths.

The **polymerase chain reaction (PCR)** replicates fragments of DNA between predetermined primers so that sufficient DNA is obtained for characterization or sequencing in the space of a few hours. For example, 20 cycles of synthesis will amplify DNA 1 millionfold. The disadvantage of PCR is that a small contamination with foreign DNA can result in an incorrect diagnosis.

Application of Molecular Biology in Clinical Genetics and Genetic Diagnosis

Genetic diagnosis can be performed by direct detection of a mutant gene or by indirect methods. Direct detection is possible only when the gene causing the disease and the nature of the mutation are known. The advantage of a diagnostic study using the direct detection of a mutant gene is that it requires the affected individual

only and need not involve the testing of other family members. The methods of direct DNA diagnosis include restriction analysis, single strand conformational polymorphism analysis, direct sequencing with assistance of PCR, heteroduplex assay, and protein truncation assay. The molecular mechanisms causing human diseases include point mutations, deletions, and insertions, and the unstable expansion of trinucleotide repeats, which leads to genetic anticipation (see previous sections and later discussion). Some disorders that may be diagnosed via direct DNA mutational analysis include Duchenne muscular dystrophy, hemophilia, some forms of craniosynostosis, cystic fibrosis, and fragile X syndrome.

Indirect detection of abnormal genes is used when the gene is known but there is extensive heterogeneity of the molecular defect between families, or when the gene responsible for a disease is unknown but its chromosome location is known.

One form of indirect analysis is the linkage method. Linkage traces the inheritance of the abnormal gene between members of a kindred. This method requires that the affected individual be studied, as well as parents and other relatives, both affected and unaffected.

Linkage analysis, is performed by using markers such as a restriction fragment length polymorphisms. Another method uses flanking microsatellite polymorphisms. An increase in density of polymorphisms discovered over the past few years allows the presence or absence of an abnormal copy of a gene in an individual to be predicted with a high degree of confidence, if the relatives have informative polymorphisms. Microsatellite polymorphisms are being used in sibling research studies to identify the multiple genes that contribute to polygenic traits such as diabetes and obesity. They are also used increasingly to identify gene changes in tumors.

Neurofibromatosis is an example of a disorder in which both the direct and indirect assay may be used. Because of the size and the heterogenous mutation pattern of the neurofibromin gene (*NFI*), the first step usually is the protein truncation assay. However, this method detects only two-thirds of affected patients, in whom a nonsense mutation exists truncating the gene message. All other cases must rely on indirect methods.

Application of Molecular Biology in Prevention of Human Diseases

Recombinant DNA technology has the potential for preventing genetic disease by facilitating the detection of carriers of defective genes and permitting prenatal diagnosis. Family studies can also clarify the mode of inheritance, thus allowing more accurate determination of recurrence risks and appropriate options. For example, differentiation of gonadal mosaicism from decreased penetrance of a dominant gene has important implications for genetic counseling. In the past, the diagnosis of a genetic disease characterized by late onset of symptoms (eg, Huntington disease) could not be made prior to the appearance of clinical symptoms. In some inborn errors of metabolism, diagnostic tests (eg, measurement of enzyme activities) could be conducted only on inaccessible tissues. Gene identification (mutation analysis) techniques can enormously enhance the ability to diagnose both symptomatic and presymptomatic individuals, heterozygous carriers of gene mutations, and affected fetuses. However, presymptomatic DNA testing is associated with psychological, ethical, and legal implications and therefore should be used only with informed consent. Formal genetic counseling is indicated to best interpret the results of molecular testing.

Application of Molecular Biology in Treatment of Human Diseases

A normal gene introduced into an individual affected with a serious inherited disorder during embryonic life (germline therapy) in principle has the potential to be transmitted to future generations, whereas its introduction into somatic cells (somatic therapy) affects only the recipient. Experimental gene therapy by bone marrow transplantation is being tried for adenosine deaminase deficiency. Recombinant enzyme replacement has been successfully applied in treating the non-neurologic form of Gaucher disease and some types of lysosomal storage disease.

PRINCIPLES OF INHERITED HUMAN DISORDERS
MENDELIAN DISORDERS

Traditionally, autosomal single gene disorders follow the principles explained by Mendel's observations. To summarize, the inheritance of genetic traits through generations relies on segregation and independent assortment. **Segregation** is the process through which gene pairs are separated during gamete formation. Each gamete receives only one copy of each gene (allele). **Independent assortment** refers to the idea that the segregation of different alleles occurs independently.

Victor McKusick's catalog, *Mendelian Inheritance in Man,* lists more than 10,000 entries in which the mode of inheritance is presumed to be autosomal dominant, autosomal recessive, X-linked dominant, X-linked recessive, and Y-linked. Single genes at specific loci on one or a pair of chromosomes cause these disorders. An understanding of inheritance terminology is helpful in approaching mendelian disorders. Analysis of the pedigree and the pattern of transmission in the family, identification of a specific condition, and knowledge of that condition's mode of inheritance usually allows for explanation of the inheritance pattern.

Terminology

The following terms are important in understanding heredity patterns.

Dominant and Recessive—As defined by Mendel, concepts for dominant and recessive refer to the **phenotypic expression** of alleles and are not intrinsic characteristics of gene loci. Therefore, it is inappropriate to discuss "a dominant locus."

Genotype—Genotype means the genetic status, that is, the alleles an individual carries.

Phenotype—Phenotype is the expression of an individual's genotype including appearance, physical features, organ structure, biochemical, and physiologic nature. It may be modified by environment.

Pleiotropy—Pleiotropy refers to the phenomenon whereby a single mutant allele can have widespread effects or expression in different tissues or organ systems. In other words, an allele may produce more than one effect on the phenotype. For example, Marfan syndrome has findings in different organ systems (skeletal, cardiac, ophthalmologic, etc) due to a single mutation within the *fibrillin* gene.

Penetrance—Penetrance refers to the proportion of individuals with a particular genotype that express the same phenotype. Penetrance is a proportion that ranges between 0 and 1.0 (or 0 and 100%). When 100% of mutant individuals express the phenotype, penetrance is **complete.** If some mutant individuals do not express the phenotype, penetrance is said to be **incomplete,** or **reduced.** Dominant conditions with incomplete penetrance, therefore, are characterized by "skipped" generations with unaffected, obligate gene carriers.

Expressivity—Expressivity refers to the variability in degree of phenotypic expression (severity) seen in different individuals with the same mutant genotype. Expressivity may be extremely variable or fairly consistent, both within and between families. Intrafamilial variability of expression may be due to factors such as epistasis, environment, genetic anticipation, presence of phenocopies, mosaicism, and chance (stochastic factors). Interfamilial variability of expression may be due to the previously mentioned factors, but may also be due to allelic or locus genetic heterogeneity.

Genetic Heterogeneity—A number of different genetic mutations may produce phenotypes that are identical or similar enough to have been traditionally considered as one diagnosis. "Anemia" or "mental retardation" are examples of this. There are two types of genetic heterogeneity, **locus heterogeneity** and **allelic heterogeneity**.

Locus Heterogeneity—Locus heterogeneity describes a phenotype caused by mutations at more than one genetic locus; that is, mutations at different loci cause the same phenotype or a group of phenotypes that appear similar enough to have been previously classified as a single disease, clinical "entity," or diagnostic spectrum. An example would be Sanfilippo syndrome (mucopolysaccharidosis III A, B, C, and D), in which the same phenotype is produced by four different enzyme deficiencies.

Allelic Heterogeneity—This term is applied to a phenotype causing different mutations at a single gene locus. As an example, cystic fibrosis may be caused by many different genetic changes, such as homozygosity for the common Δ *F 508* mutation, or Δ *F 508* and an *R117H* mutation. The latter example represents **compound heterozygosity.**

Phenotypic Heterogeneity or "Clinical Heterogeneity"—This term describes the situation in which more than one phenotype is caused by different allelic mutations at a single locus. An example of phenotypic heterogeneity is that different mutations in the *FGFR2* gene can cause different craniosynostosis disorders, including Crouzon syndrome, Jackson–Weiss syndrome, Pfeiffer syndrome, and Apert syndrome. These syndromes are clinically distinguishable and are due to the presence of a variety of genetic mutations within single genes.

Homozygous—A cell or organism that has identical alleles at a particular locus is said to be homozygous. For example, a cystic fibrosis patient with a Δ *F 508* mutation on both alleles would be called homozygous for that mutation.

Heterozygous—A cell or organism that has nonidentical alleles at a genetic locus is said to be heterozygous. In autosomal dominant conditions, a mutation of only one copy of the gene pair is all that is necessary to result in a disease state. However, an individual who is heterozygous for a recessive disorder will not manifest symptoms (see below).

Online Mendelian Inheritance in Man.
http://www.ncbi.nlm.nih.gov/entrez/query.fcgi?db=OMIM

1. Hereditary Patterns

Autosomal Dominant Inheritance

Autosomal dominant inheritance has the following characteristics:

1. Affected individuals in the same family may experience variable expressivity.
2. Nonpenetrance is common, and the penetrance rate varies for each dominantly inherited condition.
3. Both males and females can pass on the abnormal gene to children of either sex, although the manifestations may vary according to sex. For example,

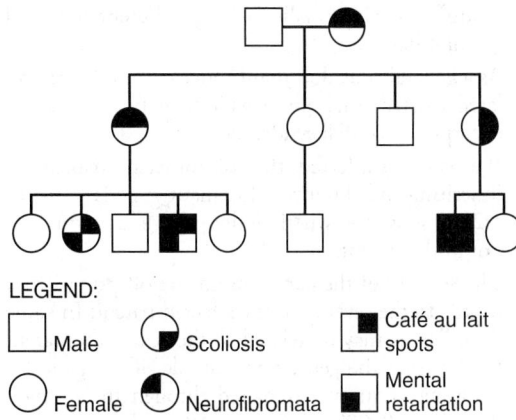

LEGEND:

☐ Male	◐ Scoliosis	◧ Café au lait spots
◯ Female	◕ Neurofibromata	◩ Mental retardation

Figure 33–6. Autosomal dominant inheritance. Variable expressivity in NF-1.

pattern baldness is a dominant trait but affects only males. In this case, the trait is said to be sex-limited.

4. Dominant inheritance is typically said to be vertical, that is, the condition passes from one generation to the next in a vertical fashion (Figure 33–6).
5. In some cases, the family history seems to be completely negative, and the patient appears to be the first affected individual. This spontaneous appearance may be caused by a new mutation. In more severe disorders, where there is a decrease in reproductive fitness, there is a high rate of new mutations. The mutation rate increases with advancing paternal age (particularly over age 40 years). Several other explanations for a negative family history are possible however, including:

   a. Nonpaternity.
   b. Decreased penetrance or mild manifestations in one of the parents.
   c. Germline mosaicism (ie, mosaicism in the germ cell line of either parent), in which case the risk of recurrence increases. Germline mosaicism may mimic autosomal recessive inheritance, because it leads to situations in which two children of completely normal parents are affected with a genetic disorder. The best example of this is osteogenesis imperfecta type II. Laboratory studies have documented germline mosaicism by finding that only one allele of the paired collagen genes is abnormal in the severe form instead of both, as would be expected in a recessive disease. The recurrence risk in this form of osteogenesis imperfecta is 7%.
   d. The abnormality present in the patient may be a phenocopy, or it may be a similar but genetically

different abnormality with a different mode of inheritance.

6. As a general rule, dominant traits are more often related to structural abnormalities of protein, as for example in Marfan syndrome.

7. If a parent is affected, the risk for each offspring of inheriting the abnormal dominant gene is 50%, or 1:2. This is true whether the gene is penetrant or not in the parent.

8. The severity of the condition in the offspring is not related to the severity in the affected parent. In some disorders, it may be related to the sex of the parent transmitting the gene. For example, if the gene for myotonic dystrophy is passed through the mother, there is a 10–20% chance that the child (regardless of sex) may have a severe congenital form of the disease. Conversely, if the gene for Huntington disease is passed through the father, the probability is 5–10% that the offspring may have the severe, rigid juvenile form. In these two conditions the inheritance of the gene is associated with expansion of the triplet repeats (see Genetic Anticipation section).

9. If an abnormality represents a new mutation of a dominant trait, the parents of the affected individual run a low risk during subsequent pregnancies, but the risk for the offspring of the affected individual is 50%. Although a mutation is thought to be new because the parents are not affected, the risk for an affected sibling is still slightly increased over the general population, because of the possibility of germline mosaicism.

10. Prevention options available for future pregnancies include prenatal diagnosis, artificial insemination, and egg or sperm donation, depending on which parent has the abnormal gene.

Autosomal Recessive Inheritance

Autosomal recessive inheritance also has some distinctive characteristics:

1. There is less variability among affected persons. Parents are carriers and are clinically normal. (There are exceptions to this rule, however. For example, carriers of sickle cell trait may become symptomatic if they become hypoxic.)

2. Males and females are affected equally.

3. Inheritance is horizontal; siblings may be affected (Figure 33–7).

4. Recessive conditions are usually rare; the rarer the condition, the more likely it is that consanguinity is present. Conversely, if a child whose parents are related presents with an unrecognized abnormality, a recessive condition must be suspected.

5. The family history is usually negative, with the exception of siblings. However, in common condi-

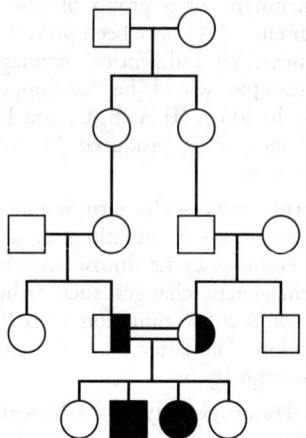

LEGEND:

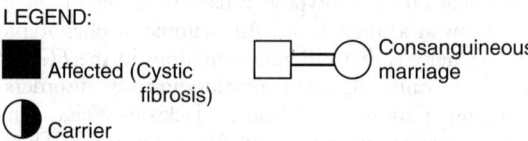

Figure 33–7. Autosomal recessive inheritance: cystic fibrosis.

tions such as cystic fibrosis, a second- or third-degree relative may be affected.

6. Recessive conditions are frequently associated with enzyme defects.

7. The recurrence risk for parents of an affected child is 25%, or 1:4 for each pregnancy. The gene carrier frequency in the general population can be used to assess the risk of having an affected child with a new partner, for unaffected siblings, and for the affected individuals themselves.

8. In rare instances, a child with a recessive disorder and a normal karyotype may have inherited both copies of the abnormal gene from one parent and none from the other. This uniparental disomy (UPD) was first described in a girl with cystic fibrosis and growth retardation. This phenomenon is of unknown frequency, but it is more likely to be present in a child with more than one autosomal recessive condition, or in a patient with unexpected and seemingly unrelated abnormalities or severe growth retardation. Molecular testing can confirm the presence of UPD. The recurrence risk is obviously lower in such a situation, although the factors predisposing to UPD are unknown. Maternal age may play a role in these situations.

9. Options available for future pregnancies include prenatal diagnosis, adoption, artificial insemination, and egg or sperm donation.

X-Linked Inheritance

When a gene for a specific disorder is on the X chromosome, the condition is said to be X-linked, or sex-linked. Females may be either homozygous or heterozygous, because they have two X chromosomes. Males, by contrast, have only one X, and a male is said to be hemizygous for any gene on his X chromosome. The severity of any disorder is greater in males than in females (within a specific family). According to the Lyon hypothesis, because one of the two X chromosomes in each cell is inactivated, and this inactivation is random, the clinical picture in females depends on the percentage of mutant versus normal alleles inactivated. The X chromosome is not inactivated until about 14 days of gestation, and parts of the short arm remain active throughout life.

X-Linked Recessive Inheritance

The following features are characteristic of X-linked recessive inheritance:

1. Males are affected, and heterozygous females are either normal or have mild manifestations.

2. Inheritance is diagonal through the maternal side of the family (Figure 33–8A).

3. A female carrier has a 50% chance that each daughter will be a carrier and a 50% chance that each son will be affected.

4. All of the daughters of an affected male are carriers, and none of his sons are affected. Because a father can give only his Y chromosome to his sons, male-to-male transmission excludes X-linked inheritance except in the rare case of UPD, in which a son receives both the X and the Y from his father.

5. The mutation rate is high in some X-linked disorders, particularly when the affected male dies or is so incapacitated by the disorder that reproduction is unlikely. In such instances, the mutation is thought to occur as a new mutation in the affected male, and in the mother, each one-third of the time and to be present in earlier generations one-third of the time. For this reason, genetic counseling may be difficult in families with an isolated case.

6. On rare occasions, a female may be fully affected. Several possible mechanisms may account for a fully affected female: (a) unfavorable lyonization; (b) 45,X karyotype; (c) homozygosity for the abnormal gene; (d) an X-autosome translocation, or other structural abnormality of one X chromosome, in which the X chromosome of normal structure is preferentially inactivated; (e) UPD; and (f) nonrandom inactivation, which may be controlled by an autosomal gene.

X-Linked Dominant Inheritance

The X-linked dominant inheritance pattern is much less common than the X-linked recessive type. Examples include incontinentia pigmenti and hypophosphatemic or vitamin D–resistant rickets.

1. The heterozygous female is symptomatic, and the disease is twice as common in females because they have two X chromosomes that can have the mutation.

2. Clinical manifestations are more variable in females than in males.

3. The risk for the offspring of heterozygous females to be affected is 50% regardless of sex.

4. All of the daughters but none of the sons of affected males will have the disorder (see Figure 33–8B).

5. Although a homozygous female is possible (particularly in an inbred population), she would be severely involved. All of her children would also be affected but more mildly.

6. Some disorders (eg, incontinentia pigmenti) are lethal in males (and in homozygous females). Affected women have twice as many daughters as sons and an increased incidence of miscarriages, because affected males will be spontaneously aborted. A 47,XXY karyotype has allowed affected males to survive.

Y-Linked Inheritance

Also known as "holandric" inheritance, these conditions are caused by genes located on the Y chromosome. These conditions are relatively rare with only about 40 entries listed in McKusick's catalog. Male-to-male transmission is seen in this category, with all sons of affected males being affected and no daughters or females being affected.

MULTIFACTORIAL INHERITANCE

Many common attributes, such as height, are familial, and are the result of the actions of multiple rather than single genes. Inheritance of these traits is described as **polygenic** or **multifactorial.** The latter term recognizes that environmental factors such as diet also contribute to these traits. Geneticists are now finding that multiple genes are often expressed in hierarchies, in which the action of a small number of genes, two or three, explains much of the variation observed within affected populations.

Studies of twins have proven useful in determining the relative importance of genetic versus environmental factors in the expression of polygenic traits. If genetic factors are of little or no importance, then the concordance between monozygotic and dizygotic twins should

A

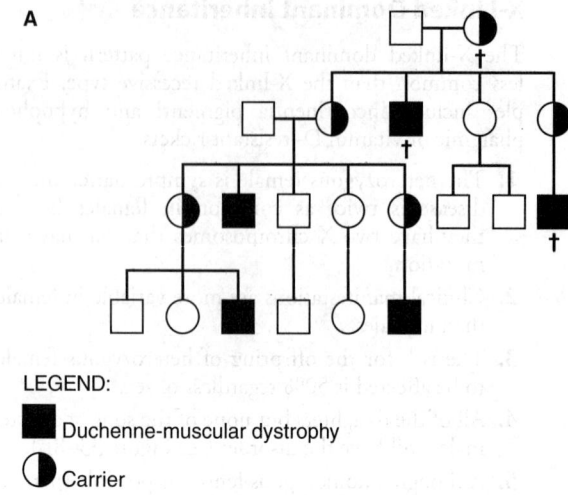

LEGEND:

■ Duchenne-muscular dystrophy

◑ Carrier

† Deceased

B

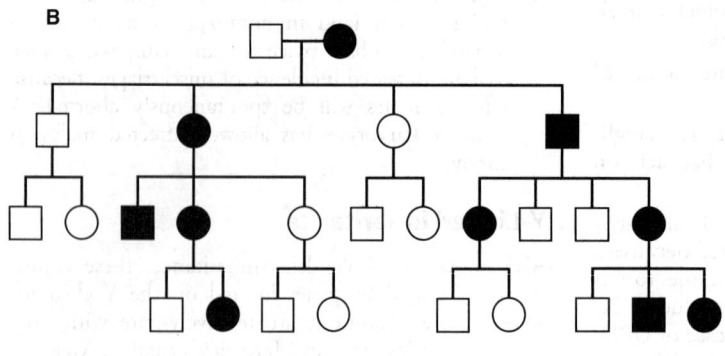

LEGEND:

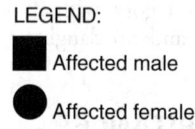

■ Affected male

● Affected female

Figure 33–8. **A:** X-linked recessive inheritance. **B:** X-linked dominant inheritance.

be the same. (Dizygotic twins are no more genetically similar to each other than to other siblings.) If an abnormality is completely genetic, the concordance between identical twins should be 100%. In polygenic conditions, the concordance rate for identical twins is usually higher than that seen in dizygotic twins but is still not 100%, indicating that both genetic and environmental factors are playing a role.

Many disorders and congenital abnormalities that are clearly familial but do not segregate as mendelian traits (eg, autosomal dominant, recessive, etc) show polygenic inheritance. For the most part, these conditions become manifest when thresholds of additive gene actions or contributing environmental factors are exceeded. Many common

disorders ranging from hypertension, stroke, and thrombophlebitis to behavioral traits such as alcoholism demonstrate multifactorial (polygenic) inheritance. Some common birth defects, including isolated congenital heart disease, cleft lip and palate, and neural tube defects, also demonstrate polygenic inheritance. Neural tube defects provide a good model for how identification of both environmental and genetic contributions to multifactorial traits can lead to preventive measures.

Polygenic or multifactorial inheritance has several distinctive characteristics:

1. The risk for relatives of affected persons is increased. The risk is higher for first-degree relatives

(those who have 50% of their genes in common) and lower for more distant relations, although the risk for the latter is higher than for the general population (Table 33–2).

2. The recurrence risk varies with the number of affected family members. For example, after one child is born with a neural tube defect, the recurrence risk is 2–3%. If a second affected child is born, the risk for any future child increases to 10–12%. This is in contrast to single gene disorders, in which the risk is the same no matter how many family members are affected.

3. The risk is higher if the defect is more severe. In Hirschsprung disease, another polygenic condition, the longer the aganglionic segment, the higher the recurrence risk.

4. Sex ratios may not be equal. If a marked discrepancy exists, the recurrence risk is higher if a child of the less commonly affected sex has the disorder. This assumes that more genetic factors are required to raise the more resistant sex above the threshold. For example, pyloric stenosis is more common in males. If the first affected child is a female, the recurrence risk is higher than if the child is a male.

5. The risk for the offspring of an affected person is approximately the same as the risk for siblings, assuming that the spouse of the affected person has a negative family history. For many conditions, however, assortative mating, "like marrying like," adds to risks in offspring.

Table 33–2. Empiric risks for some congenital disorders.

Anencephaly and spina bifida: Incidence (average) 1:1000
  One affected child: 2–3%
  Two affected children: 10–12%
  One affected parent: 4–5%
Hydrocephalus: Incidence 1:2000 newborns
  Occasional X-linked recessive
  Often associated with neural tube defect
  Some environmental etiologies (eg, toxoplasmosis)
  Recurrence risk, one affected child
    Hydrocephalus: 1%
    Some central nervous system abnormality: 3%
Nonsyndromic cleft lip and/or palate: Incidence (average) 1:1000
  One affected child: 2–4%
  One affected parent: 2–4%
  Two affected children: 10%
  One affected parent, one affected child: 10–20%
Nonsyndromic cleft palate: Incidence 1:2000
  One affected child: 2%
  Two affected children: 6–8%
  One affected parent: 4–6%
  One affected parent, one affected child: 15–20%
Congenital heart disease: Incidence 8:1000
  One affected child: 2–3%
  One affected parent, one affected child: 10%
Clubfoot: Incidence 1:1000 (male:female = 2:1)
  One affected child: 2–3%
Congenital dislocated hip: Incidence 1:1000
  (female > male) with marked regional variation
  One child affected: 2–14%
Pyloric stenosis: Incidence, males: 1:200; females: 1:1000

Male index patient	
Brothers	3.2%
Sons	6.8%
Sisters	3.0%
Daughters	1.2%
Female index patient	
Brothers	13.2%
Sons	20.5%
Sisters	2.5%
Daughters	11.1%

NONMENDELIAN INHERITANCE

Epigenetic Regulation

Although development is regulated by genes, it is initiated and sustained by nongenetic processes. Epigenetic events are points of interaction between developmental programs and the physicochemical environments in differentiating cells. Genetic imprinting and DNA methylation are examples of epigenetic processes that affect development. Certain genes important in regulation of growth and differentiation are themselves regulated by chemical modification that occurs in specific patterns in gametes. For example, genes that are methylated are "turned off" and not transcribed. The pattern of which genes are methylated may be determined or affected by the sex of the parent of origin (see Imprinting section below). Expression of imprinted genes may sometimes be limited to specific organs (eg, the brain), and imprinting may be relaxed and methyl groups lost as development progresses. Disruption of imprinting is now recognized as contributing to birth defect syndromes (described later in this chapter). Certain techniques developed to assist infertile couples (advanced reproductive technology) may affect epigenetic processes and lead to genetic disorders in the offspring conceived via these methods.

Niemitz EL, Feinberg AP: Epigenetics and assisted reproductive technology: A call for investigation. Am J Hum Genet 2004: 74:599 [PMID: 14991528].

Imprinting

Although the homologs of chromosome pairs may appear identical on routine karyotype analysis, it is now known that the parental origin of each homolog can affect which genes are actually transcribed and which are inactivated. The term "imprinting" refers to the process by which preferential transcription of certain genes takes place, depending on the parental origin, that is, which homolog (maternal or paternal) the gene is located on. Certain chromosomes, particularly chromosome X, and the autosomes 15, 11, and 7, have imprinted regions where certain genes are only read from one homolog (ie, either the maternal or paternal allele) under normal circumstances, and the gene on the other homolog is normally inactivated. Errors in imprinting may arise because of UPD (in which a copy from one parent is missing), by a chromosomal deletion causing loss of the gene normally transcribed, or by mutations in the imprinting genes that normally code for transcription or inactivation of other genes downstream. A good example of how imprinting may affect human disease is Beckwith–Wiedemann syndrome (BWS), the gene for which is located on chromosome 11p15.

Cohen MM et al: *Overgrowth Syndromes.* Oxford University Press, 2002.

Genetic Anticipation

Geneticists coined the term "anticipation" to describe an unusual pattern of inheritance in which symptoms became manifest at earlier ages and with increasing severity as traits are passed to subsequent generations. Mapping of the genes responsible for these disorders led to the discovery that certain repeat sequences of DNA at disease loci were not stable when passed through meiosis. Repeated DNA sequences, in particular triplets (eg, CGG and CAG), tended to increase their copy number. As these runs of triplets expanded, they eventually affected the expression of genes and produced symptoms. Curiously, all the disorders undergoing triplet repeat expansion detected thus far produce neurologic symptoms. Most are progressive. In general, the size of the triplet expansion is roughly correlated with the timing and severity of symptoms. The reasons for the meiotic instability of these sequences are not yet understood. The mechanisms appear to involve interactions between DNA structure (eg, formation of hairpin loops) and replication enzymes (DNA polymerase complexes) during meiosis.

Triplet repeat instability can modify the inheritance of autosomal dominant, autosomal recessive, and X-linked traits. Autosomal dominant disorders include several spinal cerebellar atrophies, Huntington disease, and myotonic dystrophy. Unstable triplet repeat expansion contributes to at least one autosomal recessive disorder, Friedreich ataxia. The most common X-linked disorder demonstrating triplet repeat instability and expansion is fragile X syndrome.

Mitochondrial Inheritance

Mitochondrial DNA is double-stranded, circular, and smaller than nuclear DNA, and is found in the cytoplasm. It codes for enzymes involved in oxidative phosphorylation, which generates adenosine triphosphate. During the last decade of the 20th century, enormous advances in technology and improved clinical documentation have led to a better understanding of the interesting disorders caused by mutations in mitochondrial DNA (mtDNA).

Mitochondrial disorders have been associated with deletions or duplications in mitochondrial DNA. Large deletions are usually sporadic, but smaller deletions may be secondary events due to defects in dominantly inherited nuclear genes. Mitochondrial dysfunction may also be caused by mutations in nuclear genes encoding mitochondrial proteins and can be inherited as dominant, recessive, or X-linked traits. Because of the difficulty in diagnosing mitochondrial disorders and the variability of the clinical course, it is often difficult to calculate specific recurrence risks.

Mitochondrial disorders have the following characteristics:

1. They show remarkable phenotypic variability.
2. They are maternally inherited, because only the egg has any cytoplasmic material, and during early embryogenesis any sperm-born mitochondrial material will be eliminated.
3. In most mitochondrial disorders, cells are heteroplasmic (Figure 33–9). That is, all cells contain both normal and mutated or abnormal mtDNA. The proportion of normal to abnormal mtDNA in the mother's egg seems to determine the severity of the offspring's disease and the age at onset in most cases.
4. Those tissues with the highest adenosine triphosphate requirements—specifically, central nervous system (CNS) and skeletal muscle—seem to be most susceptible to mutations in mtDNA.
5. Somatic cells show an increase in mtDNA mutations and a decline in oxidative phosphorylation function with age. This explains the later onset of some of these disorders and may indeed be a clue to the whole aging process.

Hayashida K et al: The sperm mitochondria—Specific translocator has a key role in maternal mitochondrial inheritance. Cell Biol Int 2005;29(6):472 [PMID: 15979907].

FAMILY HISTORY AND PEDIGREE

The first step in the collection of information regarding the genetics of a syndromic diagnosis is the construction of a family tree or pedigree. Underused by most medical personnel, the pedigree is a valuable record of genetic and medical information, which is much more

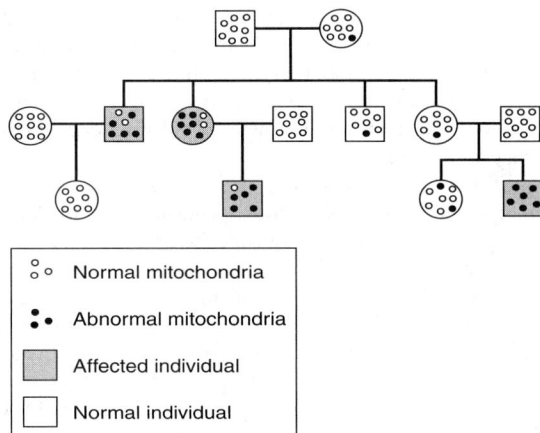

Figure 33–9. Mitochondrial inheritance. Mutations are transmitted through the maternal line.

useful in visual form than in list form. Tips for pedigree preparation include the following:

- Start with the proband—the patient's siblings and parents, and obtain a three-generational history if possible.
- Always ask about consanguinity.
- Obtain data from both sides of the family.
- Ask about spontaneous abortions, stillbirths, infertility, children relinquished for adoption, and deceased individuals.

In the course of taking the family history, one may find information that is not relevant in elucidating the cause of the patients' problem but may indicate a risk for other important health concerns. Such information should be appropriately followed and addressed. Such conditions that may arise are an overwhelming family history of early-onset breast and ovarian cancer, or multiple pregnancy losses necessitating chromosome analyses.

DYSMORPHOLOGY AND HUMAN EMBRYOLOGY

Birth defects are the leading cause of death in the first year of life. They are evident in 2–3% of newborn infants and in up to 7% of adults. Many are now detected by ultrasound prior to birth. Clinical investigation of the causes and consequences of birth defects is called dysmorphology.

MECHANISMS

Developmental Genetics

Most birth defects are multifactorial: They result from imbalances between genetic processes regulating develop-

ment and the environments in which they unfold. Specific causes of maldevelopment can be identified in about 35% of cases, but advances in developmental biology and human genetics promise better understanding. So far, single gene mutations and chromosomal abnormalities account for at least 25% of birth defects, with the numbers of specific genes and chromosome loci now being associated with recurring phenotypes, or syndromes, rapidly increasing.

Genes for the fundamental processes regulating cell division, proliferation, and those that program cell death, or apoptosis, are now being described. Both cellular proliferation and apoptosis are very active in embryogenesis and the balance between these processes is easily disrupted. Imbalances in the regulation of cell cycles are an important determinant of birth defects and may contribute to such commonly occurring problems as neural tube defects, branchial arch anomalies, limb reductions, and congenital heart disease.

Morphogenic processes and the genes that regulate them have been highly conserved through evolution. Thus, experiments in lower organisms such as *Drosophila* (fruit flies) can identify candidate genes for human birth defects. For example, mutations in *pax* genes, which are involved in eye development in *Drosophila* produce "small eye" in mice, and aniridia and other abnormalities of the anterior chamber of the eyes of humans.

Embryology and developmental biology have recently and rapidly moved from descriptive to experimental disciplines that use tools such as in situ hybridization to visualize the expression of genes in embryos, and transgenic animals in which developmentally active genes are "knocked out" to determine the contributions of specific genes to organ development. These investigations have uncovered, for example, important regulatory interactions such as the hedgehog signaling pathway, which affects morphogenesis in organs as diverse as limbs, the heart, and the CNS. Human mutations in one evolutionarily conserved gene, sonic hedgehog (*SHH*), can result in holoprosencephaly, a severe birth defect in which the CNS fails to complete its normal hemispheric division.

Cellular Interactions

The picture emerging from experimental studies of morphogenesis is one of a hierarchy of gene expression during development. Morphogenesis begins with expression of genes encoding transcription factors. These proteins bind to DNA in undifferentiated embryonic cells and recruit them into developmental fields, groups of cells primed to respond to specific signals later in development. This recruitment also establishes spatial relationships and orients cells with respect to their neighbors. As fields differentiate into identifiable tissues (eg, ectoderm, mesoderm, and endoderm), cellular proliferation, migration, and further differentiation are mediated through genes encoding cell signaling proteins.

Signaling proteins include growth factors and their receptors, cellular adhesion molecules, and extracellular matrix proteins that both provide structure and position signals within developing structures. During morphogenesis groups of primed cells repeatedly proliferate, migrate, and then differentiate in response to locally expressed growth factors or signaling proteins. Within these interactions are keys to understanding not only many human birth defects but also cancer. The genes that organize cell proliferation and differentiation during development are often precisely those that mutate during carcinogenesis.

Environmental Factors

The effects of exogenous agents during development are also mediated through genetically regulated pathways. At the cellular level, xenobiotics (compounds foreign to nature) cause birth defects either because they disrupt cell signaling and thereby misdirect morphogenesis, or because they are cytotoxic and lead to cell death in excess of the usual developmental program.

In general, drug receptors expressed in embryos and fetuses are the same molecules that mediate pharmacologic effects in adults. However, effector systems may be different, reflecting incomplete morphogenesis and differences between fetal and postnatal physiology. These circumstances allow prediction of dose-response relationships during development on the one hand, but call for caution about predicting effects on the other.

Xenobiotics must traverse the placenta to affect embryonic and fetal tissues. The human placenta is a relatively good barrier against microorganisms, but it is ineffective at excluding drugs and many chemicals. The physicochemical properties (eg, molecular size, solubility, and charge) that allow foreign chemicals to be absorbed into the maternal circulation also allow them to cross the placenta. The placenta can metabolize some xenobiotics but it is far more active against steroid hormones and low-level environmental contaminants than drugs.

The timing of xenobiotic exposures is an important determinant of their effects. Morphogenic processes express so-called critical periods, during which the organs they produce are particularly susceptible to maldevelopment. Figure 33–10 shows critical periods of development for the major organs of the fetus. Periods of susceptibility are not all confined to early gestation. Note, in particular, that the developing brain is susceptible to toxicity throughout pregnancy.

As discussed, over-the-counter, prescribed, and abused drugs that are pharmacologically active in mothers will, in general, equilibrate to the same levels across the placenta. Agents known to produce cytotoxicity at these levels in adults are therefore likely to be teratogenic (ie, cause birth defects). Abused substances such as alcohol that are toxic to adults are predictably toxic to embryos and fetuses. Drugs generally safe in adults will be generally safe for

fetuses. However, keeping in mind that embryonic and fetal physiology may differ from that of an adult in response to pharmacologic agents, some risk for abnormal development must always be considered. Risk assessment requires continuous monitoring of populations exposed to drugs during pregnancy.

Effects of toxic environmental contaminants on the embryo and fetus are also dose-dependent. Thus, the level of exposure to a toxin frequently becomes the primary determinant of its risk. Exposures producing symptoms in mothers can be assumed to be potentially toxic to the fetus.

Environmental mutagens present a special problem. Animal experiments indicate that high levels of exposure to mutagenic agents are also teratogenic. Most effects are mediated through increased apoptosis responding to DNA damage. This is especially true for the developing brain. At lower doses attempts to repair DNA damage in embryonic or fetal cells may lead to somatic mutations that can contribute to carcinogenesis or be expressed as mosaic organ dysgenesis.

Not all transplacental pharmacologic effects are toxic. The potential for therapeutic uses of drugs during pregnancy is increasing. For example, folic acid supplementation can lower risks for birth defects such as spina bifida, and maternally administered corticosteroids can induce fetal synthesis and secretion of pulmonary surfactants prior to delivery.

MECHANICAL FACTORS

Much of embryonic development and all of fetal growth occurs normally within the low pressure and space provided by amniotic fluid. Loss or inadequate production of amniotic fluid can have disastrous effects, as can disruption of placental membranes. When this occurs early in gestation, for whatever reason, major, often lethal, distortion of the embryo (early amnion disruption sequence) results. Later, deformation or even amputation of fetal extremities (amniotic band sequence) can occur.

Movement is also important for morphogenesis. Fetal movement is necessary for normal development of joints and is the principal determinant of folds and creases present at birth in the face, hands, feet, and other areas of the body. Clubfoot is an etiologically heterogeneous condition in which the foot is malpositioned at birth. It more often results from mechanical constraint secondary to intrauterine crowding, weak fetal muscles, or abnormal neurologic function than from primary skeletal maldevelopment.

Lung and kidney development are particularly sensitive to mechanical forces. Constriction of the chest through maldevelopment of the ribs, lack of surrounding amniotic fluid, or lack of movement (fetal breathing) leads to varying degrees of pulmonary hypoplasia in which lungs are smaller than normal and develop fewer alveoli. Mechanically induced pulmonary hypoplasia is a common cause of respiratory distress at birth and may be lethal.

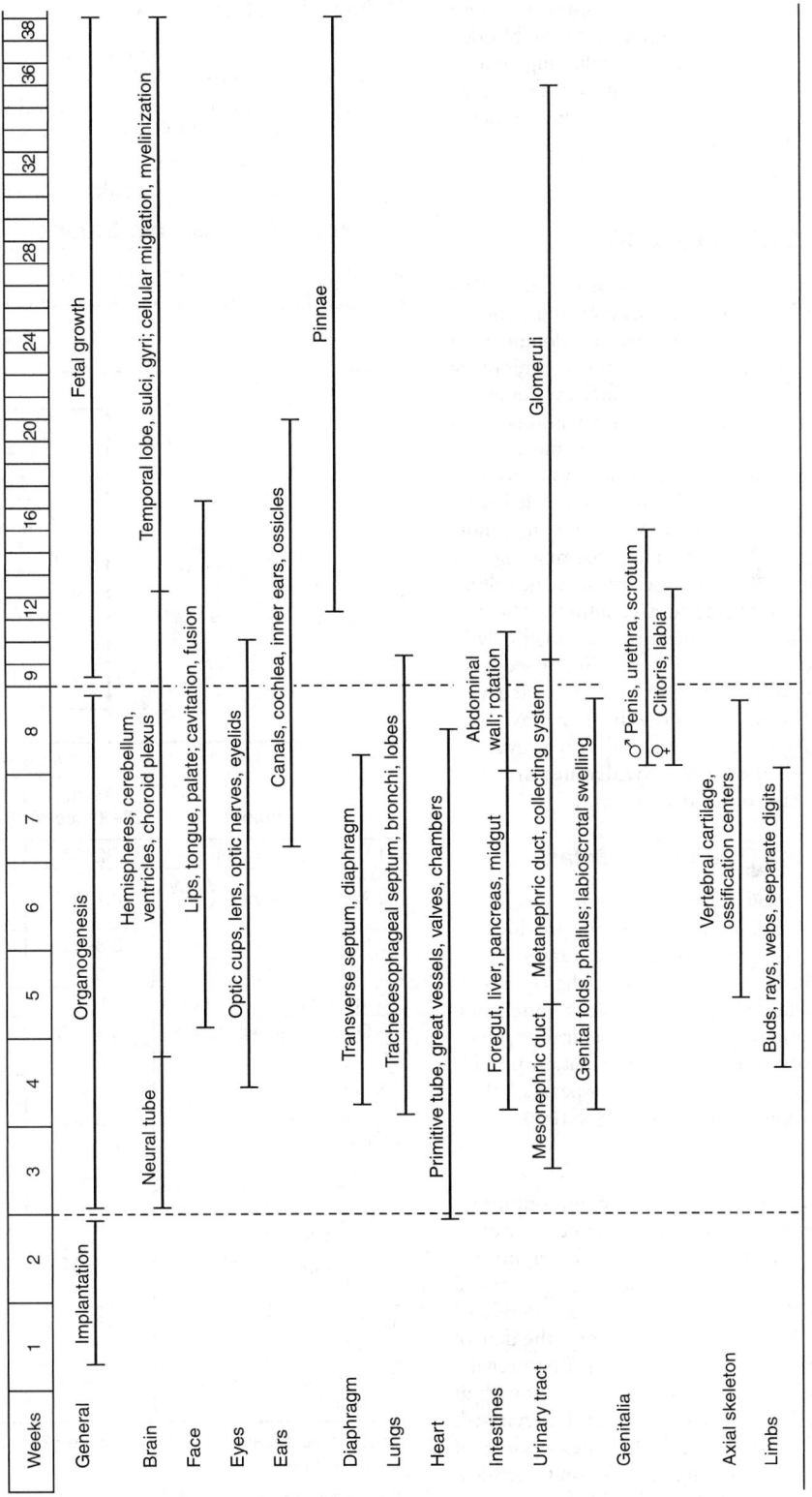

Figure 33–10. Critical periods in human gestation.

Cystic renal dysplasia commonly accompanies birth defects that obstruct ureters or outflow from the bladder. As urinary pressure within obstructed collecting systems increases it distorts cell surface interactions in developing tissues and alters histogenesis. Developing kidneys exposed to increased internal pressures for long periods eventually become nonfunctional.

CLINICAL DYSMORPHOLOGY

Classification of dysmorphic features strives to reflect mechanisms of maldevelopment. However, much of the terminology that describes abnormal development in humans remains historical and documents recognition of patterns prior to understanding of their biology. For example, birth defects are referred to as **malformations** when they result from altered genetic or developmental processes. When physical forces interrupt or distort morphogenesis, their effects are termed **disruptions** and **deformations,** respectively. The term **dysplasia** is used to denote abnormal histogenesis. Malformations occurring together more frequently than would be expected by chance alone, may be classified as belonging to **associations.** Those in which the order of maldevelopment is understood may be referred to as **sequences.** For example, Robin sequence (Pierre Robin syndrome) is used to describe cleft palate that has occurred because poor growth of the jaw (retrognathia) has displaced the tongue and prevented posterior closure of the palate. **Syndromes** are simply recurrent patterns of maldevelopment.

Evaluation of the Dysmorphic Infant

Physicians caring for infants with birth defects frequently must seek accurate diagnoses and provide care under conditions of great stress. The extent of an infant's abnormalities may not be immediately apparent, and parents who feel grief and guilt are often desperate for information. As with any medical problem, however, the history and physical examination provide most of the clues to diagnosis. Special aspects of these procedures are outlined in the following sections.

A. HISTORY

Pregnancy histories nearly always contain important clues to the diagnosis. Parental recall after delivery of an abnormal infant is better than recall after a normal birth. An obstetric wheel can help document gestational age and events of the first trimester: the last menstrual period, the onset of symptoms of pregnancy, the date of diagnosis of the pregnancy, the date of the first prenatal visit, and the physician's impressions of fetal growth at that time. Family histories should always be reviewed. Environmental histories should include descriptions of parental habits and work settings in addition to medications and use of drugs, tobacco, and alcohol.

B. PHYSICAL EXAMINATION

Meticulous physical examination is crucial for accurate diagnosis in dysmorphic infants and children. In addition to the routine procedures described in Chapter 1, special attention should be paid to the neonate's physical measurements (Figure 33–11). Photographs are helpful and should include a ruler for reference.

C. IMAGING & LABORATORY STUDIES

Radiologic and ultrasonographic examinations can be extremely helpful in the evaluation of dysmorphic infants.

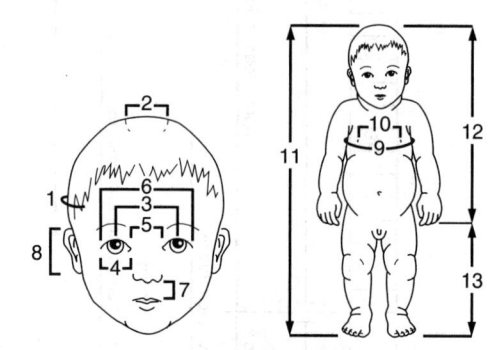

Measurement	Range (cm)	
	Term (38–40 weeks)	Preterm (32–33 weeks)
1 Head circumference	32–37	27–32
2 Anterior fontanelle $\left(\frac{L-W}{2}\right)$	0.7–3.7	. . .
3 Interpupillary distance	3.3–4.5	3.1–3.9
4 Palpebral fissure	1.5–2.1	1.3–1.6
5 Inner canthal distance	1.5–2.5	1.4–2.1
6 Outer canthal distance	5.3–7.3	3.9–5.1
7 Philtrum	0.6–1.2	0.5–0.9
8 Ear length	3–4.3	2.4–3.5
9 Chest circumference	28–38	23–29
10 Internipple distance*	6.5–10	5–6.5
11 Height	47–55	39–47
12 Ratio $\frac{\text{Upper body segment}}{\text{Lower body segment}}$ 13	1.7	. . .
14 Hand (palm to middle finger)	5.3–7.8	4.1–5.5
15 Ratio of middle finger to hand	0.38–0.48	0.38–0.5
16 Penis (pubic bone to tip of glans)	2.7–4.3	1.8–3.2

*Internipple distance should not exceed 25% of chest circumference.

Figure 33–11. Neonatal measurements.

Films of infants with apparent limb or skeletal anomalies should include views of the skull and all of the long bones in addition to frontal and lateral views of the axial skeleton. Chest and abdominal films should be obtained when indicated. The pediatrician should consult a radiologist for further work-up. Imaging by computed tomography (CT), magnetic resonance imaging (MRI), and ultrasonography are all useful diagnostic tools, but their interpretation in the face of birth defects may require considerable experience.

Cytogenetic analysis provides specific diagnoses in approximately 5% of dysmorphic infants who survive the newborn period. Chromosomal abnormalities are recognized in 10–15% of infants who die. Common disorders such as trisomy 21 and trisomy 18 can be determined rapidly through use of FISH, but this technique is limited and should always be accompanied by a complete karyotype. A normal karyotype does not rule out the presence of significant genetic disease. Any case requiring rapid diagnosis should be discussed with an experienced clinical geneticist.

D. Perinatal Autopsy

When a dysmorphic infant dies, postmortem examination can provide important diagnostic information. The pediatrician should discuss the case thoroughly with the pathologist, and photographs should always be taken. Radiologic imaging should be included whenever limb anomalies or disproportionate growth is present. Tissue, most often skin, should be submitted for cytogenetic analysis. The pediatrician and the pathologist should also consider whether samples of blood, urine, or other tissue should be obtained for biochemical analyses. Placental as well as fetal tissue can be used for viral culture.

PART II
Clinical Features of Common Genetic Disorders

■ CHROMOSOMAL DISORDERS: ABNORMAL NUMBER

ANEUPLOIDY

Trisomy 21 (Down Syndrome)

Down syndrome occurs in about 1:600 newborns; however, the incidence is greater if the mother is older than age 35 years. Mental retardation is characteristic of Down syndrome, with typical intelligence quotients (IQs) between 20 and 80 (mostly between 45 and 55). The principal physical findings include a small, brachycephalic head, characteristic facies (up-slanting palpebral fissures, epicanthal folds, midface hypoplasia, and small, dysplastic pinnae), and minor limb abnormalities. About one-third to one-half of children with Down syndrome have congenital heart disease, most often an endocardial cushion defect or other septal defect. Anomalies of the gastrointestinal tract are seen in about 15% of cases, including esophageal and duodenal atresias. Generalized hypotonia is common. Sexual development is delayed, especially in males, who are usually sterile. The affected newborn may have prolonged physiologic jaundice, polycythemia, and a transient leukemoid reaction. Later, there is an increased tendency for thyroid dysfunction, hearing loss, celiac disease, and atlanto-occipital instability. Leukemia is 12–20 times more common in Down syndrome patients than in unaffected children.

Information regarding health care guidelines for patients with Down syndrome can be found at the following website:

www.downsyn.com/guidelines/healthcare.html

Trisomy 18 Syndrome

The incidence of trisomy 18 syndrome is about 1:4000 live births, and the ratio of affected males to females is approximately 1:3. Trisomy 18 is characterized by prenatal and postnatal growth retardation that is often severe, hypertonicity, and dysmorphic features including a characteristic face and extremities (overlapping fingers and rockerbottom feet), and congenital heart disease (often ventricular septal defect or patent ductus arteriosus). To see clinical pictures of patients with trisomy 18, go to

medgen.genetics.utah.edu/photographs/pages/trisomy_18.htm

Complications are related to associated birth defects. Death is often caused by heart failure or pneumonia and usually occurs in infancy or early childhood, although a small percentage of patients reach adulthood. Surviving children show significant developmental delay and mental retardation.

Trisomy 13 Syndrome

The incidence of trisomy 13 is about 1:12,000 live births, and 60% of affected individuals are female. The symptoms and signs include prenatal and postnatal growth deficiency (although, unlike trisomy 18, infants may have a normal birth weight), CNS malformations, arrhinencephaly, eye malformations (anophthalmia, colobomas), cleft lip and palate, polydactyly or syndactyly, and congenital heart disease (usually ventricular septal defect). The facies of an infant with trisomy 13 can be viewed on the following website:

medgen.genetics.utah.edu/photographs/pages/trisomy_13.htm

Surviving children demonstrate failure to thrive, developmental retardation, apneic spells, seizures, and deafness. Death usually occurs in early infancy or by the second year of life, commonly as a result of heart failure or infection.

Treatment for Aneuploidies

No convincing documentation is available relative to the merit of any of the forms of alternative therapy that have been attempted in Down syndrome, ranging from megadoses of vitamins to amino acid solutions. However, interventions for specific issues such as surgery or medications for heart problems, antibiotics for infections and thyroid function tests, infant stimulation programs, special education, and physical, occupational, and speech therapies are all indicated. The goal of treatment is to help affected children develop to their full potential. Parents' participation in support groups such as the local chapter of the National Down Syndrome Congress should be encouraged. See the following website:

http://www.ndss.org/

There is no treatment, other than general supportive care, for trisomy 13 or 18. Because it is sometimes necessary to decide immediately after birth how extensive therapy should be for a severely malformed infant, trisomy 13 and 18 can be screened for in interphase nuclei of blood lymphocytes by FISH and confirmed by direct chromosome analysis of blood or bone marrow mitoses. A support group for families of children with trisomies 13 and 18 who survive beyond infancy is called SOFT. See the following website:

www.trisomy.org/

Genetic Counseling

Most parents of trisomic babies have normal karyotypes. The risk of having a child affected with a trisomy varies with maternal age. For trisomy 21, age-specific risks are 1:2000 for mothers younger than age 25 years; 1:200 for mothers age 35 years; and 1:100 for mothers age 40. The recurrence risk for trisomy in future pregnancies is equal to 1:100 plus the age-specific maternal risk (for example, a 40-year-old mother with a prior child with Down syndrome would have a risk of 1:100 for her age, plus 1:100 for her prior history, or 1:50).

If the child has a trisomy resulting from a translocation, and the parent has an abnormal karyotype, the risks are increased. When the mother is the carrier of a balanced 14/21 translocation, there is a 10–15% chance that the child will be affected and a 33% chance that the child will be a balanced translocation carrier. When the father is the carrier, there is a smaller than 0.5% chance of having another affected child. If the child has a 21/21 translocation and one parent has the translocation, the recurrence risk is 100%.

The recurrence risks in other trisomies are analogous to those for Down syndrome. The mother's age at the time of conception and the nature of the chromosomal abnormality are important in genetic counseling, which is indicated for prevention of all chromosomal abnormalities. Prenatal diagnosis is available.

■ SEX CHROMOSOMES

Turner Syndrome (Monosomy X, Gonadal Dysgenesis)

The incidence of Turner syndrome is 1:10,000 females. However, it is estimated that 95% of conceptuses with monosomy X are miscarried and only 5% are liveborn. Newborns with Turner syndrome may have webbed neck, edema of the hands and feet, coarctation of the aorta, and a characteristic triangular facies. Later symptoms include short stature, a shield chest with wide-set nipples, streak ovaries, amenorrhea, absence of secondary sex characteristics, and infertility. Some affected girls, particularly those with mosaicism, have only short stature and amenorrhea, without dysmorphic features. Complications relate primarily to coarctation of the aorta, when present. Rarely, the dysgenetic gonads may become neoplastic (gonadoblastoma). The incidence of malformations of the urinary tract is increased. Learning disabilities are common, secondary to difficulties in perceptual motor integration. Patients with pseudohypoparathyroidism and Noonan syndrome have a similar phenotype to patients with Turner syndrome, but have normal chromosomes.

In Turner syndrome the identification and treatment of perceptual difficulties before they become problematic is very important. Teenage patients need counseling to cope with the stigma of their condition and to understand the need for hormone therapy. Estrogen replacement therapy will permit development of secondary sex characteristics and normal menstruation and prevent osteoporosis. Growth hormone therapy has been used to increase the height of affected girls. Females with 45,X or 45,X mosaicism have a low fertility rate, and those who become pregnant have a high risk of fetal wastage (spontaneous miscarriage, approximately 30%; stillbirth, 6–10%). Furthermore, their liveborn offspring have an increased frequency of chromosomal abnormalities involving either sex chromosomes or autosomes, and congenital malformations. Thus, prenatal ultrasonography and chromosome analysis are indicated for the offspring of females with sex chromosome abnormalities.

Klinefelter Syndrome (XXY)

The incidence of Klinefelter syndrome in the newborn population is roughly 1:1000, but it is about 1% among mentally retarded males and about 3% among males seen at infertility clinics. The maternal age at birth is often advanced. Unlike Turner syndrome, Klinefelter syndrome is rarely the cause of spontaneous abortions. The diagnosis is rarely made before puberty except as a result of prenatal diagnosis, because prepubertal boys have a normal phenotype. The characteristic findings after puberty include microorchidism associated with otherwise normal external genitalia, azoospermia, sterility, gynecomastia, normal to borderline IQ, diminished facial hair, lack of libido and potency, and a tall, eunuchoid build. In chromosome variants with three or four X chromosomes (XXXY and XXXXY), mental retardation may be severe, and radioulnar synostosis may be present as well as anomalies of the external genitalia and cryptorchidism. In the XXXXY cases, these findings are especially prominent, and microcephaly, short stature, and dysmorphic features also occur. In general, the physical and mental abnormalities associated with Klinefelter syndrome increase as the number of sex chromosomes increases. Males with Klinefelter syndrome require testosterone replacement therapy. The presence of the extra X chromosome may allow expression of what might normally be a lethal X-linked disorder to occur.

XYY Syndrome

Newborns in general are normal. Affected individuals may on occasion exhibit an abnormal behavior pattern from early childhood and may have mild retardation. Fertility may be normal. Many males with an XYY karyotype are normal. There is no treatment. Long-term problems may relate to low IQ and environmental stress.

XXX Syndrome

The incidence of females with an XXX karyotype is approximately 1:1000. Females with XXX are phenotypically normal. However, they tend to be taller than usual and to have lower IQs than their normal siblings. Learning and behavioral issues are relatively common. This is in contrast to individuals with XXXX, a much rarer condition causing more severe developmental issues, and a dysmorphic phenotype reminiscent of Down syndrome.

Jones KL: *Smith's Recognizable Patterns of Human Malformation,* 6th ed. Elsevier, 2006.

MOSAICISM

Although most cases of severe chromosomal abnormality such as trisomy are lethal, some individuals may survive if the abnormality exists in mosaic form. Two examples of this include trisomy 8 and cat eye syndrome, caused by extra genetic material, which is derived from a portion of chromosome 22.

CHROMOSOMAL ABNORMALITIES: STRUCTURAL

Chromosomal abnormalities most often present in newborns as multiple congenital anomalies in association with intrauterine growth retardation. In addition to trisomies as just described, other more subtle chromosomal abnormalities are also common. In some cases, the karyotype is normal, but a subtle chromosomal rearrangement can be detected by FISH. Another new technology called comparative genomic hybridization-array, enables screening for multiple submicroscopic chromosomal abnormalities (ie, microdeletions) simultaneously, and may be a very helpful tool in the child with a suspected chromosomal abnormality.

Vissers LE et al: Array-based comparative genomic hybridization for genome-wide detection of submicroscopic chromosomal abnormalities. Am J Hum Genet 2003:73(6);1261 [PMID: 14628292].

Three common chromosomal deletion disorders that are often detected on routine karyotype analysis, and easily confirmed via FISH assay are 1p36–, Wolf-Hirschhorn syndrome (4p–), and Cri du Chat syndrome (5p–).

1p36–Syndrome

This syndrome is characterized by microcephaly and a large anterior fontanelle. Cardiac defects are common, and dilated cardiomyopathy may present in infancy. Mental retardation, hypotonia, hearing loss, and seizures are usually seen.

Wolf-Hirschhorn Syndrome

Also known as 4p– (deletion of 4p16), this syndrome is characterized by microcephaly and unusual development of the nose and orbits that produces an appearance suggesting an ancient Greek warrior's helmet. Other anomalies commonly seen include cleft lip and palate, and cardiac and renal defects. Seizure disorders are common, and the majority of patients have severe mental retardation.

Cri du Chat Syndrome

Also known as 5p– (deletion of terminal chromosome 5p), this disorder is characterized by unique facial features, growth retardation, and microcephaly. Patients have an unusual catlike cry. Most patients have major organ anomalies and significant developmental delay.

Four common contiguous gene disorders (microdeletion disorders), which are usually suspected on the basis of an abnormal phenotype and then confirmed via FISH assay, are Williams syndrome, Miller–Dieker syndrome, Smith–Magenis syndrome, and velocardiofacial syndrome.

Williams Syndrome

Williams syndrome is a contiguous gene disorder involving the elastin gene and other neighboring genes at 7q11.2. It is characterized by short stature, congenital heart disease (supravalvular aortic stenosis), coarse, elfin-like facies with prominent lips, hypercalcemia or hypercalciuria in infancy, developmental delay, and neonatal irritability evolving into an overly friendly personality. Calcium restriction may be necessary in early childhood to prevent nephrocalcinosis. The hypercalcemia often resolves during the first year of life. The natural history includes progression of cardiac disease and predisposition to hypertension and spinal osteoarthritis in adults. Most patients have mild to moderate intellectual deficits.

Miller–Dieker Syndrome

A contiguous gene syndrome involving 17p13, this abnormality is characterized by microcephaly and severe CNS dysgenesis. The most commonly seen CNS malformation is termed **lissencephaly** ("smooth brain" as the brain is lacking its normal convolutions and gyri). An unusually developed face and forehead reflect abnormal migration of neuronal germinal matrix cells. Mutations in the gene *MDS1,* which is located in the critical region, can cause isolated lissencephaly, without the full picture of Miller–Dieker. Severe cognitive and developmental delay and seizure disorders are common.

Smith–Magenis Syndrome

This syndrome is associated with microdeletion of 17p11 and is characterized by prominent forehead, deep-set eyes, cupid-shaped upper lip, self-mutilating behavior (pulling nails and hair, putting objects into body orifices), sleep disturbance, and developmental delay. Some patients also have seizure disorders. Some individuals with larger deletions involving *PMP22* can present with peripheral neuropathy.

Velocardiofacial Syndrome (Del 22q11 Syndrome)

Also known as DiGeorge syndrome, this abnormality was originally described in newborns presenting with cyanotic congenital heart disease, usually involving great vessel abnormalities; thymic hypoplasia leading to immunodeficiency; and hypocalcemia due to absent parathyroid glands. This chromosomal abnormality is associated with a highly variable phenotype. Characteristics include mild microcephaly; palatal clefting or incompetence; speech and language delays; and congenital heart disease (ventricular or atrial septal defect). Midline defects such as umbilical hernia and hypospadias can be associated anomalies. In some cases, individuals have an apparent predisposition to psychosis.

MENDELIAN DISORDERS

AUTOSOMAL DOMINANT INHERITANCE

1. Neurofibromatosis Type 1

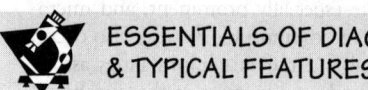

ESSENTIALS OF DIAGNOSIS & TYPICAL FEATURES

Minimal diagnostic criteria require two or more of the following:

- *Six or more café au lait macules, at least 15 mm in diameter in postpubertal and 5 mm in prepubertal individuals.*
- *Two or more neurofibromas of any type or one plexiform neurofibroma.*
- *Axillary or inguinal freckling.*
- *Two or more Lisch nodules (iris hamartomas).*
- *Optic glioma.*
- *Distinctive bony lesions such as sphenoid dysplasia or pseudarthrosis.*
- *An affected first-degree relative.*

General Considerations

Neurofibromatosis 1 (NF-1) is one of the most common autosomal dominant disorders, occurring in 1:3000 births and seen in all races and ethnic groups. In general, the disorder is progressive, with new manifestations appearing over time. Neurofibromatosis 2 (NF-2), characterized by bilateral acoustic neuromas, with minimal or no skin manifestations, is a different disease caused by a different gene.

Clinical Findings

Café au lait macules may be present at birth, and about 80% of individuals with NF-1 will have more than six by age 1 year. The typical skin lesion is 10–30 mm, ovoid, and smooth-bordered. Neurofibromas are benign tumors consisting of Schwann cells, nerve fibers, and fibroblasts; they may be discrete or plexiform. Discrete tumors are more common, are well demarcated, and can occur at any age. Plexiform neurofibromas are more diffuse and can invade normal tissue. They are congenital and are frequently detected during periods of rapid growth. If the face or a limb is involved, there may be associated hypertrophy or overgrowth. The incidence of Lisch nodules, which can be seen with a slitlamp, also increases with age.

Common features of affected individuals include a large head, bony abnormalities on radiographic studies, scoliosis, and a wide spectrum of developmental problems. The most common problems in childhood are secondary to plexiform neurofibromas and learning disabilities. Although the average IQ is within the normal range, it is lower than in unaffected family members.

Complications

Seizures, deafness, short stature, early puberty, and hypertension occur in less than 25% of persons with NF. Optic glioma occurs in about 15% of individuals with NF-1. Although the tumor may be apparent at an early age, it rarely causes functional problems and is usually nonprogressive. Patients have a slightly increased risk (5% life risk) for a variety of malignancies. Other tumors may be benign but may cause significant morbidity and mortality because of their size and location in a vital or enclosed space.

Treatment

The therapy is symptomatic. Neurofibromas can be removed if they cause discomfort or are a cosmetic problem. The most important part of therapy is close, ongoing follow-up. Because this disorder is progressive, affected individuals should be seen at regular intervals and have regular monitoring of growth parameters, orthopedic and neurologic issues, and eye examinations. Developmental screening as well as other evaluations (eg, MRI scans) are done as indicated according to symptoms. Follow-up is best done in a multidisciplinary neurocutaneous clinic. See the following website for more information:

www.nfinc.org

Prognosis

Most affected children have only skin lesions and few other problems. Severely affected individuals are rare in the pediatric age range, and close follow-up and early intervention may ameliorate some complications.

Genetic Counseling

The gene for NF-1 is on the long arm of chromosome 17 and seems to code for a protein similar to a tumor sup-

presser factor. NF results from many different mutations of this gene. Approximately 50% of all cases of NF are caused by new mutations. Careful evaluation of the parents is necessary to provide accurate genetic counseling. Recent evidence suggests that penetrance is close to 100% in those who carry the gene if individuals are examined carefully.

Differential Diagnosis

Areas of hyperpigmentation can occur in other conditions (eg, Albright, Noonan, and Leopard syndromes), but the lesions are either single or different in character. Isolated neurofibromas and familial café au lait spots as an autosomal dominant trait (fewer than six and with no other manifestations of NF) have been described. The relationship of such cases to classic NF-1 is uncertain.

2. Marfan Syndrome

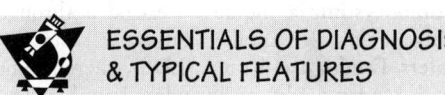

ESSENTIALS OF DIAGNOSIS & TYPICAL FEATURES

- Skeletal abnormalities, including disproportionate growth (arachnodactyly and tall stature), and joint hyperextensibility.
- Lens dislocation.
- Dilation of the aortic root.

Clinical Findings

The characteristic facies is long and thin, with downslanting palpebral fissures. The palate is high arched, and dentition is often crowded. Skeletal abnormalities are classic (arachnodactyly, tall, thin habitus, and scoliosis), and the ophthalmologic and cardiac issues are considered major criteria for making this diagnosis.

Complications

The skeletal problems including scoliosis are progressive. Myopia is very common and lens dislocation may also be progressive.

The most serious associated medical problems involve the heart. Although many patients with Marfan syndrome have mitral valve prolapse, the most serious concern is progressive aortic root dilatation, which may lead to aneurysmal rupture and death.

Treatment

Medical treatment for patients with Marfan syndrome includes appropriate management of the ophthalmologic, orthopedic, and cardiac issues. Serial echocardiograms are indicated to diagnose and follow the degree of aortic root enlargement, which can be managed medically or surgically, in more severe cases. See the following website for more information:

www.marfan.org

Genetic Counseling

The diagnosis of Marfan syndrome is still made on a clinical basis, and many cases represent sporadic new mutations. Marfan syndrome is caused by mutations in genes coding for the connective tissue protein fibrillin. However, many unique, family-specific mutations occur, making molecular confirmation difficult.

Differential Diagnosis

In individuals with marfanoid habitus and cognitive disabilities, **homocystinuria** should be excluded through careful metabolic testing. Another connective tissue disorder, **Ehlers–Danlos syndrome (EDS),** shares some features with Marfan syndrome, including joint hyperextensibility and skin fragility. The skin is the target organ for the most significant symptoms in EDS patients. At least nine forms of EDS occur, most inherited as dominant traits, but the biochemical causes have only been worked out for a few of the forms.

3. Achondroplasia

Achondroplasia, the most common form of skeletal dysplasia, is caused by a mutation in *FGFR3*.

Clinical Findings

The classic phenotype includes relative macrocephaly, midface hypoplasia, short-limbed dwarfism, and trident-shaped hands. The phenotype is apparent at birth. Individuals with achondroplasia are cognitively normal.

Treatment

Orthopedic intervention is necessary for spinal problems including severe lumbar lordosis and gibbus deformity. Long bone lengthening surgery, such as the Ilizarov procedure, are used in some centers to increase height and upper extremity function, but their use is still controversial.

Head circumference during infancy must be closely monitored and plotted on a diagnosis-specific head circumference chart.

Many patients find support through organizations such as the Little People of America, at the following website:

www.lpaonline.org

Complications

Bony overgrowth at the level of the foramen magnum may lead to progressive hydrocephalus and may warrant neurosurgical intervention.

Genetic Counseling

The vast majority of cases (approximately 90%) represent a new mutation. Two hemizygous parents with achondroplasia have a 25% risk of having a child homozygous for *FGFR 3* mutations, which is a lethal disorder.

4. Osteogenesis Imperfecta

Osteogenesis imperfecta (OI), or brittle bone disease, is a relatively common disorder, caused by mutations in type I collagen. Most patients with more severe disease represent new mutations for this disorder.

Clinical Findings

There are four types of OI.

- Type I is a mild form, with increased incidence of fracturing and blue sclerae.
- Type II is generally lethal in the newborn period with multiple congenital fractures and severe lung disease.
- Type III is the severe form causing significant bony deformity secondary to multiple fractures (many of which are congenital), blue sclerae, short stature, and mild restrictive lung disease.
- Type IV is a mild form with increased incidence of fracturing (*not* usually congenital); dentinogenesis imperfecta is common.

Treatment

A major advancement in the treatment of OI patients has been the use of Pamidronate, a bisphosphonate compound, which has been reported to lead to a reduced incidence of fracture and improvement in bone density. Patients should be followed by an experienced orthopedist, as rodding of long bones and surgery to correct scoliosis are often required. Hearing assessments are indicated, because of the association between OI and deafness. Close dental follow-up is also necessary.

Genetic Counseling

All four types of OI are associated with mutations in the gene coding for type I collagen. Collagen analysis is usually performed in skin fibroblasts to confirm the diagnosis. The milder forms may be seen as the result of dominant inheritance, while the more severe forms of OI generally result from new mutations.

5. Craniosynostoses Syndromes

The craniosynostoses disorders are common dominant disorders associated with premature fusion of cranial sutures. This class of disorders is now known to be caused by mutations in *FGFR* genes.

Clinical Findings

Crouzon syndrome is the most common of these disorders and is associated with multiple suture fusions, but with normal limbs. Other craniosynostosis disorders have limb as well as craniofacial anomalies, and include Pfeiffer, Apert, Jackson–Weiss, and Saethre–Chotzen syndromes.

Facial features associated with craniosynostosis include shallow orbits leading to proptosis, midface narrowing that may result in upper airway obstruction, and hydrocephalus that may require shunting. Children with craniosynostosis undergo multiple staged craniofacial/neurosurgical procedures to address these issues.

There are many other common autosomal dominant disorders, including Treacher-Collins syndrome, associated with a distinct craniofacial phenotype including malar and mandibular hypoplasia, and Noonan syndrome, which has a phenotype similar to Turner syndrome with short stature and a webbed neck. Two other common genetic disorders whose causative genes were recently identified and found to be dominant mutations are CHARGE syndrome and Cornelia de Lange syndrome.

6. CHARGE Syndrome

CHARGE syndrome affects structures derived from rostral neural crest cells but also includes abnormal development of the eyes and midbrain. The acronym CHARGE serves as a mnemonic for associated abnormalities that include **c**olobomas, congenital **h**eart disease, choanal **a**tresia, growth **r**etardation, **g**enital abnormalities (hypogenitalism), and **e**ar abnormalities, with deafness. Facial asymmetry is a common finding. CHARGE is now known to be caused by mutations in the CHD7 gene on chromosome 8q. A CHARGE syndrome website is available at:

http://www.chargesyndrome.org/

Vissers LE et al: Mutations in a new member of the chromodomain gene family cause CHARGE syndrome. Nat Genet 2004:36 (9):955 [PMID: 15300250].

7. Cornelia de Lange Syndrome

Cornelia de Lange syndrome is characterized by severe growth retardation; limb, especially hand, reduction

defects (50%); congenital heart disease (25%); and stereotypical facies with hirsutism, medial fusion of eyebrows (synophrys), and thin, downturned lips.

The course and severity are variable, but the prognosis for survival and normal development is poor. Chromosomal analysis is usually normal, although the phenotype of 3q duplication has many similarities.

Jones KL: *Recognizable Patterns of Human Malformation,* 6th ed. Elsevier, 2006.

8. Noonan Syndrome

Noonan syndrome is an autosomal dominant disorder characterized by short stature, congenital heart disease, abnormalities of cardiac conduction and rhythm, webbed neck, down-slanting palpebral fissures, and low-set ears. Affected children may be large at birth and have mild subcutaneous edema. The phenotype evolves with age and may be difficult to recognize in older relatives. Mild developmental delays are often present. Mutations in the gene PTPN11, mapping to chromosome 12q, cause some cases of Noonan syndrome.

AUTOSOMAL RECESSIVE DISORDERS

1. Cystic Fibrosis

The gene for cystic fibrosis (CF), *CFTR,* is found on the long arm of chromosome 7. Approximately 1 in 22 persons are carriers. Over 600 different mutations have been identified: the most common in the Caucasian population, known as Δ *F 508,* is a three-base deletion coding for phenylalanine.

Genetic Counseling

Cloning of the gene for CF and identification of the mutation in the majority of cases have completely changed genetic counseling and prenatal diagnosis for this disorder, although the sweat chloride assay is still important in confirming the diagnosis. The American College of Medical Genetics recommends the 25-mutation assay using PCR-based techniques, which can cover 85–90% of the mutations.

The identification of the mutation in the CF gene has also raised the issue of mass newborn screening, because of the high frequency of this gene in the Caucasian population. Some states, such as Colorado, have offered newborn screening by trypsinogen assay, which can detect 70% of CF patients. Although early detection can ensure good nutritional status starting at birth, newborn screening is controversial as there is no cure for CF. (For more details of medical management,

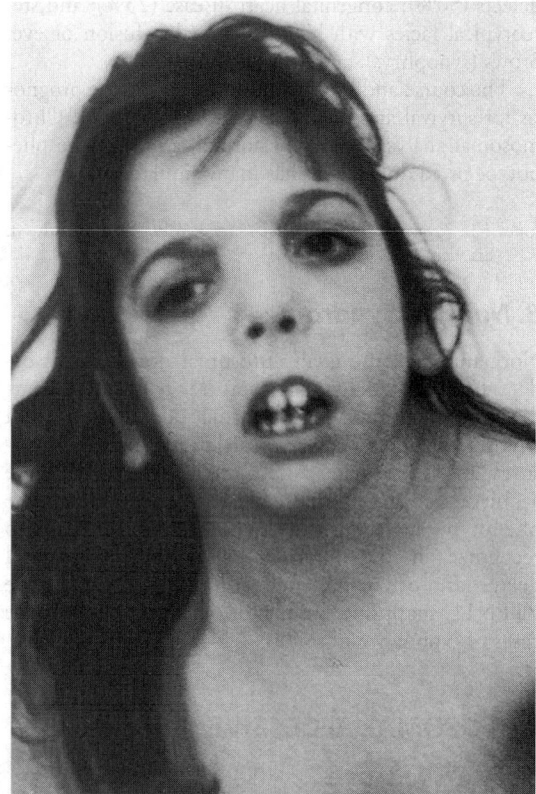

Figure 33–12. Child with Smith–Lemli–Opitz syndrome, featuring bitemporal narrowing, upturned nares, ptosis, and small chin.

please see Chapters 18 [Respiratory Tract & Mediastinum] and 20 [Gastrointestinal Tract] in this text.)

2. Smith–Lemli–Opitz Syndrome

Smith–Lemli–Opitz syndrome is caused by a metabolic error in the final step of cholesterol production, resulting in low cholesterol levels and accumulation of the precursor 7-dehydrocholesterol (7-DHC). The diagnosis can be confirmed via a simple blood test looking for the presence of the precursor, 7-DHC, which is not detectible in an unaffected individual. This blood test can only be done in special laboratories.

Clinical Findings

Patients with Smith–Lemli–Opitz syndrome present with a characteristic phenotype, including dysmorphic facial features (Figure 33–12), multiple congenital anomalies (including defects of the CNS, heart, cleft palate, cardiac system, kidneys, genitalia, and limbs), hypotonia, growth failure, and mental retardation.

Treatment

Treatment with cholesterol can ameliorate the growth failure and lead to improvement in behavior and developmental course, although treatment does not cure this complex disorder.

3. Sensorineural Hearing Loss

Although there is marked genetic heterogeneity in causes of sensorineural hearing loss, including dominant, recessive, and X-linked patterns, nonsyndromic, recessively inherited deafness is the predominant form of severe inherited childhood deafness. Of mutations known to cause sensorineural hearing loss, mutations of connexin 26 (*CX26*), a gap junction protein, are present in 49% of cases of prelingual deafness. Molecular testing is available.

Nance WE: The genetics of deafness. Ment Retard Dev Disabil Res Rev 2003:9;109 [PMID: 12784229].

4. Spinal Muscular Atrophy

Spinal muscular atrophy (SMA) is an autosomal recessive neuromuscular disorder in which anterior horn cells in the spinal cord degenerate. The mechanism for the loss of cells appears to involve apoptosis of neurons in the absence of the product of the *SMN1* (survival motor neuron) gene located on chromosome 5q. Loss of anterior horn cells leads to progressive atrophy of skeletal muscle. The disorder has an incidence of approximately 1 in 12,000, with the majority of the cases presenting in infancy. Carrier frequencies approach 1 in 50 in populations with European ancestry. Three clinical subtypes are recognized based on age of onset and rate of progression. SMA I is the most devastating. Mild weakness may be present at birth, but is clearly evident by 3 months and is accompanied by loss of reflexes and fasciculations in affected muscles. Progression of the disorder leads to eventual respiratory failure, usually by age 1 year. Symptoms of SMA II begin later, with weakness and decreased reflexes generally apparent by age 2 years. Children affected with SMA III begin to become weak as they approach adolescence.

Homozygous deletion of exon 7 of *SMN1* is detectable in approximately 95–98% of cases of all types of SMA and confirms the diagnosis. The *SMN1* region on chromosome 5q is complex and variability in presentation appears to involve expression of neighboring genes including a more centromeric *SMN2* pseudogene. Approximately 2–5% of patients affected with SMA will be compound heterozygotes in whom there is one copy of *SMN1* with exon 7 deleted and a second copy with a point mutation.

Prenatal diagnosis is available through genetic testing, but careful molecular analysis of the proband and demonstration of carrier status in parents is advised since, in addition to the problem of potential compound heterozygosity, 2% of cases occur as a result of a de novo mutation in one *SMN1* allele. In this case one of the parents is not a carrier and recurrence risks are low. Carrier testing is further complicated by a duplication of *SMN1* in 4% of the population that results in there being two *SMN1* genes on one of their chromosomes. Hence reproductive risk assessment, carrier testing and prenatal diagnosis of SMA are best undertaken in the context of careful genetic counseling.

5. Metabolic Disorders

Most inborn errors of metabolism are inherited in an autosomal recessive pattern. (See Chapter 32 in this text for detailed explanations of these disorders.)

X-LINKED INHERITANCE

1. Duchenne-Type Muscular Dystrophy

Duchenne muscular dystrophy (DMD) results from failure of synthesis of the muscle cytoskeletal protein dystrophin, whose gene is located on the X chromosome, Xp12. Approximately 1 in 4000 male children are affected. Mutations in the same gene that result in partial expression of the dystrophin protein produce a less severe phenotype, Becker muscular dystrophy (BMD). In both DMD and BMD, progressive degeneration of skeletal and cardiac muscle occurs. Boys with DMD exhibit proximal muscle weakness and pseudohypertrophy of calf muscles by age 5–6 years. Patients become nonambulatory by age 13. Serum creatine kinase levels are markedly elevated. Boys with DMD frequently die in their 20s of respiratory failure and cardiac dysfunction. The prognosis for BMD is more variable. Although corticosteroids are useful in maintaining strength, they do not slow progression of the disorder.

The gene for dystrophin is very large and a common target for mutation. Large deletions or duplications can be detected in the gene for dystrophin in 65% of cases. Methods for detecting small and even point mutations have now been developed. Mutation testing and careful clinical assessment are replacing muscle biopsies in making the diagnosis of DMD.

One-third of DMD cases presenting with a negative family history are likely to be new mutations. Genetic counseling is complicated by the fact that germline mosaicism for mutations in the dystrophin gene occur in approximately 15–20% of families. Therefore, if a mutation has been detected in a proband, prenatal diagnosis is routinely offered to his mother regardless of her apparent carrier status. It is also necessary to look for mutations in all sisters of affected boys. Since mutations are now detected in the great majority of DMD cases, there is considerably less need for estimating carrier risks based on creatine kinase levels or using genetic linkage for prenatal diagnosis. Nonetheless, counseling and prenatal diagnosis remain difficult in some families.

2. Hemophilia

Hemophilia A is an X-linked, recessive, bleeding disorder caused by a deficiency in the activity of coagulation factor VIII. Affected individuals develop a variable phenotype of hemorrhage into joints and muscles, easy bruising, and prolonged bleeding from wounds. The disorder is caused by heterogeneous mutations in the factor VIII gene, which maps to Xq28. Carrier detection and prenatal diagnosis can be done by direct detection of selected mutations, especially the inversions, the most common gene change, as well as indirectly by linkage analysis. Replacement of factor VIII is done using a variety of preparations derived from human plasma or recombinant techniques. Although replacement therapy is effective in most cases, 10–15% of treated individuals develop neutralizing antibodies that decrease its effectiveness.

3. Metabolic Disorders

Some important inborn errors are inherited as X-linked disorders, such as adrenoleukodystrophy. (See Chapter 32 in this text for more detailed descriptions.)

NONMENDELIAN INHERITANCE

DISORDERS OF IMPRINTING

1. Beckwith–Wiedemann Syndrome

The association of macrosomia (enlarged body size), macroglossia (enlarged tongue), and omphalocele constitutes the Beckwith–Wiedemann syndrome (BWS), now known to be related to abnormal expression of genes located at chromosome 11p15. Other associated findings include mild facial dysmorphism (hypertelorism, unusual ear creases), infantile hypoglycemia due to transient hyperinsulinemia, multiple congenital anomalies (cleft palate and genitourinary anomalies common), and increased risk for certain malignancies, especially Wilms tumor (7–10%).

A growth factor gene, *IGF2* is imprinted such that the maternal allele is ordinarily not expressed during intrauterine development. Chromosomal abnormalities affecting expression of this gene, such as duplication of the paternal 11p15 region, or paternal UPD, are associated with BWS. Paternal UPD may also lead to loss of expression of a tumor suppressor gene (*H19*), normally read from the maternal homolog, contributing to the increased predisposition to cancer seen in this disorder. Supporting the role of imprinting in BWS is that paternal imprinting has been documented in about 10% of BWS patients, and that about

70% of Wilms tumors from patients with BWS show loss of imprinting of the genes coding for IGF-2 and H19. Children affected with this condition should undergo tumor surveillance protocols, including an abdominal ultrasound every 3 months until they reach age 7 years, as diagnosing malignancy at early stages leads to a significant improvement in outcome.

2. Prader–Willi Syndrome

Prader–Willi syndrome results from lack of expression of a number of imprinted genes, including *SNRPn*, located on chromosome 15q11. Clinical characteristics include severe hypotonia in infancy that often necessitates placement of a feeding gastrostomy tube. In older children, characteristic facies evolve over time, including almond-shaped eyes, and frequent strabismus. Short stature, obesity, hypogenitalism, and small hands and feet with tapering fingers are now believed to be associated with growth hormone deficiency. Obsessive hyperphagia (usual onset 3–4 years) and type 2 (adult-onset) diabetes mellitus are common features.

Multiple chromosomal rearrangements and mutations have been reported to disrupt expression of the genes that contribute to this syndrome. Of these, deletion of the paternally inherited allele of chromosome 15q11 (detected by FISH) is the most common chromosomal abnormality causing Prader–Willi syndrome, followed by maternal UPD diagnosed by DNA methylation studies.

3. Angelman Syndrome

Angelman syndrome also involves imprinting and results from a variety of mutations that inactivate a ubiquitin-protein ligase gene, *UBE3A*, located in the same region of chromosome 15 as *SNRPn*, the maternally imprinted gene involved in Prader–Willi syndrome (see preceding section). *UBE3A* is paternally imprinted, and during normal development the maternal allele is expressed only in the brain. The classic phenotype includes severe mental retardation with prognathism, seizures, and marked delay in motor milestones, abnormal puppet-like gait and posturing, poor language development, and paroxysmal laughter and tongue thrusting.

Angelman syndrome is most commonly caused when sequences detectable by FISH on 15q11 are deleted from the maternal homolog. Uniparental paternal disomy 15 is the least common cause. Mutations in *UBE3A* cause the disorder in about one-fourth of cases. Imprinting errors, which may be associated with advanced reproductive techniques, may also result in Angelman syndrome.

Niemitz EL, Feinberg AP: Epigenetics and assisted reproductive technology: A call for investigation. Am J Hum Genet 2004: 74:599 [PMID: 14991528].

4. UPD 7

Certain genes on chromosome 7 are now known to be imprinted. *UPD 7* has been reported to cause CF in a child who inherited two copies of the Δ F 508 deletion from one parent. That child also had Russell–Silver syndrome, a syndrome associated with intrauterine growth failure and dwarfism. Imprinting abnormalities and UPD may prove to be associated with growth abnormalities.

DISORDERS ASSOCIATED WITH ANTICIPATION

1. (Autosomal Dominant) MYOTONIC DYSTROPHY

Most myotonic dystrophy, an autosomal dominant condition characterized by muscle weakness and tonic muscle spasms (myotonia) along with hypogonadism, frontal balding, cardiac conduction abnormalities, and cataracts, presents in adults. This disorder occurs when a CTG repeat in the *DMPK* gene on chromosome 19 expands to 50 or more copies. Normal individuals have from 5–35 CTG repeat copies. Individuals carrying 35–49 repeats are generally asymptomatic, but repeat copies greater than 35 are meiotically unstable and tend to further expand when passed to subsequent generations. Individuals with 50–100 copies may be only mildly affected (eg, cataracts). Most individuals with repeat copies greater than 100 will have symptoms or electrical myotonia as adults.

As unstable alleles continue to expand and copy numbers approach 400, symptoms become evident in children. Expansion greater than 1000 copies produces fetal and neonatal disease that can be lethal. Expansion from approximately 200–400 repeat copies produces mild, often clinically undetected symptoms, while very large copy numbers (800–2000) are associated with fetal manifestations (polyhydramnios and arthrogryposis). This occurs most frequently when the unstable repeats are passed through an affected mother. Therefore, an important component in the work-up of the floppy or weak infant is a careful neurologic assessment of both parents for evidence of weakness or myotonia. Molecular testing that measures the number of CTG repeats is diagnostic clinically and prenatally.

2. (Autosomal Recessive) FRIEDREICH ATAXIA

Symptoms of Friedreich ataxia include loss of coordination (cerebellar dysfunction) with both motor and sensory findings beginning in preadolescence and typically progressing through the teenage years. The gene involved, *FDRA*, is located on chromosome 9. Normal individuals carry 7–33 GAA repeats at this locus. Close to 96% of affected patients are homozygous for repeat expansions that exceed 66 copies. However, point mutations in the gene also occur. Meiotic instability for GAA repeats is more variable than for others and contractions occur more frequently than do expansions. Relationships between genotype and phenotype are also more complex. Molecular diagnostic testing requires careful interpretation with respect to prognosis and reproductive risks.

3. (X-Linked) FRAGILE X SYNDROME

Fragile X syndrome, present in approximately 1 in 1000 males, is the most common cause of mental retardation in males. The responsible gene is *FMR-1,* which has unstable CGG repeats at the 5′ end. Normal individuals have up to 50 CGG repeats. Individuals with 51–200 CGG repeats have a **premutation,** and may manifest symptoms including developmental, behavioral and physical traits, premature ovarian failure in a subset of females, and a progressive, neurologic deterioration in older males called FXTAS (fragile X–associated tremor-ataxia syndrome). Affected individuals with fragile X syndrome (full mutation) have greater than 200 CGG repeats and also have hypermethylation of both the CGG expansion and an adjacent CpG island. This methylation turns off the *FMR-1* gene. DNA analysis, rather than cytogenetic testing, is the method of choice for confirming the diagnosis of fragile X syndrome.

Clinical Features

Most males with fragile X syndrome present with mental retardation, oblong facies with large ears, and large testicles, especially after puberty. Other physical signs include symptoms suggestive of a connective tissue disorder (eg, hyperextensible joints or mitral valve prolapse). Many affected individuals are hyperactive and exhibit infantile autism or autistic-like behavior.

About one-half of females with the fragile X full mutation show normal intelligence, but may evidence mild learning disabilities and behavioral problems. Unlike other X-linked disorders where female heterozygotes are asymptomatic, one-half of females with the full mutation have lower IQs in the range of mental retardation and more severe behavioral problems. Females have more mild phenotypic changes than the males. Clinical expression of fragile X differs in male and female offspring depending on which parent is transmitting the gene. The premutation can change into the full mutation only when passed through a female. Identification of the abnormal DNA amplification by direct DNA analysis can confirm the diagnosis of fragile X in an affected individual and can detect asymptomatic gene carriers of both sexes. Therefore, DNA analysis is a reliable test for prenatal and postnatal diagnosis of fragile X syndrome and facilitates genetic counseling.

Hagerman PJ, Hagerman RJ: The fragile-X premutation: A maturing perspective. Am J Hum Genet 2004:74;805 [PMID: 15052536].

DISORDERS ASSOCIATED WITH MITOCHONDRIAL INHERITANCE

More than 100 point mutations and rearrangements of mtDNA have been identified, which are associated with a large number of human diseases. Symptoms of mitochondrial disorders are secondary to deficiency in the respiratory chain enzymes of oxidative phosphorylation, which supply energy to all cells. Mitochondrial diseases are usually progressive disorders with neurologic dysfunction including hypotonia, developmental delay, and seizures. Ophthalmologic issues, hearing loss, gastrointestinal tract dysfunction with growth failure, renal, endocrine, cardiac, and autonomic dysfunction are some of the many issues which can affect patients with mitochondrial diseases. The following disorders are three of the more common ones.

1. MELAS

MELAS is an acronym for **m**itochondrial **e**ncephalopathy, **l**actic **a**cidosis, and **s**trokelike episodes. Symptoms occur in the pediatric age group and include recurrent episodes resembling stroke (blindness, paralysis), headache, vomiting, weakness of proximal muscles, and elevated blood lactate. (**Note:** Lactate may be falsely elevated secondary to technical difficulties in obtaining a free-flowing blood specimen or delay in laboratory measurement.) The most common mutation causing MELAS is in the tRNA^{Leu} gene (*A3243G*).

2. MERRF

MERRF is an acronym for **m**yoclonus **e**pilepsy with **r**agged **r**ed **f**ibers. Children with MERRF present with a variety of neurologic symptoms, including myoclonus, deafness, weakness of muscles, and seizures. Eighty percent of cases are due to a missense mutation in the mitochondrial tRNA^{Lys} gene (*A8344G*).

3. Leigh Subacute Necrotizing Encephalomyelopathy

Multiple different abnormalities in respiratory chain function lead to Leigh disease, a very severe disorder associated with progressive loss of developmental milestones associated with extrapyramidal symptoms, and brainstem dysfunction. Episodes of deterioration are frequently associated with an intercurrent febrile illness. Symptoms include hypotonia, unusual choreoathetoid hand movements, feeding dysfunction with failure to thrive, and seizures. Focal necrotic lesions of the brainstem and thalamus are hallmarks on MRI scan. Mitochondrial mutations affecting the respiratory chain, especially complexes I, II and IV, and nuclear DNA mutations affecting complex II have been identified as causing Leigh disease.

Kahler SG, Fahey MC: Metabolic disorders and mental retardation. Am J Med Genet C Semin Med Genet 2003:117;31 [PMID: 12561056].

MULTIFACTORIAL INHERITANCE

CLEFT LIP & CLEFT PALATE

From a genetic standpoint, cleft lip with or without cleft palate is distinct from isolated cleft palate. The former is more common in males, the latter in females. Although both can occur in a single family, particularly in association with certain syndromes, this pattern is unusual. Racial background is a factor in the incidence of facial clefting. Among Asians, Caucasians, and blacks, the incidence is 1.61, 0.9, and 0.31, respectively, per 1000 live births.

Clinical Findings

A cleft lip may be unilateral or bilateral and complete or incomplete. It may occur with a cleft of the entire palate or just the primary (anterior and gingival ridge) or secondary (posterior) palate. An isolated cleft palate can involve only the soft palate or both the soft and hard palates. It can be a V-shaped or wide horseshoe cleft. When the cleft palate is associated with micrognathia and glossoptosis (a tongue that falls back and causes respiratory or feeding problems), it is called the **Pierre Robin sequence.** Among individuals with facial clefts—more commonly those with isolated cleft palate—the incidence of other congenital abnormalities is increased, with up to a 60% association with other anomalies or syndromes. The incidence of congenital heart disease, for example, is between 1–2% in liveborn infants, but among those with Pierre Robin sequence it can be as high as 15%. Associated abnormalities should be looked for in the period immediately after birth and before surgery.

Differential Diagnosis

A facial cleft may occur in many different circumstances. It may be an isolated abnormality or part of a more generalized syndrome. Prognosis, management, and accurate determination of recurrence risks all depend on accurate diagnosis. In evaluating a child with a facial cleft, the physician must determine if the cleft is nonsyndromic or syndromic.

Nonsyndromic

In the past, nonsyndromic cleft lip or cleft palate was considered a classic example of polygenic or multifactorial inheritance. More recently, however, this mode of inheri-

Table 33–3. Syndromic isolated cleft palate (CP) and cleft lip with or without cleft palate (CL/CP).[a]

Environmental
Maternal seizures, anticonvulsant usage (CL/CP or CP)
Fetal alcohol syndrome (CP)
Amniotic band syndrome (CL/CP)
Chromosomal
Trisomies 13 and 18 (CL/CP)
Wolf-Hirschorn or 4p– syndrome (CL/CP)
Shprintzen or 22q11.2 deletion syndrome (CP)
Single-gene disorders
Treacher Collins syndrome, AD (CP)
Stickler syndrome, AD (CP)
Smith-Lemli-Opitz, AR (CP)[b]
Unknown cause
Möbius syndrome (CP)

[a]AD = autosomal dominant.
[b]AR = autosomal recessive.

tance has been questioned, and several studies have suggested one or more major autosomal loci, both recessive and dominant (or co-dominant). Empirically, however, the recurrence risk is still in the range of 2–3% because of nonpenetrance or the presence of other contributing genes.

Syndromic

Cleft lip, with or without cleft palate, and isolated cleft palate may occur in a variety of syndromes that may be environmental, chromosomal, single gene, or of unknown origin (Table 33–3). Prognosis and accurate recurrence risks depend on the correct diagnosis.

Complications & Treatment

Problems associated with facial clefts include early feeding difficulties, which may be severe; airway obstruction necessitating tracheostomy; recurrent serous otitis media associated with fluctuating hearing; and language delays; speech problems, including language delay, hypernasality and articulation errors; and dental and orthodontic complications. Long-term management ideally should be through a multidisciplinary cleft palate clinic.

Genetic Counseling

Accurate counseling depends on accurate diagnosis and the differentiation of syndromic from nonsyndromic clefts. A complete family history must be taken, and the patient and both parents must be examined. The choice of laboratory studies is guided by the presence of other abnormalities and clinical suspicions, and may include chromosome analysis, FISH, eye examination, and radiologic studies. Clefts of both the lip and the palate can be detected on detailed prenatal ultrasound.

NEURAL TUBE DEFECTS

Neural tube defects comprise a variety of malformations, including anencephaly, encephalocele, spina bifida (myelomeningocele), sacral agenesis, and other spinal dysraphisms. Evidence suggests that the neural tube develops via closure at multiple rather than just two closure sites and that each closure site is mediated by different genes and affected by different teratogens. Hydrocephalus associated with the Arnold–Chiari type II malformation commonly occurs with myelomeningocele. Sacral agenesis, also called the caudal regression syndrome, occurs more frequently in infants of diabetic mothers.

Clinical Findings

At birth, neural tube defects can present as an obvious rachischisis (open lesion), or as a more subtle skin-covered lesion. In the latter case, MRI should be conducted to better define the anatomic defect. The extent of neurologic deficit depends on the level of the lesion and may include clubfeet, dislocated hips, or total flaccid paralysis below the level of the lesion. Hydrocephalus may be apparent at birth or may develop after the back has been surgically repaired. Neurogenic bladder and bowel are commonly seen. Other anomalies of the CNS may be present, as well as anomalies of the heart or kidneys.

Differential Diagnosis

Neural tube defects may occur in isolation (nonsyndromic) or as part of a genetic syndrome. They may result from teratogenic exposure to alcohol or the anticonvulsant valproate. Any infant with dysmorphic features or other major anomalies in addition to a neural tube defect should be evaluated by a geneticist, and a chromosome analysis should be performed.

Complications & Management

A. NEUROSURGICAL

Infants with an open neural tube defect should be placed in prone position, and the lesion kept moist with sterile dressing. Neurosurgical closure should occur within 24–48 hours after birth to reduce risk of infection. The infant should be monitored closely for signs of hydrocephalus. Shunts are required in about 85% of cases of myelomeningocele, and are associated with complications including malfunction and infection. Symptoms of the Arnold–Chiari II malformation include feeding dysfunction, abducens nerve palsy, vocal cord paralysis with stridor, and apnea. Shunt malfunction may cause an acute worsening of Arnold–Chiari symptoms that may be life-threatening.

B. ORTHOPEDIC

The child's ability to walk varies according to the level of the lesion. Children with low lumbar and sacral lesions walk with minimal support, while those with high lumbar and thoracic lesions are rarely functional walkers. Orthopedic input is necessary to address foot deformities and scoliosis. Physical therapy services are indicated.

C. UROLOGIC

Neurogenic bladders have variable presentations. Urodynamic studies are recommended early on to define bladder function, and management is guided by the results of these studies. Continence can often be achieved by the use of anticholinergic or sympathomimetic agents, clean intermittent catheterization, and a variety of urologic procedures. Renal function should be monitored regularly, and an ultrasound examination should be periodically repeated. Symptomatic infections should be treated.

Symptoms of neurogenic bowel include incontinence and chronic constipation and are managed with a combination of dietary modifications, laxatives, stool softeners, and rectal stimulation. A surgical procedure called ACE (antegrade continence enema) may be recommended for patients with severe constipation, unresponsive to conservative management.

Special Issues and Prognosis

All children requiring multiple surgical procedures (ie, patients with spina bifida or urinary tract anomalies) have a significant risk for developing hypersensitivity type I (IgE-mediated) allergic reactions to latex. For this reason, nonlatex medical products are now routinely used when caring for patients with neural tube defects.

Most individuals with spina bifida are cognitively normal, but learning disabilities are common. Individuals with encephalocele or other CNS malformations generally have a much poorer intellectual prognosis. Individuals with closed spinal cord abnormalities (eg, sacral lipomas) have more mild issues in general, and intelligence is usually normal. Problems in older patients include the development of spinal cord tethering, which usually presents with back pain, progressive scoliosis, and changes in bowel or bladder function. This often requires neurosurgical intervention.

Individuals with neural tube defects have lifelong medical issues, requiring the input of a multidisciplinary medical team. A good support for families is the national Spina Bifida Association, at the following website:

http://www.sbaa.org

Genetic Counseling

Most isolated neural tube defects are polygenic, with a recurrence risk of 2–3% in future pregnancies. The recurrence risk for siblings of the parents and siblings of the patients is 1–2%. A patient with spina bifida has a 5% chance of having an affected child. Prenatal diagnosis is possible. In fetuses with open neural tube defects, maternal serum α-fetoprotein levels measured at 16–18 weeks' gestation are elevated. α-Fetoprotein and acetylcholine esterase levels in amniotic fluid are also elevated. Ultrasound studies alone will detect approximately 90% of neural tube defects.

Prophylactic folic acid can significantly lower the incidence and recurrence rate of neural tube defects, if the intake of the folic acid starts at least 3 months prior to conception and continues for the first month of pregnancy, at a dose of 4 mg/d for women at increased risk. For women of childbearing age without a family history of neural tube defects, the dose is 0.4 mg of folic acid daily. Folic acid supplementation prior to conception may also lower the incidence of other congenital malformations such as conotruncal heart defects.

COMMON RECOGNIZABLE DISORDERS WITH VARIABLE OR UNKNOWN CAUSE

The text that follows describes several important and common human malformation syndromes. The best illustrations are in *Smith's Recognizable Patterns of Human Malformation*. An excellent Internet site at the University of Kansas Medical Center can be consulted for further information:

http://www.kumc.edu/gec/support

Arthrogryposis Multiplex

Arthrogryposis multiplex is due to lack of fetal movement. Causes most often involve constraint, CNS maldevelopment or injury, and neuromuscular disorders. Polyhydramnios is often present as a result of lack of fetal swallowing. Pulmonary hypoplasia may also be present, reflecting lack of fetal breathing. The work-up includes brain imaging, careful consideration of metabolic disease, neurologic consultation, and, in some cases, electrophysiologic studies and muscle biopsy. The parents should be examined, and a family history reviewed carefully for findings such as muscle weakness or cramping, cataracts, and early-onset heart disease, suggesting myotonic dystrophy.

Goldenhar Syndrome

Goldenhar syndrome, also known as vertebro-auriculofacial syndrome, is an association of multiple anomalies involving the head and neck. The classic phenotype includes hemifacial microsomia (one side of the face smaller than the other), with abnormalities of the pinna on the same side with associated deafness. Ear anomalies may be quite severe and include anotia. A characteristic benign fatty tumor in the outer eye, called an epibulbar dermoid, is frequently present, as are preauricular ear tags. Vertebral anomalies, particularly of the cervical vertebrae, are common. The Arnold–Chiari type I malformation (herniation of the cerebellum into the cervical spinal canal) is a common associated anomaly. Cardiac anomalies and hydrocephalus are seen in more severe cases. Most patients with Goldenhar syndrome have normal intelligence. The cause is unknown.

Kabuki Syndrome

Kabuki syndrome is a disorder of unknown cause characterized by a distinctive facial appearance (hypertelorism with long palpebral fissures, large pinnae), developmental delay, and hearing loss. Most cases are sporadic, although a few cases with dominant transmission have been reported. Anomalies of the heart and genitourinary system are occasionally seen.

Oligohydramnios Sequence (Potter Sequence)

This condition presents in newborns as severe respiratory distress due to pulmonary hypoplasia in association with positional deformities of the extremities, usually bilateral clubfeet, and typical facies consisting of suborbital creases, depressed nasal tip and low-set ears, and retrognathia. The sequence may be due to prolonged lack of amniotic fluid. Most often it is due to leakage, renal agenesis, or severe obstructive uropathy.

Opitz G/BBB

Disrupted development of midline structures is a feature of several overlapping malformation syndromes, a number of them heritable. Hypertelorism (wide set eyes), midbrain anomalies (agenesis of the corpus callosum), cardiac septal defects, and genitourinary tract anomalies (hypospadias) are the most common features. Current clinical genetic terminology refers to these conditions as Opitz G/BBB syndrome. Hypotonia and problems with swallowing and gastroesophageal reflux are hallmark symptoms. Mentation is usually subnormal. Both autosomal dominant and X-linked inheritance have been documented. Linkage studies have recently identified a candidate gene dubbed *M101* on the X chromosome. A number of patients with Opitz G/BBB syndrome have also been shown by FISH to have deletions of 22q11. Additional resources include the

Opitz Family Network and the Opitz G/BBB Family Network and the following website:

http://www.opitznet.org/joinus.html

Overgrowth Syndromes

Overgrowth syndromes are becoming increasingly recognized as important childhood conditions. They may present at birth and are characterized by macrocephaly, motor delays (cerebral hypotonia), and, in many cases, asymmetry of extremities. Bone age may be advanced. The most common overgrowth syndrome is **Sotos syndrome.** Patients with Sotos syndrome have a characteristic facies with a prominent forehead and down-slanting palpebral features. The cause of Sotos syndrome is unknown. There is a small but increased risk of cancer in patients with Sotos syndrome. Other overgrowth syndromes include **Beckwith–Wiedemann syndrome** (BWS), described in the section on imprinting, and two single gene disorders called **Simpson–Golabi–Behmel syndrome** and **Bannayan–Riley–Ruvalcaba syndrome.** Simpson–Golabi–Behmel syndrome exhibits a BWS-like phenotype, but with additional anomalies including polydactyly and more severe facial dysmorphism. Unlike patients with BWS who have normal intelligence, patients with Simpson–Golabi-Behmel syndrome often have developmental delay. It is inherited as an X-linked disorder. Patients with Bannayan–Riley–Ruvalcaba syndrome have macrosomia, macrocephaly, and unusual freckling of the penis. They have mild developmental issues. They may develop hemangiomatous/lymphangiomatous growths and have a predisposition to intestinal malignancies. The cause of Bannayan–Riley–Ruvalcaba syndrome was recently found to be a mutation of the *PTEN* gene implicated in Cowden syndrome, the association of intestinal polyposis with malignant potential.

Rubenstein–Taybi Syndrome

Rubenstein–Taybi syndrome is a genetic disorder of unknown cause, characterized by developmental delay; growth failure; and a distinctive facial dysmorphology with microcephaly, prominent nose, and small chin. Feeding problems are common. About 25% of patients have been found with a microdeletion of chromosome 16 detectable by FISH, but most patients have a normal karyotype.

Syndromic Short Stature

Short stature is an important component of numerous syndromes, or it may be an isolated finding. In the absence of nutritional deficiencies, endocrine abnormalities, evidence for skeletal dysplasia (disproportionate growth with abnormal skeletal films), or a positive family history, intrinsic short stature can be due to UPD. The phenotype of Russell–Silver syndrome—short stature with normal head growth (pseudohydrocephalus), normal development, and minor dysmorphic features (especially fifth finger clinodactyly)—has been associated in some cases with maternal UPD for chromosome 7.

VACTERL Association

VACTERL association is described by an acronym denoting the association of **v**ertebral defects (segmentation anomalies), imperforate **a**nus, **c**ardiac malformation (most often ventricular septal defect), **t**racheo-**e**sophageal fistula, **r**enal anomalies, and **l**imb (most often radial ray) anomalies. The disorder is sporadic, and some of the defects may be life-threatening. The prognosis for normal development is good. The cause is unknown, but a high association with monozygotic twinning suggests a mechanism dating back to events perhaps as early as blastogenesis. Recently, disturbance of the sonic hedgehog pathway was suggested to be part of the mechanism for VACTERL, based on a mouse model. Careful examination and follow-up are important, because numerous other syndromes with more complicated prognoses also include features present in VACTERL association. Chromosomal studies and genetic consultation are warranted.

PERINATAL GENETICS

TERATOGENS

1. Drug Abuse and Fetal Alcohol Syndrome

Fetal alcohol syndrome results from excessive exposure to alcohol during gestation and affects 30–40% of offspring of mothers whose daily intake of alcohol exceeds 3 ounces. Features of the syndrome include short stature; poor head growth (may be postnatal in onset); developmental delay; and midface hypoplasia characterized by a poorly developed long philtrum, narrow palpebral fissures, and short nose with anteverted nares. Facial findings may be subtle, but careful measurements and comparisons with standards (see Figure 33–11) are helpful. Structural abnormalities occur in half of affected children. Cardiac anomalies and neural tube defects are commonly seen. Genitourinary tract anomalies are frequent. Neurobehavioral effects also occur and may be stereotypic with poor judgment and inappropriate social interactions such as lack of stranger anxiety in toddlers commonly found. Behavioral problems may occur without other classic features of fetal alcohol syndrome.

Maternal abuse of drugs and other psychoactive substances is also associated with increased risks for adverse perinatal outcomes including miscarriage, preterm delivery, growth retardation, and increased risk for injury to the developing CNS. Methamphetamine and crack cocaine appear to be particularly dangerous. Maternal abuse of inhalants such as glue appears to be associated with findings similar to those of fetal alcohol syndrome. For most abused substances, the link between exposures and specific adverse outcomes is less well demonstrated than with alcohol. Multiple factors are probably involved, and it should be recognized that substance abuse often involves more than one drug.

Careful evaluation for other syndromes and chromosomal disorders should be included in the work-up of exposed infants. Behavioral abnormalities in older children may be the result of maternally abused substances but they may also reflect evolving psychiatric disorders. Psychiatric disorders, many recognized as heritable, affect large numbers of men and women with substance abuse problems.

2. Maternal Anticonvulsant Effects

Anticonvulsant exposure during pregnancy is associated with adverse outcomes in approximately 10% of children born to women treated with these agents. A syndrome characterized by small head circumference, anteverted nares, cleft lip and palate (occasionally), and distal digital hypoplasia was first described in association with maternal use of phenytoin but also occurs with other anticonvulsants including carbamazepine. Risks for spina bifida are increased, especially in pregnancies exposed to valproic acid.

3. Retinoic Acid Embryopathy

Vitamin A and its analogs are potent morphogens that have considerable teratogenic potential. Developmental toxicity occurs in approximately one-third of pregnancies exposed in the first trimester to the synthetic retinoid isotretinoin, commonly prescribed to treat acne. Exposure disrupts migration of rostral neural crest cells and produces CNS maldevelopment, especially of the posterior fossa; ear anomalies (often absence of pinnae); congenital heart disease (great vessel anomalies); and tracheoesophageal fistula. These findings constitute a partial phenocopy of DiGeorge syndrome and demonstrate the continuum of contributing genetic and epigenetic factors in morphogenesis. It is now recognized that vitamin A itself, when taken as active retinoic acid in doses exceeding 25,000 IU/d during pregnancy, can produce similar fetal anomalies. For safety, vitamin A intake is therefore limited to 10,000 IU/d of retinoic acid. Maternal ingestion of large amounts of vitamin A taken as retinol during pregnancy, however, does not increase risks, because conversion of this precursor to active retinoic acid is internally regulated.

ASSISTED REPRODUCTION

In vitro fertilization and other assistive reproductive technologies are now responsible for a significant number of births in the United States. Although healthy live births are accepted as the usual outcomes resulting from successful application of these procedures, questions about risks for adverse effects on development are beginning to be raised. Increased rates of twinning, both mono- and dizygotic, are well recognized while the possibility of increased rates of birth defects remains controversial. Recently, a number of geneticists have raised issues regarding abnormalities of imprinting associated with in vitro fertilization.

PRENATAL DIAGNOSIS

Prenatal screening for birth defects is now routinely offered to pregnant women of all ages. Prenatal diagnosis for specific genetic disorders is indicated in 7–8% of pregnancies. Prenatal diagnosis introduces options for management including termination of abnormal pregnancies, preparation for specialized perinatal care, and, in some cases, fetal therapies.

Methods

Prenatal assessment of the fetus includes techniques that screen maternal blood, image the conceptus, and sample fetal and placental tissues (Table 33–4).

A. MATERNAL BLOOD

Elevated levels of maternal serum α-fetoprotein correlate with open neural tube defects but low levels are associated with Down syndrome. First trimester measurements of PAPA (pregnancy-associated plasma protein A) and the free β-subunit of human chorionic gonadotropin screen for trisomy 21 and trisomy 18. In the second trimester maternal α-fetoprotein, human chorionic gonadotropin, unconjugated estradiol, and inhibin combine to estimate risks for trisomy 21 and trisomy 18. Low estradiol levels can also predict cases of Smith–Lemli–Opitz syndrome, a devastating autosomal recessive disorder discussed previously.

Fetal cells, including lymphocytes, trophoblasts, and nucleated red blood cells, circulate at low frequency in maternal blood and may eventually provide access to direct information about the conceptus.

B. FETAL SAMPLES

1. Amniocentesis—Whereas maternal blood levels are screened for fetal abnormalities, genetic amniocentesis is applied to make specific diagnoses. This procedure samples fluid surrounding the fetus and cells are cultured for cytogenetic, molecular, or metabolic analyses.

Table 33–4. Prenatal diagnostic techniques.

Maternal blood screening such as α-fetoprotein, estriol,
  hCG ("triple screen")
  Trisomies 21 and 18
  Neural tube defects
  Smith-Lemli-Opitz syndrome
Fetal cells in maternal blood (research only)
Fetal ultrasound
  Structural defects
  Fetal hydrops
  Poly- or oligohydramnios
Fetal radiograph
  Skeletal defects
Fetal MRI
Amniocentesis
  Karyotyping
  Fetal cells for molecular or metabolic studies
  Amniotic fluid α-fetoprotein level for neural tube defects
  Biochemical studies on fluid
Chorionic villus sampling
  Karyotyping
  Fetal cells for molecular or metabolic studies
Fetal tissues
  Blood by percutaneous umbilical blood sampling
  Biopsy of other fetal tissues
Direct fetal visualization via fetoscopy (rarely used today because
  of the advances in fetal visualization by ultrasound and MRI)

MRI, magnetic resonance imaging.

α-Fetoprotein and other chemical markers can also be measured. This is a safe procedure with a complication rate (primarily for miscarriage) of less than 1% in experienced hands.

2. Chorionic villus sampling (placental)—Chorionic villus sampling is now available in most perinatal centers and is generally performed at 11–12 weeks of gestation. Tissue obtained by chorionic villus sampling provides DNA for molecular analysis and contains dividing cells (cytotrophoblasts) that can be rapidly karyotyped. However, direct cytogenetic preparations may be of poor quality. In addition, chromosomal abnormalities detected by this technique may be confined to the placenta (**confined placental mosaicism**). Cultured preparations may be more relevant.

3. Fetal blood and tissue—Fetal blood can be sampled directly in late gestation through ultrasound-guided percutaneous umbilical blood sampling. A wide range of diagnostic tests ranging from biochemical to cytogenetic can be applied. Fetal urine sampled from the bladder or dilated proximal structures can provide important information about fetal renal function.

It is occasionally necessary to biopsy fetal tissues such as liver or muscle for accurate prenatal diagnosis but these procedures are available in only a few perinatal centers.

4. Embryo biopsy—With the advent of single cell PCR techniques as well as interphase FISH it is now possible to make genetic diagnoses in preimplantation human embryos by removing and analyzing blastocyst cells. How useful and accepted this technique will become remains to be seen.

C. FETAL IMAGING

Fetal ultrasonography and MRI imaging are becoming increasingly common during pregnancy while x-rays are seldom employed. Ultrasonography has joined maternal blood sampling as a screening technique for common chromosomal aneuploidies, neural tube defects, and other structural anomalies. Pregnancies at increased risk for CNS anomalies, skeletal dysplasias, and structural defects of the heart and kidneys should be monitored by careful ultrasound examinations. Although MRI has had limited use to date, it appears that there will be a definite place for it in defining abnormalities of the fetal brain.

Rimoin DL et al: *Emery and Rimoin's Principles and Practice of Medical Genetics,* 3rd ed. Churchill Livingstone, 2002.

EVALUATION OF THE DEVELOPMENTALLY DELAYED CHILD

Mental retardation or developmental delays affect 8% of the population. Disorders associated with symptoms of delayed development are heterogeneous but frequently include heritable components. Evaluation should be multidisciplinary; Table 33–5 lists its main features, emphasizing the major clinical and genetic considerations.

Obtaining a detailed history, including pertinent prenatal and perinatal events is critical. Feeding issues and slow growth velocity are seen in many genetic disorders causing developmental delay. Rate of developmental progress and particularly a history of loss of skills are important clues, as the latter might suggest a metabolic disorder with a neurodegenerative component. Family history can provide clues to suggest possible genetic etiologies, particularly if there is a history of consanguinity, or a family pattern of other affected individuals.

Physical examination provides helpful clues. Referral to a clinical geneticist is indicated whenever unusual features are encountered. Neurologic, ophthalmologic, and audiologic consultation should be sought when indicated. Brain imaging should be requested in cases involving unexplained deviations from normal head growth. Neuroimaging and skeletal studies may also be indicated when dysmorphic features are present.

Metabolic and genetic testing procedures other than those listed in the Table 33–5 may also be indicated, as

Table 33–5. Evaluation of the child with developmental delay.

History
   Pregnancy history
   Growth parameters at birth
   Neonatal complications
   Feeding history
   History of somatic growth
   Motor, language, and psychosocial milestones
   Seizures
   Loss of skills
   Abnormal movements
   Results of previous tests and examinations
Family history
   Developmental and educational histories
   Psychiatric disorders
   Pregnancy outcomes
   Medical history
   Consanguinity
Physical examination
   General pediatric examination, including growth parameters
   Focused dysmorphologic evaluation including measurement of facial features and limbs
   Complete neurologic examination
   Parental growth parameters (especially head circumferences) and dysmorphic features should also be assessed
Imaging studies
   See text
Laboratory assessment[a]
   Chromosomes (high-resolution analyses)
   Fragile X testing (analysis of *FMR1* gene for triplet repeats)
   FISH analyses guided by dysmorphic features
   Other blood analyses: complete blood count, electrolytes, liver function tests, creatinine kinase (CK), lactate, pyruvate
   Serum amino acid analysis
   Urine amino and organic acid analyses
   Urine analysis for mucopolysaccharides (if coarse features and organomegaly)

[a]In many cases, negative results may be important.
FISH, fluorescent in situ hybridization.

well as confirmatory molecular testing. Genetic consultation should be sought to coordinate these investigations.

Interpretation & Follow-Up

Clinical experience indicates that specific diagnoses can be made in approximately half of patients evaluated according to the protocol presented here. With specific diagnosis comes prognosis, ideas for management, and insight into recurrence risks. Prenatal diagnosis may also become possible.

Follow-up is important both for patients in whom diagnoses have been made and for those patients initially lacking a diagnosis. Genetic information is accumulating rapidly and can be translated into new diagnoses and better understanding with periodic review of clinical cases.

Autism

Autism is a developmental disorder comprising abnormal function in three domains: language development, social development, and behavior. The majority of patients with autism also have cognitive disabilities, and might be appropriately evaluated as per the recommendations above. However, given the enormous increase in prevalence of autism in the past decade, it is worth discussing the genetic evaluation of autism separately.

There are multiple known genetic causes of autism. Advances in molecular diagnosis, understanding of metabolic derangements, and technologies such as FISH are allowing more patients with autism to be identified with specific genetic disorders. This allows more accurate genetic counseling for recurrence risk, as well as diagnosis-specific interventions which may improve prognosis.

With this in mind, recommendations for the genetic evaluation of a child with autism include the following:

- Genetic referral if dysmorphic features or cutaneous abnormalities are present (ie, hypopigmented spots such as those seen in patients with **tuberous sclerosis**).

Laboratory testing to include the following:

- Chromosomes with high-resolution banding.
- Molecular testing for **fragile X syndrome**.
- FISH testing for 22q and 15q deletions.
- Methylation testing for UPD 15 if phenotype suggestive of **Angelman syndrome**.
- Measurement of cholesterol and 7-dehydrocholesterol if 2–3 toe syndactyly is present, to rule out mild form of **Smith–Lemli–Opitz syndrome.**
- MECP2 testing if clinical course suggestive of **Rett syndrome,** (neurodegenerative course, progressive microcephaly and seizures in a female patient).

Allergic Disorders

34

Mark Boguniewicz, MD

Allergic disorders are among the most common problems seen by pediatricians and primary care physicians, affecting over 25% of the population in developed countries. In the most recent National Health and Nutrition Examination Survey conducted in the United States between 1988 and 1994, 54% of the population had positive test responses to one more allergens. In children, the increased prevalence of asthma, allergic rhinitis, and atopic dermatitis has been accompanied by significant morbidity and school absenteeism, with adverse consequences for school performance and quality of life, as well as economic burden measured in billions of dollars. Understanding the language of allergy and the basic mechanisms involved may help physicians when treating these disorders. In this chapter, atopy refers to a genetically determined predisposition to develop IgE antibodies found in patients with asthma, allergic rhinitis, and atopic dermatitis. The "hygiene hypothesis" suggests that reduced exposure in early life to microbial organisms (or endotoxins) may account for the increase in atopic diseases. More recently, the role of reduced activity of T regulatory cells has been advanced, although both mechanisms may play a role. The Allergy Report is an easy-to-access compendium of allergic disorders that can be found on the Internet at: www.TheAllergyReport.org.

■ MAJOR ALLERGIC DISORDERS SEEN IN PEDIATRIC PRACTICE

ASTHMA

ESSENTIALS OF DIAGNOSIS & TYPICAL FEATURES

- *Episodic symptoms of airflow obstruction including wheezing, cough, and chest tightness.*
- *Airflow obstruction at least partially reversible.*
- *Exclusion of alternative diagnoses.*

General Considerations

Asthma is the most common chronic disease of childhood, affecting over 6 million children in the United States. Despite advances in the understanding of asthma, associated morbidity has increased over the past decade and mortality rates have remained relatively stable. Asthma hospitalization rates are highest in the black population, with death rates consistently highest among African Americans age 15–24 years. The reasons for this are unclear but may be related to a combination of poor access to health care and environmental factors such as smoke and perennial allergen exposure.

Up to 80% of children with asthma develop symptoms before their fifth birthday. Atopy is the strongest identifiable predisposing factor. Exposure to tobacco smoke, especially from the mother, is also a risk factor for asthma. About 40% of infants and young children who have wheezing with viral infections in the first few years of life will have continuing asthma through childhood. Sensitization to inhalant allergens increases over time and is found in the majority of children with asthma. The principal allergens associated with asthma are perennial aeroallergens such as dust mites, animal danders, cockroaches, and *Alternaria* (a soil mold). Of note, several recent studies suggest that exposure to high levels of cat allergen may have a protective effect against asthma. Rarely, foods may provoke isolated asthma symptoms. Other triggers include exercise, cold air, cigarette smoke, pollutants, strong chemical odors, and rapid changes in barometric pressure. Aspirin sensitivity is uncommon in children. Psychological factors may precipitate asthma exacerbations and place the patient at high risk from the disease.

Pathologic features of asthma include shedding of airway epithelium, edema, mucus plug formation, mast cell activation, and collagen deposition beneath the basement membrane. The inflammatory cell infiltrate includes eosinophils, lymphocytes, and neutrophils, especially in fatal asthma exacerbations. Airway inflammation contributes to airway hyperresponsiveness, airflow limitation, and disease chronicity. Persistent airway inflammation can lead to airway wall remodeling and irreversible changes.

Clinical Findings

A. SYMPTOMS AND SIGNS

Wheezing is the most characteristic sign of asthma, although it may be absent in some children, especially in those with cough-variant asthma. Patients may also have cough and shortness of breath. Complaints may include "chest congestion," prolonged cough, exercise intolerance, dyspnea, and recurrent bronchitis or pneumonia. If symptoms are absent or mild, chest auscultation during forced expiration may reveal prolongation of the expiratory phase and wheezing. As the obstruction becomes more severe, wheezes become more high-pitched and breath sounds diminished. With severe obstruction, wheezes may not be heard because of poor air movement. Flaring of nostrils, intercostal and suprasternal retractions, and use of accessory muscles of respiration are signs of severe obstruction. Flushed, moist skin may be noted, and mucous membranes may be dry. Cyanosis of the lips and nail beds may be seen with underlying hypoxia. Tachycardia and pulsus paradoxus also occur. Agitation and lethargy may be signs of impending respiratory failure.

B. LABORATORY FINDINGS

Airway hyperresponsiveness to nonspecific stimuli is a hallmark of asthma. These include inhaled pharmacologic agents such as histamine and methacholine as well as physical stimuli such as exercise and cold air. Airways may exhibit hyperresponsiveness or twitchiness even when pulmonary function tests are normal. Giving increasing amounts of a bronchoconstrictive agent to induce a decrease in lung function (usually a 20% drop in forced expiratory volume in 1 second [FEV_1]) is the most common method of testing airway responsiveness. Hyperresponsiveness in normal children younger than age 5 years is greater than in older children. The level of airway hyperresponsiveness usually correlates with the severity of asthma.

During acute asthma exacerbations, FEV_1 is diminished and the flow-volume curve shows a "scooping out" of the distal portion of the expiratory portion of the loop (Figure 34–1). The residual volume, functional residual capacity, and total lung capacity are usually increased, while the vital capacity is decreased. Reversal or significant improvement of these abnormalities in response to inhaled bronchodilator therapy alone or with anti-inflammatory therapy is observed. Increased airway resistance also results in a decreased peak expiratory flow rate (PEFR). Diurnal variation in PEFR (ie, the difference between morning and evening measurements) of greater than 15–20% has been used as a defining feature of asthma. Significant changes in PEFR may occur before symptoms become evident. In more severe cases, PEFR monitoring enables earlier recognition of suboptimal asthma control. Exercise, cold air, and methacholine or histamine challenges may help to establish a diagnosis of asthma when the history, examination, and pulmonary function tests are not definitive. Alternatively, a diagnostic trial of inhaled bronchodilators and anti-inflammatory medications may be helpful, especially in infants and young children in whom underdiagnosis and undertreatment are common. Infant pulmonary function can be measured in sedated children with compression techniques. The forced oscillation technique can be used to measure airway resistance in younger children.

Hypoxemia is present early with a normal or low P_{CO_2} level and respiratory alkalosis. Hypoxemia may be aggravated during treatment with a β_2-agonist due to ventilation–perfusion mismatch. Oxygen saturation less than 91% is indicative of significant obstruction. Respiratory acidosis and increasing CO_2 tension may ensue with further airflow obstruction and signal impending respiratory failure. Hypercapnia is usually not seen until the FEV_1 falls below 20% of predicted value. Metabolic acidosis has also been noted in combination with respi-

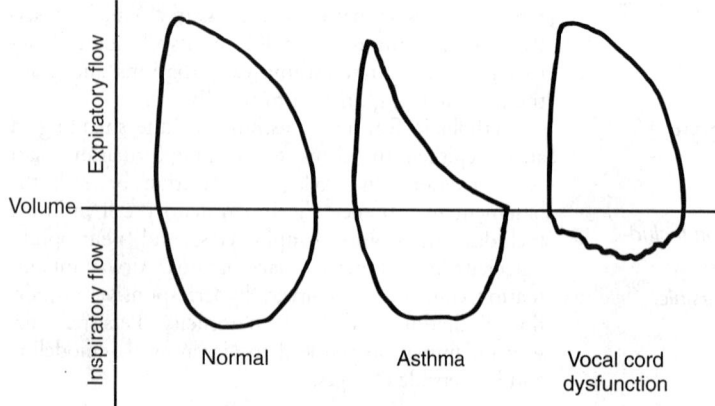

Figure 34–1. Representative flow-volume loops in persons with normal lung function, asthma, and vocal cord dysfunction.

ratory acidosis in children with severe asthma and indicates imminent respiratory failure. A Pa_{O_2} less than 60 mm Hg despite oxygen therapy and a Pa_{CO_2} over 60 mm Hg and rising more than 5 mm Hg per hour are relative indications for mechanical ventilation in a child in status asthmaticus.

Pulsus paradoxus may be present with moderate or severe asthma. In moderate asthma in a child, this may be between 10 and 25 mm Hg, and in severe asthma between 20 and 40 mm Hg. Absence of pulsus paradoxus in a child with severe asthma exacerbation may signal respiratory muscle fatigue.

Clumps of eosinophils on sputum smear and blood eosinophilia are frequent findings. Their presence tends to reflect disease activity and does not necessarily mean that allergic factors are involved. Leukocytosis is common in acute severe asthma without evidence of bacterial infection and may be more pronounced after epinephrine administration. Hematocrit can be elevated with dehydration during prolonged exacerbations or in severe chronic disease. Potential noninvasive measures of airway inflammation include serum eosinophil cationic protein levels, exhaled nitric oxide, and induced sputum. Each test has its strengths and weaknesses.

C. IMAGING

On chest radiographs, bilateral hyperinflation with flattening of the diaphragms, peribronchial thickening, prominence of the pulmonary arteries, and areas of patchy atelectasis may be present. Atelectasis may be misinterpreted as the infiltrates of pneumonia. High resolution computed tomography has been used to quantify bronchial wall thickening as a marker of airway remodeling in children with severe asthma and define peripheral airways disease and is useful in ruling out certain diagnoses in patients with difficult to manage asthma.

Allergy testing is discussed in the General measures section under Treatment, Chronic Asthma.

Differential Diagnosis

Diseases that may be mistaken for asthma are often related to the patient's age (Table 34–1). Congenital abnormalities must be excluded in infants and young children. Asthma can be confused with croup, acute bronchiolitis, pneumonia, and pertussis. Immunodeficiency may be associated with cough and wheezing. Foreign bodies in the airway may cause dyspnea or wheezing of sudden onset, and on auscultation wheezing may be unilateral. Asymmetry of the lungs secondary to air trapping may be seen on a chest radiograph, especially with forced expiration. Cystic fibrosis can be associated with or mistaken for asthma.

Table 34–1. Differential diagnosis of asthma in infants and children.

Viral bronchiolitis
Aspiration
Laryngotracheomalacia
Vascular rings
Airway stenosis or web
Enlarged lymph nodes
Mediastinal mass
Foreign body
Bronchopulmonary dysplasia
Obliterative bronchiolitis
Cystic fibrosis
Vocal cord dysfunction
Cardiovascular disease

Vocal cord dysfunction is an important masquerader of asthma, although the two occasionally coexist. It is characterized by the paradoxic closure of the vocal cords that can result in dyspnea and wheezing. Diagnosis is made by direct visualization of the vocal cords. In normal individuals, the vocal cords abduct during inspiration and may adduct slightly during expiration. Asthmatic patients may have narrowing of the glottis during expiration as a physiologic adaptation to airway obstruction. In contrast, patients with isolated vocal cord dysfunction typically show adduction of the anterior two-thirds of their vocal cords during inspiration, with a small diamond-shaped aperture posteriorly. Because this abnormal vocal cord pattern may be intermittently present, a normal examination does not exclude the diagnosis. Exercise or methacholine challenges can often precipitate symptoms of vocal cord dysfunction. The flow-volume loop may provide additional clues to the diagnosis of vocal cord dysfunction. Truncation of the inspiratory portion can be demonstrated in most patients during an acute episode, and some patients continue to show this pattern even when they are asymptomatic (see Figure 34–1). Children with vocal cord dysfunction, especially adolescents, tend to be overly competitive, primarily in athletics and scholastics. A psychiatric consultation may help define underlying psychological issues and provide appropriate therapy.

Treatment of isolated vocal cord dysfunction includes education regarding the syndrome and appropriate breathing exercises. Hypnosis, biofeedback, and psychotherapy have been effective for some patients. During an acute episode, a helium–oxygen mixture can be administered because the low density of the gas mixture facilitates movement of air through the adducted vocal cords.

Conditions That May Increase Asthma Severity

Chronic hyperplastic sinusitis is frequently found in association with asthma. Upper airway inflammation has been shown to contribute to the pathogenesis of asthma, and asthma may improve after treatment of sinusitis. However, sinus surgery is usually not indicated for initial treatment of chronic mucosal disease associated with allergy.

A significant correlation has been observed between nocturnal asthma and gastroesophageal reflux. Patients may not complain of epigastric burning or have reflux symptoms—cough may be the only sign. For patients with poorly controlled asthma, particularly with a nocturnal component, investigation for gastroesophageal reflux may be warranted even in the absence of suggestive symptoms.

The risk factors for death from asthma include psychological and sociological factors. They are probably related to the consequences of illness denial as well as to nonadherence with prescribed therapy. Recent studies have shown that less than 50% of inhaled asthma medications are taken as prescribed and that compliance does not improve with increasing severity of illness. Moreover, children requiring hospitalization for asthma, or their caregivers, have often failed to institute appropriate home treatment.

Complications

With acute asthma, complications are primarily related to hypoxemia and acidosis and can include generalized seizures. Pneumomediastinum or pneumothorax can be a complication in status asthmaticus. Recent studies point to airway wall remodeling and loss of pulmonary function with persistent airway inflammation. Childhood asthma independent of any corticosteroid therapy has been shown to be associated with delayed maturation and slowing of prepubertal growth velocity. However, attainment of final predicted adult height does not appear to be compromised.

Treatment

A. CHRONIC ASTHMA

1. General measures—Patients should avoid exposure to tobacco smoke and allergens to which they are sensitized, exertion outdoors when levels of air pollution are high, β-blockers, and sulfite-containing foods. Patients with persistent asthma should be given the inactivated influenza vaccine yearly unless they have a contraindication.

For patients with persistent asthma, the clinician should use the patient's history to assess sensitivity to seasonal allergens and *Alternaria* mold; use skin testing or in vitro testing to assess sensitivity to perennial indoor allergens; assess the significance of positive tests in the context of the patient's history; and identify relevant allergen exposures. For dust mite-allergic children, important environmental control measures include encasing the pillow and mattress in an allergen-impermeable cover and washing the sheets and blankets on the patient's bed weekly in hot water. Other measures include keeping indoor humidity below 50%, minimizing the number of stuffed toys, and washing such toys weekly in hot water. Children allergic to furred animals or feathers should avoid indoor exposure to pets, especially for prolonged periods of time. If removal of the pet is not possible, the animal should be kept out of the bedroom with the door closed. Carpeting and upholstered furniture should be removed. While a high-efficiency particle-arresting filter unit in the bedroom may reduce allergen levels, clinical symptoms may persist if the pet remains indoors. For cockroach-allergic children, control measures need to be instituted when infestation is present in the home. Poison baits, boric acid, and traps are preferred to chemical agents, which can be irritating if inhaled by asthmatic individuals. Indoor molds are especially prominent in humid environments or in homes with dampness. Measures to control dampness or fungal growth in the home may be of benefit. Patients can reduce exposure to outdoor allergens by staying in an air-conditioned environment. Allergen immunotherapy may be useful for implicated aeroallergens that cannot be avoided. However, it should be administered only in facilities staffed and equipped to treat life-threatening reactions.

The patient and family must understand the role of asthma triggers, the importance of disease activity even without obvious symptoms, how to use objective measures to gauge disease activity, and the importance of airway inflammation—and they must learn to recognize the warning signs of worsening asthma, allowing for early intervention. A stepwise care plan should be developed for all patients with asthma. This educational process extends to school personnel and all those who care for children with asthma.

Because the degree of airflow limitation is poorly perceived by many patients, peak flow meters can aid in the assessment of airflow obstruction and day-to-day disease activity. Peak flow rates may provide early warning of worsening asthma. They are also helpful in monitoring the effects of medication changes. Spacer devices optimize delivery of medication from metered-dose inhalers to the lungs and, with inhaled steroids, minimize side effects. Large-volume spacers are preferred.

Patients should be treated for rhinitis, sinusitis, or gastroesophageal reflux, if present. Treatment of upper respiratory tract symptoms is an integral part of asthma man-

Table 34–2. Stepwise approach for treating infants and young children (5 years of age and younger) with acute or chronic asthma.

Classify Severity: Clinical Features Before Treatment or Adequate Control	Symptoms/Day Symptoms/Night	Medications Required to Maintain Long-Term Control Daily Medications
Step 4: Severe persistent	Continual Frequent	Preferred treatment: 　High-dose inhaled corticosteroids 　AND 　Long-acting inhaled β_2-agonists 　AND, if needed, 　Corticosteroid tablets or syrup long term (2 mg/kg/d generally do not exceed 60 mg/d). (Make repeat attempts to reduce systemic corticosteroids and maintain control with high-dose inhaled corticosteroids.)
Step 3: Moderate persistent	Daily >1 night/wk	Preferred treatments: 　Low-dose inhaled corticosteroids and long-acting inhaled β_2-agonists 　OR 　Medium-dose inhaled corticosteroids. Alternative treatment: 　Low-dose inhaled corticosteroids and either leukotriene receptor antagonist or theophylline. If needed (particularly in patients with recurring severe exacerbations). Preferred treatment: 　Medium-dose inhaled corticosteroids and long-acting β_2-agonists. Alternative treatment: 　Medium-dose inhaled corticosteroids and either leukotriene receptor antagonist or theophylline.
Step 2: Mild persistent	>2/wk but <1/d >2 nights/mo	Preferred treatment: 　Low-dose inhaled corticosteroid (with nebulizer or MDI with holding chamber with or without face mask or DPI). Alternative treatment (listed alphabetically): 　Cromolyn (nebulizer is preferred or MDI with holding chamber) 　OR leukotriene receptor antagonist.
Step 1: Mild intermittent	≤2 d/wk ≤2 nights/mo	No daily medication needed.
All patients		Bronchodilator as needed for symptoms ≤ 2 times a week. Intensity of treatment will depend upon severity of exacerbation. 　Preferred treatment: Inhaled short-acting β_2-agonist by nebulizer or face mask and space-holding chamber 　Alternative treatment: Oral β_2-agonist With viral respiratory infection 　Bronchodilator q4–6h up to 24 h (longer with physician consult); in general no more than once every 6 wk 　Consider systemic corticosteroid if exacerbation is severe or patient has history of previous severe exacerbations Use of short-acting β_2-agonist daily indicates the need to initiate or increase long-term control therapy
Step down		Review treatment every 1–6 mos; a gradual stepwise reduction in treatment may be possible.
Step up		If control is not maintained, consider step up. First, review patient medication technique, adherence, and environmental control.

(continued)

Table 34–2. Stepwise approach for treating infants and young children (5 years of age and younger) with acute or chronic asthma. (continued)

Minimal or no chronic symptoms day or night
Minimal or no exacerbations
No limitations on activities; no school/parent's work missed
Minimal use of inhaled short-acting β_2-agonist (< 1/d, < 1 canister/mo)
Minimal or no adverse effects from medications

Notes

The stepwise approach is intended to assist, not replace, the clinical decision making required to meet individual patient needs.
Classify severity: assign patient to most severe step in which any feature occurs.
There are very few studies on asthma therapy for infants.
Gain control as quickly as possible (a course of short systemic corticosteroids may be required); then step down to the least medication necessary to maintain control.
Provide parent education on asthma management and controlling environmental factors that make asthma worse (eg, allergies and irritants).
Consultation with an asthma specialist is recommended for patients with moderate or severe persistent asthma. Consider consultation for patients with mild persistent asthma.
Reprinted, with permission, from the National Asthma Education and Prevention Program: *Expert Panel Report: Update on Selected Topics 2002.*

agement. Intranasal corticosteroids are recommended to treat chronic rhinitis in patients with persistent asthma because they reduce lower-airway hyperresponsiveness and asthma symptoms. Intranasal cromolyn reduces asthma symptoms during the ragweed season but less so than intranasal corticosteroids. Treatment of sinusitis includes medical measures to promote drainage and the use of antibiotics for acute bacterial infections. Medical management of gastroesophageal reflux includes avoiding eating or drinking 2 hours before bedtime, elevating the head of the bed with 6- to 8-inch blocks, and using appropriate pharmacologic therapy.

2. Pharmacologic therapy—A revised stepwise approach to pharmacologic therapy is recommended in the National Asthma Education and Prevention Program's *Expert Panel Report: Update on Selected Topics 2002* (www.nhlbi.nih. gov) (Tables 34–2 and 34–3). The choice of therapy is based on assessment of clinical features prior to treatment. The following key issues regarding pediatric asthma are discussed or updated compared with the 1997 guidelines:

1. Use of inhaled corticosteroids as the preferred treatment for mild or moderate persistent asthma.

2. Initiation of long-term controller therapy in infants or children who have risk factors for asthma (parental history of asthma or physician-diagnosed atopic dermatitis or two of the following: physician-diagnosed allergic rhinitis, wheezing apart from colds, or peripheral eosinophilia) with more than three episodes of wheezing over the past year that lasted longer than one day and affected sleep.

3. Benefits of inhaled corticosteroids at recommended doses (Table 34–4) versus potential risks.

4. Use of combination therapy including addition of long-acting inhaled β_2-agonists to low-to-medium doses of inhaled corticosteroids as the preferred treatment for children older than 5 years with moderate persistent asthma and either addition of long-acting inhaled β_2-agonists to a low dose of inhaled corticosteroids or medium-dose inhaled corticosteroids as monotherapy in children 5 years of age or younger. The preferred strategy is to initiate therapy at a higher level at the onset to gain prompt control and then step down, rather than gradually stepping up treatment if control is not achieved. A rescue course of systemic corticosteroids may be necessary at any step. A short course of systemic corticosteroids may be required for patients with intermittent asthma who experience infrequent but severe exacerbations—typically triggered by respiratory infections—with normal lung function between episodes.

Asthma medications are classified as long-term control medications and quick-relief medications. The former include anti-inflammatory agents, long-acting bronchodilators, and leukotriene modifiers. Inhaled corticosteroids delivered by aerosol, dry powder inhaler, or nebulizer are the most potent inhaled anti-inflammatory agents currently available. Recent data suggest that different inhaled corticosteroids are not equivalent on a per puff or microgram basis (see Table 34–4). Early intervention with inhaled corticosteroids can improve asthma control and may prevent airway remodeling. Inhaled corticosteroids may be associated with slowing of growth velocity in children, although a study of asthmatic children treated with budesonide (mean dose 412 μg/d) for a mean of 9.2 years showed no adverse

Table 34–3. Stepwise approach for managing asthma in adults and children older than 5 years of age: treatment.

Classify Severity: Clinical Features Before Treatment or Adequate Control			Medications Required to Maintain Long-Term Control
	Symptoms/Day ___ Symptoms/Night	PEF or FEV$_1$ PEF Variability	**Daily Medications**
Step 4: Severe persistent	Continual ___ Frequent	≤60% ___ >30%	**Preferred treatment:** High-dose inhaled corticosteroids AND Long-acting inhaled β$_2$-agonists AND, if needed, Corticosteroid tablets or syrup long term (2 mg/kg/d, generally do not exceed 60 mg/d). (Make repeat attempts to reduce systemic corticosteroids and maintain control with high-dose inhaled corticosteroids.)
Step 3: Moderate persistent	Daily ___ >1 night/wk	>60% – <80% ___ >30%	**Preferred treatment:** Low-to-medium dose inhaled corticosteroids and long-acting inhaled β$_2$-agonists Alternative treatment: Increase inhaled corticosteroids within medium-dose range OR Low-to-medium dose inhaled corticosteroids and either leukotriene modifier or theophylline. If needed (particularly in patients with recurring severe exacerbations): **Preferred treatment:** Increase inhaled corticosteroids within medium-dose range, and add long-acting inhaled β$_2$-agonists. Alternative treatment (listed alphabetically): Increase inhaled corticosteroids in medium-dose range, and add either leukotriene modifier or theophylline.
Step 2: Mild persistent	>2/wk but <1/d ___ >2 nights/mo	≥80% ___ 20 – 30%	**Preferred treatment:** Low-dose inhaled corticosteroids Alternative treatment (listed alphabetically): cromolyn, leukotriene modifier, nedocromil, OR sustained release theophylline to serum concentration of 5–15 µg/mL.
Step 1: Mild intermittent	≤2 d/wk ___ ≤2 nights/mo	≥80% ___ <20%	No daily medication needed. Severe exacerbations may occur, separated by long periods of normal lung function and no symptoms. A course of systemic corticosteroids is recommended.
All patients	Short-acting bronchodilator: 2–4 puffs short-acting inhaled β$_2$-agonists as needed for symptoms. Intensity of treatment will depend on severity of exacerbation: up to 3 treatments at 20-min intervals or a single nebulizer treatment as needed. Course of systemic corticosteroids may be needed. Use of short-acting inhaled β$_2$-agonists on a daily basis, or increasing use, indicates the need to initiate or increase long-term control therapy.		
Step down	Review treatment every 1–6 mos; a gradual stepwise reduction in treatment may be possible.		
Step up	If control is not maintained, consider step up. First, review patient medication technique, adherence, and environmental control.		

(continued)

Table 34–3. Stepwise approach for managing asthma in adults and children older than 5 years of age: treatment. (continued)

Minimal or no chronic symptoms day or night
Minimal or no exacerbations
No limitations on activities; no school/parent's work missed
Minimal use of inhaled short-acting β_2-agonist (< 1/d, < 1 canister/mo)
Minimal or no adverse effects from medications

Notes

The stepwise approach is intended to assist, not replace, the clinical decision making required to meet individual patient needs.

Classify severity: assign patient to most severe step in which any feature occurs (PEF is % of personal best; FEV_1 is % predicted).

Gain control as quickly as possible (consider a short course of systemic corticosteroids); then step down to the least medication necessary to maintain control.

Provide education on self-management and controlling environmental factors that make asthma worse (e.g., allergens and irritants).

Refer to an asthma specialist if there are difficulties controlling asthma or if step 4 care is required. Referral may be considered if step 3 care is required.

Reprinted with permission. (See Table 34–2).

effect on final adult height. Possible risks from inhaled corticosteroids need to be weighed against the risks from undertreated asthma. Only inhaled corticosteroids have been shown to be effective in long-term clinical studies with infants. Nebulized budesonide is approved for children as young as 12 months. The suspension (available in quantities of 0.25 mg/2 mL and 0.5 mg/2 mL) is usually administered at 0.5 mg/d, either once or twice a day in divided doses. Notably, this drug should not be given by ultrasonic nebulizer. Limited data suggest that inhaled corticosteroids may be effective even in

very young children when delivered by metered-dose inhaler with a spacer with mask.

Fewer data are available with nedocromil, although comparative data from the Childhood Asthma Management Program study showed that an inhaled corticosteroid was superior to nedocromil with respect to a number of efficacy parameters, including rate of hospitalization, symptom-free days, need for albuterol rescue, and longer time to treatment with prednisone.

Sustained-release theophylline, an alternative long-term control medication for older children, may have particular risks of adverse side effects in infants, who

Table 34–4. Estimated comparative daily dosages for inhaled corticosteroids.

Drug	Low Daily Dose Child	Medium Daily Dose Child	High Daily Dose Child
Beclomethasone CFC 42 or 84 µg/puff	84–336 µg	336–672 µg	> 672 µg
Beclomethasone HFA 40 or 80 µg/puff	80–160 µg	160–320 µg	> 320 µg
Budesonide DPI 200 µg/inhalation	200–400 µg	400–800 µg	> 800 µg
Budesonide suspension for nebulization (child dose)	0.5 mg	1.0 mg	2.0 mg
Flunisolide 250 µg/puff	500–750 µg	1000–1250 µg	> 1250 µg
Fluticasone HFA: 44, 110, or 220 µg/puff DPI: 50, 100, or 250 µg/inhalation	88–176 µg	176–440 µg	> 440 µg
Triamcinolone acetonide 100 µg/puff	400–800 µg	800–1200 µg	> 1200 µg

Mometasone DPI 220 µg/inhalation: Initial therapy 220 µg daily, up to 440 µg/day as single or divided dose; for patients on oral corticosteroids: 440 µg twice daily (maximum 880 µg/day).

frequently have febrile illnesses that increase theophylline concentrations.

Salmeterol, a long-acting β_2-agonist, is available as an inhalation powder (1 inhalation twice daily for patients age 4 years and older). Salmeterol can be used as adjunctive therapy with anti-inflammatory medications for long-term symptom control. Salmeterol should not be used for treatment of acute symptoms, and anti-inflammatory medication should not be discontinued when salmeterol is initiated, even if the patient feels better. Salmeterol, 50 µg, is available combined with fluticasone (100, 250, or 500 µg) in a dry powder inhaler. For children 12 years and older, one inhalation is taken twice daily. (**Note:** The 100/50 fluticasone/salmeterol combination is approved in children age 4 and older.) It can also be used 30 minutes before exercise (but not in addition to regularly used long-acting β_2-agonists). Formoterol is another long-acting β_2-agonist with a more rapid onset of action in a dry powder inhaler. It is approved for use in children 5 years and older, one inhalation (12 µg) twice daily. For long-term control, it should be used in combination with an anti-inflammatory agent. It can be used for exercise-induced bronchospasm in patients 5 years and older, 1 inhalation at least 15 minutes before exercise (but not in addition to regularly used long-acting β_2-agonists). Of note, the Food and Drug Administration has requested the manufacturers of Advair Diskus (salmeterol and fluticasone), Serevent Diskus (salmeterol xinafoate) and Foradil Aerolizer (formoterol fumarate) to update their product information warning sections regarding an increase in severe asthma episodes associated with these agents. This action is in response to data showing an increased number of asthma-related deaths in patients receiving long-acting β_2-agonist therapy in addition to their usual asthma care as compared to patients not receiving long-acting β_2-agonists. This notice is also intended to reinforce the appropriate use of long-acting β_2-agonists in the management of asthma. Specifically, long-acting β_2-agonist products should not be initiated as first-line asthma therapy, used with worsening wheezing, or used for acute control of bronchospasm. No data is available regarding safety concerns in patients using these products for exercise-induced bronchoconstriction. Additional information including copies of the Patient and Healthcare Professional information sheets can be found at: http://www.fda.gov/cder/drug/infopage/LABA/default.htm

Montelukast and zafirlukast are leukotriene-receptor antagonists available in oral formulations. Montelukast is given once daily and has been approved for children age 1 year and older. To date, no drug interactions have been noted. The dosage is 4 mg for children 1–5 years (oral granules are available for children 12–23 months), 5 mg for children age 6–14 years, and 10 mg for those age 15 years and older. The drug is given without regard to mealtimes, preferably in the evening. Zafirlukast is approved for patients age 5 years and older. The dose is 10 mg twice daily for 5–11 years and 20 mg twice daily for 12 years and older. It should be taken 1 hour before or 2 hours after meals. Zileuton is a 5-lipoxygenase inhibitor indicated for chronic treatment in children 12 years of age and older, 600 mg 4 times/day. Patients need to have their hepatic transaminases evaluated at initiation of therapy then once a month for the first 3 months, every 2–3 months for the remainder of the first year, and periodically thereafter for those receiving long-term zileuton therapy. Rare cases of Churg–Strauss syndrome in adult patients with severe asthma whose steroids were being tapered have been reported with concomitant treatment with leukotriene-receptor antagonists (but also with inhaled corticosteroids), and no causal link has been established. Of note, in a study of children with mild-to-moderate persistent asthma that looked at whether responses to inhaled steroids and leukotriene-receptor antagonists are concordant for individuals or whether asthmatic patients who do not respond to one medication respond to the other, response to fluticasone and montelukast were found to vary considerably. Children with low pulmonary function or high levels of markers associated with allergic inflammation responded better to the inhaled steroid.

Quick-relief medications include short-acting inhaled β_2-agonists such as albuterol, pirbuterol, or terbutaline, 1–2 puffs by inhaler. Albuterol HFA contains a nonchlorofluorocarbon propellant. Albuterol can be given by nebulizer, 0.05 mg/kg (with a minimal dose of 1.25 mg and a maximum of 2.5 mg) in 2–3 mL saline (although it is also available in a 0.63 mg/3 mL and 1.25 mg/3 mL dosing). It is better to use β_2-agonists as needed rather than on a regular basis. Increasing use, including more than one canister per month, may signify inadequate asthma control and the need to intensify anti-inflammatory therapy. Levalbuterol, the (R)-enantiomer of racemic albuterol, is available in solution for nebulization for patients age 6–11 years 0.31 mg three times a day and for patients 12 years and older 0.63–1.25 mg three times a day. It has recently become available in an HFA formulation for children 4 years and older, 2 inhalations (90 µg) every 4–6 hours as needed. Anticholinergic agents such as ipratropium, 1–3 puffs or 0.25–0.5 mg by nebulizer every 6 hours, may provide additive benefit when used together with inhaled β_2-agonists. Systemic corticosteroids such as prednisone, prednisolone, and methylprednisolone can be given in a dosage of 1–2 mg/kg, usually up to 60 mg/d in single or divided doses for 3–10 days. There is no evidence that tapering the dose following a "burst" prevents relapse.

Anti-IgE (omalizumab) is a recombinant DNA-derived humanized IgG_1 monoclonal antibody that selectively binds to human IgE. It inhibits the binding of IgE to the high-affinity IgE receptor (FcεRI) on the surface of mast cells and basophils. Reduction in surface-bound IgE on FcεRI-bearing cells limits the degree of release of mediators of the allergic response. Treatment with omalizumab also reduces the number of FcεRI receptors on basophils in atopic patients. Omalizumab is indicated for patients 12 years of age and older with moderate to severe persistent asthma who have a positive skin test or in vitro reactivity to a perennial aeroallergen with serum IgE $\leq$ 700 IU/mL and whose symptoms are inadequately controlled with inhaled corticosteroids. Omalizumab has been shown to decrease the incidence of asthma exacerbations in these patients. Dosing is based on the patient's weight and serum IgE level and is given subcutaneously every 2–4 weeks. Continual monitoring is necessary to ensure that control of asthma is achieved and sustained. Once control is established, gradual reduction in therapy is appropriate and may help determine the minimum amount of medication necessary to maintain control. Regular follow-up visits with the clinician are important to assess the degree of control and consider appropriate adjustments in therapy. At each step, patients should be instructed to avoid or control exposure to allergens, irritants, or other factors that contribute to asthma severity. Referral to an asthma specialist for consultation or co-management is recommended if there are difficulties in achieving or maintaining control or if the patient has severe persistent asthma. Referral is also recommended if allergen immunotherapy is being considered.

Referral may be considered for patients with moderate persistent asthma. For children younger than age 3 years, referral is recommended if the patient requires step 3 or 4 care and should be considered if the patient requires step 2 care (see Table 34–3).

3. Exercise-induced bronchospasm—Exercise-induced bronchospasm should be anticipated in all asthma patients. It typically occurs during or minutes after vigorous activity, reaches its peak 5–10 minutes after stopping the activity, and usually resolves over the next 20–30 minutes. Participation in physical activity should be encouraged in children with asthma, although the choice of activity may need to be modified based on the severity of illness, triggers such as cold air, and, rarely, confounding factors such as osteoporosis. Treatment immediately prior to vigorous activity or exercise is usually effective. Short-acting inhaled β_2-

agonists, cromolyn, or nedocromil can be used before exercise. The combination of a short-acting inhaled β_2-agonist with either cromolyn or nedocromil is more effective than either drug alone. Salmeterol and formoterol may block exercise-induced bronchospasm for up to 12 hours (as discussed earlier). Montelukast may be effective up to 24 hours. Occasionally an extended warm-up period may induce a refractory state, allowing patients to exercise without a need for repeat medications. If symptoms occur during usual play activities, a step-up in long-term therapy is warranted. Poor endurance or exercise-induced bronchospasm can be an indication of poorly controlled persistent asthma.

B. Acute Asthma

1. General measures—The most effective strategy in managing asthma exacerbations involves early recognition of warning signs and early treatment. For patients with moderate or severe persistent asthma or a history of severe exacerbations, this should include a written action plan. The latter usually defines the patient's peak flow zones and what steps to take if peak flows are between 50% and 80% or below 50% of personal best. The child, parents, and other caregivers must be able to assess asthma severity accurately. Prompt communication with the clinician is indicated with severe symptoms or a drop in peak flow or with decreased response to short-acting inhaled β_2-agonists. At such times, intensification of therapy may include a short course of oral corticosteroids. The child should be removed from exposure to any irritants or allergens that could be contributing to the exacerbation.

2. Management at home—Early treatment of asthma exacerbations may prevent progression to severe disease. Initial treatment should be with a short-acting inhaled β_2-agonist such as albuterol; 2–4 puffs from a metered-dose inhaler can be given every 20 minutes up to three times, or a single treatment can be given by nebulizer (0.05 mg/kg; minimum 1.25 mg, maximum 2.5 mg of 0.5% solution of albuterol in 2–3 mL saline). If the response is good as assessed by sustained symptom relief or improvement in PEFR to over 80% of the patient's best, the short-acting β_2-agonist can be continued every 3–4 hours for 24–48 hours. For patients taking inhaled corticosteroids, the dose may be doubled for 7–10 days. If the patient does not completely improve from the initial therapy, with PEFR between 50% and 80%, the β_2-agonist should be continued, an oral corticosteroid should be added, and the patient should contact the physician. If the child experiences marked distress or if PEFR persists at under 50%, the patient should repeat the β_2-agonist immediately and go to the emergency department or call 911 or another emergency number for assistance.

3. Management in the office or emergency department—Functional assessment of the patient includes obtaining objective measures of airflow limitation with PEFR or FEV_1 and monitoring the patient's response to treatment. Other tests may include oxygen saturation and blood gases. If the initial FEV_1 or PEFR is over 50%, initial treatment can be with a β_2-agonist by inhaler (albuterol, 4–8 puffs) or nebulizer (0.15 mg/kg of albuterol 0.5% solution, minimum dose 2.5 mg), up to three doses in the first hour. Oxygen should be given to maintain oxygen saturation at greater than 90%. Oral corticosteroids (1 mg/kg every 6 hours for 48 hours, then 1–2 mg/kg/d in divided doses, maximum 60 mg/d) should be instituted if the patient responds poorly to therapy or if the patient has recently been on oral corticosteroids. Sensitivity to adrenergic drugs may improve after initiation of corticosteroids. If the initial FEV_1 or PEFR is under 50%, initial treatment should be with a high-dose β_2-agonist by nebulizer every 20 minutes or continuously for the first hour (0.5 mg/kg/h). Ipratropium can be added to albuterol, 0.25 mg every 20 minutes for three doses, then every 2–4 hours. Oxygen should be given to maintain oxygen saturation at greater than 90%, and systemic corticosteroids should be instituted. For patients with severe asthma unresponsive to initial aerosolized therapy, or for those who cannot cooperate with or who resist inhalation therapy, epinephrine 1:1000 or terbutaline 1 mg/mL (both 0.01 mg/kg up to 0.3–0.5 mg) may be administered subcutaneously every 20 minutes for three doses. The role of theophylline or aminophylline remains questionable when added to optimal β_2-agonist therapy and may be associated with adverse events. For impending or ongoing respiratory arrest, patients should be intubated and ventilated with 100% oxygen and admitted to an intensive care unit. (See Asthma [life-threatening] in Chapter 13.) Further treatment is based on clinical response and objective laboratory findings. Hospitalization should be considered strongly for any patient with a history of respiratory failure.

4. Hospital management—For patients who do not respond to outpatient therapy, admission to the hospital becomes necessary for more aggressive care and support. Fluids should be given at maintenance requirements unless the patient has poor oral intake secondary to respiratory distress or vomiting, because overhydration may contribute to pulmonary edema associated with high intrapleural pressures generated in severe asthma. Potassium requirements should be kept in mind because both corticosteroids and β_2-agonists can cause potassium loss. Moisturized oxygen should be titrated by oximetry to maintain Sao_2 above 90%. Inhaled β_2-agonist should be continued by nebulization in single doses as needed or by continuous therapy, along with ipratropium and systemic corticosteroids (as discussed earlier). In addition, the role of methylxanthines in hospitalized children remains controversial. Antibiotics may be necessary to treat coexisting bacterial infection. Sedatives and anxiolytic agents are contraindicated in severely ill patients owing to their depressant effects on respiration. Chest physiotherapy is usually not recommended for acute exacerbations.

5. Patient discharge—Criteria for discharging patients home from the office or emergency department should include a sustained response of at least 1 hour to bronchodilator therapy with FEV_1 or PEFR greater than 70% and oxygen saturation greater than 90% in room air. Prior to discharge, the patient's or caregiver's ability to continue therapy and assess symptoms appropriately needs to be considered. Patients should be given an action plan for management of recurrent symptoms or exacerbations, and instructions about medications should be reviewed. The inhaled β_2-agonist and oral corticosteroids should be continued, the latter for 3–10 days. Finally, the patient or caregiver should be instructed about the follow-up visit, typically within 1 week. Hospitalized patients should receive more intensive education prior to discharge. Referral to an asthma specialist should be considered for all children with severe exacerbations or multiple emergency department visits or hospitalizations.

Prognosis

Since the 1970s, morbidity and mortality rates for asthma have increased. Mortality statistics indicate that a high percentage of deaths have resulted from underrecognition of asthma severity and undertreatment, particularly in labile asthmatic patients and in asthmatic patients whose perception of pulmonary obstruction is poor. Long-term outcome studies suggest that children with mild symptoms generally outgrow their asthma, while patients with more severe symptoms, marked airway hyperresponsiveness, and a greater degree of atopy tend to have persistent disease. In a recently published unselected birth cohort from New Zealand, more than one in four children had wheezing that persisted from childhood to adulthood or that relapsed after remission. It is possible that early intervention with anti-inflammatory therapy and environmental control measures may alter the natural history of childhood asthma. In this respect, the pediatrician or primary care provider together with the asthma specialist has a critical opportunity to affect the course of this increasingly common disease.

Resources for health care providers, patients, and families:

Asthma and Allergy Foundation of America
1233 20th St NW, Suite 402
Washington, DC 20036; (800) 7-ASTHMA
http://www.aafa.org/

Asthma and Allergy Network/Mothers of Asthmatics
2751 Prosperity Avenue, Suite 150
Fairfax, VA 22031; (800) 878-4403
http://www.aanma.org/
Lung Line (800) 222-LUNG

Bacharier LB et al; Classifying asthma severity in children. Mismatch between symptoms, medication use, and lung function. Am J Respir Crit Care Med 2004;170:426 [PMID: 15172893].

Bacharier, LB: Pets and childhood asthma—How should the pediatrician respond to new information that pets may prevent asthma? Pediatrics 2003;112:974 [PMID: 14523195].

Holgate S et al: The anti-inflammatory effects of omalizumab confirm the central role of IgE in allergic inflammation. J Allergy Clin Immunol 2005;115:459 [PMID: 15753888].

Liu AH et al: Advances in childhood asthma: Hygiene hypothesis, natural history, and management. J Allergy Clin Immunol 2003;111:S785 [PMID: 12612244].

Morgan WJ et al: Results of a home-based environmental intervention among urban children with asthma. N Engl J Med 2004; 351:1068. [PMID: 15356304].

National Asthma Education and Prevention Program: *Guidelines for the Diagnosis and Management of Asthma—Update on Selected Topics 2002.* NIH publication No. 02-5075. www.nhlbi.nih.gov

Sears MR et al: A longitudinal, population-based, cohort study of childhood asthma followed to adulthood. N Engl J Med 2003;349:1414 [PMID: 14523172].

Smith AD et al: Use of exhaled nitric oxide measurements to guide treatment in chronic asthma. N Engl J Med 2005;352:2163 [PMID; 15914548].

Spahn JD et al: Is forced expiratory volume in one second the best measure of severity in childhood asthma? Am J Respir Crit Care Med 2004;169:784 [PMID: 14754761].

Szefler SJ et al: Characterization of within-subject responses to fluticasone and montelukast in childhood asthma. J Allergy Clin Immunol 2005;115:233 [PMID: 15696076].

■ ALLERGIC RHINOCONJUNCTIVITIS

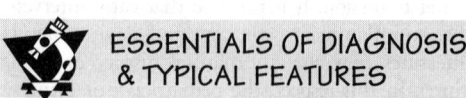

ESSENTIALS OF DIAGNOSIS & TYPICAL FEATURES

After exposure to allergen:

• *Sneezing.*

• *Itching of nose and eyes.*

• *Clear rhinorrhea or nasal congestion.*

General Considerations

Allergic rhinoconjunctivitis is the most common allergic disease and significantly affects quality of life as well as school performance and attendance. It frequently coexists with asthma and is a risk factor for subsequent development of asthma. Prevalence of this disease increases during childhood, peaking at 15% in the postadolescent years. Although allergic rhinoconjunctivitis is more common in boys during early childhood, there is little difference in incidence between the sexes after adolescence. Race and socioeconomic status are not considered to be important factors.

The pathologic changes in allergic rhinoconjunctivitis are chiefly hyperemia, edema, and increased serous and mucoid secretions caused by mediator release, all of which lead to variable degrees of nasal obstruction, pruritus, and rhinorrhea. This process may involve the eyes and other structures, including the sinuses and possibly the middle ear. Inhalant allergens are primarily responsible for symptoms, but food allergens can cause symptoms as well. Children with allergic rhinitis seem to be more susceptible to—or at least may experience more symptoms from—upper respiratory infections, which, in turn, may aggravate the allergic rhinitis.

Allergic rhinoconjunctivitis may be perennial, seasonal (hay fever), or episodic. Perennial allergic rhinitis occurs to some degree all year long but may be more severe in winter. Greater exposure to indoor allergens results from well-insulated homes, an increase in the amount of time spent indoors, and heating systems that disperse the allergens. Seasonal allergic rhinitis occurs as a result of exposure to specific aeroallergens, including pollens and molds. The major pollen groups in the temperate zones include trees (late winter to early spring), grasses (late spring to early summer), and weeds (late summer to early fall), but seasons can vary significantly in different parts of the country. Mold spores also cause seasonal allergic rhinitis, principally in the summer and fall. Seasonal allergy symptoms may be aggravated by coincident exposure to perennial allergens.

Clinical Findings

A. SYMPTOMS AND SIGNS

Patients may complain of itching of the nose, eyes, palate, or pharynx. Nasal itching can cause paroxysmal sneezing and epistaxis. Repeated rubbing of the nose (so-called allergic salute) may lead to a horizontal crease across the lower third of the nose. Nasal obstruction is associated with mouth breathing, nasal speech, allergic salute, and snoring. Nasal turbinates may appear pale blue and swollen, with dimpling, or injected, with minimal edema. Typically, clear and thin nasal secretions are increased, with anterior rhinorrhea, sniffling, postnasal drip, and congested cough. Nasal secretions often cause poor appetite, fatigue, and pharyngeal irritation. Conjunctival injection, tearing, periorbital edema, and infraorbital cyanosis (so-called allergic shiners) are frequently observed. Increased pharyngeal lymphoid tissue ("cobblestoning") from chronic drainage and enlarged tonsillar and adenoidal tissue may be present.

B. LABORATORY FINDINGS

Eosinophilia often can be demonstrated on smears of nasal secretions or blood. This is a frequent but nonspecific finding and may occur in nonallergic conditions. Although serum IgE may be elevated, measurement of total IgE is a poor screening tool owing to the wide overlap between atopic and nonatopic subjects. Skin testing to identify allergen-specific IgE is the most sensitive and specific test for inhalant allergies; alternatively, radioallergosorbent assay test (RAST), ImmunoCAP, or other in vitro tests can be done for suspected allergens.

Differential Diagnosis

Disorders that need to be differentiated from allergic rhinitis include infectious rhinitis and sinusitis. Foreign bodies and structural abnormalities such as choanal atresia, marked septal deviation, nasal polyps, and adenoidal hypertrophy may cause chronic symptoms. Overuse of topical nasal decongestants may result in rhinitis medicamentosa (rebound congestion). Use of medications such as propranolol, clonidine, and some psychoactive drugs may cause nasal congestion. Illicit drugs like cocaine can cause rhinorrhea. Spicy or hot foods may cause gustatory rhinitis. Nonallergic rhinitis with eosinophilia syndrome is usually not seen in young children. Vasomotor rhinitis is associated with persistent symptoms but without allergen exposure. Less common causes of symptoms that may be confused with allergic rhinitis include pregnancy, congenital syphilis, hypothyroidism, tumors, and cerebrospinal fluid rhinorrhea.

Complications

Sinusitis may accompany allergic rhinitis. Allergic mucosal swelling of the sinus ostia can obstruct sinus drainage, interfering with normal sinus function and predisposing to chronic mucosal disease. Nasal polyps due to allergy are unusual in children, and cystic fibrosis should be considered if they are present.

Treatment

A. GENERAL MEASURES

The value of identification and avoidance of causative allergens cannot be overstated. Reducing indoor allergens through environmental control measures as discussed in the section on asthma can be very effective. Nasal saline irrigation may be useful.

B. PHARMACOLOGIC THERAPY

1. Antihistamines—Antihistamines help control itching, sneezing, and rhinorrhea. Sedating antihistamines include diphenhydramine, chlorpheniramine, hydroxyzine, and clemastine. Sedating antihistamines may cause daytime somnolence and negatively affect school performance and other activities, especially driving. Second-generation antihistamines include loratadine, desloratadine, cetirizine, and fexofenadine. Cetirizine is approved for use in children age 6–23 months (2.5 mg daily), 2–5 years (2.5–5.0 mg/d or 2.5 mg twice a day), and 6 years or older (5–10 mg/d). Loratadine is approved for use in children age 2–5 years (5 mg/d) and 6 years or older (10 mg/d), and is available without prescription in tablet, rapidly disintegrating tablet, and liquid formulations. Desloratadine is approved for use in children age 6–11 months (1 mg/d), 1–5 years (1.25 mg/d), and for 12 years and older (5 mg/d). Fexofenadine is approved for children age 6–11 years (30 mg twice a day) and 12 years or older (60 mg twice a day or 180 mg once daily). Loratadine, fexofenadine, and cetirizine are available in combination with pseudoephedrine for patients age 12 years or older. Azelastine is available in a nasal spray and levocabastine as an ophthalmic preparation.

2. Decongestants—α-Adrenergic agents help to relieve nasal congestion. Topical decongestants such as phenylephrine and oxymetazoline should not be used for more than 4 days for severe episodes because prolonged use may be associated with rhinitis medicamentosa. Oral decongestants, including pseudoephedrine and phenylpropanolamine, are often combined with antihistamines or expectorants and cough suppressants in over-the-counter cold medications. They may cause insomnia, agitation, tachycardia, and, rarely, cardiac arrhythmias. Of note, the U.S. Food and Drug Administration has recommended the removal of phenylpropanolamine from all drug products due to a public health advisory concerning the risk of hemorrhagic stroke associated with its use.

3. Corticosteroids—Intranasal corticosteroid sprays are effective in controlling allergic rhinitis if used chronically. They are minimally absorbed in usual doses and are available in pressurized nasal inhalers and aqueous sprays. Mometasone nasal spray has been approved for use in children as young as age 2 years (1 spray in each nostril once daily) and in children 12 years or older (2 sprays/nostril once daily). Fluticasone nasal spray is approved for children 4 years or older, and budesonide and triamcinolone nasal sprays are approved for 6 years or older, 1–2 sprays/nostril once daily. Flunisolide is approved for ages 6–14 years 1 spray/nostril three times a day or 2 sprays/nostril twice a day. Side effects include nasal irritation, soreness, and bleeding, although epistaxis occurs commonly in patients with allergic rhinitis if corticosteroids are used chronically. Rarely, they can cause septal perforation. Excessive doses may produce systemic effects, especially if used together with orally inhaled steroids for asthma. Onset of action is within hours, although clinical benefit is usually not observed for a week or more. They may be effective alone or together with antihistamines.

4. Other pharmacologic agents—Montelukast is approved for perennial allergic rhinitis in children 6 months and older (4 mg/d for age 6–23 months) and seasonal allergic rhinitis in children 2 years and older in doses as discussed under the preceding section, Pharmacologic Therapy. Intranasal ipratropium can be used as adjunctive therapy for rhinorrhea. Intranasal cromolyn may be used alone or in conjunction with oral antihistamines and decongestants. It is most effective when used prophylactically, 1–2 sprays per nostril, four times a day. This dose may be tapered if symptom control is achieved. Rarely, patients complain of nasal irritation or burning. Most patients find complying with four-times-daily dosing difficult. Cromolyn is also available in an ophthalmic solution. (See also Chapter 15.) Other ophthalmic mast cell stabilizers include lodoxamide 0.1% solution, 1–2 drops four times a day, and nedocromil, 1–2 drops two times a day. Olopatadine and ketotifen ophthalmic solutions have antihistamine and mast cell-stabilizing actions and can be given to children older than age 3 years as 1 drop twice a day (8 hours apart) and every 8–12 hours, respectively.

C. SURGICAL THERAPY

Surgical procedures, including turbinectomy, polypectomy, and functional endoscopic sinus surgery, are rarely indicated in allergic rhinitis or chronic hyperplastic sinusitis.

D. IMMUNOTHERAPY

Allergen immunotherapy should be considered when symptoms are severe and due to unavoidable exposure to inhalant allergens, especially if symptomatic measures have failed. Immunotherapy is the only form of therapy that may alter the course of the disease. It should not be prescribed by sending the patient's serum to a laboratory where extracts based on in vitro tests are prepared for the patient (ie, the remote practice of allergy). Immunotherapy should be done in a facility where a physician prepared to treat anaphylaxis is present. Patients with concomitant asthma should not receive an injection if their asthma is not under good control (ie, peak flows preinjection are below 80% of personal best), and the patient should wait for 25–30 minutes after an injection before leaving the facility.

Outcomes with single allergen immunotherapy show success rates of approximately 80%. The optimal dura-

tion of therapy is unknown, but data suggest that immunotherapy for 3–5 years may have lasting benefit.

Prognosis

Perennial allergic rhinoconjunctivitis tends to be protracted unless specific allergens can be identified and eliminated from the environment. In seasonal allergic rhinoconjunctivitis, symptoms are usually most severe from adolescence through mid adult life. After moving to a region devoid of problem allergens, patients may be symptom-free for several years, but they can develop new sensitivities to local aeroallergens.

Simons FER: Advances in H1-antihistamines. N Engl J Med 2004; 351:2203 [PMID: 15548781].

■ ATOPIC DERMATITIS

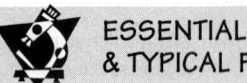

ESSENTIALS OF DIAGNOSIS & TYPICAL FEATURES

- *Pruritus.*
- *Facial and extensor involvement in infants and young children.*
- *Flexural lichenification in older children and adolescents.*
- *Chronic or relapsing dermatitis.*
- *Personal or family history of atopic disease.*

General Considerations

Atopic dermatitis is a chronically relapsing inflammatory skin disease typically associated with respiratory allergy. Over half of patients with atopic dermatitis will develop asthma and allergic rhinitis—often as they outgrow their atopic dermatitis. Atopic dermatitis may result in significant morbidity, leading to school absenteeism, occupational disability, and emotional stress. Atopic dermatitis presents in early childhood, with onset prior to age 5 years in approximately 90% of patients.

Clinical Findings

A. SYMPTOMS AND SIGNS

Atopic dermatitis has no pathognomonic skin lesions or laboratory parameters. Diagnosis is based on the clinical features, including severe pruritus, a chronically relapsing course, and typical morphology and distribution of the skin lesions. Acute atopic dermatitis is characterized by intensely pruritic, erythematous papules associated with excoriations, vesiculations, and serous exudate; subacute atopic dermatitis by erythematous, excoriated, scaling papules; and chronic atopic dermatitis by thickened skin with accentuated markings (lichenification) and fibrotic papules. Patients with chronic atopic dermatitis may have all three types of lesions present concurrently. Patients usually have dry, "lackluster" skin. During infancy, atopic dermatitis involves primarily the face, scalp, and extensor surfaces of the extremities. The diaper area is usually spared. When involved, it may be secondarily infected with *Candida*. In older patients with long-standing disease, the flexural folds of the extremities are the predominant location of lesions.

B. LABORATORY FINDINGS

Identification of allergens involves taking a careful history and performing selective immediate hypersensitivity skin tests or in vitro tests when appropriate. Negative skin tests with proper controls have a high predictive value for ruling out a suspected allergen. Positive skin tests have a lower correlation with clinical symptoms in suspected food allergen-induced atopic dermatitis and should be confirmed with double-blind, placebo-controlled food challenges unless there is a coincidental history of anaphylaxis to the suspected food. Alternatively, specific IgE levels to milk, egg, peanut, and fish proteins have been established with the Pharmacia ImmunoCAP assay correlating with a greater than 95% chance of a clinical reaction.

Elevated serum IgE levels can be demonstrated in 80–85% of patients with atopic dermatitis, and a similar number have positive immediate skin tests or in vitro tests with food and inhalant allergens. A number of well-controlled studies suggest that specific allergens can influence the course of this disease. However, triggers for clinical disease cannot be predicted simply by performing allergy testing. Double-blind, placebo-controlled food challenges show that food allergens can cause exacerbations in a subset of patients with atopic dermatitis. Although lesions induced by single positive challenges are usually transient, repeated challenges, more typical of real-life exposure, can result in eczematous lesions. Furthermore, elimination of food allergens results in amelioration of skin disease and a decrease in spontaneous basophil histamine release. Exacerbation of atopic dermatitis can occur with exposure to aeroallergens such as house dust mites, and environmental control measures have been shown to result in clinical improvement. Patients can make specific IgE directed at *Staphylococcus aureus* toxins secreted on the skin, and this correlates with clinical severity better than total serum IgE levels. Eosinophilia may occur. Routine skin biopsy does not differentiate atopic dermatitis from other eczematous processes and is not usually indicated.

Differential Diagnosis

Scabies can present as a pruritic skin disease. However, distribution in the genital and axillary areas and the presence of linear lesions as well as skin scrapings may help to distinguish it from atopic dermatitis. Seborrheic dermatitis may be distinguished by a lack of significant pruritus; its predilection for the scalp (so-called cradle cap); and its coarse, yellowish scales. Allergic contact dermatitis may be suggested by the distribution of lesions with a greater demarcation of dermatitis than in atopic dermatitis. Occasionally, allergic contact dermatitis superimposed on atopic dermatitis may appear as an acute flare of the underlying disease. Nummular eczema is characterized by coin-shaped plaques. Although unusual in children, mycosis fungoides or cutaneous T-cell lymphoma has been described and is diagnosed by skin biopsy. Eczematous rash has been reported in patients with human immunodeficiency virus (HIV) infection. Other disorders that may resemble atopic dermatitis include Wiskott–Aldrich syndrome, severe combined immunodeficiency disease, hyper-IgE syndrome, zinc deficiency, phenylketonuria, and Letterer–Siwe disease.

Complications

Ocular complications associated with atopic dermatitis can lead to significant morbidity. Atopic keratoconjunctivitis is always bilateral, and symptoms include itching, burning, tearing, and copious mucoid discharge. It is frequently associated with eyelid dermatitis and chronic blepharitis, and may result in visual impairment from corneal scarring. Vernal conjunctivitis is a severe bilateral recurrent chronic inflammatory process of the upper eyelid conjunctiva, occurring primarily in younger patients. (See Chapter 15.) It has a marked seasonal incidence, often in the spring. The associated intense pruritus is exacerbated by exposure to irritants, light, or perspiration. Examination of the eye reveals a papillary hypertrophy or cobblestoning of the upper inner eyelid surface. Keratoconus in atopic dermatitis is believed to result from persistent rubbing of the eyes in patients with atopic dermatitis and allergic rhinitis. Anterior subcapsular cataracts may develop during adolescence or early adult life.

Patients with atopic dermatitis have increased susceptibility to infection or colonization with a variety of organisms. These include viral infections with herpes simplex, molluscum contagiosum, and human papillomavirus. Of note, even a past history of atopic dermatitis is considered a contraindication for receiving the current smallpox (vaccinia) vaccine. Superimposed dermatophytosis may cause atopic dermatitis to flare.

S aureus can be cultured from the skin of more than 90% of patients with atopic dermatitis, compared with only 5% of normal subjects. Patients with atopic dermatitis often have toxin-secreting *S aureus* cultured from their skin. These patients make specific IgE antibodies directed against the toxins found on their skin. *S aureus* toxins can act as superantigens, contributing to persistent inflammation or exacerbations of atopic dermatitis. In addition, patients with atopic dermatitis may be predisposed to colonization and infections by *S aureus* and other microbial organisms due to decreased synthesis of antimicrobial peptides in the skin, which may be mediated by increased levels of TH2-type cytokines. Patients without obvious superinfection may show a better response to combined antistaphylococcal and topical corticosteroid therapy than to corticosteroids alone. Although recurrent staphylococcal pustulosis can be a significant problem in atopic dermatitis, invasive *S aureus* infections occur rarely and should raise the possibility of an immunodeficiency such as hyper-IgE syndrome.

Patients with atopic dermatitis often have a nonspecific hand dermatitis. This is frequently irritating in nature and aggravated by repeated wetting, especially in the occupational setting.

Nutritional disturbances may result from unwarranted and unnecessarily vigorous dietary restrictions imposed by physicians and parents.

Poor academic performance and behavioral disturbances may be a result of uncontrolled intense or frequent itching, sleep loss, and poor self-image. Severe disease may lead to problems with social interactions and self-esteem.

Treatment

A. GENERAL MEASURES

Patients with atopic dermatitis have a lowered threshold of irritant responsiveness. Avoidance of irritants such as detergents, chemicals, and abrasive materials as well as extremes of temperature and humidity is important in managing this disease. New clothing should be washed to reduce the content of formaldehyde and other chemicals. Because residual laundry detergent in clothing may be irritating, using a liquid rather than a powder detergent and adding an extra rinse cycle is beneficial. Occlusive clothing should be avoided in favor of cotton or cotton blends. Temperature in the home and work environments should be controlled to minimize sweating. Swimming is usually well tolerated; however, because swimming pools are treated with chlorine or bromine, patients should shower and use a mild cleanser to remove these irritating chemicals, then apply a moisturizer or occlusive agent. Sunlight may be beneficial to some patients with atopic dermatitis, but nonsensitizing sunscreens should be used to avoid sunburn. Prolonged sun exposure can cause evaporative losses, overheating, and sweating, all of which can be irritating.

In children who have undergone controlled food challenges, eggs, milk, peanuts, soy, wheat, and fish account for approximately 90% of the food allergens that exacerbate atopic dermatitis. Avoidance of foods implicated in controlled challenges can lead to clinical improvement. Extensive elimination diets, which can be nutritionally unsound and burdensome, are almost never warranted because even patients with multiple positive skin tests rarely react to more than three foods on blinded challenges.

In patients who demonstrate specific IgE to dust mite allergen, environmental control measures aimed at reducing the dust mite load improve atopic dermatitis. These include use of dust mite-proof covers on pillows and mattresses, washing linens weekly in hot water, decreasing indoor humidity levels, and in some cases removing bedroom carpeting.

Counseling may be of benefit when dealing with the frustrations associated with atopic dermatitis. Relaxation, behavioral modification, or biofeedback training may help patients with habitual scratching. Patients with severe or disfiguring disease may require psychotherapy.

Clinicians should provide the patient and family with both general information and specific written skin care recommendations. The patient or parent should demonstrate an appropriate level of understanding to help ensure a good outcome. Educational pamphlets and a video about atopic dermatitis can be obtained from the Eczema Association for Science and Education, a national nonprofit, patient-oriented organization. They can be contacted through their website at: http://www.nationaleczema.org/ or by phone: 800-818-7546.

B. HYDRATION

Patients with atopic dermatitis have evaporative losses due to a defective skin barrier, so soaking the affected area or bathing for 15–20 minutes in warm water, then applying an occlusive agent to retain the absorbed water, is an essential component of therapy. Oatmeal or baking soda added to the bath may feel soothing to certain patients but does not improve water absorption. Atopic dermatitis of the face or neck can be treated by applying a wet facecloth or towel to the involved area for 15–20 minutes. The washcloth may be more readily accepted by a child if it is turned into a mask and also allows the older patient to remain functional. Lesions limited to the hands or feet can be treated by soaking in a basin. Daily baths may be needed and increased to several times daily during flares of atopic dermatitis, while showers may be adequate for patients with mild disease. It is important to use an occlusive preparation within a few minutes after soaking the skin to prevent evaporation, which is both drying and irritating.

C. Moisturizers and Occlusives

An effective emollient combined with hydration therapy will help skin healing and can reduce the need for topical corticosteroids. Moisturizers are available as lotions, creams, and ointments. Because lotions contain more water than creams, they are more drying because of their evaporative effect. Preservatives and fragrances in lotions and creams may cause skin irritation. Moisturizers often need to be applied several times daily on a long-term basis and should be obtained in the largest size available. Crisco shortening can be substituted as an inexpensive alternative. Petroleum jelly (Vaseline) is an effective occlusive agent when used to seal in water after bathing.

D. Corticosteroids

Corticosteroids reduce the inflammation and pruritus in atopic dermatitis. Topical corticosteroids can decrease *S aureus* colonization. Systemic corticosteroids, including oral prednisone, should be avoided in the management of this chronic relapsing disease. The dramatic improvement observed with systemic corticosteroids may be associated with an equally dramatic flaring of atopic dermatitis following their discontinuation. If a short course of oral corticosteroids is given, it is usually best to prescribe a tapering dose.

Topical corticosteroids are available in a wide variety of formulations, ranging from extremely high-potency to low-potency preparations (see Table 14–3). Choice of a particular product depends on the severity and distribution of skin lesions. Patients need to be counseled regarding the potency of their corticosteroid preparation and its potential side effects. In general, the least potent agent that is effective should be used. However, choosing a preparation that is too weak may result in persistence or worsening of the atopic dermatitis. Side effects include thinning of the skin, telangiectasias, bruising, hypopigmentation, acne, and striae, although these occur infrequently when low- to medium-potency topical corticosteroids are used appropriately. In contrast, use of potent topical corticosteroids for prolonged periods—especially under occlusion—may result in significant atrophic changes as well as systemic side effects. The face (especially the eyelids) and intertriginous areas are especially sensitive to corticosteroid side effects, and only low-potency preparations should be used routinely on these areas. Because topical corticosteroids are commercially available in a variety of bases, including ointments, creams, lotions, solutions, gels, and sprays, there is no need to compound them. Ointments are most occlusive and in general provide better delivery of the medication while preventing evaporative losses. However, in a humid environment, creams may be better tolerated than ointments because the increased occlusion may cause itching or even folliculitis. Creams and lotions, while easier to spread, can contribute to skin dryness and irrita-

tion. Solutions can be used on the scalp and hirsute areas, although they can be irritating, especially to open lesions. With clinical improvement, a less potent corticosteroid should be prescribed and the frequency of use decreased. Topical corticosteroids can be discontinued when inflammation resolves, but hydration and moisturizers need to be continued.

Of note, fluticasone 0.05% cream has been shown to be safe in infants as young as 3 months of age with extensive atopic dermatitis. In addition, several studies with fluticasone 0.05% cream have shown that once atopic dermatitis is stabilized, long-term control can be maintained with twice weekly therapy. Of note, during the maintenance phase, fluticasone 0.05% cream was also applied to areas that had healed, which resulted in delayed relapses.

E. Topical Calcineurin Inhibitors

Tacrolimus and pimecrolimus are immunomodulatory agents that inhibit the transcription of proinflammatory cytokines as well as other allergic mediators and target key cells in allergic inflammation. They are available in topical formulations, and long-term studies up to 12 months have confirmed both efficacy and safety. Local burning at the site of application, which occurs more frequently with tacrolimus ointment, has been the most common side effect, although this is usually a transient problem. Tacrolimus ointment—0.03% for children 2–15 years of age and 0.1% for older patients—is approved for twice daily short-term and intermittent long-term use in moderate-to-severe atopic dermatitis. Pimecrolimus 1% cream is approved for patients 2 years of age or older who have mild-to-moderate atopic dermatitis. As a precaution, patients should wear sunscreen with both drugs. More recently, several studies in children as young as 3 months of age with all disease severities have been performed for up to 12 months with pimecrolimus 1% cream used at the earliest sign of disease activity (eg, erythema and pruritus). With this early intervention approach, the need for topical steroid rescue was significantly decreased.

While there is no evidence of a causal link between cancer and the use of topical calcineurin inhibitors, the FDA has issued a "black box" warning for pimecrolimus cream and tacrolimus ointment because of a lack of long-term safety data (see U.S. package inserts for Elidel [Novartis], and Protopic [Astellas]). The new labeling states that these drugs are recommended as second-line treatments and that their use in children under the age of 2 years is currently not recommended.

F. Tar Preparations

Tar preparations are used primarily in shampoos and rarely as bath additives. Side effects associated with tar products include skin dryness or irritation, especially if applied to inflamed skin, and, less commonly, photosensitivity reactions and folliculitis.

G. WET DRESSINGS

Wet dressings are used together with hydration and topical corticosteroids primarily for the treatment of severe atopic dermatitis. They can also serve as an effective barrier against the persistent scratching that often undermines therapy. Total body dressings can be applied by using wet pajamas or long underwear with dry pajamas or a sweat suit on top. Hands and feet can be covered by wet tube socks with dry tube socks on top. Alternatively, wet gauze with a layer of dry gauze over it can be used and secured in place with an elastic bandage. Dressings can be removed when they dry out, usually after several hours, and are often best tolerated at bedtime. Incorrect use of wet dressings can result in chilling, maceration of the skin, or secondary infection.

H. ANTI-INFECTIVE THERAPY

Systemic antibiotic therapy may be important when treating atopic dermatitis secondarily infected with *S aureus*. For limited areas of involvement, a topical antibiotic such as mupirocin may be effective. First- or second-generation cephalosporins or a semisynthetic penicillin are usually the first choice for oral therapy, as erythromycin-resistant organisms are fairly common. Maintenance antibiotic therapy is rarely indicated and may result in colonization by methicillin-resistant bacteria.

Disseminated eczema herpeticum usually requires treatment with systemic acyclovir. Patients with recurrent cutaneous herpetic lesions can be given prophylactic oral acyclovir. Superficial dermatophytosis and *Pityrosporum ovale* infection can be treated with topical or (rarely) systemic antifungal agents.

I. ANTIPRURITIC AGENTS

Pruritus is usually the least well-tolerated symptom of atopic dermatitis. Oral antihistamines and anxiolytics may be effective owing to their tranquilizing and sedating effects and can be taken mostly in the evening to avoid daytime somnolence. Nonsedating antihistamines may be less effective in treating pruritus, although beneficial effects have been reported in blinded studies. Use of topical antihistamines and local anesthetics should be avoided because of potential sensitization.

J. RECALCITRANT DISEASE

Patients who are erythrodermic or who appear toxic may need to be hospitalized. Hospitalization may also be appropriate for cases of severe disease that fail outpatient management. Marked clinical improvement often occurs when the patient is removed from environmental allergens or stressors. In the hospital, compliance with therapy can be monitored, the patient and family can receive intense education, and controlled provocative challenges can be conducted to help identify triggering factors.

Ultraviolet light therapy can be useful for chronic recalcitrant atopic dermatitis in a subset of patients under the supervision of a specialist. Photochemotherapy with oral methoxypsoralen therapy followed by UVA (ultraviolet A) has been used in a limited number of children with severe atopic dermatitis unresponsive to other therapy, and significant improvement has been noted. However, the increased long-term risk of cutaneous malignancies from this therapy prevents its widespread use.

Limited published data are available on use of the systemic immunosuppressive agent cyclosporine. In an open study, children given oral cyclosporine, 5 mg/kg daily for 6 weeks, improved significantly and tolerated the treatment well. Unfortunately, discontinuation of treatment resulted in relapse, although the relapse rate was variable. Patients treated with this agent should have their dose titrated to the lowest effective dose after the disease is brought under control with appropriate monitoring, under the care of a specialist familiar with the drug.

K. EXPERIMENTAL AND UNPROVED THERAPIES

A number of uncontrolled trials have suggested that desensitization to specific allergens may improve atopic dermatitis; however, controlled trials with standardized extracts of relevant allergens in atopic dermatitis are needed before this form of therapy can be recommended.

Traditional Chinese herbal therapy in the form of decoctions has also been proposed for atopic dermatitis. The herbs used may have antimicrobial, sedative, anti-inflammatory, and corticosteroid-like activities. Despite studies showing clinical efficacy, toxicity and idiosyncratic reactions remain a concern, and traditional Chinese herbal therapy should be considered investigational at best. Finally, although disturbances in the metabolism of essential fatty acids have been reported in patients with atopic dermatitis, well-controlled trials with fish oil and evening primrose have shown no clinical benefit.

Prognosis

Although it has been held that most children outgrow atopic dermatitis by adolescence, recent studies present less optimistic outcomes. In one study, atopic dermatitis had disappeared in only 18% of children followed from infancy until age 13 years, although the symptoms had become less severe in 65%. In a prospective study from Finland, 77–91% of adolescent patients receiving treatment for moderate or severe atopic dermatitis had persistent or frequently relapsing dermatitis as adults, although only 6% had severe disease. More than half of adolescents receiving treatment for mild dermatitis experienced a relapse of disease as adults. Adults whose childhood atopic dermatitis has been in remission for a number of years may present with hand dermatitis, especially if daily activities require repeated hand wetting.

Boguniewicz M: Atopic dermatitis: Beyond the itch that rashes. Immunol Allergy Clin North Am 2005;25:333 [PMID: 15878459].

Boguniewicz M et al: Current management of atopic dermatitis and interruption of the atopic march. J Allergy Clin Immunol 2003;112:S140 [PMID: 14657844].

Fonacier L et al: Report of the Topical Calcineurin Task Force of the American College of Allergy, Asthma and Immunology and the American Academy of Allergy, Asthma and Immunology. J Allergy Clin Immunol 2005;115:1249 [PMID: 15940142].

Leung DYM et al: Disease management of atopic dermatitis: An updated practice parameter. Ann Allergy Clin Immunol 2004; 93:S1 [PMID: 15478395].

Paul C et al: Safety and tolerability of 1% pimecrolimus cream among infants: experience with 1133 patients treated for up to 2 years. Pediatrics 2006;117:e118 [PMID: 16361223].

Williams HC: Atopic dermatitis. N Engl J Med 2005;352:2314 [PMID: 15930422].

■ URTICARIA & ANGIOEDEMA

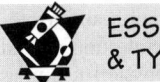

ESSENTIALS OF DIAGNOSIS & TYPICAL FEATURES

- *Urticaria: Erythematous, blanchable, circumscribed, pruritic, edematous papules ranging from 1–2 mm to several centimeters in diameter and involving the superficial dermis. Individual lesions can coalesce.*

- *Angioedema: Edema extending into the deep dermis or subcutaneous tissues.*

- *Both resolve without sequelae—urticaria usually within hours (individual lesions rarely lasting up to 24 hours), angioedema within 72 hours.*

General Considerations

Urticaria and angioedema are common dermatologic conditions, occurring at some time in up to 25% of the population. About half of patients will have concomitant urticaria and angioedema, whereas 40% will have only urticaria and 10% only angioedema. Urticarial lesions are arbitrarily designated as acute, lasting less than 6 weeks, or chronic, lasting more than 6 weeks. Acute versus chronic urticaria can also be distinguished by differences in histologic features. A history of atopy is common with acute urticaria or angioedema. In contrast, atopy does not appear to be a factor in chronic urticaria.

Mast cell degranulation, dilated venules, and dermal edema are present in most forms of urticaria or angioedema. The dermal inflammatory cells may be sparse or dense depending on the chronicity of the lesions. Mast cells are thought to play a critical role in the pathogenesis of urticaria or angioedema through release of a variety of vasoactive mediators. Mast cell activation and degranulation can be triggered by different stimuli, including cross-linking of Fc receptor-bound IgE by allergens or anti-FcεRI antibodies. Non–IgE-mediated mechanisms have also been identified, including complement anaphylatoxins (C3a, C5a), radiocontrast dyes, or physical stimuli. Chronic urticarial lesions have greater numbers of perivascular mononuclear cells, consisting primarily of T cells. There is also a marked increase in cutaneous mast cells. The cause of acute disease can be identified in about half of patients and includes allergens such as foods, aeroallergens, latex, drugs, and insect venoms. Infectious agents, including streptococci, mycoplasmas, hepatitis B virus, and Epstein–Barr virus, can cause acute urticaria. Urticaria or angioedema can occur after the administration of blood products or immunoglobulin. This results from immune complex formation with complement activation, vascular alterations, and triggering of mast cells by anaphylatoxins. Opiate analgesics, polymyxin B, tubocurarine, and radiocontrast media can induce acute urticaria by direct mast cell activation. These disorders can also occur following ingestion of aspirin or nonsteroidal anti-inflammatory agents (see section on Adverse Reactions to Drugs & Biologicals).

Physical urticarias represent a heterogeneous group of disorders in which urticaria or angioedema is triggered by physical stimuli, including pressure, cold, heat, water, or vibrations. Dermographism is the most common form of physical urticaria, affecting up to about 4% of the population and occurring at skin sites subjected to mechanical stimuli. Many physical urticarias are considered to be acute because the lesions are usually rapid in onset, with resolution within hours. However, symptoms can recur for months to years.

The cause of chronic urticaria is usually not due to allergies and typically cannot be determined. It can be associated with an underlying systemic disease such as thyroid disease. Some studies have demonstrated IgG autoantibodies directed at the high-affinity receptor for IgE or at IgE, suggesting that chronic urticaria may be an autoimmune disease.

Clinical Findings

A. SYMPTOMS AND SIGNS

Cold-induced urticaria or angioedema can occur within minutes of exposure to a decreased ambient temperature or as the skin is warmed following direct cold contact. Systemic features include headache, wheezing, and syncope. If the entire body is cooled, as may occur during swimming, hypotension and collapse can occur. Two forms of dominantly inherited cold urticaria have been described. The immediate form is known as familial cold urticaria, in which erythematous macules appear rather than wheals, along with fever, arthralgias, and leukocytosis. The delayed form consists of erythematous, deep swellings that develop 9–18 hours after local cold challenge without immediate lesions.

In solar urticaria, which occurs within minutes after exposure to light of appropriate wavelength, pruritus is followed by morbilliform erythema and urticaria.

Cholinergic urticaria occurs after increases in core body and skin temperatures and typically develops after a warm bath or shower, exercise, or episodes of fever. Occasional episodes are triggered by stress or the ingestion of certain foods. The eruption appears as small punctate wheals surrounded by extensive areas of erythema. Rarely the urticarial lesions become confluent and angioedema develops. Associated features can include one or more of the following: headache, syncope, bronchospasm, abdominal pain, vomiting, and diarrhea. In severe cases, systemic anaphylaxis may develop. In pressure urticaria or angioedema, red, deep, painful swelling occurs immediately or 4–6 hours after the skin has been exposed to pressure. The immediate form is often associated with dermographism. The delayed form, which may be associated with fever, chills, and arthralgias, may be accompanied by elevated erythrocyte sedimentation rate and leukocytosis. Lesions are frequently diffuse, tender, and painful rather than pruritic. They typically resolve within 48 hours.

B. LABORATORY FINDINGS

Laboratory tests are selected on the basis of the history and physical findings. Testing for specific IgE antibody to food or inhalant allergens may be helpful in implicating a potential cause. Specific tests for physical urticarias, such as an ice cube test or a pressure test, may be indicated. Intradermal injection of methacholine reproduces clinical symptoms locally in about one-third of patients with cholinergic urticaria. A throat culture for streptococcal infection may be warranted with acute urticaria. In chronic urticaria, selected screening studies to look for an underlying disease may be indicated, including a complete blood count, erythrocyte sedimentation rate, biochemistry panel, and urinalysis. Antithyroid antibodies may be considered. Intradermal testing with the patient's serum has been suggested as a method of detecting histamine-releasing activity, including autoantibodies. Other tests should be done based on suspicion of a specific underlying disease. If the history or appearance of the urticarial lesions suggests vasculitis, a skin biopsy for immunofluorescence is indicated. Patient diaries occasionally may be helpful to determine the cause of recurrent hives. A trial of food or drug elimination may be considered.

Differential Diagnosis

Urticarial lesions are usually easily recognized—the major dilemma is the etiologic diagnosis. Lesions of urticarial vasculitis typically last for more than 24 hours. "Papular urticaria" is a term used to characterize multiple papules from insect bites, found especially on the extremities, and is not true urticaria. Angioedema can be distinguished from other forms of edema because it is transient, asymmetrical, and nonpitting and does not occur predominantly in dependent areas. Hereditary angioedema is a rare autosomal dominant disorder caused by a quantitative or functional deficiency of C1-esterase inhibitor and characterized by episodic, frequently severe, nonpruritic angioedema of the skin, gastrointestinal tract, or upper respiratory tract. Life-threatening laryngeal angioedema may occur.

Complications

In severe cases of cholinergic urticaria, systemic anaphylaxis may develop. In cold-induced disease, sudden cooling of the entire body as can occur with swimming can result in hypotension and collapse.

Treatment

A. GENERAL MEASURES

The most effective treatment is identification and avoidance of the triggering agent. Underlying infection should be treated appropriately. Patients with physical urticarias should avoid the relevant physical stimulus. Epinephrine can be used for treatment of acute episodes, especially when laryngeal edema complicates an attack (see section on Anaphylaxis). Intubation may be indicated for life-threatening laryngeal edema.

B. ANTIHISTAMINES

For the majority of patients, H_1 antihistamines given orally or systemically are the mainstay of therapy. Antihistamines are more effective when given on an ongoing basis rather than after lesions appear. For breakthrough symptoms, the dose may need to be increased. In the case of cold urticaria, the best treatment appears to be cyproheptadine. Cholinergic urticaria can be treated with hydroxyzine and dermographism with hydroxyzine or diphenhydramine. The addition of H_2 antihistamines may benefit some patients who fail to respond to H_1-receptor antagonists alone. Second-generation antihistamines (discussed previously under Allergic Rhinoconjunctivitis) are long acting, show good tissue levels, are non- or minimally sedating at usual dosing levels, and lack anticholinergic effects.

C. CORTICOSTEROIDS

Although corticosteroids are usually not indicated in the treatment of acute or chronic urticaria, severe recalcitrant cases may require alternate-day therapy in an attempt to diminish disease activity and facilitate control with antihistamines. Systemic corticosteroids may also be needed in the treatment of urticaria or angioedema secondary to necrotizing vasculitis, an uncommon occurrence in patients with serum sickness or collagen–vascular disease.

D. OTHER PHARMACOLOGIC AGENTS

Limited studies suggest that some patients may benefit from treatment with a leukotriene-receptor antagonist. The tricyclic antidepressant doxepin blocks both H_1 and H_2 histamine receptors and may be particularly useful in chronic urticaria, although its use may be limited by the sedating side effect. A limited number of patients—including euthyroid patients—with chronic urticaria and antithyroid antibodies have improved when given thyroid hormone. Treatment of chronic urticaria with hydroxychloroquine, nifedipine, colchicine, dapsone, sulfasalazine, cyclosporine, or intravenous immune globulin should be considered investigational.

Prognosis

Spontaneous remission of urticaria and angioedema is frequent, but some patients have a prolonged course. Reassurance is important, because this disorder can cause significant frustration. Periodic follow-up is indicated, particularly for patients with laryngeal edema, to monitor for possible underlying cause.

Boguniewicz M: Chronic urticaria in children. Allergy Asthma Proc 2005;26:13 [PMID: 15813283].

ANAPHYLAXIS

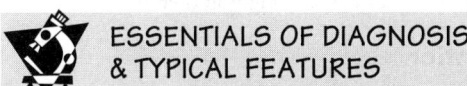

ESSENTIALS OF DIAGNOSIS & TYPICAL FEATURES

- *Rapid onset of allergic symptoms after exposure to allergen in a previously sensitized person.*
- *Generalized pruritus, anxiety, urticaria, angioedema, throat fullness, dyspnea, hypotension, and collapse.*

General Considerations

Anaphylaxis is an acute life-threatening clinical syndrome that occurs when large quantities of inflammatory mediators are rapidly released from mast cells and basophils after exposure to an allergen in a previously sensitized patient. Anaphylactoid reactions mimic anaphylaxis but are not mediated by IgE. They may be mediated by ana-

phylatoxins such as C3a or C5a or through nonimmune mast cell degranulating agents. Some of the common causes of anaphylaxis or anaphylactoid reactions are listed in Table 34–5. Idiopathic anaphylaxis by definition has no recognized external cause.

Clinical Findings

A. SYMPTOMS AND SIGNS

The symptoms and signs of anaphylaxis or anaphylactoid reactions depend on the organs affected. Onset typically occurs within minutes after exposure to the offending agent and can be short-lived, protracted, or biphasic, with recurrence after several hours despite treatment. Patients may report generalized pruritus or a feeling of impending doom. Cutaneous signs include erythema, urticaria, and angioedema. Tearing, rhinorrhea, sneezing, and nasal congestion may occur. Respiratory symptoms include a sensation of having a lump in the throat or shortness of breath; signs include uvular edema, hoarseness, dysphonia, stridor, tachypnea, and wheezing. Cardiovascular findings include tachycardia, arrhythmias, hypotension, and collapse. The patient may complain of nausea and cramping pain with associated vomiting and diarrhea. There may be anxiety or generalized seizures. Shock, upper airway edema, and bronchial obstruction are the principal life-threatening features.

B. LABORATORY FINDINGS

Tryptase released by mast cells can be measured in the serum and may remain elevated for up to 24 hours after an acute reaction. This may be helpful when the diagnosis of anaphylaxis is in question. The complete blood

Table 34–5. Common causes of systemic allergic and pseudoallergic reactions.

Causes of anaphylaxis
Drugs
Antibiotics
Anesthetic agents
Foods
Peanuts, tree nuts, shellfish, and others
Biologicals
Latex
Insulin
Allergen extracts
Antisera
Blood products
Enzymes
Insect venoms
Causes of anaphylactoid reactions
Radiocontrast media
Aspirin and other nonsteroidal anti-inflammatory drugs
Anesthetic agents

count may show an elevated hematocrit due to hemo-concentration. Elevation of serum creatine kinase, aspartate aminotransferase, and lactic dehydrogenase may be seen with myocardial involvement. Electrocardiographic abnormalities may include ST wave depression, bundle branch block, and various arrhythmias. Arterial blood gases may show hypoxemia, hypercapnia, and acidosis. The chest radiograph may show hyperinflation.

Differential Diagnosis

Although shock may be the only sign of anaphylaxis, other diagnoses should be considered, especially in the setting of sudden collapse without typical allergic findings. Other causes of shock along with cardiac arrhythmias must be ruled out. (See Chapters 11 and 13.) Respiratory failure associated with asthma may be confused with anaphylaxis. Mastocytosis, hereditary angioedema, scombroid poisoning, vasovagal reactions, vocal cord dysfunction, and anxiety attacks may cause symptoms mistaken for anaphylaxis.

Complications

Depending on the organs involved and the severity of the reaction, complications may vary from none to aspiration pneumonitis, acute tubular necrosis, bleeding diathesis, or sloughing of the intestinal mucosa. With irreversible shock, heart and brain damage can be terminal.

Treatment

A. GENERAL MEASURES

Anaphylaxis is a medical emergency that requires rapid assessment and treatment. Exposure to the triggering agent should be discontinued. Airway patency should be maintained and blood pressure and pulse monitored. The patient should be placed in a supine position with the legs elevated. Oxygen should be delivered by mask or nasal cannula with pulse oximetry monitoring. If the reaction is secondary to a sting or injection into an extremity, a tourniquet may be applied proximal to the site, briefly releasing it every 10–15 minutes.

B. EPINEPHRINE

Epinephrine 1:1000, 0.01 mL/kg to a maximum of 0.3 mL, should be injected intramuscularly, without delay. This dose may be repeated at intervals of 15–20 minutes two or three times as necessary. If the precipitating allergen has been injected intradermally or subcutaneously, absorption may be delayed by giving 0.1 mL of epinephrine subcutaneously at the injection site unless the site is a digit.

C. ANTIHISTAMINES

Diphenhydramine, an H_1-blocker, 1–2 mg/kg up to 50 mg, can be given intramuscularly or intravenously.

Intravenous antihistamines should be infused over a period of 5–10 minutes to avoid inducing hypotension. Addition of ranitidine, an H_2-blocker, 1 mg/kg up to 50 mg intravenously, may be more effective than an H_1-blocker alone, especially for hypotension.

D. FLUIDS

Treatment of persistent hypotension requires restoration of intravascular volume by fluid replacement, initially with a crystalloid solution, 20–30 mL/kg in the first hour.

E. BRONCHODILATORS

Nebulized β_2-agonists such as albuterol 0.5% solution, 2.5 mg (0.5 mL) diluted in 2–3 mL saline, may be useful for reversing bronchospasm. Intravenous methylxanthines are generally not recommended because they provide little benefit over inhaled β_2-agonists and may contribute to toxicity.

F. CORTICOSTEROIDS

Although corticosteroids do not provide immediate benefit, when given early they may prevent protracted or biphasic anaphylaxis. Intravenous methylprednisolone, 1–2 mg/kg, or hydrocortisone, 5 mg/kg, can be given every 4–6 hours.

G. VASOPRESSORS

Refractory hypotension should be treated with intravenous vasopressors such as dopamine or epinephrine. (See Chapter 13.)

H. OBSERVATION

The patient should be monitored after the initial symptoms have subsided, because biphasic or protracted anaphylaxis can occur despite ongoing therapy.

Prevention

Strict avoidance of the causative agent is extremely important. An effort to determine its cause should be made, beginning with a thorough history. Typically there is a strong temporal relationship between exposure and onset of symptoms. Testing for specific IgE to allergen with either in vitro or skin testing may be indicated. With exercise-induced anaphylaxis, patients should be instructed to exercise with another person and to stop exercising at the first sign of symptoms. If prior ingestion of food has been implicated, eating within 4 hours—perhaps up to 12 hours—before exercise should be avoided. Patients with a history of anaphylaxis should carry epinephrine for self-administration (eg, EpiPen, EpiPen Jr), and they and all caregivers should be instructed on its use. They should also carry an oral antihistamine such as diphenhydramine and wear a medical alert bracelet. Patients with idiopathic anaphylaxis may require prolonged treatment with oral corticosteroids. Specific measures for dealing with food, drug, latex, and insect venom allergies as well as radiocontrast media reactions are discussed in a later section.

Prognosis

Anaphylaxis can be fatal. In one study of children and adolescents who died from food-induced anaphylaxis (eg, from peanuts, tree nuts, or egg), treatment with epinephrine was delayed for more than 1 hour after onset. The prognosis is good when signs and symptoms are recognized promptly and treated aggressively and the offending agent is subsequently avoided. Exercise-induced and idiopathic anaphylaxis may be recurrent. Because accidental exposure to the causative agent may occur, patients, parents, and caregivers must be prepared to recognize and treat anaphylaxis.

Joint Task Force on Practice Parameters et al: The diagnosis and management of anaphylaxis: An updated practice parameter. J Allergy Clin Immunol 2005;115:S483 [PMID: 15940153].

Sampson HA: Anaphylaxis and emergency treatment. Pediatrics 2003;111:1601 [PMID: 12667272].

ADVERSE REACTIONS TO DRUGS & BIOLOGICALS

The majority of adverse drug reactions are not immunologically mediated and may be due to idiosyncratic reactions, overdosage, pharmacologic side effects, nonspecific release of pharmacologic effector molecules, or drug interactions.

Patients often describe themselves as being allergic to medications or biologicals, and clinicians may document a drug allergy in the patient's medical record based solely on this history. Adverse drug reactions are any undesirable and unintended response elicited by a drug. Allergic or hypersensitivity drug reactions are adverse reactions involving immune mechanisms. Although hypersensitivity reactions account for only 5–10% of all adverse drug reactions, they are the most serious, with 1:10,000 resulting in death.

1. Antibiotics

Antibiotics constitute the most frequent cause of allergic drug reactions. Amoxicillin, trimethoprim–sulfamethoxazole, and ampicillin are the most common causes of cutaneous drug reactions.

Most antibiotics and their metabolites are low-molecular-weight compounds that do not stimulate immunity until they have become covalently bound to a carrier protein. The penicillins and other β-lactam antibiotics, including cephalosporins, carbacephems, carbapenems, and monobactams, share a common β-lactam ring structure and a marked propensity to couple to carrier proteins. Penicilloyl is the predominant metabolite of penicillin and is called the major determinant. The other penicillin metabolites are present in low concentrations and are referred to as minor determinants. Sulfonamide reactions are mediated presumably by a reactive metabolite (hydroxylamine) produced by cytochrome P-450 oxidative metabolism. Slow acetylators appear to be at increased risk. Other risk factors for drug reactions include previous exposure, previous reaction, age (20–49 years), route (parenteral), and dose of administration (high, intermittent). Atopy does not predispose to development of a reaction, but atopic individuals have more severe reactions.

Immunopathologic reactions to antibiotics include type I (IgE-mediated) reactions resulting from a drug or metabolite interaction with preformed specific IgE bound to the surfaces of tissue mast cells or circulating basophils. Release of mediators such as histamine and leukotrienes contributes to the clinical development of angioedema, urticaria, bronchospasm, or anaphylaxis. Type II (cytotoxic) reactions involve IgG or IgM antibodies that recognize drug bound to cell membranes. In the presence of serum complement, the antibody-coated cell is either cleared or destroyed, causing drug-induced hemolytic anemia or thrombocytopenia. Type III (immune complex) reactions are caused by soluble complexes of drug or metabolite with IgG or IgM antibody. If the immune complex is deposited on blood vessel walls and activates the complement cascade, serum sickness may result. Type IV (T-cell–mediated) reactions require activated T lymphocytes that recognize a drug or its metabolite as seen in allergic contact dermatitis. Sensitization usually occurs via the topical route of administration. Immunopathologic reactions not fitting into the type I–IV classification include Stevens–Johnson syndrome, exfoliative dermatitis, and the maculopapular rash associated with penicillin or ampicillin. The prevalence of morbilliform rashes in patients given ampicillin is between 5.2% and 9.5% of treatment courses. However, patients given ampicillin during Epstein-Barr virus and cytomegalovirus infections or with acute lymphoblastic anemia have a 69–100% incidence of non-IgE-mediated rash. Serum sickness-like reactions resemble type III reactions, although immune complexes are not documented; β-lactams, especially cefaclor, and sulfonamides, have been implicated most often. They may result from an inherited propensity for hepatic biotransformation of drug into toxic or immunogenic metabolites. The incidence of "allergic" cutaneous reactions to trimethoprim–sulfamethoxazole in patients with acquired immunodeficiency syndrome (AIDS) has been reported to be as high as 70%. The mechanism is thought to relate to the severe immune dysregulation, although it may be due to glutathione deficiency resulting in toxic metabolites.

Clinical Findings

A. Symptoms and Signs

Allergic reactions can result in pruritus, urticaria, angioedema, or anaphylaxis. Serum sickness is characterized by fever, rash, lymphadenopathy, myalgias, and arthralgias. Cytotoxic drug reactions can result in symptoms and signs associated with the underlying anemia or thrombocytopenia. Delayed-type hypersensitivity may cause contact dermatitis.

B. Laboratory Findings

Skin testing is the most rapid, useful, and sensitive method of demonstrating the presence of IgE antibody to a specific allergen. Skin testing to nonpenicillin antibiotics may be difficult, however, because many immunologic reactions are due to metabolites rather than to the parent drug and because the relevant metabolites for most drugs other than penicillin have not been identified. Because metabolites are usually low-molecular-weight haptens, they must combine with carrier proteins to be useful for diagnosis. In the case of contact sensitivity reactions to topical antibiotics, a 48-hour patch test can be useful.

Solid-phase in vitro immunoassays for IgE to penicillins are available for identification of IgE to penicilloyl but are considerably less sensitive and give less information than skin testing. Assays for specific IgG and IgM have been shown to correlate with a drug reaction in immune cytopenias, but in most other instances such assays are not clinically useful. Skin testing for immediate hypersensitivity is helpful only in predicting reactions caused by IgE antibodies. Most nonpruritic maculopapular rashes will not be predicted by skin testing.

Approximately 80% of patients with a history of penicillin allergy will have negative skin tests. Penicillin therapy in patients with a history of an immediate hypersensitivity reaction to penicillin, but with negative skin tests to both penicilloyl and the minor determinant mixture, is accompanied by a 1–3% chance of urticaria or other mild allergic reactions at some time during therapy, with anaphylaxis occurring in less than 0.1% of patients. In contrast, the predictive value of a positive skin test is approximately 60%. Testing with penicilloyl linked to polylysine (PPL) alone carries about a 76% sensitivity; use of both PPL and penicillin G (used as a minor determinant) increases sensitivity to about 95%. Not using the minor determinant mixture in skin testing can result in failure to predict potential anaphylactic reactions. Unfortunately the minor determinant mixture is still not commercially available, although most academic allergy centers make their own. Approximately 4% of subjects tested with no history of penicillin allergy have positive skin tests, and most fatalities occur in patients with no prior history of reaction. Rarely, patients may have skin

test reactivity only to a specific semisynthetic penicillin. Resensitization in skin-test-negative children occurs infrequently (< 1%) after a course of oral antibiotic.

The degree of cross-reactivity of determinants formed from cephalosporins with IgE to other β-lactam drugs remains unresolved, especially because haptens that may be unique to cephalosporin metabolism remain unknown. The degree of clinical cross-reactivity is much lower than the in vitro cross-reactivity. A clinical adverse reaction rate of 3–7% for cephalosporins may be expected in patients with positive histories of penicillin allergy. Antibodies to the second- and third-generation cephalosporins appear to be directed at the unique side chains rather than at the common ring structure. The present literature suggests that a positive skin test to a cephalosporin used at a concentration of 1 mg/mL would place the patient at increased risk for an allergic reaction to that antibiotic. However, a negative skin test would not exclude sensitivity to a potentially relevant metabolite. One review concluded that there is no increased incidence of allergy to second- and third-generation cephalosporins in patients with penicillin allergy and that penicillin skin testing does not identify patients who develop cephalosporin allergy. However, another study suggested that although only 2% of penicillin-allergic patients would react to a cephalosporin, they would be at risk for anaphylaxis.

Carbacephems (loracarbef) are similar to cephalosporins, although the degree of cross-reactivity is undetermined. Carbapenems (imipenem) represent another class of β-lactam antibiotics with a bicyclic nucleus and a high degree of cross-reactivity with penicillin. In contrast, monobactams (aztreonam) contain a monocyclic rather than bicyclic ring structure and limited data suggest that aztreonam can be safely administered to most penicillin-allergic subjects.

Skin testing for non–β-lactam antibiotics is less reliable, because the relevant degradation products are for the most part unknown or multivalent reagents are unavailable.

Treatment

A. General Measures

Withdrawal of the implicated drug is usually a central component of management. Acute IgE-mediated reactions such as anaphylaxis, urticaria, and angioedema are treated according to established therapeutic guidelines that include the use of epinephrine, H_1- and H_2-receptor blocking agents, volume replacement, and systemic corticosteroids (see previous sections). Antibiotic-induced immune cytopenias can be managed by withdrawal of the offending agent or reduction in dose. Drug-induced serum sickness can be suppressed by drug withdrawal, antihistamines, and corticosteroids. Contact allergy can be managed by avoidance and treatment with antihistamines and topical corticosteroids. Reactions such as toxic epidermal necrolysis and Stevens–Johnson syndrome require immediate drug withdrawal and supportive care.

B. ALTERNATIVE THERAPY

If possible, subsequent therapy should be with an alternative drug that has therapeutic actions similar to the drug in question but with no immunologic cross-reactivity.

C. DESENSITIZATION

Administering gradually increasing doses of an antibiotic either orally or parentally over a period of hours to days may be considered if alternative therapy is not acceptable. This should be done only by a physician familiar with desensitization, typically in an intensive care setting. Of note, desensitization is only effective for the course of therapy for which the patient was desensitized, unless maintained on a chronic prophylactic dose of the medication as patients revert from a desensitized to allergic state after the drug is discontinued. In addition, desensitization does not reduce or prevent non–IgE-mediated reactions. Patients with Stevens–Johnson syndrome should not be desensitized because of the high mortality rate.

Prognosis

The prognosis is good when drug allergens are identified early and avoided. Stevens–Johnson syndrome and toxic epidermal necrolysis may be associated with a high mortality rate.

2. Latex Allergy

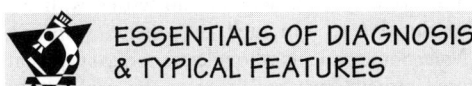

ESSENTIALS OF DIAGNOSIS & TYPICAL FEATURES

- *Immediate hypersensitivity reaction after exposure to latex, including airborne particles.*
- *Allergic contact dermatitis 24–48 hours after exposure to rubber accelerators or antioxidants.*

General Considerations

Allergic reactions to latex and rubber products have become increasingly common since the institution of universal precautions for exposure to bodily fluids. Children with spina bifida appear to have a unique sensitivity to latex, perhaps because of early and frequent latex exposure as well as altered neuroimmune interactions. Atopy—especially symptomatic latex allergy—appears to be significantly increased in patients with

spina bifida experiencing anaphylaxis during general anesthesia. Other conditions requiring chronic or recurrent exposure to latex such as urogenital anomalies and ventriculoperitoneal shunt have also been associated with latex hypersensitivity. The combination of atopy and frequent exposure seems to synergistically increase the risk of latex hypersensitivity.

Latex is the milky fluid obtained by tapping the cultivated rubber tree, *Hevea brasiliensis*. During manufacture of latex products, various antioxidants and accelerators such as thiurams, carbamates, and mercaptobenzothiazoles are added. Latex products are typically produced by dipping a porcelain mold into a tank of latex and then vulcanizing it to enhance mechanical stability. The product is washed or "leached" of excess proteins, then dry-lubricated with a powder such as corn starch.

Latex is a complex biologic mixture composed of rubber particles in a phospholipoprotein envelope and a serum containing sugars, lipids, nucleic acids, minerals, and various proteins. The protein component is thought to contain the allergenic properties. Extra leaching steps may reduce the protein content and hence the allergenicity of the final product. IgE from latex-sensitized individuals reacts with different protein components, supporting the notion that more than one clinically important latex antigen exists. New allergenic epitopes are generated during the manufacturing process. Thus, polypeptides from latex glove extracts vary both quantitatively and qualitatively with different brands and lots of gloves. Identification of the causative antigens is important because it may be possible to alter the manufacturing process to reduce the final allergen content.

Latex is ubiquitous in medical settings, and many sources may be inconspicuous. Synthetic alternatives to some latex products—including gloves, dressings, and tape—are available. Avoidance of contact with latex-containing items, however, may be insufficient to prevent allergic reactions, because lubricating powders may serve as vehicles for aerosolized latex antigens. The use of powder-free latex gloves is an important control measure for airborne latex allergen.

Nonmedical sources of latex are also common and include balloons, toys, rubber bands, erasers, condoms, and shoe soles. Pacifiers and bottle nipples have also been implicated as sources of latex allergen, although these products are molded rather than dipped, and allergic reactions to molded products are less common. Latex-allergic patients and their caregivers must be continuously vigilant for hidden sources of exposure.

Clinical Findings

A. SYMPTOMS AND SIGNS

The clinical manifestations of IgE-mediated reactions to latex can involve the full spectrum of symptoms associated with mast cell degranulation. Localized pruritus and urticaria occur after cutaneous contact; conjunctivitis and rhinitis can result from aerosol exposure or direct facial contact. Systemic reactions, including bronchospasm, laryngospasm and hypotension, may occur with more substantial exposure or in extremely sensitive individuals. Finally, vascular collapse and shock leading to fatal cardiovascular events may occur. Intraoperative anaphylaxis represents a common and serious manifestation of latex allergy.

Allergic contact dermatitis to rubber products typically appears 24–48 hours after contact. The primary allergens include accelerators and antioxidants used in the manufacturing process. The diagnosis is established by patch testing. Shoe soles are an important source of exposure. The skin lesions appear primarily as a patchy eczema on exposed surfaces, although reactions can become generalized.

B. LABORATORY FINDINGS

Epicutaneous prick testing is a rapid, inexpensive, and sensitive test that detects the presence of latex-specific IgE on skin mast cells. Obstacles to its use include lack of a standardized antigen. Reports of life-threatening anaphylactic events have been associated with skin testing to latex, and intradermal testing may be especially dangerous. A commercially available extract is pending FDA approval.

Immunoassay testing involves the in vitro measurement of specific IgE, which binds latex antigens. Antigen sources used for testing have included native plant extracts, raw latex, and finished products. When compared with a history of latex-induced symptoms or positive skin tests, the sensitivity of immunoassays testing for latex antigens ranges from 50–100% with specificity between 63% and 100%. These broad ranges may reflect the patient population studied and the source of latex antigen as well as the assay employed. A positive immunoassay test to latex in the presence of a highly suggestive latex allergy history is useful and may circumvent the potential concerns associated with prick skin testing in certain patients.

Cross-reactivity has been demonstrated between latex and a number of other antigens such as foods. Banana, avocado, and chestnut have been found to be antigenically similar to latex both immunologically and clinically.

Complications

Complications may be similar to those caused by other allergens. Prolonged exposure to aerosolized latex may lead to persistent asthma. Chronic allergic contact dermatitis, especially on the hands, can lead to functional disability.

Treatment

Avoidance remains the cornerstone of treatment for latex allergy. Prevention and supportive therapy are the most common methods for managing this problem.

Patients identified as being allergic to latex may need to have a personal supply of vinyl or latex-free gloves for use when visiting a physician or dentist. "Hypoallergenic gloves" are poorly classified with respect to their ability to induce IgE-mediated reactions; the FDA currently uses this term to designate products that have a reduced capacity to induce contact dermatitis. Gloves made from synthetic materials include Neolon (Becton-Dickinson), Tactyl 1 (Smart Practice), and Elastyren (Hermal). Autoinjectable epinephrine and medical identification bracelets may be prescribed for latex-allergic patients along with avoidance counseling.

Prophylactic premedication of latex-allergic individuals has been used in some surgical patients at high risk for latex allergy. The rationale for this therapy is derived from the pretreatment protocols developed for iodinated radiocontrast media and anesthetic reactions. Although there has been some success using this regimen, anaphylaxis has occurred despite pretreatment. This approach should not substitute for careful avoidance measures.

Prognosis

Owing to the ubiquitous nature of natural rubber, the prognosis is guarded for patients with severe latex allergy. Chronic exposure to airborne latex particles may lead to chronic asthma. Chronic dermatitis can lead to functional disability.

3. Vaccines

Mumps–measles–rubella (MMR) vaccine has been shown to be safe in egg-allergic patients (although rare reactions to gelatin or neomycin can occur). The ovalbumin content in influenza vaccine is variable, and skin testing with the specific vaccine lot is warranted in patients with egg allergy. (*Note:* Some patients who tolerate cooked egg, that is, denatured protein, may still react to the vaccine.) In addition, the newly introduced live intranasal influenza vaccine is contraindicated in egg-allergic children.

4. Radiocontrast Media

Non–IgE-mediated anaphylactoid reactions may occur with radiocontrast media with up to a 30% reaction rate on reexposure. Management involves using a low-molarity agent and premedication with prednisone, diphenhydramine, and possibly an H_2-blocker.

5. Insulin

Approximately 50% of patients receiving insulin have positive skin tests, but IgE-mediated reactions occur rarely. Insulin resistance is mediated by IgG. If less than 24 hours has elapsed after an allergic reaction to insulin, do not discontinue insulin but rather reduce the dose by one-third, then increase by 2–5 units per injection. Skin testing and desensitization are necessary if the interval between the allergic reaction and subsequent dose is greater than 24 hours.

6. Local Anesthetics

Less than 1% of reactions to local anesthetics are IgE-mediated. Management involves selecting a local anesthetic from another class. Esters of benzoic acid include benzocaine and procaine; amides include lidocaine and mepivacaine. Alternatively, the patient can be skin tested with the suspected agent, followed by a provocative challenge. To rule out paraben sensitivity, skin testing can be done with 1% lidocaine from a multidose vial.

7. Aspirin & Other Nonsteroidal Anti-Inflammatory Drugs

Adverse reactions to aspirin and nonsteroidal anti-inflammatory drugs (NSAIDs) include urticaria and angioedema; rhinosinusitis, nasal polyps, and asthma; anaphylactoid reactions; and NSAID-related hypersensitivity pneumonitis. After a systemic reaction, a refractory period of 2–7 days occurs. Most aspirin-sensitive patients tolerate sodium salicylate. All NSAIDs inhibiting cyclooxygenase cross-react with aspirin. Cross-reactivity between aspirin and tartrazine (yellow dye No. 5) has not been substantiated in controlled trials. No skin test or in vitro test is available to diagnose aspirin sensitivity. Oral challenge can induce severe bronchospasm. Desensitization and cross-desensitization to NSAIDs can be achieved in most patients and maintained long-term. Leukotriene-receptor antagonists or 5-lipoxygenase inhibitors attenuate the reaction to aspirin challenge and may be beneficial adjunct treatment in aspirin-sensitive asthmatic patients. Preliminary studies suggest that COX-2 inhibitors may be tolerated by patients with ASA-induced asthma.

8. Biological Agents

In recent years, a growing number of biological agents have become available for the treatment of autoimmune, neoplastic, cardiovascular, infectious, and allergic diseases, among others. Their use may be associated with a variety of adverse reactions including hypersensitivity reactions.

Bohlke K et al: Risk of anaphylaxis after vaccination of children and adolescents. Pediatrics 2003;112:815 [PMID: 12952113].

Centers for Disease Control and Prevention, National Immunization Program: www.cdc.gov/nip

Chiu AM et al: Anaphylaxis: Drug allergy, insect stings, and latex. Immunol Allergy Clin North Am 2005;25:389 [PMID: 15878462].

Lee SJ et al: Adverse reactions to biologic agents: Focus on autoimmune disease therapies. J Allergy Clin Immunol 2005;116:900 [PMID: 16210067].

Offit PA: Addressing parents' concerns: Do vaccines contain harmful preservatives, adjuvants, additives, or residuals? Pediatrics 2003;112:1394 [PMID: 14654615].

Pichichero ME: A review of evidence supporting the American Academy of Pediatrics recommendation for prescribing cephalosporin antibiotics for penicillin-allergic patients. Pediatrics 2005;115:1048 [PMID: 15805383].

Zeiger RS: Current issues with influenza vaccination in egg allergy. J Allergy Clin Immunol 2002;110:834 [PMID: 12373275].

FOOD ALLERGY

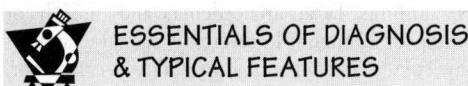

ESSENTIALS OF DIAGNOSIS & TYPICAL FEATURES

- *Temporal relationship between ingestion of a suspected food and onset of allergic symptoms.*
- *Positive prick skin test or in vitro test to a suspected food allergen confirmed by a double-blind, placebo-controlled food challenge (except in cases of anaphylaxis).*

General Considerations

Adverse reactions to foods are common in young children, especially in the first 3 years of life. The highest prevalence of food allergy is found in children with moderate-to-severe atopic dermatitis, with up to 33% affected. Up to 16% of children with asthma have been found to have food-induced wheezing in some studies. The most common food allergens in young children are eggs, milk, peanuts, soy, and wheat. In older children and adolescents, fish, shellfish, and nuts are most often involved in allergic reactions, and may prove to be a lifelong condition.

Some reactions often diagnosed by patients or physicians as food allergy involve pharmacologic or metabolic mechanisms and reactions to food toxins. Foods containing significant amounts of vasoactive amines such as chocolate, cheese, and some wines and beers may precipitate migraine headaches in some patients. Claims that dyes, sugar, and food additives may contribute to hyperactivity in children with attention-deficit/hyperactivity disorder are controversial. In the occasional case in which a child appears to benefit from a restricted diet, there is no evidence for an IgE-mediated reaction.

Clinical Findings

A. SYMPTOMS AND SIGNS

Most reactions to foods occur minutes to 2 hours after ingestion. A history of a temporal relationship between the ingestion of a suspected food and onset of a reaction—as well as the nature and duration of symptoms observed—is important in establishing the diagnosis of food allergy. With chronic atopic dermatitis or persistent urticaria, the association with food may be less obvious (see Atopic Dermatitis and Urticaria sections). At times, acute symptoms may occur, but the cause may not be obvious because of hidden food allergens. A symptom diary kept for 7–14 days may be helpful in establishing an association between ingestion of foods and symptoms and also provides a baseline observation for the pattern of symptom expression. It is important to record both the form in which the food was ingested and the foods ingested concurrently.

Hives, flushing, facial angioedema, and mouth or throat itching are common. In severe cases, angioedema of the tongue, uvula, pharynx, or upper airway can occur. Contact urticaria can occur without systemic symptoms in some children. Gastrointestinal symptoms include abdominal discomfort or pain, nausea, vomiting, and diarrhea. Children with food allergy may occasionally have isolated rhinoconjunctivitis or wheezing. Rarely, anaphylaxis to food may involve only cardiovascular collapse (see section on Anaphylaxis). Anaphylactoid reactions can occur after ingestion of foods such as certain fish containing high amounts of histamine.

B. Laboratory Findings

Typically, fewer than 50% of histories of food allergy will be confirmed by blinded challenge (although this percentage is much higher in food-induced anaphylaxis). Prick skin testing is useful to rule out a suspected food allergen, because the predictive value is high for a properly performed negative test with an extract of good quality. In contrast, the predictive value for a positive test is approximately 50%. RAST and other in vitro tests have lower specificity and positive predictive values. In contrast, specific IgE levels to milk, egg, peanut, and fish proteins have been established with the Pharmacia ImmunoCAP assay correlating with a greater than 95% chance of a clinical reaction. Measurement of IgG to foods is not clinically useful. Eosinophilia of stool mucus may be present in cases of gastrointestinal allergy; elevated circulating eosinophils may be present as well.

Double-blind, placebo-controlled food challenge is considered the standard method for diagnosing food allergy except in severe reactions. Even when multiple food allergies are suspected, most patients will be positive to three or fewer foods on blinded challenge. Therefore, extensive elimination diets are almost never indicated. Elimination without controlled challenge is a less desirable but at times more practical approach for suspected food allergy.

Differential Diagnosis

Repeated vomiting in infancy may be due to pyloric stenosis or gastroesophageal reflux. With chronic gastrointestinal symptoms, enzyme deficiency (eg, lactase), cystic fibrosis, celiac disease, chronic intestinal infections, gastrointestinal malformations, and irritable bowel syndrome should be considered.

Treatment

Treatment consists of eliminating and avoiding foods that have been documented to cause allergic reactions. This involves educating the patient, parent, and caregivers regarding hidden food allergens, the necessity for reading labels, and the signs and symptoms of food allergy and its appropriate management. Examples of ingredients that may indicate an implicated food protein include "emulsifier" (egg), "lecithin" (egg or soy), "natural flavoring" (milk), and "thickener" (soy). Consultation with a dietitian familiar with food allergy may be helpful, especially when common foods such as milk, egg, peanut, soy, or wheat are involved. Patients with a history of food-induced anaphylaxis or respiratory distress should carry epinephrine (see section on Anaphylaxis). A study of patients with peanut allergy demonstrated that treatment with monoclonal anti-IgE significantly increased the threshold of sensitivity to peanut on oral food challenge, although this treatment is currently approved only for patients with asthma (see section on Asthma).

Prognosis

The prognosis is good if the offending food can be identified and avoided. Unfortunately, accidental exposure to food allergens in severely allergic patients can result in death. Most children outgrow their food allergies to egg, milk, or soy but not to peanut or tree nuts. The natural history of food allergy to milk, egg, peanut, and fish proteins can be followed by measuring specific IgE levels by ImmunoCAP assay as discussed earlier. Approximately 2% will have food allergy as adults. Resources for food-allergic patients include the Food Allergy and Anaphylaxis Network and the National Peanut and Tree Nut Registry (800-929-4040; http://www.foodallergy.org).

Sampson HA: Update on food allergy. J Allergy Clin Immunol 2004;113:805 [PMID: 15131561].

INSECT ALLERGY

Allergic reactions to insects include symptoms of respiratory allergy as a result of inhalation of particulate matter of insect origin, local cutaneous reactions to insect bites, and anaphylactic reactions to stings. The latter are almost exclusively caused by Hymenoptera and result in approximately 40 deaths each year in the United States. The order Hymenoptera includes honey bees, yellow jackets, yellow hornets, white-faced hornets, wasps, and fire ants. Africanized honey bees, also known as killer bees, are a concern because of their aggressive behavior and excessive swarming, not because their venom is more toxic. Rarely, patients sensitized to reduviid bugs (also known as kissing bugs) may have episodes of nocturnal anaphylaxis. Lepidopterism refers to adverse effects secondary to contact with larval or adult butterflies and moths. Salivary gland antigens are responsible for immediate and delayed skin reactions in mosquito-sensitive patients.

Clinical Findings

A. SYMPTOMS AND SIGNS

Insect bites or stings can cause local or systemic reactions ranging from mild to fatal responses in susceptible persons. The frequency increases in the summer months and with outdoor exposure. Local cutaneous reactions include urticaria as well as papulovesicular eruptions and lesions that resemble delayed hypersensitivity reactions. Papular urticaria is almost always the result of insect bites, especially of mosquitoes, fleas, and bedbugs. Toxic systemic reactions consisting of gastrointestinal symptoms, headache, vertigo, syncope, convulsions, or fever can occur following multiple stings. These reactions result from histamine-like substances in the venom. In children with hypersensitivity to fire ant venom, sterile pustules occur at sting sites on a nonimmunologic basis due to the inherent toxicity of piperidine alkaloids in the venom. Mild systemic reactions include itching, flushing, and urticaria. Severe systemic reactions may include dyspnea, wheezing, chest tightness, hoarseness, fullness in the throat, hypotension, loss of consciousness, incontinence, nausea, vomiting, and abdominal pain. Delayed systemic reactions occur from 2 hours to 3 weeks following the sting and include serum sickness, peripheral neuritis, allergic vasculitis, and coagulation defects.

B. LABORATORY FINDINGS

Skin testing is indicated for children with systemic reactions. Venoms of honeybee, yellow jacket, yellow hornet, white-faced hornet, and wasp are available for skin testing and treatment. Fire ant venom is not yet commercially available, but an extract made from fire ant bodies appears adequate to establish the presence of IgE antibodies to fire ant venom. Of note, venom skin test results can be negative in patients with systemic allergic reactions, especially in the first few weeks after a sting, and the tests may need to be repeated. The presence of a positive skin test denotes prior sensitization but does not predict whether a reaction will occur with the patient's next sting, nor does it differentiate between local and systemic reactions. It is common for children who have had an allergic reaction to have positive skin tests to more than one venom. This might reflect sensitization from prior stings that did not result in an allergic reaction or cross-reactivity between closely related venoms. In vitro testing (compared with skin testing) has not substantially improved the ability to predict anaphylaxis. With venom RAST, there is a 15–20% incidence of both false-positive and false-negative results. Tests for mosquito saliva antigens or other insect allergy are not commercially available.

Complications

Secondary infection can complicate allergic reactions to insect bites or stings. Serum sickness, nephrotic syndrome, vasculitis, neuritis, and encephalopathy may be seen as late sequelae of reactions to stinging insects.

Treatment

For cutaneous reactions caused by biting insects, symptomatic therapy includes cold compresses, antipruritics (including antihistamines), and occasionally potent topical corticosteroids. Treatment of stings includes careful removal of the stinger, if present, by flicking it away from the wound and not by grasping in order to prevent further envenomation. Topical application of monosodium glutamate, baking soda, or vinegar compresses is of questionable efficacy. Local reactions can be treated with ice, elevation of the affected extremity, oral antihistamines, and NSAIDs as well as potent topical corticosteroids. Large local reactions, in which swelling extends beyond two joints or an extremity, may require a short course of oral corticosteroids. Anaphylactic reactions following Hymenoptera stings should be managed essentially the same as anaphylaxis (see section on Anaphylaxis). Children who have had severe or anaphylactic reactions to Hymenoptera stings—or their parents and caregivers—should be instructed in the use of epinephrine. Patients at risk for anaphylaxis from an insect sting should also wear a medical alert bracelet indicating their allergy. Children at risk from insect stings should avoid wearing bright-colored clothing and perfumes when outdoors and should wear long pants and shoes when walking in the grass. Patients who experience severe systemic reactions and have a positive skin test should receive venom immunotherapy. Immunotherapy is not indicated for children with only urticarial or local reactions.

Prognosis

Children generally have milder reactions than adults after insect stings, and fatal reactions are extremely rare. Patients age 3–16 years with reactions limited to the skin, such as urticaria and angioedema, appear to be at low risk for more severe reactions with subsequent stings.

Golden D: Outcomes of allergy to insect stings in children, with and without venom immunotherapy. N Engl J Med 2004;351:668 [PMID: 15306668].

Antimicrobial Therapy

35

John W. Ogle, MD

PRINCIPLES OF ANTIMICROBIAL THERAPY

Antimicrobial therapy of bacterial infections is arguably the most important scientific development of twentieth-century medicine. It contributes significantly to the quality of life of many people and reduces the morbidity and mortality due to infectious disease. The remarkable success of antimicrobial therapy has been achieved with comparatively little toxicity and expense. The relative ease of administration and the widespread availability of these drugs have led many to adopt a philosophy of broad-spectrum empiric antimicrobial therapy for many common infections.

Unfortunately this era of cheap, safe, and reliable therapy may be coming to a close owing to the increasing frequency of antimicrobial resistance in previously susceptible microorganisms. The problem of antimicrobial resistance is certainly not new—resistance was recognized for sulfonamides and penicillins shortly after their introduction. What is new is the worldwide dissemination of resistant clones of microorganisms, such as *Streptococcus pneumoniae* and *Staphylococcus aureus,* which are inherently virulent and commonly cause serious infections, not only among hospitalized patients but also among outpatients.

Until recently the recognition of new resistant clones was balanced by the promise of newer and more potent antimicrobial agents. Today, because fewer new agents are under development, clinicians are beginning to encounter limitations in their ability to treat some serious bacterial infections. Many factors contribute to the selection of resistant clones. Our success in treating chronic diseases and immune-compromising conditions, which has resulted in additional years of life for patients, has increased opportunities for selection of resistant strains in inpatient units and chronic care facilities. Overuse of antimicrobial agents by well-intentioned clinicians also contributes to the selection of resistant strains. Examples include medications for mildly ill patients with self-limited conditions such as viral infections, and administration of broad-spectrum antimicrobials for patients whose condition can be treated with narrow-spectrum agents. Similarly, failure to document infection with cultures obtained prior to starting therapy limits our willingness to stop or narrow the spectrum of antimicrobials. Little

research has been conducted to determine the necessary duration of therapy, with the result that we probably often treat longer than is necessary. Prophylactic strategies, as used for prevention of recurrent otitis media or urinary tract infection, create a selection pressure for antibiotic resistance.

The decision-making process for choosing an appropriate antimicrobial agent is summarized in Table 35–1. Accurate clinical diagnosis is based on the history, physical examination, and initial laboratory tests. The clinical diagnosis then leads to a consideration of the organisms most commonly associated with the clinical condition, the usual pattern of antimicrobial susceptibility of these organisms, and past experience with successful treatment regimens.

Cultures should be obtained in potentially serious infections. Empiric antimicrobial therapy may be initiated, then modified according to the patient's response and the culture results. Often several equally safe and efficacious antimicrobials are available. In this circumstance, the relative cost and ease of administration of the different choices should be considered.

Other important considerations include the patient's age, immune status, and exposure history. Neonates and young infants may present with nonspecific signs of infection, making the differentiation of serious disease from mild illness difficult. In older children, clinical diagnosis is more precise, which may permit avoiding therapy or use of a narrower-spectrum antibiotic. Immune deficiency may increase the number and types of potential infecting organisms that need to be considered, including organisms that are usually avirulent but that may cause infections that are serious and difficult to treat. An abnormal immune response may also diminish the severity of the clinical signs and symptoms of infection and thus lead to underestimation of the severity of illness. The exposure history may suggest the greater likelihood of certain types of infecting organisms. This history includes exposures from family members, classmates, and day care environments and exposure to unusual organisms by virtue of travel, diet, or contact with animals.

Final important considerations are the pace and seriousness of the illness. A rapidly progressive and severe illness should be treated initially with broad-spectrum antimicrobials until a specific etiologic diagnosis is

Table 35–1. Steps in decision making for use of antimicrobial agents.

Step	Action	Example
1	Determine diagnosis	Septic arthritis
2	Consider age and preexisting condition	Previously healthy 2-year-old child
3	Consider common organisms	*Staphylococcus aureus, Kingella kingae*
4	Consider organism susceptibility	Penicillin- or ampicillin-resistant, frequency MRSA[a] in community
5	Obtain proper cultures[b]	Blood, joint fluid
6	Initiate empiric therapy based on above considerations and past experience (eg, personal, literature)	Nafcillin and cefotaxime, substitute vancomycin for nafcillin if obviously ill or MRSA prevalent.
7	Modify therapy based on culture results and patient response	*S aureus* isolated. Discontinue cefotaxime. Substitute naficillin for vancomycin if susceptible.
8	Follow clinical response	Interval physical examination
9	Stop therapy	Clinically improved or well, minimum 3–4 weeks

[a]Methicillin-resistant *S aureus*.
[b]Indicated for serious or unusual infections or those with unpredictable clinical response to empiric therapy.

made. A mildly ill outpatient should receive treatment preferentially with narrow-spectrum antimicrobials.

Antimicrobial susceptibility, antimicrobial families, and dosing recommendations are listed in Tables 35–2 to 35–6.

ANTIMICROBIAL SUSCEPTIBILITY TESTING

Cultures and other diagnostic material must be obtained prior to initiating antimicrobial therapy—especially when the patient has a serious infection, initial attempts at therapy have failed, or multiagent therapy is anticipated. Whenever cultures identify the causative organism, therapy can be narrowed or optimized according to susceptibility results. Antimicrobial susceptibility testing should be done in a laboratory using carefully defined procedures (Clinical and Laboratory Standards Institute).

There are several ways to test antimicrobial susceptibility. Identification of an antibiotic-destroying enzyme (eg, β-lactamase) implies resistance to β-lactam–containing antimicrobial agents. Tube or microtiter broth dilution techniques can be used to determine the minimum inhibitory concentration (MIC) of antibiotic, which is the amount of antibiotic (in μg/mL) necessary to inhibit the organism under specific laboratory conditions. Disk susceptibility testing (also performed under carefully controlled conditions) yields similar results. The E-test is a standardized test for some organisms that correlates well with MICs. Clinical laboratories usually define antimi-crobial susceptibility (susceptible, intermediate, and resistant) in relation to levels of the test antibiotic achievable in the blood or another body fluid (CSF or urine).

Organisms are usually considered susceptible to an antibiotic if the MIC of the antibiotic for the organism is lower than levels of that agent achievable in the blood using appropriate parenteral dosages. This assumption of susceptibility should be reconsidered whenever the patient has a focus of infection (eg, meningitis, osteo-myelitis, or abscess) in which poor antibiotic penetration might occur, because the levels of antibiotic in such areas might be lower than the MIC. Conversely, although certain organisms may be reported resistant to an antibiotic because sufficiently high blood concentrations cannot be achieved, urine concentrations may be much higher. If so, a urinary tract infection might respond to an antibiotic that would not be adequate for treatment of septicemia.

Thus, antimicrobial susceptibility testing, although a very important part of therapeutic decision making, reflects assumptions that the clinician must understand, especially for serious infections. Ultimately the true test of the efficacy of therapy is patient response. Patients who do not respond to seemingly appropriate therapy may require reassessment, including reconsidering the diagnosis, reculturing, and repeat susceptibility testing, to determine whether resistant strains have evolved or superinfection with a resistant organism is present. Antimicrobial therapy cannot be expected to cure some infections unless additional supportive treatment (usually surgical) is undertaken.

Table 35–2. Susceptibility of some common pathogenic microorganisms to various antimicrobial drugs.

Organism	Potentially Useful Antibiotics[a]
Bacteria	
Anaerobic bacteria [b]	Cefoxitin,[c] cefotetan,[c] clindamycin, ertapenem,[c] imipenem,[c] meropenem, metronidazole, penicillins with or without β-lactamase inhibitor, tigecycline[c]
Bacillus anthracis	Amoxicillin, ciprofloxacin, clindamycin, doxycycline, rifampin
Bartonella henselae	Azithromycin, ciprofloxacin, clarithromycin, doxycycline, erythromycin
Bordetella pertussis	Amoxicillin, azithromycin, clarithromycin, erythromycin, trimethoprim-sulfamethoxazole
Borrelia burgdorferi	Amoxicillin, cefuroxime, cephalosporins (III),[h] clarithromycin, doxycycline
Campylobacter spp	Azithromycin, carbapenems, erythromycin, fluoroquinolones,[c,f] tetracyclines
Clostridium spp	Clindamycin, metronidazole, penicillins, tetracyclines
Clostridium difficile	Bacitracin (PO), metronidazole, vancomycin (PO)
Corynebacterium diphtheriae	Clindamycin, erythromycin, penicillins
Enterobacteriaceae[d]	Aminoglycosides,[e] ampicillin, aztreonam, cefepime, cephalosporins, ertopenem, imipenem, meropenem, fluoroquinolones,[c,f] trimethoprim-sulfamethoxazole, tigecyline
Enterococcus	Ampicillin (with aminoglycoside), carbapenems (not *E faecium*), vancomycin, linezolid, quinupristin/dalfopristin[c] (*E faecium* only), tigecycline
Haemophilus influenzae	Amoxicillin/clavulanate, ampicillin (if β-lactamase-negative),[g] cephalosporins (II and III),[h] chloramphenicol, fluoroquinolones,[c,f] rifampin, trimethoprim-sulfamethoxazole
Listeria monocytogenes	Ampicillin with aminoglycoside, trimethoprim-sulfamethoxazole, vancomycin
Moraxella catarrhalis	Amoxicillin/clavulanate, ampicillin (if β-lactamase-negative),[g] cephalosporins (II, III),[h] erythromycin, fluorquinolones, trimethoprim-sulfamethoxazole
Neisseria gonorrhoeae	Ampicillin (if β-lactamase-negative),[g] cephalosporins (II and III),[h] penicillins, selected fluoroquinolones,[c,f] spectinomycin
Neisseria meningitidis	Ampicillin, cephalosporins (II and III),[h] fluoroquinolones,[c,f] penicillins, rifampin
Nocardia asteroides	Tetracycline, trimethoprim-sulfamethoxazole (+amikacin for severe infections); meropenem or cephalosporins (II)[h] for brain abscess
Pasteurella multocida	Amoxicillin/clavulanate, ampicillins, penicillins, tetracyclines
Pseudomonas aeruginosa	Aminoglycosides,[e] anti-*Pseudomonas* penicillins,[c] aztreonam, cefepime, ceftazidime, imipenem, meropenem, ciprofloxacin[c]
Salmonella spp	Ampicillin, azithromycin, cephalosporins (III),[h] fluoroquinolones,[c,f] trimethoprim-sulfamethoxazole
Shigella spp	Ampicillin, azithromycin cephalosporins (III),[h] fluoroquinolones,[c,f] tetracyclines, trimethoprim-sulfamethoxazole
Staphylococcus aureus	Antistaphylococcal penicillins,[j] cefepime, cephalosporins (I and II), ciprofloxacin, clindamycin, erythromycin, rifampin, trimethoprim-sulfamethoxazole, vancomycin
S aureus (methicillin-resistant)	Trimethoprim-sulfomethoxaole, vancomycin, linezolid, quinupristin/dalfopristin,[c] clindamycin, daptomycin,[c] tigecyline[c]
Staphylococci (coagulase-negative)	Cephalosporins (I and II),[k] clindamycin, rifampin, vancomycin
Streptococci (most species)	Ampicillin, cephalosporins, clindamycin, enhanced fluoroquinolones,[c,n] erythromycin, meropenem, penicillins, vancomycin
Streptococcus pneumoniae[l]	Ampicillin, cephalosporins, enhanced fluoroquinolones,[c,n] erythromycin, meropenem, penicillin, vancomycin

(continued)

Table 35–2. Susceptibility of some common pathogenic microorganisms to various antimicrobial drugs. (continued)

Organism	Potentially Useful Antibiotics[a]
Intermediate organisms	
Chlamydia spp	Clarithromycin, erythromycin, levofloxacin,[c] ofloxacin,[c] tetracyclines
Mycoplasma spp	Azithromycin, clarithromycin, erythromycin, fluoroquinolones,[c,f] tetracyclines
Rickettsia spp	Fluoroquinolones,[c,f] tetracyclines
Fungi	
Candida spp	Amphotericin B, caspofungin, fluconazole, flucytosine, itraconazole, ketoconazole, voriconazole
Fungi, systemic[b]	Amphotericin B, caspofungin, fluconazole, itraconazole,[c] ketoconazole, voriconazole
Dermatophytes	Butenafine, ciclopirox olamine, clotrimazole, econozole, fluconazole, griseofulvin, itraconazole,[c] ketoconazole, miconazole, naftifine, oxiconazole, terbinafine
Pneumocystis jiroveci	Atovaquone, clindamycin+primaquin, dapsone, pentamidine, trimethoprim–sulfamethoxazole
Viruses	
Herpes simplex	Acyclovir, pencyclovir,[c] famciclovir,[c] foscarnet, trifluridine,[i] valacyclovir[c]
Human immunodeficiency virus	Four classes: (1) nucleoside reverse transcriptase inhibitor (9 drugs); (2) non-nucleoside reverse transcriptase inhibitors (3 drugs); (3) protease inhibitors (9 drugs); (4) fusion inhibitors (1 drug). Generally in combinations of ≥ 3 drugs used. (See Chapter 37: Human Immunodeficiency Virus Infection).
Influenza virus	Amantadine,[o] oseltamivir, rimantidine,[o] zanamivir
Respiratory syncytial virus	Ribavirin[m]
Varicella-zoster virus	Acyclovir, famciclovir,[c] valacyclovir[c]
Cytomegalovirus	Cidofovir, fomivireson, foscarnet, ganciclovir, valganciclovir

[a]In alphabetical order. Selection depends on patient's age, diagnosis, site of infection, severity of illness, antimicrobial susceptibility of suspected organism, and drug risk.
[b]Species-dependent.
[c]Not FDA-approved for use in children.
[d]Includes *E coli*, *Klebsiella* spp, *Enterobacter* spp, and others; antimicrobial susceptibilities should always be measured.
[e]Amikacin, gentamicin, kanamycin, tobramycin.
[f]Includes ciprofloxacin, levofloxacin, lomefloxacin, norfloxacin, ofloxacin, moxifloxacin, gatifloxacin, gemifloxacin.
[g]Also applies to amoxicillin and related compounds.
[h]Refer to second- (II) or third- (III) generation cephalosporins.
[i]Carbenicillin, mezlocillin, piperacillin, ticarcillin.
[j]Cloxacillin, dicloxacillin, methicillin, nafcillin, oxacillin.
[k]Only if the coagulase-negative *Staphylococcus* is also methicillin- or oxacillin-sensitive.
[l]Because of increasing frequency of *S pneumoniae* strains resistant to penicillin and cephalosporins, therapy for presumed severe infections (eg, meningitis) should include vancomycin until susceptibility studies are available.
[m]FDA-approved for therapy of RSV by aerosol, but clinical studies show variable efficacy.
[n]Includes levofloxacin, lomefloxacin, moxifloxacin, gatifloxacin, gemifloxacin.
[o]Influenza A only.

ALTERATION OF DOSE & MEASUREMENT OF BLOOD LEVELS

Certain antimicrobial agents have not been approved (and often not tested) for use in newborns. For those that have been approved, it is important to recognize that both dose and frequency of administration may need to be altered (see Tables 35–4 and 35–5), especially in young (7 days or younger) or low-birth-weight neonates (≤ 2000 g).

Antimicrobial agents are excreted or metabolized through various physiologic mechanisms (eg, renal,

Table 35–3. Groups of common antibacterial agents.

Group	Examples	Some Common Susceptible Organisms[a]	Common Resistant Organisms	Common or Unique Adverse Reactions
Penicillin group				
Penicillins	Penicillin G, V	*Streptococcus, Neisseria*	*Staphylococcus, Haemophilus,* Enterobacteriaceae	Rash, anaphylaxis, drug fever, bone marrow suppression
Ampicillins	Ampicillin, amoxicillin	(Same as penicillins), plus *Haemophilus* (β-lactamase negative), *Escherichia coli, Enterococcus*	*Staphylococcus,* many Enterobacteriaceae	Diarrhea
Antistaphylococcal penicillins	Cloxacillin, dicloxacillin, methicillin, nafcillin, oxacillin	*Streptococcus, Staphylococcus aureus*	Gram-negative, *Staphylococcus* (coagulase-negative), *Enterococcus*	Renal (interstitial nephritis)
Anti-*Pseudomonas* penicillins	Azlocillin, piperacillin, ticarcillin	(Same as ampicillins), plus *Pseudomonas*	(Same as ampicillins)	Decreased platelet adhesiveness, hypokalemia, hypernatremia
Penicillin and β-lactamase inhibitor combination	Amoxicillin-clavulanate, ampicillin-sulbactam, ticarcillin-clavulanate	Broad-spectrum	Some Enterobacteriaceae, *Pseudomonas*	Diarrhea
Carbapenems	Imipenem-cilastatin meropenem, ertapenem	Broad-spectrum, gram-negative rods, anaerobes, *Pseudomonas*	MRSA,[b] many enterococci	Central nervous system (CNS), seizures
Cephalosporin group				
First-generation (I)	Cefazolin, cephalexin, cephalothin, cephapirin, cephradine	Gram-positive	Gram-negative, *Enterococcus,* some *Staphylococcus* (coagulase-negative)	Rash; anaphylaxis, drug fever
Second-generation (II)	Cefaclor, cefamandole, cefprozil, cefonicid, cefuroxime, loracarbef	Gram-positive, some *Haemophilus,* some Enterobacteriaceae	*Enterococcus, Pseudomonas,* some *Staphylococcus* (coagulase-negative)	Serum sickness (cefaclor)
	Cefoxitin, cefotetan	Same as second-generation plus anaerobes		
Third-generation (III)	Cefotaxime, ceftizoxime, ceftriaxone, cefpodoxime, ceftibuten, cefdinir	*Streptococcus, Haemophilus,* Enterobacteriaceae, *Neisseria*	*Pseudomonas, Staphylococcus*	Biliary sludging (ceftriaxone) rash
	Ceftazidime, cefepime	(Same as other third-generation cephalosporins), plus *Pseudomonas*	*Staphylococcus*	
Other drugs				
Clindamycin	Clindamycin	Gram-positive, anaerobes	Gram-negative, *Enterococcus,* MRSA	Nausea, vomiting, hepatotoxicity
Vancomycin	Vancomycin	Gram-positive	Gram-negative	"Red man" syndrome, shock, ototoxicity, renal

(continued)

Table 35–3. Groups of common antibacterial agents. (continued)

Group	Examples	Some Common Susceptible Organisms[a]	Common Resistant Organisms	Common or Unique Adverse Reactions
Other drugs (*con't*)				
Macrolides and azilides	Erythromycin, clarithromycin, azithromycin	Gram-positive *Bordetella, Haemophilus, Mycoplasma, Chlamydia, Legionella*	Gram-negative	Nausea and vomiting
Monobactams	Aztreonam	Gram-negative aerobes, *Pseudomonas*	Gram-positive cocci	Rash, diarrhea
Oxazolidinones	Linezolid	Gram-positive aerobes	Gram-negative aerobes	Diarrhea, thrombocytopenia
Streptogamins	Quinupristin/dalfopristin	Gram-positive aerobes	Gram-negative aerobes	Arthralgia myalgia
Fluoroquinolones[c]	Ciprofloxacin, ofloxacin	Gram-negative, *Chlamydia, Pseudomonas* (ciprofloxacin)	*Enterococcus, Streptococcus, S pneumoniae,* anaerobes, *Staphylococcus*	Gastrointestinal (GI), rash, CNS
	Gatifloxacin, levofloxacin, moxifloxacin	Gram-negative, streptococci, *S pneumoniae,* staphylococci, anaerobes[d]	Some *Enterococcus*	GI, rash, CNS, severe hepatitis[d]
Tetracyclines	Chlortetracycline, tetracycline, doxycycline, minocycline	Anaerobes, *Mycoplasma, Chlamydia, Rickettsia, Ehrlichia*	Many Enterobacteriaceae, *Staphylococcus*	Teeth staining,[e] rash, flora overgrowth, hepatotoxicity, pseudotumor cerebri
Sulfonamides	Many	Gram-negative (urine)	Gram-positive	Rash, renal, bone marrow suppression, Stevens-Johnson syndrome
Trimethoprim-sulfamethoxazole	Trimethoprim-sulfamethoxazole	*S aureus,* gram-negative, *S pneumoniae, H influenzae*	*Streptococcus, Pseudomonas,* anaerobes	Rash, renal, bone marrow suppression, Stevens-Johnson syndrome
Rifampin	Rifampin	*Neisseria, Haemophilus, Staphylococcus, Streptococcus*	Resistance develops rapidly if used as sole agent	Rash, GI, hepatotoxicity, CNS, bone marrow suppression, alters metabolism of other drugs
Aminoglycosides	Amikacin, gentamicin, kanamycin, streptomycin, tobramycin	Gram-negative, including *P aeruginosa*	Gram-positive, anaerobes, some pseudomonads	Nephrotoxicity, ototoxicity, potentiates neuromuscular blocking agents

[a]Not all strains susceptible; always obtain antimicrobial susceptibility tests on significant isolates.
[b]MRSA = methicillin-resistant *S aureus.*
[c]Not approved for children.
[d]Trovofloxacin only.
[e]Dose-dependent in children < age 9 years.

Table 35–4. Guidelines for use of common parenteral antibacterial agents[a] in children age 1 month or older.

	Route	Dose[b] (mg/kg/d)	Maximum Daily Dose	Interval (hours)	Adjustment[c]	Blood Levels[d] (μg/mL) Peak	Trough
Amikacin	IM, IV	15–22.5	1.5 g	8	R	15–25	5–10
Ampicillin	IM, IV	100–400	12 g	4–6	R		
Aztreonam	IM, IV	90–120	6 g	6–8	R		
Cefazolin	IM, IV	50–100	6 g	8	R		
Cefepime[e]	IM, IV	100–150	4–6 g	8–12	R		
Cefotaxime	IM, IV	100–200	12 g	6–8	R		
Cefoxitin	IM, IV	80–160	12 g	4–6	R		
Ceftazidime	IM, IV	100–150	6 g	8	R		
Ceftizoxime	IM, IV	150–200	12 g	6–8	R		
Ceftriaxone	IM, IV	50–100	4 g	12–24	R		
Cefuroxime	IM, IV	100–150	6 g	6–8	R		
Cephalothin	IM, IV	75–125	12 g	4–6	R		
Cephradine	IM, IV	50–100	8 g	6	R		
Clindamycin	IM, IV	25–40	4 g	6–8	R, H		
Gentamicin	IM, IV	3–7.5	300 mg	8	R	5–10	< 2
Linezolid	IV, PO	20	1.2 g	12	R		
Meropenem	IV	60–120	2 g	8	R		
Metronidazole	IV	30	4 g	6	H		
Nafcillin	IM, IV	150	12 g	6	H		
Penicillin G	IM, IV	100,000–250,000 units/kg	20 million units	4–6	H, R		
Penicillin G (benzathine)	IM	50,000 units/kg	2.4 million units	Single dose	None		
Penicillin G (procaine)	IM	25,000–50,000 units/kg	4.8 million units	12–24	R		
Tetracycline[f]	IV[f]	20–30	2 g	12	R		
Ticarcillin	IV	200–300	24 g	4–6	R		
Tobramycin	IM, IV	3–6	300 mg	8	R	5–10	< 2
Vancomycin	IV	40–60	2 g	6	R	20–40[g]	< 5–10[g]

[a]Not including some newly released drugs, ones not recommended for use in children, or ones not widely used.

[b]Always consult package insert for complete prescribing information. Dosage may differ for alternative routes, newborns (see Table 35–6), or patients with liver or renal failure (see Adjustment column) and may not be recommended for use in pregnant women or newborns. Maximum dosage may be indicated only in severe infections or by parenteral routes.

[c]Mode of excretion (R = renal, H = hepatic) of antimicrobial agent should be assessed at the onset of therapy and dosage modified or levels determined as indicated in package insert.

[d]Suggested levels to reduce toxicity.

[e]Safety and efficacy are not established in children < age 2 months.

[f]Use with caution in children < age 9 years because of tooth staining with repeated doses.

[g]Target peak and trough vancomycin levels are not well correlated with either toxicity or outcome. Measure selectively in meningitis, impaired or changing renal function, or altered volume of distribution.

Table 35–5. Guidelines for use of common oral antibacterial agents in children age 1 month or older.

Agent[a]	Dose[b] (mg/kg/d)	Interval (hours)	Other Considerations
Amoxicillin	40	8–12	Gastrointestinal (GI) side effects
Amoxicillin[c] (high dose)	80–90	12	GI side effects
Amoxicillin-clavulanate	45	12	GI side effects
Ampicillin	50	6	GI side effects
Azithromycin	10 (first dose) then 5; 12 for pharyngitis	24	GI side effects
Cefaclor	40	8	Serum sickness–like illness
Cefadroxil	30	12	
Cefpodoxime	10	12	Taste (suspension)
Cefprozil	30	12	GI side effects
Ceftibuten	9	24	GI side effects
Cefuroxime	30–40	12	GI side effects
Cephalexin	25–50	6	
Cephradine	25–50	6	
Clarithromycin	15	12	GI side effects
Clindamycin	20–30	6	GI side effects
Cloxacillin	50–100	6	GI side effects
Dicloxacillin	12–25	6	GI side effects
Doxycycline[d]	2–4	12–24	Tooth staining < 9 years
Erythromycin[e]	20–50	6–12	GI side effects
Erythromycin-sulfisoxazole	40 (erythromycin)	6–8	
Furazolidone	5–8	6	
Linezolid	20	12	GI side effects
Loracarbef	15; 30 for otitis	12	
Metronidazole	15–35	8	
Nitrofurantoin	5–7	6	
Oxacillin	50–100	6	
Penicillin V	25–50	6	Taste (suspension)
Rifampin	10–20	12–24	
Sulfisoxazole	120–150	6	
Tetracycline[d]	25–50[c]	6	Teeth staining < 9 years
Trimethoprim-sulfamethoxazole	8–12 (TMP)	12	Stevens–Johnson syndrome

[a]Not including some newly released drugs, ones not recommended for use in children, or ones not widely used.
[b]Always consult package insert for complete prescribing information. Dosage may differ for alternative routes, newborns (see Table 35–6), or patients with liver or renal failure (see Table 35–4, Adjustment column) and may not be recommended for use in pregnant women or newborns. Maximum dosage may be indicated only in severe infections or by parenteral routes.
[c]Higher dose amoxicillin indicated for therapy of otitis media in regions where rates of penicillin-resistant *S pneumoniae* are common.
[d]Use with caution in children < age 9 years because of tooth staining with repeated doses.
[e]Preparation-dependent.

Table 35–6. Guidelines for use of selected antimicrobial agents in newborns.

	Route	Body Wt (g)	Maximum Dosage (mg/kg/d) [Frequency] < 7 Days		8–30 Days		Blood Levels (µg/mL) Peak	Trough
Amikacin[a]	IV, IM	< 2000	15	[q12h]	22.5	[q8h]	15–25	5–10
		> 2000	20	[q12h]	30	[q8h]		
Ampicillin	IV, IM	< 2000	100	[q12h]	150	[q8h]		
		> 2000	150	[q8h]	200	[q6h]		
Cefotaxime	IV, IM		100	[q12h]	150	[q8h]		
Ceftazidime	IV, IM	< 2000	100	[q12h]	150	[q8h]		
		> 2000	100	[q8h]	150	[q8h]		
Clindamycin	IV, IM, PO	< 2000	10	[q12h]	15	[q8h]		
		> 2000	15	[q8h]	20	[q6h]		
Erythromycin	PO		20	[q12h]	30	[q8h]		
Gentamicin[a]	IV, IM		5	[q12–18h]	7.5	[q8h]	5–10	< 2
Nafcillin	IV	< 2000	50	[q12h]	75	[q8h]		
		> 2000	75	[q8h]	150	[q6h]		
Oxacillin	IV, IM	< 2000	100	[q12h]	150	[q8h]		
		> 2000	50	[q8h]	200	[q6h]		
Penicillin G[b]	IV	< 2000	100,000	[q12h]	150,000	[q8h]		
		> 2000	150,000	[q8h]	200,000	[q6h]		
Ticarcillin	IV, IM	< 2000	150	[q12h]	225	[q8h]		
		> 2000	225	[q8h]	300	[q6h]		
Tobramycin[a]	IV, IM		5	[q12–18h]	7.5	[q8h]	5–10	< 2
Vancomycin[c]	IV		20	[q12h]	30	[q8h]	20–40	

[a]Neonates weighting < 1200 g may require even smaller doses. Antibiotic levels should be closely monitored.
[b]Penicillin dosages are in units/kg/d. Other preparations (eg, benzathine penicillin) may be given IM. See specific diseases for dosage.
[c]Target peak and trough vancomycin levels are not well correlated with either toxicity or outcome.

hepatic). It is important to consider these routes of excretion and alter the antimicrobial dosage appropriately in any patient with some degree of organ dysfunction. (See Chapter 41.) As indicated in Table 35–4, an assessment of renal or hepatic function may be routinely necessary for patients receiving certain drugs (eg, renal function for aminoglycosides, hepatic function for erythromycin or clindamycin); otherwise, harmful drug levels may accumulate. If significant organ dysfunction is present, drug clearance may be delayed and dosage modification may be necessary (see detailed descriptions in individual drug information packets), and measurement of drug levels may be indicated.

Serum levels of drugs posing a high risk of toxicity (eg, aminoglycosides) are ordinarily measured, and measurement of other drugs (eg, vancomycin) may be useful in selected circumstances (see following discussion). For certain other serious bacterial infections (eg, bacterial endocarditis), measurement of the serum concentration of an antimicrobial may be important to deliver optimal therapy.

Certain drug interactions may require modification of drug dosage or other therapeutic alterations. (See Chapter 41.) For example, rifampin stimulates the metabolism of warfarin, birth control pills, and anticonvulsants by stimulating the cytochrome P-450 (CYP-450) metabolic pathway. Dosage adjustments or alternative medications may be necessary to avoid significant adverse events. Another common example is erythromycin, which may inhibit the metabolism of theophylline, resulting in toxic theophylline levels. Although many drug interactions are known and well documented, it may be difficult to predict interactions that result from a combination of four, five, or more different medications. A high level of suspicion regarding adverse clinical events should be maintained.

THE USE OF NEW ANTIMICROBIAL AGENTS

New antibiotics are introduced frequently, often with claims about unique features that distinguish these usually more expensive products from existing compounds. Often, these drugs share many properties with existing drugs. The role that any new antimicrobial will play can only be determined over time, during which new or previously unrecognized side effects might be described and the clinical efficacy established. Clinical trials may not be confirmed in the larger number of patients subsequently treated in practice. Because this may take many years, a conservative approach to using new antibiotics seems fitting, especially because their costs are often higher, and appropriate antimicrobial choices for most common infections already exist. It is appropriate to ask if a new antimicrobial has been proved to be as effective as (or more effective than) the current drug of choice, and whether its side effects are comparable or less common and its cost reasonable. The withdrawal of moxalactam and caution regarding use of trovafloxacin due to unexpected serious side effects, which were not anticipated despite extensive premarket testing, highlight the caution necessary before using new antimicrobials. The heavy marketing of new cephalosporins and fluoroquinolones, which are very similar to existing drugs, is typical of the difficulty in evaluating antimicrobials.

The development of new antibiotics is important as a response to the emergence of resistant organisms and for treatment of infections that are clinically difficult to treat (eg, viruses, fungi, and some resistant bacteria). Fortunately these infections are either rare or (usually) self-limited in immunocompetent hosts.

PROPHYLACTIC ANTIMICROBIAL AGENTS

Antimicrobials can be used to decrease the incidence of postoperative infections (Table 35–7). A dose of an antimicrobial given 30 minutes to 2 hours prior to surgery can reduce postoperative wound infection. The goal is to achieve high levels in the serum at the time of incision and by this means—along with good surgical technique—to minimize bacterial contamination of the wound. During a lengthy procedure, a second dose may be given. No evidence exists that multiple subsequent doses of antimicrobials confer additional benefit. The antimicrobial(s) used for prophylaxis are directed toward the flora that most commonly cause postoperative infection at a given anatomic site. Gram-positive cocci such as *S aureus* are usually targeted, and a first-generation cephalosporin (eg, cefazolin) is a cost-effective choice. Third-generation cephalosporins and other broad-spectrum agents are more expensive and offer less benefit because they are less active than cefazolin against *S aureus*. Cefoxitin or cefotetan is useful for procedures such as colorectal surgery, although cefazolin is appropriate for most gynecologic patients. In colorectal surgery, oral antimicrobials such as neomycin and erythromycin may be as effective as parenteral therapy.

In hospitals where the predominant *S aureus* strains are methicillin-resistant or in cases where the patient is allergic to penicillin and cephalosporins, vancomycin can be considered. However, prophylactic vancomycin has caused hypotension at the time of induction of general anesthesia. Frequent use of vancomycin as a prophylactic antimicrobial will contribute to the development of vancomycin-resistant strains such as *Enterococcus faecalis*. For these reasons, vancomycin should generally not be used for prophylaxis, although it might prove useful for individual patients at extremely high risk.

Prophylactic antimicrobials are given in several other circumstances. Endocarditis prophylaxis is indicated during dental and colorectal or genitourinary procedures in patients with high-risk heart lesions, such as prosthetic cardiac valves, surgically corrected systemic pulmonary shunts, and mitral valve prolapse with regurgitation. Patients with indwelling vascular catheters, such as Broviac catheters, should receive prophylaxis during similar procedures, which are likely to induce a transient bacteremia. Prophylaxis against infection with group A streptococci reduces the recurrence rate for acute rheumatic fever. Postexposure prophylaxis is given after exposure to pertussis, *Haemophilus influenzae* type b (HIB) infection (depending on age), meningococcus, gonococcus, tuberculosis (household exposure), plague, aerosolized tularemia or anthrax, and other high-risk infections. Family or close contacts of patients with severe invasive streptococcal disease may benefit from prophylaxis. Silver nitrate, erythromycin, povidone–iodine, and tetracycline can be used in ophthalmic preparations for prevention of gonococcal ophthalmia neonatorum. Children with asplenia or sickle cell disease receive prophylactic penicillin to protect against overwhelming *S pneumoniae* sepsis, usually started immediately with the onset of fever.

Prophylactic antimicrobials are sometimes used for some children at high risk for recurrent urinary tract infection.

Table 35–7. Antimicrobial prophylaxis and preferred prophylactic agents: Selected conditions and pathogens.[a]

Pathogen (Indication)	Prophylactic Agent
Bacillus anthracis[b]	Amoxicillin (if proved susceptible), ciprofloxacin, doxycycline
Bacterial endocarditis[c]	Ampicillin, ampicillin and gentamicin, amoxicillin, or other approved regimens
Bordetella pertussis (exposure to respiratory secretions)	Azithromycin, clarithromycin, erythromycin
Chlamydia trachomatis (genital contact)	Erythromycin
Haemophilus influenzae type b[d] (household exposure)	Rifampin
Mycobacterium tuberculosis (household exposure)	Isoniazid
Neisseria meningitidis (household exposure)	Rifampin, sulfadiazine,[e] ciprofloxacin
N gonorrhoeae (ophthalmia neonatorum)	Erythromycin, silver nitrate ophthalmic
N gonorrhoeae (sexual contact)	Ceftriaxone, cefixime, cefpodoxime, fluoroquinolone
Treponema pallidum (sexual contact)	Penicillin
Streptococcus pneumoniae (sickle cell disease, asplenia)	Penicillin
Postoperative wound infection[f]	Cefazolin, other regimens[f]
Group A streptococci (rheumatic fever)[g]	Benzathine penicillin G, penicillin, sulfadiazine
Group B streptococcal sepsis	Ampicillin to mother prior to delivery
Pneumonic *Yersinia pestis*[h] (exposure)	Tetracycline[i]
Francisella tularensis[h] (aerosolized exposure)	Tetracycline[i]
Vibrio cholera	Tetracycline,[i] trimethoprim-sulfamethoxazole
Recurrent urinary tract infection	Nitrofurantoin, trimethoprim-sulfamethoxazole
Pneumocystis jiroveci (formerly *Pneumocystis carinii*)—(HIV, some immunocompromised patients)	Atovaquone, clindomycin-primaquin, dapsone, trimethoprim-sulfamethoxazole, pentamidine

[a]Decisions for prophylaxis must take a number of factors into account, including the evidence for efficacy of therapy, the degree of the exposure to an infecting agent, the risk and consequences of infection, the susceptibility of the infecting agent to antimicrobials, and the patient's ability to tolerate and comply with the antimicrobial agent. See individual chapters of the text for discussion.
[b]Decisions for prophylaxis should be made in accordance with the responsible public health department recommendations.
[c]See discussion in Chapter 19: Cardiovascular Diseases.
[d]Prophylaxis provided to family if contacts include children < age 4 years. Some experts provide prophylaxis in day care settings after one case and some after two cases of HIB.
[e]Only for known sulfadiazine-susceptible strains.
[f]Alternative regimens may be used, depending on the site of surgery and the degree of contamination.
[g]Oral prophylaxis may be indicated in some patients. Alternative regimens indicated for penicillin-allergic patients. See discussion in chapter.
[h]Prophylaxis not well established. Carefully assess risk on a case-by-case basis.
[i]Usually not indicated for children < age 9 years because of tooth staining with repeated doses.

INITIAL EMPIRIC ANTIMICROBIAL CHOICES FOR SELECTED CONDITIONS

General recommendations for specific conditions are as follows. A specific selection depends on the patient's age, diagnosis, site of infection, severity of illness, antimicrobial susceptibility of bacterial isolates, and history of drug allergy. Always consult the package insert for detailed prescribing information. Tables 35–2 to 35–6 include further information.

Neonatal Sepsis & Meningitis

The newborn with sepsis may have signs of focal infection such as pneumonia or respiratory distress syndrome or may have subtle nonfocal signs. Group

B streptococci, *Escherichia coli,* other gram-negative rods, and *Listeria monocytogenes* are commonly encountered. Ampicillin and gentamicin (or another aminoglycoside) are preferred. If meningitis is present, many clinicians substitute a third-generation cephalosporin for the aminoglycoside. *S pneumoniae* is an uncommon cause of meningitis in neonates. However, if the Gram stain shows gram-positive cocci suggesting *S pneumoniae,* substitution of vancomycin for ampicillin should be considered. In the newborn with cellulitis, *S aureus* including methicillin-resistant *S aureus* (MRSA) and group A streptococci are additional considerations. Nafcillin, oxacillin, or a first-generation cephalosporin is usually added. Vancomycin is added if MRSA is common. Omphalitis is often polymicrobial, and *Enterococcus* species, gram-negative aerobes, and anaerobes may be causative. Clindamycin, ampicillin, and an aminoglycoside or cefotaxime cover the most likely organisms; early surgical intervention is indicated.

Sepsis in an Infant

S pneumoniae and *Neisseria meningitidis* are most commonly encountered in infants. HIB infection may occur in unimmunized children. A third-generation cephalosporin is appropriate. Intermediate-level penicillin and cephalosporin resistance in *S pneumoniae* usually do not cause therapy to fail unless meningitis or another difficult-to-treat infection such as endocarditis or osteomyelitis is present.

Occult bacteremia may be encountered in young infants with high fever. Prior to immunization with vaccines effective against HIB, persistent bacteremia and complications including meningitis were seen in approximately 50% of children infected with occult HIB bacteremia. With widespread use of HIB vaccine, HIB is a very uncommon cause of occult bacteremia in young children with fever. *S pneumonia* bacteremia is demonstrated in 3–5% of infants age 3–36 months who have a fever of 39 °C or greater, no identified source for fever on examination, and a white blood cell count (WBC) = 15,000/mm^3. The risk of bacteremia increases to 6–10% in younger children with progressively high fever and high WBCs. The risk of developing meningitis due to persistent *S pneumoniae* is estimated at 3% of those who are known to be bacteremic. The risk of *S pneumoniae* bacteremia and its complications is significantly reduced in children immunized with the conjugate-7-valent pneumococcal vaccine. In clinical trials, this vaccine reduced the incidence of invasive pneumococcal diseases by approximately 90%. Observation without antimicrobials, but with appropriate plans for follow-up examinations, is appropriate for most febrile young children who are fully immunized.

Nosocomial Sepsis

Many bacterial pathogens can cause infection in hospitalized patients. Recent local experience is usually the best guide to etiologic diagnosis. For example, some intensive care units experience frequent infections due to *Enterobacter cloacae,* whereas in other units *Klebsiella pneumoniae* is the most common nosocomial isolate. Initial therapy should include antibiotics effective for MRSA and resistant *Pseudomonas aeruginosa* if these are frequent isolates. *Enterococcus faecalis* is a common cause of nosocomial bacteremia in patients with central catheters, particularly in units where cephalosporins are heavily used. Coagulase-negative staphylococci are commonly isolated from patients with indwelling central catheters. In seriously ill patients, when the local experience suggests that *Enterococcus* species or coagulase-negative staphylococci are common, the initial regimen should include vancomycin. Because *Enterococcus* species and coagulase-negative staphylococci commonly cause fever without significant morbidity or mortality, initial regimens without vancomycin are appropriate, with adjustment of treatment after susceptibility is known. If *P aeruginosa* or other resistant gram-negative rods are common, ceftazidime or cefepime should be included in initial therapy.

Meningitis

Bacterial meningitis in neonates is usually caused by infection with group B streptococci, *E coli,* or *L monocytogenes.* A combination of ampicillin and gentamicin or another aminoglycoside—or ampicillin and a third-generation cephalosporin—is started initially. In an infant or older child, *S pneumoniae* or *N meningitidis* is the most common isolate. HIB is uncommon now because of widespread immunization. Increasingly, *S pneumoniae* with multiple resistances to penicillin, cephalosporins, and other drugs is isolated. In some communities, 30–40% of *S pneumoniae* isolates have intermediate susceptibility to penicillin (MIC between 0.1 and 2 µg/mL) and 5–10% of isolates may be highly resistant to penicillin (MIC > 2 µg/mL). Resistance to a third-generation cephalosporin (MIC > 2 µg/mL) may occur in 3–5% of isolates.

In bacterial meningitis, peak cerebrospinal fluid (CSF) antimicrobial concentrations 10 or more times greater than the MIC of the organism are desirable, but this may be difficult to achieve if organisms are resistant. The therapeutic problem is complicated if dexamethasone, which reduces the entry of some antimicrobials into the CSF, is also given.

Initial therapy of bacterial meningitis in an older child thus should include vancomycin and a third-generation cephalosporin. Alternatively, clinical experience with meropenem has also been successful. A lumbar puncture should be considered 24–48 hours after the start of therapy to assess the sterility of the CSF.

Rifampin should be added if the Gram stain or cultures of CSF are positive on repeated lumbar puncture, if the child has failed to improve, or if an organism with a very high MIC to ceftriaxone is isolated. The optimal therapy of highly resistant *S pneumoniae* meningitis is not well established by clinical data.

Meningitis in a child with a ventriculoperitoneal shunt is most commonly caused by coagulase-negative staphylococci, many of which are methicillin-resistant, and *Corynebacterium* species, which are resistant to many antimicrobials. In many of these patients who are not seriously ill, therapy should be postponed while awaiting the appropriate shunt fluid for Gram stain and culture. Seriously ill patients should initially be given vancomycin and a third-generation cephalosporin, because *S aureus* and gram-negative rods are also possible and can cause serious infection.

Urinary Tract Infection

E coli is the most common isolate from the urinary tract. Outpatients with symptoms of lower urinary tract disease or with mild illness can be given ampicillin, cephalexin, or trimethoprim-sulfamethoxazole (TMP-SMX). Local experience and resistance rates should guide initial therapy. In selected patients with pyelonephritis, outpatient therapy is effective using parenteral aminoglycosides or ceftriaxone once per day. Oral cefixime has been used in place of ceftriaxone for outpatient therapy. Ciprofloxacin has been FDA-approved for therapy of urinary tract infection in children older than 1 year, but it should be reserved for complicated cases. For hospitalized patients with genitourinary tract infection and suspected bacteremia, ampicillin and gentamicin or a third-generation cephalosporin is appropriate. Gram stain should be used to guide the initial choice. For patients with known or suspected resistant organisms, such as *P aeruginosa*, or for patients with urosepsis, an aminoglycoside and ceftazidime, cefepime, or ticarcillin may be started. Unit-specific data on typical bacterial species and their patterns of susceptibility should guide the antimicrobial choice for nosocomial urinary tract infections.

BACTERIAL PNEUMONIA

Bacterial pneumonia in newborns generally should be treated with the same antimicrobial choices as sepsis. Infants and older children are frequently infected with *S pneumoniae*. Ampicillin and amoxicillin are effective in most patients eligible for outpatient therapy. Children who require hospitalization may benefit from a second- or third-generation cephalosporin. The broader initial coverage is indicated because of the greater severity of disease. A rapidly progressive pneumonia, with pneumatoceles or large pleural effusions, may be due to MRSA or group A streptococci, HIB, or another gram-

negative rod. Vancomycin should be used in addition to a third-generation cephalosporin.

Children age 6 years and older frequently have infection with *Mycoplasma pneumoniae, Chlamydia pneumoniae,* or *S pneumoniae.* Erythromycin, clarithromycin, or azithromycin is usually indicated for initial empiric therapy.

Skin and Soft Tissue Infections

S aureus and *Streptococcus pyogenes* are the most common causes of skin and soft tissue infections (SSTIs) in children. Community-acquired MRSA infections are common in many communities and complicate clinical decision making. Culture and susceptibility testing of abscesses, cellulitis, and more serious SSTIs is very important for optimal clinical management. Children with cellulitis more commonly have infection with group A streptococci, and empiric outpatient therapy with cephalexin or dicloxacillin is preferred. Children with small (< 5 cm) abscesses usually are effectively treated with incision and drainage without an antimicrobial. Outpatient therapy of large (> 5 cm) abscesses includes incision and drainage and empiric clindamycin or TMP-SMX depending on local susceptibility patterns. Group A streptococcal infections are not adequately treated with TMP-SMX. However, in many communities, 50% or greater of MRSA are also resistant to clindamycin and erythromycin. Adequate cultures, the thoroughness of drainage procedures, and careful outpatient follow-up are needed to ensure optimal outcomes.

■ SPECIFIC ANTIMICROBIAL AGENTS

PENICILLINS

1. Aminopenicillins

Penicillin remains the drug of choice for streptococcal infections, acute rheumatic fever prophylaxis, syphilis, oral anaerobic infections, dental infections, *N meningitidis* infection, leptospirosis, rat-bite fever, actinomycosis, and infections due to *Clostridium* and *Bacillus* species. For oral therapy of minor infections, amoxicillin or ampicillin is usually equivalent. For systemic therapy, aqueous penicillin G is preferable. Amoxicillin is preferred for oral therapy of Lyme disease in children. For dog or cat bites, where *Pasteurella multocida* is commonly encountered, amoxicillin–clavulanate provides good coverage of *Pasteurella* as well as *Staphylococcus*. An alternative is separate prescriptions for penicillin and an antistaphylococcal drug such as cephalexin, or clindamycin and TMP–SMX in penicillin-allergic patients. As for human bites, amoxicillin–clavulanate provides adequate therapy for *Eikenella corrodens* and other mixed oral aerobes and anaerobes. The β-lactamase inhibitor sulbactam combined with ampicillin is given parenterally for human and animal bites, and some other infections due to organisms from the oral flora where mixed aerobic and anaerobic bacteria may be resistant to ampicillin due to β-lactamase production.

2. Penicillinase-Resistant Penicillins

S aureus is usually resistant to penicillin and amoxicillin owing to penicillinase production. Nafcillin, oxacillin, methicillin, and first- and second-generation cephalosporins are stable to penicillinase and are usually equivalent for intravenous therapy. Methicillin is associated with more frequent interstitial nephritis. Oxacillin and methicillin are renally excreted, whereas nafcillin is excreted through the biliary tract. These properties are occasionally considered in children with renal or liver failure. Cost should usually be the deciding factor for choosing an agent. Often both *S aureus* and *Streptococcus pyogenes* are suspected initially (eg, in cellulitis or postoperative wound infections). The penicillinase-resistant penicillins (PRPs) and first- and second-generation cephalosporins are efficacious for most streptococcal infections, although penicillin remains the drug of choice.

MRSA is an increasingly common and serious community-acquired infection in children and may cause nosocomial infection. MRSA infections are also resistant to other PRPs and to other cephalosporins. Vancomycin is effective against MRSA and coagulase-negative staphylococci. *S aureus* infections range in severity from minor infections treated on an outpatient basis to life-threatening infections. Severe infections due to MRSA are a serious concern in many communities. It is important to culture and determine antimicrobial susceptibility of suspected *S aureus* infections in communities where MRSA is common. In communities with frequent MRSA infections in children, initial therapy of seriously ill children should include vancomycin. MRSA may also be resistant to macrolides and clindamycin by alteration in the bacterial 23S ribosomal RNA. Many strains reported as clindamycin-susceptible and erythromycin-resistant are truly resistant to clindamycin. This inducible resistance to clindamycin may be detected in erythromycin-resistant MRSA that demonstrates a D-zone in disk susceptibility testing to clindamycin. Community-acquired MRSA is more likely to be susceptible to TMP–SMX, clindamycin, and gentamicin than hospital-acquired infections.

For outpatient therapy, cloxacillin, dicloxacillin, and first- or second-generation cephalosporins are usually equally effective for infections due to susceptible *S aureus*. Cost may determine the choice between drugs.

3. Anti-Pseudomonas Penicillins

Ticarcillin, mezlocillin, and piperacillin are active intravenously against streptococci, ampicillin-susceptible enterococci, *H influenzae*, gram-negative rods (including more resistant gram-negative rods such as *Enterobacter, Proteus,* and *Pseudomonas aeruginosa*), and gram-negative anaerobes such as *Bacteroides fragilis. P aeruginosa* is inherently resistant to most antimicrobials, and high levels of these drugs are usually required. The combination of ticarcillin and an aminoglycoside is synergistic against *P aeruginosa* and many other enteric gram-negative rods. Ticarcillin in a fixed combination with clavulanic acid has activity against β-lactamase-producing strains of *Klebsiella, S aureus,* and *Bacteroides.* Piperacillin is more active in vitro against many gram-negative enteric infections and may be advantageous in some circumstances, but it is not FDA-approved in children. Piperacillin–tazobactam is another combination antimicrobial and β-lactamase inhibitor that has enhanced activity against many β-lactamase producers.

Antipseudomonal penicillins cause the same toxicities as penicillin and therefore are usually very safe. Carbenicillin, ticarcillin, and piperacillin contain large amounts of sodium, which may cause problems for some patients with cardiac or renal disease.

GLYCOPEPTIDE AGENTS

Vancomycin and teicoplanin are glycopeptide antimicrobial agents active against the cell wall of gram-positive organisms. Only vancomycin is licensed in the United States. Vancomycin is useful for parenteral therapy of resistant gram-positive cocci such as penicillin- and cephalosporin-resistant *S pneumoniae*, MRSA, methicillin-resistant coagulase-negative staphylococci, and ampicillin-resistant enterococci. Vancomycin is also used orally for therapy of colitis due to *Clostridium difficile,* although it should not be used as the drug of first choice.

The empiric use of vancomycin has increased tremendously over the last several years. As a result, vancomycin-resistant enterococci (VRE) and coagulase-negative staphylococci have become problems, particularly in inpatient units, intensive care units, and oncology wards. *S aureus* with increased MICs to vancomycin has been reported in the United States and Japan. This resistance is of concern because of the inherent virulence of many *S aureus* strains. Vancomycin use should be monitored carefully in hospitals and their intensive care units. It should not be used empirically when an infection is mild or when other antimicrobial agents are likely to be effective. Vancomycin should be stopped promptly if infection is found to be due to organisms susceptible to other antimicrobials. Infection control guidelines for prevention of spread of VRE are published by the Centers for Disease Control and Prevention.

Rapid infusion of vancomycin is associated with the "red man syndrome," characterized by diffuse red flushing, at times pruritus, and occasionally tachycardia and hypotension. As a result, vancomycin is infused slowly over 1 hour or longer in some cases. Diphenhydramine or hydrocortisone (or both) may also be used as premedication.

Measurement of peak-and-trough serum vancomycin concentrations is not necessary in most clinical situations, because the levels achieved with standard dosing are usually predictable and nontoxic. Measurement of serum concentrations is helpful in patients with abnormal or unpredictable renal function; in those with altered volume of distribution, as occurs in nephrotic syndrome or shock; and in those receiving higher-dose therapy (eg, for meningitis or other difficult-to-treat infections). For patients receiving antimicrobials for weeks to months, weekly monitoring of clinical signs and symptoms and of urinalysis, creatinine, and complete blood count will allow detection of toxicity.

OXAZOLIDINONES

Linezolid is the first drug in this new class of antimicrobials which have a distinct new mechanism of action; they bind to the 50s-ribosomal RNA subunit and prevent initiation of protein synthesis. Because of this unique mechanism, there is no cross-resistance with other classes of antimicrobials. The in vitro development of resistance has also been uncommon.

Linezolid is active against aerobic gram-positive organisms, including streptococci, staphylococci, enterococci, and pneumococci. Because linezolid is active against gram-positive organisms resistant to other antimicrobials (eg, MRSA, methicillin-resistant, coagulase-negative staphylococci, VRE, and penicillin-resistant *S pneumoniae*), it is a potentially useful rescue drug for these difficult-to-treat infections.

Linezolid is safe and well tolerated in children. Gastrointestinal symptoms are the most commonly encountered side effect. Neutropenia and thrombocytopenia have been reported, and linezolid should therefore be used with monitoring in patients at increased risk for these problems or in patients receiving therapy for 2 weeks or longer. Linezolid is an inhibitor of monoamine oxidase (MAO) and should not be used in patients taking MAO inhibitors, or in patients taking phenylpropanolamine or pseudoephedrine.

Linezolid should be used only for infections due to a proven gram-positive pathogen that is known or strongly suspected to be resistant to other available agents.

QUINUPRISTIN/DALFOPRISTIN

Quinupristin and dalfopristin are two antimicrobials of the streptogramin class, which individually are bacteriostatic but in combination are synergistic and bactericidal. These drugs are combined in a fixed ratio of 70:30, known as Synercid. Streptogramins inhibit protein synthesis by binding to the 50s ribosomal subunit. The streptogramins were discovered many years ago, but interest has increased only recently due to the activity of these agents against some very difficult-to-treat gram-positive infections.

The quinupristin/dalfopristin combination has activity against staphylococci, streptococci, pneumococci, and some enterococci. Quinupristin/dalfopristin is primarily indicated for serious infections due to vancomycin-resistant *Enterococcus faecium* and MRSA. Quinupristin/dalfopristin is not active against *E faecalis* and, therefore, differentiation of these strains from *E faecium* is important prior to initiating therapy.

Quinupristin/dalfopristin is not approved for therapy in children. Nonetheless, therapy has been initiated under a compassionate release program in some pediatric patients seriously ill with difficult-to-treat infections due to resistant organisms.

Arthralgias and myalgias have at times been severe in adult patients. Other significant side effects include elevated bilirubin and inflammation at intravenous sites.

Quinupristin/dalfopristin is a significant inhibitor of CYP-450 3A4 and, therefore, must be used with caution in patients receiving drugs metabolized by this mechanism.

The use of quinupristin/dalfopristin should be limited to serious infections due to proven *E faecium* or *S aureus* infections or infections due to proven gram-positive cocci that are resistant to other agents.

CEPHALOSPORINS

Cephalosporin agents make up a large and often confusing group of antimicrobials. Many of these drugs are similar in antibacterial spectrum and side effects and may have similar names. Clinicians should learn well the properties of one or two drugs in each class. Cephalosporins are often grouped as "generations" to signify their similar antimicrobial activity. First-generation cephalosporins such as cefazolin intravenously and cephalexin orally are useful mainly for susceptible *S aureus* infection and urinary tract infection due to susceptible *E coli*. Second-generation cephalosporins, such as cefuroxime intravenously and cefprozil and cefuroxime orally, have somewhat reduced but acceptable activity against gram-positive cocci but greater activity against some gram-negative rods compared to first generation cephalosporins. They are active against *H influenzae* and *Moraxella catarrhalis*, including strains that produce β-lactamase capable of inactivating ampicillin. Third-generation cephalosporins have substantially less activity against gram-positive cocci such as *S aureus* but greatly augmented activity against aerobic gram-negative rods. Cefotaxime and ceftriaxone are examples of intravenous drugs, whereas cefpodoxime and ceftibuten are representative oral drugs. Cefepime is a new antimicrobial often described as fourth-generation because of its broad activity against gram-positive and gram-negative organisms, including *P aeruginosa*. Cefepime is stable to β-lactamase degradation and is a poor inducer of β-lactamase. Cefepime will be most useful for organisms resistant to other drugs. Cefepime is not approved for use in children younger than age 2 months.

No cephalosporin agent has substantial activity against *L monocytogenes*, enterococci, or MRSA. The only cephalosporins useful for treating anaerobic infections are cefoxitin and cefotetan, which are second-generation cephalosporins with excellent activity against *B fragilis*. Ceftazidime is a third-generation cephalosporin with appreciable activity against *P aeruginosa*. Allergy to β-lactam antimicrobials is reported commonly by parents, but few children are not shown to be allergic when studied by skin test or oral challenge. Immediate hypersensitivity reactions, including anaphylaxis or hives, most commonly predict true allergy. In contrast, many delayed reactions and nonspecific rashes are likely due to the underlying infection or nonallergic reactions. (See Chapter 34.) Cephalosporins should be used with caution in children with immediate hypersensitivity reactions to penicillins or cephalosporins.

Resistance to cephalosporins is common among aerobic gram-negative rods. The presence of inducible cephalosporinases in the chromosome of some gram-negative rod organisms such as *P aeruginosa*, *Serratia marcescens*, *Citrobacter*, and *Enterobacter* has led to clinical failures because of the emergence of resistance during therapy. Extended spectrum β-lactamases mediate broad resistance to all penicillins, amino-penicillins, cephalosporins, and monobactams. Carbapenems, fluoroquinolones, or combinations including these drugs are used for serious infections due to gram-negative organisms with these enzymes. Active laboratory-based surveillance is necessary to detect these gram-negative organisms.

AZTREONAM

Aztreonam is the only monobactam antimicrobial agent approved in the United States. Although it is not approved for use in children less than 9 months of age, there is considerable pediatric experience with its use, including in neonates and premature infants. Aztreonam is active against aerobic gram-negative rods, including *P aeruginosa*. Aztreonam has activity against *H influenzae* and *M catarrhalis*, including those that are β-lactamase producers. Most patients with allergy to penicillin or cephalosporins are not sensitized to aztreonam, except that children with prior reactions to ceftazidime may have reactions to aztreonam because aztreonam and ceftazidime have a common side chain.

CARBAPENEMS

Meropenem, ertapenem, and imipenem are broad-spectrum β-lactam antimicrobials. Imipenem–cilastatin is a combination of an active antibiotic and cilastatin, which inhibits the metabolism of imipenem in the kidney and thereby results in high serum and urine levels of imipenem. These carbapenems are also active against *S pneumoniae*, including many penicillin-resistant and cephalosporin-resistant strains. Carbapenems have been used successfully to treat meningitis and may be considered if vancomycin is not tolerated. An increased frequency of seizures is encountered when central nervous system infections are treated with carbapenems. These agents are broadly active against streptococci, MRSA, some enterococci, and gram-negative rods such as *P aeruginosa*, β-lactamase-producing *H influenzae*, and gram-negative anaerobes. Ertapenem has less activity against *P aeruginosa*, *Acinetobacter* sp., and *Enterococcus* sp. than meropenem and imipenem. Because carbapenems are active against so many species of bacteria, there is a strong temptation to use them as single-drug empiric therapy. Units that have used carbapenems heavily have encountered resistance in many different species of gram-negative rods.

MACROLIDES & AZILIDES

Erythromycin is the most commonly used macrolide antimicrobial agent. It is active against many bacteria that are resistant to cell wall-active antimicrobials and is the drug of choice for *Bordetella pertussis*, *Legionella pneumophila*, *Chlamydia pneumoniae*, *Mycoplasma pneumoniae*, and *C trachomatis* infections (in children in whom tetracycline is not an option). Erythromycin is used for outpatient therapy of streptococcal and staphylococcal infections and in patients with penicillin allergy. More serious infections due to streptococci and staphylococci are usually treated with penicillins, clindamycin, PRPs, or cephalosporins because of a significant incidence of erythromycin resistance in both species. *S pneumoniae* resistant to erythromycin and the related macrolides are now frequent in many communities. This limits the ability of macrolide antimicrobials for therapy of otitis media and sinusitis. Gastrointestinal side effects are common. Interactions with theophylline, carbamazepine, terfenadine, cycloserine, and other drugs may require dosage modifications of erythromycin and clarithromycin. Significant interactions with azithromycin are less common.

Erythromycin is available in many formulations, including the base, estolate, ethyl succinate, and stearate. Transient hepatic toxicity occurs in adults but is much less common in children. Erythromycin base and stearate should be taken with meals for best absorption.

Clarithromycin and azithromycin, macrolide and azalide antimicrobials, respectively, are much less likely than erythromycin to cause nausea, vomiting, and diarrhea. These agents are useful in children who cannot tolerate erythromycin. Clarithromycin is more active than erythromycin against *H influenzae, M catarrhalis,* and *N gonorrhoeae* and is the drug of choice, usually in combination, for some nontuberculous mycobacterial infections. Azithromycin has a prolonged tissue half-life that achieves a prolonged antimicrobial effect. Azithromycin is dosed once daily for 5 days but must be taken 1 hour before or 2 hours after meals because food interferes with absorption. Although azithromycin is active against *H influenzae,* some authors report poor eradication of *H influenzae* from the middle ear. Azithromycin can be used for single-dose therapy of *C trachomatis* infections. It is beneficial in adolescents when compliance with erythromycin or tetracycline is a concern. Azithromycin is useful for therapy of *Shigella* and *Salmonella* infections including typhoid fever resistant to ampicillin and TMP–SMX. Alternatives include cefixime, other third-generation cephalosporins, and fluoroquinolones. Clarithromycin is effective against Lyme disease, but 7 days of azithromycin for that indication was inferior to amoxicillin. Clarithromycin and azithromycin are alternative drugs for toxoplasmosis in sulfonamide-allergic patients and as alternatives to erythromycin in legionellosis. In vitro and limited clinical experience in providing treatment to contacts of pertussis patients suggests efficacy equal to that of erythromycin. Clarithromycin and azithromycin are considerably more expensive than most erythromycin formulations, which for that reason are usually preferred, but they are advantageous by virtue of their twice-daily and once-daily dosing, respectively. Some failures of the newer macrolides have occurred in *S pneumoniae* sepsis and meningitis, perhaps because of low serum levels despite the high tissue levels achieved. High rates of resistance to macrolides and azalides have been encountered in some communities. The frequent use of azithromycin for respiratory infections and acute otitis media has contributed to selection of resistant strains.

CLINDAMYCIN

Clindamycin is active against *Staphylococcus aureus,* some MRSA, *Streptococcus pyogenes,* other streptococcal species except enterococci, and both gram-positive and gram-negative anaerobes. Clindamycin or metronidazole is frequently combined with other antimicrobials for empiric therapy of suspected anaerobic or mixed anaerobic and aerobic infections. Empiric use of clindamycin is justified in suspected anaerobic infections because cultures frequently cannot be obtained and, if obtained, may be slow in confirming anaerobic infection. Examples are pelvic inflammatory disease, necrotizing enterocolitis, other infections in which the integrity of the gastrointestinal or genitourinary tracts is compromised, and sinusitis. Clindamycin does not achieve high levels in CSF, but brain abscesses, toxoplasmosis, and other central nervous system infections, where disruption of the blood–brain barrier occurs, may be successfully treated with clindamycin. Clindamycin should be added to regimens for treatment of serious streptococcal and staphylococcal infections such as necrotizing fasciitis and toxic shock syndrome. For the usual oral anaerobes, penicillin is more active than clindamycin. Clindamycin has been associated with the occurrence of pseudomembranous colitis. Although diarrhea is a frequent side effect, pseudomembranous colitis is uncommonly due to clindamycin in children.

SULFONAMIDES

Sulfonamides—the oldest class of antimicrobials—remain useful for treatment of urinary tract infections. They are used also for other infections due to *E coli* and for *Nocardia.* Although useful for rheumatic fever prophylaxis in penicillin-allergic patients, sulfonamides fail to eradicate group A streptococci and cannot be used for treatment of acute infections.

TMP–SMX is a fixed combination that is more active than either drug alone. Gram-positive cocci, including some *S pneumoniae,* many staphylococci, *Haemophilus,* and many gram-negative rods, are susceptible. Unfortunately, resistance to TMP–SMX has developed in recent years. *S pneumoniae* resistant to penicillin and cephalosporins is often also resistant to TMP–SMX and erythromycin. In some communities, *Shigella* and *Salmonella enteritidis* strains remain susceptible, as do most *E coli.* TMP–SMX is therefore very useful for treatment of urinary tract infections and bacterial dysentery. TMP–SMX is also the drug of choice for treatment or prophylaxis against *Pneumocystis jiroveci* infection. Dermatologic and myelosuppressive side effects limit the use of TMP–SMX in some children infected with HIV.

Sulfonamide is associated with several cutaneous reactions, including urticaria, photosensitivity, Stevens–Johnson syndrome, purpura, and maculopapular rashes. Hematologic side effects such as leukopenia, thrombocytopenia, and hemolytic anemia are uncommon. Common gastrointestinal side effects are nausea and vomiting. The dermatologic and hematologic side effects are thought to be more common and more severe with TMP–SMX than with sulfonamide alone.

TETRACYCLINES

Tetracyclines are effective against a broad range of bacteria but are not commonly used in children because alternative effective drugs are available. Many different tetracycline formulations are available. Tetracyclines are effective against *Bordetella pertussis* and *E coli* and many species of *Rickettsia, Chlamydia,* and *Mycoplasma.* Doxycycline or minocycline is the drug of choice for eradication of *C trachomatis* in pelvic inflammatory disease and nongonococcal urethritis.

Staining of permanent teeth was noted in young children given repeated courses of tetracyclines. As a result, tetracyclines are generally not given to children younger than age 9 years unless alternative drugs are unavailable. A single course of tetracycline does not pose a significant risk of tooth staining. Mucous membrane candidiasis, photosensitivity, nausea, and vomiting are other common side effects. Tetracycline should be taken on an empty stomach, either 1 hour before or 2 hours after a meal. Doxycycline is well absorbed even in the presence of food; administration with food may minimize gastrointestinal side effects. Doxycycline is often preferred because it is better tolerated than tetracycline, and twice daily administration is convenient.

Tetracycline is used for therapy of rickettsial infections such as Rocky Mountain spotted fever, ehrlichiosis, rickettsialpox, murine typhus, and Q fever; as an alternative to erythromycin for *Mycoplasma pneumoniae* and *Chlamydia pneumoniae* infections; and for treatment of psittacosis, brucellosis, *Pasteurella multocida* infection, and relapsing fever.

Tigecycline is a new polyketide antimicrobial which is an analog of tetracycline and a bacteriostatic inhibitor of protein synthesis. Tigecycline is active against gram-negative aerobes, anaerobes, and many gram-positive cocci including MRSA. It is approved for intravenous therapy of adults with complicated SSTIs and complicated intra-abdominal infections.

AMINOGLYCOSIDES

The aminoglycosides bind to ribosomal subunits and inhibit protein synthesis. They are active against aerobic gram-negative rods, including *P aeruginosa.* Streptomycin was the first drug in this class, but today it is used only to treat tuberculosis and the occasional cases of plague and tularemia.

Aminoglycosides are used to treat serious gram-negative infections and are given intravenously or intramuscularly. They are also used to treat pyelonephritis, suspected gram-negative sepsis, and in other settings where *P aeruginosa* infections are common, such as cystic fibrosis and burns. Aminoglycosides have activity against gram-positive organisms and, combined with penicillin or ampicillin, may achieve synergistic killing of *L monocytogenes* and group B streptococci. Penicillin, ampicillin, or vancomycin combined with gentamicin is indicated for therapy of serious enterococcal infections, such as sepsis or endocarditis because of more rapid clinical improvement with combined therapy. Aminoglycosides have activity against *S aureus* but are always used in combination with other antistaphylococcal antibiotics.

Aminoglycosides are not active in an acidic environment and may not be effective against loculated abscesses. Aminoglycosides diffuse poorly into the CSF and achieve only about 10% of serum concentrations. As a result, a third-generation cephalosporin is preferred for treatment of bacillary meningitis.

Aminoglycosides kill bacteria in a concentration-dependent manner. They also have a prolonged suppressive effect on the regrowth of susceptible organisms (postantibiotic effect). These principles have led some investigators to establish guidelines for once-daily dosing of aminoglycosides, using larger initial doses given every 24 hours. Although aminoglycosides are associated with both renal and eighth nerve toxicity, the entry of the drug into renal and cochlear cells is saturable. It therefore was predicted that once-daily dosing would result in less toxicity than traditional twice-daily or three-times-daily dosing. Studies in adult patients confirm that once-daily dosing is as efficacious as traditional dosing and is associated with less toxicity. Although there is extensive experience with dosing intervals of 18–36 hours in premature babies, small total daily doses are customarily used (2.0–2.5 mg/kg/dose of gentamicin or tobramycin). A convenient and cost-effective approach in children is based on the experience with adult patients and uses larger daily doses (4–7 mg/kg/dose every 24 hours). Unfortunately, there is little published information on the efficacy and safety of this approach in children.

Accordingly, traditional twice-daily or three-times-daily dosing regimens of aminoglycosides, with monitoring of serum levels, are still widely used. Careful monitoring is necessary, particularly in children with abnormal or changing renal function, premature infants, and infants with rapidly changing volumes of distribution. Aminoglycosides are usually infused over 30–45 minutes, and the peak serum concentration is measured 30–45 minutes after the end of the infusion. A trough serum concentration is measured prior to the next dose. The efficacious and nontoxic serum concentrations for gentamicin and tobramycin are trough less than 2 μg/mL and peak 5–10 μg/mL; for amikacin, trough less than 10 μg/mL and peak 15–25 μg/mL (see Table 35–4). Aminoglycoside levels and creatinine levels should be measured in children expected to receive more than 3 days of therapy and weekly in children on long-term therapy even when renal function is normal and stable.

FLUOROQUINOLONES

Modification of the quinolone structure of nalidixic acid has led to many new compounds called fluoroquinolones, which are well absorbed after oral administration and possess excellent antibacterial activity against resistant gram-negative pathogens. The seven currently available fluoroquinolones vary in their activity against specific organisms. Fluoroquinolones are active against most of the Enterobacteriaceae, including *E coli, Enterobacter, Klebsiella*, in some cases *P aeruginosa*, and many other gram-negative bacteria such as *H influenzae, M catarrhalis, N gonorrhoeae*, and *N meningitidis*. Some fluoroquinolones (ofloxacin) are active against *C trachomatis*. The fluoroquinolones are active against some enterococci, *S aureus*, and coagulase-negative staphylococci but not against MRSA. The newer quinolones have good activity against penicillin and cephalosporin-resistant *Streptococcus pneumoniae*, but clinical experience in children is limited.

Ciprofloxacin and its otic and ophthalmic preparations are the only fluoroquinolone antimicrobials currently FDA-approved for use in children older than 1 year, although fluoroquinolones offer very attractive alternatives to approved agents. The objection to quinolones is based on the recognition that nalidixic acid and other quinolones cause arthropathy when used experimentally in newborn animals of many species. The fear that children would also be more susceptible than adults to cartilage injury has not been realized in clinical experience. Both retrospective long-term follow-up studies of children given nalidixic acid and prospective studies of children receiving treatment under protocols with fluoroquinolones have shown similar rates of toxicity compared with adult patients. Arthropathy occurs uncommonly, although tendon rupture is a reported rare, serious complication. For these reasons, quinolones should be considered for use in children when the benefit clearly outweighs the risk, when no alternative drug is available, and after discussion with the parents.

Ciprofloxacin is useful for oral therapy of resistant gram-negative urinary tract infections such as that caused by *P aeruginosa*. Ofloxacin, levofloxacin, ciprofloxacin, and gatifloxacin are useful for single-dose therapy of uncomplicated gonorrhea, and ofloxacin and levofloxacin are an alternative therapy for treating *Chlamydia* infections and pelvic inflammatory disease. Ciprofloxacin and ofloxacin are used as therapy of resistant cases of shigellosis. Levofloxacin and ciprofloxacin are usually the drugs of choice for treatment of traveler's diarrhea. Ciprofloxacin is useful for treatment of *P aeruginosa* infection in patients with cystic fibrosis, and as therapy for chronic suppurative otitis media. Several quinolones are used as therapy for pneumonia due to *Legionella, Mycoplasma*, or *Chlamydia pneumoniae*, although a macrolide is often preferred, and as prophylactic therapy of meningococcal infection. Ofloxacin and levofloxacin are used for treatment of some cases of *Mycobacterium tuberculosis* and some atypical mycobacterial infections.

METRONIDAZOLE

Metronidazole has excellent activity against most anaerobes, particularly gram-negative anaerobes such as *Bacteroides* and *Fusobacterium*, and against gram-positive anaerobes such as *Clostridium, Prevotella*, and *Porphyromonas*. Gram-positive anaerobic cocci such as *Peptococcus* and *Peptostreptococcus* are often more susceptible to penicillin or to clindamycin. Because metronidazole lacks activity against aerobic organisms, it is usually given with one or more other antibiotics. Metronidazole is well absorbed after oral administration and has excellent penetration into the central nervous system. Metronidazole is the drug of choice for bacterial vaginosis and for *C difficile* enterocolitis. It is active against many parasites, including *Giardia lamblia* and *Entamoeba histolytica*.

DAPTOMYCIN

Daptomycin is a newly FDA-approved antimicrobial with bactericidal activity against gram-positive cocci. Daptomycin is a lipopeptide that binds to bacterial cell membranes, resulting in membrane depolarization and cell death. Daptomycin is active against methicillin-sensitive and -resistant *Staphylococcus aureus, Streptococcus pyogenes*, and *Streptococcus agalactiae*, as well as *E faecium* (including vancomycin-resistant strains), and *E faecalis* (vancomycin-sensitive strains). Daptomycin is given as a once-daily intravenous infusion of 4 mg/kg, and is approved for therapy of complicated SSTIs, but has not been sufficiently studied in children younger than 18 years to make recommendations for dosing and use. Daptomycin therapy of pneumonia was unsuccessful in a large percentage of cases, and should not be used. Daptomycin is excreted renally, so a modification of dosing is needed in patients with impaired renal function. It has significant interactions with aminoglycosides, so monitoring serum concentrations of aminoglycosides is necessary. Nausea, constipation, and headache are the most common side effects of therapy. In patients with muscle pain, monitoring creatinine phosphokinase levels should be done.

REFERENCES

Bradley JS, Nelson JB: *Nelson's Pocketbook of Pediatric Antimicrobial Therapy*, 15th ed. Lippincott, Williams & Wilkins, 2002.

Fridkin SK et al: Methicillin-resistant *Staphylococcus aureus* disease in three communities. N Engl J Med 2005;352(4):1436 [PMID: 15814879].

Gilbert DN et al: *The Sanford Guide to Antimicrobial Therapy,* 35th ed. Antimicrobial Therapy, Inc., 2005.

Gonzalez BE et al: Pulmonary manifestations in children with invasive community-acquired staphylococcus aureus infection. Clin Infect Dis 2005;41(9):583 [PMID: 16080077].

Kaplan SL et al: Linezolid versus vancomycin for treatment of resistant gram-positive infections in children. Pediatr Infect Dis J 2003;22(8):677 [PMID: 12913766].

Mainous AG 3rd et al: Trends in antimicrobial prescribing for bronchitis and upper respiratory infections among adults and children. Am J Public Health 2003;93(11):1910 [PMID 14600065].

Pichichero ME: A review of evidence supporting the American Academy of Pediatrics recommendation for prescribing cephalosporin antibiotics for penicillin-allergic patients. Pediatrics 2005;225(4):1048 [PMID: 15805383].

Stevens DL et al: Practice guidelines for the diagnosis and management of skin and soft-tissue infections. Clin Infect Dis 2005;41:1373 [PMID: 16231249].

Websites

http://www.cdc.gov/drugresistance
http://www.cdc.gov/ncidod/guidelines/guidelines_topic_ar.htm
http://www.tufts.edu/med/apua/index.html

Infections: Viral & Rickettsial

36

Myron J. Levin, MD, & Adriana Weinberg, MD

■ I. VIRAL INFECTIONS

Viruses cause most pediatric infections. Mixed viral or viral–bacterial infections of the respiratory and intestinal tracts are rather common, as is prolonged asymptomatic shedding of some viruses in childhood. Thus, the detection of a virus is not always proof that it is the cause of a given illness. Viruses are often a predisposing factor for bacterial respiratory infections (eg, otitis, sinusitis, and pneumonia).

Many respiratory and herpes viruses can now be detected within 24–48 hours by combining culture and monoclonal antibody techniques ("rapid culture technique"). Diagnosis of many viral illnesses is also possible through antigen or nucleic acid detection techniques. These techniques are more rapid than isolation of viruses in tissue culture and in many cases are equally sensitive or more so. Polymerase chain reaction (PCR) amplification of viral genes has led to recognition of previously undetected infections. New diagnostic tests have changed some basic concepts about viral diseases and made diagnosis of viral infections both more certain and more complex. Only laboratories with excellent quality-control procedures should be used, and the results of new tests must be interpreted cautiously. The availability of specific antiviral agents increases the value of early diagnosis for some serious viral infections. Table 36–1 lists viral agents associated with common clinical signs, and Table 36–2 lists diagnostic tests. The viral diagnostic laboratory should be contacted for details regarding specimen collection, handling, and shipping. Table 36–3 lists common causes of red rashes in children that should be considered in the differential diagnosis of certain viral illnesses.

RESPIRATORY INFECTIONS

Many virus infections cause upper or lower respiratory tract signs and symptoms. Those that produce a predominance of these signs and symptoms are described in the text that follows. Many so-called respiratory viruses can also produce distinct nonrespiratory disease (eg, enteritis or cystitis caused by adenoviruses; parotitis caused by parainfluenza viruses). Respiratory viruses can cause disease in any area of the respiratory tree. Thus they can cause coryza, pharyngitis, sinusitis, tracheitis, bronchitis, bronchiolitis, and pneumonia—although certain viruses tend to be closely associated with one anatomic area (eg, parainfluenza with croup or respiratory syncytial virus [RSV] with bronchiolitis) or discrete epidemics (eg, influenza, RSV, and parainfluenza). Nevertheless, it is impossible on clinical grounds to be certain of the viral cause of an infection in a given child. This information is provided by the virology laboratory and is often important for epidemiologic, therapeutic, and preventive reasons.

VIRUSES CAUSING THE COMMON COLD

The common cold syndrome (also called upper respiratory infection) is characterized by combinations of runny nose, nasal congestion, sore throat, tearing, cough, and sneezing. Low-grade fever may be present. The causal agent is usually not sought or determined. Epidemiologic studies indicate that rhinoviruses, which are the most common cause (30–40%), are present throughout the year, but are more prevalent in the colder months in temperate climates. Adenoviruses also cause colds in all seasons, but epidemics are common. Respiratory syncytial, parainfluenza, and influenza viruses cause the cold syndrome during epidemics from late fall through winter. Coronaviruses (≈10%) also cause colds in winter, and enteroviruses cause the "summer cold." A significance of these infections is morbidity continuing for 5–7 days. It is also likely that changes in respiratory epithelium, local obstruction, and altered local immunity are sometimes the precursors of more severe illnesses such as otitis media, pneumonia, and sinusitis. During and following a cold the bacterial flora changes, and bacteria are found in normally sterile areas of the upper airway. Asthma attacks are also provoked by viruses that cause the common cold. There is no evidence that antibiotics will prevent these complications, and the unjustified widespread use of antibiotics for cold symptoms has contributed to the emergence of antibiotic-resistant respiratory flora.

Table 36–1. Some viral causes of clinical syndromes.

Rash
- Enterovirus
- Adenovirus
- Measles
- Rubella
- Human herpes virus type 6[a] or 7
- Varicella
- Parvovirus B19[b]
- Epstein-Barr virus
- Dengue
- Human immunodeficiency virus (acute syndrome)

Fever
- Enterovirus
- Epstein-Barr virus
- Human herpes virus type 6[a] or 7
- Cytomegalovirus
- Influenza
- Rhinovirus
- Most others

Conjunctivitis
- Adenovirus
- Enterovirus 70
- Measles
- Herpes simplex[c]

Parotitis
- Mumps
- Parainfluenza
- Enterovirus
- Cytomegalovirus
- Epstein-Barr virus
- Human immunodeficiency virus

Pharyngitis
- Adenovirus
- Enterovirus
- Epstein-Barr virus
- Herpes simplex virus[d]
- Influenza
- Other respiratory viruses

Adenopathy
- Epstein-Barr virus
- Cytomegalovirus
- Rubella[e]
- Human immunodeficiency virus

Croup
- Parainfluenza
- Influenza
- Adenovirus
- Other respiratory viruses

Bronchiolitis
- Respiratory syncytial virus[f]
- Adenovirus
- Parainfluenza
- Influenza
- Human metapneumovirus

Pneumonia
- Respiratory syncytial virus
- Adenovirus
- Parainfluenza
- Hantavirus
- Measles
- Varicella[g]
- Cytomegalovirus[h,i]
- Influenza
- Severe acute respiratory syndrome (SARS)

Enteritis
- Rotavirus
- Enteric adenovirus
- Enterovirus
- Astrovirus
- Calicivirus
- Novovirus
- Cytomegalovirus

Hepatitis
- Hepatitis A,[j] B, C, D, E
- Epstein-Barr virus
- Adenovirus
- Cytomegalovirus
- Varicella[k]
- Parvovirus B19

Arthritis
- Parvovirus B19
- Rubella
- Hepatitis B

Congenital or perinatal infection
- Adenovirus
- Cytomegalovirus
- Hepatitis B
- Hepatitis C[l]
- Rubella
- Human immunodeficiency virus
- Parvovirus B19
- Enterovirus
- Varicella
- Herpes simplex virus

Meningoencephalitis
- Enterovirus
- Mumps
- Arthropod-borne viruses
- Herpes simplex virus
- Cytomegalovirus
- Lymphocytic choriomeningitis virus
- Measles
- Varicella
- Adenovirus
- Human immunodeficiency virus
- Epstein–Barr virus
- Influenza
- West Nile virus

[a]Roseola agent.
[b]Erythema infectiosum agent.
[c]Conjunctivitis rare, only in primary infections; keratitis in older patients.
[d]May cause isolated pharyngeal vesicles at any age.
[e]May cause adenopathy without rash.
[f]Over 70% of cases.
[g]Immunosuppressed, pregnant, rarely other adults.
[h]Usually only in young infants.
[i]Severely immunosuppressed at risk.
[j]Anicteric cases more common in children; these may resemble viral gastroenteritis.
[k]Common, but only mild laboratory abnormalities.
[l]Especially when the mother is HIV-positive.

Table 36–2. Diagnostic tests for viral infections.

Agent	Rapid Antigen Detection (Specimen)	Tissue Culture Mean Days to Positive (Range)	Serology			Comments
			Acute	Paired	PCR[a]	
Adenovirus	+ (respiratory and enteric)	10 (1–21)	–	+	+	"Enteric" strains detected by culture on special cell line, antigen detection, or PCR
Arboviruses	–	–	+	+	RL	Acute serum may diagnose many forms
Astrovirus	–	–	–	–	RL	Diagnosis by electron microscopy
Calicivirus	–	–	–	–	RL	Diagnosis by electron microscopy
Colorado tick virus	On RBC	–	–	RL, CDC	+	
Cytomegalovirus	+ (tissue biopsy, urine, blood, respiratory secretions)	2 (2–28)	+	+	+	Diagnosis by presence of IgM antibody
Enterovirus	–	2 (2–14)	–	+	+	
Epstein-Barr virus	–	–	+	+	+	Single serologic panel defines infection status; heterophil antibodies less sensitive
Hantavirus	–	–	+	ND	RL	Diagnosis by presence of IgM antibody
Hepatitis A virus	–	–	+	ND	RL	Diagnosis by presence of IgM antibody
Hepatitis B virus	+ (blood)	–	+	ND	+	Diagnosis by presence of surface antigen or anti-core IgM antibody
Hepatitis C virus	–	–	+	ND	+	Postitive serology suggests that hepatitis C may be the causative agent. PCR is confirmatory.
Herpes simplex virus	+ (mucosa, tissue biopsy, respiratory secretions, skin)	1 (1–7)	+	+	+	Serology rarely used for herpes simplex. IgM antibody used in selected cases.
Human herpesvirus-6	+	2	+	+	+	Roseola agent
Human immunodeficiency virus	+ (blood) (acid dissociation of immune complexes)	15 (5–28)	+	ND	+	Antibody proves infection unless passively acquired (< age 15 mos); culture not widely available; PCR definitive for early diagnosis in infant
Human metapneumovirus	–	RL	–	+	+	
Influenza virus	+ (respiratory secretions)	2 (2–14)	–	+	+	Antigen detection 70–90% sensitive
Lymphocytic choriomeningitis virus	—	–	–	+	RL	Can be isolated in suckling mice
Measles virus	+ (respiratory secretions)	–	+	+	RL	Difficult to grow; IgM serology diagnostic
Mumps virus	–	> 5	+	+	RL	IgM ELISA antibody may allow single-specimen diagnosis

(continued)

Table 36–2. Diagnostic tests for viral infections. (continued)

Agent	Rapid Antigen Detection (Specimen)	Tissue Culture Mean Days to Positive (Range)	Serology			Comments
			Acute	Paired	PCR[a]	
Parvovirus B19	–	–	+	ND	+	Erythema infectiosum agent
Parainfluenza virus	+ (respiratory secretions)	2 (2–14)	–	+	+	
Rabies virus	+ (skin, conjunctiva, tissue biopsy)	–	+	+	CDC	Usually diagnosed by antigen detection
Respiratory syncytial virus	+ (respiratory secretions)	2 (2–21)	–	+	+	Rapid antigen detection; 90% sensitive
Rhinovirus	–	4 (2–7)	–	–	RL	Too many strains to type serologically
Rotavirus	+ (feces)	–	–	–	RL	Electron microscopy useful for many enteric viruses
Rubella virus	–	> 10	+	+	RL	Recommended that paired sera be tested simultaneously
SARS coronavirus	—	RL	RL	RL	+	
Varicella-zoster virus	+ (skin scraping)	3 (3–21)	RL	+	+	
West Nile virus	—	RL	+	+	+	

[a]Useful only when performed on selected specimens by qualified laboratories.

Key:

  Plus signs signify commercially or widely available; **minus signs** signify not commercially available. **Note:** Results from some commercial laboratories are unreliable.

  RL, CDC: Specific antibody titers or PCR available by arrangement with individual research laboratories or the Centers for Disease Control and Prevention.

  ND: Not done.

RBC, red blood cell; PCR, polymerase chain reaction.

In 5–10% of children, symptoms from these virus infections persist for more than 10 days. This overlap with the symptoms of bacterial sinusitis presents a difficult problem for clinicians, especially because colds can produce an abnormal computed tomography scan of the sinuses. Viruses that cause a minor illness in immunocompetent children, such as rhinoviruses, can cause severe lower respiratory disease in immunologically or anatomically compromised children.

There is no evidence that symptomatic relief for children can be achieved with oral antihistamines, decongestants, or cough suppressants. Topical decongestants provide temporary improvement in nasal symptoms.

Cohen L, Castro M: The role of viral respiratory infections in the pathogenesis and exacerbation of asthma. Semin Resp Infect 2003;18:3 [PMID: 22539104].

Greenberg SB: Respiratory consequences of rhinovirus infection. Arch Intern Med 2003;278:278 [PMID: 22466407].

Gwaltney JM Jr: Nose blowing propels nasal fluid into the paranasal sinuses. Clin Infect Dis 2000;30:387 [PMID: 10671347].

Heikkinen T, Jarvinen A: The common cold. Lancet 2003;361:51 [PMID: 22406053].

Sutter AI et al: Antihistamines for the common cold. Cochrane Database Syst Rev 2003;CD001267 [PMID: 22698575].

Taverner D et al: Nasal decongestants for the common cold. Cochrane Database Syst Rev 2000;(2):CD001953 [PMID: 10796673].

INFECTIONS DUE TO ADENOVIRUSES

Over 50 types of adenoviruses have been identified, which account for 5–10% of all respiratory illnesses in childhood, usually pharyngitis or tracheitis. Adenoviral infections are common early in life. Enteric adenoviruses are an important cause of childhood diarrhea. Epidemic respiratory dis-

Table 36–3. Red rashes in children.

Condition	Incubation Period (Days)	Prodrome	Rash	Laboratory Tests	Comments, Other Diagnostic Features
Adenovirus	4–5	URI; cough; fever	Morbilliform (may be petechial)	Normal; may see leukopenia or lymphocytosis	Respiratory symptoms are prominent. No Koplik spots. No desquamation.
Measles	9–14	Cough, rhinitis, conjunctivitis	Maculopapular; face to trunk; lasts 7–10 d; Koplik spots in mouth	Leukopenia	Toxic. Bright red rash becomes confluent, may desquamate. Fever falls after rash appears.
Rubella	14–21	Usually none	Mild maculopapular; rapid spread face to extremities; gone by day 4	Normal or leukopenia	Postauricular, occipital adenopathy common. Polyarthralgia in some older girls. Mild clinical illness.
Roseola (exanthem subitum) (HHV-6)	10–14	Fever (3–4 d)	Pink, macular rash occurs at end of illness; transient	Normal	Fever often high; disappears when rash develops; child appears well. Usually occurs in children 6 mos to 2 y of age. Seizures may complicate.
Enterovirus	2–7	Variable fever, chills, myalgia, sore throat	Usually macular, maculopapular on trunk or palms, soles; vesicles or petechiae also seen	Variable	Varied rashes may resemble those of many other infections. Pharyngeal or hand-foot-mouth vesicles may occur.
Streptococcal scarlet fever	1–7	Fever, abdominal pain, headache, sore throat	Diffuse erythema, "sandpaper" texture; neck, axillae, inguinal areas; spreads to rest of body; desquamates 7–14 d	Leukocytosis; positive group A streptococcus culture of throat or wound; positive streptococcal antigen test in pharynx	Strawberry tongue, red pharynx with or without exudate. Eyes, perioral and periorbital area, palms, and soles spared. Pastia's lines. Brief prodrome. Cervical adenopathy. Usually occurs in children 2–10y of age.
Staphylococcal scarlet fever	1–7	Variable fever	Diffuse erythroderma; resembles streptococcal scarlet fever except eyes may be hyperemic, no "strawberry" tongue, pharynx spared	Variable leukocytosis if infected	Focal infection usually present.
Staphylococcal scalded skin	Variable	Irritability, absent to low fever	Painful erythroderma, followed in 1–2 d by cracking around eyes, mouth; bullae form with friction (Nikolsky sign)	Normal if only colonized by staphylococci; leukocytosis and sometimes bacteremia if infected	Normal pharynx. Look for focal staphylococcal infection. Usually occurs in infants.
Toxic shock syndrome	Variable	Fever, myalgia, headache, diarrhea, vomiting	Nontender erythroderma; red eyes, palms, soles, pharynx, lips	Leukocytosis; abnormal liver enzymes, coagulation tests; proteinuria	Staphylococcus aureus infection; toxin-mediated multiorgan involvement. Swollen hands, feet. Hypotension or shock.

Disease	Incubation (d)	Prodrome/Symptoms	Rash	Laboratory	Comments
Erythema multiforme	—	Usually none or related to underlying cause	Discrete, red maculopapular lesions; symmetrical, distal, palms and soles; target lesions classic	Normal or eosinophilia	Reaction to drugs (especially sulfonamides), or infectious agents (mycoplasma; herpes simplex virus). Urticaria, arthralgia also seen.
Stevens-Johnson syndrome	—	Pharyngitis, conjunctivitis, fever, malaise	Bullous erythema multiforme; may slough in large areas; hemorrhagic lips; purulent conjunctivitis	Leukocytosis	Classic precipitants are drugs (especially sulfonamides), *Mycoplasma pneumoniae* and herpes simplex infections. Pneumonitis and urethritis also seen.
Drug allergy	—	None, or fever alone, or with myalgia, pruritus	Macular, maculopapular, urticarial, or erythroderma	Leukopenia, eosinophilia	Rash variable. Severe reactions may resemble measles, scarlet fever; Kawasaki disease; marked toxicity possible.
Kawasaki disease	Unknown	Fever, cervical adenopathy, irritability	Polymorphous (may be erythroderma) on trunk and extremities; red palms and soles, conjunctiva, lips, tongue, pharynx. Desquamation is common.	Leukocytosis, thrombocytosis, elevated ESR or C-reactive protein; pyuria; decreased albumin; negative cultures and streptococcal serology: resting tachycardia	Swollen hands, feet; prolonged illness; uveitis; aseptic meningitis; no response to antibiotics. Vasculitis and aneurysms of coronary and other arteries occur (cardiac ultrasound).
Leptospirosis	4–19	Fever (biphasic), myalgia, chills	Variable erythroderma	Leukocytosis; hematuria, proteinuria; hyperbilirubinemia	Conjunctivitis; hepatitis; aseptic meningitis may be seen. Rodent, dog contact.
Parvovirus (Erythema infectiosum)	10–17 (rash)	Mild (flulike)	Maculopapular on cheeks ("slapped cheek"), forehead, chin; then down limbs, trunk, buttocks; may fade and reappear for several weeks	IgM-EIA; PCR	Purpuric stocking-glove rash is rare, but distinctive; aplastic crisis for patients with chronic hemolytic anemia. May cause arthritis/arthralgia.
Ehrlichiosis (monocytic)	5–21	Fever; headache; flulike; myalgia; GI symptoms	Variable; maculopapular, petechial, scarlatiniform, vasculitic	Leukopenia, thrombocytopenia, abnormal liver function. Serology with IFA; morulae in monocytes.	Geographic distribution is a clue; seasonal; tick exposure; rash present in only 35%.
Rocky Mountain spotted fever	3–12	Headache (retroorbital); toxic; GI symptoms; high fever; flulike	Onset 2–6 d after fever; palpable maculopapular on palms, soles, extremities, with spread centrally; petechial	Leukopenia; thrombocytopenia; abnormal liver function; CSF pleocytosis; IFA or agglutination positive at 7–10 d of rash; biopsy will give earlier diagnosis	Eastern seaboard and southeastern U.S.A; April–September; tick exposure.

URI, upper respiratory infection; ESR, erythrocyte sedimentation rate; EIA, enzyme immunoassay; PCR, polymerase chain reaction; CSF, cerebrospinal fluid.

ease occurs in winter and spring, especially in closed environments such as day care centers and institutions. Because of latent infection in lymphoid tissue, asymptomatic shedding from the respiratory or intestinal tract is common.

Specific Adenoviral Syndromes

A. PHARYNGITIS

Pharyngitis is the most common adenoviral disease in children. Fever and adenopathy are common. Tonsillitis may be exudative. Rhinitis and an influenza-like systemic illness may be present. Laryngotracheitis or bronchitis may accompany pharyngitis.

B. PHARYNGOCONJUNCTIVAL FEVER

Conjunctivitis may occur alone and be prolonged, but most often is associated with preauricular adenopathy, fever, pharyngitis, and cervical adenopathy. Foreign body sensation and other symptoms last less than a week. Lower respiratory symptoms are uncommon.

C. EPIDEMIC KERATOCONJUNCTIVITIS

Symptoms are severe conjunctivitis with punctate keratitis and occasionally visual impairment. A foreign body sensation, photophobia, and swelling of conjunctiva and eyelids are characteristic. Preauricular adenopathy and subconjunctival hemorrhage are common.

D. PNEUMONIA

Severe pneumonia may occur at all ages. It is especially common in young children (< age 3 years). Chest radiographs show bilateral peribronchial and patchy ground-glass interstitial infiltrates in the lower lobes. Symptoms persist for 2–4 weeks. Adenoviral pneumonia can be necrotizing and cause permanent lung damage, especially bronchiectasis. A pertussis-like syndrome with typical cough and lymphocytosis can occur with lower respiratory tract infection.

E. RASH

A diffuse morbilliform (rarely petechial) rash resembling measles, rubella, or roseola may be present. Koplik spots are absent.

F. DIARRHEA

Enteric adenoviruses (types 40 and 41) cause 3–5% of cases of short-lived diarrhea in afebrile children.

G. MESENTERIC LYMPHADENITIS

Fever and abdominal pain may mimic appendicitis. Pharyngitis is often associated. Adenovirus-induced adenopathy may be a factor in appendicitis and intussusception.

H. OTHER SYNDROMES

Immunosuppressed patients, including neonates, may develop severe or fatal pulmonary or gastrointestinal infections or multisystem disease. Other rare complications include encephalitis, hepatitis, and myocarditis. Adenoviruses have been implicated in the syndrome of idiopathic myocardiopathy. Hemorrhagic cystitis can be a serious problem in immunocompromised children.

Diagnosis

Diagnosis is by culture of conjunctival, respiratory, or stool specimens. Several days to weeks are required for growth in conventional cultures. Viral culture using the rapid culture technique with immunodiagnostic reagents detects virus in 48 hours. Adenovirus infection can also be diagnosed using these reagents directly on respiratory secretions. This is quicker but less sensitive than the culture methods. PCR has now become an important, relatively rapid diagnostic method for adenovirus infections. Special cells are needed to isolate enteric adenoviruses. Enzyme-linked immunosorbent assay (ELISA) tests rapidly detect enteric adenoviruses in diarrheal specimens. Respiratory adenovirus infections can be detected retrospectively by comparing acute and convalescent sera, but this is not helpful during an acute illness.

Treatment

There is no specific treatment for adenovirus infections. Intravenous immune globulin (IVIG) may be tried in immunocompromised patients with severe pneumonia. There are anecdotal reports of successful treatment of immunocompromised patients with ribavirin or cidofovir, but only cidofovir inhibits adenovirus in vitro.

Chuang YY et al: Severe adenovirus infection in children. J Microbiol Immunol Infect 2003;36:37 [PMID: 22626563].

Rieger-Fackeldey E et al: Disseminated adenovirus infection in two premature infants. Infection 2000;28:237 [PMID: 10961532].

INFLUENZA

Symptomatic infections are common in children because they lack immunologic experience with influenza viruses. Infection rates in children are greater than in adults and are instrumental in initiating community outbreaks. Three main types of influenza viruses (A/H1N1, A/H3N2, B) have caused most human epidemics, with the antigenic drift ensuring a supply of susceptible hosts of all ages. Recently, avian influenza A/H5N1 caused human outbreaks in Asia. Epidemics occur in fall and winter.

Clinical Findings

Spread of influenza occurs by way of airborne respiratory secretions. The incubation period is 2–7 days.

A. SYMPTOMS AND SIGNS

Influenza infection in older children and adults produces a characteristic syndrome of sudden onset of high fever, severe myalgia, headache, and chills. These symptoms overshadow the associated coryza, pharyngitis, and cough. Usually absent are rash, marked conjunctivitis, adenopathy, exudative pharyngitis, and dehydrating enteritis. Fever, diarrhea, vomiting, and abdominal pain are common in young children. Infants may develop a sepsis-like illness and apnea. Chest examination is usually unremarkable. Unusual clinical findings or variants include croup (most severe with type A influenza), exacerbation of asthma, myositis (especially calf muscles), myocarditis, parotitis, encephalopathy (distinct from Reye syndrome), nephritis, and a transient maculopapular rash. Acute illness lasts 2–5 days. Cough and fatigue may last several weeks. Viral shedding may persist for several weeks in young children.

B. LABORATORY FINDINGS

The leukocyte count is normal to low, with variable shift. Influenza infections may be more difficult to recognize in children than in adults even during epidemics, and therefore a specific laboratory test is highly recommended. The virus may be found in respiratory secretions by direct fluorescent antibody staining of nasopharyngeal epithelial cells, ELISA, optic immunoassay, or PCR. It can also be cultured within 3–7 days from pharyngeal swabs or throat washings. Many laboratories use the rapid culture technique by centrifuging specimens onto cultured cell layers and detecting viral antigen after 48 hours. Other body fluids or tissues (except lung) rarely yield the virus in culture and are more appropriately tested by PCR, which, due to its high sensitivity, can increase influenza detection in respiratory specimens. A late diagnosis may be made with paired serology, using hemagglutination inhibition assays.

C. IMAGING

The chest radiograph is nonspecific; it may show hyperaeration, peribronchial thickening, diffuse interstitial infiltrates, or bronchopneumonia in severe cases. Hilar nodes are not enlarged. Pleural effusion is rare in uncomplicated influenza.

Differential Diagnosis

The following may be considered: all other respiratory viruses, *Mycoplasma pneumoniae* or *Chlamydia pneumoniae* (longer incubation period, prolonged illness), streptococcal pharyngitis (pharyngeal exudate or petechiae, adenitis, no cough), bacterial sepsis (petechial or purpuric rash may occur), toxic shock syndrome (rash, hypotension), and rickettsial infections (rash, different season, insect exposure). High fever, the nature of preceding or concurrent illness in family members, and the presence of influenza in the community are distinguishing features from parainfluenza or RSV infections.

Complications & Sequelae

Lower respiratory tract symptoms are most common in children younger than age 5 years. Hospitalization rates are highest in children younger than 2 years. Influenza can cause croup in these children. Secondary bacterial infections (classically staphylococcal) of the middle ear, sinuses, or lungs are most common. Of the viral infections that precede Reye syndrome, varicella and influenza (usually type B) are most notable. During an influenza outbreak, ill children who develop protracted vomiting or irrational behavior should be evaluated for Reye syndrome. (See Chapter 20.) Influenza can also cause a viral or postviral encephalitis, with cerebral symptoms much more prominent than those of the accompanying respiratory infection. Although the myositis is usually mild and resolves promptly, severe rhabdomyolysis and renal failure have been reported.

Children with underlying cardiopulmonary, metabolic, neuromuscular, or immunosuppressive disease may develop severe viral pneumonia.

Prevention

The inactivated influenza vaccine, which has been commercially available for many years, is moderately protective in older children. (See Chapter 9.) A new, live-attenuated influenza vaccine (FluMist), significantly more immunogenic in children, has been recently approved by the FDA for use in immunocompetent children 5 years of age or older. All children between 6 and 23 months of age or those at high risk of developing severe complications should be immunized. Medical staff and family members should also be immunized to protect high-risk patients. Type A infections may be prevented by amantadine or rimantadine (5 mg/kg; maximum 150 mg/d < age 10 years; 200 mg/d if older). Amantadine is divided into two daily doses; rimantadine can be given in a single dose. Both influenza A and B can be prevented with the neuraminidase inhibitors zanamivir (2 inhalations twice daily if > 7 years of age) and oseltamivir (if child < 15 kg, 30 mg twice daily; 15–23 kg, 45 mg twice daily; 23–40 kg, 60 mg twice daily; > 40 kg, 75 mg twice daily). For outbreak prophylaxis, therapy should be maintained for 2 weeks or more and 1 week after the last case of influenza is diagnosed. Chemoprophylaxis should be considered during an epidemic for high-risk children who cannot be immunized or who have not yet developed immunity (about 6 weeks after primary vaccination or 2 weeks after a booster dose).

Treatment & Prognosis

Treatment consists of general support and management of pulmonary complications, especially bacterial superinfections. Antivirals are of some benefit in immunocompetent hosts if begun within 48 hours after onset.

Studies in lung transplant patients indicate that oseltamivir might be useful for treatment of influenza in this immunocompromised population. Resistance to amantadine and rimantadine develops within a couple of days of treatment. In contrast, neuraminidase inhibitors rarely select resistant isolates.

Recovery is usually complete unless severe cardiopulmonary or neurologic damage has occurred. Fatal cases occur in immunodeficient and anatomically compromised children.

Effective treatment or prophylaxis of influenza in children markedly reduces the incidence of acute otitis media and antibiotic usage during the flu season.

Advisory Committee on Immunization Practices (Centers for Disease Control and Prevention): Prevention and control of influenza. MMWR Morb Mortal Wkly Rep 2003;52:RR–8 (RR–4):1 [PMID: 12755288].

Peltola V et al: Influenza A and B virus infection in children. Clin Infect Dis 2003;36:299 [PMID: 12539071].

Steininger C et al: Acute encephalopathy associated with influenza A virus infections. Clin Infect Dis 2003;36:567 [PMID: 12594636].

PARAINFLUENZA

Parainfluenza viruses (types 1–4) are the most important cause of croup. Most infants are infected with type 3 within the first 3 years of life, often in the first year. Infection with types 1 and 2 is experienced gradually over the first 5 years of life. Types 1 and 2 occur in the fall; type 3 appears annually, with a peak in the spring or summer. Most primary infections are symptomatic and frequently involve the lower respiratory tract.

Clinical Findings

A. SYMPTOMS AND SIGNS

Clinical diseases include febrile upper respiratory infection (especially in older children with reexposure), laryngitis, tracheobronchitis, croup, and bronchiolitis (second most common cause after RSV). The relative incidence of these manifestations is type-specific. Parainfluenza viruses (especially type 1) cause 65% of cases of croup in young children, 25% of tracheobronchitis, and 50% of laryngitis. Types 1 and 2 are more likely to cause bronchiolitis. Pneumonia occurs in infants and immunodeficient children, and it leads to particularly high mortality among stem-cell recipients. Onset is acute. Most children are febrile. Symptoms of upper respiratory tract infection often accompany croup.

B. LABORATORY FINDINGS

Diagnosis is often based on clinical findings. These viruses can be identified by conventional or rapid culture techniques (48 hours), by direct immunofluorescence on nasopharyngeal epithelial cells in respiratory secretions (< 3 hours), or by PCR (< 48 hours).

Differential Diagnosis

Parainfluenza-induced respiratory syndromes are difficult to distinguish from those caused by other respiratory viruses. Croup must be distinguished from epiglottitis caused by *Haemophilus influenzae* (abrupt onset, toxicity, drooling, dyspnea, little cough, left shift of blood smear, and a history of inadequate immunization).

Treatment

No specific therapy or vaccine is available. Croup management is discussed in Chapter 18. Ribavirin is active in vitro and has been used in immunocompromised children, but its efficacy is unproved.

Elizaga J et al: Parainfluenza virus 3 infection after stem cell transplant: Relevance to outcome of rapid diagnosis and ribavirin treatment. Clin Infect Dis 2001;32:413 [PMID: 11170949].

Mahdi SA et al. Severe lower respiratory tract infections associated with human parainfluenza viruses 1–3 in children infected and noninfected with HIV type 1. Eur J Clin Microbiol Infect Dis 2002;21:499 [PMID: 12172740].

Peltola V et al: Clinical courses of croup caused by influenza and parainfluenza viruses. Pediatr Infect Dis J 2002;21:76 [PMID: 11791108].

RESPIRATORY SYNCYTIAL VIRUS DISEASE

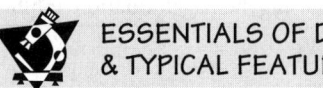

ESSENTIALS OF DIAGNOSIS & TYPICAL FEATURES

- *Diffuse wheezing and tachypnea following upper respiratory symptoms in an infant (bronchiolitis).*
- *Epidemics in late fall to early spring (January–February peak).*
- *Hyperinflation on chest radiograph.*
- *RSV antigen detected in nasal secretions.*

General Considerations

RSV is the most important cause of lower respiratory tract illness in young children, accounting for more than 70% of cases of bronchiolitis and 40% of cases of pneumonia. Outbreaks occur annually, and attack rates are high; 60% of children are infected in the first year of life, and 90% by age 2 years. During peak season (cold weather in temperate climates), the clinical diagnosis of RSV infection in infants with bronchiolitis is as accurate as most laboratory tests. Despite the presence of serum antibody, reinfection is common. Distinct genotypes predominate in a community. Yearly shift in these is a partial explanation for reinfection. However, reinfection generally causes only upper respiratory symptoms in anatomically normal children. No vaccine is available. Immunosuppressed patients may develop progressive severe pneumonia. Children with congenital heart disease with increased pulmonary blood flow, children with chronic lung disease (eg, cystic fibrosis), and premature infants younger than age 6 months are also at higher risk for severe illness.

Clinical Findings

A. SYMPTOMS AND SIGNS

Initial symptoms are those of upper respiratory infection. Low-grade fever may be present. The classic disease is bronchiolitis, characterized by diffuse wheezing, variable fever, cough, tachypnea, difficulty feeding, and, in severe cases, cyanosis. Hyperinflation, crackles, prolonged expiration, wheezing, and retractions are present. The liver and spleen may be palpable because of lung hyperinflation but are not enlarged. The disease usually lasts 3–7 days in previously healthy children. Fever is present for 2–4 days; it does not correlate with pulmonary symptoms and may be absent during the height of lung involvement.

Apnea may be the presenting manifestation, especially in premature infants, in the first few months of life; it usually resolves after a few days, often being replaced by obvious signs of bronchiolitis. No explanation for apnea has been found.

RSV infection in subsequent years is more likely to cause tracheobronchitis or upper respiratory tract infection. Exceptions are immunocompromised hosts and children with severe chronic lung or heart disease, who may have especially severe or prolonged primary infections and are subject to additional attacks of severe pneumonitis.

B. LABORATORY FINDINGS

Rapid detection of RSV antigen in nasal or pulmonary secretions by fluorescent antibody staining or ELISA requires only several hours and is more than 90% sensitive and specific. Rapid tissue culture methods take 48 hours and have comparable sensitivity.

C. IMAGING

Diffuse hyperinflation and peribronchiolar thickening are most common; atelectasis and patchy infiltrates also occur in uncomplicated infection, but pleural effusions are rare. Consolidation (usually subsegmental) occurs in 25% of children with lower respiratory tract disease.

Differential Diagnosis

Although almost all cases of bronchiolitis are due to RSV during an epidemic, other viruses, particularly human metapneumovirus, cannot be excluded. Mixed infections with other viruses, chlamydiae, or bacteria can occur. Wheezing may be due to asthma, a foreign body, or other airway obstruction. RSV infection may closely resemble chlamydial pneumonitis when fine crackles are present and fever and wheezing are not prominent. The two may also coexist. Cystic fibrosis may resemble RSV infection; a positive family history or failure to thrive associated with hyponatremia or hypoalbuminemia should prompt a sweat chloride test. Pertussis should also be considered in this age group, especially if cough is prominent and if the infant is younger than age 6 months. A markedly elevated leukocyte count should suggest bacterial superinfection (neutrophilia) or pertussis (lymphocytosis).

Complications

RSV commonly infects the middle ear. Symptomatic otitis media is more likely when secondary bacterial infection is present (usually due to pneumococci or *H influenzae*). This is the most common complication (10–20%). However, bacterial pneumonia occurs in only 0.5–1.0% of hospitalized patients. Sudden exacerbations of fever and leukocytosis should suggest bacterial infection. Respiratory failure or apnea may require mechanical ventilation, but occurs in less than 2% of hospitalized previously healthy full-term infants. Cardiac failure may occur as a complication of pulmonary disease or myocarditis. RSV—as well as parainfluenza and influenza viruses—commonly causes exacerbations of asthma. Nosocomial infection is so common during outbreaks that elective hospitalization or surgery, especially for those with underlying illness, should be postponed. Well-designed hospital programs to prevent nosocomial spread are imperative (see next section).

Treatment & Prevention

Children who are very hypoxic or cannot feed because of respiratory distress must be hospitalized and given humidified oxygen and tube or intravenous feedings. Antibiotics, decongestants, and expectorants are of no value in routine infections. Such children should be kept in respiratory isolation. Cohorting ill infants in respiratory isolation during peak season (with or without rapid diagnostic attempts) and emphasizing good hand-washing may greatly decrease nosocomial transmission.

The utility of bronchodilator therapy has not been consistently demonstrated. Often a trial of bronchodilator therapy is given to determine response and is subsequently discontinued if there is no improvement. Racemic epinephrine occasionally works when albuterol fails. The use of corticosteroids is also controversial. A meta-analysis of numerous studies indicates a significant effect on hospital stay, especially in those most ill at the time of treatment. The use of steroids in the emergency room appears to speed improvement and prevent hospitalization.

Ribavirin is the only licensed antiviral therapy used for RSV infection. It is given by continuous aerosolization (6 g in a 300-mL vial of water) by a special nebulizer for 12–18 hours of every day for 3–5 days. This agent has minimal effect on virus shedding. There is great controversy about its efficacy, and its use is infrequent in infants without significant anatomic or immunologic defects. At best, there is a very modest effect on disease severity in immunocompetent infants with no underlying anatomic abnormality. Even in high-risk infants, clinical response to ribavirin therapy was not demonstrated in several studies. Nevertheless, ribavirin is sometimes used in severely ill children who are immunologically or anatomically compromised, in those with severe cardiac disease, and in those with evidence of severe RSV infection. Bronchospasm may be exacerbated by this drug, although randomized trials do not show a deterioration of pulmonary function in patients receiving ribavirin.

Monthly intramuscular administration of humanized RSV monoclonal antibody is now recommended to prevent severe disease in high-risk patients during epidemic periods. Monthly administration should be considered during the RSV season for high-risk children, as described in Chapter 9.

Use of passive immunization for immunocompromised children is logical but not established. RSV antibody is not effective for treatment of established infection.

Prognosis

Although mild bronchiolitis does not produce long-term problems, 30–40% of patients hospitalized with this infection will wheeze later in childhood. Chronic restrictive lung disease and bronchiolitis obliterans are rare sequelae.

Black CO: Systematic review of the biology and medical management of respiratory syncytial virus infection. Resp Care 2003; 48:209 [PMID: 12667273].

Hall CB: Respiratory syncytial virus and parainfluenza virus. N Engl J Med 2001;344:1917 [PMID: 11419430].

Ogra PL: From chimpanzee to palivizumab: Changing times for respiratory syncytial virus. Pediatr Infect Dis J 2000;19:774 [PMID: 10959757].

Panitch HB: Respiratory syncytial virus bronchiolitis: Supportive care and therapies designed to overcome airway obstruction. Pediatr Infect Dis J 2003;22:S83 [PMID: 12671457].

Welliver RC: Respiratory syncytial virus and other respiratory viruses. Pediatr Infect Dis J 2003;22:S6 [PMID: 12671447].

HUMAN METAPNEUMOVIRUS

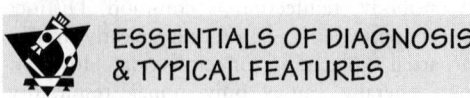

ESSENTIALS OF DIAGNOSIS & TYPICAL FEATURES

- *Cough, coryza, sore throat.*
- *Bronchiolitis.*
- *Positive hMPV PCR in respiratory secretion.*

General Considerations

After its discovery in 2001, human metapneumovirus (hMPV) was rapidly identified as a common agent of respiratory tract infections that is very similar to RSV in epidemiologic and clinical characteristics. Like RSV, parainfluenza, mumps, and measles, hMPV belongs to the paramyxovirus family. Humans are its only known reservoir. Seroepidemiologic surveys indicate that the virus has worldwide distribution. More than 90% of children contract hMPV infection by age 5 years, typically during late autumn through early spring outbreaks. hMPV accounts for 15–25% of the cases of bronchiolitis and pneumonia in children younger than 2 years of age. Older children and adults can also develop symptomatic infection.

Clinical Characteristics

A. SIGNS AND SYMPTOMS

The most common symptoms are fever, cough, rhinorrhea, and sore throat. Bronchiolitis and pneumonia occur in 40–70% of the children who acquire hMPV before the age of 2 years. Asymptomatic infection is uncommon. Other manifestations include otitis, conjunctivitis, diarrhea, and myalgia. Acute wheezing has been associated with hMPV in children of all ages, raising the possibility that this virus, like RSV, might trigger reactive airway disease. Dual infection with hMPV and RSV or other respiratory viruses seems to be a common occurrence and may increase morbidity and mortality.

B. IMAGING STUDIES

Lower respiratory tract infection frequently shows hyperinflation and patchy pneumonitis on chest radiographs.

C. LABORATORY DIAGNOSIS

The virus has very selective tissue culture tropism, which accounts for its late discovery in spite of its presence in archived specimens from the mid-1900s. The preferred method of diagnosis is PCR performed on respiratory specimens. Antibody tests are available, but are most appropriately used for epidemiologic studies.

Prognosis & Treatment

No antiviral therapies are available to treat hMPV. Children with lower respiratory tract disease may require hospitalization and ventilatory support, but less frequently than with RSV-associated bronchiolitis. Duration of hospitalization with hMPV is typically shorter than with RSV.

Boivin G et al: Virological and clinical manifestations associated with human metapneumovirus: A new paramyxovirus responsible for acute respiratory tract infections in all age groups. J Infect Dis 2002;186:1330 [PMID: 12402203].

van den Hoogen BG et al: A newly discovered human pneumovirus. Nat Med 2001;7:719 [PMID: 11385510].

SEVERE ACUTE RESPIRATORY SYNDROME (SARS)

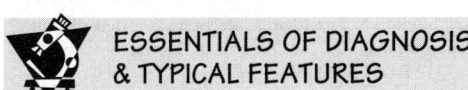

ESSENTIALS OF DIAGNOSIS & TYPICAL FEATURES

Suspected case
- *Febrile illness of unknown etiology with temperature above 38 °C.*

AND
- *One or more clinical findings of respiratory illness (eg, cough, shortness of breath (SOB), difficulty breathing, hypoxia).*

AND
- *Travel within 10 days of symptom onset to an area with documented/suspected community transmission of SARS.*

OR
- *Close contact within 10 days of onset of symptoms with a person with known or suspected SARS.*

Probable case
- *Suspected case definition plus radiographic evidence of pneumonia.*

OR
- *Autopsy evidence of acute respiratory distress syndrome or pneumonia.*

General Considerations

A new cause of atypical pneumonia arose in Asia in late 2002. Because of its severity it was named severe acute respiratory syndrome (SARS). During the following half year more than 8500 cases were documented. Many other countries reported cases from travelers, including 100 in the United States. A coronavirus (SARS-CoV) was isolated as the causative agent. This virus probably was acquired from indigenous wild animals sold in markets. Subsequent spread among close contacts, as well as within hospitals and by international travelers, extended the epidemic.

Clinical Findings

A. SYMPTOMS AND SIGNS

Initially, fever is accompanied by malaise, chills, headache, myalgia, dyspnea, and cough. Abnormal chest auscultation is noted in only 25% of cases and often is less prominent than would be expected from the chest radiograph. In two-thirds of patients the pulmonary symptoms and signs progress, hypoxia occurs, and 20–30% require intensive care. Fatal respiratory failure ensues in a third to a half of these. A watery diarrhea is prominent in one-fourth of the patients. The incubation period is 4–7 days (range is 2–10 days). The peak severity occurs at about 2 weeks after onset.

B. LABORATORY

Leukopenia, lymphopenia, and thrombocytopenia occur in many patients. Lactate dehydrogenase, aspartate aminotransferase, and creatinine phosphokinase are often elevated. However, none of these changes is diagnostic. Virus can be isolated from respiratory secretions, saliva, urine, and feces. An RT-PCR is useful for diagnosis within 5 days of onset. Antibody can be detected by immunofluorescence assay at 10–14 days and by enzyme immunoassay about a week later.

C. IMAGING

Most patients have an abnormal radiograph when first seen, typically with ground-glass opacities or focal consolidation. In severe cases this rapidly progresses to multiple bilateral consolidations.

Differential Diagnosis

The initial onset is similar to that of other causes of atypical pneumonia (eg, *Mycoplasma, Chlamydia,* Q fever, *Legionella, C psittaci,* and other viruses [especially influenza]). SARS differs from *Mycoplasma* and *Chlamydia* infections in the absence of significant coryza and sore throat. The seasonality of some viruses will suggest their exclusion from the diagnosis. The travel and contact history is a key factor in the diagnosis of SARS.

Treatment

The management is largely supportive. Since no established therapy exists, potential approaches are still evolving. A SARS-specific immunoglobulin is under study.

Prevention

Detailed surveillance and quarantine measures have evolved. These appear to have been important in limiting outbreaks. In addition, since spread within hospitals has been prominent, infection control and patient care rules for SARS are now in place.

Prognosis

Ten to twenty percent of hospitalized cases are fatal. This rate is greatest in elderly people and those with other underlying illnesses. Children have milder disease and fewer radiographic abnormalities.

Abdullah AS et al: Lessons from the severe acute respiratory syndrome outbreak in Hong Kong. Emerg Infect Dis 2003;9:1042 [PMID: 14519237].

Demmler GJ, Ligon BL: Severe acute respiratory syndrome (SARS): A review of the history, epidemiology, prevention and concerns for the future. Semin Pediatr Infect Dis 2003;14:240 [PMID: 12913837].

Peiris JSM et al: The severe acute respiratory syndrome. N Engl J Med 2003;349:2431 [PMID:14681510].

■ INFECTIONS DUE TO ENTEROVIRUSES

Enteroviruses are a major cause of illness in young children. The multiple types are physically and biochemically similar and may produce identical syndromes. The multiplicity of types makes vaccine development impractical and has hindered development of antigen detection and serologic tests. However, common RNA sequences and group antigens have led to diagnostic tests for viral nucleic acid and proteins. A PCR assay is available in many medical centers, but tissue culture is the most commonly used diagnostic method for echoviruses, polioviruses, and coxsackie B viruses. Because cultures may turn positive in 2–4 days, they should be inoculated promptly and may be clinically useful, particularly in cases of meningoencephalitis. Many coxsackie A viruses fail to grow.

Transmission is fecal–oral or from upper respiratory secretions. Multiple enteroviruses circulate in the community at any one time; summer–fall outbreaks are common in temperate climates, but infections are seen year-round. After poliovirus, coxsackie B virus is most virulent, followed by echovirus. Neurologic, cardiac, and overwhelming neonatal infections are the most severe forms of illness.

ACUTE FEBRILE ILLNESS

Accompanied by nonspecific upper respiratory or enteric symptoms, sudden onset of fever and irritability in infants or young children is often enteroviral in origin, especially in late summer and fall. More than 90% of enteroviral infections are not distinctive. Occasionally a petechial rash is seen; more often a diffuse maculopapular or morbilliform eruption (often prominent on palms and soles) occurs on the second to fourth day of fever. Rapid recovery is the rule. More than one febrile enteroviral illness can occur in the same patient in one season. The leukocyte count is usually normal. Infants, because of fever and irritability, may undergo an evaluation for bacteremia or meningitis and be hospitalized to rule out sepsis. Approximately one-half of these infants have aseptic meningitis. In the summer months enterovirus infection is more likely than human herpesvirus 6 to cause an acute medical visit for fever. Duration of illness is 4–5 days.

Sawyer MH: Enterovirus infections: Diagnosis and treatment. Semin Pediatr Infect Dis 2002;13:40 [PMID: 12118843].

Stalkup JR, Chilukuri S: Enterovirus infections: A review of clinical presentation, diagnosis, and treatment. Dermatol Clin 2002; 20:217 [PMID: 12120436].

RESPIRATORY TRACT ILLNESSES

1. Febrile Illness with Pharyngitis

This syndrome is most common in older children, who complain of headache, sore throat, myalgia, and abdominal discomfort. The usual duration is 3–4 days. Vesicles or papules may be seen in the pharynx. There is no exudate. Occasionally, enteroviruses are the cause of croup, bronchitis, or pneumonia. They may also exacerbate asthma.

2. Herpangina

Herpangina is characterized by an acute onset of fever and posterior pharyngeal grayish white vesicles that quickly form ulcers (< 20 in number), often linearly arranged on the posterior palate, uvula, and tonsillar pillars. Bilateral faucial ulcers may also be seen. Dysphagia, vomiting, abdominal pain, and anorexia also occur and, rarely, parotitis or vaginal ulcers. Symptoms disappear in 4–5 days. The epidemic form is due to a variety of coxsackie A viruses; coxsackie B viruses and echoviruses cause sporadic cases.

The differential diagnosis includes primary herpes simplex gingivostomatitis (ulcers are more prominent anteriorly, and gingivitis is present), aphthous stomatitis (fever absent, recurrent episodes, anterior lesions), trauma, hand-foot-and-mouth disease (see later discussion), and Vincent angina (painful gingivitis spreading from the gum line, underlying dental disease). If the enanthema is missed, tonsillitis might be incorrectly diagnosed.

3. Acute Lymphonodular Pharyngitis

Coxsackievirus A10 has been associated with a febrile pharyngitis characterized by nonulcerative yellow-white posterior pharyngeal papules in the same distribution as herpangina. The duration is 1–2 weeks; therapy is supportive.

4. Pleurodynia (Bornholm Disease, Epidemic Myalgia)

Caused by coxsackie B virus (epidemic form) or many nonpolio enteroviruses (sporadic form), pleurodynia is associated with an abrupt onset of unilateral or bilateral spasmodic pain of variable intensity over the lower ribs or upper abdomen. Associated symptoms include headache, fever, vomiting, myalgias, and abdominal and neck pain. Physical findings include fever, chest muscle tenderness, decreased thoracic excursion, and occasionally a friction rub. The chest radiograph is normal. Hematologic tests are nondiagnostic. The illness generally lasts less than 1 week.

This is a disease of muscle, but the differential diagnosis includes bacterial pneumonia, empyema, tuberculosis, and endemic fungal infections (all excluded radiographically and by auscultation), costochondritis (no fever or other symptoms), and a variety of abdominal problems, especially those causing diaphragmatic irritation.

There is no specific therapy. Potent analgesic agents and chest splinting alleviate the pain.

RASHES (Including Hand-Foot-and-Mouth Disease)

The rash may be macular, maculopapular, urticarial, scarlatiniform, petechial, or vesicular. One of the most characteristic is that of hand-foot-and-mouth disease (caused by coxsackieviruses, especially types A5, A10, and A16), in which vesicles or red papules are found on the tongue, oral mucosa, hands, and feet. Often they appear near the nails and on the heels. Associated fever, sore throat, and malaise are mild. The rash may appear when fever abates, simulating roseola.

Cardiac Involvement

Myocarditis and pericarditis may be caused by a number of nonpolio enteroviruses, particularly type B coxsackieviruses. Most commonly, upper respiratory symptoms are followed by substernal pain, dyspnea, and exercise intolerance. A friction rub or gallop may be detected. Ultrasound will define ventricular dysfunction, and electrocardiography may show pericarditis or ventricular irritability. Creatine kinase may be elevated. The disease may be mild or fatal; most children recover completely. In infants, other organs may be involved at the same time; in older patients, cardiac disease is usually the sole manifestation. (See Chapter 19 for therapy.) Enteroviral RNA is present in cardiac tissue in some cases of dilated cardiomyopathy or myocarditis; the significance of this finding is unknown. Epidemics of enterovirus 71, which occur in Asia, as well as sporadic cases in the United States, are associated with severe left ventricular dysfunction and pulmonary edema following typical mucocutaneous manifestations of enterovirus infection.

Severe Neonatal Infection

Sporadic and nosocomial nursery cases of severe systemic enteroviral disease occur. Clinical manifestations include combinations of fever, rash, pneumonitis, encephalitis, hepatitis, gastroenteritis, myocarditis, pancreatitis, and myositis. The infants, usually younger than 1 week old, may appear septic, with cyanosis, dyspnea, and seizures. The differential diagnosis includes bacterial and herpes simplex infections, necrotizing enterocolitis, other causes of heart or liver failure, and metabolic diseases. Diagnosis is suggested by the finding of cerebrospinal fluid (CSF) mononuclear pleocytosis and confirmed by the isolation of virus or detection of enteroviral RNA from urine, stool, CSF, or pharynx. Therapy is supportive. IVIG is often administered, but its value is uncertain. Passively acquired maternal antibody may protect newborns from severe disease. For this reason, labor should not be induced in pregnant women near term who have suspected enteroviral disease.

Huang F-L et al: Left ventricular dysfunction in children with fulminant enterovirus 71 infection: An evaluation of the clinical course. Clin Infect Dis 2002;34:1020 [PMID: 11880970].

CENTRAL NERVOUS SYSTEM ILLNESSES

1. Poliomyelitis

ESSENTIALS OF DIAGNOSIS & TYPICAL FEATURES

- Inadequate immunization or underlying immune deficiency.
- Headache, fever, muscle weakness.
- Aseptic meningitis.
- Asymmetrical, flaccid paralysis; muscle tenderness and hyperesthesia; intact sensation; late atrophy.

General Considerations

Poliovirus infection is subclinical in 90–95% of cases; it causes nonspecific febrile illness in about 5% of cases and aseptic meningitis, with or without paralytic disease, in 1–3%. In endemic areas, most older children and adults are immune because of prior inapparent infections. Occasional cases in the United States occur in patients who have traveled to foreign countries. Most cases were in immunodeficient patients who received the oral poliovirus vaccine (OPV) or were exposed to recent vaccinees. Severe poliovirus infection was a rare complication of OPV vaccination as a result of reversion of the vaccine virus. The incidence of vaccine-associated paralytic poliomyelitis (VAPP) in the United States was 1:750,000 and 1:2.4 million doses for the first and second dose of OPV, respectively. Although rare, VAPP became more common than wild-type poliomyelitis in the United States in the 1980s. This led to change in the recommended immunization regimen, substituting inactivated poliovaccine (IPV) for OPV. (See Chapter 9.)

Clinical Findings

A. SYMPTOMS AND SIGNS

The initial symptoms are fever, myalgia, sore throat, and headache for 2–6 days. In less than 10% of infected children, several symptom-free days are followed by recurrent fever and signs of aseptic meningitis: headache, stiff neck, spinal rigidity, and nausea. Mild cases resolve completely. In only 1–2% of these children does high fever, severe myalgia, and anxiety portend progression to loss of reflexes and subsequent flaccid paralysis. Sensation remains intact, although hyperesthesia of skin overlying paralyzed muscles is common and pathognomonic.

Paralysis is usually asymmetrical. Proximal limb muscles are more often involved than distal, and lower limb involvement is more common. Bulbar involvement affects swallowing, speech, and cardiorespiratory function and accounts for most deaths. Bladder distention and marked constipation characteristically accompany lower limb paralysis. Paralysis is usually complete by the time the temperature normalizes. Weakness often resolves completely. Atrophy is usually apparent by 4–8 weeks. Most improvement of muscle paralysis will take place within 6 months.

B. LABORATORY FINDINGS

In patients with meningeal symptoms, the CSF contains up to several hundred leukocytes (mostly lymphocytes) per microliter; the glucose level is normal, and protein concentration is mildly elevated. Poliovirus is easy to grow in cell culture and can be readily differentiated from other enteroviruses. It is rarely isolated from spinal fluid but is often present in the throat and stool for several weeks following infection. Paired serology is also diagnostic. Laboratory methods are available to differentiate wild from attenuated vaccine isolates.

Differential Diagnosis

Aseptic meningitis due to poliovirus is indistinguishable from that due to other viruses. Paralytic disease in the United States is usually due to nonpolio enteroviruses. Polio may resemble Guillain–Barré syndrome (variable sensory loss, symmetrical loss of function; minimal pleocytosis, high protein concentration in spinal fluid), polyneuritis (sensory loss), pseudoparalysis due to bone or joint problems (eg, trauma, infection), botulism, or tick paralysis.

Complications & Sequelae

Complications are the result of the acute and permanent effects of paralysis. Respiratory, pharyngeal, bladder, and bowel malfunction are most critical. Deaths are usually due to complications arising from respiratory dysfunction. Limbs injured near the time of infection, such as by intramuscular injections, excessive prior use, or trauma, tend to be most severely involved and have the worst prognosis for recovery (provocation paralysis). Postpolio muscular atrophy occurs in 30–40% of paralyzed limbs 20–30 years later, characterized by increasing weakness and fasciculations in previously affected, partially recovered limbs.

Treatment & Prognosis

Therapy is supportive. Bed rest, fever and pain control (heat therapy is helpful), and careful attention to progression of weakness (particularly of respiratory muscles) are important. No intramuscular injections should be given during the acute phase. Intubation or tracheostomy for secretion control and catheter drainage of the bladder may be needed. Assisted ventilation and enteral feeding may also be needed. Postpolio paralysis is mild in about 30% of patients, permanent in 15%, and results in death in 5–10%. Disease is worse in adults and pregnant women than in children.

2. Nonpolio Viral Meningitis

Nonpolio enteroviruses cause over 80% of cases of aseptic meningitis at all ages. In the summer and fall, multiple cases may be seen associated with circulation of neurotropic strains. Nosocomial outbreaks also occur.

Clinical Findings

The usual enteroviral incubation period is 4–6 days. Because many enteroviral infections are subclinical or not associated with central nervous system (CNS) symptoms, a history of contact with a patient with meningitis is unusual. Neonates may acquire infection from maternal blood, vaginal secretions, or feces at birth; occasionally the mother has had a febrile illness just prior to delivery.

A. Symptoms and Signs

Onset is usually acute with variable fever, marked irritability, and lethargy in infants. Incidence is much greater in children younger than age 1 year. Older children also describe frontal headache, photophobia, and myalgia. Abdominal pain, diarrhea, and vomiting may occur. The incidence of rash varies with the infecting strain. If rash occurs, it is usually seen after several days of illness and is diffuse, macular or maculopapular, occasionally petechial, but not purpuric. Oropharyngeal vesicles and rash on the palms and soles suggest an enterovirus. The anterior fontanelle may be full. Meningismus may be present. The illness may be biphasic, with nonspecific symptoms and signs preceding those related to the CNS. In older children, it is easier to demonstrate meningeal signs. Seizures are unusual, and focal neurologic findings, which are rare, should lead to a search for an alternative cause. Frank encephalitis, which is also uncommon at any age, occurs most often in neonates. Because of the overall frequency of enteroviral disease in children, 10–20% of all cases of encephalitis of proved viral origin are caused by enteroviruses. In some areas of the world epidemics of enterovirus 71 that begin with typical mucocutaneous manifestations of enteroviruses are complicated by severe brainstem encephalitis and polio-like flaccid paralysis. Enterovirus 70 outbreaks have resulted in hemorrhagic conjunctivitis together with paralytic poliomyelitis. Such cases of enterovirus are now appearing in the United States. Other nonpolio enteroviruses cause sporadic cases of acute motor weakness similar to that seen with poliovirus infection. Children with congenital immune deficiency, especially agammaglobulinemia, are subject to chronic enteroviral meningoencephalitis that is often fatal or associated with severe sequelae.

B. Laboratory Findings

Blood leukocyte counts are nonspecific and often normal. The spinal fluid leukocyte count is 100–1000/μL. Early in the illness, polymorphonuclear cells predominate; a shift to mononuclear cells occurs within 8–36 hours. In about 95% of cases, spinal fluid parameters include a total leukocyte count less than 3000/μL, protein less than 80 mg/dL, and glucose more than 60% of serum values. Marked deviation from any of these findings should prompt consideration of another diagnosis (see following section). The syndrome of inappropriate secretion of antidiuretic hormone may occur but is rarely clinically significant.

Culture of CSF may yield an enterovirus within a few days (< 70%); virus may be found in acellular spinal fluids. PCR for enteroviruses is a useful diagnostic method in many centers (sensitivity > 90%). This test can give an answer within 24–48 hours. Isolation of an enterovirus from throat or stool suggests but does not prove enteroviral meningitis. Vaccine poliovirus present in feces in infants being evaluated for aseptic meningitis (outside of the United States) may confuse the diagnosis but can usually be distinguished by growth characteristics.

C. Imaging

Cerebral imaging is not often indicated; if done, it is usually normal. Subdural effusions, infarcts, edema, or focal abnormalities seen in bacterial meningitis are absent except for the rare case of focal encephalitis.

Differential Diagnosis

In the prevaccine era, mumps and polio were leading causes of aseptic meningitis, but now this disease is usually caused by enteroviruses, especially in the summer and fall. Other causative viruses are mosquito-borne viruses (flavivirus and bunyavirus). These are usually considered during an investigation of encephalitis, but many of them are more likely to cause isolated meningitis and should be considered when seasonal clusters of viral meningitis occur. Primary herpes simplex infection can cause aseptic meningitis in adolescents who have a genital herpes infection. In neonates, early herpes simplex meningoencephalitis may mimic enteroviral disease (see section on Infections Due to Herpesviruses). This is an important alternative diagnosis to exclude because of the need for urgent specific therapy. Lymphocytic choriomeningitis virus causes meningitis in children in contact with rodents (pet or environmental exposure). Meningitis occurs in some patients at the time of infection with human immunodeficiency virus (HIV).

Other causes of aseptic meningitis that may resemble enteroviral infection include partially treated bacterial meningitis (recent antibiotic treatment; CSF parameters resembling those seen in bacterial disease and bacterial antigen sometimes present); parameningeal foci of bacterial infection such as brain abscess, subdural empyema, mastoiditis (predisposing factors, glucose level in CSF may be lower, focal neurologic signs, and characteristic imaging); tumors or cysts (malignant cells detected by cytologic examination, a history of neurologic symptoms, higher protein concentration or lower glucose level in CSF); trauma (presence, without exception, of red blood cells, which may be erroneously assumed to be due to traumatic lumbar puncture but are crenated and fail to clear); vasculitis (other systemic or neurologic signs, found in older children); tuberculous or fungal meningitis (see Chapters 38 and 39); cysticercosis; parainfectious encephalopathies (*Mycoplasma pneumoniae,* cat scratch disease, respiratory viruses [especially influenza]); Lyme disease; leptospirosis; and rickettsial diseases.

Treatment & Prevention

No specific therapy exists. Infants are usually hospitalized, isolated, and treated with fluids and antipyretics. Moderately to severely ill infants are given appropriate antibiotics for bacterial pathogens until cultures are negative for 48–72 hours. This practice is changing somewhat, and hospital stay shortened, in areas where the PCR assay for enteroviruses is available. If patients—especially older children—are mildly ill, antibiotics may be withheld and the child observed. The illness usually lasts less than 1 week. Codeine compounds or other strong pain relievers may be needed. C-reactive protein and lactate levels are usually low in the CSF of children with viral meningitis; both may be elevated with bacterial infection. With clinical deterioration, repeat lumbar puncture, cerebral imaging, neurologic consultation, and more aggressive diagnostic tests should be considered. Herpesvirus encephalitis is an important consideration in such cases, particularly in infants younger than age 1 month. Newborns often receive empiric acyclovir therapy until an etiologic diagnosis is made. Specific antiviral therapy (pleconaril) is under study for the treatment of severe enteroviral infections.

Measures to prevent enteroviral infection include good hygiene, scrupulous hand washing, and proper isolation in the hospital.

Prognosis

In general, enteroviral meningitis has no significant short-term neurologic or developmental sequelae. Developmental delay may follow severe neonatal infections. Unlike mumps, enterovirus infections rarely cause hearing loss.

Chang L-Y et al: Comparison of enterovirus 71 and coxsackie-virus A16 clinical illness during the Taiwan enterovirus epidemic, 1998. Pediatr Infect Dis J 1999;18:1092 [PMID: 10608631].

Romero JR, Newland JG: Viral meningitis and encephalitis: Traditional and emerging viral agents. Semin Pediatr Infect Dis 2003;14:72 [PMID: 12881794].

Stellrecht KA et al: The impact of an enteroviral RT-PCR on the diagnosis of aseptic meningitis and patient management. J Clin Virol 2002;25:S19.[PMID: 12091078].

■ INFECTIONS DUE TO HERPESVIRUSES

HERPES SIMPLEX

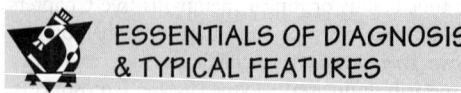

ESSENTIALS OF DIAGNOSIS & TYPICAL FEATURES

- Grouped vesicles on an erythematous base, typically in or around the mouth or genitals.

- Tender regional adenopathy, especially with primary infection.
- Fever and malaise with primary infection.
- Recurrent episodes in many patients.

General Considerations

There are two types of herpes simplex viruses. Type 1 (HSV-1) causes most cases of oral, skin, and cerebral disease. Type 2 (HSV-2) causes most (80–85%) genital and congenital infections. Latent infection in sensory ganglia routinely follows primary infection. Recurrences may be spontaneous or induced by external events (eg, fever, menstruation, or sunlight) or immunosuppression. Transmission is by direct contact with infected secretions. Herpes simplex viruses are very susceptible to antiviral drugs.

Primary infection with HSV-1 often occurs early in childhood, although many adults (20–50%) have never been infected. Primary infection with HSV-1 is subclinical in 80% of cases and causes gingivostomatitis in the remainder. HSV-2, which is transmitted sexually, is also usually (65%) subclinical or produces mild, nonspecific symptoms. Infection with one type of HSV may prevent or attenuate clinically apparent infection with the other type, but individuals can be infected at different times with both HSV-1 and HSV-2. Recurrent episodes are due to reactivation of latent HSV.

Clinical Findings

The source of primary infection is often an asymptomatic excreter. Most previously infected individuals shed HSV at irregular intervals. At any one time (point prevalence), 2–4% of normal seropositive adults excrete HSV-1 in the saliva; the percentage is higher in recently infected children. HSV-2 shedding in genital secretions occurs with a point prevalence of 8–28%, depending on the method of detection (viral isolation vs PCR). A history of contact with an active HSV infection is unusual.

A. Symptoms and Signs

1. Gingivostomatitis—High fever, irritability, and drooling occur in infants. Multiple oral ulcers are seen on the tongue and on the buccal and gingival mucosa, occasionally extending to the pharynx. Pharyngeal ulcers may predominate in older children and adolescents. Diffusely swollen red gums that are friable and bleed easily are typical. Cervical nodes are swollen and tender. Duration is 7–14 days. Herpangina, aphthous stomatitis, thrush, and Vincent angina should be excluded.

2. Vulvovaginitis or urethritis—Genital herpes (especially HSV-2) in a prepubertal child should suggest sexual abuse. Vesicles or painful ulcers on the vulva, vagina, or penis and tender adenopathy are seen. Systemic symptoms (fever, flulike illness, and myalgia) are common with the initial episode. Painful urination may cause retention. Primary infections last 10–21 days. Lesions may resemble trauma, syphilis (ulcers are painless), or chancroid (ulcers are painful and nodes are erythematous and fluctuant) in the adolescent, and bullous impetigo, trauma, and severe chemical irritation in younger children.

3. Cutaneous infections—Direct inoculation onto cuts or abrasions may produce localized vesicles or ulcers. A deep HSV infection on the fingers (called herpetic whitlow) may be mistaken for a bacterial felon or paronychia; surgical drainage is of no value and is contraindicated. HSV infection of eczematous skin may result in extensive areas of vesicles and shallow ulcers (eczema herpeticum), which may be mistaken for impetigo or varicella.

4. Recurrent mucocutaneous infection—Recurrent oral shedding is usually asymptomatic. Perioral recurrences often begin with a prodrome of tingling or burning limited to the vermilion border, followed by vesiculation, scabbing, and crusting around the lips over the next 3–5 days. Intraoral lesions rarely recur. Fever, adenopathy, and other symptoms are absent. Recurrent cutaneous herpes most closely resembles impetigo; the latter is often outside the perinasal and perioral region, responds to antibiotics, yields a positive Gram stain, and *Streptococcus pyogenes* or *Staphylococcus aureus* can be isolated. Recurrent genital disease is common after the initial infection with HSV-2. The disease is shorter (5–7 days) and milder (mean, four lesions) and is not associated with systemic symptoms.

5. Keratoconjunctivitis—Keratoconjunctivitis may be part of a primary infection due to spread from infected saliva. Most cases are caused by reactivation of virus latent in the ciliary ganglion. Keratoconjunctivitis produces photophobia, pain, and conjunctival irritation. With recurrences, dendritic corneal ulcers may be demonstrable with fluorescein staining. Stromal invasion may occur. Steroids should never be used for unilateral keratitis without ophthalmologic consultation. Other causes of these symptoms include trauma, bacterial infections, and other viral infections (especially adenovirus if pharyngitis is present; bilateral involvement makes HSV unlikely). (See Chapter 15.)

6. Encephalitis—Although unusual in infants outside the neonatal period, encephalitis may occur at any age, usually without cutaneous herpes lesions. In older children, HSV encephalitis can follow a primary infection, but often represents reactivation of latent virus. HSV is the most common cause of sporadic severe encephalitis. It is the most important because it can be treated with specific antiviral therapy. Fever, headache, behavioral changes, and neurologic deficits or focal seizures occur. Mild mononuclear pleocytosis is typically present along with an elevated protein concentration, which contin-

ues to rise on repeat lumbar punctures. In older children hypodense areas with a medial and inferior temporal lobe predilection are seen on computed tomography scan, especially after 3–5 days, but the findings in infants may be more diffuse. Magnetic resonance imaging (MRI) is more sensitive and is positive sooner. Periodic focal epileptiform discharges are seen on electroencephalograms but are not diagnostic of HSV infection. Viral cultures of CSF are rarely positive. The PCR assay to detect HSV DNA in CSF is a sensitive and specific rapid test. Without early antiviral therapy, the prognosis is poor. The differential diagnosis includes mumps, mosquito-borne and other viral encephalitides, parainfectious and postinfectious encephalopathy, brain abscess, acute demyelinating syndromes, and bacterial meningoencephalitis.

7. Neonatal infections—Infection is acquired by ascending spread prior to delivery (5–10% of cases) or at the time of vaginal delivery from a mother with genital infection. Occasionally the infection is acquired in the postpartum period from oral secretions of family members or hospital personnel. A history of genital herpes in the mother is usually absent. Within a few days and up to 4 weeks, skin vesicles (especially at sites of trauma, such as where scalp monitors were placed) appear. Some infants have infections limited to the skin, eye, or mouth. Other infants are acutely ill, presenting with jaundice, shock, bleeding, or respiratory distress. Some infants appear well initially, but dissemination of the infection to the brain or other organs becomes evident during the ensuing week if it is untreated. HSV infection (and empiric therapy) should be considered in newborns with the sepsis syndrome who are unresponsive to antibiotic therapy and have negative bacterial cultures. Skin lesions may be absent at the time of presentation. Some infected infants exhibit only neurologic symptoms at 2–3 weeks after delivery: apnea, lethargy, fever, poor feeding, or persistent overt seizures. The brain infection in these children is often diffuse and is best diagnosed by magnetic resonance imaging. The skin lesions may resemble impetigo, bacterial scalp abscesses, or miliaria; some children may fail to develop skin lesions. Skin lesions may recur over weeks or months after recovery from the acute illness. Progressive culture-negative pneumonitis is another manifestation of neonatal HSV.

B. LABORATORY FINDINGS

With multisystem disease, abnormalities in platelets, clotting factors, and liver function tests are often present. A finding of lymphocytic pleocytosis and elevated CSF protein indicates aseptic meningitis or encephalitis. Virus may be cultured from infected epithelial sites (vesicles, ulcers, or conjunctival scrapings) and from infected tissue (skin, brain) obtained by biopsy. Cultures of CSF are positive in about 50% of neonatal cases, but uncommon in older children. HSV will be detected within 2 days by rapid tissue culture methods. Isolation from throat, eye, urine, or stool of a newborn is diagnostic. Vaginal culture of the mother may offer circumstantial evidence for the diagnosis, but may be negative.

Rapid diagnostic tests include immunofluorescent stains or ELISA to detect viral antigen. The PCR assay for HSV DNA is positive ($\approx$ 95%) in the CSF when there is brain involvement. Serum is often positive in the presence of multisystem disease.

Complications, Sequelae, & Prognosis

Gingivostomatitis may result in dehydration due to dysphagia; severe chronic oral disease and esophageal involvement may occur in immunosuppressed patients. Primary vulvovaginitis may be associated with aseptic meningitis, paresthesias, autonomic dysfunction due to neuritis (urinary retention or constipation), and secondary candidal infection. Extensive cutaneous disease (as in eczema) may be associated with dissemination and bacterial superinfection. Keratitis may result in corneal opacification or perforation. Untreated encephalitis is fatal in 70% of patients and causes severe damage in most of the remainder. When acyclovir treatment is instituted early, 20% die and 40% are neurologically impaired. Disseminated neonatal infection is often fatal in spite of therapy, and survivors are often impaired.

Treatment

A. SPECIFIC MEASURES

HSV is sensitive to antiviral therapy.

1. Topical antivirals—Antivirals are most effective for corneal disease and include 1% trifluridine, 5% acyclovir, and 3% vidarabine. Trifluridine appears superior; cure rates over 95% are reported. These agents should be used with the guidance of an ophthalmologist.

2. Mucocutaneous HSV infections—These respond to administration of oral nucleoside analogs (acyclovir, valacyclovir, or famciclovir). The main indications are severe genital HSV infection in adolescents (see Chapter 40) and severe gingivostomatitis in young children. Antiviral therapy is beneficial for primary disease when begun early. Recurrent disease rarely requires therapy. Frequent genital recurrences may be suppressed by oral administration of nucleoside analogs, but this approach should be used sparingly. Other forms of severe cutaneous disease, such as eczema herpeticum, respond to these antivirals. Intravenous acyclovir may be required when disease is extensive in immunocompromised children (500 mg/m² every 8 hours). Oral acyclovir, which is available in suspension, is also used within 72–96 hours for severe primary gingivostomatitis in immunocompetent young children (10 mg/kg per dose four times a day for 5–7 days). Antiviral therapy does not alter the incidence or severity of subsequent recurrences of oral or genital infection. Development of resistance to antivirals is very rare after treating immunocompetent patients, but is increasingly reported in immunocompromised patients who receive frequent and prolonged therapy.

3. Encephalitis—This is treated with intravenous acyclovir 500 mg/m² every 8 hours for 21 days.

4. Neonatal infection—Newborns receive 20 mg/kg intravenous acyclovir every 8 hours for 21 days (14 days if infection is limited to skin, eye, or mouth).

B. GENERAL MEASURES

1. Gingivostomatitis—Gingivostomatitis is treated with pain relief and temperature control. Maintaining hydration is important because of the long duration of illness (7–14 days). Nonacidic, cool fluids are best. Topical anesthetic agents (eg, viscous lidocaine or an equal mixture of kaolin–attapulgite [Kaopectate], diphenhydramine, and viscous lidocaine) may be used as a mouthwash for older children who will not swallow it; ingested lidocaine may be toxic to infants or may lead to aspiration. Antiviral therapy is indicated in normal hosts with severe disease. Antibiotics are not helpful.

2. Genital infections—Genital infections require pain relief, assistance with voiding (warm baths, topical anesthetics, and rarely, catheterization), and psychological support. Lesions should be kept clean; drying decreases the potential for spread and may shorten the duration of symptoms. Sexual contact should be avoided during the interval from prodrome to crusting stages.

3. Cutaneous lesions—Skin lesions should be kept clean, dry, and covered if possible to prevent spread. Systemic analgesics may be helpful. Secondary bacterial infection is uncommon in patients with lesions on the mucosa or involving small areas. Secondary infection should be considered and treated if necessary (usually with an antistaphylococcal agent) in patients with more extensive lesions. Candidal superinfection occurs in 10% of women with primary genital infections.

4. Recurrent cutaneous disease—Recurrent disease is usually milder than primary infection. Sun block lip balm helps prevent labial recurrences after intense sun exposure. There is no evidence that the many popular topical or vitamin therapies are efficacious.

5. Keratoconjunctivitis—An ophthalmologist should be consulted regarding the use of cycloplegics, anti-inflammatory agents, local debridement, and other therapies.

6. Encephalitis—Extensive support will be required for obtunded or comatose patients. Rehabilitation and psychological support are often needed for survivors.

7. Neonatal infection—The affected infant should be isolated and given acyclovir. Cesarean section is indicated if the mother has obvious cervical or vaginal lesions, especially if these represent primary infection (35–50% transmission rate). With infants born vaginally to mothers who have active lesions, appropriate cultures should be obtained at 24–48 hours after birth, and the infants should be observed closely. Treatment is given to babies whose culture results are positive or who have suggestive signs or symptoms. Babies born to mothers with obvious primary genital herpes should receive therapy before the culture results are known. For women with a history of genital herpes infection, but no genital lesions, vaginal delivery with peripartum cultures of maternal cervix is the standard. Clinical follow-up of the newborn is recommended when maternal culture results are positive. Repeated cervical cultures during pregnancy are not useful.

Amir J et al: The natural history of primary herpes simplex type 1 gingivostomatitis in children. Pediatr Dermatol 1999;16:259 [PMID: 10469407].

Enright AM, Prober CG: Neonatal herpes infection: Diagnosis, treatment and prevention. Semin Neonatol 2002;7:283 [PMID: 12401298].

Kimberlin DW: Herpes simplex virus infections of the central nervous system. Semin Pediatr Infect Dis 2003;14:83 [PMID: 12881795].

Kohl S: The diagnosis and treatment of neonatal herpes simplex virus infection. Pediatr Ann 2002;31:726 [PMID: 12455481].

Whitley RJ: Herpes simplex virus infection. Semin Pediatr Infect Dis 2002;13:6 [PMID: 12118847].

VARICELLA & HERPES ZOSTER

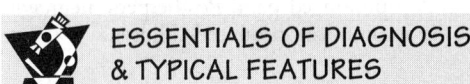

ESSENTIALS OF DIAGNOSIS & TYPICAL FEATURES

Varicella (chickenpox):

- *Exposure to varicella or herpes zoster 10–21 days previously; no prior history of varicella.*
- *Widely scattered red macules and papules concentrated on the face and trunk, rapidly progressing to clear vesicles, pustules, and then crusting, over 5–6 days. Variable fever and nonspecific systemic symptoms.*

Herpes zoster (shingles):

- *History of varicella.*
- *Local paresthesias and pain prior to eruption (more common in older children).*
- *Dermatomal distribution of grouped vesicles on an erythematous base.*

General Considerations

Primary infection with varicella-zoster virus results in varicella, which almost always confers lifelong immunity; the virus remains latent in sensory ganglia. Herpes zoster, which represents reactivation of this latent virus, occurs in 15–20% of individuals some time in their life. The incidence of herpes zoster is highest in elderly individuals and in immunosuppressed patients. Spread of varicella from a contact is by respiratory secretions or fomites from vesicles or pustules, with a greater than 90% infection rate in susceptible persons. Herpes zoster is about one-third as infectious. Over 95% of young adults with a history of varicella are immune, as are 90% of native-born Americans who are unaware of having had varicella. Many individuals from tropical or subtropical areas never have childhood exposure and are susceptible. Humans are the only reservoir.

Clinical Findings

Exposure to varicella or herpes zoster has usually occurred 14–16 days previously (range, 10–21 days). Contact may not have been recognized, since the index case is infectious 1–2 days before rash appears. Although varicella is the most distinctive childhood exanthem, inexperienced observers may mistake other diseases for varicella. A 1- to 3-day prodrome of fever, respiratory symptoms, and headache may occur, especially in older children. The preeruptive pain of herpes zoster may last several days and be mistaken for other illnesses.

A. SYMPTOMS AND SIGNS

1. Varicella—The usual case consists of mild systemic symptoms followed by crops of red macules that rapidly become small vesicles with surrounding erythema (described as a dew drop on a rose petal), form pustules, become crusted and then scab over, and leave no scar. The rash appears predominantly on the trunk and face. Lesions occur in the scalp, nose, mouth (where they are nonspecific ulcers), conjunctiva, and vagina. The magnitude of systemic symptoms usually parallels skin involvement. Up to five crops of lesions may be seen. New crops usually stop forming after 5–7 days. Pruritus is often intense. If varicella occurs in the first few months of life, it is often mild as a result of persisting maternal antibody. Once crusting begins, the patient is no longer contagious.

2. Herpes zoster—The eruption of shingles involves a single dermatome, usually truncal or cranial. The rash does not cross the midline. Ophthalmic zoster may be associated with corneal involvement. The closely grouped vesicles, which resemble a localized version of varicella or herpes simplex, often coalesce. The duration is 7–10 days before crusting. Postherpetic neuralgia is rare in children. A few vesicles are occasionally seen outside the involved dermatome. Herpes zoster is a common problem in HIV-infected or other immunocompromised children. Herpes zoster is also common in children who had varicella in early infancy or whose mothers had varicella during pregnancy.

B. LABORATORY FINDINGS

Leukocyte counts are normal or low. Leukocytosis suggests secondary bacterial infection. The virus can be identified by fluorescent antibody staining of a lesion smear. Rapid culture methods take 48 hours. Diagnosis can be made with paired serology. Serum aminotransferase levels may be modestly elevated during normal varicella.

C. IMAGING

Varicella pneumonia classically produces numerous bilateral nodular densities and hyperinflation. This is very rare in immunocompetent children. Abnormal chest radiographs are seen more frequently in adults.

Differential Diagnosis

Varicella is usually distinctive. Similar rashes include those of coxsackievirus infection (fewer lesions, lack of crusting), impetigo (fewer lesions, smaller area, no classic vesicles, positive Gram stain, perioral or peripheral lesions), papular urticaria (insect bite history, nonvesicular rash), scabies (burrows, no typical vesicles), parapsoriasis (rare in children younger than age 10 years, chronic or recurrent, often a history of prior varicella), rickettsialpox (eschar where the mite bites, smaller lesions, no crusting), dermatitis herpetiformis (chronic, urticaria, residual pigmentation), and folliculitis. Herpes zoster is sometimes confused with a linear eruption of herpes simplex or a contact dermatitis (eg, *Rhus* dermatitis).

Complications & Sequelae

A. VARICELLA

Secondary bacterial infection with staphylococci or group A streptococci is most common, presenting as impetigo, cellulitis or fasciitis, abscesses, scarlet fever, or sepsis. Bacterial superinfection occurs in 2–3% of children. Hospitalization rates associated with varicella are 1:750–1:1000 cases in children and 10-fold higher in adults.

Protracted vomiting or a change in sensorium suggests Reye syndrome or encephalitis. Because Reye syndrome usually occurs in patients who are also using salicylates, these should be avoided in patients with varicella. Encephalitis occurs in less than 0.1% of cases, usually in the first week of illness. It is usually limited to cerebellitis with ataxia, which resolves completely. Diffuse encephalitis can be severe.

Varicella pneumonia usually afflicts immunocompromised children (especially those with leukemia or lymphoma or those receiving high doses of steroids or chemotherapy) and adults; pregnant women may be at special risk. Cough, dyspnea, tachypnea, rales, and cyanosis occur several days after onset of rash. Varicella may be life-threatening in immunosuppressed patients.

Their disease is complicated by severe pneumonitis, hepatitis, and encephalitis. Varicella exposure in such patients must be evaluated immediately for postexposure prophylaxis. (See Chapter 9.)

Hemorrhagic varicella lesions may be seen without other complications. This is most often caused by autoimmune thrombocytopenia, but hemorrhagic lesions can occasionally represent idiopathic disseminated intravascular coagulation (purpura fulminans).

Neonates born to mothers who develop varicella from 5 days before to 2 days after delivery are at high risk for severe or fatal (5%) disease and must be given varicella-zoster immune globulin (VZIG) and followed closely. (See Chapter 9.)

Varicella occurring during the first 20 weeks of pregnancy may cause (2% incidence) congenital infection associated with cicatricial skin lesions, associated limb anomalies, and cortical atrophy.

Unusual complications of varicella include optic neuritis, myocarditis, transverse myelitis, orchitis, and arthritis.

B. HERPES ZOSTER

Complications of herpes zoster include secondary bacterial infection, motor or cranial nerve paralysis (1 per 200 cases in adults), encephalitis, keratitis, and dissemination in immunosuppressed patients. These complications are rare in immunocompetent children, and they do not develop prolonged pain. Postherpetic neuralgia does occur in immunocompromised children.

Treatment

A. GENERAL MEASURES

Supportive measures include maintenance of hydration, administration of acetaminophen for discomfort, cool soaks or antipruritics for itching (diphenhydramine, 1.25 mg/kg every 6 hours, or hydroxyzine, 0.5 mg/kg every 6 hours), and observance of general hygiene measures (keep nails trimmed and skin clean). Care must be taken to avoid overdosage with antihistaminic agents. Topical or systemic antibiotics may be needed for bacterial superinfection.

B. SPECIFIC MEASURES

Although acyclovir is more active against herpes simplex, it is the preferred drug for varicella and herpes zoster infections. Recommended parenteral acyclovir dosage for severe disease is 10 mg/kg (500 mg/m^2) intravenously every 8 hours, each dose infused over 1 hour. Parenteral therapy should be started early in immunosuppressed patients or high-risk infected neonates. VZIG is of no value for established disease. The effect of oral acyclovir (80 mg/kg/d, divided in four doses) on varicella in immunocompetent children was modestly beneficial and nontoxic, but only when administered within 24 hours after the onset of varicella. Oral acyclovir should be used selectively in immunocompetent children (eg, when intercurrent illness is present; possibly when second attacks occur in the household or when the patient is an adolescent—both of which are associated with more severe disease) and in children with underlying chronic illnesses. Valacyclovir and famciclovir are superior antiviral agents because of better absorption; acyclovir is available as a pediatric suspension. Herpes zoster in an immunocompromised child should be treated with intravenous acyclovir when it is severe. Oral valacyclovir or famciclovir can be used in immunocompromised children when the nature of the illness and the immune status support this decision.

Prevention

VZIG is available for postexposure prevention of varicella in high-risk susceptible persons. (See Chapter 9.) Postexposure prophylaxis with acyclovir is effective when it is started at 8 or 9 days after exposure and is continued for 7 days. The live attenuated varicella vaccine should be given as part of routine childhood immunization, and "catch-up" immunization is recommended for all other susceptible children and adults. Varicella vaccine is also useful for postexposure prophylaxis when given within 3–5 days of the exposure.

Prognosis

Except for secondary bacterial infections, serious complications are rare and recovery complete in immunocompetent hosts.

Varicella-related deaths—United States, 2002. MMWR-Morb Mortal Weekly Rep 2002;52:545 [PMID: 12803193].

ROSEOLA INFANTUM
(Exanthema Subitum)

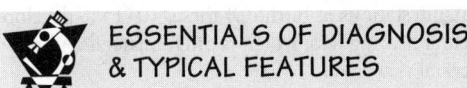

ESSENTIALS OF DIAGNOSIS & TYPICAL FEATURES

- *High fever in a child age 6–36 months.*
- *Minimal toxicity.*
- *Rose-pink maculopapular rash appears when fever subsides.*

General Considerations

Roseola infantum is a benign illness caused by human herpesviruses 6 (HHV-6) or 7 (HHV-7). HHV-6 is a major cause of acute febrile illness in young children. Its significance is its ability to mimic more serious causes of high fever and its role in inciting febrile seizures.

Clinical Findings

The most prominent historical feature is the abrupt onset of fever, often reaching 40.6 °C, which lasts up to 8 days (mean, 4 days) in an otherwise mildly ill child. The fever then ceases abruptly, and a characteristic rash may appear. Roseola occurs predominantly in children age 6 months to 3 years, with 90% of cases occurring before the second year. HHV-7 infection tends to occur somewhat later in childhood. These viruses are the most common recognized cause of exanthematous fever in this age group and are responsible for 20% of emergency room visits by children age 6–12 months.

A. SYMPTOMS AND SIGNS

Mild lethargy and irritability may be present, but generally there is a dissociation between systemic symptoms and the febrile course. The pharynx, tonsils, and tympanic membranes may be injected. Conjunctivitis and pharyngeal exudate are notably absent. Diarrhea and vomiting occur in one-third of patients. Adenopathy of the head and neck often occurs. The anterior fontanelle is bulging in one-fourth of infants infected with HHV-6. If rash appears (20–30% incidence), it begins on the trunk and spreads to the face, neck, and extremities. Rose-pink macules or maculopapules, 2–3 mm in diameter, are nonpruritic, tend to coalesce, and disappear in 1–2 days without pigmentation or desquamation. Rash may occur without fever.

B. LABORATORY FINDINGS

Leukopenia and lymphocytopenia are present early. Laboratory evidence of hepatitis occurs in some patients, especially adults.

Differential Diagnosis

The initial high fever may require exclusion of serious bacterial infection. The relative well-being of most children and the typical course and rash soon clarify the diagnosis. The erythrocyte sedimentation rate is normal. If the child has a febrile seizure, it is important to exclude bacterial meningitis. The CSF is normal in children with roseola. In children who receive antibiotics or other medication at the beginning of the fever, the rash may be attributed incorrectly to drug allergy.

Complications & Sequelae

Febrile seizures occur in 10% of patients (even higher percentages in those with HHV-7 infections). There is evidence that HHV-6 can directly infect the CNS, causing meningoencephalitis or aseptic meningitis. Multiorgan disease (pneumonia, hepatitis, bone marrow suppression, and encephalitis) may occur in immunocompromised patients.

Treatment & Prognosis

Fever is managed readily with acetaminophen and sponge baths. Fever control should be a major consideration in children with a history of febrile seizures. Roseola infantum is otherwise entirely benign.

DeAraujo T et al: Human herpesviruses 6 and 7. Dermatol Clin 2002;20:301 [PMID: 12120443].

Jackson MA, Sommerauer JF: Human herpesviruses 6 and 7. Pediatr Infect Dis J 2002;21:566 [PMID: 12182383].

CYTOMEGALOVIRUS INFECTIONS

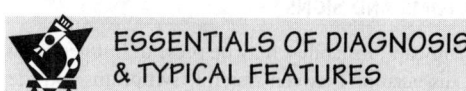

ESSENTIALS OF DIAGNOSIS & TYPICAL FEATURES

Primary infection:

- *Asymptomatic or minor illness in young children.*
- *Mononucleosis-like syndrome without pharyngitis in postpubertal individuals.*

Congenital infection:

- *Intrauterine growth retardation.*
- *Microcephaly with intracerebral calcifications and seizures.*
- *Retinitis and encephalitis.*
- *Hepatosplenomegaly with thrombocytopenia.*
- *"Blueberry muffin" rash.*
- *Sensorineural deafness.*

Immunocompromised hosts:

- *Retinitis and encephalitis.*
- *Pneumonitis.*
- *Enteritis and hepatitis.*
- *Bone marrow suppression.*

General Considerations

Cytomegalovirus (CMV) is a ubiquitous herpesvirus transmitted by many routes. It can be acquired in utero following maternal viremia or postpartum from birth canal secretions or maternal milk. Young children are infected by the saliva of playmates; older individuals are infected by sexual partners (eg, from saliva, vaginal secretions, or semen). Transfused blood products and transplanted organs can be a source of CMV infection. Clinical illness is determined largely by the patient's immune competence. Immuno-competent individuals usually develop a mild self-limited illness, whereas immunocompromised children can develop severe, progressive, often multiorgan disease. In utero infection can be teratogenic.

1. In Utero Cytomegalovirus Infection

Approximately 0.5–1.5% of children are born with CMV infections acquired during maternal viremia. CMV infection is asymptomatic in over 90% of these children, who are usually born to mothers who had experienced reactivation of latent CMV infection during the pregnancy. Symptomatic infection occurs predominantly in infants born to mothers with primary CMV infection but can also result from recurrent, most likely, reinfection during pregnancy. Even when exposed to a primary maternal infection, less than 50% of fetuses are infected, and in only 10% of those infants is the infection symptomatic at birth. Primary infection in the first half of pregnancy poses the greatest risk for severe fetal damage.

Clinical Findings

A. SYMPTOMS AND SIGNS

Severely affected infants are born ill; they are often small for gestational age, floppy, and lethargic. They feed poorly and have poor temperature control. Hepatosplenomegaly, jaundice, petechiae, seizures, and microcephaly are common. Characteristic signs are a distinctive chorioretinitis and periventricular calcification. A purpuric (so-called blueberry muffin) rash similar to that seen with congenital rubella may be present. The mortality rate is 10–20%. Survivors usually have significant sequelae, especially mental retardation, neurologic deficits, retinopathy, and hearing loss. Isolated hepatosplenomegaly or thrombocytopenia may occur. Even mildly affected children may subsequently manifest mental retardation and psychomotor delay. However, most infected infants (90%) are born to mothers with preexisting immunity who had a reactivation of latent CMV during pregnancy. These children have no clinical manifestations at birth. Of these, 10–15% develop sensorineural hearing loss, which is often bilateral and may appear several years after birth.

B. LABORATORY FINDINGS

In severely ill infants, anemia, thrombocytopenia, hyperbilirubinemia, and elevated aminotransferase levels are common. Lymphocytosis occurs occasionally. Pleocytosis and an elevated protein concentration are found in CSF. The diagnosis is readily confirmed by isolation of CMV from urine or saliva within 48 hours, using rapid culture methods combined with immunoassay. The presence in the infant of IgM-specific CMV antibodies suggests the diagnosis. Some commercial ELISA kits are 90% sensitive and specific for these antibodies.

C. IMAGING

Radiologic exams of the head may show microcephaly, periventricular calcifications, and ventricular dilation. These findings strongly correlate with neurologic sequelae and retardation. Long bone radiographs may show the "celery stalk" pattern characteristic of congenital viral infections. Interstitial pneumonia may be present.

Differential Diagnosis

CMV infection should be considered in any newborn who is seriously ill shortly after birth, especially once bacterial sepsis, metabolic disease, intracranial bleeding, and cardiac disease have been excluded. Other congenital infections to be considered in the differential diagnosis include toxoplasmosis (serology, more diffuse calcification of the CNS, specific type of retinitis, macrocephaly), rubella (serology, specific type of retinitis, cardiac lesions, eye abnormalities), enteroviral infections (time of year, maternal illness, severe hepatitis), herpes simplex (skin lesions, cultures, severe hepatitis), and syphilis (serology for both infant and mother, skin lesions, bone involvement).

Treatment & Prevention

Support is rarely required for anemia and thrombocytopenia. Most children with symptoms at birth have significant neurologic, intellectual, visual, or auditory impairment. Ganciclovir, 5 mg/kg every 12 hours, is recommended for children with severe, life- or sight-threatening disease or if end-organ disease recurs or progresses. Duration is 2–3 weeks or until symptoms resolve. This approach decreases viral shedding and limits progression of symptoms, including hearing loss, during treatment. However, the therapeutic advantage is progressively lost over time after treatment is discontinued. Children who are asymptomatic at birth have a 10–15% incidence of hearing loss but few other sequelae. There is no evidence that early treatment prevents late-onset hearing loss. Delayed development and hearing loss should be looked for and treated as soon as possible.

2. Perinatal Cytomegalovirus Infection

CMV infection can be acquired from birth canal secretions or shortly after birth from maternal milk. In some socioeconomic groups, 10–20% of infants are infected at birth and excrete CMV for many months. Infection can also be acquired in the postnatal period from unscreened transfused blood products.

Clinical Findings

A. SYMPTOMS AND SIGNS

Ninety percent of immunocompetent infants infected by their mothers at birth develop subclinical illness (ie, virus excretion only) or a minor illness within 1–3 months. The remainder develop an illness lasting several weeks and characterized by hepatosplenomegaly, lymphadenopathy, and interstitial pneumonitis in various combinations. The severity of the pneumonitis may be increased by the simultaneous presence of *Chlamydia trachomatis*. Infants who receive blood products are often premature and immunologically impaired. If they are born to CMV-negative mothers and subsequently receive CMV-containing blood, they frequently develop severe infection and pneumonia after a 2- to 6-week incubation period.

B. LABORATORY FINDINGS

Lymphocytosis, atypical lymphocytes, anemia, and thrombocytopenia may be present, especially in premature infants. Liver function is abnormal. CMV can be isolated from urine and saliva. Secretions obtained at bronchoscopy contain CMV and epithelial cells bearing CMV antigens. Serum levels of CMV antibody rise significantly.

C. IMAGING

Chest radiographs show a diffuse interstitial pneumonitis in severely affected infants.

Differential Diagnosis

CMV infection should be considered as a cause of any prolonged illness in early infancy, especially if hepatosplenomegaly, lymphadenopathy, or atypical lymphocytosis is present. This must be distinguished from granulomatous or malignant diseases and from congenital infections (syphilis, toxoplasmosis, and hepatitis B) not previously diagnosed. Other viruses (Epstein–Barr virus [EBV], HIV, and adenovirus) can cause this syndrome. CMV is a recognized cause of viral pneumonia in this age group. Because asymptomatic CMV excretion is common in early infancy, care must be taken to establish the diagnosis and to rule out concomitant pathogens such as *Chlamydia* and RSV. Severe CMV infection in early infancy may indicate that the child has a congenital or acquired immune deficiency.

Treatment & Prevention

The self-limited disease of normal infants requires no therapy. Severe pneumonitis in premature infants requires oxygen administration and often intubation. Very ill infants should receive ganciclovir (6 mg/kg every 12 hours). CMV infection acquired by transfusion can be prevented by excluding CMV-seropositive blood donors. Milk donors should also be screened for prior CMV infection. It is likely that high-risk infants receiving large doses of IVIG for other reasons will be protected against severe CMV disease.

3. Cytomegalovirus Infection Acquired in Childhood & Adolescence

Young children are readily infected by playmates, especially because CMV continues to be excreted in saliva and urine for many months after infection. The cumulative annual incidence of CMV excretion by children in day care centers exceeds 75%. In fact, young children in a family are often the source of primary CMV infection of their mothers during subsequent pregnancies. An additional peak of CMV infection takes place when adolescents become sexually active. Sporadic acquisition of CMV occurs after blood transfusion and transplantation.

Clinical Findings

A. SYMPTOMS AND SIGNS

Most young children who acquire CMV are asymptomatic or have a minor febrile illness, occasionally with adenopathy. They provide an important reservoir of virus shedders that facilitates spread of CMV. Occasionally a child may have prolonged fever with hepatosplenomegaly and adenopathy. Older children and adults, many of whom are infected during sexual activity, are more likely to be symptomatic in this fashion and can present with a syndrome that mimics the infectious mononucleosis syndrome that follows EBV infection (1–2 weeks of fever, malaise, anorexia, splenomegaly, mild hepatitis, and some adenopathy; see next section). This syndrome can also occur 2–4 weeks after transfusion of CMV-infected blood.

B. LABORATORY FINDINGS

In the CMV mononucleosis syndrome, lymphocytosis and atypical lymphocytes are common, as is a mild rise in aminotransferase levels. CMV is present in saliva and urine, and CMV DNA can be uniformly detected in plasma or blood.

Differential Diagnosis

In older children, CMV infection should be included as a possible cause of fever of unknown origin, especially when lymphocytosis and atypical lymphocytes are present. CMV infection is distinguished from EBV infection by the absence of pharyngitis, the relatively minor adenopathy, and the absence of serologic evidence of acute EBV infection. Mononucleosis syndromes are also caused by *Toxoplasma gondii*, rubella virus, adenovirus, hepatitis A virus, and HIV.

Prevention

Screening of transfused blood or filtering blood (thus removing CMV-containing white blood cells) prevents cases related to this source.

4. Cytomegalovirus Infection in Immunocompromised Children

In addition to symptoms experienced during primary infection, immunocompromised hosts develop symptoms with reinfection or reactivation of latent CMV. This is clearly seen in children with acquired immunodeficiency syndrome (AIDS), after transplantation, or with congenital immunodeficiencies. However, in most immunocompromised patients, primary infection is more likely to cause severe symptoms than is reactivation or reinfection. The severity of the resulting disease is generally proportionate to the degree of immunosuppression.

Clinical Findings

A. SYMPTOMS AND SIGNS

A mild febrile illness with myalgia, malaise, and arthralgia may occur, especially with reactivation disease. Severe disease often includes subacute onset of dyspnea and cyanosis as manifestations of interstitial pneumonitis. Auscultation reveals only coarse breath sounds and scattered rales. A rapid respiratory rate may precede clinical or radiographic evidence of pneumonia. Hepatitis without jaundice or hepatomegaly is common. Diarrhea, which can be severe, occurs with CMV colitis, and CMV can cause esophagitis with symptoms of odynophagia or dysphagia. These enteropathies are most common in AIDS, as is the presence of a retinitis that often progresses to blindness. Encephalitis and polyradiculitis also occur in AIDS.

B. LABORATORY FINDINGS

Neutropenia and thrombocytopenia are common. Atypical lymphocytosis is infrequent. Serum aminotransferase levels are often elevated. The stools may contain occult blood if enteropathy is present. CMV is readily isolated from saliva, urine, buffy coat, and bronchial secretions. Results are available in 48 hours. Interpretation of positive cultures is made difficult by asymptomatic shedding of CMV in saliva and urine in many immunocompromised patients. CMV disease correlates more closely with the presence of CMV in the blood or lung lavage fluid. Monitoring for the appearance of CMV DNA in plasma or CMV antigen in blood mononuclear cells is used as a guide to early antiviral ("preemptive") therapy.

C. IMAGING

Bilateral interstitial pneumonitis is present on chest radiographs.

Differential Diagnosis

The initial febrile illness must be distinguished from treatable bacterial or fungal infection. Similarly the pulmonary disease must be distinguished from intrapulmonary hemorrhage; drug-induced or radiation pneumonitis; pulmonary edema; and bacterial, fungal, parasitic, and other viral infection in this population. CMV infection is seen bilaterally and interstitially on chest radiographs, cough is nonproductive, chest pain is absent, and the patient is not usually toxic. *Pneumocystis jiroveci* (formerly *Pneumocystis carinii*) infection may have a similar presentation. These patients may have polymicrobial disease. It is suspected that bacterial and fungal infections are enhanced by the neutropenia that can accompany CMV infection. Infection of the gastrointestinal tract is diagnosed by endoscopy. This will exclude candidal, adenoviral, and herpes simplex infections and allows tissue confirmation of CMV-induced mucosal ulcerations.

Treatment & Prevention

Blood donors should be screened to exclude those with prior CMV infection, or blood should be filtered. Ideally, seronegative transplant recipients should receive organs from seronegative donors. Severe symptoms, most commonly pneumonitis, often respond to early therapy with intravenous ganciclovir (5 mg/kg every 12 hours for 14–21 days). Neutropenia is a frequent side effect of this therapy. Foscarnet and cidofovir are alternative therapeutic agents recommended for patients with ganciclovir-resistant virus. Prophylactic use of oral or intravenous ganciclovir may prevent CMV infections in organ transplant recipients. Preemptive therapy can be used in some high-risk transplant recipients who are monitored for CMV antigen or DNA in their plasma or mononuclear cells and who receive antivirals when the test results reach a certain threshold or rapidly increase regardless of clinical signs or symptoms. CMV-seropositive children with AIDS and low CD4 counts (< 50/µL) should have funduscopic examinations and plasma CMV DNA measurements every 3 months.

Demmler G: Congenital cytomegalovirus infection and disease. Adv Pediatr Infect Dis 1996;11:135 [PMID: 8718462].

Kimberlin DW et al: Effect of ganciclovir therapy on hearing in symptomatic congenital CMV. J Pediatr 2003;143:17 [PMID: 12915819].

Michaels M et al: Treatment of children with congenital CMV with ganciclovir. Pediatr Infect Dis J 2003;22:504 [PMID: 12799506].

INFECTIOUS MONONUCLEOSIS (Epstein–Barr Virus)

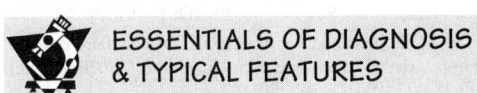

ESSENTIALS OF DIAGNOSIS & TYPICAL FEATURES

- *Prolonged fever.*
- *Exudative pharyngitis.*
- *Generalized adenopathy.*
- *Hepatosplenomegaly.*
- *Atypical lymphocytes.*
- *Heterophil antibodies.*

General Considerations

Mononucleosis is the most characteristic syndrome produced by EBV infection. Young children infected with EBV have either no symptoms or a mild nonspecific febrile illness. As the age of the host increases, EBV infection is more likely to produce the typical features of the mononucleosis syndrome in 20–25% of infected adolescents. EBV is acquired readily from asymptomatic carriers (15–20% of whom excrete the virus in saliva on any given day) and from recently ill patients, who excrete virus for many months. Young children are infected from the saliva of playmates and family members. Adolescents may be infected through sexual activity. EBV can also be transmitted by blood transfusion and organ transplantation.

Clinical Findings

A. SYMPTOMS AND SIGNS

After an incubation period of 1–2 months, a 2- to 3-day prodrome of malaise and anorexia yields, abruptly or insidiously, to a febrile illness with temperatures exceeding 39 °C. The major complaint is pharyngitis, which is often (50%) exudative. Lymph nodes are enlarged, firm, and mildly tender. Any area may be affected, but posterior and anterior cervical nodes are almost always enlarged. Splenomegaly is present in 50–75% of patients. Hepatomegaly is common (30%), and the liver is frequently tender. Five percent of patients have a rash, which can be macular, scarlatiniform, or urticarial. Rash is almost universal in patients taking penicillin or ampicillin. Soft palate petechiae and eyelid edema are also observed.

B. LABORATORY FINDINGS

1. Peripheral blood—Leukopenia may occur early, but an atypical lymphocytosis (comprising over 10% of the total leukocytes at some time in the illness) is most notable. Hematologic changes may not be seen until the third week of illness and may be entirely absent in some EBV syndromes (eg, neurologic ones).

2. Heterophil antibodies—These nonspecific antibodies appear in over 90% of older patients with mononucleosis but in fewer than 50% of children younger than age 5 years. They may not be detectable until the second week of illness and may persist for up to 12 months after recovery. Rapid screening tests (slide agglutination) are usually positive if the titer is significant; a positive result strongly suggests but does not prove EBV infection.

3. Anti-EBV antibodies—It may be necessary to measure specific antibody titers when heterophil antibodies fail to appear, as in young children. Acute EBV infection is established by detecting IgM antibody to the viral capsid antigen (VCA) or by detecting a fall over several weeks of IgG anti-VCA titers (IgG antibody peaks by the time symptoms appear).

4. EBV PCR—This assay detects EBV DNA. It is the method of choice for the diagnosis of CNS and ocular infections. Quantitative EBV PCR in peripheral blood mononuclear cells has been used to detect EBV-related lymphoproliferative disorders in transplant patients.

Differential Diagnosis

Severe pharyngitis may suggest group A streptococcal infection. Enlargement of only the anterior cervical lymph nodes, a neutrophilic leukocytosis, and the absence of splenomegaly suggest bacterial infection. Although a child with a positive throat culture result for streptococcus usually requires therapy, up to 10% of children with mononucleosis are asymptomatic streptococcal carriers. In this group, penicillin therapy is unnecessary and often causes a rash. Severe primary herpes simplex pharyngitis, occurring in adolescence, may also mimic infectious mononucleosis. In this type of pharyngitis, some anterior mouth ulcerations should suggest the correct diagnosis. EBV infection should be considered in the differential diagnosis of any perplexing prolonged febrile illness. Similar illnesses that produce atypical lymphocytosis include rubella (pharyngitis not prominent, shorter illness, less adenopathy and splenomegaly), adenovirus (upper respiratory symptoms and cough, conjunctivitis, less adenopathy, fewer atypical lymphocytes), hepatitis A or B (more severe liver function abnormalities, no pharyngitis, no lymphadenopathy), and toxoplasmosis (negative heterophil test, less pharyngitis). Serum sickness-like drug reactions and leukemia (smear morphology is important) may be confused with infectious mononucleosis. CMV mononucleosis is a close mimic except for minimal pharyngitis and less adenopathy; it is much less common. Serologic tests for EBV and CMV should clarify the correct diagnosis. The acute initial manifestation of HIV infection is a mononucleosis-like syndrome in many patients.

Complications

Splenic rupture is a rare complication, which usually follows significant trauma. Hematologic complications, including hemolytic anemia, thrombocytopenia, and neutropenia, are more common. Neurologic involvement can include aseptic meningitis, encephalitis, iso-lated neuropathy such as Bell palsy, and Guillain–Barré syndrome. Any of these may appear prior to or in the absence of the more typical signs and symptoms of infectious mononucleosis. Rare complications include myocarditis, pericarditis, and atypical pneumonia. Recurrence or persistence of EBV-associated symptoms for 6 months or longer characterizes chronic active EBV. This disease is due to continuous viral replication and warrants specific antiviral therapy. Rarely EBV infection becomes a progressive lymphoproliferative disorder characterized by persistent fever, multiple organ involvement, neutropenia or pancytopenia, and agammaglobulinemia. Hemocytophagia is often present in the bone marrow. An X-linked genetic defect in immune response has been inferred for some patients (Duncan syndrome and X-linked lymphoproliferative disorder). Children with other congenital immunodeficiencies or chemotherapy-induced immunosuppression can also develop progressive EBV infection, EBV-associated lymphoproliferative disorder or lymphoma, and other malignancies.

Treatment & Prognosis

Bed rest may be necessary in severe cases. Acetaminophen controls high fever. Potential airway obstruction due to swollen pharyngeal lymphoid tissue responds rapidly to systemic corticosteroids. Corticosteroids may also be given for hematologic and neurologic complications, although no controlled trials have proved their efficacy in these conditions. Fever and pharyngitis disappear by 10–14 days. Adenopathy and splenomegaly can persist several weeks longer. Some patients complain of fatigue, malaise, or lack of well-being for several months. Although steroids may shorten the duration of fatigue and malaise, their long-term effects on this potentially oncogenic viral infection are unknown, and indiscriminate use is discouraged. Patients with splenic enlargement should avoid contact sports for 6–8 weeks. Acyclovir, valacyclovir, penciclovir, ganciclovir, and foscarnet are active against EBV and are indicated in the treatment of chronic active EBV.

Management of EBV-related lymphoproliferative disorders relies primarily on decreasing the immunosuppression whenever possible. Adjunctive therapy with acyclovir, ganciclovir, or another antiviral active against EBV as well as CMV hyperimmune globulin has been used without scientific evidence of efficacy.

Chetham MM, Roberts KB: Infectious mononucleosis in adolescents. Pediatr Ann 1991;20:206 [PMID: 1648197].

Kanegane H et al: Increased cell-free viral DNA in fatal cases of chronic active Epstein–Barr virus infection. Clin Infect Dis 1999;28:906 [PMID: 10825059].

Weinberg A et al: Quantitative CSF PCR in Epstein–Barr virus infections of the central nervous system. Ann Neurol 2002; 52:543 [PMID: 12402250].

■ VIRAL INFECTIONS SPREAD BY INSECT VECTORS

In the United States, mosquitoes are the most common insect vectors that spread viral infections (Table 36–4). As a consequence, these infections—and others that are spread by ticks—tend to occur as summer–fall epidemics that coincide with the seasonal breeding and feeding habits of the vector, and the etiologic agent varies by region. Thus, a careful travel and exposure history is critical for correct diagnostic work-up.

ENCEPHALITIS

Encephalitis presents as fever, headache, and various combinations of sensorial or behavioral change, with or without focal neurological abnormalities. (See Chapter 23.) Evidence of meningitis is often present. CSF is abnormal, usually with mononuclear cell pleocytosis, elevated protein level, and normal sugar level. Neutrophils may be prominent in CSF early in the illness. Encephalitis is a common severe manifestation of many infections spread by insects (see Table 36–4). With many pathogens, the infection is most often subclinical, or mild CNS disease such as meningitis is present. These infections have some distinguishing features in terms of subclinical infection rate, unique neurologic syndromes, associated non-neurologic symptoms, and prognosis. The diagnosis is generally made clinically during recognized outbreaks and is confirmed by virus-specific serology. Prevention consists of control of mosquito vectors and precautions with proper clothing and insect repellents to minimize mosquito and tick bites.

1. West Nile Virus Encephalitis

This flavivirus is the most important arbovirus infection in the United States. Since it was described in 1999 in New York, it has spread to 47 states. In 2003, West Nile virus caused more than 8500 infections and 190 deaths, the largest epidemic of arboviral meningoencephalitis ever reported. Its reservoir includes more than 160 species of birds whose migration explains the rapid growth of the epidemic. During summer–fall epidemics most infected individuals are asymptomatic. Approximately 20% develop West Nile fever, which is characterized by fever, headache, retroorbital pain, nausea and vomiting, lymphadenopathy, and a maculopapular rash (20–50%). Less than 1% of infected patients develop meningitis or encephalitis, but 10% of these cases are fatal (0.1% of all infections). The major risk factor for severe disease is age older than 50 years and immune compromise, although children develop West Nile fever and occasionally have neurologic disease. The

neurologic manifestations are most often those found with other encephalitides. However, distinguishing atypical features include polio-like flaccid paralysis, movement disorders (parkinsonism, tremor, and myoclonus), brainstem symptoms, polyneuropathy, and optic neuritis. Muscle weakness, facial palsy, and hyporeflexia are common (20% of each finding). Diagnosis is best made by detecting IgM antibody (enzyme immunoassay) to the virus in CSF. This will be present by 2–3 days (95%) after onset. PCR is a specific diagnostic tool, but is less sensitive than antibody detection. Antibody rise in serum can also be used for diagnosis. Treatment is supportive, although various antivirals and specific immune globulin are being studied. The infection is not spread between contacts, but is spread by donated organs and blood and breast milk and transplacentally. The coming years will indicate if this virus will become a serious endemic problem in the United States.

Petersen LR et al: West Nile virus. JAMA 2003;290:524 [PMID: 2876096].

Solomon T et al: West Nile encephalitis. BMJ 2003;326:865 [PMID: 12702624].

DENGUE

In endemic areas 50–100 million cases of dengue occur each year, often in severe forms. In the United States, 50–150 cases are diagnosed, most often in travelers from the Caribbean or Asia and less often in those visiting Central and South America. Texas has sporadic indigenous outbreaks of dengue. The spread of dengue requires the requisite species of mosquito, which transmits virus from a reservoir of viremic humans in endemic areas. Most patients have mild disease, especially young children, who may have a nonspecific fever and rash. Severity is a function of age and prior infection with other serotypes of dengue virus, a prerequisite for severe hemorrhagic complications.

Clinical Findings

A. SYMPTOMS AND SIGNS

Dengue fever begins abruptly 4–7 days after transmission (range, 3–14 days) with fever, chills, severe retroorbital pain, severe muscle and joint pain, nausea, and vomiting. Erythema of the face and torso may occur early. After 3–4 days a centrifugal maculopapular rash appears in half of patients. The rash can become petechial, and mild hemorrhagic signs (epistaxis, gingival bleeding, or microscopic blood in stool or urine) may be noted. The illness lasts 5–7 days, although rarely fever may reappear for several additional days.

B. LABORATORY FINDINGS

Leukopenia and a mild drop in platelets are common. Liver function tests are usually normal. Diagnosis is made

Table 36–4. Some virus diseases spread by insects in the United States.

Disease	Natural Reservoir (Vector)	Geographic Distribution	Incubation Period	Clinical Presentations	Laboratory Findings	Complications, Sequelae	Diagnosis, Therapy, Comments
FLAVIVIRUSES							
St. Louis encephalitis (SLE)	Birds (*Culex* mosquitoes)	Southern Canada, central and southern United States, Caribbean, South America	2–5 d (up to 3 wk)	Abrupt onset of fever, chills, headache, nausea, vomiting; may develop generalized weakness, seizures, coma, ataxia, cranial nerve palsies. Aseptic meningitis is common in children.	Modest leukocytosis, neutrophilia, elevated liver enzymes. CSF: 100–200 WBC/µL (PMNs predominate early).	Mortality rate 2–5% in children (especially < age 5). Neurologic sequelae in 1–20%.	~35 cases a year, < 2% symptomatic. (Worse in elderly.) Therapy: supportive. Diagnosis: serology. Specific antibody often present within 5 d.
Dengue	Humans (*Aedes* mosquitoes)	Asia, Africa, Central and South America, Caribbean; rarely in southern United States	4–7 d (range 3–14 d)	Fever, headache, myalgia, joint and bone pain, retroocular pain, nausea and vomiting; maculopapular or petechial rash in 50%, sparing palms and soles; adenopathy. Meningoencephalitis in 5–10% of children.	Leukopenia, thrombocytopenia. CSF: 100–500 mononuclear cells/µL if neurologic signs are present.	Hemorrhagic fever, shock syndrome, prolonged weakness.	High infection rate. 50–150 cases occur in U.S. travelers to endemic areas. Biphasic course may occur. Therapy: supportive. Diagnosis: serology; IgM-EIA antibody by day 6.
West Nile	Birds (*Culex* mosquitoes); small mammals	N. Africa, Middle East, parts of Asia, Europe, continental United States	3–12 d	Abrupt onset of fever, headache, sore throat, myalgia, retroocular pain, conjunctivitis; 20–50% with rash; adenopathy. Encephalitis may be accompanied by muscle weakness, flaccid paralysis, or movement disorders.	Mild leukoctyosis; 10–15% lymphopenic; moderate CSF pleocytosis.	Mortality rate 10%, of those with CNS symptoms, especially in elderly; weakness and myalgia may persist for an extended period.	Most imortant mosquito-borne encephalitis in the United States. Diagnosis: IgM-EIA serology; cross-reacts with St. Louis encephalitis; positive by 2–3 d after onset of CNS symptoms. Diagnosis by PCR is less sensitive. Therapy: supportive.
ALPHA TOGA VIRUSES							
Western equine encephalitis	Birds (*Culisata* mosquitoes)	Canada, Mexico, and United States west of Mississippi River	2–5 d	Similar to that of St. Louis encephalitis. Most infections are subclinical.	Variable white counts. CSF: 10–300 WBC/µL.	Permanent brain damage, 10% overall; most severe in older adults.	No reported cases in the United States in the last several years. Case/infection is 1:1000 for older adults and 1:1 for infants. Equine illness precedes human outbreaks. Diagnosis: IgM antibody in first week. Therapy: supportive.

	Reservoir (vector)	Incubation period	Clinical findings	Laboratory findings	Complications/mortality	Epidemiology/therapy/diagnosis
Eastern equine encephalitis	Birds (*Culisata* mosquitoes)	2–5 d	Similar to that of St. Louis encephalitis but more severe. Progresses rapidly in one third to coma and death.	Leukocytosis with neutrophilia. CSF: 500–2000 WBC/µL; PMNs predominate early.	Mortality rate 20–50%; neurologic sequelae in over 50% of children.	Fewer than 10 cases a year. Only 3–10% of cases are symptomatic. Therapy: supportive. Diagnosis: serology. Titers often positive in first week. Equine deaths may signal an outbreak.
Venezuelan equine encephalitis	Horses (10 species of mosquitoes)	1–6 d	Similar to that of St. Louis encephalitis.	Lymphopenia, mild thrombocytopenia, abnormal liver function tests. CSF: 50–200 mononuclears/µL.	Severe disease more common in infants; 20% fatality rate for encephalitis.	Most infections do not cause encephalitis. No cases in the United States in recent years. Vaccination of horses will stop epidemic. Therapy: supportive. Diagnosis: IgM antibody (EIA).
BUNYAVIRUS						
California encephalitis (LaCrosse, Jamestown Canyon, California)	Chipmunks and other small mammals (*Aedes* mosquitoes)	3–7 d	Similar to that of St. Louis encephalitis; sore throat and respiratory symptoms are common; focal neurologic signs in up to 25%. Seizures prominent. Prepubertal children are most likely to have severe disease. Can mimic HSV encephalitis.	Variable white counts. CSF: 30–200 (up to 600) WBC/µL; variable PMNs; protein often normal.	Mortality rate < 1%. Seizure disorder may begin during acute illness.	About 150 cases a year in the United States, 5% symptomatic. > 10% with sequelae. Therapy: supportive. Diagnosis: serology. Up to 90% have specific IgM antibody in first week; 25% of population in certain regions has IgG antibody.
COLTIVIRUS						
Colorado tick fever	Small mammals (*Dermacentor andersoni*, or wood tick)	3–4 d (range, 2–14 d)	Fever, chills, myalgia, conjunctivitis, headache, retroorbital pain; rash in < 10%. No respiratory symptoms. Biphasic fever in 50%.	Leukopenia (maximum at 4–6 d), mild thrombocytopenia.	Rare encephalitis, coagulopathy.	Patient may have no known tick bite. Acute illness lasts 7–10 d; prolonged fatigue in adults. Therapy: supportive. Diagnosis: serology, direct FA staining of red cells for viral antigen, PCR.

CNS, central nervous system; CSF, cerebrospinal fluid; EIA, enzyme immunoassay; FA, fluorescent antibody; HSV, herpes simplex virus; PCR, polymerase chain reaction; PMN, polymorphonuclear neutrophil; WBC, white blood cells.

by viral culture of plasma (50% sensitive up to the fifth day), by detecting IgM-specific ELISA antibodies (90% sensitive at the sixth day), or by detecting a rise in type-specific antibody. PCR is available for diagnosis.

Differential Diagnosis

This diagnosis should be considered for any traveler to an endemic area who has symptoms suggestive of a systemic viral illness, although fewer than 1 in 1000 travelers to these areas develop dengue. Often the areas visited have other unique viruses circulating and are potential sources of malaria, typhoid fever, leptospirosis, and measles. EBV, influenza, enteroviruses, and acute HIV infection may produce a similar illness. An illness that starts 2 weeks after the trip ends or that lasts longer than 2 weeks is not dengue.

Complications

Rarely dengue fever is associated with meningoencephalitis (5–10%) or hepatic damage. More common in endemic areas is the appearance of dengue hemorrhagic fever, which is defined by significant thrombocytopenia, bleeding, and a plasma leak syndrome (hemoconcentration, hypoalbuminemia, and pleural or peritoneal effusions). This is the consequence of circulating antibody acquired from a prior heterotypic dengue virus infection; thus it is rarely seen in typical travelers. Failure to recognize and treat this complication may lead to dengue shock syndrome, which has a high fatality rate.

Prevention

Prevention of dengue fever involves avoiding high-risk areas and using conventional mosquito avoidance measures. The main vector is a day-time feeder.

Treatment

Dengue fever is treated by oral replacement of fluid lost from gastrointestinal symptoms. Analgesic therapy, which is often necessary, should not include drugs that affect platelet function. Recovery is complete without sequelae. The hemorrhagic syndrome requires prompt fluid therapy with plasma expanders and isotonic saline.

Gregson A, Edelman R: Dengue virus infection. Pediatr Infect Dis J 2003;22:179 [PMID:12586982].

COLORADO TICK FEVER

Colorado tick fever, a tick-borne illness, is endemic in the high plains and mountains of the central and northern Rocky Mountains and northern Pacific coast of the United States. The reservoir of the virus consists of squirrels and chipmunks. Many hundreds of cases of Colorado tick fever occur each year in visitors or laborers entering this region, primarily from May through July.

Clinical Findings

A. SYMPTOMS AND SIGNS

After a 3- to 4-day incubation period (maximum, 14 days) fever begins suddenly together with chills, lethargy, headache, ocular pain, myalgia, abdominal pain, and nausea and vomiting. Conjunctivitis may be present. A nondistinctive maculopapular rash occurs in 5–10% of patients. The illness lasts 7–10 days, and half of patients have a biphasic fever curve with several afebrile days in the midst of the illness.

B. LABORATORY FINDINGS

Leukopenia is characteristic early in the illness. Platelets are modestly decreased. Specific ELISA testing is available, but 3–4 weeks may elapse before seroconversion. Fluorescent antibody staining will detect virus-infected erythrocytes during the illness and for weeks after recovery.

Differential Diagnosis

Early findings, especially if rash is present, may suggest enterovirus, measles, or rubella infection. Enteric fever may be an early consideration because of the presence of leukopenia and thrombocytopenia. A history of tick bite, which is often obtained, information about local risk, and the biphasic fever pattern will help with the diagnosis. Because of the wilderness exposure, diseases such as leptospirosis, borreliosis, tularemia, ehrlichiosis, and Rocky Mountain spotted fever will be considerations.

Complications

Meningoencephalitis occurs in 3–7% of patients. Cardiac and pulmonary complications are rare.

Prevention & Treatment

Prevention involves avoiding endemic areas and using conventional means to avoid tick bite. Therapy is supportive. Do not use analgesics that modify platelet function.

Klasco R: Colorado tick fever. Med Clin North Am 2002;86:435 [PMID: 11982311].

OTHER MAJOR VIRAL CHILDHOOD EXANTHEMS

See Infections Due to Herpesviruses section for a discussion of varicella and roseola, two other major childhood exanthems.

ERYTHEMA INFECTIOSUM

ESSENTIALS OF DIAGNOSIS & TYPICAL FEATURES

- *Fever and rash with "slapped-cheek" appearance.*
- *Arthritis in older children.*
- *Profound anemia in patients with impaired erythrocyte production.*
- *Nonimmune hydrops fetalis.*

General Considerations

This benign exanthematous illness of school-age children is caused by the human parvovirus designated B19. Spread is respiratory, occurring in winter–spring epidemics. A nonspecific mild flulike illness may occur during the initial viremia at 7–10 days; the characteristic rash occurring at 10–17 days represents an immune response. The patient is viremic and contagious prior to—but not after—the onset of rash.

Approximately one-half of infected individuals have a subclinical illness. Most cases (60%) occur in children between ages 5 and 15 years, with an additional 40% occurring later in life. Forty percent of adults are seronegative. The disease is mildly contagious; the secondary attack rate in a school or household setting is 50% among susceptible children and 20–30% among susceptible adults.

Clinical Findings

Owing to the nonspecific nature of the exanthem and the many subclinical cases, a history of contact with an infected individual is often absent or unreliable. Recognition of the illness is easier during outbreaks.

A. SYMPTOMS AND SIGNS

Typically the first sign of illness is the rash, which begins as raised, fiery red maculopapular lesions on the cheeks that coalesce to give a "slapped-cheek" appearance. The lesions are warm, nontender, and sometimes pruritic. They may be scattered on the forehead, chin, and postauricular areas, but the circumoral region is spared. Within 1–2 days, similar lesions appear on the proximal extensor surfaces of the extremities and spread distally in a symmetrical fashion. Palms and soles are usually spared. The trunk, neck, and buttocks are also commonly involved. Central clearing of confluent lesions produces a characteristic lacelike pattern. The rash fades in several days to several weeks but frequently reappears in response to local irritation, heat (bathing), sunlight, and stress. Almost one-half of infected children have some rash remaining (or recurring) for 10 days. Fine desquamation may be present. Mild systemic symptoms occur in up to 50% of children. These symptoms include low-grade fever (38–38.5 °C), mild malaise, sore throat, and coryza. They appear for 2–3 days and are followed by a week-long asymptomatic phase before the rash appears.

Purpuric stocking-glove rashes, neurologic disease, and severe disorders resembling hemolytic–uremic syndrome have also been described in association with parvovirus B19.

B. LABORATORY FINDINGS

A mild leukopenia occurs early in some patients, followed by leukocytosis and lymphocytosis. Specific IgM and IgG serum antibody tests are available, but care must be used in choosing a reliable laboratory for this test. Nucleic acid detection tests are often definitive. The disease is not diagnosed by routine viral culture.

Differential Diagnosis

In children immunized against measles and rubella, parvovirus B19 is the most frequent agent of morbilliform and rubelliform rashes. The characteristic rash and the mild nature of the illness distinguish erythema infectiosum from other childhood exanthems. It lacks the prodromal symptoms of measles and the lymphadenopathy of rubella. Systemic symptoms and pharyngitis are more prominent with enteroviral infections and scarlet fever.

Complications & Sequelae

A. ARTHRITIS

Arthritis is more common in older patients, beginning with late adolescence. Approximately 10% of children have severe joint symptoms. Girls are affected more commonly than boys. Pain and stiffness occur symmetrically in the peripheral joints. Arthritis usually follows the rash and may persist for 2–6 weeks but resolves without permanent damage.

B. APLASTIC CRISIS

Parvovirus B19 replicates primarily in erythroid progenitor cells. Consequently, reticulocytopenia occurs for approximately 1 week during the illness. This goes unnoticed in individuals with a normal erythrocyte half-life but results in severe anemia in patients with chronic hemolytic anemia. The rash of erythema infectiosum follows the anemia in these patients.

Pure red cell aplasia, leukopenia, pancytopenia, idiopathic thrombocytopenic purpura, and a hemophagocytic syndrome have also been described. Patients with AIDS and other immunosuppressive illnesses may develop prolonged anemia or pancytopenia. Patients with hemolytic anemia and aplastic crisis or immunosuppressed patients may still be contagious and should be isolated while in the hospital.

C. OTHER END-ORGAN INFECTIONS

Parvovirus is under study as a potential cause of a variety of collagen–vascular diseases, neurologic syndromes, hepatitis, and myocarditis.

D. IN UTERO INFECTIONS

Infection of susceptible pregnant women may produce fetal infection with hydrops fetalis; fetal death occurs in about 6%, and most fatalities occur in the first 20 weeks—compared with a fetal loss of 3.5% in control subjects. The risk of fetal infection is unknown. Congenital anomalies have not been associated with parvovirus B19 infection during pregnancy.

Treatment & Prognosis

Erythema infectiosum is a benign illness for immunocompetent individuals. Patients with aplastic crisis may require blood transfusions. It is unlikely that this complication can be prevented by quarantine measures, because acute parvovirus infection in contacts is often unrecognized and is most contagious prior to the rash. Pregnant women who are exposed to erythema infectiosum or who work in a setting in which an epidemic occurs should be tested for evidence of prior infection. Susceptible pregnant women should then be followed up for evidence of parvovirus infection. Approximately 1.5% of women of childbearing age are infected during pregnancy. If maternal infection occurs, the fetus should be followed up by ultrasonography for evidence of hydrops and distress. In utero transfusion or early delivery may salvage some fetuses. Pregnancies should not be terminated because of parvovirus infection. The risk of fetal death among exposed pregnant women of unknown serologic status is less than 2.5% for women exposed in the home and less than 1.5% for exposed schoolteachers.

Intramuscular immune globulin is not protective. High-dose IVIG has stopped viremia and led to marrow recovery in some cases of prolonged aplasia. Its role in immunocompetent patients and pregnant women is unknown.

Katta R: Parvovirus B19: A review. Dermatol Clin 2002;20:333 [PMID: 12120446].

Messina MF et al: Purpuric gloves and socks syndrome caused by parvovirus B19 infection. Pediatr Infect Dis J 2003;22:755 [PMID: 12938681].

MEASLES (Rubeola)

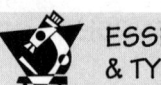

ESSENTIALS OF DIAGNOSIS & TYPICAL FEATURES

- *Exposure to measles 9–14 days previously.*
- *Prodrome of fever, cough, conjunctivitis, and coryza.*
- *Koplik spots (few to many small white papules on a diffusely red base on the buccal mucosa) 1–2 days prior to and after onset of rash.*
- *Maculopapular rash spreading down from the face and hairline to the trunk over 3 days and later becoming confluent.*
- *Leukopenia.*

General Considerations

This childhood exanthem is rarely seen in the United States because of universal vaccination (< 50 cases in 2003, all of which were imported or related to imported cases). Sporadic clusters of cases are the result of improper immunization more so than of vaccine failures, and are usually related to imported cases. It is recommended that all children be revaccinated on entrance into primary or secondary school. (See Chapter 9.) The attack rate in susceptible individuals is extremely high; spread is respiratory. Morbidity and mortality rates in the developing world are substantial because of underlying malnutrition and secondary infections. Because humans are the sole reservoir of measles, there is the potential to eliminate this disease worldwide.

Clinical Findings

A history of contact with a suspected case may be absent because airborne spread is efficient and patients are contagious during the prodrome. Contact with an imported case may not be recognized. In temperate climates, epidemic measles is a winter–spring disease. Many suspected cases are misdiagnoses of other viral infections.

A. SYMPTOMS AND SIGNS

High fever and lethargy are prominent. Sneezing, eyelid edema, tearing, copious coryza, photophobia, and harsh cough ensue and worsen. Koplik spots are white macular lesions on the buccal mucosa, typically opposite the lower molars. These are almost pathognomonic for rubeola, although they may be absent. A discrete maculopapular rash begins when the respiratory symptoms are maximal and spreads quickly over the face and trunk, coalescing to a bright red. As it involves the extremities, it fades from the face and is completely gone within 6 days; fine desquamation may occur. Fever peaks when the rash appears and usually falls 2–3 days thereafter.

B. LABORATORY FINDINGS

Lymphopenia is characteristic. Total leukocyte counts may fall to 1500/μL. The diagnosis is usually made by detection of measles IgM antibody in serum drawn at least 3 days after the onset of rash or later by detection of a significant rise in antibody. Direct detection of measles antigen by fluorescent antibody staining of nasopharyngeal cells is a useful rapid method. PCR testing of oropharyngeal secretions or urine is extremely sensitive and specific and can detect infection up to 5 days before symptoms.

C. IMAGING

Chest radiographs often show hyperinflation, perihilar infiltrates, or parenchymal patchy, fluffy densities. Secondary consolidation or effusion may be visible.

Differential Diagnosis

Table 36–3 lists other illnesses that may resemble measles.

Complications & Sequelae

A. RESPIRATORY COMPLICATIONS

These complications occur in up to 15% of patients. Bacterial superinfections of lung, middle ear, sinus, and cervical nodes are most common. Fever that persists after the third or fourth day of rash suggests such a complication, as does leukocytosis. Bronchospasm, severe croup, and progressive viral pneumonia or bronchiolitis (in infants) also occur. Immunosuppressed patients are at much greater risk for fatal pneumonia than are immunocompetent patients.

B. CEREBRAL COMPLICATIONS

Encephalitis occurs in 1 in 2000 cases. Onset is usually within a week after appearance of rash. Symptoms include combativeness, ataxia, vomiting, seizures, and coma. Lymphocytic pleocytosis and a mildly elevated protein concentration are usual CSF findings, but the fluid may be normal. Forty percent of patients so affected die or have severe neurologic sequelae.

Subacute sclerosing panencephalitis (SSPE) is a slow measles virus infection of the brain that becomes symptomatic years later in about 1 in 100,000 previously infected children. This progressive cerebral deteriora-

tion is associated with myoclonic jerks and a typical electroencephalographic pattern. It is fatal in 6–12 months. It does not occur following administration of vaccine. High titers of measles antibody are present in serum and CSF.

C. OTHER COMPLICATIONS

These include hemorrhagic measles (severe disease with multiorgan bleeding, fever, cerebral symptoms), thrombocytopenia, appendicitis, keratitis, myocarditis, and premature delivery or stillbirth. Mild liver function test elevation has been detected in up to 50% of cases in young adults; frank jaundice may also occur. Measles causes transient immunosuppression; thus, reactivation or progression of tuberculosis (including transient cutaneous anergy) occurs in untreated children.

Treatment, Prognosis, & Prevention

Recovery generally occurs 7–10 days after onset of symptoms. Therapy is supportive: eye care, cough relief (avoid opioid suppressants in infants), and fever reduction (acetaminophen, lukewarm baths; avoid salicylates). Secondary bacterial infections should be treated promptly; antimicrobial prophylaxis is not indicated. Ribavirin is active in vitro and may be useful in infected immunocompromised children. High-dose intravenous ribavirin in combination with intrathecal interferon-α has been successfully used in the management of SSPE. In malnourished children, vitamin A supplementation should be given to attenuate the illness.

The current two-dose active vaccination strategy is successful. Vaccine should not be withheld for concurrent mild acute illness, tuberculosis or positive tuberculin skin test, breast-feeding, or exposure to an immunodeficient contact. The vaccine is recommended for HIV-infected children without severe HIV complications and adequate CD4 cells (≥ 15%).

Vaccination prevents the disease in susceptible exposed individuals if given within 72 hours. (See Chapter 9.) Immune globulin (0.25 mL/kg intramuscularly; 0.5 mL/kg if immunocompromised) will prevent or modify measles if given within 6 days. Suspected cases should be diagnosed promptly and reported to the local health department.

Hosoya M et al: High-dose intravenous ribavirin therapy for subacute sclerosing panencephalitis. Antimicrob Agents Chemother 2001; 45:943 [PMID: 11181386].

van Binnendijk RS et al: Evaluation of serological and virological tests in the diagnosis of clinical and subclinical measles virus infections during an outbreak of measles in the Netherlands. J Infect Dis 2003;188:898 [PMID: 12964122].

van den Hof et al: Measles epidemic in the Netherlands 1999–2000. J Infect Dis 2002;186:1483 [PMID: 12404165].

RUBELLA

ESSENTIALS OF DIAGNOSIS & TYPICAL FEATURES

- History of rubella vaccination usually absent.
- Prodromal nonspecific respiratory symptoms and adenopathy (postauricular and occipital).
- Maculopapular rash beginning on face, rapidly spreading to the entire body, and disappearing by fourth day.
- Few systemic symptoms.
- Congenital infection.
- Retarded growth, development.
- Cataracts, retinopathy.
- Purpuric "blueberry muffin" rash at birth.
- Jaundice, thrombocytopenia.
- Deafness.
- Congenital heart defect.

General Considerations

If it were not teratogenic, rubella would be of little clinical importance. Clinical diagnosis is difficult in some cases because of its variable expression. In one study, over 80% of infections were subclinical. Because of inadequate vaccination, outbreaks most often occur in adolescents or adults. Rubella is transmitted by aerosolized respiratory secretions. Patients are infectious 5 days before until 5 days after the rash. Fewer than 10 cases were reported in the United States in 2003.

Congenital rubella, in infants both of unimmunized women and of women who have apparently been reinfected in pregnancy, is now rare (no cases in 2003).

Clinical Findings

The incubation period is 14–21 days. The nondistinctive signs may make exposure history unreliable. A history of immunization makes rubella unlikely but still possible. Congenital rubella usually follows maternal infection in the first trimester.

A. SYMPTOMS AND SIGNS

1. Infection in children—Young children may only have rash. Older patients often have a nonspecific prodrome of low-grade fever, ocular pain, sore throat, and myalgia. Postauricular and suboccipital adenopathy (sometimes generalized) is characteristic. This often precedes the rash or may occur without rash. The rash consists of erythematous discrete maculopapules beginning on the face. A "slapped-cheek" appearance or pruritus may occur. Scarlatiniform or morbilliform rash variants may occur. The rash spreads quickly to the trunk and extremities after it fades from the face; it is gone by the fourth day. Enanthema is usually absent.

2. Congenital infection—More than 80% of women infected in the first 4 months of gestation are delivered of affected infants; congenital disease occurs in less than 5% of women infected later in pregnancy. Later infections can result in isolated defects, such as deafness. The main manifestations are as follows:

a. Growth retardation—Between 50% and 85% of infants are small at birth and remain so.

b. Cardiac anomalies—Pulmonary artery stenosis, patent ductus arteriosus, ventricular septal defect.

c. Ocular anomalies—Cataracts, microphthalmia, glaucoma, retinitis.

d. Deafness

e. Cerebral disorders—Chronic encephalitis, mental retardation.

f. Hematologic disorders—Thrombocytopenia, dermal nests of extramedullary hematopoiesis or purpura ("blueberry muffin" rash), lymphopenia.

g. Others—Hepatitis, osteomyelitis, immune disorders, malabsorption, diabetes.

B. LABORATORY FINDINGS

Leukopenia is common, and platelet counts may be low. Congenital infection is associated with low platelet counts, abnormal liver function tests, hemolytic anemia, pleocytosis, and very high rubella IgM antibody titers. Total serum IgM is elevated, and IgA and IgG levels may be depressed.

C. IMAGING

Pneumonitis and bone metaphyseal longitudinal lucencies may be present in radiographs of children with congenital infection.

Diagnosis & Differential Diagnosis

Virus may be isolated from throat or urine from 1 week before to 2 weeks after onset of rash. Children with congenital infection are infectious for months. The virus laboratory must be notified that rubella is suspected. Serologic diagnosis is best made by demonstrating a fourfold rise in antibody titer between specimens drawn 1–2 weeks apart. The first should be drawn promptly, because titers increase rapidly after onset of rash. Both specimens must be tested simultaneously by a single laboratory. Specific IgM antibody can be measured by immunoassay. Because the decision to terminate a pregnancy is usually based on serologic results, testing must be done carefully.

Rubella may resemble infections due to enterovirus, adenovirus, measles, EBV, roseola, parvovirus, *Toxoplasma gondii,* and *Mycoplasma.* Drug reactions may also mimic rubella. Because public health implications are great, sporadic suspected cases should be confirmed serologically or virologically.

Congenital rubella must be differentiated from congenital CMV infection, toxoplasmosis, and syphilis.

Complications & Sequelae

A. ARTHRALGIA AND ARTHRITIS

Both occur more often in adult women. Polyarticular involvement (fingers, knees, and wrists), lasting a few days to weeks, is typical. Frank arthritis occurs in a small percentage of patients. It may resemble acute rheumatoid arthritis.

B. ENCEPHALITIS

With an incidence of about 1:6000, this is a nonspecific parainfectious encephalitis associated with a low mortality rate. A syndrome resembling SSPE (see Measles section) has also been described in congenital rubella.

C. RUBELLA IN PREGNANCY

Infection in the mother is self-limited and not severe.

Prevention

Rubella is one of the infections that could be eradicated. (See Chapter 9 for the indication and efficacy of rubella vaccine.) Standard prenatal care should include rubella antibody testing. Seropositive mothers are at no risk; seronegative mothers are vaccinated after delivery.

A pregnant woman possibly exposed to rubella should be tested immediately; if seropositive, she is immune and need not worry. If she is seronegative, a second specimen should be drawn in 4 weeks, and both specimens should be tested simultaneously. Seroconversion in the first trimester suggests high fetal risk; such women require counseling regarding therapeutic abortion.

When pregnancy termination is not an option, some experts recommend intramuscular administration of 20 mL of immune globulin within 72 hours after exposure in an attempt to prevent infection. (This negates the value of subsequent antibody testing.) The efficacy of this practice is unknown.

Treatment & Prognosis

Symptomatic therapy is sufficient. Arthritis may improve with administration of anti-inflammatory agents. The prognosis is excellent in all children and adults but poor in

congenitally infected infants, in whom most defects are irreversible or progressive. The severe cognitive defects seem to correlate closely in these infants with the degree of growth failure.

Chantler JK et al: Persistent rubella virus infection associated with chronic arthritis in children. N Engl J Med 1985;313:1117 [PMID: 4047116].

Freij BJ et al: Maternal rubella and the congenital rubella syndrome. Clin Perinatol 1988;15:247 [PMID: 3288422].

Kaplan KM et al: A profile of mothers giving birth to infants with congenital rubella syndrome: An assessment of risk factors. Am J Dis Child 1990;144:118 [PMID: 2294710].

Weber B et al: Congenital rubella syndrome after maternal reinfection. Infection 1993;21:118 [PMID: 8491520].

■ INFECTIONS DUE TO OTHER VIRUSES

HANTAVIRUS CARDIOPULMONARY SYNDROME

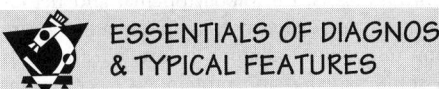

ESSENTIALS OF DIAGNOSIS & TYPICAL FEATURES

- *Influenza-like prodrome (fever, myalgia, headache, cough).*
- *Rapid onset of unexplained pulmonary edema.*
- *Residence or travel in epidemic area; exposure to aerosols from deer mouse droppings or secretions.*

General Considerations

Hantavirus cardiopulmonary syndrome is the first native bunyavirus infection endemic in this country. Hantavirus cardiopulmonary syndrome is distinctly different in mode of spread (no arthropod vector) and clinical picture from other bunyavirus diseases.

Clinical Findings

The initial cases of hantavirus pulmonary syndrome involved travel to or residence in an area where New Mexico, Colorado, Utah, and Arizona are contiguous and involved potential exposure to the habitat of the reservoir, the deer mouse. This rodent and other selected rodents that harbor related hantaviruses live in many other locales. Thus, through 2003, more than 325 cases were confirmed in 29 other states, with additional cases in Canada. Epidemics occur when environmental conditions favor large increases in the rodent population and increased prevalence of virus in this reservoir.

A. SYMPTOMS AND SIGNS

After an incubation period of 2–3 weeks, onset is sudden, with a nonspecific viruslike prodrome: fever; back, hip, and leg pain; chills; headache; and nausea and vomiting. Abdominal pain may be present. Sore throat, conjunctivitis, rash, and adenopathy are absent, and respiratory symptoms are absent or limited to a dry cough. After 1–10 days (usually 3–7), dyspnea, tachypnea, and evidence of a pulmonary capillary leak syndrome appear. This often progresses rapidly over a period of hours. Hypotension is common not only from hypoxemia but also from myocardial dysfunction. Copious, amber-colored, nonpurulent secretions are common. Decreased cardiac output and elevated systemic vascular resistance distinguish this disease from early bacterial sepsis.

B. LABORATORY FINDINGS

The hemogram shows leukocytosis with a prominent left shift and immunoblasts, thrombocytopenia, and hemoconcentration. Lactate dehydrogenase is elevated, as are liver function tests; serum albumin is low. Creatinine is elevated in some patients, and proteinuria is common. Lactic acidosis and low venous bicarbonate are poor prognostic signs. A serum IgM ELISA test is positive early in the illness. Otherwise the diagnosis is made by specific staining of tissue or PCR, usually at autopsy.

C. IMAGING

Initial chest radiographs are normal. This is followed by bilateral interstitial infiltrates with the typical butterfly pattern of acute pulmonary edema, bibasilar airspace disease, or both. Significant pleural effusions are often present. These findings contrast with those of other causes of acute respiratory distress syndrome.

Differential Diagnosis

In some geographic areas, plague and tularemia may be possibilities. Infections with viral respiratory pathogens and *Mycoplasma* have a slower tempo, do not elevate the lactate dehydrogenase, and do not cause the hematologic changes. Q fever, psittacosis, toxin exposure, legionellosis, and fungal infections are possibilities, but the history, tempo of the illness, and blood findings, as well as the exposure history, should be distinguishing features. Hantavirus cardiopulmonary syndrome is a consideration in previously healthy persons with a febrile illness associated with unexplained pulmonary edema.

Treatment & Prognosis

When given early for other bunyavirus infections, intravenous ribavirin has been effective, and hantaviruses are sensitive in vitro to ribavirin. A trial of this therapy for hantavirus cardiopulmonary syndrome was inconclusive. Management should concentrate on oxygen therapy and mechanical ventilation as required. Because of capillary leakage, Swan–Ganz catheterization to monitor cardiac output and inotropic support—rather than fluid therapy—should be used to maintain perfusion. Venoarterial extracorporeal membrane oxygenation can provide short-term support for selected patients. The virus, endemic in the US, is not spread by person-to-person contact. No isolation is required. Thus far, the case fatality rate is approximately 50%. Guidelines are available for reduction of exposure to the infectious agent.

Peters CJ, Khan AS: Hantavirus pulmonary syndrome: The new American hemorrhagic fever. Clin Infect Dis 2002;34:1224 [PMID: 11941549].

MUMPS

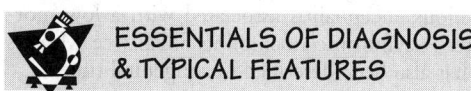

ESSENTIALS OF DIAGNOSIS & TYPICAL FEATURES

- No prior mumps immunization.
- Parotid gland swelling.
- Aseptic meningitis with or without parotitis.

General Considerations

Mumps was one of the classic childhood infections; virus spread by the respiratory route attacked almost all unimmunized children (asymptomatically in 30–40% of cases), and produced lifelong immunity. The vaccine is so efficacious that clinical disease is rare in immunized children. As a result of subclinical infections or childhood immunization, 95% of adults are immune. Infected patients can spread the infection from 1–2 days prior to the onset of symptoms and for 5 additional days. The incubation period is 14–21 days.

A history of exposure to a child with parotitis is not proof of mumps exposure. In an adequately immunized individual, parotitis is usually due to another cause. Currently in the United States less than 1 case is reported per 100,000 population.

Clinical Findings

A. SYMPTOMS AND SIGNS

1. Salivary gland disease—Tender swelling of one or more glands, variable fever, and facial lymphedema are typical. Parotid involvement is most common; signs are bilateral in 70% of patients. The ear is displaced upward and outward; the mandibular angle is obliterated. Systemic toxicity is usually absent. Parotid stimulation with sour foods may be quite painful. The orifice of the Stensen duct may be red and swollen; yellow secretions may be expressed, but pus is absent. Parotid swelling dissipates after 1 week.

2. Meningoencephalitis—Prior to widespread immunization, mumps was the most common cause of aseptic meningitis, which is usually manifested by mild headache or asymptomatic mononuclear pleocytosis. Fewer than 10% of patients have clinical meningitis or encephalitis. Cerebral symptoms do not correlate with parotid symptoms, which are absent in many patients with meningoencephalitis. Although neck stiffness, nausea, and vomiting can occur, encephalitic symptoms are rare (1:4000 cases of mumps); recovery in 3–10 days is the rule.

3. Pancreatitis—Abdominal pain may represent transient pancreatitis. Because salivary gland disease may elevate serum amylase, specific markers of pancreatic function (lipase and amylase isoenzymes) are required for assessing pancreatic involvement.

4. Orchitis, oophoritis—Involvement of the gonads is associated with fever, local tenderness, and swelling. Epididymitis is usually present. Orchitis is unusual in young children but occurs in up to one-third of affected postpubertal males. Usually it is unilateral and resolves in 1–2 weeks. Although one-third of infected testes atrophy, bilateral involvement and sterility are rare.

5. Other—Thyroiditis, mastitis (especially in adolescent females), arthritis, and presternal edema (occasionally with dysphagia or hoarseness) may be seen.

B. LABORATORY FINDINGS

Peripheral blood leukocyte count is usually normal. Up to 1000 cells/μL (predominantly lymphocytes) may be present in the CSF, with mildly elevated protein and normal to slightly decreased glucose. Viral culture of saliva, throat, urine, or spinal fluid may be positive for at least 1 week after onset. Paired sera assayed by ELISA are currently used for diagnosis. Complement-fixing antibody to the soluble antigen disappears in several months; its presence in a single specimen thus indicates recent infection.

Differential Diagnosis

Mumps parotitis may resemble the following: cervical adenitis (the jaw angle may be obliterated, but the ear does not usually protrude; the Stensen duct orifice is normal; leukocytosis and neutrophilia are observed); bacterial parotitis (pus in the Stensen duct, toxicity, exquisite tenderness); recurrent parotitis (idiopathic or associated with calculi); tumors or leukemia; and tooth infections.

Many viruses, including parainfluenza, enteroviruses, EBV, CMV, and influenza virus, can cause parotitis. Parotid swelling in HIV infection is less painful and tends to be bilateral and chronic, but bacterial parotitis occurs in some children with HIV infection.

Unless parotitis is present, mumps meningitis resembles that caused by enteroviruses or early bacterial infection. An elevated amylase is a useful clue in this situation. Isolated pancreatitis is not distinguishable from many other causes of epigastric pain and vomiting. Mumps is a classic cause of orchitis, but torsion, bacterial or chlamydial epididymitis, *Mycoplasma* infection, other viral infections, hematomas, hernias, and tumors must also be considered.

Complications

The major neurologic complication is nerve deafness (usually unilateral), which can result in inability to hear high tones. It may occur without meningitis. Permanent damage is rare, occurring in less than 0.1% of cases of mumps. Aqueductal stenosis and hydrocephalus (especially following congenital infection), myocarditis, transverse myelitis, and facial paralysis are other rare complications.

Treatment & Prognosis

Treatment is supportive and includes provision of fluids, analgesics, and scrotal support for orchitis. Systemic steroids have been used for orchitis, but their value is anecdotal. Surgery is not recommended.

Caplan CE: Mumps in the era of vaccines. Can Med Assoc J 1999;160:865 [PMID: 10189437].

Hersh BS et al: Mumps outbreak in a highly vaccinated population. J Pediatr 1991;119:187 [PMID: 1861205].

Manson AL: Mumps orchitis. Urology 1990;36:355 [PMID: 2219620].

McDonald JC, Moore DL, Quennec P: Clinical and epidemiologic features of mumps meningoencephalitis and possible vaccine-related disease. Pediatr Infect Dis J 1989;8:751 [PMID: 2594449].

RABIES

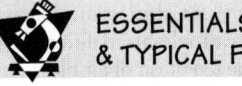 ESSENTIALS OF DIAGNOSIS & TYPICAL FEATURES

- *History of animal bite 10 days to 1 year (usually less than 90 days) previously.*
- *Paresthesias or hyperesthesia in bite area.*
- *Progressive limb and facial weakness in some patients (dumb rabies; 30%).*
- *Irritability followed by fever, confusion, combativeness, muscle spasms (especially pharyngeal with swallowing) in all patients (furious rabies).*

• *Rabies antigen detected in corneal scrapings or tissue obtained by brain or skin biopsy; Negri bodies seen in brain tissue.*

General Considerations

Rabies remains a potentially serious public health problem wherever animal immunization is not widely practiced or when humans play or work in areas with sylvan rabies. Although infection does not always follow a bite by a rabid animal (about 40% infection rate following rabid dog bites), infection is almost invariably fatal. Any warm-blooded animal may be infected, but susceptibility and transmissibility vary with different species. Bats often carry and excrete the virus in saliva or feces for prolonged periods; they are the major cause of rabies in the United States. Dogs and cats are usually clinically ill within 10 days after becoming contagious (the standard quarantine period for suspect animals). Valid quarantine periods or signs of illness are not fully known for many species. Rodents rarely transmit infection. Animal vaccines are very effective when properly administered, but a single inoculation may fail to produce immunity in up to 20% of dogs.

The risk is assessed according to the type of animal (bats always considered rabid; raccoons, skunks, and foxes in many areas); wound extent and location (infection more common after head or hand bites, or if wounds have extensive salivary contamination or are not quickly and thoroughly cleaned); geographic area (urban rabies is rare to nonexistent in U.S. cities; rural rabies is possible, especially outside the United States); and animal vaccination history (risk low if documented). Most rabies in the United States is with genotypes found in bats, yet a history of bat bite is rarely obtained. Aerosolized virus in caves inhabited by bats has caused infection.

Clinical Findings

A. SYMPTOMS AND SIGNS

Paresthesias at the bite site are usually the first symptoms. Nonspecific anxiety, excitability, or depression follows, then muscle spasms, drooling, hydrophobia, delirium, and lethargy. Swallowing or even the sensation of air blown on the face may cause pharyngeal spasms. Seizures, fever, cranial nerve palsies, coma, and death follow within 7–14 days after onset. In a minority of patients, the spastic components are initially absent and the symptoms are primarily flaccid paralysis and cranial nerve defects. The furious components appear subsequently.

B. LABORATORY FINDINGS

Leukocytosis is common. CSF is usually normal or may show elevation of protein and mononuclear cell pleocytosis. Cerebral imaging and electroencephalography are not diagnostic.

Infection in an animal may be determined by use of the fluorescent antibody test to examine brain tissue for antigen. Rabies virus is excreted in the saliva of infected humans, but the diagnosis is usually made by antigen detection in scrapings or tissue samples of richly innervated epithelium, such as the cornea or the hairline of the neck. Classic Negri cytoplasmic inclusion bodies in brain tissue are not always present. Seroconversion occurs after 7–10 days.

Differential Diagnosis

Failure to elicit the bite history in areas where rabies is rare may delay diagnosis. Other disorders to be considered include parainfectious encephalopathy; encephalitis due to herpes simplex, mosquito-borne viruses, and other viruses; and Guillain–Barré syndrome.

Prevention

See Chapter 9 for information regarding vaccination and postexposure prophylaxis. Rabies immune globulin and diploid cell vaccine have made prophylaxis more effective and minimally toxic; however, rare cases of prophylaxis failure are still being reported. Because rabies is almost always fatal, presumed exposures must be managed carefully.

Treatment & Prognosis

Survival is rare but has been reported in four patients receiving meticulous intensive care. No antiviral preparations are of proved benefit. Early diagnosis is important for the protection and prophylaxis of individuals exposed to the patient.

Jackson AC et al: Management of rabies in humans. Clin Infect Dis 2003;36:60 [PMID: 12491203].

Messenger SL et al: Emerging epidemiology of bat-associated cryptic cases of rabies in humans in the United States. Clin Infect Dis 2002;35:738 [PMID: 12203172].

■ II. RICKETTSIAL INFECTIONS

Rickettsiae are pleomorphic, gram-negative coccobacilli which are obligate intracellular parasites. Rickettsial diseases are often included in the differential diagnosis of febrile rashes, although some (notably Q fever) are not characterized by rash. Severe headache is a prominent symptom. The endothelium is the primary target tissue, and the ensuing vasculitis is responsible for severe illness.

All rickettsioses except Q fever are transmitted by cutaneous arthropod contact, either by bite or contamination of skin breaks with tick feces. Evidence of such contact by history or physical examination may be completely lacking, especially in young children. The geographic distribution of the vector is often the primary determinant for suspicion of these infections. Therapy often must be empirical. Many new broad-spectrum antimicrobials are inactive against these cell wall-deficient organisms; tetracycline is usually effective.

HUMAN EHRLICHIOSIS

Ehrlichia species are responsible for febrile pancytopenia in animals. In humans, *Ehrlichia sennetsu* is responsible for a mononucleosis-like syndrome seen in Japan and Malaysia. One agent of North American human ehrlichiosis has been identified as *E chaffeensis.* The reservoir hosts are probably wild rodents, deer, and sheep; ticks are the vectors. Most cases caused by this agent are reported in the south central and middle to southern Atlantic states. Arkansas, Missouri, Oklahoma, and North Carolina are high-prevalence areas. Almost all cases occur between March and October, when ticks are active. A second ehrlichiosis syndrome, seen in the upper Midwest and Northeast (Connecticut, Wisconsin, Minnesota, and New York are high-prevalence areas), is caused by an organism closely related to *E phagocytophila* or *E equi.* These are known large animal pathogens. *E chaffeensis* has a predilection for mononuclear cells, whereas intracytoplasmic inclusions in granulocytes are common with the *E phagocytophila* and *E equi* infections. Hence, diseases caused by these agents are referred to as human monocytic ehrlichiosis or human granulocytic ehrlichiosis, respectively. A newly discovered agent, *E ewingii,* also causes tick-borne human granulocytic ehrlichiosis. Rocky Mountain spotted fever and human monocytic ehrlichiosis share the same vector (Lone Star tick), whereas Lyme disease and human granulocytic ehrlichiosis are both spread by the deer tick. Thus, dual infections are common and should be considered in patients who fail to respond to therapy.

Clinical Findings

In approximately 75% of patients, a history of tick bite can be elicited. The majority of the remaining patients report having been in a tick-infested area. The usual incubation period is 5–21 days.

A. SYMPTOMS AND SIGNS

Fever and headache are universally present. Gastrointestinal symptoms (anorexia, nausea and vomiting) are reported in most pediatric patients. Distal limb edema may also occur in children. Chills, photophobia, conjunctivitis, myalgia, and arthralgia occur in more than half of patients. Rash occurs in one-third of patients with monocytic ehrlichiosis but is less common (< 10%) in granulocytic ehrlichiosis. Rash may be erythematous, macular, papular, petechial, scarlatiniform, or vasculitic. Meningitis occurs. Interstitial pneumonitis, adult respiratory distress syndrome, and renal failure occur in severe cases. The physical examination reveals rash, mild cervical adenopathy, and hepatomegaly. Perinatal transmission has been documented. A child without a rash may present as a case of fever of unknown origin.

B. LABORATORY FINDINGS

Laboratory abnormalities include leukopenia with left shift, lymphopenia, thrombocytopenia, and elevated aminotransferase levels. Disseminated intravascular coagulation can occur in severe cases. Anemia occurs in one-third of patients. The definitive diagnosis is made serologically. The Centers for Disease Control and Prevention uses appropriate antigens in an immunofluorescent antibody test in order to distinguish between the etiologic agents. Intracytoplasmic inclusions (morulae) may occasionally be observed in mononuclear cells in monocytic ehrlichiosis and are usually observed in polymorphonuclear cells from the peripheral blood or bone marrow in granulocytic ehrlichiosis. Specific PCR is now available for diagnosis.

Differential Diagnosis

The differential diagnosis includes septic or toxic shock, other rickettsial infections (especially Rocky Mountain spotted fever), Colorado tick fever, leptospirosis, Lyme borreliosis, relapsing fever, EBV, CMV, viral hepatitis and other viral infections, Kawasaki disease, systemic lupus erythematosus, and leukemia.

Treatment & Prognosis

Although the disease may last several weeks, it is usually self-limited. Deaths do occur in children. Doxycycline, 2–4 mg/kg/d divided every 12 hours (maximum 100 mg/dose) for 7–10 days, is the treatment of choice. Fatal disease occurs in less than 3% of cases. Immune compromise is a risk factor for severe disease.

Jacobs RF: Human monocytic ehrlichiosis: Similar to Rocky Mountain spotted fever but different. Pediatr Ann 2002;31: 180 [PMID: 11905291].

Lantos P, Krause PJ: Ehrlichiosis in children. Semin Pediatr Infect Dis 2002;13:249 [PMID: 12491230].

Singh-Behl D et al: Tick-borne infections. Dermatol Clin 2003; 21:237 [PMID: 12757245].

RICKETTSIALPOX

Rickettsia akari is transmitted by mites from infected house mice. Most cases in the United States have occurred in northeastern cities. The bite site becomes a papule, then a pustule; it ulcerates and then forms a characteristic black eschar at about the time fever develops at 9–14 days. Local adenopathy is the rule. Headache, myalgia, and photophobia are followed in 2–4 days by a generalized maculopapular rash. Palms and soles are usually spared. Vesicles develop on the papules. The fever lasts about a week. Diagnosis is established by serology.

The differential diagnosis includes varicella, enteroviral infections, other rickettsial spotted fevers, meningococcemia, and gonococcemia. Mild cases require no therapy. Tetracycline for 3 to 5 days is effective.

Paddock CD et al: Rickettsialpox in New York City: A persistent urban zoonosis. Ann N Y Acad Sci 2003;990:36 [PMID: 12860597].

ROCKY MOUNTAIN SPOTTED FEVER

Rickettsia rickettsii causes one of many similar tick-borne illnesses characterized by fever and rash that occur worldwide. Most are named for their geographic area. In all except Rocky Mountain spotted fever and murine typhus, there is a characteristic eschar at the bite site, called the *tache noire*. Dogs and rodents are reservoirs of *R rickettsii*. Rocky Mountain spotted fever is the most severe of these infections and the most important (500–1000 cases per year) in the United States. It occurs predominantly in the eastern seaboard; in the southeastern states; and in Arkansas, Texas, Missouri, Kansas, and Oklahoma—much less common to the west. Most cases occur in children exposed in rural areas from April to September. Because tick attachment lasting 6 hours or longer is needed, frequent tick removal is a preventive measure.

Clinical Findings

A. SYMPTOMS AND SIGNS

After the incubation period of 3–12 days (mean, 7 days), there is high fever (over 40 °C, often hectic), usually of abrupt onset, myalgia, severe and persistent headache (retroorbital; less obvious in infants), toxicity, photophobia, vomiting, and diarrhea. The characteristic rash occurs in 85–90% of patients and appears 2–6 days after fever onset as macules and papules, especially prominent on the palms, soles, and extremities, becoming petechial and spreading centrally. Conjunctivitis, splenomegaly, edema, meningismus, irritability, and confusion may occur.

B. LABORATORY FINDINGS

Laboratory findings are nonspecific and reflect diffuse vasculitis: thrombocytopenia, hyponatremia, early mild leukopenia, proteinuria, abnormal liver function tests, hypoalbuminemia, and hematuria. CSF pleocytosis is common. Serologic diagnosis is achieved with indirect fluorescent or latex agglutination antibody methods, but generally only 7–10 days after onset of the illness. Skin biopsy with specific fluorescent staining may give the diagnosis within the first week of the illness.

Differential Diagnosis

The differential diagnosis includes meningococcemia, measles, meningitis, staphylococcal sepsis, enteroviral infection, leptospirosis, Colorado tick fever, scarlet fever, murine typhus, Kawasaki disease, and ehrlichiosis.

Treatment & Prognosis

To be effective, therapy for Rocky Mountain spotted fever must be started early and is often based on a presumptive diagnosis in endemic areas prior to rash onset. It is important to remember that atypical presentations, such as the absence of pathognomonic rash, often lead to delay in appropriate therapy. Doxycycline is the agent of choice for children, regardless of age. Treatment should be continued for 2 or 3 days after the temperature has returned to normal for a full day. A minimum of 10 days of therapy is recommended.

Complications and death result from severe vasculitis, especially in the brain, heart, and lung. The mortality rate is 5–7%. Delay in therapy is an important determinant of mortality.

Masters EJ et al: Rocky Mountain spotted fever: A clinician's dilemma. Arch Intern Med 2003;163:769 [PMID: 12695267].

Sexton DJ, Kaye KS: Rocky Mountain spotted fever. Med Clin North Am 2002;86:351 [PMID: 11982306].

ENDEMIC TYPHUS (Murine Typhus)

Endemic typhus is present in the southern United States, mainly in southern Texas, and in Southern California. The disease is transmitted by fleas from infected rodents, from their feces in scratches or by inhalation. Domestic cats, dogs, and opossums may play a role in the transmission of suburban cases. No eschar appears at the inoculation site, which may go unnoticed. The incubation period is 6–14 days. Headache, myalgia, and chills slowly worsen. Fever may last 10–14 days. After 3–8 days, a rash appears. Truncal macules and papules spread to the extremities; the rash is rarely petechial. The location of the rash in typhus, with sparing of the palms and soles, is a distinction from Rocky Mountain spotted fever. Rash may be absent in 20–40% of patients. Hepatomegaly may be present. Intestinal and respiratory symptoms may occur. Mild thrombocytopenia and elevated liver enzymes may be present. The illness is usually self-limited and milder than epidemic typhus. More prolonged neurologic symptoms have been described. Therapy is usually not needed. Doxycycline is the drug of choice. Therapy for 3 days is usually sufficient. Fluorescent antibody and ELISA tests are available.

Fergie JE et al: Murine typhus in south Texas children. Pediatr Infect Dis J 2000;19:535 [PMID: 10877169].

Q FEVER

Coxiella burnetii is transmitted by inhalation rather than by an arthropod bite. The birth tissues and excreta of domestic animals and of some rodents are the infectious source. Unpasteurized milk from infected animals may also transmit disease. Q fever is also distinguished from other rickettsial diseases by the infrequent occurrence of cutaneous manifestations and by the prominence of pulmonary disease.

Clinical Findings

A. SYMPTOMS AND SIGNS

Many patients have a self-limited flulike syndrome of chills, fever, severe headache, and myalgia of abrupt onset occurring 10–30 days after exposure. Abdominal pain, vomiting, chest pain, and dry cough are prominent in children. Examination of the chest may produce few findings, as in other atypical pneumonias. Hepatosplenomegaly is common. The illness lasts 1–4 weeks, and frequently is associated with weight loss.

B. LABORATORY FINDINGS

Leukopenia with left shift is characteristic. Thrombocytopenia is unusual and another distinction from other symptomatic rickettsial diseases. Aminotransferase and γ-glutamyl transferase levels are elevated. Diagnosis is made by finding a complement-fixing antibody response (fourfold rise or single high titer) to the phase II organism. Chronic infection is indicated by antibody against the phase I organism. IgM ELISA and specific PCR are also available.

C. IMAGING

Pneumonitis occurs in 50% of patients. Multiple segmental infiltrates are common, but the radiographic appearance is not pathognomonic. Consolidation and pleural effusion are rare.

Differential Diagnosis

In the appropriate epidemiologic setting, Q fever should be considered in evaluating causes of atypical pneumonias such as from *Mycoplasma pneumoniae*, viruses, *Legionella*, and *Chlamydia pneumoniae*. It should also be included among the causes of mild hepatitis without rash or adenopathy in children with exposure to farm animals.

Treatment & Prognosis

Typically the illness lasts 1–2 weeks without therapy. One complication is chronic disease, which often implies myocarditis or granulomatous hepatitis. Meningoencephalitis is also a rare complication. *C burnetii* is also one of the causes of so-called culture-negative endocarditis. Both types of complication are rare. Endocarditis is difficult to treat; mortality approaches 50%. The course of the uncomplicated illness is shortened with tetracycline; doxycycline is preferred. Therapy is continued for several days after the patient becomes afebrile. Quinolones are also effective.

Maltezou HC, Raoult D: Q fever in children. Lancet Infect Dis 2002;2:686 [PMID: 12409949].

Marrie TJ, Raoult D: Update on Q fever, including Q fever endocarditis. Curr Clin Topics Infect Dis 2002;22:97 [PMID: 1250650].

Human Immunodeficiency Virus Infection

37

Elizabeth J. McFarland, MD

ESSENTIALS OF DIAGNOSIS & TYPICAL FEATURES

Children younger than age 18 months:

- *A child known to be HIV-seropositive or born to an HIV-infected mother.*

And

- *Has positive results on two separate determinations on blood or tissue (excluding cord blood) for one or more of the following HIV detection tests: HIV nucleic acid detection, HIV antigen (p24), HIV culture.*

Or

- *Meets criteria for AIDS diagnosis based on the 1987 Centers for Disease Control and Prevention (CDC) AIDS surveillance case (see Table 37–1 and CDC case definition, MMWR Morb Mortal Wkly Rep, 1994).*

Or

- *Has HIV antibody and evidence of cellular and humoral immunodeficiency (without another cause) and symptoms compatible with HIV infection.*

Children older than age 18 months:

- *HIV-seropositive by repeatedly reactive enzyme-linked immunosorbent assay and confirmatory test.*

Or

- *Meets any of the criteria listed for children younger than age 18 months.*

General Considerations

Human immunodeficiency virus (HIV) is a retrovirus that primarily infects cells of the immune system including helper T lymphocytes (CD4 T lymphocytes), monocytes, and macrophages. The function and number of CD4 T lymphocytes and other affected cells are diminished by HIV infection, with profound effects on both humoral and cell-mediated immunity. In the absence of treatment, HIV infection causes generalized immune incompetence over a period of years, leading to conditions that meet the definition of acquired immunodeficiency syndrome (AIDS), and eventually death. The clinical diagnosis of AIDS is made when an HIV-infected child develops any of the opportunistic infections, malignancies, or conditions listed in category C (Table 37–1). In adults and adolescents, the criteria for a diagnosis of AIDS also include absolute CD4 lymphocyte counts of 200/μL or less.

Combination antiretroviral treatment, available in resource-rich settings since 1996, can forestall disease progression for a prolonged period of time in many patients. The full duration of the benefits is not yet defined and it is not known whether adverse effects from the medications will impact mortality or limit use. Nevertheless, HIV infection can be considered a chronic disease for people with access to treatment rather than acutely terminal. Importantly, antiretroviral treatment for an infected woman during pregnancy and labor, with prophylactic therapy for the infant and avoidance of breast-feeding, is highly effective in preventing mother-to-infant transmission of HIV. In resource-rich countries where these interventions are routine, HIV infection in infants is rare, except when prenatal HIV testing is not performed. Access to antiretroviral therapy and infant formula is not widely available in resource-limited settings.

Mode of Transmission and Epidemiology

HIV is transmitted by sexual contact, percutaneous exposure to contaminated blood (eg, injecting drug use or transfusion with contaminated blood products), and mother-to-infant (vertical) transmission. Vertical transmission may occur in utero, at the time of delivery, or via breast-feeding. Risk factors associated with mother-to-infant transmission include high maternal plasma HIV RNA, advanced maternal disease stage, low CD4 lymphocyte count, premature delivery, and factors related to increased exposure to maternal blood or cervical secretions at the time of delivery (eg, duration of rupture of membranes, presence of blood in the infant's gastric secretions, and first-born twin delivery). Without intervention, 15–30% of infants born to HIV-infected women will be

Table 37–1. Clinical categories of children with human immunodeficiency virus (HIV) infection.

Category N: Not symptomatic
No signs or symptoms or only one of the conditions listed in category A

Category A: Mildly symptomatic
Having two or more of the following conditions:
Lymphadenopathy
Hepatomegaly
Splenomegaly
Dermatitis
Parotitis
Recurrent or persistent upper respiratory infection, sinusitis, or otitis media

Category B: Moderately symptomatic
Having symptoms attributed to HIV infections other than those in category A or C
Examples:
Anemia, neutropenia, thrombocytopenia
Bacterial meningitis, pneumonia, sepsis (single episode)
Candidiasis, oropharyngeal, persisting over 2 months
Cardiomyopathy
Cytomegalovirus infection with onset < 1 month of age
Diarrhea, recurrent or chronic
Hepatitis
Herpes simplex virus recurrent stomatitis, bronchitis, pneumonitis, esophagitis at < 1 month of age
Herpes zoster, two or more episodes or more than one dermatome
Leiomyosarcoma
Lymphoid interstitial pneumonia
Nephropathy
Nocardiosis
Persistent fever
Toxoplasmosis with onset < 1 month of age
Varicella, complicated

Category C: Severely symptomatic
Serious bacterial infections, multiple or recurrent
Candidiasis, esophageal or pulmonary
Coccidioidomycosis, disseminated
Cryptosporidiosis or isosporiasis with diarrhea > 1 month
Cytomegalovirus infection with onset > 1 month of age
Encephalopathy
Herpes simplex virus: persistent oral lesions, or bronchitis, pneumonitis, esophagitis at > 1 month of age
Histoplasmosis
Kaposi sarcoma
Lymphoma
Mycobacterium tuberculosis, extrapulmonary
Mycobacterium infection, other species, disseminated
Pneumocystis jiroveci pneumonia
Progressive multifocal leukoencephalopathy
Salmonella septicemia, recurrent
Toxoplasmosis of the brain with onset > 1 month of age
Wasting syndrome

Adapted from MMWR Morb Mortal Wkly Rep 1994;43(RR-12):6, 8.

infected. The rate of vertical transmission can be reduced to < 2% by providing combination antiretroviral treatment to the mother during pregnancy and delivery, obstetric interventions, and additional prophylaxis to the infant during the first 6 weeks after birth. In the United States, as a result of prenatal and perinatal interventions, the number of vertically acquired AIDS cases declined 83% between 1992 (907 cases) and 2001 (150 cases). Most transmissions that occur involve women not receiving therapy during pregnancy, either because the infection is undiagnosed or because of lack of prenatal care. Mother-to-infant transmission rates continue to be high in resource-limited settings where access to antiretroviral therapy is infrequent. Worldwide, an estimated 2.5 million children are infected with HIV, most of them in Africa, India, Thailand, and parts of South America. In 2004, in children younger than 15 years there were an estimated 640,000 new infections and 500,000 deaths.

Sexual activity (both heterosexual and homosexual) is the main mode of infection after puberty, with a smaller number of cases resulting from the sharing of contaminated needles. In the United States, seroprevalence rates are highest among gay men and injecting drug users. However, the proportion of new AIDS cases in 2003 acquired by heterosexual contact exceeded the proportion acquired by injecting drug use and was only slightly less than the proportion acquired by men having sex with men. Youth (ages 13–24 years) and women of color are disproportionately represented among new cases. In developing nations, heterosexual contact is the most common mode of transmission among adults, and prevalence is similar in both genders.

As a result of careful donor screening and testing of the donated blood, HIV transmission resulting from blood products is now extremely rare (1:2,000,000 transfusions). Casual, classroom, or household contact with an HIV-infected person poses no risk.

Pathogenesis

Most transmission of HIV occurs via mucosal surfaces. Virus is transported to regional lymph nodes and by approximately 48 hours after infection, replicating virus is found throughout all lymphoid tissues. Nonhuman primate models using a related virus indicate that a massive loss of CD4 T-helper lymphocytes occurs during the first days of infection. During acute infection, high levels of HIV are detected in the bloodstream. In adults, the level of viremia declines without therapy concurrent with the appearance of an HIV-specific host immune response and plasma viremia usually reaches a steady-state level about 6–12 months after primary infection. The amount of virus present in the plasma at that point and thereafter is predictive of the rate of disease progression for the individual. Despite ongoing virus replication, a period of clinical latency occurs, lasting from 1 year to more than 12 years during which the infected person is asymptomatic. The virus and anti-HIV immune responses are in a steady state, with high levels of virus production and destruction balanced against production and destruction of CD4 lymphocytes. Eventually, the balance favors the virus, and the viral burden increases as the CD4 lymphocyte count declines.

In the pre-antiretroviral treatment era, approximately 30% of infants with vertically acquired HIV infection had virus detectable in the blood at birth, presumed to be infection acquired in utero. In utero infection represents a larger fraction of vertical infections in populations where interventions to prevent transmission, often initiated during the second trimester or later, are common. The remaining infected infants (excluding those infected by breast-feeding) probably acquire HIV during labor and delivery and will test negative for HIV at birth but will soon have detectable virus, usually by 2–4 weeks. The level of viremia rises steeply, reaching a peak at age 1–2 months. In contrast with adults, infants will have a gradual decline in plasma viremia that extends beyond 2 years. Infants generally have plasma virus levels 10 times higher than those in adults. Less is known about the viral dynamics following transmission via breast-feeding.

There is a bimodal presentation of HIV disease progression in vertically infected children. Without treatment, about 20–30% of HIV-infected infants develop an AIDS-defining illness by age 1 year and die before age 2–3 years. High peak and high average levels of viremia over the first year of life characterize these rapid-progressor infants. Other predictors of rapid progression are low absolute counts of CD4 and suppressor–killer T (CD8) lymphocytes in the first 6 months. In the remainder of infants the disease progresses more slowly, with 5% progressing to AIDS or death per year and median survival of 10 years. These so-called slow-

progressors will generally have lower virus levels and a more gradual decline in CD4 lymphocyte counts. There are rare instances of children and adults with untreated infection for 8–10 years or more with no evidence of immune suppression. Studies indicate that both viral and host genetic factors, not all fully defined, play a role in determining the rate of disease progression. The initiation of antiretroviral therapy dramatically alters the natural history by slowing disease progression and permitting restoration of most immune function.

Clinical Findings

A. SYMPTOMS AND SIGNS

The manifestations described in this section are likely to be observed in children with untreated infection or in those unresponsive to therapy. Children given effective antiretroviral therapy usually have few symptoms, most of which will be from the medications.

The Centers for Disease Control and Prevention (CDC) has developed disease staging criteria for HIV-infected children (see Tables 37–1 and 37–2). The criteria incorporate clinical symptoms ranging from no symptoms to mild, moderate, and severe symptoms (categories N, A, B, and C, respectively) and age-adjusted CD4 lymphocyte counts (immunologic categories 1, 2, or 3, corresponding to none, moderate, or severe immune suppression, respectively). Each child is classified both by CD4 lymphocyte count and by clinical category. Category C diagnoses are the diseases associated with late-stage disease and confer a diagnosis of AIDS.

1. Primary acute infection—The incubation period is 2–4 weeks for primary infection acquired by adults and adolescents through high-risk behavior. Nonspecific symptoms occur in 30–90% of new infections (eg, flu- or mild mononucleosis-like illness), but may not be brought to

Table 37–2. Immunologic categories based on age-specific CD4 lymphocyte counts and percentages of total lymphocytes.

	Age of Child					
	< 12 months		1–5 years		6–12 years	
Immunologic Category	cells/μL	(%)	cells/μL	(%)	cells/μL	(%)
1. No evidence of suppression	≥ 1500	(≥ 25)	≥ 1000	(≥ 25)	≥ 500	(≥ 25)
2. Evidence of moderate suppression	750–1499	(15–24)	500–999	(15–24)	200–499	(15–24)
3. Evidence of severe suppression	< 750	(< 15)	< 500	(< 15)	< 200	(< 15)

Adapted from MMWR Morb Mortal Wkly Rep 1994;43(RR-12):4.

medical attention. However, in select cities anonymous screening of blood samples demonstrates 1% of emergency room patients have laboratory evidence of acute HIV infection. Diagnosis requires a high index of suspicion. Infected persons may present with fever, fatigue, malaise, pharyngitis, enlarged lymph nodes, and hepatosplenomegaly. Signs seen less commonly but more specific to HIV are mild oral ulcerations; a diffuse macular, erythematous rash; and mild meningitis or encephalopathy. Occasionally, thrush, *Candida* esophagitis, or genital ulcers are observed. These early symptoms of primary infection resolve spontaneously within 1–2 weeks, although some persons have fatigue and depression for weeks or months.

A primary infection syndrome is rarely recognized following perinatal acquisition. Newborns with perinatal HIV infection are rarely symptomatic at birth. Size and physical features are not different from uninfected infants. However, 75–95% will demonstrate some sign (mostly nonspecific) by age 1 year.

2. Nonspecific symptoms—These may be observed in early- or late-stage disease. Frequent illness (especially recurrent otitis media or sinusitis) is typical, in addition to poor weight gain, chronic cough, chronic diarrhea, developmental delay, unexplained fevers, night sweats, generalized lymphadenopathy, parotid swelling, or hepatosplenomegaly. Delayed growth may be observed as early as age 4 months in some infants. These common early findings may be present for years in an otherwise well child.

3. Infections related to immunodeficiency—Progressive immune dysfunction in both humoral and cell-mediated responses results in susceptibility to infections. Recurrent or serious bacterial infections are more common in children than in HIV-infected adults. Bouts of bacteremia, especially due to *Streptococcus pneumoniae*, can occur in children without suppressed CD4 T-cell counts. Infections with *Mycobacterium tuberculosis* (usually acquired from adults in the household) may be severe. Primary varicella-zoster virus (VZV) infections may be prolonged or severe. Herpes zoster (shingles), including multiple episodes, is common even in the era of combination therapy. Recurrent herpes simplex lesions may be large, painful, and persistent. Likewise, persistent aphthous ulcers may cause significant morbidity. Late-stage immunodeficiency is accompanied by susceptibility to a variety of opportunistic pathogens. Pneumonia caused by *Pneumocystis jiroveci* (formerly *Pneumocystis carinii*) is the most common AIDS-defining diagnosis in children with unrecognized HIV infection. The incidence is highest between ages 2 and 6 months and is often fatal during this period. Symptoms are difficult to distinguish from those of viral or atypical pneumonia. (See Chapter 39.) Persistent candidal mucocutaneous infections (oral,

cutaneous, and vaginal) are common. Candidal esophagitis occurs with more advanced disease. In children with severe immunosuppression, cytomegalovirus (CMV) infections may result in disseminated disease, hepatitis, gastroenteritis, retinitis, and encephalitis.

Disseminated infection with *Mycobacterium avium* complex (MAC), presenting with fever, night sweats, weight loss, diarrhea, fatigue, lymphadenopathy, hepatomegaly, anemia, and granulocytopenia occurs in infected children who have CD4 lymphocyte counts under 50–100/μL. A variety of diarrheal pathogens that cause mild, self-limited symptoms in healthy persons may result in severe, chronic diarrhea in HIV-infected persons. These include rotavirus, *Cryptosporidium parvum*, *Microsporidia*, *Cyclospora*, *Isospora belli*, *Giardia lamblia*, and bacterial pathogens. Chronic parvovirus infection manifested by anemia can occur. Reactivation of toxoplasmosis occurs rarely in children.

4. Organ system disease—HIV infection may cause a variety of organ system symptoms (encephalopathy, pneumonitis, hepatitis, diarrhea, hematologic suppression, nephropathy, and cardiomyopathy). The more common of these are described in this section. On average, HIV-infected children have lower than normal neuropsychological functioning; higher viral load correlates with more severe abnormalities. In many children, neuropsychological deficits do not normalize when antiretroviral therapy is started despite suppression of viremia. Studies are needed to determine if highly active antiretroviral therapy early in life will completely prevent the central nervous system effects of HIV. Without antiretroviral therapy, encephalopathy afflicted 20% or more of HIV-infected children. Symptoms included acquired microcephaly, progressive motor deficit, ataxia, pseudobulbar palsy, and failure to attain (or loss of) developmental milestones. Children who are older may have symptoms similar to those observed in infected adults, such as gradual mental status changes initially affecting attention span and memory.

Lymphoid interstitial pneumonitis is characterized by a diffuse peribronchial and interstitial infiltrate composed of lymphocytes and plasma cells. It may be asymptomatic or associated with dry cough, hypoxemia, dyspnea or wheezing on exertion, and clubbing of the digits. Children with this disorder frequently have enlargement of the parotid glands and generalized lymphadenopathy.

Mild to moderate elevation of liver enzymes is frequently observed, and, more rarely, overt clinical hepatitis occurs due to HIV infection itself. However, patients are often taking medications with potential hepatotoxicity, and superinfection with other pathogens (CMV, Epstein–Barr virus [EBV], MAC, hepatitis C, or hepatitis B) that affect the liver is common. Thus, the diagnosis of HIV hepatitis should be one of exclusion. Chronic diarrhea may occur with HIV infection; however, as with hepatitis, it is commonly associated with other gastrointestinal infections.

5. Malignancy—Children with HIV are at increased risk of malignancy. The most commonly occurring tumors are non-Hodgkin lymphomas. Unlike non-Hodgkin lymphomas in immunocompetent persons, these tumors commonly occur at extranodal sites (central nervous system, bone, gastrointestinal tract, liver, or lungs) and are usually high-grade and of B-cell origin. Cervical infection with human papillomavirus (HPV) is more likely to progress to neoplasia in adolescent females with HIV infection. Carcinoma due to anal HPV is also a concern. Kaposi sarcoma, a common malignancy among HIV-infected gay males, rarely occurs in children. There is an increased frequency of leiomyosarcomas.

B. LABORATORY FINDINGS

HIV antibody is measured by enzyme-linked immunosorbent assay (ELISA). A confirmatory test, usually a Western blot, must be performed because individuals occasionally have nonviral cross-reacting antibodies, which result in a false-positive ELISA. Infants born to HIV-infected mothers will have HIV antibody—regardless of infection status—owing to transplacental passage of maternal antibody. Maternal HIV antibody is lost in all children by 18 months. After that age, HIV antibody testing can be used to make the diagnosis of infection. In the early weeks after acute HIV infection acquired by risk behavior HIV antibody may be absent. Most will seroconvert by 6 weeks but occasionally the time of seroconversion is prolonged to 3–6 months. When acute HIV infection is suspected, tests for circulating virus (see below) should be obtained.

HIV nucleic acid, RNA (in plasma) or DNA (in blood cells), can be detected by a number of methods, including polymerase chain reaction, branched DNA chain assay, and nucleic acid sequence-based amplification. These tests are highly sensitive with a lower limit of detection of 20 copies/mL of plasma. An HIV protein (p24) can also be detected in plasma; the test is less costly but is less sensitive. Quantitative measures of HIV RNA in plasma are valuable in predicting rate of disease progression and are a surrogate marker of response to antiretroviral therapy.

Using nucleic acid detection, infants at risk of vertical HIV infection can be diagnosed by age 2–4 months. At birth, approximately 30% of infected infants have detectable HIV RNA and DNA. The other 70% of infected infants will have negative results for HIV RNA and DNA, due to low levels of circulating virus, probably indicating that the infection was acquired at the time of birth. Over the first 8 weeks, almost all infected infants will become positive for HIV nucleic acid. An infant who is otherwise well and has had at least two negative HIV cultures or nucleic acid detection tests, both performed after age 1 month and at least one performed after age 2–4 months, is very unlikely to be infected. The infant should be followed up for clinical symptoms and retested at ages 12, 15, and 18 months for reversion to seronegative status to confirm the absence of infection.

The hallmark of HIV disease progression is decline in the absolute number and percentage of CD4 T lymphocytes and an increasing percentage of CD8 T lymphocytes. The CD4 T-lymphocyte values are predictive of the child's risk of opportunistic infections. Healthy infants have CD4 T-lymphocyte numbers and percentages much higher than in adults; these gradually decline to adult levels by age 6 years. Hence, age-adjusted values must be used when assessing a child's CD4 T-lymphocyte parameters (see Table 37–2).

Hypergammaglobulinemia of IgG, IgA, and IgM is characteristic and may be observed as early as age 9 months. Late in the disease, some individuals may become hypogammaglobulinemic. Hematologic abnormalities (anemia, neutropenia, and thrombocytopenia) may occur due to effects of HIV disease or, more commonly, due to adverse effects of medications. With brain involvement, the cerebrospinal fluid may either be normal or the protein may be elevated and a mononuclear pleocytosis may be present.

C. IMAGING

Cerebral images can demonstrate atrophy and calcification in the basal ganglia and frontal lobes in patients with encephalopathy. Chest radiographs of children with lymphoid interstitial pneumonitis show diffuse interstitial reticulonodular infiltrates, occasionally with hilar adenopathy. The chest radiograph in *P jiroveci* pneumonia typically demonstrates perihilar infiltrates progressing to bilateral diffuse alveolar disease.

Differential Diagnosis

HIV infection should be in the differential diagnosis for children being evaluated for immunodeficiency. Depending on the degree of immunosuppression, HIV infection may present similar to B-cell, T-cell, or combined immunodeficiencies, such as hypogammaglobinemia and severe combined immunodeficiency. (See Chapter 29.) HIV infection should also be considered in the evaluation of children with failure to thrive or developmental delay. Children or adolescents with chronic HIV infection may present with generalized lymphadenopathy or hepatosplenomegaly resembling infections with viruses such as EBV or CMV. Because blood tests are definitive for the diagnosis of HIV infection, the diagnosis can be readily established or excluded. The diagnosis of chronic HIV infection is made with HIV antibody testing in a child older than age 18 months. In younger infants, a negative result usually excludes HIV infection; a positive result must be followed by testing for viral nucleic acid. In rare cases, HIV-infected children with hypogammaglobulinemia have falsely negative antibody tests. Any child suspected of having HIV infection who has negative serologic tests should be tested by a nucleic acid-based test. Absence of maternal risk factors or history of negative testing during pregnancy, particularly if documentation of the results is lacking, should not dissuade the provider from testing for HIV if the patient has signs consistent with the diagnosis.

The symptoms of acute primary infection in the adolescent may be similar to those of mononucleosis caused by EBV or CMV, toxoplasmosis, rubella, secondary syphilis, influenza, enterovirus, or viral hepatitis. In the first weeks of acute infection, HIV antibody tests will be negative. However, the diagnosis can be made by detection of HIV RNA in plasma. Seroconversion occurs over 2–6 weeks in symptomatic patients. Diagnosis of acute HIV infection has important public health benefit, as patients are highly infectious during the first months after infection. Studies are ongoing to determine if treatment during early infection improves prognosis. Thus, HIV RNA testing is warranted if the patient has a history of high-risk behavior or an alternative diagnosis is lacking.

Prevention

Vertical transmission can be substantially prevented by giving antiretroviral therapy to the mother during pregnancy and by providing prophylaxis to the newborn. Therefore, the CDC and the American College of Obstetrics and Gynecology now recommend offering HIV testing, with an option to refuse, as a part of routine prenatal care for all pregnant women irrespective of risk factors. Women who present in labor should be tested for HIV antibody using recently approved rapid tests that give results with 60 minutes. Women found to be infected should be counseled regarding all HIV-related pregnancy care issues, including the benefits and risks of therapy with antiretroviral agents. Women with access to antiretroviral therapy should receive three-drug combination regimens during pregnancy. Zidovudine should be incorporated into the regimen if possible since this is the medication with the greatest amount of efficacy and safety data. Combination therapy that results in viral suppression to less than 1000 copies/mL reduces transmission rates to less than 1%. Antiretroviral therapy begun in the last weeks of pregnancy or even within 48 hours after birth also reduces perinatal infection, although less profoundly. Such short-course treatment can reduce transmission by 30–50% for women who are diagnosed late in pregnancy or at delivery.

Elective cesarean section reduces the risk of transmission by 50% and should be offered to women who are not on antiretroviral therapy or who have viral loads over 1000 copies/mL despite treatment. Women receiving combination therapy that suppresses viral load to below 1000 copies/mL have a very low risk of transmission. For these women, the benefit and risk of cesarean section should be considered for each woman on an individual basis. Because breast milk can carry the virus, breast-feeding by HIV-infected mothers is contraindicated when access to safe formula can be ensured. In developing countries transmission via breast milk remains a major mode of pediatric HIV infection.

The only 100% effective method of avoiding sexual transmission of HIV infection is abstinence or limiting sexual contact to a mutually monogamous partner who is not HIV-infected. However, condoms—used consistently and correctly—are highly effective in preventing transmission between stable, sexually active couples in which only one partner is HIV-infected. In two studies, seroconversions occurred in 0–2% of discordant couples using condoms consistently compared with 10–15% of couples with inconsistent condom use. A third study reported 1.1 seroconversions per 100 person-years of observation among consistent condom users compared with 9.7 seroconversions among inconsistent users. The CDC provides detailed instructions on correct condom use. Prompt treatment of other sexually transmitted diseases, especially those associated with mucosal ulceration, also reduces the risk of sexual transmission.

Post-exposure prophylaxis with antiretroviral medications begun as soon as possible is recommended for people with an occupational exposure that carries a risk of HIV transmission. Prophylaxis is also recommended for people with a nonoccupational exposure that is not likely to recur (eg, sexual assault or condom rupture) who present within 72 hours of the exposure. Detailed guidelines regarding assessment of the level of risk and selection of post-exposure therapy are published by the CDC.

Treatment

HIV infection calls for specific antiretroviral treatment to prevent progressive deterioration of the immune system as well as prophylactic measures at late stages of HIV infection to prevent opportunistic infections. Whenever possible, children should be enrolled in collaborative treatment studies. Current information on clinical trials may be obtained at:

http://aidsinfo.nih.gov/clinical_trials

Guidelines for the treatment of HIV developed by a national working group of pediatric HIV specialists are published by the United States Public Health System at:

http://aidsinfo.nih.gov/guidelines

The treatment paradigm changes frequently; therefore, prior to initiating treatment, expert consultation should be obtained.

A. SPECIFIC MEASURES

1. Principles of HIV treatment

Treatment of HIV is aimed at suppressing viral replication. The rate of disease progression is directly correlated with the number of HIV copies circulating in plasma. Antiretroviral treatment that reduces HIV replication is associated with increases in CD4 T-lymphocyte counts, reconstitution of immune function, and arrest of disease progression. Children have a remarkable ability to restore normal CD4 T-cell counts, even when treatment is started at advanced disease stage. However, it is clear that even the most potent regimens fail to eradicate virus. HIV persists in long-lived resting cells and cessation of antiretroviral treatment results in resumption of viremia and decline in CD4 lymphocytes. Therefore, treatment for HIV with currently available modalities must be a lifelong endeavor.

Emergence of drug-resistant HIV during therapy is a major challenge. HIV has a high spontaneous mutation rate, and emergence of drug resistance during treatment is frequent. Many antiretroviral drugs select for resistant mutations in the virus within weeks to a few months when used as monotherapy. Prevention of resistance mutations requires complete suppression such that virus is not replicating and has no opportunity to generate new mutations. Achieving potent viral suppression requires a combination of at least three antiviral agents. Treatment with a combination of drugs with different mechanisms of action provides an additional barrier to resistance as the virus must be resistant to all the drugs in the combination. Finally, strict adherence to the prescribed treatment is critical. Studies demonstrate that more than 95% of the doses must be taken in order to maintain optimal viral suppression. Therefore programs and services that enhance adherence are essential adjuncts of any highly active antiretroviral treatment (HAART) regimen.

Determining the best time to initiate treatment is a subject of intense discussion and research. For children demonstrating HIV-related symptoms (clinical category C in Table 37–1) or evidence of immune suppression (CD4 lymphocyte counts in category 3; see Table 37–2) the consensus is that treatment should be started irrespective of age or HIV RNA level. In addition, children with a plasma HIV RNA over 100,000 copies/mL are at high risk of progression, so this is a well-accepted criterion for initiating treatment. In the United States, many experts recommend treatment for all HIV-infected infants younger than age 12 months because surrogate markers that reliably identify all infants at risk of rapid progression are lacking.

The best approach for the asymptomatic child with low or modest plasma viral load and without evidence of severe immune suppression is less clear. Such a child might live many years without HIV-related symptoms. It is possible that starting a complex medication regimen with associated toxicities and significant effect on quality of life could be delayed without detriment to the child's long-term prognosis. However, it can also be argued that early treatment will better preserve normal immune function and prevent effects on growth and development that may not be reversed when treatment is started. At present, for children older than age 12 months at diagnosis with mild to moderate clinical symptoms (clinical category A or B) or with moderate immunologic suppression (immune category 2), most experts would consider initiating therapy. For asymptomatic children, many experts favor close observation, with therapy initiated if declining CD4 lymphocyte counts or increasing HIV plasma RNA copy numbers are observed. Once therapy has been initiated, the patient should be monitored every 3 months for changes in plasma virus copy number, CD4 lymphocyte count, symptoms, and adverse drug effects.

2. Considerations in selecting antiretroviral medications

The process of selecting a combination of medications for a particular patient has become highly complex. The U.S. Food and Drug Administration (FDA) has approved 20 drugs and several fixed drug combinations from four different drug classes for the treatment of HIV (Table 37–3). The clinician must consider the potency of the drugs, tolerability, simplicity of dosing, drug interactions, prior drug therapy, and viral resistance profiles.

Potency, the intrinsic ability of the regimen to fully suppress viral replication, is foremost because without complete suppression resistant virus will emerge. Tolerability is also critical because regimens that are poorly tolerated fail due to poor adherence. When selecting a tolerable regimen, the circumstances and priorities of each individual patient and family must be considered. Certain side effects may be acceptable to one person but for another person be intolerable. Likewise, for some patients the frequency of dosing may have the greatest effect on their compliance, whereas another may be satisfied with frequent dosing provided the number or size of pills is reduced. Over the years, more drugs have become available that can be given once daily and require fewer total pills or liquids.

Drug interactions between different antiretroviral medications, and with other medications, are frequent and must be considered when selecting a combination of drugs. Most of the protease inhibitors and nonnucleoside reverse transcriptase inhibitors are metabolized by cytochrome P-450 isotypes and therefore can induce or inhibit the metabolism of other drugs that are metabolized by that pathway. Some combinations lead to significant decreases or increases in drug levels, and combined use is contraindicated. This must be considered in advance of prescribing new medications, specific for HIV or for other conditions. On the other hand, the drug interactions can be advantageous and certain

Table 37–3. Antiretroviral drugs approved by the US Food and Drug Administration.

Drug Class or Drug Name	Potential Adverse Effects[a]	Mechanism of Action
Nucleoside/nucleotide reverse transcriptase inhibitors	Lactic acidosis (rare but potentially fatal)	Chain termination of HIV DNA
Abacavir (ABC; Ziagen)	Hypersensitivity reaction	
Abacavir/lamivudine (Epzicom)	See individual drugs	
Didanosine (ddI; Videx)	Pancreatitis, peripheral neuropathy, nausea, diarrhea	
Emtricitabine (FTC; Emtriva)	Minimal toxicity	
Lamivudine (3TC; Epivir)	Minimal toxicity	
Stavudine (d4T; Zerit)	Peripheral neuropathy, lipodystrophy, pancreatitis	
Tenofovir (TDF; Viread)	Headache, nausea, diarrhea, bone demineralization, renal insufficiency (rare)	
Tenofovir/Emtricitabine (Truvada)	See individual drugs	
Zalcitabine (ddC; Hivid)	Peripheral neuropathy, stomatitis	
Zidovudine (ZDV, AZT; Retrovir)	Anemia, neutropenia, gastrointestinal intolerance, headache	
Zidovudine/lamivudine (CBV, Combivir)	See individual drugs	
Zidovudine/lamivudine/abacavir (TZV, Trizavir)	See individual drugs	
Nonnucleoside reverse transcriptase inhibitors	Rash, rarely Stevens-Johnson syndrome	Synthesis of HIV DNA inhibited
Delavirdine (Rescriptor)	Increased liver transaminases, headache	
Efavirenz (Sustiva)	Central nervous system symptoms, increased transaminases, teratogenic in monkeys	
Nevirapine (Viramune)	Hepatitis	
Protease inhibitors	Glucose intolerance, risk of bleeding in hemophilia, dyslipidemia, lipodystrophy, transaminase elevation	Production of noninfectious virions
Amprenavir (Agenerase)	Rash, oral paresthesia	
Fosamprenavir (Lexiva)		
Atazanavir (Reyataz)	Increased indirect bilirubin	
Indinavir (Crixivan)	Nephrolithiasis, increased indirect bilirubin	
Lopinavir/ritonavir (Kaletra)	Gastrointestinal intolerance	
Nelfinavir (Viracept)	Diarrhea	
Ritonavir (Norvir)	Nausea, circumoral paraesthesias, hepatitis, pancreatitis, taste perversion	
Saquinavir hard gel (Invirase)	Gastrointestinal intolerance	
Tipranovir (Aptivus)	Hepatic toxicity, rash (cross-reaction with sulfonamide)	
Fusion inhibitors		Viral entry inhibited
Enfuvirtide (Fuzeon)	Injection site reactions, increased rate of bacterial pneumonias, hypersensitivity reactions (<1%)	

[a]Relative incidence of adverse events depends on specific drug.

combinations of protease inhibitors can be used so that therapeutic plasma levels can be achieved with lower doses (and fewer pills). Drug absorption and metabolism can vary widely between individuals, especially for the protease inhibitor class. Therefore, therapeutic drug monitoring to determine the level of drug in serum and adjust doses to achieve therapeutic levels is recommended by some experts.

The potential for viral resistance should be evaluated when selecting a combination. Optimally, an initial regimen would select viral resistance mutations that do not confer cross-resistance to a large number of other drugs. This permits an opportunity to use alternative regimens if resistance to the initial regimen develops. The process is aided by laboratory methods (genotyping and phenotyping) to determine the presence of virus with specific drug resistance mutations in the patient.

3. Specific antiretroviral medications—

a. Nucleoside and nucleotide reverse transcriptase inhibitors (NRTIs)—The NRTIs act as nucleotide analogues, which are incorporated into HIV DNA during transcription by the HIV reverse transcriptase. The result is chain termination and failure to complete provirus, preventing incorporation of HIV genome into cellular DNA. The human mitochondrial DNA polymerase also has limited affinity for these analogues, the degree varying with the drug. Incorporation of the analogue into mitochondrial DNA is one mechanism thought to lead to adverse effects including pancreatitis, peripheral neuropathy, bone marrow suppression (anemia or neutropenia), and lipodystrophy (loss of peripheral fat and accumulation of visceral fat). Lactic acidosis with hepatic steatosis (fatty liver) is a rare but potentially fatal complication that may result from mitochondrial toxicity.

A hypersensitivity reaction (not related to mitochondrial toxicity) to abacavir occurs in approximately 10% of patients. The reaction, characterized by a flulike syndrome with or without rash, may be fatal with continued treatment or re-challenge. The NRTIs vary widely with regard to antiviral activity, rates at which viral resistance occurs, and adverse effects. They are dosed either once or twice daily.

b. Nonnucleoside reverse transcriptase inhibitors (NNRTIs)—NNRTIs also inhibit HIV DNA synthesis but act at a different site on the viral enzyme so no cross-resistance occurs with NRTIs. The NNRTIs have potent antiretroviral activity, but single amino acid mutations in the viral reverse transcriptase protein often induce resistance to all three drugs in this class. The most common toxicity is rash. Stevens-Johnson syndrome has been reported, but rash is usually mild and often resolves without changing therapy. Efavirenz is associated with mild central nervous system symptoms (ie, dizziness and confusion), which usually resolve after

the initial weeks of use. Inflammation of the liver, rarely fatal, may occur with any of the drugs in the class but is more common with nevirapine. The NNRTIs are dosed once or twice daily and the pills are small.

c. Protease inhibitors—Protease inhibitors (PIs) are synthetic molecules designed to bind to the HIV protease. The protease is critical for the assembly of infectious virions. In the presence of PIs, progeny virus is released from the cell but cannot infect new cells. Acute adverse effects are mainly gastrointestinal intolerance as well as other effects specific to the particular drug (see Table 37–3). All PIs are associated with a risk of glucose intolerance and for bleeding in hemophiliacs. Most are associated with dyslipidemia (elevated cholesterol and triglycerides) and may contribute to lipodystrophy. An exception is atazanavir, which is not associated with changes in serum lipids. As a rule, these drugs are highly potent and usually require multiple mutations for high-level resistance to develop. Cross-resistance is observed for some drugs in the class, but others have differing resistance mutations. Taste and pill burden limit tolerability of these medications. The PIs are metabolized by the hepatic P-450 cytochrome enzymes, resulting in many interactions with other drugs, including other antiretrovirals. Careful attention to drug interactions is necessary when treating a patient taking a PI. Regimens combining two PIs can take advantage of the drug interactions and improve the pharmacokinetic properties of the drugs.

d. Fusion inhibitors—Enfuvirtide is the first drug to be FDA-approved in this class. Enfuvirtide interferes with the fusion of the viral envelope and the cell plasma membrane, thereby preventing entry of the virus into the cell. Enfuvirtide must be administered parenterally, and local reactions at the injection site are common.

B. General Measures

1. Immunizations—Combined diphtheria–tetanus–acellular pertussis, inactivated poliovirus, conjugated *Haemophilus influenzae* type b, conjugated *Streptococcus pneumoniae*, hepatitis B, and hepatitis A vaccines should be given as recommended for healthy children. (See Chapter 9.) A dose of 23-valent polysaccharide vaccine at 2 years and a booster after 3–5 years is recommended in addition to the conjugated pneumococcal vaccine series given in infancy. Infected children and their household contacts should receive inactivated influenza vaccine annually after age 6 months. In general, live virus vaccines should be avoided. However, the risk of measles is considered greater than the potential risk of the vaccine in asymptomatic children; thus measles–mumps–rubella vaccine should be given at age 12 months, with the second dose given 1 month later, provided the child does not have evidence of severe immunosuppression (category C or category 3). Varicella vaccine, also a live virus, is recommended for asymptomatic or mildly symptomatic children without evidence of severe immunosuppression. Because antibody titers to vaccines decline with time and with progression of immune deficiency, prophylaxis with immune globulin for measles exposure and tetanus immune globulin for tetanus-prone wounds should be given regardless of immunization status. Varicella-zoster immune globulin should be considered after each varicella exposure for children with immunosuppression who have not had prior varicella or VZV vaccination.

2. Prophylaxis for infections—Children with suppressed CD4 lymphocyte numbers benefit from prophylactic treatment to prevent opportunistic infections. Children who have had their CD4 counts restored to category 1 or 2 for over 2–4 months can be taken off prophylactic treatments. Antibiotic prophylaxis for *P jiroveci* pneumonia has been extremely effective. Because this infection has its highest incidence during the first year of life, *P jiroveci* pneumonia prophylaxis is given to all infants born to HIV-infected mothers beginning at age 4–6 weeks. When tests for HIV DNA or RNA are demonstrated negative at age 3–4 months, the infant may discontinue prophylaxis. HIV-infected infants should continue on prophylactic drugs until age 12 months, when further treatment is based on assessment of symptoms and age-adjusted CD4 lymphocyte counts every 3 months. Published guidelines from the CDC for *P jiroveci* pneumonia prophylaxis are summarized in Tables 37–4 and 37–5.

Children with hypogammaglobulinemia or a history of serious or multiple bacterial infections may benefit from monthly intravenous immune globulin if they are not receiving trimethoprim–sulfamethoxazole. Clarithromycin or azithromycin reduces the frequency of disseminated MAC with a survival benefit for children with very low CD4 counts.

Recurrent mucocutaneous candidiasis can be prevented with nystatin, clotrimazole, or fluconazole. Oral antiviral prophylaxis (acyclovir, valacyclovir, or famciclovir) is effective for recurrent severe herpes simplex or VZV infections.

HIV-infected children have a higher risk of progression of infections due to *M tuberculosis*. Because the child's infection is usually acquired from adult household contacts, the child and other household members should be skin-tested for tuberculosis yearly if they belong to a population with substantial risk for exposure to *M tuberculosis*.

3. Infections and other conditions—Rates of bacteremia, especially pneumococcal bacteremia and shingles, are higher among HIV-infected children, even in the absence of severe suppression of CD4 counts. VZV and herpes simplex virus infections are treated with acyclovir since symptoms may be prolonged in children with HIV. Short courses of valacyclovir or famciclovir—drugs with

Table 37–4. *Pneumocystis jiroveci*[a] pneumonia prophylaxis for HIV-exposed and infected infants by age and HIV infection status.

Birth to 4–6 wk	No prophylaxis
4–6 wk to 2 mos	Prophylaxis
2–12 mos	
HIV-infected or indeterminate	Prophylaxis
HIV infection reasonably excluded[b]	No prophylaxis
1–5 y, HIV-infected	Prophylaxis if CD4 count < 500/µL or CD4 < 15%[c]
6–12 y, HIV-infected	Prophylaxis if CD4 count < 200/µL or CD4 < 15%[c]

[a]Formerly *Pneumocystis carinii*.
[b]Among children who have had two or more negative HIV cultures or PCR tests, at least one of which is performed after age 1 month and one of which is performed at age 2–4 months or older.
[c]Prophylaxis should be considered on a case-by-case basis for children who might otherwise be at risk for pneumocystis pneumonia, such as those with rapidly declining CD4 counts or percentages or children with category C conditions.
Adapted from 2002 USPHS/IDSA Guidelines for the Prevention of Opportunistic Infections in Persons Infected with Human Immunodeficiency Virus.
http://www.aidsinfo.nih.gov/guidelines

Table 37–5. Drug regimens for *Pneumocystis jirovaci* prophylaxis for children over age 4 weeks.

Recommended regimen
  Trimethoprim-sulfamethoxazole, 150 mg TMP/m^2/d plus 750 mg SMX/m^2/d, administered orally, divided into two doses per day 3 days a week on consecutive days
  Alternative (same total daily dosages):
    Single daily dose 3 days a week on consecutive days
    Divided twice-daily doses 7 days a week
    Divided twice-daily doses 3 days a week on alternate days
Alternative if trimethoprim–sulfamethoxazole is not tolerated[a]
  Dapsone, 2 mg/kg/d (not to exceed 100 mg) orally once daily or 4 mg/kg (not to exceed 200 mg) orally once weekly
  Aerosolized pentamidine (children over age 5 years), 300 mg via Respirgard II inhaler monthly
  Atovaquone, age 1–3 mos and > 24 mos, 30 mg/kg orally once daily; age 4–24 mos, 45 mg/kg orally once daily

[a]If dapsone, aerosolized pentamidine, or atovaquone is not tolerated, some clinicians use intravenous pentamidine 4 mg/kg every 2–4 wk.
Adapted from 2002 USPHS/IDSA Guidelines for the Prevention of Opportunistic Infections in Persons infected with Human Immunodeficiency Virus. Available at http://www.aidsinfo.nih.gov/guidelines.

good bioavailability—are also effective, although not approved for children. Aphthous ulcers also occur in children, even when on suppressive antiretroviral drug therapy. Symptomatic CMV infection is treated with ganciclovir or foscarnet and requires ongoing secondary prophylaxis if CD4 lymphocytes counts remain low. MAC requires treatment with a multidrug regimen to delay the emergence of resistance. Lymphoid interstitial pneumonitis may respond to corticosteroid therapy. Chronic parvovirus as a cause of anemia should be investigated and can be treated with intravenous immune globulin. Anemia and granulocytopenia, whether drug-induced or HIV-induced, may respond to epoetin alfa (erythropoietin) and filgrastim (granulocyte colony-stimulating factor, G-CSF), respectively. Rarely transfusions are needed; CMV-seronegative blood should be used.

4. General support—Growth failure (weight and height) is one of the earliest and most sensitive markers of disease progression. The cause is a combination of increased metabolic needs related to chronic infection and decreased caloric intake. Supplemental nutrition in the form of oral supplements may be required. Some antiretroviral drugs cause elevated cholesterol and triglycerides. A cross-sectional study found elevated serum cholesterol in 13% of children with HIV compared to 5% of uninfected pediatric controls. Although the long-term consequences of drug-induced hyperlipidemia in HIV-infected children are unknown, diet modification and exercise are recommended. Nutritional evaluation and counseling should be a part of early care and continue throughout the child's care.

Evaluation and support for psychosocial needs of HIV-affected families is imperative. As with other chronic illnesses, HIV infection affects all family members, and it also carries an additional social stigma. Emotional concerns and financial needs are more prominent than medical needs at many stages of the disease process and influence the family's ability to comply with a medical treatment regimen. HIV-infected children often have comorbid mental health conditions. Rates of attention-deficit hyperactivity disorder range from 20–50% in various studies. Hospital admissions for mental health disorders are more frequent among HIV-infected children. In one study dual diagnosis of HIV and a mental health disorder occurred in 85% of adolescents who acquired HIV infection through high-risk behaviors. Ideally, care should be coordinated by a team of caregivers that is familiar with this disease and the newest therapies and that has access to community resources.

Prognosis

Plasma viremia and age-adjusted CD4 lymphocyte count are used to assess the risk of progression and complications of HIV. Poor prognosis in perinatal infection is associated with encephalopathy, infections with *P jiroveci,* early development of AIDS, and a rapidly declining CD4 lymphocyte count. Without treatment, approximately 30% of infected infants will progress to severe symptoms (class C) or death by 1 year of age with a 5% annual risk of progression in subsequent years. With the introduction of highly active antiretroviral treatment, mortality rates for HIV-infected children in the United States declined 80% between 1994 and 1999.

Public Health Issues

In general, the infant or child who is well enough to attend day care or school should be treated no differently from other children. The exception may be a toddler with uncontrollable biting behavior or bleeding lesions that cannot be covered adequately; in these situations, the child may be withheld from group day care. Routine good hygiene used for the prevention of transmission of other infectious diseases is appropriate for the prevention of common infections, which may be severe in the HIV-infected child. Optimally the school health care provider and teacher will be aware of the diagnosis, but there is no legal requirement that any individual at the school or day care center be informed. The parents and the child may prefer to keep the diagnosis confidential, because the stigma associated with HIV infection may be difficult to overcome. Adolescents with HIV should receive counseling on the risk of transmission through sexual activity and shared needles. Programs should be made available to encourage use of barrier protection and to develop strategies for disclosure to their partners and to other friends.

Horizontal transmission (ie, in the absence of sexual contact or injecting drug use) of HIV is exceedingly rare and is associated with exposure of broken skin or mucous membranes to HIV-infected blood or bloody secretions. Because undiagnosed HIV-infected infants and children might be enrolled, all schools and day care centers should have policies with simple guidelines for using universal precautions to prevent transmission of HIV infection in these settings. Saliva, tears, urine, and stool are not contagious if there is no gross blood in these fluids. A barrier protection (eg, latex or rubber gloves or thick pads of fabric or paper) should be used when possible contact with blood or bloody body fluids may occur. Objects that might be contaminated with blood, such as razors or toothbrushes, should not be shared. No special care is required for dishes, towels, toys, or bedclothes. Blood-soiled clothing may be washed routinely with hot water and detergent. Contaminated surfaces may be disinfected easily with a variety of agents, including household bleach (1:10 dilution), some commercial disinfectants (eg, Lysol), or 70% isopropyl alcohol.

Summary

Pediatric HIV infection is a complex and multifaceted disease. Many aspects of care are under intense investigation, and recommendations for clinical care change frequently. Updated information should be sought whenever a child is diagnosed with HIV infection. With recognition of the longer survival time in most infected children, this disease is now approached as a chronic illness. Many children, infected from birth, are entering adolescence and young adulthood. The complexity of antiretroviral drug therapy requires care from a provider with HIV expertise. Primary care physicians are encouraged to participate in the care of HIV-infected children in collaboration with centers staffed by personnel with expertise in pediatric HIV issues.

REFERENCES

Abrams EJ et al: Maternal health factors and early pediatric antiretroviral therapy influence the rate of perinatal HIV-1 disease progression in children. AIDS 2003;17(6):867 [PMID: 12660534].

American Academy of Pediatrics, Committee of Pediatric AIDS and Committee on Infectious Diseases: Issues related to human immunodeficiency virus transmission in schools, child care, medical settings, the home, and community. Pediatrics 1999;104(2 Pt 1):318 [PMID: 10429018].

Bulterys M et al, for the Mother-Infant Rapid Intervention at Delivery (MIRIAD) Study Group: Rapid HIV-1 testing during labor: A multicenter study. JAMA 2004;292:219 [PMID: 15249571].

Centers for Disease Control and Prevention: 1994 Revised classification system for human immunodeficiency virus infection in children less than 13 years of age. MMWR Morb Mortal Wkly Rep 1994;43(RR-12):1 [PMID: 7908403].

European Collaborative Study: Mother-to-child transmission of HIV infection in the era of highly active antiretroviral therapy. Clin Infect Dis 2005;40:458 [PMID: 15668871].

King SM and the Committee on Pediatric AIDS: Evaluation and treatment of the human immunodeficiency virus-1-exposed infant. Pediatrics 2004;114:497 [PMID: 15286240].

Leonard EG, McComsey GA: Metabolic complications of antiretroviral therapy in children. Pediatr Infect Dis J 2003;22(1):77 [PMID: 12544413].

Magder LS et al: Risk factors for in utero and intrapartum transmission of HIV. J Acquir Immune Defic Syndr 2005;38:87 [PMID: 15608531].

McConnell MS et al, for the Pediatric Spectrum of HIV Disease Consortium: Trends in antiretroviral therapy use and survival rates for a large cohort of HIV-infected children and adolescents in the United States, 1989–2001. J Acquir Immune Defic Syndr 2005;38:488 [15764966].

Mofenson L: Tale of two epidemics—the continuing challenge of preventing mother-to-child transmission of human immunodeficiency virus. J Infect Dis 2003;187:721 [PMID: 12599044].

Nesheim S et al: Quantitative RNA testing for diagnosis of HIV-infected infants. JAIDS 2003;32(2):192 [PMID: 12571529].

Panlilio AL et al: Updated U.S. Public Health Service guidelines for the management of occupational exposures to HIV and recommendations for postexposure prophylaxis. MMWR Morb Mortal Wkly Rep 2005;54(No. RR-9):1 [PMID: 16195697].

Perinatal HIV Guidelines Working Group: Public Health Service Task Force recommendations for the use of antiretroviral drugs in pregnant women infected with HIV-1 for maternal health and interventions to reduce perinatal HIV-1 transmission in the United States. http://www.aidsinfo.nih.gov/guidelines/

Smith DK et al: Antiretroviral postexposure prophylaxis after sexual, injection-drug use, or other nonoccupational exposure to HIV in the United States: Recommendations from the U.S. Department of Health and Human Services. MMWR Morb Mortal Wkly Rep 2005;54(No. RR-2):1 [PMID: 15660015].

The Working Group on Antiretroviral Therapy and Medical Management of HIV-Infected Children: Guidelines for the use of antiretroviral agents in pediatric HIV infection. http://www.aidsinfo.nih.gov/guidelines/

Infections: Bacterial & Spirochetal

38

John W. Ogle, MD, & Marsha S. Anderson, MD

▪ I. BACTERIAL INFECTIONS

GROUP A STREPTOCOCCAL INFECTIONS

ESSENTIALS OF DIAGNOSIS & TYPICAL FEATURES

Streptococcal pharyngitis:
- *Clinical diagnosis based entirely on symptoms; signs and physical examination unreliable.*
- *Throat culture or rapid antigen detection test positive for group A streptococci.*

Impetigo:
- *Rapidly spreading, highly infectious skin rash.*
- *Erythematous denuded areas and honey-colored crusts.*
- *On culture, group A streptococci are grown in most (not all) cases.*

General Considerations

Group A streptococci (GAS) are common gram-positive bacteria producing a wide variety of clinical illnesses, including acute pharyngitis, impetigo, cellulitis, and scarlet fever, the generalized illness caused by strains that elaborate erythrogenic toxin. GAS can also cause pneumonia, septic arthritis, osteomyelitis, meningitis, and other less common infections. GAS infections may also produce nonsuppurative sequelae (rheumatic fever and acute glomerulonephritis).

The cell walls of streptococci contain both carbohydrate and protein antigens. The C-carbohydrate antigen determines the group, and the M- or T-protein antigens determine the specific type. In most strains, the M protein appears to confer virulence, and antibodies developed against the M protein are protective against reinfection with that type.

GAS are almost all β-hemolytic. These organisms may be carried without symptoms on the skin and in the pharynx, rectum, and vagina. Between 10% and 15% of school-age children in some studies are asymptomatic pharyngeal carriers of GAS. Streptococcal carriers are individuals who do not mount an immune response to the organism and are therefore believed to be at low risk for nonsuppurative sequelae. All GAS are sensitive to penicillin. Resistance to erythromycin is common in some countries and has increased in the United States.

A. CLINICAL FINDINGS

1. Respiratory infections—
a. Infancy and early childhood (< age 3 years)— The onset is insidious, with mild symptoms (low-grade fever, serous nasal discharge, and pallor). Otitis media is common. Exudative pharyngitis and cervical adenitis are uncommon in this age group.

b. Childhood type— Onset is sudden, with fever and marked malaise and often with repeated vomiting. The pharynx is sore and edematous, and generally there is tonsillar exudate. Anterior cervical lymph nodes are tender and enlarged. Small petechiae are frequently seen on the soft palate. In scarlet fever, the skin is diffusely erythematous and appears sunburned and roughened (sandpaper rash). The rash is most intense in the axillae, groin, and on the abdomen and trunk. It blanches except in the skin folds, which do not blanch and are pigmented (Pastia's sign). The rash usually appears 24 hours after the onset of fever and rapidly spreads over the next 1–2 days. Desquamation begins on the face at the end of the first week and becomes generalized by the third week. Early in the course of infection, the surface of the tongue is coated white, with the papillae enlarged and bright red (so-called white strawberry tongue). Subsequently desquamation occurs, and the tongue appears beefy red (strawberry tongue). The face generally shows circumoral pallor. Petechiae may be seen on all mucosal surfaces.

c. Adult type— The adult type of GAS is characterized by exudative or nonexudative tonsillitis with fewer systemic symptoms, lower fever, and no vomiting. Scarlet fever is uncommon in adults.

2. Impetigo— Streptococcal impetigo begins as a papule that vesiculates and then breaks, leaving a denuded area covered by a honey-colored crust. Both *Staphylococcus aureus* and GAS are isolated in some cases. The lesions spread readily and diffusely. Local lymph nodes may become swollen and inflamed. Although the child often lacks systemic symptoms, a high fever and toxicity may be present. If flaccid bullae are noted, the disease is called bullous impetigo and is caused by an epidermolytic toxin-producing strain of *S aureus*.

3. Cellulitis—The portal of entry is often an insect bite or superficial abrasion. A diffuse, rapidly spreading cellulitis occurs that involves the subcutaneous tissues and extends along the lymphatic pathways with only minimal local suppuration. Local acute lymphadenitis occurs. The child is usually acutely ill, with fever and malaise. In classic erysipelas, the involved area is bright red, swollen, warm, and very tender. The infection may extend rapidly from the lymphatics to the bloodstream.

Streptococcal perianal cellulitis is an entity peculiar to young children. Pain with defecation often leads to constipation, which may be the presenting complaint. The child is afebrile and otherwise well. Perianal erythema, tenderness, and painful rectal examination are the only abnormal physical findings. Scant rectal bleeding with defecation may occur. A perianal swab culture usually yields heavy growth of GAS. A variant of this syndrome is streptococcal vaginitis in prepubertal girls. Symptoms are dysuria and pain; marked erythema and tenderness of the introitus and blood-tinged discharge are seen.

4. Necrotizing fasciitis—This dangerous disease is reported more frequently, particularly as a complication of varicella infection. About 20–40% of cases are due to GAS; 30–40% are due to *S aureus*; and the rest are a result of mixed bacterial infections. The disease is characterized by extensive necrosis of superficial fasciae, undermining of surrounding tissue, and usually systemic toxicity. Initially the skin overlying the infection is tender and pale red without distinct borders, resembling cellulitis. Blisters or bullae may appear. The color deepens to a distinct purple or in some cases becomes pale. Tenderness out of proportion to the clinical appearance, skin anesthesia (due to infarction of superficial nerves), or "woody" induration are worrisome for necrotizing fasciitis. Involved areas may develop mild to massive edema. Early recognition and aggressive debridement of necrotic tissue are essential.

5. Group A streptococcal infections in newborn nurseries—GAS epidemics occur occasionally in nurseries. The organism may be introduced into the nursery from the vaginal tract of a mother or from the throat or nose of a mother or a staff member. The organism then spreads from infant to infant. The umbilical stump is colonized while the infant is in the nursery. Like staphylococcal infections, there may be no or few clinical manifestations while the infant is still in the nursery. Most often, a colonized infant develops a chronic, oozing omphalitis days later. The organism may spread from the infant to other family members. Serious and even fatal infections may develop, including sepsis, meningitis, empyema, septic arthritis, and peritonitis.

6. Streptococcal sepsis—Serious illness from GAS sepsis is now more common both in children and in adults. Rash and scarlet fever may be present. Prostration and shock result in high mortality rates. Pharyngitis is uncommon as an antecedent illness. Underlying disease is a predisposing factor.

7. Streptococcal toxic shock syndrome (STSS)—Toxic shock syndrome caused by GAS has been defined. Like *S aureus* associated toxic shock, multiorgan system involvement is a prominent part of the illness. The diagnostic criteria include (1) isolation of GAS from a normally sterile site, (2) hypotension or shock, and (3) at least two of the following: renal impairment (creatinine > 2 times the upper limit of normal for age), thrombocytopenia (< 100,000/mm^3), or coagulopathy, liver involvement (transaminases > 2 times normal), acute respiratory distress syndrome, generalized erythematous macular rash or soft tissue necrosis (myositis, necrotizing fasciitis, gangrene). In cases that otherwise meet clinical criteria, isolation of GAS from a nonsterile site (throat, wound, or vagina) is indicative of a probable cause.

B. LABORATORY FINDINGS

Leukocytosis with a marked shift to the left is seen early. Eosinophilia regularly appears during convalescence. Beta-hemolytic streptococci are cultured from the throat. The organism may be cultured from the skin and by needle aspiration from subcutaneous tissues and other involved sites such as infected nodes. Occasionally blood cultures are positive. Newer rapid antigen detection tests such as optical immunoassays and DNA chemiluminescence probes are very specific, and in some cases are almost as sensitive as traditional throat culture. However, sensitivity varies with the type of test used and the experience level of the lab. Many experts recommend backup throat culture in patients with negative rapid strep antigen tests. Patients with positive rapid strep antigen tests do not need a confirmation by throat culture, since the specificity of antigen tests are high.

Antistreptolysin O (ASO) titers rise about 150 units within 2 weeks after acute infection. Elevated ASO and anti-DNase B titers are useful in documenting prior throat infections in cases of acute rheumatic fever. The streptozyme test detects antibodies to streptolysin O, hyaluronidase, streptokinase, DNase B, and NADase. It is somewhat more sensitive than the measurement of ASO titers.

Proteinuria, cylindruria, and minimal hematuria may be seen early in children with streptococcal infection. True poststreptococcal glomerulonephritis is seen 1–4 weeks after the respiratory or skin infection.

Differential Diagnosis

Streptococcal infection in early childhood must be differentiated from adenovirus and other respiratory virus infections. The pharyngitis in herpangina (coxsackie A viruses) is vesicular or ulcerative. Herpes simplex also causes ulcerative lesions, which most commonly involve the anterior pharynx, tongue, and gums. In infectious mononucleosis, the pharyngitis is also exudative, but splenomegaly and generalized adenopathy are typical, and laboratory findings are often diagnostic (atypical lymphocytes, elevated liver enzymes, and a positive heterophil or other serologic test for mononucleosis). Uncomplicated streptococcal pharyngitis improves within 24–48 hours if penicillin is given and by 72–96 hours without antimicrobials.

Group G and group C streptococci are uncommon causes of pharyngitis but have been implicated in epidemics of sore throat in college students. Acute rheumatic fever does not occur following group G or group C infection, although acute glomerulonephritis is a complication. *Arcanobacterium hemolyticum* may cause pharyngitis with scarlatina-like or maculopapular truncal rash. In diphtheria, systemic symptoms, vomiting, and fever are less marked; pharyngeal pseudomembrane is confluent and adherent; the throat is less red; and cervical adenopathy is prominent. Pharyngeal tularemia causes white rather than yellow exudate. There is little erythema, and cultures for β-hemolytic streptococci are negative. A history of exposure to rabbits and a failure to respond to antimicrobials may suggest the diagnosis. Leukemia and agranulocytosis may present with pharyngitis and are diagnosed by bone marrow examination.

Scarlet fever must be differentiated from other exanthematous diseases (principally rubella), erythema due to sunburn, drug reactions, Kawasaki disease, toxic shock syndrome, and staphylococcal scalded skin syndrome (see also Table 36–3).

Complications

Suppurative complications of GAS infections include sinusitis, otitis, mastoiditis, cervical lymphadenitis, pneumonia, empyema, septic arthritis, and meningitis. Spread of streptococcal infection from the throat to other sites—principally the skin (impetigo) and vagina—is common and should be considered in every instance of chronic vaginal discharge or chronic skin infection, such as that complicating childhood eczema. Both acute rheumatic fever and acute glomerulonephritis are nonsuppurative complications of GAS infections.

A. ACUTE RHEUMATIC FEVER (SEE CHAPTER 19.)

B. ACUTE GLOMERULONEPHRITIS

Acute glomerulonephritis (AGN) can follow streptococcal infections of either the pharynx or the skin—in contrast to rheumatic fever, which follows pharyngeal infection only. AGN may occur at any age, even infancy. In most reports of AGN, males predominate by a ratio of 2:1. Rheumatic fever occurs with equal frequency in both sexes. Certain M types are associated strongly with post-

streptococcal glomerulonephritis (nephritogenic types). The serotypes producing disease on the skin often differ from those found in the pharynx.

The incidence of AGN after streptococcal infection is variable and has ranged from 0–28%. Several outbreaks of AGN in families have involved 50–75% of siblings of affected patients in 1- to 7-week periods. Second attacks of glomerulonephritis are rare. The median period between infection and the development of glomerulonephritis is 10 days. In contrast, acute rheumatic fever occurs after a median of 18 days.

Treatment

A. SPECIFIC MEASURES

Treatment is directed toward both eradication of acute infection and prevention of rheumatic fever. In patients with pharyngitis, antibiotics should be started early to relieve symptoms and should be continued for 10 days to prevent rheumatic fever. Although early therapy has not been shown to prevent AGN, it seems advisable to treat impetigo promptly in sibling contacts of patients with poststreptococcal nephritis. Neither sulfonamides nor trimethoprim–sulfamethoxazole is effective in the treatment of streptococcal infections. Although topical therapy for impetigo with antimicrobial ointments (especially mupirocin) is as effective as systemic therapy, it does not eradicate pharyngeal carriage and is less practical for extensive disease.

1. Penicillin—Except for penicillin-allergic patients, penicillin V (phenoxymethyl penicillin) is the drug of choice. Penicillin resistance has never been documented. For children weighing less than 27 kg, the regimen is 250 mg, given orally two or three times a day for 10 days. For heavier children, adolescents, or adults 500 mg two or three times a day is recommended. Giving penicillin V (250 mg) twice daily is as effective as more frequent oral administration or intramuscular therapy. Another alternative for treatment of pharyngitis and impetigo is a single dose of benzathine penicillin G, given intramuscularly (0.6 million units for children weighing < 60 lb [27.2 kg] and 1.2 million units for children weighing > 60 lb [27.2 kg]). Intramuscular delivery ensures compliance, but is painful. Parenteral therapy is indicated if vomiting or sepsis is present. Mild cellulitis due to GAS may be treated orally or intramuscularly.

Cellulitis requiring hospitalization can be treated with aqueous penicillin G (150,000 units/kg/d, given intravenously in four to six divided doses) or cefazolin (80–100 mg/kg/day, given intravenously in three divided doses) until there is marked improvement. Penicillin V (50 mg/kg/day in four divided doses) or cephalexin (50–75 mg/kg/day in four divided doses), may then be given orally to complete a 10-day course. Acute cervical lymphadenitis may require incision and drainage. Treatment of necrotizing fasciitis requires emergency surgical debridement followed by high-dose parenteral antibiotics appropriate to the organisms cultured.

2. Other antibiotics—For penicillin-allergic patients with pharyngitis or impetigo the following alternative regimens have been used: erythromycin estolate (20–40 mg/kg/d in two to four divided doses) for 10 days; clarithromycin (15 mg/kg/d in two divided doses) for 10 days; and azithromycin (12 mg/kg/d) once daily for 5 days. Erythromycin resistance, although not currently widespread in the United States, was reported in 48% of strains tested in Pittsburgh in 2001. Penicillin-allergic patients from areas with high rates of erythromycin resistance may require an alternative antibiotic. Clindamycin, cephalexin, ceftibuten, cefdinir, and cefadroxil are other effective oral antimicrobials. The dosage of clindamycin is 10–20 mg/kg/d orally in four divided doses. Each of these drugs should be given for 10 days. Patients with immediate, anaphylactic hypersensitivity to penicillin should not receive cephalosporins, because up to 15% will also be allergic to cephalosporins. In most studies, bacteriologic failures after cephalosporin therapy are less frequent than failures following penicillin. However, cephalosporins are more expensive than penicillin. Additionally, there are few conclusive data on the ability of these agents to prevent rheumatic fever. Therefore, penicillin remains the agent of choice for nonallergic patients. Many strains are resistant to tetracycline.

For infections requiring intravenous therapy, aqueous penicillin G (250,000 units/kg in six divided doses) given intravenously is usually the drug of choice. Cefazolin (100–150 mg/kg/d intravenously or intramuscularly in three divided doses); clindamycin (25–40 mg/kg/d intravenously in four divided doses); and vancomycin (40 mg/kg/d intravenously in four divided doses) are alternatives in penicillin-allergic patients. Clindamycin is preferred by many and may be superior to penicillin for necrotizing fasciitis. Clindamycin should not be used alone empirically for severe, suspected GAS infections because a small percentage of isolates in the United States are resistant to it. Some physicians use both penicillin and clindamycin in patients with STSS.

3. Serious GAS disease—Serious GAS infections, such as pneumonia, osteomyelitis, septic arthritis, sepsis, endocarditis, meningitis, and STSS, require parenteral antimicrobial therapy. Penicillin G is the drug of choice for these invasive infections. Clindamycin, in addition to penicillin G, is advocated by many experts for STSS or necrotizing fasciitis. Necrotizing fasciitis requires prompt surgical debridement. Patients with STSS need attention given to volume status and blood pressure and evaluation for a focus of infection, if not readily apparent. Intravenous immune globulin (in addition to antibiotics) has been used in severe cases.

4. Treatment failure—Even when compliance is perfect, organisms will be found cultures in 5–15% of children after cessation of therapy. Reculture is indicated only in the patient with relapse or recrudescence of pharyngitis or if the patient has a personal or family history of rheumatic fever. Repeat treatment at least once with an oral cephalosporin or clindamycin is indicated in patients with recurrent culture-positive pharyngitis.

5. Prevention of recurrences in rheumatic individuals—The preferred prophylaxis for rheumatic individuals is benzathine penicillin G, 1.2 million units intramuscularly every 4 weeks. If the risk of streptococcal exposure is high, every 3 week dosing is preferred. One of the following alternative oral prophylactic regimens may be used: sulfadiazine, 0.5 g (if < 27 kg) or 1 g (if > 27 kg)/d; penicillin V, 200,000 units twice daily; or erythromycin, 250 mg twice daily. Prophylaxis is continued for at least 5 years or until age 21 years (whichever is longer) if carditis is absent. Prophylaxis in these individuals should be continued if the risk of contact with persons with GAS is high (eg, parents of school-age children, pediatric nurses, and teachers). In the presence of carditis without residual heart or valvular disease, a minimum of 10 years (or well into adulthood, whichever is longer) is the minimum duration. If the patient has residual valvular heart disease, many recommend lifelong prophylaxis. These patients should be at least 10 years from their last episode of rheumatic disease and at least 40 years of age prior to considering discontinuation of prophylaxis. A similar approach to the prevention of recurrences of glomerulonephritis may be indicated during childhood when there is a suspicion that repeated streptococcal infections coincide with flare-ups of glomerulonephritis.

B. General Measures

Acetaminophen is useful for pain or fever. Local treatment of impetigo may promote earlier healing. Crusts should first be soaked off. Areas beneath the crusts should then be washed with soap daily.

C. Treatment of Complications

Rheumatic fever is best prevented by early and adequate penicillin treatment of the streptococcal infection.

D. Treatment of Carriers

Identification and treatment of GAS carriers is difficult. There are no established clinical or serologic criteria for differentiating carriers from the truly infected. Some children receive multiple courses of antimicrobials, with persistence of GAS in the throat, leading to a "streptococcal neurosis" on the part of families.

In certain circumstances, eradication of carriage may be desirable: (1) when a family member has a history of rheumatic fever; (2) when an episode of GAS toxic shock syndrome or necrotizing fasciitis has occurred in a household contact; (3) multiple, recurring, documented episodes of

GAS in family members despite adequate therapy; and (4) during an outbreak of rheumatic fever or GAS-associated glomerulonephritis. Clindamycin (20 mg/kg/d, given orally in three divided doses, to a maximum of 1.8 g/d) or a combination of rifampin (20 mg/kg/d, given orally for 4 days) and penicillin in standard dosage given orally has been used to attempt eradication of carriage.

Prognosis

Death is rare except in infants or young children with sepsis or pneumonia. The febrile course is shortened and complications eliminated by early and adequate treatment with penicillin.

Bisno AL et al: Practice guidelines for the diagnosis and management of group A streptococcal pharyngitis. Infectious Diseases Society of America. Clin Infect Dis 2002;35:113 [PMID: 12087516].

Gieseker K et al: Evaluating the American Academy of Pediatric diagnostic standard for *Streptococcus pyogenes* pharyngitis: Backup culture versus repeat rapid antigen testing. Pediatrics 2003; 111:e666 [PMID: 12777583].

Vincent MT, Celestin M, Hussain AN: Pharyngitis. Am Fam Physician 2004;69:1465 [PMID: 15053411].

Vinh DC, Embil JM: Rapidly progressive soft tissue infections. Lancet Infect Dis 2005;5:501 [PMID: 16048719].

The Working Group on Severe Streptococcal Infections: Defining the group A streptococcal toxic shock syndrome: Rationale and consensus definition. JAMA 1993;269:390 [PMID: 8418347].

GROUP B STREPTOCOCCAL INFECTIONS

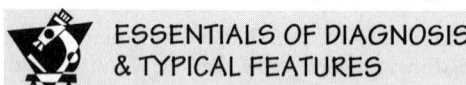

ESSENTIALS OF DIAGNOSIS & TYPICAL FEATURES

Early-onset neonatal infection:

- *Newborn younger than age 7 days, with rapidly progressing overwhelming sepsis, with or without meningitis.*
- *Pneumonia with respiratory failure frequently present; chest radiograph resembles that seen in hyaline membrane disease.*
- *Leukopenia with a shift to the left.*
- *Blood or cerebrospinal fluid (CSF) cultures growing group B streptococci.*

Late-onset infection:

- *Meningitis, sepsis, or other focal infection in a child age 1–16 weeks with blood or CSF cultures growing group B streptococci.*

General Considerations

The incidence of perinatal group B streptococci (GBS) disease has declined dramatically since screening of pregnant mothers and provision of intrapartum chemoprophylaxis began. However, neonatal infections due to GBS still occur. Although most patients with GBS disease are infants younger than age 3 months, cases are seen in infants age 4–5 months. Serious infection also occurs in women with puerperal sepsis, immunocompromised patients, patients with cirrhosis and spontaneous peritonitis, and diabetic patients with cellulitis. GBS infections occur as frequently as gram-negative infections in the newborn period. Two distinct clinical syndromes distinguished by differing perinatal events, age at onset, and serotype of the infecting strain occur in these infants.

Risk factors for early-onset group GBS disease include maternal GBS colonization, gestational age less than 37 weeks, rupture of membranes more than 18 hours prior to presentation, young maternal age, African American ethnicity, and low or absent maternal GBS anticapsular antibodies.

Clinical Findings

Early-onset illness is observed in newborns younger than 7 days old. The onset of symptoms in the majority of these infants occurs in the first 48 hours of life, and most are ill within 6 hours. Apnea is often the first sign. Sepsis, meningitis, apnea, and pneumonia are the most common clinical presentations. There is a high incidence of associated maternal obstetric complications, especially premature labor and prolonged rupture of the membranes. Newborns with early-onset disease are severely ill at the time of diagnosis, and more than 50% die. Although most infants with early-onset infections are full-term, premature infants are at increased risk for the disease. Newborns with early-onset infection acquire GBS in utero as an ascending infection or during passage through the birth canal. When early-onset infection is complicated by meningitis, more than 80% of the bacterial isolates belong to serotype III. Postmortem examination of infants with early-onset disease usually reveals pulmonary inflammatory infiltrates and hyaline membranes containing large numbers of GBS.

Late-onset infection occurs in infants between ages 7 days and 4 months (median age at onset, about 4 weeks). Maternal obstetric complications are not usually associated with late-onset infection. These infants are usually not as ill at the time of diagnosis as those with early-onset disease, and the mortality rate is lower. In recent series, about 37% of patients have meningitis and 46% have sepsis. Septic arthritis and osteomyelitis, meningitis, occult bacteremia, otitis media, ethmoiditis, conjunctivitis, cellulitis (particularly of the face or submandibular area), lymphadenitis, breast abscess, empyema, and impetigo have been described. Strains of GBS possessing the capsular type III polysaccharide antigen are isolated from more than 95% of infants with late-onset disease, regardless of clinical manifestations. The exact mode of transmission of the organisms is not well defined.

Diagnosis

Culture of GBS from a normally sterile site such as blood, pleural fluid, or cerebrospinal fluid (CSF) provides proof of diagnosis. Frequent false-positive results limit the usefulness of testing for GBS antigen in urine and CSF.

Prevention

Many women of childbearing age possess type-specific circulating antibody to the polysaccharide antigens for GBS. These antibodies are transferred to the newborn via the placental circulation. Carriers delivering healthy infants have significant serum levels of IgG antibody to this antigen. In contrast, women delivering infants who develop either early- or late-onset GBS disease rarely have detectable antibody in their sera.

Monovalent and bivalent vaccines with type II or III polysaccharide antigens have been studied in pregnant women, with 80–90% of vaccine recipients developing fourfold or greater increases in GBS capsular polysaccharide type-specific IgG. These reports are encouraging that a multivalent vaccine could be developed and given to pregnant women to prevent many cases of early-onset GBS disease.

The Centers for Disease Control and Prevention (CDC) has issued culture-based maternal guidelines for the prevention of early-onset GBS disease.

CDC Recommendations for Prevention of Perinatal GBS Disease

- All pregnant women should be screened at 35–37 weeks' gestation with a vaginal and rectal culture for GBS.

  Exceptions: Women with known GBS bacteriuria during the current pregnancy or women who have delivered a previous infant with GBS disease do not need screening—all these women need intrapartum prophylaxis.

- If GBS status is unknown at onset of labor or rupture of membranes, intrapartum chemoprophylaxis should be administered to women with any of the following:

  Gestation less than 37 weeks.

  Rupture of membranes more than 18 hours.

  Intrapartum temperature of greater than 38 °C (> 100.4 °F)

- Women with GBS colonization and a planned cesarean delivery done prior to labor and rupture of membranes do not routinely need intrapartum antibiotics (IAP).
- IAP recommendations (Table 38–1).
- Empiric treatment of a neonate whose mother received IAP for prevention of GBS (Figure 38–1).

Treatment of GBS Disease

Intravenous ampicillin and an aminoglycoside is the initial regimen of choice for newborns with presumptive invasive GBS disease. For neonates younger than 7 days of age with meningitis, the recommended ampicillin dosage is 200–300 mg/kg/d, given intravenously in three divided doses. For infants older than 7 days of age, the recommended ampicillin dosage is 300 mg/kg/d, given intravenously in four to six divided doses. Penicillin G can be used once GBS is identified and clinical and microbiologic responses have occurred. GBS are less susceptible than other streptococci to penicillin, and high doses are recommended, especially for meningitis. In infants with meningitis, the recommended dosage of penicillin G varies with age: for infants age 7 days or younger, 250,000–450,000 units/kg/d, given intravenously in three divided doses; for infants older than age 7 days, 450,000–500,000 units/kg/d, given intravenously in four to six divided doses.

A second lumbar puncture after 24–48 hours of therapy is recommended by some experts to assess efficacy. Duration of therapy is 2–3 weeks for meningitis; at least 4 weeks for osteomyelitis, cerebritis, ventriculitis, or endocarditis; and 10–14 days for most other infections. Therapy does not eradicate carriage of the organism. Ceftriaxone is active in vitro against GBS, and because of its long serum half-life it may be given once or twice daily intramuscularly or intravenously.

Ceftriaxone is sometimes used to complete a course of therapy when intravenous access has become difficult. Ceftriaxone is usually not used in newborns because of associated cholestasis.

Although streptococci have been universally susceptible to penicillins, increasing minimum inhibitory concentrations (MICs) have been observed in some isolates. In one U.S. study, 10 of 574 rectovaginal isolates obtained from pregnant women in South Carolina were not fully penicillin-susceptible. However, all isolates were vancomycin-susceptible. Resistance of isolates to clindamycin and erythromycin has increased significantly worldwide in the past few years.

Apgar BS, Greenberg G: Prevention of group B streptococcal disease in the newborn. Am Fam Physician 2005;71(5):903 [PMID: 15768620].

Baker CJ et al: Safety and immunogenicity of a bivalent group B streptococcal conjugate vaccine for serotypes II and III. J Infect Dis 2003;188(1):66 [PMID: 22708435].

Table 38–1. Centers for Disease Control and Prevention (CDC) recommended regimens for intrapartum prophylaxis for perinatal group B streptococcal (GBS) disease.[a]

Recommended	Penicillin G, 5 million units IV initial dose, then 2.5 million units IV q4h until delivery
Alternative	Ampicillin, 2 g IV initial dose, then 1 g IV q4h until delivery
If penicillin allergic[b]	
Patients not at high risk for anaphylaxis	Cefazolin, 2 g IV initial dose, then 1 g IV q8h until delivery
Patients at high risk for anaphylax[c]	
GBS susceptible to clindamycin and erythromycin[d]	Clindamycin, 900 mg IV q8h until delivery OR Erythromycin, 500 mg IV q6h until delivery
GBS resistant to clindamycin or erythromycin or susceptibility unknown	Vancomycin,[e] 1 g IV q12h until delivery

[a]Broader-spectrum agents, including an agent active against GBS, may be necessary for treatment of chorioamnionitis.
[b]History of penicillin allergy should be assessed to determine whether a high risk for anaphylaxis is present. Penicillin-allergic patients at high risk for anapylaxis are those who have experienced immediate hypersensitivity to penicillin including a history of penicillin-related anaphylaxis; other high-risk patients are those with asthma or other diseases that would make anaphylaxis more dangerous or difficult to treat, such as persons being treated with β-adrenergic-blocking agents.
[c]If laboratory facilities are adequate, clindamycin and erythromycin susceptibility testing should be performed on prenatal GBS isolates from penicillin allergic women at high risk for anaphylaxis.
[d]Resistance to erythromycin is often but not always associated with clindamycin resistance. If a strain is resistant to erythromycin but appears susceptible to clindamycin, it may have inducible resistance to clindamycin.
[e]Cefazolin is preferred over vancomycin for women with a history of penicillin allergy other than immediate hypersensitivity reactions, and pharmacologic data suggest it achieves effective intra-amniotic concentrations. Vancomycin should be reserved for penicillin-allergic women at high risk for anaphylaxis.
Reprinted, with permission, from Schrag S et al: Prevention of perinatal Group B streptococcal disease, revised guidelines from CDC. MMWR 2002;51(RR11);1.

Centers for Disease Control and Prevention: Prevention of perinatal group B streptococcal disease: Revised recommendations from CDC. MMWR Morb Mortal Wkly Rep 2002;51(No. RR-11).

Daley AJ, Garland SM: Prevention of neonatal group B streptococcal disease: Progress, challenges and dilemmas. J Paediatr Child Health 2004;40(12):664 [PMID: 15569279].

Schrag SJ et al: Group B streptococcal disease in the era of intrapartum antibiotic prophylaxis. N Engl J Med 2000;342:15 [PMID: 10620644].

STREPTOCOCCAL INFECTIONS WITH ORGANISMS OTHER THAN GROUP A OR B

Streptococci of groups other than A and B are part of the normal flora of humans and can occasionally cause disease. Group C or group G organisms occasionally produce pharyngitis (with an ASO rise) but without risk of subsequent rheumatic fever. AGN may occasionally occur. Group D streptococci and *Enterococcus* species are normal inhabitants of the gastrointestinal tract and may produce urinary tract infections, meningitis, and sepsis in the newborn, as well as endocarditis. Nosocomial infections caused by *Enterococcus* are frequent in neonatal and oncology units and in patients with central venous catheters. Nonhemolytic aerobic streptococci and β-hemolytic streptococci are normal flora of the mouth. They are involved in the production of dental plaque and probably dental caries and are the most common cause of subacute infective endocarditis. Finally, there are numerous anaerobic and microaerophilic streptococci, normal flora of the mouth, skin, and gastrointestinal tract, which alone or in combination with other bacteria may cause sinusitis, dental abscesses, brain abscesses, and intra-abdominal or lung abscesses.

Treatment

A. ENTEROCOCCAL INFECTIONS

E faecalis and *E faecium* are the two most common and most important strains causing human infections. In general, *E faecalis* is more susceptible to antibiotics than *E faecium*, but antibiotic resistance is commonly seen in both species.

1. Infections with ampicillin-susceptible enterococci—Lower tract urinary infections can be treated with oral amoxicillin. Pyelonephritis should be treated intravenously with ampicillin and gentamicin (gentamicin dosing may need to be adjusted for altered renal function). Sepsis or meningitis in the newborn should be treated intravenously with a combination of ampicillin (100–200 mg/kg/d in three divided doses) and gentamicin (3 mg/kg/d in three divided doses). Peak serum gentamicin levels of 3–5 μg/mL are adequate as gen-

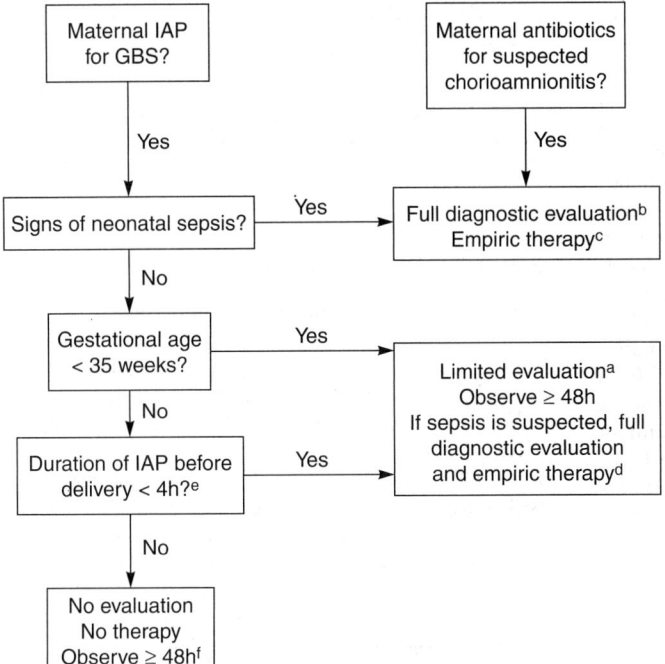

Figure 38–1. Algorithm for treatment of a newborn whose mother received intrapartum antimicrobial prophylaxis for prevention of GBS or suspected chorioamnionitis. This algorithm is not an exclusive course of management. Variations that incorporate individual circumstance or institutional preferences may be appropriate. (Reproduced, with permission, from Schrag S et al: Prevention of perinatal group B streptococcal disease, revised guidelines from CDC. MMWR Morb Mortal Wkly Rep 2002;51(RR11):1.)

[a] If no maternal intrapartum prophylaxis for GBS was administered despite an indication being present. data are insufficient on which to recommend a single management strategy.

[b] Includes complete blood cell count and differential, blood culture, and chest radiograph if respiratory abnormalities are present. When signs of sepsis are present, a lumbar puncture, if feasible, should be performed.

[c] Duration of therapy varies depending on results of blood culture, cerebrospinal fluid findings, if obtained, and the clinical course of the infant. If laboratory results and clinical course do not indicate bacterial infection, duration may be as short as 48 h.

[d] CBC with differential and blood culture.

[e] Applies only to penicillin, ampicillin, or celazoin and assumes recommended dosing regimens.

[f] A healthy-appearing infant who was 38 weeks gestation at delivery and whose mother received 4 h of intrapartum prophylaxis before delivery may be discharged home after 24 h if other discharge criteria have been met and a person able to comply fully with instructions for home observation will be present. If any one of these conditions is not met, the infant should be observed in the hospital for at least 48 h and until criteria for discharge are achieved.

tamicin is used as a synergistic agent. Endocarditis requires 4–6 weeks of intravenous treatment. Penicillin G (250,000 units/kg/d in six to eight divided doses) plus gentamicin (3 mg/kg/d in three divided doses) is most often used. Cephalosporins are not effective.

2. Infections with ampicillin-resistant or vancomycin-resistant enterococci—Ampicillin-resistant enterococci are often susceptible to vancomycin (40–60 mg/kg/d in four divided doses). Vancomycin-resistant enterococci are usually also resistant to ampicillin. Two agents are effective against vancomycin-resistant enterococci and approved for use in adults. Quinupristin/dalfopristin (Synercid) has been approved for infections with vancomycin-resistant *E faecium* (not effective against *E faeca-*

lis). Linezolid (Zyvox) is approved for vancomycin-resistant *E faecalis* and *E faecium* infections. Both agents are bacteriostatic against enterococci. Isolates resistant to these newer agents have been reported. Infectious disease consultation is recommended when use of these drugs is entertained or when vancomycin-resistant enterococcal infections are identified.

B. VIRIDANS STREPTOCOCCAL INFECTIONS (SUBACUTE INFECTIVE ENDOCARDITIS)

It is important to determine the penicillin sensitivity of the infecting strain as early as possible in the treatment of viridans streptococcal endocarditis. Resistant organisms are most commonly seen in patients receiving penicillin prophylaxis for rheumatic heart disease. Strains sensitive to penicillin G (MIC < 0.1 µg/mL) may be treated for 4 weeks with penicillin, 150,000–200,000 units/kg/d intravenously, with gentamicin (lower "synergy" dose of 1 mg/kg/dose every 8 hours in patients with normal renal function) added during the first 2 weeks. There is considerable experience with 2-week therapy in adult patients using penicillin and gentamicin. Similarly, excellent results have been obtained with ceftriaxone once daily for 4 weeks. If the MIC is 0.5 µg/mL or higher, longer therapy and higher doses of penicillin G must be used (200,000–300,000 units/kg/d intravenously in combination with gentamicin for 4–6 weeks). If the MIC is 0.1–0.5 µg/mL, penicillin G at the higher dose for a minimum of 4 weeks is recommended, with gentamicin added for the first 2 weeks. Vancomycin, 40 mg/kg/d, is usually preferred for resistant strains and patients allergic to penicillin.

Das I, Gray J: Enterococcal bacteremia in children: A review of seventy five episodes in a pediatric hospital. Pediatr Infect Dis J 1998;17:1154 [PMID: 9877366].

Giessel BE, Koenig CJ, Blake RL: Management of bacterial endocarditis. Am Fam Physician 2000;61(6):1725 [PMID: 1075-879].

Mutnick AH, Jones RN: Linezolid resistance since 2001: SENTRY Anticmibrobial Surveillance Program. Ann Pharmac 2003;37 (6):909 [PMID: 12773084].

Torres-Viera C, Embry LM: Approaches to vancomycin resistant enterococci. Curr Opin Infect Dis 2004;17(6):541 [PMID: 15640708].

Wilson WR et al: Antibiotic treatment of adults with infective endocarditis due to streptococci, enterococci, staphylococci, and HACEK microorganisms. JAMA 1995;274:1706 [PMID: 7474277].

PNEUMOCOCCAL INFECTIONS

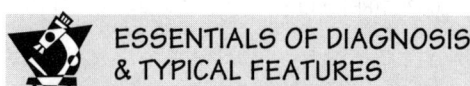

ESSENTIALS OF DIAGNOSIS & TYPICAL FEATURES

Bacteremia:
- *High fever (> 39.4 °C).*
- *Leukocytosis (> 15,000/µL).*
- *Age 6–24 months.*

Pneumonia:
- *Fever, leukocytosis, and tachypnea.*
- *Localized chest pain.*
- *Localized or diffuse rales. Chest radiograph may show lobar infiltrate (with effusion).*

Meningitis:
- *Fever, leukocytosis.*
- *Bulging fontanelle, neck stiffness.*
- *Irritability and lethargy.*

All types:
- *Diagnosis confirmed by cultures of blood, CSF, pleural fluid, or other body fluid.*

General Considerations

Sepsis, sinusitis, otitis media, pneumonitis, meningitis, osteomyelitis, cellulitis, arthritis, vaginitis, and peritonitis are all part of a spectrum of pneumococcal infection. Clinical findings that correlate with occult bacteremia in ambulatory patients include age (6–24 months), degree of temperature elevation (> 39.4 °C), and leukocytosis (> 15,000/µL). Although each of these findings is in itself nonspecific, a combination of them should arouse suspicion. This constellation of findings in a child who has no focus of infection may be an indication for blood cultures and antibiotic therapy. The cause of most of such bacteremic episodes is pneumococci.

Streptococcus pneumoniae is a common cause of acute purulent otitis media and is the organism responsible for most cases of acute bacterial pneumonia in children. The disease is indistinguishable on clinical grounds from other bacterial pneumonias. Effusions are common, although frank empyema is less common. Abscesses also occasionally occur.

Pneumococcal meningitis is still more common than *Haemophilus influenzae* type b meningitis. Pneumococcal meningitis, sometimes recurrent, may complicate serious head trauma, particularly if there is persistent leakage of CSF. This has led some physicians to recommend the prophylactic administration of penicillin or other antimicrobials in such cases.

Children with sickle cell disease, other hemoglobinopathies, congenital or acquired asplenia, and some immunoglobulin and complement deficiencies are unusually susceptible to pneumococcal sepsis and meningitis. These children often have a catastrophic illness with shock and disseminated intravascular coagulation (DIC). Even with excellent supportive care, the mortality rate is 20–50%. The spleen is important in the control of pneumococcal infection by clearing organisms from the blood and producing an opsonin that enhances phagocytosis. Autosplenectomy may explain why children with sickle cell disease are at increased risk for developing serious pneumococcal infections. Children with cochlear implants are at higher risk for pneumococcal meningitis. Children who have, or who are planning to receive, a cochlear implant should receive age-appropriate pneumococcal vaccination (> 2 weeks prior to surgery if possible).

S pneumoniae rarely causes serious disease in the neonate. Although *S pneumoniae* does not normally colonize the vagina, transient colonization does occur. Serious neonatal disease—including pneumonia, sepsis, and meningitis—may occur and clinically is similar to GBS infection.

Since being introduced in clinical medicine, penicillin has been the agent of choice for pneumococcal infections. Many strains are still highly susceptible to penicillin, and in those cases, penicillin is still the drug of choice. However, pneumococci with moderately increased resistance to penicillin are found in most communities, and reports of treatment failure, particularly in meningitis, are common. The prevalence of these relatively penicillin-resistant strains in North America varies geographically. Pneumococci with high-level resistance to penicillin and multiple other drugs are increasingly encountered throughout the United States. Pneumococci from normally sterile body fluids should be routinely tested for susceptibility to penicillin as well as other drugs.

Pneumococci have been classified into 90 serotypes based on capsular polysaccharide antigens. The frequency distribution of serotypes varies at different times, in different geographic areas, and with different sites of infection. Serotypes 4, 6B, 9V, 14, 18C, 19F, and 23F cause about 80–85% of invasive pneumococcal infections in young children. Similar serotypes—6B, 9V, 14, 19A, 19F, and 23F—are responsible for most of the penicillin-resistant isolates. A protein conjugate pneumococcal vaccine (Prevnar) is available for immunization of young children. It includes polysaccharide or oligosaccharide of seven different S pneumoniae serotypes conjugated to a protein carrier. The serotypes in the vaccine cause the bulk of pediatric invasive pneumococcal disease. The development of this vaccine is important in the prevention of pneumococcal disease because young children (< age 2 years), who are most at risk for the disease, are unable to immunologically mount a predictable response to the 23-valent polysaccharide vaccine. This vaccine is discussed further in Chapter 9. For older children and adults, the 23-valent pneumococcal vaccine is generally recommended.

Clinical Findings

A. SYMPTOMS AND SIGNS

In pneumococcal sepsis, fever usually appears abruptly, often accompanied by chills. There may be no respiratory symptoms. In pneumococcal sinusitis, mucopurulent nasal discharge may occur. In infants and young children with pneumonia, fever and tachypnea without auscultatory changes are the usual presenting signs. Respiratory distress is manifested by nasal flaring, chest retractions, and tachypnea. Abdominal pain is common. In older children, the adult form of pneumococcal pneumonia with signs of lobar consolidation may occur, but sputum is rarely bloody. Thoracic pain (from pleural involvement) is sometimes present, but is less common in children. With involvement of the right hemidiaphragm, pain may be referred to the right lower quadrant, suggesting appendicitis. Vomiting is common at onset but seldom persists. Convulsions are relatively common at onset in infants.

Meningitis is characterized by fever, irritability, convulsions, and neck stiffness. The most important sign in very young infants is a tense, bulging anterior fontanelle. In older children, fever, chills, headache, and vomiting are common symptoms. Classic signs are nuchal rigidity associated with positive Brudzinski and Kernig signs. With progression of untreated disease, the child may develop opisthotonos, stupor, and coma.

B. LABORATORY FINDINGS

Leukocytosis is often pronounced (20,000–45,000/μL), with 80–90% polymorphonuclear neutrophils. Neutropenia may be seen early in very serious infections. The presence of pneumococci in the nasopharynx is not a helpful finding, because up to 40% of normal children carry pneumococci in the upper respiratory tract. Large numbers of organisms are seen on Gram-stained smears of endotracheal aspirates from patients with pneumonia. In meningitis, CSF usually shows an elevated white blood cell (WBC) count of several thousand, chiefly polymorphonuclear neutrophils, with decreased glucose and elevated protein levels. Gram-positive diplococci may be seen on some (but not all) stained smears of CSF sediment. Antigen detection tests are not useful.

Differential Diagnosis

There are many causes of high fever and leukocytosis in young infants; 90% of children presenting with these features have a disease other than pneumococcal bacteremia such as herpesvirus 6, enterovirus, or other viral infection; urinary tract infection; unrecognized focal infection elsewhere in the body; or early acute shigellosis.

Infants with upper respiratory tract infection who subsequently develop signs of lower respiratory disease are most likely to be infected with a respiratory virus. Hoarseness or wheezing is often present. A radiograph of the chest typically shows perihilar infiltrates and increased bronchovascular markings. Viral respiratory infection often precedes pneumococcal pneumonia; therefore, the clinical picture may be mixed.

Staphylococcal pneumonia may be indistinguishable early in its course from pneumococcal pneumonia. Later, pulmonary cavitation and empyema occur. Staphylococcal pneumonia is most common in infants.

In primary pulmonary tuberculosis, children do not have a toxic appearance, and radiographs show a primary focus associated with hilar adenopathy and often with pleural involvement. Miliary tuberculosis presents a classic radiographic appearance.

Pneumonia caused by *Mycoplasma pneumoniae* is most common in children age 5 years and older. Onset is insidious, with infrequent chills, low-grade fever, prominent headache and malaise, cough, and, often, striking radiographic changes. Marked leukocytosis (> 18,000/μL) is unusual.

Pneumococcal meningitis is diagnosed by lumbar puncture. Without a Gram-stained smear and culture of CSF, it is not distinguishable from other types of acute bacterial meningitis.

Complications

Complications of sepsis include meningitis and osteomyelitis; complications of pneumonia include empyema, parapneumonic effusion, and, rarely, lung abscess. Mastoiditis, subdural empyema, and brain abscess may follow untreated pneumococcal otitis media. Both pneumococcal meningitis and peritonitis are more likely to occur independently without coexisting pneumonia. Shock, DIC, and Waterhouse–Friderichsen syndrome resembling meningococcemia are occasionally seen in pneumococcal sepsis, particularly in asplenic patients. Hemolytic–uremic syndrome may occur as a complication of pneumococcal pneumonia or sepsis.

Treatment

A. SPECIFIC MEASURES

All *S pneumoniae* isolated from normally sterile sites should be tested for susceptibility to penicillin. Susceptible strains can be treated with penicillin, ampicillin, or amoxicillin. Penicillin-intermediate or penicillin-resistant strains should be tested for susceptibility to cephalosporins, vancomycin, and selected other drugs. Therapy with penicillin, amoxicillin, or cephalosporins will usually succeed in cases of bacteremia or pneumonia due to intermediate-resistant isolates because serum levels in excess of the MIC can be achieved. Therapy of meningitis, empyema, osteomyelitis, and endocarditis due to nonsusceptible *S pneumoniae* is more difficult, because penetration of antimicrobials to these sites is limited. Vancomycin and third-generation cephalosporins are indicated in these and other serious or life-threatening infections pending susceptibility test results.

1. Bacteremia—In studies done prior to immunization of young children with conjugated pneumococcal vaccine, 3–5% of blood cultures in patients younger than 2 years of age yielded *S pneumoniae*. These percentages are expected to decrease now that an effective vaccine is available. However, pneumococcal disease will not disappear, as the vaccine prevents only 85% of invasive disease. Many experts treat suspected bacteremia with ceftriaxone (50 mg/kg, given intramuscularly or intravenously). Compared with oral amoxicillin (80–

90 mg/kg/d), ceftriaxone may reduce fever and the need for hospitalization. However, meningitis occurs with the same frequency despite presumptive therapy. All children with blood cultures that grow pneumococci should be reexamined as soon as possible. The child who has a focal infection such as meningitis or who appears septic should be admitted to the hospital to receive parenteral antimicrobials. If the child is afebrile and appears well or mildly ill, outpatient management is appropriate. If the physician is confident that close follow-up can be achieved, lumbar puncture is not mandatory.

2. Pneumonia—For infants, severely ill patients, and immunocompromised hosts with susceptible organisms appropriate regimens include aqueous penicillin G (150,000–200,000 units/kg/d, given intravenously in four to six divided doses); cefotaxime (50 mg/kg, every 8 hours); or cefuroxime (50 mg/kg, every 8 hours). If susceptibilities are not known and the patient is severely ill, vancomycin (10 mg/kg, every 6 hours) should be used as part of the regimen to provide coverage for penicillin/cephalosporin-resistant pneumococcus. Once susceptibility testing is available, the regimen can be tailored. Mild pneumonia may be treated with amoxicillin (80–90 mg/kg/d) for 7–10 days. Alternative regimens include oral macrolides and cephalosporins.

3. Otitis media—Most experts recommend oral amoxicillin (80–90 mg/kg/d, divided in two doses) as first-line therapy. The standard course of therapy is 10 days; however, many physicians have been treating uncomplicated cases for 5 days, based on recent studies. Treatment failures may be treated with amoxicillin/clavulanate (80–90 mg/kg/d of the amoxicillin component in the 7:1 formulation), intramuscular ceftriaxone, cefuroxime axetil, or cefdinir. Clarithromycin or azithromycin can also be used.

4. Meningitis—Until bacteriologic confirmation and susceptibility testing are completed, patients should receive vancomycin (60 mg/kg/d, given intravenously in four divided doses) and cefotaxime (300 mg/kg/d intravenously in four divided doses), or vancomycin (see previous dosage) and ceftriaxone (100 mg/kg/d, given intravenously in two divided doses). Corticosteroids (dexamethasone, 0.6 mg/kg/d, in four divided doses for 4 days) are recommended by many experts as adjunctive therapy for pneumococcal meningitis. However, by reducing inflammation of the meninges, steroids may reduce the entry of vancomycin into the CSF. The addition of rifampin (10 mg/kg/dose twice a day, intravenously or orally) is used by some experts if both vancomycin and steroids are given, as it penetrates CSF well and may aid in sterilization (rifampin should never be used alone for treatment of meningitis). Repeated lumbar puncture at 24–48 hours should be considered to ensure sterility of the CSF if dexamethasone is given or if resistant pneumococci are isolated. In patients not demonstrating expected improvement after 24–48 hours on therapy, a repeat lumbar puncture should be performed.

If the isolate is determined to be penicillin-susceptible, aqueous penicillin G can be administered (300,000–400,000 units/kg/d, given intravenously in four to six divided doses for 10–14 days). Use of ceftriaxone or cefotaxime is acceptable alternative therapy in penicillin and cephalosporin-susceptible isolates. Consult an infectious disease specialist or the *Red Book* (American Academy of Pediatrics, 2003) for therapeutic options for isolates that are nonsusceptible to penicillin or cephalosporins.

Prognosis

In children, case fatality rates of less than 1% should be achieved except in meningitis, in which rates of 5–20% still prevail. The presence of large numbers of organisms without a prominent CSF inflammatory response or meningitis due to a penicillin-resistant strain indicates a poor prognosis. Serious neurologic sequelae, particularly hearing loss, are frequent following pneumococcal meningitis.

Advisory Committee on Immunization Practices: Pneumococcal vaccination for cochlear implant candidates and recipients: Updated recommendations of the Advisory Committee on Immunization Practices. MMWR Morb Mortal Wkly Rep 2003;52(31):739 [PMID: 12908457].

Advisory Committee on Immunization Practices: Preventing pneumococcal disease among infants and young children. MMWR Morb Mortal Wkly Rep 2000;40:1 [PMID: 11055835].

Kaplan S: Management of pneumococcal meningitis. Pediatr Infect Dis J 2002;21(6):589 [PMID: 12182395].

Tan TQ: Antibiotic resistant infections due to *Streptococcus pneumoniae*: Impact on therapeutic options and clinical outcome. Curr Opin Infect Dis 2003;16(3):271 [PMID: 12821820].

Whitney CG et al: Decline in invasive pneumococcal disease after the introduction of protein-polysaccharide conjugate vaccine. N Engl J Med 2003;348:1737 [PMID: 12724479].

STAPHYLOCOCCAL INFECTIONS

Staphylococcal infections are common in childhood. Staphylococcal skin infections range from minor furuncles to the varied syndromes now collectively referred to as scalded skin syndrome. Staphylococci are the major cause of osteomyelitis and of septic arthritis as well as an uncommon but important cause of bacterial pneumonia. A toxin produced by certain strains causes staphylococcal food poisoning. Staphylococci are responsible for most infections of artificial heart valves. They cause toxic shock syndrome (see later discussion). Finally, they are found in infections at all ages and in multiple sites, particularly when infection is introduced from the skin or upper respiratory tract or when closed compartments become infected (pericarditis, sinusitis, cervical adenitis, surgical wounds, abscesses in the liver or brain, and abscesses elsewhere in the body).

Staphylococci that do not produce the enzyme coagulase are termed "coagulase-negative" and are seldom speciated in the clinical microbiology laboratory. Most *S aureus* strains produce coagulase. *S aureus* and coagulase-negative staphylococci are normal flora of the skin and respiratory tract. The latter rarely cause disease except in compromised hosts, the newborn, or patients with plastic indwelling lines.

Most strains of *S aureus* elaborate β-lactamase that confers penicillin resistance. This can be overcome in clinical practice by the use of a cephalosporin or a penicillinase-resistant penicillin such as methicillin, oxacillin, nafcillin, cloxacillin, or dicloxacillin. Methicillin-resistant strains of *S aureus* (MRSA) are found worldwide and are now common in certain hospitals and, increasingly, in community-acquired infections in some areas of the United States. Most MRSA retain β-lactamase production, and many are resistant to other antibiotics as well. MRSA are also resistant in vivo to all of the penicillinase-resistant penicillins and cephalosporins. Strains with intermediate susceptibility to vancomycin are occurring more frequently and occasionally vancomycin-resistant strains are isolated. The existence of such strains is of concern because of the inherent virulence of most strains of *S aureus* and because of the limited choices for therapy. *S aureus* produces a variety of exotoxins, most of which are of uncertain importance. Two toxins are recognized as playing a central role in specific diseases: exfoliatin and staphylococcal enterotoxin. The former is largely responsible for the various clinical presentations of scalded skin syndrome. Most strains that elaborate exfoliatin are of phage group II. Enterotoxin causes staphylococcal food poisoning. The exoprotein toxin most commonly associated with toxic shock syndrome has been termed TSST-1. Panton-Valentine leucocidin (PVL) is an exotoxin produced by < 5% of clinical isolates of methicillin-susceptible *S aureus* (MSSA) and MRSA strains. PVL is a virulence factor that causes leukocyte destruction and tissue necrosis. PVL-producing *S aureus* strains are often community-acquired, and have most commonly produced boils and abscesses. However, they have also been associated with severe cellulitis, osteomyelitis, and deaths from necrotizing pneumonia in otherwise healthy children and young adults.

Clinical Findings

A. SYMPTOMS AND SIGNS

1. Staphylococcal skin diseases—Dermal infection with *S aureus* causes furuncles or cellulitis. *S aureus* are often found along with streptococci in impetigo. If the strains produce exfoliatin, localized lesions become bullous (bullous impetigo).

Scalded skin syndrome is thought to be a systemic effect of exfoliatin. The initial infection may begin at any site but is in the respiratory tract in most cases. There is a prodromal phase of erythema, often beginning around the mouth, accompanied by fever and irritability. The involved skin becomes tender, and a sick infant will cry when picked up or touched. A day or so later, exfoliation begins, usually around the mouth. The inside of the mouth is red, and a peeling rash is present around the lips, often in a radial pattern. Generalized, painful peeling may follow, involving the limbs and trunk but often sparing the feet. More commonly, peeling is confined to areas around body orifices. If erythematous but unpeeled skin is rubbed sideways, superficial epidermal layers separate from deeper ones and slough (Nikolsky sign). In the newborn, the disease is termed *Ritter disease* and may be fulminant. If there is tender erythema but not exfoliation, the disease is termed *nonstreptococcal scarlet fever*. The scarlatiniform rash is sandpaper-like, but strawberry tongue is not seen, and cultures grow *S aureus* rather than streptococcus.

2. Osteomyelitis and septic arthritis—(See Chapter 24.)

3. Staphylococcal pneumonia—Staphylococcal pneumonia in infancy is characterized by abdominal distention, high fever, respiratory distress, and toxemia. It often occurs without predisposing factors or after minor skin infections. The organism is necrotizing, producing bronchoalveolar destruction. Pneumatoceles, pyopneumothorax, and empyema are frequently encountered. Rapid progression of disease is characteristic. Frequent chest radiographs to monitor the progress of disease are indicated. Presenting symptoms may be typical of paralytic ileus, suggestive of an abdominal catastrophe.

Staphylococcal pneumonia usually is peribronchial, beginning with a focal infiltrative lesion progressing to patchy consolidation. Most often only one lung is involved (80%), more often the right. Purulent pericarditis occurs by direct extension in about 10% of cases, with or without empyema.

4. Staphylococcal food poisoning—Staphylococcal food poisoning is a result of ingestion of enterotoxin produced by staphylococci growing in uncooked and poorly refrigerated food. The disease is characterized by vomiting, prostration, and diarrhea occurring 2–6 hours after ingestion of contaminated foods.

5. Staphylococcal endocarditis—*S aureus* may produce infection of normal heart valves, of valves or endocardium in children with congenital or rheumatic heart disease, or of artificial valves. About 25% of all cases of endocarditis are due to *S aureus*. The great majority of artificial heart valve infections involve either *S aureus* or coagulase-negative staphylococci. Infection usually begins in an extracardiac focus, often the skin. Involvement of the endocardium must be suspected in every case of *S aureus* bacteremia, regardless of initial signs. Suspicion must be highest in the presence of congenital heart disease, particularly ventricular septal defects with aortic insufficiency but also simple ventricular septal defect, patent ductus arteriosus, and tetralogy of Fallot.

The presenting symptoms in staphylococcal endocarditis are fever, weight loss, weakness, muscle pain or diffuse skeletal pain, poor feeding, pallor, and cardiac decompensation. Signs include splenomegaly, cardiomegaly, petechiae, hematuria, and a new or changing murmur. The course of *S aureus* endocarditis is rapid, although subacute disease occurs occasionally. Peripheral septic embolization and uncontrollable cardiac failure are common, even when optimal antibiotic therapy is administered, and may be indications for surgical intervention (see later discussion).

6. Toxic shock syndrome—Toxic shock syndrome (TSS) is characterized by fever, blanching erythroderma, diarrhea, vomiting, myalgia, prostration, hypotension, and multiorgan dysfunction. It is due to *S aureus* focal infection, usually without bacteremia. Large numbers of cases have been described in menstruating adolescents and young women using vaginal tampons. TSS has also been reported in boys and girls with focal staphylococcal infections and in individuals with wound infections due to *S aureus*. Additional clinical features include sudden onset; conjunctival suffusion; mucosal hyperemia; desquamation of skin on the palms, soles, fingers, and toes during convalescence; DIC in severe cases; renal and hepatic functional abnormalities; and myolysis. The mortality rate with early treatment is now about 2%. Recurrences are seen during subsequent menstrual periods in as many as 60% of untreated women who continue to use tampons. Recurrences occur in up to 15% of women given antistaphylococcal antibiotics who stop using tampons. The disease is caused by strains of *S aureus* that produce TSST-1 or one of the related enterotoxins.

7. Coagulase-negative staphylococcal infections—Localized and systemic coagulase-negative staphylococcal infections occur primarily in immunocompromised patients, high-risk newborns, and patients with plastic prostheses or catheters. Coagulase-negative staphylococci are the most common nosocomial pathogen in hospitalized low-birth-weight neonates in the United States. Intravenous administration of lipid emulsions and indwelling central venous catheters are risk factors contributing to coagulase-negative staphylococcal bacteremia in newborn infants. In patients with an artificial heart valve, a Dacron patch, a ventriculoperitoneal shunt, or a central venous catheter, coagulase-negative staphylococci are a common cause of sepsis or catheter infection, often necessitating removal of the foreign material and protracted antibiotic therapy. Because blood cultures are frequently contaminated by this organism, diagnosis of genuine localized or systemic infection is often difficult.

B. LABORATORY FINDINGS

Moderate leukocytosis (15,000–20,000/µL) with a shift to the left is occasionally found, although normal counts are common, particularly in infants. The sedimentation rate is elevated. Blood cultures are frequently positive in systemic staphylococcal disease and should always be obtained when it is suspected. Similarly, pus from sites of infection should always be aspirated or obtained surgically, examined with Gram stain, and cultured both aerobically and anaerobically. There are no useful serologic tests for staphylococcal disease.

Differential Diagnosis

Staphylococcal skin disease takes many forms; therefore, the differential list is long. Bullous impetigo must be differentiated from chemical or thermal burns, from drug reactions, and, in the very young, from the various congenital epidermolytic syndromes or even herpes simplex infections. Staphylococcal scalded skin syndrome may resemble scarlet fever, Kawasaki disease, Stevens–Johnson syndrome, erythema multiforme, and other drug reactions. A skin biopsy may be critical in establishing the diagnosis. Varicella lesions may become superinfected with exfoliatin-producing staphylococci and produce a combination of the two diseases (bullous varicella).

Severe, rapidly progressing pneumonia with formation of abscesses, pneumatoceles, and empyemas is typical of S aureus infection and GAS but may occasionally be produced by pneumococci, H influenzae, and GAS.

Staphylococcal food poisoning is often epidemic. It is differentiated from other common-source gastroenteritis syndromes (Salmonella, Clostridium perfringens, and Vibrio parahaemolyticus) by the short incubation period (2–6 hours), the prominence of vomiting (as opposed to diarrhea), and the absence of fever.

Endocarditis must be suspected in any instance of S aureus bacteremia, particularly when a significant heart murmur or preexisting cardiac disease is present. (See Chapter 19.)

Newborn infections with S aureus can resemble infections with streptococci and a variety of gram-negative organisms. Umbilical and respiratory tract colonization occurs with many pathogenic organisms (GBS, Escherichia coli, and Klebsiella), and both skin and systemic infections occur with virtually all of these organisms.

TSS must be differentiated from Rocky Mountain spotted fever, leptospirosis, Kawasaki disease, drug reactions, adenovirus, and measles (see also Table 36–3).

Treatment

A. SPECIFIC MEASURES

Community-acquired MRSA infections are on the rise. The incidence of community-acquired MRSA isolates varies greatly geographically. If the prevalence of MRSA isolates in the community is high or if the patient is seriously ill, vancomycin should be part of the empiric coverage until culture results and susceptibility data are known. Currently, most community-acquired MRSA strains are susceptible to trimethoprim–sulfamethoxazole (TMP–SMX) and some are susceptible to clindamycin. Less serious infections in nontoxic patients may be initially treated using one of these agents while awaiting cultures and susceptibility data.

For MSSA strains, a β-lactamase-resistant penicillin is the drug of choice (oxacillin, nafcillin, or methicillin). In serious systemic disease, in osteomyelitis, and in the treatment of large abscesses, intravenous therapy is indicated initially (oxacillin or nafcillin, 100–150 mg/kg/d in four divided doses, or methicillin, 200–300 mg/kg/d in four divided doses). When high doses over a long period are required, it is preferable not to use methicillin, because of the frequency with which interstitial nephritis occurs. In life-threatening illness, an aminoglycoside antibiotic (gentamicin or tobramycin) or rifampin may be used in addition for its possible synergistic action.

Cephalosporins may be considered for patients with a history of penicillin sensitivity unless there is a history of type 1 hypersensitivity reaction (ie, anaphylaxis, wheezing, edema, hives [cefazolin, 100–150 mg/kg/d, given intravenously in three divided doses], or cephalexin [50–100 mg/kg/d, given orally in four divided doses]) can be used once a child is able to take oral antibiotics. The third-generation cephalosporins should not generally be used for staphylococcal infections.

For nonmeningeal, suspected nosocomially acquired MRSA infections, vancomycin (40 mg/kg/d intravenously in three or four divided doses) should be used until susceptibilities are available (frequently clindamycin- and TMP–SMX-resistant). Infections due to MRSA frequently do not respond to cephalosporins despite in vitro testing that suggests susceptibility. For treatment of meningitis, vancomycin must be given in higher doses (60 mg/kg/d divided into four doses). The addition of rifampin is advocated by some (rifampin should not be used alone to treat this condition).

1. Skin infections—(See Chapter 14.)

2. Osteomyelitis and septic arthritis—Treatment should be begun intravenously, with antibiotics selected to cover the most likely organisms (staphylococci in hematogenous osteomyelitis; meningococci, pneumococci, staphylococci in children younger than age 3 years with septic arthritis; staphylococci and gonococci in older children with septic arthritis). Antibiotic levels should be kept high at all times.

In osteomyelitis, clinical studies support the use of intravenous treatment until fever and local symptoms and signs have subsided—usually after at least 3–5 days—followed by oral therapy (for susceptible strains, dicloxacillin, 100–150 mg/kg/d in four divided doses; or cephalexin, 100–150 mg/kg/d in four divided doses) for at least 3 additional weeks. Longer treatment may be required, particularly when radiographs show extensive involvement. Treatment of community-acquired MRSA osteomyelitis should be based on susceptibility results; however, isolates are frequently susceptible to TMP–SMX or clindamycin. Vancomycin can be used as part of an empiric regimen while awaiting susceptibilities in seriously ill patients or in areas where MRSA is likely as a pathogen. In arthritis, where drug diffusion into synovial fluid is good, intravenous therapy need be given only for a few days, followed by adequate oral therapy for at least 3 weeks. In all instances, oral therapy should be administered with careful attention to compliance, either in the hospital or at home. The erythrocyte sedimentation rate (ESR) is a good indicator of response to therapy. Surgical drainage of osteomyelitis or septic arthritis is often required. (See Chapter 24.)

3. Staphylococcal pneumonia—In areas of the country where MRSA is not prevalent, nafcillin and oxacillin are the usual drugs of choice. In sick patients, vancomycin can be used empirically until cultures and susceptibility results are obtained. Linezolid has recently been reported to be as efficacious as vancomycin for the treatment of resistant gram-positive pneumonia and soft tissue infections (cure rates: 95% linezolid vs 94% vancomycin).

Empyema and pyopneumothorax require drainage. The choice of chest tube versus thoracoscopic drainage depends on the practitioner's experience and skill. If staphylococcal pneumonia is treated promptly and empyema drained, resolution in children is often complete.

4. Staphylococcal food poisoning—Therapy is supportive and usually not required except in severe cases or for small infants with marked dehydration.

5. Staphylococcal endocarditis—As outlined earlier, high-dose, prolonged parenteral treatment is indicated. Methicillin-susceptible isolates are often treated with oxacillin or nafcillin. Some experts also recommend addition of gentamicin or rifampin for the first 5 days to 2 weeks. In penicillin-allergic patients (type 1 hypersensitivity or anaphylaxis) or patients with MRSA isolates, vancomycin should be used. With penicillin-sensitive organisms, penicillin G is the drug of choice. Therapy lasts in all instances for at least 6 weeks.

In some patients, medical treatment may fail. Signs of treatment failure are (1) recurrent fever without apparent treatable other cause (eg, thrombophlebitis, respiratory or

urinary tract infection, drug fever), (2) persistently positive blood cultures, (3) intractable and progressive congestive heart failure, and (4) recurrent (septic) embolization. In such circumstances—particularly (2), (3), and (4)—valve replacement becomes necessary. Antibiotics are continued for at least another 4 weeks. Persistent or recurrent infection may require a second surgical procedure.

6. Toxic shock syndrome—Treatment is aimed at expanding volume, maintaining perfusion pressure with inotropic agents as needed, prompt drainage of a focus of infection (or removal of tampons or foreign bodies), and giving intravenous antibiotics.

Vancomycin, in addition to a β-lactam antibiotic (oxacillin or nafcillin), can be used for empiric therapy. Some experts would use vancomycin and clindamycin, since clindamycin is a protein synthesis inhibitor and may turn off toxin production. Clindamycin should not be used empirically as a single agent until susceptibilities (if an isolate grows) are known; some strains of *S aureus* are clindamycin-resistant.

Intravenous immune globulin has been used as adjunctive therapy. Some experts believe that corticosteroid therapy may be effective if given to patients with severe illness early in the course of their disease. Antibiotic treatment reduces risk of recurrence.

7. Vancomycin-resistant *Staphylococcus aureus* infections (VRSA)—VRSA isolates have only been rarely reported, but are likely to increase in frequency. Such isolates are sometimes susceptible to clindamycin or TMP–SMX. If not, therapeutic options are limited and include use of quinupristin/dalfopristin, linezolid, and daptomycin. Experience is very limited with daptomycin in pediatric patients. Consultation with an infectious disease specialist is recommended.

8. Coagulase-negative staphylococcal infections—Bacteremia and other serious coagulase-negative staphylococcal infections are treated initially with vancomycin. Coagulase-negative staphylococci are uncommonly resistant to vancomycin. (See Chapter 35 for dosing.) Strains susceptible to methicillin are treated with methicillin, oxacillin, or cefazolin.

Centers for Disease Control and Prevention (CDC): Vancomycin-resistant *Staphylococcus aureus*—New York, 2004. MMWR Morb Mortal Wkly Rep 2004;53(15):322 [PMID: 15103297].

Gillet Y et al: Association between *Staphylococcus aureus* strains carrying gene for Panton-Valentine leukocidin and highly lethal necrotising pneumonia in young immunocompetent patients. Lancet 2002;359:753 [PMID: 11888586].

Kaplan SL: Use of linezolid in children. Pediatr Infect Dis J 2002;21(9):870 [PMID: 12352813].

Lowy FD: *Staphylococcus aureus* infections. N Engl J Med 1998; 339:520 [PMID: 9709046].

Marcinak JF, Frank AL: Treatment of community-acquired methicillin-resistant *Staphylococcus aureus* in children. Curr Opin Infect Dis 2003;16(3):265 [PMID: 12821819].

Reichert B, Birrell G, Bignardi G: Severe non-pneumonic necrotising infections in children caused by Panton-Valentine leukocidin producing *Staphylococcus aureus* strains. J Infect 2005; 50:438 [PMID: 15907553].

MENINGOCOCCAL INFECTIONS

 ESSENTIALS OF DIAGNOSIS & TYPICAL FEATURES

- *Fever, headache, vomiting, convulsions, shock (meningitis).*
- *Fever, shock, petechial or purpuric skin rash (meningococcemia).*
- *Diagnosis confirmed by culture of normally sterile body fluids.*

General Considerations

Meningococci (*Neisseria meningitidis*) may be carried asymptomatically for many months in the upper respiratory tract. Fewer than 1% of carriers develop disease. Meningitis and sepsis are the two most common forms of illness, but septic arthritis, pericarditis, pneumonia, chronic meningococcemia, otitis media, conjunctivitis, and vaginitis also occur. The incidence in the United States is about 1.2 cases per 100,000 people. An estimated 2400–3000 cases occur in the United States annually. The highest attack rate for meningococcal meningitis is in the first year of life. There is also an elevated attack rate during the teen years.

Meningococci are gram-negative organisms containing endotoxin in their cell walls. Endotoxins may cause capillary vascular injury and leak and may also cause DIC. The development of irreversible shock with multiorgan failure is a significant factor in the fatal outcome of acute meningococcal infections. Meningococci are classified serologically into groups: A, B, C, Y, and W-135 are the groups most commonly implicated in systemic disease. The serologic groups serve as markers for studying outbreaks and transmission of disease. Currently in the United States, serogroup B accounts for about one-third of cases. Serogroups C and Y each cause 25% of cases, and serogroup W-135 is responsible for about 15%. Serogroup A causes periodic epidemics in developing countries, but only occasionally is associated with cases of meningococcal disease in the United States. Sulfonamide resistance is common in non–serotype-A strains. *N meningitidis* with increased MICs to penicillin G are reported from South Africa and Spain. A small number of these isolates are reported in the United States. The resistance in these strains is low-level and not due to β-lactamase.

Resistant isolates are susceptible to third-generation cephalosporins. Few isolates are resistant to rifampin.

Children develop immunity from asymptomatic carriage of meningococci (usually nontypeable, nonpathogenic strains) or other cross-reacting bacteria. Patients deficient in one of the late components of complement (C6, C7, C8, or C9) are uniquely susceptible to meningococcal infection, particularly group A meningococci. Deficiencies of early and alternate pathway complement components are also associated with increased susceptibility.

Clinical Findings

A. SYMPTOMS AND SIGNS

Many children with clinical meningococcemia also have meningitis, and some have other foci of infection. All children with suspected meningococcemia should have a lumbar puncture.

1. Meningococcemia—A prodrome of upper respiratory infection is followed by high fever, headache, nausea, marked toxicity, and hypotension. Purpura, petechiae, and occasionally bright pink, tender macules or papules over the extremities and trunk are seen. The rash usually progresses rapidly. Occasional cases lack rash. Fulminant meningococcemia (Waterhouse–Friderichsen syndrome) progresses rapidly and is characterized by DIC, massive skin and mucosal hemorrhages, and shock. This syndrome also may be due to *H influenzae, S pneumoniae,* or other bacteria. Chronic meningococcemia is characterized by periodic bouts of fever, arthralgia or arthritis, and recurrent petechiae. Splenomegaly is often present. Patients may be free of symptoms between bouts. Chronic meningococcemia occurs primarily in adults and mimics Henoch–Schönlein purpura.

2. Meningitis—In many children, meningococcemia is followed within a few hours to several days by symptoms and signs of acute purulent meningitis, with severe headache, stiff neck, nausea, vomiting, and stupor. Children with meningitis generally fare better than children with meningococcemia alone, probably because they have survived long enough to develop clinical signs of meningitis.

B. LABORATORY FINDINGS

The peripheral WBC count may be either low or elevated. Thrombocytopenia may be present with or without DIC. (See Chapter 27.) If petechial or hemorrhagic lesions are present, meningococci can sometimes be demonstrated on smear by puncturing the lesions and expressing a drop of tissue fluid. CSF is generally cloudy and contains more than 1000 WBCs per microliter, with many polymorphonuclear neutrophils and gram-negative intracellular diplococci. A total hemolytic complement assay may reveal absence of late components as an underlying cause.

Differential Diagnosis

The skin lesions of *H influenzae* or pneumococci, enterovirus infection, endocarditis, leptospirosis, Rocky Mountain spotted fever, other rickettsial diseases, Henoch–Schönlein purpura, and blood dyscrasias may be similar to meningococcemia. Other causes of sepsis and meningitis are distinguished by appropriate Gram stain and cultures.

Complications

Meningitis may lead to permanent central nervous system (CNS) damage, with deafness, convulsions, paralysis, or impairment of intellectual function. Hydrocephalus may develop and requires ventriculoperitoneal shunt. Subdural collections of fluid are common but usually resolve spontaneously. Extensive skin necrosis, loss of digits or extremities, intestinal hemorrhage, and late adrenal insufficiency may complicate fulminant meningococcemia.

Prevention

Household contacts, day care center contacts, and hospital personnel directly exposed to the respiratory secretions of patients are at increased risk for developing meningococcal infection and should be given chemoprophylaxis with rifampin. The secondary attack rate among household members is 1–5% during epidemics and less than 1% in non-epidemic situations. Children between the ages of 3 months to 2 years are at greatest risk, presumably because they lack protective antibodies. Secondary cases may occur in day care centers and in classrooms. Hospital personnel are not at increased risk unless they have had contact with a patient's oral secretions, for example, during mouth-to-mouth resuscitation, intubation, or suctioning procedures. Approximately 50% of secondary cases in households have their onset within 24 hours of identification of the index case. Exposed contacts should be notified promptly. If they are febrile, they should be fully evaluated and given high doses of penicillin or another effective antimicrobial pending the results of blood cultures.

All intimate contacts should receive chemoprophylaxis for meningococcal disease. The most commonly used agent is rifampin, given orally in the following dosages twice daily for 2 days: 600 mg for adults; 10 mg/kg for children younger than 1 month old (maximum dosage 600 mg); and 5 mg/kg for infants younger than 1 month. Rifampin may stain a patient's tears (and contact lenses), sweat, and urine orange; it may also affect the reliability of oral contraceptives, and alternative contraceptive measures should therefore be employed when rifampin is administered. Rifampin should not be given to pregnant women. Instead, intramuscular ceftriaxone is the preferred agent: 125 mg given as a single dose if the patient is younger than 15 years; 250 mg given as a single dose if older than 15 years. Penicillin and most other antibiotics (even with parenteral administration) are not effective chemoprophylactic agents, because they do not eradicate upper respiratory tract carriage of meningococci. Ciprofloxacin effectively eradicates nasopharyngeal carriage in adults and children but is not approved for use in children or in pregnant women. Throat cultures to identify carriers are not useful. Meningococcal vaccine has been used increasingly for control of outbreaks. Patients with functional or anatomic asplenia, complement deficiencies, or properdin deficiency should be vaccinated.

Treatment

Blood cultures should be obtained for all children with fever and purpura or other signs of meningococcemia, and antibiotics should be administered immediately as an emergency procedure. There is a good correlation between survival rates and prompt initiation of antibiotic therapy. Purpura and fever should be considered a medical emergency.

Children with meningococcemia or meningococcal meningitis should be treated as though shock were imminent even if their vital signs are stable when they are first seen. If hypotension already is present, supportive measures should be aggressive, because the prognosis is grave in such situations. It is optimal to initiate treatment in an intensive care setting. Treatment should not be delayed for the sake of transporting the patient. Shock may worsen following antimicrobial therapy due to endotoxin release. To minimize the risk of nosocomial transmission, patients should be placed in respiratory isolation for the first 24 hours of antibiotic treatment.

A. SPECIFIC MEASURES

Antibiotics should be initiated promptly. Because other bacteria, such as *S pneumoniae, S aureus,* or other gram-negative organisms, can cause identical syndromes, initial therapy should be broadly effective. Vancomycin and cefotaxime (or ceftriaxone) are preferred initial coverage. Once *N meningitidis* has been isolated, penicillin G, cefotaxime, or ceftriaxone intravenously for 7 days are the drugs of choice. Relative penicillin resistance is uncommon but has been reported in the United States.

B. GENERAL MEASURES

Most cases of invasive meningococcal disease are treated with intravenous antibiotics for 7 days.

1. Cardiovascular—(See Chapter 11 for management of septic shock.) Corticosteroids are not beneficial. Sympathetic blockade and topically applied nitroglycerin have been used locally to improve perfusion.

2. Hematologic—Adjunctive therapy with heparin is controversial. Because hypercoagulability is frequently present in patients with meningococcemia, some experts believe heparin should be considered for those with DIC. A loading dose of 50 units/kg is followed by 15 units/kg/h as a continuous drip. The patient is monitored by following the partial thromboplastin time and heparin assay. Recombinant tissue plasminogen activator, concentrated antithrombin III, and recombinant protein C infusions have been tried experimentally to reverse coagulopathy. (See Chapter 27 for the management of DIC.)

Prognosis

Unfavorable prognostic features include shock, DIC, and extensive skin lesions. The case fatality rate in fulminant meningococcemia is over 30%. In uncomplicated meningococcal meningitis, the fatality rate is much lower (10–20%).

Vaccine

A quadrivalent polysaccharide vaccine prepared from purified meningococcal polysaccharides (A, C, Y, and W-135) is available in the United States for children older than 2 years of age. This vaccine has been used for controlling outbreak. A quadrivalent meningococcal conjugate vaccine is also available. (See Chapter 9.) This vaccine is licensed for use in children and adults between the ages of 11 and 55 years, and is preferred over the polysaccharide vaccine in the age groups for which the vaccine is licensed. Currently meningococcal conjugate vaccine is recommended for the following:

1. All children at the age 11–12-year preadolescent visit.
2. All children prior to high school entry if they have not had a previous meningococcal vaccine.
3. College students who will be residing in dormitories for the first time.
4. Patients with functional or anatomic asplenia and patients with complement or properdin deficiency.
5. Travelers to areas where meningococcal disease is endemic.
6. Microbiologists who may be working with meningococcal strains.

Campos-Outcalt D: Meningococcal vaccine: New product, new recommendations. J Fam Pract 2005;54(4):324 [PMID: 15833222].

Pathan N et al: Pathophysiology of meningococcal meningitis and septicaemia. Arch Dis Child 2003;88(7):601 [PMID: 12818907].

Recommendations of the Advisory Committee on Immunization Practices (ACIP): Meningococcal disease and college students. MMWR Morb Mortal Wkly Rep 2000;49(RR-7):11 [PMID: 10902835].

Rosenstein NE et al: Meningococcal disease. N Engl J Med 2001; 344(18):1378 [PMID:11333996].

Welch SB, Nadel S: Treatment of meningococcal infection. Arch Dis Child 2003;88(7):608 [PMID: 12818909].

GONOCOCCAL INFECTIONS

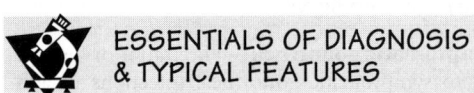

ESSENTIALS OF DIAGNOSIS & TYPICAL FEATURES

- *Purulent urethral discharge with intracellular gram-negative diplococci on smear in male patient (usually adolescent).*
- *Purulent, edematous, sometimes hemorrhagic conjunctivitis with intracellular gram-negative diplococci in infant age 2–4 days.*
- *Fever, arthritis (often polyarticular) or tenosynovitis, and maculopapular peripheral rash that may be vesiculopustular or hemorrhagic.*
- *Positive culture of blood, pharyngeal, or genital secretions.*

General Considerations

Neisseria gonorrhoeae is a gram-negative diplococcus. Although morphologically similar to other neisseriae, it differs in its ability to grow on selective media and to ferment carbohydrates. The cell wall of *N gonorrhoeae* contains endotoxin, which is liberated when the organism dies and is responsible for the production of a cellular exudate. The incubation period is short, usually 2–5 days.

Antimicrobial-resistant gonococci are a serious problem. *N gonorrhoeae* resistant to tetracyclines, penicillins, or both are common. Fluoroquinolone-resistant strains are also increasing.

Gonococcal disease in children may be transmitted sexually or nonsexually. Prepubertal gonococcal infection outside the neonatal period should be considered presumptive evidence of sexual contact or child abuse. Prepubertal girls usually manifest gonococcal vulvovaginitis because of the neutral to alkaline pH of the vagina and thin vaginal mucosa.

In the adolescent or adult, the work-up of every case of gonorrhea should include a careful and accurate inquiry into the patient's sexual practices, because pharyngeal infection must be detected if present and may be difficult to eradicate. Efforts should be made to identify and provide treatment to all sexual contacts. When prepubertal children are infected, epidemiologic investigation should be thorough.

Increasing rates of gonorrhea for the last several years are a source of concern because other sexually transmitted diseases often mirror changes in gonococcal incidence.

Clinical Findings

A. SYMPTOMS AND SIGNS

1. Asymptomatic gonorrhea—The ratio of asymptomatic to symptomatic gonorrheal infections in adolescents and adults is probably 3–4:1 in women and 0.5–1:1 in men. Asymptomatic infections are as infectious as symptomatic ones.

2. Uncomplicated genital gonorrhea—

a. Male with urethritis—Urethral discharge is sometimes painful and bloody and may be white, yellow, or green. There may be associated dysuria. The patient is usually afebrile.

b. Prepubertal female with vaginitis—The only clinical findings initially may be dysuria and polymorphonuclear neutrophils in the urine. Vulvitis characterized by erythema, edema, and excoriation accompanied by a purulent discharge may follow.

c. Postpubertal female with cervicitis—Symptomatic disease is characterized by a purulent, foul-smelling vaginal discharge, dysuria, and occasionally dyspareunia. Fever and abdominal pain are absent. The cervix is frequently hyperemic and tender when touched. This tenderness is not worsened by moving the cervix, nor are the adnexa tender to palpation.

d. Rectal gonorrhea—Rectal gonorrhea is often asymptomatic. There may be purulent discharge, edema, and pain during evacuation.

3. Pharyngeal gonorrhea—Pharyngeal infection is usually asymptomatic. There may be some sore throat and, rarely, acute exudative tonsillitis with bilateral cervical lymphadenopathy and fever.

4. Conjunctivitis and iridocyclitis—Copious exudate is characteristic of gonococcal conjunctivitis. Newborns are symptomatic on days 2–4 of life. In the adolescent or adult, infection probably is spread from infected genital secretions by the fingers.

5. Pelvic inflammatory disease (salpingitis)—The interval between initiation of genital infection and its ascent to the uterine tubes is variable and may range from days to months. Menses frequently are the initiating factor. With the onset of a menstrual period, gonococci invade the endometrium, causing transient endometritis. Subsequently salpingitis may occur, resulting in pyosalpinx or hydrosalpinx. Rarely infection progresses to peritonitis or perihepatitis. Gonococcal salpingitis occurs in an acute, subacute, or chronic form. All three forms have in common tenderness on gentle movement of the cervix and bilateral tubal tenderness during pelvic examination.

Gonococci or *Chlamydia trachomatis* are the cause of about 50% of cases of pelvic inflammatory disease. A mixed infection caused by enteric bacilli, *Bacteroides fragilis,* or other anaerobes occur in the other 50%.

6. Gonococcal perihepatitis (Fitz-Hugh and Curtis syndrome)—In the typical clinical pattern, the patient presents with right upper quadrant tenderness in association with signs of acute or subacute salpingitis. Pain may be pleuritic and referred to the shoulder. Hepatic friction rub is a valuable but inconstant sign.

7. Disseminated gonorrhea—Dissemination follows asymptomatic more often than symptomatic genital infection and often results from gonococcal pharyngitis or anorectal gonorrhea. The most common form of disseminated gonorrhea is polyarthritis or polytenosynovitis, with or without dermatitis. Monarticular arthritis is less common, and gonococcal endocarditis and meningitis are fortunately rare.

a. Polyarthritis—Disease usually begins with the simultaneous onset of low-grade fever, polyarthralgia, and malaise. After a day or so, joint symptoms become acute. Swelling, redness, and tenderness occur, frequently over the wrists, ankles, and knees but also in the fingers, feet, and other peripheral joints. Skin lesions may be noted at the same time. Discrete, tender, maculopapular lesions 5 8 mm in diameter appear that may become vesicular, pustular, and then hemorrhagic. They are few in number and noted on the fingers, palms, feet, and other distal surfaces and may be single or multiple. In patients with this form of the disease, blood cultures are often positive, but joint fluid rarely yields organisms. Skin lesions often are positive by Gram stain but rarely by culture. Genital, rectal, and pharyngeal cultures must be performed.

b. Monarticular arthritis—In this somewhat less common form of disseminated gonorrhea, fever is often absent. Arthritis evolves in a single joint. Dermatitis usually does not occur. Systemic symptoms are minimal. Blood cultures are negative, but joint aspirates may yield gonococci on smear and culture. Genital, rectal, and pharyngeal cultures must be performed.

B. LABORATORY FINDINGS

Demonstration of gram-negative, kidney-shaped diplococci in smears of urethral exudate in males is presumptive evidence of gonorrhea. Positive culture confirms the diagnosis. Negative smears do not rule out gonorrhea. Gram-stained smears of cervical or vaginal discharge in girls are more difficult to interpret because of normal gram-negative flora, but they may be useful when technical personnel are experienced. In girls with suspected gonorrhea, both the cervical os and the anus should be cultured. Gonococcal pharyngitis requires culture for diagnosis.

Cultures for *N gonorrhoeae* are plated on a selective chocolate agar containing antibiotics (eg, Thayer–Martin agar) to suppress normal flora. If bacteriologic diagnosis is critical, suspected material should be cultured on chocolate agar as well. Because gonococci are labile, agar plates should be inoculated immediately and placed without delay in an atmosphere containing CO_2 (candle jar). When transport of specimens is necessary, material should be inoculated directly into Transgrow medium prior to shipment to an appropriate laboratory. In cases of possible sexual molestation, notify the laboratory that definite speciation is needed, because nongonococcal *Neisseria* species can grow on the selective media.

Nucleic acid amplification tests on urine specimens now enable detection of *N gonorrhoeae* and *C trachomatis*. These tests have excellent sensitivity and are replacing culture in some settings. All children or adolescents with a suspected or established diagnosis of gonorrhea should have serologic tests for syphilis and human immunodeficiency virus (HIV).

Differential Diagnosis

Urethritis in the male may be gonococcal or nongonococcal (NGU). NGU is a syndrome characterized by discharge (rarely painful), mild dysuria, and a subacute course. The discharge is usually scant or moderate in amount but may be profuse. *C trachomatis* is the only proven cause of NGU. Doxycycline (100 mg orally twice a day for 7 days) is efficacious. Single-dose azithromycin, 1 g orally, may achieve better compliance. *C trachomatis* has been shown to cause epididymitis in males and salpingitis in females.

Vulvovaginitis in a prepubertal female may be due to infection caused by miscellaneous bacteria, including *Shigella* and GAS, *Candida,* and herpes simplex. Discharges may be caused by trichomonads, *Enterobius vermicularis* (pinworm), or foreign bodies. Symptom-free discharge (leukorrhea) normally accompanies rising estrogen levels.

Cervicitis in a postpubertal female, alone or in association with urethritis and involvement of Skene and Bartholin glands, may be due to infection caused by *Candida,* herpes simplex, *Trichomonas,* or discharge resulting from inflammation caused by foreign bodies (usually some form of contraceptive device). Leukorrhea may be associated with birth control pills.

Salpingitis may be due to infection with other organisms. The symptoms must be differentiated from those of appendicitis, urinary tract infection, ectopic pregnancy, endometriosis, or ovarian cysts or torsion.

Disseminated gonorrhea presents a differential diagnosis that includes meningococcemia, acute rheumatic fever, Henoch–Schönlein purpura, juvenile rheumatoid arthritis, lupus erythematosus, leptospirosis, secondary syphilis, certain viral infections (particularly rubella, but also enteroviruses and parvovirus), serum sickness, type B hepatitis (in the prodromal phase), infective endocarditis, and even acute leukemia and other types of cancer. The fully evolved skin lesions of disseminated gonorrhea are remarkably specific, and genital, rectal, or pharyngeal cultures, plus cultures of blood and joint fluid, usually yield gonococci from at least one source.

Prevention

Prevention of gonorrhea is principally a matter of sex education, condom use, and identification and treatment of contacts.

Treatment

A. UNCOMPLICATED URETHRAL, ENDOCERVICAL, OR RECTAL GONOCOCCAL INFECTIONS IN ADOLESCENTS

Ceftriaxone (125 mg intramuscularly in a single dose), cefixime (400 mg orally in a single dose), ciprofloxacin (500 mg orally in a single dose), ofloxacin (400 mg orally in a single dose), or levofloxacin (250 mg orally in a single dose) is preferred therapy. Doxycycline (100 mg orally twice a day for 7 days) or azithromycin (1 g orally in a single dose) is recommended unless *C trachomatis* is ruled out. Ceftizoxime, cefotaxime, and cefotetan parenterally are alternative single-dose therapies.

Quinolones and tetracyclines should be avoided in pregnancy. Quinolones are not approved for use in children, and repeated doses of tetracyclines may stain the teeth of young children. Erythromycin or amoxicillin is recommended for therapy of *C trachomatis* in pregnant women; azithromycin is an alternative regimen. Repeat testing 3 weeks after completion of therapy is recommended in pregnant women.

Spectinomycin (2 g intramuscularly in a single dose) is used for penicillin- and cephalosporin-allergic patients. Quinolone resistance is increasing and is common in Hawaii, Asia, the Pacific, and among men who have sex with men. Quinolones are not recommended for therapy of patients or travelers from these areas. A repeat culture after completion of therapy is not necessary in asymptomatic adolescents after the ceftriaxone–doxycycline regimen. A repeat culture after completion of therapy should be obtained from infants and children.

B. PHARYNGEAL GONOCOCCAL INFECTION

Ceftriaxone (125 mg intramuscularly in a single dose) should be used; ciprofloxacin (0.5 g orally in a single dose) is an alternative for adults and older adolescents. Neither spectinomycin nor amoxicillin is recommended. A repeat culture is recommended 4–7 days after therapy.

C. DISSEMINATED GONORRHEA

Recommended regimens include ceftriaxone (1 g intramuscularly or intravenously once daily), cefotaxime (1 g intravenously every 8 hours), ciprofloxacin (400 IV every

12 hours), ofloxacin (500 IV every 12 hours), or levofloxacin (250 IV every 24 hours). Oral therapy may follow parenteral therapy 24–48 hours after improvement. Recommended regimens include ciprofloxacin (0.5 g twice daily), ofloxacin (0.4 g twice daily), or levofloxacin (0.25 g orally once a day) to complete 7 days of therapy. Fluoroquinolones are not used for pregnant patients. If concurrent infection with *Chlamydia* is present or has not been excluded, a course of doxycycline, azithromycin, or erythromycin should also be prescribed. Total duration of therapy is 7 days for disseminated infections.

D. PELVIC INFLAMMATORY DISEASE

Doxycycline (100 mg twice a day orally) and either cefoxitin (2 g intramuscularly or intravenously every 6 hours) or cefotetan (2 g intramuscularly or intravenously every 12 hours) are given until the patient is clinically improved, then doxycycline is administered by mouth to complete 14 days of therapy. Clindamycin and gentamicin given intravenously until the patient is clinically improved may be used rather than cefoxitin. Many other regimens have been used for therapy of pelvic inflammatory disease, although comparative efficacy data are limited.

E. PREPUBERTAL GONOCOCCAL INFECTIONS

1. Uncomplicated genitourinary, rectal, or pharyngeal infections—These infections may be treated with ceftriaxone (25–50 mg/kg/d to a maximum of 125 mg intramuscularly in a single dose). Children older than age 8 years should also receive doxycycline (100 mg orally twice daily for 7 days). The physician should evaluate all children for evidence of sexual abuse and coinfection with syphilis, *Chlamydia,* and HIV.

2. Disseminated gonorrhea—This should be treated with ceftriaxone (50 mg/kg once daily parenterally for 7 days).

Benson PA, Hergenroeder AC: Bacterial sexually transmitted infections in gay, lesbian and bisexual adolescents: Medical and public health perspectives. Semin Pediatr Infect Dis 2005;16(3):181 [PMID: 16044392].

Centers for Disease Control and Prevention: Sexually transmitted diseases. www.cdc.gov/std/

Increases in fluoroquinolone-resistant *Neisseria gonorrhoeae* among men who have sex with men—United States, 2003, and revised recommendations for gonorrhea treatment, 2004. MMWR Morb Mortal Wkly Rep 2004;53(16):335 [PMID: 15123985].

BOTULISM

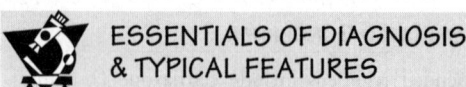

ESSENTIALS OF DIAGNOSIS & TYPICAL FEATURES

- Dry mucous membranes.
- Nausea and vomiting.
- Diplopia; dilated, unreactive pupils.
- Descending paralysis.
- Difficulty in swallowing and speech occurring within 12–36 hours after ingestion of toxin-contaminated food.
- Multiple cases in a family or group.
- Hypotonia and constipation in infants.
- Diagnosis by clinical findings and identification of toxin in blood, stool, or implicated food.

General Considerations

Botulism is a paralytic disease caused by *Clostridium botulinum,* an anaerobic, gram-positive, spore-forming bacillus normally found in soil. The organism produces an extremely potent neurotoxin. Of the seven types of toxin (A–G), types A, B, and E cause most human diseases. The toxin, a polypeptide, is so potent that 0.1 mg is lethal for humans.

Food-borne botulism usually results from ingestion of toxin-containing food. Preformed toxin is absorbed from the gut and produces paralysis by preventing acetylcholine release from cholinergic fibers at myoneural junctions. In the United States, home-canned vegetables are usually the cause. Commercially canned foods rarely are responsible. Virtually any food will support the growth of *C botulinum* spores into vegetative toxin-producing bacilli if an anaerobic, nonacid environment is provided. The food may not appear or taste spoiled. The toxin is heat-labile, but the spores are heat-resistant. Inadequate heating during processing (temperature < 115 °C) allows the spores to survive and later resume toxin production. Boiling of foods for 10 minutes or heating at 80 °C for 30 minutes before eating will destroy the toxin.

Infant botulism is seen in infants younger than age 6 months (median, 10 weeks). The initial symptoms are usually constipation and severe hypotonia. Infants younger than age 2 weeks rarely develop botulism. The toxin appears to be produced by *C botulinum* organisms residing in the gastrointestinal tract. In some instances, honey has been the source of spores. Clinical findings include constipation, weak suck and cry, pooled oral secretions, cranial nerve deficits, generalized weakness, and, on occasion, apnea. The characteristic electromyographic pattern of brief, small, abundant motor-unit action potentials (BSAP) may help confirm the diagnosis.

Annually, 10 to 15 cases of wound botulism are reported. Most cases occur in drug abusers with infection in intravenous or intramuscular injection sites.

Botulism, as a result of aerosolization of botulinum toxin, could also occur as the result of a bioterrorism event. Only three such cases of botulism have been reported; therefore, the incubation period is not well-defined, but was about 72 hours in the reported cases.

Clinical Findings

A. SYMPTOMS AND SIGNS

The incubation period for food-borne botulism is 8–36 hours. The initial symptoms are lethargy and headache. These are followed by double vision, dilated pupils, ptosis, and, within a few hours, difficulty with swallowing and speech. Pharyngeal paralysis occurs in some cases, and food may be regurgitated. The mucous membranes often are very dry. Descending skeletal muscle paralysis may be seen. Death usually results from respiratory failure.

Botulism patients present with a "classic triad": (1) afebrile; (2) symmetrical, flaccid, descending paralysis with prominent bulbar palsies; and (3) clear sensorium. Botulism is caused by a toxin, thus there is no fever unless secondary infection (eg, aspiration pneumonia) occurs. Common bulbar palsies seen include dysphonia, dysphagia, dysarthria, and diplopia (4 "Ds"). Recognition of this triad is important in making the clinical diagnosis.

B. LABORATORY FINDINGS

The diagnosis is made by demonstration of *C botulinum* toxin in stool, gastric aspirate/vomitus, or serum. Serum and stool samples can be sent for toxin confirmation (done by toxin neutralization mouse bioassay at CDC or state health departments). Foods that are suspected to be contaminated should be kept refrigerated and given to public health personnel for testing. Laboratory findings, including CSF examination, are usually normal. Electromyography suggests the diagnosis if the characteristic BSAP abnormalities are seen. A nondiagnostic electromyogram does not exclude the diagnosis.

Differential Diagnosis

Guillain–Barré syndrome is characterized by ascending paralysis, sensory deficits, and elevated CSF protein without pleocytosis.

Other illnesses that should be considered include poliomyelitis, postdiphtheritic polyneuritis, certain chemical intoxications, tick paralysis, and myasthenia gravis. The history and elevated CSF protein characterize postdiphtheritic polyneuritis. Tick paralysis presents with a flaccid ascending motor paralysis. An attached tick should be sought. Myasthenia gravis usually occurs in adolescent girls. It is characterized by ocular and bulbar symptoms, normal pupils, fluctuating weakness, absence of other neurologic signs, and clinical response to cholinesterase inhibitors.

Complications

Difficulty in swallowing leads to aspiration pneumonia. Serious respiratory paralysis may be fatal despite assisted ventilation and intensive supportive measures.

Treatment

A. SPECIFIC MEASURES

Early treatment of botulism with antitoxin (food-borne or wound botulism) or passive human botulism immune globulin (infant botulism) is beneficial. Treatment should begin as soon as the clinical diagnosis is made (prior to microbiologic or toxin confirmation).

For wound or food-borne botulism, the current form of equine, trivalent antitoxin (types A, B, and E) is given by slow intravenous infusion. Trivalent antitoxin (types A, B, and E) is available from the CDC through state health departments. All patients need to be screened for hypersensitivity to the product prior to initiating the infusion; small challenge doses are given (see package insert). Patients who have reactions to the challenge doses are desensitized prior to receiving antitoxin infusion. In addition to the antitoxin, 24-hour diagnostic consultation, epidemic assistance, and laboratory testing services are available from the CDC through state health departments.

For treatment of infant botulism, intravenous human botulism immune globulin (Baby-BIG) is approved by the U.S. Food and Drug Administration (FDA) for use. Baby-BIG is a product containing high titers of neutralizing antibodies against type A and B toxin and is made from pooled plasma of adults who were immunized with a botulism toxoid vaccine. Results of a placebo-controlled clinical trial of use in infant botulism showed reduction in the mean hospital stay (2.5 weeks as compared with the placebo group 5.5 weeks) and decrease in mechanical ventilation time in the Baby-BIG–treated group. Baby-BIG is not indicated for use in any form of botulism (wound, food-borne) other than infant botulism. Equine botulinum antitoxin should not be used to treat infant botulism.

B. GENERAL MEASURES

General and supportive therapy consists of bed rest, ventilatory support (if necessary), fluid therapy, enteral or parenteral nutrition, and administration of purgatives and high enemas. Aminoglycoside antimicrobials and clindamycin may exacerbate neuromuscular blockage and should be avoided.

Prognosis

The mortality rate has declined substantially in recent years and is currently at 6%. In nonfatal cases, symptoms subside over 2–3 months and recovery is usually complete.

Arnon SS et al: Botulinum toxin as a biological weapon. JAMA 2001;285(8):1059 [PMID: 11209178].

Centers for Disease Control and Prevention: Infant botulism—New York City, 2001–2002. JAMA 2003;289(7):834 [PMID: 12599363].

Fox CK, Keet CA, Strober JB. Recent advances in infant botulism. Pediatr Neurol 2005;32(3):149 [PMID: 15730893].

TETANUS

ESSENTIALS OF DIAGNOSIS & TYPICAL FEATURES

- *Nonimmunized or partially immunized patient.*
- *History of skin wound.*
- *Spasms of jaw muscles (trismus).*
- *Stiffness of neck, back, and abdominal muscles, with hyperirritability and hyperreflexia.*
- *Episodic, generalized muscle contractions.*
- *Diagnosis is based on clinical findings and the immunization history.*

General Considerations

Tetanus is caused by *Clostridium tetani*, an anaerobic, gram-positive bacillus that produces a potent neurotoxin. In unimmunized or incompletely immunized individuals, infection follows contamination of a wound by soil containing clostridial spores from animal manure. The toxin reaches the CNS by retrograde axon transport, is bound to cerebral gangliosides, and is thought to increase reflex excitability in neurons of the spinal cord by blocking function of inhibitory synapses. Intense muscle spasms result. Two-thirds of cases in the United States follow minor puncture wounds of the hands or feet. In many cases, no history of a wound can be obtained. Injecting substances/drug abuse may be a risk factor (in individuals who are not tetanus-immune). In the newborn, usually in underdeveloped countries, infection generally results from contamination of the umbilical cord. The incubation period typically is 4–14 days but may be longer. In the United States, cases in young children are due to failure to immunize. Eighty-five percent of cases occur in adults older than 25 years.

Clinical Findings

A. SYMPTOMS AND SIGNS

The first symptom is often mild pain at the site of the wound, followed by hypertonicity and spasm of the regional muscles. Characteristically, difficulty in opening the mouth (trismus) is evident within 48 hours. In newborns, the first signs are irritability and inability to nurse. The infant may then develop stiffness of the jaw and neck, increasing dysphagia, and generalized hyperreflexia with rigidity and spasms of all muscles of the abdomen and back (opisthotonos). The facial distortion resembles a grimace (risus sardonicus). Difficulty in swallowing and convulsions triggered by minimal stimuli such as sound, light, or movement may occur. Individual spasms may last seconds or minutes. Recurrent spasms are seen several times each hour, or they may be almost continuous. In most cases, the temperature is normal or only mildly elevated. A high or subnormal temperature is a bad prognostic sign. Patients are fully conscious and lucid. A profound circulatory disturbance associated with sympathetic overactivity may occur on the second to fourth day, which may contribute to the mortality rate. This is characterized by elevated blood pressure, increased cardiac output, tachycardia (> 20 beats/min), and arrhythmia.

B. LABORATORY FINDINGS

The diagnosis is made on clinical grounds. There may be a mild polymorphonuclear leukocytosis. The CSF is normal with the exception of mild elevation of opening pressure. Serum muscle enzymes may be elevated. Transient electrocardiographic and electroencephalographic abnormalities may occur. Anaerobic culture and microscopic examination of pus from the wound can be helpful, but *C tetani* is difficult to grow, and the drumstick-shaped gram-positive bacilli often cannot be found.

Differential Diagnosis

Poliomyelitis is characterized by asymmetrical paralysis in an incompletely immunized child. The history of an animal bite and the absence of trismus may suggest rabies. Local infections of the throat and jaw should be easily recognized. Bacterial meningitis, phenothiazine reactions, decerebrate posturing, narcotic withdrawal, spondylitis, and hypocalcemic tetany may be confused with tetanus.

Complications

Complications include sepsis, malnutrition, pneumonia, atelectasis, asphyxial spasms, decubitus ulcers, and fractures of the spine due to intense contractions. They can be prevented in part by skilled supportive care.

Prevention

A. TETANUS TOXOID

Active immunization with tetanus toxoid prevents tetanus. (See Chapter 9.) Immunity is almost always achieved after the third dose of vaccine. A booster at the time of injury is needed if none has been given in the past 10 years—or within 5 years in case of a heavily contaminated wound. Nearly all cases of tetanus (99%) in the United States are in nonimmunized or incompletely immunized individuals. Many adolescents and adults lack protective antibody.

B. TETANUS ANTITOXIN

Human tetanus immune globulin (TIG) should be used in children with fewer than three previous tetanus toxoid immunizations (DPT, DPaT, DT, Td, etc) who have "tetanus-prone wounds." These include (1) wounds contaminated with soil, saliva, debris, or feces; (2) crush wounds, puncture wounds, or wounds with avulsed or devitalized tissue; and (3) wounds due to thermal burns or frostbite. TIG should be administered to HIV-infected children with tetanus-prone wounds, regardless of their immunization history. When TIG is indicated, 250 units is given intramuscularly. If tetanus immunization is incomplete, a dose of age-appropriate vaccine should be given. When both are indicated, tetanus toxoid and TIG should be administered concurrently at different sites using different syringes.

C. TREATMENT OF WOUNDS

Proper surgical cleansing and debridement of contaminated wounds will decrease the risk of tetanus.

D. PROPHYLACTIC ANTIMICROBIALS

Prophylactic antimicrobials are useful if the child is unimmunized and TIG is not available.

Treatment

A. SPECIFIC MEASURES

Serotherapy lowers the mortality rate from tetanus, but not dramatically. Human TIG in a single dose of 3000–6000 units, intramuscularly, is given to children and adults. Doses of 500 units have been used in infants. Surgical debridement of wounds is indicated, but more extensive surgery or amputation to eliminate the site of infection is not necessary. Antibiotics are given to attempt to decrease the number of vegetative forms of the bacteria to decrease toxin production: oral metronidazole (30 mg/kg/d in four divided doses) for 10–14 days is the preferred agent.

B. GENERAL MEASURES

The patient is kept in a quiet room with minimal stimulation. Control of spasms and prevention of hypoxic episodes are crucial. Diazepam or another anxiolytic is useful (0.6–1.2 mg/kg/d intravenously in six divided doses). In the newborn, two or three divided doses should be given. Large doses (up to 25 mg/kg/d) may be required

for older children. Diazepam is given intravenously until muscular spasms become infrequent and the generalized muscular rigidity much less prominent. The drug may then be given orally and the dosage reduced as the child improves. Mechanical ventilation and muscle paralysis are necessary in severe cases. Nasogastric or intravenous feedings should be used to limit stimulation of feedings and prevent aspiration.

Prognosis

The fatality rate in newborns and heroin-addicted individuals is high. The overall mortality rate in the United States is 11%. The fatality rate depends on the quality of supportive care, the patient's age, and the patient's vaccination history. Many deaths are due to pneumonia or respiratory failure. If the patient survives 1 week, recovery is likely.

Bunch TJ et al: Respiratory failure in tetanus: Case report and review of a 25-year experience. Chest 2002;122(4):1488 [PMID: 12377887].

Centers for Disease Control and Prevention: Tetanus. www.cdc.gov/nip/publications/pink/tetanus.pdf

Pascual FB et al: Tetanus surveillance–United States, 1998–2000. MMWR Surveill Summ 2003;52(3):1 [PMID: 12825541].

Rhee P et al: Tetanus and trauma: A review and recommendations. J Trauma Injury Infect Crit Care 2005;58(5):1082 [PMID: 15920431].

GAS GANGRENE

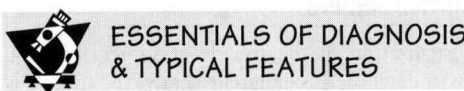

ESSENTIALS OF DIAGNOSIS & TYPICAL FEATURES

- *Contamination of a wound with soil or feces.*
- *Massive edema, skin discoloration, bleb formation, and pain in an area of trauma.*
- *Serosanguineous exudate from wound.*
- *Crepitation of subcutaneous tissue.*
- *Rapid progression of signs and symptoms.*
- *Clostridia cultured or seen on stained smears.*

General Considerations

Gas gangrene (clostridial myonecrosis) is a necrotizing infection that follows trauma or surgery and is caused by several anaerobic, gram-positive, spore-forming bacilli of the genus *Clostridium*. The spores are found in soil, feces, and vaginal secretions. In devitalized tissue, the spores germinate into vegetative bacilli that proliferate and produce toxins, causing thrombosis, hemolysis, and tissue necrosis. *Clostridium perfringens,* the species causing approximately 80% of cases of gas gangrene, produces at least eight such toxins. The areas involved most often are the extremities, abdomen, and uterus. *Clostridium septicum* may also cause myonecrosis and causes septicemia in patients with neutropenia. Nonclostridial infections with gas formation can mimic clostridial infections and are more common.

Clinical Findings

A. SYMPTOMS AND SIGNS

The onset of gas gangrene is sudden, usually 1–20 days (mean, 3–4 days) after trauma or surgery. The skin around the wound becomes discolored, with hemorrhagic bullae, serosanguineous exudate, and crepitation in the subcutaneous tissues. Pain and swelling are usually intense. Systemic illness appears early and progresses rapidly to intravascular hemolysis, jaundice, shock, toxic delirium, and renal failure.

B. LABORATORY FINDINGS

Isolation of the organism requires anaerobic culture. Gram-stained smears may demonstrate many gram-positive rods and few inflammatory cells.

C. IMAGING

Radiographs may demonstrate gas in tissues, but this is a late finding and is also seen in infections with other gas-forming organisms or may be due to air introduced into tissues during trauma or surgery.

D. OPERATIVE FINDINGS

Direct visualization of the muscle at surgery may be necessary to diagnose gas gangrene. Early, the muscle is pale and edematous and does not contract normally; later, the muscle may be frankly gangrenous.

Differential Diagnosis

Gangrene and cellulitis caused by other organisms and clostridial cellulitis (not myonecrosis) must be distinguished. Necrotizing fasciitis may resemble gas gangrene.

Prevention

Gas gangrene can be prevented by the adequate cleansing and debridement of all wounds. It is essential that foreign bodies and dead tissue be removed. A clean wound does not provide a suitable anaerobic environment for the growth of clostridial species.

Treatment

A. SPECIFIC MEASURES

Penicillin G (300,000–400,000 units/kg/d intravenously in six divided doses) should be given, usually combined with clindamycin or metronidazole. Clindamycin, metronidazole, meropenem, and imipenem–cilastatin are alternatives for penicillin-allergic patients.

B. SURGICAL MEASURES

Surgery should be prompt and extensive, with removal of all necrotic tissue.

C. HYPERBARIC OXYGEN

Hyperbaric oxygen therapy has been shown to be effective, but it is not a substitute for surgery. A patient may be exposed to 2–3 atm in pure oxygen for 1- to 2-hour periods for as many sessions as necessary until clinical remission occurs.

Prognosis

Clostridial myonecrosis is fatal if untreated. With early diagnosis, antibiotics, and surgery, the mortality rate is 20–60%. Involvement of the abdominal wall, leukopenia, intravascular hemolysis, renal failure, and shock are ominous prognostic signs.

Barnes C et al: *Clostridium septicum* myonecrosis in congenital neutropenia. Pediatrics 2004;114(6):e757 [PMID: 15574607].

Brook I: Microbiology and management of infectious gangrene in children. J Pediatr Orthop 2004;24(5):587 [PMID: 15308913].

DIPHTHERIA

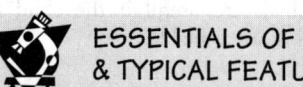

ESSENTIALS OF DIAGNOSIS & TYPICAL FEATURES

- *A gray, adherent pseudomembrane, most often in the pharynx but also in the nasopharynx or trachea.*
- *Sore throat, serosanguineous nasal discharge, hoarseness, and fever in a nonimmunized child.*
- *Peripheral neuritis or myocarditis.*
- *Positive culture.*
- *Treatment should not be withheld pending culture results.*

General Considerations

Diphtheria is an acute infection of the upper respiratory tract or skin caused by toxin-producing *Corynebacterium diphtheriae*. Diphtheria in the United States is rare; one case was reported in 2003–2005, and only 48 cases were reported from 1980–1997. However, significant numbers of elderly adults and unimmunized children are susceptible to infection. Diphtheria still occurs in epidemics in countries where immunization is not universal. Travelers to these areas may acquire the disease. *Corynebacteria* are gram-positive, club-shaped rods with a beaded appearance on Gram stain.

The capacity to produce exotoxin is conferred by a lysogenic bacteriophage and is not present in all strains of *C diphtheriae*. In immunized communities, infection probably occurs through spread of the phage among carriers of susceptible bacteria rather than through spread of phage-containing bacteria themselves. Diphtheria toxin kills susceptible cells by irreversible inhibition of protein synthesis.

The toxin is absorbed into the mucous membranes and causes destruction of epithelium and a superficial inflammatory response. The necrotic epithelium becomes embedded in exuding fibrin and red and white blood cells, forming a grayish pseudomembrane over the tonsils, pharynx, or larynx. Any attempt to remove the membrane exposes and tears the capillaries, resulting in bleeding. The diphtheria bacilli within the membrane continue to produce toxin, which is absorbed and may result in toxic injury to heart muscle, liver, kidneys, and adrenals, and is sometimes accompanied by hemorrhage. The toxin also produces neuritis, resulting in paralysis of the soft palate, eye muscles, or extremities. Death may occur as a result of respiratory obstruction or toxemia and circulatory collapse. The patient may succumb after a somewhat longer time as a result of cardiac damage. The incubation period is 2–7 days.

Clinical Findings

A. SYMPTOMS AND SIGNS

1. Pharyngeal diphtheria—Early manifestations of diphtheritic pharyngitis are mild sore throat, moderate fever, and malaise, followed fairly rapidly by prostration and circulatory collapse. The pulse is more rapid than the fever would seem to justify. A pharyngeal membrane forms and may spread into the nasopharynx or the trachea, producing respiratory obstruction. The membrane is tenacious and gray and is surrounded by a narrow zone of erythema and a broader zone of edema. The cervical lymph nodes become swollen, and swelling is associated with brawny edema of the neck (so-called bull neck). Laryngeal diphtheria presents with stridor, which can progress to obstruction of the airway.

2. Other forms—Cutaneous, vaginal, and wound diphtheria account for up to one-third of cases and are characterized by ulcerative lesions with membrane formation.

B. LABORATORY FINDINGS

Diagnosis is clinical. Direct smears are unreliable. Material is obtained from the nose, throat, or skin lesions, if present, for culture, but specialized culture media are

required. Between 16 and 48 hours is required before identification of the organism. A toxigenicity test is then performed. Cultures may be negative in individuals who have received antibiotics. The WBC count is usually normal, but hemolytic anemia and thrombocytopenia are frequent.

Differential Diagnosis

Pharyngeal diphtheria resembles pharyngitis secondary to β-hemolytic streptococcus, Epstein–Barr virus, or other viral respiratory pathogens. A nasal foreign body or purulent sinusitis may mimic nasal diphtheria. Other causes of laryngeal obstruction include epiglottitis and viral croup. Guillain–Barré syndrome, poliomyelitis, or acute poisoning may mimic the neuropathy of diphtheria.

Complications

A. MYOCARDITIS

Diphtheritic myocarditis is characterized by a rapid, thready pulse; indistinct heart sounds, ST-T wave changes, conduction abnormalities, dysrhythmias, or cardiac failure; hepatomegaly; and fluid retention. Myocardial dysfunction may occur from 2–40 days after the onset of pharyngitis.

B. POLYNEURITIS

Neuritis of the palatal and pharyngeal nerves occurs during the first or second week. Nasal speech and regurgitation of food through the nose are seen. Diplopia and strabismus occur during the third week or later. Neuritis may also involve peripheral nerves supplying the intercostal muscles, diaphragm, and other muscle groups. Generalized paresis usually occurs after the fourth week.

C. BRONCHOPNEUMONIA

Secondary pneumonia is common in fatal cases.

Prevention

A. IMMUNIZATION

Immunization with diphtheria toxoid combined with pertussis and tetanus toxoids (DTP) should be used routinely for infants and children. (See Chapter 9.)

B. CARE OF EXPOSED SUSCEPTIBLES

Children exposed to diphtheria should be examined, and nose and throat cultures obtained. If signs and symptoms of early diphtheria are found, antibiotic treatment should be instituted. Immunized asymptomatic individuals should receive diphtheria toxoid if a booster has not been received within 5 years. Unimmunized close contacts should receive either erythromycin orally (40 mg/kg/d in four divided doses) for 7 days or benzathine penicillin G intramuscularly (25,000 units/ kg), active immunization with diphtheria toxoid, and observation daily.

Treatment

A. SPECIFIC MEASURES

1. Antitoxin—To be effective, diphtheria antitoxin should be administered within 48 hours. (See Chapter 9.)

2. Antibiotics—Penicillin G (150,000 units/kg/d intravenously) should be given for 10 days. For penicillin-allergic patients, erythromycin (40 mg/kg/d) is given orally for 10 days.

B. GENERAL MEASURES

Bed rest in the hospital for 10–14 days is usually required. All patients must be strictly isolated for 1–7 days until respiratory secretions are noncontagious. Isolation may be discontinued when three successive nose and throat cultures at 24-hour intervals are negative. These cultures should not be taken until at least 24 hours have elapsed since the cessation of antibiotic treatment.

C. TREATMENT OF CARRIERS

All carriers should receive treatment. Erythromycin (40 mg/kg/d orally in three or four divided doses), penicillin V potassium (50 mg/kg/d for 10 days), or benzathine penicillin G (600,000–1,200,000 units intramuscularly) should be given. All carriers must be quarantined. Before they can be released, carriers must have three negative cultures of both the nose and the throat taken 24 hours apart and obtained at least 24 hours after the cessation of antibiotic therapy.

Prognosis

Mortality varies from 3–25% and is particularly high in the presence of early myocarditis. Neuritis is reversible; it is fatal only if an intact airway and adequate respiration cannot be maintained. Permanent damage due to myocarditis occurs rarely.

Centers for Disease Control and Prevention: Diphtheria. www.cdc.gov/nip/publications/pink/dip.pdf

Fatal respiratory diphtheria in a U.S. traveler to Haiti—Pennsylvania, 2003. MMWR Morb Mortal Wkly Rep 2004;52–53: 1285 [PMID: 14712177].

Lumio J et al: Fatal case of diphtheria in an unvaccinated infant in Finland. Pediatr Infect Dis J 2003;22(9):844 [PMID: 14515838].

Munford L et al: Cardiac diphtheria in a previously immunized individual. J Natl Med Assoc 2003;95(9):875 [PMID: 14527057].

Sing A, Heesemann J: Imported cutaneous diphtheria, Germany, 1997–2003 [Letter]. Emerg Infect Dis 2005;Feb. http:// www.cdc.gov/ncidod/EID/vol11no02/04-0560.htm [PMID: 15759338].

INFECTIONS DUE TO ENTEROBACTERIACEAE

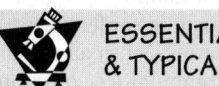

ESSENTIALS OF DIAGNOSIS & TYPICAL FEATURES

- *Diarrhea by several different mechanisms due to Escherichia coli.*
- *Hemorrhagic colitis and hemolytic–uremic syndrome.*
- *Neonatal sepsis or meningitis.*
- *Urinary tract infection.*
- *Opportunistic infections.*
- *Diagnosis confirmed by culture.*

General Considerations

Enterobacteriaceae are a family of gram-negative bacilli that are normal flora in the gastrointestinal tract and are also found in water and soil. They cause gastroenteritis, urinary tract infections, neonatal sepsis and meningitis, and opportunistic infections. *Escherichia coli* is the organism in this family that most commonly causes infection in children, but *Klebsiella, Morganella, Enterobacter, Serratia, Proteus,* and other genera are also important, particularly in the compromised host. *Shigella* and *Salmonella* are discussed in separate sections.

E coli strains capable of causing diarrhea were originally termed enteropathogenic (EPEC) and were recognized by serotype. It is now known that *E coli* may cause diarrhea by several distinct mechanisms. Classic EPEC strains cause a characteristic histologic injury in the small bowel termed "adherence and effacement." Enterotoxigenic *E coli* (ETEC) causes a secretory, watery diarrhea. ETEC adheres to enterocytes and secretes one or more plasmid-encoded enterotoxins. One of these, heat-labile toxin, resembles cholera toxin in structure, function, and mechanism of action. Enteroinvasive *E coli* (EIEC) is very similar to *Shigella* in pathogenetic mechanism. Enterohemorrhagic *E coli* (EHEC) is the cause of hemorrhagic colitis and the hemolytic–uremic syndrome. The most common EHEC serotype is 0157:H7, although several other serotypes cause the same syndrome. These strains elaborate one of several cytotoxins, closely related to Shiga toxin produced by *S dysenteriae*. Outbreaks of hemolytic— uremic syndrome associated with EHEC have followed consumption of inadequately cooked ground beef. Thorough heating to 68–71 °C is necessary. Unpasteurized fruit juice, various uncooked vegetables, and contaminated water have also caused infections and epidemics. The common source for EHEC in all of these foods and water is the feces of cattle. Person-to-person spread including spread in day care centers by the fecal–oral route has been reported.

E coli that aggregate on the surface of hep cells in tissue culture are termed *enteroaggregative (EAggEC) E coli*. EAggEC cause diarrhea by a distinct but unknown mechanism.

Eighty percent of *E coli* strains causing neonatal meningitis possess specific capsular polysaccharide (K1 antigen), which, alone or in association with specific somatic antigens, confers virulence. Approximately 90% of urinary tract infections in children are caused by *E coli*. *E coli* binds to the uroepithelium by P-fimbriae, which are present in more than 90% of *E coli* that cause pyelonephritis. Other bacterial cell surface structures, such as O and K antigens, and host factors are also important in the pathogenesis of urinary tract infections.

Klebsiella, Enterobacter, Serratia, and *Morganella* are normally found in the gastrointestinal tract and in soil and water. *Klebsiella* may cause a bronchopneumonia with cavity formation. *Klebsiella, Enterobacter,* and *Serratia* are often hospital-acquired opportunists associated with antibiotic usage, debilitated states, and chronic respiratory conditions. They frequently cause urinary tract infection or sepsis. In many newborn nurseries, nosocomial outbreaks caused by antimicrobial-resistant *Klebsiella* or *Enterobacter* spp. are a major problem.

Many of these infections are difficult to treat because of antibiotic resistance. Antibiotic susceptibility tests are necessary. Parenteral third-generation cephalosporins are usually more active than ampicillin, but resistance due to high-level production of chromosomal cephalosporinase may occur. *Enterobacter* and *Serratia* strains broadly resistant to cephalosporins also cause infections in hospitalized newborns and children. Aminoglycoside antibiotics are usually effective but require monitoring of serum levels to ensure therapeutic and nontoxic levels.

Clinical Findings

A. SYMPTOMS AND SIGNS

1. *E coli* gastroenteritis—*E coli* may cause diarrhea of varying types and severity. ETEC usually produce mild, self-limiting illness without significant fever or systemic toxicity, often known as traveler's diarrhea. However, diarrhea may be severe in newborns and infants, and occasionally an older child or adult will have a cholera-like syndrome. EIEC strains cause a shigellosis-like illness, characterized by fever, systemic symptoms, blood and mucus in the stool, and leukocytosis, but currently are uncommon in the United States. EHEC strains cause hemorrhagic colitis. Diarrhea is initially watery, and fever is usually absent. Abdominal pain and cramping occur, and diarrhea progresses to blood streaking or grossly bloody stools. Hemolytic–uremic syndrome occurs within a few days of diarrhea in 2–5% of children and is characterized by microangiopathic hemolytic anemia, thrombocytopenia, and renal failure. (See Chapter 22.)

2. Neonatal sepsis—Findings include jaundice, hepatosplenomegaly, fever, temperature lability, apneic spells, irritability, and poor feeding. Meningitis is associated with sepsis in 25–40% of cases. Other metastatic foci of infection may be present, including pneumonia and pyelonephritis. Sepsis may lead to severe metabolic acidosis, shock, DIC, and death.

3. Neonatal meningitis—Findings include high fever, full fontanelles, vomiting, coma, convulsions, pareses or paralyses, poor or absent Moro reflex, opisthotonos, and occasionally hypertonia or hypotonia. Sepsis coexists or precedes meningitis in most cases. Thus, signs of sepsis often accompany those of meningitis. CSF usually shows a cell count of over 1000/μL, mostly polymorphonuclear neutrophils, and bacteria on Gram stain. CSF glucose concentration is low (usually less than half that of blood), and the protein is elevated above the levels normally seen in newborns and premature infants (> 150 mg/dL).

4. Acute urinary tract infection—Symptoms include dysuria, increased urinary frequency, and fever in the older child. Nonspecific symptoms such as anorexia, vomiting, irritability, failure to thrive, and unexplained fever are seen in children younger than age 2 years. Young infants may present with jaundice. As many as 1% of girls of school age and 0.05% of boys have asymptomatic bacteriuria. Screening for and treatment of asymptomatic bacteriuria is not recommended.

B. LABORATORY FINDINGS

Because *E coli* are normal flora in the stool, a positive stool culture alone does not prove that the *E coli* in the stool are causing disease. Serotyping, tests for enterotoxin production or invasiveness, and tests for P-fimbriae are performed in research laboratories. MacConkey agar with sorbitol substituted for lactose (SMAC agar) is useful to screen stool for EHEC. Serotyping and testing for enterotoxin are available at many state health departments. Blood cultures are positive in neonatal sepsis. Cultures of CSF and urine should also be obtained. The diagnosis of urinary tract infections is discussed in Chapter 22.

Differential Diagnosis

The clinical picture of EPEC infection may resemble that of salmonellosis, shigellosis, or viral gastroenteritis.

Neonatal sepsis and meningitis caused by *E coli* can be differentiated from other causes of neonatal infection only by blood and CSF culture.

Treatment

A. SPECIFIC MEASURES

1. *E coli* gastroenteritis—Gastroenteritis due to EPEC seldom requires antimicrobial treatment. Fluid and electrolyte therapy, preferably given orally, may be required to avoid dehydration. Bismuth subsalicylate reduces stool volume by about one-third in infants with watery diarrhea, probably including ETEC. In nursery outbreaks, *E coli* gastroenteritis has been treated with neomycin (100 mg/kg/d orally in three divided doses for 5 days). Clinical efficacy is not established. Traveler's diarrhea may be treated with TMP–SMX in children and with fluoroquinolones in adults. The risk of hemolytic–uremic syndrome increases following treatment of EHEC colitis, and antimicrobials should be withheld in suspected cases.

2. *E coli* sepsis, pneumonia, or pyelonephritis—The drugs of choice are ampicillin (150–200 mg/kg/d, given intravenously or intramuscularly in divided doses every 4–6 hours), cefotaxime (150–200 mg/kg/d, given intravenously or intramuscularly in divided doses every 6–8 hours), ceftriaxone (50–100 mg/kg/d, given intramuscularly as single dose or in two divided doses), and gentamicin (5.0–7.5 mg/kg/d, given intramuscularly or intravenously in divided doses every 8 hours). Treatment is continued for 10–14 days. Amikacin or tobramycin may be used instead of gentamicin if the strain is susceptible. Third-generation cephalosporins are often an attractive alternative as single-drug therapy and do not require monitoring for toxicity.

3. *E coli* meningitis—Third-generation cephalosporins such as cefotaxime (200 mg/kg/d intravenously in four divided doses) are given for a minimum of 3 weeks. Ampicillin (200–300 mg/kg/d intravenously in four to six divided doses) and gentamicin (5.0–7.5 mg/kg/d intramuscularly or intravenously in three divided doses) are also effective. Treatment with intrathecal and intraventricular aminoglycosides does not improve outcome. Serum levels need to be monitored.

4. Acute urinary tract infection—(See Chapter 22.)

Prognosis

Death due to gastroenteritis leading to dehydration can be prevented by early fluid and electrolyte therapy. Neonatal sepsis with meningitis is still associated with a mortality rate of over 50%. Most children with recurrent urinary tract infections do well if they have no underlying anatomic defects. The mortality rate in opportunistic infections usually depends on the severity of infection and the underlying condition.

Bonsu BK et al: Susceptibility of recent bacterial isolates to cefdinir and selected antibiotics among children with urinary tract infections. Acad Emerg Med 2005;Dec 19 [PMID: 16365328].

Centers for Disease Control and Prevention: Diarrheagenic *Escherichia coli*. www.cdc.gov/ncidod/dbmd/diseaseinfo/diarrecoli_t.htm

Ladhani S, Gransden W: Increasing antibiotic resistance among urinary tract isolates. Arch Dis Child 2003;88(5):444 [PMID: 12716722].

Lutter SA et al: Antibiotic resistance patterns in children hospitalized for urinary tract infections. Arch Pediatr Adolesc Med 2005;159(10):992 [PMID: 16203936].

Ochoa TJ, Cleary TG: Epidemiology and spectrum of disease of *Escherichia coli* 0157. Curr Opin Infect Dis 2003;16(3):259 [PMID: 12821818].

Outbreaks of *Escherichia coli* 0157:H7 associated with petting zoos—North Carolina, Florida and Arizona, 2004 and 2005. MMWR Morb Mortal Wkly Rep 2005;54(50):1277 [PMID: 16371942].

PSEUDOMONAS INFECTIONS

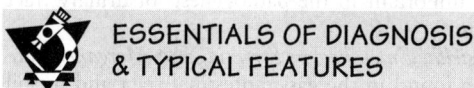

ESSENTIALS OF DIAGNOSIS & TYPICAL FEATURES

- *Opportunistic infection.*
- *Confirmed by cultures.*

General Considerations

Pseudomonas aeruginosa is an aerobic gram-negative rod with versatile metabolic requirements. *P aeruginosa* may grow in distilled water and in commonly used disinfectants, complicating infection control in medical facilities. *P aeruginosa* is both invasive and destructive to tissue, and toxigenic due to secreted exotoxins, all factors that contribute to virulence. Other genera previously classified as *Pseudomonas* occasionally cause nosocomial infections. *Stenotrophomonas maltophilia* (previously *P maltophilia*) and *Burkholderia cepacia* (previously *P cepacia*) are the most frequent.

P aeruginosa is an important cause of infection in children with cystic fibrosis, neoplastic disease, neutropenia, or extensive burns and in those receiving antibiotic therapy. Infections of the urinary and respiratory tracts, ears, mastoids, paranasal sinuses, eyes, skin, meninges, and bones are seen. *Pseudomonas* pneumonia is a common nosocomial infection in patients receiving assisted ventilation.

P aeruginosa sepsis may be accompanied by characteristic peripheral lesions called ecthyma gangrenosum. Ecthyma gangrenosum also may occur by direct invasion through intact skin in the groin, axilla, or other skinfolds. *P aeruginosa* is an infrequent cause of sepsis in previously healthy infants and may be the initial sign of underlying medical problems. *P aeruginosa* osteomyelitis often complicates puncture wounds of the feet. *P aeruginosa* is a frequent cause of malignant external otitis media and of chronic suppurative otitis media. Outbreaks of vesiculopustular skin rash have been associated with exposure to contaminated water in whirlpool baths and hot tubs.

P aeruginosa infects the tracheobronchial tree of nearly all patients with cystic fibrosis. Mucoid exopolysaccharide, an exuberant capsule, is characteristically overproduced by isolates from patients with cystic fibrosis. Although bacteremia seldom occurs, patients with cystic fibrosis ultimately succumb to chronic lung infection with *P aeruginosa*. Infection due to *B cepacia* has caused a rapidly progressive pulmonary disease in some colonized patients and may be spread by close contact.

Clinical Findings

The clinical findings depend on the site of infection and the patient's underlying disease. Sepsis with these organisms resembles gram-negative sepsis with other organisms, although the presence of ecthyma gangrenosum suggests the diagnosis. The diagnosis is made by culture. *Pseudomonas* infection should be suspected in neonates and neutropenic patients with clinical sepsis. A severe necrotizing pneumonia occurs in patients on ventilators.

Patients with cystic fibrosis have a persistent bronchitis that progresses to bronchiectasis and ultimately to respiratory failure. During exacerbations of illness, cough and sputum production increase with low-grade fever, malaise, and diminished energy.

The purulent aural drainage without fever in patients with chronic suppurative otitis media is not distinguishable from that due to other causes.

Prevention

A. INFECTIONS IN DEBILITATED PATIENTS

Colonization of extensive second- and third-degree burns by *P aeruginosa* can lead to fatal septicemia. Aggressive debridement and topical treatment with 0.5% silver nitrate solution, 10% mafenide cream, or silver sulfadiazine will greatly inhibit *P aeruginosa* contamination of burns. (See Chapter 11 for a discussion of burn wound infections and prevention.)

B. NOSOCOMIAL INFECTIONS

Faucet aerators, communal soap dispensers, disinfectants, improperly cleaned inhalation therapy equipment, infant incubators, and many other sources have all been associated with *Pseudomonas* epidemics. Infant-to-infant transmission by nursery personnel carrying *Pseudomonas* on the hands is frequent in neonatal units. Careful maintenance of equipment and enforcement of infection control procedures are essential to minimize nosocomial transmission.

C. PATIENTS WITH CYSTIC FIBROSIS

Chronic infection of the lower respiratory tract occurs in nearly all patients with cystic fibrosis. The infecting organism is seldom cleared from the respiratory tract, even with intensive antimicrobial therapy, and the resultant injury to the lung eventually leads to pulmonary insufficiency. Treatment is aimed at controlling signs and symptoms of the infection.

Treatment

P aeruginosa is inherently resistant to many antimicrobials and may develop resistance during therapy. Mortality rates in hospitalized patients exceed 50%, owing both to the severity of underlying illnesses in patients predisposed to *Pseudomonas* infection and to the limitations of therapy. Antibiotics effective against *Pseudomonas* include the aminoglycosides, ureidopenicillins (ticarcillin and piperacillin), β-lactamase inhibitor with a ureidopenicillin (ticarcillin–clavulanate and piperacillin–tazobactam), expanded-spectrum cephalosporins (ceftazidime and cefepime), imipenem, meropenem, and ciprofloxacin. Antimicrobial susceptibility patterns vary from area to area, and resistance tends to appear as new drugs become popular. Treatment of infections is best guided by clinical response and susceptibility tests.

Gentamicin or tobramycin (5.0–7.5 mg/kg/d, given intramuscularly or intravenously in three divided doses) or amikacin (15–22 mg/kg/d, given in two or three divided doses) in combination with ticarcillin (200–300 mg/kg/d, given intravenously in six divided doses) or with another antipseudomonal β-lactam antibiotic is recommended for treatment of serious *Pseudomonas* infections. Ceftazidime (150–200 mg/kg/d, given in four divided doses) or cefepime (150 mg/kg/d, given in three divided doses) has excellent activity against *P aeruginosa*. Treatment should be continued for 10–14 days. Treatment with two active drugs is recommended for all serious infections.

Pseudomonas osteomyelitis requires thorough surgical debridement and antimicrobial therapy for 2 weeks. *Pseudomonas* folliculitis does not require antibiotic therapy.

Oral or intravenous ciprofloxacin is also effective against susceptible *P aeruginosa*, but is approved by the FDA for use in children except in the case of urinary tract infection. Nonetheless, in some circumstances of antimicrobial resistance, or when the benefits clearly outweigh the small risks, ciprofloxacin may be used.

Chronic suppurative otitis media responds to intravenous ceftazidime (150–200 mg/kg/d in three or four divided doses) given until the drainage has ceased for 3 days. Twice-daily ceftazidime with aural debridement and cleaning given on an outpatient basis has also been successful. Swimmer's ear may be caused by *P aeruginosa* and responds well to topical drying agents (alcohol–vinegar mix) and cleansing.

Prognosis

Because debilitated patients are most frequently affected, the mortality rate is high. These infections may have a protracted course, and eradication of the organisms may be difficult.

Blumer JL et al: The efficacy and safety of meropenem and tobramycin vs ceftazidime and tobramycin in the treatment of acute pulmonary exacerbations in patients with cystic fibrosis. Chest 2005;128(4):2336 [PMID: 16236892].

Korvoca J et al: Bacteraemia due to *Pseudomonas putida* and other *Pseudomonas* non-*aeruginosa* in children J Infect 2005;51(1):81 [PMID: 15979496].

Sims EJ et al, Steering Committee of the UK Cystic Fibrosis Database: Neonatal screening for cystic fibrosis is beneficial even in the context of modern treatment. J Pediatr 2005;147(3 Suppl):S42 [PMID: 16202781].

Wisplinghoff H et al: Nosocomial bloodstream infections in pediatric patients in United States hospitals: Epidemiology, clinical features and susceptibilities. Pediatr Infect Dis J 2003;22 (8):686 [PMID: 1291376].

SALMONELLA GASTROENTERITIS

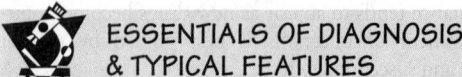

ESSENTIALS OF DIAGNOSIS & TYPICAL FEATURES

- *Nausea, vomiting, headache, meningismus.*
- *Fever, diarrhea, abdominal pain.*
- *Culture or organism from stool, blood, or other specimens.*

General Considerations

Salmonellae are gram-negative rods that frequently cause food-borne gastroenteritis and occasionally bacteremic infection of bone, meninges, and other foci. Three species—*Salmonella typhi, Salmonella choleraesuis,* and *Salmonella enteritidis*—and approximately 2000 serotypes are recognized. *S typhimurium* is the most frequently isolated serotype in most parts of the world. An estimated 4 million cases of salmonellosis occur yearly in the United States, but only 40,000 are reported.

Salmonellae are able to penetrate the mucin layer of the small bowel and attach to epithelial cells. Organisms penetrate the epithelial cells and multiply in the submucosa. Infection results in fever, vomiting, watery diarrhea, and occasionally mucus and polymorphonuclear neutrophils in the stool. Although the small intestine is generally regarded as the principal site of infection, colitis also occurs. *S typhimurium* frequently involves the large bowel.

Salmonella infections in childhood occur in two major forms: (1) gastroenteritis (including food poisoning), which may be complicated by sepsis and focal suppurative complications; and (2) enteric fever (typhoid fever and paratyphoid fever) (see next section). Although the incidence of typhoid fever has decreased in the United States, the incidence of *Salmonella* gastroenteritis has greatly increased in the past 15–20 years. The highest attack rates occur in children younger than age 6 years, with a peak in the age group from 6 months to 2 years.

Salmonellae are widespread in nature, infecting domestic and wild animals. Fowl and reptiles have a particularly high carriage rate. Transmission results primarily from ingestion of contaminated food. Transmission from human to human occurs by the fecal–oral route via contaminated food, water, and fomites. Numerous foods, including meats, milk, cheese, ice cream, and chocolate, are associated with outbreaks. Contaminated egg powder and frozen whole egg preparations used to make ice cream, custards, and mayonnaise are responsible for outbreaks. Eggs with contaminated shells that are consumed raw or undercooked have been incriminated in outbreaks and sporadic cases.

Because salmonellae are susceptible to gastric acidity, the elderly, infants, and patients taking antacids or H_2-blocking drugs are at increased risk for infection. Most cases of *Salmonella* meningitis (80%) and bacteremia occur in infancy. Newborns may acquire the infection from their mothers during delivery and may precipitate outbreaks in nurseries. Newborns are at special risk for developing meningitis.

Clinical Findings

A. SYMPTOMS AND SIGNS

Infants usually develop fever, vomiting, and diarrhea. The older child may also complain of headache, nausea, and abdominal pain. Stools are often watery or may contain mucus and, in some instances, blood, suggesting shigellosis. Drowsiness and disorientation may be associated with meningismus. Convulsions occur less frequently than with shigellosis. Splenomegaly is occasionally noted. In the usual case, diarrhea is moderate and subsides after 4–5 days, but it may be protracted.

B. LABORATORY FINDINGS

Diagnosis is made by isolation of the organism from stool, blood, or, in some cases, from urine, CSF, or pus from a suppurative lesion. The WBC count usually shows a polymorphonuclear leukocytosis but may show leukopenia. *Salmonella* isolates should be reported to public health authorities for epidemiologic purposes. Stool cultures are rarely positive when obtained from children who develop diarrhea after 3 days of hospitalization.

Differential Diagnosis

In staphylococcal food poisoning, the incubation period is shorter (2–4 hours) than in *Salmonella* food poisoning (12–24 hours). Fever is absent, and vomiting rather than diarrhea is the main symptom. In shigellosis, many pus cells are likely to be seen on a stained smear of stool and there is more apt to be a marked shift to the left in the peripheral white count, although some cases of salmonellosis are indistinguishable from shigellosis. *Campylobacter* gastroenteritis commonly resembles salmonellosis clinically. Culture of the stools is necessary to distinguish the causes of bacterial gastroenteritis.

Complications

Unlike most types of infectious diarrhea, salmonellosis is frequently accompanied by bacteremia, especially in newborns and infants. Septicemia with extraintestinal infection is seen, most commonly with *S choleraesuis* but also with *S enteritidis, S typhimurium,* and *S paratyphi* B and C. The organism may spread to any tissue and may cause arthritis, osteomyelitis, cholecystitis, endocarditis, meningitis, pericarditis, pneumonia, or pyelonephritis. Patients with sickle cell anemia or other hemoglobinopathies have a predilection for the development of osteomyelitis. Severe dehydration and shock are more likely to occur with shigellosis but may occur with *Salmonella* gastroenteritis.

Prevention

Measures for the prevention of *Salmonella* infections include thorough cooking of foodstuffs derived from contaminated sources, adequate refrigeration, control of infection among domestic animals, and meticulous meat and poultry inspections. Raw and undercooked fresh eggs should be avoided. Food handlers and child care workers with salmonellosis should have three negative stool cultures before resuming work. Asymptomatic children, who have recovered from *Salmonella* infection, do not need exclusion.

Treatment

A. SPECIFIC MEASURES

In uncomplicated *Salmonella* gastroenteritis, antibiotic treatment does not shorten the course of the clinical illness and may prolong convalescent carriage of the organism. Colitis or secretory diarrhea due to *Salmonella* may improve with antibiotic therapy.

Because of the higher risk of sepsis and focal disease, antibiotic treatment is recommended in infants younger than age 3 months; in severely ill children; and in children with sickle cell disease, liver disease, recent gastrointestinal surgery, cancer, depressed immunity, or chronic renal or cardiac disease. Infants younger than age 3 months with positive stool cultures or suspected salmonellosis sepsis should be admitted to the hospital, evaluated for focal infection including cultures of blood and CSF, and given

treatment intravenously. A third-generation cephalosporin is recommended due to frequent resistance to ampicillin and TMP–SMX. Older patients developing bacteremia during the course of gastroenteritis should receive parenteral treatment initially, and a careful search should be made for additional foci of infection. After signs and symptoms subside, these patients should receive oral medication. Parenteral and oral treatment should last a total of 7–10 days. Longer treatment is indicated for specific complications. If susceptibility tests indicate resistance to ampicillin, third-generation cephalosporins or TMP–SMX should be given. Fluoroquinolones also are efficacious but are not approved for administration to children. Fluoroquinolones are used for strains resistant to multiple other drugs.

Salmonella meningitis is best treated with ampicillin (200–300 mg/kg/d intravenously in four to six divided doses) and a third-generation cephalosporin (cefotaxime, ceftriaxone) for 3 weeks. If the child improves rapidly and the CSF is sterile, treatment may be completed with a single drug, the choice guided by results of susceptibility tests.

Outbreaks on pediatric wards are difficult to control. Strict hand washing, cohorting of patients and personnel, and ultimately closure of the unit may be necessary.

B. TREATMENT OF THE CARRIER STATE

About half of patients may have positive stool cultures after 4 weeks. Infants tend to remain convalescent carriers for up to a year. Antibiotic treatment of carriers is not effective.

C. GENERAL MEASURES

Careful attention must be given to maintaining fluid and electrolyte balance, especially in infants.

Prognosis

In gastroenteritis, the prognosis is good. In sepsis with focal suppurative complications, the prognosis is more guarded. The case fatality rate of *Salmonella* meningitis is high in infants. There is a strong tendency to relapse if treatment is not continued for at least 14–21 days.

Amieva MR: Important bacterial gastrointestinal pathogens in children: A pathogenesis perspective. Pediatr Clin North Am 2005;52(3):749, vi. [PMID: 15925661].

Centers for Disease Control and Prevention: *Salmonella* infection (salmonellosis). www.cdc.gov/ncidod/diseases/submenus/sub_salmonella.htm

Centers for Disease Control and Prevention (CDC): Salmonellosis associated with pet turtles—Wisconsin and Wyoming, 2004. MMWR Morb Mortal Wkly Rep 2005;54(9):223 [PMID: 15758895].

Fisker N et al: Clinical review of nontyphoid *Salmonella* infections from 1991 to 1999 in a Danish county. Clin Infect Dis 2003;37(4):e47 [PMID: 12905152].

Zaidi MB et al: Nontyphoidal *Salmonella* from human clinical cases, asymptomatic children, and raw retail meats in Yucatan Mexico. Clin Infect Dis 2006;42(1):21. Epub 2005 Nov 29. [PMID: 16323087].

TYPHOID FEVER & PARATYPHOID FEVER

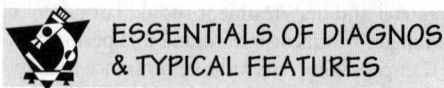

ESSENTIALS OF DIAGNOSIS & TYPICAL FEATURES

- Insidious or acute onset of headache, anorexia, vomiting, constipation or diarrhea, ileus, and high fever.
- Meningismus, splenomegaly, and rose spots.
- Leukopenia; positive blood, stool, bone marrow, and urine cultures.

General Considerations

Typhoid fever is caused by the gram-negative bacillus *Salmonella typhi*. Paratyphoid fevers, which are usually milder but may be clinically indistinguishable, are caused by *Salmonella paratyphi* A, *Salmonella schottmülleri*, or *Salmonella hirschfeldii* (formerly *Salmonella paratyphi* A, B, and C). Children have a shorter incubation period than do adults (usually 5–8 days instead of 8–14 days). The organism enters the body through the walls of the intestinal tract and, following a transient bacteremia, multiplies in the reticuloendothelial cells of the liver and spleen. Persistent bacteremia and symptoms then follow. Reinfection of the intestine occurs as organisms are excreted in the bile. Bacterial emboli produce the characteristic skin lesions (rose spots). Symptoms in children may be mild or severe, but children younger than age 5 years rarely have severe typhoid fever.

Typhoid fever is transmitted by the fecal–oral route and by contamination of food or water. Unlike other *Salmonella* species, there are no animal reservoirs of *S typhi*; each case is the result of direct or indirect contact with the organism or with an individual who is actively infected or a chronic carrier.

About 250 cases per year are reported in the United States, 80% of which are acquired during foreign travel.

Clinical Findings

A. SYMPTOMS AND SIGNS

In children, the onset of typhoid fever is apt to be sudden rather than insidious, with malaise, headache, crampy abdominal pains and distention, and sometimes constipation followed within 48 hours by diarrhea, high

fever, and toxemia. An encephalopathy may be seen with irritability, confusion, delirium, and stupor. Vomiting and meningismus may be prominent in infants and young children. The classic lengthy three-stage disease seen in adult patients is often shortened in children. The prodrome may last only 2–4 days, the toxic stage only 2–3 days, and the defervescence stage 1–2 weeks.

During the prodromal stage, physical findings may be absent, or there may merely be some abdominal distention and tenderness, meningismus, mild hepatomegaly, and minimal splenomegaly. The typical typhoidal rash (rose spots) is present in 10–15% of children. It appears during the second week of the disease and may erupt in crops for the succeeding 10–14 days. Rose spots are erythematous maculopapular lesions 2–3 mm in diameter that fade on pressure. They are found principally on the trunk and chest, and they generally disappear within 3–4 days. The lesions usually number fewer than 20.

B. LABORATORY FINDINGS

Typhoid bacilli can be isolated from many sites, including blood, stool, urine, and bone marrow. Blood cultures are positive in 50–80% of cases during the first week and less often later in the illness. Stool cultures are positive in about 50% of cases after the first week. Urine and bone marrow cultures are also valuable. Most patients will have negative cultures (including stool) by the end of a 6-week period. Serologic tests (Widal reaction) are not as useful as cultures because both false-positive and false-negative results occur. Leukopenia is common in the second week of the disease, but in the first week, leukocytosis may be seen. Proteinuria, mild elevation of liver enzymes, thrombocytopenia, and DIC are common.

Differential Diagnosis

Typhoid and paratyphoid fevers must be distinguished from other serious prolonged fevers. These include typhus, brucellosis, malaria, tularemia, miliary tuberculosis, psittacosis, vasculitis, lymphoma, mononucleosis, and Kawasaki disease. The diagnosis of typhoid fever is often made clinically in developing countries, but the accuracy of clinical diagnosis is variable. In developed countries, where typhoid fever is uncommon and physicians are unfamiliar with the clinical picture, the diagnosis is often not suspected until late. Positive cultures confirm the diagnosis.

Complications

The most serious complications of typhoid fever are gastrointestinal hemorrhage (2–10%) and perforation (1–3%). They occur toward the end of the second week or during the third week of the disease.

Intestinal perforation is one of the principal causes of death. The site of perforation generally is the terminal ileum or cecum. The clinical manifestations are indistinguishable from those of acute appendicitis, with pain, tenderness, and rigidity in the right lower quadrant.

Bacterial pneumonia, meningitis, septic arthritis, abscesses, and osteomyelitis are uncommon complications, particularly if specific treatment is given promptly. Shock and electrolyte disturbances may lead to death.

About 1–3% of patients become chronic carriers of *S typhi*. Chronic carriage is defined as excretion of typhoid bacilli for more than a year, but carriage is often lifelong. Adults with underlying biliary or urinary tract disease are much more likely than children to become chronic carriers.

Prevention

Routine typhoid vaccine is not recommended in the United States but should be considered for foreign travel to endemic areas. An attenuated oral typhoid vaccine produced from strain Ty21a has better efficacy and causes minimal side effects but is not approved for children younger than age 6 years. A capsular polysaccharide vaccine (ViCPS) requires one intramuscular injection and may be given to children age 2 years and older. (See Chapter 9.)

Treatment

A. SPECIFIC MEASURES

Antimicrobial susceptibility testing and local experience are used to guide therapy. Equally effective regimens for susceptible strains include the following: TMP–SMX (10 mg/kg trimethoprim and 50 mg/kg sulfamethoxazole per day orally in two or three divided doses), amoxicillin (100 mg/kg/d orally in four divided doses), and ampicillin (100–200 mg/kg/d intravenously in four divided doses). Aminoglycosides and first- and second-generation cephalosporins are clinically ineffective regardless of in vitro susceptibility results. Third-generation cephalosporins are used for resistant strains. Ceftriaxone and cefotaxime may be used parenterally. Ciprofloxacin or other fluoroquinolones are efficacious but not approved in children, but may be used for multiply resistant strains. Occasionally the presence of multiply resistant strains requires the use of chloramphenicol (50–100 mg/kg/d orally or intravenously in four doses). Treatment duration is 14–21 days. Patients remain febrile for 3–5 days even with appropriate therapy.

B. GENERAL MEASURES

General support of the patient is exceedingly important and includes rest, good nutrition, and careful observation, with particular regard to evidence of intestinal bleeding or perforation. Blood transfusions may be needed even in the absence of frank hemorrhage.

Prognosis

A prolonged convalescent carrier stage may occur in children. Three negative cultures after all antibiotics have been stopped are required before contact precautions are stopped. With early antibiotic therapy, the prognosis is excellent, and the mortality rate is less than 1%. Relapse occurs 1–3 weeks later in 10–20% of patients despite appropriate antibiotic treatment.

Bhan MK, Bahl R, Bhatnagar S: Typhoid and paratyphoid fever. Lancet 2005;366(9487):749 [PMID: 16125594].

Frenck RW Jr et al: Short-course azithromycin for the treatment of uncomplicated typhoid fever in children and adolescents. Clin Infect Dis 2004;38(7):951. Epub 2004 March 12. [PMID: 15034826].

Mai NL et al: Persistent efficacy of Vi conjugate vaccine against typhoid fever in young children. N Engl J Med 2003;349 (14):1390 [PMID: 14523155].

Olsen SJ et al: Outbreaks of typhoid fever in the United States, 1960–99. Epidemiol Infect 2003;130(1):13 [PMID: 12613741].

Thaver D et al: Fluoroquinolones for treating typhoid and paratyphoid fever (enteric fever). Cochrane Database Syst Rev 2005;(2):CD004530 [PMID: 15846718].

SHIGELLOSIS (Bacillary Dysentery)

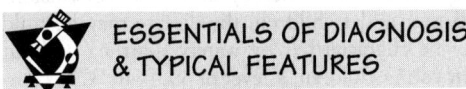

ESSENTIALS OF DIAGNOSIS & TYPICAL FEATURES

- *Cramps and bloody diarrhea.*
- *High fever, malaise, convulsions.*
- *Pus and blood in diarrheal stools examined microscopically.*
- *Diagnosis confirmed by stool culture.*

General Considerations

Shigellae are nonmotile gram-negative rods of the family Enterobacteriaceae and are closely related to *E coli*. The genus *Shigella* is divided into four major groups, A–D, representing *Shigella dysenteriae*, *Shigella flexneri*, *Shigella boydii*, and *Shigella sonnei*, respectively. Approximately 30,000 cases of shigellosis are reported each year in the United States. *S sonnei* followed by *S flexneri* are the most common isolates.

S dysenteriae, which causes the most severe diarrhea of all species and the greatest number of extraintestinal complications, accounts for fewer than 1% of all *Shigella* infections in the United States.

Shigellosis may be a serious disease, particularly in young children, and without supportive treatment an appreciable mortality rate results. In older children and adults, the disease tends to be self-limited and milder. *Shigella* is usually transmitted by the fecal–oral route. Food- and water-borne outbreaks are increasing in occurrence, but are less important overall than person-to-person transmission. The disease is very communicable—as few as 200 bacteria can produce illness in an adult. The secondary attack rate in families is high, and shigellosis is a serious problem in day care centers and custodial institutions. *Shigella* organisms produce disease by invading the colonic mucosa, causing mucosal ulcerations and microabscesses. A plasmid-encoded gene is required for enterotoxin production, chromosomal genes are required for invasiveness, and smooth lipopolysaccharides are required for virulence. An experimental vaccine is under development and is safe and immunogenic in young children.

Clinical Findings

A. SYMPTOMS AND SIGNS

The incubation period of shigellosis is usually 2–4 days. Onset is abrupt, with abdominal cramps, urgency, tenesmus, chills, fever, malaise, and diarrhea. Hallucinations and seizures sometimes accompany high fever. In severe forms, blood and mucus are seen in small stools (dysentery), and meningismus and convulsions may occur. In older children, the disease may be mild and may be characterized by watery diarrhea without blood. In young children, a fever of 39.4–40 °C is common. Rarely there is rectal prolapse. Symptoms generally last 3–7 days.

B. LABORATORY FINDINGS

The total WBC count varies, but often there is a marked shift to the left. The stool may contain gross blood and mucus, and many neutrophils are seen if mucus from the stool is examined microscopically. Stool cultures are usually positive; however, they may be negative because the organism is somewhat fragile and present in small numbers late in the disease, and because laboratory techniques are suboptimal for the recovery of shigellae.

Differential Diagnosis

Diarrhea due to rotavirus infection is a winter rather than a summer disease. Usually children with rotavirus infection are not as febrile or toxic as those with shigellosis, and in rotavirus infection, stool does not contain gross blood or neutrophils. Intestinal infections caused by *Salmonella* or *Campylobacter* are differentiated by culture. Grossly bloody stools in a patient without fever or stool leukocytes suggest *E coli* 0157:H7 infection. Amebic dysentery is diagnosed by microscopic examination of fresh stools or sigmoidoscopy specimens. Intussusception is characterized by an abdominal mass, so-called currant jelly stools without leukocytes, and absence of fever. Mild shigellosis is not distinguishable clinically from other forms of infectious diarrhea.

Complications

Dehydration, acidosis, shock, and renal failure are the major complications. In some cases, a chronic form of dysentery occurs, characterized by mucoid stools and poor nutrition. Bacteremia and metastatic infections are rare but serious complications. Febrile seizures are common. Fulminating fatal dysentery and hemolytic–uremic syndrome occur rarely.

Treatment

A. SPECIFIC MEASURES

Resistance to TMP–SMX (10 mg/kg/d trimethoprim and 50 mg/kg/d sulfamethoxazole, given in two divided doses orally for 5 days) is now commonly encountered in many communities and limits the use of this otherwise effective drug to cases where results of susceptibility testing are known. Amoxicillin is not effective. Ampicillin (100 mg/kg/d, given in four divided doses) is also efficacious if the strain is sensitive. Parenteral ceftriaxone and oral cefixime are both effective, although cefixime is now unavailable, and experience with other third-generation oral cephalosporins is limited. Azithromycin (12 mg/kg/d on day 1, then 6 mg/kg/d for four days) was superior to cefixime in one study. Ciprofloxacin (500 mg, given twice daily for 5 days) is efficacious in adults but is not approved for use in children. However, it may be used in children who remain symptomatic and in need of therapy, and when multiply resistant strains limit other preferred choices. Successful treatment reduces the duration of fever, cramping, and diarrhea and terminates fecal excretion of *Shigella*. Tetracycline and chloramphenicol are also effective, but resistance is common. Presumptive therapy should be limited to children with classic shigellosis or known outbreaks. Afebrile children with bloody diarrhea are more commonly infected with EHEC. Antimicrobial therapy of EHEC may increase the likelihood of hemolytic uremic syndrome.

B. GENERAL MEASURES

In severe cases, immediate rehydration is critical. A mild form of chronic malabsorption syndrome may supervene and require prolonged dietary control.

Prognosis

The prognosis is excellent if vascular collapse is treated promptly by adequate fluid therapy. The mortality rate is high in very young, malnourished infants who do not receive fluid and electrolyte therapy. Convalescent fecal excretion of *Shigella* lasts 1–4 weeks in patients not receiving antimicrobial therapy. Long-term carriers are rare.

Ashkenazi S: *Shigella* infections in children: New insights. Semin Pediatr Infect Dis 2004:15(4):246 [PMID: 15494948].

Greenberg D et al: *Shigella* bacteremia: A retrospective study. Clin Pediatr (Phila) 2003;42(5):411 [PMID: 12862343].

Jain SK et al: Antimicrobial-resistant *Shigella sonnei:* Limited antimicrobial treatment options for children and challenges of interpreting in vitro azithromycin susceptibility. Pediatr Infect Dis J 2005;24(6):494 [PMID: 15933557].

CHOLERA

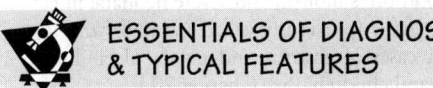

ESSENTIALS OF DIAGNOSIS & TYPICAL FEATURES

- *Sudden onset of severe watery diarrhea.*
- *Persistent vomiting without nausea or fever.*
- *Extreme and rapid dehydration and electrolyte loss, with rapid development of vascular collapse.*
- *Contact with a case of cholera or with shellfish, or the presence of cholera in the community.*
- *Diagnosis confirmed by stool culture.*

General Considerations

Cholera is an acute diarrheal disease caused by the gram-negative organism *Vibrio cholerae*. It is transmitted by contaminated water or food, especially contaminated shellfish. Typical disease is generally so dramatic that in endemic areas the diagnosis is obvious. Individuals with mild illness and young children may play an important role in transmission of the infection.

Asymptomatic infection is far more common than clinical disease. In endemic areas, rising titers of vibriocidal antibody are seen with increasing age. Infection occurs in individuals with low titers. The age-specific attack rate is highest in children younger than age 5 years and declines with age. Cholera is unusual in infancy.

Cholera toxin is a protein enterotoxin that is primarily responsible for symptoms. Cholera toxin binds to a regulatory subunit of adenylyl cyclase in enterocytes, causing increased cyclic adenosine monophosphate and an outpouring of NaCl and water into the lumen of the small bowel.

Nutritional status is an important factor determining the severity of the diarrhea. Duration of diarrhea is prolonged in adults and children with severe malnutrition.

Cholera is endemic in India and southern and Southeast Asia and in parts of Africa. The most recent pandemic, caused by the El Tor biotype of *V cholerae*

01, began in 1961 in Indonesia. Epidemic cholera spread in Central and South America, with a total of 1 million cases and 9500 deaths reported through 1994. Cases in the United States occurred in the course of foreign travel or as a result of consumption of contaminated imported food. Cholera is increasingly associated with consumption of shellfish. Interstate shipment of oysters has resulted in cholera in several inland states.

Several recent studies provide evidence that *V cholerae* is a natural inhabitant of shellfish and copepods in estuarine environments. Seasonal multiplication of *V cholerae* may provide a source of outbreaks in endemic areas. Chronic cholera carriers are rare. The incubation period is short, usually 1–3 days.

Clinical Findings

A. SYMPTOMS AND SIGNS

Many patients infected with *V cholerae* have mild disease, with 1–2% developing severe diarrhea. During severe cholera, there is a sudden onset of massive, frequent, watery stools, generally light gray in color (so-called rice-water stools) and containing some mucus but no pus. Vomiting may be projectile and is not accompanied by nausea. Within 2–3 hours, the tremendous loss of fluids results in life-threatening dehydration, hypochloremia, and hypokalemia, with marked weakness and collapse. Renal failure with uremia and irreversible peripheral vascular collapse will occur if fluid therapy is not administered. The illness lasts 1–7 days and is shortened by appropriate antibiotic therapy.

B. LABORATORY FINDINGS

Markedly elevated hemoglobin (20 g/dL) and marked acidosis, hypochloremia, and hyponatremia are seen. Stool sodium concentration may range from 80 mEq/L to 120 mEq/L. Cultural confirmation using thiosulfate-citrate-bile salt-sucrose agar takes 16–18 hours for a presumptive diagnosis and 36–48 hours for a definitive bacteriologic diagnosis.

Prevention

Cholera vaccine is available and provides 50% efficacy. Protection lasts 3–6 months. Cholera vaccine is not generally recommended for travelers. Tourists visiting endemic areas are at little risk if they exercise caution in what they eat and drink and maintain good personal hygiene. In endemic areas, all water and milk must be boiled, food protected from flies, and sanitary precautions observed. Simple filtration of water is highly effective in reducing cases. Thorough cooking of shellfish prevents transmission. All patients with cholera should be isolated.

Chemoprophylaxis is indicated for household and other close contacts of cholera patients. It should be initiated as soon as possible after the onset of the disease in the index patient. Tetracycline (500 mg/d for 5 days) is effective in preventing infection. TMP–SMX may be substituted in children.

Treatment

Physiologic saline or lactated Ringer solution should be administered intravenously in large amounts to restore blood volume and urine output and prevent irreversible shock. Potassium supplements are required. Sodium bicarbonate, given intravenously, may also be needed initially to overcome profound acidosis. Moderate dehydration and acidosis can be corrected in 3–6 hours by oral therapy alone, because the active glucose transport system of the small bowel is normally functional. The optimal composition of the oral solution (in mEq/L) is as follows: Na^+, 90; Cl^-, 80; and K^+, 20 (with glucose, 110 mmol/L).

Treatment with tetracycline (50 mg/kg/d orally in four divided doses for 2–5 days) or azithromycin (10 mg/kg/d in one dose for 1–5 days) shortens the duration of the disease in children and prevents clinical relapse but is not as important as fluid and electrolyte therapy. Tetracycline resistance occurs in some regions, and ciprofloxacin may be used depending on local resistance patterns. TMP–SMX should be used in children younger than age 9 years.

Prognosis

With early and rapid replacement of fluids and electrolytes, the case fatality rate is 1–2% in children. If significant symptoms appear and no treatment is given, the mortality rate is over 50%.

Ali M et al: Herd immunity conferred by killed oral cholera vaccines in Bangladesh: A reanalysis. Lancet 2005;366(9479):7 [PMID: 15993232].

Colwell RR et al: Reduction of cholera in Bangladeshi villages by simple filtration. Proc Natl Acad Sci U S A 2003;100(3):1051 [PMID: 12529505].

O'Ryan M, Prado V, Pickering LK: A millennium update on pediatric diarrheal illness in the developing world. Semin Pediatr Infect Dis 2005;16(2):125 [PMID: 15825143].

Saha D et al: Single-dose ciprofloxacin versus 12-dose erythromycin for childhood cholera: A randomized controlled trial. Lancet 2005;366(9491):1085 [PMID: 16182896].

CAMPYLOBACTER INFECTION

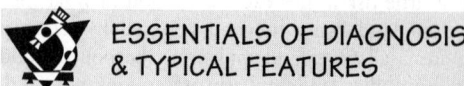

ESSENTIALS OF DIAGNOSIS & TYPICAL FEATURES

- *Fever, vomiting, abdominal pain, diarrhea.*
- *Presumptive diagnosis by darkfield or phase contrast microscopy of stool wet mount or modified Gram stain.*
- *Definitive diagnosis by stool culture.*

General Considerations

Campylobacter species are small gram-negative, curved or spiral bacilli that are commensals or pathogens in many animals. *Campylobacter jejuni* frequently causes acute enteritis in humans. In the 1990s, *C jejuni* was responsible for 3–11% of cases of acute gastroenteritis in North America and Europe. In many areas, enteritis due to *C jejuni* is more common than that due to *Salmonella* or *Shigella*. *Campylobacter fetus* causes bacteremia and meningitis in immunocompromised patients. *C fetus* may cause maternal fever, abortion, stillbirth, and severe neonatal infection. *Helicobacter pylori* (previously called *Campylobacter pylori*) causes most cases of gastritis and peptic ulcer disease in both adults and children. (See Chapter 20.)

Campylobacter colonizes in domestic and wild animals, especially poultry. Numerous cases have been associated with sick puppies or other animal contacts. Contaminated food and water, improperly cooked poultry, and person-to-person spread by the fecal–oral route are common routes of transmission. Outbreaks associated with day care centers, contaminated water supplies, and raw milk have been reported. Newborns may acquire the organism from their mothers at delivery.

Clinical Findings

A. SYMPTOMS AND SIGNS

C jejuni enteritis can be mild or severe. In tropical countries, asymptomatic stool carriage is common. The incubation period is usually 1–7 days. The disease usually begins with sudden onset of high fever, malaise, headache, abdominal cramps, nausea, and vomiting. Diarrhea follows and may be watery or bile-stained, mucoid, and bloody. The illness is self-limiting, lasting 2–7 days, but relapses occur in 15–25% of cases. Without antimicrobial treatment, the organism remains in the stool for 1–6 weeks.

B. LABORATORY FINDINGS

The peripheral WBC count generally is elevated, with many band forms. Microscopic examination of stool reveals erythrocytes and pus cells.

Isolation of *C jejuni* from stool is not difficult but requires selective agar, incubation at 42 °C rather than 35 °C, and incubation in an atmosphere of about 5% oxygen and 5% CO_2 (candle jar is satisfactory).

Differential Diagnosis

Campylobacter enteritis may resemble viral gastroenteritis, salmonellosis, shigellosis, amebiasis, or other infectious diarrheas. Because it also mimics ulcerative colitis,

Crohn disease, intussusception, and appendicitis, mistaken diagnosis can lead to unnecessary surgery.

Complications

The most common complication is dehydration. Other uncommon complications include erythema nodosum, convulsions, reactive arthritis, bacteremia, urinary tract infection, and cholecystitis. Guillain-Barré syndrome may follow *C jejuni* infection by 1–3 weeks.

Prevention

No vaccine is available. Hand washing and adherence to basic food sanitation practices help prevent disease. Hand washing and cleaning of kitchen utensils after contact with raw poultry are important.

Treatment

Treatment of fluid and electrolyte disturbances is important. Antimicrobial treatment with erythromycin in children (30–50 mg/kg/d orally in four divided doses for 5 days), or with azithromycin or ciprofloxacin in adults terminates fecal excretion and may prevent relapses. Fluoroquinolone-resistant *C jejuni* are now common worldwide. Therapy given early in the course of the illness will shorten the duration of symptoms but is unnecessary if given later. Antimicrobials used for shigellosis, such as TMP–SMX and ampicillin, are inactive against *Campylobacter*. Supportive therapy is sufficient in most cases.

Prognosis

The outlook is excellent if dehydration is corrected and misdiagnosis does not lead to inappropriate diagnostic or surgical procedures.

Butzler JP: Campylobacter, from obscurity to celebrity. Clin Microbiol Infect 2004;19(10):868 [PMID: 15370134].

Centers for Disease Control and Prevention: *Campylobacter* infections. www.cdc.gov/ncidod/dbmd/diseaseinfo/campylobacter_g.htm

Shea KM; American Academy of Pediatrics Committee on Environmental Health; American Academy of Pediatrics Committee on Infectious Diseases: Nontherapeutic use of antimicrobial agents in animal agriculture: Implications for pediatrics. Pediatrics 2004;114(3):862 [PMID: 15342867].

TULAREMIA

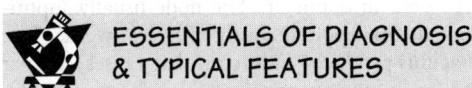

ESSENTIALS OF DIAGNOSIS & TYPICAL FEATURES

- *A cutaneous or mucous membrane lesion at the site of inoculation and regional lymph node enlargement.*
- *Sudden onset of fever, chills, and prostration.*
- *History of contact with infected animals, principally wild rabbits, or history of tick exposure.*
- *Positive culture or immunofluorescence from mucocutaneous ulcer or regional lymph nodes.*
- *High serum antibody titer.*

General Considerations

Tularemia is caused by *Francisella tularensis,* a gram-negative organism usually acquired directly from infected animals (principally wild rabbits) or by the bite of an infected tick. Occasionally infection is acquired from infected domestic dogs or cats; by contamination of the skin or mucous membranes with infected blood or tissues; by inhalation of infected material; by bites of fleas or deer flies that have been in contact with infected animals; or by ingestion of contaminated meat or water. The incubation period is short, usually 3–7 days, but may vary from 2–25 days.

Ticks are the most important vector of tularemia and rabbits are the classic vector. It is important to seek a history of rabbit hunting, skinning, or food preparation in any patient who has a febrile illness with tender lymphadenopathy, often in the region of a draining skin ulcer.

Clinical Findings

A. SYMPTOMS AND SIGNS

Several clinical types of tularemia occur in children. Sixty percent of infections are of the ulceroglandular form and start as a reddened papule that may be pruritic, quickly ulcerates, and is not very painful. Soon, the regional lymph nodes become large and tender. Fluctuance quickly follows. There may be marked systemic symptoms, including high fever, chills, weakness, and vomiting. Pneumonitis occasionally accompanies the ulceroglandular form or may be seen as the sole manifestation of infection (pneumonic form). A detectable skin lesion may be absent, and localized lymphoid enlargement may exist alone (glandular form). Oculoglandular and oropharyngeal forms also occur. The latter is characterized by tonsillitis, often with membrane formation, cervical adenopathy, and high fever. In the absence of a primary ulcer or localized lymphadenitis, a prolonged febrile disease reminiscent of typhoid fever can occur (typhoidal form). Splenomegaly is common in all forms.

B. LABORATORY FINDINGS

F tularensis can be recovered from ulcers, regional lymph nodes, and sputum of patients with the pneumonic form. However, the organism grows only on an enriched medium (blood-cystine-glucose agar), and laboratory handling is dangerous owing to the risk of airborne transmission to laboratory personnel. Immunofluorescent staining of biopsy material or aspirates of involved lymph nodes is diagnostic, although it is not widely available.

The WBC count is not remarkable. Agglutinins are present after the second week of illness, and in the absence of a positive culture their development confirms the diagnosis. An agglutination titer of 1:160 or higher is considered positive.

Differential Diagnosis

The typhoidal form of tularemia may mimic typhoid, brucellosis, miliary tuberculosis, Rocky Mountain spotted fever, and mononucleosis. Pneumonic tularemia resembles atypical or mycotic pneumonitis. The ulceroglandular type of tularemia resembles pyoderma caused by staphylococci or streptococci, plague, anthrax, and cat-scratch fever. The oropharyngeal type must be distinguished from streptococcal or diphtheritic pharyngitis, mononucleosis, herpangina, or other viral pharyngitides.

Prevention

Children should be protected from insect bites, especially those of ticks, fleas, and deer flies, by the use of proper clothing and repellents. Because rabbits are the source of most human infections, the dressing and handling of such game should be performed with great care. If contact occurs, thorough washing with soap and water is indicated.

Treatment

A. SPECIFIC MEASURES

Historically, streptomycin was the drug of choice (30 mg/kg/d, given intramuscularly in two divided doses, to a maximum dose of 1 g). Gentamicin and amikacin are also efficacious, more available, and familiar to clinicians. Doxycycline is effective, but relapse rates are higher. Chloramphenicol therapy is also associated with a higher relapse rate. Failures occur with ceftriaxone.

B. GENERAL MEASURES

Antipyretics and analgesics may be given as necessary. Skin lesions are best left open. Glandular lesions occasionally require incision and drainage.

Prognosis

The prognosis is excellent in cases of tularemia that are recognized early and treated appropriately.

Ellis J et al: Tularemia. Clin Microbiol Rev 2002;15(4):631 [PMID: 12364373].

Parola P, Raoult D: Ticks and tickborne bacterial diseases in humans: An emerging infectious threat. Clin Infect Dis 2001; 32(6):897 [PMID: 11247714].

PLAGUE

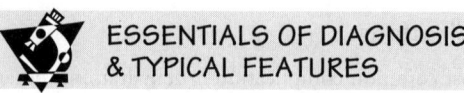

ESSENTIALS OF DIAGNOSIS & TYPICAL FEATURES

- *Sudden onset of fever, chills, and prostration.*
- *Regional lymphadenitis with suppuration of nodes (bubonic form).*
- *Hemorrhage into skin and mucous membranes and shock (septicemia).*
- *Cough, dyspnea, cyanosis, and hemoptysis (pneumonia).*
- *History of exposure to infected animals.*

General Considerations

Plague is an extremely serious acute infection caused by a gram-negative bacillus, *Yersinia pestis.* It is a disease of rodents that is transmitted to humans by flea bites. Plague bacilli have been isolated from rodents in 15 of the western states in the United States. Direct contact with rodents, rabbits, or domestic cats may transmit fleas infected with plague bacilli. Most cases occur from June through September. Human plague in the United States appears to occur in cycles that reflect cycles in wild animal reservoirs.

Clinical Findings

A. SYMPTOMS AND SIGNS

Plague assumes several clinical forms; the two most common are bubonic and septicemic. Pneumonic plague, the form that occurs when organisms enter the body through the respiratory tract, is uncommon.

1. Bubonic plague—Bubonic plague begins after an incubation period of 6 days with a sudden onset of high fever, chills, headache, vomiting, and marked delirium or clouding of consciousness. A less severe form also exists, with a less precipitous onset, but with progression over several days to severe symptoms. Although the flea bite is rarely seen, the regional lymph node, usually inguinal and unilateral, is painful and tender, 1–5 cm in diameter. The node usually suppurates and drains spontaneously after 1 week. The plague bacillus produces endotoxin that causes vascular necrosis. Bacilli may overwhelm regional lymph nodes and enter the circulation to produce septicemia. Severe vascular necrosis results in widely disseminated hemorrhage in skin, mucous membranes, liver, and spleen. Myocarditis and circulatory collapse may result from damage by the endotoxin. Plague meningitis or pneumonia may occur following bacteremic spread from an infected lymph node.

2. Septicemic plague—Plague may initially present as septicemia without evidence of lymphadenopathy. In some series, 25% of cases are initially septicemic. Septicemia plague carries a worse prognosis than bubonic plague, largely because it is not recognized and treated early. Patients may present initially with a nonspecific febrile illness characterized by fever, myalgia, chills, and anorexia. Plague is frequently complicated by secondary seeding of the lung causing plague pneumonia.

3. Primary pneumonic plague—Inhalation of *Y pestis* bacilli causes primary plague pneumonia. This form of plague has been transmitted to humans from cats with pneumonic plague and would be the form of plague most likely seen after aerosolized release of *Y pestis* in a bioterrorist incident. After an incubation of 1–6 days, the patient develops fever, cough, shortness of breath, and the production of bloody, watery, or purulent sputum. Gastrointestinal symptoms are sometimes prominent. Because the initial focus of infection is the lung, buboes are usually absent; occasionally cervical buboes may be seen.

B. LABORATORY FINDINGS

Aspirate from a bubo contains bipolar staining gram-negative bacilli. Pus, sputum, and blood all yield the organism. Rapid diagnosis can be made with fluorescent antibody detection or polymerase chain reaction (PCR) on clinical specimens. Confirmation is made by culture or serologic testing. Laboratory infections are common enough to make bacterial isolation dangerous. Cultures are usually positive within 48 hours. Paired acute and convalescent sera may be tested for an antibody rise in those cases with negative cultures.

Differential Diagnosis

The septic phase of the disease may be confused with illnesses such as meningococcemia, sepsis, and rickettsioses. The bubonic form resembles tularemia, anthrax, cat-scratch fever, streptococcal adenitis, and cellulitis. Primary gastroenteritis and appendicitis may have to be distinguished.

Prevention

Proper disposal of household and commercial wastes and chemical control of rats are basic elements of plague prevention. Flea control is instituted and maintained with liberal use of insecticides. Children vacationing in remote camping areas should be warned not to handle dead or dying animals. Domestic cats that roam freely in suburban areas may contact infected wild animals and acquire infected fleas. There is no commercially available vaccine for plague.

Treatment

A. SPECIFIC MEASURES

Streptomycin (20–40 mg/kg/d intramuscularly) or gentamicin (7.5 mg/kg/d) in three divided doses for 7–10 days after defervescence is effective. For patients not requiring parenteral therapy, doxycycline may be given. Doxycycline is not usually recommended for children younger than 8 years of age unless benefits of use outweigh the risk of dental staining. Plague bacilli that are multiply resistant to antimicrobials are uncommon but of serious concern.

Mortality is extremely high in septicemic and pneumonic plague if specific antibiotic treatment is not started in the first 24 hours of the disease.

Every effort should be made to effect resolution of buboes without surgery. Pus from draining lymph nodes should be handled with gloves.

B. GENERAL MEASURES

Pneumonic plague is highly infectious, and droplet isolation is required until the patient has been on effective antimicrobial therapy for 48 hours. All contacts should receive prophylaxis with oral doxycycline 2.2 mg/kg/dose (maximum dose 100 mg) given twice a day for 7 days. State health officials should be notified immediately about suspected plague cases.

Prognosis

The mortality rate in untreated bubonic plague is about 50%. The mortality rate for treated pneumonic plague is 50–60%. Recent mortality rates in New Mexico were 3% for bubonic plague and 71% for the septicemic form.

Centers for Disease Control and Prevention: Plague. http://www.cdc.gov/ncidod/dvbid/plague

Dennis DT, Chow CC: Plague. Pediatr Infect Dis J 2004;23(1):69 [PMID: 14743050].

Inglesby T et al: Plague as a biological weapon: Medical and public health management. JAMA 2000;283(17):2281 [PMID: 10807389].

HAEMOPHILUS INFLUENZAE TYPE B INFECTIONS

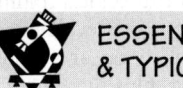

ESSENTIALS OF DIAGNOSIS & TYPICAL FEATURES

- *Purulent meningitis in children younger than age 4 years with direct smears of CSF showing gram-negative pleomorphic rods.*
- *Acute epiglottitis: High fever, drooling, dysphagia, aphonia, and stridor.*

- Septic arthritis: Fever, local redness, swelling, heat, and pain with active or passive motion of the involved joint in a child age 4 months to 4 years.
- Cellulitis: Sudden onset of fever and distinctive cellulitis in an infant, often involving the cheek or periorbital area.
- In all cases, a positive culture from the blood, CSF, or aspirated pus confirms the diagnosis.

General Considerations

H influenzae type b (Hib) has become uncommon because of widespread immunization in early infancy. The 99% reduction in incidence seen in many parts of the United States is due to high rates of vaccine coverage and reduced nasopharyngeal carriage after vaccination. Forty percent of cases occur in children younger than 6 months who are too young to have completed a primary immunization series. Hib may cause meningitis, bacteremia, epiglottitis (supraglottic croup), septic arthritis, periorbital and facial cellulitis, pneumonia, and pericarditis.

Disease due to *H influenzae* types A, C, D, E, F, or unencapsulated strains is rare, but it now accounts for a larger proportion of positive culture results. Third-generation cephalosporins are preferred for initial therapy of Hib infections. Ampicillin is adequate for culture-proved Hib susceptible strains.

Unencapsulated, nontypeable *H influenzae* frequently colonize the mucous membranes and cause otitis media, sinusitis, bronchitis, and pneumonia in children and adults. Bacteremia is uncommon. Neonatal sepsis similar to early-onset GBS is recognized. Obstetric complications of chorioamnionitis and bacteremia are usually the source of neonatal cases.

Ampicillin resistance occurs in 25–40% of nontypeable *H influenzae*.

Clinical Findings

A. Symptoms and Signs

1. Meningitis—Infants usually present with fever, irritability, lethargy, poor feeding with or without vomiting, and a high-pitched cry.

2. Acute epiglottitis—The most useful clinical finding in the early diagnosis of Hib epiglottitis is evidence of dysphagia, characterized by a refusal to eat or swallow saliva and by drooling. This finding, plus the presence of a high fever in a "toxic" child—even in the absence of a cherry-red epiglottis on direct examination—should strongly suggest the diagnosis and lead to prompt intubation. Stridor is a late sign. (See Chapter 17.)

3. Septic arthritis—Hib is a common cause of septic arthritis in unimmunized children younger than age 4

years in the United States. The child is febrile and refuses to move the involved joint and limb because of pain. Examination reveals swelling, warmth, redness, tenderness on palpation, and severe pain on attempted movement of the joint.

4. Cellulitis—Cellulitis due to Hib occurs almost exclusively in the age group from 3 months to 4 years but is now uncommon as a result of immunization. Fever is usually noted at the same time as the cellulitis, and many infants appear toxic. The cheek or periorbital (preseptal) area is usually involved.

B. Laboratory Findings

The WBC count in Hib infections may be high or normal with a shift to the left. Blood culture is frequently positive. Positive culture of aspirated pus or fluid from the involved site proves the diagnosis. In untreated meningitis, CSF smear may show the characteristic pleomorphic gram-negative rods.

C. Imaging

A lateral view of the neck may suggest the diagnosis in suspected acute epiglottitis, but misinterpretation is common. Intubation should not be delayed to obtain radiographs. Haziness of maxillary and ethmoid sinuses occurs with orbital cellulitis.

Differential Diagnosis

A. Meningitis

Meningitis must be differentiated from head injury, brain abscess, tumor, lead encephalopathy, and other forms of meningoencephalitis, including mycobacterial, viral, fungal, and bacterial agents.

B. Acute Epiglottitis

In croup caused by viral agents (parainfluenza 1, 2, and 3, respiratory syncytial virus, influenza A, adenovirus), the child has more definite upper respiratory symptoms, cough, hoarseness, slower progression of obstructive signs, and lower fever. Spasmodic croup usually occurs at night in a child with a history of previous attacks. Sudden onset of choking and paroxysmal coughing suggests foreign body aspiration. Retropharyngeal abscess may have to be differentiated from epiglottitis.

C. Septic Arthritis

Differential diagnosis includes acute osteomyelitis, prepatellar bursitis, cellulitis, rheumatic fever, and fractures and sprains.

D. Cellulitis

Erysipelas, streptococcal cellulitis, insect bites, and trauma (including popsicle panniculitis or other types of freezing injury) may mimic Hib cellulitis. Periorbital cellulitis must be differentiated from paranasal sinus disease without cellulitis, allergic inflammatory disease of the lids, conjunctivitis, and herpes zoster infection.

Complications

A. Meningitis (See Chapter 23.)

B. Acute Epiglottitis

The disease may rapidly progress to complete airway obstruction with complications owing to hypoxia. Mediastinal emphysema and pneumothorax may occur.

C. Septic Arthritis

Septic arthritis may result in rapid destruction of cartilage and ankylosis if diagnosis and treatment are delayed. Even with early treatment, the incidence of residual damage and disability after septic arthritis in weight-bearing joints may be as high as 25%.

D. Cellulitis

Bacteremia may lead to meningitis or pyarthrosis.

Prevention

The risk of invasive Hib disease is highest in unimmunized, or partially immunized, household contacts who are younger than 4 years of age. The following situations require rifampin chemoprophylaxis of all household contacts to eradicate potential nasopharyngeal colonization with Hib and limit risk of invasive disease: (1) families where at least one household contact is younger than 4 years of age and either unimmunized or incompletely immunized against Hib; (2) an immunocompromised child (of any age or immunization status) resides in the household; or (3) a child younger than 12 months of age resides in the home and has not received three doses of the Hib vaccine. Preschool and day care center contacts may need prophylaxis if more than one case has occurred in the center in the previous 60 days (discuss with state health officials). The index case also needs chemoprophylaxis unless treated with ceftriaxone or cefotaxime (both are effective in eradication of Hib from the nasopharynx). Household contacts and index cases who are younger than 1 month of age needing chemoprophylaxis should be given rifampin, 20 mg/kg/dose (maximum adult dose 600 mg), orally, once daily for 4 successive days. Persons younger than 1 month of age should be given oral rifampin 10 mg/kg/dose once daily for 4 days. Rifampin should not be used in pregnant females.

Treatment

All patients with bacteremic or potentially bacteremic Hib diseases require hospitalization for treatment. The drugs of choice in hospitalized patients are a third-generation cephalosporin (cefotaxime or ceftriaxone) until the sensitivity of the organism is known.

A. Meningitis

Therapy is begun as soon as bacterial meningitis has been identified and CSF, blood, and other appropriate cultures have been obtained. Therapy is begun with cefotaxime (50 mg/kg intravenously every 6 hours) or ceftriaxone (50 mg/kg intravenously every 12 hours). If the organism is sensitive to ampicillin, it is the drug of choice. Therapy should preferably be given intravenously for the entire course. Ceftriaxone may be given intramuscularly if venous access becomes difficult.

Duration of therapy is 10 days. Longer treatment is reserved for children who respond slowly or in whom septic complications have occurred.

Repeated lumbar punctures are usually not necessary in Hib meningitis. They should be obtained in the following circumstances: unsatisfactory or questionable clinical response, seizure occurring after several days of therapy, and prolonged (7 days) or recurrent fever if the neurologic examination is abnormal or difficult to evaluate. Dexamethasone given immediately after diagnosis and continued for 2–4 days may reduce the incidence of hearing loss in children with Hib meningitis. The use of dexamethasone is controversial, but when it is used the dosage is 0.6 mg/kg/d in four divided doses for 4 days.

B. Acute Epiglottitis (See Chapter 17.)

C. Septic Arthritis

Initial therapy should include an effective antistaphylococcal antibiotic and cefotaxime or ceftriaxone (dosage as for meningitis). If the isolate is sensitive to ampicillin, it is given in a dosage of 200–300 mg/kg/d intravenously in four divided doses. If a child is improved following initial intravenous therapy, oral amoxicillin (75–100 mg/kg/d in four divided doses every 6 hours) may be administered under careful supervision to complete a 2-week course. Alternative oral agents for ampicillin-resistant organisms include amoxicillin–clavulanic acid or second- or third-generation cephalosporins. Ideally, susceptibility to these agents should be proved prior to use. Drainage of infected joint fluid is an essential part of treatment. In joints other than the hip, this can often be accomplished by one or more needle aspirations. In hip infections—and in arthritis of other joints where treatment is delayed or clinical response is slow—surgical drainage is advised. The joint should be immobilized.

D. Cellulitis, Including Orbital Cellulitis

Initial therapy should include an agent effective against staphylococci in combination with cefotaxime or ceftriaxone. Ampicillin may be used if the isolate is susceptible. Therapy is given parenterally for 3–7 days, followed by oral treatment as for septic arthritis, and supportive and symptomatic treatment as required. There is usually marked improvement after 72 hours of treatment. Antibiotics should be given for 10–14 days.

Prognosis

The case fatality rate for Hib meningitis is less than 5%. Young infants have the highest mortality rate. One of the most common neurologic sequelae, developing in 5–10% of patients with Hib meningitis, is sensorineural hearing loss. Patients with Hib meningitis should have their hearing checked during the course of the illness or shortly after recovery. Children in whom invasive Hib infection develops despite appropriate immunization should have tests to investigate immune function and to rule out HIV. The case fatality rate in acute epiglottitis is 2–5%. Deaths are associated with bacteremia and the rapid development of airway obstruction. The prognosis for the other diseases requiring hospitalization is good with the institution of early and adequate antibiotic therapy.

Vaccines

Four separate carbohydrate protein conjugate Hib vaccines are currently available. (See Chapter 9.)

Heath PT et al: Non-type b *Haemophilus influenzae* disease: Clinical and epidemiologic characteristics in the *Haemophilus influenzae* type b vaccine era. Pediatr Infect Dis J 2001; 20:300.

Leibovitz E, Jacobs MR, Dagan R: *Haemophilus influenzae:* A significant pathogen in acute otitis media. Pediatr Infect Dis J 2004;23(12):1142 [PMID: 15626953].

Rosenstein N, Perkins B: Update of *Haemophilus influenzae* serotype B and meningococcal vaccines. Pediatr Clin North Am 2000;47(2):337 [PMID: 10761507].

PERTUSSIS (Whooping Cough)

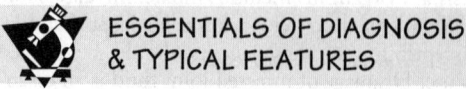

ESSENTIALS OF DIAGNOSIS & TYPICAL FEATURES

- Prodromal catarrhal stage (1–3 weeks) characterized by mild cough, coryza, without fever.
- Persistent staccato, paroxysmal cough ending with a high-pitched inspiratory "whoop."
- Leukocytosis with absolute lymphocytosis.
- Diagnosis confirmed by PCR or culture of nasopharyngeal secretions.

General Considerations

Pertussis is an acute, highly communicable infection of the respiratory tract caused by *Bordetella pertussis* and characterized by severe bronchitis. Children usually acquire the disease from symptomatic family contacts. Adults who have mild respiratory illness, not recognized as pertussis, frequently are the source of infection. Asymptomatic carriage of *B pertussis* is not recognized. Infectivity is greatest during the catarrhal and early paroxysmal cough stage (for about 4 weeks after onset).

Pertussis cases have increased in the United States since 1980. In 2004 and 2005, about 20,000 cases were reported. The morbidity and mortality of pertussis is greatest in young children. Fifty percent of children younger than age 1 year with a diagnosis of pertussis are hospitalized.

The duration of active immunity following natural pertussis is not known. Reinfections are usually milder. Immunity following vaccination wanes in 5–10 years. The majority of young adults in the United States are susceptible to pertussis infection, and disease is probably common but unrecognized.

Bordetella parapertussis causes a similar but milder syndrome.

B pertussis organisms attach to the ciliated respiratory epithelium and multiply there; deeper invasion does not occur. Disease is due to several bacterial toxins, the most potent of which is pertussis toxin, which is responsible for lymphocytosis and many of the symptoms of pertussis.

Clinical Findings

A. SYMPTOMS AND SIGNS

The onset of pertussis is insidious, with catarrhal upper respiratory tract symptoms (rhinitis, sneezing, and an irritating cough). Slight fever may be present; temperature greater than 38.3 °C suggests bacterial superinfection or another cause of respiratory tract infection. After about 2 weeks, cough becomes paroxysmal, characterized by 10–30 forceful coughs ending with a loud inspiration (the whoop). Infants and adults with otherwise typical severe pertussis often lack characteristic whooping. Vomiting commonly follows a paroxysm. Coughing is accompanied by cyanosis, sweating, prostration, and exhaustion. This stage lasts for 2–4 weeks, with gradual improvement. Cough suggestive of chronic bronchitis lasts for another 2–3 weeks. Paroxysmal coughing may continue for some months and may worsen with intercurrent viral respiratory infection. In adults, older children, and partially immunized individuals, symptoms may consist only of irritating cough lasting 1–2 weeks. In the younger unimmunized child, symptoms of pertussis last about 8 weeks or longer. Clinical pertussis is milder in immunized children.

B. LABORATORY FINDINGS

WBC counts of 20,000–30,000/μL with 70–80% lymphocytes typically appear near the end of the catarrhal stage. Severe pulmonary hypertension and hyperleukocytosis are associated with severe disease and death in young children with pertussis. Many older children and adults with mild infections never demonstrate lymphocytosis. The blood picture may resemble lymphocytic leukemia or leukemoid reactions. Identification of *B pertussis* by culture or PCR from nasopharyngeal swabs or nasal wash specimens proves the diagnosis. The organism may be found in the respiratory tract in diminishing numbers beginning in the catarrhal stage and ending about 2 weeks after the beginning of the paroxysmal stage. After 4–5 weeks of symptoms, cultures and fluorescent antibody tests are almost always negative. Charcoal agar containing an antimicrobial should be inoculated as soon as possible; *B pertussis* does not tolerate drying or prolonged transport. PCR detection is replacing culture in most pediatric centers because of improved sensitivity, decreased time to diagnosis, and cost. Enzyme-linked immunosorbent assays (ELISA) for detection of antibody to pertussis toxin or filamentous hemagglutinin may be useful for diagnosis but are currently not widely available, and interpretation of antibody titers may be difficult in previously immunized patients. The chest radiograph reveals thickened bronchi and sometimes shows a "shaggy" heart border.

Differential Diagnosis

The differential diagnosis of pertussis includes bacterial, tuberculous, chlamydial, and viral pneumonia. Cystic fibrosis and foreign body aspiration may be considerations. Adenoviruses and respiratory syncytial virus may cause paroxysmal coughing with an associated elevation of lymphocytes in the peripheral blood, mimicking pertussis.

Complications

Bronchopneumonia due to superinfection is the most common serious complication. It is characterized by abrupt clinical deterioration during the paroxysmal stage, accompanied by high fever and sometimes a striking leukemoid reaction with a shift to predominantly polymorphonuclear neutrophils. Atelectasis is a second common pulmonary complication. Atelectasis may be patchy or extensive and may shift rapidly to involve different areas of lung. Intercurrent viral respiratory infection is also a common complication and may provoke worsening or recurrence of paroxysmal coughing. Otitis media is common. Residual chronic bronchiectasis is infrequent despite the severity of the illness. Apnea and sudden death may occur during a particularly severe paroxysm. Seizures complicate 1.5% of cases, and encephalopathy occurs in 0.1%. The encephalopathy frequently is fatal. Anoxic brain damage,

cerebral hemorrhage, or pertussis neurotoxins are hypothesized, but anoxia is most likely the cause. Epistaxis and subconjunctival hemorrhages are common.

Prevention

Active immunization (see Chapter 9) with DTaP vaccine should be given in early infancy. The recent increase in incidence of pertussis is primarily due to increased recognition of disease in adolescents and adults. A booster dose of vaccine in adolescents between the ages of 11 and 18 is recommended.

Chemoprophylaxis with azithromycin or erythromycin should be given to exposed family and hospital contacts, particularly those younger than age 2 years. Hospitalized children with pertussis should be isolated because of the great risk of transmission to patients and staff. Several large hospital outbreaks have been reported.

Treatment

A. SPECIFIC MEASURES

Antibiotics may ameliorate early infections but have no effect on clinical symptoms in the paroxysmal stage. Erythromycin is the drug of choice because it promptly terminates respiratory tract carriage of *B pertussis*. Resistance to macrolides has been rarely reported. Patients should be given erythromycin estolate (40–50 mg/kg/24 h in four divided doses for 14 days). A recent study suggests that 7 days and 14 days of treatment are equally effective. Treatment with clarithromycin for 7 days and azithromycin for 5 days was equal to erythromycin for 14 days, with fewer gastrointestinal side effects. Ampicillin (100 mg/kg/d in four divided doses) may also be used for erythromycin-intolerant patients. Household or other close contacts (eg, in day care centers) should be given erythromycin to reduce secondary transmission. This prophylaxis should be used regardless of age or immunization status.

Corticosteroids reduce the severity of disease but may mask signs of bacterial superinfection. Albuterol (0.3–0.5 mg/kg/d in four doses) has reduced the severity of illness, but tachycardia is common when the drug is given orally, and aerosol administration may precipitate paroxysms.

B. GENERAL MEASURES

Nutritional support during the paroxysmal phase is important. Frequent small feedings, tube feeding, or parenteral fluid supplementation may be needed. Minimizing stimuli that trigger paroxysms is probably the best way of controlling cough. In general, cough suppressants are of little benefit.

C. TREATMENT OF COMPLICATIONS

Respiratory insufficiency due to pneumonia or other pulmonary complications should be treated with oxygen and assisted ventilation if necessary. Convulsions are treated with oxygen and anticonvulsants. Bacterial pneumonia or otitis media requires additional antibiotics.

Prognosis

The prognosis for patients with pertussis has improved in recent years because of excellent nursing care, treatment of complications, attention to nutrition, and modern intensive care. However, the disease is still very serious in infants younger than age 1 year; most deaths occur in this age group. Children with encephalopathy have a poor prognosis.

Cherry JD: The epidemiology of pertussis: A comparison of the epidemiology of the disease pertussis with the epidemiology of *Bordetella pertussis* infection. Pediatrics 2005;115(5):1422 [PMID: 15867059].

Halasa NB et al: Fatal pulmonary hypertension associated with pertussis in infants: Does extracorporeal membrane oxygenation have a role? Pediatrics 2003;112(6):1274 [PMID: 14654596].

LISTERIOSIS

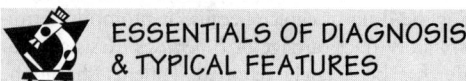

ESSENTIALS OF DIAGNOSIS & TYPICAL FEATURES

Early-onset neonatal disease:
- *Signs of sepsis a few hours after birth in an infant born with fetal distress and hepatosplenomegaly; maternal fever.*

Late-onset neonatal disease:
- *Meningitis, sometimes with monocytosis in the CSF and peripheral blood. Onset at age 9–30 days.*

General Considerations

Listeria monocytogenes is a gram-positive, non–spore-forming aerobic rod distributed widely in the animal kingdom and in food, dust, and soil. It causes systemic infections in newborn infants and immunosuppressed older children. In pregnant women, infection is relatively mild, with fever, aches, and chills, but is accompanied by bacteremia and sometimes results in intrauterine or perinatal infection with grave consequences for the fetus or newborn. One-fourth of cases occur in pregnant women, and 20% of their pregnancies end in stillbirth or neonatal death. *Listeria* is present in the stool of approximately 10% of the healthy population. Persons in contact with animals are at greater risk. Outbreaks of listeriosis have been traced to contaminated cabbage in coleslaw, soft cheese, hot dogs, luncheon meats, and milk. *Listeria* infections have decreased since the adoption of strict regulations for ready-to-eat foods.

Like GBS infections, *Listeria* infections in the newborn can be divided into early and late forms. Early infections are more common, leading to a severe congenital form of infection. Later infections are often characterized by meningitis.

Clinical Findings

A. SYMPTOMS AND SIGNS

In the early neonatal form, symptoms of listeriosis usually appear on the first day of life and always by the third day. Fetal distress is common, and infants frequently have signs of severe disease at birth. Respiratory distress, diarrhea, and fever occur. On examination, hepatosplenomegaly and a papular rash are found. A history of maternal fever is common. Meningitis may accompany the septic course. The late neonatal form usually occurs after age 9 days and can occur as late as 5 weeks. Meningitis is common, characterized by irritability, fever, and poor feeding.

Listeria infections are rare in older children and are usually associated with immunodeficiency. Several recent cases are associated with tumor necrosis factor-α neutralizing agents. Signs and symptoms are those of meningitis, usually with insidious onset.

B. LABORATORY FINDINGS

In all patients except those receiving white cell depressant drugs, the WBC count is elevated, with 10–20% monocytes. When meningitis is found, the characteristic CSF cell count is high (> 500/µL) with a predominance of polymorphonuclear neutrophils in 70% of cases. Monocytes may predominate in up to 30% of cases. Gram-stained smears of CSF are usually negative, but short gram-positive rods may be seen. The chief pathologic feature in severe neonatal sepsis is miliary granulomatosis with microabscesses in liver, spleen, CNS, lung, and bowel.

Cultures are frequently positive from multiple sites, including blood from the infant and the mother.

Differential Diagnosis

Early-onset neonatal disease resembles hemolytic disease of the newborn, GBS sepsis or severe cytomegalovirus infection, rubella, or toxoplasmosis. Late-onset disease must be differentiated from meningitis due to echovirus and coxsackievirus, GBS, and gram-negative enteric bacteria.

Prevention

Immunosuppressed, pregnant, and elderly patients can decrease the risk of *Listeria* infection by avoiding soft cheeses, by thoroughly reheating or avoiding delicatessen and ready-to-eat foods, by avoiding raw meat and milk, and by thoroughly washing fresh vegetables.

Treatment

Ampicillin (150–300 mg/kg/d q6h intravenously) is the drug of choice in most cases of listeriosis. Gentamicin (2.5 mg/kg every 8 hours intravenously) has a synergistic effect with ampicillin and should be given in serious infections and to patients with immune deficits. If ampicillin cannot be used, TMP–SMX is also effective. Cephalosporins are not effective. Treatment of severe disease should continue for at least 2 weeks.

Prognosis

In a recent outbreak of early-onset neonatal disease, the mortality rate was 27% despite aggressive and appropriate management. Meningitis in older infants has a good prognosis. In immunosuppressed children, prognosis depends to a great extent on that of the underlying illness.

Braden CR: Listeriosis. Pediatr Infect Dis J 2003;22(8):745 [PMID: 12913780].

Centers for Disease Control and Prevention: Listeriosis. www.cdc.gov/ ncidod/dbmd/disease info/listeriosis_g.htm

Gottlieb SL et al: Multistate outbreak of listeriosis linked to turkey deli meat and subsequent changes in US regulatory policy. Clin Infect Dis 2006;42(1):29. Epub 2005 Nov 23. [PMID: 16323088].

TUBERCULOSIS

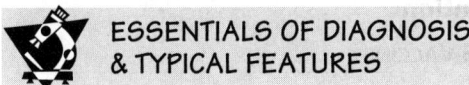

ESSENTIALS OF DIAGNOSIS & TYPICAL FEATURES

- *All types: Positive tuberculin test in patient or members of household, suggestive chest radiograph, history of contact, and demonstration of organism by stain and culture.*
- *Pulmonary: Fatigue, irritability, and undernutrition, with or without fever and cough.*
- *Glandular: Chronic cervical adenitis.*
- *Miliary: Classic snowstorm appearance of chest radiograph; choroidal tubercles.*
- *Meningitis: Fever and manifestations of meningeal irritation and increased intracranial pressure. Characteristic CSF.*

General Considerations

Tuberculosis is a granulomatous disease caused by *Mycobacterium tuberculosis*. It is a leading cause of death throughout the world. Children younger than age 3 years are most susceptible. Lymphohematogenous dissemination through the lungs to extrapulmonary sites, including the brain and meninges, eyes, bones and joints, lymph nodes, kidneys, intestines, larynx, and skin, is more likely to occur in infants. Increased susceptibility occurs again in adolescence, particularly in girls within 2 years of menarche. Following substantial increases in disease during the 1980s, tuberculosis incidence has decreased since 1992 due to increased control measures. More than 10,000 new cases were reported in 2005. High-risk groups include ethnic minorities, foreign-born persons, prisoners, residents of nursing homes, indigents, migrant workers, and health care providers. However, 50% of cases occurred in U.S.-born persons. HIV infection is an important risk factor for both development and spread of disease. Pediatric tuberculosis incidence mirrors the trends seen in adults.

Exposure to an infected adult is the most common risk factor in children. The primary complex in infancy and childhood consists of a small parenchymal lesion in any area of the lung with caseation of regional nodes and calcification. Postprimary tuberculosis in adolescents and adults occurs in the apices of the lungs and is likely to cause chronic progressive cavitary pulmonary disease with less tendency for hematogenous dissemination. *Mycobacterium bovis* infection is clinically identical to *M tuberculosis*. *M bovis* may be acquired from unpasteurized dairy products obtained outside the United States.

Clinical Findings

A. SYMPTOMS AND SIGNS

1. Pulmonary—(See Chapter 18.)

2. Miliary—Diagnosis is usually based on the classic "snowstorm" or "millet seed" appearance of lung fields on radiograph, although early in the course of disseminated tuberculosis the chest radiograph may show no or only subtle abnormalities. The majority of patients have a fresh primary complex and pleural effusion. Choroidal tubercles are sometimes seen on funduscopic examination. Other lesions may be present and produce osteomyelitis, arthritis, meningitis, tuberculomas of the brain, enteritis, or infection of the kidneys and liver.

3. Meningitis—Symptoms include fever, vomiting, headache, lethargy, and irritability, with signs of meningeal irritation and increased intracranial pressure, cranial nerve palsies, convulsions, and coma.

4. Lymphatic—The primary complex may be associated with a skin lesion drained by regional nodes or chronic cervical node enlargement or infection of the tonsils. Involved nodes may become fixed to the overlying skin, suppurate, and drain.

B. LABORATORY FINDINGS

The Mantoux test (0.1 mL of intermediate-strength purified protein derivative [PPD] [5 TU] inoculated intradermally) is positive at 48–72 hours if there is significant induration (Table 38–2). Parental reporting of skin test results is often inaccurate. All tests should be read by professionals trained to interpret Mantoux tests. False-negative results occur in malnourished patients, in those with overwhelming disease, and in 10% of children with isolated pulmonary disease. Temporary suppression of tuberculin reactivity may be seen with viral infections (eg, measles, influenza, varicella, and mumps), after live virus immunization, and during corticosteroid or other immunosuppressive drug therapy. For these reasons, a negative Mantoux test does not exclude the diagnosis of tuberculosis. When tuberculosis is suspected in a child, household members and adult contacts (eg, teachers and caregivers) should also be tested immediately. Multiple puncture tests (tine tests) should not be used because they are associated with false-negative and false-positive reactions, and because standards for interpretation of positive results do not exist. The ESR is usually elevated. Cultures of pooled early morning gastric aspirates from three successive days will yield *M tuberculosis* in about 40% of cases. Biopsy may be necessary to establish the diagnosis. Therapy should not be delayed in suspected cases. The CSF in tuberculous meningitis shows slight to moderate pleocytosis (50–300 WBCs/µL, predominantly lymphocytes), decreased glucose, and increased protein.

The direct detection of mycobacteria in body fluids or discharges is best done by staining specimens with auramine-rhodamine and examining them with fluorescence microscopy; this method is superior to the Ziehl–Neelsen method.

C. IMAGING

Chest radiograph should be obtained in all children with suspicion of tuberculosis at any site or with a positive skin test. Segmental consolidation with some volume loss and hilar adenopathy are common findings in children. Pleural effusion also occurs with primary infection. Cavities and apical disease are unusual in children but are common in adolescents and adults.

Differential Diagnosis

Pulmonary tuberculosis must be differentiated from fungal, parasitic, mycoplasmal, and bacterial pneumonias; lung abscess; foreign body aspiration; lipoid pneumonia; sarcoidosis; and mediastinal cancer. Cervical lymphadenitis is most likely due to streptococcal or staphylococcal infections. Cat-scratch fever and infection with atypical mycobacteria may need to be distinguished from tuberculous lymphadenitis. Viral meningoencephalitis, head trauma (child abuse), lead poisoning, brain abscess, acute bacterial meningitis, brain tumor, and disseminated fungal infections must be excluded in tuberculous meningitis. The skin test in the patient or family contacts is frequently valuable in differentiating these conditions from tuberculosis.

Prevention

A. BCG VACCINE

Bacille Calmette–Guérin (BCG) vaccines are live-attenuated strains of *M bovis*. Although neonatal and childhood administration of BCG is carried out in countries with a high prevalence of tuberculosis, protective efficacy varies greatly with vaccine potency and method of delivery. Because the great majority of children who have received BCG still have negative Mantoux tests, the past history of BCG vaccination should be ignored in interpreting the skin test. In the United States, BCG vaccination is not recommended.

B. ISONIAZID CHEMOPROPHYLAXIS

Daily administration of isoniazid (10 mg/kg/d orally; maximum 300 mg) is advised for children who are exposed by prolonged close or household contact with adolescents or adults with active disease. Isoniazid is given until 3 months after last contact. At the end of this time, a Mantoux test should be done, and therapy should be continued for an additional 6 months if the test is positive.

C. OTHER MEASURES

Tuberculosis in infants and young children is evidence of recent exposure to active infection in an adult, usually a

Table 38–2. Interpretation of tuberculin skin test reactions.[a]

Degree of Risk	Risk Factors	Positive Reaction
High	Recent close contact with a case of active tuberculosis; chest x-ray compatible with tuberculosis; immunocompromise; HIV infection	≥ 5 mm induration
Medium	Current or previous residence in high-prevalence area (Asia, Africa, Latin America); skin test converters within past 2 years; intravenous drug use; homelessness or residence in a correctional institution; recent weight loss or malnutrition; leukemia, Hodgkin disease, diabetes mellitus; age < 4 years	≥ 10 mm induration
Low	Children ≥ 4 years without any risk factor	≥ 15 mm induration

[a]Standard intradermal Mantoux test, 5 test units.

family member or household contact. The source contact (index case) should be identified, isolated, and given treatment to prevent other secondary cases. Reporting cases to local health departments is essential for contact tracing. Exposed tuberculin-negative children should usually receive isoniazid chemoprophylaxis. If a repeated skin test is negative 2–3 months following the last exposure, isoniazid may be stopped. Routine tuberculin skin testing is not recommended for children without risk factors who reside in communities with a low incidence of tuberculosis. Children with no personal risk for tuberculosis but who reside in communities with a high incidence of tuberculosis should be given a skin test at school entry and then again at age 11–16 years. Children with a risk factor for acquiring tuberculosis should be tested every 2–3 years. Incarcerated adolescents and children living in a household with HIV-infected persons should have annual skin tests.

Children who immigrate from a country with a high incidence of infection should receive a skin test on entry to the United States or upon presentation to health care providers. A past history of BCG vaccine should not delay skin testing.

Treatment

A. SPECIFIC MEASURES

Most children with tuberculosis in the United States are hospitalized initially. If the infecting organism has not been isolated from the presumed contact for susceptibility testing, reasonable attempts should be made to obtain it from the child using morning gastric aspirates, sputum, bronchoscopy, thoracentesis, or biopsy when appropriate. Unfortunately, cultures are frequently negative in children, and the risk of these procedures must be weighed against the yield. Therapy is given daily for 2–4 weeks and then reduced to 2–3 times per week for the duration of the course. Directly observed administration of all doses of antituberculosis therapy by a trained health care professional is essential to ensure compliance with therapy.

All children with positive skin tests (see Table 38–2) without evidence of active disease have latent tuberculosis and should receive 9 months of isoniazid (10 mg/kg/d orally; maximum 300 mg) therapy. In children with active pulmonary disease, therapy for 6 months using isoniazid (10 mg/kg/d), rifampin (15 mg/kg/d), and pyrazinamide (25–30 mg/kg/d) in a single daily oral dose for 2 months, followed by isoniazid plus rifampin (either in a daily or twice-weekly regimen) for 4 months appears effective for eliminating isoniazid-susceptible organisms. For more severe disease, such as miliary or CNS infection, duration is increased to 12 months or more, and a fourth drug (streptomycin or ethambutol) is added for the first 2 months. In communities with resistance rates greater than 4%, initial therapy should usually include four drugs.

1. Isoniazid—The hepatotoxicity from isoniazid seen in adults and some adolescents is rare in children. Transient elevation of aminotransferases (up to three times normal) may be seen at 6–12 weeks, but therapy is continued unless clinical illness occurs. Routine monitoring of liver function tests is unnecessary unless prior hepatic disease is known or the child is severely ill. Peripheral neuropathy associated with pyridoxine deficiency is rare in children, and it is not necessary to add pyridoxine unless significant malnutrition coexists.

2. Rifampin—Although it is an excellent bactericidal agent, rifampin is never used alone owing to rapid development of resistance. Hepatotoxicity may occur but rarely with recommended doses. The orange discoloration of secretions is benign but may stain contact lenses or clothes.

3. Pyrazinamide—This excellent sterilizing agent is most effective during the first 2 months of therapy. With the recommended duration and dosing, it is well tolerated. Although pyrazinamide elevates the uric acid level, it rarely causes symptoms of hyperuricemia in children. Use of this drug is now common for tuberculous disease in children, and resistance is almost unknown. Oral acceptance and CNS penetration are good.

4. Ethambutol—Because optic neuritis is the major side effect in adults, ethambutol has usually been given only to children whose vision can be reliably tested for loss of color differentiation. Optic neuritis is rare and usually occurs in those receiving more than the recommended dosage of 25 mg/kg/d. Documentation of optic toxicity in children is lacking despite considerable worldwide experience. Therefore, many four-drug regimens for children now include ethambutol.

5. Streptomycin—Streptomycin (20–30 mg/kg/d, given intramuscularly in one or two doses) should be given for 1 or 2 months in severe disease. The child's hearing should be tested periodically during use as ototoxicity is common.

B. CHEMOTHERAPY FOR DRUG-RESISTANT TUBERCULOSIS

The incidence of drug resistance is increasing and reaches 10–20% in some areas of the United States. Transmission of multiply drug-resistant strains to contacts has occurred in some epidemics. All patients with resistant strains should be given at least two effective drugs. In areas with rates of resistance greater than 4%, initial therapy should include four drugs pending susceptibility testing. Consultation with local experts in treating tuberculosis is important in these difficult cases. Therapy should continue for 12 months or longer.

C. GENERAL MEASURES

1. Corticosteroids—These drugs may be used for suppressing inflammatory reactions in meningeal, pleural, and pericardial tuberculosis and for the relief of bronchial obstruction due to hilar adenopathy. Prednisone is given orally, 1 mg/kg/d for 6–8 weeks, with gradual withdrawal at the end of that time. The use of corticosteroids may mask progression of disease. Accordingly, the clinician needs to be sure that an effective regimen is being used.

Prognosis

If bacteria are sensitive and treatment is completed, most children are cured with minimal sequelae. Repeat treatment is more difficult and less successful. With antituberculosis chemotherapy (especially isoniazid), there should now be nearly 100% recovery in miliary tuberculosis. Without treatment, the mortality rate in both miliary tuberculosis and tuberculous meningitis is almost 100%. In the latter form, about two-thirds of patients receiving treatment survive. There may be a high incidence of neurologic abnormalities among survivors if treatment is started late.

American Thoracic Society, CDC, Infectious Diseases Society of America: Treatment of tuberculosis. MMWR Recomm Rep 2003;52(RR-11):1 [PMID: 12836625].

Centers for Disease Control and Prevention (CDC): *Mycobacterium tuberculosis* transmission in a newborn nursery and maternity ward—New York City, 2003. MMWR Morb Mortal Wkly Rep 2005;54(50):1280 [PMID: 16371943].

Khan K et al: Global drug-resistance patterns and the management of latent tuberculosis infection in immigrants to the United States. N Engl J Med 2002;347(23):1850 [PMID: 12466510].

Taylor Z, Nolan CM, Blumberg HM; American Thoracic Society; Centers for Disease Control and Prevention; Infectious Diseases Society of America: Controlling tuberculosis in the United States. Recommendations from the American Thoracic Society, CDC, and the Infectious Diseases Society of America. MMWR Morb Mortal Wkly Rep 2005;54(RR-12):1 [PMID: 16267499].

Young J, O'Connor ME: Risk factors associated with latent tuberculosis infection in Mexican American children. Pediatrics 2005;115(6):e647 [PMID: 15930191].

INFECTIONS WITH NONTUBERCULOUS MYCOBACTERIA

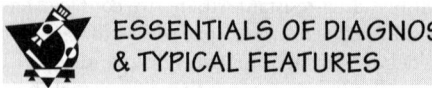

ESSENTIALS OF DIAGNOSIS & TYPICAL FEATURES

- Chronic unilateral cervical lymphadenitis.
- Granulomas of the skin.
- Chronic bone lesion with draining sinus (chronic osteomyelitis).
- Reaction to PPD-S (standard) of 5–8 mm, negative chest radiograph, and negative history of contact with tuberculosis.
- Diagnosis by positive acid-fast stain or culture.
- Disseminated infection in patients with AIDS.

General Considerations

Various species of acid-fast mycobacteria other than *Mycobacterium tuberculosis* may cause subclinical infections and occasionally clinical disease resembling tuberculosis. Strains of nontuberculous mycobacteria are common in soil, food, and water. Organisms enter the host by small abrasions in skin, oral mucosa, or gastrointestinal mucosa. Strain cross-reactivity with *M tuberculosis* can be demonstrated by simultaneous skin testing (Mantoux) with PPD-S (standard) and PPD prepared from one of the atypical antigens. Unfortunately, reagents prepared for routine nontuberculosis skin testing are not available to clinicians.

The Runyon classification of mycobacteria includes the following:

Group I. Photochromogens (PPD-Y): (*M kansasii* and *M marinum*) Yellow color develops on exposure to light in previously white colony grown 2–4 weeks in the dark.

Group II. Scotochromogens (PPD-G): (*M scrofulaceum*) Colonies are definitely yellow-orange after incubation in the dark. Organisms may be found in small numbers in the normal flora of some human saliva and gastric contents. Subclinical infection is widespread in the United States, but clinical disease appears rarely.

Group III. Nonphotochromogens (PPD-B): "Battey avian-swine group" grows as small white colonies after incubation in the dark, with no significant development of pigment on exposure to light. Infection with *Mycobacterium avium* complex (MAC) is prevalent on the East Coast of the United States, particularly the Southeast, and in patients with AIDS.

Group IV. "Rapid growers": (*M fortuitum, M chelonei*) Within 1 week after inoculation they form colonies closely resembling *M tuberculosis* morphologically.

Clinical Findings

A. SYMPTOMS AND SIGNS

1. Lymphadenitis—In children, the most common form of infection due to mycobacteria other than *M tuberculosis* is cervical lymphadenitis. MAC is the most common organism. A submandibular or cervical node swells slowly and is firm and initially somewhat tender. Low-grade fever may occur. Over time, the node suppurates and may drain chronically. Nodes in other areas of the head and neck and elsewhere are sometimes involved.

2. Pulmonary disease—In the western United States, pulmonary disease is usually due to *M kansasii*. In the eastern United States, it may be due to MAC. In other countries, disease is usually caused by MAC. In adults, there is usually underlying chronic pulmonary disease. Immunologic deficiency may be present. Presentation is clinically indistinguishable from that of tuberculosis. Adolescents with cystic fibrosis may be infected with nontuberculous mycobacteria.

3. Swimming pool granuloma—This is due to *M marinum.* A solitary chronic granulomatous lesion with satellite lesions develops after minor trauma in infected swimming pools. Minor trauma in home aquariums or other aquatic environments also may lead to infection.

4. Chronic osteomyelitis—Osteomyelitis is caused by *M kansasii, M fortuitum,* or other rapid growers. Findings include swelling and pain over a distal extremity, radiolucent defects in bone, fever, and clinical and radiographic evidence of bronchopneumonia. Such cases are rare.

5. Meningitis—Disease is due to *M kansasii* and may be indistinguishable from tuberculous meningitis.

6. Disseminated infection—Rarely, apparently immunologically normal children develop disseminated infection due to nontuberculous mycobacteria. Children are ill, with fever and hepatosplenomegaly, and organisms are demonstrated in bone lesions, lymph nodes, or liver. Chest radiographs are usually normal. Between 60% and 80% of patients with AIDS will acquire MAC infection, characterized by fever, night sweats, weight loss, and diarrhea. Infection usually indicates severe immune dysfunction and is associated with CD4 lymphocyte counts less than 50/μL.

B. LABORATORY FINDINGS

In most cases, there is a small reaction (< 10 mm) when Mantoux testing is done. Larger reactions may be seen. The chest radiograph is negative, and there is no history of contact with tuberculosis. Needle aspiration of the node excludes bacterial infection and may yield acid-fast bacilli on stain or culture. Fistulization should not be a problem because total excision is usually recommended for infection due to atypical mycobacteria. Cultures of any normally sterile body site will yield MAC in immunocompromised patients with disseminated disease. Blood cultures are positive, with a large density of bacteria.

Differential Diagnosis

See section on differential diagnosis in the previous discussion of tuberculosis and in Chapter 18.

Treatment

A. SPECIFIC MEASURES

The usual treatment of lymphadenitis is complete surgical excision. Occasionally excision is impossible because of proximity to branches of the facial nerve. Chemotherapy may then be necessary. Response of extensive adenopathy

or other forms of infection varies according to the infecting species and susceptibility. Usually, combinations of two to four medications administered for months are required. Isoniazid, rifampin, and ethambutol (depending on sensitivity to isoniazid) will result in a favorable response in almost all patients with *M kansasii* infection. Chemotherapeutic treatment of MAC is much less satisfactory because resistance to isoniazid, rifampin, and pyrazinamide is common. Susceptibility testing is necessary to optimize therapy. Most clinicians favor surgical excision of involved tissue if possible and treatment with at least three drugs to which the organism has been shown to be sensitive. Disseminated disease in patients with AIDS calls for a combination of three or more active drugs. Clarithromycin and ethambutol, in addition to one or more of the following drugs, is started: ethionamide, capreomycin, amikacin, rifabutin, or ciprofloxacin. *M fortuitum* and *M chelonei* are usually susceptible to amikacin plus cefoxitin followed by erythromycin, clarithromycin, azithromycin, or doxycycline and may be successfully treated with such combinations. Swimming pool granuloma due to *M marinum* is usually treated with doxycycline (in children > age 9 years) or rifampin, plus ethambutol, clarithromycin, or TMP–SMX for a minimum of 3 months. Surgery may also be beneficial.

B. GENERAL MEASURES

Isolation of the patient is usually not necessary. General supportive care is indicated for the child with disseminated disease.

Prognosis

The prognosis is good for localized disease, although fatalities occur in immunocompromised children who have disseminated disease.

Albright JT, Pransky SM: Nontuberculous mycobacterial infections of the head and neck. Pediatr Clin North Am 2003; 59(2):503 [PMID: 12809337].

Lindeboom JA et al: Cervicofacial lymphadenitis in children caused by mycobacterium haemophilum. Clin Infect Dis 2005;41 (11):1569. Epub 2005 Oct 28 [PMID: 16267728].

Loeffler AM: Treatment options for nontuberculous mycobacterial adenitis in children. Pediatr Infect Dis J 2004;23(10):957 [PMID: 15602198].

Vu TT, Daniel SJ, Quach C: Nontuberculous mycobacteria in children: A changing pattern. J Otolaryngol 2005;34(Suppl 1):S40 [PMID: 16089239].

LEGIONELLA INFECTION

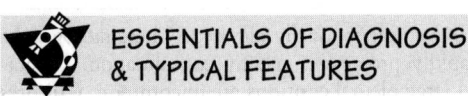

ESSENTIALS OF DIAGNOSIS & TYPICAL FEATURES

- *Severe progressive pneumonia in a child with compromised immunity.*

- *Diarrhea and neurologic signs are common.*
- *Positive culture requires buffered charcoal yeast extract media and proves infection.*
- *Direct fluorescent antibody staining of respiratory secretions proves infection.*

General Considerations

Legionella pneumophila is a ubiquitous gram-negative bacillus that causes two distinct clinical syndromes: Legionnaire disease and Pontiac fever. Usually Legionnaire disease is an acute, severe pneumonia that is frequently fatal in immunocompromised patients. Pontiac fever is a mild, flulike illness that spares the lungs and is characterized by fever, headache, myalgia, and arthralgia. The disease is self-limited and is described in outbreaks in otherwise healthy adults.

Over 40 species of *Legionella* have been discovered, but not all cause disease in humans. *L pneumophila* causes most infections. *Legionella* is present in many natural water sources as well as domestic water supplies (faucets and showers). Contaminated cooling towers and heat exchangers have been implicated in several large institutional outbreaks. Person-to-person transmission has not been documented.

Few cases of Legionnaire disease have been reported in children. Most were in children with compromised cellular immunity. In adults, risk factors include smoking, underlying cardiopulmonary or renal disease, alcoholism, and diabetes.

L pneumophila is thought to be acquired by inhalation of a contaminated aerosol. The bacteria are phagocytosed but proliferate within macrophages. Cell-mediated immunity is necessary to activate macrophages to kill intracellular bacteria.

Clinical Findings

A. SYMPTOMS AND SIGNS

Onset of fever, chills, anorexia, and headache is abrupt. Pulmonary symptoms appear within 2–3 days and progress rapidly. The cough is nonproductive early. Purulent sputum occurs late. Hemoptysis, diarrhea, and neurologic signs (including lethargy, irritability, tremors, and delirium) are seen.

B. LABORATORY FINDINGS

The WBC count is usually elevated. Chest radiographs show rapidly progressive patchy consolidation. Cavitation and large pleural effusions are uncommon. Cultures from sputum, tracheal aspirates, or bronchoscopic specimens, when grown on buffered yeast charcoal extract media, are positive in 70–80% of patients at 3–7 days.

Direct fluorescent antibody staining of sputum or other respiratory specimens is only 50–70% sensitive but 95% specific. A negative culture or direct fluorescent antibody staining of sputum or tracheal secretions does not rule out disease due to *Legionella*. PCR of respiratory secretions for *Legionella* is available at some centers. A urine immunoassay for *Legionella* antigen is more sensitive than the immunoassay using respiratory secretions and is highly specific. Serologic tests are available, but a maximum rise in titer may require 6–8 weeks.

Differential Diagnosis

Legionnaire disease is usually a rapidly progressive pneumonia in a patient who appears very ill with unremitting fevers. Other bacterial pneumonias, viral pneumonias, *Mycoplasma* pneumonia, and fungal disease are all possibilities and may be difficult to differentiate clinically in an immunocompromised patient.

Complications

In sporadic untreated cases, mortality rates are 5–25%. In immunocompromised patients with untreated disease, mortality approaches 80%. Hematogenous dissemination may result in extrapulmonary foci of infection, including pericardium, myocardium, and kidneys. *Legionella* may be the cause of culture-negative endocarditis.

Prevention

No vaccine is available. Hyperchlorination and periodic superheating of water supplies in hospitals have been shown to reduce the number of organisms and the risk of infection.

Treatment

Intravenous azithromycin 10 mg/kg/d given as a once-daily dose (maximum dose 500 mg) is the drug of choice. Rifampin (20 mg/kg/d divided in two doses) may be added to the regimen in gravely ill patients. Ciprofloxacin and levofloxacin are effective in adults, but are not approved for use in children. Duration of therapy is 5–10 days if azithromycin is used; for other antibiotics a 14–21-day course is recommended. Oral therapy may be substituted for intravenous therapy as the patient's condition improves.

Prognosis

Mortality rate is high if treatment is delayed. Malaise, problems with memory, and fatigue are common after recovery.

Fields BS, Benson RF, Besser R: *Legionella* and Legionnaires' disease: 25 years of investigation. Clin Microbiol Rev 2002;15(3):506 [PMID: 12097254].

Roig J et al: *Legionella* spp.: Community acquired and nosocomial infections. Curr Opin Infect Dis 2003;16(2):145 [PMID: 12734447].

PSITTACOSIS (Ornithosis) & *CHLAMYDIA PNEUMONIAE* INFECTION

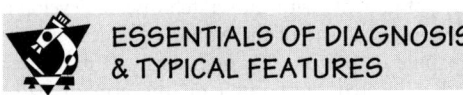

ESSENTIALS OF DIAGNOSIS & TYPICAL FEATURES

- Fever, cough, malaise, chills, headache.
- Diffuse rales; no consolidation.
- Long-lasting radiographic findings of bronchopneumonia.
- Isolation of the organism or rising titer of complement-fixing antibodies.
- Exposure to infected birds (ornithosis).

General Considerations

Psittacosis is caused by *Chlamydia psittaci*. When the agent is transmitted to humans from psittacine birds (parrots, parakeets, cockatoos, and budgerigars), the disease is called psittacosis or parrot fever. However, other avian genera (eg, pigeons and turkeys) are common sources of infection in the United States, and the general term "ornithosis" is often used. The agent is an obligate intracellular parasite. Human-to-human spread rarely occurs. The incubation period is 5–14 days. The bird from which the disease was transmitted may not be clinically ill.

C pneumoniae may cause atypical pneumonia similar to that due to *M pneumoniae*. Transmission is by respiratory spread. Infection appears to be most prevalent during the second decade; half of surveyed adults are seropositive. Only a small percentage of infections result in clinical pneumonia. The disease may be more common than atypical pneumonia due to *M pneumoniae*. Lower respiratory tract infection due to *C pneumoniae* is uncommon in infants and young children.

Clinical Findings

A. SYMPTOMS AND SIGNS

1. *C psittaci*—The disease is extremely variable but tends to be mild in children. The onset is rapid or insidious, with fever, chills, headache, backache, malaise, myalgia, and dry cough. Signs include pneumonitis, alteration of percussion note and breath sounds, and rales. Pulmonary findings may be absent early. Dyspnea and cyanosis may occur later. Splenomegaly, epistaxis,

prostration, and meningismus are occasionally seen. Delirium, constipation or diarrhea, and abdominal distress may occur.

2. *C pneumoniae*—Clinically, *C pneumoniae* infection is similar to *M pneumoniae* infection. Most are mild upper respiratory infections. Lower respiratory tract infection is characterized by fever, sore throat (perhaps more severe with *C pneumoniae*), cough, and bilateral pulmonary findings and infiltrates.

B. LABORATORY FINDINGS

1. *C psittaci*—In psittacosis, the WBC count is normal or decreased, often with a shift to the left. Proteinuria is frequently present. *C psittaci* is present in the blood and sputum during the first 2 weeks of illness and can be isolated by inoculation of specimens into mice or embryonated eggs, but culture is available only in research laboratories. A fourfold rise in complement fixation titers in specimens obtained at least 2 weeks apart or a single titer above 1:32 is considered evidence of infection. The titer rise may be blunted or delayed by therapy. Infection with *C pneumoniae* may lead to diagnostic confusion because cross-reactive antibody may cause falsely positive *C psittaci* titers. Microimmunofluorescence and PCR assays are specific but usually not available for *C psittaci*.

2. *C pneumoniae*—A fourfold rise in IgG titer (microimmunofluorescence antibody test) or an IgM above 16 is evidence of infection. IgG antibody peaks 6–8 weeks after infection. *C pneumoniae* can be isolated from nasal wash or throat swab specimens after inoculation into cell culture. A PCR assay is also available.

C. IMAGING

The radiographic findings in psittacosis are those of central pneumonia, which later becomes widespread or migratory. Psittacosis is indistinguishable from viral pneumonias by radiograph. Signs of pneumonitis may appear on radiograph in the absence of clinical suspicion of pulmonary involvement.

Differential Diagnosis

Psittacosis can be differentiated from viral or mycoplasmal pneumonias only by the history of contact with potentially infected birds. In severe or prolonged cases with extrapulmonary involvement the differential diagnosis is broad, including typhoid fever, brucellosis, and rheumatic fever.

Complications

Complications of psittacosis include myocarditis, endocarditis, hepatitis, pancreatitis, and secondary bacterial pneumonia. *C pneumoniae* infection may be prolonged or may recur.

Treatment

Doxycycline should be given for 14 days after defervescence to patients older than age 8 years with psittacosis. Alternatively, erythromycin, azithromycin, or clarithromycin may be used in younger children. Supportive oxygen may be needed. The patient should be kept in isolation. *C pneumoniae* responds to macrolides or doxycycline: a 14-day course is recommended.

Centers for Disease Control and Prevention: Compendium of measures to control *Chlamydia psittaci* infection among humans (psittacosis) and pet birds (avian chlamydiosis), 2000. MMWR Morb Mortal Wkly Rep 2000;49(RR-8):3.

File TM Jr et al: The role of atypical pathogens: *Mycoplasma pneumoniae, Chlamydia pneumoniae,* and *Legionella pneumophila* in respiratory infection. Infect Dis Clin North Am 1998;12:569.

Tsai MH et al: Chlamydial pneumonia in children requiring hospitalization: Effect of mixed infection on clinical outcome. J Microbiol Immunol Infect 2005;38(2):117 [PMID: 15843856].

CAT-SCRATCH DISEASE

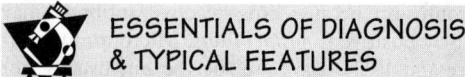

ESSENTIALS OF DIAGNOSIS & TYPICAL FEATURES

- *History of a cat scratch or cat contact.*
- *Primary lesion (papule, pustule, or conjunctivitis) at site of inoculation.*
- *Acute or subacute regional lymphadenopathy.*
- *Aspiration of sterile pus from a node.*
- *Laboratory studies excluding other causes.*
- *Biopsy of node or papule showing histopathologic findings consistent with cat-scratch disease and occasionally characteristic bacilli on Warthin–Starry stain.*
- *Positive cat-scratch serology (antibody to Bartonella henselae).*

General Considerations

The causative agent of cat-scratch disease is *Bartonella henselae,* a gram-negative bacillus that also causes bacillary angiomatosis. Cat-scratch disease is a benign, self-limited form of lymphadenitis. Patients often report a cat scratch (67%) or contact with a cat or kitten (90%). The cat almost invariably is healthy. The clinical picture is that of a regional lymphadenitis associated with an erythematous papular skin lesion without intervening lymphangitis. The disease occurs worldwide and is more common in the fall and winter. It is estimated that more than 20,000 cases per year occur in the

United States. The most common systemic complication is encephalitis.

Clinical Findings

A. SYMPTOMS AND SIGNS

About 50% of patients with cat-scratch disease develop a primary lesion at the site of the wound. The lesion usually is a papule or pustule that appears 3–10 days after injury and is located most often on the arm or hand (50%), head or leg (30%), or trunk or neck (10%). The lesion may be conjunctival (10%). Regional lymphadenopathy appears 10–50 days later and may be accompanied by mild malaise, lassitude, headache, and fever. Multiple sites are seen in about 10% of cases. Involved nodes may be hard or soft and 1–6 cm in diameter. They are usually tender, and 10–20% of them suppurate. The overlying skin may be inflamed. Lymphadenopathy usually resolves in about 2 months but may persist for up to 8 months.

Unusual manifestations include erythema nodosum, thrombocytopenic purpura, conjunctivitis (Parinaud oculoglandular fever), parotid swelling, pneumonia, osteolytic lesions, mesenteric and mediastinal adenitis, neuroretinitis, peripheral neuritis, hepatitis, granulomata of the liver and spleen, and encephalitis.

Immunocompetent patients may develop an atypical systemic form of cat-scratch disease. These patients have prolonged fever, fatigue, and malaise. Lymphadenopathy may be present. Hepatosplenomegaly or low-density hepatic or splenic lesions visualized by ultrasound or computed tomography scan are seen in some patients.

Infection in immunocompromised individuals may take the form of bacillary angiomatosis, presenting as vascular tumors of the skin and subcutaneous tissues. Immunocompromised patients may also have bacteremia or infection of the liver (peliosis hepatis).

B. LABORATORY FINDINGS

Serologic evidence of *Bartonella* infection by indirect fluorescent antibody or ELISA with a titer above 1:64 is supportive of the diagnosis. PCR assays are available. Cat-scratch skin test antigens are not recommended.

Histopathologic examination of involved tissue may show pyogenic granulomas or bacillary forms demonstrated by Warthin–Starry silver stain. There is usually some elevation in the ESR. In patients with CNS involvement, the CSF is usually normal but may show a slight pleocytosis and modest elevation of protein.

Differential Diagnosis

Cat-scratch disease must be distinguished from pyogenic adenitis, tuberculosis (typical and atypical), tularemia, plague, brucellosis, lymphoma, primary toxoplasmosis, infectious mononucleosis, lymphogranuloma venereum, and fungal infections.

Treatment

Treatment of cat-scratch disease adenopathy is controversial because the disease usually resolves without therapy and the patient is typically not exceedingly ill. Treatment of typical cat-scratch disease with a 5-day course of azithromycin has been shown to speed resolution of lymphadenopathy in some patients. The best therapy is reassurance that the adenopathy is benign and will subside spontaneously with time (mean duration of illness is 14 weeks). In cases of suppuration, node aspiration under local anesthesia with an 18- to 19-gauge needle relieves the pain. Excision of the involved node is indicated in cases of chronic adenitis. In some reports, gentamicin, ciprofloxacin, and TMP–SMX have been useful. Immunocompromised patients with evidence of infection should be treated with antibiotics: long-term therapy (months) in these patients with azithromycin, erythromycin, or doxycycline is often needed to prevent relapses.

Prognosis

The prognosis is good if complications do not occur.

Bass JW et al: Prospective randomized double blind placebo-controlled evaluation of azithromycin for treatment of cat scratch disease. Pediatr Infect Dis J 1998;17:447 [PMID: 9655532].

Lamps LW, Scott MA: Cat-scratch disease: Historic, clinical, and pathologic perspectives. Am J Clin Pathol 2004;121(Suppl):S71 [PMID: 15298152].

Schutze GE: Diagnosis and treatment of *Bartonella henselae* infections. Pediatr Infect Dis J 2000;19:1185 [PMID: 11144381].

■ II. SPIROCHETAL INFECTIONS

SYPHILIS

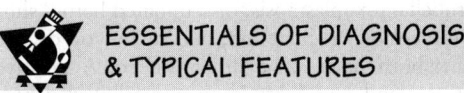

ESSENTIALS OF DIAGNOSIS & TYPICAL FEATURES

Congenital:

- *All types: History of untreated maternal syphilis, a positive serologic test, and a positive darkfield examination.*
- *Newborn: Hepatosplenomegaly, characteristic radiographic bone changes, anemia, increased nu-*

cleated red cells, thrombocytopenia, abnormal spinal fluid, jaundice, edema.

- *Young infant (3–12 weeks): Snuffles, maculopapular skin rash, mucocutaneous lesions, pseudoparalysis (in addition to radiographic bone changes).*
- *Children: Stigmata of early congenital syphilis, interstitial keratitis, saber shins, gummas of nose and palate.*

Acquired:

- *Chancre of genitals, lip, or anus in child or adolescent. History of sexual contact.*

General Considerations

Syphilis is a chronic, generalized infectious disease caused by a spirochete, *Treponema pallidum*. In the acquired form, the disease is transmitted by sexual contact. Primary syphilis is characterized by the presence of an indurated painless chancre, which heals in 7–10 days. A secondary eruption involving the skin and mucous membranes appears in 4–6 weeks. After a long latency period, late lesions of tertiary syphilis involve the eyes, skin, bones, viscera, CNS, and cardiovascular system.

Congenital syphilis results from transplacental infection. Infection may result in stillbirth or produce illness in the newborn, in early infancy, or later in childhood. Syphilis occurring in the newborn and young infant is comparable to secondary disease in the adult but is more severe and life-threatening. Late congenital syphilis (developing in childhood) is comparable to tertiary disease.

Congenital syphilis is increasing in the United States due to increasing primary and secondary syphilis in women of childbearing age, and perhaps due to inadequate diagnosis and treatment of syphilis in prenatal care programs.

Clinical Findings

A. SYMPTOMS AND SIGNS

1. Congenital syphilis
a. Newborns—Most newborns with congenital syphilis are asymptomatic. If not detected and treated, symptoms develop within weeks to months. When clinical signs are present, they usually consist of jaundice, anemia with or without thrombocytopenia, increase in nucleated red blood cells, hepatosplenomegaly, and edema. Overt signs of meningitis (bulging fontanelle or opisthotonos) may be present, but subclinical infection with CSF abnormalities is more likely.

b. Young infants (3–12 weeks)—The infant may appear normal for the first few weeks of life only to develop mucocutaneous lesions and pseudoparalysis of the arms or legs. Shotty lymphadenopathy may be felt. Hepatomegaly is universal, with splenomegaly in 50% of patients. Other signs of disease similar to those seen in the newborn may be present. Anemia has been reported as the only presenting manifestation of congenital syphilis in this age group. "Snuffles" (rhinitis), characterized by a profuse mucopurulent discharge is present in 25% of patients. A syphilitic rash is common on the palms and soles but may occur anywhere on the body. The rash consists of bright red, raised maculopapular lesions that gradually fade. Moist lesions occur at the mucocutaneous junctions (nose, mouth, anus, and genitals) and lead to fissuring and bleeding.

Syphilis in the young infant may lead to stigmata recognizable in later childhood, such as rhagades (scars) around the mouth or nose, a depressed bridge of the nose (saddle nose), and a high forehead (secondary to mild hydrocephalus associated with low-grade meningitis and frontal periostitis). The permanent upper central incisors may be peg-shaped with a central notch (Hutchinson teeth), and the cusps of the sixth-year molars may have a lobulated mulberry appearance.

c. Children—Bilateral interstitial keratitis (at age 6–12 years) is characterized by photophobia, increased lacrimation, and vascularization of the cornea associated with exudation. Chorioretinitis and optic atrophy may also be seen. Meningovascular syphilis (at age 2–10 years) is usually slowly progressive, with mental retardation, spasticity, abnormal pupillary response, speech defects, and abnormal CSF. Deafness sometimes occurs. Thickening of the periosteum of the anterior tibias produces saber shins. A bilateral effusion into the knee joints (Clutton joints) may occur but is not associated with sequelae. Gummas may develop in the nasal septum, palate, long bones, and subcutaneous tissues.

2. Acquired syphilis—The primary chancre of the genitals, mouth, or anus may occur as a result of intimate sexual contact. If the chancre is missed, signs of secondary syphilis, such as rash, fever, headache, and malaise, may be the first manifestations.

B. LABORATORY FINDINGS

1. Darkfield microscopy—Treponemes can be seen in scrapings from a chancre and from moist lesions.

2. Serologic tests for syphilis—There are two general types of serologic tests for syphilis: treponemal and nontreponemal. The latter (Venereal Disease Research Laboratory, or VDRL) is useful for screening and follow-up of known cases. A rapid test (the rapid plasma reagin, or RPR) is useful for screening, but positive sera should be examined further by quantitative nontreponemal and treponemal tests. Positive nontreponemal tests are confirmed with more specific fluorescent treponemal antibody absorbed, or FTA-ABS, test. False-

positive FTA-ABS tests are uncommon except with other spirochetal disease.

One or two weeks after the onset of primary syphilis (chancre), the FTA-ABS test becomes positive. The VDRL or a similar nontreponemal test usually turns positive a few days later. By the time the secondary stage has been reached, virtually all patients show both positive FTA-ABS and positive nontreponemal tests. During latent and tertiary syphilis, the VDRL may become negative, but the FTA-ABS test usually remains positive. The quantitative VDRL or a similar nontreponemal test should be used to follow-up treated cases (see following discussion).

Positive serologic tests in cord sera may represent passively transferred antibody rather than congenital infection and therefore must be supplemented by a combination of clinical and laboratory data. Elevated total cord IgM is a helpful but nonspecific finding. A specific IgM–FTA-ABS is available, but negative results are not conclusive and should not be relied on. Demonstration of characteristic treponemes by darkfield examination of material from a moist lesion (skin; nasal or other mucous membranes) is definitive. Serial measurement of quantitative VDRL is also very useful, because passively transferred antibody in the absence of active infection should decay with a normal half-life of about 18 days.

In one study, 15% of infants with congenital syphilis had negative cord blood serology, presumably due to maternal infection late in pregnancy.

C. IMAGING

Radiographic abnormalities are present in 90% of infants with symptoms of congenital syphilis and in 20% of asymptomatic infants. Metaphyseal lucent bands, periostitis, and a widened zone of provisional calcification may be present. Bilateral symmetrical osteomyelitis with pathologic fractures of the medial tibial metaphyses (Wimberger sign) is almost pathognomonic.

Differential Diagnosis

A. CONGENITAL SYPHILIS

1. Newborns—Sepsis, congestive heart failure, congenital rubella, toxoplasmosis, disseminated herpes simplex, cytomegalovirus infection, and hemolytic disease of the newborn have to be differentiated. A positive Coombs test and blood group incompatibility distinguish hemolytic disease.

2. Young infants—Injury to the brachial plexus, poliomyelitis, acute osteomyelitis, and septic arthritis must be differentiated from pseudoparalysis. Coryza due to viral infection often responds to symptomatic treatment. Rash (ammoniacal diaper rash) and scabies may be confused with a syphilitic eruption.

3. Children—Interstitial keratitis and bone lesions of tuberculosis are distinguished by positive tuberculin reaction and chest radiograph. Arthritis associated with syphilis is unaccompanied by systemic signs, and joints are nontender. Mental retardation, spasticity, and hyperactivity are shown to be of syphilitic origin by strongly positive serologic tests.

B. Acquired Syphilis

Herpes genitalis, traumatic lesions, and other venereal diseases must be differentiated.

Prevention

A serologic test for syphilis should be performed at the initiation of prenatal care and repeated at delivery. In mothers at high risk for syphilis, repeated tests may be necessary. Serologic tests may be negative on both the mother and baby at the time of birth if the mother acquires syphilis near term. Adequate treatment of mothers with secondary syphilis before the last month of pregnancy reduces the incidence of congenital syphilis from 90% to less than 2%. Examination and serologic testing of sexual partners and siblings should also be done.

Treatment

A. Specific Measures

Penicillin is the drug of choice for *T pallidum* infection. If the patient is allergic to penicillin, erythromycin or one of the tetracyclines may be used.

1. Congenital syphilis—Infants born to seropositive mothers require careful examination and quantitative antitreponemal (VDRL, RPR) syphilis testing. The same quantitative antitreponemal test should be done on the infant as the one done on the mother so the titers can be compared. Maternal records regarding the diagnosis of syphilis, treatment, and follow-up titers should be reviewed. Infants should be further evaluated for congenital syphilis for any of the following circumstances:

- The maternal titer has increased fourfold.
- The infant's titer is at least fourfold greater than the maternal titer.
- Signs of syphilis are found on examination.
- Maternal syphilis was not treated or inadequately treated during pregnancy.
- Maternal treatment of syphilis with a nonpenicillin regimen, or the regimen or dose of medication is undocumented.
- Maternal syphilis treated during pregnancy, but therapy completed less than 4 weeks prior to delivery.

- Maternal syphilis treated appropriately during pregnancy, but without the appropriate decrease in maternal nontreponemal titers after treatment.

The complete evaluation of an infant for possible congenital syphilis includes complete blood count, liver function tests, long bone radiographs, CSF examination (cell counts, glucose, and protein), CSF VDRL, and quantitative serologic tests. In addition, the placenta and umbilical cord should be examined pathologically using fluorescent antitreponemal antibody.

Treatment for congenital syphilis is indicated for infants with physical signs, umbilical cord or placenta positive for DFA-TP staining or darkfield examination, abnormal radiographs, elevated CSF protein or cell counts, reactive CSF VDRL, or serum quantitative nontreponemal titer that is more than fourfold higher than the maternal titer (using same test). Infants with proved or suspected congenital syphilis should receive either (1) aqueous crystalline penicillin G, 50,000 units/kg/dose intravenously every 12 hours (if < 1 week old) or every 8 hours (if 1–4 weeks old) for 10 days; or (2) aqueous procaine penicillin G, 50,000 units/kg/dose intramuscularly once daily for 10 days. All infants diagnosed after age 4 weeks receive 50,000–60,000 units/kg/dose aqueous crystalline penicillin intravenously every 6 hours for 10 days.

Additionally, treatment should be given to infants whose mothers have inadequately treated syphilis, to those whose mothers received treatment less than 1 month before delivery, to those whose mothers have undocumented or inadequate serologic response to therapy, and to those whose mothers were given nonpenicillin drugs to treat syphilis. In these instances, if the infant is asymptomatic, has a normal physical exam, normal CSF parameters, nonreactive CSF VDRL, normal bone films, quantitative nontreponemal titer less than fourfold of the mother's titer, and good follow-up is certain, some experts would give a single dose of penicillin G benzathine 50,000 units/kg intramuscularly. If there is any abnormality in the preceding evaluation or if the CSF testing is not interpretable, the full 10 days of intravenous penicillin should be given. Close clinical and serologic monthly follow-up is necessary.

Asymptomatic, seropositive, infants with normal physical examinations born to mothers who received adequate syphilis treatment (completed > 4 weeks prior to delivery) and whose mothers have an appropriate serologic response (fourfold or greater decrease in titer) to treatment may be at lower risk for congenital syphilis. Some experts believe complete laboratory and radiographic evaluation in these infants (CSF and long bone films) is not necessary. Infants who meet the preceding criteria, have nontreponemal titers less than fourfold higher than maternal titers, and for whom follow-up is certain can be given benzathine penicillin G, 50,000 units/kg, administered intramuscularly in a single dose. Infants should be followed with quantitative serologic tests and physical examinations until the nontreponemal serologic test is negative (see follow-up section below). Rising titers or clinical signs usually occur within 4 months in infected infants, requiring a full evaluation (including CSF studies and long bone radiographs) and institution of intravenous penicillin therapy.

a. Follow-up for congenital syphilis—Children treated for congenital syphilis need physical examinations at 1 and 2 months after completion of therapy, and both physical examinations and quantitative VDRL or RPR tests should be performed at 3, 6, and 12 months after the end of therapy or until the tests become nonreactive. Repeat CSF examination, including a CSF VDRL test, every 6 months until normal is indicated for infants with a positive CSF VDRL reaction. A reactive CSF VDRL test at the 6-month interval is an indication for re-treatment. Titers decline with treatment and are usually negative by 6 months. Repeat treatment is indicated for children with rising titers or stable titers that do not decline.

2. Acquired syphilis of less than 1 year's duration—Benzathine penicillin G (50,000 units/kg, given intramuscularly, to a maximum of 2.4 million units) is given to adolescents with primary, secondary, or latent disease of less than 1 year's duration. All children should have a CSF examination (with CSF VDRL) prior to commencing therapy, to exclude neurosyphilis. Adolescents and adults need a CSF examination if clinical signs or symptoms suggest neurologic involvement.

3. Syphilis of more than 1 year's duration (late latent disease)—Syphilis of more than 1 year's duration (without evidence of neurosyphilis) requires weekly intramuscular benzathine penicillin G therapy for 3 weeks. CSF examination and VDRL test should be done on all children and patients with coexisting HIV infection or neurologic symptoms. In addition, patients who have failed treatment or who were previously treated with an agent other than penicillin need a CSF examination and CSF VDRL.

4. Neurosyphilis—Aqueous crystalline penicillin G is recommended, 200,000–300,000 U/kg/d in four to six divided doses, given intravenously for 10–14 days. The maximum adult dose is 4 million units/dose. This regimen should possibly be followed by an intramuscular course of benzathine G penicillin, 50,000 U/kg given once a week for 3 consecutive weeks, to a maximum dose of 2.4 million units.

B. GENERAL MEASURES

Penicillin treatment of early congenital or secondary syphilis may result in a Jarisch–Herxheimer reaction.

Treatment is symptomatic, with careful follow-up. Transfusion may be necessary in infants with severe hemolytic anemia.

Prognosis

Severe disease, if undiagnosed, may be fatal in the newborn. Complete cure can be expected if the young infant is given penicillin. Serologic reversal usually occurs within 1 year. Treatment of primary syphilis with penicillin is curative. Permanent neurologic sequelae may occur in meningovascular syphilis.

Carey JC: Congenital syphilis in the 21st century. Curr Women Health Rep 2003;3(4):299 [PMID: 12844452].

Centers for Disease Control and Prevention: Congenital syphilis—United States, 2000. JAMA 2001;286(5):529 [PMID: 11508285].

Goldmeier D, Guallar C: Syphilis: An update. Clin Med 2003;3 (3):209 [PMID: 12848252].

Guidelines for treatment of sexually transmitted diseases. MMWR Morb Mortal Wkly Rep 1998;47(RR-1):28.

RELAPSING FEVER

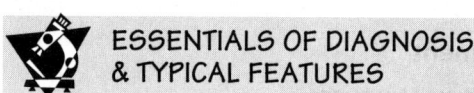

ESSENTIALS OF DIAGNOSIS & TYPICAL FEATURES

- *Episodes of fever, chills, malaise.*
- *Occasional rash, arthritis, cough, hepatosplenomegaly, conjunctivitis.*
- *Diagnosis confirmed by direct microscopic identification of spirochetes in smears of peripheral blood.*

General Considerations

Relapsing fever is a vector-borne disease caused by spirochetes of the genus *Borrelia*. Epidemic relapsing fever is transmitted to humans by body lice (*Pediculus humanus*) and endemic relapsing fever by soft-bodied ticks (genus *Ornithodoros*). Tick-borne relapsing fever is endemic in the western United States. Transmission usually takes place during the warm months, when ticks are active and recreation or work brings people into contact with *Ornithodoros* ticks. Infection is often acquired in mountain camping areas and cabins. The ticks are nocturnal feeders and remain attached for only 5–20 minutes. Consequently, the patient seldom remembers a tick bite. Rarely, neonatal relapsing fever results from transplacental transmission of *Borrelia*. Both louse-borne and tick-borne relapsing fever may be acquired during foreign travel.

Clinical Findings

A. SYMPTOMS AND SIGNS

The incubation period is 4–18 days. The attack is sudden, with high fever, chills, tachycardia, nausea and vomiting, headache, myalgia, arthralgia, bronchitis, and a dry, nonproductive cough. Hepatomegaly and splenomegaly appear later. Meningeal irritation may be present. An erythematous rash may be seen over the trunk and extremities, and petechiae may be present. After 3–10 days, the fever falls. Jaundice, iritis, conjunctivitis, cranial nerve palsies, and hemorrhage occur more commonly during relapses.

The disease is characterized by relapses at intervals of 1–2 weeks and lasting 3–5 days. The relapses duplicate the initial attack but become progressively less severe. In louse-borne relapsing fever, there is usually a single relapse. In tick-borne infection, two to six relapses occur.

B. LABORATORY FINDINGS

During febrile episodes, the patient's urine contains protein, casts, and occasionally erythrocytes; a marked polymorphonuclear leukocytosis is present; and, about 25% of patients have a false-positive serologic test for syphilis. Examination of the peripheral blood smear is the diagnostic test of choice. Spirochetes can be found in the peripheral blood by direct microscopy in approximately 70% of cases by darkfield examination or by Wright, Giemsa, or acridine orange staining of thick and thin smears. Spirochetes are not found during afebrile periods. Immunofluorescent antibody (or ELISA confirmed by Western blot) can sometimes help establish the diagnosis serologically. However, high titers of *Borrelia hermsii* can cross-react with *Borrelia burgdorferi* (the agent in Lyme disease) in immunofluorescent antibody assay, ELISA, and Western blots. Serologic specimens can be sent to the Division of Vector-Borne Infectious Diseases, Centers for Disease Control and Prevention, Fort Collins, CO 80522.

Differential Diagnosis

Relapsing fever may be confused with malaria, leptospirosis, dengue, typhus, rat-bite fever, Colorado tick fever, Rocky Mountain spotted fever, collagen vascular disease, or any fever of unknown origin.

Complications

Complications include facial paralysis, iridocyclitis, optic atrophy, hypochromic anemia, pneumonia, nephritis, myocarditis, endocarditis, and seizures. CNS involvement occurs in 10–30% of patients.

Treatment

For children younger than age 8 years who have tick-borne relapsing fever, standard dosages of penicillin or

erythromycin should be given for 10 days. Older children may be given doxycycline. Chloramphenicol is also efficacious and was often used in the past.

Severely ill patients should be hospitalized. Antibiotic treatment should be started after the fever has dropped, to reduce the risk of severe Jarisch–Herxheimer reaction. Isolation precautions are not necessary for relapsing fever. Contact precautions are recommended for patients with louse infestations.

Prognosis

The mortality rate in treated cases of relapsing fever is very low, except in debilitated or very young children. With treatment, the initial attack is shortened and relapses prevented. The response to antimicrobial therapy is dramatic.

Cadavid D, Barbour AG: Neuroborreliosis during relapsing fever: Review of the clinical manifestations, pathology, and treatment of infections in humans and experimental animals. Clin Infect Dis 1998;26:151 [PMID: 9455525].

Centers for Disease Control and Prevention: Tickborne relapsing fever outbreak after a family gathering—New Mexico, August 2002. MMWR Morb Mortal Wkly Rep 2003;52(34):809 [PMID: 12944877].

LEPTOSPIROSIS

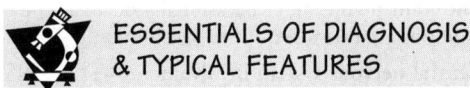

ESSENTIALS OF DIAGNOSIS & TYPICAL FEATURES

- Biphasic course lasting 2 or 3 weeks.
- Initial phase: high fever, headache, myalgia, and conjunctivitis.
- Apparent recovery for 2–3 days.
- Return of fever associated with meningitis.
- Jaundice, hemorrhages, and renal insufficiency (severe cases).
- Culture of organism from blood and CSF (early) and from urine (later), or direct microscopy of urine or CSF.
- Positive leptospiral agglutination test.

General Considerations

Leptospirosis is a zoonosis caused by many antigenically distinct but morphologically similar spirochetes. The organism enters through the skin or respiratory tract. Classically the severe form (Weil disease), with jaundice and a high mortality rate, was associated with infection with *Leptospira icterohaemorrhagiae* after immersion in water contaminated with rat urine. It is now known that a variety of animals (eg, dogs, rats, and cattle) may serve as reservoirs for pathogenic *Leptospira*, that a given serogroup may have multiple animal species as hosts, and that severe disease may be caused by many different serogroups.

In the United States, leptospirosis usually occurs after contact with dogs. Cattle, swine, or rodents may transmit the organism. Sewer workers, farmers, abattoir workers, animal handlers, and soldiers are at risk for occupational exposure. Outbreaks have resulted from swimming in contaminated streams and harvesting field crops. In the United States, about 100 cases are reported yearly, and about one-third are in children.

Clinical Findings

A. SYMPTOMS AND SIGNS

1. Initial phase—The incubation period is 4–19 days (mean, 10 days). Chills, fever, headache, myalgia, conjunctivitis (episcleral injection), photophobia, cervical lymphadenopathy, and pharyngitis commonly occur. The initial leptospiremic phase lasts for 3–7 days.

2. Phase of apparent recovery—Symptoms typically (but not always) subside for 2–3 days.

3. Systemic phase—Fever reappears and is associated with headache, muscular pain and tenderness in the abdomen and back, and nausea and vomiting. Lung, heart, and joint involvement occasionally occurs. These manifestations are due to extensive vasculitis.

    a. Central nervous system involvement—The CNS is involved in 50–90% of cases. Severe headache and mild nuchal rigidity are usual, but delirium, coma, and focal neurologic signs may be seen.

    b. Renal and hepatic involvement—In about 50% of cases, the kidney or liver is affected. Gross hematuria and oliguria or anuria is sometimes seen. Jaundice may be associated with an enlarged and tender liver.

    c. Gallbladder involvement—Leptospirosis may cause acalculous cholecystitis in children, demonstrable by abdominal ultrasound as a dilated, nonfunctioning gallbladder. Pancreatitis is unusual.

    d. Hemorrhage—Petechiae, ecchymoses, and gastrointestinal bleeding may be severe.

    e. Rash—A rash is seen in 10–30% of cases. It may be maculopapular and generalized or may be petechial or purpuric. Occasionally erythema nodosum is seen. Peripheral desquamation of the rash may occur. Gangrenous areas are sometimes noted over the distal extremities. In such cases, skin biopsy demonstrates the presence of severe vasculitis involving both the arterial and the venous circulations.

B. LABORATORY FINDINGS

Leptospires are present in the blood and CSF only during the first 10 days of illness. They appear in the urine during the second week, where they may persist for 30 days or longer. The organism can be isolated from blood inoculated into Fletcher's semisolid medium or Ellinghausen–McCullough–Johnson–Harris semisolid medium, but culture techniques are slow (7–10 days), difficult, and not generally available.

The WBC count is often elevated, especially when there is liver involvement. Serum bilirubin levels usually remain below 20 mg/dL. Other liver function tests may be abnormal, although the aspartate transaminase usually is elevated only slightly. An elevated serum creatine kinase is frequently found. CSF shows moderate pleocytosis (< 500/μL)—predominantly mononuclear cells—increased protein (50–100 mg/dL), and normal glucose. Urine often shows microscopic pyuria, hematuria, and, less often, moderate proteinuria (++ or greater). The ESR is elevated markedly. Chest radiograph may show pneumonitis.

Serologic antibodies measured by enzyme immunoassay may be demonstrated during or after the second week of illness. The serologic test of choice is a microscopic agglutination test using live organisms (performed at the CDC). Leptospiral agglutinins generally reach peak levels by the third to fourth week. A 1:100 titer is considered suspicious; a fourfold or greater rise is diagnostic. A PCR assay may be available at specialized research centers or through the CDC.

Differential Diagnosis

Fever and myalgia associated with the characteristic episcleral injection should suggest leptospirosis. During the prodrome, malaria, typhoid fever, typhus, rheumatoid arthritis, brucellosis, and influenza may be suspected. Later, depending on the organ systems involved, a variety of other diseases need to be distinguished, including encephalitis, viral or tuberculous meningitis, viral hepatitis, glomerulonephritis, viral or bacterial pneumonia, rheumatic fever, subacute infective endocarditis, acute surgical abdomen, and Kawasaki disease (see Table 36–3).

Prevention

Preventive measures include avoidance of contaminated water and soil, rodent control, immunization of dogs and other domestic animals, and good sanitation. Immunization or antimicrobial prophylaxis with doxycycline may be of value to certain high-risk occupational groups.

Treatment

A. SPECIFIC MEASURES

Aqueous penicillin G (150,000 units/kg/d, given in four to six divided doses intravenously for 7–10 days) should be given when the diagnosis is suspected. Studies in severely ill patients indicate a benefit even if treatment is started 4 days after onset. A Jarisch–Herxheimer reaction may occur. Oral doxycycline may be used for mildly ill patients.

B. GENERAL MEASURES

Symptomatic and supportive care is indicated, particularly for renal and hepatic failure and hemorrhage.

Prognosis

Leptospirosis is usually self-limiting and not characterized by jaundice. The disease usually lasts 1–3 weeks but may be more prolonged. Relapse may occur. There are usually no permanent sequelae associated with CNS infection, although headache may persist. The mortality rate in the United States is 5%, usually from renal failure. The mortality rate may reach 20% or more in elderly patients who have severe kidney and hepatic involvement.

Bharti AR et al. Peru-United States Leptospirosis Consortium. Leptospirosis: A zoonotic disease of global importance. Lancet Infect Dis 2003;3(12):757 [PMID: 14652202].

Levett PN: Leptospirosis. Clin Microbiol Rev 2001;14:296 [PMID: 11292640].

Plank R, Dean D: Overview of the epidemiology, microbiology, and pathogenesis of *Leptospira* spp. in humans. Microbes Infect 2000;2:1265 [PMID: 11008116].

LYME DISEASE

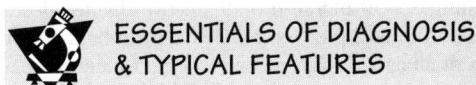

ESSENTIALS OF DIAGNOSIS & TYPICAL FEATURES

- *Characteristic skin lesion (erythema migrans) 3–30 days after tick bite.*
- *Arthritis, usually pauciarticular, occurring about 4 weeks after appearance of skin lesion. Headache, chills, and fever.*
- *Residence or travel in an endemic area during the late spring to early fall.*

General Considerations

Lyme disease is a subacute or chronic spirochetal infection caused by *Borrelia burgdorferi* and transmitted by the bite of an infected deer tick (*Ixodes* species). The disease was known in Europe for many years as tick-borne encephalomyelitis, often associated with a characteristic rash (erythema migrans). Discovery of the agent and vector followed investigation of an outbreak of pauciarticular arthritis in Lyme, Connecticut, in 1977.

Although cases are reported from many countries, the most prominent endemic areas in the United States include the Northeast, upper Midwest, and West Coast. The northern European countries also have high rates of infection. More than 20,000 cases were reported in the United States in 2005. The disease is spreading as a result of increased infection in and distribution of the tick vector. Most cases with rash are recognized in spring and summer, when most tick bites occur; however, because the incubation period for joint and neurologic disease may be months, cases may present at any time. *Ixodes* ticks are very small, and their bite is often unrecognized.

Clinical Findings

A. SYMPTOMS AND SIGNS

Erythema chronicum migrans, the most characteristic feature of Lyme disease, develops in 60–80% of patients. Between 3 and 30 days after the bite, a ring of erythema develops at the site and spreads over days. It may attain a diameter of 20 cm. The center of the lesion may clear (resembling tinea corporis), remain red, or become raised (suggesting a chemical or infectious cellulitis). Many patients are otherwise asymptomatic. Some have fever (usually low-grade), headache, and myalgias. Multiple satellite skin lesions, urticaria, or diffuse erythema may occur. Untreated, the rash lasts days to 3 weeks.

In up to 50% of patients, arthritis develops several weeks to months after the bite. Recurrent attacks of migratory, monarticular, or pauciarticular arthritis involving the knees and other large joints occur. Each attack lasts for days to a few weeks. Fever is common and may be high. Complete resolution between attacks is typical. Chronic arthritis develops in less than 10% of patients, more often in those with the DR4 haplotype.

Neurologic manifestations develop in up to 20% of patients and usually consist of Bell palsy, aseptic meningitis (which may be indistinguishable from viral meningitis), or polyradiculitis. Peripheral neuritis, Guillain–Barré syndrome, encephalitis, ataxia, chorea, and other cranial neuropathies are less common. Seizures suggest another diagnosis. Untreated, the neurologic symptoms are usually self-limited but may be chronic or permanent. Although fatigue and nonspecific neurologic symptoms may be prolonged in a few patients, Lyme disease is not proved to be a cause of chronic fatigue syndrome. Self-limited heart block or myocardial dysfunction occurs in about 5% of patients.

B. LABORATORY FINDINGS

Most patients with only rash have normal laboratory tests. Children with arthritis may have moderately elevated ESRs and WBC counts; the antinuclear antibodies and rheumatoid factor tests are negative or nonspecific;

streptococcal antibodies are not elevated. Circulating IgM cryoglobulins may be present. Joint fluid may show up to 100,000 cells with a polymorphonuclear predominance, normal glucose, and elevated protein and immune complexes; Gram stain and culture are negative. In patients with CNS involvement, the CSF may show lymphocytic pleocytosis and elevated protein; the glucose and all cultures and stains are normal or negative. Abnormal nerve conduction may be present with peripheral neuropathy.

Diagnosis

Lyme disease is a clinical diagnosis. History, physical examination, and laboratory features are important to consider. The causative organism is difficult to culture. Serologic testing may support the clinical diagnosis. Antibody testing should be performed in experienced laboratories. Serologic diagnosis of Lyme disease is based on a two-test approach: an ELISA and an immunoblot to confirm a positive or indeterminate ELISA. Antibodies may not be detectable until several weeks after infection has occurred; therefore, serologic testing in children with a typical rash is not recommended. Therapy early in disease may blunt antibody titers. Recent studies have shown considerable intralaboratory and interlaboratory variability in titers reported. Overdiagnosis of Lyme disease based on atypical symptoms and positive serology appears to be common. Sera from patients with syphilis, HIV, and leptospirosis may give false-positive results. Patients who receive appropriate treatment for Lyme disease may remain seropositive for years. Diagnosis of CNS disease requires objective abnormalities of the neurologic examination, laboratory or radiographic studies, and consistent positive serology.

Differential Diagnosis

Aside from the disorders already mentioned, the rash may resemble pityriasis, erythema multiforme, a drug eruption, or erythema nodosum. Erythema chronicum migrans is nonscaly, minimally tender or nontender, and persists longer in the same place than many of the more common childhood erythematous rashes. The arthritis may resemble juvenile rheumatoid arthritis, reactive arthritis, septic arthritis, reactive effusion from a contiguous osteomyelitis, rheumatic fever, leukemic arthritis, systemic lupus erythematosus, and Henoch–Schönlein purpura. Spontaneous resolution in a few days to weeks helps differentiate Lyme disease from juvenile rheumatoid arthritis, in which arthritis lasting a minimum of 6 weeks is required for diagnosis. The neurologic signs may suggest idiopathic Bell palsy, viral or parainfectious meningitis or meningoencephalitis,

lead poisoning, psychosomatic illness, and many other conditions.

Prevention

Prevention consists of avoidance of endemic areas, wearing long sleeves and pants, frequent checks for ticks, and application of tick repellents. Ticks usually are attached for 24–48 hours before transmission of Lyme disease occurs. Ticks should be removed with a tweezer by pulling gently without twisting or excessive squeezing of the tick. Permethrin sprayed on clothing decreases tick attachment. Repellents containing high concentrations of DEET may be neurotoxic and should be used cautiously and washed off when tick exposure ends. The CDC does not recommend prophylactic antibiotics for tick bites in asymptomatic individuals.

A Lyme vaccine was licensed for use in persons between the ages of 15 and 70 years, but was withdrawn and is not available.

Treatment

Antimicrobial therapy is beneficial in most cases of Lyme disease. It is most effective if started early. Prolonged treatment is important for all forms. Relapses occur in some patients on all regimens.

A. RASH, OTHER EARLY INFECTIONS

Amoxicillin, 25–50 mg/kg/d orally in two divided doses (to a maximum of 2 g/d) for 14–21 days can be used for children of all ages. Doxycycline (100 mg, orally twice a day) for 14–21 days may be used for children older than age 8 years. Erythromycin (30 mg/kg/d) or cefuroxime is used in penicillin-allergic children, although erythromycin may be less effective than amoxicillin.

B. ARTHRITIS

The amoxicillin or doxycycline regimen (same dosage as for the rash) should be used, but treatment should continue for 4 weeks. Parenteral ceftriaxone (75–100 mg/kg/d) or penicillin G (300,000 units/kg/d, given intravenously in four divided doses for 2–4 weeks) is used for persistent arthritis.

C. BELL PALSY

The same oral drug regimens may be used for 3–4 weeks.

D. OTHER NEUROLOGIC DISEASE OR CARDIAC DISEASE

Parenteral therapy for 2–3 weeks is recommended with either ceftriaxone (75–100 kg/d in one daily dose) or penicillin G (300,000 units/kg/d intravenously in four divided doses).

Centers for Disease Control and Prevention: Lyme disease. http://www.cdc.gov/ncidod/dvbid/lyme

DePietropaolo DL et al: Diagnosis of Lyme disease. Am Fam Physician 2005;72(2):297 [PMID: 16050454].

Eppes SC: Diagnosis, treatment and prevention of Lyme disease in children. Paediatr Drugs 2003;5(6):363 [PMID: 12765486].

Magaldi JA: Bell's palsy. N Engl J Med 2005;351(13):1323 [PMID: 15675099].

Moses JM, Riseberg RS, Mansbach JM: Lyme disease presenting with persistent headache. Pediatrics 2003;112(6 Pt 1):e477 [PMID: 14654649].

Pickering LK et al (editors): *2003 Red Book: Report of the Committee on Infectious Diseases,* 26th ed. American Academy of Pediatrics, 2003.

Vazquez M et al: Long-term neuropsychologic and health outcomes of children with facial nerve palsy attributable to Lyme disease. Pediatrics 2003;112(2):e93 [PMID: 12897313].

Infections: Parasitic & Mycotic

39

Adriana Weinberg, MD, & Myron J. Levin, MD

◾ PARASITIC INFECTIONS

Parasitic diseases are common and may present clinically in a variety of ways (Table 39–1). Although travel to endemic areas suggests particular infections, many are transmitted through fomites or acquired from contact with human carriers and can occur anywhere. Some of the less common parasitic infections and those seen primarily in the developing world are presented in abbreviated form in Table 39–2.

Selection of Patients for Evaluation

The incidence of parasitic infections varies greatly with geographic area. Children who have traveled or lived in areas where parasitic infections are endemic are at risk for infection with a variety of intestinal and tissue parasites. Children who have resided only in developed countries are usually free of tissue parasites (except *Toxoplasma*). Searching for intestinal parasites is expensive for the patient and time-consuming for the laboratory. More than 90% of ova and parasite examinations performed in most hospital laboratories in the United States are negative; many have been ordered inappropriately. An approach to determining which children with diarrhea need such examinations is presented in Figure 39–1. It can be more cost-effective to treat symptomatic U.S. immigrants with albendazole or nitazoxanide, broad-spectrum antiparasitic drugs, and to investigate only those whose symptoms persist.

Immunodeficient children are very susceptible to protozoal intestinal infections. Multiple opportunists are frequently identified, and the threshold for ordering tests should be low for these children.

Specimen Processing

For tissue parasites, contact the laboratory for proper collection procedures. Diarrheal stools may contain trophozoites that die rapidly during transport. The specimen should be either examined immediately or placed in a stool fixative such as polyvinyl alcohol. Fixative vials for home collection of stool are available. They may contain toxic compounds, so they should be stored safely. Fixed specimens are stable at room temperature. Formed stools usually contain cysts that are more stable. It is best to fix these also after collection, but they may be reliably examined after transport at room temperature.

Eosinophilia & Parasitic Infections

Although parasites commonly cause eosinophilia, in developed countries other causes are much more common and include allergies, drugs, and other infections. Heavy intestinal nematode infections cause eosinophilia; they are easily detected on a single ova and parasite examination. Light nematode infections and common protozoal infections—giardiasis, cryptosporidiosis, and amebiasis—rarely cause eosinophilia. Eosinophilia is also unusual or minimal in more serious infections such as amebic liver abscess, toxoplasmosis, and malaria.

The most common parasitic infection in the United States that causes significant eosinophilia with negative stool examination is toxocariasis. In a young child with unexplained eosinophilia and a negative stool examination, a serologic test for *Toxocara* may be the next appropriate test. Trichinosis is a rare cause of marked eosinophilia; strongyloidiasis is a cause of eosinophilia that may be difficult to diagnose with stool examinations. The differential diagnosis of eosinophilia is broad for patients who have been in developing countries.

Cohen SA: Use of nitazoxanide as a new therapeutic option for persistent diarrhea: pediatric perspective. Curr Med Res Opin 2005;21:999 [PMID: 16004666].

◾ PROTOZOAL INFECTIONS

SYSTEMIC INFECTIONS

1. Malaria

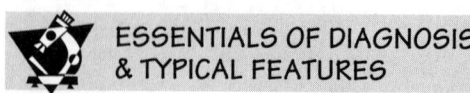

ESSENTIALS OF DIAGNOSIS & TYPICAL FEATURES

• *Residence in or travel to an endemic area.*

Table 39–1. Signs and symptoms of parasitic infection.

Sign/Symptom	Agent	Comments[a]
Abdominal pain	*Anisakis*	Shortly after raw fish ingestion.
	Ascaris	Heavy infection may obstruct bowel, biliary tract.
	Clonorchis	Heavy, early infection. Hepatomegaly later.
	Entamoeba histolytica	Hematochezia, variable fever, diarrhea.
	Fasciola hepatica	Diarrhea, vomiting.
	Hookworm	Iron deficiency anemia with heavy infection.
	Strongyloides	Eosinophilia, pruritus. May resemble peptic disease.
	Trichinella	Myalgia, periorbital edema, eosinophilia.
	Trichuris	Diarrhea, dysentery with heavy infection.
Cough	*Ascaris*	Wheezing, eosinophilia during migration phase.
	Paragonimus westermani	Hemoptysis; chronic. May mimic tuberculosis.
	Strongyloides	Wheezing, pruritus, eosinophilia during migration or dissemination.
	Toxocara	Affects ages 1–5 y; hepatosplenomegaly; eosinophilia.
	Tropical eosinophilia	Pulmonary infiltrates, eosinophilia.
Diarrhea	*Blastocystis*	Possibly with heavy infection in immunosuppressed or immunocompetent individuals.
	Cryptosporidium	Watery; prolonged in normals, chronic in immunosuppressed individuals.
	Dientamoeba fragilis	Only with heavy infection.
	Entamoeba histolytica	Hematochezia, variable fever; no eosinophilia.
	Giardia	Afebrile, chronic; anorexia; no hematochezia or eosinophilia.
	Schistosoma	Chronic; hepatosplenomegaly (some types).
	Strongyloides	Abdominal pain; eosinophilia.
	Trichinella	Myalgia, periorbital edema, eosinophilia.
	Trichuris	With heavy infection.
Dysentery	*Balantidium coli*	Swine contact.
	Entamoeba histolytica	Few to no leukocytes in stool; fever; hematochezia.
	Schistosoma	During acute infection.
	Trichuris	With heavy infection.
Dysuria	*Enterobius*	Usually girls with worms in urethra, bladder; nocturnal, perianal pruritus.
	Schistosoma	Hematuria. Exclude bacteriuria, stones (some types).
Headache (and other cerebral symptoms)	*Angiostrongylus*	Eosinophilic meningitis.
	Naegleria	Fresh-water swimming; rapidly progressive meningoencephalitis.
	Plasmodium	Fever, chills, jaundice, splenomegaly. Cerebral ischemia (with *P falciparum*).
	Taenia solium	Cysticercosis. Focal seizures, deficits; hydrocephalus, aseptic meningitis.
	Toxoplasma	Meningoencephalitis (especially in the immunosuppressed); hydrocephalus in infants.
	Trypanosoma	African forms. Chronic lethargy (sleeping sickness).

(continued)

Table 39–1. Signs and symptoms of parasitic infection. (continued)

Sign/Symptom	Agent	Comments[a]
Pruritus	*Ancylostoma braziliense*	Creeping eruption; dermal serpiginous burrow.
	Enterobius	Perianal, nocturnal.
	Filaria	Variable; seen in many filarial diseases.
	Hookworm	Local at penetration site in heavy exposure.
	Strongyloides	Diffuse with migration; may be recurrent.
	Trypanosoma	African forms; one of many nonspecific symptoms.
Fever	*Entamoeba histolytica*	With acute dysentery or liver abscess.
	Leishmania donovani	Hepatosplenomegaly, anemia, leukopenia.
	Plasmodium	Chills, headache, jaundice; periodic.
	Toxocara	Cough, hepatosplenomegaly, eosinophilia.
	Toxoplasma	Generalized adenopathy; splenomegaly.
	Trichinella	Myalgia, periorbital edema, eosinophilia.
	Trypanosoma	Early stage, African forms; lymphadenopathy.
Anemia	*Diphyllobothrium*	Megaloblastic due to B_{12} deficiency; rare.
	Hookworm	Iron deficiency.
	Leishmania donovani	Fever, hepatosplenomegaly, leukopenia (kala-azar).
	Plasmodium	Hemolysis.
	Trichuris	Heavy infection; due to iron loss.
Eosinophilia	*Angiostrongylus*	Eosinophilic meningitis.
	Fasciola	Abdominal pain.
	Filaria	Microfilariae in blood. Lymphadenopathy.
	Onchocerca	Skin nodules, keratitis.
	Schistosoma	Chronic; intestinal or genitourinary symptoms.
	Strongyloides	Abdominal pain, diarrhea.
	Toxocara	Hepatosplenomegaly, cough; affects ages 1–5 y.
	Trichinella	Myalgia, periorbital edema.
	Tropical pulmonary eosinophilia	Cough.
Hematuria	*Schistosoma*	*S haematobium.* Bladder, urethral granulomas. Exclude stones, bacteriuria.
Hemoptysis	*Paragonimus westermani*	Lung fluke. Variable chest pain; chronic.
Hepatomegaly	*Clonorchis*	Heavy infection. Tenderness early; cirrhosis late.
	Echinococcus	Chronic; cysts.
	Entamoeba histolytica	Toxic hepatitis or abscess. No eosinophilia.
	Leishmania donovani	Splenomegaly, fever, pancytopenia.
	Schistosoma	Chronic; hepatic fibrosis, splenomegaly (some types).
	Toxocara	Splenomegaly, eosinophilia, cough; no adenopathy.

(continued)

Table 39–1. Signs and symptoms of parasitic infection. (continued)

Sign/Symptom	Agent	Comments[a]
Splenomegaly	*Leishmania donovani*	Hepatomegaly, fever, anemia.
	Plasmodium	Fever, chills, jaundice, headache.
	Schistosoma	Hepatomegaly.
	Toxocara	Eosinophilia, hepatomegaly.
	Toxoplasma	Lymphadenopathy, other symptoms.
Lymphadenopathy	Filaria	Inguinal typical; chronic.
	Leishmania donovani	Hepatosplenomegaly, pancytopenia, fever.
	Schistosoma	Acute infection; fever, rash, arthralgia, hepatosplenomegaly.
	Toxoplasma	Cervical common; may involve single site; splenomegaly.
	Trypanosoma	Localized near bite or generalized; hepatosplenomegaly (Chagas disease); generalized (especially posterior cervical) in African forms.

[a]Symptoms usually related to degree of infestation. Infestation with small numbers of organisms is often asymptomatic.

- Cyclic paroxysms of chills, fever, and intense sweating.
- Headache, backache, cough, abdominal pain, nausea, vomiting, diarrhea.
- Coma, seizures.
- Splenomegaly, anemia.
- Malaria parasites in peripheral blood smear.

General Considerations

Malaria kills a million children worldwide each year and is undergoing a resurgence in areas where it was previously controlled. Approximately 1000 imported cases are diagnosed in the United States each year, but local transmission may also occasionally take place. The female anopheline mosquito transmits the parasites—*Plasmodium vivax* (most common), *P falciparum* (most virulent), *P ovale* (similar to *P vivax*), and *P malariae*. The gametocytes ingested from an infected human form sporozoites in the mosquito; when inoculated into a susceptible host, these sporozoites infect hepatocytes. The preerythrocytic phase (hepatic) is about 1–2 weeks for all but *P malariae* infection (3–5 weeks), but the initial symptoms may be delayed for up to a year in *P falciparum*, 4 years in *P vivax*, and decades in *P malariae* infections. Merozoites released into the circulation from hepatocytes infect red cells (young cells by *P vivax* and *P ovale*, old cells by *P malariae*, and all cells by *P falciparum*) and begin the synchronous erythrocytic cycles, rupturing the infected cells at regular 48- or 72-hour

intervals. Asynchronous cycles causing daily fevers are most common in early stages of infection. Survival is associated with a progressive decrease in intensity of cycles; relapses years later may occur from persistent hepatic infection, which occurs in *P vivax* and *P ovale* infections. Infection acquired congenitally or from transfusions or needlesticks does not result in a hepatic phase.

Susceptibility varies genetically; certain red cell phenotypes are partially resistant to *P falciparum* infection (hemoglobin S, hemoglobin F, thalassemia, and possibly glucose-6-phosphate dehydrogenase deficiency). The worldwide distribution of the four species is determined to some extent by host genetic factors. The absence of *P vivax* from Africa reflects the lack of specific Duffy blood group substances among most native Africans. Recurrent infections result in some natural species-specific immunity; this does not prevent infection but does decrease parasitemia and symptoms. Normal splenic function is an important factor because of the immunologic and filter function of the spleen. Asplenic persons develop rapidly progressive malaria with many circulating infected erythrocytes (including mature forms of *P falciparum*). Maternal immunity protects the neonate.

Clinical Findings

A. Symptoms and Signs

Clinical manifestations vary according to species, strain, and host immunity. The infant presents with recurrent bouts of fever, irritability, poor feeding, vomiting, jaundice, and splenomegaly. Rash is usually absent, which

Table 39–2. Some parasitic infections seen less commonly in developed regions.

Agent (Disease)	Geographic Region	Vector	Symptoms and Signs	Laboratory Findings	Diagnosis	Therapy and Comments
Trypanosoma cruzi (Chagas disease)	South and Central America, Mexico	Reduviid bug	Acute: painful red nodule at bite site, conjunctivitis, periorbital edema (Romaña sign), fever, local ± generalized adenitis. Late: myocarditis, megaesophagus, megacolon.	Mononuclear leukocytosis	Organisms in peripheral blood. Positive serology.	Nifurtimox or benznidazole may help early. No therapy for late disease. May be transmitted by blood transfusion or congenitally.
Trypanosoma brucei (sleeping sickness)	Africa	Tsetse fly	Hepatosplenomegaly, adenopathy. Nodule at bite site (resolves). Recurrent fever, headache, myalgia, progressive encephalitis.	Elevated ESR, anemia, CSF pleocytosis	Organisms in blood, CSF, marrow, nodes. Positive serology.	Suramin, eflornithine, fentamidine, melarsoprol.
Leishmania donovani (kala-azar)	Mideast, India, Mediterranean, South and Central America	Sandfly	Fever, generalized adenopathy, hepatosplenomegaly weeks to months after infection.	Pancytopenia, hypergammaglobulinemia	Organisms in marrow, nodes, spleen. Positive serology.	Sodium stibogluconate, meglumine antimonate, pentamidine, amphotericin B.
Leishmania tropica (Oriental sore)	Asia, India, North Africa	Sandfly	Papule at bite site (usually on face, limbs) develops after weeks to months, then ulcerates and scars.	—	Organisms in skin biopsy. Positive skin test, serology.	Same as for *L donovani*.
Leishmania braziliensis, *L mexicana* (chiclero ulcer)	South America	Sandfly	Painful mucocutaneous ulcers or granulomas. Nasolabial lesions common.	—	Skin biopsy. Positive skin test, serology.	Same as for *L donovani*; ketoconazole.

Organism (disease)	Distribution	Source	Clinical	Eosinophilia	Diagnosis	Treatment/Comments
Wuchereria, Brugia (filariasis)	Tropics, subtropics	Mosquito	Chronic adenopathy, often inguinal. Obstructive lymphedema.		Concentrated blood smears for larvae. Positive serology.	Ivermectin, diethylcarbamazine kill larvae. Surgery for lymphatic obstruction.
Angiostrongylus cantonensis (eosinophilic meningitis)	Hawaii, Asia, Pacific Islands	Snails, slugs	Ingestion (usually inadvertent) followed in 1–4 wk by meningitis of variable severity. Paresthesias.	Eosinophils in CSF and blood	Positive serology. Larvae may be present in CSF.	Fever absent or low. No focal lesions on CNS imaging. No specific therapy. Steroids may be beneficial. Mebendazole may help.
Paragonimus westermani (lung fluke infection)	Asia, South America, Africa	Raw crabs, crustaceans	Cough, hemoptysis. Rarely seizures, other CNS signs if migration to brain occurs.	—	Large ova in concentrated specimens, feces. Cystic nodular lesions on chest radiograph or CNS imaging.	Resembles pulmonary tuberculosis. Praziquantel very effective.
Clonorchis sinensis (liver fluke infection)	Asia	Raw fish	Adult flukes obstruct biliary tree. Acute: hepatomegaly, fever, jaundice, urticaria. Late: cirrhosis, carcinoma.	Variable liver function abnormalities	Ova in feces.	Praziquantel. Advanced disease not treatable. Liver transplant.

CNS, central nervous system; ESR, erythrocyte sedimentation rate; CSF, cerebrospinal fluid.

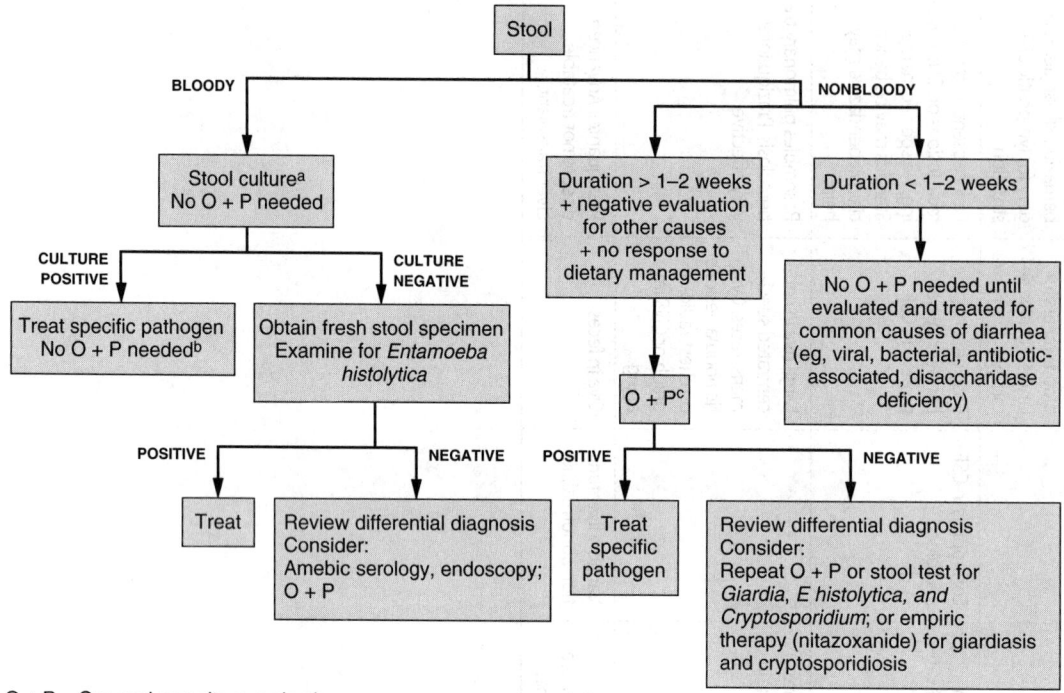

O + P = Ova and parasite examination.
a *Shigella*, *Salmonella*, *Campylobacter*, *E coli* (*Escherichia coli*) O157, *Yersinia*; assay for *Clostridium difficile* toxin
if recent antimicrobial use.
b Unless critically ill, from endemic area for amebiasis, or unresponsive to standard therapy.
c Include examination for *Cryptosporidium* and *Cyclospora*; immediate stool fixation needed if stool is diarrheal.

Figure 39–1. Parasitologic evaluation of acute diarrhea.

helps distinguish malaria from viral infections in patients presenting with similar symptoms. In older children, the pathognomonic constellation of headache, backache, chills, myalgia, and fatigue is more easily elicited. Fever may be cyclic (every 48 hours for all but *P malariae* infection, in which it occurs every 72 hours) or irregular (most commonly observed with *P falciparum*). Between attacks, patients may look quite well. If the disease is untreated, relapses cease within a year in *P falciparum* and within several years in *P vivax* infections but may recur decades later with *P malariae* infection. Infection during pregnancy often causes intrauterine growth restriction or premature delivery but rarely true fetal infection.

Physical examination in patients with uncomplicated cases may show only mild splenomegaly and anemia.

B. LABORATORY FINDINGS

The diagnosis of malaria relies on detection of one or more of the four human plasmodia in blood smears. Most acute infections are caused by *P vivax*, *P ovale*, or *P falciparum*, although 5–7% are due to multiple species. Giemsa-stained thick smears offer the highest diagnostic accuracy for malaria parasites. Identification of the *Plasmodium* species relies on morphologic criteria (Table 39–3) and requires an experienced observer.

Alternative techniques of similar or higher diagnostic accuracy for *P falciparum* include enzyme-linked immunosorbent assay (ELISA), DNA hybridization, and polymerase chain reaction (PCR). A unique feature of the microscopic examination is the semiquantitative estimate of the parasitemia, which is best done on thin smears. This information is particularly useful in the management of infections caused by *P falciparum,* in which high parasitemia (more than 10% infected erythrocytes or more than 500,000 infected erythrocytes/μL) is associated with high morbidity and mortality and requires hospitalization. Treatment response of *P falciparum* and chloroquine-resistant *P vivax* infections is best monitored by daily parasitemia assays. Constant or increased number of infected erythrocytes after 48 hours of treatment or after the second hemolytic crisis suggests an inadequate therapeutic response. Other laboratory findings that reflect the severity of hemolysis include decreased hematocrit, hemoglobin, and haptoglobin levels; increased reticulocyte count; and hyper-

Table 39–3. Differentiation of malaria parasites on blood smears.

	Plasmodium falciparum	P vivax, P ovale
Multiple infected erythrocytes	Common	Rare
Mature tropho-zoites or schizonts	Absent[a]	Common
Schüffner dots	Absent	Common
Enlarged erythro-cytes	Absent	Common
Banana-shaped ga-metocytes	Common	Absent

[a]Usually sequestered in the microcirculation. Rare cases with circulating forms have extremely high parasitemia and a poor prognosis.

bilirubinemia and increased lactate dehydrogenase. Thrombocytopenia is common, but the incidence of leukocytosis is variable.

Differential Diagnosis

Relapsing fever may be associated with borreliosis, brucellosis, sequential common infections, Hodgkin disease, juvenile rheumatoid arthritis, rat-bite fever, or one of the idiopathic periodic fevers. Other common causes of high fever and headache include influenza, *Mycoplasma pneumoniae* or enteroviral infection, sinusitis, meningitis, enteric fever, tuberculosis, occult pneumonia, or bacteremia. Fever, headache, and jaundice in a patient returning from tropical areas indicate that leptospirosis and yellow fever should be included in the differential diagnosis. Malaria may also coexist with other diseases.

Complications & Sequelae

Severe complications are limited to *P falciparum* infection and result from microvascular obstruction and tissue ischemia. Impaired consciousness and seizures are the most common complications of malaria in children. In addition, respiratory failure, renal impairment, severe bleeding, and shock are associated with a poor prognosis. Among the laboratory abnormalities, hypoglycemia, acidosis, elevated aminotransferases, and parasitemia greater than 10% characterize severe malaria.

Prevention

Malaria chemoprophylaxis should be instituted 2 weeks (weekly regimens) to 2 days (daily regimens) before traveling to an area of endemic infection to permit changes if the drug is not tolerated. Because the antimalarial drugs recommended for prophylaxis do not kill sporozoites, therapy should be continued for 1 week (atovaquone/proguanil) or 4 weeks (all other regimens) after returning from an endemic area to cover infection acquired at departure.

Chloroquine is the drug of choice for prophylaxis of *P vivax*, *P ovale*, *P malariae*, and chloroquine-sensitive *P falciparum* (Table 39–4). Chloroquine is safe for all ages and during pregnancy. Side effects (dizziness, blurred vision, and headache) can be reduced by administering half of the weekly dose twice per week. Effects of chloroquine on heart rhythm are infrequent and are typically associated with rapid intravenous infusion or overdosage. Chloroquine has immunosuppressive properties and has been reported to impair immunization against rabies but not against yellow fever.

For chloroquine-resistant *P falciparum*, the regimens of choice are weekly mefloquine, daily doxycycline, or daily atovaquone/proguanil. The side effects of mefloquine are headache, dizziness, and blurred vision. This drug is now considered safe during pregnancy but is not used in children weighing less than 15 kg. Daily doxycycline is recommended for patients older than age 8 years who are unable to tolerate mefloquine. Women on prolonged doxycycline therapy tend to develop yeast vaginitis, and it is advisable to supply them with nystatin suppositories. Atovaquone/proguanil is better tolerated than mefloquine. For optimal absorption, this drug should be administered with food or no later than 45 minutes after a meal. Daily primaquine is also effective. Primaquine is also used to prevent relapse of *P vivax* or *P ovale* infections. Primaquine is contraindicated for patients with glucose-6-phosphate dehydrogenase deficiency, in whom it induces hemolysis. Less effective alternatives include chloroquine plus proguanil or chloroquine alone, with one therapeutic dose of pyrimethamine/sulfadoxine made available for self-treatment in the advent of potential breakthrough, signaled by fever, in areas where medical attention is not readily available.

No drug regimen guarantees protection against malaria. If fever develops within 1 year (particularly within 2 months) after travel to an endemic area, patients should be advised to seek medical attention. Insect repellents, insecticide-impregnated bed nets, and proper clothing are important adjuncts for malaria prophylaxis.

Treatment

Treatment for malaria includes a variety of supportive strategies in addition to the antimalarial drugs. It is advisable to hospitalize nonimmune patients infected with *P falciparum* until a decrease in parasitemia is demonstrated, indicating that treatment is effective and severe complications are unlikely to occur.

Partially immune patients with uncomplicated *P falciparum* infection and nonimmune persons infected with *P vivax*, *P ovale*, or *P malariae* can receive treatment as out-

Table 39–4. Chemoprophylaxis of malaria.[a]

Drug	Dosage
Chloroquine-sensitive areas[b]	
Chloroquine	5 mg base/kg/wk up to 300 mg (adult dose)
Chloroquine-resistant areas	
Mefloquine	0.25 tablet (62.5 mg) once a week (15–19 kg)
	0.5 tablet (125 mg) (20–30 kg)
	0.75 tablet (187.5 mg) (31–45 kg)
	1 tablet (250 mg) (> 45 kg)
Doxycycline	2 mg/kg/d (age > 8 years) up to 100 mg (adult dose)
Atovaquone/proguanil	11–20 kg: 62.5 mg/25 mg daily
	21–30 kg: 125 mg/50 mg
	31–40 kg: 187.5 mg/75 mg
	> 40 kg: 250 mg/100 mg
Primaquine	0.5 mg/kg base daily up to 30 mg (adult dose)
Chloroquine	As above
plus	
Proguanil	50 mg daily (age <2 y)
	100 mg (age 2–6 y)
	150 mg (age 7–10 y)
	200 mg (age > 10 y)
or	
Pyrimethamine-sulfadoxine for presumptive treatment (carry a single dose for self-treatment of febrile illness when medical care is not immediately available)	< 1 y: 1/4 tablet
	1–3 y: 1/2 tablet
	4–8 y: 1 tablet
	9–14 y: 2 tablets
	> 14 y: 3 tablets
Relapse of *P vivax* or *P ovale*[c]	
Primaquine	0.3 mg base/kg/d up to 15 mg (adult dose) during the last 2 wk of prophylaxis

[a]Updated malaria chemoprophylaxis information may be obtained by calling the Centers for Disease Control and Prevention Hot Line at 404-332-4555 or on the web at http://www.cdc.gov.
[b]Chloroquine-resistant *Plasmodium falciparum* has not yet been identified in Central America west of the Panama Canal zone, Haiti, Dominican Republic, Mexico, and most of the Middle East.
[c]Optional. Observation and prompt initiation of treatment when relapse occurs is sufficient.

patients if follow-up is reliable. For children, hydration and treatment of hypoglycemia are of utmost importance. Anemia, seizures, pulmonary edema, and renal failure require conventional management. Corticosteroids are contraindicated for cerebral malaria because of increased mortality. In severe malaria, exchange transfusion can be life-saving, particularly in nonimmune persons with parasitemia greater than 15%.

Chloroquine is the drug of choice for treatment of infection with chloroquine-sensitive plasmodia (Table 39–5). For patients unable to take oral medication, intravenous chloroquine or quinidine can be administered with careful monitoring for potential arrhythmogenic effects. Therapy can later be converted to oral chloroquine. For chloroquine-resistant *P falciparum* infection, oral therapy includes quinine with pyrimethamine/sulfadoxine, tetracycline, doxycycline, or clindamycin. Two-drug treatment shortens the quinine course from 7 to 3 days unless the malaria is severe or was acquired in areas of multidrug-resistant *P falciparum* (South America and Southeast Asia). Other options are mefloquine, halofantrine, and atovaquone/proguanil. Artemether and artesunate are very effective against *P falciparum,* including quinine-resistant strains (but note that these two agents are not licensed for use in the U.S.). Their use as monotherapy is associated with development of resistance. However, in combination with clindamycin, amodiaquin, chloroquine, piperaquine, lumefantrine, or mefloquine they are highly effective and well tolerated. If chemoprophylaxis failed to protect the patient, the same drug should not be used for treatment. Halofantrine should not be used as treatment for persons who failed mefloquine chemoprophylaxis, because the two drugs exhibit cross-resistance. Patients infected with chloroquine-resistant *P falciparum* who cannot take oral medication should receive intravenous quinidine, which is two or three times more active than quinine. Serum levels of quinidine can be measured in most North American hospitals. Chloroquine-resistant *P vivax* infection, which has been identified in Papua New Guinea, Irian Jaya (in Indonesia), India, Brazil, and Colombia, can be treated with mefloquine or halofantrine. *P vivax* or *P ovale* infections in persons living in nonendemic areas are usually treated with primaquine to prevent late relapse.

Baird JK, Hoffman SL: Primaquine therapy for malaria. Clin Infect Dis 2004;39:1336 [PMID: 15494911].

Centers for Disease Control and Prevention Web site: www.cdc.gov

Kremsner PG, Krishna S: Antimalarial combinations. Lancet 2004; 364:285 [PMID: 15262108].

Stauffer W et al: Diagnosis and treatment of malaria in children. Clin Infect Dis 2003;37:1340 [PMID: 14583868].

2. Babesiosis

Babesia microti is a malarialike protozoan that infects and lyses erythrocytes of wild and domestic animals in North

Table 39–5. Treatment of malaria.

Drug	Dosage
Chloroquine-sensitive plasmodia	
Chloroquine	10 mg base/kg up to 600 mg, followed either by 5 mg base/kg after 6, 24, and 48 h, or 5 mg base/kg after 12, 24, and 36 h
Chloroquine-resistant *P falciparum*	
A. Oral regimens	
1. Quinine sulfate	25 mg/kg/d up to 2g/d in three doses for 3–7 d
plus	
Pyrimethamine-sulfadoxine	$^1/_4$ tablet on the last day of quinine (age < 1 y)
	$^1/_2$ tablet (age 1–3 y)
	1 tablet (age 4–8 y)
	2 tablets (age 9–14 y)
	3 tablets (age > 15 y)
or	
Tetracycline	20 mg/kg/d up to 1 g/d in four doses for 7 d
or	
Doxycycline	3 mg/kg/d up to 100 mg as single daily dose for 7 d
or	
Clindamycin	20–40 mg/kg/d up to 2700 mg in three doses for 3 d
2. Mefloquine	25 mg/kg up to 1250 mg as a single dose
3. Halofantrine	8 mg/kg up to 500 mg every 6 h for three doses; repeat in 1 wk
4. Atovaquone/proguanil	11–20 kg: 1 tablet (250 mg/100 mg daily for 3 d)
	21–30 kg: 2 tablets
	31–40 kg: 3 tablets
	> 40 kg: 4 tablets
B. Parenteral regimen	
Quinidine gluconate	10 mg/kg up to 600 mg as loading dose IV in normal saline slowly over 1–2 h followed by continuous infusion of 0.02 mg/kg/min until oral therapy can be started
Chloroquine-resistant *P vivax*	
Mefloquine	25 mg/kg up to 1250 mg in a single dose
Halofantrine	8 mg/kg up to 500 mg/kg every 6 h for three doses; repeat in 1 week
Prevention of relapse with *P vivax* or *P ovale*	
Primaquine phosphate[a]	0.3 mg base/kg/d up to 15 mg base/d for 14 d

[a]Screen for glucose-6-phosphate dehydrogenase deficiency.

America and Europe. In the United States, human babesiosis has been identified in the coastal areas of New England, northern California and Washington State, and in the lakes region of the upper Midwest. Humans accidentally enter the cycle when bitten by *Ixodes scapularis,* one of the intermediate hosts and vectors of *B microti.* After inoculation, the protozoan penetrates the erythrocytes and starts an asynchronous cycle that causes hemolysis.

Clinical Findings

The incubation period is 1–3 weeks but may extend up to 6 weeks. Many times the tick bite is unnoticed. Symptoms are nonspecific and include sustained or cyclic fever up to 40 °C, shaking chills, malaise, myalgias, headache, and dark urine. Hepatosplenomegaly is an uncommon finding. The disease is usually self-limited, but severe cases have been described in asplenic patients and immunocompromised hosts. Because *Babesia* and *Borrelia burgdorferi* share another vector, *Ixodes dammini,* dual infection may occur.

Diagnosis

Microscopic evaluation of thin or thick blood smears reveals the intraerythrocytic organisms that resemble *P falciparum* ring forms. Specific serology is also available through the Centers for Disease Control and Prevention. IgG titers greater than or equal to 1:1024 are diagnostic of acute infection.

Treatment

Clindamycin (20 mg/kg/d, up to 900 mg every 8 hours) or azithromycin (500 mg on the first day, followed by 250 mg/d) in combination with quinine (25 mg/kg/d, up to 650 mg every 6–8 hours) or azithromycin and atovaquone (750 mg bid) for 7–10 days is the treatment of choice. Other antimalarial drugs, including chloroquine, have been unsuccessful.

Krause PJ et al: Atovaquone and azithromycin for the treatment of babesiosis. N Engl J Med 2000;343:1454 [PMID: 11078770].

Lantos PM et al: Babesiosis: Similar to malaria but different. Pediatr Ann 2002;31:192 [PMID: 11905293].

3. Toxoplasmosis

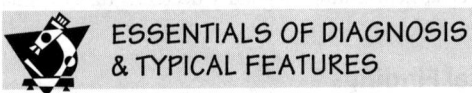 **ESSENTIALS OF DIAGNOSIS & TYPICAL FEATURES**

- *Congenital toxoplasmosis: chorioretinitis, microphthalmia, strabismus, microcephaly, hydrocephaly, convulsions, psychomotor retardation, intracranial calcifications, jaundice, hepatosplenomegaly, abnormal blood cell counts.*

- Acquired toxoplasmosis in an immunocompetent host: lymphadenopathy, hepatosplenomegaly, rash.
- Acquired or reactivated toxoplasmosis in an immunocompromised host: encephalitis, chorioretinitis, myocarditis, and pneumonitis.
- Ocular toxoplasmosis: chorioretinitis.
- Serologic evidence of infection with Toxoplasma gondii or demonstration of the agent in tissue or body fluids.

General Considerations

Toxoplasma gondii is a worldwide parasite of animals and birds. Felines, the definitive hosts, excrete oocysts in their feces. Ingested mature oocysts or tissue cysts lead to tachyzoite invasion of the intestinal cells. Intracellular replication of the tachyzoites cause cell lysis and spread of the infection to adjacent cells or to other tissues via the bloodstream. In chronic infection, T gondii appears as bradyzoite-containing tissue cysts that do not trigger an inflammatory reaction. In immunocompromised hosts, tachyzoites are released from the cysts and begin a new cycle of infection. The two major routes of Toxoplasma transmission to humans are oral (including pica) and congenital. Oocysts survive for up to 18 months in moist soil. Oral infection occurs after ingestion of cyst-containing undercooked meat or other food products. Oocyst survival is limited in dry, very cold, or very hot conditions, and at high altitude, which probably accounts for the lower incidence of toxoplasmosis in these climatic regions. In the United States, less than 1% of cattle and 25% of sheep and pigs are infected with toxoplasmosis. In humans, depending on geographic area, seropositivity increases with age from nil–10% in children younger than age 10 years to 3–70% in adults. Congenital transmission occurs during acute infection of pregnant women; this occurs in 0.2–1% of all pregnancies in the United States. Rarely, fetal infection has been documented in immunocompromised mothers who have chronic toxoplasmosis. The rate of vertical transmission in patients with untreated toxoplasmosis increases from 10% in the first trimester to 60% in the third. Symptomatic disease, however, is more likely to follow infection in early gestation (20–25%) compared with late gestation (less than 11%). Treatment during pregnancy decreases transmission by 60%.

Clinical Findings

A. CONGENITAL TOXOPLASMOSIS

Congenital toxoplasmosis has a variety of manifestations, including miscarriage, prematurity, and stillbirth. Most frequently, symptomatic infants present with a combination of fever, microcephaly or hydrocephaly, hepatosplenomegaly, jaundice, chorioretinitis, convulsions, abnormal cerebrospinal fluid (CSF) (xanthochromia and mononuclear pleocytosis), and cerebral calcifications. Other findings include strabismus, eye palsy, maculopapular rash, pneumonitis, myocarditis, thrombocytopenia, lymphocytosis and monocytosis, and an erythroblastosis-like syndrome. The overall mortality rate for congenital toxoplasmosis, which is approximately 10%, is higher in neonates who are symptomatic at birth. Congenital toxoplasmosis must be differentiated from cytomegalovirus infection, rubella, herpes simplex infection, syphilis, Lyme disease, listeriosis, erythroblastosis, and the encephalopathies that accompany degenerative diseases.

B. ACQUIRED TOXOPLASMA INFECTION IN THE IMMUNOCOMPETENT HOST

Only 10–20% of acute Toxoplasma infections produce symptoms. Patients usually present with lymphadenopathy without fever. The nodes are discrete, variably tender, and do not suppurate. Cervical lymph nodes are most frequently involved, but any nodes may be enlarged. Less common findings include fever, malaise, myalgias, fatigue, hepatosplenomegaly, low lymphocyte counts (usually less than 10%), and liver enzyme elevations. Unilateral chorioretinitis may occur. The disease is self-limited, although lymph node enlargement may persist or may wax and wane for a few months to 1 or even more years. Rarely, an apparently healthy child may develop severe disseminated disease associated with myocarditis, pneumonitis, or encephalitis.

Toxoplasmic lymphadenitis must be distinguished from other causes of infectious mononucleosis-like syndromes (< 1% are caused by Toxoplasma).

C. ACUTE TOXOPLASMOSIS IN THE IMMUNODEFICIENT HOST

Patients with human immunodeficiency virus (HIV), lymphoma, leukemia, or transplantation are at high risk for developing severe disease (encephalitis, chorioretinitis, myocarditis, or pneumonitis) following acute infection or reactivation. Children born to HIV- and Toxoplasma-infected mothers may acquire both pathogens in utero.

D. OCULAR TOXOPLASMOSIS

In active congenital toxoplasmosis, chorioretinitis is usually bilateral and shows acute inflammatory foci on funduscopic examination. This generally resolves, leaving depigmented scars of the retina surrounded by areas of hyperpigmentation. Chorioretinitis may reactivate in a single eye later in life. The appearance of the ocular lesion is not specific and mimics other granulomatous ocular diseases.

Diagnosis

Active infection is diagnosed by demonstration of *T gondii* or its DNA in blood or body fluids; seeing tachyzoites in histologic sections or cytology preparations; cysts in placenta or fetal tissues; characteristic lymph node histology; or typical serology (most commonly used). IgG antibodies, measured by the Sabin-Feldman dye test, immunofluorescence, ELISA, or particle agglutination, become detectable 1–2 weeks after infection, peak at 1–2 months, and after decreasing at variable speed, persist for life. IgM antibodies, measured by ELISA or particle agglutination, appear earlier and decline faster than IgG antibodies. Absence of both serum IgG and IgM virtually rules out the diagnosis of toxoplasmosis. Acute toxoplasmosis in an immunocompetent host is best documented by analyzing IgG and IgM in paired blood samples drawn 3 weeks apart. Because high antibody titers (IgM or IgG) can persist for several months after acute infection, a single high-titer determination is nonspecific. However, seroconversion or a fourfold increase in titer confirms the diagnosis.

In the immunocompromised host, serology is not sensitive, and active infection is documented by PCR or finding tachyzoites by histologic examination.

Patients with *Toxoplasma* chorioretinitis typically have low levels of specific IgG and absent IgM. The diagnosis can be confirmed by demonstrating high antibody titers in aqueous fluid.

Congenital infection is documented by anti-*Toxoplasma* IgM or IgA antibodies in the blood of the neonate. Prenatal diagnosis of congenital infection requires a combination of ultrasonography (to detect ventricle enlargement) and amniotic fluid PCR or cord blood serology. Amniotic fluid PCR is highly sensitive and carries fewer risks than cord puncture.

Differential Diagnosis

Congenital infection may resemble that due to cytomegalovirus, syphilis, rubella, or herpes simplex. Acquired infection mimics viral, bacterial, or lymphoproliferative disorders.

Prevention

Pregnant women and immunocompromised patients should wash hands thoroughly after handling raw meat, cook meat to 66 °C or greater, wash fruits and vegetables before consumption, and avoid contact with cat feces. Serologic screening of pregnant women is warranted in areas of high prevalence. A first test should be performed by 10–12 weeks of pregnancy. Seronegative patients should be retested at 20–22 weeks' gestation and near term. Seroconverters require specific therapy.

Treatment

Treatment does not reverse central nervous system (CNS) damage in neonates but does markedly decrease late sequelae. A year of treatment is recommended for all congenitally infected infants; symptomatic patients receive 6 months of pyrimethamine and sulfadiazine, followed by alternating spiramycin and pyrimethamine-sulfadiazine monthly for the next 6 months. Subclinical infection is treated with pyrimethamine and sulfadiazine for 6 weeks, followed by alternating spiramycin for 6 weeks with pyrimethamine-sulfadiazine for 4 weeks.

Oral pyrimethamine at 1 mg/kg/d (maximum 25 mg) causes gastrointestinal upset, leukopenia, thrombocytopenia, and rarely, agranulocytosis. Frequent blood counts should be performed to guide therapy. Leucovorin calcium (folinic acid), 5 mg given intramuscularly every 3 days, decreases myelotoxicity. The dosage of sulfadiazine is 40–45 mg/kg twice a day orally (maximum 8 g/d). Clindamycin can be substituted for sulfadiazine in patients who cannot tolerate sulfonamides. Spiramycin and trimethoprim-sulfamethoxazole are less active.

In acquired infection, usually self-limited, the potentially toxic therapy should be prescribed with discretion, only if the illness is complicated.

In chorioretinitis, antimicrobial therapy is used for 4 weeks. A course of corticosteroids (prednisone, 1.5 mg/kg up to 75 mg) is recommended when lesions involve the macula or the optic nerve. Lesions tend to improve after 10 days of therapy.

In primary infection during pregnancy, spiramycin is started immediately. Pyrimethamine plus sulfadiazine, alternating every 3 weeks with spiramycin, are used when fetal infection has been documented.

Montoya JG et al: Diagnosis and management of toxoplasmosis. Clin Perinatol 2005;32:705 [PMID: 16085028].

GASTROINTESTINAL INFECTIONS

1. Amebiasis

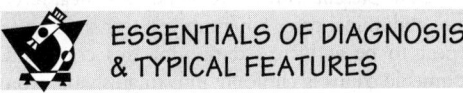

ESSENTIALS OF DIAGNOSIS & TYPICAL FEATURES

- *Acute dysentery: diarrhea with blood and mucus, abdominal pain, tenesmus.*

or

- *Chronic nondysenteric diarrhea.*

or

- *Hepatic abscess.*

- Amebas or cysts in stool or abscesses; amebic antigen in stool.
- Serologic evidence of amebic infection.

General Considerations

Amebiasis, caused by *Entamoeba histolytica,* is a common problem in areas with poor hygiene. An estimated 10% of the world's population is infected with *E histolytica* or *Entamoeba dispar,* and an estimated 100,000 people die of amebic infection each year. Amebiasis should be suspected in patients with a history of travel to, or contact with individuals who may be asymptomatic carriers from, endemic areas. In the United States, amebiasis may occur in homes for the handicapped, where poor hygiene fosters the spread of enteric pathogens. *E histolytica* has been found in the stools of as many as 30% of homosexual men. Individuals of any age may be infected. Transmission is usually fecal-oral, often from asymptomatic carriers who pass cysts. Trophozoites are killed by stomach acid and are not infectious. Infection with *E dispar,* which is morphologically identical to *E histolytica* but results only in asymptomatic carriage, is ten times more common than infection with *E histolytica.* Furthermore, only 10% of *E histolytica* infections result in gastrointestinal or other symptoms.

Clinical Findings

Patients with intestinal amebiasis can have asymptomatic cyst passage, or be symptomatic with acute amebic proctocolitis, chronic nondysenteric colitis, or ameboma. Because all *E dispar* infections and up to 90% of *E histolytica* infections are asymptomatic, carriage is the most common manifestation of amebiasis. Patients with acute amebic colitis typically have a 1- to 2-week history of watery stools containing blood and mucus, abdominal pain, and tenesmus. A minority of patients are febrile or dehydrated. Abdominal examination may reveal pain over the lower abdominal quadrants. Fulminant colitis is an unusual complication of amebic dysentery and is associated with a grave prognosis (more than 50% mortality). Patients with fulminant colitis present with severe bloody diarrhea, fever, and diffuse abdominal pain. Children younger than age 2 years appear to be at increased risk for this condition. Chronic amebic colitis is clinically indistinguishable from idiopathic inflammatory bowel disease; patients present with recurrent episodes of bloody diarrhea over a period of years. Ameboma is a localized amebic infection, usually in the cecum or ascending colon, which presents as a painful abdominal mass.

The most common complication of intestinal amebiasis is intestinal perforation and peritonitis. Perianal ulcers, a less common complication, are painful, punched-out lesions that usually respond to medical therapy. Infrequently, colonic strictures may develop following colitis.

Extraintestinal amebiasis can result in liver, lung, and cerebral abscesses, and rarely genitourinary disease. Patients with amebic liver abscess, the most common form of extraintestinal amebiasis, present with recent-onset fever and right upper quadrant tenderness. The pain may be dull or pleuritic or referred to the right shoulder. Physical examination reveals liver enlargement in less than 50% of affected patients. Some patients have a subacute presentation lasting 2 weeks to 6 months. In these patients, hepatomegaly, anemia, and weight loss are common findings, and fever is less common. Jaundice and diarrhea are rarely associated with an amebic liver abscess.

The most common complication of amebic liver abscess is pleuropulmonary amebiasis due to rupture of a right liver lobe. Lung abscesses may occur from hematogenous spread. Cough, dyspnea, and pleuritic pain can also be caused by the serous pleural effusions and atelectasis that frequently accompany amebic liver abscesses. Rupture of hepatic abscesses can lead to peritonitis and more rarely to pericarditis. Cerebral amebiasis is an infrequent manifestation. Genitourinary amebiasis, which is also uncommon, results from rupture of a liver abscess, hematogenous dissemination, or lymphatic spread.

Diagnosis

Intestinal amebiasis is diagnosed by detecting the parasite on stool examination or mucosal biopsy. The clinical differential diagnosis of acute amebic colitis includes bacillary diarrhea and perhaps infection with *Balantidium coli* and *Dientamoeba fragilis,* which have occasionally been associated with acute diarrhea but whose pathogenic role remains controversial. Chronic amebic colitis has to be distinguished from inflammatory bowel disease, *Cyclospora,* and perhaps *B coli.* Occult blood is present in virtually all cases of amebic colitis and can be used as an inexpensive screening test. Fecal leukocytes are uncommon. The presence of hematophagous trophozoites in feces indicates pathogenic *E histolytica* infection.

Ideally, a wet mount of the stool should be examined no longer than 20 minutes after collection to detect motile trophozoites. Otherwise, specimens should be fixed with polyvinyl alcohol or refrigerated to avoid disintegration of the trophozoites. The use of three separate stool examinations has 90% sensitivity for the diagnosis of amebic dysentery. However, infection of the ascending colon, amebomas, and extraintestinal infections frequently yield negative stool examinations. The antigen detection test for stool is very sensitive and more specific, because it detects *E histolytica*–specific antigens that do not cross-react with *E dispar.* Colonoscopy and biopsy are most helpful in diagnosing amebic colitis when stool samples lack ova or parasites. Barium studies are contraindicated for patients with suspected acute amebic colitis because of the risk of perforation.

The presence of antibodies against *E histolytica* can differentiate *E histolytica* from *E dispar* infections. The antibody response follows both intestinal and extraintestinal invasive amebiasis and can be used for diagnostic purposes. ELISA and indirect hemagglutination assays are positive in 85–95% of invasive *E histolytica* colitis or amebic abscess. However, these antibodies persist for years, and a positive result does not distinguish between acute and past infection. Noninvasive imaging studies have greatly improved the diagnosis of hepatic abscesses. Ultrasonographic examination and computed tomography (CT) are sensitive techniques that can guide fine-needle aspiration to obtain specimens for definitive diagnosis. Because an amebic abscess may take up to 2 years to completely resolve on CT scans, imaging techniques are not recommended for therapeutic evaluation.

Treatment & Prevention

Treatment of amebic infection is complex because different agents are required for eradicating the parasite from the bowel or tissue (Table 39–6). Whether treatment of asymptomatic cyst passers is indicated is a controversial issue. The prevalent opinion is that asymp-

Table 39–6. Treatment of amebiasis.

Type of Infection	Drug of Choice	Dosage
Asymptomatic	Iodoquinol	30–40 mg/kg/d up to 2 g/d in three doses for 20 d
	or	
	Paromomycin	25–35 mg/kg/d in three doses for 7 d
	or	
	Diloxanide furoate[a]	20 mg/kg/d up to 1.5 g/d in three doses for 10 d
Intestinal disease and hepatic abscess[b]	Metronidazole	35–50 mg/kg/d up to 2.25 g/d in three doses for 10 d
	or	
	Tinidazole[c]	50 or 60 mg/kg up to 2 g/d for 3 d

[a]Diloxanide furoate is available from the CDC Drug Service, 404-639-3670.
[b]Treatment should be followed by iodoquinol or another intraluminal cysticidal agent.
[c]Not marketed in the United States; higher dosage is for hepatic abscess.

tomatic infection with *E histolytica,* as evidenced by amebic cysts in the stool and a positive serologic test, should be treated in nonendemic areas. If serology is negative, the cysts are more likely to represent infection with the nonpathogenic *E dispar,* which does not require treatment. Among the drugs active against intraluminal cysts, iodoquinol is the most readily available but also the most toxic (causing prominent gastrointestinal side effects, interfering with thyroid function, and causing dose-dependent optic neuritis). Paromomycin, a nonabsorbable aminoglycoside, can be used safely during pregnancy and has only mild intestinal side effects, including flatulence and increased number of stools. Diloxanide furoate is relatively nontoxic and used widely outside the United States. The treatment of invasive amebiasis requires metronidazole. Metronidazole has a disulfiramlike effect and should be avoided in patients receiving ethanol-containing medications. Tinidazole, a more potent nitroimidazole against amebic infection, can be used for shorter treatment courses and is well tolerated in children.

In patients who cannot tolerate metronidazole or tinidazole, erythromycin and tetracycline are active against intestinal trophozoites but are inactive against trophozoites in liver abscesses. Conversely, chloroquine is active only against hepatic amebiasis. Treatment of invasive amebiasis should always be followed with an intraluminal cysticidal agent, even if the stool examination is negative. Patients with large, thin-walled hepatic abscesses may need therapeutic aspiration to avoid abscess rupture. Patients with amebiasis should be placed under enteric precautions. Travelers to endemic areas need to follow the precautions designed to prevent enteric infections—drink bottled or boiled water and eat cooked or peeled vegetables and fruits.

Tanyuksel M et al: Comparison of two methods (microscopy and enzyme-linked immunosorbent assay) for the diagnosis of amebiasis. Exp Parasitol 2005;110:322 [PMID: 15955332].

Thielman NM et al: Acute infectious diarrhea. N Engl J Med 2004;350:38 [PMID: 14702426].

2. Giardiasis

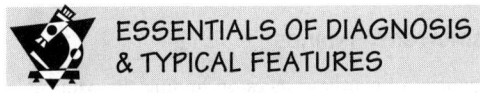

ESSENTIALS OF DIAGNOSIS & TYPICAL FEATURES

- *Chronic relapsing diarrhea, flatulence, bloating, anorexia, poor weight gain.*
- *Absence of fever and hematochezia.*
- *Detection of trophozoites, cysts, or Giardia antigens in stool.*

General Considerations

Giardiasis, caused by *Giardia lamblia*, is the most common intestinal protozoal infection in children in the United States and in most of the world. Endemic worldwide, the infection is classically associated with drinking contaminated water, either in rural areas or in areas with faulty purification systems. But even ostensibly clean urban water supplies can be contaminated intermittently. Persons have acquired the infection in swimming pools. Fecal-oral contamination allows person-to-person spread. Day care centers have become a major source of infection, with an incidence of up to 50% reported in some centers. No symptoms occur in 25% of infected persons, facilitating spread to household contacts. Food-borne outbreaks also occur. Although infection is rare in neonates, giardiasis may occur at any age.

Clinical Findings

A. SYMPTOMS AND SIGNS

Giardia infection is followed by asymptomatic cyst passage, acute self-limited diarrhea, or a chronic syndrome of diarrhea, malabsorption, and weight loss. Acute diarrhea occurs 1–2 weeks after infection and is characterized by abrupt onset of diarrhea with greasy, malodorous stools; malaise; flatulence; bloating; and nausea. Fever and vomiting occur in a minority of patients. Urticaria, reactive arthritis, biliary tract disease, gastric infection, and constipation have occasionally been reported. The disease has a protracted course (> 1 week) and frequently leads to weight loss. Patients who develop chronic diarrhea complain of profound malaise, lassitude, headache, and diffuse abdominal pain in association with bouts of diarrhea—most typically foul-smelling, greasy stools—intercalated with periods of constipation or normal bowel habits. This syndrome can persist for months until specific therapy is administered or until it subsides spontaneously. Chronic diarrhea frequently leads to malabsorption, steatorrhea, vitamin A and vitamin B_{12} deficiencies, and disaccharidase depletion. Lactose intolerance, which develops in 20–40% of patients, can persist for several weeks after treatment and needs to be differentiated from relapsing giardiasis or reinfection.

B. LABORATORY FINDINGS

The diagnosis of giardiasis relies on finding the parasite in stool or duodenal aspirates or detecting *Giardia* antigen in feces. For ova and parasite examination, a fresh stool provides the best results. Liquid stools have the highest yield of trophozoites, which are more readily found on wet mounts. With semiformed stools, the examiner should look for cysts in fresh or fixed specimens, preferably using a concentration technique. When these techniques are applied carefully, one examination has a 50–70% sensitiv-ity; three examinations increase the sensitivity to 90%. Antigen assays detect *Giardia* by means of immunofluorescence or ELISA. They are comparable in cost to a stool ova and parasite examination and are 85–90% sensitive and 95–100% specific. With a careful stool ova and parasite examination or with the use of a new antigen test, direct sampling of the duodenal contents should be restricted to particularly difficult cases. Three methods are currently available: the string test (Entero-Test), duodenal aspiration, and duodenal biopsy.

Treatment & Prevention

Metronidazole and nitazoxanide are the drugs of choice for treatment of giardiasis. When given at 5 mg/kg (up to 250 mg) three times daily for 5 days, metronidazole has 80–95% efficacy. The drug is well tolerated in children. It has a disulfiram-like effect and should be avoided in patients receiving ethanol-containing medication. Metronidazole can be administered safely during pregnancy. Nitazoxanide is available in liquid formulation and reduces the duration of treatment to 3 days. Recommended doses are 100 mg (5 mL) every 12 hours for children 12–47 months of age and 200 mg (10 mL) for 4- to 11-year-olds. Furazolidone is sometimes used in children because it is available in suspension. Administered at 1.5 mg/kg (up to 100 mg) four times daily for 7–10 days, it has only 80% efficacy. Furazolidone may cause gastrointestinal side effects, turn urine red, and cause mild hemolysis in patients with glucose-6-phosphate dehydrogenase deficiency. For patients who do not respond to metronidazole or furazolidone or who suffer relapse, a second course with the same drug or switching to the other drug is equally effective. In cases of repeated treatment failure, albendazole (400 mg/d for 5–10 days), although not specifically recommended in the U.S. for the treatment of giardiasis, is an effective option. Tinidazole, which is not available in the U.S., and the recently FDA-approved broad-spectrum antiparasitic nitazoxanide have higher efficacy than any of the drugs already mentioned.

The prevention of giardiasis requires proper treatment of water supplies and interruption of person-to-person transmission. Travelers to developing countries or wilderness areas should halogenate or boil (for over 10 minutes) drinking water and avoid uncooked foods that might have been washed with contaminated water. Sexual transmission is prevented by avoiding oral-anal and oral-genital sex. Interrupting fecal-oral transmission requires strict hand washing. However, outbreaks of diarrhea in day care centers might be particularly difficult to eradicate, and reinforcing hand-washing and treating the disease in both symptomatic and asymptomatic carriers may be necessary.

Ochoa TJ et al: Nitazoxanide for the treatment of intestinal parasites in children. Pediatr Infect Dis J 2005;24:641 [PMID: 15999008].

Thielman NM et al: Acute infectious diarrhea. N Engl J Med 2004;350:38 [PMID: 14702426].

3. Cryptosporidiosis

Cryptosporidium parvum is an intracellular protozoan that has gained importance because it causes severe diarrhea in patients with acquired immunodeficiency syndrome (AIDS) and in other immunodeficient persons. The parasite is ubiquitous and infects and reproduces in the epithelial cell lining of the digestive and respiratory tracts of humans and most other vertebrate animals. Humans acquire the infection from contaminated water supplies or from close contact with infected humans or animals.

Clinical Findings

A. SYMPTOMS AND SIGNS

Immunocompetent persons infected with *Cryptosporidium* usually develop self-limited diarrhea (2–26 days) with or without abdominal cramps. Diarrhea is intermittent and scant or continuous, watery, and voluminous. Low-grade fever, nausea, vomiting, loss of appetite, and malaise may accompany the diarrhea. Young children (< age 2 years) appear more susceptible to infection than older children. Immunocompromised patients (either cellular or humoral deficiency) tend to develop prolonged disease, which usually subsides only after the immunodeficiency is corrected. Other clinical manifestations associated with cryptosporidiosis in immunocompromised hosts include cholecystitis, pancreatitis, hepatitis, and respiratory symptoms.

B. LABORATORY FINDINGS

Cryptosporidiosis has no characteristic laboratory features other than identification of the microorganism in feces or on biopsy. ELISA and PCR tests are more sensitive than staining of stool specimens or concentrates.

Treatment & Prevention

Immunocompetent patients and those with temporary immunodeficiencies respond to treatment with nitazoxanide, antidiarrheal agents, and hydration. Immunocompromised patients usually require more intense supportive care with parenteral nutrition in addition to hydration and nonspecific antidiarrheal agents. Octreotide acetate, a synthetic analogue of somatostatin that inhibits secretory diarrhea, has been associated with symptomatic improvement, but not with parasitologic cure. Among the antiparasitic agents, nitazoxanide, paromomycin/azithromycin, rifabutin, and hyperimmune bovine colostrum, in that order, have met with success. For patients with AIDS, institution of effective antiretroviral therapy eliminates symptomatic cryptosporidiosis. Prevention of *Cryptosporidium* infection is limited by oocyst resistance to some of the standard water purification procedures and to common disinfectants. Enteric precautions are recommended for infected persons. Boiled or bottled drinking water may be considered for those at high risk for developing chronic infection (eg, patients with AIDS).

Chen X et al: Cryptosporidiosis. N Engl J Med 2002;346:1723 [PMID: 12037153].

Goh S et al: Sporadic cryptosporidiosis decline after membrane filtration of public water supplies, England, 1996-2002. Emerg Infect Dis 2005;11:251 [PMID: 15752443].

Insulander M et al: An outbreak of cryptosporidiosis associated with exposure to swimming pool water. Scand J Infect Dis 2005;37:354 [PMID: 16051572].

4. Cyclosporiasis

Cyclospora is a coccidian that infects both humans and animals with worldwide distribution. It causes food-associated outbreaks, characterized by an incubation period of 2–11 days followed by watery diarrhea in relapsing patterns, sometimes alternating with constipation. Other symptoms include profound fatigue, vomiting, and myalgias. Although the illness is self-limited, it may last for several weeks. Diagnosis is based on finding oocysts 8–10 mm in diameter on examination of stool specimens stained with acid-fast stain. The treatment of choice is trimethoprim-sulfamethoxazole for 7 days.

Herwaldt BL: Cyclospora cayetanensis: A review, focusing on the outbreaks of cyclosporiasis in the 1990s. Clin Infect Dis 2000;31:1040 [PMID: 11049789].

5. Free-Living Amebas

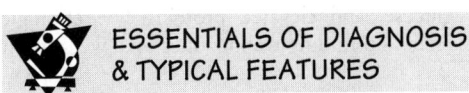

ESSENTIALS OF DIAGNOSIS & TYPICAL FEATURES

- *Acute meningoencephalitis: fever, headache, meningismus, acute mental deterioration.*
- *Swimming in warm, fresh water in endemic areas.*
- *Chronic granulomatous encephalitis: insidious onset of focal neurologic deficits.*
- *Keratitis: pain, photophobia, conjunctivitis, blurred vision.*

General Considerations

Infections with free-living amebas are uncommon. *Naegleria* species, *Acanthamoeba* species, and *Balamuthia* (previously called leptomyxid) amebas have been associated with human disease.

Acute meningoencephalitis, caused by *N fowleri,* occurs mostly in children and young adults. Patients present with abrupt fever, headache, nausea and vomiting, meningismus, and decreased mental status a few days to 2 weeks after swimming in warm freshwater lakes. Swimming history may be absent. CNS invasion occurs after nasal inoculation of *N fowleri.* The disease is rapidly progressive, and death ensues within 1 week of onset.

Chronic granulomatous encephalitis, caused by *Acanthamoeba* or *Balamuthia,* occurs most commonly in patients who are immunocompromised from corticosteroid use, chemotherapy, or AIDS. There is no association with freshwater swimming. This disease has an insidious onset of focal neurologic deficits, and approximately 50% of patients present with headache. Skin, sinus, or lung infections with *Acanthamoeba* precede many of the CNS infections and may still be present at the onset of neurologic disease. The granulomatous encephalitis progresses to fatal outcome over a period of weeks to months (average 6 weeks).

Acanthamoeba keratitis is a corneal infection associated with minor trauma or use of soft contact lenses in otherwise healthy persons. Frequently misdiagnosed as herpes simplex or bacterial keratitis, *Acanthamoeba* keratitis has a characteristic dendritiform epithelial pattern that suggests the diagnosis.

Diagnosis

Amebic encephalitis should be included in the differential diagnosis of acute meningoencephalitis in children with a history of recent freshwater swimming. The CSF is usually hemorrhagic, with leukocyte counts that may be normal early in the disease, but later range from 400–2600/μL with neutrophil predominance, low to normal glucose, and elevated protein. The etiologic diagnosis relies on finding trophozoites on a wet mount of the CSF.

Granulomatous encephalitis is diagnosed by brain biopsy of CT-identified nonenhancing lucent areas. The CSF of these patients is usually nondiagnostic with intermediate white blood cell counts, elevated protein, and decreased glucose. *Acanthamoeba* or leptomyxid amebas have not been found in the CSF; however, they can be visualized in biopsies or grown from brain or other infected tissues.

Acanthamoeba keratitis is diagnosed by finding the trophozoites in corneal scrapings or by isolating the parasite from corneal specimens or contact lens cultures.

Treatment & Prevention

The few patients who have survived acute amebic meningoencephalitis received high-dose intravenous and intrathecal amphotericin B, accompanied by miconazole, rifampin, and sulfisoxazole in some cases. The first

two cases of successful treatment of *Balamuthia* encephalitis were reported after combination therapy with flucytosine, pentamidine, fluconazole, sulfadiazine, and a macrolide.

Acanthamoeba keratitis responds well to surgical debridement followed by 3–4 weeks of topical 1% miconazole; 0.1% propamidine isethionate; and polymyxin B sulfate, neomycin, and bacitracin (Neosporin).

Because primary amebic meningitis occurs infrequently, active surveillance of lakes for *N fowleri* is not warranted. However, in the presence of a documented case, it is advisable to close the implicated lake to swimming. *Acanthamoeba* keratitis can be prevented by heat disinfection of contact lenses, by storage of lenses in sterile solutions, and by not wearing lenses when swimming in fresh water.

Deetz TR et al: Successful treatment of *Balamuthia* amoebic encephalitis: Presentation of two cases. Clin Infect Dis 2003; 37:1304 [PMID: 14583863].

Kumar R et al: Recent advances in the treatment of *Acanthamoeba* keratitis. Clin Infect Dis 2002;35:434 [PMID: 12145728].

McKee T et al: Primary amebic meningoencephalitis—Georgia, 2002. MMWR Morb Mortal Wkly Rep 2003;52:962 [PMID: 14534512].

TRICHOMONIASIS

Trichomonas vaginalis is discussed in Chapter 40.

■ METAZOAL INFECTIONS

NEMATODE INFECTIONS

1. Enterobiasis (Pinworms)

ESSENTIALS OF DIAGNOSIS & TYPICAL FEATURES

- *Anal pruritus.*
- *Worms in the stool or eggs on perianal skin.*

General Considerations

This worldwide infection is caused by *Enterobius vermicularis.* The adult worms are about 5–10 mm long and live in the colon; females deposit eggs on the perianal area, primarily at night, causing intense pruritus. Scratching contaminates the fingers and allows transmission back to the host (autoinfection) or to contacts.

Clinical Findings

A. SYMPTOMS AND SIGNS

Although blamed for myriad symptoms, pinworms are definitely associated only with localized pruritus. Adult worms may migrate within the colon or up the urethra or vagina in girls. They can be found within the bowel wall, in the lumen of the appendix (usually an incidental finding by the pathologist), in the bladder, and even in the peritoneal cavity of girls. The granulomatous reaction that may be present around these ectopic worms is usually asymptomatic. Worm eradication may correspond with the cure of recurrent urinary tract infections in some young girls.

B. LABORATORY FINDINGS

The usual diagnostic test consists of pressing a piece of transparent tape on the child's anus in the morning prior to bathing, then placing it on a drop of xylene on a slide. Microscopic examination under low power usually demonstrates the ova. Occasionally eggs or adult worms are seen in fecal specimens. Parents may also notice adult worms.

Differential Diagnosis

Nonspecific irritation or vaginitis, streptococcal perianal cellulitis (usually painful with marked erythema), and vaginal or urinary bacterial infections may at times resemble pinworm infection, although the symptoms of pinworms are often so suggestive that a therapeutic trial is justified without a confirmed diagnosis.

Treatment

A. SPECIFIC MEASURES

Treat all household members at the same time to prevent reinfections. Because the drugs are not active against the eggs, therapy should be repeated after 2 weeks to kill the recently hatched adults.

Pyrantel pamoate is given as a single dose (11 mg/kg, maximum 1 g); it is safe and very effective. Mebendazole (100 mg) and albendazole (400 mg) in a single dose are highly effective for this infection at all ages.

B. GENERAL MEASURES

Personal hygiene must be emphasized. Nails should be kept short and clean. Children should wear undergarments to bed to diminish contamination of fingers; bedclothes should be laundered frequently. Although eggs may be widely dispersed in the house and multiple family members infected, the disease is mild and treatable. Avoid creating in the parents an excessive concern with contamination.

St Georgiev V: Chemotherapy of enterobiasis (oxyuriasis). Expert Opin Pharmacother 2001;2:267 [PMID: 11336585].

2. Ascariasis

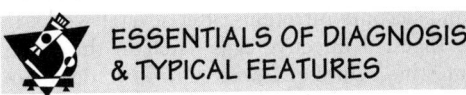

ESSENTIALS OF DIAGNOSIS
& TYPICAL FEATURES

- *Abdominal cramps and discomfort.*
- *Large, white or reddish, round worms, or ova in the feces.*

General Considerations

Ascaris lumbricoides is a worldwide human parasite. Ova passed by carriers may remain viable for months under the proper soil conditions. The ova contaminate food or fingers and are subsequently ingested by a new host. The larvae hatch, penetrate the intestinal wall, enter the venous system, reach the alveoli, are coughed up, and return to the small intestine, where they mature. The female lays thousands of eggs daily.

Clinical Findings

A. SYMPTOMS AND SIGNS

Infections usually remain asymptomatic; severe cases, however, can be associated with pain, weight loss, anorexia, diarrhea, or vomiting. Adult worms may be seen in feces or vomitus. Rarely, they perforate or obstruct the small bowel, biliary system, or appendix. Large numbers of larvae migrating through the lungs may cause an acute, transient eosinophilic pneumonia (Löffler syndrome).

B. LABORATORY FINDINGS

The diagnosis is made by observing the large roundworms in the stool or by microscopic detection of the ova.

Treatment

Because the adult worms live less than a year, asymptomatic infection need not be treated. Mebendazole (100 mg twice daily for 3 days), pyrantel pamoate (a single dose of 11 mg/kg, maximum 1 g), and albendazole (400 mg in a single dose) are highly and equally effective. In cases of intestinal or biliary obstruction, piperazine (150 mg/kg initially, followed by six doses of 65 mg/kg every 12 hours by nasogastric tube) is recommended because it narcotizes the worms and helps relieve obstruction. However, surgical removal is occasionally required.

3. Trichuriasis (Whipworm)

Trichuris trichiura is a widespread human and animal parasite common in children living in warm, humid areas conducive to survival of the ova. The adult worms live in the cecum and colon; the ova are passed and become infectious after several weeks in the soil. Ingested infective eggs hatch in the upper small intestine. Unlike *Ascaris*, *Trichuris* does not have a migratory tissue phase. Symptoms are not present unless the infection is severe, in which case pain, diarrhea, and mild abdominal distention are present. Massive infections may also cause rectal prolapse and dysentery. Detection of the characteristic barrel-shaped ova in the feces confirms the diagnosis. Adult worms may be seen in the prolapsed rectum or at proctoscopy; their thin heads are buried in the mucosa, and the thicker posterior portions protrude. Mild to moderate eosinophilia may be present.

Mebendazole (100 mg orally twice daily for 3 days) or albendazole (400 mg in a single dose) improves gastrointestinal symptoms and terminates constitutional symptoms.

Crompton DW et al: Nutritional impact of intestinal helminthiasis. Ann Rev Nutr 2002;22:35 [PMID: 12055337].

4. Hookworm

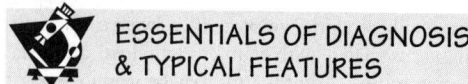

ESSENTIALS OF DIAGNOSIS & TYPICAL FEATURES

- *Iron deficiency anemia.*
- *Abdominal discomfort, weight loss.*
- *Ova in the feces.*

General Considerations

The common human hookworms are *Ancylostoma duodenale* and *Necator americanus*. Both are widespread in the tropics and subtropics. The larger *A duodenale* is more pathogenic because it consumes more blood, up to 0.5 mL per worm per day.

The adults live in the jejunum. Eggs are passed in the feces and develop and hatch into infective larvae in warm, damp soil within 2 weeks. The larvae penetrate human skin on contact, enter the blood, reach the alveoli, are coughed up and swallowed, and develop into adults in the intestine. The adult worms attach with their mouth parts to the mucosa, from which they suck blood. Blood loss is the major sequela of infection. Infection rates reach 90% in areas without sanitation.

A separate species, *A braziliense* (dog or cat hookworm), causes creeping eruption (cutaneous larva

migrans). This disease occurs mainly on the warmwater American coasts.

Clinical Findings

A. SYMPTOMS AND SIGNS

The larvae usually penetrate the skin of the feet and cause intense local itching (ground itch). This subsides as the larvae continue their migration. Löffler syndrome may supervene during lung migration. In creeping eruption, the nonhuman *Ancylostoma* larvae migrate blindly in the skin before dying, creating serpiginous burrows.

Mild intestinal infections produce no symptoms. Severe infections cause iron deficiency anemia and malnutrition. Occasionally abdominal pain and diarrhea may be observed.

B. LABORATORY FINDINGS

The large ova of both species of hookworm are found in feces and are indistinguishable. Microcytic anemia, hypoalbuminemia, eosinophilia, and hematochezia occur in severe cases.

Prevention

Fecal contamination of soil and skin contact with potentially contaminated soil should be avoided.

Treatment

A. SPECIFIC MEASURES

Mebendazole (100 mg orally twice daily for 3 days) and pyrantel pamoate (11 mg/kg, maximum 1 g, daily for 3 days) are the drugs of choice. Topical thiabendazole or albendazole or oral thiabendazole are useful for creeping eruption.

B. GENERAL MEASURES

Iron therapy may be as important as worm eradication.

Prognosis

The outcome is usually excellent.

Caumes E: Treatment of cutaneous larva migrans. Clin Infect Dis 2000;30:811 [PMID: 10816151].

5. Strongyloidiasis

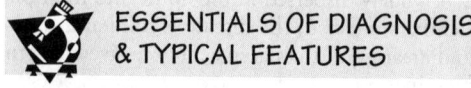

ESSENTIALS OF DIAGNOSIS & TYPICAL FEATURES

- *Abdominal pain, diarrhea.*
- *Eosinophilia.*

- *Larvae in stools and duodenal aspirates.*
- *Serum antibodies.*

General Considerations

Strongyloides stercoralis is unique in having both parasitic and free-living forms; the latter can survive in the soil for several generations. The parasite is found in most tropical and subtropical regions of the world. The adults live in the submucosal tissue of the duodenum and occasionally elsewhere in the intestines. Eggs deposited in the mucosa hatch rapidly; the first-stage (rhabditiform) larvae, therefore, are the predominant form found in duodenal aspirates and feces. The larvae mature rapidly to the tissue-penetrating filariform stage and initiate internal autoinfection. The filariform larvae also inhabit the soil and can penetrate the skin of another host, subsequently migrating into veins and pulmonary alveoli, reaching the intestine when coughed up and swallowed.

Older children and adults are infected more often than are young children. Even low worm burden can result in significant clinical symptoms. Infestations due to poor sanitation and hygiene are noteworthy. Immunosuppressed patients may develop fatal disseminated strongyloidiasis, known as the hyperinfection syndrome.

Clinical Findings

A. SYMPTOMS AND SIGNS

At the site of the skin penetration, a pruritic rash may occur. Large numbers of migrating larvae can cause wheezing, cough, and hemoptysis. Although one-third of intestinal infections are asymptomatic, the most prominent features of strongyloidiasis include abdominal pain, distention, diarrhea, vomiting, and occasionally malabsorption.

Patients with cellular immunodeficiencies and those on steroid therapy may develop disseminated infection involving the intestine, the lungs, and the meninges. Gram-negative sepsis may complicate disseminated strongyloidiasis.

B. LABORATORY FINDINGS

Finding larvae in the feces, in duodenal aspirates, on a string test (Entero-Test), or in sputum is diagnostic. IgG antibodies measured by ELISA or immunoblot are sensitive and specific for *Strongyloides*. These persist after successful therapy. Marked eosinophilia is common.

Differential Diagnosis

Strongyloidiasis should be differentiated from peptic disease, celiac disease, regional or tuberculous enteritis, hookworm infection, and other causes of intestinal symptoms or malabsorption. The pulmonary phase may mimic

asthma or bronchopneumonia. Patients with severe infection can present with an acute abdomen.

Treatment & Prevention

Thiabendazole (25 mg/kg orally twice daily for 2 days; maximum 3 g/d) and ivermectin (200 mg/kg/d for 1 or 2 days) are the drugs of choice. Relapses are common. In the hyperinfection syndrome, 2–3 weeks of therapy may be necessary. Patients from endemic areas should be tested for specific antibodies and receive treatment before undergoing immunosuppression.

Keiser PB et al: *Strongyloides stercoralis* in the immunocompromised population. Clin Microbiol Rev 2004;17:208 [PMID: 14726461].

6. Visceral Larva Migrans (Toxocariasis)

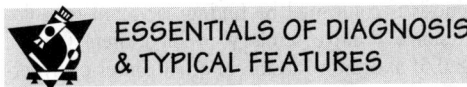

ESSENTIALS OF DIAGNOSIS & TYPICAL FEATURES

- *Visceral involvement including hepatomegaly, marked eosinophilia, and anemia.*
- *Posterior or peripheral ocular inflammatory mass.*
- *Elevated antibody titers in serum or aqueous fluid; demonstration of* Toxocara larvae *on biopsy.*

General Considerations

Visceral larva migrans is a worldwide disease. The agent is the cosmopolitan intestinal ascarid of dogs and cats, *Toxocara canis* or *Toxocara cati*. The eggs passed by infected animals contaminate parks and other areas that young children frequent. Children with pica are at increased risk. In the United States, seropositivity ranges from 2.8% in unselected populations to 23% in southern states to 54% in rural areas. Ingested eggs hatch and penetrate the intestinal wall, then migrate to the liver, lungs, eyes, and other organs, where they die and incite a granulomatous inflammatory reaction.

Clinical Findings & Diagnosis

A. VISCERAL LARVA MIGRANS

Toxocariasis is usually asymptomatic, but young children (age 1–5 years) sometimes present with anorexia, fever, fatigue, pallor, abdominal distention, abdominal pain, nausea, vomiting, and cough. Hepatomegaly is common, splenomegaly is unusual, and adenopathy is absent. Lung involvement, usually asymptomatic, can be demonstrated readily by radiologic examination. Seizures are common, but more severe neurologic abnormalities are infrequent. Eosinophilia with leukocytosis, anemia, and elevated liver function tests are typical laboratory findings. ELISA is sensitive, specific, and useful in confirming the clinical diagnosis. Most patients recover spontaneously, but disease may last up to 6 months.

B. OCULAR LARVA MIGRANS

This condition occurs in older children and adults who present with a unilateral posterior or peripheral inflammatory mass. History of visceral larva migrans and eosinophilia are typically absent. Anti-*Toxocara* antibody titers are low in the serum and high in vitreous and aqueous fluids.

Diagnosis

Hypergammaglobulinemia and elevated isohemagglutinins sometimes result from cross-reactivity between *Toxocara* antigens and human group A and B blood antigens. The diagnosis is confirmed by finding larvae in granulomatous lesions. Positive serology in high titers (optical density ≥ 0.5) and the exclusion of other causes of hypereosinophilia allow a presumptive diagnosis to be made in typical cases.

Differential Diagnosis

Diseases associated with hypereosinophilia must be considered. These include trichinosis (enlarged liver not common; muscle tenderness common), eosinophilic leukemia (rare in children; eosinophils are abnormal in appearance), collagen-vascular disease (those associated with eosinophilia are rare in young children), strongyloidiasis (no organomegaly; enteric symptoms are common), early ascariasis, tropical eosinophilia (occurring mainly in India), allergies, and hypersensitivity syndromes.

Treatment & Prevention

A. SPECIFIC MEASURES

The clinical benefit of specific anthelmintic therapy is not defined. Treatment with thiabendazole (25 mg/kg—maximum 3 g/d orally twice a day for 5–7 days), diethylcarbamazine (2 mg/kg three times a day orally for 7–10 days), albendazole (400 mg twice a day for 3–5 days), or mebendazole (100–200 mg twice a day for 5 days) is indicated for severe complications of brain, lung, or heart.

B. GENERAL MEASURES

Treating any cause of pica, such as iron deficiency, is important. Corticosteroids are used to treat marked inflammation of lung, eye, or other organs. Pets should be dewormed routinely. Other children in the household may be infected. Mild eosinophilia and positive serologic tests may be the only clue to their infection. Therapy is not necessary for these individuals.

7. Trichinosis

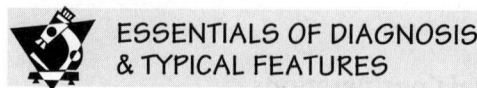

ESSENTIALS OF DIAGNOSIS & TYPICAL FEATURES

- *Vomiting, diarrhea, and pain within 1 week of eating infected meat.*
- *Fever, periorbital edema, myalgia, and marked eosinophilia.*

General Considerations

Trichinella spiralis is a small roundworm that inhabits hogs and several other meat-eating animals. The human cycle begins with ingestion of viable larvae in undercooked meat. In the intestine, the larvae develop into adult worms that mate and produce hundreds of larvae. The larvae enter the bloodstream and migrate to the striated muscle where they continue to grow and eventually encyst. Symptoms are caused by the inflammatory response in the intestines or muscle.

Clinical Findings

A. SYMPTOMS AND SIGNS

Most infections are asymptomatic. The initial bowel penetration may cause nausea, vomiting, diarrhea, and cramps within 1 week after ingestion of contaminated meat. This may progress to the classic myopathic form, which consists of fever, periorbital edema, myalgia, and weakness. Many organs may be infected by the migrating larvae: diaphragm, heart, lungs, kidneys, spleen, skin, and brain. Severe cerebral involvement may be fatal. Myocarditis may also be severe or fatal. Symptoms usually peak after 2–3 weeks but may last months.

B. LABORATORY FINDINGS

Marked eosinophilia is the rule. Serology confirms the diagnosis. Muscle biopsy is rarely necessary.

Differential Diagnosis

The classic symptoms are pathognomonic if one is aware of this disease. It has to be distinguished from dermatomyositis, typhoid fever, sinusitis, influenza with myopathy, and angioneurotic edema.

Prevention

Because a microscopic examination must be performed, meat in the United States is not inspected for trichinosis. Although all states require the cooking of hog swill, hog-to-hog or hog-to-rat cycles may continue. All pork and sylvatic meat (eg, bear or walrus) should be heated to at least 65 °C. Freezing meat to at least –15 °C for 3 weeks may also prevent transmission. Animals used for food should not be fed or allowed access to raw meat.

Treatment

Mebendazole has activity against the intestinal, circulating, and tissue stages of infection. The adult dose is 200–400 mg three times daily for 3 days followed by 400–500 mg three times daily for 10 days. Pediatric dosing has not been standardized. Concurrent corticosteroids are used in an attempt to prevent the Herxheimer reaction associated with treatment.

Prognosis

Death may occur within the first weeks, but most infections are self-limited.

Bruschi F et al: New aspects of human trichinellosis: The impact of new *Trichinella* species. Postgrad Med J 2002;78:15 [PMID: 11796866].

8. Raccoon Roundworm Infections

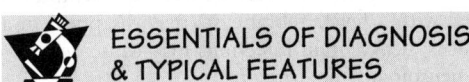

ESSENTIALS OF DIAGNOSIS & TYPICAL FEATURES

- *Eosinophilic meningoencephalitis or encephalopathy.*
- *Ocular larva migrans.*
- *Contact with raccoons and/or raccoon latrines.*

General Considerations

Human infections with *Baylisascaris procyonis,* the raccoon roundworm, have been increasingly recognized, particularly in children. The definitive host of this ascarid is the raccoon. Humans who ingest the eggs excreted in raccoon feces become intermediate hosts when the larvae penetrate the gut and disseminate via the bloodstream to the brain, eyes, viscera, and muscles. Young age, pica, and exposure to raccoon feces (eg, while camping) represent the main risk factors for this infection. Most of the infections are asymptomatic, but cases of severe encephalitis and endophthalmitis occur. Symptoms typically begin 2–4 weeks after inoculation. CNS infections characteristically present as acute rapidly progressive encephalitis with eosinophilic pleocytosis of the CSF. Both CNS and ocular infections resemble other larva migrans infections such as toxocariasis, and therefore *B procyonis* should be

considered in the differential diagnosis of these infections with negative *Toxocara* serology. The diagnosis of *B procyonis* is established by encountering the larvae in tissue biopsies or by serology. Treatment consists of anthelmintics and corticosteroid anti-inflammatory drugs. Prognosis is reserved, since complete resolution of symptoms has not been achieved thus far.

Murray JW, Kazacos KR: Raccoon roundworm encephalitis. Clin Infect Dis 2004;39:1484 [PMID: 15546085].

CESTODE INFECTIONS (Flukes)

1. Taeniasis & Cysticercosis

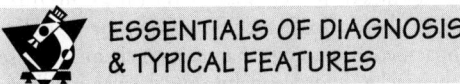

ESSENTIALS OF DIAGNOSIS & TYPICAL FEATURES

- *Mild abdominal pain; passage of worm segments (taeniasis).*
- *Focal seizures, headaches (neurocysticercosis).*
- *Cysticerci present in biopsy specimens, on plain films (as calcified masses), or on CT scan or magnetic resonance imaging.*
- *Proglottids and eggs in feces; specific antibodies in serum or CSF.*

General Considerations

Both the beef tapeworm (*Taenia saginata*) and the pork tapeworm (*Taenia solium*) cause taeniasis. The adults live in the intestines of humans; the egg-laden distal segments, or proglottids, break off and are passed in feces, disintegrating and releasing the ova in the soil. After ingestion in food or water by cattle or pigs, the eggs hatch and the larvae migrate to and encyst in skeletal muscle. Encysted larvae in meat ingested by humans mature into adult tapeworms.

Humans can be an intermediate host for *T solium* (but not *T saginata*), and the larvae released from ingested eggs encyst in a variety of tissues, especially muscle and brain. Full larval maturation occurs in 2 months, but the cysts cause little inflammation until they die months to years later. Inflammatory edema ensues with calcification or disappearance of the cyst. A slowly expanding mass of sterile cysts at the base of the brain may cause obstructive hydrocephalus (racemose cysticercosis).

Both parasites are distributed worldwide. Contamination of foods by eggs in human feces allows infection without exposure to meat or travel to endemic areas. Asymptomatic cases are common, but neurocysticercosis is a leading cause of seizures in endemic areas.

Person-to-person spread may occur, resulting in infection of individuals with no exposure to infected meat.

Clinical Findings

A. SYMPTOMS AND SIGNS

1. Taeniasis—In most tapeworm infections, the only clinical manifestation is the passage of fecal proglottids, which are white, motile bodies 1–2 cm in size. They occasionally crawl out onto the skin and down the leg, especially the larger *T saginata*. Children may harbor the adult worm for years and complain of abdominal pain, anorexia, and diarrhea.

2. Cysticercosis—Most cases are asymptomatic. Subcutaneous nodules of 1–2 cm may be the only sign. After several years, the cysticerci calcify and appear as radiographic opacities. Brain cysts may remain silent or cause seizures, headache, hydrocephalus, and basilar meningitis. Rarely, the spinal cord is involved. Neurocysticercosis manifests an average of 5 years after exposure but may cause symptoms in the first year of life. In the eye, cysts cause bleeding, retinal detachment, and uveitis. Definitive diagnosis requires histologic demonstration of larvae or cyst membrane. Presumptive diagnosis is often made by the characteristics of the cysts seen on CT scan or magnetic resonance imaging; the differential diagnosis may include tuberculoma, brain abscess, arachnoid cyst, and tumor. The presence of *T solium* eggs in feces is uncommon but supports the diagnosis.

B. LABORATORY FINDINGS

Eggs or proglottids may be found in feces or on the perianal skin (using the tape method employed for pinworms). Eggs of both *Taenia* species are identical. The species are identified by examination of proglottids.

Peripheral eosinophilia is minimal or absent. CSF eosinophilia is seen in 10–75% of cases of neurocysticercosis; its presence supports an otherwise presumptive diagnosis.

ELISA antibody titers are eventually positive in up to 98% of serum specimens and over 75% of CSF specimens from patients with neurocysticercosis. Solitary cysts are associated with seropositivity less often than are multiple cysts. High titers tend to correlate with more severe disease. CSF titers are higher if cysts are near the meninges.

Treatment

A. TAENIASIS

Praziquantel (5–10 mg/kg once) and albendazole are equally effective. Feces free of segments or ova for 3 months suggest cure.

B. CYSTICERCOSIS

Specific treatment is reserved for patients with meningitis or parenchymal cysts. In contrast, those with inactive disease require only symptomatic treatment (anticonvulsants). Praziquantel and albendazole cause disappearance of noninflamed cysts and possibly more rapid resolution of inflamed ring-enhancing cysts. Albendazole, 15 mg/kg divided into three doses daily for 8 days, is the treatment of choice. Larval death may result in clinical worsening because of inflammatory edema. A short course of dexamethasone may decrease these symptoms. Giant subarachnoidal cysts may require more than one cycle of therapy or surgery (or both). Follow-up scans every several months help assess the response to therapy. Treatment of patients with calcified lesions and seizure disorder results in a decrease of generalized seizures.

Prevention

The incidence in the United States is low, because beef and pork are inspected for taeniasis. Prevention requires proper cooking of meat, careful washing of raw vegetables and fruits, treatment of intestinal carriers, avoiding the use of human excrement for fertilizer, and providing proper sanitary facilities.

Prognosis

The prognosis is good in intestinal taeniasis. Symptoms associated with a few cerebral cysts may disappear in a few months; heavy brain infections may cause death or chronic neurologic impairment.

Garcia HH et al: A trial of antiparasitic treatment to reduce the rate of seizures due to cerebral cysticercosis. N Engl J Med 2004; 350:249 [PMID: 14724304].

Singhi P et al: One week versus four weeks of albendazole therapy for neurocysticercosis in children: a randomized placebo-controlled double blind trial. Pediatr Infect Dis J 2003;22:268 [PMID: 12634590].

2. Hymenolepiasis

Hymenolepis nana, the cosmopolitan human tapeworm, is a common parasite of children; *Hymenolepis diminuta*, the rat tapeworm, is rare. The former is capable of causing autoinfection. Larvae hatched from ingested eggs penetrate the intestinal wall and then reenter the lumen to mature into adults. Their eggs are immediately infectious for the same or a new host. The adult is only a few centimeters long. Finding the characteristic eggs in feces is diagnostic.

H diminuta has an intermediate stage in rat fleas and other insects; children are infected when they ingest these insects.

Light infections with either tapeworm are usually asymptomatic; heavy infection can cause diarrhea and abdominal pain. Therapy is with praziquantel (25 mg/kg once).

3. Echinococcosis

ESSENTIALS OF DIAGNOSIS & TYPICAL FEATURES

- Cystic tumors of liver, lung, kidney, bone, brain, and other organs.
- Eosinophilia.
- Urticaria and pruritus if cysts rupture.
- Protoscoleces or daughter cysts in the primary cyst.
- Positive serology.
- Epidemiologic evidence of exposure

General Considerations

Dogs, cats, and other carnivores are the hosts for *Echinococcus granulosus*. Endemic areas include Australia, New Zealand, and the southwestern United States, including Native American reservations where shepherding is practiced. The adult tapeworm lives in sheep intestines, and eggs are passed in the feces. When ingested by humans, the eggs hatch, and the larvae penetrate the intestinal mucosa and disseminate in the bloodstream. The larvae produce cysts; the primary sites of involvement are the liver (60–70%) and the lungs (20–25%). A unilocular cyst is most common. Over years, the cyst may reach 25 cm in diameter, although most are much smaller. The cysts of *Echinococcus multilocularis* are multilocular and demonstrate more rapid growth.

Clinical Findings

A. Symptoms and Signs

Clinical disease is due to pressure from the enlarging cysts, vessel erosion, and sensitization to cyst or worm antigens. Liver cysts present as slowly expanding tumors that may cause biliary obstruction. Most are in the right lobe and extend inferiorly; 25% are on the upper surface and may be asymptomatic for years. Omental torsion or hemorrhage from vessel erosion may occur.

Rupture of a pulmonary cyst causes coughing, dyspnea, wheezing, urticaria, chest pain, and hemoptysis; cyst and worm remnants are found in sputum. Brain cysts may cause focal neurologic signs and convulsions; renal cysts cause pain and hematuria; bone cysts cause pain.

B. Laboratory Findings

Presumptive diagnosis is made by a combination of radiographic or ultrasonographic and serologic findings. ELISA, which is the method most widely used for antibody testing, is highly sensitive but has only limited specificity.

Confirmation may be obtained by ultrasonography-guided fine-needle aspiration coupled with parasitologic exam for protoscoleces, rostellar hooks, antigens, or DNA. Eosinophilia is variable and may be absent. Serologic tests are useful for diagnosis and follow-up of therapy.

C. Imaging

Pulmonary or bone cysts may be visible on plain films. Other imaging techniques are preferred for cysts in other organs. Visualization of daughter cysts is highly suggestive of echinococcosis.

Differential Diagnosis

Tumors, bacterial or amebic abscess, and tuberculosis (pulmonary) must be considered.

Complications

Sudden cyst rupture with anaphylaxis and death is the worst complication. If the patient survives, secondary infections from seeding of daughter cysts may occur. Segmental lung collapse, secondary bacterial infections, effects of increased intracranial pressure, and severe renal damage due to renal cysts are other potential complications.

Treatment

Definitive therapy of *E multilocularis* requires meticulous surgical removal of the cysts, preceded by careful injection of the cyst with formalin, iodine, or 95% alcohol solution to sterilize infectious protoscoleces, freezing the cyst wall and injecting silver nitrate prior to its removal, or puncture-aspiration/injection-reaspiration technique, which is best suited for treatment of multiple cysts. A surgeon familiar with this disease should be consulted. Medical therapy may be of additional benefit, particularly in disseminated disease. Albendazole (15 mg/kg/d for 28 days with repeat courses as necessary following a 14-day rest period) is effective in many cases of *E granulosus* infection (hydatid disease). If the cyst leaks or ruptures, the allergic symptoms must be managed immediately.

Prognosis

Patients with large liver cysts may be asymptomatic for years. Surgery is often curative for lung and liver cysts but not always for cysts in other locations. Secondary disease has a much worse prognosis; about 15% of patients with this disease die.

Eckert J et al: Biological, epidemiological, and clinical aspects of echinococcosis, a zoonosis of increasing concern. Clin Microbiol Rev 2004;17:107 [PMID: 14726458].

Smego RA et al: Percutaneous aspiration–injection–reaspiration drainage plus albendazole or mebendazole for hepatic cystic echinococcosis: A meta-analysis. Clin Infect Dis 2003;37:83 [PMID: 14523772].

TREMATODE INFECTIONS

1. Schistosomiasis

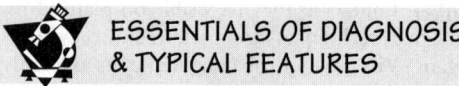

ESSENTIALS OF DIAGNOSIS & TYPICAL FEATURES

- *Transient pruritic rash after exposure to fresh water.*
- *Fever, urticaria, arthralgias, cough, lymphadenitis, and eosinophilia.*
- *Weight loss, anorexia, hepatosplenomegaly.*
- *Hematuria, dysuria.*
- *Eggs in stool, urine, or rectal biopsy specimens.*

General Considerations

One of the most common serious parasitic diseases, schistosomiasis, is caused by several species of *Schistosoma* flukes. *Schistosoma japonicum, S mekongi,* and *S mansoni* involve the intestines and *S haematobium* the urinary tract. The first two are found in eastern and southeastern Asia; *S mansoni* in tropical Africa, the Caribbean, and parts of South America; and *S haematobium* in northern Africa.

Infection is caused by free-swimming larvae (cercariae), which emerge from the intermediate hosts, certain species of freshwater snails. The cercariae penetrate human skin, migrate to the liver, and mature into adults, which then migrate through the portal vein to lodge in the bladder veins (*S haematobium*), superior mesenteric veins (*S mekongi* and *S japonicum*), or inferior mesenteric veins (*S mansoni*). Clinical disease results primarily from inflammation caused by the many eggs that are laid in the perivascular tissues or that embolize to the liver. Escape of ova into bowel or bladder lumen allows microscopic visualization and diagnosis from stool or urine specimens, as well as contamination of fresh water and infection of the snail hosts that ingest them.

Clinical Findings

Much of the population in endemic areas is infected but asymptomatic. Only heavy infections produce symptoms.

A. SYMPTOMS AND SIGNS

The cercarial penetration may cause a pruritic rash; larval migration may cause fever, urticaria, and cough; the maturation phase may cause tender hepatosplenomegaly followed by days to weeks of fever and malaise as the worms migrate to their final destination. Bladder infection results

in dysuria, hematuria, reflux, stones, and incontinence. Secondary pyelonephritis and ureteral obstruction may occur. Intestinal infection is usually asymptomatic. The final stages of disease are characterized by hepatic fibrosis, portal hypertension, splenomegaly, ascites, and bleeding from esophageal varices. The chronic inflammation in the urinary tract associated with *S haematobium* infections may result in obstructive uropathy, stones, infection, bladder cancer, fistulas, and anemia due to chronic hematuria. Spinal cord granulomas and paraplegia due to egg embolization into the Batson plexus have been reported.

B. LABORATORY FINDINGS

The diagnosis is made by finding the species-specific eggs in feces (*S japonicum, S mekongi, S mansoni,* and occasionally *S haematobium*) or urine (*S haematobium* and occasionally *S mansoni*). A rectal biopsy may reveal *S mansoni* and should be done if other specimens are negative. Peripheral eosinophilia is common, and eosinophils may be seen in urine.

Prevention

The best prevention is to avoid contact with contaminated fresh water in endemic areas. Efforts to destroy the snail hosts have been successful in areas of accelerated economic development.

Treatment

A. SPECIFIC MEASURES

Praziquantel is the treatment of choice for schistosomiasis. A dosage of 40 mg/kg/d in two divided doses (*S mansoni* or *S haematobium*) or 20 mg/kg three times in 1 day (*S japonicum* or *S mekongi*) is very effective and nontoxic. Oxamniquine (20 mg/kg/d in two doses once per day) is an alternative regimen for treatment of *S mansoni* infection. Artemether, 6 mg/kg every 3 weeks, may prevent new infections or reinfection after curative treatment.

B. GENERAL MEASURES

Medical therapy of nutritional deficiency or secondary bacterial infections may be needed. The patient's urinary tract should be evaluated carefully in *S haematobium* infection; reconstructive surgery may be needed. Hepatic fibrosis requires careful evaluation of the portal venous system and surgical management of portal hypertension when appropriate.

Prognosis

Medical therapy decreases the worm infection and liver size, despite continued exposure in endemic areas. Early disease responds well to therapy, but once significant scarring or severe inflammation has occurred, eradication of the parasites is of little benefit.

Corachan M: Schistosomiasis and international travel. Clin Infect Dis 2002;35:446 [PMID: 12145730].

Utzinger J et al: Oral artemether for prevention of *Schistosoma mansoni* infection: Randomised controlled trial. Lancet 2000; 355:1320 [PMID: 10776745].

■ MYCOTIC INFECTIONS

Fungi can be classified as yeasts, which are unicellular and reproduce by budding; as molds, which are multicellular and consist of tubular structures (hyphae) and grow by elongation and branching; or as dimorphic fungi, which can exist either as yeasts or molds depending on environmental conditions. Fungal infections can be categorized as shown in Table 39–7.

In the United States, systemic disease in normal hosts is commonly caused by three organisms—*Coccidioides, Histoplasma,* and *Blastomyces*—which are restricted to certain geographic areas. Prior residence in or travel to these areas, even for a brief time, is a prerequisite for inclusion in a differential diagnosis. Of these three, *Histoplasma* most often relapses years later in patients who are immunosuppressed.

Immunosuppression, foreign bodies (eg, central catheters), ulceration of gastrointestinal and respiratory mucosa, broad-spectrum antimicrobial therapy, malnutrition, HIV infection, and neutrophil defects or depletion are major risk factors for opportunistic fungal disease.

Laboratory diagnosis may be difficult because of the small number of fungi present in some lesions, slow growth of some organisms, and difficulty in distinguishing normal colonization of mucosal surfaces from infection. A tissue biopsy with fungal stains and culture is the best method for diagnosing systemic disease with some fungi. Repeat blood cultures may be negative even in the presence of intravascular infections. Serology is useful for diagnosing coccidioidomycosis and histoplasmosis, and antigen detection is useful for diagnosing histoplasmosis and cryptococcosis.

Susceptibility testing of *Candida* species with some drugs is now available, but testing of other organisms, especially molds, and testing with additional antifungal agents is not well standardized.

The common superficial fungal infections of the hair and skin are discussed in Chapter 14.

BLASTOMYCOSIS

General Considerations

The causative fungus, *Blastomyces dermatitidis,* is found in soil primarily in the Mississippi and Ohio River valleys, additional southeastern and south central states, and the states bordering the Great Lakes. Transmission is by inha-

lation of spores. Subclinical disease is common. Severe disease is much more common in adults and males. In children, infection rates are similar in both sexes.

Clinical Findings

A. SYMPTOMS AND SIGNS

Primary infection is unrecognized or produces pneumonia. Acute symptoms include cough, chest pain, headache, weight loss, and fever occurring several weeks to months after inoculation. Infection is usually self-limited in immunocompetent patients (50%). In some patients an indolent progressive pulmonary disease occurs after an incubation period of 30–45 days. Cutaneous lesions usually represent disseminated disease; local primary inoculation is rare. Slowly progressive ulcerating lesions with a sharp, heaped-up border or verrucous lesions occur. Bone disease resembles other forms of chronic osteomyelitis. Lytic skull lesions in children are typical, but long bones, vertebrae, and the pelvis may be involved. Extrapulmonary disease occurs in 25–40% of patients. A total body radiographic examination is advisable when blastomycosis is diagnosed in the skin or another nonpulmonary site. The genitourinary tract involvement characteristic of dissemination in adults is rare in prepubertal children. Lymph nodes, brain, and kidneys may be involved.

B. LABORATORY FINDINGS

Diagnosis requires isolation or visualization of the fungus. Pulmonary specimens (sputum, tracheal aspirates, or lung biopsy) may be positive with conventional stains or fungal cell wall stains. An initial suppurative response is followed by an increase in the number of mononuclear cells, and then formation of noncaseating granulomas. On microscopic examination, the budding yeasts are thick-walled, have refractile walls, and are very large and distinctive. Sputum specimens are positive in 50–80% of cases and skin lesions are positive in 80–100%. The fungus can be grown readily in most laboratories, but 2–4 weeks are required. Serologic tests are generally not helpful for diagnosis. An ELISA antigen detection method, similar to that used for histoplasmosis, is under study, utilizing urine, serum, and other body fluids.

C. IMAGING

Radiographic consolidation and fibronodular interstitial and alveolar infiltrates are typical; effusions, hilar nodes, and cavities are less common. The paucity of cavitation distinguishes acute blastomycosis from histoplasmosis and tuberculosis. Miliary patterns also occur with acute infection. Chronic disease can develop in the upper lobes, with cavities and fibronodular infiltrations similar to those seen in tuberculosis, but unlike in tuberculosis or histoplasmosis, these lesions rarely caseate or calcify.

Table 39–7. Pediatric fungal infections.

Type	Agents	Incidence	Diagnosis	Diagnostic Tests	Therapy	Prognosis
Superficial	*Candida* Dermatophytes *Malassezia*	Very common	Simple	KOH prep	Topical	Good
Subcutaneous	*Sporothrix*[b]	Uncommon	Simple[a]	Culture	Oral	Good
Systemic: normal host	*Coccidioides* *Histoplasma* *Blastomyces*	Common: regional	Often presumptive	Chest radiograph Serology, antigen detection (histo- plasmosis) Histology Culture of body fluids or tissue	None[c] or systemic	Good
Systemic: opportunistic infection	*Candida*[b] *Pneumocystis*[d] *Aspergillus* *Mucorales* *Malassezia* *Pseudallescheria* *Cryptococcus*	Uncommon	Difficult[e]	Tissue biopsy, cul- ture, antigen de- tection (crypto- coccosis)	Systemic, prolonged	Poor if therapy is delayed and in severely immu- nocompromised patients

KOH, potassium hydroxide.
[a]Sporotrichosis may require biopsy for diagnosis.
[b]*Candida* and *Sporothrix* in immunocompromised patients may cause severe, rapidly progressive disease and require systemic therapy.
[c]Often self-limited in normal host.
[d]Now reclassified as a fungus. May infect many normal hosts.
[e]Except *Cryptococcus,* which is often diagnosed by antigen detection.

Differential Diagnosis

Primary pulmonary infection resembles acute viral, bacterial, or mycoplasmal infections. Blastomycosis should be considered when a significant pulmonary infection in an endemic area fails to respond to antibiotic therapy. Subacute infection mimics tuberculosis, histoplasmosis, and coccidioidomycosis. Chronic pulmonary or disseminated disease must be differentiated from cancer, tuberculosis, or other fungal infections.

Treatment

Mild pulmonary blastomycosis does not require treatment; indeed, it is rarely recognized. Recommended therapy for life-threatening (especially in the immunocompromised patient) or CNS infections is amphotericin B (0.7–1.0 mg/kg intravenously for a total of 1.5–2.0 g). Itraconazole (6–8 mg/kg/d for 6 months) is preferred for other forms of blastomycosis. Bone disease may require a full year of itraconazole therapy. Surgical debridement is required for devitalized bone, drainage of large abscesses, and pulmonary lesions not responding to medical therapy.

Bradsher RW et al: Blastomycosis. Infect Dis Clin North Am 2003;17:21 [PMID: 12751259].

CANDIDIASIS

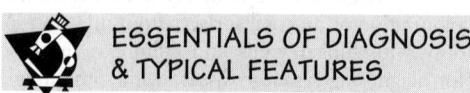 **ESSENTIALS OF DIAGNOSIS & TYPICAL FEATURES**

- *In normal or immunosuppressed individuals: superficial infections (oral thrush or ulcerations; vulvovaginitis; erythematous intertriginous rash with satellite lesions); fungemia related to intravascular devices.*

- *In immunosuppressed individuals: systemic infections (renal, hepatic, splenic, pulmonary, or cerebral abscesses); cotton-wool retinal lesions; cutaneous nodules.*

- *In either patient population: budding yeast and pseudohyphae are seen in biopsy specimens, body fluids, or scrapings of lesions; positive culture.*

General Considerations

Disease due to *Candida* is caused by *Candida albicans* in 60–80% of cases; similar systemic infection may be due to *C tropicalis, C parapsilosis, C glabrata,* and a few other *Candida* species. Speciation is important because of differences in pathogenicity and response to azole therapy. In tissue, pseudohyphae or budding yeast (or both) are seen. *Candida* grows on routine media more slowly than bacteria; growth is usually evident on agar after 2–3 days and in blood culture media in 2–7 days.

C albicans is ubiquitous and often present in small numbers on skin, mucous membranes, or in the intestinal tract. Normal bacterial flora, intact epithelial barriers, neutrophils and macrophages in conjunction with antibody and complement, and normal lymphocyte function (manifested by skin test reactivity) are factors in preventing invasion. Disseminated infection is almost always preceded by prolonged broad-spectrum antibiotic therapy, instrumentation (including intravascular catheters), or immunosuppression. Patients with diabetes mellitus are especially prone to superficial *Candida* infection; thrush and vaginitis are most common. *Candida* is the third most common blood isolate in hospitals in the United States and is a common cause of catheter-related urinary tract infection.

Clinical Findings

A. Symptoms and Signs

1. Oral candidiasis (thrush)—Adherent creamy white plaques on the buccal, gingival, or lingual mucosa are seen. These may be painful. Lesions may be few and asymptomatic, or they may be extensive, extending into the esophagus. Thrush is very common in otherwise normal infants in the first weeks of life; it may last weeks despite topical therapy. Spontaneous thrush in older children is unusual unless they have recently received antimicrobials. Steroid inhalation for asthma predisposes patients to thrush. HIV infection should be considered if there is no other reason for oral thrush, or if it is persistent or recurrent. Angular cheilitis is the name given to painful erythematous fissures caused by *Candida* at the corners of the mouth, often in association with a vitamin or iron deficiency.

2. Vaginal infection—Vulvovaginitis occurs in sexually active girls, in diabetic patients, and in girls receiving antibiotics. Thick, odorless, cheesy discharge with intense pruritus is typical. The vagina and labia are usually erythematous and swollen. Outbreaks are more frequent before menses.

3. Skin infection—

    a. Diaper dermatitis—Diaper dermatitis is often due entirely or partly to *Candida.* Pronounced erythema with a sharply defined margin and satellite lesions is typical. Pustules, vesicles, papules, or scales may be seen. Weeping, eroded lesions with a scalloped border are common. Any moist area, such as axillae or neck folds, may be involved.

    b. Congenital skin lesions—These lesions may be seen in infants born to women with *Candida* amnionitis. A red maculopapular or pustular rash is seen. Dis-

semination may occur in premature babies or infants after prolonged rupture of membranes.

    c. Scattered red papules or nodules—Such findings may represent cutaneous dissemination.

    d. Paronychia and onychomycosis—These conditions occur in immunocompetent children but are often associated with immunosuppression, hypoparathyroidism, or adrenal insufficiency (*Candida* endocrinopathy syndrome). The selective absence of specific T-cell responses to *Candida* can lead to marked, chronic skin and nail infections called chronic mucocutaneous candidiasis.

    e. Chronic draining otitis media—This problem may occur in patients who have received multiple courses of antibiotics and are superinfected with *Candida.*

4. Enteric infection—Esophageal involvement in immunosuppressed patients is the most common enteric manifestation. It is manifested by substernal pain, dysphagia, painful swallowing, and anorexia. Nausea and vomiting are common in young children. Most patients do not have thrush. Stomach or intestinal ulcers also occur. A syndrome of mild diarrhea in normal individuals who have predominant *Candida* on stool culture has also been described, although *Candida* is not considered a true enteric pathogen. Its presence more often reflects recent antimicrobial therapy.

5. Pulmonary infection—Because the organism frequently colonizes the respiratory tract, it is commonly isolated from respiratory secretions. Thus demonstration of tissue invasion is needed to diagnose *Candida* pneumonia or tracheitis. It is rare, being seen in immunosuppressed patients and patients intubated for long periods, usually while taking antibiotics. The infection may cause fever, cough, abscesses, nodular infiltrates, and effusion.

6. Renal infection—Candiduria may be the only manifestation of disseminated disease. More often, candiduria is associated with instrumentation, an indwelling catheter, or anatomic abnormality of the urinary tract. Symptoms of cystitis may be present. Masses of *Candida* may obstruct ureters and cause obstructive nephropathy. *Candida* casts in the urine suggest renal tissue infection.

7. Other infections—Endocarditis, myocarditis, meningitis, and osteomyelitis usually occur only in immunocompromised patients or neonates.

8. Disseminated candidiasis—Skin and mucosal colonization precedes but does not predict dissemination. Too often, dissemination is confused with bacterial sepsis. This occurs in neonates—especially premature infants—in an intensive care unit setting, and is recognized when the infant fails to respond to antibiotics or when candidemia is documented. These infants often have unexplained feeding intolerance, cardiovascular instability, apnea, new or worsening respiratory failure, glucose intolerance, thrombocytopenia, or hyperbilirubinemia. A careful search should be carried out for lesions suggestive of disseminated *Candida* (retinal cotton-wool spots or nodular dermal abscesses). If these findings are absent, diagnosis is often based presumptively on the presence of a compatible illness in an immunocompromised patient, a burn patient, or a patient with prolonged postsurgical or intensive care unit course who has no other cause for the symptoms; who fails to respond to antimicrobials; and who usually has *Candida* colonization of mucosal surfaces. Treatment for presumptive infection is often undertaken because candidemia is not identified antemortem in many such patients.

Hepatosplenic candidiasis occurs in immunosuppressed patients. The typical case consists of a severely neutropenic patient who develops chronic fever, variable abdominal pain, and abnormal liver function tests. No bacteria are isolated, and there is no response to antimicrobials. Symptoms persist even when neutrophils return. Ultrasound or CT scan of the liver and spleen demonstrates multiple round lesions. Biopsy is needed to confirm the diagnosis.

B. Laboratory Findings

Budding yeast cells are easily seen in scrapings or other samples. A wet mount of vaginal secretions is 40–50% sensitive; this is increased to 50–70% with the addition of 10% potassium hydroxide. The use of a gram-stain smear is 70–100% sensitive. The presence of pseudohyphae suggests tissue invasion. Culture is definitive. Ninety-five percent of positive blood cultures will be detected within 3 days, but cultures may remain negative (10–40%), even with disseminated disease or endocarditis. *Candida* should never be considered a contaminant in cultures from normally sterile sites. *Candida* in any number in appropriately collected urine suggests true infection. Antigen tests are not sensitive or specific enough for clinical use. Antibody tests are not useful. The ability of yeast to form germ tubes when incubated in human serum gives a presumptive speciation for *C albicans*.

Differential Diagnosis

Thrush may resemble formula (which can be easily wiped away with a tongue blade or swab, revealing normal mucosa without underlying erythema or erosion), other types of ulcers (including herpes), burns, or oral changes induced by chemotherapy. Skin lesions may resemble contact, allergic, chemical, or bacterial dermatitis; miliaria; folliculitis; or eczema. Candidemia and systemic infection should be considered in any seriously ill patient with the risk factors previously mentioned.

Complications

Failure to recognize disseminated disease early is the greatest complication. Arthritis and meningitis occur more often in neonates than in older children. Blindness from retinitis, massive emboli from large vegetations of endocarditis, and abscesses in any organ are other complications; the greater the length or degree of immunosuppression and the longer the delay before therapy, the more complications are seen.

Treatment

A. Oral Candidiasis

In infants, oral nystatin suspension (100,000 units four to six times a day in the buccal fold after feeding until resolution) usually suffices. Nystatin must come in contact with the lesions because it is not absorbed systemically. Older children may use it as a mouthwash (200,000–500,000 units four times a day), although it is poorly tolerated because of its taste. Clotrimazole troches (10 mg) four times a day are an alternative in older children. Prolonged therapy with either agent or more frequent dosing may be needed. Painting the lesions with a cotton swab dipped in gentian violet (0.5–1%) is visually dramatic and messy but may help refractory cases. Eradication of *Candida* from pacifiers, bottle nipples, toys, or the mother's breasts (if the infant is breast feeding and there is candidal infection of the nipples) may be helpful.

Oral azoles—fluconazole (6 mg/kg/d)—is effective in older children with candidal infection refractory to nystatin. Discontinuation of antibiotics or corticosteroids is advised when possible.

B. Skin Infection

Cutaneous infection usually responds to a cream or lotion containing nystatin, amphotericin B, or an azole. Associated inflammation, such as severe diaper dermatitis, is also helped by concurrent use of a topical mild corticosteroid cream, such as 1% hydrocortisone. One approach is to keep the involved area dry; a heat lamp and nystatin powder may be used. Cornstarch is a yeast nutrient and should not be used as a drying agent.

Suppression of intestinal *Candida* with nystatin and eradicating thrush may speed recovery and prevent recurrence of the diaper dermatitis.

C. Vaginal Infections

Vaginal infection (see Chapter 40) is treated with clotrimazole, miconazole, triazoles, or nystatin (cheapest if generic is used) suppositories or creams, usually applied once nightly for 3–7 days. In general, nystatin is less effective and longer therapy is required. A high-dose clotrimazole formulation need be given for only a single night. *Candida* balanitis in sexual partners should be treated. Oral azole therapy is equally effective. A single 150-mg oral dose of fluconazole is effective for vaginitis. It is more expensive but very convenient. No controlled study has shown that treating colonization of male sexual partners prevents recurrence in females. Frequent recurrent infections may require elimination of risk factors, the use of oral therapy, or some prophylactic antifungal therapy, such as a single dose of fluconazole weekly.

D. RENAL INFECTION

Candiduria limited to the bladder may be treated with amphotericin B bladder irrigation (if a catheter is already in place). A more effective approach is a 7- to 14-day course of fluconazole, which is concentrated in the urine. Renal abscesses or ureteral fungus balls require systemic antifungal therapy. Surgical debridement may be required. Removal of an indwelling catheter is imperative. Amphotericin B may improve poor renal function caused by renal candidiasis, even though the drug is nephrotoxic.

E. SYSTEMIC INFECTION

Systemic infection is dangerous and resistant to therapy. Surgical drainage of abscesses and removal of all infected tissue (eg, a heart valve) are required for cure. Hepatosplenic candidiasis should be treated until all lesions have disappeared or are calcified on imaging studies. Treatment of systemic infection has traditionally utilized amphotericin B or a lipid formulation. Lipid forms of amphotericin B retain the antifungal potency of the free drug but are much better tolerated. Although they are much more expensive than amphotericin B, they are indicated for patients who are intolerant of conventional therapy, for those whose infection is refractory to treatment, or for those who have a high likelihood of developing renal toxicity from such therapy. Fluconazole and the newer azole drugs, such as itraconazole and voriconazole, and a new class of drugs, echinocandins (caspofungin), are now being used interchangeably with amphotericin; in general these are less toxic. The new drugs also are often effective against fluconazole-resistant candidal infection.

Correction of predisposing factors is important (eg, discontinuing antibiotics and immunosuppressives, and improving control of diabetes). Addition of flucytosine (50–75 mg/kg/d orally in four doses; keep serum levels below 75 μg/mL) may be additive or synergistic to amphotericin B. This is frequently added to treat neonatal infections, but clinical outcome seems to be similar when amphotericin B is used alone. Unlike amphotericin B, flucytosine penetrates tissues well. It should not be used as a single agent in serious infections because resistance develops rapidly.

Fluconazole, itraconazole, and voriconazole are acceptable alternatives for serious *C albicans* infections in non-neutropenic patients and are often effective as first-line therapy in immunocompromised patients. However, the decision to use systemic azole therapy should include consideration of the local experience with azole-resistant *Candida*. Susceptibility testing for *Candida* species is now available to guide this decision. *C glabrata* and *C krusei* are common isolates that may be resistant to fluconazole; these may be susceptible to the newer azoles and caspofungin. Infected central venous lines must be removed immediately; this alone often is curative. Persistent fever and candidemia suggest infected thrombus, endocarditis, or tissue infection. If the infection is considered limited to the line and environs, a 14-day course (after the last positive culture) of a systemic antifungal agent following line removal is recommended for immunocompromised patients. Systemic azole therapy should also be considered for immunocompetent patients with candidemia, because of the late occurrence of focal *Candida* infection in some cases.

Fluconazole is well absorbed (oral and intravenous therapy are equivalent), reasonably nontoxic, and effective for a variety of *Candida* infections. Fluconazole dosage is 8–12 mg/kg/d in a single daily dose for initial therapy of severely ill children. Selected patients with prolonged immunosuppression (eg, after bone marrow transplantation) should receive fluconazole, itraconazole, or intermittent amphotericin B prophylaxis. These drugs are less expensive than the lipid formulations of amphotericin and are becoming first-line alternatives.

Prognosis

Superficial disease in normal hosts has a good prognosis; in abnormal hosts, it may be refractory to therapy. Early therapy of systemic disease is often curative if the underlying immune response is adequate. The outcome is poor when therapy is delayed or when host response is inadequate.

Bendel CM: Nosocomial neonatal candidiasis. Pediatr Infect Dis J 2005;24:831 [PMID: 16148852].

Chapman RL: *Candida* infections in the neonate. Curr Opin Pediatr 2003;15:97 [PMID: 12544279].

Kalfa VC et al: The syndrome of chronic mucocutaneous candidiasis with selective antibody deficiency. Ann Allergy Asthma Immunol 2003;90:259 [PMID: 12602677].

Pappas PG et al: Guidelines for treatment of candidiasis. Clin Infect Dis 2004;38:161 [PMID: 14699449].

Segal E: Candida, still number one—what do we know and where are we going from there? Mycoses 2005;48(Suppl 1):3 [PMID: 15887329].

Williams K et al: Lipid amphotericin preparations. Pediatr Infect Dis J 2000;19:567 [PMID: 10877175].

COCCIDIOIDOMYCOSIS

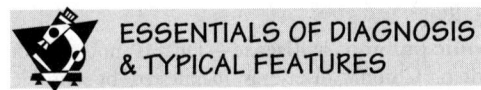

ESSENTIALS OF DIAGNOSIS & TYPICAL FEATURES

- *Residence in or travel to an endemic area.*
- *Primary pulmonary form: fever, chest pain, cough, anorexia, weight loss, and often a macular rash or erythema nodosum or multiforme.*

- *Primary cutaneous form: trauma followed in 1–3 weeks by an ulcer and regional adenopathy.*
- *Spherules seen in pus, sputum, CSF, joint fluid; positive culture.*
- *Appearance of precipitating (early) and complement-fixing antibodies (late).*

General Considerations

Coccidioidomycosis is caused by the dimorphic fungus *Coccidioides immitis,* which is endemic in the Sonoran Desert areas of western parts of Texas, southern New Mexico and Arizona, southern California, northern Mexico, and South America. Infection results from inhalation or inoculation of arthrospores (highly contagious and readily airborne in the dry climate). Even brief travel in or through an endemic area, especially during windy seasons, may allow infection. Human-to-human transmission does not occur. More than half of all infections are asymptomatic, and fewer than 5–10% are associated with significant pulmonary disease. Chronic pulmonary disease or dissemination occurs in less than 1% of cases.

Clinical Findings

A. SYMPTOMS AND SIGNS

1. Primary disease—The incubation period is 10–16 days (range, 7–28 days). Symptoms vary from those of a mild fever and arthralgia to severe influenzalike illness with high fever, nonproductive cough, pleurisy, myalgias, arthralgias, headache, night sweats, and anorexia. Upper respiratory tract signs are not common. Severe pleuritic chest pain suggests this diagnosis. Signs vary from none to rash, rales, pleural rubs, and signs of pulmonary consolidation. Weight loss may occur.

2. Skin disease—Up to 10% of children develop erythema nodosum or multiforme. These manifestations imply a favorable host response to the organism. Less specific maculopapular eruptions occur in a larger number of children. Skin lesions can occur following fungemia. Primary skin inoculation sites develop indurated ulcers with local adenopathy. Contiguous involvement of skin from deep infection in nodes or bone also occurs. The presence of chronic skin lesions with this fungus should lead to a search for other areas of infection (eg, lung).

3. Chronic pulmonary disease—This is uncommon in children. Chronic disease is manifested by chronic cough (occasionally with hemoptysis), weight loss, pulmonary consolidation, effusion, cavitation, or pneumothorax.

4. Disseminated disease—This is less common in children than adults. It is more common in infants, neonates, pregnant women (especially during the third trimester), blacks, Filipinos, American Indians, and patients with HIV or other types of immunosuppression. One or more organs may be involved. The most common sites involved are bone or joint (usually a single bone or joint; subacute or chronic swelling, pain, redness), nodes, meninges (slowly progressive meningeal signs, ataxia, vomiting, headache, and cranial neuropathies), and kidney (dysuria and urinary frequency). As with most fungal diseases, the evolution of the illness is usually slow.

B. LABORATORY FINDINGS

Direct examination of respiratory secretions, pus, CSF, or tissue may reveal large spherules (30–60 μm) containing endospores. These are the product of coccidioidal spores germinating in tissue. Phase-contrast microscopy is useful for demonstrating these refractile bodies; Gram or methylene blue stains are not helpful, but periodic acid-Schiff reagent, methenamine silver, and calcofluor stains are. Fluffy, gray-white colonies grow within 2–5 days on routine fungal and many other media. They are highly infectious. CSF cultures are often negative.

Routine laboratory tests are nonspecific. The sedimentation rate is usually elevated. Eosinophilia may occur, particularly prior to dissemination, and is more common in coccidioidomycosis than in many other conditions with similar symptoms. Meningitis causes a mononuclear pleocytosis (70% with eosinophils) with elevated protein and mild hypoglycorrhachia.

Within 2–21 days, most patients develop a delayed hypersensitivity reaction to coccidioidin skin test antigen (Spherulin 0.1 mL, intradermally, should produce 5-mm induration at 48 hours). Erythema nodosum predicts strong reactivity; when this reaction is present the antigen should be diluted 10–100 times before use. The skin test may be negative in immunocompromised patients or in those with disseminated disease. Positive reactions may remain for years and do not prove active infection.

Antibodies consist of precipitins (usually measurable by 2–3 weeks in 90% of cases and gone by 12 weeks) and complement-fixing antibodies (delayed for several weeks; appear as the precipitins are falling and disappear by 8 months, unless dissemination or chronic infection occurs). The extent of the complement-fixing antibody response reflects the severity of infection. Persistent high levels suggest dissemination. Serum precipitins usually indicate acute infection. Excellent ELISA assays are now available to detect IgM and IgG antibodies against the precipitin and complement-fixing antigens. The presence of antibody in CSF indicates CNS infection.

C. IMAGING

Approximately half of symptomatic infections are associated with abnormal chest radiographs—usually infiltrates with hilar adenopathy. Pulmonary consolidation, effusion, and thin-walled cavities may be seen. About 5% of infected patients have asymptomatic nodules or cysts after recovery. Unlike reactivation tuberculosis, apical disease is not prominent. Bone infection causes osteolysis that enhances with technetium. Cerebral imaging may show hydrocephalus and meningitis; intracranial abscesses and calcifications are unusual. Radiographic evolution of all lesions is slow.

Differential Diagnosis

Primary pulmonary infection resembles acute viral, bacterial, or mycoplasmal infections; subacute presentation mimics tuberculosis, histoplasmosis, and blastomycosis. Chronic pulmonary or disseminated disease must be differentiated from cancer, tuberculosis, or other fungal infections.

Complications

Dissemination of primary pulmonary disease is associated with ethnic background, prolonged fever (> 1 month), a negative skin test, high complement-fixation antibody titer, and marked hilar adenopathy. Local pulmonary complications include effusion, empyema, and pneumothorax. Cerebral infection can cause noncommunicating hydrocephalus due to basilar meningitis.

Treatment

A. SPECIFIC MEASURES

Mild pulmonary infections in most normal hosts require no therapy. These patients should be assessed for 1–2 years to document resolution and to identify any complications early. Antifungal therapy is used for prolonged fever, weight loss (> 10%), prolonged duration of night sweats, severe pneumonitis (especially if persisting for 4–6 weeks), or any form of disseminated disease. Neonates, those with genetic risk factors, pregnant women, and those with high antibody titer also receive treatment. Therapy is often utilized for pregnant women and subjects with high-risk racial origins.

Amphotericin B is used to treat severe disease (1 mg/kg/d until better, then reduce dose; total duration, 2–3 months). Lipid formulations are used at 2–5 mg/kg/d. In general, the more rapidly progressing the infection, the more compelling the case for amphotericin B therapy. For less severe disease and for meningeal disease, fluconazole or itraconazole are preferred (duration of therapy is more than 6 months, and is indefinite for meningeal disease). Measurement of serum levels is suggested to monitor therapy. Chronic fibrocavitary pneumonia is treated for at least 12 months. Lifelong suppressive therapy is recommended after treating coccidioidal meningitis. Itraconazole may be

superior to fluconazole. Refractory meningitis may require prolonged intrathecal or intraventricular amphotericin B therapy. Pregnant patients should not receive azoles.

B. GENERAL MEASURES

Most pulmonary infections require only symptomatic therapy, self-limited activity, and good nutrition. They are not contagious.

C. SURGICAL MEASURES

Excision of chronic pulmonary cavities or abscesses may be needed. Infected nodes, sinus tracts, and bone are other operable lesions. Azole therapy should be given prior to surgery to prevent dissemination; it is continued for 4 weeks arbitrarily or until other criteria for cure are met.

Prognosis

Most patients recover. Even with amphotericin B, however, disseminated disease may be fatal, especially in those racially predisposed to severe disease. Reversion of the skin test to negative or a rising complement-fixing antibody titer are ominous signs. Individuals who later in life undergo immunosuppressive therapy or develop HIV may experience reactivation of dormant disease. Thus, some programs determine prior infection by serology and either provide prophylaxis or observe patients closely during periods of intense immune suppression.

Cortez KJ et al: Successful treatment of coccidioidal meningitis with voriconazole. Clin Infect Dis 2003;36;1619 [PMID: 12802765].

Galgiani JN et al: Coccidioidomycosis. Clin Infect Dis 2005;41: 1217 [PMID: 16206093].

CRYPTOCOCCOSIS

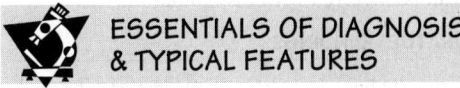

ESSENTIALS OF DIAGNOSIS & TYPICAL FEATURES

- *Acute pneumonitis in immunocompetent individuals.*
- *Immunosuppressed patients especially vulnerable to CNS infection (headache, vomiting, cranial nerve palsies, meningeal signs; mononuclear cell pleocytosis).*
- *Cryptococcal antigen detected in CSF; also in serum and urine in some patients.*
- *Readily isolated on routine media.*

General Considerations

Cryptococcus neoformans is a ubiquitous soil yeast. It appears to survive better in soil contaminated with bird excrement, especially that of pigeons. However, most infections in humans are not associated with a history of significant contact with birds. Inhalation is the presumed route of inoculation. Infections in children are rare, even in heavily immunocompromised patients such as those with HIV infection. Immunocompetent individuals can also be infected. Asymptomatic carriage does not occur.

Clinical Findings

A. SYMPTOMS AND SIGNS

1. Pulmonary disease—Pulmonary infection precedes dissemination to other organs. It is frequently asymptomatic (most older children and adults have serologic evidence of prior infection) and less often clinically apparent than cryptococcal meningitis. Pneumonia is the primary manifestation in one-third of patients and CNS disease in 50%; cryptococcal pneumonia may coexist with cerebral involvement. Symptoms are nonspecific and subacute—cough, weight loss, and fatigue. The fungus can persist in a latent form in subpleural granulomas.

2. Meningitis—The most common clinical disease is meningitis, which follows hematogenous spread from a pulmonary focus. Symptoms of headache, vomiting, and fever occur over days to months. Meningeal signs and papilledema are common. Cranial nerve dysfunction and seizures may occur.

3. Other forms—Cutaneous forms are usually secondary to dissemination. Papules, pustules, and ulcerating nodules are typical. Bones (rarely joints) may be infected; osteolytic areas are seen, and the process may resemble osteosarcoma. Many other organs, especially the eye, can be involved with dissemination.

B. LABORATORY FINDINGS

The CSF usually has a lymphocytic pleocytosis; it may be completely normal in immunosuppressed patients who have cryptococcal meningitis. Direct microscopy may reveal organisms in sputum, CSF, or other specimens. The capsular antigen can be detected by latex agglutination or ELISA, which are both sensitive (> 90%) and specific. Serum, CSF, and urine may be tested. The serum may be negative if the only organ infected is the lung. False-negative CSF tests have been reported. The organism grows well after several days on many routine media; for optimal culture, collecting and concentrating a large amount of CSF (≤ 10 mL) is recommended, because the number of organisms may be low.

C. IMAGING

Radiographic findings are usually lower lobe infiltrates or nodular densities; less often effusions; and rarely cavitation, hilar adenopathy, or calcification. Single or multiple focal mass lesions (cryptococcoma) may be detected in the CNS on CT or magnetic resonance imaging scan.

Differential Diagnosis

Cryptococcal meningitis may mimic tuberculosis, viral meningoencephalitis, meningitis due to other fungi, or a space-occupying CNS lesion. Lung infection is difficult to differentiate from many causes of pneumonia.

Complications

Hydrocephalus may be caused by chronic basilar meningitis. Symptomatic intracranial hypertension is common. Significant pulmonary or osseous disease may accompany the primary infection or dissemination.

Treatment

Patients with symptomatic pulmonary disease should receive fluconazole for 3–6 months. All immunocompromised patients should have a lumbar puncture to rule out CNS infection; this should also be done for immunocompetent patients with cryptococcal antigen in the serum. Severely ill patients should instead receive amphotericin B (0.7 mg/kg/d). Meningitis is treated with amphotericin B and flucytosine (100 mg/kg/d). The combination is synergistic and allows lower doses of amphotericin B to be used. Therapy is usually 6 weeks for cerebral infections (or for 1 month after sterilization) and 8 weeks for osteomyelitis. An alternative is to substitute fluconazole after 2 weeks of the combination therapy and continue fluconazole alone for 8–10 weeks. Fluconazole is the preferred maintenance therapy to prevent relapses in high-risk (HIV) patients. CSF antigen levels should be checked after 2 weeks of therapy. Intracranial hypertension is treated by frequent spinal taps or a lumbar drain.

Prognosis

Treatment failure, including death, is common in immunosuppressed patients, especially those with AIDS. Lifelong maintenance therapy is required in these patients. Poor prognostic signs are the presence of extrameningeal disease; fewer than 20 cells/μL of initial CSF; and initial CSF antigen titer greater than 1:32.

Lindell RM et al: Pulmonary cryptococcosis. CT findings in immunocompetent patients. Radiology 2005;236:326 [PMID: 15987984].

Pappas PG: Managing cryptococcal meningitis is about handling the pressure. Clin Infect Dis 2005;40:480 [PMID: 15668875].

Perfect TF, Casadevall A: Cryptococcosis. Infect Dis Clin North Am 2002;16:837 [PMID: 12512184].

HISTOPLASMOSIS

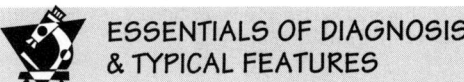

ESSENTIALS OF DIAGNOSIS & TYPICAL FEATURES

- *Residence in or travel to endemic areas.*
- *Pneumonia with flulike illness.*
- *Hepatosplenomegaly, anemia, leukopenia if disseminated.*
- *Histoplasmal antigen in urine, blood, or CSF.*
- *Detection of the organism in smears or tissue or by culture.*

General Considerations

The dimorphic fungus *Histoplasma capsulatum* is found in the central and eastern United States (Ohio and Mississippi River valleys), Mexico, and most of South America. Soil contamination is enhanced by the presence of bat or bird feces. The small yeast form (2–4 μm) is seen in tissue, especially within macrophages. Infection is acquired by inhaling spores that transform into the pathogenic yeast phase. Infections in endemic areas are very common at all ages and are usually asymptomatic. Over two-thirds of children are infected in these areas. Reactivation is very rare in children; it may occur years later, usually owing to significant immunosuppression. Reinfection also occurs. The extent of symptoms with primary or reinfection is influenced by the size of the infecting inoculum.

Clinical Findings

Because human-to-human transmission does not occur, infection requires exposure in the endemic area—usually within prior weeks or months. Congenital infection does not occur.

A. SYMPTOMS AND SIGNS

1. Asymptomatic infection (50% of infections)— Asymptomatic histoplasmosis is usually diagnosed by the presence of scattered calcifications in lungs or spleen and a positive skin test. The calcification may resemble that caused by tuberculosis but may be more extensive than the usual Ghon complex.

2. Pneumonia—Approximately 45% of patients have mild to moderate disease. Most of these patients are not recognized as having a histoplasmal infection. Acute pulmonary disease may resemble influenza, with fever, myal-

gia, arthralgia, and cough occurring 1–3 weeks after exposure; the subacute form resembles infections such as tuberculosis, with cough, weight loss, night sweats, and pleurisy. Chronic disease is unusual in children. Physical examination may be normal, or rales may be heard. A small number of patients may have immune-mediated signs such as arthritis, pericarditis, and erythema nodosum. The usual duration of the disease is less than 2 weeks, followed by complete resolution. Symptoms may last several months and still resolve without antifungal therapy.

3. Disseminated infection (5% of infections)— Fungemia during primary infection probably occurs in the first 2 weeks of all infections, including those with minimal symptoms. Transient hepatosplenomegaly may occur, but resolution is the rule in immunocompetent individuals. Heavy exposure, severe underlying pulmonary disease, and immunosuppression are risk factors for progressive reticuloendothelial cell infection, with anemia, fever, weight loss, organomegaly, bone marrow involvement, and death. Dissemination may occur in otherwise immunocompetent children; usually they are younger than age 2 years.

4. Other forms—Ocular involvement consists of multifocal choroiditis. This usually occurs in immunocompetent adults who exhibit other evidence of disseminated disease. Brain, heart valve, pericardium, intestine, and skin (oral ulcers and nodules) are other involved sites. Adrenal gland involvement is common with systemic disease.

B. LABORATORY FINDINGS

Routine tests are normal or nonspecific in the benign forms. Pancytopenia is present in many patients with disseminated disease. The diagnosis can be made by demonstrating the organism by histology or culture. Tissue yeast forms are small and may be mistaken for artifact. They are usually found in macrophages, occasionally in peripheral blood leukocytes in severe disease, but rarely in sputum, urine, or CSF. Cultures of infected fluids or tissues may yield the organism after 1–6 weeks of incubation on fungal media, but even cultures of bronchoalveolar lavage or transbronchial biopsy specimens in immunocompromised patients are often negative (15%). Thus bone marrow and tissue specimens are needed. Detection of histoplasmal antigen in blood, urine, CSF, and bronchoalveolar lavage fluid is probably the most sensitive diagnostic test (90% positive in the urine with disseminated disease; 75% positive with acute pneumonia). The level of antigen correlates with the extent of the infection, and antigen levels can be used to follow the response to therapy and to indicate low-grade infection persisting after completion of therapy (eg, in a child with HIV infection).

Antibodies may be detected by immunodiffusion, complement fixation, and precipitation; the latter two measures rise in the first 2–6 weeks of illness and fall unless dissemination occurs. Cross-reactions occur with some other endemic fungi. A single high titer or rising titer indicates a high likelihood of disease. Antigen detection has replaced serology as a rapid diagnostic test.

C. IMAGING

Scattered pulmonary calcifications in a well child are typical of past infection. Bronchopneumonia (focal mid-lung infiltrates) occurs with acute disease, often with hilar and mediastinal adenopathy, occasionally with nodules, but seldom with effusion. Apical cavitation occurs with chronic infection, often on the background of preexisting pulmonary infection.

Differential Diagnosis

Pulmonary disease resembles viral infection, tuberculosis, coccidioidomycosis, and blastomycosis. Systemic disease resembles disseminated fungal or mycobacterial infection, leukemia, histiocytosis, or cancer.

Treatment

Mild infections do not require therapy. Treatment is indicated for severe pulmonary disease (diffuse radiographic involvement); disseminated disease; when endovascular, CNS, or chronic pulmonary disease is present; and for children younger than age 1 year. Treatment should also be considered for patients who show no clinical improvement after 1 month. Disseminated disease in infants may respond to as few as 10 days of amphotericin B, although 4–6 weeks (or 30 mg/kg total dosage) is usually recommended. Amphotericin B is the preferred therapy for moderately severe forms of the disease. Patients with severe disease may benefit from a short course of steroid therapy (see also section on *Pneumocystis jiroveci*). Surgical excision of chronic pulmonary lesions is rarely required. Itraconazole (3–5 mg/kg/d for 6–12 weeks; achieve peak serum level of > 1.0 μg/mL) appears to be equivalent to amphotericin B therapy for mild disease and can be substituted for amphotericin B in severe disease after a favorable initial response has occurred. With chronic pulmonary, CNS, or disseminated disease, therapy may be required for prolonged periods.

Quantification of fungal antigen is useful for directing therapy. Histoplasmosis can reactivate in previously infected individuals who subsequently become immunosuppressed. Chronically immunosuppressed patients (eg, those with HIV) may require lifelong maintenance therapy with an azole.

Prognosis

Mild and moderately severe infections have a good prognosis. With early diagnosis and treatment, infants with disseminated disease usually recover; the prognosis worsens if the immune response is poor.

Silveira F, Paterson DL: Pulmonary fungal infections. Curr Opin Pulm Med 2005;11:242 [PMID: 15818187].

Wheat LJ, Kauffman CA: Histoplasmosis. Infect Dis Clin North Am 2003;17:1 [PMID: 1271258].

SPOROTRICHOSIS

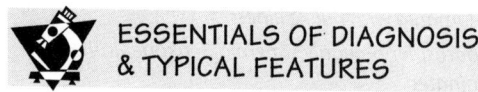

ESSENTIALS OF DIAGNOSIS & TYPICAL FEATURES

- *Subacute cutaneous ulcers.*
- *New lesions appearing proximal to existing lesions along a draining lymphatic.*
- *Absence of systemic symptoms.*
- *Isolation of Sporothrix schenckii from wound drainage or biopsy.*

General Considerations

Sporotrichosis is caused by *Sporothrix schenckii*, a dimorphic fungus present as a mold in soil, plants, and plant products from most areas of North and South America. Spores of the fungus can cause infection when they breach the skin at areas of minor trauma. Sporotrichosis has been transmitted from cutaneous lesions of pets.

Clinical Findings

Cutaneous disease is by far the most common manifestation. Typically at the site of inapparent skin injury an initial papular lesion will slowly become nodular and ulcerate. Subsequent new lesions develop in a similar fashion proximally along lymphatics draining the primary lesion. This sequence of developing painless, chronic ulcers in a linear pattern is strongly suggestive of the diagnosis. Solitary lesions may exist and some lesions may develop a verrucous character. Systemic symptoms are absent and laboratory evaluations are normal, except for acute phase reactants. The fungus rarely disseminates in immunocompetent hosts, but bone and joint infections have been described. Cavitary pneumonia is an uncommon manifestation when patients inhale the spores. Immunocompromised patients, especially those with HIV infection, may develop multiorgan disease and extensive pneumonia.

Diagnosis

The differential diagnosis of nodular lymphangitis (sporotrichoid infection) includes other endemic fungi and some bacteria, especially atypical mycobacteria. Diagnosis is made by culture. Biopsy of skin lesions will demonstrate a suppurative response with granulomas and provides the best source for laboratory isolation. Occasionally the characteristic yeast will be seen in the biopsy.

Treatment & Prognosis

Treatment is with itraconazole (100 mg/d or 5 mg/kg/d) for 3–6 months. Prognosis is excellent with lympho-cutaneous disease in immunocompetent children. Pulmonary or osteoarticular disease, especially in immunocompromised individuals, requires longer therapy, and surgical debridement may be required.

Burch JM et al: Unsuspected sporotrichosis in childhood. Pediatr Infect Dis J 2001;20:442 [PMID: 11332673].

Pang KR et al: Subcutaneous fungal infections. Dermatol Ther 2004;17:523 [PMID 15571502].

Queiroz-Telles F et al: Subcutaneous mycoses. Infect Dis Clin North Am 2003;17;59 [PMID: 12751261].

OPPORTUNISTIC FUNGAL INFECTIONS

These infections occur most commonly when therapy with steroids, antineoplastic drugs, or radiation is used for treatment, thereby reducing the number or function of neutrophils and competent lymphocytes. Inborn errors in immune function (combined immune deficiency or chronic granulomatous disease) may also be complicated by these fungal infections. Infection is also facilitated by altering the normal flora with antibiotics and by disruption of mucous membranes or skin with antineoplastic therapy and with indwelling lines and tubes.

Table 39–8 indicates that filamentous fungi are prominent causes of severe systemic fungal disease in immunocompromised patients. *Aspergillus* species (usually *fumigatus*) and Zygomycetes (usually Mucorales) cause subacute pneumonia and sinusitis and should be considered when these conditions do not respond to antibiotics in immunocompromised patients. Mucormycosis is especially likely to produce severe sinusitis in patients with chronic acidosis, usually because of poorly controlled diabetes. This fungus may invade the orbit and cause brain infection. Mucormycosis also occurs in patients receiving iron chelation therapy. These fungal infections may disseminate widely. Imaging procedures may suggest these infections, but they are best diagnosed by aspiration or biopsy of infected tissues. *Cryptococcus*, which can cause disease in the immunocompetent host, is more likely to be clinically apparent and severe in immunocompromised patients. This yeast causes pneumonia and is a prominent cause of fungal meningitis. *Candida* species in these patients cause

fungemia and multiorgan disease, with lung, esophagus, liver, and spleen frequently affected.

Malassezia furfur is a yeast that normally causes the superficial skin infection known as tinea versicolor (see Chapter 14). This organism is considered an opportunist when it is associated with prolonged intravenous therapy, especially central lines used for hyperalimentation. The yeast, which requires skin lipids for its growth, can infect lines when lipids are present in the infusate. Some species will grow in the absence of lipids. Unexplained fever and thrombocytopenia are common. Pulmonary infiltrates may be present. The diagnosis is facilitated by alerting the bacteriology laboratory to add olive oil to culture media. The infection will respond to removal of the line or the lipid supplement. Amphotericin B may hasten resolution.

Opportunistic fungal infections are always in the differential diagnosis for immunocompromised patients with unexplained fever or pulmonary infiltrates. These pathogens should be aggressively pursued with imaging studies and with tissue sampling when clues are available. These infections are difficult to treat. Amphotericin B and appropriate triazole drugs are usually indicated. Caspofungin, the first echinocandin, and voriconazole, a new triazole, are now available to treat *Candida* and *Aspergillus* infections. Combinations of current antifungal drugs are being tested in order to improve the outcome. Many children who will have depressed phagocytic and T-cell–mediated immune function for long periods should receive antifungal prophylaxis, most often itraconazole.

Marr KA et al: *Aspergillus* pathogenesis, clinical manifestations, and therapy. Infect Dis Clin North Am 2002;16:875 [PMID: 12512185].

Spellberg B et al: Novel perspectives on mucormycosis: pathophysiology, presentation, and management. Clin Microbiology Rev 2005;18:556 [PMID: 16020690].

PNEUMOCYSTIS JIROVECI INFECTION

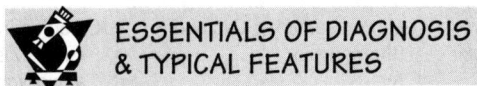

ESSENTIALS OF DIAGNOSIS & TYPICAL FEATURES

- *Significant immunosuppression.*
- *Fever, tachypnea, cough, dyspnea.*
- *Hypoxemia; diffuse interstitial infiltrates.*

General Considerations

Although classified as a fungus on the basis of structural and nucleic acid characteristics, *Pneumocystis* responds readily to antiprotozoal drugs and antifols. It is a ubiqui-

Table 39–8. Unusual fungal infections in children.

Organism	Predisposing Factors	Route of Infection	Clinical Disease	Diagnostic Tests	Therapy and Comments
Aspergillus species	None	Inhalation of spores	Allergic bronchopulmonary aspergillosis; wheezing, cough, migratory infiltrates, eosinophilia.	Organisms in sputum; positive skin test; specific IgE antibody; elevated IgE levels.	Hypersensitivity to fungal antigens. Use steroids. Antifungals may not be needed.
	Immunosuppression	Inhalation of spores	Progressive pulmonary disease: consolidation, nodules, abscesses. Sinusitis. Disseminated disease: usually lung, brain; occasionally intestine, kidney, heart, bone. Invades blood vessels.	Demonstrate fungus in tissues by stain or culture; septate hyphae branching at 45-degree angle.	Amphotericin B, voriconazole, and oral caspofungin are equally effective; these can be used in combination.
Malassezia furfur, M pachydermatis	Central venous catheter, usually lipid infusion (can occur in the absence of lipid)	Line infection from skin colonization	Sepsis; pneumonitis, thrombocytopenia.	Culture of catheter or blood on lipid-enriched media (for *M furfur; M pachydermatis* does not need lipid). Fungus may be seen in buffy coat.	Discontinuation of lipid may be sufficient. Remove catheter. Short-term amphotericin B may be added. Organism ubiquitous on normal skin; requires long-chain fatty acids for growth.
Mucorales (*Mucor, Rhizopus, Absidia*)	Immunosuppression, diabetic acidosis, iron chelation therapy	Inhalation, mucosal colonization	Rhinocerebral: sinus, nose, necrotizing vasculitis; central nervous system spread. Pulmonary. Disseminated: any organ.	Broad aseptate hyphae branching at 90-degree angles demonstrates fungus in tissues by stain. Culture: rapidly growing, fluffy fungus.	Amphotericin B, surgical débridement; voriconazole may be a second agent for combined therapy. Poor prognosis.
Pseudallescheria boydii	Immunosuppression	Inhalation	Disseminated abscesses (lung, brain, liver, spleen, other).	Culture of pus or tissue.	Surgical drainage; voriconazole or caspofungin.
	Minor trauma	Cutaneous	Mycetoma (most common).	Yellow-white granules in pus. Culture.	Aggressive surgery. Amputation may be needed.
Sporothrix schenckii	Minor trauma (thorns, splinters)	Cutaneous	Chronic skin ulcers, subcutaneous nodules along lymphatics. Rarely pneumonia, osteomyelitis, arthritis. Disseminated disease in immunocompromised host.	Gram or fungal stain of pus or tissue may show "hockey stick" organisms. Culture of pus, tissue.	Itraconazole, drainage, débridement.

tous pathogen. Initial infection was presumed to occur asymptomatically via inhalation, usually in early childhood, and to become a clinical problem upon reactivation during immune suppression. There is now evidence that person-to-person transmission may contribute to symptomatic disease. Nevertheless, it appears that in the normal host clinical disease rarely occurs. A syndrome of afebrile pneumonia similar to that caused by *Chlamydia trachomatis* in normal infants has been described but is rarely diagnosed. Whether by reactivation or new exposure, severe signs and symptoms occur chiefly in patients with abnormal T-cell function such as occurs with HIV infection, hematologic malignancies, and organ transplantation. Prolonged, high-dose corticosteroid therapy for any condition is a risk factor; onset of illness as steroids are tapered is a typical presentation. Severely malnourished infants with no underlying illness may also develop this infection, as can those with congenital humoral or cellular immune deficiency. The incubation period is usually at least 1 month after onset of immunosuppression.

Pneumocystis pneumonia is a common complication of advanced HIV infection and is one of the diseases that defines AIDS. Prophylaxis usually prevents this infection (see Chapter 37).

Infection is generally limited to the lower respiratory tract. In advanced disease, spread to other organs occurs.

Clinical Findings

A. SYMPTOMS AND SIGNS

In most patients, a gradual onset of fever, tachypnea, dyspnea, and mild, nonproductive cough occurs over 1–4 weeks. Initially the chest is clear, although retractions and nasal flaring are present. At this stage the illness is nonspecific. Hypoxemia out of proportion to the clinical and radiographic signs is an early finding, however, and even minimally decreased arterial oxygen pressure values should suggest this diagnosis in immunosuppressed children. Tachypnea, nonproductive cough, and dyspnea progress. Respiratory failure and death occur without treatment. In some children with AIDS or severe immunosuppression from chemotherapy or organ transplantation, the onset may be abrupt and progression more rapid. Acute dyspnea with pleuritic pain may indicate the related complication of pneumothorax.

The general examination is unremarkable except for tachypnea and tachycardia. There are no upper respiratory signs, conjunctivitis, organomegaly, enanthem, or rash.

B. LABORATORY FINDINGS

Laboratory findings reflect the individual child's underlying illness and are not specific. Serum lactate dehydrogenase levels may be elevated markedly as a result of pulmonary damage. In moderately severe cases, the arterial oxygen pressure is less than 70 mm Hg or the alveolar-arterial gradient is less than 35 mm Hg.

C. IMAGING

Early chest radiographs are normal. The classic pattern in later films is that of bilateral, interstitial, lower lobe alveolar disease starting in the perihilar regions, without effu-sion, consolidation, or hilar adenopathy. High resolution CT may reveal extensive ground-glass attenuation or cystic lesions. Older HIV-infected patients present with other patterns, including nodular infiltrates, lobar pneumonia, cavities, and upper lobe infiltrates.

Diagnosis

Diagnosis requires finding characteristic round (6–8 mm) cysts in a lung biopsy specimen, bronchial brushings, alveolar washings, induced sputum, or tracheal aspirates. The latter specimens are less sensitive but are more rapidly and easily obtained. They are more often negative in children with leukemia compared with those with HIV infection; presumably, greater immunosuppression results in larger numbers of organisms. Because pneumonia in immunosuppressed patients may have many causes, negative results from tracheal secretions should prompt more aggressive diagnostic attempts. Bronchial washing using fiberoptic bronchoscopy is usually well tolerated and rapidly performed.

Several rapid stains—as well as the standard methenamine silver stain—are useful. The indirect fluorescent antibody method is most sensitive. These methods require competent laboratory evaluation, because few organisms may be present and many artifacts may be found.

Differential Diagnosis

In immunocompetent infants, *C trachomatis* pneumonia is the most common cause of the afebrile pneumonia syndrome described for *Pneumocystis*. In older immunocompromised children, the differential diagnosis includes influenza, respiratory syncytial virus, cytomegalovirus, adenovirus, and other viral infections; bacterial and fungal pneumonia; pulmonary emboli or hemorrhage; congestive heart failure; and *Chlamydia pneumoniae* and *Mycoplasma pneumoniae* infections. Lymphoid interstitial pneumonitis, which occurs in older infants with HIV infection, is more indolent and the patient's lactate dehydrogenase level is normal (see Chapter 37). *Pneumocystis* pneumonia is uncommon in children who are complying with prophylactic regimens.

Prevention

Children at high risk for developing *Pneumocystis* infection should receive prophylactic therapy. Children at risk include those with hematologic malignancies or for other reasons are receiving intensive chemotherapy or high-dose corticosteroids, and children with organ transplants or advanced HIV infection. All children born to HIV-infected mothers should receive prophylaxis against *Pneumocystis* starting at age 6 weeks. Prophylaxis should be maintained until HIV infection has been ruled out, or if the infant is infected, until the patient's immunologic status has been clarified (see Chapter 37). The prophylaxis of choice is trimethoprim-sulfamethoxazole (150 mg/m²/d of trimethoprim and 750 mg/m²/d of sulfamethoxazole) for 3 consecutive days of each week. Alternatives to this prophylaxis regimen are described in Chapter 37.

Treatment

A. GENERAL MEASURES

Supplemental oxygen and nutritional support may be needed. Bronchodilators may be tried but are usually not helpful. The patient should be in respiratory isolation.

B. SPECIFIC MEASURES

Trimethoprim-sulfamethoxazole (20 mg/kg/d of trimethoprim and 100 mg/kg/d of sulfamethoxazole in four divided doses intravenously or orally if well tolerated) is the treatment of choice. Improvement may not be seen for 3–5 days. Duration of treatment is 3 weeks in HIV-infected children. Methylprednisolone (2–4 mg/kg/d in four divided doses intravenously) should also be given to HIV-infected patients with moderate to severe infection for the first 5 days of treatment. The dosage is reduced 50% for the next 5 days, and further reduced by 50% until antibiotic treatment is completed. If trimethoprim-sulfamethoxazole is not tolerated or there is no clinical response in 5 days, pentamidine isethionate (4 mg/kg once daily by slow intravenous infusion) should be given. There is growing concern that antimicrobial resistance may be developing in some locations. Clinical efficacy is similar with pentamidine, but adverse reactions are more common. These reactions include dysglycemia, pancreatitis, nephrotoxicity, and leukopenia. Other effective alternatives in adults include atovaquone, trimethoprim-dapsone, and primaquine plus clindamycin.

Because of the exuberant response to the organism (especially noted in non–HIV infected patients), corticosteroids are added in patients with hypoxemia (partial oxygen pressure < 70 mm Hg or alveolar-arterial gradient > 35).

Prognosis

The mortality rate is high in immunosuppressed patients who receive treatment late in the illness.

Hidalgo A et al: Accuracy of high-resolution CT in distinguishing between *Pneumocystis carinii* pneumonia and non-*Pneumocystis carinii* pneumonia in AIDS patients. Eur Radiol 2003;13:1179 [PMID: 12695843].

LaRocque RC et al: The utility of sputum induction for diagnosis of *Pneumocystis* pneumonia in immunocompromised patients without human immunodeficiency virus. Clin Infect Dis 2003;37:1380 [PMID: 1453873].

Mahindra AD, Grossman SA: *Pneumocystis carinii* pneumonia in HIV negative patients with primary brain tumors. J Neurooncol 2003;63:263 [PMID: 12892232].

REFERENCES

Parasitic Infections

Drugs for parasitic infections. Med Lett Drugs Ther 1998;40:1 [PMID: 9442765].

Liu LY, Weller PF: Antiparasitic drugs. N Engl J Med 1996; 334:1178 [PMID: 8602186].

Mycotic Infections

Antachopoulos C, Walsh TJ: New agents for invasive mycoses in children. Curr Opin Pediatr 2005;17:78 [PMID: 15659969].

Deresinski SC, Stevens DA: Caspofungin. Clin Infect Dis 2003; 36:1445 [PMID: 12766841].

Krcmery VC Jr: Antifungal chemotherapeutics. Med Princ Pract 2005;14:125 [PMID: 15863983].

Kyle AA, Dahl MV: Topical therapy for fungal infections. Am J Clin Derm 2004;5:443 [PMID: 15663341].

Johnson LB, Kauffman CA: Voriconazole: A new triazole antifungal agent. Clin Infect Dis 2003;36:630 [PMID: 12594645].

Silveira F, Paterson DL: Pulmonary fungal infections. Curr Opin Pulm Med 2005;11:242 [PMID: 15818187].

Steinbach WJ: Antifungal agents in children. Pediatr Clin North Am 2005;52:895 [PMID: 15925667].

Sexually Transmitted Infections 40

Ann-Christine Nyquist, MD, Eric J. Sigel, MD, & Myron J. Levin, MD

The rate of sexually transmitted infections (STIs) acquired during adolescence remains high despite widespread educational programs and increased access to health care. The highest age-specific rates for gonorrhea, chlamydia, and human papillomavirus infection occur in adolescents and young adults. By age 18 years, half of youth will have had sexual intercourse. One-quarter of those having intercourse will develop an STI—an estimated 3 million teenagers per year. Adolescents contract STIs at a higher rate than adults because of sexual risk-taking, age-related biologic factors, and barriers to health care access. Providers need to comply with state-sanctioned confidentiality laws covering STI-related services, while recognizing the importance of confidentiality to adolescents. Except in a few states, adolescents can provide consent for the diagnosis and confidential treatment of STIs without parental consent or knowledge. In many states, adolescents can also provide consent for human immunodeficiency virus (HIV) counseling and testing.

Providers should screen sexually experienced adolescents for STIs and use this opportunity to discuss risk reduction. Health education counseling should be nonjudgmental and appropriate for the developmental level, yet sufficiently thorough to identify risk behaviors because many adolescents may not readily acknowledge engaging in these behaviors.

ADOLESCENT SEXUALITY

The spectrum of sexual behavior includes romance—holding hands and kissing; touching, including mutual masturbation; oral-genital contact; and vaginal and anal intercourse. Each has its associated risks. A small but statistically significant trend has occurred in the epidemiology of sexual risk taking toward less sexual involvement and later onset of vaginal intercourse. The most recent Youth Risk Behavior Survey (2003) reports that 47% of high school students have had vaginal intercourse during their lifetime; down slightly from 50% in 1999. Seven percent of teenagers have initiated sex by age 13. Significant racial and gender differences exist, with 19% of black students (32% of males and 7% of females), 8% of Hispanics, and 4% of whites initiating sex by age 13. Thirty-three percent of students have had

sex in the last 3 months—49% of twelfth-graders and 21% of ninth-graders. Condom use has increased, with 63% of youth reporting that either they or their partner had used a condom during their last sexual intercourse, compared with 42% in 1999. Paradoxically, condom use decreases with age—69% of ninth-graders report condom use at last intercourse compared with 49% of twelfth-graders.

Oral sex has not been as well studied. A recent study reports that 38% of boys and 42% of girls in the tenth grade engaged in oral sex, with only 17% using any protection.

A significant number of teenagers exhibit higher-risk sexual behavior: 20% of high school seniors have had four or more sexual partners. One million teenagers become pregnant annually. Eight percent of students have had sex forced on them—10% of females and 5% of males. Anal intercourse occurs in both heterosexual and homosexual populations.

Adolescents may not yet identify themselves as gay, lesbian, or bisexual, but continue to question and to engage in high-risk behaviors with multiple partners. Anywhere from 10% to 30% of males experiment with same-sex partners in some fashion, with 4–10% practicing anal sex. Frequently teenage males have their first same-sex experience with partners who are significantly older, which puts them at higher risk for STIs. Lesbians often experiment with male partners during their teen years as they sort out their sexual orientation, placing them at increased risk for pregnancy and STIs.

Impaired judgment related to alcohol or drug use creates an environment for unsafe sexual experimentation. Eighty-two percent of high school students have experimented with alcohol; 50% of high school senior boys have been drunk in the last 30 days. Nationwide, among students who were currently having sexual intercourse, one-fourth (25%) used alcohol or drugs the last time they had sex. This additional barrier to decision-making ability results in decreased condom use and an increased incidence of forced sex.

RISK FACTORS

Certain behaviors and experiences put the adolescent at higher risk for developing STIs. These include early age at sexual debut, lack of condom use, multiple partners, prior STI, history of STI in a partner, and sex with a partner who is 3 or more years older. The type of sex affects risk as well, with intercourse being riskier than oral sex. Other risk-taking behaviors associated with STIs in adolescents are smoking, alcohol use, drug use, dropping out of school, pregnancy, and watching X-rated movies.

Biologically the adolescent female is predisposed to chlamydia, gonorrhea, and human papillomavirus (HPV) infection because the cervix during adolescence has an exposed squamocolumnar junction. The rapidly dividing cells in this area are especially susceptible to microorganism attachment and infection. During early to midpuberty this junction slowly invaginates as the uterus and cervix mature, and by the late teens to early 20s the squamocolumnar junction is inside the cervix.

Centers for Disease Control and Prevention: Surveillance Summaries. Youth risk behavior surveillance, United States 2003. MMWR Morb Mortal Wkly Rep 2004;53:(SS-2) [PMID: 15460738].

Duncan P et al: Childhood and adolescent sexuality. Pediatr Clin North Am 2003;50:765 [PMID: 12964693].

Halpern-Flesher BL et al: Oral versus vaginal sex among adolescents: perceptions, attitudes, and behavior. Pediatrics 2005;115:845 [PMID: 15805354].

Prinstein MJ et al: Adolescent oral sex, peer popularity, and perceptions of best friend's sexual behavior. J Pediatr Psychol 2003;28:243 [PMID: 22616299].

Risser WL et al: The epidemiology of sexually transmitted infections in adolescents. Semin Pediatr Infect Dis 2005;16:160 [PMID: 16044389].

PREVENTION OF SEXUALLY TRANSMITTED INFECTIONS

Efforts to reduce STI risk behavior should begin before the onset of sexual experimentation, first by helping youth personalize their risk for STIs and encouraging positive behaviors that minimize these risks, and then by enhancing communication skills with sexual partners about STI prevention, abstinence, and condom use.

Primary prevention focuses largely on education and risk-reduction techniques. Health care providers should routinely discuss these as part of well adolescent checkups. Nationwide, more than 90% of students have been taught about acquired immunodeficiency syndrome (AIDS) or HIV infection in school. Although adolescents may be aware of HIV/AIDS or other STIs, they still have a difficult time personalizing risk. Discussing prevalence, symptoms, and sequelae of STIs can raise awareness and help teenagers make informed decisions about initiating sexual activity and the use of safer sex techniques. Making condoms available reiterates the message that safer sex is vital to health. Discussing condoms, dental dams, and the proper use of lubrication also facilitates safer sex practices.

Condoms prevent infections with HIV, gonorrhea, *Chlamydia,* and herpes simplex. They are probably effective in preventing other STIs as well.

Secondary prevention requires identifying and treating STIs (see section on screening) before infected individuals transmit infection to others. Access to medical care is critical to this objective. Identifying and treating STIs in partners are essential in limiting the spread of these infections. Cooperation with the state or county health department is valuable, because these agencies assume the responsibility for locating the contacts of infected persons and ensuring appropriate treatment.

Tertiary prevention is directed toward complications of a specific illness. Examples of tertiary prevention would be treating pelvic inflammatory disease (PID) before infertility develops; following the serologic response to syphilis to prevent late-stage syphilis; treating cervicitis to prevent PID; or treating a chlamydial infection before epididymitis ensues.

Finally, preexposure vaccination against hepatitis B or hepatitis A reduces the risk for these preventable STIs. All adolescents should have prior or current immunization against hepatitis B. However, because hepatitis B infection is frequently sexually transmitted, this vaccine is especially critical for all unvaccinated patients being evaluated for an STI. Hepatitis A vaccination is recommended for men who have sex with men and for injection drug users.

DiClemente RJ et al: A programmatic and methodologic review and synthesis of clinic-based risk-reduction interventions for sexually transmitted infections: research and practice implications. Semin Pediatr Infect Dis 2005;16:199 [PMID: 16044394].

SCREENING FOR SEXUALLY TRANSMITTED INFECTIONS

An essential part of screening is by history. Teenagers should be asked open-ended questions about their sexual experiences to assess their risk for STIs. The ability of the health care provider to obtain an accurate sexual history is crucial in prevention and control efforts. Questions must be explicit and understandable to the youth. If the adolescent has ever engaged in sexual activity, the provider needs to determine what kind of sexual activity (mutual masturbation or oral, anal, or vaginal sex); whether it has been heterosexual, homosexual, or both; whether birth control and condoms were used; and whether it has been consensual or forced. During the interview the clinician should take the opportunity to discuss risk-reduction techniques regardless of the history obtained from the youth. Importantly, female health care providers are twice as likely as male providers to screen female teenagers for STIs, so male health care providers need to better use screening opportunities.

A routine laboratory screening process is warranted if the patient has engaged in intercourse, presents with STI symptoms, or reports a partner with an STI. The availability of nucleic acid amplification tests (NAAT), primarily for *Chlamydia* and *Neisseria gonorrhoeae*, has changed the nature of STI screening and intervention. These amplification tests are more than 95% sensitive and more than 99% specific, using either urine or cervical/urethral swabs.

Initial screening for urethritis in males begins with a physical exam. If there are no signs (urethral discharge/lesions) or symptoms, then a first-catch urine sample (the first 10–40 mL of voided urine collected after not voiding for 2 hours) should be sent for *Chlamydia* and *Neisseria gonorrhoeae* testing. If signs or symptoms are present, then either the urine or a urethral swab should be sent to test for both *N gonorrhoeae* and *Chlamydia*. A wet prep should then be done on a spun urine sample or from urethral discharge, evaluating for the presence of *Trichomonas vaginalis*.

For females, screening asymptomatic patients has become more complicated because a variety of approaches are available. Generally, either a first-void urine specimen or a cervical swab is used to screen for *Chlamydia* and *N gonorrhoeae* by NAAT. When screening for *N gonorrhoeae*, it is important to recognize that certain NAATs are less sensitive when using urine compared with a cervical swab, and the specific test available should guide the screening procedure. A wet mount of the vaginal secretions should be performed annually to check for bacterial vaginosis and trichomoniasis, and a potassium hydroxide (KOH) preparation done to screen for yeast infections. The Papanicolaou (Pap) smear serves to evaluate the cervix for the presence of HPV or other cervical cytopathology. Availability of ThinPrep, which accomplishes HPV typing, along with an increased understanding of the progression of abnormal cervical changes, has led to a change in the recommendations for performing Pap smears. An initial Pap smear does not need to be done until 3 years after initiation of sexual intercourse, or by age 21.

For both sexes if high-risk behavior is present (three or more partners in the last 6 months or more than two partners per year for several years), then screening for hepatitis B surface antigen is warranted if not fully immunized prior to initiation of sexual intercourse. The presence of hepatitis B surface antigen indicates either the carrier state or active infection. Presence of only hepatitis B surface antibody identifies vaccinated individuals, whereas hepatitis B core antibody identifies individuals with past infection (see Chapter 21).

In urban areas with a relatively high rate of syphilis or in men who have sex with men, an RPR/VDRL (rapid plasma reagin/Venereal Disease Research Laboratory) test should be drawn yearly. RPR should be done in all cases in which a concomitant STI is present. HIV antibody determination should be considered for every sexually active adolescent and is strongly recommended for patients engaging in high-risk behaviors.

Gaydos CA: Nucleic acid amplification tests for gonorrhea and chlamydia: practice and applications. Infect Dis Clin North Am 2005;19:367 [PMID: 15963877].

Olshen E, Shrier LA: Diagnostic tests for chlamydial and gonorrheal infections. Semin Pediatr Infect Dis 2005;16:192 [PMID: 16044393].

SIGNS & SYMPTOMS

For males, the most common symptoms are dysuria and penile discharge resulting from urethral inflammation. Less common symptoms are scrotal pain, hematuria, proctitis, and pruritus in the pubic region. Signs include epididymitis, orchitis, and urethral discharge. Rarely do males develop systemic symptoms. For females, the most common symptoms are vaginal discharge and dysuria. Vaginal itching and irregular menses or spotting are also common. Abdominal pain, fever, and vomiting, though less common, are signs of PID. Pain in the genital region and dyspareunia may be present.

Signs that can be found in both males and females with an STI include genital ulcerations, adenopathy, and genital warts.

■ THE MOST COMMON ANTIBIOTIC-RESPONSIVE SEXUALLY TRANSMITTED INFECTIONS

Chlamydia trachomatis and *Neisseria gonorrhoeae* are sexually transmitted infections that are epidemic in the United States and are readily treated when appropriate antibiotics are administered in a timely fashion.

CHLAMYDIA TRACHOMATIS INFECTION

General Considerations

Chlamydia trachomatis is the most common bacterial cause of STIs in the United States. Three million cases are estimated to occur annually in adolescents and young adults. *Chlamydia trachomatis* is an obligate intracellular bacterium that replicates within the cytoplasm of host cells. Destruction of *Chlamydia*-infected cells is mediated by host immune responses.

Clinical Findings

A. SYMPTOMS AND SIGNS

Clinical infection in females manifests as dysuria, urethritis, vaginal discharge, cervicitis, or PID. The presence of mucopus at the cervical os (mucopurulent cervicitis) is a sign of *Chlamydia* infection or gonorrhea. *Chlamydia* infection is asymptomatic in 75% of females.

Chlamydial infection may be asymptomatic in 70% of males or manifest as dysuria, urethritis, or epididymitis. Some patients complain of urethral discharge. On clinical exam a clear white discharge may be found after milking the penis. Proctitis or proctocolitis from *Chlamydia* may occur in adolescents practicing receptive anal intercourse.

B. LABORATORY FINDINGS

NAAT (polymerase or ligase chain reaction) is the most sensitive (92–99%) way to detect *Chlamydia*. Enzyme-linked immunosorbent assay or direct fluorescent antibody tests are less sensitive but may be the only testing option in some centers. Culture is mandated for sexual abuse cases.

A cervical swab, using the manufacturer's swab provided with the specific test, or first-void urine specimen should be obtained. Often a single swab can be used to collect both the *Chlamydia* and *N gonorrhoeae* specimen. To optimize detection of *Chlamydia* from the cervix, columnar cells need to be collected by inserting the swab in the os and rotating it 360 degrees. If rectal symptoms are present, a rectal specimen should be obtained.

The first-void urine test for leukocyte esterase was previously used for screening asymptomatic, sexually active males. Due to the high false-positive rate this screening technique is now less commonly used. In symptomatic males, examination of the urine sediment for white blood cells (WBCs) can provide evidence of urethritis, though it is often impractical to perform in a clinical setting. In general, a first-void urine sample, or urethral swab for NAAT should be done at least annually. Some studies suggest that more frequent screenings—every 6 months—in higher-prevalence populations can decrease the rate of chlamydial infection. Evaluation of the symptomatic male patient or an asymptomatic contact for *Chlamydia* is the same.

For both males and females, testing urine allows for more frequent screening and simplifies screening in schools, the military, or other groups.

Complications

Epididymitis is a complication in males. Reiter syndrome occurs in association with chlamydial urethritis (see Chapter 26). This should be suspected in male patients who are sexually active and present with low back pain (sacroiliitis), arthritis (polyarticular), characteristic mucocutaneous lesions, and conjunctivitis. PID is an important complication in females.

Treatment

Infected patients and their contacts, regardless of the extent of signs or symptoms, need to receive treatment (Table 40–1). Because adolescents have a high risk of acquiring a repeat *Chlamydia* infection within several months of the first infection, all infected females should be rescreened 3–4 months after treatment.

Watson EJ et al: The accuracy and efficacy of screening tests for *Chlamydia trachomatis:* A systematic review. J Med Microbiol 2002:51;1021 [PMID: 22354463].

NEISSERIA GONORRHOEAE INFECTION

General Considerations

Gonorrhea is the second most prevalent bacterial STI. Rates, however, are at their lowest point ever, with 113.5 cases per 100,000 detected in 2004, with the exception of men who have sex with men, for whom there has been an increase in rates of gonorrhea. Among 15- to 19-year-old-males, for instance, the gonorrhea rate declined by 21.1% from 320.6 in 2000 to 252.9 in 2004. Sites of infection include the cervix, urethra, rectum, and pharynx. In addition, gonorrhea is a cause of PID. Humans are the natural reservoir. Gonococci are present in the exudate and secretions of infected mucous membranes.

Clinical Findings

A. SYMPTOMS AND SIGNS

In uncomplicated gonococcal cervicitis, females may be symptomatic between 23% and 57% of the time, presenting with vaginal discharge and dysuria. Urethritis and pyuria may also be present. Mucopurulent cervicitis with a yellowish discharge may be found, and the cervix may be edematous and friable. Other symptoms include abnormal menstrual periods and dyspareunia. Approximately 15% of women with endocervical gonorrhea will have signs of involvement of the upper genital tract. Compared with *Chlamydia* infection, pelvic inflammation with gonorrhea often has a shorter duration, but an increased intensity of symptoms, and is more often associated with fever. Older studies in males indicated that more than 95% of males had symptoms, usually a yellowish-green urethral discharge and burning on urination. Recent studies, however, have reported that the majority (55–67%) of males with *N gonorrhoeae* appear to be asymptomatic. Both males and females can develop gonococcal proctitis and pharyngitis after appropriate exposure.

B. LABORATORY FINDINGS

A cervical swab from females should be sent for NAAT or cultured on Thayer-Martin agar. Obtaining specimens from the rectum or pharynx when clinically indicated will increase the likelihood of positive results. Pharyngeal infection requires more intensive therapy. Nongonococcal *Neisseria* species reside in the vagina, thereby negating the value of the Gram stain in a female. NAAT screening

Table 40–1. Treatment regimens.

Disease	Recommended Regimens	Pregnancy[a] [Category]
Pelvic inflammatory disease (PID) Inpatient therapy regimen A *Note:* Therapy should be continued for 24–48 h after the patient has improved; therapy can then be switched to either oral regimen to complete a 14-d course.	Cefotetan, 2 g IV q6 h or Cefoxitin, 2 g IV q12 h plus Doxycycline, 100 mg IV or PO bid	Safe [B] Safe [B] Contraindicated [D]
Inpatient therapy regimen B *Note:* Once clinically improved for 48 h, patients can be discharged and continue doxycycline 100 mg PO bid for 14 days total.[b]	Clindamycin, 900 mg IV q8 h plus Gentamicin, 2 mg/kg IV loading dose, then 1.5 mg/kgIV q8 h	Safe [B] Safe [B]
Alternative parenteral regimens	Ofloxacin, 400 mg IV q12 h[c] or Levofloxacin, 500 mg IV once daily[c] with or without Metronidazole, 500 mg IV q8 h or Ampicillin/sulbactam, 3 g IV q6 h plus Doxycycline, 100 mg IV or PO q12 h	Contraindicated [C] Contraindicated [C] Safe[d] [B] Safe[d] [A] Contraindicated [D]
Outpatient therapy regimen A	Ofloxacin, 400 mg PO bid for 14 d[c] or Levofloxacin, 500 mg PO, once a day for 14 d[c] with or without metronidazole, 500 mg PO bid for 14 d	Contraindicated [C] Contraindicated [C] Safe [B]
Outpatient therapy regimen B *Note:* Pregnant patients with PID should be hospitalized and given parenteral antibiotics.[b]	Ceftriaxone, 250 mg IM once or Cefoxitin, 2 g IM once plus probenicid, 1 g PO or Third-generation cephalosporin plus Doxycycline, 100 mg, PO bid for 14 d with or without Metronidazole, 500 mg PO bid for 14 d	Safe [B] Safe [B] Safe [B] Contraindicated [D] Safe[d] [B]
Gonorrhea, uncomplicated Cervicitis, urethritis *Note:* Empiric treatment for *Chlamydia trachomatis* with azithromycin or doxycycline is recommended due to coexisting infection in 20–40% of patients with gonorrhea infection if chlamydial infection is not ruled out.	Cefixime, 400 mg PO as single dose or Ceftriaxone, 125 mg IM as single dose or Ciprofloxacin, 500 mg PO as single dose or Ofloxacin, 400 mg PO as single dose[c] or Levofloxacin, 250 mg PO as single dose[c]	Safe [B] Safe [B] Contraindicated [C] Contraindicated [C] Contraindicated [C]
Pharyngitis	Ceftriaxone, 125 mg IM once or Ciprofloxacin, 500 mg PO once[c]	Safe [B] Contraindicated [C]

(continued)

Table 40–1. Treatment regimens. (continued)

Disease	Recommended Regimens	Pregnancy[a] [Category]
Gonorrhea disseminated **Note:** Treat IV until clinically improved (usually 48h; then switch to PO); complete at least a 7-d course with cefixime, 400 mg PO bid.	Ceftriaxone, 1 g IV or IM every 24 h	Safe [B]
	or	
	Ceftizoxime, 1 g IV every 8 h	Safe [B]
	or	
	Ciprofloxacin, 400 mg IV every 12 h	Contraindicated [C]
	or	
	Ciprofloxacin, 500 mg PO bid	Contraindicated [C]
	or	
	Ofloxacin, 400 mg PO bid	Contraindicated [C]
	or	
	Levofloxacin, 500 mg PO once daily	Contraindicated [C]
Nongonococcal, nonchlamydial urethritis	Azithromycin, 1 g PO as single dose	
	or	
	Doxycycline, 100 mg PO bid for 7 d	
Alternative regimens	Erythromycin base, 500 mg PO qid for 7 d	
	or	
	Erythromycin ethylsuccinate, 800 mg PO qid for 7 d	
	or	
	Ofloxacin, 300 mg PO bid for 7 d[c]	
	or	
	Levofloxacin, 500 mg PO once daily for 7 d[c]	
Recurrent or persistent urethritis	Metronidazole, 2 g PO as single dose	
	plus	
	Erythromycin base, 500 mg PO qid for 7 d	
	or	
	Erythromycin ethylsuccinate, 800 mg PO qid for 7 d	
Proctitis, proctocolitis, and enteritis	Ceftriaxone 125 mg IM	Safe [B]
	plus	
	Doxycycline, 100 mg PO bid for 7 d	Contraindicated [D]
***Trichomonas vaginalis* vaginitis or urethritis**	Metronidazole, 2 g PO as single dose	Safe[d] [B]
	or	
	Metronidazole, 500 mg PO bid for 7d	Safe[d] [B]
	or	
	Tinidazole, 2 g PO as simple dose	Contraindicated [C]
Bacterial vaginosis	Metronidazole, 500 mg PO bid for 7 d	Safe[d] [B]
	or	
	Metronidazole, 0.75% gel, 5 g intravaginally once a day for 5 d	Safe[d] [B]
	or	
	Clindamycin cream, 2%, one applicator intravaginally at bedtime for 5 d	Safe [B]
Alternative regimen	Metronidazole, 2 g PO as single dose	Safe[d] [B]
	or	
	Clindamycin, 300 mg PO bid for 7 d	Safe [B]
	or	
	Clindamycin ovule 100 mg intravaginally once at bedtime for 3 d	

(continued)

Table 40–1. Treatment regimens. (continued)

Disease	Recommended Regimens	Pregnancy[a] [Category]
Vulvovaginal candidiasis	Butoconazole, clotrimazole, miconazole, terconazole or tioconazole, intravaginally for 1, 3, or 7 d	Safe [B]
	Butoconazole sustained-release, 5 g once intravaginally	Safe [B]
	or	
	Fluconazole, 150 mg oral tablet, in single dose	Contraindicated [C]
Syphilis Early (primary, secondary, or latent < 1 y)	Benzathine penicillin G, 2.4 million units IM (for patients > 40 kg)	Safe [B]
	Benzathine penicillin G, 50,000 units/kg IM (for patients < 40 kg); up to 2.4 million units in one dose	Safe [B]
	or	
	Doxycycline, 100 mg PO bid for 14 d	Contraindicated [D]
Late (more than 1 y duration)	Benzathine penicillin G, 2.4 million units IM (for patients > 40 kg) once a week for 3 consecutive weeks	Safe [B]
	or	
	Benzathine penicillin G, 50,000 units/kg IM (for patients < 40 kg) once a week for 3 consecutive weeks; up to 2.4 million units in one dose	
	or	
	Doxycycline, 100 mg PO bid for 4 wk	Contraindicated [D]
Epididymitis Most likely caused by gonococcal or chlamydial infection	Ceftriaxone, 250 mg IM as single dose plus Doxycycline, 100 mg PO bid for 14 d	
Most likely caused by enteric organisms; patient older than 35 y old or allergies to cephalosporins and/or tetracyclines	Ofloxacin, 300 mg PO bid for 14 d or Levofloxacin, 500 mg PO once daily for 14 d	
Chlamydia trachomatis Cervicitis or urethritis	Azithromycin, 1 g PO as single dose	Safe [B]
	or	
	Erythromycin, 500 mg PO qid for 7 d	Safe [B]
Alternative regimen[b]	Doxycycline, 100 mg PO bid for 7d	Contraindicated [D]
	or	
	Ofloxacin, 300 mg PO bid for 7 d	Contraindicated [C]
	or	
	Levofloxacin 500 mg PO once daily for 7 d	Contraindicated [C]
Granuloma inguinale	Doxycycline, 100 mg PO bid for 3 wk or longer	Contraindicated [D]
	or	
	Trimethoprim–sulfamethoxazole, one double-strength tablet PO bid for 3 weeks or longer	Safe [B]

(continued)

Table 40–1. Treatment regimens. (continued)

Disease	Recommended Regimens	Pregnancy[a] [Category]
Alternative regimen	Ciprofloxacin, 750 mg PO bid for at least 3 wk	Contraindicated [C]
	or	
	Erythromycin base, 500 mg PO four times daily for at least 3 wk	Safe [B]
	or	
	Azithromycin, 1 g PO once per week for at least 3 wk	Safe [B]
Lymphogranuloma venereum	Doxycycline, 100 mg PO bid for 3 wk	Contraindicated [D]
	or	
	Erythromycin, 500 mg PO qid for 3 wk	Safe [B]
Herpes simplex First episode, genital	Acyclovir, 400 mg PO tid for 7–10 d	Safe [B]
	or	
	Famciclovir, 250 mg PO tid for 7–10d	Safe [B]
	or	
	Valacyclovir, 1 g PO bid for 7–10 d	Safe [B]
Recurrent	Acyclovir, 400 mg PO tid for 5 d	
	or	
	Acyclovir, 800 mg PO bid for 5 d	
	or	
	Famciclovir, 125 mg PO bid for 5 d	
	or	
	Valacyclovir, 500 mg PO bid for 3–5 d	
	or	
	Valacyclovir, 1 g PO once a day for 5 d	
Suppression	Acyclovir, 400 mg PO bid	Safe [B]
	or	
	Famciclovir, 250 mg PO bid	
	or	
	Valacyclovir, 500 mg PO daily (if < 10 recurrences per year; if ≥ 10 recurrences use 1 g daily)	
Chancroid	Azithromycin, 1 g PO as single dose	Safe [B]
	or	
	Ceftriaxone 250 mg IM once	Safe [B]
	or	
	Ciprofloxacin, 500 mg PO bid for 3 d	Contraindicated [D]
	or	
	Erythromycin, 500 mg PO tid for 7 d	Safe [B]
Human papillomavirus External lesions *Note:* Topical therapies usually require weekly treatments for 4 consecutive weeks	Podophyllin, 25% in benzoin tincture applied directly to warts; wash off in 1–4 h [contraindicated for urethral or intravaginal lesions]	Contraindicated [X]
	or	
	Trichloroacetic acid (85%); apply directly to warts; wash off in 6–8 h	Safe
	or	

(continued)

Table 40–1. Treatment regimens. (continued)

Disease	Recommended Regimens	Pregnancy[a] [Category]
	Podofilox, 0.5% solution; apply bid for 3 d; used by the patient at home; practitioner needs to demonstrate how compound is applied (to be used only on external lesions)	Contraindicated [C]
	or	
	Imiquimod 5% cream, applied three times per week overnight (maximum of 16 weeks)	Contraindicated [B]
	Cryotherapy: liquid nitrogen, cryoprobe	Safe
	Laser surgery	
Ectoparasitic infections **Pediculosis pubis**[e]	Permethrin 1% creme rinse: wash off after 10 min	Safe [B]
	or	
	Lindane 1% shampoo: apply for 4 min, then wash off	Contraindicated [B]
	or	
	Pyrethins with piperonyl butoxide: apply, wash off after 10 min	Safe [B]
Scabies	Permethrin creme 5%: apply to entire body from the neck down, wash off after 8 h	Safe [B]
	or	
	Ivermectin 200 mcg/kg orally, repeat in 2 weeks	Contraindicated [C]

[a]FDA use in pregnancy ratings: [A]*Controlled studies show no risk.* Adequate, well-controlled studies in pregnant women have failed to demonstrate a risk to the fetus in any trimester of pregnancy. [B]*No evidence of risk in humans.* Adequate, well-controlled studies in pregnant women have not shown increased risk of fetal abnormalities despite adverse findings in animals, or, in the absence of adequate human studies, animal studies show no fetal risk. The chance of fetal harm is remote but remains a possibility. [C]*Risk cannot be ruled out.* Adequate, well-controlled human studies are lacking, and animal studies have shown a risk to the fetus or are lacking as well. There is a chance of fetal harm if the drug is administered during pregnancy; but the potential benefits outweigh the potential risk. [D]*Positive evidence of risk.* Studies in humans, or investigational or post-marketing data, have demonstrated fetal risk. Nevertheless, potential benefits from the use of the drug may outweigh the potential risk. For example, the drug may be acceptable if needed in a life-threatening situation or serious disease for which safer drugs cannot be used or are ineffective. [X]*Contraindicated in pregnancy.* Studies in animals or humans, or despite adverse findings in animals, or investigational or post-marketing reports have demonstrated positive evidence of fetal abnormalities or risk that clearly outweighs any possible benefit to the patient.
[b]Doxycycline is contraindicated in pregnancy. Alternative therapies during pregnancy which include erythromycin, azithromycin, and amoxicillin are not as effective, but are clinically useful if the recommended regimens cannot be used due to allergy or pregnancy.
[c]Quinolones should not be used in areas with increased prevalence of quinolone resistance (ie, Asia, the Pacific, Hawaii, California) or to treat proven or suspected gonococcal infections in men who have sex with men.
[d]Previously metronidazole was contraindicated in the first trimester.
[e]Bedding and clothing need to be decontaminatedby washing in hot water or by dry cleaning. Regimen may be repeated in 1 week if complete response is not achieved.

of female urine can be used; however, polymerase chain reaction is less sensitive (83%) compared to ligase chain reaction (99%).

Culture or NAAT for *N gonorrhoeae* in males can be achieved with a swab of the urethra or first-void urine. Urethral culture is less sensitive (85%) compared with the 95–99% sensitivity using NAAT methods on either urethral or urine specimens. Gram stain of urethral discharge showing gram-negative intracellular diplococci indicates gonorrhea in a male.

If proctitis is present, appropriate cultures should be obtained and treatment for both gonorrhea and *Chlamydia* infection given. If oral exposure to gonorrhea is suspected, cultures should be taken and the patient given empiric treatment.

Differential Diagnosis

Gonococcal pharyngitis needs to be differentiated from streptococcal infection, herpes simplex pharyngitis, and infectious mononucleosis. *Chlamydia* infection needs to be differentiated from gonococcal infection.

Complications

Disseminated gonococcal infection occurs in a minority (0.5–3%) of patients with untreated gonorrhea. Hematogenous spread most commonly causes arthritis and dermatitis. The joints most frequently involved are the wrist, metacarpophalangeal joints, knee, and ankle. Skin lesions are typically tender, with hemorrhagic or necrotic pustules or bullae on an erythematous base occurring on the distal extremities. Disseminated disease occurs more frequently in women than in men. Risk factors include pregnancy and gonococcal pharyngitis. Gonorrhea is complicated occasionally by perihepatitis and very rarely by endocarditis or meningitis.

Treatment

Historically, patients diagnosed with gonorrhea were treated for chlamydia as well. As chlamydia testing has become more sensitive, the Centers for Disease Control and Prevention suggests that treatment for coinfection is not necessary if testing for chlamydia has been done by NAAT. Their guidelines also state that *N gonorrhoeae* and *C trachomatis* do not require tests of cure when they are treated with first-line medications, unless the patient remains symptomatic. If retesting is indicated it should be delayed for 1 month after completion of therapy if NAATs are used to document a test of cure. Retesting might also be considered for sexually active adolescents likely to be reinfected. Patients should be advised to abstain from sexual intercourse until both they and their partners have completed a course of treatment. Treatment for disseminated disease may require hospitalization (see Table 40–1). Fluoroquinolone resistance is high in Hawaii and California and among men who have sex with men. Failure of initial treatment should prompt reevaluation of the patient and consideration of retreatment with ceftriaxone.

■ THE SPECTRUM OF SEXUALLY TRANSMITTED INFECTIONS

The patient presenting with an STI usually has one or more of the signs or symptoms described in this section. Management considerations for STIs include assessing the patient's adherence to therapy and ensuring follow-up, treating STIs in partners, and determining pregnancy risk. Treatment of each STI is detailed in Table 40–1.

MUCOPURULENT CERVICITIS

General Considerations

Mucopurulent cervicitis (MPC) is caused by *C trachomatis* or *N gonorrhoeae* approximately 30% of the time. Herpes simplex virus and *Mycoplasma genitalium* are less common causes. MPC can also be present without an STI.

Clinical Findings

A. SYMPTOMS AND SIGNS

MPC is often asymptomatic, but many women have an abnormal vaginal discharge or postcoital bleeding. MPC is characterized by a purulent or mucopurulent endocervical exudate visible in the endocervical canal or on an endocervical swab specimen. The cervix is often friable with easily-induced bleeding.

B. LABORATORY FINDINGS

Although endocervical Gram stain may show an increased number of polymorphonuclear leukocytes, it has a low positive predictive value and is not recommended for diagnosis. Patients who have MPC should be tested for *C trachomatis* and *N gonorrhoeae* by using the most sensitive and specific tests available at the site.

Complications

Persistent MPC is difficult to manage and requires reassessment of the initial diagnosis. MPC can persist despite repeated courses of antimicrobial therapy. Presence of a large ectropion can contribute to persistent MPC.

Treatment

Empiric treatment for both gonorrhea and chlamydial infection is recommended when the prospect of follow-up is questionable or the patient is part of a high-risk population. If the patient is asymptomatic except for MPC, then treatment may wait until diagnostic tests are back (see Table 40–1). Follow-up is recommended if symptoms persist. Patients should be instructed to abstain from sexual intercourse until they and their sex partners are cured and treatment is completed.

Marrazzo JM: Mucopurulent cervicitis: no longer ignored, but still misunderstood. Infect Dis Clin North Am 2005;19:333 [PMID: 15963875].

PELVIC INFLAMMATORY DISEASE

General Considerations

Pelvic inflammatory disease (PID) is defined as inflammation of the upper female genital tract and may include endometritis, salpingitis, tubo-ovarian abscess, and pelvic peritonitis. It is the most common gynecologic disorder necessitating hospitalization for women of reproductive age in the United States. Over 1 million women develop PID annually, and 275,000 are hospitalized. The incidence is highest in the teen population. Teenage girls who are sexually active have a high risk (1 in 8) of developing PID, whereas women in their 20s have one-tenth the risk. Predisposing risk factors include multiple sexual partners, younger age of initiating sexual intercourse, prior history of PID, and lack of condom use. Lack of protective antibody from previous exposure to sexually transmitted organisms and cervical ectopy contribute to the development of PID. Many adolescents with subacute or asymptomatic disease are never identified.

PID is often polymicrobial. Causative agents include *N gonorrhoeae, Chlamydia,* anaerobic bacteria that reside in the vagina, and genital mycoplasmas. Vaginal douching and other mechanical factors such as an intrauterine device or prior gynecologic surgery increase the risk of PID by providing access of lower genital tract organisms to pelvic organs. Recent menses and bacterial vaginosis have been associated with the development of PID.

Clinical Findings

A. SYMPTOMS AND SIGNS

Acute PID is difficult to diagnose because of the wide variation in the symptoms and signs. No single historical, clinical, or laboratory finding has both high sensitivity and specificity for the diagnosis. Diagnosis of PID is usually made clinically (Table 40–2). Typical patients have lower abdominal pain, nausea, vomiting, and fever. However, the patient may be afebrile. Vaginal discharge is variable. Cervical motion tenderness, uterine or adnexal tenderness, or signs of peritonitis are often present. Mucopurulent cervicitis is present in 50% of patients. Tubo-ovarian abscesses can be detected by careful physical examination (feeling a mass or fullness in the adnexa).

Laparoscopy is the gold standard for detecting salpingitis; it can be used if the diagnosis is in question or to help differentiate PID from an ectopic pregnancy, ovarian cysts, or adnexal torsion. The clinical diagnosis of PID has a positive predictive value for salpingitis of 65–90% in comparison with laparoscopy. Pelvic ultrasonography also is helpful in detecting tubo-ovarian abscesses, which are found in almost 20% of teens with PID. Transvaginal ultrasound is more sensitive than abdominal ultrasound.

B. LABORATORY FINDINGS

Laboratory findings include elevated WBCs with a left shift and elevated acute-phase reactants (erythrocyte sedimentation rate or C-reactive protein). A positive test for *N gonorrhoeae* or *C trachomatis* is supportive, although

Table 40–2. Diagnostic criteria for pelvic inflammatory disease (PID).

Minimum criteria
Empiric treatment of PID should be initiated in sexually active young women and others at risk for sexually transmitted infections if all the following minimum criteria are present and no other cause(s) for the illness can be identified:
> Lower abdominal tenderness
> Uterine adnexal tenderness
> Cervical motion tenderness

Additional supportive criteria
Oral temperature > 38.3 °C (101 °F)
Abnormal cervical or vaginal mucopurulent discharge
Presence of white blood cells on saline microscopy of vaginal secretions
Elevated erythrocyte sedimentation rate or elevated C-reactive protein
Laboratory documentation of infection with *N gonorrhoeae* or *C trachomatis*

Definitive criteria [selected cases]
Histopathologic evidence of endometritis on endometrial biopsy
Tubo-ovarian abscess on sonography or other radiologic tests
Laparoscopic abnormalities consistent with PID

Adapted, with permission, from Centers for Disease Control and Prevention. Sexually transmitted diseases treatment guidelines 2002. MMWR Morb Mortal Wkly Rep 2002;51(No. RR-6).

25% of the time neither of these bacteria is detected. Pregnancy needs to be ruled out, because patients with an ectopic pregnancy can present with abdominal pain.

Differential Diagnosis

Differential diagnosis includes other gynecologic illnesses (ectopic pregnancy, threatened or septic abortion, adnexal torsion, ruptured and hemorrhagic ovarian cysts, dysmenorrhea, endometriosis, or mittelschmerz); gastrointestinal illnesses (appendicitis, cholecystitis, hepatitis, gastroenteritis, or inflammatory bowel disease); and genitourinary illnesses (cystitis, pyelonephritis, or urinary calculi).

Complications

Scarring of the fallopian tubes is one of the major sequelae of PID. With one episode of PID, 17% of patients become infertile, 17% develop chronic pelvic pain, and 10% will have an ectopic pregnancy. Infertility rates increase with each episode of PID; three episodes of PID result in a 73% infertility rate. Fitz-Hugh-Curtis syndrome is inflammation of the liver capsule (perihepatitis) from either hematogenous or lymphatic spread of organisms from the fallopian tubes. This results in right upper quadrant pain and elevation of liver function tests.

Treatment

The objective of treatment is both to achieve a clinical cure and prevent long-term sequelae. The success of various therapeutic regimens in preventing sequelae has not been determined. PID is frequently managed at the outpatient level, although some clinicians argue that all adolescents with PID should be hospitalized because of the rate of complications. Severe systemic symptoms and toxicity, signs of peritonitis, inability to take fluids, pregnancy, and elevated WBCs and erythrocyte sedimentation rate support hospitalization. In addition, if the health care provider believes that the patient will not comply with treatment, hospitalization is warranted. Surgical drainage may be required to ensure adequate treatment of tubo-ovarian abscesses.

The treatment regimens described in Table 40–1 are broad spectrum to cover the numerous microorganisms associated with PID. Outpatient treatment should be reserved for compliant patients who have classic signs of PID without systemic symptoms. Patients with PID who receive treatment as outpatients should be reexamined within 24–48 hours, with phone contact in the interim, to detect persistent disease or treatment failure. Patients should have substantial improvement within 48–72 hours. An adolescent should be reexamined 7–10 days after the completion of therapy to ensure the resolution of symptoms.

Banikarim C, Chacko MR: Pelvic inflammatory disease in adolescents. Semin Pediatr Infect Dis 2005;16:175 [PMID: 16044391].

Centers for Disease Control and Prevention: Sexually Transmitted Disease Surveillance 2003 Supplement, Division of STD Prevention, November 2004. http://www.cdc.gov/std/GISP2003/GISP2003.pdf

Eissa MA, Cromwell PF: Diagnosis and management of pelvic inflammatory disease in adolescents. J Pediatr Health Care 2003;17:145 [PMID: 22620085].

Ness RB et al: Effectiveness of treatment strategies of some women with pelvic inflammatory disease: a randomized trial. Obstet Gynecol 2005;106:573 [PMID: 16135590].

URETHRITIS

General Considerations

Common bacterial causes of urethritis in men are *N gonorrhoeae* and *C trachomatis*. Additionally, *Trichomonas vaginalis*, herpes simplex virus (HSV), *Ureaplasma urealyticum*, and *Mycoplasma genitalium* cause urethritis. Approximately 20% of nongonococcal, nonchlamydial urethritis can be attributed both to *Mycoplasma genitalium* and *Ureaplasma urealyticum*. Coliforms may cause urethritis in men practicing insertive anal intercourse. Mechanical manipulation or contact with irritants can also cause transient urethritis.

Women often present with symptoms of a urinary tract infection from which no enteric bacterial pathogens are isolated. These women often have urethritis caused by the organisms just mentioned.

Clinical Findings

A. SYMPTOMS AND SIGNS

Men present most commonly with a clear or purulent discharge from the urethra and dysuria. Hematuria and associated inguinal adenopathy can occur. Most infections caused by *C trachomatis* and *T vaginalis* are asymptomatic, while 70% of men with *M genitalium* and 23–90% with gonococcal urethritis are symptomatic.

B. LABORATORY FINDINGS

In a symptomatic male a positive leukocyte esterase test on first-void urine, or microscopic examination of first-void urine demonstrating more than 10 WBCs per high-power field, is suggestive of urethritis. Gram stain of urethral secretions demonstrating more than 5 WBCs per high-power field is also suggestive. Gonococcal urethritis is established by documenting the presence of WBCs containing intracellular gram-negative diplococci. Urethral swab or first-void urine for culture or NAAT should be sent to the laboratory to detect *N gonorrhoeae* and *C trachomatis*. Evaluation for *T vaginalis* by a wet preparation of either urethral discharge or spun urine should be considered when the other test results are negative. Additionally polymerase chain reaction testing is more sensitive for *T vaginalis* than culture or direct microscopy. Specific polymerase chain reaction testing of urine is available for *Mycoplasma* and *Ureaplasma*, though it is not often clinically utilized.

Complications

Complications include recurrent or persistent urethritis or epididymitis.

Treatment

Patients with evidence of urethritis should receive empiric treatment for gonorrhea and *Chlamydia* infection. If the infection is unresponsive and NAAT-negative, trichomoniasis should be ruled out, and nongonococcal, nonchlamydial urethritis should be suspected, and treated appropriately. Patients should be instructed to return for evaluation if symptoms persist or recur after completion of initial empiric therapy. Symptoms alone, without documentation of signs or laboratory evidence of urethral inflammation, are not a sufficient basis for retreatment (see Table 40–1). Azithromycin is the initial recommended therapy for persistence of symptoms and urethritis.

Falk L et al: Symptomatic urethritis is more prevalent in men infected with *Mycoplasma genitalium* than with *Chlamydia trachomatis*. Sexually Transm Infect 2004;80:289 [PMID: 15295128].

Simpson T, Oh MK: Urethritis and cervicitis in adolescents. Adolesc Med Clin 2004;15:253 [PMID: 15449844].

EPIDIDYMITIS

General Considerations

Epididymitis is most often caused by *C trachomatis* or *N gonorrhoeae*. Epididymitis caused by *Escherichia coli* occurs among homosexual men who are the insertive partners during anal intercourse and in men who have urinary tract abnormalities.

Clinical Findings

A. SYMPTOMS AND SIGNS

Epididymitis is associated with unilateral testicular pain and tenderness. Palpable, tender swelling of the epididymis is usually present. Often these symptoms are accompanied by asymptomatic urethritis.

B. LABORATORY FINDINGS

Diagnosis is made clinically. Additional evaluation is similar to that described for suspected urethritis (see section on urethritis).

Differential Diagnosis

Acute epididymitis associated with sexual activity must be distinguished from orchitis due to infarct, testicular torsion, or viral infection.

Complications

Infertility is rare, and chronic local pain is uncommon.

Treatment

Empiric therapy is indicated before culture results are available. As an adjunct to therapy, bed rest, scrotal elevation, and analgesics are recommended until fever and local inflammation subside. Lack of improvement of swelling and tenderness within 3 days requires reevaluation of both the diagnosis and therapy (see Table 40–1).

PROCTITIS, PROCTOCOLITIS, & ENTERITIS

General Considerations

Proctitis occurs predominantly among persons who participate in anal intercourse. Enteritis occurs among those whose sexual practices include oral-fecal contact. Proctocolitis can be acquired by either route depending on the pathogen. Common sexually transmitted pathogens causing proctitis or proctocolitis include *C trachomatis*, *Treponema pallidum*, HSV, *N gonorrhoeae*, *Giardia lamblia*, and enteric organisms.

Clinical Findings

A. SYMPTOMS AND SIGNS

Proctitis, defined as inflammation limited to the distal 10–12 cm of the rectum, is associated with anorectal pain, tenesmus, and rectal discharge. Acute proctitis among persons who have recently practiced receptive anal intercourse is most often sexually transmitted. The symptoms of proctocolitis combine those of proctitis, plus diarrhea or abdominal cramps (or both), because of inflamed colonic mucosa more than 12 cm from the anus. Enteritis usually results in diarrhea and abdominal cramping without signs of proctitis or proctocolitis.

B. LABORATORY FINDINGS

Evaluation may include anoscopy or sigmoidoscopy, stool exam, and culture for appropriate organisms and serology for syphilis.

Treatment

Management will be determined by the etiologic agent. (See Table 40–1 and Chapters 20 and 38.) Reinfection may be difficult to distinguish from treatment failure.

Klausner JD et al: Etiology of clinical proctitis among men who have sex with men. Clin Infect Dis 2004;38:300 [PMID: 14699467].

Rompalo AM: Diagnosis and treatment of sexually acquired proctitis and proctocolitis: An update. Clin Infect Dis 1999;28(Suppl 1):S84 [PMID: 99152439].

VAGINAL DISCHARGE

Adolescent girls may have a normal physiologic leukorrhea, secondary to turnover of vaginal epithelium. Infectious causes of discharge include *T vaginalis*, *C trachomatis*, *N gonorrhoeae*, and bacterial vaginosis pathogens. Candidiasis is a yeast infection that produces vaginal discharge, but is not usually sexually transmitted. Vaginitis is characterized by vaginal discharge, vulvar itching, and irritation; the discharge may be foul-smelling. Discharge may be white, gray, or yellow. Physiologic leukorrhea is usually white, homogeneous, and not associated with itching, irritation, or foul odor. Mechanical, chemical, allergic, or other noninfectious irritants of the vagina may cause vaginal discharge.

1. Bacterial Vaginosis

General Considerations

Bacterial vaginosis (BV) is a polymicrobial infection of the vagina caused by an imbalance of the normal bacterial vaginal flora. The altered flora has a paucity of hydrogen peroxide–producing lactobacilli and increased concentrations of *Mycoplasma hominis* and anaerobes, such as *Gardnerella vaginalis* and *Mobiluncus*. It is unclear whether BV is sexually transmitted, but it is associated with having multiple sex partners.

Clinical Findings

A. SYMPTOMS AND SIGNS

The most common symptom is a heavy, malodorous, homogeneous gray-white vaginal discharge. Patients may report vaginal itching or dysuria. The fishy odor may be more noticeable after intercourse or during menses, when the high pH of blood or semen volatilizes the amines.

B. LABORATORY FINDINGS

BV is most often diagnosed by the use of clinical criteria, which include (1) presence of gray-white discharge; (2) fishy (amine) odor before or after the addition of 10% KOH (whiff test); (3) pH of vaginal fluid greater than 4.5 determined with narrow-range pH paper; and (4) presence of greater than 20% "clue cells." Clue cells are squamous epithelial cells that have multiple bacteria adhering to them, making their borders irregular and giving them a speckled appearance. Diagnosis requires three out of four criteria, although many women who fulfill these criteria have no discharge or other symptoms.

Complications

BV during pregnancy is associated with adverse outcomes such as premature labor, preterm delivery, and postpartum endometritis. In the nonpregnant individual, it may be associated with PID and urinary tract infections.

Treatment

All women who have symptomatic disease should receive treatment to relieve vaginal symptoms and signs of infection (see Table 40–1). Additional goals for pregnant women include prevention of adverse outcomes of pregnancy. Treatment for patients who do not complain of vaginal discharge or itching, but who demonstrate BV on routine pelvic examination, is unclear. Because some studies associate BV and PID, the recommendation is to have a low threshold for treating asymptomatic BV. Follow-up visits are unnecessary if symptoms resolve. Recurrence of BV is not unusual. Follow-up examination 1 month after treatment for high-risk pregnant women is recommended.

Males do not develop infection equivalent to BV. Treatment of male partners has no effect on the course of infection in females.

Koumans EH et al: Indications for therapy and treatment recommendations for bacterial vaginosis in nonpregnant and pregnant women: A synthesis of data. Clin Infect Dis 2002;35:S152 [PMID: 12353202].

O'Brien RF: Bacterial vaginosis: many questions—any answers? Curr Opin Pediatr 2005;17:473 [PMID: 16012258].

Wilson J: Managing recurrent bacterial vaginosis. Sex Transm Infect 2004;80:1 [PMID: 14755028].

2. Trichomoniasis

General Considerations

Trichomoniasis is caused by *Trichomonas vaginalis*, a flagellated protozoan that infects 2.5–3 million people annually.

Clinical Findings

A. SYMPTOMS AND SIGNS

Fifty percent of females with trichomoniasis develop a symptomatic vaginitis with vaginal itching, a green-gray malodorous frothy discharge, and dysuria. Occasionally postcoital bleeding and dyspareunia may be present. The vulva may be erythematous and the cervix friable.

B. LABORATORY FINDINGS

Mixing the discharge with normal saline facilitates detection of the flagellated protozoan on microscopic examination (wet preparation). The infection may be detected by the pathologist when reviewing the Pap smear. The InPouch TV system is available for culture when the diagnosis is unclear. Culture, antigen detection, and polymerase chain reaction are sensitive, but expensive and not readily available. Trichomonal urethritis frequently causes a positive urine leukocyte esterase test or WBCs on urethral smear.

Complications

Male partners of females diagnosed with trichomoniasis have a 22% chance of having trichomoniasis. Half of men with trichomoniasis will have urethritis. *Trichomonas* infection in women has been associated with adverse pregnancy outcomes.

Treatment

See Table 40–1 for treatment recommendations.

Schwebke JR, Burgess D: Trichomoniasis. Clin Microbiol Rev 2004;17:794 [PMID: 15489349].

Schwebke JR, Hook EW 3rd: High rates of *Trichomonas vaginalis* among men attending a sexually transmitted diseases clinic: Implications for screening and urethritis management. J Infect Dis 2003;188:465 [PMID: 22751764].

3. Vulvovaginal Candidiasis

General Considerations

Vulvovaginal candidiasis is caused by *Candida albicans* in 85–90% of cases. Most women will have at least one episode of vulvovaginal candidiasis, and almost half will have two or more episodes. The highest incidence is between ages 16 and 30 years. Predisposing factors include recent use of antibiotics, diabetes, pregnancy, and HIV. Risk factors include vaginal intercourse, use of oral contraceptives, and use of spermicide. This is rarely a sexually transmitted infection. Recurrences generally reflect reactivation of colonization.

Clinical Findings

A. SYMPTOMS AND SIGNS

Typical symptoms include pruritus and a white, cottage cheese–like vaginal discharge without odor. The itching is more common midcycle and shortly after menses. Other symptoms include vaginal soreness, vulvar burning, vulvar edema and redness, dyspareunia, and dysuria (especially after intercourse).

B. LABORATORY FINDINGS

The diagnosis is usually made by visualizing yeast or pseudohyphae with 10% KOH (90% sensitive) or Gram stain (77% sensitive) in the vaginal discharge. Fungal culture can be used if symptoms and microscopy are not definitive or if disease is unresponsive or recurrent, although colonization is common in asymptomatic women. Vaginal pH is normal with yeast infections.

Complications

The only complication of vulvovaginal candidiasis is recurrent infections (ie, four or more episodes annually).

Treatment

Topical formulations effectively treat vaginal yeast infections. The topically-applied azole drugs are more effective than nystatin. Treatment with azoles results in relief of symptoms and negative cultures in 80–90% of patients who complete therapy. Oral fluconazole as a one-time dose is an effective oral medication. Patients should be instructed to return for follow-up visits only if symptoms persist or recur. Six-month prophylaxis regimens have been effective in many women with persistent or recurrent yeast infection. Recurrent disease is usually due to *C albicans* that remains susceptible to azoles, and should be treated for 14 days with oral azoles. Some non-albicans *Candida* will respond to itraconazole or boric acid capsules (600 mg daily for 14 days) intravaginally. Treatment of sex partners is not recommended but may be considered for women who have recurrent infection (see Table 40–1).

Nyirjesy P, Sobel JD: Vulvovaginal candidiasis. Obstet Gynecol Clin North Am 2003;30:671 [PMID: 14719844].

Sobel JD: Management of patients with recurrent vulvovaginal candidiasis. Drugs 2003;63:1059 [PMID: 22635335].

GENITAL ULCERATIONS

In the United States, young, sexually active patients who have genital ulcers have genital herpes, syphilis, or chancroid. The relative frequency of each disease differs by geographic area and patient population; however, in most areas of the United States, genital herpes is the most prevalent of these diseases. More than one of these diseases could be present in a patient with genital ulcers. All ulcerative diseases are associated with an increased risk for HIV infection. The acute retroviral syndrome of HIV infection may be accompanied by oral and genital ulcers.

Ulcers are vaginal, vulvar, or cervical in females, and on any part of the penis in males. Oral lesions may occur concomitantly with genital ulcerations in HSV and syphilis. Each etiologic agent has specific characteristics that are described in the following sections. Lesion pain, inguinal lymphadenopathy, and urethritis may be found in association with the ulcers.

1. Herpes Simplex Virus

General Considerations

HSV is the most common cause of visible genital ulcers. At least 50 million people are infected with genital herpes in the U.S. Approximately 0.5–1.5 million new cases occur each year. Approximately one-third of herpetic genital lesions are caused by HSV-1, and the rest by HSV-2. As with oral HSV infections, many primary genital infections are asymptomatic (60–80%) or not recognizable as herpetic in origin.

Clinical Findings

A. SYMPTOMS AND SIGNS

Symptomatic initial HSV infection causes vesicles of the external genitalia, quickly followed by shallow, painful ulcerations. These may occur in the vulva, vagina, cervix, penis, rectum, or urethra. Atypical presentation of HSV infection includes vulvar erythema and fissures. Urethritis may occur. Initial infection can be severe, lasting up to 3 weeks, and be associated with fever and malaise, as well as localized tender adenopathy. The pain and dysuria can be extremely uncomfortable, requiring sitz baths, topical anesthetics, and occasionally catheterization for urinary retention.

Symptoms tend to be more severe in females. Recurrence in the genital area with HSV-2 is likely (65–90%). Recurrent genital herpes is of shorter duration (7–10 days), with fewer lesions and usually no systemic symptoms. Prodromal pain in the genital, buttock, or pelvic region is common prior to recurrences. HSV-1, which accounts for 30% of first-episode genital herpes infections, is usually the consequence of oral-genital sex. Primary HSV-1 infection is as severe as HSV-2 infection, and treatment is the same. Recurrence of HSV-1 happens in 10–55% of patients.

B. Laboratory Findings

Diagnosis of genital HSV is often made presumptively, but in one large series this diagnosis was incorrect for 20% of cases. Culture or antigen testing of the vesicles can confirm the diagnosis, but sensitivity decreases with advancing age of the ulcer. Several serologic tests with sensitivities between 80% and 90% are available and can distinguish between HSV-1 and HSV-2, which is important for prognosis. Recurrent genital ulceration is suggestive of HSV infection.

Differential Diagnosis

Any genital ulcer should be cultured for HSV and differentiated from syphilis and chancroid ulcers. The character of the ulcers and inguinal nodes differ in these diseases. (See sections on chancroid and syphilis).

Complications

Complications, usually with the first episode of genital HSV, include viral meningitis, urinary retention, transmission to newborns at birth, and pharyngitis.

Prevention

All patients with active lesions should be counseled to abstain from sexual contact. Almost all patients have periodic asymptomatic shedding of HSV, and many cases of genital HSV are transmitted by persons who are unaware that they have the infection or are asymptomatic when transmission occurs. Reactivation can occur in individuals who never had symptomatic disease. Individuals with prior HSV infection should be encouraged to always use condoms to protect susceptible partners. Antiviral prophylaxis of infected individuals reduces shedding and significantly reduces the chance of transmission to their sexual partners.

Treatment

Antivirals administered within the first 5 days of primary infection decrease the duration and severity of HSV infection (see Table 40–1). The effect of antivirals on the severity or duration of recurrent disease is limited. For best results, therapy should be started with the prodrome or during the first day of the attack. Patients should have a prescription at home to initiate treatment. If recurrences are frequent and cause significant physical or emotional discomfort, patients may elect to take antiviral prophylaxis on a daily basis to reduce the frequency (75% decrease) and duration of recurrences. Treatment of first or subsequent attacks will not prevent future attacks, but recurrence frequency decreases in many individuals over time.

Corey L: Challenges in genital herpes simplex virus management. J Infect Dis 2002;186(Suppl):S29 [PMID: 22239185].

Whitley RJ: Herpes simplex virus infection. Semin Pediatr Infect Dis 2002;13:6 [PMID: 22409051].

2. Syphilis

General Considerations

Syphilis is an acute and chronic STI caused by infection with *Treponema pallidum*. The overall rate of syphilis has increased annually after reaching an all time low in 2000. Increases have only been observed in men, with rates nearly doubling, from 2.4/100,000 in 2000 to 4.7/100,000 in 2004, predominantly in men who have sex with men. The male:female prevalence ratio of syphilis is 5.2:1. Unlike other STIs, rates of syphilis remain relatively low in the adolescent population, 1.7/100,000, with only a slight increased incidence in males. The South and certain urban areas continue to have high rates of syphilis.

Clinical Findings

A. Symptoms and Signs

Skin and mucous membrane lesions characterize the acute phase of primary and secondary syphilis. Lesions of the bone, viscera, aorta, and central nervous system predominate in the chronic phase (tertiary syphilis) (see Chapter 38). Prevention of syphilis is also important because syphilitic mucosal lesions facilitate transmission of HIV.

Primary syphilis usually presents as a solitary chancre—a painless ulcer with an indurated base and associated nontender, firm adenopathy. The chancre appears 10–90 days after exposure and resolves spontaneously 4–8 weeks later. Because it is painless, it may go undetected, especially if the lesion is within the vagina. Chancres may occur on the genitalia, lips, or anus. Secondary syphilis occurs 4–10 weeks after the chancre appears, with generalized malaise, adenopathy, and a nonpruritic maculopapular rash that often includes the palms and soles. Secondary syphilis resolves in 1–3 months but can recur. Verrucous lesions known as condyloma lata may develop on the genitalia. These must be distinguished from genital warts.

B. LABORATORY FINDINGS

If the patient has a suspect primary lesion, is at high risk, is a contact, or may have secondary syphilis, a nontreponemal serum screen—either RPR or VDRL—should be performed. If the nontreponemal test is positive, then a specific treponemal test, a fluorescent treponemal antibody-absorbed (FTA-ABS) or microhemagglutination–*Treponema pallidum* (MHA-TP) test, is done to confirm the diagnosis. An additional diagnostic tool is darkfield microscopy, which can be used to detect spirochetes in scrapings of the chancre base. Darkfield examinations and direct fluorescent antibody tests of lesion exudate or tissue are the definitive methods for diagnosing early syphilis.

If a patient is engaging in high-risk sexual behavior or is living in an urban area in which syphilis is endemic, RPRs should be drawn yearly to screen for asymptomatic infection. Syphilis is reportable to state health departments, and all contacts need to be evaluated. Patients also need to be evaluated for other STIs, including HIV.

Complications

Untreated syphilis can lead to tertiary complications with serious multiorgan involvement, including aortitis and neurosyphilis. Transmission to the fetus can occur from an untreated pregnant woman (see Chapters 1 and 38).

Treatment

See Table 40–1. Patients should be reexamined clinically and serologically with nontreponemal tests at 6 months and 12 months after treatment. If signs or symptoms persist or recur, or patients do not have a fourfold decrease in their nontreponemal test titer, they should be considered to have failed treatment or be reinfected and need retreatment.

Golden MR et al: Update on syphilis: Resurgence of an old problem. JAMA 2003;290;1510 [PMID: 13129993].

Primary and secondary syphilis–United States, 2002. MMWR Morb Mortal Wkly Rep 2003;52:1117 [PMID: 14627949].

Zeltser R, Kurban AK: Syphilis. Clin Dermatol 2004;22:481 [PMID: 15596319].

3. Chancroid

General Considerations

Chancroid is caused by *Haemophilus ducreyi*. It is relatively rare, but endemic in some urban areas, and has been associated with HIV infection, drug use, and prostitution. Ten percent of patients with chancroid are coinfected with HSV or syphilis.

Clinical Findings

A. SYMPTOMS AND SIGNS

The typical lesion begins as a papule that erodes after 24–48 hours into an ulcer. The ulcer has ragged, sharply demarcated edges and a purulent base, is painful (unlike syphilis), solitary, and somewhat deeper than HSV infection. Tender, fluctuant (unlike syphilis and HSV) inguinal adenopathy is present in one-third of patients. A painful ulcer in combination with suppurative inguinal adenopathy is very often chancroid.

B. LABORATORY FINDINGS

Gram stain shows gram-positive cocci arranged in a boxcar formation. Culture can be performed on special media that is available in academic centers. Other causes of genital ulceration should be excluded.

Differential Diagnosis

Chancroid is distinguished from syphilis by the painful nature of the ulcer and the associated tender suppurative adenopathy. HSV vesicles often produce painful ulcers, but these are multiple, smaller, and shallower than chancroid ulcers. Adenopathy associated with initial HSV infection does not suppurate. A presumptive diagnosis of chancroid should be considered in a patient with typical painful genital ulcers and regional adenopathy, if the test results for syphilis and HSV are negative.

Treatment

Symptoms improve within 3 days after therapy (see Table 40–1). Most ulcers resolve in 7 days, although large ulcers may take 2 weeks to heal. All sexual contacts need to be examined and given treatment, even if asymptomatic.

Lewis DA: Chancroid: Clinical manifestations, diagnosis, and management. Sex Transm Infect 2003;79:68 [PMID: 12576620].

4. Other Ulcerations

Lymphogranuloma venereum (LGV), caused by *Chlamydia trachomatis* serovars L1, L2, or L3, is rare in the United States although some communities of men who have sex with men have seen increased rates of disease. Patients with LGV present with a painless vesicle or ulcer that heals spontaneously, followed by development of tender adenopathy, either unilateral or bilateral. A classic finding is the groove sign—an inguinal crease created by concomitant involvement of inguinal and femoral nodes. These become matted and fluctuant and may rupture. LGV can cause proctocolitis, fistulas, and strictures in patients with anal involvement. Diagnosis can be made by culturing a node aspirate for *Chlamydia* or by serology. Differential diagnosis during the adenopathy phase includes bacterial adenitis, lymphoma, and cat-scratch disease. Differential diagnosis during the ulcerative phase encompasses all causes of genital ulcers. Treatment is with doxycycline, 100 mg twice daily for 21 days.

Granuloma inguinale, or donovanosis, is caused by *Klebsiella granulomatis* (formerly *Calymmatobacterium granulomatis*), a gram-negative bacillus that is rare in the U.S. An indurated subcutaneous nodule erodes to form a painless, friable ulcer with granulation tissue. Diagnosis is based on clinical suspicion and supported by a Wright or Giemsa stain of the granulation tissue that reveals intracytoplasmic rods (Donovan bodies) in mononuclear cells. See Table 40–1 for treatment recommendations.

Mabey D, Peeling RW: Lymphogranuloma venereum. Sex Transm Dis 2002;78:90 [PMID: 22075989].

GENITAL WARTS
(Human Papillomavirus)

General Considerations

Condylomata acuminata, or genital warts, are caused by human papillomavirus (HPV), which can also cause cervical dysplasia. Estimates suggest that 32–50% of adolescent females having sexual intercourse in the U.S. have HPV infections, though only 1% may have visible lesions. HPV is transmitted sexually: 30–60% of males whose partners have HPV have evidence of condylomata on examination.

Up to 100 serotypes of HPV have been identified. Types 6 and 11 are detected most frequently in genital warts, whereas 16 and 18 cause more than 70% of cervical dysplasia. The infection is more common in persons with multiple partners and in women who have previously had an abnormal Pap smear or genital warts. Cervical HPV is relatively more common in the adolescent population because of increased susceptibility of the cervical transition zone.

The American Cancer Society indicates that there is little risk of missing an important cervical lesion until 3–5 years after initiation of intercourse. Pap smears should be obtained after this time or by age 21. Thereafter, annual cervical screening should be performed using conventional Pap smears or every 2 years if using liquid-based cytology (ThinPrep), which can type HPV.

Clinical Findings

A. SYMPTOMS AND SIGNS

For males, verrucous lesions are found on the shaft or corona of the penis. Lesions also may develop in the urethra or rectum. Lesions do not produce discomfort. They may be single or found in clusters. Females develop verru-

cous lesions on any genital mucosal surface, either internally or externally. In women, cervical HPV infection may only be detected by cytology.

B. LABORATORY FINDINGS

External, visible lesions have unique characteristics that make the diagnosis straightforward. Condylomata acuminata can be distinguished from condylomata lata (syphilis), skin tags, and molluscum contagiosum by application of 5% acetic acid solution. Aceto-whitening is used to indicate the extent of cervical infection.

Pap smears detect cervical abnormalities. HPV infection is the most frequent cause of an abnormal smear. Pap smear findings are graded by the atypical nature of the cervical cells. These changes range from atypical squamous cells of undetermined significance (ASCUS) to low-grade squamous intraepithelial lesions (LSIL) and high-grade squamous intraepithelial lesions (HSIL). LSIL encompasses cellular changes associated with HPV and mild dysplasia. HSIL includes moderate dysplasia, severe dysplasia, and carcinoma in situ.

Follow-up for ASCUS is controversial, as only 25% progress to dysplasia, and the remainder are unchanged or regress. If ASCUS is present, the laboratory should be instructed to do HPV typing on ThinPrep Pap smears. If HSIL is found, colposcopy should be performed. If LSIL is detected, colposcopy is not needed, but a repeat Pap smear should be done in 1 year and if LSIL or HSIL are subsequently detected, the patient should be referred for colposcopy for direct visualization or biopsy of the cervix (or both). If a Pap smear shows signs of inflammation only, and concomitant infection such as vaginitis or cervicitis is present, the smear should be repeated after the infection has cleared.

Differential Diagnosis

The differential diagnosis includes normal anatomic structures (pearly penile papules, vestibular papillae, and sebaceous glands), molluscum contagiosum, seborrheic keratosis, and syphilis.

Complications

Because genital warts can proliferate and become friable during pregnancy, many experts advocate their removal during pregnancy. HPV types 6 and 11 can cause laryngeal papillomatosis in infants and children. Complications of appropriate treatment include scarring with changes in skin pigmentation or chronic pain at the treatment site. Cervical cancer is the most common and important sequela of HPV.

Prevention

The use of condoms may reduce, but does not eliminate, the risk for transmission to uninfected partners.

Treatment

All penile and external vaginal or vulvar lesions can be treated topically. Treatment may need to occur weekly for 4–6 weeks. An experienced practitioner should treat internal and cervical lesions (see Table 40–1). Treatment may clear the visible lesions, but may not reduce the presence of virus, nor is it clear whether transmission of HPV is reduced.

Warts may resolve or remain unchanged if left untreated or they may increase in size or number. Treatment can induce wart-free periods in most patients. Most recurrences occur within the 3 months following completion of a treatment regimen. Appropriate follow-up of abnormal Pap smears is essential to detect any progression to malignancy.

Gravitt PE, Jamshidi R: Diagnosis and management of oncogenic cervical human papillomavirus infection. Infect Dis Clin North Am 2005;19:439 [PMID: 15963882].

Kahn JA, Hillard PA: Human papillomavirus and cervical cytology in adolescents. Adolesc Med Clin 2004;15:301 [PMID: 15473368].

Lacey CJ: Therapy for genital human papillomavirus-related disease. J Clin Virol 2005;32(Suppl 1):S82 [PMID: 15753016].

Saslow D et al: American Cancer Society Guideline for the early detection of cervical neoplasia and cancer. CA Cancer J Clin 2002;52:342 [PMID: 12469763].

Shew ML, Fortenberry JD: HPV infection in adolescents: natural history, complications, and indicators for viral typing. Semin Pediatr Infect Dis 2005;16:168 [PMID: 16044390].

OTHER VIRAL INFECTIONS

1. Hepatitis (See Chapters 21 & 36.)

General Considerations

Hepatitis B and hepatitis C are often STIs. Hepatitis B is at least 10 times more common than HIV in the adolescent population. Since 1998, sexual transmission has accounted for approximately 50% of the estimated 181,000 new hepatitis B infections that occur annually in the United States. Heterosexuals who have unprotected sex with multiple partners and men who have sex with men are the groups at highest risk for sexual transmission.

Hepatitis C generally is transmitted through blood products and shared intravenous needles, although about 10% of hepatitis C infections have been linked to sexual transmission. Hepatitis C needs to be considered in teenagers who are symptomatic and engage in high-risk sexual behavior or intravenous drug use. Outbreaks of sexually transmitted hepatitis A infection have occurred among men who have sex with men, although the efficiency of sexual transmission is low.

Clinical Findings

A. SYMPTOMS AND SIGNS

Symptoms, diagnosis, and treatment are described in Chapter 36.

B. LABORATORY FINDINGS

Adolescents with high-risk behaviors need to be screened for hepatitis B virus (see section on screening). If hepatitis B surface antigen is present, the patient should be followed to distinguish acute from chronic infection and to provide appropriate management of chronic infection.

Complications

Hepatocellular carcinoma and chronic liver disease are complications of hepatitis B and C infections.

Prevention

Hepatitis B vaccination is the most effective means of preventing infection. All unvaccinated youth should be immunized. A simpler two-dose regimen is available for this age group. Universal vaccination for hepatitis A virus is recommended for young children and for travelers to high-prevalence areas, intravenous drug users, men who have sex with men, and individuals with chronic liver disease of other etiologies.

Treatment

See Chapters 21 and 36.

2. Human Immunodeficiency Virus (See Chapter 37.)

General Considerations

One in four new HIV infections in the United States is acquired by a person age 22 years or younger. Each hour two new young people in the U.S. become infected with HIV. Because of the long latency period between infection with HIV and progression to AIDS, it is felt that many HIV-positive young adults contracted HIV during adolescence. The number of females who become HIV-positive has increased dramatically, representing almost half of teenagers with HIV infection.

Risk factors for contracting HIV include a prior STI, infrequent condom use, practicing insertive or receptive anal sex (both males and females), practicing survival sex (ie, trading sex for money or drugs), intravenous drug or crack cocaine use, crystal methamphetamine use, homelessness, and being the victim of sexual abuse (males). HIV infection should be considered in any sexual risk-taking youths, whether they are practicing heterosexual or homosexual sex.

Clinical Findings

A. SYMPTOMS AND SIGNS

Adolescents may be asymptomatic with recent HIV infection or may present with the acute retroviral syndrome, which is evident 2–6 weeks after exposure. Fever, malaise, lymphadenopathy, rash, upper respiratory symptoms, oral and genital ulcerations, aseptic meningitis, and thrush may occur. If HIV infection is suspected, diagnosis is made in the acute period by HIV RNA polymerase chain reaction or p24 antigen detection.

B. LABORATORY FINDINGS

Screening for HIV by serology should include risk-taking youths and those with any STI. Adolescents may also present to the office requesting an HIV test. In either case, a careful history of sexual behavior should be obtained to assess risk and intervene with risk-reduction counseling. It is also necessary to determine how teens may respond to being told they are HIV-positive and what support systems they have in place. If an adolescent is homeless; does not have emotional support from family, friends, or a counselor; or threatens suicide or homicide in response to the idea of being HIV-positive, then testing should be deferred until the health care provider is confident that the youth will be safe if the test is positive.

Treatment

Many experts recommend aggressive antiretroviral treatment of patients diagnosed with acute retroviral syndrome.

Guidelines for the Use of Antiretroviral Agents in HIV-Infected Adults and Adolescents: http://www.aidsinfo.nih.gov

Futterman DC: HIV and AIDS in adolescents. Adolesc Med Clin 2004;15:369 [PMID: 15449850].

3. Human Immunodeficiency Virus Post–Sexual Exposure Prophylaxis

The risk of acquiring HIV infection through sexual assault or abuse is low but present. The risk for HIV transmission per episode of receptive penile-anal sexual exposure is estimated at 0.1–0.3%; the risk per episode of receptive vaginal exposure is estimated at less than 0.1–0.15%. For males practicing vaginal intercourse, the risk is somewhat less (0.03–0.1%). HIV transmission also occurs from receptive oral exposure, but the risk is unknown.

Health care providers who consider offering postexposure therapy should take into account the likelihood that exposure to HIV occurred, the potential benefits and risks of such therapy, and the interval between the exposure and initiation of therapy. It will be helpful to know the HIV status of the sexual contact. In general, postexposure therapy is not recommended for exposures to noninfectious fluids or exposures to intact skin and when more than 72 hours has passed since exposure. If the patient decides to take postexposure therapy, clinical management should be implemented according to published Centers for Disease Control and Prevention guidelines.

Havens PL et al: Postexposure prophylaxis in children and adolescents for nonoccupational exposure to human immunodeficiency virus. Pediatrics 2003;111:1475 [PMID: 22662832].

Olshen E et al: Postexposure prophylaxis: an intervention to prevent human immunodeficiency virus infection in adolescents. Curr Opin Pediatr 2003;15:379 [PMID: 12891049].

ECTOPARASITIC INFECTIONS

1. Pubic Lice

Pthirus pubis, or pubic lice, lives in the pubic hair. The louse or the nits can be transmitted by close contact from person to person. Patients complain of itching, and they may report having seen the insect. Examination of the pubic hair may reveal the louse crawling around or attached to the hair. Closer inspection may reveal the nit or sac of eggs, which is a gelatinous material (1–2 mm) stuck to the hair shaft.

2. Scabies

Sarcoptes scabiei, or scabies, is an organism smaller than the louse. It can be identified by the classic burrow, which is created by the organism laying eggs and traveling just below the skin surface. Scabies can be sexually transmitted by close skin-to-skin contact and can be found in the pubic region, groin, lower abdomen, or upper thighs. The rash is intensely pruritic, especially at night, erythematous, and scaly.

See Table 40–1 for treatment options. The entire area needs to be covered with the lotion or shampoo for the time specified by the manufacturer. One treatment usually clears the infestation, although a second treatment may be necessary. Bed sheets and clothes must be washed in hot water. Both sexual and close personal or household contacts within the preceding month should be examined and treated.

Orion E et al: Ectoparasitic sexually transmitted diseases: scabies and pediculosis. Clin Dermatol 2004;22:513 [PMID: 15596323].

Wendel K, Rompalo A: Scabies and pediculosis pubis: An update of treatment regimens and general review. Clin Infect Dis 2002;35:S146 [PMID: 12353201].

EVALUATION OF SEXUALLY TRANSMITTED INFECTIONS IN SEXUAL ABUSE AND ASSAULT

Sexual abuse is common: 25% of females and 12% of males will have suffered some form of sexual violence by age 18 years. Half of rape victims are younger than age 18 years. Rape is both a medical and a psychological emergency. Evaluation and treatment after sexual abuse or assault depends on the patient's age, his or her ability to communicate what occurred, and the timing of the abuse.

Teenagers usually can describe the kind of abuse (eg, oral, anal, vaginal; receptive or insertive), and evaluation needs to be directed accordingly. If the abuse has occurred in the preceding 72 hours, most states require for legal purposes that a rape kit be used. All practitioners should have access to a rape kit, which guides the practitioner through a stepwise collection of evidence and cultures. A thorough physical examination is indicated to evaluate for other signs of trauma.

Beyond 72 hours, evaluation is tailored to the history provided. The involved orifices should be cultured for *Neisseria gonorrhoeae* and *Chlamydia trachomatis* (NAAT is not admissible in court), and vaginal secretions evaluated for *Trichomonas*. RPR, hepatitis B, and HIV serology should be drawn at baseline and repeated in 2–3 months. Pregnancy testing should be done as indicated.

Trichomoniasis, BV, chlamydia, and gonorrhea are the most frequently diagnosed infections among women who have been sexually assaulted. Because the prevalence of these STIs is substantial among sexually experienced women, their presence after an assault does not necessarily signify acquisition during the assault.

Prophylactic therapy should be offered when patients present within the incubation time of any of the disease processes: oral ceftriaxone for gonorrhea and azithromycin or doxycycline for *Chlamydia* infection. If a person is exposed and does not have anti-hepatitis B surface antibody, give hepatitis B immune globulin and vaccine. The efficacy of hepatitis B immune globulin for sexual exposure is diminished if delay is greater than 7 days after exposure, and the value after 14 days is uncertain. No effective prophylaxis is available for hepatitis C. Evaluating the perpetrator for STI, if possible, can help determine risk exposure and guide prophylaxis. HIV prophylaxis should be considered in certain circumstances (discussed earlier). Emergency contraception should be given if the abuse occurred within 72 hours. Psychological assessment at the time of presentation, as well as over the next several months, is a top priority. Any suspected abuse must reported to the local authorities.

All younger children should be referred to child abuse multidisciplinary teams that help with the psychological aspects of the abuse and are well versed in helping children communicate what may have occurred. Colposcopic examination is critical in determining the extent of damage and provide documentation for the legal system.

Although it is often difficult for persons to comply with follow-up examinations weeks after an assault, such examinations are essential to detect new infections, complete immunization with hepatitis B vaccination if needed, and continue psychological support.

American Academy of Pediatrics: Committee on Adolescence: Care of the adolescent sexual assault victim. Pediatrics 2001; 107:1476 [PMID: 21293379].

REFERENCES

Burstein GR, Workowski KA: Sexually transmitted disease treatment guidelines. Curr Opin Pediatr 2003;15:391 [PMID: 12891051].

Centers for Disease Control and Prevention Sexually Transmitted Infections: http://www.cdc.gov/std/

Centers for Disease Control and Prevention: Sexually transmitted diseases treatment guidelines 2002. MMWR Morb Mortal Wkly Rep 2002;51(No. RR-6):1 [PMID: 12184549]. http://www.cdc.gov/std/treatment/

Fluid, Electrolyte, & Acid-Base Disorders & Therapy

Douglas M. Ford, MD

REGULATION OF BODY FLUIDS, ELECTROLYTES, & TONICITY

Total body water (TBW) constitutes 50–75% of the total body mass, depending on age, sex, and fat content. After an initial postnatal diuresis, the TBW slowly decreases to the adult range near puberty (Figure 41–1). TBW is divided into the intracellular and extracellular spaces. Intracellular fluid (ICF) accounts for two-thirds of the TBW, or roughly 50% of total body mass. Extracellular fluid (ECF) constitutes one-third of the TBW and 25% of total body mass. The ECF is further compartmentalized into plasma (intravascular) volume and interstitial fluid (ISF).

The principal constituents of plasma are sodium, chloride, bicarbonate, and protein (primarily albumin). The ISF is similar to plasma but lacks significant amounts of protein (Figure 41–2). Conversely, the ICF is rich in potassium, magnesium, phosphates, sulfates, and protein.

An understanding of osmotic shifts between the ECF and ICF is fundamental to understanding disorders of fluid balance. Iso-osmolality is generally maintained between fluid compartments. Because the cell membrane is water-permeable, abnormal fluid shifts occur if the concentration of solutes that cannot permeate the cell membrane in the ECF does not equal the concentration of such solutes in the ICF. Thus, NaCl, mannitol, and glucose (in the setting of hyperglycemia) remain restricted to the ECF space and contribute effective osmoles by obligating water to remain in the ECF compartment. In contrast, a freely permeable solute such as urea does not contribute effective osmoles because it is not restricted to the ECF and readily crosses cell membranes. Tonicity, or effective osmolality, differs from measured osmolality in that it accounts only for osmotically active impermeable solutes rather than all osmotically active solutes, including those that are permeable to cell membranes. Osmolality may be estimated by the following formula:

$$mOsm/kg = 2(Na^+, mEq/L) + \frac{Glucose, mg/dL}{18} + \frac{BUN, mg/dL}{2.8}$$

Although osmolality and osmolarity differ, the former being an expression of osmotic activity per weight (kg) and the latter per volume (L) of solution, for clinical purposes they are similar and occasionally used interchangeably. Oncotic pressure represents the osmotic activity of macromolecular constituents such as albumin in the plasma and body fluids.

The principal mechanisms that regulate ECF volume and tonicity are antidiuretic hormone (ADH), thirst, aldosterone, and atrial natriuretic factor (ANF).

Antidiuretic Hormone

In the kidney, ADH increases water reabsorption in the cortical and medullary collecting ducts, leading to formation of a concentrated urine. In the absence of ADH, a dilute urine is produced. Under normal conditions, ADH secretion is regulated by the tonicity of body fluids rather than the fluid volume and becomes detectable at a plasma osmolality of 280 mOsm/kg or greater. However, tonicity may be sacrificed to preserve ECF volume, as in the case of hyponatremic dehydration, wherein ADH secretion and renal water retention are maximal.

Thirst

Water intake is commonly determined by cultural factors rather than by thirst. Thirst is not physiologically stimulated until plasma osmolality reaches 290 mOsm/kg, a level at which ADH levels are sufficient to induce maximal antidiuresis. Thirst provides control over a wide range of fluid volumes and can even be a response to absence of ADH with attendant production of copious and dilute urine. One who cannot perceive thirst develops profound problems with fluid balance.

Aldosterone

Aldosterone—released from the adrenal cortex in response to decreased effective circulating volume and stimulation of the renin-angiotensin-aldosterone axis or in response to increasing plasma K^+—enhances renal tubular reabsorption of Na^+ in exchange for K^+ and to a lesser degree, H^+. At a constant osmolality, retention of

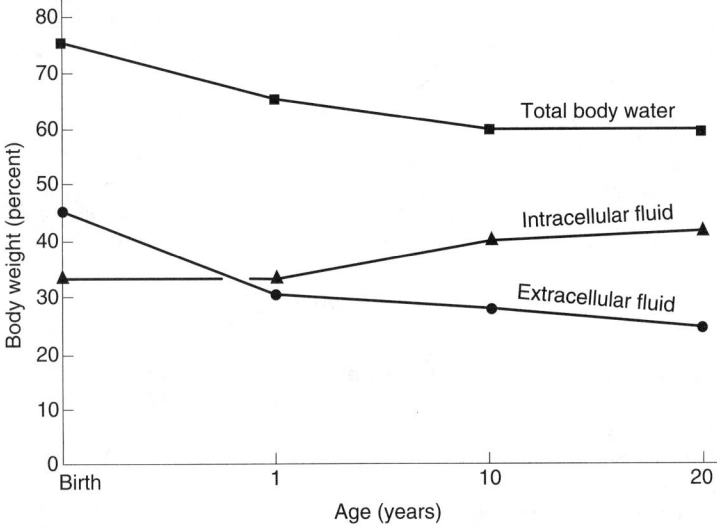

Figure 41–1. Body water compartments related to age. (Modified, with permission, from Friis-Hansen B: Body water compartments in children: Changes during growth and related changes in body composition. Pediatrics 1961;28:169 [PMID: 13702099].)

Na^+ leads to expansion of ECF volume and suppression of aldosterone release.

Atrial Natriuretic Factor

ANF, a polypeptide hormone secreted principally by the cardiac atria in response to atrial dilation, plays an important role in regulation of blood volume and blood pressure. ANF inhibits renin secretion and aldosterone synthesis and causes an increase in glomerular filtration rate and renal sodium excretion. ANF also guards against excessive plasma volume expansion in the face of increased ECF volume by shifting fluid from the vascular to the interstitial compartment. ANF inhibits angiotensin II– and norepinephrine-induced vasoconstriction and acts in the brain to decrease the desire for salt and inhibit the release of ADH. Thus the net effect of ANF is a decrease in blood volume and blood pressure associated with natriuresis and diuresis.

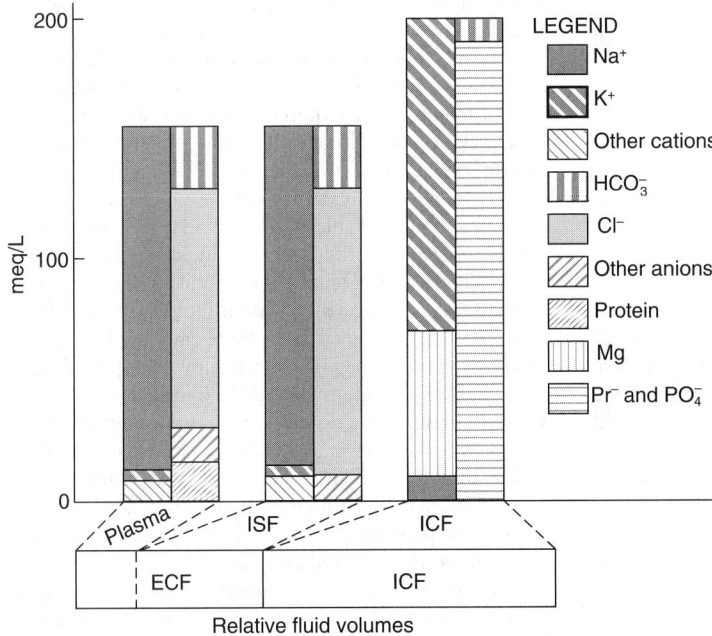

Figure 41–2. Composition of body fluids. ECF, extracellular fluid; ICF, intracellular fluid; ISF, interstitial fluid.

ACID-BASE BALANCE

The pH of arterial blood is maintained between 7.38 and 7.42 to ensure that pH-sensitive enzyme systems function normally. Acid-base balance is maintained by interaction of the lungs, kidneys, and systemic buffering systems. Over 50% of the blood's buffering capacity is provided by the carbonic acid/bicarbonate system, roughly 30% by hemoglobin, and the remainder by phosphates and ammonium. The carbonic acid/bicarbonate system, depicted chemically as:

$$CO_2 + H_2O \rightleftharpoons H_2CO_3 \leftrightarrow H^+ + HCO_3$$

interacts with the lungs, kidneys, and nonbicarbonate systems to stabilize systemic pH. The concentration of dissolved CO_2 in blood is established by the respiratory system and that of HCO_3^- by the kidneys. Disturbances in acid-base balance are initially stabilized by chemical buffering, compensated for by pulmonary or renal regulation of CO_2 or HCO_3^-, and ultimately corrected when the primary cause of the acid-base disturbance is eliminated.

Renal regulation of acid-base balance is accomplished by the reabsorption of filtered HCO_3^- and the excretion of H^+ or HCO_3^- to match the net input of acid or base. When urine is alkalinized, HCO_3^- enters the kidney and is ultimately lost in the urine. Alkalinization of the urine may occur when an absolute or relative excess of bicarbonate exists. However, urinary alkalinization will not occur if there is a deficiency of Na^+ or K^+, because HCO_3^- must also be retained to maintain electroneutrality. In contrast, the urine may be acidified if an absolute or relative decrease occurs in systemic HCO_3^-. In this setting, proximal tubular HCO_3^- reabsorption and distal tubular H^+ excretion are maximal. Some of the processes involved in acid-base regulation are shown in Figure 41–3.

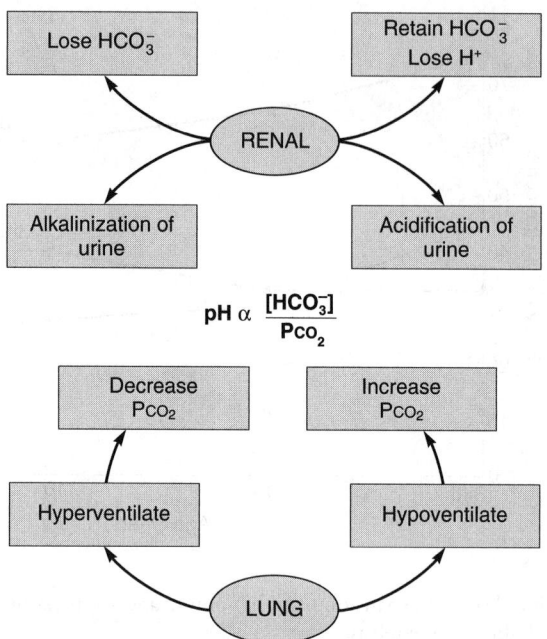

$$pH \propto \frac{[HCO_3^-]}{Pco_2}$$

Figure 41–3. Maintaining metabolic stability via compensatory mechanisms.

FLUID & ELECTROLYTE MANAGEMENT

Therapy of fluid and electrolyte disorders is directed toward providing maintenance fluid and electrolyte requirements, replenishing prior losses, and replacing persistent abnormal losses. Therapy should be phased to (1) rapidly expand the ECF volume and restore tissue perfusion, (2) replenish fluid and electrolyte deficits while correcting attendant acid-base abnormalities, (3) meet the patient's nutritional needs, and (4) replace ongoing losses.

The cornerstone of therapy involves an understanding of maintenance fluid and electrolyte requirements. Maintenance requirements call for provision of enough water, glucose, and electrolytes to prevent deterioration of body stores. During short-term parenteral therapy, sufficient glucose is provided to prevent ketosis and limit protein catabolism, although this is usually little more than 20% of the patient's true caloric needs. Prior to the administration of maintenance fluids, it is important to consider the patient's volume status and to determine whether intravenous fluids are needed at all.

Various models have been devised to facilitate calculation of maintenance requirements based on body surface area, weight, and caloric expenditure. A system based on caloric expenditure is most helpful, because 1 mL of water is needed for each kilocalorie expended. The system presented in Table 41–1 is based on caloric needs and is applicable to children weighing more than 3 kg.

As depicted in Table 41–1, a child weighing 30 kg would need 1700 kcal and 1700 mL of water daily. If the child received parenteral fluids for 2 days, the fluid would usually contain 5% glucose, which would provide 340 kcal/d, or 20% of the maintenance caloric needs. Maintenance fluid requirements take into account normal insensible water losses and water lost in sweat, urine, and stool, and assume the patient to be afebrile and relatively inactive. Maintenance requirements are greater for low-birth-weight and preterm infants. Table 41–2 lists other factors that commonly alter fluid and caloric needs.

Electrolyte losses occur primarily through the urinary tract and to a lesser degree via the skin and stool. Although

Table 41–1. Caloric and water needs per unit of body weight.

Body Weight (kg)	kcal/kg	mL of Water/kg
3–10	100	100
11–20	1000 kcal + 50 kcal/kg for each kg > 10 kg	1000 mL + 50 mL/kg for each kg > 10 kg
> 20	1500 kcal + 20 kcal/kg for each kg > 20 kg	1500 mL + 20 mL/kg for each kg > 20 kg

Adapted, with permission, from Holliday MA, Segar WE: The maintenance need for water in parenteral fluid therapy. Pediatrics 1957;19:823.

maintenance electrolyte estimates vary, reasonable approximations for maintenance needs are 3 mEq Na^+/100 kcal and 2 mEq K^+/100 kcal or 30 mEq Na^+/L and 20 mEq K^+/L, respectively, of intravenous fluid.

It is helpful to monitor the patient's daily weight, urinary output, fluid input, and urine specific gravity. If fluid or electrolyte balance is abnormal, serial determination of electrolyte concentrations, blood urea nitrogen, and creatinine may be necessary. In patients with significant burns, anuria, oliguria, or persistent abnormal losses (eg, from a stoma, or polyuria secondary to a renal concentrating defect), it is important to measure output, and if needed its components, so that appropriate replacement can be provided.

DEHYDRATION

Depletion of body fluids is one of the most commonly encountered problems in clinical pediatrics. Children

Table 41–2. Alterations of maintenance fluid requirements.

Factor	Altered Requirement
Fever	12% per degree C[a]
Hyperventilation	10–60 mL/100 kcal
Sweating	10–25 mL/100 kcal
Hyperthyroidism	Variable: 25–50%
Gastrointestinal loss and renal disease	Monitor and analyze output. Adjust therapy accordingly.

[a]Do not correct for 38 °C; correct 24% for 39 °C.

have a high incidence of gastrointestinal diseases, including gastroenteritis, and may demonstrate gastrointestinal symptoms in nongastrointestinal conditions. Infants and young children often decrease their oral intake when ill, and their high ratio of surface area to weight promotes significant evaporative losses. Renal concentrating mechanisms do not maximally conserve water in early life, and fever may significantly increase fluid needs. Dehydration decreases ECF volume, leading to decreased tissue perfusion, impaired renal function, compensatory tachycardia, and lactic acidosis. The clinical effects of dehydration relate to the degree of dehydration and to the relative amounts of salt and water lost. Caregivers must be particularly aware of dehydration occurring in breast-fed newborn infants who go home soon after birth and whose mothers fail to produce enough milk. This problem is more common in the hot summer months and has been associated with severe dehydration, brain damage, and death.

The clinical evaluation of a child with dehydration should focus on the composition and volume of fluid intake; the frequency and amount of vomiting, diarrhea, and urine output; the degree and duration of fever; the nature of any administered medications; and the existence of underlying medical conditions. A recently recorded weight, if known, can be very helpful in calculating the magnitude of dehydration. Important clinical features in estimating the degree of dehydration include the capillary refill time, postural blood pressure, and heart rate changes; dryness of the lips and mucous membranes; lack of tears; lack of external jugular venous filling when supine; a sunken fontanelle in an infant; oliguria; and altered mental status (Table 41–3). Children generally respond to a decrease in circulating volume with a compensatory increase in pulse rate and may maintain their blood pressure in the face of severe dehydration. A low or falling blood pressure is, therefore, a late sign of shock in children, and when present should prompt emergent treatment. Salient laboratory parameters include a high urine specific gravity (in the absence of an underlying renal concentrating defect), a relatively greater elevation in blood urea nitrogen than in creatinine, a low urinary $[Na^+]$ excretion (< 15 mEq/L), and an elevated hematocrit or serum albumin level secondary to hemoconcentration.

Emergent intravenous therapy is indicated when there is evidence of compromised perfusion (inadequate capillary refill, tachycardia, poor color, oliguria, or hypotension). The initial goal is to rapidly expand the plasma volume and to prevent circulatory collapse. A 20 mL/kg bolus of isotonic fluid should be given intravenously as rapidly as possible. Either colloid (5% albumin) or crystalloid (normal saline or Ringer lactate) may be used. Colloid is particularly useful in hypernatremic patients in shock, in malnourished infants, and in neonates. If no intravenous site is available, fluid may be administered intraosseously through the mar-

Table 41–3. Clinical manifestations of dehydration.

Clinical Signs	Degree of Dehydration		
	Mild	**Moderate**	**Severe**
Decrease in body weight	3–5%	6–10%	11–15%
Skin			
Turgor	Normal (+/–)	Decreased	Markedly decreased
Color	Normal	Pale	Markedly decreased
Mucous membranes	Dry ⟶		Mottled or gray; parched
Hemodynamic signs			
Pulse	Normal	Slight increase	Tachycardia
Capillary refill	2–3 s	3–4 s	> 4 s
Blood pressure	Normal ⟶		Low
Perfusion	Normal ⟶		Circulatory collapse
Fluid loss			
Urinary output	Mild oliguria	Oliguria	Anuria
Tears	Decreased ⟶		Absent
Urinary indices			
Specific gravity	> 1.020 ⟶		Anuria
Urine [Na⁺]	> 20 mEq/L ⟶		Anuria

row space of the tibia. If there is no response to the first fluid bolus, a second bolus may be given. When adequate tissue perfusion is demonstrated by improved capillary refill, decreased pulse rate and urine output, and improved mental status, deficit replacement may be instituted. If adequate perfusion is not restored after 40 mL/kg of isotonic fluids, other pathologic processes must be considered such as sepsis, occult hemorrhage, or cardiogenic shock. Isotonic dehydration may be treated by providing half of the remaining fluid deficit over 8 hours and the second half over the ensuing 16 hours in the form of 5% dextrose with 0.2–0.45% saline containing 20 mEq/L KCl. In the presence of metabolic acidosis, potassium acetate may be considered. Maintenance fluids and replacement of ongoing losses should also be provided. Typical electrolyte compositions of various body fluids are depicted in Table 41–4, although it may be necessary to measure the specific constituents of a patient's fluid losses to guide therapy. If the patient is unable to eat for a prolonged period, nutritional needs must be met through hyperalimentation or enteral tube feedings.

Oral rehydration may be provided to children with mild to moderate dehydration. Clear liquid beverages found in the home, such as broth, soda, juice, and tea, are inappropriate for the treatment of dehydration. Commercially available solutions provide 45–75 mEq/L of Na⁺, 20–25 mEq/L of K⁺, 30–34 mEq/L of citrate or bicarbonate, and 2–2.5% glucose. Frequent small aliquots (5–15 mL) should be given to provide approximately 50 mL/kg over 4 hours for mild dehydration and up to 100 mL/kg over 6 hours for moderate dehydration. Oral rehydration is contraindicated in children with altered levels of consciousness or respiratory distress who cannot drink freely; in children suspected of having an

Table 41–4. Typical electrolyte compositions of various body fluids.

	Na⁺ (mEq/L)	K⁺ (mEq/L)	HCO₃⁻ (mEq/L)
Diarrhea	10–90	10–80	40
Gastric	20–80	5–20	0
Small intestine	100–140	5–15	40
Ileostomy	45–135	3–15	40

Adapted, with permission, from Winters RW: *Principles of Pediatric Fluid Therapy.* Little,Brown, 1973.

Table 41–5. Estimated water and electrolyte deficits in dehydration (moderate to severe).

Type of Dehydration	H₂O (mL/kg)	Na⁺ (mEq/kg)	K⁺ (mEq/kg)	Cl⁻ and HCO₃⁻ (mEq/kg)
Isotonic	100–150	8–10	8–10	16–20
Hypotonic	50–100	10–14	10–14	20–28
Hypertonic	120–180	2–5	2–5	4–10

Adapted, with permission, from Winters RW: *Principles of Pediatric Fluid Therapy.* Little, Brown, 1982.

acute surgical abdomen; in infants with greater than 10% volume depletion; in children with hemodynamic instability; and in the setting of severe hyponatremia ($[Na^+]$ < 120 mEq/L) or hypernatremia ($[Na^+]$ > 160 mEq/L). Failure of oral rehydration due to persistent vomiting or inability to keep up with losses mandates intravenous therapy. Successful oral rehydration requires explicit instructions to caregivers.

The type of dehydration is characterized by the serum $[Na^+]$. If relatively more solute is lost than water, the $[Na^+]$ falls, and hyponatremic dehydration ($[Na^+]$ < 130 mEq/L) ensues. This is important clinically because hypotonicity of the plasma contributes to further volume loss from the ECF into the intracellular space. Thus tissue perfusion is more significantly impaired for a given degree of hyponatremic dehydration than for a comparable degree of isotonic or hypertonic dehydration. It is important to note, however, that significant solute losses also occur in hypernatremic dehydration. Furthermore, because plasma volume is somewhat protected in hypernatremic dehydration, it poses the risk of underestimating the severity of dehydration. Typical fluid and electrolyte losses associated with each form of dehydration are shown in Table 41–5.

HYPONATREMIA

Hyponatremia may be factitious in the presence of high plasma lipids or proteins, which decrease the percentage of plasma volume that is water. Hyponatremia in the absence of hypotonicity also occurs when an osmotically active solute, such as glucose or mannitol, is added to the ECF. Water drawn from the ICF dilutes the serum $[Na^+]$ despite isotonicity or hypertonicity.

Patients with hyponatremic dehydration generally demonstrate typical signs and symptoms of dehydration (see Table 41–3), because the vascular space is compromised as water leaves the ECF to maintain osmotic neutrality. The treatment of hyponatremic dehydration is fairly straightforward. The magnitude of the sodium deficit may be calculated by the following formula:

$$Na^+ \text{ deficit} = (Na^+ \text{ desired} - Na^+ \text{ observed}) \times \text{Body weight (kg)} \times 0.6$$

One-half of the deficit is replenished in the first 8 hours of therapy, and the remainder is given over the following 16 hours. Maintenance and replacement fluids should also be provided. The deficit plus maintenance calculations generally approximate 5% dextrose with 0.45% saline. The rise in serum $[Na^+]$ should not exceed 2 mEq/L/h. The dangers of too rapid correction of hyponatremia include cerebral dehydration and injury due to fluid shifts from the ICF compartment.

Hypovolemic hyponatremia also occurs in cerebral salt wasting associated with central nervous system (CNS) insults, a condition characterized by high urine output and elevated urinary $[Na^+]$ (> 80 mEq/L) due to an increase in ANF. This must be distinguished from the syndrome of inappropriate secretion of ADH (SIADH), which may also become manifest in CNS conditions and certain pulmonary disorders. In contrast to cerebral salt wasting, SIADH is characterized by euvolemia or mild volume expansion and relatively low urine output due to ADH-induced water retention. Urinary $[Na^+]$ is high in both conditions, though generally not as high as in SIADH. It is important to distinguish between these two conditions, because the treatment of the former involves replacement of urinary salt and water losses, whereas the treatment of SIADH involves water restriction.

In cases of severe hyponatremia (serum $[Na^+]$ < 120 mEq/L) with CNS symptoms, intravenous 3% NaCl may be given over 1 hour to raise the $[Na^+]$ to 120 mEq/L, to alleviate CNS manifestations and sequelae. In general, 6 mL/kg of 3% NaCl will raise the serum $[Na^+]$ by 5 mEq/L. If 3% NaCl is administered, estimated Na^+ and fluid deficits should be adjusted accordingly. Further correction should proceed slowly, as outlined earlier.

Hypervolemic hyponatremia may occur in edematous disorders such as nephrotic syndrome, congestive heart failure, and cirrhosis, wherein water is retained in excess of salt. Treatment involves restriction of Na^+ and water and correction of the underlying disorder. Hypervolemic hyponatremia due to water intoxication is characterized by a maximally dilute urine (specific gravity < 1.003) and is also treated with water restriction.

HYPERNATREMIA

Although diarrhea is commonly associated with hyponatremic or isonatremic dehydration, hypernatremia may develop in the presence of persistent fever or decreased fluid intake or in response to improperly mixed rehydration solutions. Extreme care is required to treat hypernatremic dehydration appropriately. If the serum [Na$^+$] falls precipitously, the osmolality of the ECF drops more rapidly than that of the CNS. Water shifts from the ECF compartment into the CNS to maintain osmotic neutrality. If hypertonicity is corrected too rapidly (a drop in [Na$^+$] of greater than 0.5–1 mEq/L/h), cerebral edema, seizures, and CNS injury may occur. Thus, following the initial restoration of adequate tissue perfusion using isotonic fluids, a gradual decrease in serum [Na$^+$] is desired (10–15 mEq/L/d). This is commonly achieved using 5% dextrose with 0.2% saline to replace the calculated fluid deficit over 48 hours. Maintenance and replacement fluids should also be provided. If the serum [Na$^+$] is not correcting appropriately, the free water deficit may be estimated as 4 mL/kg of free water for each milliequivalent of serum [Na$^+$] above 145 and provided as 5% dextrose over 48 hours. If metabolic acidosis is also present, it must be corrected slowly to avoid CNS irritability. Potassium is provided as indicated—as the acetate salt if necessary. Electrolyte concentrations should be assessed every 2 hours in order to control the decline in serum [Na$^+$]. Elevations of blood glucose and blood urea nitrogen may worsen the hyperosmolar state in hypernatremic dehydration and should also be monitored closely. Hyperglycemia is often associated with hypernatremic dehydration and may necessitate lower intravenous glucose concentrations (eg, 2.5%).

Patients with diabetes insipidus, whether nephrogenic or central in origin, are prone to develop profound hypernatremic dehydration as a result of unremitting urinary free water losses (urine specific gravity < 1.010), particularly during superimposed gastrointestinal illnesses associated with vomiting or diarrhea. Treatment involves restoration of fluid and electrolyte deficits as described earlier as well as replacement of excessive water losses, with subsequent water deprivation testing during daylight hours to distinguish responsiveness to ADH. The evaluation and treatment of nephrogenic and central diabetes insipidus are discussed in detail in Chapters 22 and 30, respectively.

Hypervolemic hypernatremia (salt poisoning), associated with excess total body salt and water, may occur as a consequence of providing improperly mixed formula, excessive NaCl or NaHCO$_3$ administration, or as a feature of primary hyperaldosteronism. Treatment includes the use of diuretics, and potentially, concomitant water replacement or even dialysis.

POTASSIUM DISORDERS

The predominantly intracellular distribution of potassium is maintained by the actions of Na$^+$-K$^+$-ATPase in the cell membranes. Potassium is shifted into the ECF and plasma by acidemia and into the ICF in the setting of alkalosis, hypochloremia, or in conjunction with insulin-induced tissue glucose uptake. The ratio of intracellular to extracellular K$^+$ is the major determinant of the cellular resting membrane potential and contributes to the action potential in neural and muscular tissue. Abnormalities of K$^+$ balance are potentially life-threatening. In the kidney, K$^+$ is filtered at the glomerulus, reabsorbed in the proximal tubule, and excreted in the distal tubule. Distal tubular K$^+$ excretion is regulated primarily by aldosterone. Renal K$^+$ excretion continues for significant periods even after the intake of K$^+$ is decreased. Thus, by the time urinary [K$^+$] decreases, the systemic K$^+$ pool has been depleted significantly.

The causes of net K$^+$ loss are primarily renal in origin. Gastrointestinal losses through nasogastric suction or vomiting reduce total body K$^+$ to some degree. However, the attendant volume depletion results in an increase in plasma aldosterone, promoting renal excretion of K$^+$ in exchange for Na$^+$. Diuretics (especially thiazides), mineralocorticoids, and intrinsic renal tubular diseases (eg, Bartter syndrome) enhance the renal excretion of K$^+$. Clinically, hypokalemia is associated with neuromuscular excitability, decreased peristalsis or ileus, hyporeflexia, paralysis, rhabdomyolysis, and arrhythmias. Electrocardiographic changes include flattened T waves, a shortened PR interval, and the appearance of U waves. Arrhythmias associated with hypokalemia include premature ventricular contractions; atrial, nodal, or ventricular tachycardia; and ventricular fibrillation. Hypokalemia increases responsiveness to digitalis and may precipitate overt digitalis toxicity. In the presence of arrhythmias, extreme muscle weakness, or respiratory compromise, intravenous K$^+$ should be given. If the patient is hypophosphatemic ([PO$_4^{-3}$] < 2 mg/dL), a phosphate salt may be used. The first priority in the treatment of hypokalemia is the restoration of an adequate serum [K$^+$]. Providing maintenance amounts of K$^+$ is usually sufficient; however, when the serum [K$^+$] is dangerously low and K$^+$ must be administered intravenously, it is imperative that the patient have a cardiac monitor. Intravenous K$^+$ should generally not be given faster than at a rate of 0.5 mEq/kg/h. Oral K$^+$ supplements may be needed for weeks to replenish depleted body stores.

Hyperkalemia—due to decreased renal K$^+$ excretion, mineralocorticoid deficiency or unresponsiveness, or K$^+$ release from the ICF compartment—is characterized by muscle weakness, paresthesias, and tetany; ascending paralysis; and arrhythmias. Electrocardiographic changes associated with hyperkalemia include peaked T waves, widening of the QRS complex, and arrhythmias such as sinus bradycardia or sinus arrest, atrioventricular block, nodal or idioventricular rhythms, and ventricular tachycardia or fibrillation. The severity of hyperkalemia depends on the electrocardiographic changes, the status of the other electrolytes, and the stability of the underlying disorder. A rhythm strip should be obtained when significant hyperkalemia is suspected. If the serum [K^+] is less than 6.5 mEq/L, discontinuing K^+ supplementation is usually sufficient. If the serum [K^+] is greater than 7 mEq/L or if potentiating factors such as hyponatremia, digitalis toxicity, and renal failure are present, more aggressive therapy is needed. If electrocardiographic changes or arrhythmias are present, treatment must be initiated promptly. Intravenous 10% calcium gluconate (0.2–0.5 mL/kg over 2–10 minutes) will rapidly ameliorate depolarization and may be repeated after 5 minutes if electrocardiographic changes persist. Calcium should be given only with a cardiac monitor in place and should be discontinued if bradycardia develops. The intravenous administration of a diuretic that acts in the loop of Henle, such as furosemide (1–2 mg/kg), will augment renal K^+ excretion and can be very helpful in lowering serum and total body [K^+]. Administering Na^+ and increasing systemic pH with bicarbonate therapy (1–2 mEq/kg) will shift K^+ from the ECF to the ICF compartment, as will therapy with a β-agonist such as albuterol. In nondiabetic patients, 0.5 g/kg of glucose over 1–2 hours will enhance endogenous insulin secretion, lowering serum [K^+] 1–2 mEq/L. Administration of intravenous glucose and insulin may be needed as a simultaneous drip (0.5–1 g/kg glucose and 0.3 units of regular insulin per gram of glucose) given over 2 hours with monitoring of the serum glucose level every 15 minutes.

The therapies outlined provide transient benefits. Ultimately, K^+ must be reduced to normal levels by reestablishing adequate renal excretion using diuretics or optimizing urinary flow using ion exchange resins such as sodium polystyrene sulfonate orally or as a retention enema (0.2–0.5 g/kg orally or 1 g/kg as an enema), or by dialysis.

ACID-BASE DISTURBANCES

When evaluating a disturbance in acid-base balance, the systemic pH, partial carbon dioxide pressure (P_{CO_2}), serum [HCO_3^-], and anion gap must be considered. The anion gap, $Na^+ - (Cl^- + HCO_3^-)$, is an expression of the unmeasured anions in the plasma and is normally 12 ± 4 mEq/L. An increase above normal suggests the presence of an unmeasured anion, such as occurs in diabetic ketoacidosis, lactic acidosis, salicylate intoxication, and so on. Although the base excess (or deficit) is also used clinically, it is important to recall that this expression of acid-base balance is influenced by the renal

response to respiratory disorders and cannot be interpreted independently (as in a compensated respiratory acidosis, wherein the base excess may be quite large).

METABOLIC ACIDOSIS

Metabolic acidosis is characterized by a primary decrease in serum [HCO_3^-] and systemic pH due to the loss of HCO_3^- from the kidneys or gastrointestinal tract, the addition of an acid (from external sources or via altered metabolic processes), or the rapid dilution of the ECF with non-bicarbonate–containing solution (usually normal saline). When HCO_3^- is lost through the kidneys or gastrointestinal tract, Cl^- must be reabsorbed with Na^+ disproportionately, resulting in a hyperchloremic acidosis with a normal anion gap. Thus a normal anion gap acidosis in the absence of diarrhea or other bicarbonate-rich gastrointestinal losses suggests the possibility of renal tubular acidosis and should be evaluated appropriately. (See Chapter 22.) In contrast, acidosis that results from addition of an unmeasured acid is associated with a widened anion gap. Examples are diabetic ketoacidosis, lactic acidosis, starvation, uremia, toxin ingestion (salicylates, ethylene glycol, or methanol), and certain inborn errors of organic or amino acid metabolism. Dehydration may also result in a widened anion gap acidosis as a result of inadequate tissue perfusion, decreased O_2 delivery, and subsequent lactic and keto acid production. Respiratory compensation is accomplished through an increase in minute ventilation and a decrease in P_{CO_2}. The patient's history, physical findings, and laboratory features should lead to the appropriate diagnosis.

The ingestion of unknown toxins or the possibility of an inborn error of metabolism (see Chapter 32) must be considered in children without an obvious cause for a widened anion gap acidosis. Unfortunately, some hospital laboratories fail to include ethylene glycol or methanol in their standard toxicology screens, so that these toxins must be requested specifically. This is of grave importance when therapy with ethanol must be considered for either ingestion—and instituted quickly to head off profound toxicity. Ethylene glycol (eg, antifreeze) is particularly worrisome because of its sweet taste and accounts for a significant number of toxin ingestions. Screening by fluorescence of urine under a Wood lamp is relatively simple but does not replace specific laboratory assessment. Salicylate intoxication has a stimulatory effect on the respiratory center of the CNS; thus patients may initially present with respiratory alkalosis or mixed respiratory alkalosis and widened anion gap acidosis.

Most types of metabolic acidosis will resolve with correction of the underlying disorder, improved renal perfusion, and acid excretion. Intravenous $NaHCO_3$

administration may be considered in the setting of metabolic acidosis when the pH is less than 7.0 or the $[HCO_3^-]$ is less than 5 mEq/L, but only if adequate ventilation is ensured. The dose (in milliequivalents) of $NaHCO_3$ may be calculated as:

$$\text{Weight (kg)} \times \text{Base deficit} \times 0.3$$

and given as a continuous infusion over 1 hour. The effect of $NaHCO_3$ in lowering serum potassium and ionized calcium concentrations must also be considered and monitored.

METABOLIC ALKALOSIS

Metabolic alkalosis is characterized by a primary increase in $[HCO_3^-]$ and pH resulting from a loss of strong acid or gain of buffer base. The most common cause for a metabolic alkalosis is the loss of gastric juice via nasogastric suction or vomiting. This results in a Cl^--responsive alkalosis, characterized by a low urinary $[Cl^-]$ (< 20 mEq/L) indicative of a volume-contracted state that will be responsive to the provision of adequate Cl^- salt (usually in the form of normal saline). Cystic fibrosis is also commonly associated with a Cl^--responsive alkalosis due to the high losses of $NaCl$ through the sweat, whereas congenital Cl^--losing diarrhea is a rare cause of Cl^--responsive alkalosis. Chloride-resistant alkaloses are characterized by a urinary $[Cl^-]$ greater than 20 mEq/L and include Bartter syndrome, Cushing syndrome, and primary hyperaldosteronism, conditions associated with primary increases in urinary $[Cl^-]$, or volume-expanded states lacking stimuli for Cl^- reabsorption. Thus the urinary $[Cl^-]$ is helpful in distinguishing the nature of a metabolic alkalosis, but must be specifically requested in many laboratories because it is not routinely included in urine electrolyte screens. The serum $[K^+]$ is also low in these settings (hypokalemic metabolic alkalosis) owing to a combination of increased mineralocorticoid activity associated with volume contraction, the shift of K^+ to the ICF compartment, preferential reabsorption of Na^+ rather than K^+ to preserve intravascular volume, or primary mineralocorticoid excess.

RESPIRATORY ACIDOSIS

Respiratory acidosis develops when alveolar ventilation is decreased, increasing Pco_2 and lowering systemic pH. The kidneys compensate for a respiratory acidosis by increasing HCO_3^- reabsorption, a process that takes several days to manifest. Patients with acute respiratory acidoses frequently demonstrate air hunger with retractions and the use of accessory respiratory muscles. Respiratory acidoses occur in upper or lower airway obstruction, ventilation-perfusion disturbances, CNS depression, and neuromuscular defects. Hypercapnia is not as detrimental as the hypoxia that usually accompanies these disorders. The goal of therapy is to correct or compensate for the underlying pathologic process, to improve alveolar ventilation. Bicarbonate therapy is not indicated in a pure respiratory acidosis, because it will worsen the acidosis by shifting the equilibrium of the carbonic acid–bicarbonate buffer system to increase Pco_2.

RESPIRATORY ALKALOSIS

Respiratory alkalosis occurs when hyperventilation results in a decrease in Pco_2 and an increase in pH. Patients may experience tingling, paresthesias, dizziness, palpitations, syncope, or even tetany and seizures due to the associated decrease in ionized calcium. Causes of respiratory alkalosis include psychobehavioral disturbances, CNS irritation from meningitis or encephalitis, and salicylate intoxication. Therapy is directed toward the causal process. Rebreathing into a paper bag will decrease the severity of symptoms in acute hyperventilation.

REFERENCES

Adrogue JA, Madias NE: Management of life-threatening acid–base disorders: Parts 1 and 2. N Engl J Med 1998;338:26, 107 [PMID: 9414329].

Avner ED: Clinical disorders of water metabolism: Hyponatremia and hypernatremia. Pediatr Ann 1995;24:23 [PMID: 7715960].

Fall PJ: A stepwise approach to acid-base disorders. Practical patient evaluation for metabolic acidosis and other conditions. Postgraduate Med 2000;107:249 [PMID: 10728149].

Finberg L et al: *Water and Electrolytes in Pediatrics: Physiology, Pathophysiology and Treatment,* 2nd ed. WB Saunders, 1993.

Hellerstein S: Fluids and electrolytes: Physiology. Pediatr Rev 1993;14:70 [PMID: 8493184].

Jospe N, Forbes G: Fluids and electrolytes: Clinical aspects. Pediatr Rev 1996;17:395 [PMID: 8937172].

Kappy MS, Ganong CA: Cerebral salt wasting in children: The role of atrial natriuretic hormone. Adv Pediatr 1996;43:271 [PMID: 8794180].

Liebelt EL: Clinical and laboratory evaluation and management of children with vomiting, diarrhea, and dehydration. Curr Opin Pediatr 1998;10:461 [PMID: 9818241].

McDonald RA: Disorders of potassium balance. Pediatr Ann 1995;24:31 [PMID: 7715961].

Roberts KB: Fluid and electrolytes: parenteral fluid therapy. Pediatr Rev 2001;22:380 [PMID: 11691948].

Watkins SL: The basics of fluid and electrolyte therapy. Pediatr Ann 1995;24:16 [PMID: 7715959].

Information Technology in Pediatrics

Carol S. Kamin, MS, EdD

Increasing numbers of physicians and patients are taking advantage of technologic resources, especially those available on the Internet. Nearly 100% of physicians report access to the Internet through office, hospital, or home connections. In a survey of British physicians conducted in June 2000, 88% of pediatricians reported using the Internet, with 50% using it both at work and at home (www.rsm.ac.uk/new/websurvey.htm). Technology is impacting general pediatric practices in many ways but especially in the areas of lifelong learning, clinical support, and patient education.

Note: When typing the address of a website into your browser, always use the site's exact designation, which may or may not start with "www." Websites listed in this chapter that omit "www." should be typed exactly that way, as in pediatrics.about.com. Your browser will automatically add the familiar tag, "http://."

LIFELONG LEARNING

Staying up to date in medicine has become much more complicated with the rapid acquisition of new information. The traditional avenues of staying up to date have included continuing medical education (CME), which includes approved conferences and self-study. Both of these are increasingly supported by technology. Consultations with other providers have also been facilitated with Internet technology.

Continuing Medical Education Online

The numbers of CME websites and continuing education online providers are increasing (Table 42–1). In 2000, 96 CME sites were available; in 2001 this number increased to 200. By 2004, one website linked to 270 online CME sites with more than 12,000 courses (www.cmelist.com/list.htm). Accreditation Council for Continuing Medical Education requirements are still grounded in conferences and have been slow to adopt regulations regarding CME credit for computer-based educational materials. In addition, limited educational strategies have been applied to those that are available. For the most part, existing programs and lectures have been transferred to the Internet without much thought about how the medium could best be used to improve the instruction, as evidenced by the fact that most CME websites are text-based with only 20% containing interactive components. Cases and tutorials on CD-ROMs can provide more interactivity and video images than the Internet bandwidth can currently manage, but this is changing quickly as broadband access spreads.

In a 2002 survey of 2200 U.S. office-based physicians, the most common reason physicians look for Internet-based CME is to solve a specific patient problem. They expect these programs to be easy to use, relevant, and credible. An example of the potential for case-based CME is an award-winning CME program on genetic counseling produced by the Dartmouth Interactive Media Laboratory and distributed by the American College of Medical Genetics for $25.00 at www.acmg.net/resources/cd-rom-01/intro.asp. This highly interactive program incorporates multiple learning strategies with rich video cases.

Casebeer L et al: Physician Internet medical information seeking and online continuing education use patterns. J Contin Educ Health Prof 2002;22:33 [PMID: 12004639].

Conferences

There are several website directories of medical meetings. One example is the Physician's Guide to the Internet, at www.physiciansguide.com. In addition to announcements of CME events and national conferences, this site contains sections on professional opportunities, clinical practice guidelines, and practical advice (eg, repaying medical loans).

However, today's busy clinical practice makes it difficult to attend local and national conferences. The Internet offers opportunities to make conference materials available to those unable to attend. These include PowerPoint slides with audio tracks, streaming video, or papers. You can see an example of streaming video at the University of Nebraska site that has a Grand Round lecture series (www.unmc.edu/Pediatrics/GrandRounds/home.htm).

A new trend in technology which may make conferences or even university grand rounds more available to

Table 42–1. Continuing medical education (CME) resources.

See CME finder at Pedialink sponsored by the American Academy of Pediatrics	https://www.pedialink.org/index.cfm
Pediatric emergency medicine site with cases of the week	www.pediatric-emergency.com
CME web	www.cmeweb.com
Pediatric development and behavior; click on Learning	www.dbpeds.org
CME super site, portal affiliated with the Health Channel	www.cmeweb.com
Pediatrics in Review CME	pedsinreview.aapjournals.org/cme
Contemporary Pediatrics with CME, puzzlers, journals, and forums	www.contemporarypediatrics.com/contpeds/static/staticHtml.jsp?id=100016
Links to 200 CME sites, up to 4000 courses and 8000 Accreditation Council for Continuing Medical Education accredited hours	www.cmelist.com
Electronic CME: online and software resources	www.medicalcomputingtoday.com/0listcme.html
CME at the Virtual Lecture Hall	www.vlh.com
E-mail alerts with CME in areas of interest	www.medscape.com/pediatricshome
Online Education for the Pediatric Professional	www.pedseducation.org/main/
The American Medical Association's CME Locater	http://www.ama-assn.org/ama/pub/category/2797.html

the private practitioner is called podcasting. Podcasting is a method of publishing audio broadcasts via the Internet, allowing users to subscribe to a feed of new files (usually MP3s). It became popular in late 2004, largely due to automatic downloading of audio onto portable players or personal computers. The popularity of iPods and other MP3 players makes it possible to download these files and listen to talks wherever you like and the audio is far superior to that of audiotapes.

Self-Study

Scientific information is growing exponentially, and most physicians have difficulty managing and evaluating this abundance of information. The Internet provides access to tools to help the practitioner manage the information overload. In addition to exclusively online journals, many print journals now have subscription online versions that can be searched by keywords (Table 42–2). Electronic newsletters inform subscribers of the latest research findings. Abstracts on topics the subscriber selects can be sent to an e-mail account. You can find the latest pediatric practice guidelines online (Table 42–3). Do you have questions about a new drug? Information on specific drugs is available online. In fact, some websites have e-detailing, which provides multimedia presentations of new drugs. If you still have questions about the drug, you can create an online request for a call from a drug representative.

A service being subscribed to by individual practitioners and institutions is UpToDate (www.uptodate.com).

Over 3000 authors contribute to this growing database of expert clinical information. Some studies report that this resource is used more frequently than any other electronic clinical reference. It can also be accessed on wireless PDAs. CME credit is available.

A bulletin from the National Library of Medicine in June 2005 announced that PubMed is offering RSS 2.0 (Really Simple Syndication) feeds. RSS is a Web standard for the delivery of news and other frequently updated content provided by websites. An RSS reader is required to use this service on your computer and retrieve new items from PubMed. There are numerous RSS readers from which to choose and many are available to download free from the Web. You can find out more about this PubMed service at www.nlm.nih.gov/pubs/techbull/mj05/mj05_rss.html.

The pressure to practice evidence-based medicine (EBM) is growing, by integrating individual clinical expertise with the best available external clinical evidence from systematic research. Clinical databases like PubMed (www.ncbi.nlm.nih.gov/PubMed), a Web-based resource of Medline, is a service of the National Library of Medicine and can offer access to over 11 million citations. Before conducting your search, identify key concepts you are interested in and consider alternative phrasing of those concepts. Next, limit your search by refining the dates, gender and age if possible, and the type of publication (clinical trials, editorials, letters, meta-analyses, practice guidelines, randomized controlled trials, or reviews). Boolean logic represents the

Table 42–2. Journal web sites.

American Academy of Pediatrics News	www.aapnews.org
Archives of Pediatrics and Adolescent Medicine	archpedi.ama-assn.org
Journal of the American Medical Association	jama.ama-assn.org
Journal of Pediatrics	www2.us.elsevierhealth.com/scripts/om.dll/serve? action=searchDB&searchDBfor=home&id=pd
Journal of the American Academy of Child and Adolescent Health	www.jaacap.com
Pediatrics	www.aappublications.org/
Pediatrics subspecialty collections	www.pediatrics.org/collections
The New England Journal of Medicine	www.nejm.org
Pediatric Research	www.pedresearch.org
British Medical Journal	www.bmj.com/index.dtl
Morbidity and Mortality Weekly Report	www.cdc.gov/mmwr
Annals of Internal Medicine	www.annals.org

relationship between more than one keyword. Use AND (in all caps) to retrieve citations that contain all of the search terms. Use OR to retrieve citations that contain at least one of the search terms. Use NOT to exclude the retrieval of terms from your search (eg, lead poisoning NOT adults). Under clinical queries, you can use filters to limit your search to therapy, etiology, diagnosis, or prognosis. An example of results using these strategies for a search on attention-deficit disorder is found in Table 42–4. What you hope to find is a manageable number of articles that match your clinical question as closely as possible. You still must evaluate the studies and determine whether they offer any new information for your patients.

Table 42–3. Online clinical practice guidelines.

American Academy of Pediatrics Clinical Practice Guidelines	aap.org/policy/paramtoc.html
Agency for Health Care Policy and Research	www.ahrq.gov
Bright Futures	www.brightfutures.org
Centers for Disease Control Prevention Guidelines	www.phppo.cdc.gov/cdcRecommends/AdvSearchV.asp
National Guideline Clearinghouse	www.guideline.gov
American College of Emergency Physicians Practice Resources	www.acep.org/webportal/PracticeResources
American Heart Association Guidelines	www.americanheart.org
Society for Adolescent Medicine Position Statements	www.adolescenthealth.org
National Cancer Institute (includes clinical trials)	cancernet.nci.nih.gov
Agency for Healthcare Research and Quality Clinical Practice Guidelines	www.ahrq.gov/clinic/cpgsix.htm
American Medical Association Policy Finder	www.ama-assn.org/apps/pf_online/pf_online
American Medical Association Practice Management Tools	www.ama-assn.org/ama/pub/category/4555.html
U.S. Preventive Services Task Force Guidelines	www.ahrq.gov/clinic/uspstfix.htm

Table 42–4. Sample PubMed search results on attention-deficit disorder.

Search Terms and Limits	Number of Citations
Attention-deficit disorder (no limits)	9285
Limit to 6–12 years of age, English	6083
Attention-deficit disorder (using Clinical Query–Therapy, Specific)	489
Limit to 2000–2005	155
Copy and paste search query into Clinical Query for Systematic Review	7
Limit to meta-analyses	1

Systematic reviews and meta-analyses of the literature are available in evidence-based medicine databases that have been compiled by EBM experts. Most of these services require a fee. However, as medical schools struggle to enhance clinical sites to provide experience to students and residents, one of the fringe benefits increasingly provided to preceptors is access to library resources that may include EBM databases. Critically-appraised topics (CATS) websites offer opportunities to read others' appraisals of the literature or tools to contribute your own. Additional EBM resources are listed in Table 42–5.

Sackett D et al: Evidence-based medicine: What it is and what it isn't (editorial). Br Med J 1996;312:71 [PMID: 8555924].

CONSULTATION

With electronic access to experts and colleagues readily available, it is not surprising that clinicians and patients seek advice over the Internet. This may be done directly by e-mail or as part of an asynchronous discussion group or listserv. To have e-mail service, you must have an account with an Internet service provider who has an address (a server) or mailbox where you receive incoming mail. Listservs use e-mail technology to allow users to subscribe to discussion groups (Table 42–6). If you subscribe to a listserv, you receive a copy of every message sent to the group. Some of these services offer the option of receiving messages in a digest form that compiles several messages into one. Some of them also keep an archive of old messages that can be searched by keywords. A listserv may be moderated to ensure that messages are appropriate for its audience. Discussion groups are slightly different from listservs. The messages are posted on restricted (password-protected) websites. Users log on to the site to read or add messages. Younger age, urban setting, private practice, and infrequent consultation with colleagues were found to be the most common characteristics of the users of the discussion groups on Physicians' Online, an Internet-based information and communication network with more than 200,000 members.

A weblog, or blog, is a new form of website that allows the owner the opportunity to post writings on any topic imaginable. Some sites offer opportunities for readers to respond. Most blog software is free. There are a few hundred weblogs authored by physicians and the number is growing. There is even a medlog aggregator hosted at www.medlogs.com/. Currently, the use is similar to posting editorial comments and debating.

Angelo SJ, Citkowitz E: An electronic survey of physicians using online clinical discussion groups. Conn Med 2001;65:135 [PMID: 11291565].

Conn J: Blogging offers doctors outlet for opinions. Modern Physician, 2004. Accessed August 31, 2005 at http://www.kevinmd.com/modphysician.htm.

CLINICAL SUPPORT

E-mail

Corresponding with patients and their families through e-mail is becoming commonplace in clinical practice communication. The utility of e-mail is its asynchronous

Table 42–5. Evidence-based medicine (EBM) resources.

PubMed tutorial	www.nlm.nih.gov/bsd/pubmed_tutorial/m1001.html
Critically-appraised topics (CAT) in pediatrics	PedsCCM.wustl.edu/EBJ/EB_Resources.html www.med.umich.edu/pediatrics/ebm.htm
CAT Tool	www.cebm.net/cats.asp
EBM (benefit vs. harm) tool	www.hsc.usf.edu/~bdjulbeg/Programs/evidencetable.htm
Series of online articles on EBM	www.cmaj.ca/
Resources for practicing EBM at IntensiveCare.com	Pedsccm.wustl.edu/EBJ/EB_Resources.html

Table 42–6. Listservs and discussion groups.

Listing of parent discussion groups	www-med.stanford.edu/touchstone/listserv.html
PedTalk: for general pediatric discussions	www.pcc.com/lists/pedtalk/
This is a site with many different types of forums or discussion groups including those for pediatricians	Pediatrics.about.com/mpboards.htm
Celiac-wheat and gluten intolerance discussion group	www.alamoceliac.org/acforums.html
Spina bifida/hydrocephalus discussion group	www.sbaa.org/site/PageServer?pagename= ecommunities or www.geocities.com/HotSprings/Spa/3247/ spinabifida.html
Cystic fibrosis list	esiason.org/newsResourcesMail.html
Diabetes list	www.lsoft.com/scripts/wl.exe?SL1=SP-DIABETES-LIST&H=LISTSERV.BUFFALO.EDU
Disability and medical-related discussion lists	www.makoa.org/listserv.htm

nature. It provides a permanent form of documentation and helps prevent "telephone tag." The use of e-mail has dramatically increased, with over 100 million users in 2000 in the United States. E-mail communication is being used for consultation, patient communication, and practice management. With the growing use of e-mail in clinical practice, the American Medical Informatics Association has published guidelines for the use of electronic mail with patients for clinical purposes:

- Establish a set turnaround time for messages. Do not use e-mail for urgent matters.
- Inform patients about privacy issues.
- Determine who besides the addressee on the receiving end processes messages.
- Include messages as part of the medical record.
- Establish acceptable types of transactions (eg, prescription refills or appointment scheduling) and discourage e-mail communications on sensitive matters (eg, HIV or mental health issues).
- Instruct patients to put the type of transaction in the subject line to allow prioritizing (eg, "prescription," "appointment," "medical advice," or "billing question").
- Request that patients put their name and medical record or patient identification number in the body of the message.
- Configure an automatic reply to acknowledge receipt of messages.
- Print all messages with replies and confirmation of receipt and place the e-mail in the patient's paper chart.
- Send a message to inform the patient of completion of the request.

- Request that the patients reply to the provider's message to acknowledge receipt.
- Configure e-mail messages so that when broadcasting to a group of patients, individual recipient names are not visible to others on the mailing list.
- Pay attention to the tone of your message. Avoid anger, sarcasm, or harsh criticism.

In addition, the American Medical Informatics Association recommended the following medicolegal and administrative guidelines:

- Consider obtaining the patient's informed consent for the use of e-mail. The consent form should include the communication guidelines, provide instructions for when and how to escalate to phone calls and office visits, describe security mechanisms that are in place, indemnify the health care institution for information lost due to technical failures, and waive encryption requirements, if any, at the patient's insistence.
- Use password-protected workstations in the clinical setting.
- Never forward patient-identifying information to a third party without the patient's express permission.
- Never use the patient's e-mail address for marketing.
- Use encrypted secure e-mail that is user friendly and practical.
- Regularly back up e-mail onto long-term storage.

E-mail is used for patient education, including distribution of disease-specific "handouts," and for conveying medication information, gathering references for current medical research, and sharing Internet resources. It is used for monitoring such markers of chronic illness as peak flow measurements, weight, blood pressure, and glucose levels. Finally, e-mail is used for administrative information including requests for referrals, address changes, and other demographic updates along with requests for prescription refills, laboratory test results, and reminders about appointments and vaccinations.

As the volume of e-mail begins to increase, providers may resist the burden of this new form of communication. It is not known if physicians will begin to provide e-mail care that is reimbursable.

Kane B, Sands DZ: Guidelines for the clinical use of electronic mail with patients: The AMIA Internet Working Group, Task Force on Guidelines for the Use of Clinic-Patient Electronic Mail. J Am Med Inform Assoc 1998;5:104 [PMID: 9452989].

Kohn L et al (editors): To Err Is Human: Building a Safer Health System. Committee on Quality of Health Care in America. Institute of Medicine. National Academy Press, 1999.

Electronic Medical Records

Electronic medical record systems, also known as digital health records, are computer-based systems that provide quicker retrieval of patient data with the potential for greater accuracy. President George W. Bush established the National Health Information Technology Office within the Health and Human Services Department. Dr. David Brailer was appointed as the coordinator and charged with developing national uniform technical standards and infrastructure.

In a recent study in Nottingham, researchers compared electronic versus paper medical records in primary care practices. They found that electronic records contained significantly more words and abbreviations than paper records. They were more legible, easier to understand, and contained more diagnoses, medications, and details of referrals. Electronic medical records systems will continue to evolve, driven both by the technology and the public's need for access to personal health care information.

The Institute of Medicine (IOM) has produced two companion reports. The first, entitled "To Err Is Human: Building a Safer Health System," concluded that "reorganization and reform are urgently needed to fix what is now a disjointed and inefficient health care system." Studies estimate that between 44,000 and 98,000 patients die each year as a result of medical errors, and preventable medication errors occur in 7.3% of hospital admissions. Even using the lower estimate for deaths, more people die in a given year as a result of medical errors than from motor vehicle crashes, breast cancer, or the acquired immunodeficiency syndrome. The decentralized and fragmented nature of the health care delivery system contributes to unsafe conditions for patients, and serves as an impediment to efforts to improve safety.

The second IOM report, "Crossing the Quality Chasm: A New Health System for the Twenty-First Cen-

tury," calls for action to improve health care over the next decade and emphasizes the use of information technology as key to a comprehensive strategy. The IOM committee believes that "information technology must play a central role in the redesign of the health care system if substantial improvement in quality is to be achieved in the coming decade." Health care delivery has been relatively untouched by the revolution in information technology that has been transforming nearly every other aspect of society. Health care organizations are only beginning to apply technologic advances. Patient information typically is dispersed in a collection of paper records, which often are poorly organized, illegible, and not easy to retrieve, making it nearly impossible to manage various chronic illnesses that require frequent monitoring and ongoing patient support.

Growth in clinical knowledge and technology has been profound, yet many health care settings lack basic computer systems to provide clinical information or support clinical decision making. The implementation of an electronic clinical information system offers the potential for improved patient safety, efficiency, and effectiveness. Standardized data collection can assist in implementing consistent care pathways and eliminating the need for data interpretation after the fact. The general attributes of a computer-based patient record should include the following:

- Problem list
- Measurement and recording of health status and functional level
- Statements about the logical basis for all diagnoses and conclusions
- Linkage with all of the patient's clinical records across settings and time periods
- Assurance of confidentiality
- Widespread accessibility
- Selective retrieval and formatting
- Linkage to local and remote knowledge sources
- Structured data collection using a defined vocabulary
- Expandability to meet evolving needs

Features specific for pediatrics include the following:

- The ability to calculate, display, and compare a child's growth percentiles and body mass index with normal ranges
- Special terminology and information to document developmental milestones and physical findings in infants and children
- Age-based normal ranges for vital signs and other physiologic parameters
- Prescribing medications based on age, weight, and body surface area of the child

Tools such as clinical alerts, ordering guidelines, care paths, and structured clinical documentation can provide clinicians with assistance in ordering and delivering health care. Clinical data repositories designed to capture, store, and analyze extensive patient information can form the foundation for effective care decisions. When automated documentation becomes part of the workflow, effective data collection becomes a byproduct rather than an additional task.

Although all-inclusive, computer-based patient records are still rare, especially outside the area of primary care, the benefits of an electronic patient record system are significant:

- Convenient access to patient data from a variety of locations, whenever it is needed; with the advent of the Internet, remote access to clinical data has been further simplified.

- Electronic access to clinical data allows for rapid filtering, sorting, and searching for specific information. Numeric data such as height, weight, and blood pressure can be graphed.

- Automated alerts, reminders, and suggestions can be built into clinical orders and decision points.

- Population-based data are available for clinical research, epidemiologic studies, and the development of quality measures.

- Clinical patient records offer the potential of coordinated information collected at all points of care, incorporating primary care, consultation, hospitalization, laboratory and radiology data, transcription, rehabilitation, and home care.

Bates DW et al: Relationship between medication errors and adverse drug events. J Gen Intern Med 1995;10:199 [PMID: 7790981].

Committee on Quality of Health Care in America: *Crossing the Quality Chasm: A New Health System for the 21st Century.* National Academy Press, 1999.

Dick RS et al (editors): *The Computer Based Patient Record: An Essential Technology for Health Care.* The Institute of Medicine. National Academy Press, 1997.

Hippisley-Cox J et al: The electronic patient record in primary care—regression or progression? A cross sectional study. BMJ 2003;326:1439 [PMID: 12829558].

Kaushal R et al: Medication errors and adverse drug events in pediatric inpatients. JAMA 2001;285:2114 [PMID: 11311101].

Special Requirements for the Electronic Medical Records Systems in Pediatrics—American Academy of Pediatrics: Task Force on Medical Informatics. Pediatrics 2001;108:513 [PMID: 11483828].

Personal Digital Assistants

PDAs, also know as palm-tops or handheld computers, have grown in popularity, and as they have so have their software applications for medical providers. A 2003 Forrester Research Study stated that more than 40% of physicians owned a PDA compared to 8% of all consumers. There are many drug references and other clinical ebooks such as the Redbook 2003 available for the PDA (see a review at www.pedspalm.com/files/ebooks/redbook2003.html).

Sittig and colleagues conducted a study to determine what physicians wanted from a PDA. Important tasks cited included checking drug information and treatment regimens, viewing patient data, and looking up diagnostic codes and laboratory values. The Riley Kidometer received five thermometers from pdaMD.com. Designed for pediatricians, it has database-driven tools for basic vital signs, lab values for all ages, growth and development tools, vaccine recommendations, electrocardiographic findings, resuscitation dosage codes, and more (see www.kidometer.com). PediSuite, a suite of seven modules providing calculations and other information, recently won the PDA Cortex Golden Software Award. Downloadable database programs using JFile or HanDBase can be found at www.keepkidshealthy.com/pediatricpilotpage/jfile.html. To find out more about pediatric-specific PDA software, see the comprehensive website at www.pediatricsonhand.com, where software is organized by subspecialty and other specific areas of interest.

The new multipurpose PDAs that include cameras, cell phones, and other features are driving the single-purpose PDAs out of the market. With a wireless access service, many of these multipurpose PDAs can access the Internet including e-mail accounts. One study found that physician response time decreased when pagers were replaced with PDA-mobile devices. Wireless users can also subscribe to channels of information. For information about software for physicians in any specialty, check out PdaMD.com.

Programs like PatientKeeper (patientkeeper.com/index.html) and PocketChart (www.caretools.com/) enable physicians to create, enter, update, and access their patients' medical record data with a few taps of a pen. A feature on PatientKeeper's Mobile Dictation application also lets you dictate notes into your PDA and send them via the Internet to a transcription service. PDAs can record dictation in real time over a secure and wireless network with the voice files transmitted directly to the server without being stored on the PDA. You can pause, rewind, and even save a draft. Another feature in Patient-Keeper is the ePrescription, in which you can forward accurate prescriptions electronically to pharmacies, saving the patient time and eliminating potential errors.

Many software developers creating medical applications for the PDA are developing companion products for patients. One example includes award-winning PediSuite by Medical Wizards, who have also created

PediParents. Instead of keeping paper diaries, physicians can monitor electronic diaries kept by their patients with diabetes or asthma on PDAs and specialized software (eg, the diabetes application at www.HealthEngage.com). In a randomized trial, children with arthritis and headaches reported recurrent pain and recorded it on electronic and paper formats. The e-diary group had significantly fewer errors and omissions compared to the group with the paper diaries. Boys demonstrated greater compliance with the e-diary format than girls.

Johns Hopkins Department of Pediatrics describes their progress in the use of PDAs as well as some of the clinical applications they have developed at www.welch.jhu.edu/about/mac2002_pdas.pdf.

Palermo TM et al: A randomized trial of electronic versus paper pain diaries in children: Impact on compliance, accuracy and acceptability. Pain 2004;107:213 [PMID: 14736583].

Sittig DF et al: Techniques for identifying the applicability of new information management technologies in the clinical setting: An example focusing on handheld computers (Proceedings). AMIA Symposium 2000;20(Suppl):804 [PMID: 11079995].

Telemedicine

Telemedicine uses telecommunications technology for medical diagnostic, monitoring, and therapeutic purposes when distance separates the users. There are three general categories of telemedicine: (1) store-and-forward, (2) self-monitoring and testing, and (3) clinical interactive services. Store-and-forward telemedicine services collect data, store it, and then forward it for interpretation later. The store-and-forward system eliminates the need for the patient and clinician to be available at the same time and place. It is generally used in clinical consultation. Self-monitoring and testing enable providers to monitor physiologic measurements, test results, images, and sounds, usually collected in another care facility or the patient's residence. This modality is used to monitor patients with chronic illnesses and those whose conditions limit their mobility. In the United States more than 450 telemedicine programs exist to provide clinical interactive services. The most common activities are consultation or second opinions, diagnostic test interpretation, chronic disease management, and posthospitalization or postoperative follow-up.

Telemedicine is being used in a wide variety of clinical settings, some examples of which are disasters and emergencies; home care and home nursing; new neurologic outpatient referrals; psychiatric and neuropsychological evaluation; hypertension and diabetes management; and surgical consultation. In addition to a growing number of programs in Western countries, it is being used to assist in delivering health services in other parts of the globe, such as northwest Russia, Bangladesh, Thailand, Taiwan, and Africa.

In pediatrics, telemedicine is being used in a range of subspecialties for consultation. Among these is remote echocardiographic diagnosis of congenital heart defects. In one 2-year study in Halifax, the telemedicine network saved a necessary patient transfer in 31 cases and avoided over $100,000 in additional costs. Use of the Internet and telemedicine has been studied as an adjunct in improving care for high-risk infants. The technology was used to enhance interactions among families, staff, and community providers. A video conferencing module allowed for virtual visits and distance learning from a family's home during an infant's hospitalization, as well as for virtual house calls and remote monitoring after discharge. In a randomized study of very low-birth-weight infants, the study group (Baby CareLink) reported a higher overall quality of care and greater satisfaction. Although the length of hospitalization was similar between the study and control groups, all of the study infants were discharged directly to home, whereas 20% of the control infants were transferred to a community hospital before discharge.

A number of questions remain for clinical telemedicine consultation and monitoring. What are the geographic limits for reimbursement? Which practitioners are eligible to present patients? Which practitioners are eligible to act as consultants? What teleconsultation services will be covered? What technologies will be covered? One reason for the lack of coverage of telemedicine has been uncertainty about its efficacy and cost. In a systematic review of clinical outcomes resulting from telemedicine interventions commissioned by the U.S. Health Care Financing Agency and the Agency for Healthcare Research and Quality, evidence concerning the benefits of its use exists in only a small number of health care areas despite widespread use of telemedicine.

Reimbursement for telemedicine services varies among states and insurers. Presently in the U.S., at least 18 states are allowing reimbursement through Medicaid for services provided via telemedicine, for reasons that include improved access to specialists for rural communities and reduced transportation costs.

With faster and less expensive computers and greater access to high bandwidth, telemedicine should continue to improve in quality and ease of use. As the use of telemedicine matures, essential elements to improve performance will include the following:

1. Licensing and credentialing. Telemedicine overcomes geographic boundaries but may be constrained by state laws.

2. Data security and privacy. Telemedicine consultation records need to be stored to document clinical decisions, especially for risk management.

3. Informed consent.

4. Peer-reviewed quality assessment.

Hersh WR et al: Clinical outcomes resulting from telemedicine interventions: A systematic review. BMC Med Inform Decis Mak 2001;1:5. Epub 2001 Nov 26 [PMID: 11737882].

Security

Although the principles of protecting the confidentiality and privacy of medical records apply to all forms of personally identifiable information, whether communicated on paper, orally, or electronically, the electronic dissemination of patient data is of special concern. Computerization makes it much easier to acquire, manipulate, and disseminate vast amounts of personal health information rapidly. Highly sensitive health data flow through employer-sponsored health plans, managed care organizations, hospitals, pharmacies, laboratories, and physicians' offices. These data are used for numerous health-related purposes, including clinical care, quality assurance, utilization review, reimbursement, research, and public health. In 1996, the Health Insurance Portability and Accountability Act (HIPAA) authorized the federal government to establish a national standard for medical record privacy either by legislative or regulatory action. In 1999, the Department of Health and Human Services published regulations to guarantee patients new rights and protections against the misuse or disclosure of their health records. The regulations apply to what are called "covered entities": health care providers, health plans, and health care clearinghouses that transmit health information in electronic form. The regulations are made up of three distinct parts: transaction standards, privacy, and security. The transactions standards call for use of common electronic claims standards, common code sets, and unique identifiers for all health care payers and providers. The privacy rules govern the release of individually identifiable health information, specifying how health providers must provide notice of privacy policies and procedures to patients and obtain consent and authorization for use of information; tell how information is generally shared; and tell how patients can access, inspect, copy, and amend their own medical records. The security regulations dictate the kind of administrative procedures and physical safeguards covered entities must have in place to ensure the confidentiality and integrity of protected health information. All medical records and other individually identifiable health information used or disclosed by a covered entity in any form, whether electronically, on paper, or orally, are covered by the new rule. Providers and health plans are required to give patients a clear written explanation of how their health data may be used and their health information disclosed. In general, the disclosure of health information is limited to the minimum amount necessary for the purposes of the disclosure. In very limited circumstances, health information may be disclosed in emergencies, for public health concerns, and for research when a waiver of authorization is independently approved by a privacy board or institutional review board.

PATIENT EDUCATION

Patients are accessing many kinds of websites that offer information about their conditions. Home use of the Internet is more common among highly educated and wealthier individuals, with no difference based on gender or community size. However, there is a "gray gap" with many elderly who shun the Internet. Sixty-three percent of women and 46% of male Internet users use the Internet to get medical information on a regular basis (www.pewtrusts.com/index.cfm). How might this change the patient-physician relationship? A study of patients with breast cancer who participated in online education and support groups reported that patients increased their confidence in their physicians and their competence to participate in their own care. A Harris online poll found that patients who used the Internet to look for health information were more likely to ask informed questions of their physicians and were more likely to comply with prescribed treatment plans. Similar results have been reported in studies of patients with cystic fibrosis and amyotrophic lateral sclerosis.

In addition to changing the relationship between physician and patient, patient outcomes can improve as a result of online patient education. In a study of patients participating in an online diabetes education and support group, patients lowered their blood glucose level more than the control group.

Social networks have steadily increased on the Internet. Women in particular are interested in this facet of the technology. It should be no surprise then that there are a number of Internet "communities" built around medical problems (see Table 42–6).

Though the Internet has an abundance of information, navigating its terrain is problematic. Increasingly, sites are being created as indexes of multiple websites of interest to a particular population (eg, www.generalpediatrics.com). Keeping these indexes current is a endless task since new sites are added daily and old sites may be removed or changed. However, this changing Internet landscape can provide opportunities to improve health by supporting and educating both providers and patients.

Physicians can help their patients evaluate the accuracy of information found on the Web and provide links to reliable patient education resources. General sites, like Medline Plus (www.nlm.nih.gov/medlineplus), provide a great deal of reliable information indexed at one site by the National Library of Medicine. A recent review of online pediatric patient education materials suggests that the majority of materials are not written at an appropriate reading level for the average adult (eighth to ninth grade). If your practice is interested in hosting a patient education website, consider the following guidelines:

- Write patient guidelines clearly, make them highly visible, and ensure that all parties read and understand them before they use the resource.
- Present a statement about the intent and limitations of the resource, and provide contact information should the user have questions.
- Address concerns about privacy; identify possible security breaches and the steps users must take to protect their information.
- Define and clarify which areas of the resource are for posting private messages to providers containing health information, and which areas are public.
- Define the patient's rights and responsibilities, and provide examples of queries that should be posted and those situations that require more immediate medical attention.
- Define the provider's responsibilities.

Because a mixture of high-quality and low-quality resources are available for patients on the Web, it is important that physicians are aware of Web-based resources and have reliable sites to recommend to an increasingly sophisticated population.

Technology and the Internet are changing our culture as well as medical education and health care delivery.

Properly implemented and adopted, these new applications offer physicians the opportunity to harness the technology for better and more efficient patient care.

Alessandro DM et al: The readability of pediatric patient education materials on the World Wide Web. Arch Pediatr Adolesc Med 2001;155:807 [PMID: 11434848].

Characteristics and Choices of Internet Users: Report to the Ranking Minority Member Subcommittee on Telecommunications Committee on Energy and Commerce, House of Representatives. United States General Accounting Office, February 2001.

Feenberg AL et al: The online patient meeting. J Neurol Sci 1996;139(Suppl):129 [PMID: 8899672].

Gustafson DH et al: Effect of computer support on younger women with breast cancer. J Gen Intern Med 2001;16:435 [PMID: 11520380].

Harris Interactive: The increasing impact of eHealth on consumer behavior. Health Care News 2001;1:1.

Johnson KB et al: Hopkins Teen central: Assessment of an Internet-based support system for children with cystic fibrosis. Pediatrics 2001;107:E24 [PMID: 11158498].

McKay HG et al: The diabetes network Internet-based physical activity intervention: A randomized pilot study. Diabetes Care 2001;24:1328 [PMID: 11473065].

Prady SL et al: Expanding the guidelines for electronic communication with patients. JAMA 2001;8:344 [PMID: 11418540].

Chemistry & Hematology Reference Intervals

43

Georgette Siparsky, PhD, & Frank J. Accurso, MD

Laboratory tests provide valuable information necessary to evaluate a patient's condition and to monitor recommended treatment. Chemistry and hematology test results are compared to those of healthy individuals or those undergoing similar therapeutic treatment to determine clinical status and progress. In the past, the term "normal ranges" was ambiguous since statistically, the term "normal" also implied a specific (gaussian or normal) distribution, and epidemiologically it implied the state of the majority, which is not necessarily the desirable or target population. This is most apparent in cholesterol levels, where values greater than 200 mg/dL are common but not desirable. Use of the term "reference range" or "reference interval" is therefore recommended by the International Federation of Clinical Chemistry and the Clinical and Laboratory Standards Institute (CLSI, formerly the National Committee for Clinical Laboratory Standards) to indicate that the values relate to a reference population and clinical condition.

Reference ranges are established for a specific age (eg, α-fetoprotein), gender, and level of sexual maturity (eg, luteinizing hormone and testosterone); they are also defined for a specific pharmacologic status (eg, taking cyclosporine), dietary restriction (eg, phenylalanine), and stimulation protocol (eg, growth hormone). Similarly, diurnal variation is a factor (eg, cortisol), as is degree of obesity (eg, insulin). Some reference ranges are particularly meaningful when combined with other results (eg, parathyroid hormone and calcium), or when an entire set of analytes is evaluated (eg, lipid profile: triglyceride, total cholesterol, high-density lipoprotein cholesterol, and low-density lipoprotein cholesterol).

Laboratory tests are becoming more specific and measure much lower concentrations than ever before. Therefore reference ranges should reflect the analytic procedure, as well as reagents and instrumentation used for a specific analysis. As test methodology continues to evolve, reference ranges are modified and updated.

THE CHALLENGE OF DETERMINING & INTERPRETING PEDIATRIC REFERENCE INTERVALS

The pediatric environment is particularly challenging for the determination of reference intervals since growth and developmental stages do not have distinct and finite boundaries by which test results can be tabulated. Reference ranges may overlap, and in many cases complicate diagnosis and treatment. Collection and allocation of test results by age for the purpose of establishing a reference range is a convenient and manageable way to report them, but caution is needed in their interpretation and clinical correlation.

A particular difficulty lies in establishing reference ranges for analytes whose levels are changed under scheduled stimulation conditions. The common glucose tolerance test is one example, but more complex endocrinologic tests (eg, stimulation by clonidine and cosyntropin) require skill and extensive experience to interpret. Reference ranges for these serial tests are established over a long period of time and are not easily transferable between test methodologies. Changing analytical technologies adds a new dimension to the challenges of establishing pediatric reference ranges.

Guidelines for Data Used for a Reference Range Study

The College of American Pathologists provides guidelines for the adoption of reference ranges used in hospitals and commercial clinical laboratories. It recognizes the enormous task of establishing a laboratory's own reference ranges, and recommends alternatives to the process. A laboratory may acquire reference ranges by:

1. Conducting its own study to evaluate a statistically significant number of "healthy" volunteers. It is a monumental task for a laboratory to develop its own

pediatric reference ranges, since parental consent and procedural approval by review boards need to be addressed. The numerous age categories to be evaluated also add to the complexity and size of the study.

2. Adopting ranges established by the manufacturer of a particular analytical instrument. The laboratory must validate the data by analyzing a sample of 20 reference subjects (patients representing that specific population) to confirm that the adopted range is truly representative of that group.

3. Using reference data in the general medical literature and conferring with physicians to make sure the data agree with their clinical experience. A validation study is also recommended.

4. Analyzing hospital patient data. Laboratory test results from hospital patients have been used to compute reference ranges provided they fulfill stated clinical criteria. Patient records need to indicate that his or her specific medical condition does not influence the analyte whose reference range is being determined. For example, a child undergoing surgery for bone fracture repair is expected to have normal electrolytes and thyroid function, whereas a child examined for precocious puberty should not be included in a reference range study for luteinizing hormone. Grossi et al chose the "inclusion criterion," whereby tests that have a single laboratory measurement were used; justification was based on the fact that persons with repeated testing had a higher probability of being diseased and their results should be excluded from the study.

Statistically, the sample size of a hospital patient study should be considerably larger than that of a healthy group. A study from a healthy population may require 20 subjects to be statistically significant, whereas a hospital population should evaluate a minimum of 120 patients. At Children's Hospital in Denver, the free thyroxine reference range was recently established using 1480 clinic and hospital patient results in this manner.

Statistical Computation of Reference Intervals

The establishment of reference intervals is based on a statistical distribution of test results obtained from a representative population. The CLSI recommendation for data collection and statistical analysis provides guidelines for managing the data. For clinicians, it is not important that they can reproduce the calculation. It is far more critical to understand the benefits and restrictions provided by the described statistical approaches, and to evaluate patient results with these limitations in mind.

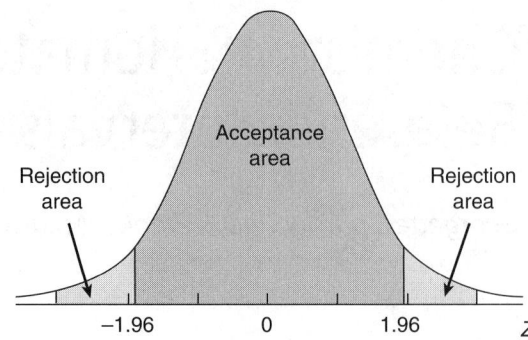

Figure 43–1. Gaussian distribution and parametric calculation using x ± 1.96s to define the range.

A. Parametric Method of Computation

The parametric method of establishing reference intervals is simple, though not always representative, since it is based on the assumption that the data has a gaussian distribution. A mean (x) and standard deviation (s) are calculated; test results of 95% of that specific population will fall within the mean ±1.96s, as shown in Figure 43–1.

Where the distribution is not gaussian, a mathematical manipulation of the values (for example, plotting the log of the value, instead of the value itself) may give a gaussian distribution. The mean and standard deviation are then converted back to give a usable reference range.

B. Nonparametric Method of Computation

The nonparametric method of establishing reference ranges is currently recommended by CLSI since it defines outliers as those in the extreme 2.5 percentiles of the upper and lower limits of data. The number of data points excluded at the limits depends on the skew of the curve, and so the computation accommodates a nongaussian distribution. A histogram depicting the nongaussian distribution of data from a free thyroxine reference range study conducted at The Children's Hospital in Denver is shown in Figure 43–2.

In reviewing the statistics, 95% of all results will be inherently included in the reference range. Note that 5% of that population will have "abnormal" results, when in fact they are "healthy" and an integral part of the reference group study. Similarly an equivalent 5% of the "ill" population will have laboratory results within the reference range. These are inherent features of the statistical computation. Taking that analysis one step further, the probability of a healthy patient having a test result within a calculated reference range is

$$P = 0.95$$

When multiple tests or panels of tests are used, the combined probability of all the test results falling in their

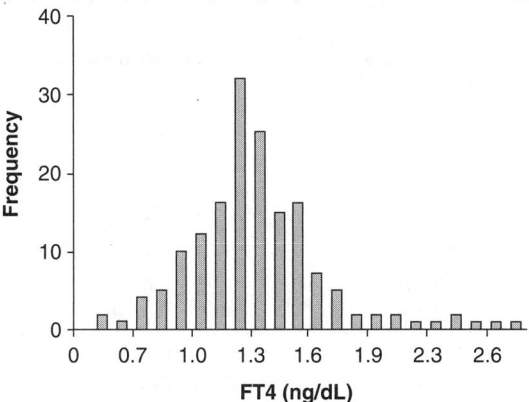

Figure 43–2. Histogram of free thyroxine using clinic and hospital patients at Children's Hospital in Denver.

respective reference ranges drops dramatically. For example, the probability of all results from 10 tests in the "complete metabolic panel" being in the reference range is

$$P = (0.95)^0 = 0.60$$

Therefore, about one-third of healthy patients will have one test result in the panel that is outside the reference range.

Why Reference Intervals Vary

Recent modifications to reference ranges are due to the introduction of new and improved analytic procedures, advanced automated instrumentation, and standardization of reagents and reference materials. Reference ranges are also affected by preanalytic variations that can occur during sample collection, processing, and storage.

Preanalytic variations of biological origin include situations in which specimens are drawn in the morning versus those drawn in the evening, and hospitalized recumbent patients versus ambulatory outpatients. The variation may also be caused by metabolic and homodynamic factors. Preanalytical factors may be a product of the socioeconomic environment or ethnic background (eg, genetic or dietary).

Analytic variations are caused by differences in analytic measurements, and depend on the analytic tools as well as the inherent variability in obtaining a quantitative value. Furthermore, scientific progress is constantly introducing new reagents, instruments, and improved testing procedures to the clinical laboratory, and each tool adds an element of variability between tests.

1. Antigen-antibody reactions have revolutionized clinical chemistry, but have also added a degree of variability because biologically-derived reagents have different specificities and sensitivities. In addition to the targeted analyte, some of its metabolites are also measured, and these may or may not be biologically active.

2. Reference materials continue to be reviewed and evaluated by organizations such as the World Health Organization and the National Institute for Standards and Technology. A new standard was recently established for troponin I and reference ranges were modified to reflect the new standard.

3. Analytic instrumentation with advanced electronics and robotics has improved accuracy of results and increased throughput. However, they have added an element of variability between instruments from different manufacturers.

4. Analytic detection methods have also made great strides as they have expanded from simple ultraviolet-visible spectrophotometry, to fluorescence, nephelometry, radioimmunoassay, and chemiluminescence studies. For example, the third-generation thyroid-stimulating hormone assays can now measure concentrations as low as 0.001 μIU/mL and the reference range was recently modified to reflect the improved sensitivity of the assay.

Clinical laboratory data are frequently interpreted with a dynamic approach rather than a static state, so that each value is compared to another, instead of a strict reference range. In this case, time series analysis of relative values may provide more important information than comparison to a reference range. Examples include the evaluation of enzyme activity over time and various stimulation studies for endocrine assessment. Drug monitoring is also a dynamic process.

The establishment of reference ranges is a complex process. Assumptions are made in the management of data processes, regardless of whether "healthy" individuals or hospital patients are used for the accumulation of test results. Analytic instrument manufacturers conduct large studies to identify reference intervals for each specific analyte, and pediatric values have always been the most challenging. Some of the manufacturers' recommended reference intervals are listed in Table 43–1 for general chemistry, Table 43–2 for endocrinology, and Table 43–3 for hematology. The interpretation of chemistry and hematology laboratory results is equally complex and poses a continuing challenge for physicians and the medical community at large.

REFERENCES

Bishop M, Fody E, Schoeff L: *Clinical Chemistry, Principles and Procedures,* 5th ed. Lippincott Williams & Wilkins, 2005.

Clinical and Laboratories Standards Institute (CLSI) (formerly the National Committee for Clinical Laboratory Standards): How to Define and Determine Reference Intervals in the Clinical Laboratory. Approved Guidelines, Second Edition. NCCLS Document C28-A2, June 2000. http://www.clsi.org/es/source/orders

Table 43–1. General chemistry.

Analyte, Units, Specimen Type	Age	Male Range	Female Range
Albumin (g/dL) S, P	1–7 d	2.4–3.9	1.9–4.0
	8–30 d	2.1–4.5	1.9–4.4
	31–90 d	2.1–4.8	2.0–4.2
	3–6 mo	2.2–4.9	2.3–4.4
	6 mo–1 y	2.2–4.7	2.3–4.7
	1–3 y	3.5–4.2	3.5–4.7
	4–6 y	3.6–5.2	3.6–5.2
	7 y–Adult	3.8–5.6	3.8–5.6
Alkaline phosphatase (U/L) S, P	1–7 d	121–351	107–357
	8–30 d	138–486	107–474
	31–90 d	101–467	125–547
	4–6 mo	94–425	125–449
	7–12 mo	101–394	101–431
	1–3 y	185–383	185–383
	4–6 y	191–450	191–450
	7–9 y	218–499	218–499
	10–11 y	174–624	169–657
	12–13 y	245–584	141–499
	14–15 y	169–618	103–283
	16–19 y	98–317	82–169
Alanine amino trasferase (U/L) S, P	1–7 d	20–54	21–54
	8–30 d	24–54	22–46
	1–3 mo	27–54	26–61
	4–6 mo	26–55	26–51
	7–12 mo	26–59	26–55
	1–3 y	19–59	24–59
	4–6 y	24–49	24–49
	10–11 y	24–49	24–44
	12–13 y	24–68	24–44
	14–15 y	24–59	19–44
	16–19 y	24–54	19–49
Ammonia (μmol/L)	All Ages	< 51	< 51
Amylase (U/L) S, P	1–30 d	< 18	< 18
	31–182 d	< 43	< 43
	183–365 d	< 81	< 81
	1 y–Adult	< 106	< 106
Aspartate aminotransferase (U/L) S, P	1–7 d	26–98	20–93
	8–30 d	16–67	20–69
	1–3 mo	16–60	16–61
	4–6 mo	16–62	16–60
	7–12 mo	16–52	16–60
	1–3 y	16–57	16–57
	5–6 y	10–47	10–47
	7–9 y	10–36	5–36
	12–13 y	10–36	5–26
	16–19 y	10–41	0–26

(continued)

Table 43–1. General chemistry. (continued)

Analyte, Units, Specimen Type	Age	Male Range	Female Range
Blood urea nitrogen (mg/dL) S, P	0–4 d	3–19	3–19
	5 d–2 y	6–17	6–17
	3–12 y	8–18	8–18
	13–18 y	9–21	9–21
C3 (mg/dL) S	0–6 mo	38–100	39–91
	6 mo–3 y	58–119	49–109
	4–6 y	68–127	65–122
	7–9 y	78–140	70–124
	10–12 y	75–107	74–127
	13–15 y	66–134	75–118
	16–18 y	77–125	62–120
C4 (mg/dL) S	0–6 mo	13–30	14–28
	6 mo–3 y	17–48	17–43
	4–6 y	23–47	21–42
	7–9 y	21–37	20–42
	10–12 y	21–38	18–47
	13–15 y	21–51	20–38
	16–18 y	21–39	15–41
Calcium (mg/dL) S, P	0–7 d	7.6–11.3	7.8–11.2
	8–30 d	8.8–11.6	8.6–11.8
	31–90 d	8.7–11.2	8.2–11.0
	91–180 d	8.5–11.3	8.0–11.4
	181–365 d	8.0–10.9	8.1–11.0
	1–3 y	8.9–9.9	8.9–9.9
	4–11 y	9.0–10.1	9.0–10.1
	12–13 y	9.0–10.6	9.0–10.6
	14 y–Adult	9.3–10.7	9.3–10.7
Chloride (mmol/L) S, P	0–6 mo	97–108	97–108
	6 mo–1 y	97–106	97–106
	> 1 y	97–107	97–107
Cholesterol (mg/dL) S, P	0–1 mo	38–174	56–195
	2–6 mo	53–194	59–216
	7–12 mo	83–205	68–216
	1–3 y	37–178	37–178
	4–6 y	103–184	103–184
	7–9 y	107–245	107–245
	10–11 y	120–228	122–242
	12–13 y	122–228	120–211
	14–15 y	101–222	125–211
	16–18 y	105–218	101–215
Creatine kinase (U/L) S, P	0–90 d	29–303	43–474
	3–12 mo	25–172	27–242
	13–24 mo	28–162	25–177
	2–10 y	31–152	25–177
	11–14 y	31–152	31–172
	15–18 y	34–147	28–142

(continued)

Table 43–1. General chemistry. (continued)

Analyte, Units, Specimen Type	Age	Male Range	Female Range
Cardiac troponin I (ng/mL) S, P	0–30 d	0–8.4	0–8.4
	31–90 d	0–0.7	0–0.7
	3–6 mo	0–0.5	0–0.5
	7–12 mo	0–0.3	0–0.3
	1–18 y	< 0.1	< 0.1
Creatinine (mg/dL) S, P	0–7 d	0.7–1.2	0.7–1.2
	7 d–1 mo	0.3–0.8	0.3–0.8
	1 mo–1 y	0.2–0.5	0.2–0.5
	1–3 y	0.2–0.8	0.2–0.8
	10–12 y	0.5–1.1	0.5–1.1
Gamma-glutamyl transferase (U/L) S, P	1–7 d	25–168	18–148
	8–30 d	23–174	16–140
	1–3 mo	16–147	16–140
	4–6 mo	5–93	13–123
	7–12 mo	8–38	8–59
	1–3 y	2–15	2–15
	4–6 y	5–17	5–17
	7–9 y	9–20	9–20
	10–11 y	12–25	12–23
	12–13 y	12–39	10–20
	14–15 y	8–29	10–22
	16–19 y	6–30	6–23
Glucose (mg/dL) S, P	0–1 y	36–110	36–89
	1–7 y	47–110	47–110
	> 7 d	54–117	54–117
Glucose-CSF (mg/dL)	Neonate	41–84	41–84
	16 y	41–84	41–84
Glucose-urine (mg/dL)	Neonate	6–19	6–19
High-density lipoprotein cholesterol (mg/dL) S, P	0–< 2 y	12–60	12–60
	2–< 7 y	26–68	16–62
	7–< 12 y	28–76	26–77
	12–15 y	22–73	28–79
	16–19 y	28–72	24–74
IgA (mg/dL) S, P	1–30 d	0–11	0–10
	31–182 d	0–40	0–42
	183–365 d	1–82	6–68
	1–3 y	9–137	15–111
	4–6 y	44–187	33–166
	7–9 y	58–204	28–180
	10–12 y	46–218	55–193
	13–15 y	29–251	62–241
	16–18 y	68–259	69–262

(continued)

Table 43–1. General chemistry. (continued)

Analyte, Units, Specimen Type	Age	Male Range	Female Range
IgG (mg/dL) S, P	1–30 d	197–833	162–872
	31–182 d	140–533	311–664
	183–365 d	130–156	325–647
	1–3 y	413–1112	451–1202
	4–6 y	468–1328	560–1319
	7–9 y	582–1441	485–1473
	10–12 y	685–1620	586–1609
	13–15 y	590–1600	749–1640
	16–18 y	522–1703	804–1817
IgM (mg/dL) S, P	1–30 d	0–65	1–57
	31–182 d	6–84	0–127
	183–365 d	15–117	0–130
	1–3 y	30–146	35–184
	4–6 y	31–151	42–184
	7–9 y	21–140	30–165
	10–12 y	27–151	42–211
	13–15 y	26–184	34–225
	16–18 y	18–179	45–224
Iron (µg/dL) S, P		Males and females (5–11 AM)	Males and females (5–11 PM)
	0–24 mo	20–105	20–140
	2–9 y	20–105	20–145
	10–Adult	20–100	20–145
Lactate dehydrogenase (U/L) S, P	1–30 d	178–629	187–600
	1–3 mo	158–373	452–353
	4–6 mo	135–376	158–353
	7–12 mo	129–367	152–327
	1–3 y	164–286	164–286
	4–6 y	155–280	155–280
	7–9 y	141–237	141–237
	10–11 y	141–231	129–222
	12–13 y	141–231	129–205
	16–19 y	117–217	117–213
Magnesium (mg/dL) S, P	7–30 d	1.3–2.7	1.3–2.7
	1 mo–1 y	1.7–2.7	1.7–2.7
	1–3 y	1.6–2.5	1.6–2.5
	4–6 y	1.7–2.4	1.7–2.4
	13–15 y	1.6–2.4	1.6–2.3
Potassium (m/mol/L) S, P	0–7 d	3.2–5.7	3.2–5.7
	7–30 d	3.4–6.2	3.4–6.2
	1–6 mo	3.5–5.8	3.5–5.8
	6 mo–1 y	3.5–6.3	3.5–6.3
	>1 y	3.3–4.7	3.3–4.7

(continued)

Table 43–1. General chemistry. (continued)

Analyte, Units, Specimen Type	Age	Male Range	Female Range
Prealbumin (mg/dL) S, P	0–5 d	8.6–23.2	8.6–23.2
	6 d–1 y	9.6–32.0	9.6–32.0
	2–5 y	16.4–32.0	16.4–32.0
	6–9 y	17.3–34.9	17.3–34.9
	10–13 y	22.2–37.8	22.2–37.8
	14–19 y	24.2–46.6	24.2–46.6
Phosphorus (mg/dL) S, P	0–30 d	2.8–7.0	3.1–7.7
	31–90 d	3.1–6.6	3.1–7.2
	3–12 mo	3.1–6.6	3.1–6.8
	13–24 mo	3.1–6.2	3.1–6.3
	2–12 y	3.1–5.9	3.1–5.9
	13–15 y	3.1–5.3	3.1–5.5
	16–18 y	3.1–5.1	3.1–4.8
Protein–CSF (mg/dL)	0–14 d	15–100	15–153
	15–30 d	15–96	15–100
	31–90 d	15–48	15–93
	3–5 mo	15–48	15–44
	7–24 mo	15–50	15–48
	2–7 y	15–45	15–45
	8–19 y	15–40	15–45
Sodium (mmol/L) S, P	0–7 d	131–144	131–144
	7–31 d	132–142	132–142
	1 mo–1 y	131–140	131–140
	> 1 y	132–141	132–141
Total bilirubin (mg/dL) S, P	0–1 d	< 5.1	< 5.1
	1–2 d	<7.2	<7.2
	3–5 d	< 10.3	< 10.3
	1 mo–adult	< 0.8	< 0.8
Thyroxine (µg/dL) S, P	1–30 d	3.4–14.5	3.5–13.5
	1–12 mo	5.6–16.4	5.0–13.5
	1–5 y	5.9–11.6	6.7–12.9
	6–10 y	5.7–10.8	5.6–11.0
	11–15 y	4.9–10.5	5.3–10.2
	16–18 y	5.2–9.1	5.5–10.2
Total protein (g/dL) S, P	1–60 d	4.0–7.6	3.6–7.0
	61–180 d	4.0–7.0	4.0–7.6
	181 d–1 y	4.2–7.9	4.6–7.8
	1–3 y	6.0–8.0	6.0–7.8
	7–9 y	6.3–8.1	6.3–8.1
	10–19 y	6.4–8.6	6.4–8.6

(continued)

Table 43–1. General chemistry. (continued)

Analyte, Units, Specimen Type	Age	Male Range	Female Range
Triglycerides (mg/dL) S, P	0–7 d	19–174	26–159
	8–30 d	37–279	33–270
	31–90 d	42–279	34–340
	1–3 y	25–119	25–119
	4–6 y	30–110	30–110
	7–9 y	26–123	26–123
	10–11 y	22–131	37–134
	12–13 y	22–138	35–124
	14–15 y	32–158	36–129
	16–19 y	32–134	35–134
Total carbon dioxide (mmol/L) S, P	0–7 d	13–21	13–21
	7 d–1 mo	13–22	13–22
	1–6 mo	13–23	13–23
	6 mo–1 y	14–23	14–23
	> 1 y	16–25	16–25
Uric acid (mg/dL) S, P	0–15 y	2.2–7.0	2.2–7.0
	16 y–Adult	4.0–8.7	2.4–6.8

B, whole blood; CSF, cerebrospinal fluid; P, plasma; S, serum; U, urine.
All data reproduced, with permission, from Ghoshal AK, Soldin SJ: Evaluation of the Dade Behring Dimension RxL: integrated chemistry system—pediatric reference ranges. Clin Chim Acta 2003; 331:135.

Table 43–2. Endocrine chemistry.

Analyte, Units, Specimen Type	Age	Methodology	Male Range	Female Range
Cortisol (μm/dL) S	< 2 y	DPC Immulite	1.1–33.0	1.1–29.0
	2–11 y		1.1–31.9	1.1–23.2
	11–18 y		1.1–27.2	1.1–20.3
Estradiol (ng/mL) S	Prepuberty	Esoterix	< 1.5	< 1.5
	Tanner I		0.5–1.1	0.5–2.0
	Tanner II		0.5–1.6	1.0–2.4
	Tanner III		0.5–2.5	0.7–6.0
	Tanner IV		1.0–3.6	2.1–8.5
	Tanner V		1.0–3.6	3.4–17
Follicle-stimulating hormone (mIU/mL) S	0–2 years	DPC Immulite	0.1–0.8	0.1–5.9
	2–5 years		0.1–0.4	10.1–3.6
	6–10 years		0.1–0.3	0.1–1.7
	11–18 years		0.1–7.5	0.1–7.4
	Tanner I		0.16–3.5	0.38–3.6
	Tanner II		0.44–6.0	1.25–8.9
	Tanner III		0.44–6.0	1.25–8.9
	Tanner IV		1.40–11.8	1.65–9.1
	Tanner V		1.28–14.9	1.20–12.3
Growth hormone (ng/mL) S	Tanner I	DPC Immulite	0.12–2.8	0.24–5.4
	Tanner II		0.10–5.7	0.13–8.5
	Tanner III		0.10–5.7	0.13–8.5
	Tanner IV		0.07–7.9	0.14–13.4
	Tanner V		0.10–15.1	0.24–9.9
Insulin-like growth factor-1 (ng/mL) S, P	0–7 d	DPC Immulite	1–26	1–26
	8–15 d		11–41	11–41
	16 d–1 y		55–327	55–327
	1 y		55–327	55–327
	2 y		51–303	51–303
	3 y		49–289	49–289
	4 y		49–283	49–283
	5 y		50–286	50–286
	6 y		52–297	52–297
	7 y		57–316	57–316
	8 y		64–345	64–345
	9 y		74–388	74–388
	10 y		88–452	88–452
	11 y		111–551	111–551
	12 y		143–693	143–693
	13 y		183–850	183–850
	14 y		220–972	220–972
	15 y		237–996	237–996
	16 y		226–903	226–903
	17 y		193–731	193–731
	18 y		163–584	163–584
	19 y		141–483	141–483
	20 y		127–424	127–424

(continued)

Table 43–2. Endocrine chemistry. (continued)

Analyte, Units, Specimen Type	Age	Methodology	Male Range	Female Range
Insulin-like growth factor–binding protein 3 (μg/mL) S, P	0–7 d	DPC Immulite	0.1–0.7	0.1–0.7
	8–15 d		0.5–1.4	0.5–1.4
	16 d–1 y		0.7–3.6	0.7–3.6
	1 y		0.7–3.6	0.7–3.6
	2 y		0.8–3.9	0.8–3.9
	3 y		0.9–4.3	0.9–4.3
	4 y		1.0–4.7	1.0–4.7
	5 y		1.1–5.2	1.1–5.2
	6 y		1.3–5.6	1.3–5.6
	7 y		1.4–6.1	1.4–6.1
	8 y		1.6–6.5	1.6–6.5
	9 y		1.8–7.1	1.8–7.1
	10 y		2.1–7.7	2.1–7.7
	11 y		2.4–8.4	2.4–8.4
	12 y		2.7–8.9	2.7–8.9
	13 y		3.1–9.5	3.1–9.5
	14 y		3.3–10	3.3–10
	15 y		3.5–10	3.5–10
	16 y		3.4–9.5	3.4–9.5
	17 y		3.2–8.7	3.2–8.7
	18 y		3.1–7.9	3.1–7.9
	19 y		2.9–7.3	2.9–7.3
	20 y		2.9–7.2	2.9–7.2
Luteinizing hormone (mIU/mL) S	0.1–1.5 y	DPC Immulite	ND–4.1	ND–2.3
	1.6–9 y		ND–3.8	ND–1.3
	Tanner I		0.7–1.2	0.7–2.0
	Tanner II		0.3–4.4	0.4–11
	Tanner III		0.3–4.4	0.4–11
	Tanner IV		0.5–4.7	0.9–13
	Tanner V		0.7–10.6	1.1–19
Free thyroxine (ng/dL) Sa	0–1 d	DPC Immulite	0.8–1.9	0.8–1.9
	1–7 d		1.2–2.5	1.2–2.5
	8 d–Adult		0.8–1.7	0.8–1.7
Thyroid-stimulating hormone (μIU/mL) S	1 y	DPC Immulite	0.40–8.6	0.40–8.6
	2 y		0.36–7.6	0.36–7.6
	3 y		0.33–6.7	0.33–6.7
	4 y		0.33–6.3	0.33–6.3
	5 y		0.34–6.1	0.34–6.1
	6 y		0.34–6.0	0.34–6.0
	7 y		0.35–5.8	0.35–5.8
	8–12 y		0.35–5.7	0.35–5.7
	9 y		0.35–5.6	0.35–5.6
	10 y		0.36–5.5	0.36–5.5
	11 y		0.36–5.5	0.36–5.5
	12 y		0.36–5.4	0.36–5.4

(continued)

Table 43–2. Endocrine chemistry. (continued)

Analyte, Units, Specimen Type	Age	Methodology	Male Range	Female Range
Total testosterone (ng/dL) S	Premature	DPC Immulite	37–198	5–22
	Newborn		75–400	20–64
	Prepubertal		2–30	1–20
	Tanner I		2–23	2–10
	Tanner II		5–70	5–30
	Tanner III		15–280	10–30
	Tanner IV		105–545	15–40
	Tanner V		265–800	10–40

B, whole blood; CSF, cerebrospinal fluid; P, plasma; RBC, red blood cells; S serum; U, urine.

[a]Data from Children's Hospital, Denver, Colorado.

All other data reproduced, with permission, from Soldin SJ, Brugnara SJ, Wong EC: *Pediatric Reference Ranges*, 4th ed. American Association for Clinical Chemistry Press, 2003; and Werner Kuhnell: DPC Immulite Reference Range Compendium. http://www.dpconline.com/documents/medical/reference_ranges/ZB197-A.pdf

Table 43–3. Hematology.

Analyte, Units, Specimen Type	Age	Male Range	Female Range
White blood cells (× 10⁹/L) EDTA whole blood	Newborn	9.0–32.0	9.0–32.0
	1–24 mo	5–13.0	5–13.0
	2–10 y	4–12.0	4–12.0
	10–17 y	4–10.5	4–10.5
	Adult	4–10.5	4–10.5
Red blood cells (× 10¹²/L) EDTA whole blood	Newborn	4.6–6.7	4.6–6.7
	1–24 mo	3.8–5.4	3.8–5.4
	2–10 y	4.0–5.3	4.0–5.3
	10–17 y	4.2–5.6	4.2–5.6
	Adult	4.7–6.0	4.2–5.4
Hemoglobin (g/dL) EDTA whole blood	Newborn	13–22	13–22
	1–24 mo	9.5–14.0	9.5–14.0
	2–10 y	11.5–14.5	11.5–14.5
	10–17 y	12.5–16.1	12–15
	Adult	13.5–18	12.5–16.0
Hematocrit (%) EDTA whole blood	Newborn	42–70	42–70
	1–24 mo	30–41	30–41
	2–10 y	33–43	33–43
	10–17 y	36–47	35–45
	Adult	42–52	37–47
Mean corpuscular volume (fL) EDTA whole blood	Newborn	90–115	90–115
	1–24 mo	70–90	70–90
	2–10 y	76–90	76–90
	10–17 y	78–95	78–95
	Adult	78–100	78–100
Polymorphonuclear leukocytes (absolute) EDTA whole blood	Newborn	6–23.5	6–23.5
	1–24 mo	1.1–6.6	1.1–6.6
	2–10 y	1.4–6.6	1.4–6.6
	10–17 y	1.5–6.6	1.5–6.6
	Adult	1.5–6.1	1.5–6.6
Band cells (absolute) EDTA whole blood	Newborn	< 3.5	< 3.5
	1–24 mo	< 1.0	< 1.0
	2–10 y	< 1.0	< 1.0
	Adult	< 1.0	< 1.0
Lymphocytes (absolute) EDTA whole blood	Newborn	2.5–10.5	2.5–10.5
	1–24 mo	1.8–9.0	1.8–9.0
	2–10 y	1.0–5.5	1.0–5.5
	10–17 y	1.0–3.5	1.0–3.5
	Adult	1.5–3.5	1.5–3.5
Monocytes (absolute) EDTA whole blood	Newborn	< 2.0	< 2.0
	1 mo–Adult	< 1.0	< 1.0
Eosinophils (absolute) EDTA whole blood	Newborn	< 2.0	< 2.0
	1–24 mo	< 0.7	< 0.7
	2–10 y	< 0.7	< 0.3
	10–17 y	< 0.3	< 0.3
	Adult	< 0.3	< 0.7

(continued)

Table 43–3. Hematology. (continued)

Analyte, Units, Specimen Type	Age	Male Range	Female Range
Basophils (absolute) EDTA whole blood	Newborn	< 0.4	< 0.4
	1–24 mo	< 0.1	< 0.1
Platelets (× 109/L) EDTA whole blood	Newborn	2.5–10.5	2.5–10.5
	1–24 mo	1.8–9.0	1.8–9.0
	2–10 y	1.0–5.5	1.0–5.5
	10–17 y	1.0–3.5	1.0–3.5
	Adult	1.5–3.5	1.5–3.5

All data reproduced, with permission, from Oski N: *Hematology of Infancy and Childhood.* Saunders, 1987.

College of American Pathology Commission of Laboratory Accreditation: Laboratory Accreditation Program. Chemistry and Toxicology Checklist, March 30, 2005. http://www.cap.org/apps/docs/laboratory_accreditation/checklists/chemistry_and_toxicology_march2005.pdf

Cornell University: Clinical Pathology Laboratory–Reference Intervals. http://www.diaglab.vet.cornell.edu/clinpath/reference/

Frazer CG: *Biological Variations from Principles to Practice.* American Association for Clinical Chemistry Press, 2001.

Ghoshal AK, Soldin SJ: Evaluation of the Dade Behring Dimension RxL: integrated chemistry system–pediatric reference ranges. Clin Chim Acta 2003;331:135 [PMID: 12691874].

Grossi E et al: The REALAB Project: A new method for the formulation of reference intervals based on current data. Clin Chem 2005;51:1232 [PMID: 15919879].

International Federation of Clinical Chemistry and Laboratory Medicine: http://www.ifcc.org/ifcc.asp

Kairisto V: Reference Values and Clinical Interpretation of Laboratory Data. Prepared for Internet Publication by Veli Kairisto, University of Turku, Department of Clinical Chemistry. http://www.med.utu.fi/clinchem/tempus/dl/lessons.htm

National Institute of Standards and Technology: Standard for human cardiac troponin complex. https://srmors.nist.gov/view_detail.cfm?srm=2921

Oski N: *Hematology of Infancy and Childhood.* Saunders, 1987.

Soldberg H: Establishment and use of reference values. In: *Tiez Textbook of Clinical Chemistry.* WB Saunders, 1999.

Soldberg H: Using a hospitalized population to establish reference intervals. Pros and cons. Clin Chem 1994;40:2205 [PMID: 7988005].

Soldin SJ, Brugnara SJ, Wong EC: *Pediatric Reference Ranges,* 4th ed. American Association for Clinical Chemistry Press, 2003.

Spencer CA, Schwarzbein D, Guttler RB, LoPresti JS: Thyrotropin (TSH)-releasing hormone stimulation test responses employing third and fourth generation TSH assays. J Clin Endocrinol Metab 1993;76:494 [PMID: 8432796]. http://www.thyroidmanager.org/Chapter4/4-frame.htm

Werner Kuhnel: DPC Immulite Reference Range Compendium. http://www.dpconline.com/documents/medical/reference_ranges/ZB197-A.pdf

Index

NOTE: A *t* following a page number indicates tabular material, and an *f* following a page number indicates a figure.